Pulmonary Pathology

Second Edition

David H. Dail   Samuel P. Hammar

Editors

Pulmonary Pathology

Second Edition

With 1,517 Illustrations in 1,989 Parts

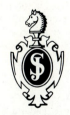

Springer-Verlag

New York Berlin Heidelberg London Paris
Tokyo Hong Kong Barcelona Budapest

1994

DAVID H. DAIL, MD
Department of Pathology, The Virginia Mason Clinic, Seattle, WA 98101, USA

SAMUEL P. HAMMAR, MD
Diagnostic Specialties Laboratory, Bremerton, WA 98310, USA

Library of Congress Cataloging-in-Publication Data
Pulmonary pathology / David H. Dail and Samuel P. Hammar, editors.—
  2nd ed.
     p. cm.
   Includes bibliographical references and index.
   1. Lungs—Histopathology. 2. Lung—Diseases. I. Dail, David H.
II. Hammar, Samuel P.
   [DNLM: 1. Lung Diseases—pathology.   WF 600 P98378]
RC711.P83   1993
616.2′407—dc20   92-2383

Production managed by Bill Imbornoni; manufacturing supervised by Rhea Talbert.
Typeset by ATLIS Graphics & Design, Inc., Mechanicsburg, PA.
Printed and bound by Universitätsdruckerei Stürtz AG, Würzburg, Federal Republic of Germany.

9 8 7 6 5 4 3 2 1

ISBN 0-387-97897-6 Springer-Verlag New York Berlin Heidelberg
ISBN 3-540-97897-6 Springer-Verlag Berlin Heidelberg New York

To all those who have
contributed to the field of
pulmonary pathology—
past and present

Preface

The first edition of *Pulmonary Pathology* was dedicated to two giants in the field, Drs. Averill Liebow and Herbert Spencer. The current edition is dedicated to all those who have contributed and are contributing to the field, those whose individual contributions and queries create its rich fabric. It is our pleasure and honor to summarize the work of many of these individuals.

Changes since the first edition have been significant. New entities are discussed, further elaboration offered, and adjustments made to those in the first edition. In response to our readers' requests, we have added some new chapters. **Lung Defenses** have been added as Chapter 3. Some authors have asked, How do we begin? Chapter 4, **Common Pathways and Patterns of Injury,** discusses this. The pulmonary pathology of AIDS, which is certainly significant today, is discussed in multiple sites, and now is also reviewed in Chapter 6, **Introduction to AIDS Pathology. Transplantation Pathology** has been added as Chapter 24 and **Metastases to and from the Lung** has been added as Chapter 35.

New authorship has added enrichment to several topics previously discussed, including **Bacterial** and **Mycobacterial Infections, Mycoplasmal, Chlamydial and Rickettsial Pneumonias, Rheumatic Connective Tissue Diseases, Iatrogenic Injury: Radiation and Drug Effects, Asbestos,** and **Vasculitis.** Several other adjustments have been made. **Extrinsic Allergic Alveolitis** and **Pulmonary Histiocytosis X (Pulmonary Langerhans' Cell Granulomatosis)** each is now discussed in its own chapter. Large specimen preparation, formerly appended as the last chapter, has been integrated into the first chapter. Edema emboli and vascular anomalies are now discussed in conjunction with hypertension and low flow states in the chapter called

Vascular Diseases. Vasculitis is so complex as to continue to warrant a separate chapter.

Each chapter has been updated and revised. Extensive expansion has occurred in **Bacterial Infections, Rheumatic Connective Tissue Diseases, Asbestos, Vasculitis, Common Neoplasms, Uncommon Lung Tumors** and **Pleural Diseases.** Despite feeling these were moderately complete in the first edition, among them there has been a 56% increase in illustrations, a 91% increase in text, and a 160% increase in references. In **Uncommon Lung Tumors** alone, there are about 500 new references, 100 new illustrations, and discussion of 16 additional entities. Updated critical review of the vast literature on **Common Neoplasms** has been incorporated, while still trying to maintain some sense of readable length.

The general organization of the chapters follows that in the first edition: Chapters 1–6, introduction and assorted diseases; Chapters 7 and 8, congenital and pediatric diseases; Chapters 9–15, infections; Chapters 16–22, allergic and/or immunological reactions; Chapters 23 and 24, therapeutic injuries; Chapters 25–28, effects of dust inhalation; Chapters 29–30, vascular diseases; and Chapters 31–35, neoplasms.

Our goals remain to present the reader with an authoritative yet readable text which hopefully answers questions that might arise in facing problem cases and to offer the reader appropriate review of particular areas within the field of pulmonary pathology. We have attempted to maintain some reasonable size and, with the expansions previously noted, no longer felt we could be "all things to all people." We therefore have deferred our three correlations chapters to other very worthy and thorough separate sources. Clinical correlations are well-defined in comprehensive books such as *Pulmonary Diseases and Disorders* by Fishman, *Textbook of Pulmonary Diseases* by Baum and Wolinsky, and *Textbook of Respiratory Medicine* by Murray and Nadel. Several additional compendiums are due out soon. Radiographic correlations are well-handled in the now classic issues of *Diagnosis of Diseases of the Chest* by Fraser, Paré, Paré, Fraser, and Genereau, and *The Lung: Radiologic-Pathologic Correlations* by Heitzman. Cytological correlations are readily available in the multi-contributor *Comprehensive Cytopathology* by Bibbo and *Diagnostic Cytology* by Koss. To complement this listing, there are of course other good pathology reviews reviewing many of the same topics covered here. Spencer's four editions of *Pathology of the Lung* have been the classic standard and still represent an excellent source of detail, and prove particularly valuable in tracing the history of many of the diseases. Some of our favorite sources in pulmonary pathology include the Armed Forces Institute of Pathology Fascicles on *Lung Tumors*, now approaching its third edition; Katzenstein and Askin's *Surgical Pathology of Non-Neoplastic Lung Disease*, Marchevsky's *Surgical Pathology of Lung Neoplasms*, Thurlbeck's *Pathology of the Lung*, Corrin's *The Lung*, Mackay, Lukeman, and Or-

donez's *Tumors of the Lung*, Henderson et al.'s *Malignant Mesothelioma*, Roggli, Greenberg, and Pratt's *Pathology of Asbestos-Associated Diseases*. Of course, other good sources are also available and others will be forthcoming.

As in the preface of our first edition, the following stands as true today as then: "Our contributors have tolerated admirably the many deadlines and details imposed on them. The luxury of time is evasive. We appreciate the extra energy put into producing manuscripts during the course of a busy day or under the handicap of limited resources."

We have benefited greatly from the input of our readers and reviewers. We welcome any such input directly. If anyone has an outstanding example he or she would like to contribute to future editions, we shall make every effort to properly credit this contribution. Many of the outstanding examples currently used have been contributed by interested pathologists. We continue to strive to make this as valuable a resource as we can for our readers and would appreciate any help you may offer to achieve this.

DAVID H. DAIL
SAMUEL P. HAMMAR

Individual Authors' Dedications and Acknowledgments

Often in a multi-contributor book, individual authors do not have a chance to express appreciation to those who have been important to them in both their personal lives and in the composition of their chapters. Such an opportunity is given here.

Dedications

Chapter 1/D.H.D.—Kim Dail, Holly Dail

Chapter 2/N.-S.W.—William M. Thurlbeck, Huai-San Lin, and Shu-Wen How

Chapter 3/J.L. and J.H.S.—Patients of the University of Nebraska and Jennifer Larsen

Chapter 4/S.A.M.—Charles Carrington and all my teachers in pathology

Chapter 5/D.H.D.—Evalyn Dail, Phyllis and Ray Lindquist

Chapter 6/D.H.D.—Kristen, Mary, and Jane Lindquist

Chapter 7/J.T.S.—Patty, Rick, Dave, and Meg

Chapter 8/J.T.S. and L.P.D.—Jake and Arlene Stocker and Becky, Rebecca, and Rachel Dehner

Chapter 9/W.C.W. and F.W.C.—John Craighead and A. Bleakley Chandler and Mr. and Mrs. Francis W. Chandler, Sr.

Chapter 10/R.H.H. and G.M.H.—Zdenek, Jarmila, and Claire Hruban and Loretta Hutchins and Our Children

Chapter 11/F.W.C. and J.C.W.—Gloria, Cathy, and Melinda Chandler and Ann, Jennifer, and Kristen Watts

Chapter 12/W.C.W. and D.H.W.—David E. Smith, John M. Kissane and Joe Grisham and Franz von Lichtenberg

Chapter 13/D.H.W.—Marjorie Walker

Chapter 14/R.E.S.—Lynne Sobonya, Jack M. Layton, and Ronald S. Weinstein

Chapter 15/J.K.B., R.C.N., and A.M.M.—Wayne M. Meyers, Chapman H. Binford, and William Lamar Chester

Chapter 16/D.H.D.—Don Bauermeister, Susan Patterson, and John Bolan

Chapter 17/S.P.H.—Judy Hammar, Lisa Hammar, and Mike Hammar

Chapter 18/S.P.H.—Ella and Samuel Hammar and James C. O'Bryan

Chapter 19/Y.R.—Valentin A. Yermakov, Harold A. Lyons, and Gordon R. Hennigar

Chapter 20/S.P.H.—Irene and Douglas Howe

Chapter 21/J.T.L.—Margaret R. Lie

Chapter 22/D.H.D.—Katherine Galagan, Marla Fenske, and Dail Doucette

Chapter 23/R.A.S.—Beth, Laurel, and Jennifer Schmidt

Chapter 24/D.W.C.—Joel D. Cooper

Chapter 25/R.A.H.—Averill Liebow, Charles Carrington, and Gordon Hennigar

Chapter 26/P.C.P.—Arnold R. Rich

Chapter 27/V.L.R. and J.D.S.—Linda and Heather Roggli and Kerri, Mark, and Katherine Shelburne

Chapter 28/S.P.H. and R.F.D.—Pat Skerbeck and Mr. and Mrs. Benjamin F. Dodson

Chapter 30/W.D.T. and M.N.K.—Lois B. Travis, David M. Travis, and Jeanne D. Travis, Mary and Leon Koss and Linda Koss

Chapter 32/S.P.H.—Dawn Bockus, Franque Remington, and Susie Friedman

Chapter 33/D.H.D.—Kip Richards

Chapter 34/S.P.H.—N. Karle Mottet

Chapter 35/D.H.D.—Lorraine Blackburn, Pat Kipper, and Sandi Jorgenson

Acknowledgments

Chapter 1/Susan Kreml, Jean Engler, and Deb Gallant

Chapter 2/Stephanie Ching, Catherine Reynolds, and Teresa Espinosa

Chapter 3/Valorie Gunderson and Anthony G. Moss

Chapter 5/Taylor Ubben, John Horman, and Sandy Bjorgen

Chapter 6/Bob Riedlinger, Michelle Martinez, and Jeff Williams

Chapter 9/Judy Kessler and Beverly Chandler

Chapter 10/Claire E. Hruban, Amy Pielert, and J. Stephen Dumler

Chapter 11/Melita R. Posey

Chapter 12/Judy Kessler

Chapter 13/Rose Herndon

Chapter 14/Samuel P. Hammar

Chapter 15/Roger G. Thorpe, Leo O. Lanoie, and L. Arden Almquist

Chapter 16/Ann Robertson, Dani Haas, and Beth Levine

Chapter 17/Richard A. Schlag

Chapter 18/Dawn Bockus

Chapter 19/Herbert A. Fischler

Chapter 20/Franque Remington

Chapter 22/Kathy Rohrback, Joyce Higashi, and Patti Stewart

Chapter 23/Jake Van Dyck, Sheri Storey, and Melinda Ogilvie

Chapter 25/Librarians of the University of Kentucky Tobacco and Health Research Institute and of the Medical University of South Carolina

Chapter 27/Marjorie, Penny, and Susan Embry, and Walter Fennell, Jr., and Eva Whalin

Chapter 28/Pat Skerbeck, Carolyn Tuley, Carolyn Corn, and Michael O'Sullivan

Chapter 30/Richard Dreyfuss, J.T. Lie, MD, and Ralph L. Isenberg, and L. Duckett

Chapter 32/Pat Skerbeck and Harrison Memorial Hospital Library

Chapter 33/Dawn Oakes, Denise DeRouchey, and Mike Dorval

Chapter 34/Susie Friedman and Pat Skerbeck

Chapter 35/Sorena Thamert, Shiloh Lee, and Theresa Merrill

Contents

Contributors

J. KEVIN BAIRD, M.S.
Parasitology Division, US Naval Medical Research
Unit #2, Jakarta, Indonesia, Box 3—American
Embassy, APO AP 96520-5000

DEAN W. CHAMBERLAIN, M.D.
Department of Pathology, University of
Toronto/Toronto Hospital, Toronto, Ontario M5G
2C4, Canada

FRANCIS W. CHANDLER, D.V.M., PH.D.
Department of Pathology, Medical College of
Georgia, Augusta, GA 30912, USA

THOMAS V. COLBY, M.D.
Department of Pathology, Mayo Clinic, Rochester,
MN 55905, USA

DAVID H. DAIL, M.D.
Department of Pathology, The Virginia Mason
Clinic, Seattle, WA 98101, USA

LOUIS P. DEHNER, M.D.
Anatomic Pathology, Barnes Hospital, St. Louis,
MO 63110, USA

RONALD F. DODSON, PH.D.
Department of Cell Biology and Environmental
Sciences, The University of Texas Health Center
at Tyler, Tyler, TX 75710, USA

SAMUEL P. HAMMAR, M.D.
Diagnostic Specialties Laboratory, 700 Lebo
Boulevard, Bremerton, WA 98310, USA

RUSSELL A. HARLEY, JR., M.D.
Pathology Department, Medical University
Hospital of South Carolina, Charleston, SC 29425,
USA

RALPH H. HRUBAN, M.D.
Pathology Department, Johns Hopkins Hospital,
Baltimore, MD 21205, USA

GROVER M. HUTCHINS, M.D.
Pathology Department, Johns Hopkins Hospital,
Baltimore, MD 21205, USA

MICHAEL N. KOSS, M.D.
Pulmonary and Mediastinal Branch, Armed Forces
Institute of Pathology, Washington, DC
20306-6000, USA

J.T. LIE, M.D.
Division of Anatomic Pathology, University of
California Davis Medical Center, Sacramento, CA
95817, USA

J. LINDER, M.D.
Department of Pathology, University of Nebraska
Medical Center, Omaha, NE 68198-3135, USA

AILEEN M. MARTY, M.D.
Department of Infectious and Parasitic Diseases
Pathology, Armed Forces Institute of Pathology,
Washington, DC 20306-6000, USA

W.J. MOOI, M.D., PH.D.
Department of Tumor Pathology, Free University,
Amsterdam, and Department of Pathology,
Netherlands Cancer Institute, Plesmanlaan 121,
1066 CX Amsterdam, The Netherlands

JEFFREY L. MYERS, M.D.
Department of Pathology and Laboratory
Medicine, Mayo Clinic, Rochester, MN 55905,
USA

RONALD C. NEAFIE, M.S.
Department of Infectious and Parasitic Diseases
Pathology, Armed Forces Institute of Pathology,
Washington, DC 20306-6000, USA

PHILIP C. PRATT, M.D.
Department of Pathology, Duke University Medical
Center, Durham, NC 27710, USA

VICTOR L. ROGGLI, M.D.
Laboratory Services, Durham Veteran's
Administration Medical Center, Durham, NC
27710, USA

Y. ROSEN, M.D.
Department of Pathology, Winthrop University
Hospital, Mineola, NY 11501, USA

RODNEY A. SCHMIDT, M.D., PH.D.
Department of Pathology, University of
Washington Medical Center, Seattle, WA 98195,
USA

JOHN D. SHELBURNE, M.D., PH.D.
Laboratory Services, Durham Veteran's
Administration Medical Center, Durham, NC
27710, USA

J.H. SISSON, M.D.
Department of Pulmonary Pathology, University of
Nebraska Medical Center, Omaha, NE
68198-3135, USA

RICHARD E. SOBONYA, M.D.
Department of Pathology, University of Arizona
College of Medicine, Tucson, AZ 85724, USA

J. THOMAS STOCKER, COL, MC, USA
Armed Forces Institute of Pathology, Washington,
DC 20306-6000, USA

WILLIAM D. TRAVIS, M.D.
Department of Pathology, National Institutes
Health Laboratory of Pathology, Bethesda, MD
20892, USA

C.A. WAGENVOORT, M.D.
Department of Pathology, Erasmus University of
Rotterdam, 3000 DR Rotterdam, The Netherlands

DAVID H. WALKER, M.D.
Department of Pathology, University of Texas,
Medical Branch at Galveston, Galveston, TX
77550, USA

NAI-SAN WANG, M.D.
Department of Pathology, University of California
Irvine Medical Center, Orange, CA 92668, USA

JOHN C. WATTS, M.D.
Department of Anatomic Pathology, William
Beaumont Hospital, Royal Oak, MI 48073, USA

WASHINGTON C. WINN, JR., M.D.
Department of Pathology, Medical Center Hospital
of Vermont, University of Vermont, Burlington,
VT 05401, USA

SAMUEL A. YOUSEM, M.D.
Department of Pathology, Montefiore University
Hospital, Pittsburgh, PA 15213-3241, USA

CHAPTER 1

Tissue Sampling

DAVID H. DAIL

The continuous development of new clinical, radiologic, surgical, and pathologic techniques highlights an ever-changing practice of pathology. With reference to many locations in the body, and certainly in the lung, the pathologist is being asked to be more diagnostic with smaller and smaller samples. Immunohistochemistry, DNA probes, polymerase chain reactions, and other newer techniques entering diagnostic practice may lead to a diagnosis based on only a few cells. As in electron microscopy, the challenge will be to judge whether such samples are truly representative and whether the changes observed account for the patient's disease. Pattern recognition on tissue sections is still valuable (see Chapter 4), but is being supplemented and in part replaced with some of these newer techniques.

Because tissue samples start with the smallest, least invasive ones, it is important to know when more tissue must be obtained. Surgical pathology and cytology techniques are discussed first in this chapter, followed by discussion of samples in immunocompromised hosts, concentrating on non-AIDS types of immunosuppression in this chapter. A separate chapter is devoted to AIDS (see Chapter 6), and other chapters cover other aspects of AIDS. At the end of this chapter is a special section on large specimen preparations that will be of use in preparing teaching specimens and museum specimens or in examining certain diseases such as emphysema and vascular hypertension or vascular anomalies.

Standard thoracotomies are now used only for therapeutic resections. Use of the minithoracotomy for diffuse lung disease diagnosis was introduced by Klassen[1] in 1949. This technique involves entering the anterior fourth or fifth intercostal space, and with slight modifications has led the way to replacing a full thoracotomy for diagnostic purposes. Several variations of the minithoracotomy have been developed. One alternative approach is a mini-anterior thoracotomy through the second or third intercostal space (modified Chamberlain type).[2,3] Another alternative is a slightly larger incision entering through the posterior auscultatory triangle. Some advantages and disadvantages are inherent with each technique. In biopsies done for more limited disease, compared to the greater choice of open biopsy sites in diffuse lung disease, the approach is usually dictated by the distribution of the disease. Thorascopy-directed biopsies are currently gaining favor, as they cause less morbidity and are done through a small incision. These are reliable for sampling peripheral diffuse lung diseases, and techniques even are evolving for excising nodules.

The results from rigid bronchoscopy with generously sized biopsies were well outlined by the serial reports of Andersen of 13 patients in 1965,[4] 450 patients in 1972,[5] and 939 in 1978.[6] Rigid bronchoscopy is still used for excisions or laser procedures of central endobronchial lesions, removal of foreign bodies, dilatation of stricture, placement of airway stints, management of massive hemoptysis,[7] or to obtain bigger biopsies of difficult central lesions.

To better reach the upper lobes by the transbronchial route and to enter more distal bronchi, flexible fiberoptic bronchoscopy is now widely accepted worldwide: its use in North America was reviewed in 1991.[8] It was developed in Japan between 1964 and 1966 by Ikeda[9,10] and was introduced in the United States in 1969. Its original smaller channel biopsy forceps has been replaced by a larger channel (2.6-mm) crocodile forceps allowing capture of samples in the range of 1 to 2 mm. Using the standard 5.2-mm external dimension flexible bronchoscope, Kovnat and associates[10] noted they

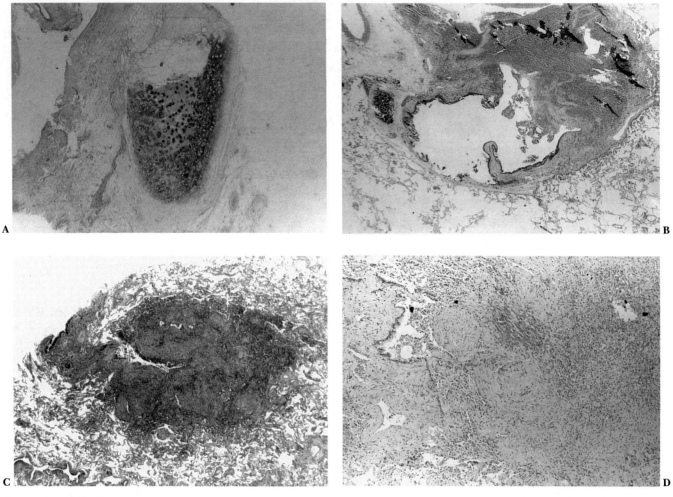

Fig. 1–1 A–D. Transbronchial biopsy sites. **A.** The biopsy forceps sometimes bite through native bronchial cartilage. H and E, × 40. **B.** Two days postbiopsy show area of perforation of bronchiole with adjacent hemorrhage. H and E, × 20. **C.** Healing of transbronchial biopsy site near a bronchioalveolar tumor is seen at 10 days. H and E, × 30. **D.** High-power view of biopsy site in **C** shows remnant bronchial wall to left and scarring fibrosis, inflammation and hemorrhage in biopsy site in middle of field and to the right. H and E, × 200.

could obtain direct cannulation of all third-order, 74% of fourth-order, and 38% of fifth-order, bronchi. They could directly visualize all fourth-order, 86% of fifth-order, and 56% of sixth-order bronchi. Biopsies are obtained more distally in a blind fashion, forcing the open-jawed biopsy forceps beyond the visual field of the scope. Such areas of sampling are shown in Fig. 1–1. Fluoroscopic guidance has helped localize the endoscope into the abnormal lung regions and, with experience gained from taking multiple biopsies, the limited invasiveness and relative safety of the flexible bronchoscope have made it the standard biopsy technique today.

Complications of this procedure in a large user survey conducted by Herf et al.[11] showed a 5.5% incidence of pneumothorax, a 1.3% incidence of greater than 50 ml of bleeding, and a mortality of 0.24%. A literature review by Zavala[12] found corresponding incidences of 4% pneumothorax, 9% hemorrhage (averaging 25–100 ml where specified), and a mortality of 0.23%, mostly in those with a bleeding tendency. Bleeding was increased in immunosuppressed (29%) and uremic (45%) patients.

Transthoracic large-core needle biopsies were generally fraught with difficulties of low biopsy yield and high pneumothorax rate. Although the cutting needle has been widely used in other organs since its introduction in 1938,[13] its yield in the lung is low because the lung is both rubbery and delicate and because of the patchiness of some diseases such as Kaposi's sarcoma. Thus, this use has largely disappeared from practice today. The high-speed rotary drill or trephine biopsies obtained better tissue samples, but could not reduce the 30%–40% incidence of pneumothorax and consequently have also fallen into general disuse. There is an excellent review of these techniques and their results by Gaensler.[14] These procedures have generally been replaced with transbronchial biopsies, with brushings, washings, and collection of lavage fluids for cytologic review. Transtracheal or transbronchial needle aspirations are used to help diagnose peripheral masses, submucosal and peribronchial lesions, and mediastinal tumor spread.[15–18] So far these have not obtained a high yield but if positive are helpful.[7,8] Transthoracic fine-needle aspirations are used mainly to cytologically diagnose malignancy but may also be helpful in cases of infection.

Oropharyngeal contamination has been a problem when using transbronchial routes to obtain material for culture,[19] but quantitative sample techniques similar to urine techniques have been developed.[20] Bacteria in the lung usually become coated with antibody, apparently indicating a degree of immune response, and this test helps confirm that the sample is of lung origin.

The diagnoses considered on small bits of tissue obtained in the laboratory should reflect the clinical and radiologic impressions. After all, a radiologist is an expert three-dimensional gross pathologist in his or her own media. A skilled clinician is best able to understand whether a suggested diagnosis is consistent with the patient's history, physical examination, and laboratory findings. If either or both suggest a proposed pathologic diagnosis is unlikely, careful reconsideration by the pathologist is warranted if the pathology is not absolutely diagnostic. A descriptive diagnosis with discussion may replace an attempted definitive pathologic diagnosis in such cases.

Tissue Techniques

Transbronchial Biopsies

The most common pulmonary tissue specimens received in the histology laboratory are transbronchial biopsies obtained through the flexible bronchoscope. Our pulmonologists usually submit four to seven specimens, each about 1–2 mm in diameter, in a fixative appropriate for routine light microscopy. This fixative currently is chosen to be the best available for immunoperoxidase. They may submit two to four additional specimens in a fixative appropriate for electron microscopy. All pulmonologists should be encouraged to obtain multiple and generous samples to increase their

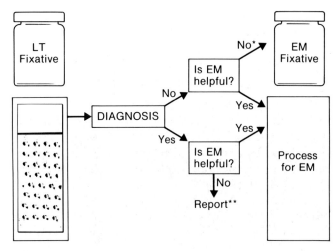

Fig. 1–2. Handling of small tissue biopsies. *, Process EM fixative for light; **, EM fixative stored for 2 years.

diagnostic yield. To obtain the most information from these small specimens for light microscopy, the following steps are employed in our laboratory (Fig. 1–2).

1. The samples fixed for light microscopy are serially sectioned, and approximately 80 sections are placed on a total of three slides and stained with hematoxylin and eosin (H and E). As they are serially sectioned from the paraffin block, the paraffin strips are placed across the minor dimension of the glass slide, as shown in Fig. 1–2. The pathologist may sample these by reading the midportion of tissue across the longer dimension. The fragments on either side may be referred to as necessary if abnormalities are detected and each represents the adjacent step section. If need be, all sections may be examined.

2. Between about every 20–30 sections, several unstained sections are placed on each of two slides, and are held as unstained slides. A total of approximately two-thirds of the tissue in the paraffin block is sectioned for light microscopy as H and E-stained and unstained slides as noted in steps 1 and 2; the other third is held in the paraffin block for further sections as necessary.

3. Special stains, such as for infective organisms, mucin, or specific antigens by immunoperoxidase technique, can be done on the unstained slides and the remaining tissue in the block. If more than two stains are needed, those judged most helpful or most critical should be done on the first two unstained slides prepared from representative samples from the first two-thirds of the tissue; the others are done on slides cut from the remaining tissue in the block.

4. Any material obtained electron microscopic fixative may then be stored if not needed for immediate

diagnosis, or processed for light or electron microscopy as judged most appropriate.

Open Lung Biopsies

Samples from different institutions and different surgeons vary. Chest surgeons at our institutions like to use a limited posterior thoracotomy and sample two or three lobes on one side, each specimen being approximately 3–4 × 2 × 1 cm, covered by pleura on two sides, and usually stapled at the line of excision. The newer thoroscopic directed biopsies are usually smaller. By whichever route, the samples should be selected by the surgeon to cover different degrees of involvement by disease. Choosing only the most involved area has been shown to be inappropriate.[21]

When received in the surgical pathology laboratory, the following questions, as outlined in Fig. 1–3, are considered and appropriate action taken.

1. Representative areas are selected and sterile tissue is set aside for culture, if not already obtained. This should be from one or more representative areas. As culture material in most microbiology laboratories is homogenized, an adequate sample free of staples is supplied. Collections of samples for microbiology may vary, but in our laboratory these are routinely done by the pathologist who first samples the tissue and who then hand-carries them to the microbiology laboratory. Routine anaerobic and aerobic bacterial, mycobacterial, and fungal smears and cultures are done on all tissue samples. Viral cultures are done with some frequency, and mycoplasma exams are available through outside laboratories. Representative samples are put in appropriate holding medium in cases in which these examinations are needed. Routine Gram stains, fluorescent mycobacteria stains, and fluorescent calcofluor stains for direct fungal examination are reported from the microbiology laboratory. The use of fluorescent antipneumocystic specific antibodies on smears has greatly reduced the yield of identifying both cysts and trophozoites and significantly reduced our need for rapid Gomori methenamine silver (GMS) stains. We are now taking advantage of the nonspecific but intense immunofluorescence staining of fungal walls by calcofluor white, and this has mostly replaced our potassium hydroxide (KOH) techniques for lung specimens.
2. Each handling of unfixed tissue subjects the tissue to further artefact. As we are aware of this, after gentle palpation a sharp scalpel or razor blade is carefully used to section parts of the specimen. Representative samples may be submitted for frozen section exami-

Is culture needed?
Do frozen section?
Is specimen adequate?
Touch-smear preps helpful?
Special fixatives needed?
Retain a frozen sample?
Do STAT special stains?
Inflate remaining tissue?

Fig. 1–3. Considerations in handling open lung biopsies.

nation to be sure (a) the specimen contains diagnostic material, (b) to get some impression of the process to see that appropriate fixatives and preparations are done, and (c) to obtain a diagnostic impression for the clinicians. Unless there is a solid mass or the lung is dense, you can expect fairly poor quality frozen sections because the less involved lung cuts poorly and retains its shape with difficulty; also, the elastic tissue does not stain well.

3. Depending on the problem or differential diagnosis, appropriate fixatives are chosen and smear preparations made or tissue retained frozen. Rapid stains, particularly a rapid GMS (see Appendix at end of chapter), and stains for other infective organisms can be done on frozen sections and smear preparations. Material is kept frozen if lymphocyte markers are to be done or if possibly helpful for specific problems, as for immunofluorescence in Good pasture's disease. The lung has such abundant autofluorescence that often immunofluorescent exams are imperfect.
4. The remaining tissue is gently inflated with a small-gauge needle and appropriate fixative. This may require multiple injections with small volumes (1 ml^3 or so) to avoid overdistension. Fixatives vary in different laboratories between aldehydes and heavy metals; some fixatives may use combined bases. The inflated sample is submerged in the chosen fixative and sectioned for routine processing after appropriate fixation. As has been described by several authors[21–27] and as is apparent with experience, the difference between collapsed and more normally distended lung will make a significant difference in the ease, and often the accuracy, of interpretation in such specimens (see Fig. 1–4).

Resection Specimens

Larger specimens of segments, lobes, or lungs may be handled in several ways. These may be combined diagnostic and therapeutic operations. Initially the surgeon

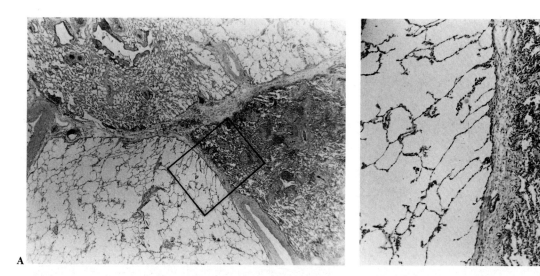

Fig. 1–4 A,B. Variable inflation of lung causes significant differences in appearance. **A.** Low power. H and E, × 100. **B.** Higher magnification of boxed area in **A.** H and E, × 100.

is usually interested in the nature (if unknown) and extent of the disease. Further proper handling of the tissue and of the operation requires knowledge of the type of disease. If this disease has not been previously diagnosed, a frozen section of the primary process may be requested. Pathways of handling the tissue from this point differ depending on whether it is infectious, malignant, or not clearly diagnostic on frozen section. For malignant disease, the bronchial line of excision and any close borders are usually sampled for frozen section. Further mediastinal node samplings are usually obtained by the surgeon if the lesion is a possible primary lung cancer. For infectious processes, sterile culture material must be collected before contamination of the specimen. It is often necessary to be sure this procedure has been done, and if not, to collect it at this time, as noted was for lung biopsies. For processes that are unclear, both cultures and assorted special fixatives and preparations are usually necessary. If tissue digestion for asbestos fibers is requested, it is helpful to be sure you have enough tissue; 2–5 g per site sampled is ideal (see Chapter 28).

All these requirements and the need for special fixatives as outlined in the following section may mean the specimen is at least partially dissected in the fresh state for examination purposes. Research requests for fresh tissue, such as to develop monoclonal antibodies, may require further divisions of samples. For these reasons it is rare, at least in our laboratory, to be able to inflate and fix an intact specimen before dissection.

Inflation techniques, where possible, work well and certainly allow the best demonstration of the locations, associations, and connections of the diseased areas of the lung. This allows the best pathologic descriptions, tissue sampling, and photographs. Inflation may be done by occluding the main bronchial resection line(s) around a catheter, tube, or graduated attachment connected to a tank of fixative with a water pressure of approximately 25–30 cm. It is usually necessary to move the connector about to inflate all bronchi, and a tight seal is necessary to maintain pressure during inflation. Some clamp this line of excision after inflation, but this may not be required.[27] Obstructing masses and/or prior incisions as required in the fresh state may prevent proper inflation of critical areas. Smaller inflation devices may be used, either a smaller catheter connected to the main tank or more often a syringe, to inflate identified more distal bronchi or to inject the tissue as in open lung biopsies. After appropriate fixation, the tissue is further sectioned. Fixation for 24 h is recommended but even distended fixation for a few hours is helpful in preserving the architecture. The latter allows processing the same day and is used if inflation has been done, particularly to study the appearance of the surrounding less involved lung tissue.

Considering the possibilities for a specimen before inflation, the pathologist may choose to use several different fixatives and inject several different areas with each, selecting each area for excision and submersion in the respective fixatives. Such localized inflation can also be done for more normal lung sampling, and may preclude the need for generalized inflation. This is particularly valuable when the lung has been extensively sectioned in the fresh state and different fixatives are desired.

An inflated fixed specimen may be sectioned in sev-

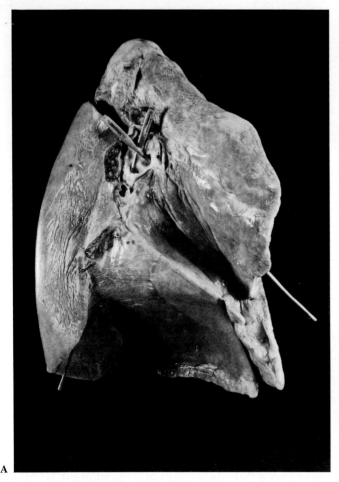

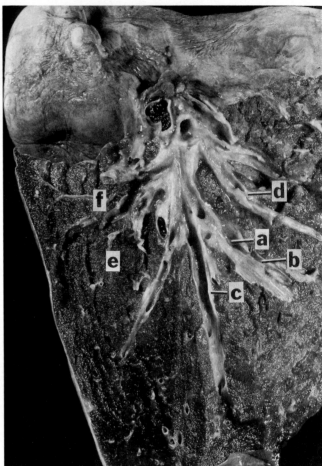

A

B

Fig. 1–5 A,B. Sectioning of larger specimens. **A.** Probes may be used as guides to sectioning, or scissors may be used to channel along bronchi, followed by planing off tissue between channels. **B.** Whichever method is used, common artifacts may occur; a and b, high and low sectioning of same bronchus gives thick and thin appearance; c, overhanging edge needs to be trimmed slightly to prevent shadow; d, smaller bronchus needs opening; e, irregular cut marks distract from "flat face" appearance; f, superior segment has been supported from underneath to more approximate basilar segment plane. (Photography by Taylor Ubben, Mason Clinic, Seattle, Washington.)

eral ways (Fig. 1–5). The first consists of placing two metal probes into adjacent bronchi in a plane of the pertinent lesion. Penetrating the pleura with these probes helps to anchor them. A large sharp knife is angled 45° against the probes, and pressure is applied from the proximal to the distal end of the probes, ideally extending through the pleura. There is a tendency to come off the plane of the probed bronchi, at least along one probe, and to follow principally the other probe, and to have other artifacts as mentioned next. Practice and care will reduce these difficulties.

The second technique involves channeling down the two desired bronchi with scissors while pulling up on the bronchi or perhaps supporting them from underneath with a hand. The remaining wedge of tissue between two adjacent channels may then be carefully planed off with a knife, scalpel, or scissors, giving a flat

plane similar to the first process. Adjacent bronchi are chosen and the process is repeated. Further scissor trimming of bronchi and careful trimming of broad pieces of tissue may make an excellent photographic surface.

With either technique, a lesion that extends into a different plane from the major plane may also be sampled. From the plane of the first section, the probe or scissors technique may be used in the second plane, such as in the superior segment of the lower lobe (see Fig. 1–5B). If the lesion is soft, this new area may be artifactually supported from underneath the specimen with towels, tissue, or other material to achieve a flat face, and trimming of the apex between the two planes may almost make a flat surface of the junction between the two planes. This does not work well for a stiff lesion, such as a solid tumor, and photographic views in several planes may be necessary to adequately demonstrate these specimens.

Several artifacts often occur with sectioning inflated specimens. These may not be serious, but the more of them that can be eliminated the better the focus of the viewer on the pathology. As shown in Fig. 1–5B, irregular cutting pressure along the same bronchus may result in cutting at different heights, giving adjacent wide (a) and narrow (b) portions. In areas (c) and (b), the bronchi may need further opening to allow light to expose their depths. Scissors can usually do this quite effectively. Usually the top half to two-thirds of an exposed bronchus needs to be removed to avoid shadows from its overhanging edges. Orienting the specimen to the source of the photographic light may complement this. In area (e), knife marks ("hash," hesitation, or "stutter" marks) detract from the best demonstration. This is most common in the usually more elastic peripheral lung. A smooth cutting action and careful fine trimming, with practice, will help perfect your technique.

Another technique for sectioning inflated and fixed specimens, especially whole lungs, consists of cutting slabs of lung in 1- to 2-cm slices. This technique is especially used in autopsy material because this is the most common source of whole lung specimens. This consists of trimming the mainstem bronchus, then placing the lung hilar surface down and cutting with a long sharp knife along an established plane (usually a cutting board), making the most even slices possible. Sometimes this is aided by placing the specimen between two measured supports (1 cm or more high) and proceeding with full-length sectioning. Special cutting boards may be developed for this purpose. Such lung slabs are often sectioned in the anterior-to-posterior, apical-to-inferior dimension, showing a maximum face of lung. As one slice is removed, the process is repeated until the whole lung is sectioned. The thinner the slices, the more thorough the examination, but the more technically difficult it becomes. Such slabs may also be used for Gough sections.

Fixatives

Most laboratories have a choice of fixatives for special occasions. We use formalin as our routine fixative for most larger specimens such as covered under *Resection Specimens*, but have three other fixatives for special needs. One of our most frequently used alternate fixatives is a modified Carnoy's solution. This modification, which consists of substituting methyl alcohol for ethyl alcohol in the standard Carnoy's solution, is named methacarn. Methacarn fixative is not as good as formalin for kappa or lambda light chains or quite as good for S-100 protein staining. For routine histology, methacarn is less desirable for most silver stains and Congo red stain than formalin. Special techniques such as for viral identification in paraffin blocks may not work with these alternate fixatives. Both fixatives require special disposal, the methacarn more so than formalin. Methacarn causes a more intense staining reaction on H and E and several other stains using standard techniques for these stains, and at times this may be more or less desirable.

When we can use only one fixative for small biopsies, such as with transbronchial lung biopsies, we choose methacarn to get the best immunoperoxidase results currently available. Small biopsies are rapidly and firmly fixed with methacarn, which allows them to be serially sectioned without difficulty. To avoid having to use alternate fixatives, and for use in studying older tissues already fixed in formalin, more and more antibodies are being developed for immunoperoxidase identification of various antigens in formalin-fixed tissues. As yet no fixative is ideal for all purposes, nor is it likely that one ever will be.

Our choice for electron microscopy is Karnovsky's fixative, which is a mixture of paraform aldehyde and glutaraldehyde. For transbronchial biopsies, as noted, samples of tissue are submitted in this fixative. Open lung biopsy and larger section samples are carefully cut no more than 1 mm thick. This may either be as wider but thin slabs up to 3–6 mm across, or may be as 1 × 1 mm cubes or rectangles. At times, focal injection of a larger specimen with Karnovsky fixative helps to stiffen the tissue, especially if it fixes for a short time before thin slicing.

For possible lymphoproliferative diseases in the lung, we also employ B5 fixative. In addition, we save an adequate sample of frozen tissue for possible lymphocyte cell marker studies. As has been noted, on special occasions such as study for Goodpasture's disease by immunofluorescent techniques, material is saved frozen. At other times frozen tissue is saved for possible future research purposes.

Discussion

Clinical evaluation is often quite competent in diagnosing many pulmonary problems. Some disorders escape a specific diagnosis, and eventually biopsies are necessary. In one series of 106 open lung biopsies, the first clinical impression was different from the pathologic diagnosis in 53% of the cases, and the correct diagnosis was not even suspected in a third of these.[28] In a series of 462 open lung biopsies for chronic interstitial disease read by a single skilled pulmonary pathologist (C. B. Carrington), a confident single diagnosis could be made in only one-half of the cases.[14,29] Likewise, in immuno-compromised hosts, open lung biopsies confirmed the favored clinical diagnosis in only 44% of cases.[30]

Lung biopsies submitted for diagnosis generally fall into the two groups of patients: (1) immunocompromised and (2) nonimmunocompromised.

Biopsies in Immunocompromised Patients

Lung diseases in the immunocompromised host today generally fall into two groups, autoimmunodeficiency syndrome (AIDS) and non-AIDS cases. The acute and chronic conditions for the latter are discussed here. A good general review of lung problems in both AIDS and non-AIDS was compiled by McLoud and Naidich[31] and specific reviews, mostly toward the spectrum of *Pneumocystis carinii* pneumonia (PCP) in AIDS compared to non-AIDS patients, are also available.[32,33] Some reviews cover non-AIDS PCP in the AIDS era.[34,35]

A few generalities will serve to highlight some of the differences in these two settings. Non-AIDS patients are often leukopenic and have low polymorphonuclear neutrophil leukocytes (PMNs); because their lymphocytes are not as profoundly affected as in AIDS, their spectrum of disease is somewhat different. Certainly the profound lymphocyte suppression in AIDS has brought new attention to the whole spectrum of opportunistic infections, and these are often multiple; they are seen not only by the pathologists and cytologists but also by the microbiology laboratory. Some new ones such as respiratory cryptosporidiosis appear limited to lung involvement in AIDS patients only.

Pneumocystis pneumonia has gained renewed attention. In AIDS cases, there are more PCP organisms than in non-AIDS , so much so that induced sputum is a worthwhile procedure, whereas in non-AIDS it has a very low yield. All the atypical features of PCP, including apical predominance, nodular and/or granulomatous presentation, calcification, fibrosis, cyst formation, pneumothorax, and systemic spread, have been noted in non-AIDS cases but certainly are more frequent in AIDS cases. (See Chapter 6 for contrasting PCP effects in both groups.) Systemic PCP in non-AIDS and AIDS has nicely been reviewed by Raviglione.[36] In contrast, and for reasons that are not understood, PCP develops more rapidly in non-AIDS compared to AIDS patients, in one series being 5 days versus 28 days.[32] Also, CMV, *Aspergillus, Legionella,* and many of the other bacterial infections do not have the same incidence of involvement or severity in AIDS as in non-AIDS patients, but on the other hand new malignancies are more frequently seen in AIDS patients whereas recurrent malignancies are sought in non-AIDS patients initially treated for malignancy. The noninfectious effects of chemotherapy or radiotherapy are more prevalent in the non-AIDS group, yet nonspecific pneumonitis is prevalent in both groups.

Because of the importance and prevalence of AIDS pulmonary pathology, a separate chapter (Chapter 6) is devoted to an introduction to AIDS pulmonary diseases. Common problems in AIDS and non-AIDS patients are further discussed in Chapter 3, **Lung Defenses**; Chapter 4, **Common Pathways and Patterns of Injury**; Chapter 8, **Acquired Neonatal and Pediatric Diseases**; and the infectious groups of Chapter 9, **Bacterial Infections**; Chapter 10, **Mycobacterial Infections**; Chapter 11, **Fungal Infections**; Chapter 12, **Viral Infections**; Chapter 14, **Pneumocystis**; and Chapter 15, **Parasitic Infections**. Therapeutic injury is further discussed in Chapter 23, **Iatrogenic Injury**, and in Chapter 24, **Transplantation Pathology**; and neoplasms in the two groups are further discussed in Chapter 31, **Lymphoproliferative Disorders**, and in Chapter 33, **Uncommon Lung Tumors**; and, in the non-AIDS group, in Chapter 35, **Metastases to and from the Lung**. The remaining discussion of immunosuppressive lung disease in this chapter is concerned with non-AIDS immunocompromised hosts.

The cause of non-AIDS immunocompromise in patients varies; it most often results from primary malignancies involving the host response, such as leukemia or lymphoma, from cytotoxic drug therapies for these and other malignancies, or from cytotoxic drug or steroid therapies for assorted benign diseases such as interstitial pulmonary fibrosis, collagen vascular disease, nephritis, and hepatitis. Congenital immunodeficiencies, which are also important, are covered in Chapters 7 and 8. Transplantation pathology, as was noted, is discussed further in Chapter 24.

The most frequently and intensively studied subgroup in non-AIDS immunocompromised patients consists of those under treatment for acute leukemia. Leukemic patients, along with bone marrow transplant recipients, have the greatest immunosuppression and therefore have the highest incidence of problems. Acute leukemic patients with fever and pulmonary infiltrates have a higher mortality (62%) than those with fever but without pulmonary infiltrates (9%).[37] Pulmonary infiltrates are often detected acutely and accompanied by fever. Fever itself is not always helpful in separating infectious from noninfectious causes. Presenting complaints, physical and radiographic findings, white blood cell counts, and knowledge of the type(s) and extent of therapy are not very helpful in making such a distinction.[38–43] Pneumonias in this setting may develop with devastating rapidity.[44] Sputum and other aspiration samples may help identify an infective cause.

Blood cultures do not always correlate with tissue cultures.[45]

Patients are often empirically placed on broad-spectrum antibiotics, often including treatment for *Pneumocystis carinii,* and are frequently on antifungal agents by the time biopsies are done. An illustrative series is from Stanford University in Palo Alto, California, by McCabe and associates.[46] Fifteen acute leukemic patients with pulmonary infiltrates, fever, and neutropenia had open lung biopsies. They averaged 20 days in the hospital before this procedure: 1 patient had two antibiotics, 12 had three, and 4 had 4 during this time. One-third had either pentamidine or trimethoprim/sulfamethoxazole. Nine (67%) were on amphotercin for a mean of 22 days. Biopsies showed 4 patients with fungi, including 3 with *Aspergillus;* 2 had leukemia, and 9 (60%) had nonspecific changes. Of 60% with nonspecific changes, 89% had continued broad-spectrum antibiotic coverage after biopsy. Eighty-six percent had continued amphotercin, and the 4 on antipneumocystis medications continued these drugs. This group received an average of 4.3 antimicrobial agents before biopsy and 3.9 afterward. Eight of 15 died while in the hospital. Of those with fungi diagnosed at open lung biopsy, 3 were not receiving amphotercin but later responded well to this drug and were discharged; 1 had been on this medication for 15 days and was continued on it for 3 more days until his death by *Pseudomonas* sepsis. Two of those dying with nonspecific changes had invasive *Aspergillus* at autopsy; 1 had been on amphotercin for 21 days, the other for 90 days.

The reader is referred to the appropriate chapters for more detail on drug and other therapy effects (Chapter 23) and for more information about specific infectious organisms (Chapters 9–15). Several other good reviews are available,[31,47,48] including pulmonary drug toxicity,[49–53] radiotherapy effects,[54,55] and opportunistic infections.[56] Careful search for *Pneumocystis carinii* is often necessary, and some more recent reviews of PCP in non-AIDS patients are suggested.[32–35] Advance consideration of all possibilities will assure proper handling of the tissue. Bacteria in this setting are often gram negative, and *Aspergillus* leads the group of possible fungi. Mycobacteria and, occasionally, parasites must also be considered.

As one might suspect, increasingly invasive techniques yield more and more accurate diagnoses. When clinical, radiographic, sputum cytologic, and microbiologic exams fail to give the answer, transbronchial biopsies, often with brush and wash cytologic specimens, are obtained. Lavage specimens are particularly helpful for rapid *Pneumocystis* and fungal diagnoses. Transtracheal and transbronchial aspirations are gaining acceptance, and transthoracic fine-needle aspirations are used to obtain malignant or infectious material.

Several transbronchial biopsies series concentrating on non-AIDS immunocompromised hosts are available.[57–69] These biopsies generally produced diagnoses in 32%–85%. When only diagnoses of treatable infection in malignancy are considered, these percentages were 32%–50%. Transbronchial biopsies in general have their highest yield in infectious and diffuse lung diseases. Most consider lung parenchyma necessary to judge a specimen "satisfactory." However, there is no good judge of adequacy of bronchial biopsies if lung parenchyma is present and no specific diagnosis is available.[70]

Many series of biopsies of immunocompromised patients combined transbronchial biopsy findings with open biopsies or consisted of open biopsies only (see Table 1–1).* These series differ somewhat from each other depending on the amount, type, and length of prebiopsy treatment with antibiotics, the inclusion or exclusion of other potentially diagnostic specimens before, during, or after the biopsy, and the patient populations. The poorest survival is, of course, obtained in the sickest patients with the worst diseases. Some series tend to concentrate on one or more techniques for diagnosis, such as culture and cytology specimens along with biopsies. Other review biopsies only. Some do not allow comparison of data, as in determining effect of biopsy results on survival. Also, the types of pathology included in the "nonspecific" category vary in different series. Most define "specific diagnosis" as those for which there are specific treatments. Many of these include infectious and malignant causes. Viral changes and/or hemorrhage may or may not fall within the "treatable" definition. Some authors consider beneficial effect to include withdrawal of potentially harmful therapy where pertinent. As reviewed by Rosenow et al.,[47] pulmonary hemorrhage may be present in 43%–88% of cases, but may not be accepted as a diagnosis until autopsy.

One series worthy of detailed comment is that by Tenholder and Hooper,[80] who studied 98 pulmonary infiltrate episodes in 139 cases of adult leukemic patients, of whom 61% had acute leukemia. They divided their patients into those with pulmonary infiltrates before and up to 3 days of instigation of chemotherapy and those with infiltrates occurring later in the course of chemotherapy. Seventeen episodes of pulmonary infiltrates with fever in the "pretreatment" group and 81 episodes in the "during treatment" group were studied. The cause of the infiltrates was determined in 94% of

---

* References: 30, 44–46, 71–85.

Table 1–1. Open lung biopsy series in immunocompromised hosts[a]

Reference	Episodes/Patients (% with malignancy)	Infection (%)	Tumor[b] (% of all 1% with malignancy)	Nonspecific (%) (nontreatable and/or nondiagnostic)	Mortality (%)
Roback et al., 1973[71c]	46/40 (55)	41	7/14	52	—
Greenman et al., 1975[30]	95/78 (64)	27	29/41	35	49
Rosen et al., 1975[72]	52 (92)	44	10	35	74
Nelems et al., 1976[73]	28 (39)	46[d]	14/36	39[e]	57
Pennington and Feldman, 1977[74]	47/43 (100)	57	3	22	45[f]
Wolff et al., 1977[75]	24 (96)	96	4	0[g]	—
Leight and Michaelis, 1978[76]	42 (74)	48	7/10	29	31
Singer et al., 1979[77]	44 (99)	48	14	39	52
Rossiter et al., 1979[78]	83 (96)	18	42/51	45	25[h]
Toledo-Peyera et al., 1980[79]	20 (100)	25	40	24	10–15
Tenholder and Hooper, 1980[80]	98/?# (100)	46	8	40	50[i]
Waltzer et al., 1980[81]	23/22 (0)	73	0[j]	35	23
Jaffee and Maki, 1981[44]	53 (74)	33	13/23	45	23
Hiatt et al., 1982[45]	68 (53)	21	12/22	48	63
Canham et al., 1988[82]	57/48 (92)	25	10	41	44
McKenna et al., 1984[83]	64 (95)	10	25	66	—
Prober et al., 1984[84c]	46/44 (59)	72	4/7	24	—
McCabe et al., 1985[46]	15 (100)	33	13	47	60
Cockerill et al., 1985[85]	90 (60)	55	20/33	43	38

[a] May include transbronchial biopsies (TBB) but excludes TBB only series.

[b] Single percentage (%) given in predominantly malignant series. Percentage (%) of those with malignancy originally is second number.

[c] Roback et al.,[71] Wolff et al.,[75] and Prober et al.[84] are pediatric series.

[d] Nelems et al.[73] Includes four viral; some infections are multiple (with tumor and infection).

[e] Nelems et al.[73] Includes four viral as nontreatable.

[f] Pennington and Feldman.[74] Worse with neutropenia (55%) or acute leukemia (67%).

[g] Wolff et al.[75] 83% of children had pneumocystis.

[h] Rossiter et al.[78] 25% hospital mortality, 40% late mortality (mean, 9.7 months).

[i] Tenholder and Hooper.[80] 45 patients died of 139 (32%) followed, but 98 episodes of infiltrate were evaluated in unidentified number of patients (estimated, 50%).

[j] Waltzer et al.[81] Renal transplant series.

the "pretreatment" group. Many of these were localized and proved to be bacterial. No opportunistic infections were identified in this group and survival was good. Tenholder and Hooper's "during treatment" group had 31 episodes of local infiltrates and 50 episodes of diffuse infiltrates. The cause of the localized infiltrate subgroup was determined in 90%, and of these 82% were infectious, again mostly bacterial. However, 13% of this group had opportunistic infections. The cause was identified in 80% of the diffuse group during treatment, but was infectious in only 35%, the other 65% being assorted diagnoses as hemorrhage, edema, fibrosis, and persistent leukemia. Ninety-three percent of the identified infections in the diffuse "during treatment" group were opportunistic infections. These authors suggested pursuing a final diagnosis in this last group while giving a trial of broad-spectrum antibiotics in the "pretreatment" and localized infiltrate "during treatment" subgroups.

Validity of Biopsies in Immunosuppressed Patients

How good are biopsy techniques at diagnosing the patient's problem, or does it matter? As noted in Table 1–1 and excluding the one series by Wolff et al.,[75] nonspecific findings were present in 22%–66% of the open lung biopsy series, averaging 37%. A high percentage of similar findings are present in AIDS biopsies (see Chapter 6). These nonspecific findings included diffuse alveolar damage, nonspecific cellular infiltrates, and interstitial thickening or fibrosis. Some of these changes may result from drug, oxygen, or radiotherapy, a few from graft-versus-host disease where appropriate, and some from infections, possibly viral. The significance of documenting specific versus nonspecific findings varies in immunosuppressed patients in different series. Some investigators reported with documenting a specific diagnosis, a better* or a worse prognosis[44,61,73] or no change,† in patients who have a specific or treatable diagnosis.

In caring for patients, we sometimes pursue answers supposing the answers will help the patient. In the case of obtaining a specific diagnosis in such patients, one might assume specific therapy will be beneficial. As noted, several series support this, but more and more

---

* References 37, 65, 72, 79–82.

† References: 45, 46, 78, 80.

show that despite such knowledge and application of appropriate therapy, these patients do no better than those without a specific diagnosis or treatable disease. Finding persistent primary malignancy usually indicates treatment failure.[82] Several editorials[86–90] have questioned the benefit of a specific diagnosis. A prospective trial is needed to randomize such patients post biopsy to "treatment" versus "nontreatment" groups, but such a trial is unlikely, because to not treat a patient with a potentially treatable disease is untenable to most clinicians.[90]

The hospital mortality for many acutely ill patients in the immunocompromised group is high (see Table 1–1). Some benefit may ensue from discontinuing potentially harmful and unnecessary therapies. Biopsy findings are probably most helpful in those groups with better prognoses who have a better chance of responding to therapy or of surviving nonspecific findings.

Biopsies in Nonimmunocompromised Hosts

This group is sometimes referred to as the "non-critically ill" group.[91] It covers almost everything else for which a lung tissue diagnosis is required. In the series of Ray et al.[92] of 416 open lung biopsies, symptoms were cough (71%), dyspnea (61%), chest pain (40%), and weight loss (40%). These patients have chest radiographs that show a mass effect, persistent localized infiltrate, or diffuse interstitial disease.

In the large and progressive series by Carrington and Gaensler,[21] Gaensler and Carrington,[22,29] Gaensler et al.,[28] and Wall et al.,[93] about one-third of the patients with diffuse infiltrative diseases required lung biopsy for diagnosis, often to distinguish the 200 or so "interstitial" diseases.[21,29] Buechner[94] noted about 100 miliary diseases in the lung, of which 40 or so are confined to this system. Occasionally open lung biopsies are necessary for those with symptoms but with normal radiographs.[95] In this group, changes of desquamative interstitial pneumonia or extrinsic allergic alveolitis were most often found.[29,95] Open lung biopsies in those with chronic interstitial disease occurred on average 1.53 years after the first documented radiographic change.[28] The diseases most frequently diagnosed in this setting are sarcoid, pneumoconiosis, interstitial pneumonia,[21,29] interstitial fibrosis,[96] and, depending on the series, extrinsic allergic alveolitis and malignancy.[21,29]

A large percentage of masses are potentially malignant, and transbronchial specimens may be quite beneficial in establishing a diagnosis.[97] Even when transbronchial biopsy under fluoroscopic guidance is used, and even when multiple biopsies are taken, often only small portions of the multiple pieces may be positive, and one at times makes essentially a cytologic diagno-

sis.[70] Fechner et al.[70] proposed that the biopsy forceps may not penetrate a peripheral mass and may only obtain tissue on its edge. If tumor has extended into the edge, the sample may be diagnostic, but one must be aware of nonspecific changes around such masses. Bronchial brush, needle, and wash specimens help increase this yield. Very few clinicians will stop investigating a suspicious mass and will usually pursue potential resection after appropriate staging procedures, bypassing a mini-open lung biopsy.

Transbronchial biopsies are most diagnostic in diffuse interstitial disease. Pattern recognition also becomes more important in many chronic diseases in this diffuse group, and this may be a reason for part of the failure rate obtained with small fragments of tissue. These patients are not often acutely ill and so infections, at least acute infections with easily identified organisms, are not as significant a part of the findings as they are in the immunocompromised group. It may still be necessary to culture both the transbronchial and open lung biopsies for fungi, mycobacteria, viruses, and possibly *Mycoplasma*.

When typical lesions present, transbronchial biopsies may adequately allow diagnosis of various diseases such as sarcoid, tuberculosis, an assortment of fungal diseases, esoinophilic pneumonia, eosinophilic granuloma, aspiration, alveolar proteinosis, and amyloid. The granulomas of sarcoid are often multifocal with frequent bronchial mucosal involvement, and so should be one of the more diagnostic groups for comparison. Transbronchial biopsies are positive for noncaseating granulomata in 57%–90% of cases.[93,98–100] In a series by Wall et al.,[93] 67% of transbronchial biopsies recognized sarcoid when it was the final diagnosis. However, in one-third of the patients in whom the clinical picture was most suggestive of sarcoid, an open lung biopsy yielded a different diagnosis. Among those who were eventually diagnosed as having sarcoid, a different clinical picture was suggested in 48% (see Chapter 19).

Wall and associates[93] extended their earlier series by comparing their open lung biopsies with their transbronchial biopsies. When characteristic changes of tumor, sarcoid, or infection were present, a diagnosis was given and no further tissue was obtained. This occurred in 38% of the cases. Twenty-five percent of their transbronchial biopsies were either insufficient because lung parenchyma was not obtained or contained only normal lung. Others have reported this combination for transbronchial biopsies in from 9% to 32%.*

As in the transbronchial biopsies of immunocompromised patients, biopsies in the noncompromised group included a large number with nonspecific findings,

---

* References: 6, 57, 98, 101, 102.

varying between 31% and 59% in different series.† Wall et al.[93] found a diagnosis was rendered in 97% of the open lung biopsies and that there was poor correlation with semi- or nonspecific findings on transbronchial biopsies. For example, the degree of fibrosis in fibrotic lung disease could not be estimated on transbronchial biopsy. This is partly because of the variability of this disease and partly the nonspecific increased fibrous tissue near bronchioles.

In one series by Wilson and associates,[91] 127 noncritically ill patients were studied; transbronchial biopsy was diagnostic of neoplasm, granulomatous inflammation, or pneumonia in 23% with mass effect, 21% with localized infiltrate, and 62% with diffuse infiltrate. The addition of cytologic specimens obtained during this time added 17%, 8%, and 6%, respectively, to the diagnostic yields. In their series, approximately 51% had nonspecific findings, and of these 92% became better and the others experienced a worsening course and had neoplastic disease diagnosed on open lung biopsy. Those in the nonimmunosuppressed group with nonspecific findings certainly fared better than those immunocompromised discussed in the previous section.

Because dust diseases are an important part of the chronic non-immunosuppressed group of lung biopsies, the International Labour Organization and Union Internationale Contre le Cancer developed a combined radiographic rating scale in 1971, known as the ILO U/C.[103,104] This has been reviewed with correlative pathology by McLoud et al.[105] (See also Chapters 27 and 28.)

Choice of Biopsy Site

There has been a debate as to whether the easily accessible and resectable tip of lingula or right-middle lobe, or any edge or tip for that matter, is adequate and represents a site for biopsy for diffuse lung disease. Because of its distance and circuitous route, some have noted a nonspecific increase in inflammation, scarring, and vascular thickening.‡ Others disagree,[109,110] and as long as the area is representative, this is probably acceptable. Our surgeons use a limited posterior approach that gives them good access to much of the midlung and hilum, so we have not studied this problem. It seems that if the disease biopsied is quite recognizable and is distinct from the nonspecific findings described above, and the lingula appears to be involved with the rest of the lung by a diffuse process, this might

---

† References: 5, 57, 59, 64, 91, 98, 101.
‡ References: 14, 21, 22, 29, 92, 106–108.

suffice. The inability to sample different areas in too limited an approach and an increase in nonspecific findings may be expected.

Some surgeons plan their approach to sample the worst area, which can lead to nonrepresentative samples. For example, the degree of honeycombing, other scarring, or necrosis in the sample may not be compatible with life! More intermediate activity samples better help to define the pathologic processes.[21,28,96,111] Surgeons should attempt to sample several areas of varying intensity of involvement, which may include but not exclusively contain the worst areas.

Open lung biopsies in the nonimmunocompromised group, as in the immunocompromised group, should be directed toward patients with potentially treatable diseases. For example, older people with end-stage fibrosis or honeycombing of the lungs may be excluded as there is no effective therapy, but younger people with less advanced disease should be biopsied.

Search for Infective Organisms in Tissue Samples

The question pathologists often ask themselves is, "How long do I search special stains of tissue for infective organisms?" The answer to this question should be "Until the pathologist is sure, to the best of his or her ability, there are no organisms present." Another guideline of ours is, "If another competent pathologist carefully searches this specimen, I know (s)he will either (a) be extremely lucky or (b) will have to work long and hard if (s)he diagnoses a specific infection and I don't." Pathologists should not be proven wrong by their microbiology laboratory too often. There is no absolute answer to what is required to reach this end. In small biopsies, such as on transbronchial biopsies, a careful search of H and E sections for viral inclusions and special stains for organisms may be conducted in a few minutes. On open lung tissue, such a search of multiple stains requiring 15 min may not be unreasonable. The pathologist must be wary of fatigue, and if he is highly suspicious of scant organisms, such as acid-fast bacilli, he might, as we do, review slides at two separate times, such as in the afternoon of one day and first thing in the morning of the next day. In handling such stains, the first rule is to slow down and carefully search tissue under high dry microscopy, using oil microscopy for anything suspicious or for part of routine surveillance in suspicious areas.

In nonimmunocompromised persons, fungi and acid-fast bacilli are usually found in the centers of necrosis when necrotic granulomata are found.[112] In immunocompromised hosts, the typical reactive patterns of infection may not be present.[67] In this group one should establish a routine of using at least acid-fast (AFB) and methenamine (GMS) stains and perhaps also immunofluorescence-specific antibodies to search for organisms, even in the absence of the usual histologic changes. One must then be diligent in carefully reviewing these stains because the areas of reaction cannot be selected for review. We routinely do GMS stains for any debris in the alveoli, including early hyaline membranes.[113]

It has been stated traditionally that microbiology is better than histology at detecting fungi or mycobacteria, but this has been questioned.[112] Certainly most pathologists can remember identifying fungi on tissue sections when none were cultured. Perhaps these represent dead organisms. Also, some other organisms may be seen on smears but are culture negative. Culture, smear, and special stains of tissue should all complement each other.

Large Specimen Techniques

Many special techniques have been developed to study particular problems in anatomy and its alteration by disease processes in the lung and elsewhere. This part of Chapter 1 does not attempt to be panoramic or extremely detailed in its presentation but does describe some highlights of these preparations as they particularly apply to the lung. The reader is referred to the original articles for many of the details with cross reference to other publications on the subjects.[114,115] Other techniques have been described in this volume: formalin fume inflation under positive internal pressure or negative external pressure has been used by others in preparing beautiful dry preparations, and freeze-drying, as illustrated in Chapter 26. Such dry specimen techniques have been most effectively used in studying emphysema[116–119] and correlative radiographic appearances of lung disease.[120–122] Some pulmonary functions can even be done on excised lungs.[123] Illustrations of many of the procedures discussed here are drawn from examples offered in the chapters that follow.

Other special procedures for solving unusual problems are described. Use of serial sections is outlined in Chapter 1 for handling small biopsies, particularly transbronchial biopsies. Point counting has been used in defining emphysema (Chapter 26) and in quantitating lung development.

Destruction of lung tissue is sometimes necessary for more exact quantification of some abnormalities, especially those caused by dusts. Analysis of asbestos fibers is still most quantitative when done after complete diges-

tion of tissue (Chapter 28). Bronchopulmonary lavage may emerge as a less invasive technique for such quantification. Other mineral analysis in the past has used incineration of tissue, but newer techniques nicely detailed in Chapter 27 and summarized in Table 27–6 have replaced destructive techniques in current usage. Some of these sublight microscopic techniques can be applied to tissue sections, including old ones, and can be used in correlation with light and scanning electron microscopy.

Thick and thin sections for light microscopy have special applications. The adjective *thick* has been applied to some of the preparations in this chapter, such as Gough–Wentworth sections (100–500 μm), thick microscopic slides (8–100 μm), and to tissues being prepared for electron microscopy (1 μm). *Thin* is applied to routine histology (2–3 μm) in paraffin-embedded tissue, in plastic-embedded light microscopy (1–2 μm), and in the final preparations for electron microscopy (0.06–0.09 μm).

Some special photographic techniques have been useful to this author. For projection purposes tissue samples may be stained with hematoxylin and eosin (H and E) or the stain of your choice, mounted on 35-mm (2 × 2 in.) glass plates, covered with either a thin 35-mm coverslip or a similar 35-mm mounting glass, and projected in a manner similar to other 35-mm slides. For this purpose, tissues benefit from slightly thicker sectioning (6–10 μm) and some overstaining. These give beautiful low-power detail when projected; however, the subjects must be chosen carefully if they are to illustrate a specific process at such a fixed low power. In formal presentations, higher resolution photomicrography is often necessary to complement these initial slides.

Either these 35-mm-type histologic slides or routine histologic slides may be mounted directly into a photographic enlarger and projected onto direct positive black-and-white film. Magnification is limited by the height and resolution of the enlarger; such preparations may range from 1 to 17 power in this author's enlarger. Again, very crisp detail is available at low magnification, which helps cover this particularly awkward area of magnification for microphotography.

Gough–Wentworth Sections

Large portions of lung, either whole lungs, lobes, or other significant portions, can be sliced on a giant microtome and then mounted as a wet preparation between glass or plastic plates or dry mounted on paper. This technique was originally described in the late 1940s by Gough and Wentworth.[124,125] The thickness may vary, but is usually in the range of 100 to 500 μm.

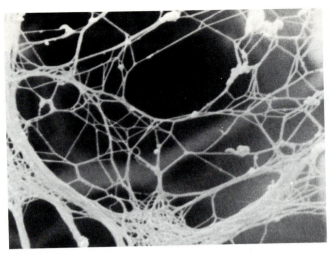

Fig. 2–18. Portion of alveolar wall digested with 0.1 *N* NaOH shows fine network of elastic fibers arising from relatively thick orifice bundle. Rabbit. SEM, ×11,000. (From Am Rev Respir Dis 1977;115:449 with permission.)

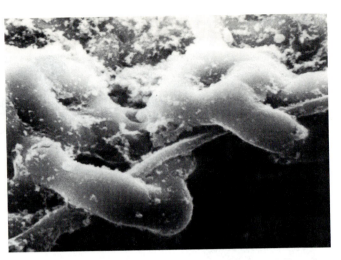

Fig. 2–19. Interwoven pattern of capillary loops and fibroelastic fibers is best shown at edge of alveolus. Capillary was filled with fine latex beads and alveolus digested with 0.1 *N* NaOH. Hamster, SEM, ×1,600. (From Scan Electron Microsc 1976;II:233 with permission.)

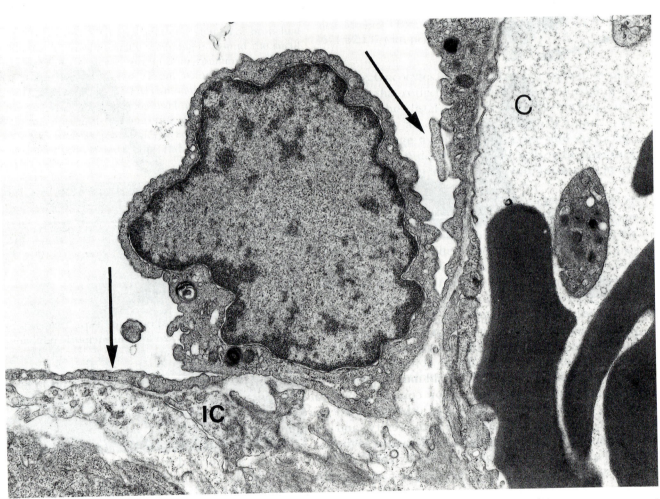

Fig. 2–20. Type I alveolar lining cell has a relatively large nucleus and thin, widely stretched cytoplasm (*arrows*). Thickened portion of alveolar wall contains an interstitial cell (IC) but air–blood barrier is very thin. Red blood cells and platelet in capillary (C). Mouse. TEM, ×15,000. (From Fraser and Paré: Diagnosis of diseases of the chest, Vol. 1. 2d Ed. Philadelphia: WB Saunders, Co. 1977:24 with permission.)

elastic fibers, including the fine meshwork of the alveolus, are interconnected in all directions to form an integrated elastic network that is fundamental to the uniform expansion and elastic retraction of the lung in respiration.

The Alveolar Lining Cells

There are two types of alveolar lining cells. The *type I* alveolar lining cell, which lies on the alveolar wall like a fried egg, has a central flattened nucleus and a peripheral cytoplasm that reaches 50 μm in diameter and is as thin as 0.1 μm (Fig. 2–20); these cells constitute 40% of the alveolar lining cells but cover 90% of the alveolar surface. (See Table 20–2.) The type I cells are joined by tight junctions, underlined by a well-developed basal lamina, but have sparse surface microvilli and cytoplasmic organelles (Figs. 2–20 and 2–21).

The *type II* alveolar lining cell, a cuboidal cell with diameter up to 15 μm, is characterized by a large basal nucleus with a prominent nucleolus, and abundant osmiophilic lamellar inclusion bodies, the precursors of the surfactant (Figs. 2–22 and 2–23). It constitutes 60% of the surface cells but covers only some 5% of the surface. It has many stubby microvilli on the alveolar surface (Figs. 2–21 through 2–23), well-formed tight junctions with the adjacent type I cell, a basement membrane, and abundant cytoplasm with well-developed endoplasmic reticulum and Golgi apparatus. Besides secreting surfactant, the type II alveolar lining cell also serves as the reserve cell, maturing into the type I cell normally. The type II alveolar lining cell becomes hyperplastic in response to alveolar damage; it may also become dysplastic.

Surfactant

The type II alveolar cell secretes its osmiophilic lamellar inclusion bodies into the alveolar space (Figs. 2–22 and 2–23) to form a partially crystallized hypophase of tubular myelin, which then spreads out into a thin layer of surfactant (Fig. 2–24). *Surfactant* is formed mainly by phospholipids, especially dipalmitoyl lecithin, with the addition of glycoprotein components. When the alveolus deflates, the phospholipids are compressed and aligned into a layer with hydrophilic and hydrophobic ends on each side at the air–liquid interface. This arrangement reduces the surface tension and prevents the collapse of the alveolus. At alveolar inflation, the orderly arrangement of the phospholipids molecules is disrupted, and the resulting increase in the surface tension assists the elastic recoil of the alveolus in expiration. The replenishment of surfactant about the alveolus and its presumed ascending flow toward the bron-

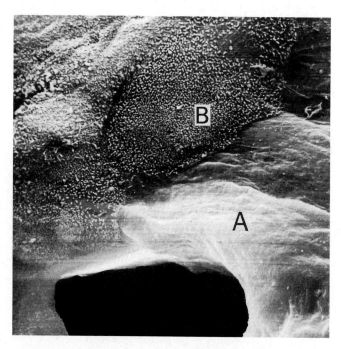

Fig. 2–21. Surface of type II cell (B) shows abundant stubby microvilli. Microvilli sparse on type I cell (A) around alveolar pore. Human. SEM, ×1,200.

chiole is also helpful in alveolar clearance. Surfactant, therefore, plays several important roles in the stability and function of the alveolus.

Insufficient production of surfactant in prematurity results in hyaline membrane disease with alveolar collapse and pulmonary edema. In diffuse alveolar damage syndrome at any age, excessive leakage of fibrin and other capillary contents into the alveolar space interferes with the action of surfactant despite a normal or even increased amount of surfactant in the alveolus.

Air–Blood Barrier

For the most efficient exchange of oxygen and carbon dioxide between air spaces and red blood cells, the alveolar arrangement is nearly perfect. The alveolar interstitial cells and interstitial fibers are minimal (see Fig. 2–17), and a rich interanastomosing network of capillaries bulges into adjacent air spaces[16] (Figs. 2–19 and 2–25). It is estimated that 85%–95% of the approximately 140 m^2 of alveolar surface is covered with the pulmonary capillary network, giving an air–blood interface of about 126 m^2, a surface area about 70 times that of the skin.

The endothelial and epithelial alveolar type I cell cytoplasm is spread as thinly as possible and the basal laminas are fused, leading to an air–blood barrier with a mean thickness of 0.6 μm. Plasma and other red cells may increase this distance in reality (see Fig. 2–20).

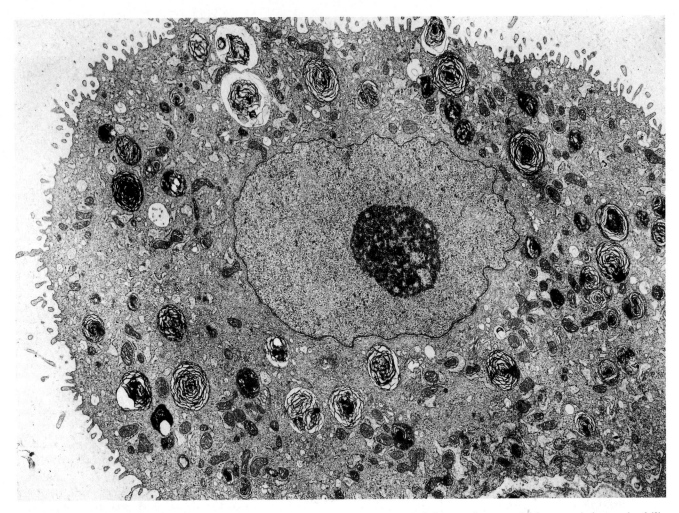

Fig. 2–22. Type II alveolar lining cell is cuboidal with large nucleus and nucleolus, many stubby microvilli, and abundant cytoplasmic organelles including mitochondria, endoplasmic reticulum, Golgi apparatus, and characteristic osmiophilic lamellar inclusion bodies. Human. TEM, ×5,000.

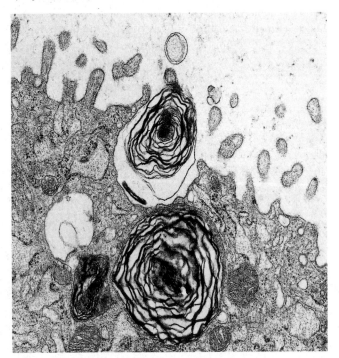

Fig. 2–23. Precursor of surfactant is being released from type II alveolar cell. Human. TEM, ×15,500.

◁————————————————

————————————————▷

Fig. 2–24. Surfactant on alveolar surface has thin surface layer (top) and crystallized hypophase material with tubular myelin figure. Mouse. TEM, ×45,000.

Fig. 2–25 A–D. Rich capillary plexus of alveolar septa **A.** Latex-injected, 0.1 *N* NaOH digested human lung. SEM, ×250; scale = 50 μm. (Reprinted from Am Rev Respir Dis 1977;115:449–460 with permission.) **B.** Histological section shows capillary supply radiating about center of photo. H and E, ×400. **C.** Note interconnections in this thin section (1 μm) between capillaries on opposite sides of same alveolar septum. Toluidine blue, ×400. (Courtesy of H. Spencer Pulmonary Collection, London.) **D.** En face view of histological section of congested alveolar septum. H and E, ×400.

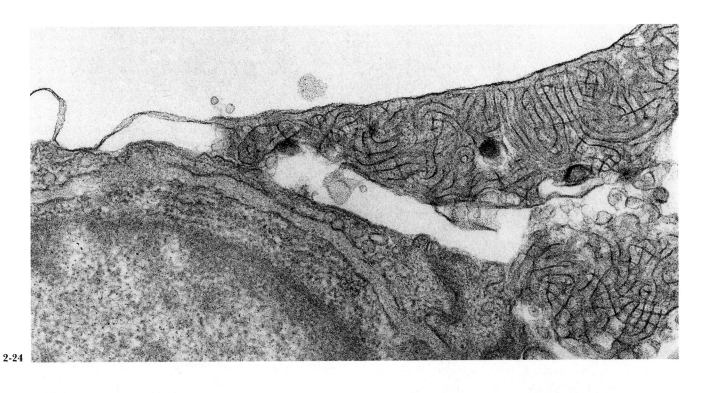

2-24

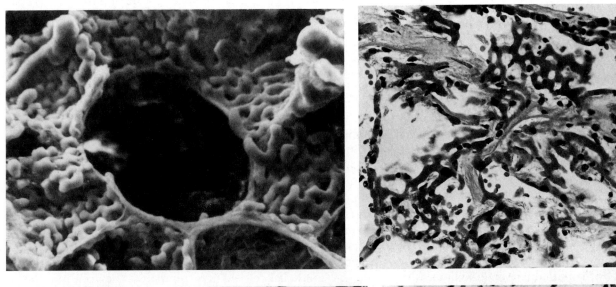

2-25A

2-25B

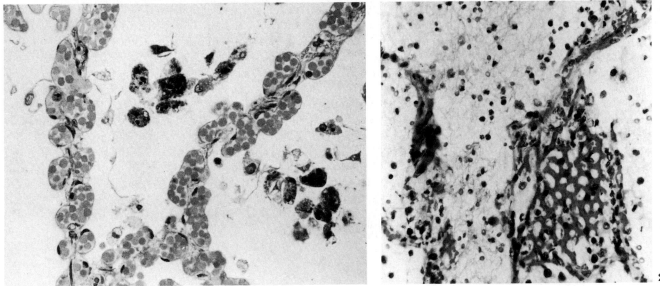

2-25C

2-25D

Considering that a red blood cell has an average diameter of 7 μm, one can appreciate the delicacy of these interfaces as well as how easily they might be damaged.

About 200 ml of blood are within the capillary network at a given time. Spread over 126 m^2, this is equivalent to about 1.6 ml of blood (1/3 teaspoon) spread over 1 m^2! Only about a third of the capillary network is functioning in the resting state, but it opens up extensively with exercise. The blood passes this capillary bed in 0.75 s, and the flow must continue to move to handle the entire cardiac output. The combined weight of the two lungs in vivo are approximately 1000 g, of which half consists of blood in the arteries, capillaries, and veins.

The Capillary Endothelium

The pulmonary endothelium of the alveolus, which occupies a surface area of more than 140 m^2, is the largest and most dense vascular bed in the human body (see Fig. 2–25). The fine structure and permeability of the *alveolar capillary endothelium* is similar to that of the capillary endothelium elsewhere in the body.

Besides serving as a barrier and actively regulating gas, water, and solute transport, the pulmonary endothelium also selectively processes and modifies a wide range of substances. A classic example is the conversion of angiotensin I to angiotensin II and the inactivation of bradykinin by the angiotensin-converting enzyme; this reaction occurs in caveolae (pinocytic vesicles) and the microvilli of the luminal cytoplasmic membrane. The endothelium also clears serotonin, norepinephrine, prostaglandin E and F, adenine nucleotides, and some hormones and drugs, and releases angiotensin II, adenosine, some prostaglandins, and previously accumulated drugs and metabolites. It is of note that angiotensin II, epinephrine, and prostaglandins A and I$_2$ are not altered by the pulmonary endothelium.

The endothelia of pulmonary arteries and veins differ from the capillary endothelium in that the pulmonary arteries and veins are subjected to much greater changes in the vascular inner surface area than is the capillary. In resting or low-pressure conditions, the endothelium of pulmonary arteries appears elliptical with the long axis of cell arranged parallel to the direction of the blood flow: the endothelium of pulmonary veins appears polygonal. Both of them have more surface microvilli and cytoplasmic organelles than the capillary endothelium, particularly on rod-shaped, membrane-bound structures (Weibel–Palade bodies), which probably are the storage site of the coagulation Factor VIII.

Other Cells and Structures in the Alveolar Wall

Mesenchymal cells, including fibroblasts, pericytes of capillaries, and myofibroblasts (*contractile interstitial cells*), are present in the alveolar septum opposite the alveolar surface of the capillary. They are responsible for the maintenance and metabolism of the elastic and collagen fibers and proteoglycans in the alveolar walls. *Collagen* fibers, the rigid structural components of the lung (as opposed to its elastic fibers), are present mainly in the bronchovascular bundles and lobar and lobular septi and pleura. As the delicate collagen fibers in the normal alveolar wall can only be seen by electron microscopy, collagen fibers in alveolar walls that are apparent by light microscopy are abnormal. Contractile cells participate in the regulation of blood flow (see next section).

Neutrophils, eosinophils, lymphocytes, plasma cells, basophils or *mast cells*, and fixed or migratory macrophages are present in small numbers in the alveolar wall and bronchial interstitial space. Neutrophils are most frequently found within the alveolar capillaries. Heavy sequestration and degranulation of neutrophils in the alveolar capillary may be responsible for insidious tissue lysis, such as elastolysis in pulmonary emphysema. An increase in the number of mast cells and eosinophiles occurs in bronchial asthma or other hypersensitivity diseases.

Alveolar Regulation of Capillary Flow

The pulmonary blood flow is regulated mainly by small pulmonary arteries, especially in hypoxia. Local regulation of the blood flow in the alveolar wall occurs via several possible mechanisms. The contractile interstitial cells are attached between adjacent endothelial and epithelial cells. When stimulated, they contract to distort and disrupt the capillary flow. The detailed control mechanisms, the mediators that induce their contraction, and the physiologic importance of this mechanism are not clear.

Another regulatory mechanism of the alveolar capillary flow is related to the interweaving of the elastocollagen fibers and the capillaries (see Fig. 2–19). The capillary flow is disrupted at the extremes of inflation or deflation because of interlocking or pinching of both structures in many places. If widespread, prolonged diffuse collapse or hyperinflation of the lung is incompatible with life. Interruption of blood flow to focally collapsed or overinflated alveoli, however, is efficient and beneficial.

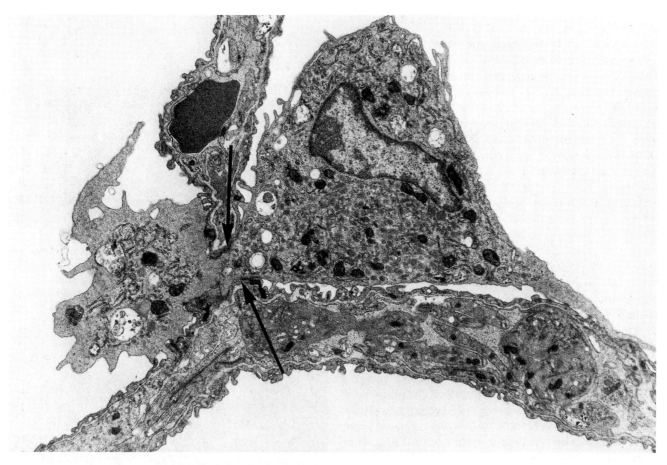

Fig. 2–26. Macrophage crossing pore of Kohn (*arrows*) has elongated cell processes and abundant cytoplasmic dense bodies containing lysosomes, phagosomes, etc. Mouse. TEM, ×8,500. (From Thurlbeck and Wang: MTP International Review of Sciences. Physiology, Ser. 1, Vol. 1. 1974:2 with permission.)

Alveolar Pores (of Kohn), Fenestrae, and Collateral Ventilation

Communications between adjacent alveoli are not present in the fetal lung. *Pores* 2–10 μm or more in size start to appear in the alveolar wall soon after birth and appear to increase in number with age (see Fig. 2–17). Normal alveolar pores are filled with surfactant, thus blocking the airflow between adjacent alveoli. No normal function of the alveolar pores is known, but macrophages may wander through them (Fig. 2–26). In classic lobar pneumonia, edema fluid, fibrin, and bacteria spread rapidly between alveoli through the alveolar pores, and at times tumor extends through them (see Figs. 33–136 and 33–137).

Alveolar pores larger than 15 μm, which are considered abnormal, are called fenestrae (see Chapter 24). Alveoli distal to an obstructed airway can receive collateral ventilation through fenestrae from alveoli venti-lated by a nearby unobstructed bronchiole. Other collateral ventilation channels include communications between alveolar ducts or small bronchioles, and between bronchioles and alveoli (canal of Lambert). These structures are found most often in aged adult lungs, especially in diseased lungs such as those of miners.

The Vasculature of the Lung

The lung has dual blood supplies: the *pulmonary* or *minor circulation system* and the *bronchial* or *nutritional system*. The former (pulmonary) is a low-pressure system that accommodates total systemic venous return and is prepared structurally to absorb a large change of the flow volume with a minimal change in pressure. The latter (bronchial system), a part of the systemic circulation, has high pressure and high oxygen content.

Pulmonary Arteries and Veins

The pulmonary trunk arises from the right ventricle and almost immediately divides into left and right main *pulmonary arteries;* these further divide into *lobar* arteries before entering left and right lungs with the lobar bronchi. Intrapulmonary arteries follow and divide with bronchi and bronchioles, roughly in the same frequency and in similar diameters, out to the bronchioloalveolar junctions. From here the blood flows into the alveolar capillary network and the air diffuses into the alveoli.

The wall of a pulmonary artery that is greater than 0.5 cm in external diameter is thinner than that of a systemic artery of corresponding size and has less smooth muscle cells but more elastic fibers. The normal systolic and diastolic pressures in the main pulmonary artery are approximately 20 and 10 mm Hg, respectively (mean, 14 mm Hg), as compared to 120 and 80 (mean, 90 mm Hg) in the systemic circulation. Doubling of the resting flow volume only raises the pulmonary systolic pressure by 5 mm Hg.

The *pulmonary venules* collect the capillary blood into the lobular septum. The small venules and lobular veins converge toward the hilum, forming larger pulmonary veins in the subsegmental septa. They group with the bronchi and pulmonary arteries at the segmental level, and proceed in their company to the hilum. The muscle layer of the pulmonary vein is scarce and irregularly arranged. The portion of the extrapulmonary vein near the left atrium is surrounded by cardiac muscle. Although less obvious in gross and light microscopic sections, the intrapulmonary arrangement of pulmonary arteries and veins and bronchial arteries resembles, in principle, that of the portal and the hepatic veins and hepatic artery in the liver.

Bronchial Arteries and Veins

The origin of the *bronchial artery* varies considerably among individuals. It is usually located near the descending portion of the aortic arch or at the origin of one of its major branches. Classically the bronchial artery is the fused first pair of the intercostal arteries, which then descends along and enters the wall of the lower trachea (Fig. 2–27A). The bronchial artery follows and nourishes the bronchial tree as far as the respiratory bronchiole. These vessels may increase their flow in response to any injury (Fig. 2–27B). At the hilum, branches of the bronchial artery also radiate out and supply most portions of the mediastinal visceral pleura. The bronchial artery characteristically has only an internal elastica in contrast to the internal and external elastica in the pulmonary arteries of similar size.

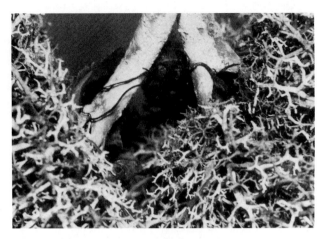

A

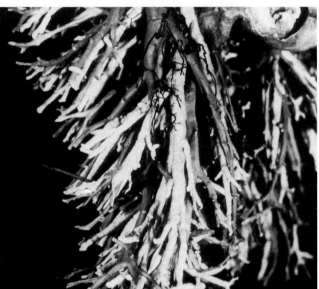

B

Fig. 2–27 A,B. Bronchial artery supply (black fine branches) demonstrated by corrosion cast techniques (see Chapter 34). **A.** Normal supply shown by branches entering lungs along right and left major bronchi. **B.** Increased bronchial artery supply in mild bronchiectasis. (**A** and **B**, courtesy of A. A. Liebow pulmonary collection, San Diego.)

The *bronchial veins* mainly follow the course of the large bronchial arteries and drain into azygos or hemiazygos. The dilated, prevenous capillaries in the bronchial wall are frequently fenestrated, as are those in the submucosa of the upper airway.

Vascular Shunts

Communications exist between all arteries and veins of the pulmonary and bronchial systems. The best documented communication is that between bronchial and pulmonary capillaries and small veins. It has been proposed that the thick-walled blockade or "sperr arteries" connect bronchial and pulmonary arteries. These probably do exist but their documentation has been difficult. Such an artery would be closed normally but would open during pulmonary arterial insufficiency, as with an acute pulmonary embolism, to perfuse the ischemic lung tissue. The extent of shunting in the normal lung has been estimated to be less than 3% or up to 10% of the total cardiac output.

With each injury, repair or neoplastic proliferation, the altered tissue is vascularized by the bronchial artery and more shunting channels are created. The left-to-right shunt in the lung, therefore, increases with age and can be substantial in patients with neoplasm or chronic destructive lung diseases such as tuberculosis and bronchiectasis. Vascular shunts in the lung also induce clubbing of fingers (an arteriovenous shunt in the distal digits) and hypertrophic pulmonary osteoarthropathy, a process presumably mediated through humoral factors.

Lymphatics

The lung has extensive networks of lymphatics, which are divided into the pleural or superficial plexus in the visceral pleura and the deep or parenchymal plexus in the bronchovascular bundles and the lobar and lobular septa. The two systems communicate with each other at the boundaries between lobes or lobules and the pleura, but both systems primarily drain separately toward hilar nodes in large lymphatic channels equipped with valves.

Lymphatic channels following the bronchovascular bundle start at the level of the respiratory bronchiole. Alveolar walls do not have lymphatic spaces, although juxtaalveolar lymphatics in the small or distal bronchovascular bundle are partly facing and in contact with the basal surface of the adjacent alveolar type I cells.[17]

Lymphatic capillaries are lined by large flattened endothelial cells with few organelles. Although all types of intercellular junctions are present, focally open or movable junctions devoid of the basal lamina are unique to lymphatic capillaries. The collecting lymphatic channels resemble thin-walled veins with funnel-shaped, rather than bicuspid, valves. These valves may, however, appear bicuspid in histologic section.

Clasically, it is said that the lymphatics of the right lung and left-lower lobes drain into the right thoracic duct and those of the left-upper lobe drain into the left thoracic duct. The thoracic ducts drain into the brachiocephalic vein on the corresponding side. Because of the intermixture of lymph flow in the interconnecting mediastinal lymphatic pathways, cross-drainage is frequent.

Lymphoid cells may accumulate in the bronchial musosa [bronchus-associated lymphoid tissue (BALT)] and protrude toward the lumen as do mucosal nodules in the ileum. These lymphoid cell collections are more frequent in chronically infected animal lungs. *Lymph nodes* are found along the lymphatic pathways in the lung (intrapulmonary), hilum (hilar), carina (superior and inferior tracheobronchial), and along the trachea (paratracheal). Scalene lymph nodes in the supraclavicular space are frequently involved by metastatic lung cancer, either through lymphatic connections with the paratracheal lymph nodes or through direct extension from the visceral to the parietal pleural lymphatics through adhesions, especially as they occur at the apex of the lung.

Although the maximum draining capacity of the lymphatic system in the lung is not clearly defined, lymphatic fluid in high-pressure pulmonary edema accumulates first in the interstitium of the bronchovascular bundle before flooding back into the alveolar space. Normal pressure pulmonary edema, on the other hand, is caused by damage and destruction of the alveolar and capillary barriers from a variety of noxious agents.

The lymphatic pressure is usually low and the network of channels extensive. The direction of the lymph flow is, therefore, readily subjected to modification. The diffuse lymphangitic spread of cancer (lymphangitis carcinomatosa) is not from massive hilar node metastases and obstruction with retrograde spread, as previously believed, but represents multiple lymphangitic invasions following a widespread vascular dissemination of tumor cells.

Pulmonary Alveolar Macrophages

All pulmonary macrophages originate from the monocytic series derived from the bone marrow. Most of them, especially in acute irritation, emerge directly from the circulation and traverse bronchial or alveolar walls to enter the air space. Some of them, mainly in a chronic stage of injury, divide and emerge from the residential population of mesenchymal or monocytic cells that arrived and settled earlier in the alveolar wall. Macrophages have elongated cellular processes called pseudopods, a well-developed endoplasmic reticulum and Golgi apparatus, membrane-bound structures that contain inflammatory mediators, and primary and secondary lysosomes.

The macrophages move around on the alveolar and bronchial surfaces, may trespass the alveolar pore, and usually engulf exogenous and endogenous tissues and debris (Figs. 2–26 and 2–28). Once in the airspace, and especially after engulfing all the debris, macrophages

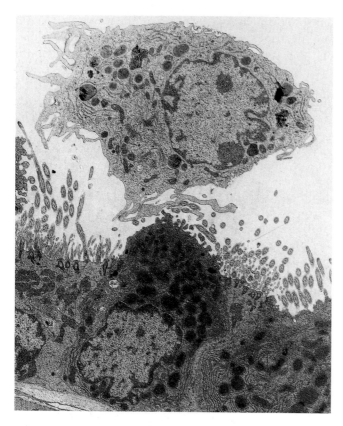

Fig. 2–28. Macrophage on surface of bronchiole on top of Clara and ciliated cells. Mouse. TEM, ×6,500. (From Thurlbeck and Wang: MTP International Review of Science. Physiology, Ser. 1, Vol. 2. 1974:18 with permission.)

cannot migrate through the intact alveolar or bronchial epithelial layer back into the interstitium. Intravascular macrophages, along with BALT, are rare in human lungs, and probably represent intravascular and submucosal clearance of noxious agents following the breakdown of the normal epithelial and endothelial barriers by massive exposures. Alveolar macrophages either move by amoeboid motion or drift with the alveolar surfactant or fluid to reach the terminal bronchiole, and then are swept up with the surface fluid by cilia in the bronchus, to be finally swallowed or expectorated.

Clearance of Inhaled Particles in the Lung

Depending on their sizes, inhaled particles in the lung are trapped by impaction, sedimentation, diffusion, or Brownian movements. Particles larger than 10 μm are mostly deposited by impaction on the mucous blanket of the upper airway. Particles of 2–10 μm settle out mainly in the peripheral air spaces. Particles less than 0.2 μm are not deposited readily and are mostly exhaled while still suspended in air. All deposited particles in the bronchus and bronchioles are cleared either by the mucociliary movement, which is most efficient in the upper airway, or through lymphatic drainage if particles have penetrated the bronchial wall through endocytosis by the epithelial cells or through mucosal defects. In addition to particle size, the chemical nature, concentration, and duration of exposure are all important in assessing the retention of particles and damage of the lung from such exposures.

Particles deposited on the alveolar surface are cleared by three mechanisms: centripetal, mainly by macrophages to the terminal bronchiole; centrifugal, to reach the pleura or septum; and transmural, through the alveolar wall and capillaries. Because one terminal bronchiole collects and concentrates the content of approximately 10,000 alveoli, the small airway is frequently damaged by inhaled toxins or other causes of irritations. Ample examples of such changes include the "alveolar ductitis" of young cigarette or marihuana smokers, small-airways disease in the early stage of pneumoconiosis or cystic fibrosis, and bronchiolitis obliterans or incompletely resolved pneumonia from a variety of causes.

The centrifugal removal of particles probably occurs mainly when the centripedal pathway is disturbed or overburdened. The clearance of particles and macrophages in this direction is less efficient as it is more circumferential, and foreign particles frequently accumulate in the pleura and septum to cause local fibrosis. Clearance of particles through the alveolar wall and capillaries also occurs when exposures are excessive. Both type I and II alveolar lining cells engulf particles in those conditions, as do the bronchial epithelial cells via forced phagocytosis, and release them either into the interstitium or back into the air space. Those released into the interstitial space may enter the capillaries, engulfed by monocytic cells (intravascular macrophages) or, if close to the terminal airways, be engulfed by interstitial macrophages and drain into the lymphatics. Those in the alveolar space may reach the juxtaalveolar lymphatics through the type I cell cytoplasm. Following heavy exposures, asbestos fibers several microns in length can be recovered in hilar lymph nodes and also in distant organs such as spleen, bone marrow, and liver.

Nerves and Humoral Controls

The sympathetic and parasympathetic nervous systems form the pulmonary plexus at the hilum and then distribute around and along the airways and pulmonary vessels to reach the alveoli and pleura.

The *parasympathetic* system has both sensory and mo-

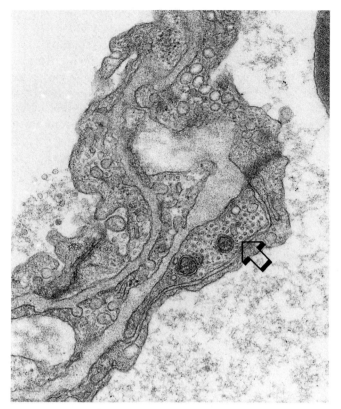

Fig. 2–29. Nerve ending with small empty vesicles and mitochondria, representing afferent cholinergic nerve ending, in alveolar wall (*arrow*). Human. TEM, ×45,000.

tor nerves. Its afferent sensory nerve endings are present in the bronchial and alveolar walls (Fig. 2–29) and pleura (as stretch receptors) and the bronchial mucosa (as irritant receptors). The ganglia, located in the bronchial wall, reflexly integrate the local input and output. Its preganglionic afferent fibers, in the vagus nerve, reach the sensory vagal nuclei in medulla near the respiratory center. The central vagal nuclei also receive impulses from the chemoreceptors in carotid and aortic bodies and the pressor receptors in the carotid sinus and aortic arch. Moreover, impulses from nose and upper airways arrive through the trigeminal and glossopharyngeal nerves, and all are integrated in the respiratory center.

The preganglionic efferent fibers of the parasympathetic system arise from the motor vagal nuclei in the medulla. The postganglionic motor fibers, which are cholinergic, innervate and stimulate contraction of bronchial and bronchiolar muscle cells, cause secretion of the bronchial gland, and stimulate vasodilatation.

The *sympathetic* system is mainly efferent. Its preganglionic fibers, from the central nervous system, emerge from the second to sixth thoracic segments of the spinal cord to reach ganglions in the sympathetic trunk along each side of the vertebral column. The postganglionic fibers and endings are adrenergic and have two types of receptors. The *alpha-adrenergic* stimulation induces constriction of bronchial and vascular smooth muscle cells. The *beta-adrenergic* stimulation induces bronchodilatation and decreases secretion of the bronchial gland. The roles of the afferent sympathetic system are not well defined.

Although the functions of the two major autonomic nervous systems are fairly well defined, the distribution of the sympathetic and parasympathetic systems and their subtype fibers varies in the large and small bronchi. A third nonadrenergic inhibitory or *purinergic* system has also been suggested, even though its distribution and function are not completely clear. Afferent and efferent nerve endings with dense core granule-containing cells have been identified in the paracrine system. Mast cells, macrophages, and other mononuclear cells in the bronchial and alveolar walls also release a variety of mediators, including serotonin and prostaglandins, which among their many effects also alter muscle tone. The bronchial muscle and pulmonary vascular reactivities are monitored by many neural and humoral pathways and are influenced by both central and local factors; thus, they are very complex. Their responses to stimuli in disease are frequently unpredictable.

The Thorax

The Thoracic Cage

The skeletal elements of the *thorax* consist of 12 thoracic *vertebrae*, 12 pairs of *ribs*, and the *sternum*. The *clavicle* is positioned above and in front of the first rib to protect the thoracic inlet and its major vessels and other vital structures. The adjacent vertebral bodies are interposed by fibroelastic cartilaginous *disks* bound together by heavy ligaments and are further reinforced and made flexible by paravertebral muscles.

The rib is a semicircular, slightly angulated blade of bone that forms a joint with the body and the transverse process of the vertebra (the *costovertebral joints*). The anterior ends of the first 10 ribs are joined to the sternum by cartilage, the first 7 directly and the next 3 indirectly; the last 2 ribs usually remain unattached. The costovertebral joints allow the anteriorly slanted ribs with attached mediastinum to elevate at inspiration and fall back passively at expiration.

The *intercostal muscles* seal the space between the ribs and costal cartilages. They contract with each respiratory movement to prevent the intercostal pleural membrane from sinking in with inspiration or blowing out with expiration. The external oblique components of the intercostal muscle also lift up the thoracic cage to increase the anterior posterior and transverse dimensions while the diaphragm contracts to lengthen the thoracic cage. Accessory inspiratory muscles include the sternocleidomastoid and scalenus muscles, which elevate the sternum and upper ribs in strenuous breathing. Expiration in quiet breathing is a passive relaxation of inspiratory muscles aided by the recoil of the stretched elastic fiber network and changes in surfactant. Additional expiratory effect is achieved by contraction of the internal oblique components of the intercostal and abdominal muscles.

The Diaphragm

The *diaphragm* is a dome-shaped muscle plate with a central tendon and peripheral radiating muscle fibers that cover the floor of the thoracic cage and are divided into three main parts. The sternal part usually forms two strips and attaches to the posterior surface of the xyphoid process. The costal part attaches to the inner surface of the last six costal cartilages and ribs bilaterally. The lumbar portion fuses into left and right crura and attaches to the upper lumbar vertebral bodies. The central tendon is also divided into three leaflets, which lie in front of and on either side of the vertebral column.

The left and right *phrenic* nerves come mainly from the fourth *cervical* nerve and descend from the cervical plexus over the surface of the pericardium to innervate the diaphragm. Unilateral elevation of diaphragm can occur from phrenic nerve damage along its long course.

The dome of the diaphragm, in its relaxed state at expiration, reaches to the *xyphoid process* level. With contraction, it flattens and lowers the diaphragm as much as 8.3 cm on the right and 10.7 cm on the left. The diaphragm has to move incessantly with the lung for life. It is uncertain whether the skeletal muscles, capillaries, and patterns of the blood flow in the diaphragm are different from those of other skeletal muscles. The diaphragm can become hypertrophic in the early stage of chronic obstructive lung disease but tends to become atrophic and flattened by the hyperinflated lung in the advanced stage of disease.

The Mediastinum

The *mediastinum* is the intrathoracic, midline, pliable soft-tissue compartment bordered laterally by left and right pleural cavities and lungs, anteriorly by sternum, and posteriorly by the vertebrae. The mediastinum can be pushed away from either side by pleural effusion, tension pneumothorax, or other increases in the pleural

contents, and can be pulled toward the same side in atelectasis, fibrosis, or surgical excision.

The mediastinum traditionally is separated into superior, anterior, and posterior parts, the middle part containing heart and pericardium serving as the reference unit. This classification is simple and useful in the differential diagnosis of mediastinal lesions: lymphomas and thymic and thyroid tumors occur more frequently in the superior and anterior parts, neural tumors in the posterior and lymph nodes, and metastatic tumors in the lateral portions of the middle mediastinum.

The Pleural Cavity and Mesothelial Cells

The primitive body cavity or *coelom*, lined by mesothelial cells, appears early in the embryo. All constantly moving organs such as the lung, heart, and intestines subsequently develop into this cavity and are enveloped by the mesothelial cell layer as they do so. This arrangement renders all these organs not only readily movable but also pliable in size and shape during maturation.

The *pleural* and *peritoneal* cavities are normally completely separated. They communicate with each other only indirectly through lymphatics. The pleural cavity is a potential space between the *visceral* pleura, which covers the entire surface of the lung including the interlobar fissures, and the *parietal* pleura, which covers the inner surface of the thoracic cage, mediastinum, and diaphragm. The visceral pleura reflects at the hilum to continue as the parietal pleura. The opposing two layers of mesothelial cells are separated only by a layer of hyaluronic acid-rich fluid less than 20 μm thick. The pleural recesses or sinuses are acutely angled portions of parietal pleura at the costophrenic or costomediastinal junctions. At the end of normal expiration (functional reserve capacity), the costophrenic sinus is a potential space that may extend up to the sixth or seventh intercostal space at the posterior axillary line. In inspiration, the lungs expand into this space. A needle introduced into the pleural space at these levels, especially at expiration, may easily go through the two apposing layers of parietal pleura at the same time and enter the liver or other abdominal organs.

The gross appearance of the pleura is smooth, glistening, and semitransparent. By light microscopy the pleura is typically divided into (1) a mesothelial layer, (2) a thin submesothelial connective tissue layer, (3) a superficial elastica layer, (4) a loose subpleural connective tissue layer, and (5) a deep dense fibroelastic layer. The presence and thickness of each layer varies regionally. The loose layer (fourth) is the plane of cleavage for decortication. The fifth layer frequently adheres tightly

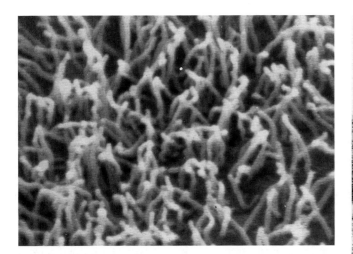

Fig. 2–30. Mesothelial cells with abundant "bushy" microvilli 0.1 μm in diameter and up to 3 μm in length. Rabbit. SEM, ×11,700. (From Am Rev Respir Dis 1974;110:623 with permission.)

or blends into the parenchyma of the lung or the chest wall.

The mesothelial cells are stretchable and range in size from 16.4 ± 6.8 to 41.9 ± 9.5 μm. They may appear flat, cuboidal, or columnar. Generally speaking cuboidal or columnar cells indicate either that their substructures are loose and fatty, as in the pleural recesses, or that the cells are metabolically active. Flattened cells either are stretched quiescent cells on the visceral surface or cover a very rigid substructure such as a rib.

Mesothelial cells are characterized ultrastructurally by an abundance of elongated bushy microvilli 0.1 μm in diameter and up to 3 or more μm in length (Fig. 2–30).[18] The microvilli trap hyaluronic acid, which acts as a lubricant to lessen the friction between the moving lung and the chest wall. The cytoplasm is rich in pinocytic vesicles, mitochondria, and other organelles and prekeratin fibrils (Fig. 2–31). The presence of dominant bushy microvilli (by electron microscopy) and of prekeratin fibrils (by immunochemistry), and absence of epithelial markers such as carcinoembryonic antigen, have been useful in differentiating mesothelioma from metastatic adenocarcinoma in the pleural space.

The secretion and absorption of pleural fluid is governed by Starling's law. Large particles and cells such as fibrin molecules or macrophages are removed from preformed stomas directly connecting the pleural cavity with the lymphatics (Fig. 2–32). The stomas are found only in specific areas of the parietal pleura including mediastinal and infracostal regions, especially in the lower thorax. The entry of large particles into a dilated lymphatic lacuna through the stoma is facilitated by the respiratory movement (Fig. 2–33). The roof of the

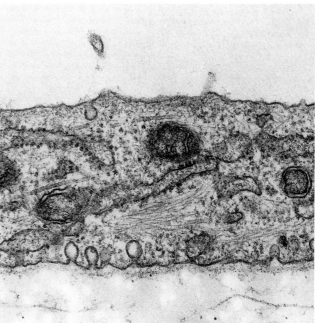

Fig. 2–31. Cytoplasm of mesothelial cells is rich in mitochondria, prekeratin fibrils, and other organelles in addition to elongated bushy microvilli. Rabbit. TEM, ×12,600. (From Am Rev Respir Dis 1974;110:623 with permission.)

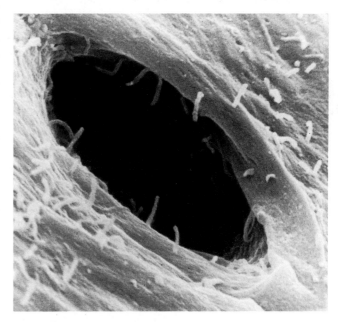

Fig. 2–32. Preformed stoma on parietal pleura of lower thorax. Mesothelial cells extend into stoma. Mouse. SEM, ×25,800. (From Chrétien J, Hirsch A, eds: Diseases of the pleura. Masson, 1983:10 with permission.)

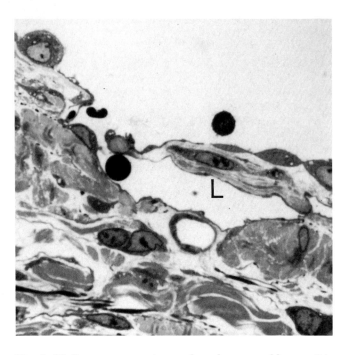

Fig. 2–33. Stoma communicates pleural space and lacuna (L), a dilated lymphatic space. Red blood cell is present at stoma. Particles as large as macrophages (two dark cells) are removed from pleural cavity through this passage. Rabbit. LM, ×1,000. (From Am Rev Respir Dis 1975;111:12 with permission.)

lacuna is formed by a network of thick collagen bundles that is covered by mesothelial cells on the pleural and endothelial cells on the lacuna side. These two layers of cells rupture readily in disease to increase the route of pleural clearance.

References

1. Hayek vH. The human lung. (Krahl VE, transl.) New York: Hafner, 1960.
2. Nagaishi C. Functional anatomy and histology of the lung. Tokyo: Igaku Shoin, 1972.
3. Murray JF. The normal lung. 2d Ed. Philadelphia: WB Saunders, 1986.
4. Weibel ER. Lung cell biology. In: Handbook of physiology: The respiratory system I. Washington D.C. 1990:47–91.
5. Thurlbeck WM, Wang NS. The structure of the lungs. In: Widdicombe JG, ed. Respiratory physiology. Physiology series 1, Vol. 2. MTP International Review of Science, 1974:1–30.
6. Kuhn C. Ciliated and Clara cells. In: Bouhuys A, ed. Lung cells in disease. Amsterdam: North-Holland, 1976:91–108.
7. Crapo JD, Barry BE, Gehr P, Bachofen M, Weibel ER. Cell number and cell characteristics of the normal human lung. Am Rev Respir Dis 1982;125:740–745.
8. Gail DB, Lenfant DJM. Cells of the lung: Biology and clinical implication. Am Rev Respir Dis 1983;127:366–367.
9. Gehr P, Bachofen M, Weibel ER. The normal human lung: Ultrastructure and morphometric estimation of diffusing capacity. Respir Physiol 1978;32:121–140.
10. Macklem PT. Airway obstructive and collateral ventilation. Physiol Rev 1971;51:368–431.
11. Ryan US. Structural bases for metabolic activity. Annu Rev Physiol 1982;44:22–239.
12. Meyrick B, Reid L. The alveolar wall. Br J Dis Chest 1970;64:121–140.
13. Wang NS. Scanning electron microscopy of the lung. In: Schraufnagel DE, Lenfant C, eds. Lung biology in health and disease, Vol. 48. New York: Marcel Dekker, 1990:517–555.
14. Newman SL, Michel RP, Wang NS. Lingular lung biopsy: Is it representative. Am Rev Respir Dis 1985;125:1084–1086.
15. Lauweryns JM, Peuskens JC. Neuroepithelial bodies (neuroreceptor or secretory organs?) in human infant bronchial and bronchiolar epithelium. Anat Rec 1972;172:471–482.
16. Ryan SF. The structure of the intraalveolar septum of the mammary lung. Anat Rec 1969;165:467–484.
17. Lauweryns IM, Baert IH. Alveolar clearance and the role of the pulmonary lymphatics. Am Rev Respir Dis 1977;115:625–683.
18. Wang NS. Anatomy and physiology of the pleural space. In: Light RW, ed. Symposium on pleural diseases. Philadelphia: WB Saunders, 1985:3–16.

CHAPTER 3

Lung Defenses

J. LINDER and J.H. SISSON

The lung is unique among the visceral organs because it is exposed to the external environment. Remarkably, there is continuity between the tip of the nostril and the most distal alveoli. Thousands of cubic feet of air pass through the airways each day, air that contains noxious gases, dusts, particulate material, and microbial organisms that alone or in combination can damage the lung. Fortunately, the lung has multiple defense mechanisms that protect against potentially injurious agents.

Some defenses are inherent in the anatomic configuration of the lung. The branching of the tracheobronchial tree, for example, traps much of the particulate matter in the upper airways before it reaches the alveoli. The lung also has unique mechanical functions, such as the mucociliary escalator and the cough reflex, that help to remove material from large airways.

Conceptually, it is worthwhile to distinguish nonspecific from specific defenses. Nonspecific defenses include the anatomic configuration of the airway, antioxidants, and substances within the epithelial lining fluid that accelerate bacterial phagocytosis. Much of the phagocytic activity by neutrophils or pulmonary macrophages, such as the ingestion of particulate debris and microorganisms, is nonspecific. Other phagocytic activity and immune defense mechanisms are target specific, recapitulating the general immunologic defenses that function throughout the body.

The relative importance of different defense mechanisms depends on the level of the respiratory tract. For example, in the upper airways the mechanical barrier provided by the mucous membranes and by sneezing, coughing, and mucociliary clearance are the first line of defense; in the bronchioli and alveoli, phagocytic cells are critical for defense against invading microorganisms.[1]

The functions of the different pulmonary defense mechanisms are the topic of this chapter.

Defense Mechanisms

Anatomic

The configuration of the upper respiratory tract is the first line of defense for the lung. Of fundamental importance is the closure of the glottis and larynx during swallowing. A closed glottis prevents contamination of the lung by oral secretions and ingested materials. In individuals with dysfunctional pharyngeal musculature or anatomic malformations that impair closure of the glottis, the importance of this defense mechanism is apparent. These persons have repeated bacterial pneumonias because of chronic aspiration. Closure of the glottis is also important in the cough reflex, as is discussed momentarily.

Aside from its role in supporting eyeglasses, the nose filters and humidifies inspired air. The anatomy of the nasal cavity causes turbulence of the airstream, which increases the time that inspired air is in contact with nasal secretions and ciliated epithelial cells. This assists filtration of any particulate matter that may be present. Filtration is also aided by humidification of the air. Small particles coalesce into larger particles because of their hydroscopic properties. Larger particulates are more likely to be deposited in the upper airways rather than passing into the distal alveoli.

Respiratory Secretions

Secretions produced by cells that cover the upper airways (nose, nasopharynx, trachea) and lower airways (bronchi, bronchioles, and alveoli) are a significant nonspecific defense mechanism. Most of these secretions are gelatinous, which aids the entrapment of particulate material. The turbulence of inspired air resulting from the anatomic configuration of the airways increases the contact of particles with respiratory secretions. Once trapped in the secretions, particles are removed by the mucociliary escalator, which is discussed in detail shortly.

Secretions are a critical component of the lung's protection from gaseous injury. Free radicals such as O_2^-, superoxide, and oxides of nitrogen are highly reactive with cell membranes and DNA, which can cause oxidative tissue injury or cell death. A major mechanism of protecting respiratory tissues from oxidative gases is the enzyme superoxide dismutase. This enzyme catalyzes the conversion of the superoxide ion to hydrogen peroxide and water. The bronchial and epithelial lining fluid also contain proteins and mucopolysaccharides that contribute to the protection of airways. Proteins have buffering effects, and substances such as transferrin and lactoferrin can reduce oxidative ions. Unfortunately, the capability of our respiratory defenses has not kept pace with the development of our industrialized society: Industrial gases and pollutants are a major cause of asthma and chronic bronchitis.

Fluid coating the airways also contributes to antibacterial protection. In experimental systems, lipopolysaccharides in respiratory surfactant fluid increase the permeability of bacterial cell walls, making the organisms more susceptible to cytolysis. Lipopolysaccharide-mediated bactericidal activity has been observed with pneumococci and several nonpneumococcal gram-positive bacteria, including *Streptococcus viridans*, *Streptococcus pyogenes*, *Streptococcus bovis*, and *Bacillus* spp. For example, a palmitoyl lysophosphatidylcholine-like material was observed to support autolysin-mediated pneumococcal lysis, altered cell membrane permeability, and antibacterial activity against several gram-positive bacteria.[2] Other authors, however, have questioned the significance of this mechanism in humans.[3]

The epithelial lining fluid also contains dissolved immunoglobulins. IgG and IgA may aid the neutralization of microorganisms by facilitation of phagocytosis. Immunoglobulins can also bind to inspired antigens, muting immunologic responses by preventing the interaction of these antigens with mast cells.

Perhaps the most significant substances in epithelial lining field are alpha-1-antitrypsin and transferrin. These serve to inhibit proteases that are released from neutrophils and macrophages during phagocytosis. Antiproteases protect the lung from autolytic damage. The functions of alpha-1-antitrypsin, and the conse-

quences of alpha-1-antitrypsin deficiency, are discussed in Chapter 26.

Alveolar Macrophages

The alveolar macrophage plays at a pivotal role in the scheme of lung defenses. Chemotactic factors produced directly by the alveolar macrophages or secondarily through activation of the complement system are essential in initiating the influx of neutrophils into the alveolar space. Coupling phagocytosis (afferent function) with its capacity to secrete several kinds of effector molecules (chemotactic factors, complement components, leukotrienes, and platelet-activating factor), the alveolar macrophage controls the overall regulation of the inflammatory reaction.[4,5]

In the distal airways, the alveolar macrophage is particularly significant in defense of the lung against inhaled pathogens. These cells have been observed in vitro to move chemotactically in response to many types of attractants that may be present on the lung's surface during a bacterial or particulate challenge.[6] Cigarette smoking may impair the chemotactic responses of macrophages[7] (see Chapter 25).

Defense against fungal and bacterial organisms is an important function of pulmonary macrophages. Macrophages function in concert with T lymphocytes to provide cell-mediated immunity to *Candida* sp. *Aspergillus* sp., and other fungi.[8]

Aspergillus is one of the most significant pathogens of immunocompromised individuals. Consequences of aspergillus exposure range from allergic conditions (asthma, hypersensitivity pneumonitis), to colonization with or without an allergic component (allergic bronchopulmonary aspergillosis, aspergilloma, saprophytic involvement of infarcted tissue), to invasion and destruction of lung parenchyma (invasive aspergillosis, chronic necrotizing pulmonary aspergillosis). The development of lung infection or disease depends on interaction among three factors: the characteristics of the fungus (virulence factors), the status of host defense mechanisms, and the type of exposure.[9] Macrophages are the final effector cells in the defenses against these organisms. However, some fungi can escape destruction by phagocytic cells by virtue of their cell wall or capsule. The clearest example is the polysaccharide capsule of *Candida neoformans*, which diminishes the adherence of phagocytes to the fungus, thus impeding phagocytosis.[10] In other circumstances, capsular material may be chemotactic for inflammatory cells.[11]

With respect to bacteria, lung phagocytic defenses against aerosolized *Streptococcus aureus* challenges are provided solely by the alveolar macrophage in the absence of inflammation. Endotoxin, however, can cause a significant decrease in pulmonary bactericidal activity, indicating a defect in alveolar macrophage function.[12] Macrophages do not uniformly protect against bacteria. For example, alveolar macrophages are not capable of limiting the growth of *Legionella* spp. Instead, the alveolar macrophages appear to be the primary site of *Legionella* spp. multiplication. Although alveolar macrophages may participate in other aspects of pulmonary immunity to the *Legionella* spp., these data indicate that the alveolar macrophage alone does not act as an effector cell in cell-mediated immunity to the organism.[13] Macrophages are also not completely effective in controlling mycobacterial infection. The mycolic acids within the mycobacterial cell wall protect the organism from destruction by lysosomal enzymes, allowing the organisms to persist for long periods within the macrophage cytoplasm.

A number of studies have been directed toward understanding the influence of cytokines on macrophage function, an interest partly the result of the therapeutic potential of aersolized cytokines.[14] This approach was based on the observation that recombinant cytokine interferon (rIFN gamma and tumor necrosis factor (TNF) alpha stimulate several macrophage-mediated functions important in host defense. Adminstration in this fashion causes minimal host toxicity. Aerosolized cytokines appear to stimulate alveolar macrophage and blood monocyte function, and may induce an inflammatory response in the lungs of normal rats. Aerosolized murine rIFN-gamma or recombinant human TNF-alpha increased IL-1 production by both alveolar macrophages and blood monocytes for at least 5 days after administration. Also, murine rIFN-gamma increased the expression of Ia antigen on alveolar macrophages, and human rTNF-alpha increased alveolar macrophage- and blood monocyte-mediated tumor lysis. Sequential aerosolization of IFN-gamma and TNF-alpha significantly increased both IL-1 release and Ia expression compared to either cytokine administered alone. In the experimental systems, aerosolized cytokines did not induce lung edema or an inflammatory cell infiltrate within the airways or alveoli. Aerosol administration of IFN-gamma or TNF-alpha enhanced both pulmonary and systemic monocyte function, and the combination of IFN-gamma and TNF-alpha produced additive or synergistic effects; aerosolized TNF-alpha produced high cytokine levels in the lung but very low uptake into the circulation.

Mucociliary Clearance

Mucociliary clearance is an important host defense mechanism responsible for clearing the airways of environmental toxins, inhaled particles, and aspirated microorganisms. Substances deposited on the mucous lining of the airways are propelled cephalad to the hypopharynx by the "escalator" function of the lining cells of the trachea and bronchi. Effective mucociliary clearance depends on the propulsion of airway mucus by the coordinated beating of cilia. The role that airway mucus secretion plays in normal airway function and disease is discussed elsewhere in this chapter. This section focuses on the role that normal airway cilia function has in the process of mucociliary clearance, and discusses cilia abnormalities that are associated with airway disease.

The upper respiratory tract is populated with ciliated epithelial cells.[15] The relative density of ciliated cells varies from as high as 50%–80%, on the luminal surface of the trachea, to the respiratory bronchioles, which are only sparsely ciliated. Cilia are not present in the terminal air spaces.

Individual cilia are finger-like organelles that extend from the cell surface into the lumen and number 200 cilia/cell or more. Human respiratory cilia are 3–6 μm in length and 0.25 μm in diameter. The cytoskeletal framework or axoneme of the cilium is enveloped in an extension of the cell membrane and internally consists of the structural and enzymatic elements required for motility (Fig. 3–1) (also see Chapter 2). Much of the mechanical force required for normal cilia motion is generated by the protein complexes called dynein arms. The dynein complexes consist of multiple distinct peptides including at least two or three different high molecular weight peptides with ATPase activity. Through the dynein-directed hydrolysis of ATP, high-energy phosphate bonds are transduced into motor activity in the form of cilia bending.

The physical orientation of cilia is directed to promote the flow of mucus toward the oropharynx. In the case of the tracheobronchial tree, the flow is cephalad, and in the case of the nasal passages, caudad. This orientation is apparent on examination of axonemal direction in neighboring cilia. The central microtubular pairs of adjoining cilia are coplanar with one another and perpendicular to the direction of mucus flow. In normal airway cells, neighboring axonemes are typically oriented within 30° of one another. In addition to orientation, other factors such as cilia coordination contribute to the effective propulsion of mucus by cilia.

Cilia motion in neighboring cilia is carefully synchronized so that sequential cilia bending produces waves that continually move across the epithelial surface toward the oropharynx. The inter- and intracellular coordination of adjacent cilia to produce propulsive waves is called metachronism. Effective clearance, therefore, requires that individual cilia are motile and that adjacent motile cilia beat metachronically.

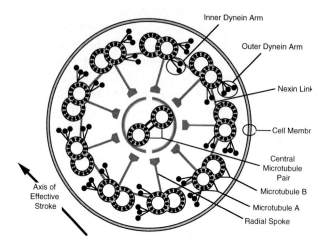

Inner Dynein Arm

Outer Dynein Arm

Nexin Link

Cell Membr.

Central
Microtubule
Pair

Microtubule B

Microtubule A

Radial Spoke

Axis of
Effective
Stroke

Table 3–1. Factors that alter cilia beat frequency or mucus velocity

Factor[a]	Cilia beat frequency	Mucus velocity
Beta agonists[66–68]	↑	↑
Histamine[69–71]	±	↑
Bradykinin[72–74]	↑↑	↑
Neurokinin A[75]	↑	?
Angiotensin II[76]	↑	?
Substance P[77,78]	↑	↑
Serotonin[79]	↑	↑
Prostaglandins E[69,80–82]	↑	—
Leukotriene C4[69,81]	±	?

[a] Superscripted numbers are cited references for this study.

Fig. 3–1. Cross-sectional representation of cilia axoneme when viewed from the base of the cilium, looking toward the tip. The axoneme consists of an outer ring of nine microtubule doublets surrounding an inner central pair of microtubules. The axis drawn between the central pair of microtubules is perpendicular to the direction of mucus flow (*arrow*). The outer nine microtubule pairs are linked circumferentially to one another by nexin links and tethered radially to the central microtubule pair by the radial spokes. The outer microtubule doublets are decorated with inner and outer dynein arms, which extend from the microtubule A of one pair to the microtubule B of an adjacent pair. The entire axoneme is enveloped by the cell membrane. The precise location of each of these cytoskeletal elements is crucial to normal cilia motility. (From Sisson, Thompson, and Schultz: Airway mucociliary clearance. In Bone (ed) *Pulmonary and Critical Care Medicine*. St. Louis: Mosby-Yearbook Publishers, 1993, with permission.)

Airway mucus conventionally has been thought to be a thin "blanket" that covers the entire epithelial surface of the airways.[16] This concept has been challenged, however, on the basis of both theoretical considerations and observations made in animal studies. An alternative hypothesis proposes that mucus forms and travels in small droplets less that 4 μm in diameter in the small airways.[17] These droplets progressively aggregate as the mucus is propelled proximally such that large semi-confluent aggregates are observed in the upper airways. In either case, it is agreed that the cilia are bathed in a thin watery "periciliary" fluid that is of low viscosity and that the mucus-containing region rests on top of this fluid. The cilia tips, which contain barbed hook-like structures, directly brush the mucus-containing region only during full extension of the axoneme. This phase of cilia bending is termed the forward or effective stroke. In contrast, during the backward or relaxation stroke, the cilia do not directly touch the mucus-containing region. This intermittent, ratchet-like interaction between cilia and the mucus-containing region

promotes unidirectional mucous flow across the epithelial surface.

Human proximal airway cilia normally beat at a frequency between 15 and 20 Hz at normal body temperature. Although the cilia beat frequency (CBF) has not been studied in vivo in man at different regions of the tracheobronchial tree, the frequency presumably varies depending on the zone of the airways examined.[18] Animal studies have demonstrated that the CBF is slower in the peripheral airways (≈7 Hz) compared to proximal airways (≈18 Hz).[18] A similar gradient from small to large airways has been observed in animals for the rate of mucus movement. Mucus velocity has been observed to be as slow as 0.4–1.6 mm/min in the smallest bronchiole and as fast as 11.5–12.6 mm/min in lobar bronchi and trachea.[18] Most factors that alter CBF also similarly alter mucus velocity, but the relationship between CBF and mucus transport is not precisely defined. Factors that have been observed to alter CBF or mucus velocity are summarized in Table 3–1. The best way to understand the role mucociliary clearance plays in maintenance of normal host defenses is to examine the natural history of individuals who have genetically defective cilia. These conditions are discussed next.

Immunologic Defense Mechanisms

Cell-mediated immunity is important for the defense of the airways against many viral, fungal, and mycobacterial infections.[19] The role of cell-mediated immunity in protection against opportunistic pathogens has been reviewed by Lipscomb.[20]

It is widely believed that cell-mediated immunity and the associated ability of macrophages to destroy or inhibit the bacillus are all that are required to control pulmonary tuberculosis. However, although cell-mediated immunity is a major host defense against the tubercle bacillus, it is fully effective only in one of the four stages of the disease. The delayed-type hypersensitivity reaction (producing tissue necrosis) greatly benefits the host by arresting the logarithmic growth of bacilli within immature macrophages.[21]

Recipients of lung/heart allografts may be particularly prone to pulmonary infection because of systemic immunosuppression and the fact that defense mechanisms in the transplanted lung may be further impaired through tissue incompatibility and the effects of surgery. In a recent study, the prevalence of *Pneumocystis* infection was 88%.[22] The total number of cells recovered from the lung by bronchoalveolar lavage (BAL), the proportion of T lymphocytes, and the numbers of cytotoxic/suppressor and helper/inducer cells were elevated during infection with *Pneumocystis* when these parameters were compared before and after transplantation. Spontaneous and interleukin-2-induced proliferation of BAL cells in vitro was also higher during infection, suggesting that there was an increased number of activated T lymphocytes in the air spaces of the infected allograft. BAL cells cultured with irradiated spleen cells from the donor proliferated at higher levels when obtained after *Pneumocystis* infection than when obtained before or during infection, even for subclinical infections. These results indicate that in the absence of prophylaxis the prevalence of *Pneumocystis* infestation is very high after lung/heart transplantation. Impaired defense of the transplanted lung does not seem to stem from the inability of activated T lymphocytes to accumulate in the allograft. Alveolar macrophage migration is not impaired in lung allograft recipients without apparent signs of infection or rejection, and is in fact increased during periods of possible macrophage activation (shortly after transplantation and during chronic rejection).[23]

Bronchus-associated lymphoid tissue (BALT) is considered to play an important role in the local immunologic defense mechanisms in the respiratory tract. Experimental studies suggest that BALT regulates the local immune responses against chronic pulmonary infection caused by *Pneumocystis aeruginosa*.[24]

Impaired Defense Mechanisms

Anatomic

As mentioned previously, the impairment of oropharyngeal musculature that may accompany cerebral palsy, multiple sclerosis, or other neurodegenerative conditions is a major risk factor for pulmonary infection.[25] Chronic aspiration may also occur in individuals with anatomic defects of the oropharynx, or in those with tracheoesophageal fistulae or other more subtle conditions (see Chapter 5). Mechanical factors such as pulmonary atelectasis predispose the lung to infection. The phagocytic activity against *Pseudomonas aeruginosa*

of alveolar macrophages harvested by bronchoalveolar lavage from collapsed segments for as long as 24 h is progressively depressed in vitro.[26] Reexpansion of the atelectatic lobes with mechanical ventilation and 100% oxygen supplementation for 4 h after 6 h of atelectasis resulted in reversal of the impaired alveolar macrophage phagocytic activity.

Congenital Impairment

One of the most compelling examples of impaired pulmonary defenses is seen in the cystic fibrosis patient. Mucoid *P. aeruginosa* is the primary pathogen in perhaps 90% of these patients, causing chronic pulmonary obstruction and infection. No defect in systemic host defense has been elucidated; however, several mechanisms contribute to the breakdown in host defenses that allow persistence of this organism in the endobronchial space. *P. aeruginosa* adapts to the host by expressing a mucoid exopolysaccharide capsule and a less virulent form of lipopolysaccharide. These features make the pathogen less likely to cause sytemic infection but still enable it to resist local host defenses. Mucociliary clearance becomes impaired because of abnormal viscoelastic properties of sputum, squamous metaplasia of the respiratory epithelium, and bronchiectasis. Despite a brisk antibody response to a variety of *Pseudomonas* antigens, several defects in antibody-mediated opsonophagocytosis have been identified, including (1) development of antibody isotypes that are suboptimal at promoting phagocytosis, (2) formation of immune complexes that inhibit phagocytosis, and (3) proteolysis of endobronchial immunoglobulins. Complement-mediated opsonophagocytosis is also compromised by proteolytic cleavage of complement receptors from the cell surface of neutrophils and complement opsonins from the surface of *Pseudomonas*.[27]

Several genetically transmitted cilia defects can impair the function of the mucociliary escalator. The syndrome of bronchiectasis, sinusitis, and situs inversus was described originally by Siewert in 1904[28] and further characterized by Kartagener in 1933.[29] Afzelius observed in 1976[30] that several individiuals with Kartagener's syndrome had immotile sperm and cilia, absent mucociliary clearance, and ultrastructurally abnormal cilia axonemes. This collection of findings was termed the "immotile cilia syndrome," but it is now recognized that some individuals with this syndrome have motile cilia but ineffective cilia function. The term "primary cilia dyskinesia" is more descriptive and best describes this group of findings. It must be emphasized that primary cilia dyskinesia (PCD) is a *syndrome* and not a specific disease. This is apparent on consideration of the ever-increasing number of distinct axoneme ultrastructural abnormalities that have been described in

Table 3–2. Cilia axoneme ultrastructural abnormalities in primary cilia dyskinesia

Axoneme defect	References cited
Absent inner and outer arms	30, 33, 83
Absent outer arms	30, 33
Absent inner arms	30, 33
Absent radial spokes	33, 84
Microtubular transposition	33, 85
Absent central core structures	31
Basal body orientation	86

individuals with largely the same clinical findings (Table 3–2). The original description of absent dynein arms in affected individuals remains the most common ultrastructural axoneme abnormality observed.[31] Alterations of almost all the other axonemal elements, however, have now been described in individuals with the signs and symptoms of PCD. Thus, when discussing PCD it should be emphasized that the term encompasses a family of related but distinct cilia-related disorders.[32]

PCD is an hereditary group of disorders with autosomal recessive inheritance, an estimated prevalence of approximately 1 in 16,000, and a calculated heterozygote frequency of 1 in 60.[33] On the basis of numerous family studies, it appears that only about 50% of affected individuals have the classic Kartagener's triad including situs inversus.[33] The widely held explanation of this apparent random association of situs inversus with PCD has been that visceral orientation is a cilia-directed event during embryogenesis.[34] The absence of functioning cilia, therefore, results in a random occurrence of either situs inversus or situs solitus. In addition to the random association of situs inversus with PCD, it is important to note that only approximately 25% of individuals with situs inversus have PCD and its associated respiratory complications. This means that (1) the absence of situs inversus does not exclude PCD, and that (2) the presence of situs inversus does not establish PCD.

The clinical manifestations of PCD are easily understood when the normal locations of ciliated epithelial cells are considered. Table 3–3 lists the important locations of ciliated epithelia and the associated problems encountered in individuals with PCD. Although multiple organs in the body can be affected, impaired cilia function results in a predominance of upper respiratory problems. Affected individuals typically have a history of lifelong productive cough and sinus drainage. Recurrent and sometimes life-threatening respiratory infections are common, usually leading to bronchiectasis by the second or third decade. Nasal obstruction and impaired sinus drainage associated with recurrent sinusitis frequently necessitate surgical drainage of the sinuses. Despite these serious upper respiratory problems, individuals with PCD often have normal life spans, especially when infectious complications are adequately treated.

There are several important reasons to establish the diagnosis of an inherited cilia disorder: (1) PCD is frequently complicated by serious infections, and knowledge of the syndrome by both patient and physician will expedite prevention or early treatment of infectious sequelae such as pneumonia and empyema; (2) when the diagnosis of PCD has been established, alternative explanations of cough, sinusitis, and infertility may not need to be pursued; (3) genetic counseling of affected individuals may be advisable concerning fertility and the probability of PCD in siblings.

The diagnosis of PCD remains challenging, and first requires a high index of suspicion. Any individual with lifelong productive cough, recurrent respiratory tract infections, chronic sinusitis, bronchiectasis, or immotile sperm should be suspected as having PCD. Other diseases with similar manifestations, such as cystic fibrosis, immune deficiencies, or allergies, should be excluded. A family history of similar problems including situs inversus should also be sought.

The diagnosis of PCD ideally should include all the following: (1) the presence of the clinical findings of impaired cilia function previously described (see Table 3–3); (2) the demonstration of impairment of cilia or sperm function in vivo or in vitro, with functional tests of cilia motility including the measurement of nasal

Table 3–3. Association of cilia or axoneme locations and clinical manifestations in primary cilia dyskinesia[a]

Cilia or Axoneme Location	Clinical Manifestation
Tracheobronchial epithelium	Chronic cough, bronchitis, and bronchiectasis
Nasal and sinus epithelium	Sinusitis
Middle ear	Otitis media and hearing loss
Vestibular hair cells	Impaired equilibrium and vertigo
Brain ependyma	Headaches and impaired spinal fluid circulation
Ductuli efferentes (testes/epididymis)	Epididymal obstruction and oligospermia
Endometrial lining of cervix and oviducts	Female fertility decreased
Spermatozoa	Male infertility

[a]Summarized from reference 30.

mucociliary transit time by the saccharine test or radio-nucleotide lung clearance studies; (3) absent or altered motility of cilia from fresh nasal or tracheal scrapings and sperm (if available); and finally (4) the presence of cilia or sperm ultrastructural abnormalities confirmed by electron microscopy (see Table 3–2 and Fig. 3–1). It must be emphasized that the absence of ultrastructural abnormalities does not exclude PCD, because it is difficult to avoid artifact when handling ciliated tissues and there is potential for sampling error when only small numbers of axonemes are examined.

Other cilia-related disorders distinct from PCD should also be considered in individuals with recurrent airway infections. Young's syndrome (also known as Berry–Perkins–Young syndrome) consists of azoospermia associated with lung defects including bronchitis and bronchiectasis. Individuals with this syndrome have reduced mucociliary clearance as measured by radioaerosol clearance technique and experience recurrent chest infection. Unlike those with PCD, individuals with Young's syndrome typically have ultrastructurally normal sperm axoneme architecture.[35]

Polynesian bronchiectasis is a syndrome describing the bronchiectasis seen with high frequency among natives of several Pacific islands including Samoa, Tonga, and New Zealand. Mucociliary clearance is either reduced or absent in affected individuals. Although a wide variety of ultrastructural cilia abnormalities have been observed in these individuals, including partial or complete absence of dynein arms, the etiology of this syndrome is unknown and it is assumed to be genetic.[36]

Congenital abnormal monocyte/macrophage function may result from genetic or developmental disorders. Because of the central role of monocytes and macrophages in host defense (in inflammatory responses, antigen presentation, and immunoregulatory networks), monocyte/macrophage dysfunction may result in one or more pathophysiologic consequences: defects in monocyte maturation, deficiencies in the clearance of physiologic substrates in lysosomal diseases (e.g., Gaucher's disease, mucopolysaccharidoses, osteopetrosis, metachromatic leukodystrophy), decreased synthesis and secretion of mediators (complement component deficiencies), defects in microbicidal activity (chronic granulomatous disease), and defects that are acquired following infection and during chemotherapy [e.g., acquired immunodeficiency syndrome (AIDS)].[37]

Infections

The function of pulmonary defense mechanisms against infection have been eloquently described by Quie.[38]

"The human lung has an exquisitely effective and complex defense against infections. Mucus prevents attachment of bacteria to the epithelium, and those bacteria that cannot cross the mucus are cleared by exhalation or by the mucus-ciliary escalator. Alveolar macrophages dispatch microbes that reach the peripheral barriers of the lung. The pulmonary phagocytic system immobilizes, kills, and walls off invading bacteria. The phagocytic system, developed in bone marrow, includes alveolar macrophages, granulocytes, and monocytes. The phagocytic system is amplified by humoral factors, including inflammatory mediators, acute-phase reactants, and opsonins that allow rapid engulfment and killing of microbes. Highly mobile polymorphonuclear granulocytes reinforce the macrophages when invading organisms reach tissue. Sterility of the lower respiratory tract in the normal host is evidence that the defense systems of the lung are highly effective and potently bactericidal. The oxidative and nonoxidative microbicidal mechanisms of alveolar macrophages and granulocytes are lethal for most ordinary microbes."

However, certain pathogens have means of preventing phagocytosis, and obligate intracellular species have evolved mechanisms of intracellular survival. Oftentimes, systemic infection can impair lung defense mechanisms.[39] Successful biologic detente between microbe and host is the usual situation in the normal human lung, but the relationship is unfortunately short lived in patients with cystic fibrosis: Mucus is not an adequate barrier in these patients. Bacterial pathogens colonize respiratory tissue and, as a consequence, compromise lung function. Better understanding of local defenses in normal human lungs and of the defects in lung defenses in patients with cystic fibrosis should lead to methods that will provide these patients with successful defense against invading microbes.

In experimental systems, systemic endotoxin significantly impairs lung host defenses against intrapulmonary bacterial challenges. Tumor necrosis factor-mediated events may play a central role.[40] The interaction between neutrophils and pulmonary macrophages would appear to be important in providing a front-line defense against microorganisms. For example, alveolar macrophages release neutrophil chemotactic factor (NCF) when incubated with *P. aeruginosa*, an important step in initiating the neutrophil-dependent defense system against the organism.[41]

Macrophages may activate neutrophils through the elaboration of polypeptides such as neutrophil-activating factor (NAF), a polypeptide which in vitro enhances the ability of neutrophils to kill target cells, presumably through greater release of superoxide anion on their subsequent stimulation by either bacterial phagocytosis or by phorbol myristate acetate.[42]

Acquired ciliary defects, which can be broadly de-

Table 3–4. Acquired cilia disorders affecting the upper respiratory tract[a]

Clinical setting	Abnormality
Cigarette-smoke exposure	Ciliostasis
	Cilia swelling
	Supernumerary microtubules
	Deficient microtubules
	Ciliated cell loss
Aldehyde exposure	Ciliostasis
	Dynein ATPase inhibition
Sulfur dioxide exposure	Cilia detachment
Bronchopneumonia	Supernumerary microtubules
Pseudomonas infection	Ciliostasis
	Cilia detachment
Viral infection	Cilia loss
Mycoplasma infection	Cilia loss
Topical anesthetic exposure	Ciliostasis
Ionizing radiation	Cilia tip swelling
Perennial rhinitis	Flaccid matted cilia
Allergic reactions	Cilia loss and detachment
Vitamin A deficiency	Ciliated cell replacement

[a] Summarized from references 32, 58, 87, and 88.

fined as impairments of mucociliary function that are not inherited, are very important because of their high prevalence. This results from the association of cilia injury with such common disorders as viral respiratory tract infections, allergic disorders, and exposure to cigarette smoke and other pollutants. From a clinical perspective, acquired ciliary disorders present with many of the same manifestations as those described in individuals with PCD, with several notable differences. First, the clinical manifestations can appear at any stage of life whereas PCD is present at birth. Second, the manifestations are usually limited to one or two organ systems such as the upper respiratory tract, whereas PCD usually involves many organ systems. Finally, acquired cilia disorders are often reversible once the etiologic factor has been removed whereas PCD persists throughout life. A summary of some of the clinical settings in which acquired cilia abnormalities have been described is provided in Table 3–4.

Much of the known information about acquired cilia defects is based on morphologic studies of tissue by electron microscopy. The types of ultrastructural defects described range from total detachment of the ciliated epithelium to the formation of compound cilia or the scattered loss of inner and outer dynein arms on selected axonemes. The large variation of acquired ultrastructural defects described in the literature must be interpreted with caution. The same preparation artifacts and sampling errors encountered when examining tissue from individuals with suspected PCD must also be considered when a acquired ciliary disorder is suspected.[43] The morphologic findings in PCD usually include a specific defect restricted to a particular axoneme element that is present in all or most of the cilia examined. In contrast, acquired defects tend to be scattered in distribution, to involve multiple axonemal elements, and frequently to affect entire cilia of groups of cilia.

Acquired cilia defects such as those abnormalities observed following viral upper respiratory tract infection can be completely reversible. The natural history of most acquired cilia defects, however, is not known. Also, very little is known about the prevention or possible treatments of acquired cilia disorders. Because acquired cilia abnormalities affect most people at some point in their lives, cilia abnormalities have a major impact on societal health and warrant further extensive investigation.

Immunodeficiency

Pulmonary defenses are also affected by the overall immunocompetence of the individual It is well known that immunocompromised hosts are susceptible to a variety of pulmonary complications.[44] Although AIDS is the most contemporary example of immunodeficiency (see Chapter 6), immune pulmonary defenses can be impaired by factors such as drug therapy, protein calorie malnutrition, and generalized immunodeficiency diseases. In the rat, for example, malnutrition has been shown to slow the clearance of microorganisms from the respiratory tract.[45] It seems likely that the human respiratory tract is similarly affected, given the known relationship between human immunity and malnutrition. Some examples include the role of T cells in the defense against certain types of infection, such as *Pneumocystis carinii*[46]; also, compromise of B-cell function as seen in hemorrhage or other severe injuries may produce marked alterations in pulmonary B-cell populations, which may contribute to postinjury abnormalities in host defenses.[47]

Human immunodeficiency virus (HIV) infection stimulates the phagocytic capacity of pulmonary alveolar macrophages, suggesting that these cells may be activated by this retroviral infection. Patients with AIDS who develop pneumonia, especially smokers, show a significant decrease in the number, viability, and phagocytic capacity of these cells.[48]

Functional immunodeficiency can occur in patients with autoimmune disorders in which macrophage dysfunction has been observed, such as systemic lupus erythematosus.[49] Patients with lung carcinoma may have impaired natural killer cell activity, which contributes to their increased risk of infection.[50]

Metabolic Impairment

Pulmonary defense mechanisms may be interdependent with other organ systems. For example, the pathogenesis of the adult respiratory distress syndrome may be linked to the pulmonary macrophage and to liver function. Endotoxin [lipopolysaccharide (LPS)] and tumor necrosis factor (TNF-alpha) have been implicated in the pathogenesis of sepsis-induced adult respiratory distress syndrome. In hepatic failure, however, LPS spillover to the lung may promote adult respiratory distress syndrome by inducing unregulated TNF-alpha production within the pulmonary microenvironment.[51] Diabetic patients with hyperglycemia are persistently at risk for pulmonary and other infections.[52] Impaired humoral host defense includes such varied neutrophil functions as adhesion, chemotaxis, and phagocytosis. In addition, binding of glucose to the biochemically active site of the third component of complement C3 inhibits the attachment of this protein to the microbial surface and thereby impairs opsonization. *Candida albicans* expresses a glucose-inducible protein that is structurally and functionally homologous to a complement receptor on mammalian phagocytes, and this protein promotes adhesion in the yeast and subverts phagocytosis by the host.[53]

The functions of cells obtained from diabetic BB rats have been studied. The impaired phagocytotic and bactericidal functions of alveolar macrophages appeared to be caused by a cellular abnormality associated with the degree of insulin deficiency.[54]

Pulmonary clearance of pneumococci was observed to be reduced in experimental models of rats with cirrhosis and ascites.[55] Similar impairment may occur in humans with liver disease, explaining their susceptibility to respiratory infection. Patients with adult respiratory distress syndrome are at high risk for pulmonary infection, which is related to defects in neutrophil superoxide anion production and chemotaxis.[56]

Finally, stress may impair leukocyte function; in experimental animals, the generation of superoxide anion by neutrophils was diminished for a period of time after stress.[57]

Injurious Agents and Therapeutic Drugs

Cigarette smoke is the agent most commonly responsible for impairment of pulmonary defense mechanisms. As discussed by Sisson et al.,[58] the motility of cilia is dramatically impaired by even brief exposure to smoke.

This can significantly compromise the mucociliary escalator.

Short-term exposures to ozone (O_3) impair pulmonary antibacterial defenses and alveolar macrophage (AM) phagocytosis in a dose-related manner.[59]

Therapeutic drugs may impair pulmonary defenses by compromising the function of pulmonary macrophages or neutrophils. For example, aminophylline, commonly used to treat obstructive lung diseases, has been shown in experimental systems to compromise the bactericidal activity of polymorphonuclear leukocytes.[60] Erythromycin has been observed to inhibit normal neutrophil migration into the alveoli in response to a bacterial challenge.[61] Drugs may also render the lung more susceptible to oxidative injury. For example, halothane and isofluorane thus enhance the sensitivity of pulmonary endothelial cells to injury by stimulated neutrophils.[62]

Adverse Effects of Defense Mechanisms

Although the inflammatory reaction in the lung is critical for defense against infectious agents, there are numerous examples in which the inflammatory response in the lung causes harm. Moreover, as discussed by Reynolds,[63] excessive or poorly regulated inflammation can destroy tissue, thus contributing to many disease processes that can lead to fibrosis and impaired gas exchange. Examples include asthma, chronic bronchitis, interstitial lung diseases, and acute lung injury leading to adult respiratory distress syndrome in which neutrophils and their breakdown products and enzymes are enough to amplify local destruction of alveolar tissue.

Another adverse effect of oxygen may be the suppression of macrophage proliferation. A high concentration of oxygen can impede the intraalveolar proliferation of lung macrophages.[64] This observation implies that there is a delicate balance between the needs of individuals requiring respiratory support and the potential risk of infection.

For optimal phagocytosis, antibodies and complement are needed; phagocytic cells possess receptors for the Fc fragment of the immunoglobulin (IgG) molecule and complement. Receptors for cytokines are also present. These cytokines are important for activating the alveolar macrophage and recruiting other phagocytic cells and lymphocytes to the site of infection. Alveolar macrophages also contain cytophilic antibodies, IgG molecules that are bound to the cell via the F(ab)$_2$ fragments. These cytophilic antibodies can interfere with the process of phagocytosis. They can bind to bacteria containing an Fc receptor (e.g., *Staphylococcus aureus* protein A) and therefore provide the alveolar macrophage with a means to bind and digest staphylococci. Pulmonary surfactant proteins enhance the uptake of bacteria and viruses by alveolar macrophages and viruses. Thus, surfactant contributes to the defense mechanisms of the lung. Phagocytic cells can injure alveoli; during phagocytosis, toxic oxygen species and enzymes needed for killing bacteria are produced. These toxic substances may leak out of the cell and damage the surrounding tissues. All these phenomena contribute to the processes of inflammation. The function of phagocytic cells, crucial for the elimination of microorganisms, is decreased in smokers and by certain air pollutants.

Alpha-1 antitrypsin (alpha-1AT) is important for protecting the lung from the effects of neutrophil elastase. Individuals with alpha-1AT deficiency develop emphysema. Yeast-produced recombinant alpha-1AT (rAAT) has normal antielastase function but is associated with high renal clearance, thus making it unsuitable for chronic intravenous administration. Aerosol administration of rAAT to alpha-1AT-deficient individuals have been attempted. After aerosol administration of single doses of 10 200 mg of rAAT, epithelial lining fluid (ELF) alpha-1AT antineutrophil elastase defenses were augmented in proportion to the dose of rAAT administered. ELF alpha-1AT levels and antineutrophil elastase capacity 4 h after 200 mg rAAT aerosol were increased 40 fold over preaerosol levels, and were 5 fold increased over baseline at 24 h after aerosol administration. rAAT was detectable in serum after aerosol, indicating that the lower respiratory tract epithelium may be permeable to rAAT, and that aerosolized rAAT is capable of gaining access to lung interstitium. No adverse clinical effects were noted. These observations demonstrate that aerosol administration of rAAT is safe and results in significant augmentation of lung antineutrophil elastase defenses, suggesting this method is a feasible approach to therapy.[65]

References

1. Verhoef J. Host–pathogen relationships in respiratory tract infections. Clin Ther 1991;13(1):172–180.
2. Coonrod JD, Rehm SR, Yoneda K. Pneumococcal killing in the alveolus. Evidence for a nonphagocytic defense mechanism for early clearance. Chest 1983;83 (Suppl.):895–905.
3. Jonsson S, Musher DM, Goree A, Lawrence EC. Human alveolar lining material and antibacterial defenses. Am Rev Respir Dis 1986;133(1):136–140.
4. Reynolds HY. Lung inflammation: Role of endogenous chemotactic factors in attracting polymorphonuclear granulocytes. Am Rev Respir Dis 1983;127(2):S16–S25.
5. Sibille Y, Reynolds HY. Macrophages and polymorphonuclear neutrophils in lung defense and injury. Am Rev Respir Dis 1990;141(2):471–501.
6. Fisher ES, Lauffenburger DA, Daniele RP. The effect of alveolar macrophage chemotaxis on bacterial clearance from the lung surface. Am Rev Respir Dis 1988; 137(5):1129–1134.
7. Valberg PA, Jensen WA, Rose RM. Cell organelle motions in bronchoalveolar lavage macrophages from smokers and nonsmokers. Am Rev Respir Dis 1990;141:1272–1279.
8. Waldorf AR, Levitz SM, Diamond RD. In vivo bronchoalveolar macrophage defense against *Rhizopus oryzae* and *Aspergillus fumigatus*. J Infect Dis 1984;150(5):752–760.
9. Elstad MR. Aspergillosis and lung defenses. Semin Respir Infect 1991;6(1):27–36.
10. Flesch IE, Schwamberger G, Kaufmann SH. Fungicidal activity of IFN-gamma-activated macrophages. Extracellular killing of *Cryptococcus neoformans*. J Immunol 1989;142(9):3219–3224.
11. Tuomanen E, Rich R, Zak O. Induction of pulmonary inflammation by components of the pneumococcal cell surface. Am Rev Respir Dis 1987;135(4):869–874.
12. Harris SE, Nelson S, Astry CL, Bainton BG, Summer WR. Endotoxin-induced suppression of pulmonary antibacterial defenses against *Staphylococcus aureus*. Am Rev Respir Dis 1988;138(6):1439–1443.
13. Levi MH, Pasculle AW, Dowling JN. Role of the alveolar macrophage in host defense and immunity to *Legionella micdadei* pneumonia in the guinea pig. Microb Pathog 1987;2(4):269–282.
14. Debs RJ, Fuchs HJ, Philip R, et al. Lung-specific delivery of cytokines induces sustained pulmonary and systemic immunomodulation in rats. J Immunol 1988; 140(10):3482–3488.
15. Rhodin AJ. The ciliated cell. Ultrastructure and function of the human tracheal mucosa. Amer Ref Resp Dis 1966;93:1–15.
16. Dalhamn T. Mucus flow and ciliary activity in the trachea of healthy rats and rats exposed to respiratory irritant gases. Acta Physiol Scand (Suppl. 123) 1956;36:1–163.
17. Iravani J, Van As A. Mucus transport in the tracheobronchial tree of normal and bronchitic rats. J Pathol 1972;106:81–93.
18. Sleigh MA. The nature and action of respiratory tract cilia. In: Brain J, Proctor D, Reid L, ed. Respiratory defense mechanisms. New York: Dekker, 1977:247–289.
19. Fick RB, Jr. Cell-mediated antibacterial defenses of the distal airways. Am Rev Respir Dis 1985;131(5):543–548.
20. Lipscomb MF. Lung defenses against opportunistic infections. Chest 1989;96(6):1393–1399.
21. Dannenberg AJ. Delayed-type hypersensitivity and cell-mediated immunity in the pathogenesis of tuberculosis. Immunol Today 1991;12(7):228–233.
22. Gryzan S, Paradis IL, Zeevi A, et al. Unexpectedly high incidence of *Pneumocystis carinii* infection after lung-heart transplantation. Implications for lung defense and allograft survival. Am Rev Respir Dis 1988;137(6):1268–1274.

23. Hoffman RM, Dauber JH, Paradis IL, Griffith BP, Hardesty RL. Alveolar macrophage migration after lung transplantation. Am Rev Respir Dis 1991;143:834–838.

24. Iwata M, Sato A. Morphological and immunohistochemical studies of the lungs and bronchus-associated lymphoid tissue in a rat model of chronic pulmonary infection with *Pseudomonas aeruginosa*. Infect Immun 1991;p59(4):1514–1520.

25. Toews GB, Hansen EJ, Strieter RM. Pulmonary host defenses and oropharyngeal pathogens. Am J Med 1990;88(5A):205–245.

26. Shennib H, Mulder DS, Chiu RC. The effects of pulmonary atelectasis and reexpansion on lung cellular immune defenses. Arch Surg 1984;119(3):274–277.

27. Marshall BC, Carroll KC. Interaction between *Pseudomonas aeruginosa* and host defenses in cystic fibrosis. Semin Respir Infect 1991;6(1):11–18.

28. Siewert A. Uber einen fall von bronchiectasie bei einem patienten mit situs inversus viscerum. Berl Klin Wochenschr 1904;41:139–141.

29. Kartagener M. Zur pathogenese der bronchiektasien. I. Mitteilung: Bronchiektasien bei situs viscerum inversus. Beitr Klin Tuberk 1933,83:498–501.

30. Afzelius BA. A human syndrome caused by immotile cilia. Science 1976;193:317–319.

31. Afzelius BA, Eliasson R. Flagellar mutants in man: On the heterogeneity of the immotile-cilia syndrome. J Ultrastruct Res 1979;69:43–52.

32. Afzelius BA. The immotile cilia syndrome and other ciliary diseases. Int Rev Exp Pathol 1979;19:1–43.

33. Sturgess J, Thompson M, Czegledy-Nagy E, Turner J. Genetic aspects of immotile cilia syndrome. Am J Med Genet 1986;25:149–160.

34. Afzelius BA. Disorders of ciliary motility. Hosp Pract 1986;21(3):73–80.

35. Pavia D, Agnew JE, Bateman JRM, et al. Lung mucociliary clearance in patients with Young's syndrome. Chest 1981;80:892–893.

36. Waite DA, Wakefield SJ, Mackay JB, Ross IT. Mucociliary transport and ultrastructural abnormalities in Polynesian bronchiectasis. Chest 1981;80(Suppl):896–898.

37. Douglas SD, Musson RA. Phagocytic defects—monocytes/macrophages. Clin Immunol Immunopathol 1986;40(1):62–68.

38. Quie PG. Lung defense against infection. J Pediatr 1986;108:813–816.

39. White JC, Nelson S, Winkelstein JA, Booth FV, Jakab GJ. Impairment of antibacterial defense mechanisms of the lung by extrapulmonary infection. J Infect Dis 1986;153(2):202–208.

40. Nelson S, Chidiac C, Bagby G, Summer WR. Endotoxin-induced suppression of lung host defenses. J Med (Westbury) 1990;21(1–2):85–103.

41. Ozaki T, Maeda M, Hayashi H, et al. Role of alveolar macrophages in the neutrophil-dependent defense system against *Pseudomonas aeruginosa* infection in the lower respiratory tract. Amplifying effect of muramyl dipeptide analog. Am Rev Respir Dis 1989;140(6):1595–1601.

42. Pennington JE, Rossing TH, Boerth LW, Lee TH. Isolation and partial characterization of a human alveolar macrophage-derived neutrophil-activating factor. J Clin Invest 1985;75(4):1230–1237.

43. Ehouman A, Pinchon MC, Escudier E, Bernaudin JF. Ultrastructural abnormalities of respiratory cilia. Virchows Arch B Cell Pathol 1985;48:87–95.

44. Rosenow EC, III, Wilson WR, Cockerill FR, III. Pulmonary disease in the immunocompromised host. 1. Mayo Clin Proc 1985;60(7):473–487.

45. Martin TR, Altman LC, Alvares OF. The effects of severe protein-calorie malnutrition on antibacterial defense mechanisms in the rat lung. Am Rev Respir Dis 1983;128(6):1013–1019.

46. Shellito J, Suzara VV, Blumenfeld W, Beck JM, Steger HJ, Ermak TH. A new model of *Pneumocystis carinii* infection in mice selectively depleted of helper T lymphocytes. J Clin Invest 1990;85(5):1686–1693.

47. Robinson A, Abraham E. Hemorrhage in mice produces alterations in pulmonary B cell repertoires. J Immunol 1990;145(11):3734–3739.

48. Musher DM, Watson DA, Nickeson D, Gyorkey F, Lahart C, Rossen RD. The effect of HIV infection on phagocytosis and killing of *Staphylococcus aureus* by human pulmonary alveolar macrophages. Am J Med Sci 1990;299(3):158–163.

49. Wallaert B, Aerts C, Bart F, et al. Alveolar macrophage dysfunction in systemic lupus erythematosus. Am Rev Respir Dis 1987;136(2):293–297.

50. Weissler JC, Nicod LP, Toews GB. Pulmonary natural killer cell activity is reduced in patients with bronchogenic carcinoma. Am Rev Respir Dis 1987;135(6):1353–1357.

51. Callery MP, Kamei T, Mangino MJ, Flye MW. Organ interactions in sepsis. Host defense and the hepatic-pulmonary macrophage axis. Arch Surg 1991;126(1):28–32.

52. Waldorf AR, Ruderman N, Diamond RD. Specific susceptibility to mucormycosis in murine diabetes and bronchoalveolar macrophage defense against *Rhizopus*. J Clin Invest 1984;74(1):150–160.

53. Hostetter MK. Handicaps to host defense. Effects of hyperglycemia on C3 and *Candida albicans*. Diabetes 1990;39(3):271–275.

54. Sima AA, O'Neill SJ, Naimark D, Yagihashi S, Klass D. Bacterial phagocytosis and intracellular killing by alveolar macrophages in BB rats. Diabetes 1988;37(5):544–549.

55. Mellencamp MA, Preheim LC. Pneumococcal pneumonia in a rat model of cirrhosis: Effects of cirrhosis on pulmonary defense mechanisms against *Streptococcus pneumoniae*. J Infect Dis 1991;163(1):102–108.

56. Martin TR, Pistorese BP, Hudson LD, Maunder RJ. The function of lung and blood neutrophils in patients with the adult respiratory distress syndrome. Implications for the pathogenesis of lung infections. Am Rev Respir Dis 1991;144(2):254–262.

57. Binkhorst GJ, Henricks PA, VD Inghts, Hajer R, Nijkamp FP. The effect of stress on host defense system and on lung damage in calves experimentally infected with

Pasteurella haemolytica type A1. Zentralbl Veterinaemed Reihe A 1990;37(7):525–536.

58. Sisson JH, Tuma DJ, Rennard SI. Acetaldehyde-mediated cilia dysfunction in bovine bronchial epithelial cells. Am J Physiol 1991;260:L29–L36.

59. Gilmour MI, Hmieleski RR, Stafford EA, Jakab GJ. Suppression and recovery of the alveolar macrophage phagocytic system during continuous exposure to 0.5 ppm ozone. Exp Lung Res 1991;17(3):547–588.

60. Nelson S, Summer WR, Jakab GJ. Aminophylline-induced suppression of pulmonary antibacterial defenses. Am Rev Respir Dis 1985;131(6):923–927.

61. Nelson S, Summer WR, Terry PB, Warr GA, Jakab GJ. Erythromycin-induced suppression of pulmonary antibacterial defenses. A potential mechanism of superinfection in the lung. Am Rev Respir Dis 1987;136(5):1207–1212.

62. Shayevitz JR, Varani J, Ward PA, Knight PR. Halothane and isoflurane increase pulmonary artery endothelial cell sensitivity to oxidant-mediated injury. Anesthesiology 1991;74(6):1067–1077.

63. Reynolds HY. Lung Inflammation: Normal host defense or a complication of some diseases? Annu Rev Med 1987;38(1):295–323.

64. Sherman MP, Evans MJ, Campbell LA. Prevention of pulmonary alveolar macrophage proliferation in newborn rabbits by hyperoxia. J Pediatr 1988;112(5):782–786.

65. Hubbard RC, McElvaney NG, Sellers SE, Healy JT, Czerski DB, Crystal RG. Recombinant DNA-produced alpha 1-antitrypsin administered by aerosol augments lower respiratory tract antineutrophil elastase defenses in individuals with alpha-1-antitrypsin deficiency. J Clin Invest 1989;84(4):1349–1354.

66. Sanderson M, Dirksen E. Mechanosensitive and beta-adrenergic control of the ciliary beat frequency of mammalian respiratory tract cells in culture. Am Rev Respir Dis 1989;139:432–440.

67. Yeates D, Spektor D, Pitt B. Effect of orally administered orciprenaline on tracheobronchial mucociliary clearance. Eur J Respir Dis 1986;69:100–108.

68. Foster WM, Langenback E, Bohning DE, Bergofsky EH. Quantitation of mucus clearance in peripheral lung and comparison with tracheal and bronchial mucus transport velocities in man: Adrenergics return depressed clearance and transport velocities in asthmatics to normal. Am Rev Respir Dis 1978;177(Suppl.):337 (abstr.).

69. Wanner A, Maurer D. Abraham W, Szepfalusi Z, Sielczak M. Effects of chemical mediators of anaphylaxis on ciliary function. J Allergy Clin Immunol 1983;72:663–667.

70. Mussatto D, Lourenco R. The effect of inhaled histamine on human tracheal mucus velocity and bronchial mucociliary clearance. Am Rev Respir Dis 1988;138:775–779.

71. Bisgaard H, Pedersen M. SRS-A leukotrienes decreases the activity of human respiratory cilia. Clin Allergy 1987;17:95–103.

72. Tamaoki J, Kobayaski K, Sakai N, Chiyotani A, Kanemura T, Takizawa T. Effect of bradykinin on airway ciliary motility and its modulation by neutral endopeptidase. Am Rev Respir Dis 1989;140:430–435.

73. Lindberg S, Mercke U. Bradykinin accelerates mucociliary activity in rabbit maxillary sinus. Acta Otolaryngol (Stockh) 1988;101:114–121.

74. Wong L, Miller I, Yeates D. Regulatory pathways for the stimulation of canine tracheal ciliary beat frequency by bradykinin. J Physiol (London) 1990;422:421–431.

75. Kondo M, Tamaoki J, Takizawa T. Neutral endopeptidase inhibitor potentiates the tachykinin-induced increase in ciliary beat frequency in rabbit trachea. Am Rev Respir Dis 1990;142:403–406.

76. Kobayashi K, Tamaoki J, Sakai N, Kanemura T, Horii S, Takizawa T. Angiotensin II stimulates airway ciliary motility in rabbit cultured tracheal epithelium. Acta Physiol Scand 1990;138:497–502.

77. Khan A, Bengtsson B, Lindberg S. Influence of substance P on ciliary beat frequency in airway isolated preparations. Eur J Pharmacol 1986;130:91–96.

78. Lindberg S, Mercke U, Uddman R. The morphological basis for the effect of substance P on mucociliary activity in rabbit maxilliary sinus. Acta Otolaryngol (Stockh) 1986;101:314–319.

79. Dadaina J, Yin S, Laurenzi G. Studies of mucus flow in the mammalian respiratory tract. Am Rev Respir Dis 1971;103:808–815.

80. Verdugo P. Calcium-dependent hormonal stimulation of ciliary activity. Nature (London) 1980;283:764–765.

81. Wanner A, Sielczak M, Mella J, Abraham W. Ciliary responsiveness in allergic and nonallergic airways. J Appl Physiol 1986;60:1967–1971.

82. Villalon M, Hinds T, Verdugo P. Stimulus-response coupling in mammalian ciliated cells. Demonstration of two mechanisms of control for cytosolic [Ca^{2+}]. Biophys J 1989;56:1255–1258.

83. Jonsson MS, McCormick JR, Gillies CG, Gondos B. Kartagener's syndrome with motile spermatozoa. N Engl J Med 1982;307:1131–1133.

84. Sturgess JM, Chao J, Wong J, Aspin N, Turner JAP. Cilia with defective radial spokes—A cause of human respiratory disease. N Engl J Med 1979;300:53–56.

85. Sturgess JM, Chao J, Turner JA. Tranposition of ciliary microtubules. Another cause of impaired ciliary motility. N Engl J Med 1980;303:318–322.

86. Schneeberger EE, McCormack J, Issenberg HJ, Schuster SR, Gerald PS. Heterogeneity of ciliary morphology in the immotile-cilia syndrome in man. J Ultrastruct Res 1980;73:34–43.

87. Afzelius BA, Camner P, Mossberg B. Acquired ciliary defects compared to those seen in the immotile-cilia syndrome. Eur J Respir Dis 1983;64:5–10.

88. Carson JL, Collier AM. Ciliary defects: Cell biology and clinical perspectives. Adv Pediatr 1988;35:139–165.

CHAPTER 4

Common Pathways and Patterns of Injury

Jeffrey L. Myers, Thomas V. Colby, and Samuel A. Yousem

Pulmonary diseases often affect the lung parenchyma in a relatively specific and predictable distribution. In addition, a striking or predominant histopathologic feature (e.g., nonnecrotizing granulomas in sarcoidosis) frequently provides an important clue to the diagnosis. Recognition of the resulting patterns of lung injury at low magnification can be extremely useful in limiting diagnostic considerations. Thus, two important questions to address in histologically categorizing lung lesions are (1) which compartments are primarily affected (i.e., what is the distribution of the changes?), and (2) what is the nature of the predominant tissue reaction (e.g., acute/chronic inflammatory infiltrate, proliferation of fibroblasts, collagen deposition, granulomatous inflammation, lung necrosis, neoplastic proliferation, etc.)? This scheme of "pattern recognition" can greatly facilitate histopathologic analysis of a surprisingly large number of lung diseases. This chapter provides a general summary of anatomic features important in biopsy and autopsy diagnosis of a wide range of pulmonary conditions, reviews some of the shortcomings in using pattern recognition as a diagnostic approach, and emphasizes examples of classical patterns of acute and chronic lung injury. For more detailed discussions concerning clinical and pathologic features of the specific diseases illustrated in this section, the reader is referred to corresponding chapters elsewhere in this volume.

Summary of Lung Anatomy

The lung comprises several distinct anatomic compartments: airways, alveolar spaces, interstitium, and pleura (see Chapter 2). Many conditions that affect the lung tend to preferentially involve one or more of these compartments.

Conducting airways include the larger cartilage-containing bronchi as well as the smaller bronchioles. Small bronchioles can be identified by their muscular coats and the presence of an accompanying pulmonary artery. Respiratory bronchioles have incomplete muscular walls and are partially alveolated. Alveolar ducts, which have incomplete walls with regular outpouchings of alveolar sacs, represent a transition zone between airways and air spaces. Alveolar spaces or sacs account for the bulk of the lung's volume. The interstitial compartment is the structural matrix of the lung, which is bounded by basal lamina underlying bronchial, bronchiolar, and alveolar epithelium. The interstitium can be divided into peribronchial/peribronchiolar matrix, alveolar septal matrix, interlobular septa, and visceral pleura, each characterized by a unique and complex arrangement of collagen fibers, inflammatory and mesenchymal cells, blood vessels, and lymphatics.

Pulmonary vasculature includes pulmonary arteries and arterioles, capillaries, pulmonary veins, and the bronchial circulation. Arteries and arterioles are part of the bronchovascular bundles and accompany bronchi, bronchioles, and alveolar ducts, while pulmonary veins are located within interlobular septa. The visceral pleura includes the connective tissue covering of the lung and is separated from the remainder of the interstitial compartment by an elastic lamina.

Bronchocentric and bronchiolocentric lesions have a peribronchial, peribronchiolar, or intraluminal distribution at low magnification and can affect large airways, small airways, or both. Secondary changes resulting from airway obstruction occur in the distal lung parenchyma (e.g., endogenous lipid pneumonia) and

57

sometimes represent the major, albeit secondary, finding in open lung biopsy specimens. Bronchiolocentric lesions are centered on distal conducting and respiratory bronchioles. Elastic tissue stains are useful to highlight bronchiole walls and the accompanying pulmonary arteries. Lesions in this category are frequently associated with secondary changes that affect the peribronchiolar interstitium and peribronchiolar alveolar spaces.

Vasocentric processes can preferentially target arteries, veins, or capillaries, and therefore can have different low-magnification distributions. Conditions in this category include variants of hypertensive pulmonary vasculopathy, vasculitides, and some malignant neoplasms.

Air space-filling processes often affect distal airways (respiratory bronchioles) as well as alveolar ducts and alveolar spaces. Alveolar filling results in a solid appearance at low magnification, and most conditions in this category have a patchy distribution. Patchy air space-filling processes often show a distinctively bronchiolocentric orientation.

Pattern Recognition as a Diagnostic Approach

The term diffuse interstitial lung disease is usually used in a clinicoradiologic context to refer to conditions that cause diffuse radiographic abnormalities and which typically are associated with physiologic deficits. Diffuse interstitial diseases account for perhaps the greatest number of difficulties in diagnostic pathology of lung disease. This reflects, in part, the large number of etiologically diverse conditions included under this heading. It also reflects the fact that certain morphologically similar conditions can be separated into distinct categories only after correlation of the anatomic changes with clinical and radiographic findings. The main pathologic abnormalities in most of these entities include expansion of the interstitium by inflammation, fibrosis, or a combination of the two, and associated secondary changes in the air spaces. The interstitial changes may diffusely involve all segments of the interstitial compartment or may preferentially affect a specific compartment such as peribronchiolar matrix, interlobular septa, or visceral pleura.

Low-magnification examination is critical in evaluating interstitial lung diseases.[1,2] Interstitial lesions can be either *diffuse* or *patchy* in distribution. (It should be emphasized that clinically and radiologically diffuse lesions can be either diffuse or patchy at the light microscopic level). Hereafter, diffuse is used in a histological sense to refer to those processes that tend to involve the lung parenchyma in a relatively uniform fashion; that is, each low-magnification field is uniformly abnormal, and each field examined tends to look like the next. Patchy lesions have a heterogeneous appearance at low magnification, and one microscopic field may not resemble the next. Patchy processes may affect the interstitium in a random or a more ordered distribution.

Temporal relationships are also important in evaluating interstitial lung diseases. Temporally *homogeneous* lesions appear as if the lung had sustained a single insult at a single point in time. The abnormal areas show qualitatively similar degrees of inflammation, fibroblast proliferation, and collagen deposition. Temporally *heterogeneous* conditions are those in which the abnormal foci show a spectrum of changes ranging from acute lung injury to dense collagen scarring, as if various parts of the lung had been injured at different points in time over an extended period.

Attempts to simplify diagnosis of inflammatory lung diseases using a pattern recognition algorithm underscore the difficulty in categorizing a diverse number of conditions on the basis of only a few parameters.[1,2] Although low-magnification distribution is the key to recognizing certain lesions, in other lesions individual histologic features of tissue response overshadow the importance of anatomical compartmentalization. The most common patterns of injury (Table 4–1) are discussed next.

Common Patterns of Injury

Acute Lung Injury Patterns

Acute lung injury patterns is a term recently coined by Katzenstein and Askin[3] to refer to a group of morphologically distinct tissue response patterns that occur after a wide range of acute pulmonary insults. The entities included under this heading are diffuse alveolar damage, acute interstitial pneumonia, and bronchiolitis obliterans with organizing pneumonia. Although each of these represents a distinct morphologic pattern, they share certain light microscopic features: temporal uniformity and fibroblast proliferation. Temporal uniformity means that the pathologic changes appear to represent a response to a single injury that occurred at a single point in time; that is, the histopathologic changes tend to look the same from one low-magnification field to the next and are evenly distributed within each higher magnification field. The fibrosis that occurs in each of these conditions consists mainly of fibroblast proliferation rather than the collagen deposition seen in many other fibrosing lung diseases.

Table 4–1. Common patterns of injury in lung disease

Affected compartment	Pattern	Examples
Interstitium: alveolar septal matrix	Acute lung injury	Diffuse alevolar damage
		Acute interstitial pneumonia
		Bronchiolitis obliterans organizing pneumonia
	Chronic interstitial	Usual interstitial pneumonia
		Desquamative interstitial pneumonia
		Nonclassifiable chronic interstitial pneumonia
Interstitium: peribronchiolar matrix	Peribronchiolar	Extrinsic allergic alveolitis
		Eosinophilic granuloma
		Respiratory bronchiolitis-associated interstitial lung disease
Interstitium: arteries/veins/capillaries	Vasocentric	1° Pulmonary arteriopathy
		Pulmonary veno-occlusive disease
		Capillary hemangiomatosis
		Necrotizing capillaritis
		Angiocentric lymphoma
Interstitium: lymphatics/interlobular septa	Lymphangitic	Lymphangitic carcinomatosis
		Sarcoidosis
		Lymphangioleiomyomatosis
Alveolar space	Air space filling	Bronchopneumonia
		Eosinophilic pneumonia
		Alveolar hemorrhage
		Pulmonary edema
		Pulmonary alveolar proteinosis
Large airways	Bronchocentric	Bronchiectasis
		Bronchitis
Visceral pleura	Pleural	Eosinophilic pleuritis
Interstitium and air spaces	Nodules/masses	Hyalinizing granuloma

Diffuse Alveolar Damage

Diffuse alveolar damage is the pathologic lesion that occurs in patients with adult respiratory distress syndrome (ARDS), a syndrome characterized by acute respiratory failure associated with diffuse lung infiltrates on chest roentgenograms.[4,5] The causes of diffuse alveolar damage are, therefore, analagous to the causes of ARDS and include a large number of catastrophic insults (Table 4–2).[5] Histologically, diffuse alveolar damage begins with an acute or exudative stage that is followed by a proliferative or organizing stage.[4] The changes that characterize these two stages represent a continuum of acute lung injury with no sharp line of demarcation between them. The histologic hallmark of the acute stage is the presence of eosinophilic hyaline membranes; interstitial and intraalveolar edema, patchy hyperplasia of type II pneumocytes, and a relatively scant interstitial infiltrate of mononuclear inflammatory cells also occur. At low magnification, the changes can be extremely subtle in the early phase, including delicate diffuse alveolar septal thickening with hyperplasia of cuboidal type II pneumocytes (Fig. 4–1). In autopsy material the hyperplastic pneumocytes often appear to separate from the alveolar septa and may provide the only clue to the diagnosis. Hyaline membranes appear within about 48 h of the insult and tend to be accentuated along alveolar ducts (Fig. 4–2). The hyaline membranes appear to be plastered against

Table 4–2. Causes of diffuse alveolar damage

Infections
  Pneumocystis carinii
  Viruses (influenza, cytomegalovirus, varicella, adenovirus)
  Fungi (blastomycosis, aspergillus)
  Legionella sp.
Toxins
  Inhaled toxins (e.g., O_2, NO_2, household ammonia and bleach, mercury vapor)
  Ingested toxins (e.g., paraquat)
Drugs
  Cytotoxic (azathioprine, carmustine [BCNU], bleomycin, busulfan, lomustine [CCNU], cyclophosphamide, melphalan, methotrexate, mitomycin, procarbazine, teniposide, vinblastine, zinostatin)
  Noncytotoxic (amiodarone, amitriptyline, colchicine, gold salts, hexamethonium, nitrofurantoin, penicillamine, streptokinase, sulfathiazole)
  Ilicit (heroin)
Shock
  Traumatic
  Septic
  Cardiogenic
Radiation
Miscellaneous
  Acute pancreatitis

the interstitium and are vaguely refractile and brightly eosinophilic. As the lesion progresses, alveolar septal thickening becomes more marked and begins to dominate the histologic picture.

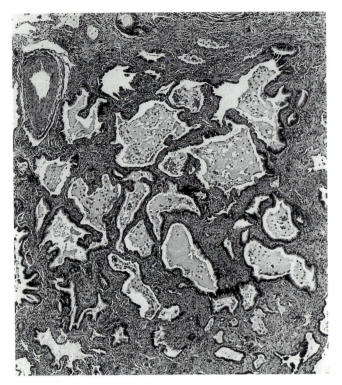

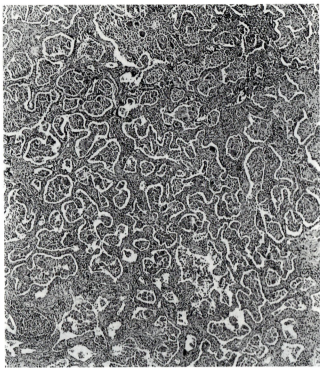

Fig. 4–11. Low-magnification photomicrograph shows honeycomb change in usual interstitial pneumonia. Remodeled cystic air spaces are lined by bronchiolar epithelium and contain mucinous debris.

Fig. 4–12. Low-magnification photomicrograph of desquamative interstitial pneumonia shows diffuse, uniform changes that include alveolar septal thickening and air space filling, imparting solid appearance to tissue.

Ultrastructural studies of usual interstitial pneumonia have demonstrated focal areas of acute lung injury with epithelial necrosis.[27] Immunohistochemical studies have also identified foci of intraluminal fibrosis that appear to be incorporated back into the interstitium in a manner analogous to the sequence described for acute lung injury patterns.[8] These findings indicate a certain degree of morphologic overlap between usual interstitial pneumonia and the various forms of acute lung injury, and suggest common pathways of tissue injury and repair. The key histopathologic and ultrastructural feature that separates usual interstitial pneumonia from acute lung injury patterns is temporal heterogeneity, as if small portions of the lung have been injured over long periods of time, eventually causing extensive lung scarring.

Desquamative Interstitial Pneumonia

Morphologically, desquamative interstitial pneumonia is a distinct entity that differs substantially from usual interstitial pneumonia.[2,3,28] The changes in desquamative interstitial pneumonia differ mainly in that they affect the lung parenchyma in a much more uniform pattern and lack the variegated appearance typical of

usual interstitial pneumonia. The combination of uniform thickening of alveolar septa and uniform filling of alveolar spaces by macrophages at low magnification is pathognomonic of desquamative interstitial pneumonia (Fig. 4–12).[2,3] The alveolar septa are thickened by a sparse inflammatory infiltrate that often includes plasma cells and occasional eosinophils, and are lined by plump cuboidal pneumocytes. The most striking feature, perhaps, is the presence of numerous alveolar macrophages within most of the distal air spaces (Fig. 4–13). The macrophages usually have lightly pigmented dusty brown cytoplasm, a finding undoubtedly related to the observation that nearly all affected patients are cigarette smokers.[28,29]

Desquamative interstitial pneumonia (DIP) is similar to usual interstitial pneumonia in that it represents a distinct pattern of chronic lung injury. As with usual interstitial pneumonia, however, it represents a specific clinicopathologic entity only when it is seen in the appropriate clinical setting (i.e., idiopathic pulmonary fibrosis). A pattern indistinguishable from idiopathic desquamative interstitial pneumonia can also occur in rare examples of drug toxicity and in asbestosis. A "DIP-like pattern" can also occur as a patchy finding in a variety of other conditions, notably respiratory bronchiolitis and pulmonary eosinophilic granuloma.[30]

Nonclassifiable Chronic Interstitial Pneumonia

Lung biopsies occasionally show chronic interstitial pneumonias affecting alveolar septal matrix that lack any distinctive pathologic features to allow classification into a specific category such as usual interstitial pneumonia or desquamative interstitial pneumonia. These lesions are often characterized by a relatively uniform appearance at low magnification caused by a cellular alveolar septal infiltrate of mononuclear inflammatory cells associated with varying degrees of interstitial fibrosis.[3] Examples of this condition have undoubtedly been included in studies of idiopathic pulmonary fibrosis as "early" or "cellular" usual interstitial pneumonia. This type of tissue response may be seen as a manifestation of collagen vascular disease or drug-induced lung disease, and may also occur as an idiopathic lesion. There are no good data to establish this latter group as a specific nosologic entity, and the precise therapeutic and prognostic implications of this diagnosis are uncertain.

Peribronchiolar Lesions in Diffuse Lung Disease

A number of conditions that present with clinical features of diffuse lung disease are characterized by a peribronchiolar pattern of lung injury, meaning that the histopathologic changes preferentially involve peribronchiolar interstitium. Extrinsic allergic alveolitis, pulmonary eosinophilic granuloma, and respiratory bronchiolitis-associated interstitial lung disease are the most important members of this group. Low-magnification recognition of a peribronchiolar pattern can be extremely useful in separating these entities from the chronic interstitial pneumonias.

Extrinsic Allergic Alveolitis

Extrinsic allergic alveolitis, also called hypersensitivity pneumonia, is an inflammatory lung disorder that results from sensitization to a variety of inhaled organic dusts (see Chapter 18).[2,3,31,32] Granulomatous interstitial pneumonia is the lesion most frequently described in extrinsic allergic alveolitis. At low magnification there is a cellular interstitial infiltrate distributed in a bronchiolocentric pattern (Fig. 4–14); it is this bronchi-

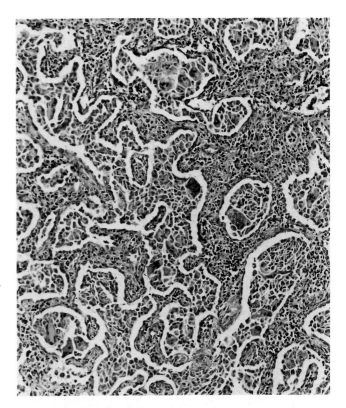

Fig. 4–13. Higher magnification photomicrograph of desquamative interstitial pneumonia. Alveolar septa are thickened by inflammatory infiltrate and hyperplasia of cuboidal type II pneumocytes; alveolar spaces contain closely packed macrophages with scattered multinucleated giant cells.

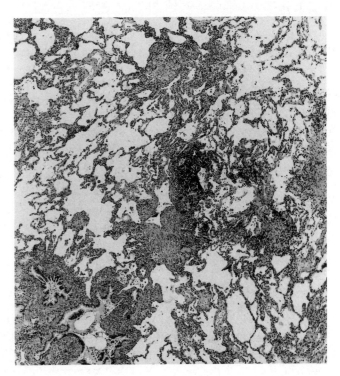

————————————————▷

Fig. 4–14. Low-magnification photomicrograph of extrinsic allergic alveolitis (hypersensitivity pneumonia). Interstitial infiltrate of chronic inflammatory cells is distributed in distinctly bronchiolocentric pattern.

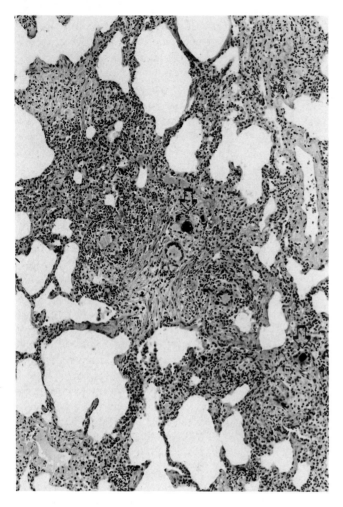

Fig. 4–15. Higher magnification photomicrograph of extrinsic allergic alveolitis (hypersensitivity pneumonia) shows prominent multinucleated giant cells, some of which contain calcified cytoplasmic inclusions (*arrows*), a nonspecific finding.

olocentric distribution that is the tip-off to the diagnosis at low magnification.[31,32] The interstitial infiltrate is composed mainly of lymphocytes, plasma cells, and histiocytes, which are occasionally admixed with eosinophils and neutrophils. Epithelioid histiocytes, including multinucleated giant cells, are usually present and impart a granulomatous appearance to the inflammatory infiltrate (Fig. 4–15). The giant cells may contain a variety of nonspecific cytoplasmic inclusions, such as asteroid bodies, Schaumann bodies, and birefringent calcium oxalate crystals. Well-formed nonnecrotizing granulomas are also seen and, in a minority of cases, may represent a striking feature. Bronchiolitis obliterans is an associated finding in about half the cases and is characterized by the presence of polypoid plugs of fibroblastic tissue within bronchioles and alveolar ducts. In advanced cases, the changes are less characteristic

and consist mainly of bland interstitial fibrosis and honeycomb change.

The differential diagnosis on biopsy specimens often includes chronic interstitial pneumonias, particularly usual interstitial pneumonia. The features that are most helpful in distinguishing extrinsic allergic alveolitis from chronic interstitial pneumonias are the peribronchiolar accentuation of the interstitial lesion, the presence of granulomatous inflammation, and the frequent coexistence of bronchiolitis obliterans in the former. Recognition of these features is important because of significant differences in treatment and prognosis. Coleman and Colby[31,32] have shown that the presence of these histologic features usually is associated with a good prognosis regardless of whether one is able to serologically demonstrate an offending antigen. When well-formed granulomas are prominent, extrinsic allergic alveolitis is sometimes confused with sarcoidosis. An interstitial pneumonia accentuated around bronchioles in extrinsic allergic alveolitis, and the "lymphangitic" distribution of granulomas characteristically seen in sarcoidosis are features that should help distinguish these conditions. In rare cases it may be exceedingly difficult or impossible to distinguish these conditions on the basis of morphology alone; indeed, the possibility of extrinsic allergic alveolitis should always be considered in patients thought to have sarcoidosis limited to the lungs.

Pulmonary Eosinophilic Granuloma

Primary pulmonary eosinophilic granuloma, also called Langerhans' granulomatosis or histiocytosis X, is an interstitial lesion of uncertain etiology characterized by an abnormal proliferation of modified histiocytes (see Chapter 17).[2,3,33–35] While pulmonary eosinophilic granuloma shares many histologic features with the disseminated forms of histiocytosis X, it differs in that pulmonary involvement is the sole or predominant manifestation of disease.

Pathologically, eosinophilic granuloma is characterized by patchy interstitial nodules that often have a stellate configuration at low magnification (Fig. 4–16).[2,3] The nodules are distributed in a peribronchiolar fashion, a feature best appreciated in cases with small early cellular lesions. Larger nodules may show central cavitation. At higher magnification, the nodules contain a mixed inflammatory infiltrate including eosinophils, lymphocytes, plasma cells, and diagnostic histiocytes, so-called Langerhans cells. The proportion and number of inflammatory cell types contained within the nodules varies, and accurate diagnosis depends on recognition of pathognomonic Langerhans cells (see Chapter 17). Langerhans cells have character-

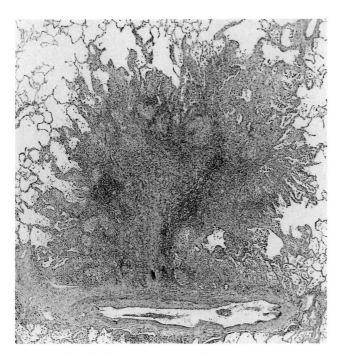

Fig. 4–16. Scanning magnification photomicrograph of pulmonary eosinophilic granuloma. Stellate nodule resembling starfish is situated adjacent to pulmonary artery (lower portion of photomicrograph) indicating bronchiolocentric location. Periphery of nodule shows radiating tentacles contiguous with alveolar septa.

istic convoluted nuclei with bland, evenly dispersed chromatin, inconspicuous nucleoli, and abundant eosinophilic cytoplasm with indistinct borders. The convoluted nuclei have a grooved appearance that distinguishes them from other histiocytes.

The diagnosis of eosinophilic granuloma usually can be made on the basis of light microscopy alone. Ultrastructurally Langerhans cells contain unique pentalaminar inclusions (Birbeck or Langerhans granules) within their cytoplasm, and for this reason electron microscopy has long been considered the method of choice for establishing the diagnosis of eosinophilic granuloma in difficult cases. More recently it has been shown that Langerhans cells react with commercially available antibodies to S-100 protein, HLA-DR, and OKT6.[36–38] Immunoperoxidase staining, a procedure that is easily applied to even small specimens, has thus become an important tool that largely replaces the need for electron microscopy in selected cases.[39,40] The results of these procedures must be interpreted in the context of the clinical and pathologic findings, however, because Langerhans cells may be present in small numbers normally and have also been demonstrated in a variety of neoplastic and nonneoplastic lung conditions.[41,42] Interestingly, increased numbers of Langerhans cells

have also been demonstrated in cigarette smokers, providing additional evidence that pulmonary eosinophilic granuloma may be linked to cigarette smoking.[43,44]

As the lesions of pulmonary eosinophilic granuloma become less cellular, they also become more fibrotic and may be confused with the chronic interstitial pneumonias. It is imperative to distinguish these conditions because of marked differences in prognosis and treatment. At low magnification the first clue to the diagnosis of eosinophilic granuloma is the relatively symmetrical and often stellate configuration of the nodules coupled with a peribronchiolar distribution.[2,3] This contrasts with the patchy, asymmetrical interstitial fibrosis in usual interstitial pneumonia, which is often accentuated in subpleural and paraseptal zones. Alveolar spaces surrounding the nodules of eosinophilic granuloma frequently contain clusters of lightly pigmented macrophages, thus imparting a DIP-like appearance to the lesion. Desquamative interstitial pneumonia differs from eosinophilic granuloma in that the changes affect the interstitium in a diffuse and uniform manner. Eosinophilic pneumonia is predominantly an air space rather than an interstitial process, and is characterized by the presence of a mixture of eosinophils and macrophages within alveolar spaces. Reactive eosinophilic pleuritis is an unusual but nonspecific inflammatory response that occurs in about a third of patients with spontaneous pneumothorax.[45] It is frequently mentioned in the differential diagnosis of eosinophilic granuloma because the inflammatory infiltrate includes eosinophils and histiocytes. The majority of patients with reactive eosinophilic pleuritis, however, lack clinical, radiographic, and pathologic evidence of interstitial lung disease and are unlikely to be confused with eosinophilic granuloma (see also Chapter 34).

Respiratory Bronchiolitis-Associated Interstitial Lung Disease

Respiratory ("smoker's") bronchiolitis is a lesion of cigarette smokers in which the respiratory bronchioles and adjacent alveolar spaces are filled with lightly pigmented macrophages (Fig. 4–17).[29,46–48] Respiratory bronchiolitis can cause clinically detectable interstitial lung disease in some individuals, a condition referred to as respiratory bronchiolitis-associated interstitial lung disease.[29,47,48] There is some evidence to suggest that desquamative interstitial pneumonia and respiratory bronchiolitis-associated interstitial lung disease are related entities; however, the precise relationship between these conditions is not known. The main distinguishing histologic feature is the distribution of the changes at low magnification, which is exquisitely bronchiolocentric in respiratory bronchiolitis as opposed to

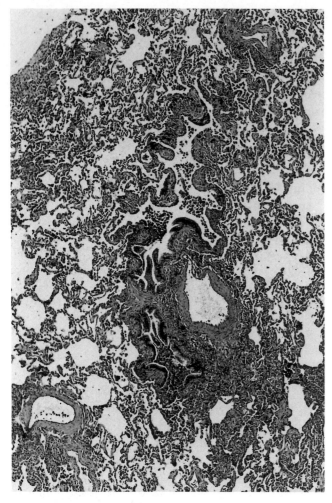

Fig. 4–17. Low-magnification photomicrograph shows respiratory bronchiolitis. Bronchiole in center shows mild thickening of peribronchiolar interstitium associated with clusters of intraluminal macrophages.

the diffuse abnormalities in desquamative interstitial pneumonia.

Vasocentric Diseases

Arteries and veins can be the main target for a number of neoplastic and nonneoplastic pulmonary conditions. The resulting patterns of injury depend, to some extent, on which vessels are primarily affected (i.e., large or small arteries, capillaries, veins, or a combination). Vascular changes can be extremely subtle, and the possibility of vascular disease should always be considered in open lung biopsies initially interpreted as being within normal limits.

Hypertensive Pulmonary Vasculopathy

The clinical syndrome of primary pulmonary hypertension is associated with a number of morphologic pat-

terns that can be separated into three main groups: primary pulmonary arteriopathy, pulmonary venoocclusive disease, and capillary hemangiomatosis (see Chapter 29).[49] Primary pulmonary arteriopathy comprises plexogenic as well as thromboembolic forms of pulmonary arteriopathy, both of which preferentially affect small muscular arteries. Pulmonary veno-occlusive disease differs in that the changes are centered on pulmonary veins located within interlobular septa, with relative sparing of muscular arteries. Capillary hemangiomatosis, as the name implies, is characterized by proliferation of capillaries within alveolar septa and along bronchovascular bundles.

Necrotizing Capillaritis

Necrotizing capillaritis is a subtle pathologic finding that is nearly always superimposed on a background of diffuse alveolar hemorrhage (see Chapter 30).[50–54] Mark and Ramirez[50] emphasized several histopathologic criteria for diagnosis: (1) focal necrosis of alveolar septa, (2) a concomitant alveolar septal infiltrate of necrotic neutrophils characterized by the presence of pyknosis and karyorrhexis ("nuclear dust"), and (3) spilling of necrotic neutrophils, fibrin, and erythrocytes into adjacent alveolar spaces. Other less specific changes include the presence of fibrin thrombi within alveolar septal capillaries as well as intersitial hemorrhage and hemosiderin. Although capillaritis is not pathognomonic of any one disorder, it can be useful in limiting the differential diagnosis of pulmonary hemorrhage.[52,53]

Angiocentric Lymphoma and Intravascular Lymphomatosis

Pulmonary lymphomas frequently show striking vascular involvement (see Chapter 31).[55] In most circumstances, however, vascular involvement does not occur as a pure pattern but is associated with nodules and masses. Lymphomas with prominent vascular infiltration have been referred to by a number of terms including lymphomatoid granulomatosis,[3,56] lymphomatoid granulomatosis-lymphoma,[3] angiocentric lymphoma,[2] and angiocentric immunoproliferative lesions[57,58] (see Chapter 31). Intravascular lymphomatosis is a rare condition in which the lymphoid infiltrate is exquisitely intravascular with little or no involvement of other anatomic compartments.[59–60]

Lymphangitic Patterns

Pulmonary lymphatics are distributed within bronchovascular bundles, interlobular septa, and visceral

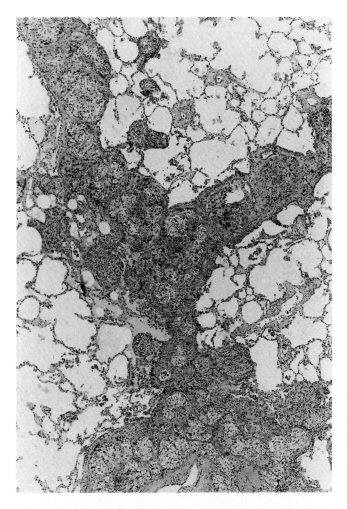

Fig. 4–18. Low-magnification photomicrograph of metastatic prostatic adenocarcinoma distributed in "lymphangitic" pattern. Lymphatic spaces are filled with clusters of tumor cells, causing distension and accentuation of interlobular septa.

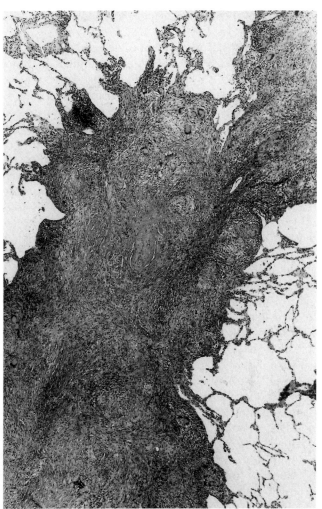

Fig. 4–19. Low-magnification photomicrograph of sarcoidosis shows characteristic "lymphangitic" distribution of granulomas associated with dense collagen fibrosis, resulting in thickening of interlobular septa similar to that seen in lymphangitic carcinomatosis (see Fig. 4–18).

pleura. A number of conditions are characterized by histopathologic changes that tend to follow these lymphatic pathways resulting in a "lymphangitic pattern" of injury.[2] The classical example is, of course, lymphangitic carcinomatosis, in which metastatic carcinoma cells are limited to lymphatic channels (Fig. 4–18). A number of other conditions, including sarcoidosis and lymphangioleiomyomatosis, are also distinguished by a lymphangitic pattern of injury.

Sarcoidosis

Sarcoidosis is a disease of undetermined etiology characterized by the presence of nonnecrotizing granulomas in multiple organs and perpetuated by the presence of activated T lymphocytes within the involved sites[61] (see Chapter 19). Nonnecrotizing granulomas are characteristic of sarcoidosis. The granulomas are

compact, well-circumscribed collections of plump epithelioid histiocytes and multinucleated giant cells surrounded by a rim of lymphocytes and collagen fibrosis. A small proportion of the granulomas may show central pyknosis and karyorrhexis as well as small foci of eosinophilic necrosis. The granulomas tend to be distributed along bronchovascular bundles, interlobular septa, and visceral pleura, resulting in a lymphangitic distribution at low magnification.[2,3] The presence of well-formed granulomas distributed in this distinctive manner results in a nearly pathognomonic pattern of lung injury (Fig. 4–19). Coalescence of granulomas combined with dense collagen fibrosis can cause macroscopically apparent nodules in a minority of cases and is responsible for examples of so-called nodular sarcoidosis.

Granulomatous involvement of vessel walls occurs in nearly 70% of cases of sarcoidosis examined by open lung biopsy, and is usually seen in cases with extensive parenchymal involvement.[62] The granulomas may be localized to either the intima or the media of affected vessels, and either arteries or veins may be involved. The granulomatous inflammation may lead to extensive destruction of the vessel wall and even total occlusion of the vascular lumen; however, true vessel wall necrosis is not seen. Despite the frequency of granulomatous vasculitis in sarcoidosis, hemodynamically significant pulmonary hypertension is rare except in patients with advanced disease characterized by extensive pulmonary fibrosis and honeycomb change.[63,64]

The differential diagnosis includes mainly granulomatous infection, chronic berylliosis, and extrinsic allergic alveolitis. Special stains and cultures should always be done to rule out mycobacterial and fungal infections. Chronic berylliosis, a systemic illness caused by hypersensitivity to beryllium, may be clinically, radiographically, and pathologically indistinguishable from sarcoidosis.[65] Necrosis and granulomatous vasculitis occur more frequently in sarcoidosis and may be helpful in distinguishing these conditions. Hyalinized fibrotic nodules resembling silicotic nodules are seen in a minority of patients with chronic berylliosis, and may also be helpful in differential diagnosis. Recognition of berylliosis is ultimately predicated on an appropriate occupational history and tissue analysis. The difficulties of distinguishing extrinsic allergic alveolitis from sarcoidosis were discussed earlier.

Lymphangioleiomyomatosis

Lymphangioleiomyomatosis, also called lymphangiomyomatosis, is a rare condition that exclusively affects women, usually in the reproductive age group (see Chapter 33).[66,67] The main pathologic abnormality in lymphangioleiomyomatosis is a disorderly proliferation of atypical smooth muscle cells along lymphatic pathways with extension into bronchiole walls, veins, and small air spaces. The proliferating cells tend to be spindled in shape, although plump epithelioid forms also occur and even predominate in some cases. This proliferation results in a characteristic low-magnification pattern characterized by the presence of randomly distributed cystic "emphysematous" spaces (Fig. 4–20); indeed, the presence of cystic spaces overshadows the lymphangitic distribution of spindled cells as a low magnification marker for lymphangioleiomyomatosis.[66,67] The intervening lung parenchyma often looks remarkably normal. At higher magnification the cystic

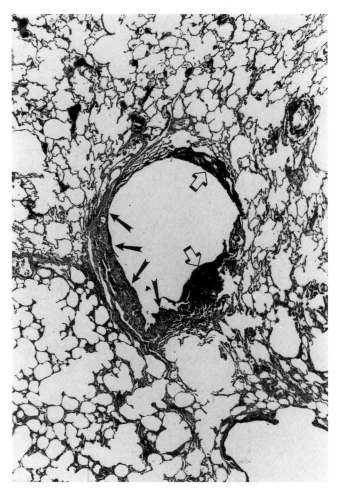

Fig. 4–20. Low-magnification photomicrograph of lymphangioleiomyomatosis. Cystic air spaces, separated by relatively normal pulmonary parenchyma, show walls focally thickened by abnormal spindle cells (*solid arrows*). Evidence of associated hemorrhage is also seen (*open arrows*).

spaces contain nodular smooth muscle bundles within at least a portion of their walls. Hemosiderin often is present within surrounding air spaces and attests to pulmonary hemorrhage in these patients.

The differential diagnosis of lymphangioleiomyomatosis is limited. So-called benign metastasizing leiomyoma is a rare condition characterized by the presence of multiple circumscribed nodules of cytologically bland smooth muscle cells within the lungs. The nodules differ from the lesions of lymphangioleiomyomatosis in that they are usually solid and well circumscribed, and frequently have a "biphasic" appearance because of the entrapped alveolar epithelial cells. Hemosiderin pigment deposition can be a prominent feature of lymphangioleiomyomatosis and may lead to confusion with pulmonary hemorrhage syndromes, particularly idiopathic pulmonary hemosiderosis. The presence of cystic spaces coupled with foci of neoplastic spindled cells in lymphangioleiomyomatosis should serve to distinguish these conditions.

Air Space Filling

The previously described patterns of lung injury primarily affect components of the interstitial compartment. Certain conditions are characterized by abnormalities of alveolar spaces with relative sparing of the interstitial compartment, resulting in an air space-filling pattern of injury. Alveolar spaces may contain cellular exudates, as in acute bronchopneumonia, or relatively acellular debris (e.g., pulmonary edema). Regardless of the nature of the air space-filling material, the result is the presence of patchy areas of solid-appearing lung parenchyma.

Eosinophilic Pneumonia

Eosinophilic pneumonia, defined in purely histopathologic terms, occurs in a variety of clinical contexts (see Chapter 16).[2,3] The histologic features of eosinophilic pneumonia are relatively constant regardless of the clinical context. The major abnormality is filling of distal air spaces by a cellular exudate composed of eosinophils and histiocytes including multinucleated giant cells (Fig. 4–21). The relative proportions of the two cell types is variable, and histiocytes may predominate in some areas. Necrosis of the alveolar exudate results in formation of eosinophilic abscesses. Alveolar septa are thickened and contain a similar inflammatory infiltrate associated with hyperplasia of type II pneumocytes. Bronchiolitis obliterans with organizing pneumonia is a frequent associated finding; indeed, there is significant clinical and pathological overlap between idiopathic BOOP and chronic eosinophilic pneumonia.

Diffuse Alveolar Hemorrhage

Pulmonary hemorrhage may be the presenting manifestation of a variety of conditions.[51,68–74] Potential etiologies include immunologically mediated and nonimmunologically mediated disorders as well as illnesses of unknown pathogenesis. The clinical presentation is similar regardless of the underlying etiology. The most consistent features include a combination of hemoptysis, anemia, and diffuse pulmonary infiltrates. Evidence of concomitant glomerulonephritis is also present in the majority of adult patients (i.e., pulmonary-renal syndrome).[70,74] Diagnostic considerations in this setting include antiglomerular basement membrane disease (Goodpasture's syndrome), idiopathic pulmonary hemosiderosis, systemic lupus erythematosus, Wegener's

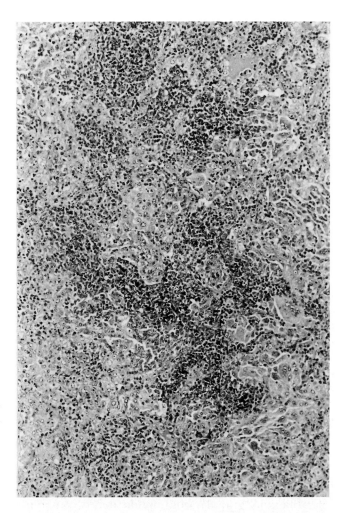

Fig. 4–21. Photomicrograph of eosinophilic pneumonia in open lung biopsy from patient with chronic eosinophillic pneumonia. Lung architecture is largely obscured by dense air space infiltrate of histiocytes and eosinophils. Relative proportion of histiocytes and eosinophils varies throughout field; most darker smaller cells are eosinophils.

granulomatosis, and nonclassifiable systemic necrotizing vasculitis. Most of these conditions have characteristic extrapulmonary manifestations or unique laboratory findings and are diagnosed without lung biopsy. Occassionally, however, the clinical syndrome is not specific, and an open lung biopsy is required for diagnosis.

The histopathologic features of diffuse alveolar hemorrhage are relatively constant regardless of the underlying cause. The presence of an associated vasculitis, including necrotizing capillaritis, can be helpful in limiting the differential diagnosis (see Chapter 30). The main change in diffuse alveolar hemorrhage is filling of alveolar spaces by a combination of erythrocytes, fibrin, and hemosiderin-laden macrophages. Air space filling tends to be uniform and generally lacks a bronchiolocentric distribution. The presence of fibrin, areas of early organization, and hemosiderin pigment are helpful in separating clinically significant alveolar hemorrhage from traumatic bleeding secondary to the biopsy procedure. Organizing hemorrhage can lead to formation of intraluminal plugs of fibroblastic tissue identical to those seen in bronchiolitis obliterans with organizing pneumonia. The presence of hemosiderin pigment, as well as a clinical history suggestive of pulmonary hemorrhage, can be important clues to the diagnosis in such cases. Chronic recurrent pulmonary hemorrhage results in dramatic hemosiderin deposition including encrustation of vascular elastic lamina with associated fibrosis and a giant cell reaction (i.e., endogenous pneumoconiosis).[75] In this late stage of alveolar hemorrhage, the interstitial changes may overshadow the air space filling component.

Pulmonary Alveolar Proteinosis

Pulmonary alveolar proteinosis, more recently called pulmonary alveolar lipoproteinosis or phospholipoproteinosis, is a distinctive lesion characterized by the presence of amorphous granular eosinophilic debris within alveolar spaces.[2,3,76–79] This tissue response can be seen in various clinical contexts and can be categorized into primary (idiopathic) and secondary forms[76,78] (see Chapter 22). The morphologic changes are similar regardless of the underlying cause, and consist of alveolar filling by granular eosinophilic debris containing cholesterol casts and cellular "ghosts" (Fig. 4–22). The result is patchy consolidation of the lung by an eosinophilic alveolar exudate. The interstitium is usually relatively unaffected, although associated alveolar septal fibrosis has been described in rare examples. Ultrastructural studies reveal free lamellar bodies as well as tubular myelin and myelin structures which are thought to represent surfactant breakdown products.[78,80,81]

Bronchocentric Lesions

Inflammatory lesions of the large airways are relatively uncommon and are usually associated with secondary abnormalities of distal lung parenchyma. Occasionally, however, acute and chronic inflammatory infiltrates are limited to the peribronchial interstitium and bronchial lumens. Bronchiectasis from any cause, including cystic fibrosis, causes acute and chronic bronchitis characterized by dense cuffs of peribronchial infiltrates at low magnification. The peribronchial inflammation is often associated with epithelial alterations including necrosis, ulceration, and metaplasia. True bronchial dilatation is

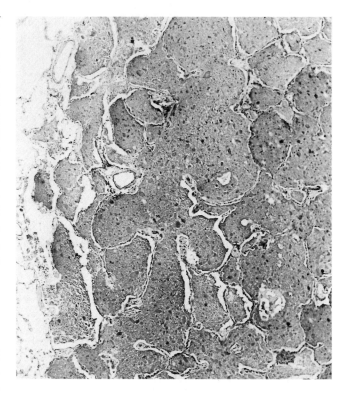

Fig. 4–22. Low-magnification photomicrograph shows pulmonary alveolar proteinosis. Alveolar spaces are filled with amorphous eosinophilic material containing cellular debris. Alveolar septa remain thin and delicate.

difficult to evaluate on lung biopsies, and the presence of acute and chronic bronchitis may be the only clue to the diagnosis of bronchiectasis in these specimens.

Pleural Lesions

Inflammatory conditions limited to the visceral pleura, with relative preservation of underlying lung parenchyma, rarely present as diagnostic problems. Malignant lymphomas, pulmonary amyloidosis, sarcoidosis, and asbestosis occasionally show prominent visceral pleural involvement, but there are nearly always associated parenchymal abnormalities. Reactive eosinophilic pleuritis is a nonspecific pleuritis that results from pneumothorax.[45] At low magnification the resulting pattern is visceral pleural thickening due to a dense inflammatory infiltrate. At higher magnification the inflammatory infiltrate includes prominent numbers of eosinophils as well as mononuclear inflammatory cells. The presence of eosinophils is nonspecific and has no connotations concerning potential etiologies. Distinguishing reactive eosinophilic pleuritis from eosinophilic granuloma was discussed earlier.

Nodules/Masses

Nodules or masses are the primary abnormality in a number of neoplastic and nonneoplastic lung diseases. In general, nodules and masses do not respect anatomic compartments and show "cross-country" destruction of interstitial and air space compartments. Nodules and masses may be distributed in a predictable pattern (i.e., bronchiolocentric nodules in pulmonary eosinophilic granuloma) or may be randomly distributed throughout the lung tissue.

Pulmonary Hyalinizing Granuloma

Pulmonary hyalinizing granuloma is an uncommon condition characterized histologically by the low-magnification appearance of multiple fibrotic nodules resembling ancient granulomas[2,3,82] (see Chapter 33). The nodules are randomly distributed and are composed of dense hyalinized collagen bundles arranged in a concentric whorled pattern. The collagen bundles are often associated with a patchy infiltrate of lymphocytes and plasma cells.

References

1. Colby TV. Anatomic distribution and histopathologic patterns in interstitial lung disease. In: Schwarz MI, King TE, eds. Interstitial lung disease, 2d Ed. Philadelphia: BC Decker, 1992;59–77.
2. Colby TV, Lombard C, Yousem SA, Kitaichi M. Atlas of pulmonary surgical pathology. Philadelphia: WB Saunders, 1991.
3. Katzenstein AA, Askin FB. Surgical pathology of non-neoplastic lung disease, 2d Ed. Philadelphia: WB Saunders, 1990.
4. Katzenstein AA, Bloor CM, Leibow AA. Diffuse alveolar damage—The role of oxygen, shock, and related factors. Am J Pathol 1976;85:210–224.
5. Murray JF, Matthay MA, Luce JM, Flick MR. An expanded definition of the adult respiratory distress syndrome. Am Rev Respir Dis 1988;138:720–723.
6. Fukuda Y, Ishizaki M, Masuda Y, Kimurda G, Kawanami O, Masugi Y. The role of intraalveolar fibrosis in the process of pulmonary structural remodeling in patients with diffuse alveolar damage. Am J Pathol 1987;126:171–182.
7. Fukuda Y, Ferrans VJ, Schoenberger CI, Rennard SI, Crystal RG. Patterns of pulmonary structural remodeling after experimental paraquat toxicity: The morphogenesis of intraalveolar fibrosis. Am J Pathol 1985;118:452–475.
8. Kuhn C, Boldt J, King TE, Crouch E, Vartio T, McDonald JA. An immunohistochemical study of architectural remodeling and connective tissue synthesis in pulmonary fibrosis. Am Rev Respir Dis 1989;140:1693–1703.
9. Katzenstein AA, Myers JL, Mazur MT. Acute interstitial pneumonia: A clinicopathologic, ultrastructural, and cell

kinetic study. Am J Surg Pathol 1986;10:256–267.
10. Olson J, Colby TV, Elliott CG. Hamman-Rich syndrome revisited. Mayo Clin Proc 1990;65:1538–1548.
11. Katzenstein AA. Pathogenesis of "fibrosis" in interstitial pneumonia: An electron microscopic study. Hum Pathol 1985;16:1015–1024.
12. Myers JL, Colby TV. Bronchiolitis obliterans with organizing pneumonia and constrictive bronchiolitis: Comparative analysis of two distinct entities. Prog Surg Pathol 1991;12:167–180.
13. Epler GR, Colby TV. The spectrum of bronchiolitis obliterans. Chest 1983;83:161–162.
14. van Thiel RJ, van der Burg S, Groote AD, Nossent GD, Wills SH. Bronchiolitis obliterans organizing pneumonia and rheumatoid arthritis. Eur Respir J 1991;4:905–911.
15. Epler GR, Colby TV, McLoud TC, Carrington CB, Gaensler EA. Bronchiolitis obliterans organizing pneumonia. N Engl J Med 1985;312:152–158.
16. Cordier JF, Loire R, Brune J. Idiopathic bronchiolitis obliterans organizing pneumonia: Definition of characteristic clinical profiles in a series of 16 patients. Chest 1989;96:999–1004.
17. Bartter T, Irwin RS, Nash G, Balikian JP, Hollingsworth HH. Idiopathic bronchiolitis obliterans organizing pneumonia with peripheral infiltrates on chest roentgenogram. Arch Intern Med 1989;149:273–279.
18. Davison AG, Heard BE, McAllister WAC, Turner-Warwick MEH. Cryptogenic organizing pneumonitis. QJ Med 1983;207:382–394.
19. Katzenstein AA, Myers JL, Prophet WD, Corley LS, Shin SM. Bronchiolitis obliterans and usual interstitial pneumonia. Am J Surg Pathol 1986;10:373–381.
20. Gosink BB, Friedman PJ, Liebow AA. Bronchiolitis obliterans: Roentgenologic pathologic correlation. AJR 1973;117:816–832.
21. Guerry-Force ML, Müller NL, Wright JL, et al. A comparison of bronchiolitis obliterans with organizing pneumonia, usual interstitial pneumonia, and small airways disease. Am Rev Respir Dis 1987;135:705–712.
22. Alegre-Martin J, Fernandez de Sevilla T, Garcia F, Falcó V, Martinez-Vazquez JM. Three cases of idiopathic bronchiolitis obliterans with organizing pneumonia. Eur Respir J 1991;4:902–904.
23. Myers JL, Katzenstein AA. Ultrastructural evidence of alveolar epithelial injury in idiopathic bronchiolitis obliterans-organizing pneumonia. Am J Pathol 1988;132:102–109.
24. Basset F, Ferrans VJ, Soler P, Takemura T, Fukuda Y, Crystal RG. Intraluminal fibrosis in interstitial lung disorders. Am J Pathol 1986;122:443–461.
25. Liebow AA. Definition and classification of interstitial pneumonias in human pathology. Prog Respir Res 1975;8:1–33.
26. Ohori NP, Sciurba FC, Owens GR, Hodgson MJ, Yousem SA. Giant-cell interstitial pneumonia and hard-metal pneumoconiosis: A clinicopathologic study of four cases and review of the literature. Am J Surg Pathol 1989;13:581–587.
27. Myers JL, Katzenstein AA. Epithelial necrosis and alveo-

lar collapse in the pathogenesis of usual interstitial pneumonia. Chest 1988;94:1309–1311.

28. Carrington CB, Gaensler EA, Coutu RE, FitzGerald MX, Gupta RG. Natural history and treated course of usual and desquamative interstitial pneumonia. N Engl J Med 1978;298:801–809.

29. Yousem SA, Colby TV, Gaensler EA. Respiratory bronchiolitis-associated interstitial lung disease and its relationship to desquamative interstitial pneumonia. Mayo Clin Proc 1989;64:1373–1380.

30. Bedrossian CWM, Kuhn C, Luna MA, Conklin RH, Byrd RB, Kaplan PD. Desquamative interstitial pneumonia-like reaction accompanying pulmonary lesions. Chest 1977;72:166–169.

31. Coleman A, Colby TV. Histologic diagnosis of extrinsic allergic alveolitis. Am J Surg Pathol 1988;12:514–518.

32. Colby TV, Coleman A. The histologic diagnosis of extrinsic allergic alveolitis and its differential diagnosis. Prog Surg Pathol 1989;10:11–25.

33. Basset F, Corrin B, Spencer H, et al. Pulmonary histiocytosis X. Am Rev Respir Dis 1978;118:811–820.

34. Friedman PJ, Liebow AA, Sokoloff J. Eosinophilic granuloma of lung: Clinical aspects of primary pulmonary histiocytosis in the adult. Medicine (Baltimore, 1981;60:385–396.

35. Colby TV, Lombard C. Histiocytosis X in the lung. Hum Pathol 1983;14:847–856.

36. Webber D, Tron V, Askin F, Churg A. S-100 staining in the diagnosis of eosinophilic granuloma of lung. Am J Clin Pathol 1985;84:447–453.

37. Flint A, Lloyd RV, Colby TV, Wilson BW. Pulmonary histiocytosis X. Arch Pathol Lab Med 1986;110:930–933.

38. Cagle PT, Mattioli CA, Truong LD, Greenberg SD. Immunohistochemical diagnosis of pulmonary eosinophilic granuloma on lung biopsy. Chest 1988;94:1133–1137.

39. Mierau GW, Favara BE. S-100 protein immunohistochemisty and electron microscopy in the diagnosis of Langerhans' cell proliferative disorders: A comparative assessment. Ultrastruct Pathol 1986;10:303–309.

40. Ye F, Huang S, Dong H. Histiocytosis X. S-100 protein, peanut agglutinin, and transmission electron microscopy study. Am J Clin Pathol 1990;94:627–631.

41. Hammar S, Bockus D, Remington F, Bartha M. The widespread distribution of Langerhans' cells in pathologic tissues: An ultrastructural and immunohistochemical study. Hum Pathol 1986;17:894–905.

42. Kawanami O, Basset F, Ferrans VJ, Soler P, Crystal RG. Pulmonary Langerhans' cells in patients with fibrotic lung disorders. Lab Invest 1981;44:227–233.

43. Casolaro MA, Bernaudin J, Saltini C, Ferrans VJ, Crystal RG. Accumulation of Langerhans' cells on the epithelial surface of the lower respiratory tract in normal subjects in association with cigarette smoking. Am Rev Respir Dis 1988;137:406–411.

44. Soler P, Moreau A, Basset F, Hance AJ. Cigarette smoking-induced changes in the number and differentiated state of pulmonary dendritic cells/Langerhans' cells. Am Rev Respir Dis 1989;139:1112–1117.

45. McDonnell TJ, Crouch EC, Gonzalez JG. Reactive eosino-

philic pleuritis: A sequela of pneumothorax in pulmonary eosinophilic granuloma. Am J Clin Pathol 1989;91:107–111.

46. Niewoehner DE, Kleinerman J, Rice DB. Pathologic changes in the peripheral airways of young cigarette smokers. N Engl J Med 1974;291:755–758.

47. Myers JL, Veal CF, Shin MS, Katzenstein AA. Respiratory bronchiolitis causing interstitial lung disease: A clinicopathologic study of six cases. Am Rev Respir Dis 1987;135:880–884.

48. Myers JL. Respiratory bronchiolitis with interstitial lung disease. Semin Respir Med 1991;13:134–139.

49. Pietra GG, Edwards WD, Kay JM, et al. Histopathology of primary pulmonary hypertension: A qualitative and quantitative study of pulmonary blood vessels from 58 patients in the national heart, lung, and blood institute, primary pulmonary hypertension registry. Circulation 1989;80:1198–1206.

50. Mark EJ, Ramirez JF. Pulmonary capillaritis and hemorrhage in patients with systemic vasculitis. Arch Pathol Lab Med 1985;109:413–418.

51. Travis WD, Colby TV, Lombard CL, Carpenter HA. A clinicopathologic study of 34 cases of diffuse pulmonary hemorrhage with lung biopsy confirmation. Am J Surg Pathol 1990;14:1112–1125.

52. Myers JL, Katzenstein AA. Wegener's granulomatosis presenting with massive pulmonary hemorrhage and capillaritis. Am J Surg Pathol 1987;11:895–898.

53. Myers JL, Katzenstein AA. Microangiitis in lupus-induced pulmonary hemorrhage. Am J Clin Pathol 1986;85:552–556.

54. Imoto EM, Lombard CM, Sachs DPL. Pulmonary capillaritis and hemorrhage. Chest 1989;96:927–928.

55. Colby TV, Carrington CB. Pulmonary lymphomas simulating lymphomatoid granulomatosis. Am J Surg Pathol 1982;6:19–32.

56. Katzenstein AA, Carrington CB, Liebow AA. Lymphomatoid granulomatosis: A clinicopathologic study of 152 cases. Cancer 1979;43:360–373.

57. Jaffe ES. Pulmonary lymphocytic angiitis: A nosologic quandry. Mayo Clin Proc 1988;63:411–413.

58. Lipford EH, Margolick JB, Longo DL, Fauci AS, Jaffe ES. Angiocentric immunoproliferative lessions: A clinicopathologic spectrum of post-thymic T-cell proliferations. Blood 1988;72:1674–1681.

59. Yousem SA, Colby TV. Intravascular lymphomatosis presenting in the lung. Cancer 1990;65:349–353.

60. Snyder LS, Harmon KR, Estensen RD. Intravascular lymphomatosis (malignant angioendotheliomatosis) presenting as pulmonary hypertension. Chest 1989;96:1199–1200.

61. Thomas PD, Hunninghake GW. Current concepts of the pathogenesis of sarcoidosis. Am Rev Respir Dis 1987;135:747–760.

62. Rosen Y, Moon S, Huang C, Gourin A, Lyons HA. Granulomatous pulmonary angiitis in sarcoidosis. Arch Pathol Lab Med 1977;101:170–174.

63. Smith LJ, Lawrence JB, Katzenstein AA. Vascular sarcoidosis: A rare cause of pulmonary hypertension. Am J

Med Sci 1983;285:38–44.

64. Hoffstein V, Ranganathan N, Mullen JBM. Sarcoidosis simulating pulmonary veno-occlusive disease. Am Rev Respir Dis 1986;134:809–811.

65. Colby TV. Berylliosis. In: Churg A, Green FHY, eds. Pathology of occupational lung disease. New York: Igaku-Shoin, 1988: 73–87.

66. Templeton PA, McLoud TC, Müller NL, Shepard JO, Moore EH. Pulmonary lymphangioleiomyomatosis: CT and pathologic findings. J Comput Assist Tomogr 1989; 13:54–57.

67. Taylor JR, Ryu J, Colby RV, Raffin TA. Lymphangioleiomyomatosis: Clinical course in 32 patients. N Engl J Med 1990;323:1254–1260.

68. Albelda SM, Gefter WB, Epstein DM, Miller WT. Diffuse pulmonary hemorrhage: A review and classification. Radiology 1985;154:289–297.

69. Leatherman JW, Davies SF, Hoidal JR. Alveolar hemorrhage syndromes: Diffuse microvascular lung hemorrhage in immune and idiopathic disorders. Medicine (Baltimore) 1984;63:343–361.

70. Bonsib SM, Walder WP. Pulmonary-renal syndrome: Clinical similarity amidst etiologic diversity. Mod Pathol 1989;2:129–137.

71. Morgan PGM, Turner-Warwick M. Pulmonary haemosiderosis and pulmonary haemorrhage. Br J Dis Chest 1981;75:225–242.

72. Leatherman JW. Immune alveolar hemorrhage. Chest 1987;91:891–897.

73. Lombard CM, Colby TV, Elliott CG. Surgical pathology of the lung in antibasement membrane antibody-associated Goodpasture's syndrome. Hum Pathol 1989;20: 445–451.

74. Young KR. Pulmonary-renal syndromes. Clin Chest Med 1989;10:655–675.

75. Walford RL, Kaplan L. Pulmonary fibrosis and giant-cell reaction with altered elastic tissue. AMA Arch Pathol 1957;63:75–90.

76. Bedrossian CWM, Luna MA, Conklin RH, Miller WC. Alveolar proteinosis as a consequence of immunosuppression: A hypothesis based on clinical and pathologic observations. Hum Pathol 1980;11:527–535.

77. Kariman K, Kylstra JA, Spock A. Pulmonary alveolar proteinosis: Prospective clinical experience in 23 patients for 15 years. Lung 1984;162:223–231.

78. Prakash UBS, Barham SS, Carpenter HA, Dines DE, Marsh HM. Pulmonary alveolar phospholipoproteinosis: Experience with 34 cases and a review. Mayo Clin Proc 1987;62:499–518.

79. Rubinstein I, Mullen JBM, Hoffstein V. Morphologic diagnosis of idiopathic pulmonary alveolar lipoproteinosis—revisited. Arch Intern Med 1988;148:813–816.

80. Hook GER, Gilmore LB, Talley FA. Multilamellated structures from the lungs of patients with pulmonary alveolar proteinosis. Lab Invest 1984;50:711–725.

81. Hook GER, Gilmore LB, Talley FA. Dissolution and reassembly of tubular myelin-like multilamellated structures from the lungs of patients with pulmonary alveolar proteinosis. Lab Invest 1986;55:194–208.

82. Yousem SA, Hochholzer L. Pulmonary hyalinizing granuloma. Am J Clin Pathol 1987;87:1–6.

CHAPTER 5

Bronchial and Transbronchial Diseases

DAVID H. DAIL

The disorders that are discussed in this chapter include aspiration, abscess, bronchostenosis, bronchial mucocele, bronchorrhea, bronchiectasis, broncholithiasis, bronchial fistulae, cystic fibrosis in adults, obstruction, bronchiolitis obliterans, BOOP, diffuse panbronchiolitis, atelectasis, organizing pneumonia, gangrene, and torsion. Disorders of bronchia often overlap with similar involvements in the trachea, and tracheobronchomalacia (polychondritis), tracheobronchopathia osteochondroplastica, and tracheobronchial amyloid are discussed in Chapter 22, **Metabolic Diseases**. Tumors of the trachea overlap somewhat with mainstem bronchi and are discussed in Chapter 32, **Common Neoplasms**, in Chapter 33, **Uncommon Tumors**, and even in endobronchial metastases in Chapter 35. Other bronchial wall and luminal diseases such as asthma, mucoid impaction, or bronchocentric granulomatosis are discussed in Chapter 16, **Eosinophilic Infiltrates**. The pediatric counterparts of all these and some unique bronchial and transbronchial disorders in younger patients are discussedin Chapter 7, **Congenital and Developmental Diseases**, and in Chapter 8, **Acquired Neonatal and Pediatric Diseases**. Ciliary dyskinesia is covered with anatomy in Chapter 2. Infections such as viral-induced bronchiolitis are discussed in their respective areas. The bronchial effects of tobacco are discussed in Chapter 25, **Tobacco Injury**, and in Chapter 26, **Emphysema and Small and Large Airways Diseases**. Dust effects are covered in Chapters 27 and 28. The conducting airways are also considered in Chapter 2, **Anatomy**; Chapter 3, **Lung Defenses**; Chapter 4, **Common Pathways and Patterns of Injury**; and Chapter 19, **Sarcoid**.

Aspiration

Aspiration is the inhalation of liquid or solid materials into the lower respiratory tract, usually from the oral or nasal cavities, oropharynx, esophagus, or stomach. Elsewhere in this volume, inhalation of allergens (Chapters 16–19), and dusts and fumes (Chapters 25–28) are discussed.

Logically, the course of aspiration is determined by such laws of physics as inertia and gravity. Larger, more solid materials, and finer, or more liquid materials, all follow the straightest and most dependent course after they enter the trachea. As explained in Chapter 2, the right mainstem bronchus continues a straighter course (20°–30° off center compared to 40°–60° for left mainstem bronchus); the more acute angle of the left is necessary to reach around the heart. Larger, more solid objects that pass the larynx often impact in the right mainstem bronchus, and smaller solid objects most often enter the right basilar bronchus.[1] This has been well demonstrated in aspiration of foreign objects in children, generally in the age group of 1–3 years.[2] During this age range, children examine almost everything by putting the items into their mouths. In both children and adults, larger objects are sometimes stopped at the larynx and may be expelled by strong coughing. In adults, this is most frequently a *cafe coronary*[3] in which food impacts in the larynx.

More than 80% of aspirated foreign bodies occur in children[4] and in either age group, only 5% are spontaneously expectorated.[5] Sharper objects may perforate a bronchus and cause bleeding, or even penetrate the

79

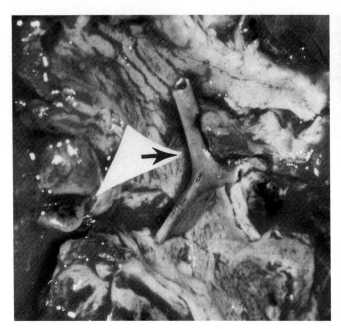

Fig. 5–1. Foreign-body aspiration. Fragment of chicken bone (*arrow*) wedged into junction of lobar bronchi has caused acute hemorrhage and was reason for emergency resection before bronchoscopic diagnosis.

pleural cavity and cause pneumothorax.[6] A foreign body may move around in the chest and cause wandering infiltrates.[7]

Young children most frequently aspirate peanuts, beads, and other fragments of wooden or plastic toys. Peanuts and sunflower seeds lead the list in Western countries, whereas in Arabic countries children most often aspirate melon seeds.[6] Older children may inhale flowering grass fragments, which because of their spikelet arrangements work their way into more distal bronchi and resist expectoration. In any age, teeth, fragments of bone (Fig 5–1), food, blood clots, tissue fragments, nasal pack components, lipids from oily nosedrops or orally administered cathartics, bacterial fragments, and gastric contents most commonly enter the lung. Noguchi et al.[8] reported a subacute reaction to mud aspiration. Drowning, often thought of as occurring in fresh or salt water, has also occurred in large vats of beer, liquid chocolate, and other interesting concoctions.

Brock[9,10] beautifully illustrated the logic of aspiration in 1942 with aspiration-induced abscess formation, which most often followed the dependent course described. Finer and more fluid ingredients not only follow the straighter course, but flow into the first dependent orifices after they enter the lung. In the supine position, these are most often the posterior segment of the upper lobe and superior segment of the lower lobes (Fig. 5–2). In the more upright position, this

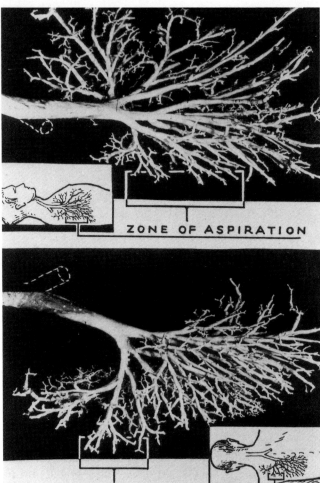

Fig. 5–2. Routes of aspiration. Corrosion cast and diagram of bronchial tree show left lung to illustrate effects of position on eventual course of aspiration. In addition to zone of aspiration marked, dependent upper-lobe posterior segment is common site of involvement, as would be more obvious on cast of right lung. (Reproduced with permission from Brock, RC. *Lung Abscess.* Springfield, IL: Charles C. Thomas, Publisher, 1952, p. 10.)

material flows into the superior segment and basilar segments on the lower lobes. The basilar segments divide rather evenly, and localization within these segments is not as discrete as in other areas of the lung. When a person is in the lateral decubitus position, the axillary branches of the subsegments of apical and posterior upper lobe bronchi are favored. The more anterior portions of the lung are usually spared the effects of aspiration, unless aspiration occurs in the prone position, as in near drowning.

Aspiration need not only be from external sources. Figure 5–3 illustrates a necrotizing tuberculous reaction breaking open from an apical cavity (Fig. 5–3A) with

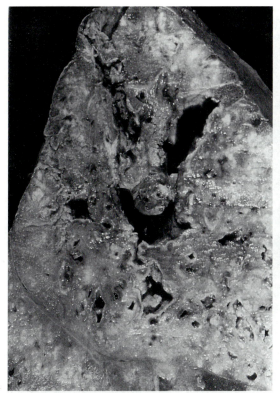

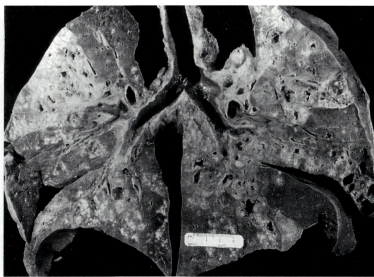

Fig. 5–3. Internal aspiration. **A.** A tuberculous cavity in the upper lobe has broken open. **B.** Its contents have been aspirated into both lungs in zones that appear positional.

internal aspiration transbronchially into dependent zones (Fig. 5–3B). Sudden rupture of large fluid-filled abscess cavities or other cysts might cause a similar reaction and an aspirated broncholith is illustrated later in this chapter (see Fig. 5–29, p. 101).

The most common conditions predisposing to aspiration include some alterations of consciousness, most frequently from alcohol, drugs, and anesthesia, followed by central nervous system disorders or neuromuscular disorders; these are followed by aspiration secondary to obstructing masses or other functional defects in the esophagus or stomach. Episodes of aspiration that are eventually proven have been documented in 85% of children;[2] they have been proven in a lesser number (some 30%) of adults.[11] The difference in statistics is probably related to the altered level of consciousness in adults causing temporary amnesia. Aspiration is two or more times as common in males, either boys or men, than in females. This frequency may be explained because men are more often in higher risk groups of alcohol or drug abuse and are more subject to the greater risks of physical extremes of the environment. Boys may be more willing to take risks or may have a less well-developed swallowing and/or cough response as compared to girls. Of interest in children, the wheezing that is sometimes associated with aspirated foreign bodies many times is improved with

theophylline, leading to more diagnostic confusion with asthma.[12]

Several experimental studies with animals, starting in the 1920s,[13,14] proved that regular aspiration of material into the lungs occurred when materials were placed in the nares or accessory sinuses of animals during anesthesia. Myerson[15] found blood immediately postoperatively in the tracheobronchial tree in 79 to 100 human patients who underwent tonsillectomy, including those under general or local anesthetic. The early history of aspirated infected material from the upper airway, covered in the abscess section of this chapter, supports these findings. Several experimental studies have proven that normal adults aspirate with some regularity. Quinn and Meyer[16] in 1929 introduced lipiodal (iodinated poppy seed oil) into the noses of sleeping subjects and found the material often entered the lungs. Amberson[17] in 1937 reported placing barium in the mouths of normal subjects during sleep with similar results. Radiologists often observe aspiration while performing upper gastrointestinal tract barium studies. As reviewed by Bartlett,[18] various markers placed in the stomach the night before surgery have been documented as being in lungs sampled during surgery the next day in 7%–16% of patients.[19,20] Nasogastric and oropharyngeal tubes, including endoscopes and tracheostomies, increase the rate of aspiration.

with those products that disperse most easily, specifically those that cause the greatest decrease in surface tension, or have the least viscosity or the highest volatility.[28]

Although ingestion precedes aspiration, Eade and associates[29] nicely reviewed the reasons that aspiration is the most important toxic pathway of injury: Symptoms develop rapidly and radiographs often show localized pulmonary infiltrates, often in the aspiration zones mentioned earlier; experimentally, the lethal dose by ingestion alone is much higher than that usually ingested by sick persons; sizable doses of distillates have been placed in the stomachs of experimental animals whose esophagi were ligated, and these animals did not suffer pulmonary toxicity.

The pulmonary changes, almost identical to those of gastric acid aspiration, include diffuse congestion, hemorrhage, edema, hyaline membrane formation, and bronchopneumonia. Atelectasis occurs early, apparently by direct toxic effect of these light hydrocarbons on surfactant.[30]

About 75% of involved children have abnormal chest radiographs, but only 25%–40% have pulmonary symptoms or signs.[31] In the past, death has been reported in some 2%–10% of cases,[31] but in two larger more recent series it was reported in 0.3%[29] and 1%.[31] Death, if it occurs, usually happens within 24 h of exposure, and most who survive do so with few sequelae.

Food

Various food particles, such as skeletal muscle, fat tissue, or fragments of bone, may be aspirated. Cooking or digestion may result in poorly defined particles that appear foreign but escape further definition. As was well demonstrated by Knoblich,[32] portions of legume seeds are one of the better markers of food aspiration. The legumes most commonly eaten are various peas, beans, and peanuts; because they are relatively inexpensive and nutritious, they occur in many products. (The word "lentil" is sometimes used in this reference, but it is also the name of a specific type of bean.) The legume seed (Fig. 5–6) consists of a thick cellulose outer coat, the cellulose walls of the inner food storage compartments, and the starch cells contained within these food compartments. Cooking softens the outer shell and cell walls of the beans or peas and allows easy disruption of the contents, with a resulting jelling effect of the starch particles (called "thickening" in cooking). The cellulose walls of the outer coat and starch compartments are more difficult to totally disrupt or digest, and therefore act as both a chronic irritant and a good marker of aspiration.

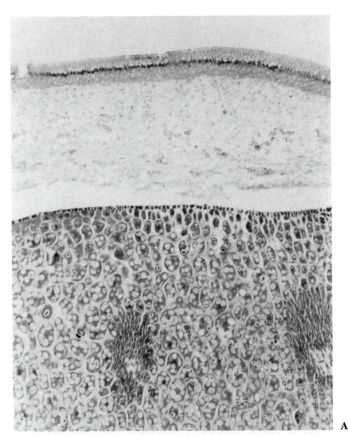

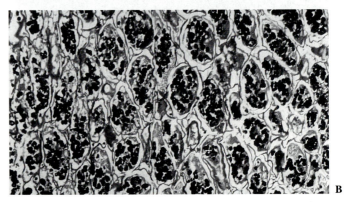

Fig. 5–6A,B. Lentil bean. **A.** At top is thick outer coat; below, cotyledon compartments with starch cells. H and E, ×100. **B.** PAS stain highlights glycogen granules shown as clear spaces in **A.** PAS, ×250.

Aspiration of these fragments in both experimental animals and humans produces an acute exudative response within 24 h (Fig. 5–7), followed by a foreign-body giant cell reaction (Fig. 5–8). These cell wall fragments are GMS positive; the glycogen compartments, when intact, are vividly PAS positive (Fig. 5–8; also see Fig. 5–6B). At about 10 days (experimentally) an organized granulomatous reaction occurs around

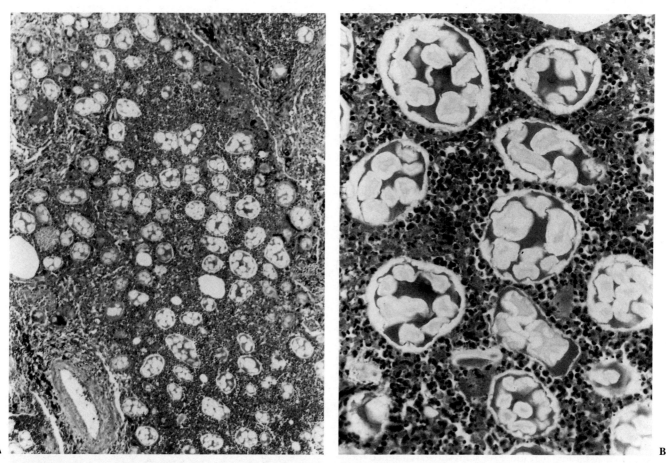

Fig. 5–7A,B. Aspirated legume ("lentil bean") pneumonia. Starch cells, liberated from bean by cooking, cause acute exudative response. **A.** Low power. H and E, ×100. **B.** High power. H and E, ×400.

the aspirated particles, and eventually the starch cells disappear, leaving only the cellulose fragments.

The walls of carrots, onions, and most nonlegumes digest more readily and do not give rise to as much chronic reactions as seen with legumes. They do, however, undergo the same type of early changes if aspirated, with acute and subacute pneumonia during digestion of the starch cells. Some of the most offensive aspirated food fragments have undergone alterations in preparation, and some of the worst combinations are cooking oils and salts, as, for example, an aspirated potato chip (Fig. 5–9).

Eventually these areas become small fibrotic nodules; some calcify and at times appear almost as parasites (Fig. 5–10). They may appear as small hyalinized granulomas or possibly as entrapped calcospherites,[32] usually within a fibrous stroma. At times the conditions for aspiration are chronic, and recurrent aspiration leads to the acute and chronic changes together or in close proximity in the same specimen. Other nonfood material taken orally, such as barium, may be also aspirated and at times elicits little host response (Fig. 5–11).

Oil Aspiration or Exogenous Lipid Pneumonia

Oils that may be aspirated include mineral oils such as used in nosedrops and cathartics, vegetable oils used in cooking, and animal oils such as cod liver oil or fat-soluble vitamin preparations. Oil aspiration was first described by Laughlen[33] in 1925 in a child who received oily oral and pharyngeal preparations for diphtheria; it was confirmed by him experimentally. The role of oil-based contrast media used for bronchoscopy reviewed was well by Spencer.[34] Animal oils cause a worse reaction than mineral or vegetable oils, and this difference appears related to the number of free fatty acids[35] and increased viscosity of each oil.[28,36] Mineral oils are fairly inert, as they have no fatty acids, and are rapidly emulsified and consumed by pulmonary macrophages. Vegetable oil droplets may remain in alveoli for months without eliciting much reaction, but because of their low-grade but chronic irritation they eventually do cause scarring. Animal oils elicit a very active inflammatory response. Animal and mineral oils, but only rarely vegetable oils, may be seen in regional nodes.[35]

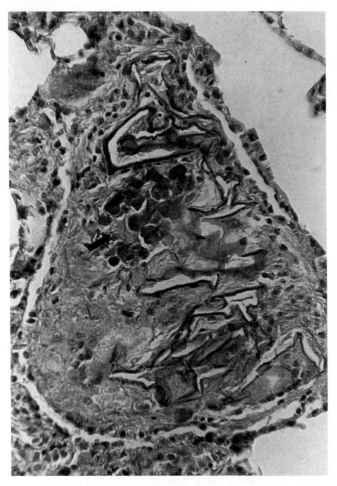

Fig. 5–8. Aspirated legume. PAS stain shows darkened (positive staining) glycogen packets (*arrow*) with dissociated cell wall, beginning foreign-body response. PAS, ×600.

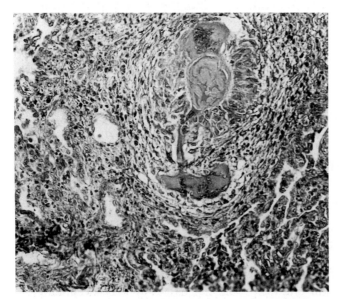

Fig. 5–9. Aspirated potato chip. Remnant starch cell elicits abundant response, considering its size. Oils used in cooking and added salt probably caused this accentuated host response. H and E, ×250.

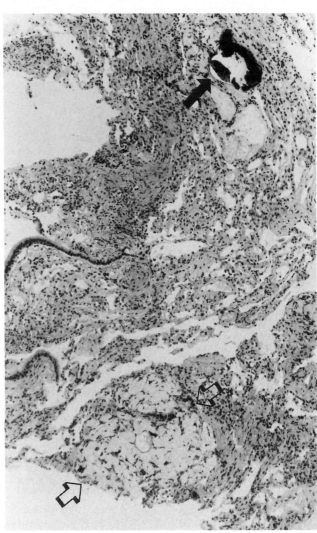

Fig. 5–10. Chronic reaction from aspirated lentil beans. Two older areas remain calcified spherule (*black arrow*) and fragment of collapsed cotyledon skeleton with absent starch (*open arrow*). Latter appearance may be mistaken for parasites. Terminal bronchiole at left. H and E, ×100.

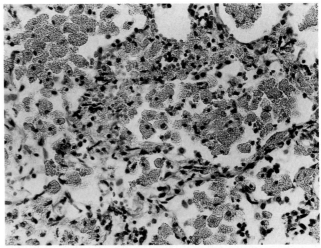

Fig. 5–11. Barium aspiration. Macrophages are distended with glistening granular barium particles. H and E, ×400.

Aspiration of oils commonly occurs in older individuals, who may take their oily nosedrops or cathartics at bedtime. Aspiration most frequently occurs in the basilar segments of the lower lobe,[37] suggesting these patients usually sleep in a more upright position or experience aspiration before lying down. Chronic aspiration of these oils is often undetected; only 2 of 14 autopsy cases documenting exogenous lipid pneumonia at autopsy had reported significant clinical symptoms during life.[38] Because these oils float in the stomach, it is possible they also are aspirated via reflux from the stomach.[18,38] In unselected autopsy series, oil aspiration has been documented in 2.5%[38]–14.6%[39] of adults.

Other oily products that have been incriminated as being aspirated in the lung include fragments of lip balm,[40] burning fats (an occupational exposure),[41] a rapid drying agent in spray enamel paint,[42] oils applied to tobacco products (black fat tobacco),[43] and possibly hair spray.[44] Children may aspirate oily medications if they are force-fed these while resisting and crying violently.[45] Atypical mycobacteria have been reported associated with oil aspiration pneumonia.[46–50]

Grossly, lungs affected by oil aspiration are often grey to yellow and rather solid. Occasionally oily droplets exude from the cut surface. Microscopically, the lipid droplets are often dissolved by tissue processing.[35] One exception is cod liver oil, which remains as salmon-colored droplets on hematoxylin and eosin stain after tissue processing. Fats may be seen with rapid water-soluble or oil red O stains on frozen section (Fig. 5–12); varyingly sized fat droplets and varying numbers of multinucleate giant cells may be seen (Fig. 5–13A,B). When only a small amount of fat has been aspirated, the reaction may be contained in alveolar macrophages. This is most commonly seen in mild degrees of aspiration with a diluted fatty substance, as might be seen with milk aspiration. When larger doses of thicker and more toxic oils are aspirated or when oil aspiration is repeated, the areas become densely fibrotic with reduction of the background lung architecture (Fig. 5–13C). Occasionally, cor pulmonale results.[51,52] Transbronchial biopsies may provide enough tissue to make this diagnosis.

In the differential diagnosis is artifactual collapse of lung around remnant air bubbles (Fig. 5–13D). Also, this entity histologically can usually be distinguished from endogenous lipid pneumonia by subdivisions within fat droplets, multinucleated foreign-body giant cell response, and, and, in more chronic cases, a greater degree of chronic inflammation and fibrosis with destruction of background lung parenchyma in exogenous lipid pneumonia. At times some fat is incorporated/entrapped in the interstitium (Fig. 5–14), crossing over with a similar appearance in diffuse panbronchiolitis and xanthomatous bronchiolitis obliterans

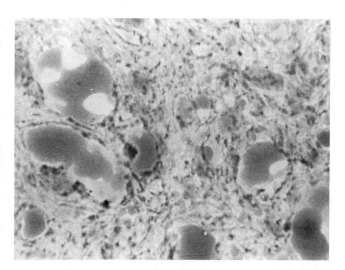

Fig. 5–12. Oil aspiration. With rare exceptions, most aspirated oils are dissolved on tissue processing. Oil red O stain may be used to demonstrate oil droplets on frozen tissue. ×400.

(see following). Diffuse panbronchiolitis is centered more on terminal-respiratory bronchioles and is composed mostly of finely vaculated fat (see Fig. 5-43; p. 111, later in chapter).

Sputum cytology or cytologic aspiration specimens have been used to confirm this diagnosis. In 1950, Losner et al.,[53] using oil stains, found lipid-rich macrophages in 19 of 20 suspected cases in contrast to 2 of 45 control patients. More recently, Corwin and Irwin[54] restudied this possibility using bronchoalveolar lavage in various lung diseases including aspiration, hemoptysis, cancer in the lung (either primary or secondary), bronchiectasis, interstitial fibrosis, and cases of sarcoid. When compared to normal lungs, samples from diseased lungs contained increased fat-filled macrophages. These authors warned that the simple presence of fatty macrophages in these preparations is not diagnostic of lipoid pneumonia; however, the quantity of lipid was more abundant in aspirators than in these other groups. Their "aspirator" group consisted mainly of patients with a history of upper gastrointestinal tract disease, including reflux in most. Corwin and Irwin[54] emphasized that the size of the fat droplets in lavage fluid cannot be used to distinguish endogenous from exogenous lipid pneumonia.

Abscess

Wherever it occurs, an abscess is an accumulation of inflammatory cells, initially having abundant polymorphonuclear cells, that is usually accompanied by tissue destruction. In the lungs, "cross-country" necrosis occurs during the formation of an abscess[55] (Fig. 5–15 through 5–18). This type of necrosis involves destruc-

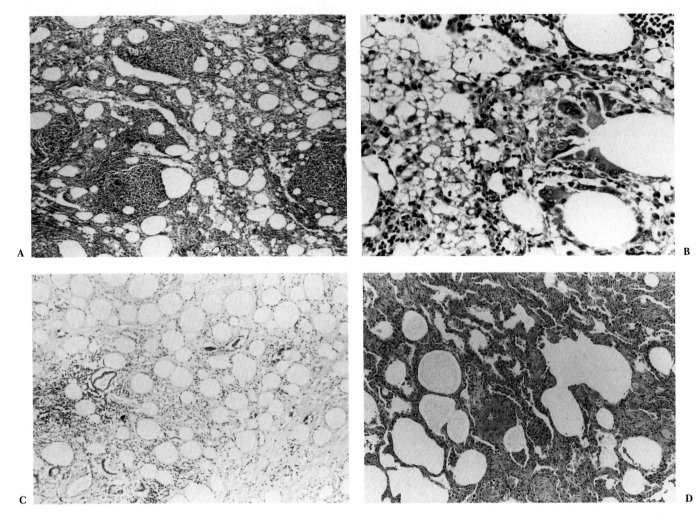

Fig. 5–13 A–D. Oil aspiration. **A.** Subacute effects of oil aspiration show varyingly sized fat droplets, inflammation, and fibrosis. Most of lung architecture has been oblitered. H and E, ×100. **B.** Higher power view shows foamy lipid-filled macrophages to left and multinucleate foreign-body cells to right. H and E, ×400. **C.** In chronic state, oil droplets are still seen with encasement by fibrous tissue. Cellular inflammatory response is less in this stage than in earlier stages. H and E, ×25. **D.** Entrapped air bubble surrounded by collapsed lung on biopsy can be mistaken for lipid aspiration. Note absence of giant cells or other inflammatory reaction. H and E, ×400.

tion of lung parenchyma, bronchi, and arteries. In contrast, cavities that are more chronic and more slowly formed, such as tuberculous cavities, often leave remnants of fibrotic bronchopulmonary rays coursing through the cavity itself (see Chapter 10). Some more slowly forming nontuberculous abscesses can do this, but most of the abscesses in the lung have an acute initial phase that destroys most of the tissue in the area although exceptions occur in each case (Fig. 5–17B). As lung tissue is permeated by the breathing tubes, some of these bronchi frequently connect with abscess cavities, and often some of the necrotic material is drained, leaving an empty (Figs. 5–17A and 5–19) or partially empty cavity with or without an air/fluid level on chest radiograph. Occasionally inflammation seals off all such bronchial connections, resulting in a solid mass that may be suspected of being a tumor (Fig. 5–20).

Adjacent organization in acute and subacute abscesses (Fig. 5–21) often accounts for an enlarged surrounding radiographic density.

There are many etiologies for cavity formation in the lung, and abscess formation is but one of them. Other causes include cavitary tumor, cystic spaces of assorted etiologies, cavitary fungal (see Fig. 5–18) and mycobacterial infections, and necrotizing pneumonia. In 1922, Lockwood[56] reviewed the early history of lung abscesses dating from Hippocrates. Many of the conditions and factors in pulmonary abscess formation, which were already well known by 1922, were summarized in this review. By 1936, 2,114 cases had been published.[57]

Aspiration is the most common cause of lung abscess. Other instigators of this type of damage include penetrating trauma, postoperative states, obstruction, hemorrhage or infarction, necrotizing pneumonia, infected

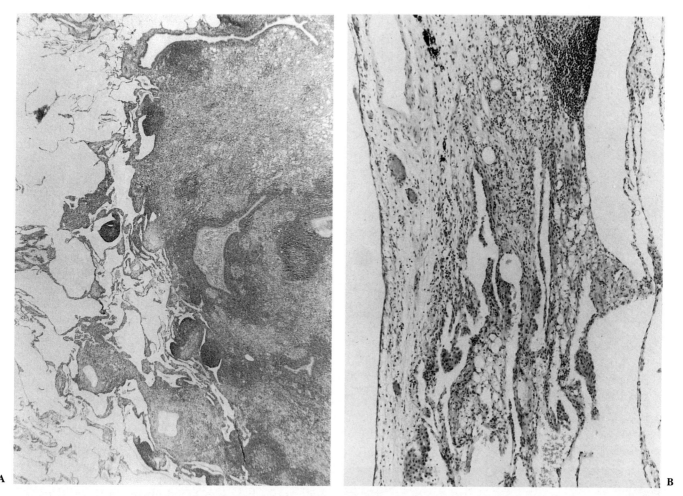

Fig. 5–14 A,B. Aspirated lipid. **A.** Lower power view shows focal areas of confluence inflammatory reaction around lipid droplets. H and E, ×100. **B.** Interstitial foamy cells are seen focally near these areas. H and E, ×400.

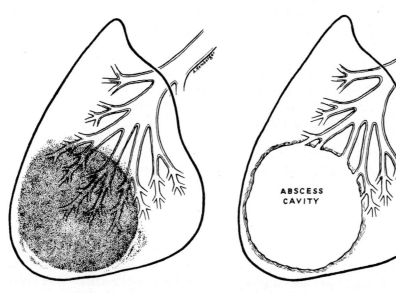

Fig. 5–15. Abscess cavity formation. "Cross-country" necrosis often occurs in abscess formation. Multiple bronchi often open into such a cavity. (From Glenn WWL, Liebow AA, Lindskog GE. Thoracic and cardiovascular surgery with related pathology. 3d Ed. Norwalk: Appleton-Lange. 1975:166, with permission.)

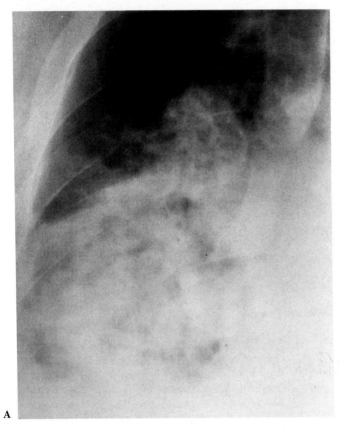

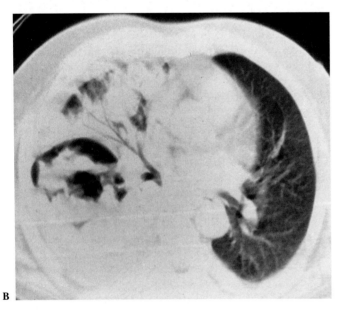

Fig. 5–16 A,B. Necrotizing pneumonia converting to abscess. Necrosis and abscess formation with *Legionella pneumophilia* is unusual but in this case has led to almost complete necrosis of the lower lobe. **A.** Plain film of right-lower lobe shows many cavities. **B.** CT scan shows midlateral cavity forming with dense areas of pneumonia anterior and posterior. Note patent bronchi draining some of these cavities. (Courtesy of Dr. Ellen Hauptmann, Virginia Mason Clinic, Seattle, Washington.)

emboli, infection of a preexistent cyst or bulla, or extension from nearby infected areas in the mediastinum, chest wall or diaphragm, or below the diaphragm. Nonaspiration types of pulmonary abscesses of course do not follow the aspiration patterns of distribution, but occur as their coexistent factors dictate. For example, if there is an infarct or an obstructing tumor, infection would occur in the affected areas. Septic emboli are hematogenously spread and are often multiple and small.

As aspiration is the number one cause of pulmonary abscess formation, it is reasonable that conditions that favor abscess formation are identical to those favoring aspiration. The locations are similar; men are more frequently affected than women, and the right lung is involved twice as often as the left.[58–62] The posterior segments of the right-upper lobe and superior segments of the right-lower lobe are involved most frequently, followed by the corresponding parts on the left side.[62] The single most commonly associated event is an alteration of consciousness; the second most frequent association is with poor dental hygiene; and the third is a defect in immunocompetence.

Poor dental hygiene was noted in cases without other apparent causes of pulmonary abscess in the studies in 1927–1936.[62–67] The spectrum of bacteria involved in abscess formation is almost identical to that in the mouth, as is discussed later. Another supporting argument for this relationship is that children and edentulous older people do not often have lung abscesses.[68] Some series have described abscesses in children[69,70] and adolescents,[71] but one must try to separate those cases caused by aspiration from other cases of cavitary necrosis, such as primary staphylococcal pneumonia in children.[70]

Other upper airway material may be aspirated and so carry bacteria into the lungs (see preceding, **Aspiration**). Nasal, oral, and oropharyngeal operations, especially tonsillectomies when these were done in an upright position, were noted in earlier years as being associated with lung abscesses.[56,72,73]

Infected abscess material is often composed of anaerobic and mixed flora that are quite similar to the spectrum of bacteria in the mouth.[74–77] Special care must be taken in collecting and culturing anaerobic bacteria, as these must not be contaminated with air. However, even in earlier studies the role of anaerobic bacteria was emphasized.[64] In two of the better more recent series, Bartlett et al.[78] prospectively cultured lung abscesses and found anaerobic cultures in 24 of 26 samples, and Gonzales and Calia[79] found anaerobes in all of their series. Anaerobic bacteria are the only organisms cultured in about one-half to two-thirds of lung abscesses; the others are aerobic, facultative aerobic bacteria, or no bacteria are cultured.[80]

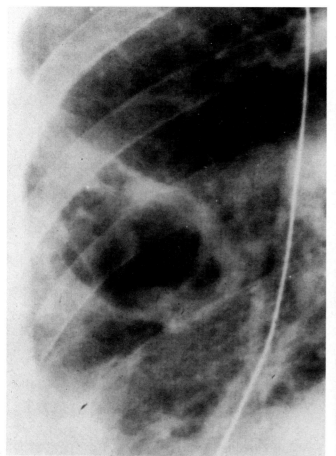
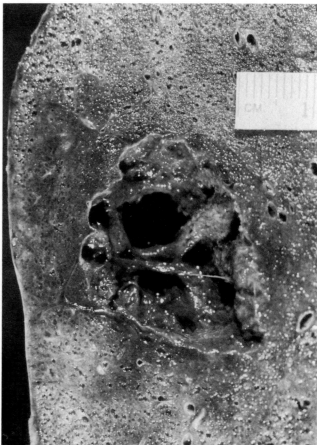

A

B

Fig. 5–17 A,B. Acute abscess cavity. **A.** Chest radiograph shows cavity with loss of parenchymal detail internally from drainage of necrotic debris. Note variable thickness of reaction in surrounding lung. Radiodense line is radiographic marker on tube. **B.** Gross specimen. Note cavity is mostly drained, with fresh-appearing, thin lining without fibrous wall. Note also persistence of some trabeculae, presumed bronchopulmonary rays, and variable but narrow surrounding inflammatory reaction.

The anaerobic bacteria most frequently found are *Fusobacterium nucleatum, Bacteroides melaninogenicus,* and anaerobic gram-positive peptostreptococci. *Bacteroides fragilis* is also found in 14%–21% of cases which is interesting as it is not part of the normal mouth flora.[81] Its origin in lung abscesses is unclear, but is probably still related to aspirated mouth contents. The two most extensive and most current series studying anaerobic infections of lung are by Bartlett[81] and Finegold et al.[82] and have been compared by Bartlett.[81] Spirochetes were described morphologically in earlier studies[64] and seemed to be significant, as they were present in the growing rims of necrosis; however, they have not been mentioned much recently, perhaps because they are difficult to culture.[80]

About half of cultures with anaerobes also contained aerobic bacteria capable of necrosis, specifically *Staphylococcus, Steptrococcus, Haemophilus, Pseudomonas, Klebsiella,* and *Escherichia* spp.[83] Patients with predominantly anaerobic pulmonary abscesses often present with indolent symptoms, in contrast to those with necrotizing aerobic abscesses. Immunocompromised patients often acquire gram-negative necrotizing pneumonias and vasoinvasive necrotizing fungal pneumonias, both of which may lead to cavitation. One clue to aspirated bacteria in lung abscesses is finding mixed-type organisms on smear Gram stain, tissue Gram stain, or culture. The oral cavity abounds with mixed bacteria and is estimated to contain some 200 different types of organisms.[80] This is one reason sputum cultures are notoriously difficult to interpret, and why even oral contamination of a bronchoscope interferes with most lung cultures.[83] Transtracheal and transthoracic needle aspirations correlate well with blood culture results.[81,84]

Saliva is estimated to contain 10^6–10^9 bacteria per milliliter. Gingival crevices are estimated to contain 10 to 1,000 times that amount, in the range of 10^8–10^{12} bacteria/ml. The higher figures approach counts for pure bacteria, and were found on more recent studies with better techniques. The ratio of anaerobic to aerobic

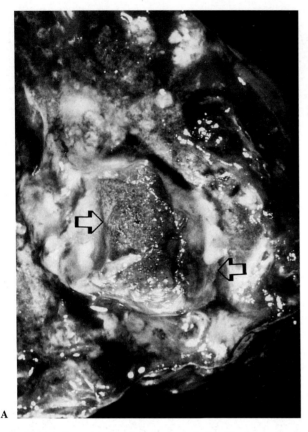 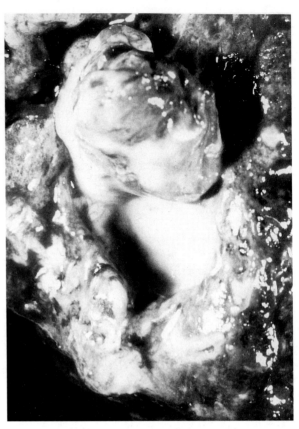

Fig. 5–18 A,B. Lung cavity in evolution. *Aspergillus* has caused necrotizing reaction in lung. **A.** Still partially attached but necrotic lung (*arrows*) sits within cavity. **B.** This portion of focally attached necrotic lung is elevated, exposing cavity partially filled with white pus.

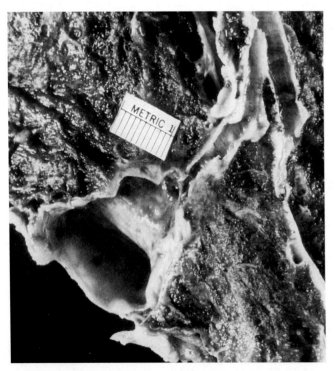

bacteria in saliva is about 3:1 to 5:1, whereas in the gingival crevices it is 1000:1.[80]

Pus from a patient with pyorrhea was used to produce pulmonary abscesses in mice, guinea pigs, and rabbits in the 1920s.[63] Eight to 14 days after this material was placed in anesthetized animal tracheas, 30% of the animals developed typical pulmonary abscesses. Those animals that did not develop abscesses were thought to have natural resistance, or good recovery, or not to have had sufficient depth of anesthesia to allow these organisms to settle in the lungs. The time course in humans is almost identical. In the same experimental animal studies mentioned earlier, it was proven that a mixture of at least four anaerobic bacteria species was necessary to establish an abscess. Putrid breath appears to be a good indicator of putrefaction of tissue and a reliable indicator of anaerobic lung abscess. This has been docu-

Fig. 5–19. Empty chronic abscess cavity. Note fibrotic but thin lined wall and patent connection with bronchus allowing complete drainage of cavity. (Courtesy of A.A. Liebow Pulmonary Pathology collection, San Diego, California.)

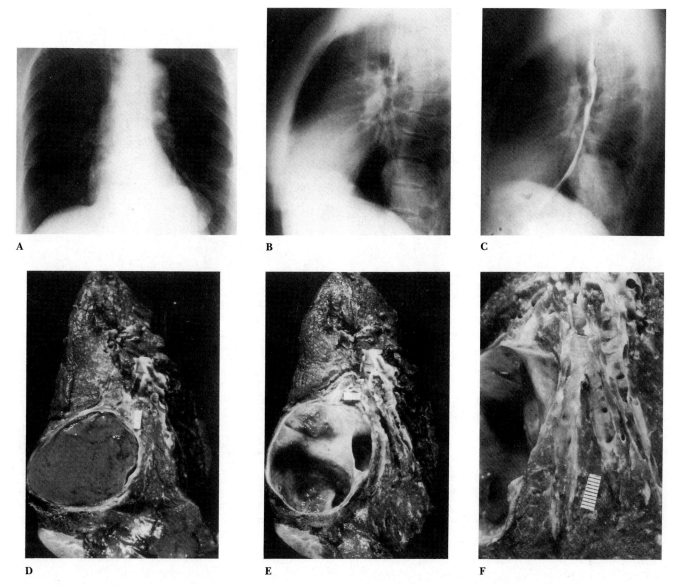

Fig. 5–20 A–F. Radiographs show chronic sealed-off abscess cavity. Retrocardiac (**A**) and posterior basal segment mass (**B**) without esophageal connections (**C**). **D.** Gross specimen. Coagulum of necrotic debris fills space. **E.** Capsule is thin and fibrotic. **F.** No definite bronchial attachments remain. (Courtesy of A.A. Liebow Pulmonary Pathology collection, San Diego, California.)

mented in 60% of such cases in a large review of 19 series by Bartlett.[80] Empyema in those not previously exposed to surgery was found to result from anaerobic infections in 75% of cases.[80] Necrotizing pneumonias are also often anaerobic. Other good reviews of anaerobic pleural pulmonary infections are by Bartlett and Finegold.[85,86] These authors stated "Anaerobic bacteria are undoubtedly the most overlooked bacterial pathogens of the lower respiratory tracts."[85] Another good general review is by Pennza.[87]

The third most frequent factor in abscess formation is host response. Factors that compromise normal host defenses include alcohol ingestion, diabetes mellitus, renal failure, malnutrition, malignancy, and other debilitations, along with treatment with immunosuppressive agents for any reason (see Chapter 1). Patients with these factors do more poorly with pulmonary abscesses (and most other insults) than those without.[87–89]

Pathologically, acute cavities have only a thin transition zone into the reactive adjacent lung parenchyma (see Fig. 5–17), and do not have the thicker capsules of subacute or some chronic cavities. They show variable numbers of polymorphonuclear neutrophil leukocytes (PMNs), macrophages, and tissue necrosis, and the nearby lung parenchyma has variable findings depending on the rapidity of spread. The rapidly growing

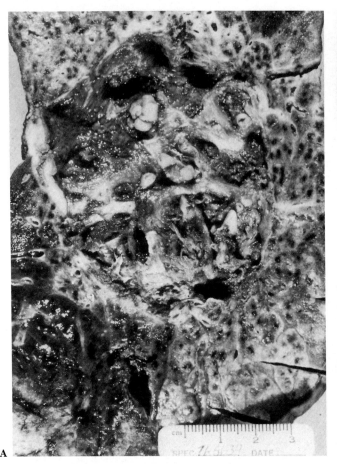

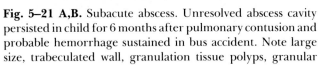

A

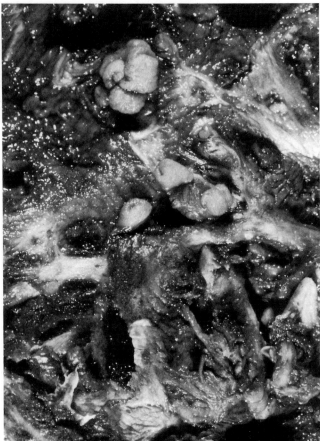

B

Fig. 5–21 A,B. Subacute abscess. Unresolved abscess cavity persisted in child for 6 months after pulmonary contusion and probable hemorrhage sustained in bus accident. Note large size, trabeculated wall, granulation tissue polyps, granular reepithelialized surface (seen better in **B**), extensive surrounding lung parenchymal changes of golden or obstructive pneumonia, and fibrosis. Least involved zones are at top right and bottom left of **A.**

cavities necrose nearby lung parenchyma, destroying any early attempts at organization. There may be adjacent hemorrhage, exudate, and fibrin extravasation. In those that are slightly more stable, beginning organization occurs in the surrounding lung parenchyma, along with varying degrees of chronic inflammation outside the areas of acute inflammation. Collagen becomes deposited at this junction, first as a confluent organizing pneumonia, and later as a capsule.

A subacute to chronic cavity, shown in Fig. 5–21, persisted for 6 months in a child who had been in a bus accident. The capsule and trabeculae in the wall have varying degrees of thickness, and granulation tissue polyps extend into the cavity. The contents have been evacuated, and nearby lung parenchyma shows mostly atelectasis and obstructive changes. Sometimes chronic cavities heal with a thin fibrous border (see Fig. 5–19) and may retain a coagulum of necrotic debris in their lumen (see Fig. 5–20). This apparently indicates that the nearby bronchi, which are sometimes excised for possible malignancy, have been sealed off. Chronic cavities may resolve by collapse and fibrosis, or may remain open. In the open variety they may become reepithelialized, first with a squamous lining and then with respiratory ciliated lining.[90] In the latter case, the differential between bronchiectasis and bronchocele may be somewhat confusing, but multiple bronchial connections in chronic abscess cavity formation distinguish these.

Spontaneous healing may occur, but healing is greatly aided by appropriate antibiotic dosage, often in the range of 1.2–10 million units of penicillin per day for 4 weeks or more. Weiss[91] noted in appropriately treated and followed cavities that 13% of cavities disappeared by 2 weeks of therapy, 44% by 4 weeks, 59% by 6 weeks, and 70% by 3 months.

Most chest physicians consider 6 (sometimes up to 8) weeks of persistent cavitation bothersome. Indications for surgery include: (1) persistent sepsis and/or toxicity; (2) a large (greater than 6 cm) persistent cavity despite adequate antibiotic coverage; (3) evidence of chronic obstructive changes of thick-walled cavities, adjacent chronic atelectasis, fibrosis, or bronchiectasis; (4) hemoptysis of significant amounts; (5) occurrence of bronchopulmonary fistula and/or empyema; and (6) concern about malignancy.

When cavitation is first suspected, bronchoscopy is recommended to (1) attempt to exclude malignancy because 8%–17% of pulmonary cavities can contain malignancy,[59,92,93] (2) establish exact localization for future postural drainage, (3) attempt a quantitative culture (see Chapter 1 and preceding discussion), and (4) establish drainage if the bronchus is not open, sometimes with the aid of a cardiac catheter.[59,94] Transthoracic tube drainage is considered inappropriate because of the risk of empyema. Long-standing cavities run the risk of being superinfected by *Aspergillus spp.* and other fungi. A case of radiographic pseudoabscess of lung was reported related to a particular connector on some tracheostomy equipment.[95]

The incidence of abscess formation has greatly decreased during the past 40 years, partly because antibiotics are available and frequently used early in pulmonary infections, and partly because factors leading to abscess formation are better understood; for example, we avoid surgery in the upright position or on patients with gastric material in the stomach. An excellent sequence of 796 cases of pulmonary abscess from one institution (Massachusetts General Hospital), covering 1909–1923,[96] 1924–1932,[72] 1933–1937,[73] 1938–1942,[97] and 1943–1956,[61] demonstrated this change. In the preantibioic era approximately 345 of the patients treated either conservatively or by surgery died,[57] and another one-third had chronic residual lung disease. More recently the prognosis is much better, but the mortality associated with established abscess formation remains in the range of 25%.[58]

Bronchiectasis

Bronchiectasis refers to dilatation of bronchi. If acute and reversible, it is usually a radiographic finding in atelectasis[98,99] or pneumonia.[100–104] The usual type seen by the pathologist, however, is the chronic irreversible form.

The two basic subdivisions of either acute or chronic forms are (1) obstructive and (2) nonobstructive types. The obstructive type is most commonly seen beyond tumors (Fig. 5–22), but foreign bodies, concretions such as broncholiths, secretions such as inspissated mucus in mucoid impaction and allergic bronchopulmonary aspergillosis (Chapter 16), or compression as by tumor or enlarged nodes or stricture may play a role. Rarely, lack

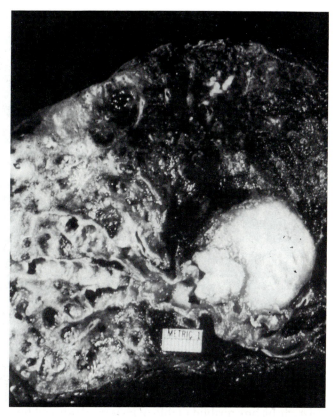

Fig. 5–22. Tumor causing obstructive bronchiectasis. Slowly growing tumor has caused typical changes distally. (Courtesy of A.A. Liebow Pulmonary Pathology Collection, San Diego, California.)

of cartilaginous support with airway collapse, bronchial atresia, or mucosal webs may also play a role.

The obstructive type occurs anywhere obstruction occurs, but there are some localizing factors in a few of these conditions; for example, the upper lobes in allergic aspergillosis, most primary epithelial tumors, which are more common in the upper lobes unless related to asbestos (Chapter 28), middle-lobe syndrome with its tendency toward middle-lobe compression (see Chapter 2 and following), and the more usual routes of aspiration (covered earlier in this chapter). There are many exceptions, and bronchoscopy is usually indicated in both children and adults to diagnose the type of obstruction.

The nonobstructive type of bronchiectasis is usually more widespread in the lung than is the obstructive type. It occurs most frequently in the basilar segment of the lower lobes, often sparing the superior segment and the anterior basal segment. It is found more than twice as frequently in the left-lower lobe as in the right.[105–107] Next in frequency are the right-middle lobe and its counterpart, the lingula. These may represent those areas of lung with the worst drainage. The upper lobes

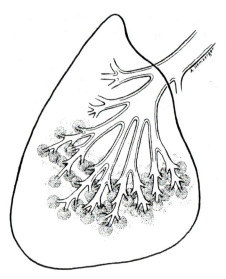
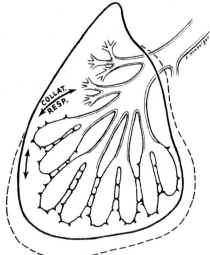

Fig. 5–24. Diagram of probable role of infection in formation of bronchiectasis. Left: Infection involves areas adjacent to bronchi and more distal connections. Right: With resolution and scarring, involved areas contract and pull against bronchi and cause their dilatation and overall lung contraction (*dotted line*). (From Glenn WWL, Liebow AA, Lindskog GE. Thoracic and cardiovascular surgery with related pathology. 3d Ed. Norwalk: Appleton-Lange, 1975:191, with permission.)

degree of bronchiectasis in the usual case of interstitial fibrosis and honeycombing, but it is usually not as marked as in the entity just discussed. Localized bronchiectasis may occur in any scarred zone, and in interstitial fibrosis is most severe in the peripheral subpleural zone. It seems very reasonable to this author that the young age of first infection and recurrent infections during childhood in bronchiectasis lead to some significant differences in the zones of the lung involved in these two diseases. Continued lung growth and expansion in the involved areas of children's lungs are probably influenced by such tissue loss, and possibly this accounts for at least a part of the simplification of the bronchial system as described in bronchiectasis.[112] The more diffuse suppurative nature of bronchiectasis may also play a role compared to the low-grade but chronic scarring of interstitial fibrosis, where only focal PMNs occur in mucous collections in dilated peripheral bronchioles (see Chapter 20).

Grossly, the involved lung tissue is usually atelectastic, grey-blue, shrunken, and rubbery. There may be zones of golden or obstructive pneumonia, and sometimes these layer around the dilated bronchial tubes. It may be difficult or impossible to adequately inflate such a chronically contracted specimen. The involved bronchi are dilated instead of following their smoothly contoured courses as they extend peripherally. These dilated bronchi extend almost to the pleural surface and run in a somewhat parallel or radial fashion; although expanded, they do not have connections with each other. Partially or totally circumferential thin folds in mucosa extend out from the wall and are seen as transverse infolded pleats on the bronchial cast (Fig. 5–23A). These give the appearance of webs or bands of mucosa. There are varyingly sized outpouchings, larger ones between the remnant bronchial cartilages, and dilated smaller pits that appear to be dilated submucosal glands. Grossly, elastic fibers can be seen still running through the wall, but these are more widely separated than is normal because of the stretched diameter of the bronchus. In wet bronchiectasis there is thickening of the wall, and mucinous, granular, semisolid material can accumulate in the bronchus, perhaps related to poor drainage. Occasionally this material hardens and even calcifies (see following broncholithiasis section). In dry bronchiectasis the wall is thin, almost translucent, and grey-pink without wall thickening.

Microscopically the respiratory mucosa may be intact, show squamous metaplasia (Fig. 5–26), and be ulcerated or inflamed. The bronchial walls are usually chronically inflamed. Submucosal glands and surface goblet cells are not prominent and may decrease, although they may occasionally increase. Elastic tissue is preserved. Smooth muscle is usually present and often shows some degree of hypertrophy; occasionally this is atrophic. Cartilage seems less obvious as an artefact of dilatation, and occasionally is eroded, but most often appears normal histologically. Polymorphonuclear cells, macrophages, and desquamative and mucinous debris is present in the bronchial lumen in wet atelectasis. Acute inflammatory cells may be in the bronchial wall or in the adjacent lung parenchyma, depending on

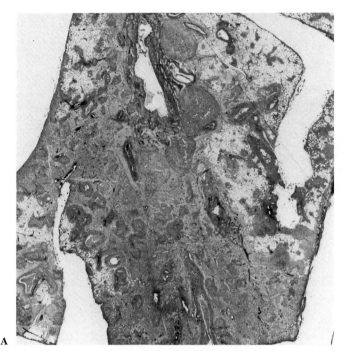

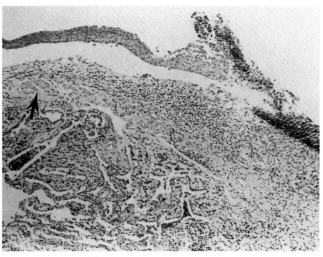

Fig. 5–26. Bronchiectatic wall. A few muscle bundles mark remnant wall (*arrow*). Exudate lines bronchus at right; squamous metaplasia lines it at left. Note inflammatory cell infiltration into adjacent lung parenchyma. H and E, ×100.

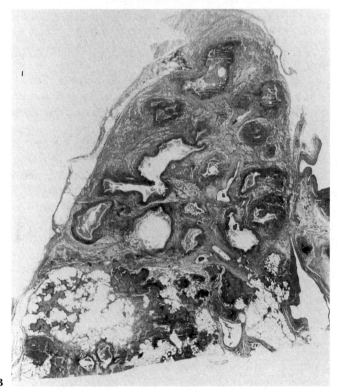

Fig. 5–25 A,B. Two cases of tuberculosis illustrate role of infection in bronchiectasis. **A.** Gough section of extensive transbronchial spread of tuberculosis from open cavity (cavity not shown). **B.** Later stage with inflammatory consolidation, scarring, and contraction of lung tissue. Note also Fig. 5–3A. (Courtesy of A.A. Liebow Pulmonary Pathology Collection, San Diego, California.)

the degree of acute inflammation occurring at the time of resection. As these patients are subject to recurrent infections, acute pneumonia may also be present.

Lymphocytes and plasma cells usually predominate in bronchial wall and surrounding lung tissue (Fig. 5–26). There may be a degree of obstructive pneumonia correlating with the gross yellow color. Small granulomas are present in a few cases, apparently as a reaction to some of the inspissated material in the bronchi. If granulomas are extensive or in the adjacent lung parenchyma, in more normally contoured segmental and subsegmental bronchi, or in nodes, one must consider fungal or mycobacterial infections. If granulomas are just in the injured areas, one must also consider aspiration. Bronchioles are dilated and sometimes mucus filled (Fig. 5–27), probably because of their obstruction at the junction with the larger bronchi. Foci of carcinoid atypical proliferation (tumorlets) occur with some frequency in bronchiectasis (see Chapter 32). Bronchial arteries respond here as they do to other forms of damage, and may enlarge to more than 1 mm in diameter.[138] Ulceration of these arteries may account for bright-red bleeding that is sometimes seen in these patients. As noted in Chapter 2, bronchial arteries have only an internal elastic membrane as compared to the internal and external elastic membranes of pulmonary arteries. Also, pulmonary artery branches are usually not seen in bronchial walls.

Middle-Lobe Syndrome

The right-middle lobe especially, and occasionally its left-sided counterpart, the lingula, have lobar bronchi

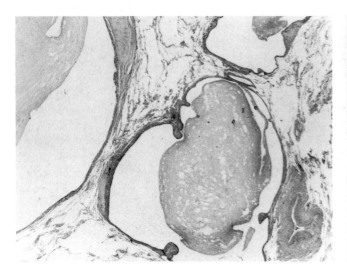

Fig. 5–27. Bronchiolectasis. Bronchioles are dilated and filled with secretions. H and E, ×50.

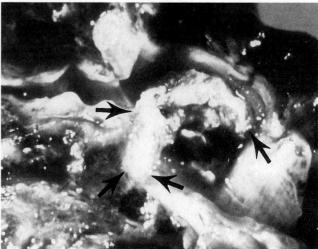

Fig. 5–28. Broncholith. Calcified crescent-shaped material (*arrows*) has partially eroded into bronchial lumen in patient with history of histoplasmosis.

that come off their parent supply at a more acute angle than most other dividing bronchi. They are relatively narrow, and there are frequently moderately prominent nodes in these angles that further complicate the situation. The subcarinal node may even approach this angle, at least on the right. Several authors[139,140] have also suggested there is less effective collateral ventilation here than in the adjacent upper lobe. Because of both these effects there is a greater tendency toward atelectasis, inflammation, nonspecific scarring broncholith formation, and bronchiectasis in these regions, and this has been called the *middle lobe syndrome.* A concise but relative thorough review is that by Banyai.[141]

Broncholithiasis

Broncholiths represent calcified material in the airways.[142–148] They most commonly are calcified lymph nodes that can compress bronchi[145] and either partially (Fig. 5–28) or completely erode through the bronchial walls. They then may be expectorated (lithopytsis) or aspirated (Fig. 5–29), and cause hemorrhage or obstructive changes, including cough, atelectasis, pneumonia, abscess formation, and bronchiectasis or air trapping. They form less often from chronic reaction to retained aspirated material or eroded fragments of calcified or ossified bronchial cartilage.[110] They may also occur with retained mucus as in bronchiectasis.[110] Historically, "spitting stones" dates back to descriptions by Aretaeus, Galen, and Aristotle.[146] Although usually less than 1 cm in diameter, a record-sized stone of 139 g (⅓ lb.) occurred in a patient who also had produced

multiple sand-like or melon-seed-sized calcified particles.[142] The pathognomonic finding of lithoptysis is fairly rare and was seen in only 5% (2 of 43) cases by Faber et al.[146] and 15% (6 of 41) cases by Schmidt et al.[144]

The regional nodes usually calcify from old granulomatous disease, and tuberculosis is the most common etiology worldwide while histoplasmosis is the most common etiology in the United States. Other infections include *Coccidioides, Cryptococcus,*[147,148] *Actinomyces,* or *Nocardia.*[149] The latter two organisms may represent supra infections of necrotic debris.[150] Silicosis may also cause a similar reaction.[151,152] Men and women are about equally involved,[145,153] and although calcified nodes may occur at any junction of the bronchial tree they are 2–6.5 times as common[153] on the right side, and favor the anterior superior segment of the upper lobe and the bronchus intermedius, along with the right-middle-lobe bronchus, where they may produce the middle-lobe syndrome.[153] The superior segment of the lower lobes is also a site of occurrence. Occasionally, erosive calcified nodes may cause bronchopleural fistula,[154] and of interest (in a similar fashion), the most common cause of esophageal fistulae are erosions from calcified or necrotic nodes.[154–156] Retraction diverticula of the esophagus may also occur by similar mechanism of nearby calcified nodes-broncholiths.[146,157]

Calcified nodes have been studied with CT scans, and in one retrospective series by Conces et al.,[153] 15 patients with proven broncholiths had calcified nodes near bronchi that were identified on chest radiographs in 11 of 15 (73%) of cases while calcified intraparchymal nodules were seen on similar radiographs in only 4

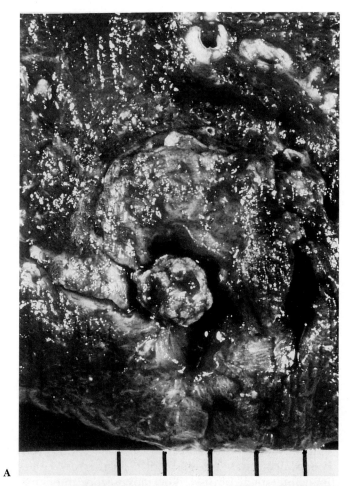

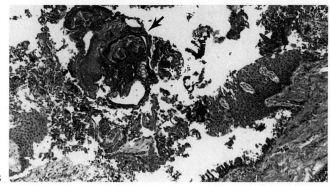

Fig. 5–29 A,B. Aspirated broncholith. **A.** Impacted or eroded lith is seen in distal lung. Note it has formed its own cavity in the surrounding inflammatory reaction. Also note small size of bronchi superiorly, suggesting this has progressed peripherally through erosion. **B.** Microscopy of portion of broncholith (*arrow*). Note squamous metaplasia of wall. H and E, ×100.

(27%). All 15 cases had calcified bronchial nodes by CT scan. Bronchoscopy was less accurate detecting these in some 28%–56% of cases. Rarely, calcifying tumors such as an ossifying bronchial carcinoid can cause confusion.[158]

Bronchial Fistula

Within the chest, fistula may be bronchopleural, bronchocutaneous, bronchomediastinal, or bronchoesophageal in their connections; outside the chest, they may connect with liver, pancreas, and assorted sites. Of these, bronchopleural fistula are most common and often are secondary to surgery, most often from a leaking postoperative bronchial stump; other causes are necrotizing pneumonia or abscess, penetrating wounds, eroding granulomatous disease, penetrating broncholiths, or malignancies. See Chapter 7 for congenital causes.

Bronchial Stenosis

Bronchial stenosis has assorted causes, including congenital, malignant, inflammatory, postinflammatory, and traumatic causes including postoperative changes. As noted in the introduction to this chapter, causes such as congenital and pediatric are covered in Chapters 7 and 8; amyloid, chondomalacia, and tracheobronchopathia, osteochondroplastica overlap with those described in the trachea in Chapter 22, **Metabolic and Other Diseases**. Allergic bronchial compromise is covered in Chapter 16, **Eosinophilic Infiltrates**. The effects of stenosis may be irritative with a cough and hemoptysis or obstructive changes. With partial obstruction, there may be hyperinflation, and with complete obstruction may occur atelectasis, recurrent postobstructive pneumonia, abscess formation, bronchiectasis, fistulization, or mucocele affect (see following section).

Bronchial Mucocele—Bronchocele—Bronchial Atresia

Bronchocele means one or more dilated bronchi are filled with fluid, which may be mucinous (bronchomucele) or consist of pus (bronchopyocele).[159] This condition is caused by stenosis or occlusion of the proximal end of dilated sac(s), and therefore differs from bronchectasis and mucoid impaction, whose proximal ends are generally still patent. It may be either congenital, or early or late acquired, usually of postinflammatory nature but sometimes of malignant nature.[160] Usually, associated localized emphysema occurs around this area, which may be caused either by inflammation early in lung growth with continued traction-type effects on nearby lung, or by ongoing air-trapping disease.[159,161,162] Some cases are reported as bronchial atresia.[163]

Bronchocele may be a relative of the racemose form of bronchectasis and may be the etiology for some intraparechmal bronchogenic cysts (see following and Chapter 8).[164] Mucoid impaction is related to an allergic effect, often to noninvasive *Aspergillus* (see Chapter 16), usually does not have proximal bronchial stenosis-occlusion, and has more eosinophils and cellular debris in the mucus, in addition to intramural hyphal elements.

Bronchogenic Cysts

Bronchogenic cysts are closed sacs lined by respiratory mucosa, usually with bronchial glands, smooth muscle, and cartilage. They often represent congenital fragments that "drop off" or are remnants of the original budding of the lungs off the primative endodermal canal. They are most common in the mediastinum where they account for 10%–15% of all primary mediastinal masses,[165] but can be seen as isolated mass(es) in the lung. In the lung itself, some may form as bronchoceles as discussed previously. A nice series of 86 cases of bronchogenic cysts, 66 (77%) in the mediastinum and 20 (23%) in the lung, was presented by St. Georges et al.[165] from Montreal. Of interest, 90% of those in the lung were symptomatic at the time of operation, most often because of infection, and although suspected, a preoperative diagnosis was not correctly made in any case in this large series.[165] Most (65%) occurred in the lower lobes but some occurred in each other lobe. They are uncommon in adults and are further discussed in children in chapter 7.

Bronchorrhea

Bronchorrhea is arbitrarily defined as production of more than 100 ml of sputum per day.[166] Although it is a clinical symptom, pathologists may ponder the differential diagnosis if faced with this history on a specimen request card. Bronchorrhea may be idiopathic,[167] secondary to chronic bronchitis,[168] bronchiectasis, or scleroderma,[169] asthma,[166] mucinous bronchioloalveolar carcinoma,[170] tuberculosis,[171] or polychondritis.[172] Cytology exams, cultures and/or transbronchial biopsies may help sort out at least some of these possibilities.

Cystic Fibrosis (Mucoviscidosis) in Adults

More patients with cystic fibrosis are living into adulthood. The median life expectancy of such children born in 1990 is projected to be 40 years, twice that of those born in 1970.[173] The number of children with this disease is expected to remain stable while those surviving into adulthood increases, principally because of better care. Also, there is no evidence of this increased survivorship plateauing.[172,173] diSant' Agnese and Davis[174] contributed 75 cases and reviewed 232 cases in adults aged 18–47 years, and found the same, eventually terminal course as in children. In 22% of their patients, the diagnosis of mucoviscidosis was made after the age of 15 years, and pancreatic insufficiency was present but was less symptomatic than in children.

All cystic fibrosis cases will eventually develop pulmonary disease.[174] The effects of mucus stasis include recurrent pneumonia, bacterial colonization, bronchectasis, and interstitial pneumonia. Some will develop only localized pulmonary disease, most often to the right-upper lobe,[175] but most will suffer more widespread disease. CT scanning in this disease details mucus plugging in bronchectasis more accurately than routine chest radiographs.[176]

Bronchiectasis is a prevalent problem. Esterly and Oppenheimer[177] have shown that bronchiectasis always accompanies mucoviscidosis. Their pathologic study in young children showed no bronchiectasis present in the first month of life, but it was noted in 58% of patients aged 1–6 months, and was documented in 100% of children older than 6 months. Bedrossian et al.[178] found no bronchiectasis in the first 4 months of life, but all patients aged over 2 years in their study had the disease, and it progressed with further aging.

Bronchiectasis in this disease occurs in upper lobes with equal frequency as lower lobes, and as mentioned earlier, unexplained bronchiectasis in the upper lobes alone should alert the investigator to study the patient for possible mucoviscidosis. Systemic amyloid occurs in some of the young adults with this disease.[179]

In an autopsy study of 43 cases of cystic fibrosis, Tomashefski et al.[180] found 9 (21%) with grossly identified interstitial fibrosis. The most severe interstitial fibrosis was in the lower lobes, posterior basal segments, and upper lobes anterior segments. These patients were from 17 to 28 years old at the time of death; all had clinically severe lung disease and *Pseudomonas aeruginousa* colonization for a mean duration of 12.4 ± 14.1 years, and 8 of the 9 were colonized with *Pseudomonas cepacia*.[180,181]

Grossly, many bronchi are seen to be filled with mucinous material (Fig. 5–30), and histologically an admixture of exudate, polymorphonuclear cells, and often colonies of *Staphylococcus aureus*, and as noted, *Pseudomonas aeruginosa* or *Pseudomonas cepacia*, particularly mucoid colony-forming types, occur within these masses. A similar kind of reaction spills into adjacent lung parenchyma. (Figures 5–31 and 5–32 correlate the gross and histologic appearance with the radiographic appearance. As noted, patchy interstitial pneumonia and/or fibrosis is present in some cases.

---→

Fig. 5–31. Mucoviscidosis (cystic fibrosis). Bronchus (BR), bronchioles (B), and terminal bronchioles (T) are distended with mucopus. Spillage or spread into lung parenchyma is seen next to terminal bronchioles (T) and as pneumonia (P). (**A**), pulmonary artery; (V), vein. H and E, ×10.

Obstruction

In this section, obstruction of both large and small breathing tubes is considered. Obstruction of bronchi or bronchioles may be partial or complete. Partial obstructoin may lead to air trapping with overdistension of the distal air parenchyma, as in asthma (Chapter 16), mucoviscidosis (Chapter 8 and this chapter), or unilateral hyperlucent lung (Chapter 8), among other diseases. If complete, it may lead to atelectasis. Collateral ventilation, both in and out of the affected areas, may alter some of the observed effects, and if complete obstruction occurs in segmental or smaller size bronchi, atelectasis may occur (see end of this chapter). Obstruction may also lead to pneumonia, abscess formation, and bronchiectasis. Obstructive pneumonia changes may occur as a result of either small or large airway occlusion.

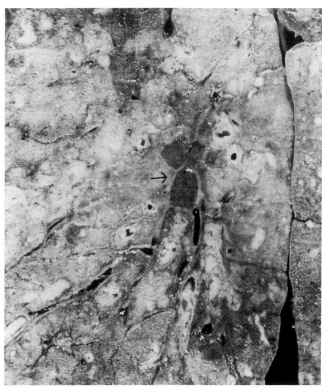

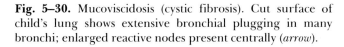

Fig. 5–30. Mucoviscidosis (cystic fibrosis). Cut surface of child's lung shows extensive bronchial plugging in many bronchi; enlarged reactive nodes present centrally (*arrow*).

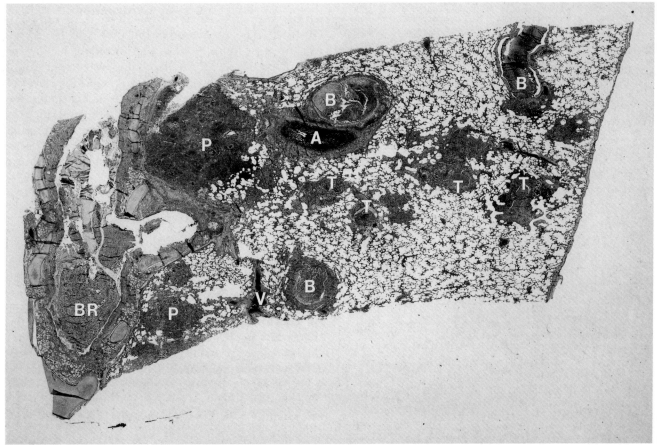

5-31

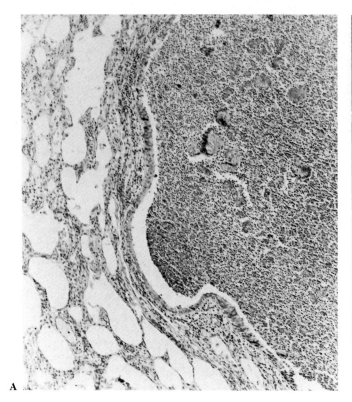

A

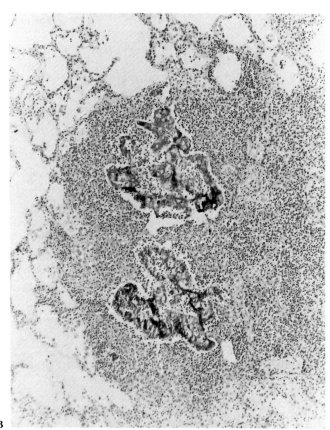

B

Fig. 5–32 A,B. Mucoviscidosis (cystic fibrosis). Granular masses of mucoid *Pseudomonas* are present in mucopus in (**A**) distending terminal bronchiole (H and E, ×250) and extending into (**B**) adjacent lung (H and E, ×400).

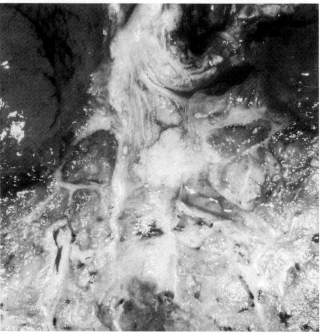

Fig. 5–33. Obstructive pneumonia. Squamous carcinoma in 69-year-old man presenting with endobronchial mass has caused endogenous lipoid (postobstructive, golden, or cholesterol) pneumonia. Some distal bronchiectasis and more proximal mucosal and submucosal spread of cancer cause blurring of elastic fiber bundle detail.

Larger Airway Obstruction

Obstruction here is caused by the same type of obstructive forces as those listed in the preceding section for obstructive bronchiectasis. In adults, obstruction is most frequently caused by primary tumors of lung, most of which cause obstruction by endobronchial extension (Fig. 5–33). Some tumors compromise the lumen by wall infiltration or constriction. Eighty percent of aspirated foreign bodies occur in children,[182] and is an important cause of obstruction in this age group, but it may also occur in adults.

Obstructive Pneumonia

The entity of obstructive, golden, or endogenous lipid pneumonia is most commonly seen secondary to tumor obstruction. The obstructive effect accounts for a much larger infiltrate on the usual chest radiograph than is caused by tumor alone. Any of the causes of obstruction can lead to obstructive pneumonia. The involved area is that supplied by the affected bronchus, and the larger the obstructed bronchus the greater the area involved. However, even in the smallest bronchioles, there may be a focal obstructive effect in the central acinar regions. The involved lung is reduced in size, but not as much as one would expect in simple atelectasis. The difference

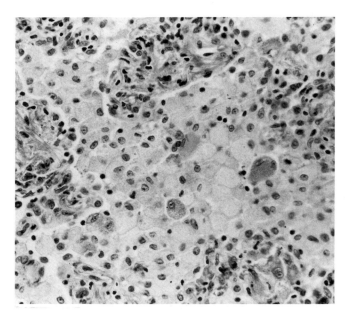

Fig. 5–34. Obstructive pneumonia. Air space occupying much of center of field is filled with finely vacuolated, foamy macrophages. H and E, ×400.

results from its infiltration by abundant inflammatory cells.

The microscopic hallmark of obstructive pneumonia is a flooding of airspaces by fat-filled, finely vacuolated or foamy alveolar macrophages (Fig. 5–34). Cholesterol crystals may form, and there may be a few lymphocytes and plasma cells. The lipid content of the macrophages accounts for the gross creamy-tan to golden-yellow color, the latter color accounting for the term "golden pneumonia." Obstructed secretions and increased cell breakdown products, and possible leakage from vessels and interstitium, may give rise to the fat seen in this characteristic reaction. As these products are derived from the lung, this is called endogenous lipid pneumonia. Early in its course the alveolar outlines are well defined even though alveoli are flooded with foamy macrophages. If the pneumonia is rapidly reversed, lung function may return. Over time, some permanent damage may take place, including fibrosis and vascular sclerosis, and it is then harder to restore functional lung even though the obstruction may eventually be reversed (see Chapter 2). Although some degree of intraalveolar organization is possible it is usually remarkably absent.

In contrast to exogenous lipid pneumonia (aspiration), in endogenous lipid pneumonia the fat is finely vaculated, and there is usually no foreign body response and much less inflammatory and fibrous obliteration of the background lung architecture. Sometimes there are changes that suggest pulmonary alveolar lipoproteinosis in post obstructive lipid pneumonia.[183] At times parenchymal changes very similar to those just described may be present although no obstruction of bronchus can be identified, as described next.

Chronic Organizing Pneumonia

This grouping covers several entities that may be related. In 1954, Ackerman et al.[184] described 15 cases that suggested lobar pneumonia or cancer, all of whom were chronically ill with weight loss. Of the 15, 13 (87%) were men, and 14 of 15 (93%) were over age 40; hilar mass effect was present in 10 of the 15 (67%), and there was frequent overlying pleural fibrosis adhesion with the adjacent chest wall. In these cases, disease was confined to the upper lobes in 11 (67%), most often in the right-upper lobe, and there was no evidence of bronchiectasis.

Ackerman et al.[184] attributed the original pathology description to the German literature, as reviewed by Floyd in 1922.[185] Bronchi were inflamed, some early cavitation was present, and grossly the involved areas were grey-red to light yellow. Microscopically there was organizing exudate in lung and bronchi (see following sections) rich in mononuclear cells including lymphocytes and plasma cells, and in cases with necrosis, PMNs were noted. The degree of interstitial fibrosis and organizing intraalveolar fibrous polyps varied. There were rarely scattered single giant cells, but no aspirated foreign material was identified. Foamy macrophages were minimal. No mention of asbestos fiber detection or asbestos exposure was noted. Some cases may represent rounded atelectasis, as discussed in Chapter 34.

In 1948, Robbins and Sniffen[186] described 11 cases of chronic nonobstructive cholesterol pneumonia, 10 of which (91%) occurred in men aged 32–67 years, the only female being a 12-year-old girl. In size, 5 of their cases involved most of the lobe and 6 cases included a portion of one or more segments, often with pleural adhesions; some had small abscess cavities. The involved areas were wedge shaped with their bases on the pleura and were described as bright yellow; they were accounted for histologically by abundant, finely vacuolated foamy macrophages, but otherwise these areas presented as mass effects as described by Ackerman et al.[184] Mucoid or mucopurulent exudate filled some bronchioles and bronchi, but no other cause of obstruction was present. Bronchectasis was absent, although focal necrotizing bronchitis was noted. The lobar distribution was not documented. These authors argued against aspiration as they noted the usual aspiration to be more diffuse, often multifocal, and more often seen in lower lobes. Lawler[187] in 1977 summarized the literature on 50 such cases; most were in the age range 30 to 67 and occurred in men (90%), most were in a single location (78%), and 40% in the right-upper lobe were followed by multifocal involvement in 23% and left-upper lobe involvement in 18%. Some cases of nonobstructive cholesterol pneumonia have similar changes in bronchioles.[188]

Bulmer et al.[189] studying a series of 30 cases of unresolved pneumonia, confirmed identifiable foreign material in 11 (37%) and strongly suspected aspiration in another 6 for a total of 57% in this series. All except two cases (82%) of confirmed aspiration were solitary lesions. It seems reasonable that at least some of both chronic organizing pneumonia and idiopathic lipid pneumonias, even when not so confirmed, may be secondary to aspiration, usually involving ingredients other than exogenous lipid that should be more easily identified (see discussion of aspiration earlier in this chapter).

Bronchiolitis Obliterans and BOOP

Certainly some small airway damage occurs by lack of support of surrounding tissue, as in emphysema (Chapter 26), inflammation in small-airways disease (Chapter 26), or mucus stasis as in bronchiolectasis mentioned earlier. Bronchiolitis obliterans (or obliterative bronchiolitis) has a distinctive meaning, although it may have many causes and therefore is a common injury effect and not a separate disease. As with a larger breathing tube obstruction, the obstruction may be partial and air trapping is possible, as in the Swyer–James[190]–MacLeod[191] syndrome or unilateral hyperlucent lung (Fig. 5–35),[192,192a] or it may be complete, leading to small foci of obstructive pneumonia or possibly atelectasis.

Grossly, these lungs may be hyperinflated, but more often at biopsy they contain focal nodules, often 1–2 mm in diameter or sometimes larger. The lung tissue may not deflate in the expected time after biopsy, surgical resection, or remal at autopsy. The typical histologic appearance is that of organizing fibroblastic polyps, usually extending from one side wall of a respiratory and possibly terminal bronchiole, and sometimes extending into adjacent alveolar ducts and sacs (Fig. 5–36). Lymphocytes and plasma cells are sometimes mixed with these (Fig. 5–36). Elastic stains may help define the injured edge of bronchial wall (Figs. 5–36 through 5–39). Sometimes bronchioles show apparent destruction by PMNs (Fig. 5–37), obliteration by confluent fibrosis (Fig. 5–38), and/or narrowed persistent or recanalized lumen (Fig. 5–39). These latter two changes may be prominent in patients having undergone lung transplantation (Fig. 5–38B) or those with collagen vascular disease. Individual fibroblastic polyps are frequently present in nearby alveoli (Figs. 5–40 and Fig. 41), and when extensive Epler and associates[193] called

this association "bronchiolitis obliterans with patchy organizing pneumonia" or BOOP (see Chapter 4). The ultrastructural characteristics of BOOP have been examined by Myers and Katzenstein.[194] At times bronchi are also involved,[195–197] and Yamanaka et al.[198] have suggested calling this combination bronchobronchiolitis obliterans. These cases appear to have a worse prognosis; some occur in children and some in adults.

The organizing fibroblastic polyps in alveoli are somewhat similar to intraalveolar Masson bodies in an organizing alveolar pneumonia, but usually they are not as admixed with inflammatory or other stages of organization. Some are associated with chronic inflammatory cells in the interstitium (Fig. 5–40), while others are but remnants of a past reaction without much remaining interstitial or alveolar inflammatory cells (Fig. 5–42). When present either solely as organizing pneumonia or together with bronchiolitis obliterans, the microscopic nodules in each location are of about the same age, suggesting a common insult dating from the same time (see Fig. 5–42).

The etiologic agents of bronchiolitis obliterans must be able to carry their damage into the most terminal airways. Katzenstein and Askin[199] listed the etiologic agents under the following groups: (1) infections, particularly viral, especially adenovirus and respiratory syncytial virus (mycoplasma, and less often bacterial, fungal, and mycobacterial infections, can also cause this reaction); (2) toxic fumes, as in nitrogen dioxide, acid fumes, ammonia inhalation, or other toxic or hot gas inhalation; (3) obstructive; (4) aspiration; (5) collagen vascular diseases, especially rheumatoid arthritis, possibly related to penicillamine treatment[200,201]; and (6) unknown (in 30%–40% of cases). This reaction has also been observed in bone marrow transplant[202–205] and heart/lung transplant patients,[206] in both situations possibly related to graft-versus-host disease. (See Chapter 24.) It has also been described in AIDS cases[207] and after radiation,[208] along with other assorted conditions.[209,210] The role of infectious etiologies in these cases cannot be excluded. The entity of bronchiolitis obliterans has been extensively reviewed in 1989 by King.[206]

In the large series by Epler and associates,[193] 50 of 94 cases were not associated with any known cause or disease, and these occurred with the patchy organizing pneumonia peripherally. A cough or flu-like illness was noted 4–10 weeks before the diagnosis, clinically suggesting a slowly resolving viral infection. Radiographs showed patchy ground-glass densities. Pulmonary function tests demonstrated restriction in 72% of cases and impaired diffusing capacity in 86% of those tested. Men and women were equally represented; most were 40–60 years of age, and half were nonsmokers. Admin-

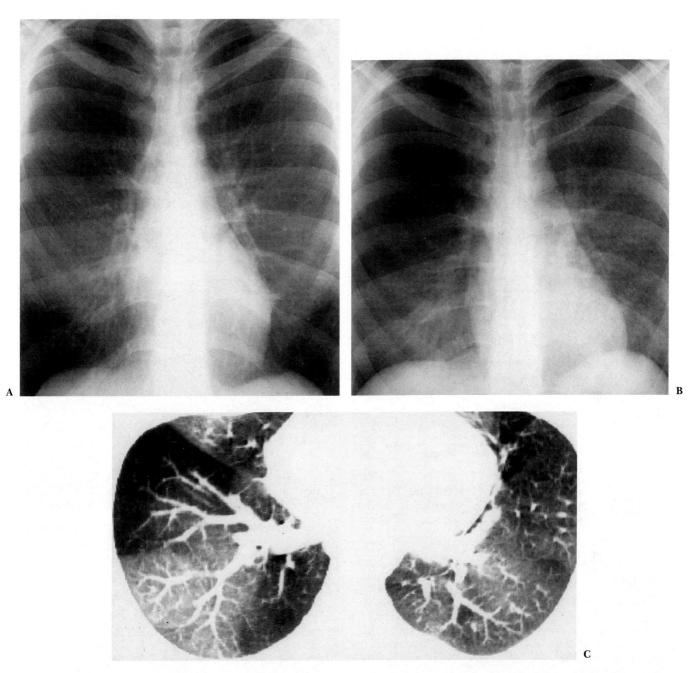

Fig. 5–35 A–C. Swyer–James–MacLeod syndrome. **A.** Chest radiograph made in inspiration shows slight hyperlucency and diminished vascularity of right lung. **B.** Chest radiograph made in expiration shows persistent hyperlucency of right-lung apex, but normal increase in radiopacity of left lung and medial basal right lung. **C.** High-resolution CT scan made in expiration shows abnormal patchy bilateral hyperlucency indicating air trapping. (Reproduced with the permission of the American Roentgen Ray Society from Moore ADA, Godwin JD, Dietrich PA, Verschakelen JA, Henderson WR, Jr. Swyer–James syndrome: CT findings in eight patients. AJR 1992;158:1211–1215.)

istration of steroids led to complete recovery in 65% of cases. These changes should be distinguished from interstitial fibrosis, which has a poor overall prognosis. Cordier et al.[211] classified 16 cases as solitary or multifocal pneumonia-like or diffuse interstitial lung disease-like patterns. The solitary ones were usually excised to exclude malignancy; the multifocal ones responded well to steroids but relapsed if treatment was stopped too soon; about half of the interstitial group responded to steroids and half did not, perhaps indicating a

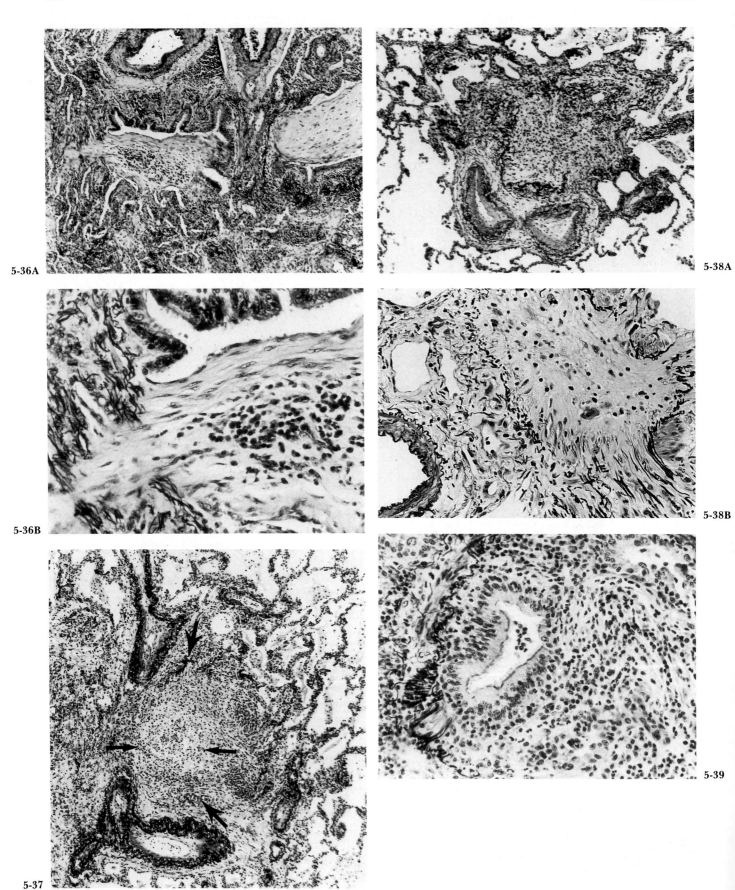

5-36A

5-36B

5-37

5-38A

5-38B

5-39

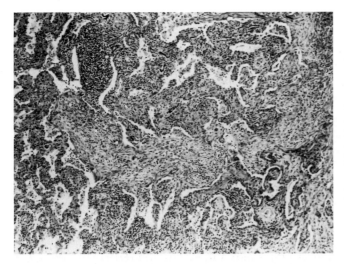

Fig. 5–40. Organizing pneumonia with cellular interstitial inflammation. Note polyps of organizing tissue and increased numbers of interstitial lymphocytes, including one nodule to upper left. H and E, ×100.

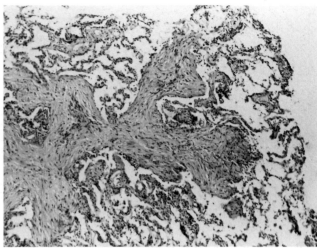

Fig. 5–41. Patchy organizing pneumonia. Fibrosis with only mild cellular component may be present in pattern suggesting alveolar duct, or at least with confluent involvement of adjacent alveoli. H and E, ×100.

greater degree of irreversible fibrosis. A variant rich in xanthoma cells has been described with cholesterol pneumonia.[188]

The radiographic appearance of bronchiolitis obliterans has been well explored by Gosink et al. In their

◁————————————————

Fig. 5–36 A,B. Bronchiolitis obliterans. **A.** Polyps of organizing inflammatory reaction in terminal bronchioles. Movat pentachrome, ×100. **B.** Higher power view of left side shows respiratory ciliated mucosa at top. Elastic fibers that appear disrupted by polyp of fibrous tissue are at left with entrapped plasma cells and rare lymphocytes. Movat pentachrome, ×400.

Fig. 5–37. Necrotizing reaction in bronchiole. Lining and much of wall have been replaced by inflammatory reaction with PMNs (*smaller arrows*) surrounded by chronic inflammation. Remnant bronchiole is identified by position next to pulmonary artery and by remnant elastic tissue (*larger arrows*). Movat pentachrome, ×100.

Fig. 5–38 A,B. Bronchiolitis obliterans. **A.** Total obliteration by fibrous tissue with some chronic inflammatory cells. Movat pentachrome, ×100. **B.** Total chronic fibrous obliteration marks area of bronchiolitis obliterans in this patient 6 months after single lung transplant with chronic rejection. Movat pentachrome, ×100. (Courtesy of Dr. Dean Chamberlain, Toronto General Hospital, Toronto, Ontario.)

Fig. 5–39. Stenosing bronchiolitis. Persistent but small lumen (or possible recanalized lumen) shows great narrowing of expected diameter compared to general contour of bronchiolar elastic tissue. Movat pentachrome, ×400.

series, twice as many had an alveolar pattern of opacities (Fig. 5–43) as had nodular densities, and the right lung was involved four times as frequently as the left, especially in the right-upper lobe.

Some of the patients in the Gosink et al.[212] series had a fibrosing obliterative process of the terminal bronchioles that appeared more permanent than the usual bronchiolitis obliterans. This has also been described in the background of rheumatoid arthritis and possible penicillamine therapy by Geddes et al.[200] Dense scarring is seen (see Fig. 5–38) with small persistent lumens or perhaps eventual attempts at recanalization (see Fig. 5–39). Whether such patients had rheumatoid arthritis or associated collagen vascular disease in Gosink's series is not specified.

Diffuse Panbronchiolitis

This is a disease that appears to occur most frequently in the Orient and in patients of Oriental descent, but can occur in others.[213,214] It occurs in adults, usually those over the age of 40, and favors men twice as often as women. Lesions are usually widespread and diffuse but are often worse in the lower lobes. They appear as small, less than 2-mm-diameter, nodules on chest radiographs, and CT scans show bronchiolar wall thickening, along with some cyst formation.[215] Air trapping may lead to hyperinflation, and pulmonary function tests usually show obstructive changes; however, some show restrictive defects, some both, and some have gas diffusion abnormalities. This is a protracted disease and symptoms are often of chronic cough, productive sputum, and dyspnea.

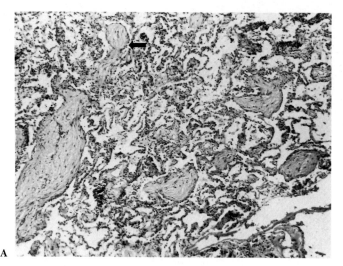

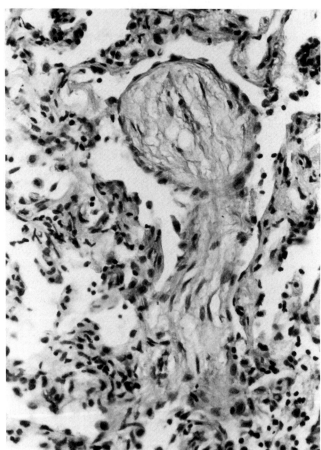

Fig. 5–42 A,B. Patchy organizing pneumonia. **A.** Multiple smaller areas of lesser involvement may be present as well as larger areas of organization such as in Fig. 5–40. Note all areas of organization appear to be of same age. H and E, ×100. **B.** High-power view of polyp at *arrow* tip in **A.** H and E, ×400.

As nicely reviewed by Homma et al.,[216] superinfection may occur with *Pseudomonas* organisms in about two-thirds of cases that have positive bacterial cultures. Mean survival is 21.1 years from beginning of productive cough, 7.7 years from onset of dyspnea, and 2.9 years from documenting colonization by *Pseudomonas* organisms.[213] Therefore, *Pseudomonas* is a late finding.[216] Chronic sinusitis occurs in more than three-fourths of patients, but a few cases have been associated with ulcerative colitis,[217] allergic angiitis and granulomatosis,[218] adult T-cell lymphoma, or adult T-cell leukemia[219] and non-Hodgkins lymphoma.[220] Of interest, there is no association with tobacco exposure.[216] Prognosis is better in those under age 40 and those without sinusitis.[221] Family occurrences have been documented, and there is an increased occurrence in the HLA BW54[222–224] haplotype, a type confined to those of Japanese, Chinese, or Korean descent, perhaps accounting for the apparent racial selection.[224]

Pathologically, multiple small grey-white to yellow-tan nodules have seen confined to respiratory bronchioles in the transition zone between the end of the conducting system, the membranous bronchioles, and the air-exchange sacs more peripherally. There is at times more proximal bronchiolectasis. All layers of the walls of the delicate respiratory bronchioles are involved, and therefore the term pan- is used in panbronchiolitis. Abundant chronic inflammation is noted with lymphocytes, plasma cells, and histiocytes at this location (Fig. 5–44) and in the lumens of the bronchioles; PMNs or mucus may be identified. More distally, a peculiar finding is of interstitial foaming macrophages,[216] a finding only rarely seen elsewhere, as in aspiration (see Fig. 5–14). BAL samples show increased number of PMNs and decreased number of alveolar macrophages,[225] probably reflecting the PMNs in the respiratory bronchioles and the effect of occlusion thereof. The work of Kudoh et al., as cited by Izumi,[226] noted that the usual antibiotic therapies are ineffective but that treatment with low doses of erythromycin in subtherapeutic doses (400–600 mg/day for at least 4 weeks) is beneficial; however, the mechanism for this action is unclear. With the high incidence of sinusitis, it is wondered whether this might be a relative of ciliary dyskinesia, but this has not been proven. Aspiration of sinus drainage is a possible mechanism. As yet there is no definite primary infection, and colonies may show *Pseudomonas, Staphylococcus, Streptococcus,* or *Hemophilus* organisms, probably representing suprainfections.

Atelectasis

Atelectasis is the collapse of aerating lung. Most often it is caused by internal bronchial obstruction of the air

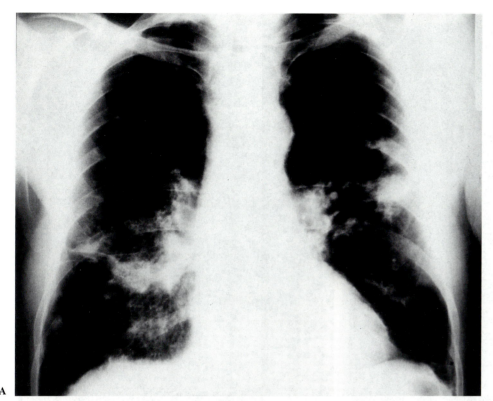

Fig. 5–43 A,B. Bronchiolitis obliterans organizing pneumonia (BOOP). **A.** Note bilateral patchy dense infiltrates here in both perihilar and peripheral locations. **B.** CT scan shows patchy, peripheral, dense air space consolidation containing a few air bronchograms. (Courtesy of Dr. Ingrid Peterson, Virginia Mason Clinic, Seattle, Washington.)

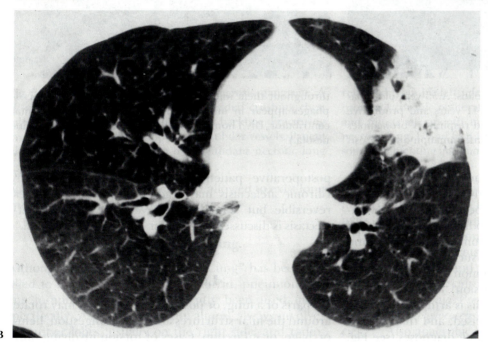

flow (Figs. 16–1 and 16–2 are examples), but it may result from external compression on the lung, such as by empyema or mesothelioma or other constricting scars or tumor masses, or by internal compression within the lung itself, as when adjacent to a bleb, tumor, or other space-occupying lesion. It may also be caused by a change in metabolism or surface-wetting balance such as with hyaline membrane disease, infection, or gastric acid or other aspiration. It may also be vascular, as with embolism and hypoxia, or neuromuscular such as postoperative, with obesity (Pickwickian syndrome) nerve or muscle dysfunction of diaphragm or chest wall.

When in the upper lobes, it appears to progress through necrotizing pneumonia with thrombosis of arteries and veins.[231]

Although not strictly abiding by the foregoing definition (of localization in upper lobe), in one case a total unilateral lung gangrene was attributed to hilar vessel involvement following treatment of a massive hilar recurrence of Hodgkins disease.[234] I have seen a similar case in a 32-year-old man who survived massive left chest trauma, with multiple rib fractures compressing hilar vessels and causing thrombosis and necrosis (Fig. 5–45).

References

1. Ross AHM, McCormack RJM. Foreign body inhalation. J R Coll Surg Edinb 1980;25:104–109.
2. Kim IG, Brummitt WM, Humphry A, Siomra SW, Wallace WB. Foreign body in the airway: A review of 202 cases. Laryngoscope 1973;83:347–354.
3. Haugen RK. The cafe coronary: sudden deaths in restaurants. JAMA 1963;186:142–143.
4. Glenn WWL, Leibson AA, Lindskog GE. Thoracic and cardiovascular surgery with related pathology. 3d Ed. New York: Appleton-Century-Crofts, 1975:113.
5. Jackson C, Jackson CL. Bronchoscopy, esophagoscopy and gastroscopy. Philadelphia: Saunders, 1934:185.
6. Anonymous. Inhaled foreign bodies. Br Med J 1981; 282:1649–1650.
7. Hargis JL, Hiller C, Bone RC. Migratory pulmonary infiltrates secondary to aspirated foreign body. JAMA 1978;240:2469.
8. Noguchi M, Kimula Y, Ogata T. Muddy lung. Am J Clin Pathol 1985;83;240–244.
9. Brock RC. Observations on the anatomy of the bronchial tree, with special reference to the surgery of lung abscess. Guy's Hospital Reports 1942;91:111–130.
10. Brock RC, Hodgkiss F, Jones HO. Bronchial embolism and posture in relation to lung abscess. Guy's Hospital Reports 1942;91:131–139.
11. Abdulmajid OA, Ebeid AM, Motawek MM, Kleibo IS. Aspirated foreign bodies in the tracheobronchial tree: report of 250 cases. Thorax 1976;31:635–640.
12. Çaglayan S, Erkin S, Coteli I, Oniz H. Bronchial foreign body vs. asthma. Chest 1989;96:509–511.
13. Mullin WV, Ryder CT. Studies on the lymph drainage of the accessory nasal sinuses. Laryngoscope 1921; 31:158–178.
14. Corper HJ, Robin HA. The pulmonary aspiration of particulate matter. Am Rev Tuberc 1922;6:813–850.
15. Myerson MC. Pulmonary aspects of tonsillectomy under general anesthesia. Laryngoscope 1922;32:929–942.
16. Quinn LH, Meyer OO. The relationship of sinusitis and bronchiectasis. Arch Otolaryngol 1929;10:152–165.
17. Amberson JB Jr. Aspiration bronchopneumonia. Internat Clin 1937;3:126–138.
18. Bartlett JG. Aspiration pneumonia. In: Baum GL, Wolinsky E, eds. Textbook of pulmonary diseases. 4th Ed. Boston: Little, Brown, 1989:531–543.
19. Berson W, Adriani J. "Silent" regurgitation and aspiration of gastric content during anesthesia. Anesthesiology 1954;15:644–649.
20. Gardner AMN. Aspiration of food and vomit. QJ Med 1958;27:227–242.
21. Huxley EJ, Viroslav J, Gray WR, Pierce AK. Pharyngeal aspiration in normal adults and patients with depressed consciousness. Am J Med 1978;64:564–568.
22. Hamelberg WV, Bosomworth PP. Aspiration pneumonitis. Springfield: Thomas, 1968.
23. Mendelson CL. The aspiration of stomach contents into the lungs during obstetrical anesthesia. Am J. Obstet Gynecol 1946;52:191–205.
24. Bynum LJ, Pierce AK. Pulmonary aspiration of gastric contents. Am Rev Respir Dis 1976;114:1129–1136.
25. Hiebert CA, Belsey R. Incompetency of the gastric cardia without radiologic evidence of hiatus hernia: The diagnosis and management of 71 cases. J Thorac Cardiovasc Surg 1961;42:352–362.
26. Mays EE, Dubois JJ, Hamilton GB. Pulmonary fibrosis associated with tracheobronchial aspiration: A study of the frequency of hiatal hernia and gastroesophageal reflux in interstitial pulmonary fibrosis of obscure etiology. Chest 1976;69:512–515.
27. Allen CJ, Craven MA, Waterfall WE, Newhouse MT. Gastroesophageal reflux and chronic respiratory disease. In: Baum GL, Wolinsky E. Textbook of pulmonary diseases. 4th Ed. Boston: Little, Brown, 1989: 1471–1486.
28. Gerarde HW. Toxicological studies on hydrocarbons: V. Kerosene. Toxicol Appl Pharmacol 1959;1:462–474.
29. Eade NR, Taussig IM, Marks MI. Hydrocarbon pneumonitis. Pediatrics 1974;54:351–357.
30. Giammona ST. Effects of furniture polish on pulmonary surfactant. Am J Dis Child 1967;113:658–663.
31. Brünner S, Rovsing H, Wulf H. Roentgenographic changes in the lungs of children with kerosene poisoning. Am Rev Respir Dis 1964;89:250–254.
32. Knoblich R. Pulmonay granulomatosis caused by vegetable particles: So-called lentil pulse pneumonia. Am Rev Respir Dis 1969;99:380–389.
33. Laughlen GF. Pneumonia following nasopharyngeal injections of oil. Am J Pathol 1925;1:407–414.
34. Spencer H. Pathology of the lung. 4th Ed. Oxford: Pergamon, 1985:527–525.
35. Pinkerton H. The reaction to oils and fats in the lungs. AMA Arch Pathol 1928;5:380–401.
36. Gerarde HW. Toxicological studies on hydrocarbon: IX. The aspiration hazard and toxicity of hydrocarbons and hydrocarbon mixtures. Arch Environ Health 1963;6:329–341.
37. Fox M, Bartlett JG. Lipoid pneumonia. In: Baum GL, Wolinsky E, eds. Textbook of pulmonary diseases. 3d Ed. Boston: Little, Brown, 1983:605–612.

38. Greenridge HW, Tuttle MJ. Lipoid pneumonia in a veterans' hospital. Ann Intern Med 1955;43:1259–1268.

39. Volk BW, Nathanson L, Losner S, Slade WR, Jacobi M. Incidence of lipoid pneumonia in a survey of 389 chronically ill patients. Am J Med 1951;10:316–324.

40. Hurwitz SA. Lipoid pneumonia: A new etiology. J Thorac Cardiovasc Surg 1972;63:551–552.

41. Oldenburger D, Maurer WJ, Beltaos E, Magnin GE. Inhalation lipoid pneumonia from burning fats. A newly recognized industrial hazard. JAMA 1972;222:1288–1289.

42. Baron HC, Shafiroff BGP. Acute lipoid pneumonitis due to aspiration of pressurized paint droplets. Dis Chest 1959;36:434–437.

43. Miller GJ, Ashcroft MT, Beadnell HMSG, Wagner JC, Pepys J. The lipoid pneumonia of black fat tobacco smokers in Guyana. QJ Med 1971;40:457–470.

44. Wright JL, Cockcroft DW. Lung disease due to abuse of hair spray. Arch Pathol Lab Med 1981;105:363–366.

45. Nagrath SD, Sapru RP. Lipoid pneumonia: Review of the literature with a case report. J Indian Med Assoc 1964;42:453–456.

46. Gibson JB. Infection of lungs by "saprophytic" mycobacteria in achalasia of cardia, with report of fatal cases showing lipoid pneumonia due to milk. J Pathol Bacteriol 1953;65:239–251.

47. Corpe RF, Smith CE, Sterg I. Death due to *Mycobacterium foritutum*.. JAMA 1961;177:262–263.

48. Guest JL Jr, Arean VM, Brenner HA. Group IV atypical mycobacterium infection occurring in association with mineral oil granulomas of lung. Am Rev Respir Dis 1967;95:656–662.

49. Hutchins GM, Boitnott JK. Atypical mycobacterial infection complicating mineral oil pneumonia. JAMA 1978; 240:539–541.

50. Hughes RL, Craig RM, Freilich RA, Moran JM, Bytell DE. Aspiration and occult esophageal disorders. Chest 1981;80:489–495.

51. Steinberg I, Finby N. Lipoid (mineral oil) pneumonia and cor pulmonale due to cardiospasm. Report of a case. AJR 1956;76:108–114.

52. Casey JF. Chronic cor pulmonale associated with lipoid pneumonia. JAMA 1961;177:896–898.

53. Losner S, Volk BW, Slade WR, Nathanson L, Jacobi M. Diagnosis of lipoid pneumonia by examination of the sputum. Am J Pathol 1950;20:539–545.

54. Corwin RW, Irwin RS. The lipid-laden alveolar macrophage as a marker of aspiration in parenchymal lung disease. Am Rev Respir Dis 1985;132:576–581.

55. Liebow AA. Pulmonary abscess. In: Glenn WWL, Liebow AA, Lindskog GE, eds. Thoracic and cardiovascular surgery with related pathology. 3d Ed. New York: Appleton-Century-Crofts, 1975:166–182.

56. Lockwood AL. Abscess of the lung. Surg Gynecol Obstet 1922;35:461–492.

57. Allen CI, Blackman JF. Treatment of lung abscesses with report of 100 consecutive cases. J Thorac Surg 1936;6:156–172.

58. Hagan JL, Hardy JD. Lung abscess revisited: A survey of 184 cases. Ann Surg 1983;197:755–761.

59. Estrada AS, Platt MR, Mills LJ, Shaw RR. Primary lung abscess. J Thorac Cardiovasc Surg 1980;79;275–282.

60. Chidi CC, Mendelsohn HJ. Lung abscess: A study of the results of treatment based on 90 consecutive cases. J Thorac Cardiovasc Surg 1974;68:168–172.

61. Schweppe HI, Knowles JH, Kane L. Lung abscess: An analysis of the Massachusetts General Hospital cases from 1943 through 1956. N Engl J Med 1961;265:1039–1043.

62. Brock RC. Lung abscess. London: Blackwell, 1952.

63. Smith DT. Experimental aspiration abscess. Arch Surg 1927;14:231–239.

64. Smith DT. Fuso-spirochaetal diseases of the lungs. Tubercle 1928;9:420–437.

65. Stern L. Putrid abscess of the lung following dental operations. J Thorac Surg 1935;4:547–557.

66. Stern L. Etiologic factors in the pathogenesis of putrid abscess of the lung. J Thorac Surg 1936;6:202–211.

67. Touroff ASW, Moolten SE. The symptomatology of putrid abscess of the lung. J Thorac Surg 1935;4:558–572.

68. Amberson JB. A clinical consideration of abscesses and cavities of the lung. Bull Johns Hopkins Hosp 1954;94:227–237.

69. Mark PH, Turner JAP. Lung abscess in childhood. Thorax 1968;23:126–220.

70. Groff DB, Rapkin RH. Primary lung abscess in childhood. J Med Soc NJ 1974;71:649–652.

71. Levine MM, Ashman R. Heald F. Anaerobic (putrid) lung abscess in adolescence. Am J Dis Child 1976;130:77–81.

72. King DS, Lord FT. Certain aspects of pulmonary abscess from analysis of 210 cases. Ann Intern Med 1934;8:468–474.

73. Sweet RH. Lung abscess: analysis of Massachusetts General Hospital cases from 1933 through 1937. Surg Gynecol Obstet 1940;70:1011–1021.

74. Gibbons RJ, Socransky SS, Sawyer S, Kapsimalis B, McDonald JB. The microbiota of the gingival crevice area of man–II: The predominant cultivable organisms. Arch Oral Biol 1963;8:281–289.

75. Socransky SS, Gibbons RJ, Dale AC, Bortnick L, Rosenthal E, McDonald JB. The microbiota of the gingival crevice area in man–I: Total microscopic and viable counts and counts of specific organisms. Arch Oral Biol 1963;8:275–280.

76. Loesche WJ. Dental infections. In: Balows A, DeHaan RM, Dowell VR Jr, Guze LB, eds. Anaerobic bacteria: Role in disease. Springfield: Thomas, 1974:409–434.

77. Rosebury T. Microorganisms indigenous to man. New York: McGraw-Hill, 1966:314, 331.

78. Bartlet JG, Gorbach SL, Tally FP, Finegold SM. Bacteriology and treatment of primary lung abscess. Am Rev Respir Dis 1974;109:510–518.

79. Gonzales-C CL, Calia FM. Bacteriologic flora of aspiration-induced pulmonary infections. Arch Intern Med 1975;135:711–714.

80. Bartlett JG. Lung abscess. In: Baum GL, Wolinsky E, eds. Textbook of pulmonary disease. 4th Ed. Boston: Little, Brown, 1989:545–555.

81. Bartlett JG. Anaerobic bacterial infections of the lung. Chest 1987;91:901–909.

82. Finegold SM, George WL, Mulligan ME. Anaerobic infections. DM 1985;31:8–77.

83. Bartlett JG, Alexander J, Mayhew J, Sullivan-Sigler M, Gorbach SL. Should fiberoptic bronchoscopy aspirates be cultured? Am Rev Respir Dis 1976;110:73–78.

84. Bartlett JG. Diagnostic accuracy of transtracheal aspiration bacteriologic studies. Am Rev Respir Dis 1977; 115:777–782.

85. Bartlett JG, Finegold SM. Anaerobic infections of the lung and pleural space. Am Rev Respir Dis 1974; 110:56–77.

86. Bartlett JG, Finegold SM. Anaerobic pleuropulmonary infections. Medicine (Baltimore) 1972;51:413–450.

87. Pennza PT. Aspiration pneumonia, necrotizing pneumonia, and lung abscess. Emerg Med Clin North Am 1989;7:279–307.

88. Perlman LV, Lerner GE, D'Esopo N. Clinical classification and analysis of 97 cases of lung abscess. Am Rev Respir Dis 1969;99:390–398.

89. Pohlson EC, McNamara JJ, Char C, Kurata L. Lung abscess: A changing pattern of disease. Am J Surg 1985;150:97–101.

90. Pryce DM. The lining of healed but persistent abscess cavities in the lung with epithelium of the ciliated columnar type. J Pathol Bacteriol 1948;60:259–264.

91. Weiss W. Cavity behavior in acute, primary nonspecific lung abscess. Am Rev Respir Dis 1973;108:1273–1275.

92. Bernhard WF, Malcolm JA, Wylie RH. The carcinomatous abscess: A clinical paradox. N Engl J Med 1962;266:914–919.

93. Maxwell J. Lung abscess, with special reference to causation and treatment. QJ Med 1934;3:467–522.

94. Connors JP, Roper CL, Ferguson TB. Transbronchial catheterization of pulmonary abscess. Ann Thorac Surg 1975;19:254–260.

95. Nakao MA. "Pseudoabscess" of the lung—misinterpretation of a novel piece of medical apparatus. Crit Care Med 1990;18:248.

96. Lord FT. Certain aspects of pulmonary abscess from analysis of 227 cases. Boston Med Surg J 1925;192: 785–788.

97. Sweet RH. Analysis of Massachusetts General Hospital cases of lung abscess from 1938 through 1942. Surg Gynecol Obstet 1945;80:568–574.

98. Jennings GH. Reexpansion of atelectatic lower lobe and disappearance of bronchiectasis. Br Med J 1937; 2:963–965.

99. Blades B, Duncan DJ. Pseudobronchiectasis. J Thorac Surg 1944;13:40–48.

100. Opie EL. The pathologic anatomy of influenza. Based chiefly on American and British sources. Arch Pathol 1928;5:285–303.

101. Bachman AL, Hewitt WR, Beekley HC. Bronchiectasis: A bronchographic study of 60 cases of pneumonia. Arch Intern Med 1953;91:78–96.

102. Pontius JR, Jacobs LG. The reversal of advanced bronchiectasis. Radiology 1957;68:204–208.

103. Nelson SW, Christoforidis A. Reversible bronchiectasis. Radiology 1958;72:375–382.

104. Smith KR, Morris JF. Reversible bronchial dilatation: A report of a case. Dis Chest 1962;42:652–656.

105. Whitwell F. Study of pathology and pathogenesis of bronchiectasis. Thorax 1952;7:213–239.

106. Ogilvie AG. The natural history of bronchiectasis. A clinical, roentgenologic and pathologic study. Arch Intern Med 1941;68:395–465.

107. Perry KMA, King DS. Bronchiectasis: A study of prognosis based on a follow-up of 400 cases. Am Rev Tuberc 1940;41:531–548.

108. Graham EA, Singer JJ, Balcon HC. Surgical diseases of the chest. Philadelphia: Lea and Febiger, 1935.

109. Glenn WWL, Liebow AA, Lindskog GE. Thoracic and cardiovascular surgery with related pathology. 3d Ed. New York: Appleton-Century-Crofts, 1975;183–203.

110. Spencer H. Pathology of the lung. 4th Ed. Oxford: Pergamon, 1985:147–165.

111. Thurlbeck WM. Chronic airflow obstruction in lung disease. Philadelphia: Saunders, 1976:60–73.

112. Reid IM. Reduction in bronchial subdivision in bronchiectasis. Thorax 1950;5:233–247.

113. Thurlbeck WM. Chronic airflow obstruction. In: Thurlbeck WM, ed. Pathology of the lung. New York: Thieme, 1988:519–575.

114. Davis AL. Bronchiectasis. In: Fishman AD, ed. Pulmonary diseases and disorders. New York: McGraw-Hill, 1980:1209–1219.

115. Baum GL, Hershko EP. Bronchiectasis. In: Baum GL, Wolinsky E, eds. Textbook of pulmonary diseases. 3d Ed. Boston: Little Brown, 1983:615–633.

116. Katzenstein A-L A, Askin FB. Surgical pathology of non-neoplastic lung disease. Philadelphia: Saunders, 1982:392–395.

117. Boyd GL. Bronchiectasis in children. Can Med Assoc J 1931;25:174–182.

118. Erb IH. Pathology of bronchiectasis. Arch Pathol 1933;15:357–386.

119. Robinson WL. Bronchiectasis: Study of pathology of 16 surgical lobectomies for bronchiectasis. Br J Surg 1933;21:302–312.

120. Warner WP. Factors causing bronchiectasis: Their clinical application to diagnosis and treatment. JAMA 1935;105:1666–1670.

121. Lisa JR, Rosenblatt MB. Bronchiectasis. New York: Oxford, 1943.

122. Kenney WM. Bronchiectasis: A neglected disease. Dis Chest 1947;13:33–47.

123. Fine A, Baum GL. Long-term follow-up of bronchiectasis. J Lancet 1966;85:505–507.

124. Barker AF, Bardana EJ, Jr. Bronchiectasis: Update of an orphan disease. Am Rev Respir Dis 1988;137:969–978.

125. Opie EL, Freeman AW, Blake FG, Small JC, Rivers TM. Pneumonia following influenza (at Camp Pike,

Ark). JAMA 1919;72:556–565.

126. Crofton J. Respiratory tract disease. Diagnosis and treatment of bronchiectasis. I. Diagnosis. Br Med J 1966;1:721–723.

127. Crofton J. Respiratory tract disease. Bronchiectasis. II. Treatment and prevention. Br Med J 1966;1:783–785.

128. MacFarlane PS, Sommerville RG. Non-tuberculous juvenile bronchiectasis: A viral disease? Lancet 1957; i:770–771.

129. Becroft DM. Bronchiolitis obliterans, bronchiectasis, and other sequelae of adenovirus 21 infections in young children. J Clin Pathol 1971;24:72–82.

130. Datau G, Icart J, Delsol G. Bronchiectasies secondaires a une adénovirose: Étude radiologique, virologique et anatomique d'une observation. Rev Fr Mal Respir 1977;5:533–542.

131. Laraya-Cuasay LR, DeForest A, Huff D, Lischner H, Huang NN. Chronic pulmonary complications of early influenza virus infection in children. Am Rev Respir Dis 1977;116:617–625.

132. Simila S, Linna O, Lanning P, Heikkinen E, Ala-Houhala M. Chronic lung damage caused by adenovirus type 7: A ten-year follow-up study. Chest 1981;80:127–131.

133. Glauser EM, Cook CD, Harris GBC. Bronchiectasis: A review of 187 cases in children with follow-up pulmonary function studies in 58. Acta Paediatr Scand [Suppl] 1966;165:1–16.

134. Kass I, Zamel N, Dobry CA, Hulzer M. Bronchiectasis following ammonia burns of the respiratory tract: A review of two cases. Chest 1972;62:282–285.

135. Sobonya R. Fatal anhydrous ammonia inhalation. Hum Pathol 1977;8:293–299.

136. Hoeffler HB, Schweppe I, Greenberg SD. Bronchiectasis following pulmonary ammonia burn. Arch Pathol Lab Med 1982;106:686–687.

137. Slutzker AD, Kinn R, Said SI. Bronchiectasis and progressive respiratory failure following smoke inhalation. Chest 1989;95:1349–1350.

138. Liebow AA, Hales MR, Lindskog GE. Enlargement of the bronchial arteries and their anastomoses with the pulmonary arteries in bronchiectasis. Am J Pathol 1949;25:211–231.

139. Culiner MM. The right middle lobe syndrome, a nonobstructive complex. Dis Chest 1966;50:57–66.

140. Inners CR, Terry PB, Traystman RJ, Menkes HA. Collateral ventilation and the right middle lobe syndrome. Am Rev Respir Dis 1978;118:305–310.

141. Banyai AL. The middle lobe syndrome and its quasi variants. Chest 1974;65:135.

142. Lloyd JJ. Broncholiths. Am J Med Sci 1930;179:694–699.

143. Bech K. Broncholithiasis. Nord Med 1946;30:810–812.

144. Schmidt HW, Clagett OT, McDonald JR. Broncholithiasis. J Thorac Surg 1950;19:226–245.

145. Arrigoni MG, Bernatz PE, Donaghue FE. Broncholithiasis. J Thorac Cardiovasc Surg 1971;62:231–237.

146. Faber LP, Jensik RJ, Chawla SK, Kittle CF. The surgical implication of broncholithiases. J Thorac Cardiovasc Surg 1975;70:779–789.

147. Kelly WA. Bronchiolithiasis. Postgrad Med 1979;66: 81–90.

148. Igoe D, Lynch V, McNicholas WT. Bronchiolithasis: Bronchioscopic vs. surgical management. Respir Med 1990;80:163–165.

149. Weed LA, Anderson HA. Etiology of bronchiolithiasis. Chest 1960;37:270–277.

150. Hirschfield LS, Graver LM, Isenberg HD. Bronchiolithiasis due to *Histoplasma capsulatum* subsequently infected by *Actinomyces*. Chest 1989;96:218–219.

151. Sartorelli E. Letter: Broncholithiasis is silicosis. Am Rev Respir Dis 1974;105:687.

152. Cahill BC, Harmon KR, Shumway SJ, Mickman JR, Hertz MI. Tracheobronchial obstruction due to silicosis. Am Rev Respir Dis 1992;145:719–721.

153. Conces DJ, Jr., Tarver RD, Vix VA. Bronchiolithiasis: CT features in 15 patients. AJR 1991;157:249–253.

154. Carasso B, Couropmitree C, Heredia R. Egg-shell silicotic calcification causing bronchoesophageal fistula. Am Rev Respir Dis 1973;108:1384–1387.

155. Davis EW, Katz S, Peabody JW. Broncholithiasis: A neglected cause of bronchoesophageal fistula. JAMA 1956;160:555–557.

156. Anderson RP, Sabiston DC Jr. Acquired bronchoesophageal fistula of benign origin. Surg Gynecol Obstet 1965;121:261–266.

157. Kutty CP, Carstens SA, Funahashi A. Traction diverticula of the esophagus in the middle lobe syndrome. Can Med Assoc J 1981;124:1320–1322.

158. Shin MS, Berland LL, Myers JL, Clary G, Zorn GL. CT demonstration of an ossifying bronchial carcinoid simulating broncholithiasis. AJR 1989;153:51–52.

159. Lemire P, Trepanier A, Hebert G. Bronchiolcele and blocked bronchiectasis. Am J Roentgenol Radium Ther Nucl Med 1970;110:687–693.

160. Talner LB, Gmelich JT, Liebow AA, Greenspan RH. The syndrome of bronchial mucocele and regional hyperinflation of the lung. AJR 1970;110:675–686.

161. Mayer E, Rappaport A. Developmental origin of cystic, bronchiectatic and emphysematous changes in lungs; new concept. Dis Chest 1952;21:146–160.

162. Tsuji S, Heki S, Kobara Y, Sato A. The syndrome of bronchial mucocele and regional hyperinflation of lung: Report of four cases. Chest 1973;64:444–447.

163. Curry TS, III, Curry GC. Atresia of bronchus to apical posterior segment of left upper lobe. AJR 1966;98: 350–353.

164. Ramsay H, Byron F., Mucocele, congenital bronchiectasis and bronchogenic cyst. J Thoracic Surg 1953;26:21–30.

165. St-Georges R, Deslauriers J, Duranceau A, et al. Clinical spectrum of bronchogenic cysts of the mediastinum and lung in the adult. Ann Thorac Surg 1991;52:6–13.

166. Keal EE. Biochemistry and rheology of sputum in asthma. Postgrad Med J 1971;47:171–177.

167. Hartley PHS, Davies J. A case of pituitous catarrh. Br Med J 1923;1:1052–1053.

168. Calin A. Bronchorrhea. Br Med J 1972;4:274–275.

169. Crofton J, Douglas A. Respiratory diseases. Oxford: Blackwell, 1981.

170. Spiro SG, Lopez-Vidriero MT, Charmann J, Das I, Reid L. Bronchorrhea in a case of alveolar cell carcinoma. J Clin Pathol 1975;28:60–65.

171. So SY, Lam WK, Sham MK. Bronchorrhoea—a presenting feature of active endobronchial tuberculosis. Chest 1983;84:635–636.

172. Chan HS, Pang J. Relapsing polychrondritis presenting with bronchorrhea. Respir Med 1990;84:341–343.

173. Elborn JS, Shale DJ, Britton JR. Cystic fibrosis: Current survival and population estimates to the year 2000. Thorax 1991;46:881–885.

174. di Sant' Agnese PA, Davis PB. Cystic fibrosis in adults: 75 cases and a review of 343 cases in the literature. Am J Med 1979;66:121–132.

175. Smith MB, Hardin WD, Dressel DA, Beckerman RC, Moynihan PC. Predicting outcome following pulmonary resection in cystic fibrosis patients. J Pediatr Surg 1991;26:655–659.

176. Bhalla M, Turcios N, Aponte V, et al. Cystic fibrosis: Scoring system with thin-section CT. Radiology 1991;179:783–788.

177. Esterly JR, Oppenheimer EH. Observations in cystic fibrosis of the pancreas. 3. Pulmonary Lesions. Johns Hopkins Med J 1968;122:94–101.

178. Bedrossian CWM, Greenberg SD, Singer DB, Hansen JJ, Rosenberg HS. The lung in cystic fibrosis: A quantitative study including prevalence of pathologic findings among different age groups. Hum Pathol 1976; 7:195–204.

179. McGlennen RC, Burke BA, Dehner LD. Systemic amyloidosis complicating cystic fibrosis. Arch Pathol Lab Med 1986;110:879–884.

180. Tomashefski JF, Jr., Konstan MW, Bruce MC, Abramowsky CR. The pathologic characteristics of interstitial pneumonia in cystic fibrosis: A retrospective autopsy study. Am J Clin Pathol 1989;91:522–530.

181. Tomashefski JF, Jr., Thomassen MJ, Bruce MC, Goldberg HI, Konstan MW, Stern RC. *Pseudomonas cepacia*-associated pneumonia in cystic fibrosis. Relation of clinical features to histopathologic patterns of pneumonia. Arch Pathol Lab Med 1988;112:166–172.

182. Glenn WWL, Liebow AA, Lindskog GE. Thoracic and cardiovascular surgery with related pathology. 3d Ed. New York: Appleton-Century-Crofts, 1975:85–117.

183. Verbeken EK, Demedts M, Vanwing J, Deneffe G, Lauweryns JM. Pulmonary phospholipid accumulation distal to an obstructed bronchus. Arch Pathol Lab Med 1981;113:886–890.

184. Ackerman LV, Elliott GV, Alanis M. Localized organizing pneumonia: Its resemblance to carcinoma. A review of its clinical, roentgenographic and pathologic features. AJR 1954;71:988–996.

185. Floyd R. Organization of pneumonic exudates. Am J Med Sci 1922;163:527–548.

186. Robbins LL, Sniffen RC. Correlation between the roentgenologic and pathologic findings in chronic pneumonitis of the cholesterol type. Radiology 1949; 53:187–202.

187. Lawler W. Idiopathic cholesterol pneumonitis. Histopathology 1977;1:385–395.

188. Hefflefinger SC, Weilbaecher DG, Lawrence EC, Johnson EH, Greenberg DS. Xanthromatous bronchiolitis obliterans with cholesterol pneumonia. Arch Pathol Lab Med 1988;112:650–653.

189. Bulmer SR, Lamb D, McCormack RJM, Walbaum PR. Aetiology of unresolved pneumonia. Thorax 1978; 33:307–314.

190. Swyer PR, James GCW. A case of unilateral pulmonary emphysema. Thorax 1953;8:133–136.

191. MacLeod WM. Abnormal transradiancy of one lung. Thorax 1954;9:147–153.

192. Moore ADA, Godwin JD, Dietrich PA, Verschakelen JA, Henderson WR, Jr. Swyer–James syndrome: CT findings in eight patients. AJR 1992;158:1211–1215.

192a. Moore ADA, Godwin JD, Dietrich PA, Verschakelen JA, Henderson WR, Jr. Swyer–James syndrome: CT findings in eight patients. AJR 1992;158:1211–1215.

193. Epler GR, Colby TV, McLoud TC, Carrington CB, Gaensler EA. Bronchiolitis obliterans organizing pneumonia. N Engl J Med 1985;312:152–158.

194. Myers JL, Katzenstein A-LA. Ultrastructural evidence of alveolar epithelial injury in idiopathic bronchiolitis obliterans-organizing pneumonia. Am J Pathol 1988; 132:102–109.

195. Kargi HA, Kuhn C. Bronchiolitis obliterans: Unilateral obliterans of the lumen of bronchi with atelectasis. Chest 1988;93:1107–1108.

196. Azizird H, Polzar G, Brons PF, Chatten J. Bronchiolitis obliterans. Clin Pediatr 1975;14:572–584.

197. Tsunoda N, Iwanaga T, Saito T, Kitamura S, Saito K. Rapidly progressive bronchiolitis obliterans associated with Stevens–Johnson syndrome. Chest 1990;98:243–245.

198. Yamanaka A, Maeda M, Yamamoto R. Bronchobronchiolitis obliterans. Jpn J Chest Dis 1986;45:540–554.

199. Katzenstein A-L A, Askin FB. Surgical pathology of non-neoplastic lung disease. Philadelphia: Saunders, 1982:349–356.

200. Geddes DM, Corrin B, Brewerton DA, Davies RJ, Turner-Warwick M. Progressive airway obliteration in adults and its association with rheumatoid disease. QJ Med 1977;46:427–444.

201. Murphy KC, Atkins CJ, Offer RC, Hugg JC, Stein HB. Obliterative bronchiolitis in two rheumatoid arthritis patients treated with penicillamine. Arthritis Rheum 1981;24:557–560.

202. Link H, Reinhard D, Neithammer D. Obstructive ventilation disorders as a severe complication of chronic graft-versus-host disease after bone marrow transplantation. Exp Hematol 1982;10:92–93.

203. Roca J, Granena A, Rodriguez-Roisin J, Alvarez P, Agusti-Vidal A, Rozman C. Fatal airway disease in an adult with chronic graft-versus-host disease. Thorax 1982;37:77–78.

204. Ralph DD, Springmeyer SC, Sullivan KM. Rapidly progressive airflow obstruction in marrow transplant

recipients: possible association between obliterative bronchiolitis and graft-versus-host disease. Am Rev Respir Dis 1984;129:641–643.

205. Ostrow D, Buskard N, Hill RS, Vickars L, Churg A. Bronchiolitis obliterans complicating bone marrow transplantation. Chest 1985;87:828–830.

206. Burke CM, Theodore J, Dawkins KD, et al. Post-transplant obliterative bronchiolitis and other late sequelae in human heart-lung transplantation. Chest 1984;86:824–829.

207. Allen JN, Wewers MD. HIV-associated bronchiolitis obliterans organizing pneumonia. Chest 1989;96:197–198.

208. Kaufman J, Komorowski R. Bronchiolitis obliterans: A new clinical-pathologic complication of irradiation pneumonitis. Chest 1990;97:1243–1244.

209. Hardy KA, Schidlow DV, Zaeri N. Obliterative bronchiolitis in children. Chest 1988;93:460–466.

210. King TE, Jr. Bronchiolitis obliterans. Lung 1989;167:69–93.

211. Cordier J-F, Loire R, Brune J. Idiopathic bronchiolitis obliterans organizing pneumonia. Definition of characteristic clinical profiles in a series of 16 patients. Chest 1989;96:999–1004.

212. Gosink BB, Friedman PJ, Liebow AA. Bronchiolitis obliterans: Roentgenologic-pathologic correlations. AJR 1973;117:816–832.

213. Randhawa P, Hoaglund MH, Yousem SA. Diffuse panbronchiolitis in North America: Report of three cases and review of the literature. Am J Surg Pathol 1991;15:43–47.

214. Poletti V, Patelli M, Poletti G, Bertanti T, Spiga L. Diffuse panbronchiolitis observed in an Italian. Chest 1990;98:515–576.

215. Akira M, Kitatani F, Yong-Sik L, et al. Diffuse panbronchiolitis: Evaluation with high-resolution CT. Radiology 1988;168:433–438.

216. Homma H, Yamanaka A, Tanimoto S, et al. Diffuse panbronchiolitis: A disease of the transitional zone of the lung. Chest 1983;83:63–69.

217. Desai SJ, Gephardt GN, Stoller JK. Diffuse panbronchiolitis preceding ulcerative colitis. Chest 1989;45:1342–1344.

218. Saito S, Mori M, Kawamura O, Umegai T, Kurosawa M, Kobayashi S. A case of allergic granulomatosis angiitis (Churg-Strauss) associated with diffuse panbronchiolitis [in Japanese]. Nippon Naika Gakkai Zasshi 1988;77:445–446.

219. Ono K, Shimamoto Y, Matsuzaki M, et al. Diffuse panbronchiolitis as a pulmonary complication with adult T cell leukemia. Am J Hematol 1989;30:86–90.

situ after detorsion (letter). J Thorac Cardiovasc Surg 1990;99:1112–1114.

229. Ghio AJ, Elliott G, Crapo RO, Collins MP, Tocino I. A migratory infiltrate in a patient with hemoptysis and chest pain. Chest 1989;96:195–196.

230. Shirakusa T, Motonaga R, Takada S, Sakuragi T, Dan K. Lung lobe torsion following lobectomy. Am Surg 1990;56:639–642.

231. Phillips LG, Rao KVS. Gangrene of the lung. J Thorac Cardiovasc Surg 1989;97:114–118.

232. Osler W. Gangrene of the lung. In: The principles and practice of medicine. 5th Ed. New York: Appleton, 1984:660–662.

233. O'Reilly GV, Dee PM, Otteni GV. Gangrene of the lung: Successful medical management of three patients. Radiology 1978;126:575–579.

234. Juettner FM, Arian-Schad K, Kraus I, Gallofer G, Popper H, Friehs G. Total unilateral lung gangrene in Hodgkin's disease: Treatment by thoracostomy. Am Thorac Surg 1991;51:302–303.

220. Mimura T, Yoshimura K, Nakamori Y, Nakata K, Tanimoto H. Non Hodgkin lymphoma associated with diffuse panbronchiolitis [in Japanese; abstract in English]. Nippon Kyobu Shikkan Gakkai Zasshi 1987;25:1211–1218.

221. Chonabayashi N, Yoahimura K, Nakatani T, Nakamori Y, Nakata K, Tanimoto H. Prognosis of diffuse panbronchiolitis [in Japanese; abstract in English]. Nippon Kyobu Shikkan Gakkai Zasshi 1986;245:1088–1095.

222. Danbara T, Matsuoka R, Nukiwa T, Natori H, Arai T, Kira S. Familial occurrence of diffuse panbronchiolitis accompanied by evolution of cold agglutinin titer in a father and his two daughters [in Japanese;abstract in English]. Nippon Kyobu Shikkan Gakkai Zasshi 1982;20:597–603.

223. Sugiyama Y, Takeuchi K, Yotsumoto H, Takaku F. A case of diffuse panbronchiolitis in a second generation Korean male [in Japanese; abstract in English]. Nippon Kyobu Shikkan Gakkai Zasshi 1986;24:183–187.

224. Sugiyama Y, Kudoh S, Maeda H, Suzaki H, Takaku F. Analysis of HLA antigens in patients with *diffuse panbronchiolitis*. Am Rev Respir Dis 1990;141:1459–1462.

225. Ichikawa Y, Koga H, Tanaka M, Nakamura M, Tokunaga N, Kaji M. Neutrophilia in bronchoalveolar lavage. Chest 1990;98:917–923.

226. Izumi T. Diffuse panbronchiolitis. Chest 1991;100:596–597.

227. Jamieson WG, Lansing AM. Bacteriological studies in pulmonary atelectasis. Arch Surg 1963;87:200–204.

228. Fu J-J, Chen C-L, Wu J-Y. Lung torsion: Survival of a patient whose hemorrhagic infarcted lung remained in

CHAPTER 6

Introduction to AIDS Pathology

DAVID H. DAIL

Acquired immunodeficiency syndrome (AIDS) was first described in the United States in 1981[1–3] following several unusual outbreaks of community-acquired *Pneumocystis* pneumonia in homosexual men. This disease has now become a terror known around the world, and much has been learned about it in the short time since its original description. The medical literature and lay press daily add voluminous amounts of literature, often repetitive and often prematurely hopeful. Politicians are faced with the need for greater and greater commitments toward attempts at preventing or curing this disease. Its terrible toll, often on individuals in the prime of their lives including working men and women, mothers, and children, its (so far) universal fatality, its increasing drain on health care resources—financial, workforce, and facilities—and its increasing spread are all well known.

This chapter serves as an introduction to discussions of AIDS pathology elsewhere in this volume. The reader is referred specifically to Chapter 8, **Acquired Neonatal Pediatric Diseases;** the infection group, including Chapter 9, **Bacterial,** Chapter 10, **Mycobacterial,** Chapter 11, **Fungal,** Chapter 12, **Viral,** Chapter 14 **Pneumocystis,** and Chapter 15, **Parasitic.** Chapter 31, **Lymphoproliferative Disorders,** and Chapter 33, **Uncommon Lung Tumors,** provide further detail, and non-AIDS immunosuppressive diseases are further addressed in Chapter 1, **Tissue Handling.** Chapter 23, **Iatrogenic Injury,** and Chapter 24, **Transplantation Pathology,** complement discussions of immunosuppressive disorders. The few illustrations in this chapter are intended to complement and not to duplicate those offered in other chapters, but some overlap in both illustration and discussion is inevitable.

As is also well known, attempts at preventing the spread of AIDS have been unsuccessful. Currently, it is estimated that in the United States 0.02%–0.04% of random blood donors are human immunodeficiency virus (HIV) positive and that 1.5% of civilian recruits to military service are so involved.[4] Several other prevalence studies have found a 3% HIV positivity rate in critically ill patients in emergency rooms who were not previously known to be HIV positive.[5] Within high-risk groups, it has been estimated that 50% of drug abusers, 65% of San Francisco homosexual men, and 70% of hemophiliacs requiring Factor VIII transfusions are HIV positive. In several cohort studies of male HIV-positive homosexuals in San Francisco,[4,6] 15% are diagnosed with AIDS by 60 months, 24% by 72 months, and 36% by 88 months after becoming HIV positive. Of the San Francisco group with HIV for at least 11 years,[6] 49% have died, 10% have AIDS, 19% have AIDS-related complex, 3% have persistent generalized lymphadenopathy, and 19% remain symptom free.

Several significant studies offer some horrifying predictions as to AIDS spread in the 1990s. A new study by 30 epidemiologists conducted through Harvard University, which is not yet published although abstracts are available, offers somewhat higher predictions than those currently offered by the World Health Organization (WHO).[7] According to this study, about 2.6 million people worldwide were expected to have AIDS (WHO estimate, 1.5 million) and 13 million to be HIV positive (WHO estimate, 9–11 million) by 1992. By the year 2000 as many as 120 million will be HIV positive (WHO estimate, 30–40 million) and by then 24 million adults and several million children will have AIDS. The percentage of women with AIDS will rise from 25% in 1990 to 40% in the year 2000. In the 1990s, mothers or both parents of more than 1 million children will have died of HIV infection/AIDS.[8]

No country will escape the AIDS epidemic. Since

Table 6–1. 1987 Revision of case definition for AIDS for surveillance purposes[a]

For national reporting, a case of AIDS is defined as an illness characterized by one or more of the following "indicator" diseases, depending on the status of laboratory evidence of HIV infection, as shown below.

I. Without laboratory evidence regarding HIV infection: If laboratory tests for HIV were not performed or gave inconclusive results and the patient had no other cause of immunodeficiency listed in Section I.A, below, then any disease listed in Section I.B indicates AIDS if it was diagnosed by a definitive method.

  A. Causes of immunodeficiency that disqualify diseases as indicators of AIDS in the absence of laboratory evidence for HIV infection.

    1. High-dose or long-term systemic corticosteroid therapy or other immunosuppressive-cytotoxic therapy $\leq$3 months before the onset of the indicator disease.

    2. Any of the following diseases diagnosed $\leq$3 months after diagnosis of the indicator disease: Hodgkins' disease, non-Hodgkin's lymphoma (other than primary brain lymphoma), lymphocytic leukemia, multiple myeloma, any other cancer of lymphoreticular or histiocytic tissue, or angioimmunoblastic lymphadenopathy.

    3. A genetic (congenital) immunodeficiency syndrome or an acquired immunodeficiency syndrome atypical of HIV infection, such as one involving hypogammaglobulinemia.

  B. Indicator diseases diagnosed definitively.

    1. Candidiasis of the esophagus, trachea, bronchi, or lungs.

    2. Cryptococcosis, extrapulmonary.

    3. Cryptosporidiosis with diarrhea persisting >1 month.

    4. Cytomegalovirus disease of an organ other than liver, spleen, or lymph nodes in a patient >1 month of age.

    5. Herpes simplex virus infection causing a mucocutaneous ulcer that persists longer than >1 month; or bronchitis, pneumonitis, or esophagitis for any duration affecting a patient >1 month of age.

    6. Kaposi's sarcoma affecting a patient <60 years of age.

    7. Lymphoma of the brain (primary) affecting a patient >60 years of age.

    8. Lymphoid interstitial pneumonia and/or pulmonary lymphoid hyperplasia (LIP/PLH complex) affecting a child <13 years of age.

    9. *Mycobacterium avium* complex or *M. kansasii* disease, disseminated (at a site other than or in addition to lungs, skin, or cervical or hilar lymph nodes).

    10. *Pneumocystis carinii* pneumonia.

    11. Progressive multifocal leukoencephalopathy.

    12. Toxoplasmosis of the brain affecting a patient >1 month of age.

II. With laboratory evidence for HIV infection: Regardless of the presence of other causes of immunodeficiency (I.A.), in the presence of laboratory evidence for HIV infection any disease listed above (I.B.) or below (II.A or II.B) indicates a diagnosis of AIDS

  A. Indicator diseases diagnosed definitively.

    1. Bacterial infections, multiple or recurrent (any combination of at least two within a 2-year period), of the following types affecting a child <13 years of age: septicemia, pneumonia, meningitis, bone or joint infection, or abscess of an internal organ or body cavity (excluding otitis media or superficial skin or mucosal abscesses), caused by *Haemophilus*, *Streptococcus* (including *Pneumococcus*), or other pyogenic bacteria.

    2. Coccidioidomycosis, disseminated (at a site other than or in addition to lungs or cervical or hilar lymph nodes).

    3. HIV encephalopathy (also called HIV dementia, AIDS dementia, or subacute encephalitis due to HIV).

    4. Histoplasmosis, disseminated (at a site other than or in addition to lungs or cervical or hilar lymph nodes).

    5. Isosporiasis with diarrhea persisting >1 month.

    6. Kaposi's sarcoma at any age.

    7. Lymphoma of the brain (primary) at any age.

    8. Other non-Hodgkin's lymphoma of B-cell or unknown immunologic phenotype and the following histologic types:

      a. Small noncleaved lymphoma (either Burkitt or non-Burkitt type).

      b. Immunoblastic sarcoma (equivalent to any of the following, although not necessarily all in combination: immunoblastic lymphoma, large-cell lymphoma, diffuse histiocytic lymphoma, diffuse undifferentiated lymphoma, or high-grade lymphoma).

      NOTE: Lymphomas are not included here if they are of T-cell immunologic phenotype or their histologic type is not described or is described as "lymphocytic," "lymphoblastic," or "small cleaved," or "plasmacytoid lymphocytic."

    9. Any mycobacterial disease caused by mycobacteria other than *M. tuberculosis*, disseminated (at a site other than or in addition to lungs, skin, or cervical or hilar lymph nodes).

    10. Disease caused by *M. tuberculosis*, extrapulmonary (involving at least one site outside the lungs, regardless of whether there is concurrent pulmonary involvement).

    11. Salmonella (nontyphoid) septicemia, recurrent.

    12. HIV wasting syndrome (emaciation, "slim disease").

  B. Indicator diseases diagnosed presumptively (without histopathology or culture).

    1. Candidiasis of the esophagus.

    2. Cytomegalovirus retinitis with loss of vision.

    3. Kaposi's sarcoma.

    4. Lymphoid interstitial pneumonia and/or pulmonary lymphoid hyperplasia (LIP/PLH complex) affecting a child <13 years of age.

Table 6–1. *Continued*

    5. Mycobacterial disease (acid-fast bacilli with species not identified by culture), disseminated (involving at least one site other than or in addition to lungs, skin, or cervical or hilar lymph nodes).

    6. *Pneumocystis carinii* pneumonia.

    7. Toxoplasmosis of the brain affecting a patient >1 month of age.

III. With laboratory evidence against HIV infection: With laboratory test results negative for HIV infection a diagnosis of AIDS for surveillance purposes is ruled out unless:

    A. All the other causes of immunodeficiency listed above, in Sec. I.A, are excluded and

    B. The patient has had either:

        1. *Pneumocystis carinii* pneumonia diagnosed by a definitive method or

        2. a. Any of the other diseases indicative of AIDS listed above in Sec. I.B diagnosed by a definitive method and

            b. A T-helper/inducer (CD4) lymphocyte count <400 per cubic millimeter.

a Source: Centers for Disease Control. MMWR (Suppl. 1S)36:3S–15S, 1987.

1985, the number of HIV-infected individuals in Africa alone has tripled and was expected to be over 7.5 million by 1992. The infection is spreading explosively in Asia, and it is predicted that by the year 2000, 42% of the total HIV-positive population in the world will reside in Asia, surpassing 31% in sub-Saharan Africa.[7] In fact, 90% of HIV-positives are predicted to be in developing countries, specifically sub-Sahara Africa, Southeast Asia, Latin America, and the Caribbean.[8] The amount of money per year per resident currently being invested in these areas to prevent AIDS is estimated (in U.S. dollars) to be $2.70 in North America, $1.18 in Europe, $.07 in Africa, and $.03 in Latin America![7]

In the United States, the Centers for Disease Control (CDC) have carefully followed the AIDS epidemic and have helped organize criteria and disseminate information. The 1987 list of index diagnoses for AIDS (Table 6–1)[4,9] includes infectious and noninfectious categories. The predominant virus so far described is HIV-1, but HIV-2[10] is just now being described and appears to function in much the same way in the human host. It would be expected that other serotypes of HIV and perhaps other non-HIV but similar viruses will be discovered in the future that can also cause profound immunosuppression with many of the same effects as listed in Table 6–1. Not all items listed in Table 6–1 are of equal importance; for example, *Pneumocystis* pneumonia (PCP) is the AIDS-defining diagnosis in 65% of cases.[11] The CDC has also recently expanded its surveillance to include HIV-infected people with evidence of severe immunosuppression, specifically CD4+ lymphocyte counts of less than 200 per micrometer (0.2 × 10⁹/liter).[12,13] As HIV infection primarily affects the T-lymphocyte helper cells (CD4+), this is reasonable, Farizo et al.[12] noted that of 7,634 HIV-positive individuals receiving health care, 2 additional persons needed care for each 1 meeting the AIDS criteria. Moss et al.[14] has shown linear deterioration in HIV-infected CD4+ cells during a 3-year period of observation; the cell counts

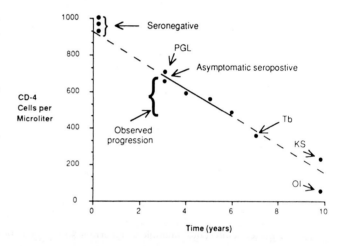

Fig. 6–1. Progressive decline in CD4+ lymphocytes with time in patients with human immunodeficiency virus (HIV) infection. Data represented by *solid line* are from Moss et al. Br Med J 1988;296:745–750. Extrapolation and other data are from Hopewell PC. Semin Respir Infect 1989;4:73–74. PGL, progressive generalized lymphadenopathy; Tb, tuberculosis; KS, Kaposi's sarcoma; OI, opportunistic infection.

deteriorated approximately 65–70 cells per year, as was nicely illustrated by Hopewell (Fig. 6–1).[15] This rather linear effect helps clinicians estimate longevity of infection and prospects for the future, specifically the time and the course of disease. Some exceptions of course occur, and it should be emphasized that although the slope of the terminal portion of the CD4+ cell deterioration is not known with assurance, this is the time when many infections and malignancies occur.

The interested reader is referred, in addition to discussions elsewhere in this volume, to some excellent reviews and large series: the general aspects of AIDS by Ioachim[16] and Garay,[4] clinical aspects by White and Stover,[17] Stover et al.,[18] and Murray and associates,[19,20] opportunistic infections in chest by Murray and

Table 6–2. Differential diagnosis of commonly observed chest radiographic patterns in patients with HIV infection[a]

Pattern	Diseases
Diffuse reticulonodular infiltration	*Pneumocystis carinii* pneumonia
	Disseminated tuberculosis
	Disseminated histoplasmosis
	Disseminated coccidioidomycosis
	Lymphocytic interstitial pneumonitis
Focal airspace consolidation	Bacterial pneumonia
	Kaposi's sarcoma
	Cryptococcosis
Normal	*Pneumocystis carinii* pneumonia
	Disseminated *Mycobacterium avium* complex
	Disseminated histoplasmosis
Adenopathy	Tuberculosis
	Kaposi's sarcoma
	Disseminated *Mycobacterium avium* complex
	Non-Hodgkin's lymphoma
Pleural effusion	Kaposi's sarcoma
	Tuberculosis
	Non-Hodgkin's lymphoma
	Pyogenic empyema

[a] From Murray JF, Mills JL. Am Rev Respir Dis 1990;141:1356–1372, with permission.

Mills,[21,22] noninfectious involvement by White and Matthay,[23] general and radiologic review by McLoud and Naidich,[24] and pulmonary pathology by Gal,[25] with autopsy pathology findings by Guarda et al.,[26] Moskowitz et al.,[27] Welch et al.,[28] Niedt and Schinella,[29] Marchevsky et al.[30] Wallace and Hannah,[31] and McKenzie et al.[32] Mitchell[33] and Mitchell and Miller[34] have provided recent reviews in the British literature. Radiographic chest patterns may overlap (Table 6–2).

The pulmonary system has a high incidence of involvement in AIDS, in one series,[18] 8% of AIDS cases presented with pulmonary involvement and eventually 47% were so involved. In another multicenter study,[19] 41% of cases had significant pulmonary abnormalities, and *Pneumocystis carinii* pneumonia (PCP) represented an index diagnosis for AIDS in 67% of cases.[11] It is not clear why AIDS infections center on the lung,[4] but several have suggested that the lungs represent a source of reactivation and, being in contact with the environment, often also represent the source of a new infection. AIDS patients often associate or commune with other AIDS cases, and transmission of infections within immunosuppressed high-risk groups is likely. In the latter situation, tuberculosis may be the main, and perhaps only, such truly communicable disease in AIDS (see following).[35]

Many of the aspects of infectious and noninfectious complications of AIDS have been described in other immunosuppressed situations preceding the onset of the AIDS epidemic. However, AIDS has certainly refocused attention on these conditions, and their prevalence in many cases appears to be greater than those seen in non-AIDS immunosuppression. This is perhaps caused more profound degree of immunosuppression in AIDS than in other conditions, and as current therapies prolong the course of AIDS, it is predicted that there will be more unusual or atypical manifestations of these diseases.[22] It is common for multiple infectious and noninfectious complications of AIDS to occur (see Table 6–1) either sequentially or concurrently, and many of the infections are recurrent and often are never truly cured. Also, therapies vary in effectiveness and have a higher incidence of adverse reactions, probably because polyclonal disorders are associated with malregulation of B lymphocytes, by deficient T lymphocytes.[36–42] We are destined to learn more about the effects of immunosuppression, host responses, and oncogenesis through the AIDS epidemic, but at a terrible price. The most common cause of death in AIDS is related to respiratory tract involvement, which is estimated to occur in 50% of cases.[27,32]

The following discussions center first on infections in AIDS and are followed by noninfectious AIDS complications. Again, the reader is referred to reviews given in each section and discussions elsewhere in this volume for more information. The following discussions are meant to be complementary to other sources and some are highly selective.

Pneumocystis carinii Pneumonia

Pneumocystis carinii pneumonia (PCP) is the most prevalent infection observed in AIDS patients, being also the most common serious complication of AIDS, whether infectious or malignant.[22,43–45] As reviewed by Murray and Mills,[22] PCP occurs as a primary diagnosis in 64% of AIDS patients, occurring at least once in 80%; in 15%–28% of first episodes it is fatal. Therefore, it is the single most important/frequent index diagnosis or indicator disease in AIDS. This section reviews some features that are particularly noted in AIDS patients. (More information is available in Chapter 14.) A 1988 review by Levine and White[43] estimated that the typical chest radiographic appearance of PCP, which in early stages is bilateral ground-glass perihilar infiltrates similar to pulmonary edema and later spreads to more diffuse interstitial alveolar infiltrates, is present in 48%–86% of cases of AIDS–PCP patients. Normal or near-normal chest radiographs were seen in 6%–25%,[43,46] some of whom had positive gallium scans.[15,47]

Patients with AIDS who have PCP have a more insidious onset of symptoms, averaging 28 days versus 5 days for PCP in non-AIDS patients.[4] The symptoms are usually fever, nonproductive cough, and dyspnea; shaking chills and pleuritis should suggest other infectious diagnoses. AIDS patients also have a slower response to therapy, a higher incidence of adverse reactions to systemic therapy, and a greater residual and recurrent infectious rate, averaging 20%–30% in 6–9 months.[48] They also have a higher incidence of atypical features. Although many of these features have been described in pre-AIDS cases, they are much more prevalent in AIDS cases; those further discussed here include upper-lobe predominant disease, pulmonary alveolar septal, pleural, and vascular invasive PCP, cyst formation, pneumothorax, and extrapulmonary dissemination. Minor atypical histologic appearances of granulomatous inflammation, fibrosis, desquamative interstitial pneumonitis (DIP) like appearance and dystrophic calcification are also briefly discussed. Rare atypical clinical features including hilar or mediastinal node enlargement,[48,49] pleural effusions, usually small,[50–53] focal,[54] or localized lobar,[55] parenchymal disease, normal chest radiographs,[46,56] endobronchial spread,[57] and unilateral hyperlucent lung[56] are not further discussed here but have been referenced for the interested reader. Several good reviews address the pathology of atypical PCP in AIDS cases.[58–63]

Travis et al.[59] conducted a detailed histologic review of 123 biopsies from 76 patients with AIDS PCP at the U.S. National Institutes of Health (NIH); atypical features were interstitial fibrosis (63%), intraluminal fibrosis (36%), absence of intraalveolar "exudate" (19%) (which was only noted on transbronchial biopsies, not open lung biopsies), DIP-like reaction (9%), granulomas (5%), hyaline membranes (4%), marked cellular interstitial pneumonitis (2%), interstitial microcalcifications (2%), cysts (2%), spontaneous pneumothorax (2%), minimal histologic reaction (2%), and vascular invasion-vasculitis (1%) and dissemination (1%). Travis et al.[59] found associated infections in about 10% of these cases and malignancies in only 1%, in contrast to the multi-institute series in which Murray et al.[19] found 27% incidence of coinfection and 8% of associated malignancy. Other clinical and radiographic reviews are incorporated in the excellent general reviews referred to in the introduction of this chapter and as applied to the special situations to follow.

To alert the pathologist to treatments and their effects on pathology, a brief introduction is in order. The mainstay of treatment of PCP is trimethoprim-sulfamethoxazol (co-trimoxazole) and pentamidine. The former, at least in Caucasian AIDS patients, has a higher incidence of adverse side reaction.[64,65] Pentamidine by semimonthly or monthly aerosolized administration has become the prophylactic drug of choice. Aerosolized prophylactic pentamidine has been shown to reduce the incidence of PCP in AIDS cases to approx-

imately 20% of that otherwise expected over the course of a year.[24] In the work of Masur et al.,[66] only 4.3% of PCP cases occurred when CD4+ cells were higher than 200/ml[3], and aerosolized pentamidine is suggested by the CDC in HIV+ cases where the CD4+ count is less than 200/mm[3] or these cells account for 20% or less of the total lymphocytes.[67] The normal range is 800–1200 CD4+ helper lymphocytes/mm[3].

It is predicted that the character of PCP in AIDS cases will change with continued prophylaxis, and some of the atypical findings described here may be evidence of this. Other drugs being considered for PCP treatment in AIDS are Dapsone (diamino-diphenylsulfone, an antileprosy drug), DFMO (difluoromethylornithine, also called eflornithine, used to treat trypanosomiasis), and trimetrexate (a methotrexate analog).[4,22] Several other combinations are trimethoprine-dapsone and primaquine-clindamycin. In Great Britain an experimental drug, BW566, shows some promise.[34,45] Some patients become worse in the first 3–5 days of therapy, but then respond. Others progress to respiratory failure; steroids have proven helpful in some of these cases.[22,45] Because inflammatory cells do not occur frequently in PCP, steroids may work by other routes. As with non-AIDS cases, the persistent use of corticosteroids unleashes its own cascade of other opportunistic infections and other complications. Earlier reported cases of respiratory failure in AIDS were usually fatal,[19,68–70] but more recently about 20%–30% of the patients have survived.[69,71–73]

Although PCP infection in AIDS is considered a reactivation of latent infection (see introduction), a study performed in San Francisco[74] of sudden deaths in AIDS cases not otherwise caused by AIDS infections or AIDS-associated malignancies, and several other specific studies to evaluate background findings of PCP in AIDS cases during life[75–80] and at autopsy,[81] found no evidence of detectable "background" PCP organisms in lung samples or their fluids. Therefore the use of pentamidine is truly prophylactic, and the carrier state–reactivation route is yet to be proven for PCP, although serologic evidence indicates a high incidence of early childhood exposure.[22] Perhaps we do not know enough about the life cycle of this organism; there may be a form not yet detected that is present in the carrier state that our tests do not detect. The route of transmission of this organism is unknown but is most likely aerogenous. The natural reservoir is unknown, even whether it be in the environment or in humans.

Tissue Invasion

Although extrapulmonary spread was already documented in PCP in pre-AIDS cases,[82] it is much more commonly seen in AIDS. Extrapulmonary spread is

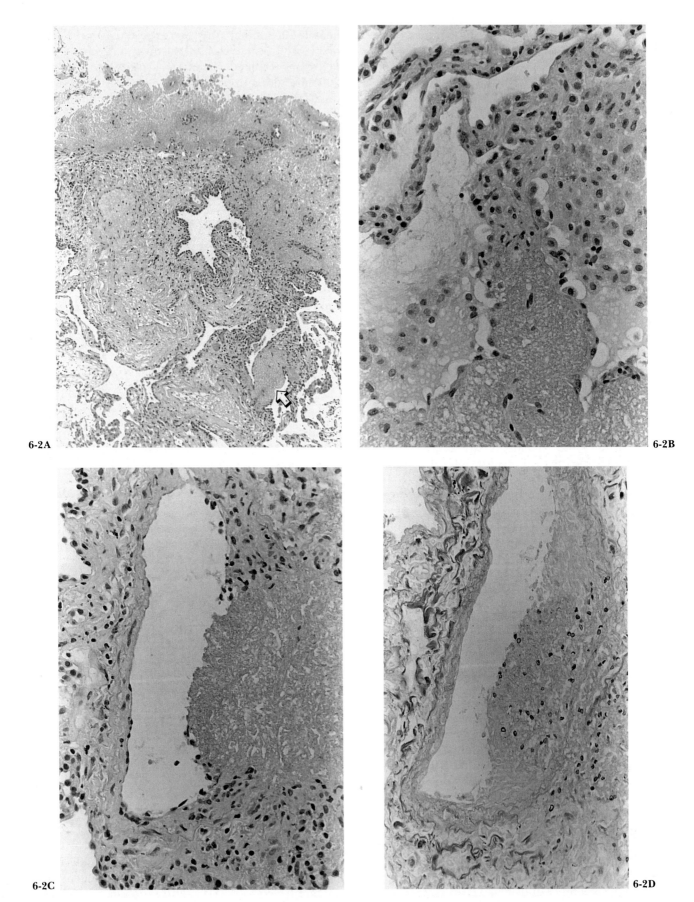

6-2A

6-2B

6-2C

6-2D

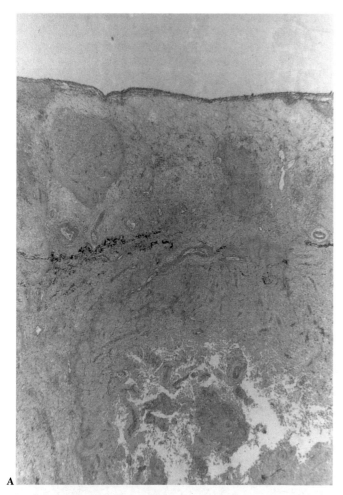

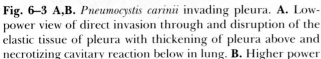

Fig. 6–3 A,B. *Pneumocystis carinii* invading pleura. **A.** Low-power view of direct invasion through and disruption of the elastic tissue of pleura with thickening of pleura above and necrotizing cavitary reaction below in lung. **B.** Higher power view shows no resistance to PCP extending across pleural elastic tissue. Same case as shown in Fig. 6–2. VVG stain. (Original contributor, D. Bauermeister, M.D., Virginia Mason Clinic, Seattle, Washington.)

reasonably thought to follow tissue invasion in lungs,[59] and like its upper-lobe predominence[83–86] it is thought to occur predominently in those receiving aerosolized pentamidine. As discussed next, cyst formation and pneumatoceles are also related to tissue invasion. Because PCP has so often been considered a disease limited to the air spaces, such infiltration is rather startling (Fig. 6–2). Direct vascular invasion may also be seen (Fig. 6–2 C,D) along with pleural invasion (Fig.

◁————————————————————

Fig. 6–2 A–D. Invasive *Pneumocystis carinii.* **A.** Edge of cyst wall at top shows confluent zone of organisms; separate focus of invasion is shown at *arrow.* **B.** Organisms invading from bottom of field, discretely in interstitium. **C.** PCP organisms extend directly through arterial wall into vascular lumen. H and E. **D.** Same field as in **C,** stained with GMS. (Original contributor, D. Bauermeister, M.D., Virginia Mason Clinic, Seattle, Washington.)

6–3).[87–90] Silver stains highlight scattered cyst walls (Fig. 6–2 D), and much of the fine vacuolization is caused by nonstaining cyst walls or trophozoites highlighted by immunoperoxidase stains or Giemsa stains.[87]

Vascular invasion has been described in both children and adults in both non-AIDS[91–97] and AIDS cases.[59,90,98–104] It has also been described in extrapulmonary sites, including dermal vessels,[99,100] and in embolic intravascular material.[101] Vascular invasion is a logical source of sepsis in dissemination, either by directly invading the blood vessels (Fig. 6–2 C,D) or via lymphatic drainage; the latter is proven as a route of spread by the fact that nodal spread is the most common site of extrapulmonary pneumocystosis, seen in 11 of 16 (69%) of non-AIDS cases and 12 of 34 (35%) of AIDS cases in the review by Raviglione.[82] Also, when only one extrapulmonary site is involved it is most often the hilar, and sometimes in the mediastinal nodes draining the lung.[82]

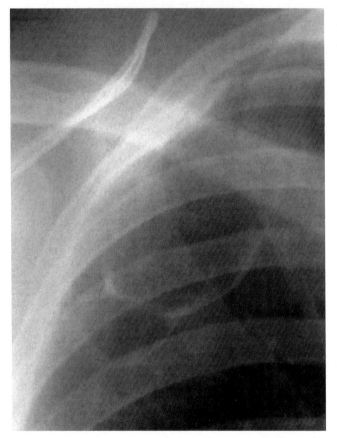

Fig. 6–4. Chest radiograph of invasive *Pneumocystis carinii* with cyst formation. Same case as shown in 6-2 and 6-3. These cysts later ruptured leading to specimens obtained for histology. (Courtesy of E. Hauptmann, Virginia Mason Clinic, Seattle, Washington.)

Cyst Formation

Although pulmonary cystic-cavitary lesions have rarely been described in pre-AIDS cases,[105–107] in AIDS patients such lesions in PCP are becoming commonly recognized.* Although visible in some patients on plain films (Fig. 6–4), CT scanning better delineates these (Fig. 6–5). The incidence of cysts in different series in AIDS PCP is 10% (10 of 100 cases[114] and 10 of 104 cases[48]), 20% (8 of 40)[113] and 42% (23 of 55).[51] Kuhlman et al.[105] contrasted their 42% of pulmonary cysts in cases with AIDS with a controlled series of 16% cysts (8 of 50) in non-AIDS neutropenic patients with acute leukemia. These incidences were compared to occurrence rates of pneumatoceles in children in a series of 5,000 pediatric autopsies by Boisset[118] in which sub-

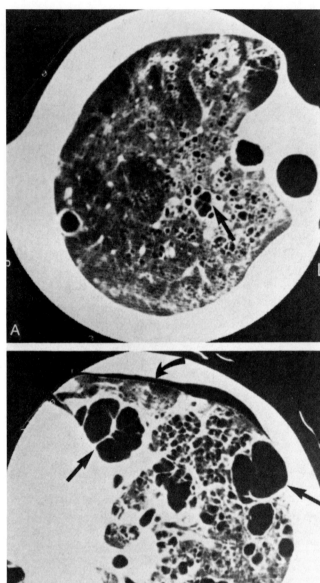

Fig. 6–5 A,B. Cystic *Pneumocystis carinii* pneumonia by high-resolution CT scans, both **A** and **B** show progressive evolution of cysts from small areas of consolidation to large cysts, becoming odd shaped in **B** (*straight arrows*). Curved arrow on **B** indicates pneumothorax. (From McLoud TC, Naidich DP. Radiol Clin North AM 1992;30:525–554, with permission.)

---

*References: 48, 50, 51, 104, 105, 108–117.

pleural air collections were observed in 65 of 595 (11%) of children dying of staphylococcal pneumonia, in 10 of 42 (23%) dying of measles pneumonia, and 21 of 273 (7%) of those children dying of tuberculosis. Similar postinfarction cysts can occur in children[119] (see Chapter 8).

For reference for the pathologist, the Fleischner Society,[115,120,121] composed of those interested in chest radiology, defines *air cyst* as any thin-walled space 1 or more cm in diameter, a *bulla* as air cyst with a thin wall less than 1 mm thick, a *bleb* as similar to a bulla but within the adjacent opposed pleural leaves of the major fissure, a *pneumatocele* as a thin-walled air cyst usually associated with acute pneumonia and usually transient, and a *cavity* as an air-filled space with a wall of variable thickness located within an area of density, such densities being described as consolidation, mass, or nodule. Others use the term bulla to indicate an air-filled cavity that does not change over 6 months and a pneumatocele as a cavity more likely to show change during this time. Others note cavitary lesions have thicker walls and usually have debris in their lumens. Cavitary AIDS–PCP has been described,[122–126] and occasionally others use the term bullous emphysema.[105]

These cysts seem to have a strong association with PCP. Sandhu and Goodman[114] found 8 of their 10 cases (80%) had cysts appear concurrent with PCP and in 6 of these 10 cases, only PCP was documented, the other 4 each having one other organism, either *Candida, Aspergillus, Mycobacterium avium-intracellulare,* or cytomegalovirus, all types of infections usually not associated with thin-walled cavities. In the series of Delorenzo et al.,[48] all 6 of the 104 AIDS cases who had cavities also had PCP. Kuhlman et al.[105] found a statistical signifi-

cance ($p < .05$) between cysts occurring and patients with documented pulmonary infections (6 of 23, or 70%), of whom 14 of 23 (61%) had PCP, while only 13% had no prior history of lung infection. In contrast, 12 of their 32 (38%) AIDS cases without pulmonary cysts had a prior history of pulmonary infection, 10 of these with PCP. Although cysts have been seen in drug abuse (see Chapter 23) and there is a high incidene of tobacco smoking in AIDS, Kuhlman et al.[105] found no significant difference in the prevalence of cysts with histories of smoking or drug abuse.

These cysts are often in the range of 1–3 cm in diameter, but have been described from quite small to 8.5 cm.[54] Their evolution from focal areas of consolidation to small cysts to more confluent cysts to subpleural bulla has been traced radiographically by McLoud and diagramed by Feuerstein et al.[104] (Fig. 6–6). PCP has been found lining the borders of these cysts (see Fig. 6–2A) in some pathologic studies, and in others there is fibrous tissue and chronic inflammation. PCP organisms sometimes are rare in these cyst walls and a careful search must be conducted to document or exclude their presence. Occasionally other infections coexist in these same cyst walls (see MAI in **Mycobacteria**). Radiographically some of these pneumatoceles-cysts have been shown to regress or disappear with appropriate therapy[52]; others have gone on to rupture and cause pneumothorax.

Pneumothorax

Rupturing pulmonary cysts can lead to spontaneous pneumothorax in 13%[105] to 30%[114] of AIDS-PCP cases.

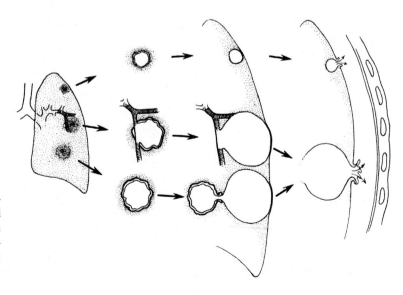

Fig. 6–6. Diagram of progressive cystic *Pneumocytis carinii* shows attachment both to bronchus and primarily in lung parenchyma, with evolution toward enlarging cysts and eventual pneumothorax. (From Feuerstein et al. Radiology 1990; 174:697–702, with permission.)

AIDS, PCP, and pneumothorax have been associated by others** (Fig. 6–5B). In an excellent review of this problem by Beers et al.[136] a total of 38 cases were reviewed from the literature from 1984 to 1989 and, as with cyst formation, PCP was the major organism identified in the majority. In two abstracted series this was seen in patients on aerosolized pentamidine, occurring in 10 of 256 (4%)[130] and 8 of 327 (2%)[132] patients some 3–13 months into prophylactic therapy. In one of these series,[132] 75% had evidence of active PCP at or near the time of pneumothorax; pneumothorax occurs during active infection and not as a late sequela.[136] Cyst formation is also a risk for accidentally induced pneumothorax during procedures such as placement of central intravenous lines or bronchoscopy with or without transbronchial biopsies.

The mechanism of cyst formation extending to pneumothorax appears to be infiltration with invasion and weakening of interalveolar septa and anchoring subpleural attachments[136] (see Fig. 6–2). PCP can directly invade the pleura, destroying its elastic tissue and other supporting structures. When PCP begins infiltrating tissue, it seems to continue through fibrous and elastic tissue with little resistance (see Fig. 6–3).

Recurrent or bilateral pneumothoraces are seen in a significant number of AIDS–PCP cases. In the literature reviewed by Beers et al.,[136] 38% were thus involved while the other 62% had insufficient follow-up after the first event. In another abstracted series by Mann et al.[131] of 22 patients with spontaneous pneumothorax in AIDS patients with PCP, 68% had bilateral or recurrent pneumothoraces. Of interest in this latter series, in about half the cases with pneumothorax in AIDS PCP was not documented, probably partially related to the extent to which these patients are evaluated for active disease. In a series by McClellan et al.,[135] pneumothorax occurred in 9% (8 of 89) of AIDS–PCP cases but in none (0 of 45) of AIDS without PCP. The occurrence of one or more pneumothoraces is usually a poor prognostic sign; 57.5% of the 40 patients in the literature reviewed by Beers et al.[136] died within 8 weeks of the initial event. One patient reported by Eng et al.[63] had seven episodes of pneumothorax. Multiple pneumothoraces may be on the same side or bilateral, either synchronous or asynchronous. Some patients respond well and others poorly to closed chest tube suction.

The possible mechanisms of cyst formation have been reviewed by Panicek.[115] These include inflammation with protease-antiprotease, elastase, and antielastase imbalances, effects of accelerated aging, tobacco smoke

and i.v. drug abuse, direct cytotoxic effect of HIV, or perhaps via a co-agent recently named "virus-like infectious agent."[137,138] The latter agent could help explain cysts and pneumothoraces in AIDS patients whose PCP is not documented. It has also been proposed that there is a possible check valve mechanism in the bronchus with hyperinflation, but endobronchial involvement is only rarely documented.[57] Tracing evolution of these cysts radiographically through small areas of consolidation to small cysts to confluence of cysts to subpleural spread would do credence to the necrotizing effect of PCP, and invasion of the interlobular septa, vessels, and pleura, with weakening of their supporting structures, appears to be the most likely mechanism. PCP is seen in the surrounding walls of some of these cysts, and in others there are fibrous linings. In some of these, PCP may be missed because the observer is concentrating on the fibrous reaction or DIP-like reaction. Certainly trophozoites must be present in some cases in which cysts are missed on GMS stain. No doubt some are remnants of past infection for which the organisms can no longer be identified.

Other Tissue Patterns

The variations of fibrosis, nodules, granulomas, and calcification are discussed together as there is some overlap among these. The careful histologic review by Travis et al.[59] is used for rough incidence figures. Fibrosis may be more widespread and interstitial; it was seen in the Travis et al.[59] series in 63% but was patchy in 36%. Whether widespread or patchy, fibrosis suggests that there has been either a focal or more widespread disruption of basal lamina. Nodules may have varying mixture of fibrosis, PCP organisms, chronic inflammation, or granulomas with or without giant cells. Cavitation as described here, sometimes with cysts, can occur within a granulomatous reaction[124] or with other nodular PCP. Pulmonary granulomatous PCP has been described in non-AIDS,[94,139–144] and AIDS–PCP,[145–150] and in the series of Travis et al.[59] was seen in 5% of the cases. It was noted in about one-half the nodular cases of PCP reviewed by Saldana and Moines.[60] Granuloma formation has been described with extrapulmonary pneumocystosis in both non-AIDS† and in AIDS.[151,152]

Dystrophic calcification occurs in some cases of PCP, both in non-AIDS‡ and in AIDS.§ It is sometimes so

---

†References: 94, 96, 140, 144, 150.
‡References: 94, 96, 142, 153, 154.
§References: 29, 59, 60, 62, 104, 123, 130, 146, 155.

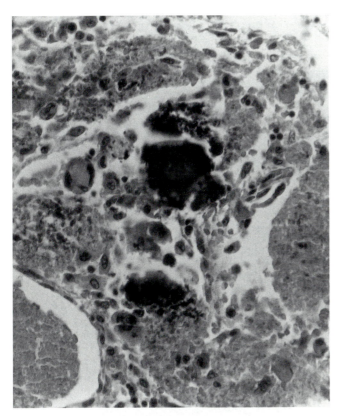

Fig. 6–7. *Pneumocystis carinii* with darkly stained plate-like calcifications and small multinucleated giant cell.

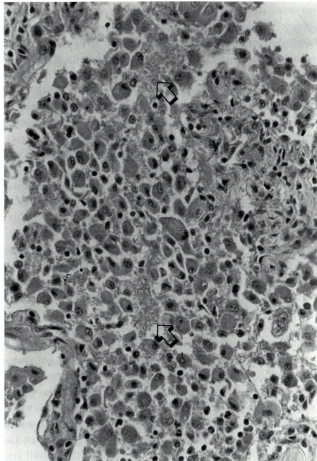

Fig. 6–8. *Pneumocystis carinii* in desquamative interstitial pneumonitis (DIP) appearance. Among abundant alveolar macrophages are multiple cysts of pneumocystis; largest clumps indicated by *arrows*.

extensive as to show up vividly on CT scans of lung,[156] hilar nodes,[157] and elsewhere.[158–160] Lee and Schinella[155] have conducted the largest single histological study of calcification in 13 cases of AIDS–PCP. The incidence of calcification of 3.1% in their series; Travis et al.[59] found 2%. Lee and Schinella[155] described four microscopic patterns of calcification: that occurring most frequently is bubbly, forming around cyst in pneumocystis; plate-like and elongate calcification occurs less frequently, either with or without bubbly calcification (Fig. 6–7), and conchoidal calcification was rarely seen. Elongate calcification resembled fungal hyphae. The plate-like calcification was usually seen in large areas of fibrosis and therefore is probably a late form. In none of their cases was the calcification intense enough to be noted radiographically, and no patient had an altered course from calcification when compared with noncalcifying PCP control patients. Calcification can also be seen associated with granulomatous PCP.§§ Rarely, a des-

quamative intersitital pneumonitis (DIP) pattern is seen. The number of pulmonary alveolar macrophages may distract the observer from the intervening of PCP (Fig. 6–8).

Extrathoracic and Disseminated Pneumocystosis

Spread of *Pneumocystis carinii* to extrapulmonary sites have been documented in non-AIDS and AIDS cases. As already discussed, systemic spread of PCP is thought to follow both hematogenous and lymphatic routes.[94] The abbreviation PCP is inappropriate for this spread because the last "P" of PCP stands for pneumonia, and the term extrapulmonary pneumocystosis has been suggested instead.[82] Anderson and Barrie[161] described the

_____
§§References: 59, 62, 96, 149, 155.

been observed to be associated with T-cell defects. *Nocardia asteroides* was reported in 21 AIDS cases from one institution,[180] and the radiographic appearance is as varied in AIDS[180] as in non-AIDS, immunosuppressed patients.[181] *Nocardia* may present as lobar or multilobar consolidation (52%), a solitary mass (24%), reticulonodular infiltrates (33%) with pleural fusion (33%), cavitation (62%), and upper-lobe distribution (71%). Non-typhae *Salmonella* has been considered an opportunistic infection in this setting.[182] In pre-AIDS days, *Salmonella* pneumonia or pleuritis was rare.[183] Bacillary angiomatosis, now thought to be caused by *Rochalimaea henselae*,[184,185] has only recently been described in the bronchi in AIDS,[186] but most certainly will soon also be described in the lung.

The interested reader is referred to the reviews cited for other less common bacterial organisms identified in AIDS cases.

Fungus

Invasive fungal pneumonias occur in less than 5% of AIDS patients.*** A good general review of fungal infections in AIDS is that by Macher et al.[187] These pneumonias do not occur as frequently in AIDS cases as in other leukopenic immunocompromised hosts, such as those undergoing therapy for leukemia or solid tumors, nor are they as frequent as in patients treated with steroids for other reasons, but fungi remain a significant pathogen. In general AIDS patients with fungal pneumonia often have dissemination, may initially respond to amphotericin but frequently recur, and have a high mortality. In non-AIDS immunocompromised hosts, invasive *Aspergillus*, is the most common fungal infection, but in AIDS, fungal pneumonias, *Cryptoccus neoformans, Histoplasma capsulatum, Coccidiodes immitus,* and even *Candida albicans* are more common than Aspergillus.[24] Much more elaborate detail on each of these fungi is available in Chapter 11, **Fungal Infections;** these introductory comments are related to the more common fungi seen in association with AIDS; less common fungal pneumonias as seen in AIDS are discussed in the reviews cited and in Chapter 11.

Cryptococcus

Cryptococcus neoformans is the most common invasive fungal pneumonia in AIDS cases, occurring in 2%–13.3% of cases,[192–201] and reaching 7% in one composite series of 16,000 AIDS cases.[201] As reviewed by

***References: 22, 24, 170, 187–193.

Fels,[170] clinically 67%–85% of these patients present with cryptococcal meningoencephalitis,[193,196] and about one-third of these have concurrent pulmonary involvement.[193] Some 4%–6% present with pulmonary involvement, and in one series of 12 such cases all went on to disseminate.[197] Because one-third to one-half of all cases of cryptococcal infection in AIDS progress to dissemination, the lungs are frequently involved secondarily.[196] The overall mortality is 60% despite therapy.[198] Transbronchial biopsies, BAL, and brush samples provide a high diagnostic yield.[197,199] Cryptococcal pulmonary disease usually presents as interstitial organisms but may present as endobronchial disease[197] or pleural disease effusion.[200]

Histoplasma

Histoplasma capsulatum is the most common endemic fungal disease in the United States, estimated to infect 25%–75% of the endemic population.[191,202–204] The lungs are its primary route of infection. In AIDS cases, therefore, it is seen as a reactivated disease, although new infection cannot be excluded. It becomes disseminated in almost all cases,[191,205] although rare examples are confined to the lung.[191] As summarized by Fels,[170] lung involvement is documented in 69% of those patients in whom the disease disseminates.[191,204,206] Johnson et al.[202] provided a single large series of 125 cases of disseminated histoplasmosis in AIDS cases.

Coccidioidomycosis

Coccidioides immitus is the second most common endemic fungal infection in the United States, and again the respiratory tract is its usual portal of entry. As with histoplasmosis, immunosuppression, including AIDS, may lead to reactivation and dissemination, but primary infection can also occur.[188,207–212] In one study,[188] in the midst of an endemic area (Phoenix, Arizona) 27% of AIDS cases had disseminated coccidioidomycosis. When dissemination occurs, rapid deterioration occurs in more than half the affected patients despite therapy.[208,209]

Aspergillus

Invasive *Aspergillus* is only rarely reported in AIDS cases and usually occurs late in the course of AIDS, often in those patients who have been treated with broad-spectrum antibiotics or steroids or who are otherwise neutropenic.[213] Good series, of 13 patients by Denning et al.[213] and 10 patients by Klapholz et al.,[214] are available. It usually coexists with other AIDS-associated infections or malignancies by the time of its detection.[214] The prognosis therefore is quite poor. Because *Aspergillus* infection occurs late, in a period of severe immunosuppression, it should not be considered an AIDS-related opportunistic infection.[215]

Candida

Although this is the most frequent fungal infection in any site in AIDS cases, it is most often confined to the mucous membranes and often heralds conversion of pre-AIDS to AIDS. In one autopsy series of 56 AIDS patients, Neidt and Schinella[29] observed that 61% had oral candidiasis and 21% had *Candida* esophagitis. It is rarely a cause of pulmonary infection, but when it does occur it is difficult to diagnose during life; dissemination is frequent, occurring in an autopsy series in 90% of cases.[170]

Mycobacteria

This section introduces three causes of mycobacterial infection: *Mycobacterium tuberculosis, Mycobacterium avium-intracellulare* (MAI), and other myocobacteria (see also Chapter 10). Tuberculosis is discussed first. The incidence of tuberculosis in the United States had been decreasing (see Fig. 6–10), but the rate of decrease has flattened out since 1984 with most of this change attributed to HIV infection.[216] In other portions of the world where tuberculosis is more prevalent, most of the population is exposed at an earlier age and some 90% of those infected go into latent phase, 5% reactivate early (within 5 years, also called early progression), and an additional 5% reactinate later (late progression). The rate of progression from infection to disease in HIV-positive people is 30%, or sixfold that of HIV-negative people, making HIV infection the greatest acquired risk factor to be developed in clinical tuberculosis, far beyond the risk factors of diabetes melitus, Hodgkin's disease, steroid administration, gastrectomy, or silicosis.[216] *M. tuberculosis* is one of the more virulent latent infections in humans, and when immunosuppression occurs it is one of the first infections to reactivate. In HIV-infected patients, this usually occurs before reactivation of pneumocystis, CMV, or toxoplasma (see Fig. 6–1).

The lungs are the primary portal of entry for the organisms and therefore also a major source of reactivation. Tuberculosis was reported in about 4% of cases as of 1984[19]; in other series, it was 4.8%–35% in HIV-positive patients.[216–225] The risk now of developing active tuberculosis in AIDS is approaching 8% per year.[223] In a study of close immunocompetent contacts

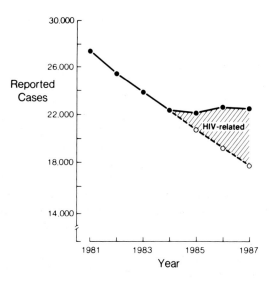

Fig. 6–10. Number of tuberculosis cases in United States, 1981–1987; cases in shaded area attributed to HIV infection. (From Murray. Am Rev Resp Dis 1989;140:1788–1795, with permission.)

of active non-AIDS tuberculosis cases, about 50% converted their skin test, suggesting new infection.[226] Because of close contact and poor immunity among high-risk AIDS patients, who often aggregate together, the risk must be even higher. Spread as in non-AIDS cases is usually by droplet nuclei, making the lungs the most important portal of entry. Current concern is for increased drug resistance, for reasons that appear also related to HIV infection.

In HIV-infected individuals, tuberculosis occurs in two fairly distinct forms.[21,225,227] In early HIV infection when immunity is not so suppressed, tuberculosis may reactivate in a classical pattern as seen in non-HIV-infected individuals: upper-lobe infiltrate predominance, cavitation, fibrosis, large nodes, positive skin tests, active histologic granuloma formation, and, in 15%–20% of cases, extrapulmonary manifestations. Later in the course of HIV infection, often preceding a definitive AIDS diagnosis, immunosuppression is enough to lead to a different progression: only about half of patients react to skin tests, one half present with extrapulmonary disease, most often have nodal spread, chest radiographs are atypical with infrequent upper-lobe disease and infrequent cavitation,[224] and a greater toxic effect from drug therapy and need for treatment for longer periods of time, less granuloma formation, greater number of organisms, and a greater chance for drug resistance to evolve. Patients presenting in this later phase have a poor prognosis, and in one study patients died 7.4 months after diagnosis, although usually of other AIDS complications.[225] As

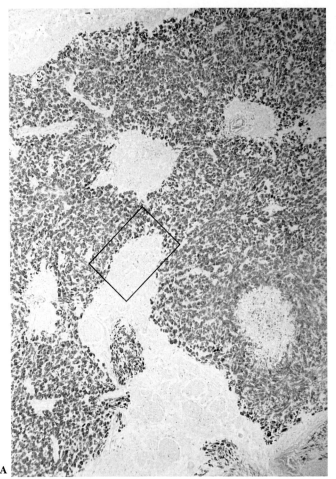

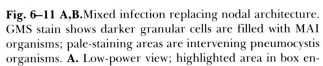

A

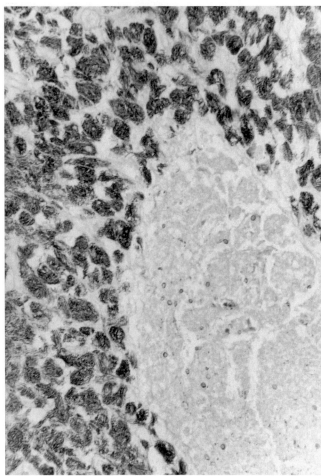

B

Fig. 6–11 A,B. Mixed infection replacing nodal architecture. GMS stain shows darker granular cells are filled with MAI organisms; pale-staining areas are intervening pneumocystis organisms. **A.** Low-power view; highlighted area in box en-

larged in **B. B.** High-power view shows diffuse staining of pneumocystis organisms in cleared zones. (Courtesy of William Travis, National Institutes of Health, Bethesda, Maryland; represents same case as Figs. 6–9 and 6–12.)

noted in the introduction, enlarged hilar nodes in AIDS cases are often result from tuberculosis, *M. avium-intracellulare*, Kaposi's sarcoma, and, less often, lymphoma and fungi.[228]

Mycobacterium avium-intracellulare (MAI) is a complex of two closely related organisms, *M. avium* and *M. intracellulare*. This complex is composed of ubiquitous organisms that occur in water and soil and infect birds, some mammals,[229] and humans with portals of entry through both the lungs and the gastrointestinal (GI) tract.[230] In AIDS cases it is proposed that sexual intercourse may also be a route of spread.[231] Before AIDS, only 78 cases of disseminated nontuberculous mycobacterial infections were reported,[229] of which 37 (47%) cases were disseminated MAI.[229,232] During the time period 1981–1987, 2,269 cases of nontuberculous mycobacteria were reported in 41,349 cases of AIDS for an incidence of 5.5%; of these, 1,906 or 96.1% were

MAI.[233] The incidence of this disease in AIDS appears to be decreasing.[233] MAI is usually not an index case for AIDS; in contrast to *M. tuberculosis*, it often occurs late in the course of AIDS after an AIDS diagnosis is made.

In life, MAI has been estimated to occur in several AIDS series, in 14%[229] to 17%,[19] whereas in autopsy series it has been reported in 53%[234] to 56%[235] of cases. It is usually disseminated and most often involves lymph nodes, spleen, bone marrow, and GI tract; sepsis is common, resulting in a high percentage of blood culture positivity.[236,237] The pathology of this disease in one autopsy series[238] of 12 cases (of 116 AIDS autopsies) showed that when MAI was present it involved lymph nodes in 100% (Fig. 6–11), spleen in 92%, liver in 83%, GI tract in 58%, bone marrow in 50%, adrenal gland in 33%, and lung (Fig. 6–12) in only 17% of cases. It may be seen within blood vessels or lymphatic spaces (Fig. 6–12C). The miliary lesions/granulomas varied between 0.1 and 1.8 cm, most about 0.4 cm, and varied in color from yellow to tan to white, but in this series more than half were "lemon yellow."[238] In any location the typical histologic appearance was pale blue-gray striated histiocytes, appearing to be pseudo-Gaucher cells, and sometimes considered pseudo-Whipple-like (Fig. 6–12). In the series by Klatt et al.[238] these were seen in 90% of cases of the positive cases, as were epithelioid histiocytes in 33%, lymphocytic infiltrate, 31%, necrosis, 21%, and granulomas with fibrosis, 17%; infrequently, calcification (4%) and Langhans' giant cells (2%) were seen. MAI organisms histologically stain positive with any of the acid-fast stains, but they also stain positive with GMS, PAS, and tissue Gram stains. With the collage of infections that AIDS patients are subject to at a time when they may also have MAI, multiple infections are common. In none of the cases reported by Klatt et al.[238] was there skin involvement: this finding helps to differentiate this infection from leprosy.

Although sepsis occured in 85% in one series[239] and widespread and extensive tissue involvement can occur, MAI is only infrequently thought to contribute directly to death, and death in AIDS cases is often from other intercurrent/concurrent infections or nonspecific processes leading to respiratory failure, as is discussed later. The series by Modilevsky et al.[239] is of note as it directly compares the clinical features of 39 cases of *M. tuberculosis* infection with 55 cases of MAI in HIV patients.

It is unknown why MAI accounts for such a high percentage (96.1%) of disseminated nontuberculous mycobacteria in AIDS. Other nontuberculous/atypical mycobacteria are seen in AIDS. In the large number reviewed by Horsburg and Selik[233] 2.9% of infections were caused by *M. kansasii*, 0.6% to *M. gordonae*, and 0.3% each to *M. fortuitum* and *M. chelonei*. Rare invasions by *M. xeropi* and *M. bovim* have also been identified in disseminated AIDS cases, and localized disease has been reported involving *M. scrofulaceum, M. szulgai, M. flavescens, M. asiaticum, M. malmoense,* and *M. xenopi*.[240]

Mycobacterium kansasii deserves a few comments. One series of HIV-infected individuals described 19 patients in one institution between 1985 and 1990[241] with docu-

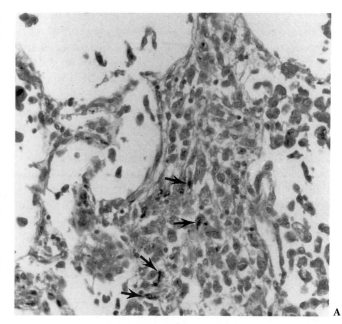

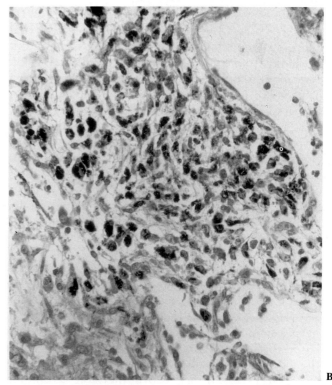

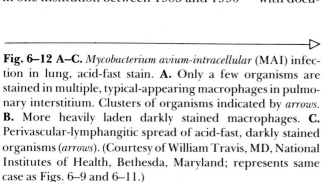

Fig. 6–12 A–C. *Mycobacterium avium-intracellular* (MAI) infection in lung, acid-fast stain. **A.** Only a few organisms are stained in multiple, typical-appearing macrophages in pulmonary interstitium. Clusters of organisms indicated by *arrows.* **B.** More heavily laden darkly stained macrophages. **C.** Perivascular-lymphangitic spread of acid-fast, darkly stained organisms (*arrows*). (Courtesy of William Travis, MD, National Institutes of Health, Bethesda, Maryland; represents same case as Figs. 6–9 and 6–11.)

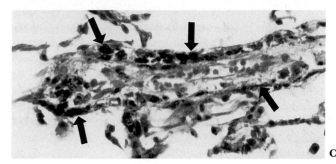

mented *M. kansasii* infection, of which 14 (74%) had exclusive pulmonary infection, 3 (16%) had pulmonary and extrapulmonary, and only 2 (11%) had exclusive extrapulmonary infection. Chest radiograph showed focal upper-lobe infiltrates (42%), diffuse interstitial disease (50%), or thin-walled cavities (50%). Two untreated patients had progressive cavitary disease and died of this infection but others responded well to therapy. Unlike other nontuberculous mycobacteria isolated in AIDS and non-AIDS cases, this organism is virtually never a contaminant and always causes disease.[242] Why some infections in AIDS cases such as *M. kansasii* remain mostly oriented toward the lungs and others such as MAI remain mostly disseminated and extrapulmonary is unknown. See further corresponding details in Chapter 10.

Viral Infections

Some interesting relationships of viruses and AIDS have been noted. Despite the occurrence of latent viral infections from childhood on in all of us, significant morbidity from viral infections is not frequent in AIDS cases for reasons that are unclear; viral infections seem to be more important in other non-AIDS immunosuppressive disorders.[243,244] See also Chapters 1, 12, and 24.

Cytomegalovirus (CMV) is the most prevalent of the viral infections noted in AIDS cases. However, most infections are not associated with significant morbidity or mortality, in contrast to such infections in bone marrow transplants. Some 25%–90% of children are infected in early childhood,[21] and transmission can be via sexual intercourse. By the ages 30–40, about 50%–95% of people are infected with CMV,[21] and CMV infection in AIDS cases therefore usually represents reactivation. CMV infection is present in more than 99% of sexually active homosexual men, both those that are HIV negative and those HIV positive.[245] Unlike herpes simplex, varicella zoster, and Epstein–Barr viruses, the CMV genome does not appear to specify a thymidine kinase enzyme necessary to activate the more common antiviral drug acyclovir, therefore accounting for the insensitivity of CMV to this drug.[21] In AIDS cases, CMV may cause infection of the gastrointestinal tract, retina, or kidney in a small percentage of cases. It is present in 30%–40% of cases of AIDS pneumonia of any etiology,[19,246] and at autopsy may be noted in 69%–90% cases of AIDS, with the lung being most commonly involved.†† However, the clinical course

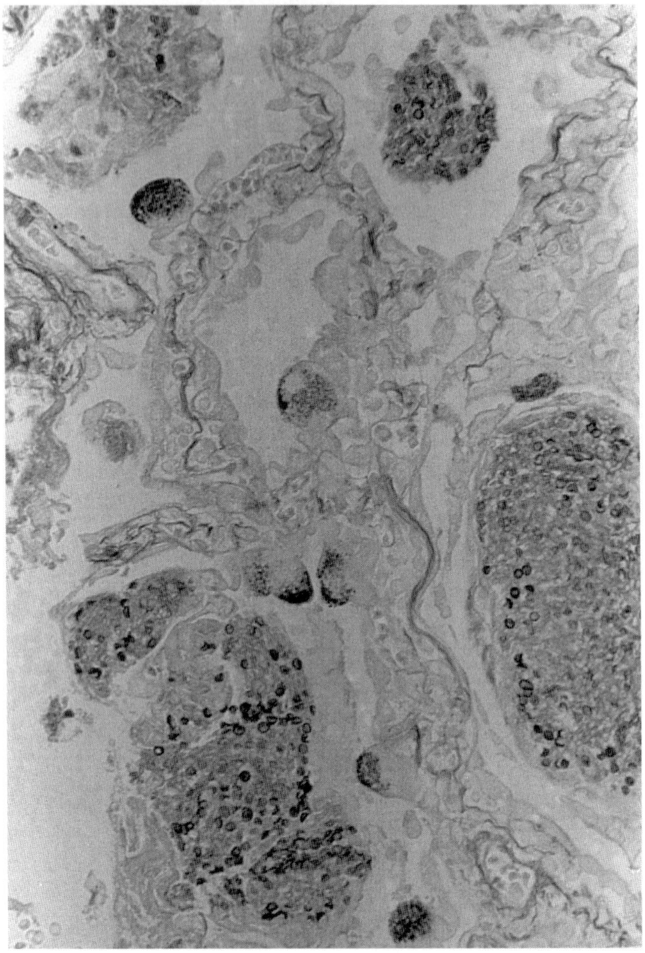

Fig. 6–13. Coexistent *Pneumocystis carinii* pneumonia (PCP) and cytomegalovirus (CMV). PCP cysts shown intraalveolar with GMS silver stain. Cytoplasmic CMV inclusions also stain with silver stain; six are seen toward the center between PCP cysts. (Provided by John Bolen, M.D., Virginia Mason Clinic, Seattle, Washington.)

does not seem to differ with and without AIDS,[249–253] and in a detailed inquiry into causes of death in HIV patients[32] CMV was noted in 81% of cases, in 59% of the total in the lung, and was much more frequently diagnosed at autopsy than during life, not infrequently coexisting with other infections (Fig. 6–13). Only two cases with more than 80% destruction of the adrenal cortex appear to be directly related to death of AIDS cases.[32] Again, see Chapter 12 for further details.

Other pulmonary viral infections such as herpes simplex are only occasionally reported in AIDS.[19,54,108] Varicella-zoster pneumonia is infrequent although 11 cases of disseminated disease have been reported.[254] The role of Epstein–Barr virus is discussed in lymphocytic interstitial pneumonitis. Other reported incidences of viruses such as influenza in AIDS appear to

---

††References: 28, 31, 54, 247, 248.

reflect background coincidence. Little association with adenoviruses disease has been proven.[255] However, respiratory syncytial virus and parainfluenza virus may cause prolonged or severe illnesses in AIDS.[256–258]

Parasitic Infections

This section concentrates on the role of *Toxoplasma*, *Cryptosporidium*, and *Strongyloides* in AIDS. Respiratory cryptosporidia receives major attention here, but the interested reader is referred to more thorough discussions of other parasites in Chapter 15.

Toxoplasma gondii has been found in 3%–40% of AIDS series[182,259–261] and is the most common cause of brain lesions in AIDS cases, while pulmonary involvement has been reported less frequently.[19,262–264] In a series of 14 cases of toxoplasmic encephalitis, extracerebral spread was seen in 6, in 5 of whom the lung was involved (42%).[259] Because the lung is frequently involved with extracerebral spread, it has been considered as a possible site of biopsy but the pulmonary lesions are so focal that this may not be fruitful.[259,265] Pulmonary involvement is occasionally diagnosed by BAL samples.[19,262,264] It may be responsible for death in AIDS cases because of cerebral involvement, as in 75% of one series,[32] but usually death is not caused by pulmonary involvement. Other causes of cerebral death in AIDS are multifocal leukoencephalopathy, tuberculous, cryptococcal or histoplasma meningitis, or complications of diagnostic procedures.[32]

When the lungs are involved, there usually are multiple, confluent, gray-red areas of consolidation and necrosis and microscopically vague granuloma formation or focal areas of injury, fibrin, hemorrhage, and diffuse interstitial inflammation.[259,265–267] Cysts, bradyzoites, and tachyozoites may be found; of these, the cyst is of course most easily identified, and cysts are also frequently found in the heart at autopsy. Differentiation of the cysts from CMV cytoplasmic inclusions cut at such a plane that the nucleus with its CMV intranuclear inclusion is not identified can be done with a PAS stain, as the CMV cytoplasmic inclusions are PAS positive. Direct immunofluorescence or immunoperoxidase is also possible, and of course finding typical isolated cysts in brain or heart is also helpful.

As reviewed in the series by Garcia et al.[267] Luft and Remington,[260] and Yermakov et al.,[261] disseminated disease in both AIDS and non-AIDS is often diagnosed only at autopsy.[268–273] In contrast, in a series of 70 cases of AIDS toxoplasmic encephalitis,[260] many brain tissue specimens failed to show cysts but all showed positive staining of free tachyzoites by immunoperoxidase techniques. In contrast to normal hosts, typical toxoplasma

lymphadenitis was not seen but cysts were easily identified in nodes and in other involved organs, such as esophagus, stomach, small bowel, colon, pancreas, heart, lungs, trachea, testes, epididymis, prostate, thyroid gland, adrenal gland, and bone marrow.[267] At autopsy, the central nervous system, (CNS), heart, and lungs are most frequently involved.

Strongyloides stercoralis hyperinfection can occur in AIDS cases; a nice review is that by Maayan et al.[274] This infection is endemic in tropical and subtropical zones and in the southeast portion of the United States, although migrant and immigrant populations can experience reactivation of this disease even 30 years after leaving endemic zones.[275] This may be a sexually transmitted disease in homosexual men, often through oral–anal contact.[276] Filariform larvae penetrate small and large intestinal mucosa and lodge in pulmonary capillaries (Fig. 6–14), where they migrate through alveolar septa, causing small focal areas of hemorrhage, and then ascend to the alveolar surfaces to the bronchiolar routes (see Fig. 6–14) and there ascend the mucociliary blanket to be aspirated back into the GI tract to complete their maturation cycle. The most common complications are gram-negative bacterial meningitis and septicemia, thought to result from associated contamination of the migratory organisms by large intestinal bacteria.[277,278] Purtilo et al.[279] provided an extensive review in non-AIDS cases. Of interest in AIDS, only 4 cases of extraintestinal strongyloidiasis occurred in the first 13,042 cases of AIDS in the United States, while on the basis of a 3.9% incidence in sexually active American homosexual men[276] more than 370 homosexual AIDS patients presumably were at risk during this time although only 4 cases were reported.

In endemic zones, visceral leishmaniasis in HIV and AIDS populations has been described; the largest series is by Peters et al.[280] who reviewed 47 reported cases and compared HIV-positive and HIV-negative presentations. Leishmania was seen in only one BAL sample and one postmortem lung case in this series.

Cryptosporidia has gained a notoriety among parasites in the AIDS epidemic, and thus is emphasized here. (The interested reader is also referred to Chapter 15, **Parasitic Infections**.) *Cryptosporidium* sp., an intestinal parasite closely related to other coccidia such as *Isospora belli* and *Toxoplasma gondi*,[281] was first described by Tyzzer in 1907[282] and is a frequent cause of diarrhea in mammals such as calves, lambs, pigs, guinea pigs, and mice, and also in birds and reptiles. The first two cases in humans were described in 1976, one in an immunocompetent host[283] and the other in an immunosuppressed host.[284] With better techniques of diagnosis, it is now being found more regularly in humans in cases of short-term diarrhea, in day nurseries, and among trav-

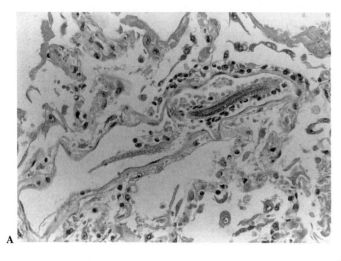
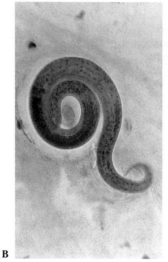
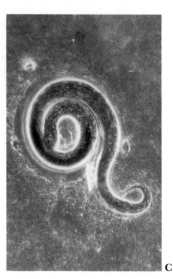
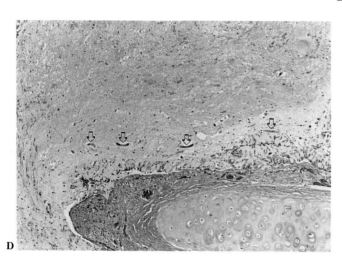
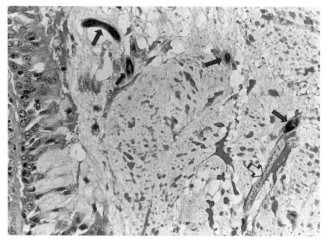

Fig. 6–14 A–E. *Strongyloides stercoralis.* **A.** Filaria is in lung capillary ready to penetrate into alveolar space. **B** and **C.** Sputum of organisms from this patient: **B,** by routine light microscopy showing presumed eggs inside organism and **C,** by highlighting of parasite wall by dark-field microscopy. **D, E.** Migration in bronchi. **D.** Low power. Note partial sections of parasites near mucosa (*arrows*) and filling of dilated bronchus with mucus. **E.** High power shows partial sections of microfilaria (*solid arrows*), one of which has presumed eggs (*open arrow*). (Provided by M. Mauney, M.D., and T. Gleason, M.D., Group Health Cooperative Medical Center, Seattle, Washington.)

elers.[285] In AIDS cases it most often involves the GI tract, and diarrhea is its common symptom. In a detailed series by Godwin,[286] it was found in the bowel in 13 of 183 (7%) of AIDS autopsies, specifically, in descending order of frequency, in small intestine, extrahepatic and intrahepatic bile ducts, large intestine, stomach, and esophagus. No mention of respiratory tract infection was noted in the large series by Godwin.[286]

Respiratory tract involvement has been documented in fowl, notably turkeys,[287] chickens,[288] quail,[289] and peacocks.[282] By 1991, 17 cases have been described in AIDS patients involving respiratory tract, but only 7 were tissue diagnosed,[290–295] the others having been diagnosed by cytologic examination of sputum,[294,296] bronchoalveolar lavage,[297,298] tracheal aspirate,[299] and touch preparation of tissue.[294] It can also cause laryngitis,[299] pharyngitis,[299] and sinusitis.[300] Most human cases occur among AIDS patients, although other immunodeficiency states, such as in children,[299] and cases secondary to other adult immunodeficiency[281,291,297,301] have been described.

Cryptosporidial infection so far has been described in various organs in the human only in direct connection with the GT tract in patients with gastrointestinal symptoms, usually watery diarrhea. Therefore, direct surface spread seems to be the favored route of infection, although inhalation, aspiration, fecal–oral, and hematogenous routes have been suggested. In the lung as elsewhere it is usually found on the surface of the glands (Fig. 6–15) or on ciliated surfaces often affected by squamous metaplasia, and only rarely in macrophages or as focal or mild interstitial pneumonia.[294] It causes mild inflammation and is often found in AIDS cases in association with other infections or malignancies. In cytologic specimens, it is acid fast but this is not so in tissue sections for unknown reasons.[281] Also in the stool and other smear preparations, modified cold Kinyoun and hemacolor stains also help. In lung smears, *Pneumocystis* and *Toxoplasma* do not stain with modified cold Kinyoun stain although cryptosporidia do.[294] In tissues it is seen best on H and E, PAS, or Giemsa stains, but is also weakly GMS positive and can be detected using immunohistochemical techniques[302] and electron microscopy.[303–305] It does not readily cause significant disease or death by itself.[281]

Lymphocytic Interstitial Pneumonia

The entity lymphocytic interstitial pneumonia (LIP) represents widespread ("diffuse") interstitial lymphocytic, plasmacytic, and immunoblastic infiltration in lung tissue, often without nodal enlargement or pleural effusion. See Chapter 31 in this text and the excellent reviews by White and Matthay[23] and by Teirstein and Rosen.[306] As noted in non-AIDS cases (Chapter 31), this disease in the past has been described mostly in middle-aged women with Sjögren's syndrome, systemic lupus erythematosis, myastemia gravis, pernicious anemia, autoerythrocytic anemia, and chronic active hepatitis.[24] Also as noted in Chapter 31, many of the past cases have been unrecognized small lymphocytic lymphomas, but this is not as much a problem in AIDS cases. LIP became an AIDS-defining diagnosis in 1987 in children under age 13 (see Table 6–1). In this age group, it overlaps with the separately described entity of pulmonary lymphoid hyperplasia (PLH),[307,308] and some combine these terms as PLH/LIP complex.[23,306,309] The majority of patients with AIDS who are younger than 16 years, including infants,[310,311] have the entity LIP.[312] As such, LIP is particularly important in pediatric cases of possible AIDS and is further discussed in this age group in Chapter 8 and in a separate review of AIDS pulmonary disease in infants and children by Rubenstein et al.[308] In children, there is also an apparent increase in occurrence of desquamative interstitial pneumonitis (DIP) (see Fig. 6–8) in AIDS cases.[23,307,308] Less common in

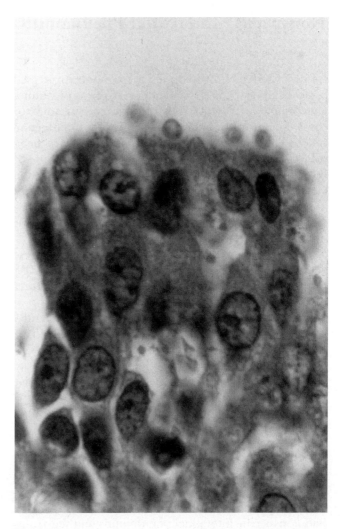

Fig. 6–15. Cryptosporidiosis seen as small round parasites on surface of bronchial mucosa. (Courtesy of W. Travis, MD, National Institutes of Health, Bethesda, Maryland.)

adults, in one series DIP was found in 3% of adult AIDS autopsies.

As nicely reviewed by White and Matthay,[23] HIV infection itself has been documented in lungs and their secretions and it is wondered whether LIP could be a primary immunologic response to this virus.[313–315] Likewise, it has been wondered whether Epstein–Barr virus may cause or be related to LIP.[316–319] Of interest, Epstein–Barr virus-infected cells are especially susceptible to HIV infection.[320] BAL studies may refer to the entity of "lymphocytic alveolitis," when they are not accompanied by tissue confirmation.[321] A LIP diagnosis requires tissue diagnosis by either transbronchial biopsy or open lung biopsy because an increased number of lymphocytes in BAL is nonspecific. Lymphocytic bronchiolitis is also associated with HIV infection.[322]

Nonspecific Interstitial Pneumonitis

Kaposi's Sarcoma

As discussed in lung biopsies in immunosuppressed hosts (Chapter 1), this is a common pathway of pulmonary injury in patients with respiratory symptoms or chest radiography abnormalities in whom no infection can be documented. These patients may have been subject to other identifiable infections preceding or following the biopsy or an assortment of drugs, antibiotics, oxygen treatment, and coexistent diseases before biopsy. This was seen in pre-AIDS era and defined by Fanta and Pennington[323] using the term "nonspecific interstitial pneumonitis."

In a large series, Suffredini et al.[324] noted these changes in 32% of all episodes of pneumonitis in AIDS cases who were referred at the U.S. National Institutes of Health either before or within 48 h of institution of antimicrobial therapy. By their definition, this entity consists of "diffuse alveolar damage of varying degrees in association with increased number of macrophages, alveolar hemorrhage, or lymphoid aggregates, and no associated microbial pathogens on the bronchoalveolar lavage stains or culture or on histologic tissues sections." Most of these did not show progression of the pulmonary abnormalities, even when antibiotics were discontinued, and this was true even of those that persisted through time of death. The radiographic and histologic findings in this group of 41 patients was compared with 21 patients with follow-up after initial episode of pneumocystis pneumonia; 100% of the follow-up patients had nonspecific interstitial pneumonitis on their transbronchial biopsies despite histologic clearance of infectious organisms as far as could be detected by special stains. Of note, more than 50% of patients with nonspecific interstitial pneumonitis have a normal chest radiograph. In AIDS cases, the effects seen in other immunocompromised hosts, such as drug toxicities from chemotherapeutic agents, radiation, and oxygen toxicity, are often not present and so cannot be implicated. It is again wondered whether it is caused primarily by the HIV infection, Epstein–Barr virus, other viruses such as preinclusion CMV, effects of therapy, associated toxins, or other agents. At the same institution as the study just mentioned, Ognibene et al.[77] studied the incidence of *Pneumocystis carinii* pneumonia in asymptomatic HIV-positive patients without pulmonary manifestations of AIDS or with low CD4+ count and found no detectable PCP in BAL or transbronchial biopsy specimens; in 11 of 23 patients (48%), however, there was evidence of chronic nonspecific interstitial pneumonitis.

The history of disseminated Kaposi's sarcoma is interesting, and its occurrence in AIDS cases with severe immunosuppression was foretold in the early days of organ transplantation, especially kidney transplantation (see Chapter 33). Kaposi's sarcoma is the most common malignancy in HIV-positive patients.[325] Most patients have extrapulmonary Kaposi's sarcoma (KS), particularly of skin, before they have disseminated disease. Of the first 1,000 reported cases of AIDS, KS was the initial manifestation of the disease in one-third[326] and was noted[327] 1 month after the two original reports of unusual clusters of pneumocystis pneumonia in homosexual patients.[1-3] Pulmonary KS occurs in about 20%–25% of those AIDS cases with cutaneous KS.[29,328,329]

The high incidence of KS in AIDS patients is unexplained, but is thought perhaps to be caused by a cofactor such as cytomegalovirus (CMV) infection.[23] The incidence of both KS and CMV is declining for unknown reasons in AIDS patients,[23] and KS is now the basis for initial diagnosis of AIDS in only 10% versus 33% initially[326] and is seen in the course of AIDS illness in only 20% (versus 60% in earlier years).[330] Patients with pulmonary KS may present with violaceous plaques in their bronchi, on their pleura, sometimes with bloody pleural effusion, or with diffuse interstitial infiltrates that follow interlobular septa. Kaposi's sarcoma is rather unique in that it is a lymphangitic sarcoma which especially well demonstrated in the lung (see Chapter 33). When in the lungs, it presents with respiratory symptoms in some 21%–40% of patients.[18,329,331,332] Many cases are undetected during life, but as seen in autopsy series the incidence of pulmonary KS is about 50%, varying between 38% and 75%.[171,333,334]

Symptoms of KS include nonproductive cough and occasionally a fever, which appears to be related in some patients to KS only, and about the only symptom that is fairly specific is hemoptysis. Pleural effusions have been recorded in 15%–66% of cases,[18,329,332,335,336] with bilateral effusions reported most often in association with pulmonary infiltrates but occasionally as its sole manifestation of pulmonary KS.[329,335] Thoracic lymph node enlargement has not been noted in some series[325,329,331,333] but was found in 23%–63% of patients in others.[331,332,335-338] Although the yield of transbronchial biopsy is variable, if the clinician sees a violaceous plaque and uses a large alligator forceps, it is increasingly easy to make this diagnosis (see Chapter 33). Of interest, even open lung biopsies miss some cases that were confirmed shortly thereafter at autopsy.[29,175,329] Most patients with pulmonary KS do not die of this disease but of other complications of AIDS.

Lymphomas

An increased number of non-Hodgkin's lymphomas[339–349] were noted early in the course of AIDS, and a series of 90 cases was published in 1984.[347] It is now the second most common cause of AIDS malignancy.[325] Most of these are high-grade B cell lymphomas, often (about 80%)[348] extranodal, usually with widespread dissemination with an increasing percentage occuring in the brain.[325,349,350] Presence of any high-grade lymphoma in association with HIV represents a diagnostic criterion for AIDS (see Table 6–1).

The most common sites for these lymphomas are the central nervous system, gastrointestinal tract, liver, spleen, bone marrow, and skin[342–344] but unusual sites have also been identified. Most patients have died of opportunistic infections rather than directly of lymphomas.[351] Chemotherapy or corticosteroids used to treat the lymphomas may further enhance opportunistic infections and provides one of the instances of invasive *Aspergillus* being identified in AIDS cases (see earlier).

Hodgkin's disease does occur but is not common and is infrequent enough as to not represent a defining diagnosis of AIDS. Intrathoracic lymphomas may present with nodal spread, but Kaposi's sarcoma or mycobacterial or fungal infections should also be considered; in one series of 22 AIDS cases with hilar and/or mediastinal adenopathy, 95% were caused by infection.[108]

More information is available in Chapter 31 and in the excellent review by White and Matthay.[23]

References

1. Gottlieb MS, Schanker H, Fan P, Saxon A, Weisman JD. Pneumocystis pneumonia—Los Angeles. MMWR 1981;30:250–252.
2. Gottlieb MS, Schroff R, Schanker HM, et al. *Pneumocystis carinii* pneumonia and mucosal candidiasis in previously healthy homosexual men. Evidence of a new acquired cellular immunodeficiency. N Engl J Med 1981;305:1425–1431.
3. Masur H, Michelis MA, Green JB, et al. An outbreak of community-acquired *Pneumocystis carinii* pneumonia. N Engl J Med 1981;305:1431–1438.
4. Garay SM. The acquired immunodeficiency syndrome. In: Fishman AP, ed. Pulmonary diseases and disorders, 2d Ed. New York: McGraw-Hill, 1988:1683–1705.
5. Baker JL, Kelen GD, Silverson KT, Quinn TC. Unsuspected human immunodeficiency virus in critically ill emergency patients. JAMA 1987;275:2609–2611.
6. Rutherford GW, Lifson AR, Hersol NA. Course of HIV-1 infection in a cohort of homosexual and bisexual men: An 11-year follow up study. Br Med J 1990;301:1183–1188.
7. AIDS 'out of control', will strike everywhere. Am Med News June 22, 1992:35.
8. Update: Acquired immunodeficiency syndrome—United States, 1981–1990. MMWR 1991;40:358–369.
9. Centers for Disease Control: Revision of the CDC surveillance case definition for acquired immunodeficiency syndrome. MMWR (Suppl. IS) 1987;36:3S–15S.
10. O'Brien TR, George R, Holmberg SD. Human immunodeficiency virus type 2 infections in the United States: Epidemiology, diagnosis and public health implications. JAMA 1992;267:2775–2779.
11. Centers for Disease Control: HIV/AIDS Surveillance Report, January 1991;1–22.
12. Farizo KM, Buehler JW, Chamberland ME, et al. Spectrum of disease in persons with human immunodeficiency virus infection in the United States. JAMA 1992;267:1798–1805.
13. 1992 Revised classification system for HIV infection and expanded AIDS surveillance case definition for adolescents and adults. Atlanta, Georgia: Centers for Disease Control, 1991. (Draft issued for public comment, November 1991. Final pending.)
14. Moss AR, Bacchetti P, Osmond D, et al. Most men seropositive for HIV will progress to AIDS or ARD: Three-year follow-up of the San Francisco General Hospital cohort. Br Med J 1988;296:745–750.
15. Hopewell PC. Human immunodeficiency virus-associated lung disease: an overview. Semin Respir Infect 1989;4:73–74.
16. Ioachim HL. Pathology of AIDS: Color atlas and textbook. Philadelphia: Lippincott, 1988.
17. White DA, Stover DE. Pulmonary effects of AIDS. Clin Chest Med 1988;9:363–537.
18. Stover DE, White DA, Romano PA, Gellene RA, Robeson WA. Spectrum of pulmonary diseases associated with the acquired immune deficiency syndrome. Am J Med 1985;78:429–437.
19 Murray JF, Felton CP, Garay S, et al. Pulmonary complications of the acquired immunodeficiency syndrome. Report of a National Heart, Lung, and Blood Institute Workshop. N Engl J Med 1984;310:1682–1688.
20. Murray JF, Garay SM, Hopewell PC, Mills J, Snider GL, Stover DE. Pulmonary complications of the acquired immunodeficiency syndrome: An update. Am Rev Respir Dis 1987;135:504–509.
21. Murray JF, Mills JL. Pulmonary infectious complications of human immunodeficiency virus infection: Part 1. Am Rev Respir Dis 1990;141:1356–1372.
22. Murray JF, Mills JL. Pulmonary infectious complications of human immunodeficiency virus infection: Part 2. Am

Rev Respir Dis 1990;141:1582–1598.

23. White DA, Matthay RA. Noninfectious pulmonary complications of infection with the human immunodeficiency virus. Am Rev Respir Dis 1989;140:1763–1787.

24. McLoud TC, Naidich DP. Thoracic disease in the immunocompromised patient. Radiol Clin North Am 1992;30:525–554.

25. Gal AA, Hartman B, Koss MN, Stringle S. A review of pulmonary pathology in the acquired immune deficiency syndrome. Surg Pathol 1988;1:325–346.

26. Guarda L, Luna MA, Smith JL, Jr., Mansell PWA, Gyorkey F, Roca AN. Acquired immune deficiency syndrome: Postmortem findings. Am J Clin Pathol 1984;81:549–558.

27. Moskowitz L, Hensley GT, Chan JC, Adams K. Immediate causes of death in acquired immunodeficiency syndrome. Arch Pathol Lab Med 1985;109:735–738.

28. Welch K, Finkbeiner W, Alpers CE, et al. Autopsy findings in the acquired immune deficiency syndrome. JAMA 1984;252:1152–1159.

29. Niedt GW, Schinella RA. Acquired immunodeficiency syndrome. Arch Pathol Lab Med 1985;109:727–734.

30. Marchevsky A, Rosen MJ, Chrystal G, Kleinerman J. Pulmonary complications of the acquired immunodeficiency syndrome: A clinicopathologic study of 70 cases. Hum Pathol 1985;16:659–670.

31. Wallace JW, Hannah JB. Pulmonary disease at autopsy in patients with the acquired immunodeficiency syndrome. West J Med 1988;149:167–171.

32. McKenzie R, Travis WD, Dolan SA, et al. The causes of death in patients with human immunodeficiency syndrome: A clinical and pathologic study with emphasis on the role of pulmonary diseases. Medicine (Baltimore) 1991;70:326–343.

33. Mitchell DM. Diagnostic problems in AIDS and the lung. Respir Med 1989;83:9–14.

34. Mitchell DM, Miller RF. Recent developments in the management of the pulmonary complications of HIV disease. Thorax 1992;47:381–390.

35. Heckbert SR, Elarth A, Nolan CM. The impact of human immunodeficiency virus infection on tuberculosis in young men in Seattle-King County, Washington. Chest 1992;102:433–437.

36. Lane HC, Masur M, Edgar LC, et al. Abnormalities of B-cell activation and immunoregulation in patients with the acquired immunodeficiency syndrome. N Engl J Med 1983;309:453–458.

37. Ammann AJ, Schiffman G, Abrams D, Volberding P, Ziegler J, Conant M. B-cell immunodeficiency in acquired immune deficiency syndrome. JAMA 1984;251:1447–1449.

38. Pahwa SG, Quilop MTJ, Lange M, Pahwa RN, Grieco MH. Defective B-lymphocyte function in homosexual men in relation to the acquired immunodeficiency syndrome. Ann Intern Med 1984;101:757–763.

39. Simberkoff MS, El Sadr W, Schiffman G, Rahal JJ, Jr. Streptococcus pneumoniae infections and bacteremia in patients with acquired immunodeficiency syndrome with report of a pneumococcal vaccine failure. Am Rev

Respir Dis 1984;130:1174–1176.

40. Schnittman SM, Lane HC, Higgins SE, Folks T, Fauci AS. Direct polyclonal activation of human B-lymphocytes by the acquired immunodeficiency syndrome virus. Science 1986;233:1084–1086.

41. Seligmann M, Pinching AJ, Rosen FS, et al. Immunology of human immunodeficiency virus infection and the acquired immunodeficiency syndrome: An update. Ann Intern Med 1987;107:234–242.

42. Janoff EN, Douglas JM, Jr., Gabriel M, et al. Class-specific antibody response to pneumococcal polysaccharides in men infected with human immunodeficiency virus type 1. J Infect Dis 1988;158:983–990.

43. Levine SJ, White DA. *Pneumocystis carinii*. Clin Chest Med 1988;9:395–423.

44. Bedrossian CWM, ed. *Pneumocystis carinii* infection. Semin Diagn Pathol 1989;6:191–312.

45. Miller RF, Mitchell DM. *Pneumocystis carinii* pneumonia. Thorax 1992;42:305–314.

46. Rosen MJ, Tow TW, Tierstein AS, Chuang MT, Marchevsky A, Boltone EJ. Diagnosis of pulmonary complications of the acquired immune deficiency syndrome. Thorax 1985;40:571–575.

47. Charron M, Ackerman ES, Kolodny GM, Rosenthal L. Focal lung uptake of gallium-67 in patients with acquired immunodeficiency syndrome secondary to *Pneumocystis carinii* pneumonia. Eur J Nucl Med 1988;14:424–426.

48. DeLorenzo LJ, Huang CT, Maguire GP, Stone DJ, Rosen MJ. Roentgenographic patterns of *Pneumocystis carinii* pneumonia in 104 patients with AIDS. Chest 1987;91:323–327.

49. Afessa B, Green WR, Williams WA, et al. *Pneumocystis carinii* complicated by lymphadenopathy and pneumothorax. Arch Intern Med 1988;148:2651–2654.

50. Bergin CJ, Wirth RL, Berry GJ, et al. *Pneumocystis carinii* pneumonia: CT and HRCT observations. J Comput Assist Tomogr 1990;14:756–759.

51. Kuhlman JE, Kavaro M, Fishman EK, et al. *Pneumocystis carinii* pneumonia: spectrum of parenchymal CT findings. Radiology 1990;175:711–714.

52. Nadich DP, McGuinness G. Pulmonary manifestations of AIDS: Radiographic CT correlation. Radiol Clin North Am 1991;29:999–1017.

53. Gamsu G, Hecht ST, Birnberg FA, Coleman DI, Golden JA. *Pneumocystis carinii* pneumonia in homosexual men. AJR 1982;139:647–651.

54. Cohen BA, Pomeranz S, Rabinowitz JG, et al. Pulmonary complications of AIDS: Radiologic features. AJR 1984;143:115–122.

55. Molthrop DC, Thiele JS, Cook EW, Faust BF. Unusual *Pneumocystis carinii* pneumonia in an AIDS patient. J La State Med Soc 1987;139:63–65.

56. Stokes DC, Shenep JL, Horowitz ME, Hughes WT. Presentation of *Pneumocystis carinii* pneumonia as unilateral hyperlucent lung. Chest 1988;94:201–202.

57. Gagliardi AJ, Stover DE, Zaman MK. Endobronchial *Pneumocystis carinii* infection in a patient with the acquired immune deficiency syndrome. Chest 1987;91:

463–464.

58. Travis WD, Lack EE, Ognibene FP, Suffredini AF, Shelhamer JH. Lung biopsy interpretation in the acquired immunodeficiency syndrome (AIDS). Review of the National Institutes of Health experience with literature review. Prog AIDS Pathol 1989;1:51–84.

59. Travis WD, Pittaluga S, Lipschitz GY, et al. Atypical pathologic manifestations of *Pneumocystis carinii* pneumonia in the acquired immune deficiency syndrome. Review of 123 lung biopsies from 76 patients with emphasis on cysts, vascular invasion, vasculitis, and granulomas. Am J Surg Pathol 1990;14:615–625.

60. Saldana MJ, Mones J. Cavitation and other atypical manifestations of *Pneumocystis carinii* pneumonia. Semin Diagn Pathol 1989;6:273–286.

61. Saldana MJ, Mones JM, Martinez GR. The pathology of treated *Pneumocystis carinii* pneumonia. Semin Diagn Pathol 1989;6:300–312.

62. Gal AA, Koss MN, Strigle S, Angritt P. *Pneumocystis carinii* infection in the acquired immune deficiency syndrome. Semin Diagn Pathol 1989;6:287–299.

63. Eng RHK, Bishburg E, Smith SM. Evidence of destruction of lung tissue during *Pneumocystis carinii* infection. Arch Intern Med 1987;147:746–749.

64. Hazel E, Sethi N, Jacquette G, Dobkin J. Diminished sulfa-trimethoprim toxicity in blacks treated for *Pneumocystis carinii* pneumonia. In: Proceedings, Third International Conference on AIDS, Washington, DC, 1987:208 (abstr.).

65. Gordin FM, Simon GL, Wofsy CB, Mills J. Adverse reactions to trimethoprim-sulfamethoxazole in patients with the acquired immunodeficiency syndrome. Ann Intern Med 1984;100:495–499.

66. Masur J, Frederick P, Ognibene FP, et al. CD4 counts as predictors of opportunistic pneumonias in human immunodeficiency virus (HIV) infection. Ann Intern Med 1989;111:223–231.

67. Centers for Disease Control. Guidelines for prophylaxis against *Pneumocystis carinii* pneumonia for persons with human immunodeficiency virus infection. MMWR 1989;38:1–8.

68. Kovacs JA, Heimenz JW, Macher AM, et al. *Pneumocystis carinii* pneumonia: A comparison between patients with the acquired immunodeficiency syndrome and patients with other immunodeficiencies. Ann Intern Med 1984;100:663–671.

69. Wachter RM, Luce JM, Hopewell PC. Critical care of patients with AIDS. JAMA 1992;267:541–547.

70. Wachter RM, Luce JM, Turner J, Volberding P, Hopewell PC. Intensive care of patients with the acquired immunodeficiency syndrome. Am Rev Respir Dis 1986;134:891–896.

71. Kovacs JA. Diagnosis, treatment and prevention of *Pneumocystis carinii* pneumonia in HIV-infected patients. AIDS Updates March/April 1989;2:1–12.

72. Wachter RM, Russi MB, Hopewell PC, Luce JM. The improving survival rate after intensive care for *P. carinii* pneumonia and respiratory failure. In: Fifth International Conference on AIDS, Montreal, Canada, 1989:201 (abstr.).

73. Efferen LS, Nadarajah D, Palat DS. Survival following mechanical ventilation for *Pneumocystis carinii* pneumonia in patients with acquired immunodeficiency syndrome: A different perspective. Am J Med 1989; 87:401–404.

74. Coleman DL, Luce JM, Wilber JC, et al. Antibody to the retrovirus associated with acquired immunodeficiency syndrome (AIDS). Presence in presumably healthy San Franciscans who died unexpectedly. Arch Intern Med 1986;146:713–715.

75. Blumenfeld W, McCook O, Holodniy M, Katzenstein DA. Correlation of morphologic diagnosis of *Pneumocystis carinii* with the presence of *Pneumocystis* DNA amplified by the polymerase chain reaction. Mod Pathol 1992;5:103–106.

76. Lundgren JD, Orholm M, Nielsen TL, Iversen J, Hertz J, Nielsen JO. Bronchoscopy of symptom free patients infected with human immunodeficiency virus for detection of pneumocystosis. Thorax 1989;44:68–69.

77. Ognibene FP, Masur H, Rogers P, et al. Nonspecific interstitial pneumonitis without evidence of *Pneumocystis carinii* in asymptomatic patients infected with human immunodeficiency virus (HIV). Ann Intern Med 1988;109:874–879.

78. Millard PR, Heryet AR. Observation favoring *Pneumocystis carinii* pneumonia as a primary infection: A monoclonal antibody study on paraffin sections. J Pathol 1988;154:365–370.

79. Wakefield AE, Pixley FJ, Banerji S, et al. Detection of *Pneumocystis carinii* with DNA amplification. Lancet 1990;336:451–453.

80. Wakefield AE, Guiver L, Miller RF, Hopkin JM. DNA amplification on induced sputum samples for diagnosis of *Pneumocystis carinii* pneumonia. Lancet 1991;337: 1378–1379.

81. Peters SE, Wakefield AE, Sinclair K, Millard PR, Hopkin JM. A search for *Pneumocystis carinii* in post mortem lungs by DNA amplification. J Pathol 1992;166:195–198.

82. Raviglione MC. Extrapulmonary pneumocystosis: The first 50 cases. Rev Infect Dis 1990;12:1127–1138.

83. Milligan SA, Stulbarg MS, Gamsu G, Golden JA. *Pneumocystis carinii* pneumonia radiographically simulating tuberculosis. Am Rev Respir Dis 1985;132:1124–1126.

84. Abd AG, Nierman DM, Ilowite JS, Pierson RN, Bell ALL. Bilateral upper lobe *Pneumocystis carinii* pneumonia in a patient receiving inhaled pentamidine prophylaxis. Chest 1988;94:329–331.

85. Scannel KA. Atypical presentation of *Pneumocystis carinii* pneumonia in a patient receiving inhalational pentamidine. Am J Med 1988;85:881–884.

86. Conces DJ, Jr., Kraft JL, Vix V, Tarver RD. Apical *Pneumocystis carinii* pneumonia after inhaled pentamidine prophylaxis. AJR 1989;152:1193–1194.

87. Murray CE, Schmidt RA. Tissue invasion by *Pneumocystis carinii*: A possible cause of cavitary pneumonia and pneumothorax. Hum Pathol 1992;23:1380–1387.

88. Balachandran I, Jones DB, Humphrey DM. A case of

Pneumocystis carinii in pleural fluid with cytologic, histologic and ultrastructural documentation. Acta Cytol
1990;34:486–490.

89. Mariuz P, Raviglione MC, Gould IA, Mullen MP. Pleural
Pneumocystic carinii infection. Chest 1991;99:774–776.

90. Dyner TS, Lang W, Busch DF, Gordon PR. Intravascular and pleural involvement by *Pneumocystis carinii* in a
patient with the acquired immunodeficiency syndrome
(AIDS). Ann Intern Med 1989;111:94 (letter).

91. Zandanell E. Pneumozystisbefund ausserhalb der lunge
bei interstitieller plasmazellularer pneumoniae der
sauglinge und fruhgerburtern. Zentralbl Allg Pathol
1954;92:74–80.

92. Doppman JL, Geelhoed GW, DeVita, VT. Atypical radiographic features in *Pneumocystis carinii* pneumonia.
Radiology 1975;114:39–44.

93. Paldy L, Ivady G. Roentgenologic diagnosis of interstitial plasma cell pneumonia in infancy. Natl Cancer Inst
Mongt 1976;43:99–118.

94. Barnett RN, Hull JG, Vortel V, et al. *Pneumocystis carinii*
in lymph nodes and spleen. Arch Pathol 1969;88:175–
180.

95. Awen CF, Baltzan MA. Systemic dissemination of *Pneumocystis carinii* pneumonia. Can Med Assoc J 1971;
104:809–812.

96. LeGolvan DP, Heidelberger KP. Disseminated granulomatous *Pneumocystis carinii* pneumonia. Arch Pathol
1973;95:344–348.

97. Henderson DW, Humeniuk V, Meadows R, Forbes IJ.
Pneumocystis carinii pneumonia with vascular and lymph
nodal involvement. Pathology 1974;6:235–241.

98. Case Records of the Massachusetts General Hospital,
Case 9-1989. N Engl J Med 1989;320:582–587.

99. Liu YC, Tomashefski JF, Tomford JW, Green H. Necrotizing *Pneumocystis carinii* vasculitis associated with lung
necrosis. Arch Pathol Lab Med 1989;113:494–497.

100. Grimes MM, LaPook JD, Bar MH, Wasserman HS,
Dwork A. Disseminated *Pneumocystis carinii* infection in a
patient with acquired immunodeficiency syndrome.
Hum Pathol 1987;18:307–308.

101. Davey RT, Jr., Margolis D, Kleiner D, Deyton L, Travis
W. Digital necrosis and disseminated *Pneumocystis carinii*
infection after aerosolized pentamidine prophylaxis.
Ann Intern Med 1989;111:681–682.

102. Coulman CU, Green I, Archibald RWR. Cutaneous
pneumocystosis. Ann Intern Med 1987;106:396–398.

103. Unger PD, Rosenblum M, Krown SE. Disseminated
Pneumocystis carinii infection in a patient with acquired
immunodeficiency syndrome. Hum Pathol 1989;19:
113–116.

104. Feuerstein IM, Archer A, Pluda J, et al. Thin-walled
cavities and pneumothorax in patients with *Pneumocystis
carinii* pneumonia: CT demonstration. Radiology
1990;174:697–702.

105. Kuhlman JE, Knowles MC, Fishman EK, Siegelman SS.
Premature bullous pulmonary damage in AIDS: CT
diagnosis. Radiology 1989;173:23–26.

106. Luddy RE, Champion LAA, Schwartz AD. *Pneumocystis
carinii* pneumonia with pneumatocele formation. Am J
Dis Child 1977;131:470 (letter).

107. Seigel R, Wolson AH. The radiographic manifestations
of chronic *Pneumocystis carinii* pneumonia. AJR 1977;
128:150–152.

108. Suster B, Akerman M, Orenstein M, Wax MR. Pulmonary manifestations of AIDS: Review of 106 episodes.
Radiology 1986;161:87–93.

109. Goodman PC, Daley C, Minagi H. Spontaneous pneumothorax in AIDS patients with *Pneumocystis carinii*
pneumonia. AJR 1986;147:29–31.

110. Naidich DP, Garay SM, Leitman BS, McCauley DI,
Radiographic manifestations of pulmonary disease in
the acquired immunodeficiency syndrome (AIDS).
Semin Roentgenol 1987;22:14–30.

111. Pincus PS, Sandler MA, Kallenback JM, et al. Multiple
pulmonary cavities—an unusual complication of *Pneumocystis carinii* pneumonia. S Afr Med J 1987;72:871–
872.

112. Gronbeck C, III. *Pneumocystis carinii* pneumonia presenting as cavitary lung disease. Milit Med 1988;153:
314–316.

113. Gurney JW, Bates FT. Pulmonary cystic disease: Comparison of *Pneumocystis carinii* pneumatoceles and bullous emphysema due to intravenous drug abuse. Radiology 1989;173:27–31.

114. Sandhu JS, Goodman PC. Pulmonary cysts associated
with *Pneumocystis carinii* pneumonia in patients with
AIDS. Radiology 1989;173:33–35.

115. Panicek DM. Cystic pulmonary lesions in patients with
AIDS. Radiology 1989;173:12–14.

116. Godwin JD, Webb WR, Savoca CJ, Gamsu G, Goodman
PC. Multiple thin-walled cystic lesions of the lung. AJR
1980;135:593–604.

117. Jules-Elysee KM, Stover DE, Zaman MB, Bernard EM,
White DA. Aerosolized pentamidine: Effect on diagno-
sis and presentation of *Pneumocystis carinii* pneumonia.
Ann Intern Med 1990;112:750–757.

118. Boisset GF. Subpleural emphysema complicating staphylococcal and other pneumonias. J Pediatr 1972;
81:259–266.

119. Stocker JT, McGill LC, Orsini EN. Postinfarction peripheral cysts of the lung in pediatric patients: A possible
cause of idiopathic spontaneous pneumothorax. Pediatr
Pulmonol 1985;1:7–18.

120. Tuddenham WJ. Glossary of terms for thoracic radiology: Recommendations of the Nomenclature Committee of the Fleischner Society. AJR 1984;143:509–517.

121. Austin J, Simon M, Trapnell D, Fraser RG. The
Fleischner Society Glossary: Critique and revisions. AJR
1985;145:1096–1098.

122. Chechani V, Zaman MK, Finch PJP. Chronic cavitary
Pneumocystis carinii pneumonia in a patient with AIDS.
Chest 1989;95:1347–1348.

123. Barrio JL, Suarez M, Rodriguez JL, Saldana MJ, Pitchenik AE. *Pneumocystis carinii* pneumonia presenting as
cavitating and noncavitating solitary pulmonary nodules
in patients with the acquired immunodeficiency syndrome. Am Rev Respir Dis 1986;134:1094–1096.

124. Klein JS, Warnock M, Webb WR, Gamsu G. Cavitating
and noncavitating granulomas in AIDS patients with
Pneumocystis pneumonitis. AJR 1989;152:753–754.

125. Stein DS, Weems JJ. Cavitary *Pneumocystis carinii* pneumonia in patients receiving aerosol pentamidine prophylaxis. South Med J 1991;84:273–275.

126. Conetta R, Kilstein S, Chitkara RK. Cavitation as an unusual roentgenographic manifestation of *Pneumocystis carinii* pneumonia in a patient with acquired immunodeficiency syndrome. NY State J Med 1988;88:652–653.

127. Wolschlager CM, Kahn FA, Chitkara RK, Shivaram U. Pulmonary manifestations of the acquired immunodeficiency syndrome (AIDS). Chest 1984;85:197–202.

128. Byrnes TA, Brevig JK, Yeoh CB. Pneumothorax in patients with acquired immunodeficiency syndrome. J Thorac Cardiovasc Surg 1989;98:546–550.

129. Joe L, Gordin F, Parker RH. Spontaneous pneumothorax with *Pneumocystis carinii* infection: Occurrence in patients with acquired immunodeficiency syndrome. Arch Intern Med 1986;146:1816–1817.

130. Leuong GS, Wardlaw L, Montgomery AB, Abrams DJ, Feigal DW. Pneumothorax in patients receiving aerosol pentamidine for *Pneumocystis carinii* pneumonia prophylaxis. In: Proceedings, Fifth International Conference on AIDS, Montreal, Canada, 1989:299 (abstr.).

131. Mann J, Montgomery AB, Luce JM, et al. Spontaneous pneumothorax in patients with *P. carinii* pneumonia. Am Rev Respir Dis 1989;139:A148.

132. Newsome GS, Ward DJ, Pierce PF. Spontaneous pneumothorax in AIDS patients on prophylactic aerosolized pentamidine. In: Proceedings, Fifth International Conference on AIDS, Montreal, Canada, 1989:256 (abstr.).

133. Shanley DJ, Luyckx BA, Haggerty MF, Murphy TF. Spontaneous pneumothorax in AIDS patients with recurrent *Pneumocystis carinii* pneumonia despite aerosolized pentamidine. Chest 1991;99:502–504.

134. Bevan JS, Doshi M, Grocutt M, Scott CD, Lloyd JH. AIDS-related *Pneumocystis carinii* pneumonia. Respir Med 1989;83:245–246.

135. McClellan ND, Miller SB, Parsons PE, Cohn DL. Pneumothorax with *Pneumocystis carinii* pneumonia in AIDS. Incidence and clinical features. Chest 1991;100:1224–1228.

136. Beers MF, Sohn M, Swartz M. Recurrent pneumothorax in AIDS patients with pneumocystis pneumonia: A clinicopathologic report of three cases and review of the literature. Chest 1990;98:266–270.

137. Lo SC, Shih JWK, Yang NY, Ou CY, Wang RYH. A novel virus-like infectious agent in patients with AIDS. Am J Trop Med Hyg 1989;40:213–226.

138. Lo SC, Wang RYH, Newton PB, III, Yang NY, Sonoda MA, Shih JWK. Fatal infection of silvered leaf monkeys with a virus-like infectious agent (VLIA) derived from a patient with AIDS. Am J Trop Med Hyg 1989;40:399–409.

139. Schmid KO. Studien zur Pneumocystis-Erkrankung des Menschen. I. Frankfurt Z Pathol 1964;74:121–145.

140. Arean VM. Pulmonary pneumocystosis, pathology of protozoal and helminthic diseases. In: Marcial-Rojas RA, ed. Pathology of protozoal and helminthic diseases with clinical correlation. Baltimore: Williams & Wilkins, 1971:307.

141. Cruickshank B. Pulmonary granulomatous pneumocystosis following renal transplantation: Report of a case. Am J Clin Pathol 1975;63:384–390.

142. Weber WR, Askin FB, Dehner LP. Lung biopsy in *Pneumocystis carinii* pneumonia: A histopathologic study of typical and atypical features. Am J Clin Pathol 1977;67:11–19.

143. Cupples JB, Blackie SP, Road JD. Granulomatous *Pneumocystis carinii* pneumonia mimicking tuberculosis. Arch Pathol Lab Med 1989;113:1281–1284.

144. Rahimi SA. Disseminated *Pneumocystis carinii* in thymic almphoplasia. Arch Pathol 1974;97:162–165.

145. Hartz JW, Geisinger KR, Scharyj M, Muss HB. Granulomatous pneumocystosis presenting as a solitary pulmonary nodule. Arch Pathol Lab Med 1985;109:466–469.

146. Bier S, Halton K, Krivisky B, Leonidas J. Pneumocystis pneumonia presenting as a single pulmonary nodule. Pediatr Radiol 1986;16:59–60.

147. Bleiweiss IJ, Jagirdar JS, Klein MJ, et al. Granulomatous *Pneumocystis carinii* pneumonia in three patients with the acquired immune deficiency syndrome. Chest 1988;94:580–583.

148. Bhatt M, Muller M, Sabatini M. Solitary pulmonary granulomatous pneumocystosis. Ann Intern Med 1988;109:343–344.

149. Blumenfeld W, Basgoz N, Owen WF, Schmidt D. Granulomatous pulmonary lesions in patients with the acquired immunodeficiency syndrome (AIDS) and *Pneumocystis carinii* infection. Ann Intern Med 1988;109:505–507.

150. Pilon VA, Echols RM, Celo JS, Elmendorf SL. Disseminated *Pneumocystis carinii* infection in AIDS. N Engl J Med 1987;316:1410–1411 (letter).

151. Schinella RA, Breda SD, Hammerschlag PE. Otic infection due to *Pneumocystis carinii* in an apparently healthy man with antibody to the human immunodeficiency virus. Ann Intern Med 1987;106:399–400.

152. Carter TR, Cooper PH, Petri WA, Jr., Kim CK, Walzer PD, Guerrant RL. *Pneumocystis carinii* infection of the small intestine in a patient with acquired immunodeficiency syndrome. Am J Clin Pathol 1988;89:679–683.

153. Dutz W. *Pneumocystis carinii* pneumonia. Pathol Annu 1970;5:309–341.

154. Burke BA, Good RA. *Pneumocystis carinii* infection. Medicine (Baltimore) 1973;52:23–51.

155. Lee MM, Schinella RA. Pulmonary calcification caused by *Pneumocystis carinii* pneumonia. A clinicopathological study of 13 cases in acquired immune deficiency syndrome patients. Am J Surg Pathol 1991;15:376–380.

156. Srivatsu SS, Burger CD, Douglas WW. Upper lobe pulmonary parenchymal calcification in a patient with AIDS and *Pneumocystis carinii* pneumonia receiving aerosolized pentamidine. Chest 1992;101:266–267.

157. Groskin SA, Massi AF, Randall PA. Calcified hilar and mediastinal lymph nodes in an AIDS patient with *Pneumocystis carinii* infaction. Radiology 1990;175:345–346.

158. Radin DR, Baker EL, Klatt EC, et al. Visceral and nodal calcification in patients with AIDS-related *Pneumocystis carinii* infection. AJR 1990;154:27–31.

159. Lubat E, Megibow AJ, Balthazar EJ, Goldenberg AS,

Birnbaum BA, Bosniak MA. Extrapulmonary *Pneumocystis carinii* infection in AIDS: CT findings. Radiology 1990;174:157–160.

160. Bargman JM, Wagner C, Cameron R. Renal cortical nephrocalcinosis: A manifestation of extrapulmonary *Pneumocystic carinii* infection in the acquired immunodeficiency syndrome. Am J Kid Dis 1991;17:712–715.

161. Anderson CD, Barrie HJ. Fatal pneumocystis pneumonia in an adult. Report of a case. Am J Clin Pathol 1960;34:365–370.

162. Shami MJ, Freeman W, Friedberg D, Siderides E, Listhous A, Ai E. A multicenter study of pneumocystic choroidopathy. Am J Ophthalmol 1991;112:15–22.

163. Pavlica F. Erste beobachfung von angeborener pneumozystenpneumonie bei einem reifen, ausgetragenen totgeborenen kind. Zentralbl Allg Pathol 1962;103:236–241.

164. Coker RJ, Clark D, Clayton EL, et al. Disseminated *Pneumocystis carinii* infection in AIDS. J Clin Pathol 1991;44:820–823.

165. Cote RJ, Rosenblum M, Telzak EE, May M, Unger PD, Cartum RW. Disseminated *Pneumocystis carinii* infection causing extrapulmonary organ failure: Clinical, pathologic, and immunohistochemical analysis. Mod Pathol 1990;3:25–30.

166. Telzak EE, Cote RJ, Gold JWM, Campbell SW, Armstrong D. Extrapulmonary *Pneumocystis carinii* infections. Rev Infect Dis 1990;12:380–386.

167. Walzer PD. *Pneumocystis carinii*. In: Mandell GL, Douglas RG, Jr., Bennett JE, eds. Principles and practice of infectious diseases. New York: Churchill Livingstone, 1990:2103–2110.

168. Harris JE. Improved short-term survival of AIDS patients initially diagnosed with *Pneumocystis carinii* pneumonia, 1984 through 1987. JAMA 1990;263:397–401.

169. Lemp GF, Payne SF, Neal D, Temelso T, Rutherford GW. Survival trends for patients with AIDS. JAMA 1990;263:402–406.

170. Fels AOS. Bacterial and fungal pneumonias. Clin Chest Med 1988;9:449–457.

171. Cohn DL. Bacterial pneumonia in the HIV-infected patient. Infect Dis Clin North Am 1991;5:485–507.

172. Polsky B, Gold JWM, Whimbey E, et al. Bacterial pneumonia in patients with the acquired immunodeficiency syndrome. Ann Intern Med 1986;104:38–41.

173. Witt DJ, Craven DE, McCabe WR. Bacterial infections in adult patients with the acquired immunodeficiency syndrome (AIDS) and AIDS-related complex. Am J Med 1987;82:900–906.

174. Fels AOS, Sourour MS, Stover DE. Pulmonary disease in AIDS patients with lymphoma. (In manuscript.)

175. Nash G, Fligiel S. Pathologic features of the lung in the acquired immune deficiency syndrome (AIDS): An autopsy study of seventeen homosexual males. Am J Clin Pathol 1984;81:6–12.

176. Murata GH, Ault MJ, Meyer RD. Community-acquired bacterial pneumonias in homosexual men: presumptive evidence for a defect in host resistance. AIDS Res 1984–5;1:379–393.

177. Whimbey E, Gold JWM, Polsky B, et al. Bacteremia and fungemia in patients with the acquired immunodeficiency syndrome. Ann Intern Med 1986;104:511–514.

178. Levine SJ, White DA, Fels AD. The incidence and significance of *Staphylococcus aureus* in respiratory cultures from patients infected with the human immunodeficiency virus. Am Rev Respir Dis 1990;141:89–93.

179. Allam AA, Kamholz SL. Legionella pneumonia and AIDS. Chest 1989;95:707–708.

180. Kramer MR, Uttamchandani RB. The radiographic appearance of pulmonary nocardiosis associated with AIDS. Chest 1990;98:382–385.

181. Feign DS. Nocardiosis of the lung: Chest radiographic finding in 21 cases. Radiology 1986;159:9–14.

182. Blaser MJ, Cohn DL. Opportunistic infections in patients with AIDS: Clues to the epidemiology of AIDS and the relative virulence of pathogens. Rev Infect Dis 1986;8:21–30.

183. Blaser MJ, Newman LS. A review of human salmonellosis. I. Infective dose. Rev Infect Dis 1982;4:1096–1106.

184. Regnery RL, Anderson BE, Clarridge JE, III, Rodriguez-Barradas MC, Jones DC, Carr JH. Characterization of a novel *Rochalimaea* species, *R. henselae* sp. nov., isolated from blood of a febrile, human immunodeficiency virus-positive patient. J Clin Microbiol 1992;30:265–274.

185. Slater LN, Welch DF, Min KW. *Rochalimaea henselai* causes bacillary angiomatosis and peliosis hepatis. Arch Intern Med 1992;152:602–606.

186. Slater LN, Min K-W. Polyploid endobronchial lesions. A manifestation of bacillary angiomatosis. Chest 1992;102:972–974.

187. Macher AM, De Vinatea ML, Tuur SM, Angritt P. AIDS and the mycoses. Infect Dis Clin North Am 1988;2:827–839.

188. Bronnimann DA, Adam RD, Galgiani JN, et al. Coccidiomycosis in the acquired immunodeficiency syndrome. Ann Intern Med 1987;106:372–379.

189. Mandell W, Goldberg DM, Neu HC. Histoplasmosis in patients with the acquired immune deficiency syndrome. Am J Med 1986;81:974–978.

190. Miller WT, Jr., Edelman JM, Miller WT. Cryptococcal pulmonary infection in patients with AIDS: Radiographic appearance. Radiology 1990;175:725–728.

191. Wheat LJ, Slama TG, Zeckel ML. Histoplasmosis in the acquired immune deficiency syndrome. Am J Med 1985;78:203–210.

192. Eng RHK, Bishburg E, Smith SM, Kapila R. Cryptococcal infections in patients with acquired immune deficiency syndrome. Am J Med 1986;81:19–23.

193. Zuger A, Louie E, Holzman RS, Simberkoff MS, Rahal JJ. Cryptococcal disease in patients with the acquired immunodeficiency syndrome. Ann Intern Med 1986;104:234–240.

194. Lerner CW, Tapper ML. Opportunistic infection complicating acquired immune deficiency syndrome: clinical features of 25 cases. Medicine (Baltimore) 1984;63:155–164.

195. Snider WD, Simpson DM, Nielson S, Gold JW, Metroka GE, Posner JB. Neurological complications of acquired immune deficiency syndrome: analysis of 50 patients.

Ann Neurol 1983;14:403–418.

196. Kovacs JA, Kovacs AA, Polis M, et al. Cryptococcosis in the acquired immunodeficiency syndrome. Ann Intern Med 1985;103:533–538.

197. Chechani V, Kamholz SL. Pulmonary manifestations of disseminated cryptococcus in patients with AIDS. Chest 1990;98:1060–1066.

198. Grant IH, Armstrong D. Fungal infections in AIDS: Cryptococcus. Infect Dis Clin North Am 1988;2:457–464.

199. Gal AA, Koss MN, Hawkins J, Evans S, Einstein H. The pathology of pulmonary cryptococcal infections in the acquired immunodeficiency syndrome. Arch Pathol Lab Med 1986;110:502–507.

200. Katz AS, Neisenbaum L, Mass B. Pleural effusion as the initial manifestation of disseminated cryptococcosis in acquired immune deficiency syndrome: Diagnosis by pleural biopsy. Chest 1989;96:440–441.

201. Devita VT, Jr., Broder S, Fauci AS, Kovacs JA, Chabner BA. Developmental therapeutics and the acquired immunodeficiency syndrome. Ann Intern Med 1987; 106:568–581.

202. Johnson PC, Hamil RJ, Sarosi GA. Clinical review: Progressive disseminated histoplasmosis in the AIDS patient. Semin Respir Infect 1989;4:139–146.

203. Bartholomew C, Raju C, Patrick A, Penco F, Jankey N. AIDS on Trinidad. Lancet 1984;1:103 (letter)

204. Bonner JR, Alexander J, Dismukes WE, et al. Disseminated histoplasmosis in patients with the acquired immune deficiency syndrome. Arch Intern Med 1984; 144:2178–2181.

205. Taylor MN, Baddour LM, Alexander JR. Disseminated histoplasmosis associated with acquired immune deficiency syndrome. Am J Med 1984;77:579.

206. Salzman SH, Smith RL, Aranda CP. Histoplasmosis in patients with risk factors for the acquired immunodeficiency syndrome (AIDS). Am Rev Respir Dis 1986; 135:A171.

207. Abrams DI, Robia M, Blumenfeld W, Simonson J, Choen MD, Hadley WK. Disseminated coccidioidomycosis in AIDS. N Engl J Med 1984;310:986–987.

208. Ampel NM, Ryan KJ, Carry PJ, Wieden MA, Schifman RB. Fungemia due to Coccidioides immitis: An analysis of 16 episodes in 15 patients and review of the literature. Medicine (Baltimore) 1986;65:312–321.

209. Roberts CJ. Coccidioidomycosis in acquired immune deficiency syndrome. Am J Med 1984;76:734.

210. Kovacs A, Forthal DN, Kovacs JA, Overturf GD. Disseminated coccidioidomycosis in a patient with acquired immune deficiency syndrome. West J Med 1984; 140:447–449.

211. Macher AM, DeVinatea ML, Koch Y, Bernard LR, Rivers R. Disseminated coccidioidomycosis in a patient with AIDS. Milit Med 1986;151:M57–M64.

212. Wolf JE, Little JR, Pappagianis D, Kobayashi GS. Disseminated coccidioidomycosis in a patient with the acquired immune deficiency syndrome. Diagn Microbiol Infect Dis 1986;5:331–336.

213. Denning DW, Follansbee SE, Scolaro M, Norris S, Edelstein H, Stevers DA. Pulmonary aspergillosis in the acquired immunodeficiency syndrome. N Engl J Med 1991;324:654–662.

214. Klapholz A, Salomon N, Perlman DC, Talavera W. Aspergillosis in the acquired immunodeficiency syndrome. Chest 1991;100:1614–1618.

215. Singh N, Yu VL, Rihs JD. Invasive aspergillosis in AIDS. South Med J 1991;84:822–827.

216. Murray JF. The white plague: Down and out, or up and coming. Am Rev Respir Dis 1989;140:1788–1795.

217. Styblo K. Epidemiology of tuberculosis. Jena, GDR: Gustav Fischer Verlag, 1984:1–161.

218. Jacobson MA. Mycobacterial diseases: Tuberculosis and Mycobacterium avium complex. Infect Dis Clin North Am 1988;2:465–474.

219. Centers for Disease Control. Tuberculosis and acquired immunodeficiency syndrome—Florida. MMWR 1986;35:587–590.

220. Louie E, Rice LB, Holzman RS. Tuberculosis in non-Haitian patients with acquired immunodeficiency syndrome. Chest 1986;90:542–545.

221. Handwerger S, Mildvan D, Senie R, McKinley FW. Tuberculosis and the acquired immunodeficiency syndrome at a New York City Hospital: 1978–1985. Chest 1987;91:176–180.

222. Sunderam G, McDonald RJ, Maniatis T, et al. Tuberculosis as a manifestation of the acquired immunodeficiency syndrome (AIDS). JAMA 1986;256:362–366.

223. Barnes PF, Bloch AB, Davidson PT, Snider DE, Jr. Tuberculosis in patients with human immunodeficiency virus infection. N Engl J Med 1991;324:1644–1650.

224. Pitchenik AE, Robinson HA. The radiographic appearance of tuberculosis in patients with the acquired immune deficiency syndrome (AIDS) and pre-AIDS. Am Rev Respir Dis 1985;131:393–396.

225. Chaisson RE, Schecter GR, Theuer CP, Rutherford GW, Echenberg DF, Hopewell PC. Tuberculosis in patients with the acquired immunodeficiency syndrome. Clinical features, response to therapy, and survival. Am Rev Respir Dis 1987;136:570–574.

226. Rouillon A, Pedrizet S, Parrot R. Transmission of tubercle bacilli: The effects of chemotherapy. Tubercle 1976;57:275–299.

227. Hopewell PC. Tuberculosis and the human immunodeficiency virus infection. Semin Respir Infect 1989; 4:111–112.

228. Hewlett D, Jr., Duncanson FP, Jagadha V, Lieberman J, Lenox TH, Wormser GP. Lymphadenopathy in an inner-city population consisting principally of intravenous drug abusers with suspected acquired immunodeficiency syndrome. Am Rev Respir Dis 1988;137:1275–1279.

229. Wolinsky E. Nontuberculous mycobacteria and associated diseases. Am Rev Respir Dis 1979;119:107–159.

230. MacDonnell KB, Glassroth J. Mycobacterium avium complex and other nontuberculous mycobacteria in patients with HIV infection. Semin Respir Infect 1989;4:123–132.

231. Damsker B, Bottone EF. Mycobacterium avium-Mycobacterium intracellulare from the intestinal tracts of patients with the acquired immunodeficiency syndrome: Con-

Cryptosporidium in paraffin-embedded tissue sections with the use of a monlconal antibody. Am J Clin Pathol 1989;91:206–209.

303. Current WL, Reese NC, Ernst JV, Bailey WS, Heyman MB, Weinstein WM. Human cryptosporidiosis in immunocompetent and immunodeficient persons: Studies of an outbreak and experimental transmissions. N Engl J Med 1983;308:1252–1257.

304. Guarda LA, Stein SA, Cleary KA, Ordonez NG. Human cryptosporidiosis in the acquired immunodeficiency syndrome. Arch Pathol Lab Med 1983;107:562–566.

305. Lefkowitch JH, Krumholz S, Feng-Chen KC, Griffin P, Despommier D, Brasitus TA. Cryptosporidiosis of the human small intestine: A light and electron microscopic study. Hum Pathol 1984;15:746–752.

306. Teirstein AS, Rosen MJ. Lymphocytic interstitial pneumonia. Clin Chest Med 1988;467–471.

307. Joshi VV, Oleske JM, Minnefor AB, et al. Pathologic pulmonary findings in children with the acquired immunodeficiency syndrome: A study of ten cases. Hum Pathol 1985;16:241–246.

308. Rubinstein A, Morecki R, Goldman H. Pulmonary disease in infants and children. Clin Chest Med 1988;507–517.

309. Joshi VV, Oleske JM. Pulmonary lesions in children with the acquired immunodeficiency syndrome: A reappraisal based on data in additional cases and follow-up study of previously reported cases. Hum Pathol 1986;17:641–642 (letter).

310. Kornstein MJ, Peitra GG, Hoxie JA, Conley ME. The pathology and treatment of interstitial pneumonitis in two infants with AIDS. Am Rev Respir Dis 1986;133:1196–1198.

311. Scott GB, Buch BE, Leterman JG, et al. Acquired immunodeficiency in infants. N Engl J Med 1984;310:76–81.

312. Lin RY, Gruber PJ, Saunders R, Perla, EN. Lymphocytic interstitial pneumonitis in adult HIV infection. NY State J Med 1988;88:273–276.

313. Resnick L, Pitchenik AE, Fisher E, Croney R. Detection of HTLV-III/LAV-specific IgG and antigen in bronchoalveolar lavage fluid from two patients with lymphocytic interstitial pneumonitis associated with AIDS-related complex. Am J Med 1987;82:553–558.

314. Ziza JM, Brun-Vezinet F, Venet A, et al. Lymphadenopathy-associated virus isolated from bronchoalveolar lavage fluid in AIDS-related complex with lymphoid interstitial pneumonitis. N Engl J Med 1985;313:183 (letter).

315. Chayt KJ, Harper ME, Marselle LM, et al. Detection of HTLV-III RNA in lungs of patients with AIDS and pulmonary involvement. JAMA 1986;156:2356–2359.

316. Andiman WA, Martin K, Rubinstein A, et al. Opportunistic lymphoproliferations associated with Epstein-Barr viral DNA in infants and children with AIDS. Lancet 1985;ii:1390–1393.

317. Pahwa S, Kaplan M, Fikrig S, et al. Spectrum of human T-cell lymphotropic virus type III infection in children. Recognition of symptomatic, asymptomatic, and seronegative patients. JAMA 1986;255:2299–2310.

318. Rubinstein A, Morecki R, Silverman B, et al. Pulmonary disease in children with acquired immune deficiency syndrome and AIDS-related complex. J Pediatr 1986; 108:498–503.

319. Fackler JC, Nagel JE, Adler WH, Mildvan PT, Ambinder RF. Epstein-Barr virus infection in a child with acquired immunodeficiency syndrome. Am J Dis Child 1985;139:1000–1004.

320. Montagnier L, Gruest J, Charmaret S, et al. Adaptation of lymphadenopathy associated virus (LAV) to replication in EBV-transformed B lymphoblastoid cell lines. Science 1984;225:63–66.

321. Guillon J-M, Autran B, Denis M, et al. Human immunodeficiency virus-related lymphocytic alveolitis. Chest 1988;94:1264–1270.

322. Ettensohn DB, Mayer KH, Kessimian N, Smith PS. Lymphocytic bronchiolitis associated with HIV infection. Chest 1988;93:201–202.

323. Fanta CH, Pennington JE. Fever and new lung infiltrates in the immunocompromised host. Clin Chest Med 1981;2:19–39.

324. Suffredini AF, Ognibene FP, Lack EE, et al. Nonspecific interstitial pneumonitis: A common cause of pulmonary disease in the acquired immunodeficiency syndrome. Ann Intern Med 1987;107:7–13.

325. Kaplan MH, Susin M, Pahwa SG, et al. Neoplastic complications of HTLV-III infection. Lymphomas and solid tumors. Am J Med 1987;82:389–396.

326. Des Jariais DC, Stoneburner R, Thomas P, Friedman SR. Declines in proportion of Kaposi's sarcoma among cases of AIDS in multiple risk groups in New York City. Lancet 1987;ii:1024–1025.

327. Centers for Disease Control: Kaposi's sarcoma and *Pneumocystis* pneumonia among homosexual men—New York City and California. MMWR 1981;30:305–308.

328. Ognibene FP, Shelhamer JH. Kaposi's sarcoma. Clin Chest Med 1988;9:459–465.

329. Ognibene FP, Steis RG, Macher AM, et al. Kaposi's sarcoma causing pulmonary infiltrates and respiratory failure in the acquired immunodeficiency syndrome. Ann Intern Med 1985;102:471–475.

330. Rutherford GW, Schwarcz SK, Lemp GF, et al. The epidemiology of AIDS-related Kaposi's sarcoma in San Francisco. J Infect Dis 1989;569–572.

331. Zibrak JD, Silvestri RC, Costello P, et al. Bronchoscopic and radiologic features of Kaposi's sarcoma involving the respiratory system. Chest 1986;90:476–479.

332. Garay SM, Belenko M, Fazzini E, Schinella R. Pulmonary manifestations of Kaposi's sarcoma. Chest 1987; 91:39–43.

333. Meduri GU, Stover DE, Lee M, Myskowski PL, Caravelli JF, Zaman MB. Pulmonary Kaposi's sarcoma in the acquired immune deficiency syndrome. Am J Med 1986;81:11–18.

334. Lemlich G, Schwam L, Lebwohl M. Kaposi's sarcoma and acquired immunodeficiency syndrome. Postmortem findings in twenty-four cases. J Am Acad Dermatol 1987;16:319–325.

335. Davis SD, Henschke CI, Chamides BK, Westcott JL. Intrathoracic Kaposi sarcoma in AIDS patients: Radiographic-pathologic correlation. Radiology 1987;163: 495–500.

336. Gill PS, Akil B, Colletti P, et al. Pulmonary Kaposi's sarcoma: Clinical findings and results of therapy. Am J Med 1989;87:57–61.

337. Kaplan LD, Hopewell PC, Jaffe H, Goodman PC, Bottles K. Volberding PA. Kaposi's sarcoma involving the lung in patients with the acquired immunodeficiency syndrome. J Acquir Immune Defic Syndr 1988;1:23–30.

338. Sivit CJ, Schwartz AM, Rockoff SD. Kaposi's sarcoma of the lung in AIDS: Radiologic-pathologic analysis. AJR 1987;148:25–28.

339. Ziegler JL, Miner RC, Rosenbaum ET, et al. Outbreak of Burkitt's-like lymphoma in homosexual men. Lancet 1982;ii:631–633.

340. Ahmed T, Wormser GP, Stahl RE, et al. Malignant lymphomas in a population at risk for acquired immune deficiency syndrome. Cancer (Philadelphia) 1987;60:719–723.

341. Beckhardt RN, Farady N, May M, Torres RA, Strauchen JA. Increased incidence of malignant lymphoma in AIDS: A comparison of risk groups and possible etiologic factors. Mt Sinai J Med (NY) 1988;55:383–389.

342. DiCarlo EF, Amberson JB, Metroka CE, Balard P, Moore A, Mouradian JA. Malignant lymphomas and the acquired immunodeficiency syndrome. Evaluation of 30 cases using a working formulation. Arch Pathol Lab Med 1986;110:1012–1016.

343. Ioachim HL, Cooper MC, Hellman GC. Lymphomas in men at high risk for acquired immune deficiency syndrome (AIDS). A study of 21 cases. Cancer (Philadelphia) 1985;56:2831–2842.

344. Kalter SP, Riggs SA, Cabanilla F, et al. Aggressive non-Hodgkin's lymphomas in immunocompromised homosexual males. Blood 1985;66:655–659.

345. Khojasteh A, Reynolds RD, Khojasteh CA. Malignant lymphorecticular lesions in patients with immune disorders resembling acquired immunodeficiency syndrome (AIDS): Review of cases. South Med J 1986;79:1070–1075.

346. Levine AM, Meyer PR, Begandy MK, et al. Development of B-cell lymphoma in homosexual men: Clinical and immunologic findings. Ann Intern Med 1984;100:7–13.

347. Ziegler JL, Beckstead JA, Volberding PA, et al. Non-Hodgkin's lymphoma in 90 homosexual men. Relation to generalized lymphadenopathy and the acquired immunodeficiency syndrome. N Engl J Med 1984;311:565–570.

348. Polish LB, Cohn DL, Ryder JW, Myers AM, O'Brien RF. Pulmonary non-Hodgkin's lymphoma in AIDS. Chest 1989;96:1321–1326.

349. Kaplan LD, Abrams DI, Feigal E, et al. AIDS-associated non-Hodgkin's lymphoma in San Francisco. JAMA 1989;261:719–724.

350. Knowles DM, Chamulak GA, Subar M, et al. Lymphoid neoplasia associated with the acquired immunodeficiency syndrome (AIDS). Ann Intern Med 1988;108:744–753.

351. Lowenthal DA, Strauss DJ, Campbell SW, Gold JWM, Clarkson BD, Koziner B. AIDS-related lymphoid neoplasia: The Memorial Hospital experience. Cancer (Philadelphia) 1988;61:2325–2337.

CHAPTER 7

Congenital and Developmental Diseases

J. Thomas Stocker*

The pathology of infectious diseases of the lung is, for the most part, similar in adults and children. However, a number of other disorders either are seen almost exclusively in the pediatric age group (e.g., congenital anomalies) or occur in circumstances peculiar to this age group (e.g., hyaline membrane disease and bronchopulmonary dysplasia). Congenital anomalies of the lung are usually noted within the first weeks to months of life but may not be discovered until later in childhood or, in some cases such as bronchogenic cysts, until adulthood. A knowledge of the development of the lung is important in the understanding of the morphologic features of these anomalies.

Development of the Lung

The *embryonic period* of lung development covers the period from 4 to 6 weeks in utero (Table 7–1).[1,2] The lung arises in the 3-mm-long embryo in the fourth week of gestation as a ventral outpouching of the foregut forming the laryngotracheal groove. A single lung bud forms from the groove late in the fourth week of gestation and divides into two primary bronchial buds, the forerunners of the right and left lobes (Fig. 7–1). The primary bronchi divide during the fifth week, forming lobar bronchi which by the end of the sixth week have given rise to the segmental bronchi (10 on the right and 8–9 on the left). These primitive airways are

composed of a central core of glycogen-rich epithelial cells lying on a thin basement membrane and surrounded by loose mesenchyme rich in mucopolysaccharides. The mesenchymal cells are round to oval with little or no evidence of differentiation to smooth muscle, fibroblasts, or cartilage. Widely separated capillaries can be found within the mesenchyme. Late in the embryonic period, the sixth aortic arches give rise to the primitive pulmonary arteries.[3] The primitive pulmonary veins appear as evaginations of the left atrium in the fourth week and unite with the mesenchymal capillary plexus early in the fifth week.[4]

With completion of proximal airway formation, the embryonic period ends and the *pseudoglandular period*, covering the period from 6 to 16 weeks of gestation, begins. Within this 10-week period all the conducting airways are formed through repeated branching of bronchial buds (Fig. 7–2). Subsequent growth of these airways is in size only.[5] Cilia can be seen on the surface of the pseudostratified columnar epithelium of the trachea and mainstream bronchi at 10 weeks of gestation and are present in the epithelial cells of the peripheral airways by 13 weeks. Goblet cells appear in bronchial epithelium at 13–14 weeks, and submucosal glands arise as solid buds from basal layers of surface epithelium at 15–16 weeks. Smooth muscle cells derived from the primitive mesenchyme surrounding the airways can be seen at the end of the seventh week and by the twelfth week from the posterior wall of large bronchi.[6] Lymphatics appear first in the hilar region of the lung in the eighth week and in the lung itself by the tenth week.[7]

The *acinar or canalicular period* follows at 17–28 weeks of gestation, during which time the basic structure of the gas-exchanging portion of the lung is formed and

---

*The opinions or assertions contained herein are the private views of the author and are not to be construed as official or reflecting the views of the Department of the Army or the Department of Defense.

Table 7–1. Phases of intrauterine lung development[a]

Phase	Gestation period	Major event
Embryonic	26 days–6 weeks	Development of major airways
Pseudoglandular	6–16 weeks	Development of airways to terminal bronchioles
Acinar or canalicular	16–28 weeks	Development of acinus and its vascularization
Saccular	28–34 weeks	Subdivision of saccules by secondary crests
Alveolar	34 weeks to term (and beyond)	Alveolar acquisition

[a] Adapted from Langston C. Prenatal lung growth and pulmonary hypoplasia. In: Stocker JT, ed. Pediatric pulmonary disease. Washington, DC: Hemisphere, 1989:2.

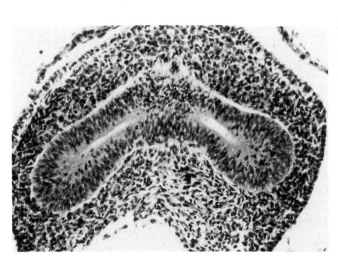

Fig. 7–1. Embryonic period. Lung in this 4-week-gestation embryo consists of right and left mainstem bronchi surrounded by undifferentiated mesenchyme. H and E, ×20 (AFIP Neg. 86-5323).

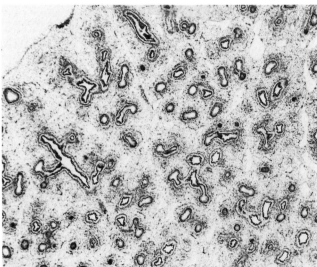

A

B

Fig. 7–2 A,B. Pseudoglandular period. **A.** At 10 weeks gestation, evenly distributed glandular structures, the primitive conducting airways, lie in loose mesenchymal tissue containing irregular clear spaces representing vascular channels. H and E, ×50 (AFIP Neg. 86-5324). **B.** Primitive airways are lined by tall columnar epithelial cells with apical nuclei and vacuolated basal cytoplasm rich in glycogen. Note early "condensation" of mesenchymal cells around airways as smooth muscle and fibroblasts differentiate. H and E, ×400 (AFIP Neg. 86-5325).

vascularized.[8] Beginning as smooth-walled, blind-ending channels lined by cuboidal epithelium and continuing through multiple subdivisions, acini take on an irregular internal configuration (Fig. 7–3). By 20 weeks, the cuboidal cells lining these potential gas-exchanging structures develop lamellar and multivesicular bodies associated with surfactant synthesis and can be identified as type II (alveolar) lining cells. At the same time, type I (alveolar) cells differentiate through flattening of the epithelial cells in the proximal portion of the acinus, forming the thin air–blood interface needed for gas exchange. The interstitium, which is thick and sparsely cellular during the early portion of this period, thins somewhat to allow some of the capillaries of the rapidly

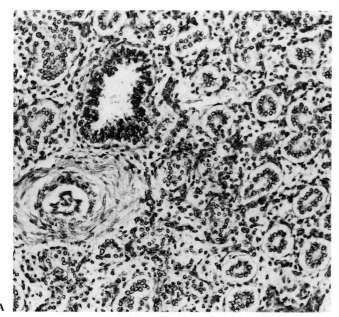

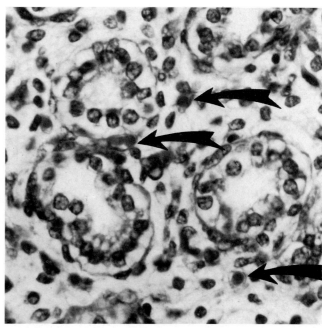

Fig. 7–3 A,B. Acinar (canalicular) period. **A.** Midway through acinar period, lung of 21-week-gestation fetus displays bronchiole and pulmonary artery (left) surrounded by primitive respiratory bronchioles and alveolar ducts lined by cuboidal epithelial cells. H and E, ×180 (AFIP Neg. 75-9743). **B.**

Capillaries (*arrows*) within loose interstitial tissue lie adjacent to basement membrane of primitive ducts but still are too far away from potential air spaces for effective gas exchange. H and E, ×575 (AFIP Neg. 76-7878).

increasing vasculature to be directly beneath the thinned type I cells. Submucosal glands in the trachea and bronchi progress from tubules to mucus-containing acini. Cartilage development in these same structures is complete by the twenty-fourth week.

The *saccular period* is from 28 to about 34 weeks of gestation, ending between 32 and 36 weeks, and is characterized by the development of lateral projections (secondary crests) that extend from the air space walls and divide the distal air spaces, or saccules, into smaller units (Fig. 7–4). At the same time a marked decrease in the interstitial tissue and concomitant increase in the capillary bed produces a distinct, double interwoven capillary network in the walls of the saccules.[9,10] Although cuboidal epithelial cells progressively decrease in proportion during this period, they still constitute the dominant cell of the more distal air spaces.

During the final phase of lung development, the *alveolar period*, formation of alveoli begins as early as 32 weeks and is present in all lungs by 36 weeks.[8] Alveoli develop as flask-shaped or multifaceted polygonal structures with thin walls with a double capillary network that meshes to appear as a single capillary bed (Fig. 7–5). Alveolar type I cells attenuate to form an extremely thin layer that, with the underlying basement membrane and endothelial cell cytoplasm of the capillary, measures approximately 0.2 μm, a thickness well

suited for gas exchange. Alveolar acquisition continues from late gestation through the neonatal period and early childhood until 18–24 months after birth.

The vascular supply of the lung changes significantly in late gestation and infancy. The bronchial arterial circulation, arising from the aortic arch and supplying the bronchi, bronchioles, and interlobular septa in older children and adults, also contributes significantly (in utero and early infancy) to the circulation to the alveolar ducts and alveoli in the central portions of the lung.[4]

Bronchial arteries at this stage have direct anastomotic connections with pulmonary arteries, and some of these connections are maintained into adulthood. The bronchial arteries directly supply pulmonary alveolar capillary beds at this time (Fig. 7–6).[11] Lymphatic channels at term have attained their adult distribution around pulmonary arteries, bronchi, bronchioles, and in interlobular septa anastomosing over the surface of the lung within the pleura. Lymphatic spaces do not exist between alveoli.

As these morphologic changes progress, quantitative changes occur as well. Between 20 and 32 weeks of gestation, the air space wall thickness decreases from 45 to 20 μm. This is accompanied by a proportional increase in air space volume and gas-exchanging surface area. At 28 weeks gestation, surface area is approxi-

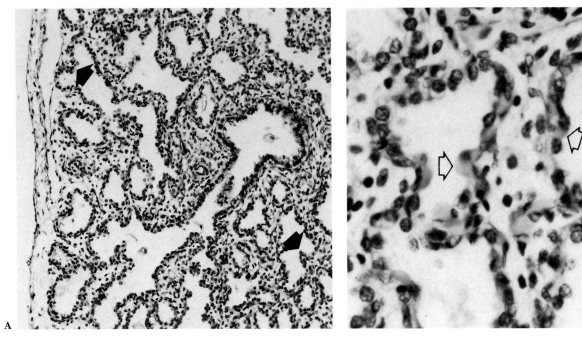

Fig. 7–4 A,B. Saccular period. **A.** Early in saccular period (28 weeks), secondary crests are present along air space walls (*arrowheads*) dividing saccules into smaller units. H and E, ×145 (AFIP Neg. 76-5079). **B.** Capillaries (*open arrowheads*) have pushed between alveolar lining cells in many areas to lie within 1–2 μm of airspace lumen. Interstitial space, while narrow, is still readily visible. H and E, ×615 (AFIP Neg. 76-5082).

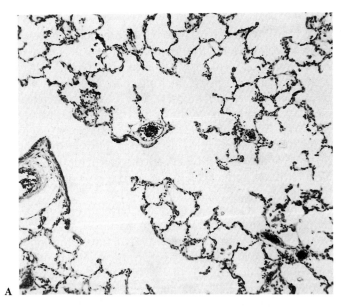

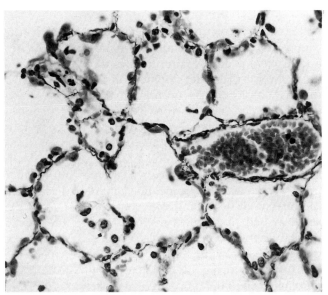

Fig. 7–5 A,B. Alveolar period. **A.** Lung of this 1-month-old infant resembles that of adult. H and E, ×100 (AFIP Neg. 76-7871). **B.** Alveolar walls display fine meshwork of capillaries beneath attenuated cytoplasm of type I alveolar lining cells. EVG, ×350 (AFIP Neg. 76-7873).

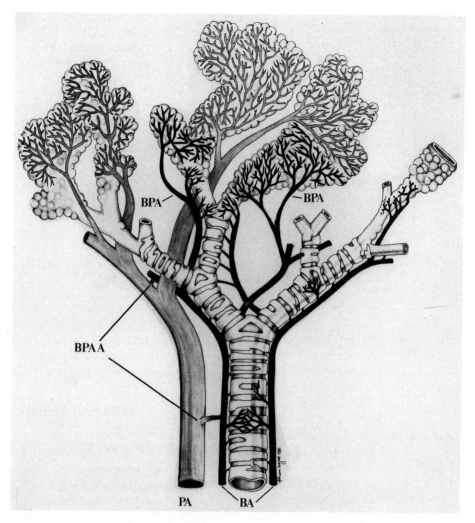

Fig. 7–6. Diagram of arterial supply to lung. Pulmonary artery (PA) is primary supply to alveolar ducts, alveolar saccules, and alveoli (left). Bronchial artery (BA) supplies bronchi and bronchioles to level of respiratory bronchioles (right). In utero and in infancy, bronchopulmonary arteries (BPA) can directly supply alveolar capillary bed along with bronchopulmonary arterial anastomoses (BPAA) that exist throughout life, providing direct connections between systemic and pulmonary arterial circulation. (From Stocker JT, McGill LC, Orsini EN. Postinfarction peripheral cysts of the lung in pediatric patients: A possible cause of idiopathic spontaneous pneumothorax. Pediatric Pulmonology 1985;1:7–18, with permission.)

mately 1 m², having increased only slightly since 20 weeks of gestation. By term, however, surface area is about 4 m², spread among an average of 55 million alveoli (range, 10–150 million). Alveoli increase in number after birth but alveolar development to the adult average of 300 million is usually complete by 2 years of age. Lung volume and alveolar size gradually increase throughout childhood with males attaining larger lung volumes than females.

Malformations of the Trachea

Laryngotracheoesophageal Cleft

Separation of the trachea from the esophagus occurs by 35 days of gestation with the formation of a septum derived from mesoderm that eventually forms the fused cricoid cartilage and arytenoid cartilage and tissue. Failure of formation of this septum leads to the

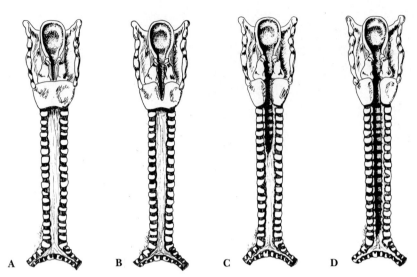

Fig. 7–7 A–D. Types of laryngotracheosophageal cleft. **A.** Supraglottic interaytenoid cleft. **B.** Partial cricoid cleft. **C.** Total cricoid cleft. **D.** Complete cleft to level of carina. (From Stocker JT. The respiratory tract. In: Stocker JT, Dehner LP, eds. Pediatric pathology. Philadelphia: Lippincott, 1992:511–519, with permission.)

development of one of the forms of laryngotracheoesophageal cleft (Fig. 7–7).

Infants present shortly after birth with respiratory distress, excessive oral mucus, and cyanosis and choking when feeding.[12–14] Other anomalies noted in more than 45% of cases include esophageal atresia, tracheoesophageal fistula (see following), and congenital heart malformations, all components of the VATER association. Pulmonary hypoplasia, extrophy of the bladder, polysplenia, the G syndrome, and facial anomalies have been described. Familial occurrence has also been reported.[15] Nearly 50% of the lesions are limited to a cleft of the supraglottic interarytenoid region, sparing the cricoid cartilage and trachea (Fig. 7–7A).

Tracheal Agenesis

Tracheal agenesis is a rarely occurring entity that is usually associated with tracheo- or bronchoesophageal fistula. Approximately 40 cases, both with and without fistulous connection to the esophagus, have been reported.[16–24] A classification scheme (Fig. 7–8)[25] identifying seven types of tracheal ageneses proposed by Faro et al. in 1979[19] was based largely on the locations and size of the tracheo- or bronchoesophageal fistula. Only their types A and B have no communication with the esophagus, encompassing both cases of total pulmonary agenesis as well as cases of tracheal agenesis without esophageal fistula. Only 6 cases of tracheal agenesis with no esophageal connection (Fig. 7–8F) have been reported, including 2 seen by the authors.[16,21–23] Both of these were premature infants (26 weeks gestation), a stillborn girl and a boy who survived only a few minutes. Both infants displayed other anomalies (ventricular septal defect, syndactyly) as well as lungs that grossly and histologically were virtually identical to cases of

extralobar sequestration. Associated anomalies, many part of the VATER association, are seen in 75% of infants with all forms of tracheal agenesis.[17,20] Survival beyond the first week of life is rare, and no survivors beyond 6 weeks of age have been reported.[19]

Tracheal Stenosis

While subglottic stenosis is often seen in the neonatal period as an acquired lesion related to intubation and, recently, high-frequency jet ventilation, congenital stenosis of the trachea is rare. Three forms are described: (1) generalized hypoplasia; (2) funnel-like narrowing, usually tapering to a tight stenosis just above the carina; and (3) segmental stenosis of various lengths occurring at any level.[26,27] Complete tracheal cartilage rings can produce a "napkin-ring" stenosis.[28] Extrinsic compression of the trachea may be produced by abnormally placed or abnormally large blood vessels such as a vascular ring caused by a right or double aortic arch, an aberrant right subclavian artery, an anomalous left carotid or innominate artery, and a "sling" retrotracheal left pulmonary artery.[29] Bronchial abnormalities and pulmonary agenesis have been seen in association with tracheal stenosis.[26,30] Tracheal compression by a dilated esophagus has been noted in a 7-year-old boy.[31]

Tracheomalacia

Congenital tracheomalacia ("soft or collapsing" trachea) is an exceedingly rare entity that overlaps considerably with tracheal stenosis secondary to cartilage plate deficiency.[27] Although isolated cases of diffuse tracheomalacia have been reported in infants with polychondritis[32] and various chondrodystrophies (Ellis–van Creveld syndrome, Langer-type mesomelic dwarfism,

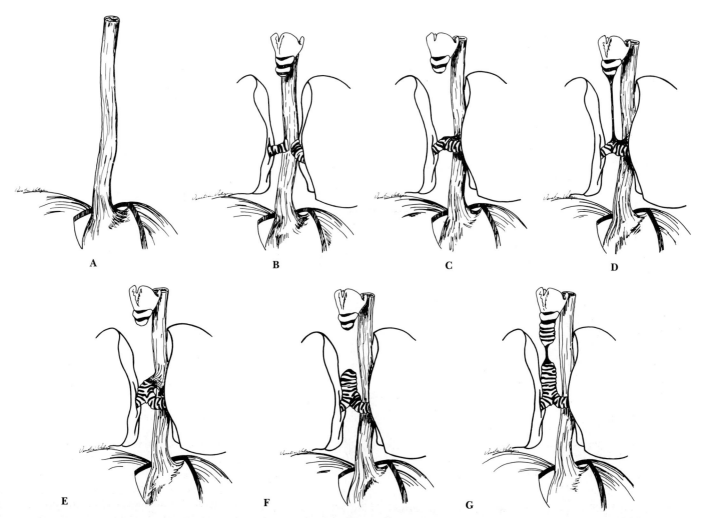

Fig. 7–8 A–G. Types of tracheal agenesis. **A.** Total pulmonary agenesis (8% of cases). **B.** Tracheal agenesis with main bronchi arising directly from esophagus (10%). **C.** Tracheal agenesis with fused main bronchi and bronchoesophageal fistula (56%). **D.** Tracheal agenesis with larynx joined by atretic strand to distal trachea, which has fistulous connection with esophagus (10%). **E.** Upper tracheal agenesis with large direct tracheoesophageal communication (5%). **F.** Tracheal agenesis with no communication with esophagus. **G.** Short segment tracheal agenesis (5%). (From Stocker JT. The respiratory tract. In: Stocker JT, Dehner LP, eds. Pediatric pathology. Philadelphia: Lippincott, 1992:511–519, with permission.)

diastrophic dwarfism),[27] and an animal model has been described,[33] most clinical cases of tracheomalacia in which the trachea can be examined have cartilage plate deficiency rather than cartilage with an abnormally pliant matrix. Acquired tracheomalacia is discussed in Chapters 8 and 22.

Tracheobronchiomegaly

An entity of unknown cause closely related to tracheomalacia is tracheobronchiomegaly or Mounier–Kuhn syndrome.[34] This disorder, usually involving males in the third and fourth decade, has been reported in children and has been shown to have a familial occurrence suggesting an autosomal recessive type of inher-itance.[35–37] Bronchography may display outpouching of the tracheal lumen between tracheal cartilage rings that produces multiple diverticula. The disorder has been noted in a child with cutis laxa[35] and an adult with Ehler–Danlos syndrome,[38] leading to the hypothesis that tracheobronchiomegaly results from a congenital defect in the development of the connective tissue elements in the trachea and mainstream bronchi.

Tracheoesophageal Fistula and Esophageal Atresia

Tracheoesophageal fistula is seen most frequently in association with esophageal atresia, although approxi-mately 10% of infants with esophageal atresia will have

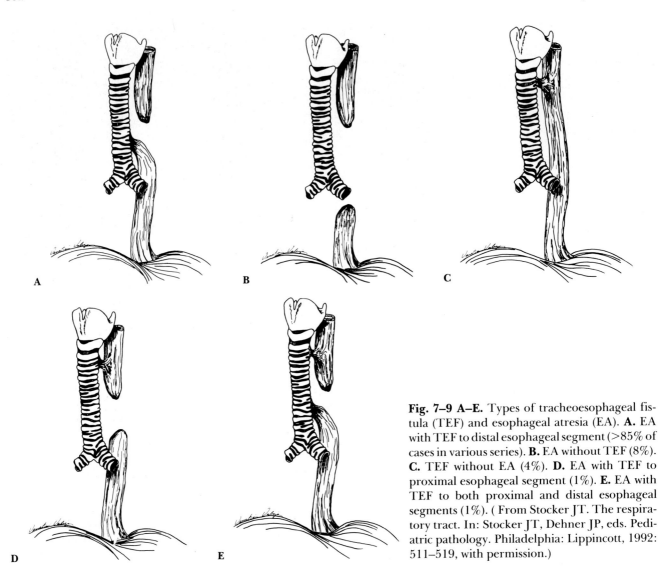

Fig. 7–9 A–E. Types of tracheoesophageal fistula (TEF) and esophageal atresia (EA). **A.** EA with TEF to distal esophageal segment (>85% of cases in various series). **B.** EA without TEF (8%). **C.** TEF without EA (4%). **D.** EA with TEF to proximal esophageal segment (1%). **E.** EA with TEF to both proximal and distal esophageal segments (1%). (From Stocker JT. The respiratory tract. In: Stocker JT, Dehner JP, eds. Pediatric pathology. Philadelphia: Lippincott, 1992: 511–519, with permission.)

no communication between the esophagus and tracheobronchial tree. Esophageal atresia, with or without tracheoesophageal fistula, should be suspected if maternal polyhydramnios is present, the infant has excessive oral and pharyngeal secretion, or if choking, cyanosis, or coughing occurs with an attempt at feeding.[39,40] Five to eight types have been described (Fig. 7–9 A–E); the most frequently occurring type is esophageal atresia with tracheoesophageal fistula to the distal esophageal segment.[41] (Fig. 7–10).

An associated anomaly may be found in up to 70% of infants with esophageal atresia, with multiple anomalies present in 57% of cases.[42] Musculoskeletal, cardiovascular, or gastrointestinal anomalies are seen most frequently (>20%) (Table 7–2).[41–44] A nonrandom association of tracheoesophageal fistula with other malformations has been recognized and given the acronym of VATER, VACTER, or VACTERL (Vertebral, Anal, Cardiac, Tracheo Esophageal, Renal, or Radial

and Limb).[45–49] Tracheoesophageal fistula may recur in nearly 10% of cases after surgical repair.[50] Mild obstruction at the level of the trachea may persist for years.[51]

Tracheoesophageal fistula can be most readily recognized at autopsy by removing the esophagus and the trachea en bloc, then opening the esophagus lengthwise along its posterior or dorsal margin. Esophageal atresia will be readily apparent, but a small fistula between the anterior or ventral esophagus and the trachea can also be demonstrated, as can the rare esophagobronchial fistula.[52] Histologically, squamous metaplasia of the trachea and bronchi may be seen in 80% of cases, primarily in the posterior muscular wall of the trachea but frequently extending around the entire internal surface of the trachea and into the bronchi.[53] Pulmonary changes associated with aspiration of gastric contents may also be present, including pneumonia and foreign-body giant cell reaction with aspirated material.

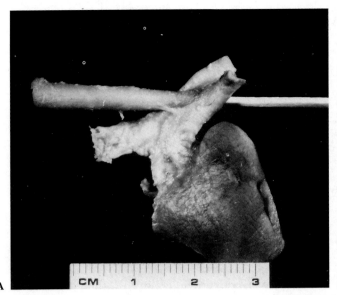

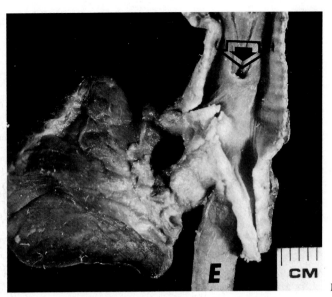

Fig. 7–10 A,B. Tracheoesophageal fistula. **A.** Wooden probe inserted into esophagus at its point of origin from lower trachea. Left mainstem bronchus is present below esophagus.

Right lung is attached to right bronchus. (AFIP Neg. 75-8595-1.) **B.** Opening (*arrow*) to esophagus (E) is present above carina. (AFIP Neg. 75-8595-4.)

Table 7–2. Anomalies most frequently associated with esophageal atresia and tracheoesophageal fistula

Organ system	Incidence (%)	Most frequent example
Musculoskeletal	14.7–24	Vertebral defects, rib defects, radial amelia, caudal dysgenesis
Cardiovascular	22.8	Ventricular septal defect, patent ductus arteriosus, right aortic arch
Gastrointestinal	20.3	Imperforate anus, malrotation, duodenal atresia
Genitourinary	12.2–50	Renal malposition, renal cysts or agenesis, ureteral duplication
Craniofacial	9.7	Choanal stenosis, ear malformations, micrognathia
Central nervous system	7.2	Hydrocephalus
Pulmonary	2.1	Congenital cystic adenomatoid malformation, pulmonary hypoplasia

Abnormalities of Bronchi

Bronchial development, as previously mentioned, occurs between the fifth and sixteenth weeks of gestation. By this time, all conducting airways are present, and subsequent growth is limited to increase in the size of bronchi. Congenital anomalies of bronchi involve abnormalities of origin or location, of size or components, or of connection (Table 7–3).

Abnormality of Origin or Location

Bronchial isomerism yields symmetric lobar bronchial patterns (i.e., bilateral right or left lung), and is seen in association with five types of polysplenia/asplenia syndromes as described by Landing.[54]

Type 1.   Ivemarks asplenia syndrome, a nonfamilial malformation complex involving bilateral right-sidedness, absence of the spleen, intestinal malrotation, sym-

Table 7–3. Bronchial abnormalities

Abnormality of origin or location
  Tracheal bronchus
  Preparterial bronchus
  Additive bronchus
  Isomerism
  "Bridging" bronchus
Abnormal size or component
  Bronchial stenosis or atresia
  Bronchiectasis
  Bronchomalacia
Abnormal connection
  Bronchobiliary fistula
  Bronchoesophageal fistula
"Bronchogenic cysts"

metric liver, bilateral three-lobed "right" lungs with bronchi for both lungs, and a variety of cardiac malformations including right aortic arch, symmetric venae cavae, transposition of the great vessels, and total anomalous pulmonary venous return.

Type 2.   M-anisosplenia, a complex in males with one or more larger and one or more smaller spleens who also have congenital heart malformations, bilateral three-lobed "right" lungs, and relatively normal visceral situs.

Type 3.   Polysplenia syndrome, a complex involving bilateral two-lobed "left" lung bronchial pattern with intestinal malrotation, symmetric liver, congenital heart malformations and 4–14 uniform small spleens.

Type 4.   F-anisosplenia, a complex in females with no splenic tissue who have bilateral two-lobed "left" lungs and congenital heart malformations, particularly double-outlet right ventricle.

Type 5.   O-anisosplenia, a complex equally seen in males and females involving bilateral two-lobed "left" lungs and multiple spleens, congenital heart malformations, particularly double-outlet right ventricle or ostium atrioventricular commune, and a 50% incidence of intestinal malrotation.

Normal bronchial branching but with externally bilobed "left" lungs is part of a polysplenia syndrome including congenital heart malformations, intestinal malformations, and a short pancreas.[55] Left pulmonary isomerism has also been noted in two adults with normal cardiac and abdominal organs. Each, however, displayed bilateral hyparterial upper-lobe bronchi.[56] Symmetrical bronchi were seen in an infant with trisomy 21, tracheostenosis, normal atrial arrangement of the heart, and anomalous thoracic vessels.[57]

Tracheal bronchus usually refers to a "displaced" bronchus arising from the trachea; when involving the right-upper-lobe apical segment bronchus, it is called a preeparterial bronchus. A tracheal bronchus is found in 2% of children requiring bronchoscopy and may be associated with recurrent pneumonia, stridor, and respiratory distress.[58] Other anomalies are frequently seen (78%) in patients with a tracheal bronchus.[59] An unusual origin of the bronchi to the right-middle and lower lobes has been described; a branch arising from the left-mainstem bronchus "bridged" the mediastinum before entering the right lung.[60] This infant also had partial anomalous pulmonary venous return. Wells et al.[61] described two forms of retrotracheal or "sling" left pulmonary artery, one with a normal tracheobronchial pattern and a second with a "bridging" bronchus. The abnormal bronchus was either a branch of the left main bronchus supplying the right-middle or -lower lobes or, in cases with no right bronchial tree, a bridging bronchus from the left main bronchus supplied the entire right lung.

Abnormal Size or Intrinsic Component

Bronchial atresia in association with infantile (congenital) lobar emphysema (see following) is seen with some frequency in infants but has also been reported in adults in the third and fourth decade. While the majority of adults are asymptomatic and the condition discovered only incidentally by radiography, others may present with respiratory distress, recurrent infections, or cough.

Bronchial obstruction, either partial or complete, may be produced by intrinsic or extrinsic mechanisms. Intrinsic bronchial stenosis may be produced by circumferential or eccentric fibrosis, possibly secondary to in utero inflammation, or by an intraluminal mass such as aspirated meconium, bronchial adenoma, ectopic thyroid tissue, or bronchial mucosal web.[62,63] Extrinsic causes of stenosis include enlarged or abnormally located pulmonary arteries and parabronchial masses such as teratoma and bronchogenic cyst.

Bronchiectasis associated with congenital conditions is seen most frequently in children with cystic fibrosis, the immotile cilia syndrome (Kartagener syndrome), and the Williams–Campbell syndrome. It may also occur with various deficiency states such as alpha-1 antitrypsin, IgG, IgA, neutrophil, or complement deficiency.

The Williams–Campbell syndrome is a condition in which cartilage is absent, markedly diminished, or soft in the more proximal bronchi, extending from the fourth to eighth generations.[64,65] In contradistinction to the immunodeficiency states, the presence of chronic inflammation is not thought to play a major role in the destruction of bronchial cartilage; rather, a true congenital defect in cartilage development occurs in a symmetric distribution.[66] Grossly, segmental bronchi are normal but by the second or third division the bronchi become soft and easily compressible, resembling blood vessels. Microscopically subsegmental bronchi are enlarged and show a marked and progressive decrease in the number and size of cartilage plates. The muscular wall is present, but may be attenuated in dilated areas. Chronic inflammation of submucosal connective tissue is present in varying degrees.[64] The peripheral lung displays obliterative bronchiolitis and focal emphysema.[65]

Cystic fibrosis, the most prevalent lethal genetic disease of the white population, is frequently associated with bronchietasis and bronchiolitis. Chronic pulmonary disease is the most important cause of morbidity and mortality in cystic fibrosis. No airway lesion specific for cystic fibrosis has been found,[67,68] although mucus stasis in bronchi and pseudomonas pneumonia are frequently seen.

Familial situs inversus with bronchiectasis and sinusitis, known as Kartagener's syndrome or immotile cilia syndrome, is associated with ciliary immobility resulting from absence of the ciliary dynein arms of respiratory and other epithelial cells (see Chapter 2). This lack of ciliary motility decreases clearance of inhaled material, leading to repeated infections and eventual bronchiectasis.[69,70]

Bronchomalacia

Congenital bronchomalacia is a rare disorder in which there is abnormal development of bronchial cartilage (usually that of the left mainstem bronchus), leading to collapse of the lumen and development of secondary pneumonia.[71,72] This condition has been reported as part of a familial syndrome of cryptorchidism, chest deformity, muscular hypoplasia, dolichocephaly, and severe mental retardation.[73]

In histological appearance, the affected bronchus is decreased in size with the usual cartilage plates replaced by scattered small islands of immature-appearing cartilage. The lung distal to the collapsed bronchus may show evidence of pneumonia or be distended in a pattern typical of infantile lobar emphysema.

Bronchomalacia and tracheobronchomalacia are most frequently seen in infants treated for prolonged periods with mechanical ventilation (see Chapters 8 and 32).

Abnormal Connection

Congenital communication between bronchi and structures outside the respiratory tree is limited to bronchoesophageal and bronchobiliary fistulae, both exceedingly unusual occurrences. A bronchoesophageal fistula probably represents an "extended" tracheoesophageal fistula, but a bronchobiliary fistula[52] is believed to represent a duplication of the upper gastrointestinal tract from its junction with the airway to the level of the ampulla of Vater.[74,75] Tracheoesophageal and bronchobiliary fistulas have been seen in the same patient.[76]

Infants with bronchobiliary fistula present in the first few days of life with patchy atelectasis, emphysema, pneumonia, and a cough productive of yellow or green sputum. Characteristically the fistula arises from the proximal portion of the right mainstem bronchus just distal to the carina, accompanies the esophagus through the diaphragm, and joins the biliary tree at the level of the left hepatic duct. The tract in its proximal portion resembles a bronchus, with cartilage rings and ciliated pseudostratified columnar epithelium, and in its distal portion resembles a bile duct or esophagus with foci of squamous or columnar epithelium and/or more prominent muscularis mucosa.[70] Bronchobiliary fistula has also been reported in association with biliary atresia.[77]

Bronchogenic Cyst

A bronchogenic cyst is a discrete extrapulmonary spherical mass filled with fluid that is composed of a wall of fibromuscular tissue, contains islands of cartilage and seromucinous glands, and is lined by ciliated cuboidal to pseudostratified columnar epithelium. It is located most frequently in the hilar or middle mediastinal region, but may be found in a midline location from beneath the diaphragm to the hypopharynx that includes presenting as cysts in the skin and subcutaneous tissue. Connection to the normal tracheobronchial tree is unusual. This definition excludes cases of "intrapulmonary" or "peripheral" bronchogenic cysts, which are often described as multicystic and probably represent cases of congenital cystic adenomatoid malformation or postinfectious cysts.

Bronchogenic cysts are seen in infants, children, and young adults with no sexual predominance.[78,79] Intrathoracic bronchogenic cysts may present as acute respiratory distress in the newborn period if they compress a major airway, but in older patients may present with symptoms related to secondary infection of the cyst, including fever, hemorrhage, or perforation.[80] More than 15% are asymptomatic, and are seen as incidental findings at surgery or autopsy. On radiography, most cysts in the mediastinum appear as homogeneous water-density masses with smooth margins.[81] Bronchogenic cysts of the skin and subcutaneous tissues usually are discovered at birth as a swelling or draining sinus, most frequently at or in the vicinity of the suprasternal notch and manubrium sterni.[82]

Intrathoracic bronchogenic cysts may be found anywhere along the midline, but in infants are most frequently seen adjacent to the trachea, carina, or left mainstem bronchus as a smooth-to-irregular spheroid cystic mass of 1–4 cm (Figs. 7–11 and 7–12) that is attached to but rarely communicates with the tracheobronchial tree.[83–86] A bronchogenic cyst at the level of

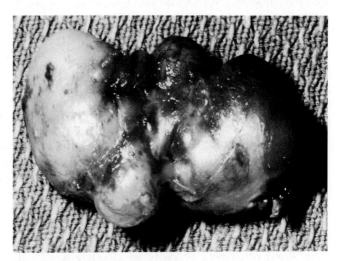

Fig. 7–11. Bronchogenic cyst. Irregular cystic mass was present beneath, and to right of, carina in 10-year-old boy. (AFIP Neg. 86-5326.)

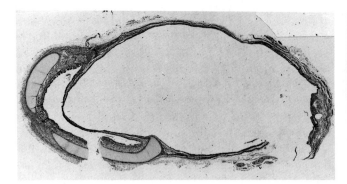

Fig. 7–12. Bronchogenic cyst. This fluid-filled bronchogenic cyst compressed and obstructed right mainstem bronchus (left with cartilage plates), causing severe respiratory distress and death in newborn male. H and E, ×4 (AFIP Neg. 76-1117).

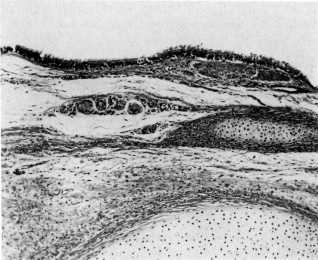

Fig. 7–13. Bronchogenic cyst. Ciliated pseudostratified columnar epithelium overlies fibromuscular wall containing cartilage plate and seromucinous glands. H and E, ×110 (AFIP Neg. 76-1120).

the carina was diagnosed by sonography in a female of 23 weeks of gestation.[87] Polyhydramnios was present along with a hyperexpanded left lung secondary to compression of the left mainstem bronchus.

Bronchogenic cysts usually contain clear serous fluid, but if infected they may contain turbid, viscid, or hemorrhagic fluid. In older patients the cysts may reach 8–10 cm in diameter, and in addition to appearing paratracheally or parabronchially may be found behind the heart,[88] within the diaphragm,[89] or adjacent to the esophagus.[90] Extrathoracic cysts as previously noted are seen most frequently in and beneath the skin of the anterior chest wall.[82]

Microscopically, the cysts are lined by ciliated cuboidal-to-pseudostratified columnar epithelium overlying a fibrous connective tissue wall containing seromucinous glands and cartilage plates (Figs. 7–12 and 7–13).[88] Smooth muscle may also be present in the wall, but large amounts of smooth and/or striated muscle in a cyst partially lined with squamous epithelium probably represent an esophageal cyst. Bronchogenic cysts may also be confused with enteric cysts that are normally lined by mucus-secreting columnar epithelium and whose walls may contain gastric glands and parietal cells. Bronchogenic cysts as well as esophageal and enteric cysts may display squamous metaplasia, inflammation, ulceration, or complete necrosis of the mucosal lining and wall, making diagnosis of the origin of the cysts as bronchogenic, esophageal, or enteric difficult or impossible.[88,91]

The presence of pulmonary parenchyma (bronchioles, alveolar ducts and alveoli) may rarely be seen in true bronchogenic cysts (i.e., located separate from the normal lung) but even then may represent an extralobar sequestration with "bronchiectasis." Bronchogenic cysts, however, have been seen in association with an extralobar sequestration, usually situated between the sequestration and the midline and probably represent-

ing a remnant of the abortive foregut branch that gave rise to the extralobar sequestration.[92,93] This association of extralobar sequestration with bronchogenic cysts is seen only in older infants and in children, indicating that a certain time is needed for the "bronchogenic" cells to develop into a cyst large enough to be recognized. Bronchogenic cysts have also been seen in association with infantile or congenital lobar emphysema both as a cause of the emphysema[94] and coexisting with an infantile lobar emphysema resulting from bronchial atresia.[95]

Abnormalities of Pulmonary Parenchyma

Abnormalities of size and shape of the lung vary from total absence of the lung (bilateral agenesis) to mild variations in the lobation of the lung and location of fissures. Abnormalities of lobation are usually inconsequential clinically unless associated with other anomalies, such as pulmonary isomerism associated with the asplenia/polysplenia syndrome.[27] Abnormalities of size, on the other hand, often have profound clinical implications resulting from the amount of absent tissue, as in bilateral pulmonary agenesis, or from the associated anomalies so frequently seen, as in pulmonary hypoplasia with bilateral renal agenesis.

Horseshoe Lung

A rare congenital abnormality of lung lobation is the "horseshoe lung," analagous to the horseshoe kidney, in which the right and left lungs are fused in the midline behind the heart. Bronchial supply to both lungs is anatomically normal although the bronchi may be decreased in size to one side.[96] Abnormalities usually exist in pulmonary arterial supply and venous drainage.[97,98] Four of five children reported by Freedem et al.[99] and 11 of 14 cases reported or reviewed by Frank et al.[100] occurred in conjunction with the scimitar syndrome: hypoplasia of the right lung, anomalous right pulmonary venous return, and anomalous arterial supply to the right lung. Surgical separation of the lobes is recommended, but the anomalous vascular patterns may lead to infarction of portions of the lung.[97]

Herniation of the Lung—"Ectopic Lung"

Herniation of the lung outside the thoracic cavity, although unusual,[74] may be seen in adults with emphysema, chronic cough, or bronchial asthma.[101] Herniation in the newborn period is much more unusual but upward herniation into the neck has been reported with iniencephalus, the Klippel–Feil syndrome, and the cri du chat syndrome.[102–104] Herniation through the diaphragm and intercostal spaces may also occur.[74]

Agenesis of Lung

Pulmonary agenesis is the complete absence of lung tissue beyond the trachea or mainstem bronchus. Agenesis may be unilateral, bilateral, or rarely lobar. Bilateral pulmonary agenesis is a rare anomaly (fewer than 10 cases have been reported) that is obviously incompatible with life. Associated anomalies, which are frequent, include absent pulmonary arteries and veins, tracheoesophageal fistula, imperforate anus, and renal dysgenesis or agenesis.[105–108]

Unilateral pulmonary agenesis is seen frequently, and more than 250 cases have been reported. In the absence of other severe anomalies, it is compatible with longterm survival. There is a slight female predominance (1.3 : 1)[109] and a suggestion that an autosomal recessive mode of inheritance may be involved in some cases.[110] The right or left lung is absent with equal frequency, but right-lung agenesis appears to be associated with a higher mortality rate, possibly because of the more frequent association of right-lung agenesis with cardiovascular anomalies.[111,112] Associated anomalies frequently seen in some 75% of cases involve, in decreasing order of frequency, the heart and great vessels, skeleton, urogenital system, and gastrointestinal tract. Cardiovascular malformations most often encountered include septal defects, patent ductus arteriosus, and anomalous pulmonary venous return.[113] Radial aplasia, imperforate anus, and tracheoesophageal fistula have also been seen in association with unilateral pulmonary agenesis, suggesting that some of these cases may be part of the VACTERL or VATER association.[46,47,114] Osborne et al.[115] noted unilateral pulmonary agenesis in 6 children with vertebral, rib, or limb abnormalities (the limb anomalies occurred on the same side as the pulmonary agenesis) and suggested a neural crest injury, primarily at the T_2–T_4 level.

In pulmonary agenesis, the larynx and upper trachea are usually well formed, although total absence of the trachea may be seen with bilateral agenesis.[106] With unilateral agenesis, the lower trachea may continue directly into the existing lung as a tracheobronchus or bifurcate at the carina, giving rise to a rudimentary, blind-ending bronchus to one side and a normal bronchus to the other. Bronchomalacia of the bronchus to the existing lung may be present.[116] Rarely, true agenesis of a single bronchus and lobe is found with normal development of the remaining ipsilateral lobes and contralateral lung.[117] The pulmonary artery to the side with agenesis will be hypoplastic or absent as will the pulmonary veins.[118] Mediastinal shift is usually present, and in instances of right-lung agenesis dextrocardia may be noted. The existing lung may be enlarged, particularly in patients surviving beyond the newborn period. Quantitative studies of the existing lung have displayed an absolute increase in alveolar number, representing the normal total number of alveoli for age, despite a reduced number of bronchial generations and pulmonary artery branches.[119]

Pulmonary Hypoplasia

Pulmonary hypoplasia is the incomplete or defective development of the lung, which results in diminished size because of the diminished numbers of units.

Pulmonary hypoplasia can be determined by a variety of methods (see Table 7–4), of which the simplest is the direct measurement of lung weight and comparison of that weight with expected values as done by Potter and Craig[120] and Gruenwald and Minh.[121] Lung weight can also be compared with body weight; the expected normal lung weight to body weight ratio for term and near-term infants is 0.022 ± 0.002.[122] The radial alve-

Table 7–4. Methods of determining pulmonary hypoplasia

Lung weight: direct comparison with expected values
Lung weight/body weight ratio
Radial alveolar count
Alveolar count per unit volume
Lung volume measurement and correlation with crown rump length
Airway branching count using latex injection
DNA content

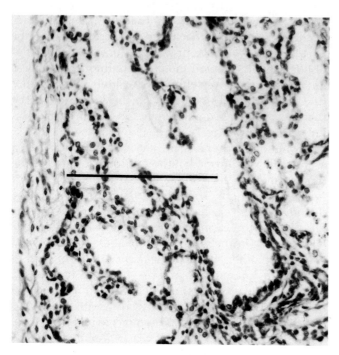

Fig. 7–14. Pulmonary hypoplasia, radial alveolar count. *Line* drawn from terminal bronchiole perpendicular to pleural surface intersects two alveolar septa in this hypoplastic lung (normal is 4.4 ± 0.9). H and E, ×250 (AFIP Neg. 86-5010).

olar count method of Emery and Methal[123] utilizes a line intersect method in which a line is drawn from a terminal bronchiole perpendicular to the nearest septal division or pleural surface (see Fig. 7–14). The number of alveolar septa intersected by that line constitutes the count with the mean for term infants of 4.4 ± 0.9.[123,124]

Alveolar counting and lung volume measurement require closely controlled preparation of the tissue. Distension of the lung with 10% formalin maintained at a transpulmonary pressure of 25 cm of water pressure for 24 h can produce accurate results if carefully controlled. Distended lungs are weighed in air and by displacement of water, and are considered hypoplastic when the measured volume is less than 69% of predicted volume.[125,126] Alveoli are counted per square centimeter in similarly prepared sections to determine the number of alveoli per unit volume.[9] Lung volume may also be correlated with crown rump length.

The airway branching count requires injection of the lung with a latex solution that forms a cast of the airways. The lung tissue is then removed by dissolving it in acid so that the number of branches can be counted. The most sophisticated method for assessing lung growth is the determination of cell population by measuring the DNA content of the lung. Hypoplasia is present when the lung DNA is less than 100 mg/kg body weight.[127]

Table 7–5. Etiologic factors in pulmonary hypoplasia

Limitation of available space
    Intrathoracic lesions
    Thoracic constriction secondary to malformed thorax
    Thoracic constriction secondary to disturbance of amniotic
       and lung fluid volume
    Diaphragmatic elevation
Abnormal or absent fetal breathing movements
Environmental agents
Primary mesodermal defect
Unknown

While they may be determined easily, and in most cases quite accurately, lung weight and lung weight to body weight ratio can be significantly distorted by various conditions such as pneumonia, pulmonary hemorrhage or edema, hyaline membrane disease, and anasarca. Alveolar count, lung volume, airway branching, and DNA content are accurate and reproducible methods but require special equipment and techniques not generally available in most laboratories. The radial alveolar count, however, is readily performed and is only mildly influenced by pathologic conditions, including pneumonia and hemorrhage, or fixation artifact, such as uneven distension or focal atelectasis.[128,129] Diffuse or severe atelectasis, however, may distort the count and make interpretation difficult in the absence of control cases.[2,130]

The etiologic factors that cause pulmonary hypoplasia are outlined in Table 7–5. In 60%–75% of cases, pulmonary hypoplasia is a deformity readily attributable to an associated malformation that has directly or indirectly compromised the thoracic space available for lung growth (Fig. 7–15).[131] The cause of decreased thoracic space may be either intrathoracic, as with abdominal contents herniated through a defective diaphragm, pleural effusion, or intrathoracic extralobar sequestration, or extrathoracic, as in oligohydramnios with uterine fetal "compression."[132–134] This also encompasses defects in the thorax itself such as arthrogryposis multiplex and osteogenesis imperfecta. Abnormal or absent fetal breathing has also been implicated in producing hypoplasia of the lungs, but this may indirectly be related to decreased volume of the thorax in the nonbreathing state.[135] Pulmonary hypoplasia associated with right-sided congenital heart defects has prompted the suggestion that pulmonary blood flow may be an important factor in normal lung development. A primary generalized mesodermal defect may be the factor producing hypoplasia in infants with chromosomal or genetic abnormalities such as Trisomy 13, 18, and 21 in which no obvious factor such as thoracic compression or mass is present. The pulmonary hypoplasia associated with Down's syndrome (Tri-

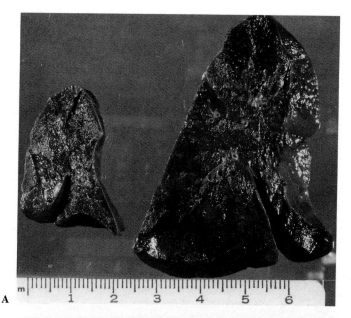

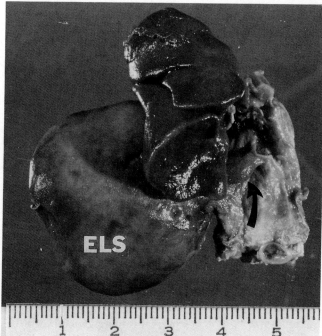

Fig. 7–15 A,B. Pulmonary hypoplasia. **A.** Left lung from infant with left-sided diaphragmatic hernia is obviously hypoplastic. Also, right lung was only 60% of expected weight. (AFIP Neg. 86-5327.) **B.** Large extralobar sequestration (ELS) is noted behind hypoplastic right lung that was 35% of expected weight. Second, much smaller ELS is present medial to lower lobe (*arrow*). Scale in centimeters. (AFIP Neg. 86-5328.)

Table 7–6. Anomalies associated with pulmonary hypoplasia[a]

Common
    Diaphragmatic hernia
    Renal agenesis, bilateral
    Renal dysgenesis, bilateral
    Obstructive uropathy
    Polycystic renal disease (Potter, type I)
    Large abdominal wall defects
Infrequent
    Diaphragmatic hypoplasia or eventration
    Hemolytic disease of the newborn
    Pleural effusion, as with nonimmune fetal hydrops
    Musculoskeletal abnormalities such as thoracic dystrophies
    Anencephaly
    Scimitar syndrome
    Chromosomal anomalies, including trisomy 13, 18, and 21
Rare
    Abdominal pregnancy
    Ascites secondary to congenital cytomegalovirus infection
    Cloacal dysgenesis
    Congenital hydropericardium
    Down's syndrome (probably postnatal "hypoplasia")
    Glutaric acidemia, type II
    Laryngotracheoesophageal cleft
    Neonatal hypophosphatasia
    Pena–Shokeir I syndrome
    Phrenic nerve agenesis
    Right-sided cardiovascular malformation as with hypoplastic right heart
    Thoracic neuroblastoma
    Upper cervical spinal cord
    Extralobar sequestration

[a] From Stocker JT. The respiratory tract. In: Stocker JT, Dehner LP, eds. Pediatric pathology. Philadelphia: Lippincott, 1992:524, with permission.

prominent in children and adults. Enlarged alveoli and peripheral cysts (see Chapter 8) are frequently present in older patients with Down's syndrome.[137,138]

Pulmonary hypoplasia can occur in the absence of any other anomaly and usually presents clinically as respiratory distress in full-term infants within minutes after delivery. As in instances of pulmonary hypoplasia secondary to other anomalies, these infants are exceedingly difficult to ventilate, and episodes of interstitial emphysema and pneumothoraces are common. The death of these infants from progressive hypoxemia is not uncommon.[131,138,139]

Pulmonary hypoplasia may be present in more than 10% of neonatal autopsies, and more than 85% of those cases will display significant associated anomalies.[131] Most of these lesions will be diaphragmatic or renal but musculoskeletal, cardiovascular, chromosomal, central nervous system, and gastrointestinal malformations may also be present (Table 7–6).[140–146]

somy 21) is seen only after the neonatal period. Late intrauterine growth of the lung is normal, but decreased acinar complexity including reduced number of alveoli is noted by 4 months of age and is most

Scimitar Syndrome

A disorder worth special mention, in which the right lung is hypoplastic, is the scimitar syndrome. There is systemic arterial supply to the right lung, dextroposition of the heart, and anomalous right pulmonary venous drainage to the inferior vena cava; this vein is visible radiographically as a band-like shadow parallel to the right boundary of the heart, broadening in the direction of the diaphragm in a configuration reminiscent of the curved Turkish saber, the scimitar.[147]

Hypoplasia or absence of the right-upper-lobe bronchus may also be present. Other anomalies include horseshoe lung (see earlier), accessory diaphragm, atrial or ventricular septal defect, and phrenic cyst.[148,149] Familial occurrence in an autosomal dominant inheritance pattern has been reported.[150] The presence of an anomalous systemic arterial supply has led many authors to include this syndrome in the category of intralobar sequestration, a distinctly separate entity probably not congenital in origin (see Chapter 8).

Extralobar Sequestration

Extralobar sequestration is a mass of pulmonary parenchyma not connected to the tracheobronchial tree that lies outside the normal investment of the visceral pleura. Extralobar sequestration is believed to arise from an outpouching of the foregut, separate from the normally developing lung that later becomes partially or completely separated from its foregut source.

Extralobar sequestration is seen most frequently in the first 6 months of life (61%) (Table 7–7), often presenting in the first day of life with dyspnea, cyanosis, and feeding difficulties.[92] Anasarca or localized edema and maternal polyhydramnios may be present, and pleural effusion may be found.[151–153] Extralobar sequestration may be seen in older children as well, but rarely in adults; male predominance is three or four to one.[154] The ectopic pulmonary parenchyma is usually within the thorax in 85% of cases, most frequently (63%) between a lower lobe and the diaphragm. Extrathoracic lesions are found within or beneath the diaphragm and are rarely symptomatic.[155] Systemic arteries supply the extralobar sequestration in 95% of cases, either directly from the thoracic or abdominal aorta (80%) or from smaller arteries such as the splenic or subclavian arteries.[156] The pulmonary artery, or rarely a pulmonary and systemic artery, supply the extralobar sequestration in 5% of cases. Venous drainage is primarily through the systemic system (>80%), but partial or complete drainage through the pulmonary veins occurs in nearly 25%.[154]

Associated anomalies, including some that are multiple, are present in more than 65% of patients with extralobar sequestration.[92] Diaphragmatic hernia is

Table 7–7. Extralobar sequestration (ELS): summary of findings in 52 cases[a]

	Number of cases
Age	
<1 month	30
1–6 months	5
6 months–2 years	7
2–5 years	3
>5 years	7
Sex	
Male	39
Female	13
Location of lesion	
Right side	17
Left side	35
Upper thorax	7
Midthorax	6
Between lower lobe and diaphragm	31
Partially within diaphragm	3
Infradiaphragmatic	5
Vascular supply	
Arterial	
Thoracic aorta	27
Abdominal aorta	13
Pulmonary artery	6
Subclavian artery	1
Not stated	5
Venous	
Pulmonary vein	3
Azygos vein	1
Subclavian vein	2
Portal vein	1
Outcome	
Alive and well following resection	31
Died of causes not related to ELS	12
Died of causes related to ELS	9

[a] From Stocker JT. The respiratory tract. In: Stocker JT, Dehner LP, eds. Pediatric Pathology. Philadelphia: Lippincott, 1992:519, with permission.

found in 16% of cases, and pulmonary hypoplasia, either secondary to the diaphragmatic hernia or to the mass effect of the extralobar sequestration, is seen in more than 25%.[131] Other anomalies include bronchogenic cyst, cardiovascular malformations, bronchopulmonary foregut connection, and pectum excavatum.

Extralobar sequestration is usually a single pyramidal to round or ovoid lesion ranging from 0.5 to 15 cm in largest diameter (see Fig. 7–5B). It is covered by a smooth to finely wrinkled pleura beneath which a fine recticular pattern of lymphatics may be visible in some cases. If previously infected, it may be encased in connective tissue or adherent to the lung, diaphragm, or mediastinal tissue. On cut section, homogenous pink-to-tan tissue resembling normal pulmonary parenchyma is seen, although well-formed bronchi are infrequent (Fig. 7–16). A "hilar" region containing vessels and irregular bronchi may be present near a margin,

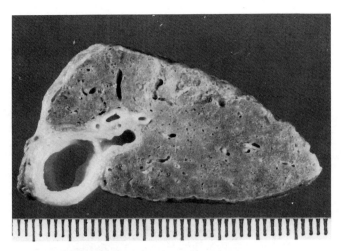

Fig. 7–16. Extralobar sequestration. On cut section, dilated cyst-like bronchus (left) blends with normal-appearing pulmonary parenchyma. (AFIP Neg. 86-5329.)

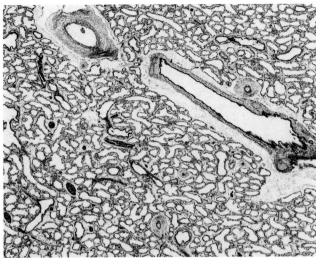

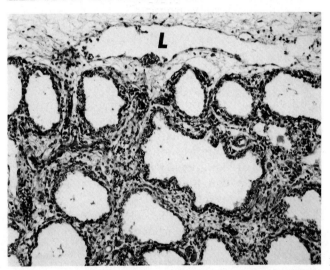

Fig. 7–17 A,B. Extralobar sequestration. **A.** Uniformly dilated bronchioles, alveolar ducts, and alveoli are seen throughout lesion. Bronchus at center right contains only a few cartilage plates within its wall. H and E, ×25 (AFIP Neg. 86-8330). **B.** Alveolar ducts and alveoli are lined by cuboidal cells resembling embryonal epithelial cells. Thick alveolar septa reflect general immaturity of pulmonary tissue from this 950-g fetus. Note dilated lymphatic (L) within pleural connective tissue. H and E, ×160 (AFIP Neg. 85-10041).

and prominent lymphatic channels may be visible in this area and beneath the pleura.[116,151]

Microscopically the lesion consists of uniformly dilated bronchioles, alveolar ducts, and alveoli (Fig. 7–17A). A well-formed bronchus may be present but dilated bronchial structures line by ciliated pseudostratified columnar epithelium overlying a fibromuscular wall, containing only an isolated cartilage plate, are more frequently seen. Bronchioles are tortuous with undulating cuboidal-to-columnar epithelium. Alveolar ducts and alveoli are two to five times normal size and are lined by flattened epithelial cells or, in some areas, vacuolated cuboidal cells that are rich in glycogen and resemble embryonal epithelial cells (Fig. 7–17B). Lymphatics may be unremarkable but occasionally are diffusely dilated and increased in number beneath the pleura and around bronchovascular bundles, severely enough in some cases to resemble congenital pulmonary lymphangiectasis. Superimposed conditions within an extralobar sequestration, such as infarction, arteritis, inflammation, and congenital cystic adenomatoid malformation (CCAM), may alter the microscopic features.[157–159] Lesions resembling CCAM type II (see following) with back-to-back bronchiolar-like structures may occupy part of or all the sequestration in approximately 25% of cases.[25] Immature infants with extralobar sequestration who develop hyaline membrane disease may display no hyaline membrane formation or other features of the disease within the extralobar sequestration.[87]

Infantile (Congenital) Lobar Emphysema

Infantile lobar emphysema, the most frequently occurring congenital lung malformation, is characterized by overinflation of the pulmonary parenchyma (alveolar ducts and alveoli) of a lobe secondary to obstruction, either intrinsic or extrinsic, of the bronchus to that lobe.[160] Infantile lobar emphysema may rarely be an acquired lesion as with aspiration of meconium.

Infantile lobar emphysema occurs more frequently in boys than girls (1.8 : 1) and presents within the first few weeks to months of life, rarely after 6 months,[161] as mild respiratory distress or dyspnea gradually increasing over a period of days to weeks.[160] Other symptoms less frequently seen include cyanosis, respiratory infections,

Table 7–8. Causes of infantile lobar emphysema

Congenital
    Bronchial stenosis
    Bronchial atresia
    Abnormal origin of bronchus
        Tracheal
        Eparterial
Obstruction by vascular anomaly
    Pulmonary artery sling
    Anomalous pulmonary venous return
Obstruction by external mass
    Bronchogenic cyst
Pulmonary hyperplasia
Acquired
    Aspirated meconium
    Mucous plug
    Granulation tissue
    Torsion of bronchus
    Bronchial mucosal folds

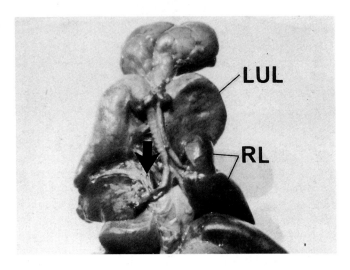

Fig. 7–18. Infantile lobar emphysema. Viewed from posterior surface, enormously enlarged left-upper lobe (LUL) has herniated across midline and is compressing right lung (RL). *Arrow* indicates atretic area of bronchus to left-upper lobe. (AFIP Neg. 86-5331.)

vomiting, choking, and feeding difficulties. Infantile lobar emphysema may rarely be asymptomatic. Radiographically, it may produce an overdistended hyperlucent lobe with mediastinal shift, herniation of the lung across the anterior mediastinum, depression of the diaphragm, and compression of the uninvolved lobes. Infantile lobar emphysema has been described in a mother and a daughter, both of whom had right-middle-lobe involvement.[162]

Infantile lobar emphysema most frequently is caused by stenosis or atresia of a bronchus or abnormal origin of the bronchus, such as tracheal or eparterial bronchus,[163,164] but may also be secondary to external compression of the bronchus or internal obstruction of a normal lumen (Table 7–8). External compression may occur by anomalous vessels, as with a pulmonary artery "sling"[165] or anomalous pulmonary venous return,[166] or by mediastinal masses such as bronchogenic cysts.[26] Aspirated meconium or granulation tissue formed in response to repeated mechanical trauma of endotracheal suctioning may produce a partial or complete lumenal obstruction leading to infantile lobar emphysema.[167] Rotation of a lobe producing torsion and obstruction of the bronchus has also been seen.[168]

Infantile lobar emphysema rarely may be treated surgically by correcting the cause of the bronchial obstruction, as with bronchogenic cysts or a mucous plug, but most often requires resection of the lobe along with the stenotic or atretic bronchus.[169] Nonsurgical management may be successful in exceptional cases.[170–172] Follow-up studies of children who had had a lobectomy for infantile lobar emphysema showed near-normal total lung capacity in nearly all cases.[173,174]

Associated anomalies are noted in more than 40% of patients with infantile lobar emphysema.[160,175] Nearly 70% of these anomalies are cardiovascular; the most common are tetralogy of Fallot, ventricular septal defect, and patent ductus arteriosus.[176–178]

Infantile lobar emphysema involves the left-upper lobe in 50% of cases, the right-middle lobe in 24%, and the right-upper lobe in 18%.[160] The lower lobes are thus involved in less than 10% of cases. The resected lobe is usually overinflated and characteristically fails to deflate after excision. The pleural is smooth, and individual alveoli can be identified grossly (Fig. 7–18). Multiple lobe involvement is rare.

Microscopically, alveolar ducts and alveoli are distended, often as much as 3- to 10-fold normal size (Fig. 7–19). (See exceptions later: pulmonary hyperplasia.) The alveolar walls may show focal disruption, but inflammation, necrosis, or alveolar fibrosis is rare.[179] The major pathologic changes lie in the bronchus to the affected lobe. Elegant dissections and staining studies of the tracheobronchial tree by Campbell[180] and by Landing and Wells[26] have demonstrated decreased amounts of cartilage within the wall of bronchi of the affected lobe. The deficiency of cartilage may be focal or diffuse and results in a flaccid bronchial wall prone to collapse. Bronchial stenosis or atresia may also be seen with collagen and fibroblasts present in the narrowed or atretic area. Both bronchial atresia and abnormal cartilage may be seen in an individual case.[181] Whether this represents an inherent cartilage and/or connective tissue defect or is the result of an in utero inflammatory process is, at present, impossible to determine.

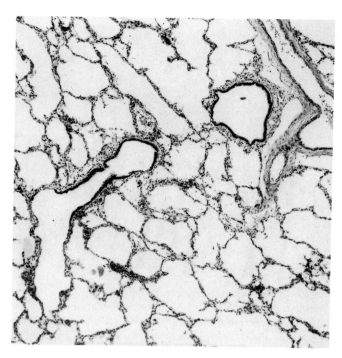

Fig. 7–19. Infantile lobar emphysema. Alveolar ducts and alveoli are markedly distended but otherwise unremarkable. H and E, ×60 (AFIP Neg. 86-5007).

Pulmonary Hyperplasia

Polyalveolar lobe or pulmonary hyperplasia is a congenital malformation of the lung having clinical features similar to infantile lobar emphysema but in which a distinct abnormality of the alveolar parenchyma, an increase in the absolute numbers of alveoli, can be identified.[182–184] The alveoli individually are normal in size and shape but are three- to fivefold increased in number; in the affected lobe, this produces a lobar volume 1.5 to 3 times normal that leads, as with infantile lobar emphysema, to compression of the adjacent lung and mediastinal shift.

Congenital Pulmonary Lymphangiectasis

Congenital pulmonary lymphangiectasis is a rare, usually fatal disorder characterized by dilated and increased numbers of subpleural, septal, and peribronchial lymphatics that occurs most frequently in association with obstructive cardiovascular lesions, but may be seen as part of a generalized lymphangiectasis or rarely as an isolated pulmonary lesion.[160,185,186] While occurring in stillborns in 10% of cases, it more frequently presents in the first hours of life as acute respiratory distress. Congenital pulmonary lymphangiectasis may also present at birth with pleural effusion, chylothorax, or maternal polyhydramnios.[187,188] In utero diagnosis of pleural effusion has been reported in an infant with congenital pulmonary lymphangiectasis.[189] Interstitial pulmonary emphysema and pneumothorax are seen in infants subsequently believed to have congenital pulmonary lymphangiectasis,[190] but extreme care must be made in diagnosing congenital pulmonary lymphangiectasis in the presence of a history of interstitial pulmonary emphysema or pneumothorax (see following).

Radiographs demonstrate prominent interstitial and subpleural lymphatics known as Kerley "B" lines, along with diffuse hyperlucency of the pulmonary parenchyma, overexpansion of the thorax, and depression of the diaphragm.[160] Patients occasionally survive, but in most cases progressive respiratory failure leads to death in the first days to weeks of life. The male/female ratio is approximately 1.5 : 1. Although most cases of congenital pulmonary lymphagiectasis are isolated instances, familial occurrence in two of three female infants in one family has been reported.[191] Review of the photomicrographs of the lungs of these two infants suggested that one case may represent interstitial pulmonary emphysema and the other appears to be congenital pulmonary lymphangiectasis.

Multiple anomalies, particularly cardiovascular lesions, are frequently seen (>80%) in patients with congenital pulmonary lymphangiectasis.[160,192] Association with the asplenia syndrome and its severe cardiovascular anomalies is noted in nearly 30% of cases.[193] The most common lesions include total anomalous pulmonary venous connection (43%),[194] atrioventricular communis (18%), and septal defects (7%). Noncardiac lesions include renal malformations and ichthyosis congenita.[195]

The lungs in congenital pulmonary lymphangiectasis are often bulky and noncompressible and display a prominent network of dilated subpleural lymphatics diffusely spread over the surface. This diffuse involvement of subpleural lymphatics helps distinguish congenital pulmonary lymphangiectasis from acute interstitial pulmonary emphysema, with which it is frequently confused. As noted in Chapter 8, interstitial pulmonary emphysema is largely limited to the interlobular septa, rarely extending laterally beneath the pleural surface.

Microscopically, congenital pulmonary lymphangiectasis is characterized by dilated lymphatics surrounding bronchovascular bundles within the interlobular septa and beneath the pleura, both in areas adjacent to and separate from the interlobular septa (Fig. 7–20). The lymphatics are increased in number, uniformly dilated, lined by endothelial cells, and separated by loose-to-dense connective tissue often containing foci of extramedullary hematopoiesis (Fig. 7–21). The lym-

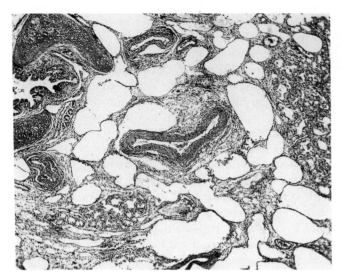

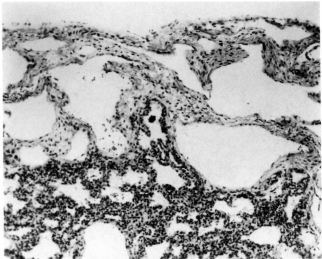

Fig. 7–20. Congenital pulmonary lymphangiectasis. Numerous uniformly dilated lymphatics surround and partially compress pulmonary artery (center) of bronchovascular bundle within interlobular septum. H and E, ×42 (AFIP Neg. 76-3428).

Fig. 7–21. Congenital pulmonary lymphangiectasis. Dilated subpleural lymphatics are lined by endothelial cells and separated from each other by fibrous connective tissue. Alveolar septa (lower left) of premature infant are unremarkable. H and E, ×110 (AFIP Neg. 76-273).

phatics are usually empty but may contain faintly eosinophilic material or red blood cells. Interstitial pulmonary emphysema, on the other hand, is characterized by larger air-containing cysts without a discernible (or at best an intermittent) endothelial cell lining. The cysts of interstitial pulmonary emphysema extend to the subpleural space along interlobular septa, but rarely extend laterally beneath the pleura as do the lymphatic channels of congenital pulmonary lymphangiectasis.

Congenital Cystic Adenomatoid Malformation

Although it was originally described by Chin and Tang[196] in 1949 as a rare lesion occurring in premature or stillborn infants with anasarca, congenital cystic adenomatoid malformation has come to encompass all congenital cystic lung lesions characterized by the presence of abnormal bronchiolar structures of varying sizes and/or distribution. Current classifications are based primarily on the size of the cysts at the time of initial clinical or pathologic examination of the surgical or autopsy specimen.[159,197]

Congenital cystic adenomatoid malformation of the lung is a relatively common hamartomatous lesion of which approximately 95% of cases can be separated into three types on the basis of clinical, radiographic, and pathologic features (Fig. 7–22).[159,198] (See later for proposed additional types 0 and 4.) The three types occurring most frequently include the common diagnostic feature of multiple, irregular, variably sized,

bronchiolar-like cystic structures lined by cuboidal-to-ciliated pseudo-stratified columnar epithelium. The presence of acute or chronic inflammation[199] or fibrosis precludes the diagnosis of congenital cystic adenomatoid malformation, because normal repair mechanisms following necrosis of pulmonary tissue result in cystic spaces lined by cuboidal, columnar, or pseudostratified columnar epithelium.

Congenital cystic adenomatoid malformation of these three types displays a slight male predominance (Table 7–9), but no racial predilection has been noted. The lesion is seen most frequently in newborns, occurring almost equally in premature and term infants. Congenital cystic adenomatoid malformation has been described in older paients, including two men 24 and 35 years of age,[200] but most (80%–85%) are seen in the first 2 years of life.[201–218]

Respiratory distress including cyanosis, retractions, and grunting is the presenting symptom in 67%–85% of cases; cough, fever, and/or repeated respiratory infections are seen in 10%–20%.[159,201] Vomiting or chest pain may rarely be seen, and occasional cases are asymptomatic. The severity of the symptoms and the time of presentation is directly related to the size of the lesion or the size to which individual cysts within the lesion may expand. Anasarca and maternal polyhydramnios, which occurred relatively frequently in earlier reports, was noted in about 5% of recently reported cases (Table 7–10).

Radiographically, congenital cystic adenomatoid malformation may display a multicystic appearance, a

TYPE 1   TYPE 2   TYPE 3

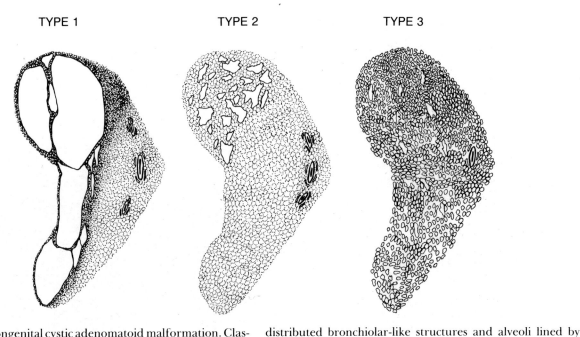

Fig. 7–22. Congenital cystic adenomatoid malformation. Classification: type 1 is composed of single or multiple large cysts (3–7 cm in diameter) surrounded by smaller collapsed cysts; type 2 contains smaller more uniform cysts (0.5–2.0 cm in diameter) and is associated with increased incidence of other anomalies; type 3 occupies large portion of lobe or occasionally entire lung on one side and is composed of randomly distributed bronchiolar-like structures and alveoli lined by cuboidal epithelium. Cysts are usually less than 0.5 cm in diameter but if expanded by air may reach 1.5 cm. (From W.B. Saunders Co. Stocker JT, Madewell JE, Drake RM. Congenital cystic adenomatoid malformation of the lung: Classification and morphologic spectrum. Human Pathology 1977;8: 155–171, with permission.)

Table 7–9. Clinical features of 82 cases of congenital cystic adenomatoid malformation (published 1977–1985)

Sex			
Male	44		
Female	36		
Not stated	2		
Age			
Birth–2 months	50		
2 months–2 years	12		
2–10 years	18		
Not stated	2		
Location			
RUL	11	LUL	17
RML	5		
RLL	19	LLL	22
More than one lobe			
R Lung	1		
L Lung	2		
Bilateral	1		
Within an ELS	5[a]		
Not stated	1		

[a] Three were in an extralobar sequestration (ELS) alone; two were in an ELS and another lobe of lung.

dominant cyst in a multicystic background, or a solid homogeneous mass.[198] This appearance, however, is dependent not only on the size of cysts within the lesion but also on the presence of fluid within the cysts. For example, a type 1 or large cyst lesion (as described below) with cysts filled with fluid may present radiographically as a solid mass similar to that seen with the type 3 or adenomatoid lesion. Many initially "solid" lesions may, over the course of days to weeks, become cystic as fluid clears from the cysts.[198,202]

Surgical resection of the lesion is indicated, and care must be taken to include small or collapsed cysts adjacent to the obvious large ones. Lobar resection is recommended to ensure that all the lesion is removed. With adequate resection, more than 85% of patients will survive (see Table 7–11). Long-term follow-up has shown lung volumes of nearly 90% of predicted normal values.[174] Congenital cystic adenomatoid malformation, particularly type 2, is associated with other anomalies in 20% of cases. Some of these are so severe (Table 7–11) as to make resection of the lesion impractical in these instances. One such example is bilateral renal agenesis.

Congenital cystic adenomatoid malformation is a unilateral lesion in more than 98% of cases and involves a single lobe in more than 95% of cases. Right and left lung are affected almost equally (see Table 7–9), with lower lobe involvement slightly more prominent (55%). Congenital cystic adenomatoid malformation has also been noted within extralobar sequestrations.[159,201]

The type 1 lesion is characterized by a single or more frequently multiple intercommunicating cysts 3–10 cm

Table 7–10. Treatment and survival in 62 cases of congenital cystic adenomatoid malformation (published 1977–1985)

Total	Resected, alive and well	Resected, died	No survery, died	Associated anomalies	Material polyhydramnios
Type 1 40 (64%)	31 (77.5%)	4 (10%)	5 (12.5%)	5 (12.5%)	4 (10%)
Type 2 14 (23%)	9 (64%)	2 (14%)	3 (22%)	7 (50%)	0
Type 3 8 (13%)	6 (75%)		2 (25%)	0	0

Table 7–11. Anomalies reported in association with congenital cystic adenomatoid malformation

Bilateral renal agenesis/ dysgenesis	6
Extralobar sequestration	5
Diaphragmatic hernia	3
Cardiovascular malformation	3
Skeletal malformation	1
Hydrocephalus/macrocephaly	2
Jejunal atresia	1
Bilateral nephromegaly	1
Pierre Robin syndrome	1
Pulmonary hypoplasia	1

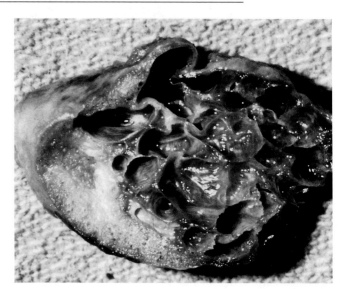

A

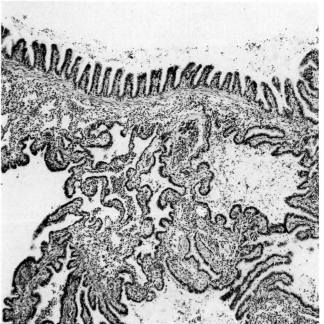

B

Fig. 7–23 A, B. Congenital cystic adenomatoid malformation, type 1. **A.** Large intercommunication cysts are separated by thin delicate membranes. Compressed normal lung is at left. (AFIP Neg. 86-5332). **B.** Ciliated pseudostratified columnar epithelium with polypoid projections lines surface of large cyst (top). Small cysts lined by cuboidal and columnar epithelium are present beneath wall of larger cyst. H and E, ×60 (AFIP Neg. 86-5340).

in diameter and surrounded by smaller cysts (Fig. 7–23A; Table 7–12). The cysts, when expanded by air or fluid, produce mediastinal shift in 75% of cases and compress the lung adjacent to the lesions as well as the lung on the contralateral side. Thin delicate membranes separate the cysts, and vascular structures can be seen beneath their smooth surface.

The large cysts are lined by ciliated pseudostratified columnar epithelium, which displays numerous polypoid projections when the cysts are partially collapsed (Fig. 7–23B). A thick fibromuscular layer underlies the epithelium, and a rare cartilage plate may be present within the wall (Fig. 7–24A). Cartilage plates, noted primarily in the type 1 lesion (5%–10% of cases), are usually present as widely scattered isolated plates but cases with cartilage throughout the lesion have been reported.[217] The cysts lie back to back, often separated by a common fibromuscular wall or by structures resembling dilated alveolar ducts and alveoli. Smaller cysts partially or completely lined by ciliated cuboidal to tall columnar epithelium are present near the periphery of the lesion or interspersed among the larger cysts. Mucus-producing cells, seen only in type 1 lesions, are present along short segments of the wall of cysts or within alveolus-like structures in about one-third of cases (Fig. 7–24B). Elastic tissue in amounts greater than normal can be seen immediately beneath the epithelium throughout the lesions.

The type 2 lesion, generally smaller than types 1 and 3, is composed of multiple evenly distributed cysts 0.5–2.0 cm in diameter; rarely, a larger cyst may be present. Mediastinal shift is seen less frequently (12%) than with type 1 lesions, probably because of the smaller

Table 7–12. Pathologic features of congenital cystic adenomatoid malformation

	Type 0	Type 1	Type 2	Type 3	Type 4
Approximate frequency (%)	1–3	>65	20–25	8	2–4
Cyst size (maximum, cm)	0.5	10.0	2.5	1.5	7
Epithelial lining (cysts)	Ciliated Pseudostratified Tall columnar with goblet cells	Ciliated Pseudostratified Tall columnar	Ciliated Cuboidal or columnar	Ciliated Cuboidal	Flattened Alveolar lining cells
Muscular wall thickness (μm) of cysts	100–500	100–300	50–100	0–50	25–100
Mucous cells	Present in all cases	Present (33% of cases)	Absent	Absent	Absent
Cartilage	Present in all cases	Present (5–10% cases)	Absent	Absent	Rare
Skeletal muscle	Absent	Absent	Present (5% of cases)	Absent	Absent

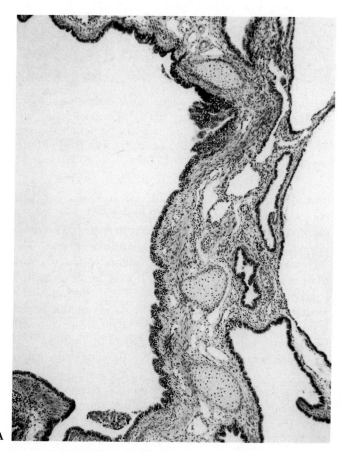

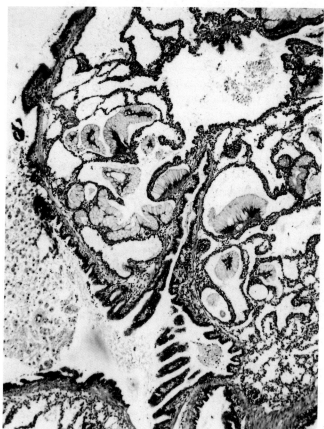

Fig. 7–24 A, B. Congenital cystic adenomatoid malformation, type 1. **A.** Isolated cartilage plates are present within wall of large cyst. H and E, ×60 (AFIP Neg. 86-5342). **B.** Clusters of mucous cells fill alveolus-like structures adjacent to epithelium-lined cysts. H and E, ×60 (AFIP Neg. 86-5341).

size overall of the type 2 lesions. On cut section the lesion blends with the adjacent normal parenchyma; cysts and normal bronchi and bronchioles are often indistinguishable (Fig. 7–25). The type 2 cysts are lined by cuboidal-to-columnar epithelium, rarely displaying pseudostratification (Fig. 7–26). A thin fibromuscular layer underlies larger cysts but is absent in smaller ones. The entire lesion may be composed of dilated bronchiolar-like structures lying back to back and separated only by scattered alveolar ducts (Fig. 7–27). Mucus-

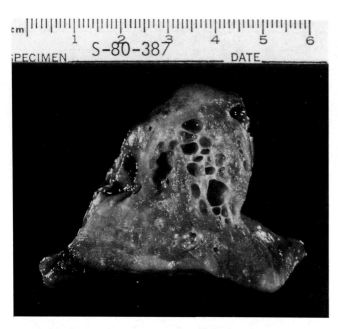

Fig. 7–25. Congenital cystic adenomatoid malformation, type 2. Thin-walled cysts (0.2–1.0 cm in diameter) blend with adjacent normal parenchyma. (AFIP Neg. 86-5333.)

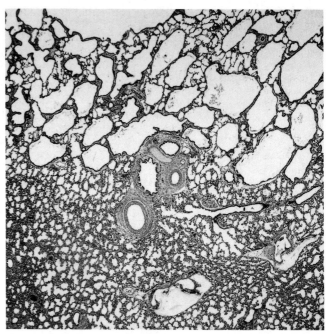

Fig. 7–26. Congenital cystic adenomatoid malformation, type 2. Multiple cysts resembling terminal bronchioles abut and partially surround normal bronchovascular bundle (center). There is no distinct capsule between lesion (bottom) and normal lung (top). H and E, ×15 (AFIP Neg. 85-9544).

producing cells are not present, and cartilage plates are noted only in association with "entrapped" normal bronchi usually near the periphery of the lesion.

A peculiar subgroup of the type 2 lesion contains strands of striated muscle fibers throughout the lesion, both in association with the cysts and also between alveolar ducts and around blood vessels (Fig. 7–27B).[159,219,220] Rhabdomyosarcoma arising in a congenital cystic adenomatoid malformation has been noted in two instances, possibly derived from the skeletal muscle of this subtype.[221,222] Associated anomalies, often severe (see Table 7–11), are seen in more than 50% of infants with this type 2 lesion. Congenital cystic adenomatoid malformation, when present in an extralobar sequestration, is of the type 2 variety.

The type 3 lesion accounts for about 10% of all cases and is often a large bulky lesion occupying an entire lobe or even an entire lung, producing mediastinal shift in nearly all cases (Fig. 7–28). The rubbery, noncrepitant mass may contain small, evenly distributed cysts, but they rarely exceed 0.2 cm in diameter. Microscopically the lesion is composed of randomly distributed irregular bronchiolar-like structures lined by cuboidal-to-low-columnar epithelium and separated by masses of alveolus-sized structures lined by cuboidal epithelium, a true "adenomatoid" malformation (Fig. 7–29A). A thin fibromuscular layer may be present beneath the epithe-

lium of the "bronchioles," but mucous cells, cartilage plates, and striated muscle fibers are absent, and if unexpanded the lesion may have the appearance of an immature lung of the pseudoglandular phase. The "alveolar septa" are wider and more poorly vascularized than in the normal lung, which may be present in a subpleural location at the periphery of the lesion. Ultrastructurally the cysts and pseudoglands of the type 3 lesion are lined by alveolar type II pneumocytes with prominent villi and lamellar inclusion bodies.[201,204] Tonofilaments have also been described in these cells.[203]

Recently described, less commonly occurring malformations of the pulmonary acinus might be included in an expanded classification based on the area of the tracheobronchial tree involved by the malformation. Rutledge and Jensen[223] described a malformation of the proximal tracheobronchial tree composed of bronchial-like structures with respiratory epithelium surrounded by a wall containing smooth muscle, glands, and numerous cartilage plates. These bronchial-like structures and, rarely, structures resembling proximal bronchioles were surrounded by mesenchymal tissue containing thin-walled vascular channels, collections of amorphous basophilic debris, and foci of extramedullary hematopoiesis (Fig. 7–30). We have subsequently seen two additional cases in term and preterm infants

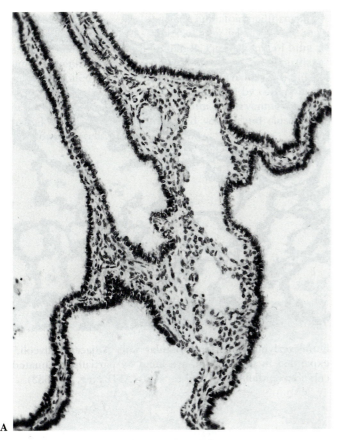

A

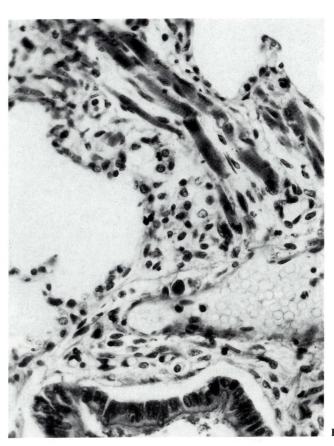

B

Fig. 7–27 A, B. Congenital cystic adenomatoid malformation, type 2. **A.** Back-to-back cysts lined by ciliated cuboidal to low columnar epithelium are separated by a few alveolus-like structures. H and E, ×165 (AFIP Neg. 75-6825). **B.** Skeletal muscle fibers with distinct cross striations lie in loose connective tissue between alveolus-like structures (left center and upper right) and columnar epithelial-lined cyst (bottom). H and E, ×350 (AFIP Neg. 75-6821).

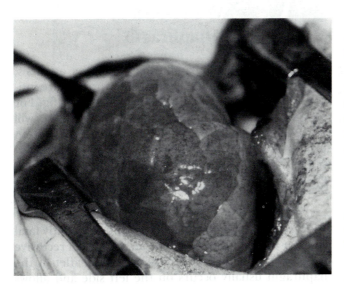

Fig. 7–28. Congenital cystic adenomatoid malformation, type 3. Enlarged bulky lobe protrudes from opened chest. Individual cysts are not visible. (AFIP Neg. 86-5334.)

who were cyanotic at birth and survived only a few hours. One of these infants also had dermal hypoplasia.

These cases of acinar dysplasia or dysgenesis as described by Rutledge and Jensen[223] might be included as CCAM, type 0 (Fig. 7–31) reflecting an abnormality of the proximal tracheobronchial tree with types 1, 2, and 3 representing malformations of the proximal acinus (bronchial/bronchiolar), midacinus (bronchiolar), and alveolar duct/alveolar saccular regions, respectively.

We have noted another cystic lesion of the lung that appears to represent a malformation of the most distal portion of the acinus and could be included in the classification of CCAM as type 4 (Fig. 7–31). These large thin-walled cystic lesions are equally seen in males and females from birth to 4 years of age who may be asymptomatic, display mild respiratory distress, or present with sudden respiratory distress from tension pneumothorax. Radiographically, large air-filled cysts of one or two lobes produce mediastinal shift and

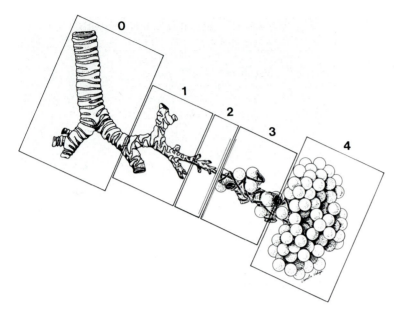

Fig. 7–31. Expanded classification of congenital cystic adenomatoid malformation based on hamartomatous components of each lesion. Type 0, composed of bronchial-like structures, appears to be malformation of proximal tracebronchial tree. Type 1, composed of bronchial-like structures and proximal bronchiolar-like structures, mimicks distal bronchial tree and proximal acinus. Type 2, composed of bronchiolar-like structures, resembles bronchiolar section of acinus. Type 3, composed of structures resembling terminal bronchioles and alveolar ducts, suggests midacinar malformation. Type 4, composed of thin-walled structures lined by alveolar lining cells, suggests origin from distal components of acinus.

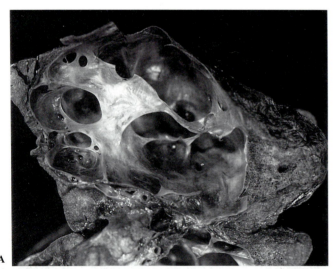

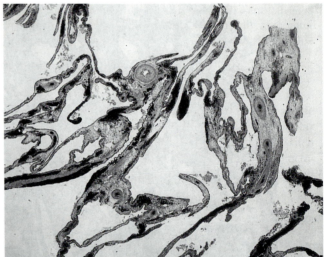

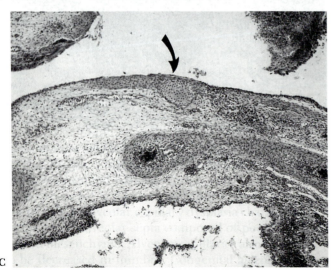

Fig. 7–32 A–C. Congenital cystic adenomatoid malformation, Type 4. **A.** Large intercommunicating smooth-walled cysts compress adjacent normal-appearing pulmonary parenchyma. **B.** Cyst walls are composed of loose mesenchymal tissue containing scattered thick walled vessels. (H and E, ×15.) **C.** Cysts are lined by indistinct layer of epithelial cells (type 1 alveolar lining cells). Note thick-walled vessel (center) and isolated island of cartilage (*arrow*). (H and E, ×75.)

positioning the liver to help occlude the opening, postoperative cardiopulmonary problems related to the pulmonary hypoplasia frequently cause death.[231,232]

Accessory Diaphragm

An accessory diaphragm is a rare congenital malformation in which incomplete descent of the septum transversum results in the division of a hemithorax into an upper and lower compartment by an incomplete shelf-like muscular platform. The accessory diaphragm, always unilateral, and right-sided in more than 90% of cases, occupies the anterior and lateral portion of the thorax but is incomplete dorsomedially to allow passage of the hilar structures.[233,234] The lesion can present as respiratory distress in infants, but may be asymptomatic; it is seen incidentally in adults, the oldest patient being 57 years old. Associated anomalies that are seen frequently include cardiovascular anomalies, pulmonary hypoplasia, and ipsilateral diaphragmatic hernia.[235] The diagnosis of accessory diaphragm can readily be made from routine posterolateral and lateral chest radiographs. Removal of the aberrant tissue, which morphologically resembles normal diaphragm, allows expansion of the lung and usually alleviates the symptoms.[236]

Diaphragmatic Hernia

As diaphragmatic hernia occurs once in every 2000–5000 births, it is one of the most frequent congenital anomalies of the lungs and thorax.[237,238] This defect, resulting from failure of closure of the posterolateral pleuroperitoneal folds at the eighth to ninth week of gestation, allows herniation of the abdominal contents, especially the liver, intestine, and spleen, into the thoracic cavity. Clinical presentation is greatly influenced by the size of the defect and whether it is on the left side (65%–80%) or right side (20%–35%). Large left-sided diaphragmatic defects allow herniation of abdominal contents into the thorax, which inhibits lung development with resultant severe pulmonary hypoplasia.[131,138,239] In right-sided hernias, the liver may "occlude" the diaphragmatic defect. Infants present clinically with severe respiratory distress in the first minutes to hours after birth. Mortality, in fact, is directly related to age at presentation and is greatest (18%–60%) in those who develop symptoms within the first 24 hours.[240–242] Aggressive postoperative medical treatment and the use of extracorporeal membrane oxygenation have led to a significant increase in survival (82%) in recent years.[237]

Patients with right-sided diaphragmatic hernia usually present considerably past the newborn period

Table 7–13. Anomalies associated with diaphragmatic hernia

Pulmonary
  Hypoplasia
  Extralobar sequestration
  Tracheoesophageal fistula
  Congenital cystic adenomatoid malformation
Cardiovascular
  Tetralogy of Fallot
  Endocardial cushion defect
  Atrial and ventricular septal defects
  Ectopia cordis
  Coarctation of the aorta
  Pulmonic stenosis
Gastrointestinal
  Imperforate anus
  Omphalocele
  Pyloric stenosis
  Stomach duplication
  Malrotation of bowel
Genitourinary
  Hydronephrosis
  Multicystic kidney
  Duplicated collecting system
Chromosomal
  Trisomy 18 and 21
Other
  Cleft lip and palate
  Meningomyelocele
  Hemivertebrae
  Fetal alcohol syndrome
  Cornelia de Lange syndrome
  Syndactyly

(75%) with mild respiratory symptoms, such as chest pain and recurrent upper respiratory infections, or with symptoms of acute intestinal obstruction or strangulation, such as abdominal pain or vomiting.[243] Such patients may be asymptomatic, and the hernias are discovered incidentally on chest films with a mass of distorted liver in the right hemithorax. "Delayed" presentation of right-sided hernias has been noted in association with Group B streptococcus infection in the newborn.[244] The delay may be related to a splinting effect of the liver in combination with a lung that is less than normally compliant as the result of the streptococcal pneumonia.

Associated anomalies, aside from the pulmonary hypoplasia present in most infants with diaphragmatic hernia, are noted in about 25% of cases. Cardiovascular abnormalities account for the majority of anomalies (Table 7–13) and may significantly influence survival.[237,245]

Diaphragmatic Eventration

Congenital eventration of the diaphragm, either partial or complete, is caused by aplasia of diaphragmatic muscle. Acquired eventration may be seen with injury to the phrenic nerve, which produces paralysis and elevation of the entire diaphragm.[246] Congenital eventration is noted more frequently in males (62%). Partial involvement is seen in 65% of cases, most frequently on the right side, and unilateral eventration (right side, 67%; left side, 33%) accounts for more than 85% of cases.[247,248] Presenting symptoms are usually respiratory in nature with repeated upper respiratory tract infection or pulmonary consolidation, but because nearly half of patients have mild or no symptoms, only 38% of cases will be recognized in the neonatal period in contrast to more than 90% of diaphragmatic hernia.[249] Plication of the involved segment of the diaphragm is recommended in symptomatic patients. The morphology of the involved segments includes normal parietal pleural thoracic and abdominal layers separated by delicate fibrovascular connective tissue either devoid of skeletal muscle or with only a few scattered muscle fibers present. Associated anomalies similar to those seen in patients with diaphragmatic hernia (see Table 7–13) are present in about one-third of patients..

The Lung in Children with Selected Genetically Inherited Systemic Disorders

Cystic fibrosis, as previously mentioned, displays no specific pulmonary lesion but is frequently associated with bronchiectasis.[67] Chronic granulomatous disease of childhood, an X-linked chromosome disorder, results in the inability of phagocytes to kill microorganisms; resultant localized infections are characterized by suppurative inflammation, granuloma formation, necrosis, and accumulation of pigmented histiocytes.[250] Lung involvement begins in the peribronchial or perivascular areas as microabscesses that undergo coagulative necrosis, enlarging to areas of massive necrosis. Aggregation of macrophages at the periphery of abscesses or areas of necrosis produces the granulomas from which this entity derives its name. Giant cells of both the foreign-body and Langhan's types are seen infrequently.

Alpha-1-antitrypsin deficiency usually manifests itself as neonatal jaundice and hepatic cirrhosis in childhood, but may rarely present as bronchiectasis and panlobular emphysema in the older child.[74]

Numerous genetic disorders that produce bronchiectasis or pneumonia as a result of a defective immune system include Chediak–Higashi syndrome, severe combined immunodeficiency, Bloom's syndrome, and ataxia-telangiectasis.[251] Inherited neuromuscular disorders and chest wall deformities can produce pulmonary hypoplasia, but also lead to pulmonary infections, largely because of the inability to adequately clear secretions and inhaled organisms.

References

1. Inselman LS, Mellins RB. Growth and development of the lung. J Pediatr 1981;98:1–15.
2. Langston C. Prenatal lung growth and pulmonary hypoplasia. In: Stocker JT, ed. Pediatric pulmonary disease. Washington, DC: Hemisphere, 1989:1.
3. Hislop A, Reid L. Fetal and childhood development of the intra-pulmonary veins in man—branching pattern and structure. Thorax 1973;28:313–319.
4. Hislop A, Reid L. Intrapulmonary arterial development during life—branching pattern and structure. J Anat 1972;113:35–48.
5. Kitterman JA. Fetal lung development. J Dev Physiol 1984;6:67–82.
6. Avery ME, Fletcher DB, William RG. The lung and its disorders in the newborn infant. 4th Ed. Philadelphia: WB Saunders. 1981:3–27.
7. Lauweryns JM. The blood and lymphatic microcirculation of the lung. Pathol Annu 1971;6:365–415.
8. Langston C, Thurlbeck WM. Lung growth and development in late gestation and early postnatal life. Perspect Pediatr Pathol 1982;7:203–235.
9. Langston C, Kida K, Reed M, Thurlbeck WM. Human lung growth in late gestation and in the neonate. Am Rev Respir Dis 1984;129:607–613.
10. Robertson B. The normal intrapulmonary arterial pattern of the human late fetal and neonatal lung. Acta Paediatr Scand 1967;56:349–364.
11. Stocker JT, McGill LC, Orsini EN. Post-infarction peripheral cysts of the lung in pediatric patients: A possible cause of idiopathic spontaneous pneumothorax. Pediatr Pulmonol 1985;1:7–18.
12. Benjamin B, Inglis A. Minor congenital laryngeal clefts: Diagnosis and classification. Ann Otol Rhinol Laryngol 1989;98:417–420.
13. Burroughs N, Leape LL. Laryngotracheoesophageal cleft: Report of a case successfully treated and review of the literature. Pediatrics 1974;53:516–522.
14. Delahunty JE, Cherry J. Congenital laryngeal cleft. Ann Otol Rhinol Laryngol 1969;78:96–106.
15. Phelan PD, Stocks JG, William HE, Danks DM. Familial occurrence of congenital laryngeal clefts. Arch Dis Child 1973;48:275–277.
16. Payne WA. Congenital absence of the trachea. Brooklyn Med J 1900;14:568.
17. Effman EL, Spackman TJ, Berden WE, Kuhn JP, Leonidas JC. Tracheal agenesis. AJR 1975;125:767–781.
18. Warfel KA, Schulz DM. Agenesis of the trachea. Arch Pathol Lab Med 1976;100:357–359.
19. Faro RS, Goodwin CD, Organ CH, et al. Tracheal agenesis. Ann Thorac Surg 1979;28:295–299.
20. Milstein JM. Tracheal agenesis in infants with VATER association. Am J Dis Child 1985;139:77–80.
21. Milles G, Dorsey DB. Intra-uterine respiration-like movements in relation to development of the fetal vascular system. Am J Pathol 1950;26:411–425.
22. Eimer H. Aplasia of the trachea in a newborn. Zentralbl Gynaekol 1969;91:1614–1616.
23. Morison JE Congenital malformations in one of

monozygotic twins. Arch Dis Child 1949;24:214–218.

24. Brichard B, Smeets E, Withofs L, et al. Tracheal agenesis: An exceptional cause of neonatal respiratory distress. Pediatr Pulmonol 1990;9:119–120.

25. Stocker JT. The respiratory tract. In: Stocker JT, Dehner LP, eds. Pediatric pathology. Philadelphia: Lippincott, 1992:511–519.

26. Harrison MR, Heldt GP, Brusch RG, DeLorimer AA, Gregory GA. Resection of distal tracheal stenosis in a baby with agenesis of the lung. J Pediatr Surg 1980;15:938–943.

27. Landing BH, Wells TR. Tracheobronchial anomalies in children. Perspect Pediatr Pathol 1973;1:1–32.

28. Berdon WE. Complete cartilage-ring tracheal stenosis associated with anomalous left pulmonary artery: The ring-sling complex. Radiology 1984;152:57–64.

29. Smith RJG, Smith MCF, Glossop LP, Bailey CM, Evans JNG. Congenital vascular anomalies causing tracheoesophageal compressions. Arch Otolaryngol 1984;110:82–87.

30. Nelson CS, McMillan IKR, Bharucha PK. Tracheal stenosis, pulmonary agenesis, and patent ductus arteriosis. Thorax 1967;22:7–12.

31. Chapman S, Weller PH, Campbell CA, Buick RG. Tracheal compression caused by achalasia. Pediatr Pulmonol 1989;7:49–51.

32. Johner CH, Szanto PA. Polychondritis in a newborn presenting as tracheomalacia. Ann Otol Rhinol Laryngol 1970;79:1114–1116.

33. Seegmiller R, Fraser FC, Ferguson CC, Sheldon H. Studies on cartilage. VI. A genetically determined defect in tracheal cartilage. J Ultrastruct Res 1972;38:288–301.

34. Katz I, Levine M, Herman P. Tracheobronchiomegaly: The Mounier-Kuhn syndrome. AJR 1962;88:1084–1094.

35. Wanderer AA, Ellis EF, Goltz RW, Cotton EK. Tracheobronchiomegaly and acquired cutis laxa in a child. Pediatrics 1969;44:709–715.

36. Hunter TB, Kuhns LR, Roloff MA, Holt JF. Tracheobronchiomegaly in an 18-month-old-child. AJR 1975;123:687–690.

37. Johnston RF, Green RA. Tracheobronchiomegaly: Report of 5 cases and demonstration of familial occurrence. Am Rev Respir Dis 1965;91:35–50.

38. Aaby GV, Blake HA. Tracheobronchiomegaly. Ann Thorac Surg 1966;2:64–70.

39. Avery ME, Fletcher BD, Williams RG. The lung and its disorders in the newborn infant. 4th Ed. Philadelphia: WB Saunders, 1981:150–154.

40. Sankaran K, Bhagirath CP, Bingham WT, Hjertaas R, Haight K. Tracheal atresia, proximal esophageal atresia and distal tracheoesophageal fistula: Report of two cases and review of literature. Pediatrics 1983;71:81–823.

41. Holder TM, Cloud DT, Lewis JE, Pilling GB. Esophageal atresia and tracheoesophageal fistula. Pediatrics 1964;35:542–549.

42. German JC, Mahour GH, Woolley MM. Esophageal atresia and associated anomalies. J Pediatr Surg 1976;11:299–306.

43. Greenwood RD, Rosenthal A. Cardiovascular malformations associated with tracheoesophageal fistula and esophageal atresia. Pediatrics 1976;57:87–91.

44. Atwell JD, Beard RC. Congenital anomalies of the upper urinary tract associated with esophageal atresia and tracheoesophageal fistula. J Pediatr Surg 1974;9:825–831.

45. Quan L, Smith DW. The VATER association, Vertebral defects, Anal atresia, T-E fistula with esophageal atresia, Radial and Renal dysplasia: A spectrum of associated defects. J Pediatr 1973;82:104–107.

46. Temtamy SA, Miller JD. Extending the scope of the VATER association: Definition of the VATER syndrome. J. Pediatr 1974;85:345–349.

47. Nora AH, Nora JJ. A syndrome of multiple congenital anomalies associated with teratogenic exposure. Arch Environ Health 1975;30:17–21.

48. Khoury MJ, Cordero JF, Greenberg F, James LM, Erickson JD. A population study of the VACTERL association: Evidence for its etiologic heterogeneity. Pediatrics 1983;71:815–820.

49. Uehling DT, Gilbert E, Chesney R. Urologic implications of the VATER association. J Urol 1983;129:352–354.

50. Ein SH, Stringer DA, Stephens CA, Shandling B, Simpson J, Filler RM. Recurrent tracheoesophageal fistulas: Seventeen-year review. J Pediatr Surg 1983;18:436–441.

51. Couriel JM, Hibbert M, Olinsky A, Phelan PD. Long-term pulmonary consequences of oesophageal atresia with tracheo-oesophageal fistula. Acta Paediatr Scand 1982;71:973–978.

52. Becher RM, Lesperance R, Despas P, Wilson JAS. Congenital esophagobronchial fistula in a 62-year-old woman. Chest 1976;69:110–112.

53. Emery JL, Haddadin AJ. Squamous epithelium in respiratory tract of children with tracheo-oesophageal fistula. Arch Dis Child 1971;46:236–242.

54. Landing BH. Five syndromes (malformation complexes) of pulmonary symmetry, congenital heart disease, and multiple spleens. Pediatr Pathol 1984;2:125–151.

55. Hatayoma C, Wells TR. Syndrome of externally bilobed lungs with normal bronchial branch pattern, congenital heart disease, multiple spleens, intestinal malrotation and short pancreas: An apparently hitherto undefined malformation complex. Pediatr Pathol 1984;2:127–133.

56. Escarous A. Left pulmonary isomerism with normal arrangement of the heart and abdominal organs. Computed tomography of two adults. Int J Cardiol 1989;24:118–120.

57. Devine WA, Debich DE, Taylor SR. Symmetrical bronchial pattern with normal atrial morphology. Int J Cardiol 1988;20:395–398.

58. McLaughlin FJ, Strieder DJ, Harris GBC, Vawter GP, Eraklis AJ. Tracheal bronchus: association with respiratory morbidity in childhood. J Pediatr 1985;106:751–755.

59. Atwell SW. Major anomalies of the tracheobronchial tree with a list of minor anomalies. Dis Chest 1967;52:611–615.

60. Gonzalez-Crussi F, Padilla L, Miller JK, Grosfeld JL. "Bridging bronchus." Am J Dis Child 1976;130:1015–1018.

61. Wells TR, Gwinn JL, Landing BH, Stanley P. Reconsideration of the anatomy of sling left pulmonary artery; the association of one form with bridging bronchus and imperforate anus. Anatomic and diagnostic aspects. J Pediatr Surg 1988;23:892–898.

62. Gleason IO, Tildon TT, Rosen VJ. Ectopic thyroid tissue causing bronchial obstruction. Ann Thorac Surg 1967;3:151–153.

63. Patronas NJ, MacMahon H, Variakojis D. Bronchial web diagnosed by bronchiography. Radiology 1976; 121:526.

64. Williams H, Campbell P. Generalized bronchiectasis associated with deficiency of cartilage in the bronchial tree. Arch Dis Child 1960;35:182–191.

65. Mitchell RE, Bury RG. Congenital bronchiectasis due to deficiency of bronchial cartilage (Williams-Campbell syndrome). J Pediatr 1975;87:230–234.

66. Davis PB, Hubbard VS, McCoy K, Taussig LM. Familial bronchiectasis. J Pediatr 1983;102:177–185.

67. Oppenheimer EH. Similarity of the tracheobronchial mucous glands and epithelium in infants with and without cystic fibrosis. Hum Pathol 1981;12:36–48.

68. Simel DL, Mastin JP, Pratt PC, et al. Scanning electron microscopic study of the airways in normal children and in patients with cystic fibrosis and other lung diseases. Pediatr Pathol 1984;2:47–64.

69. Pysher TJ, Neustein HB. Ciliary dysmorphology. Perspect Pediatr Pathol 1984;8:101–131.

70. Turner JAP, Corkey CWB, Lee JYV, Levison H, Sturgess K. Clinical expressions of immotile cilia syndrome. Pediatrics 1981;67:805–810.

71. MacMahon HE, Ruggieri J. Congenital segmental bronchomalacia. Am J Dis Child 1969;118:923–926.

72. Chandra Mohan Cupta TG, Goldberg SJ, Lewis E, Fonkalsurd EW. Congenital bronchiomalacia. Am J Dis Child 1968;115:88–90.

73. Van Benthem LHBM, Driessin O, Haneveld GT, Rietema HP. Cryptorchidism, chest deformities and other congenital anomalies in three brothers. Arch Dis Child 1970;45:143–144.

74. Landing BH. Congenital malformations and genetic disorders of the respiratory tract. Am Rev Respir Dis 1979;120:151–185.

75. Sane SM, Steber WK, Girdany BR: Congenital bronchobiliary fistula. Surgery 1971;69:599–608.

76. Kalayoglu M, Olcay I. Congenital bronchiobiliary fistula associated with esophageal atresia and tracheo-esophageal fistula. J Pediatr Surg 1976;11:463–464.

77. Chan YT, Ng WD, Mak WP, Kwong ML, Chow CB. Congenital bronchiobiliary fistula associated with ciliary atresia. Br J Surg 1984;71:240–241.

78. Buntain WL, Isaacs H, Payne VC, Lindesmith GG, Rosenkrantz JG. Lobar emphysema, cystic adenomatoid malformation, pulmonary sequestration, and bronchogenic cyst in infancy and childhood: A clinical group. J Pediatr Surg 1974;9:85–93.

79. Ramenofsky ML, Leape LL, McCauley RGK. Bronchogenic cyst. J Pediatr Surg 1979;14:219–224.

80. Sirivella S, Ford WB, Zikria EA, Miller WH, Samadani SR, Sullivan ME. Foregut cysts of the mediastinum. J Thorac Cardiovasc Surg 1985;90:776–782.

81. Katzenstein AA, Askin FB. Pediatric disorders. I. Congenital malformations. In: Surgical pathology of non-neoplastic lung disease. Philadelphia: WB Saunders, 1982;314–337.

82. Fraga S, Helwig EB, Rosen SH. Bronchogenic cysts in the skin and subcutaneous tissue. Am J Clin Pathol 1971;56:230–238.

83. Eraklis AJ, Griscom NT, McGovern JB. Bronchogenic cysts of the mediastinum in infancy. N Engl J Med 1969;281:1150–1155.

84. Touloukian RJ. Air-filled bronchogenic cyst presenting as a cervical mass in the newborn. J Pediatr Surg 1982;17:311–312.

85. Canty TG, Hendren WH: Upper airway obstruction from foregut cysts of the hypopharynx. J Pediatr Surg 1975;10:807–812.

86. Alshakbhoun S, Starkey GWB, Asnes RA. Bronchogenic cysts of the mediastinum in infancy. Ann Thorac Surg 1967;4:532–541.

87. Young G, L'Heureux RR, Krueckeberg ST, Swanson DA. Mediastinal bronchogenic cyst: Prenatal sonographic diagnosis. AJR 1989;152:125–127.

88. Reed JC, Sobonya RE. Morphologic analysis of foregut cysts in the thorax. AJR 1974;120:851–860.

89. Aaron BL. Intradiaphragmatic cyst: a rare entity. J Thorac Cardiovasc Surg 1965;49:531–534.

90. Harmand D, Grosdidier J, Hoeffel JC. Multiple bronchogenic cysts of the esophagus. Am J Gastroenterol 1981;75:321–323.

91. Houser WC, Dorff GJ, Rosenweig DY, Aussem JW. Mycobacterial infection of a congenital bronchogenic cyst. Thorax 1980;35:312–313.

92. Stocker JT, Kagan-Hallet K. Extralobar pulmonary sequestration: analysis of 15 cases. Am J Clin Pathol 1979;72:917–925.

93. Black TL, Fernandes ET, Wrenn EL, Jr., Magill HL. Extralobar pulmonary sequestration and mediastinal bronchogenic cyst. J Pediatr Surg 1988;23:999–1001.

94. Weichert RF, Lindsey ES, Pearce CW, Waring WW. Bronchogenic cyst with unilateral obstructive emphysema. J. Thorac Cardiovasc Surg 1970;59:287–291.

95. Williams AJ, Schuster SR. Bronchial atresia associated with a bronchogenic cyst: evidence of early appearance of atretic segments. Chest 1985;87:396–398.

96. Cipriano P, Sweeney LJ, Hutchins GM, Rosenquist GC. Horseshoe lung in an infant with recurrent pulmonary infections. Am J Dis Child 1975;129:1343–1345.

97. Orzem F, Angelini P, Oglietti J, Leachman RD, Cooley DA. Horseshoe lung: report of two cases. Am Heart J 1977;93:501–505.

98. Dische MR. Horseshoe lung associated with a variant of the "scimitar" syndrome. Br Heart J 1974;36:617–620.

99. Freedem RM, Burrows PE, Moes CAF. "Horseshoe" lung: Report of five new cases. AJR 1986;146:211–215.

100. Frank JL, Poole CA, Rosas G. Horseshoe lung: Clinical, pathologic, and radiologic features and a new plain film finding. AJR 1986;146:217–226.

101. Siegelman SS, Shanser JD, Attai LA. Cervical herniation of the lung associated with transient venous occlusions. Dis Chest 1968;53:785–787.

102. Chaurasia BD, Singh MP. Ectopic lungs in a human fetus with Klippel-Feil syndrome. Anat Anz 1977;142:205–208.

103. Chaurasia BD, Wagh KV. Iniencephalus with ectopic lungs. Anat Anz 1974;136:447–452.

104. Cunningham MD, Peters ER. Cervical hernia of the lung associated with cri du chat syndrome. Am J Dis Child 1969;118:769–771.

105. Ostor AG, Stillwell R, Fortune DW. Bilateral pulmonary agenesis. Pathology 1978;10:243–248.

106. Devi B, More JRS. Total tracheopulmonary agenesis. Acta Pediatr Scand 1966;55:107–116.

107. Claireaux AE, Ferreira HP. Bilateral pulmonary agenesis. Arch DisChild 1958;33:364–366.

108. Tuyman PE, Gardner LW. Bilateral aplasia of the lung. Arch Pathol Lab Med 1952;54:306–313.

109. Schechter DC. Congenital absence or deficiency of lung tissue. Ann Thorac Surg 1968;6:286–313.

110. Mardini MK, Nyhan WL. Agenesis of the lung: report of four patients with unusual anomalies. Chest 1985;87:522–527.

111. Booth JB, Berry CL. Unilateral pulmonary agenesis. Arch Dis Child 1967;42:361–374.

112. Maltz DL, Nadas AS. Agenesis of the lung. Pediatrics 1968;42:175–188.

113. Boxer RA, Hayes CJ, Hordof AJ, Mellins RB. Agenesis of the left lung and total anomalous pulmonary venous connection. Chest 1978;74:106–109.

114. Mygind H, Paulsen SM. Agenesis of the right lung. Arch Pathol Lab Med 1980;104:444.

115. Osborne J, Masel J, McCredie J. A spectrum of skeletal anomalies associated with pulmonary agenesis: Possible neural crest injuries. Pediatr Radiol 1989;19:425–432.

116. Harrison MR, Hendren WH. Agenesis of the lung complicated by vascular compression and bronchomalacia. J Pediatr Surg 1975;10:813–817.

117. Storey CF, Marrangoni AG. Lobar agenesis of the lung. J Thorac Surg 1954;28:536–543.

118. Sbokos CG, McMillan. Agenesis of the lung. Br J Dis Chest 1977;71:183–197.

119. Ryland D, Reid L. Pulmonary aplasia—a quantitative analysis of the development of the single lung. Thorax 1971;26:602–609.

120. Potter EL, Craig JM. Pathology of the fetus and infant. 3d ed. Chicago: Year Book Medical, 1975:21.

121. Gruenwald P, Minh HN. Evaluation of body and organ weights in perinatal pathology. Am J Clin Pathol 1960;34:247–253.

122. Reale FR, Esterly JR. Pulmonary hypoplasia: a morphometric study of the lungs of infants with diaphragmatic hernia, anencephaly, and renal malformations. Pediatrics 1973;51:91–96.

123. Emery JL, Mithal A. The number of alveoli in the terminal respiratory unit of man during late intrauterine life and childhood. Arch Dis Child 1960;35:544–547.

124. Askenazi SS, Perlman M. Pulmonary hypoplasia: lung weight and radial alveolar count as criteria of diagnosis. Arch Dis Child 1979;54:614–618.

125. Scherle W. A simple method for volumetry of organs in quantitative sterology. Mikroskopie 1970;26:57–60.

126. Thurlbeck WM. Postmortem lung volumes. Thorax 1979;34:735–739.

127. Wigglesworth JS, Desai R. Use of DNA estimation for growth assessment in normal and hypoplastic fetal lungs. Arch Dis Child 1981;56:601–605.

128. Cooney TD, Thurlbeck WM. The radial alveolar count method of Emery and Mithal: a reappraisal. 2. Intrauterine and early postnatal lung growth. Thorax 1982;37:580–583.

129. Cooney TD, Thurlbeck WM. The radial alveolar count of Emery and Mithal: a reappraisal. I. Postnatal lung growth. Thorax 1982;37:572–579.

130. George DK, Cooney TP, Chiu BK, Thurlbeck WM. Hypoplasia and immaturity of the terminal lung unit (acinus) in congenital diaphragmatic hernia. Am Rev Respir Dis 1987;136:947–950.

131. Page DN, Stocker JT. Anomalies associated with pulmonary hypoplasia. Am Rev Respir Dis 1982;125:216–221.

132. Nakayama DK, Gluk PL, Harrison MR, Villa RL, Noall R. Experimental pulmonary hypoplasia due to oligohydramnios and its reversal by relieving thoracic compression. J Pediatr Surg 1983;18:347–353.

133. Perlman M, Williams F, Hirsch W. Neonatal pulmonary hypoplasia after prolonged leakage of amniotic fluid. Arch Dis Child 1976;51:349–353.

134. Thomas IT, Smith DW. Oligohydramnios, cause of the nonrenal features of Potter's syndrome, including pulmonary hypoplasia. J Pediatr 1974;84:811–814.

135. Goldstein JD, Reid LM. Pulmonary hypoplasia resulting from phrenic nerve agenesis and diaphragmatic amyoplasia. J Pediatr 1980;97:282–287.

136. Cooney TP, Wentworth PJ, Thurlbeck WM. Diminished radial count is found only postnatally in Down's syndrome. Pediatr Pulmonol 1988;5:204–209.

137. Gonzalez OR, Gomez IG, Recaldi AL, Landing BH. Postnatal development of the cystic lung lesion of Down syndrome: Suggestion that the cause is reduced formation of peripheral air spaces. Pediatr Pathol 1991;4:623–633.

138. Swischuk LE, Richardson CJ, Nichols MM, Ingman MJ. Bilateral pulmonary hypoplasia in the neonate. AJR 1979;133:1057–1063.

139. Swischuk LE, Richardson CJ, Nichols MM, Ingman MJ. Primary pulmonary hypoplasia in the neonate. J Pediatr 1979;95:573–577.

140. Hislop A, Hey E, Reid L. The lungs in congenital bilateral renal agenesis and dysplasia. Arch Dis Child 1979;54:32–38.

141. Stocker JT. Congenital cytomegalovirus infection presenting as massive ascites with secondary pulmonary hypoplasia. Hum Pathol 1985;16:1173–1175.

142. Novak RM. Laryngotracheoesophageal cleft and unilat-

eral pulmonary hypoplasia in twins. Pediatrics 1981;67:732–734.

143. Symonds DA, Driscoll SC. Massive fetal ascites, urethral atresia and cytomegalic inclusion disease. Am J Dis Child 1974;127:895–897.

144. Ellis MI, Hey EN, Walker W. Neonatal death in babies with rhesus isoimmunization. Q J Med 1979;190:211–225.

145. Wigglesworth JS, Winston RML, Barttett K. Influence of the CNS in fetal lung development. Arch Dis Child 1977;52:965–967.

146. Pena SDJ, Shokeir MHK. Syndrome of camptodactly, multiple ankylosis, facial anomalies, and pulmonary hypoplasia: a lethal condition. J Pediatr 1974;85:373–375.

147. Derksen OS. Scimitar syndrome and pulmonary sequestration. Radiol Clin North Am 1977;46:81–93.

148. Felson B. Pulmonary agenesis and related anomalies. Semin Roentgenol 1972;7:17–30.

149. Farnsworth AE, Ankeney JL. The spectrum of the scimitar syndrome. J Thorac Cardiovasc Surg 1974;68:37–42.

150. Neil CA, Ferencz C, Sabiston DC, Sheldon H. The familial occurrence of hypoplastic right lung with systemic arterial supply and venous drainage. "Scimitar syndrome." Bull Johns Hopkins Hosp 1960;107:1–15.

151. Dresler S. Massive pleural effusion and hypoplasia of the lung accompanying extralobar pulmonary sequestration. Hum Pathol 1981;12:862–864.

152. Lucaya J, Garcia-Conesa JA, Bernado L. Pulmonary sequestration associated with unilateral pulmonary hypoplasia and massive pleural effusion. Pediatr Radiol 1984;14:228–229.

153. Turkel SB. Conditions associated with non-immune hydrops fetalis. Clin Perinatol 1982;9:613–625.

154. Stocker JT. Sequestration of the lung. Semin Diagn Pathol Path 1986;3:106–121.

155. Savic B, Birtel FJ, Tholen W, Funke HD, Knoche R. Lung sequestration: Report of seven cases and review of 540 published cases. Thorax 1979;34:96–101.

156. Kaude JV, Laurin S. Ultrasonographic demonstration of systemic artery feeding extrapulmonary sequestration. Pediatr Radiol 1984;14:226–227.

157. Mahadevia PS. Necrotizing vasculitis in an extralobar sequestered lung. Arch Pathol Lab Med 1980;104:114.

158. Maull KI, McElvein RB. Infarcted extralobar pulmonary sequestration. Chest 1975;68:98–99.

159. Stocker JT, Madewell JE, Drake RM. Congenital cystic adenomatoid malformation of the lung: Classification and morphologic spectrum. Hum Pathol 1977;8:155–171.

160. Stocker JT, Drake RM, Madewell JE. Cystic and congenital lung diseses in the newborn. Perspect Pediatr Pathol 1978;4:93–154.

161. Adeyemo AO, Omole CO, Oyedeyi GA. Congenital lobar emphysema of left upper lobe: A case report. Scand J Thorac Cardiovasc Surg 1983;17:57–59.

162. Wall MA, Eisenberg JD, Campbell JR. Congenital lobar emphysema in a mother and daughter. Pediatrics 1982;70:131–133.

163. Iancur T, Boyanova Y, Eilam N, Eilan E, Lerner MA. Infantile sub-lobar emphysema with tracheal bronchus. Acta Paediatr Scand 1975;64:551–554.

164. Keller MS. Congenital lobar emphysema with tracheal bronchus. J Can Assoc Radiol 1983;34:306–307.

165. Capitano MA, Ramos R, Kirkpatrick JA. Pulmonary sling. AJR 1971;112:28–34.

166. Sulayman R, Thilenius O, Replogle R, Arcilla RA. Unilateral emphysema in total anomalous pulmonary venous return. J Pediatr 1975;87:433–435.

167. Miller KE, Edwards DK, Hilton S, Collins D, Lynch F, Williams R. Acquired lobar emphysema in premature infants with bronchopulmonary dysplasia: An iatrogenic disease? Radiology 1981;138:589–592.

168. Hislop A, Reid L. New pathological findings in emphysema of childhood: 2. Overinflation of a normal lobe. Thorax 1971;26:190–194.

169. Schneider JR, St Cyr JA, Thompson TR, Johnson DE, Burke BA, Foker JE. The changing spectrum of cystic pulmonary lesions requiring surgical resection in infants. J Thorac Cardiovasc Surg 1985;89:332–339.

170. Man DWK, Handy MH, Hendry GMA, Bisset WH, Forfar JO. Congenital lobar emphysema: Problems in diagnosis and management. Arch Dis Child 1983;58:709–712.

171. Morgan WJ, Lemen RJ, Rojas R. Acute worsening of congenital lobar emphysema with subsequent spontaneous improvement. Pediatrics 1983;71:844–848.

172. Robotham JL, Menkes HA, Chipps BE, et al. A physiologic assessment of segmental bronchial atresia. Am Rev Respir Dis 1980;121:533–540.

173. McBride JT, Wohl MEB, Strieder DJ, et al. Lung growth and airway function after lobectomy in infancy for congenital lobar emphysema. J Clin Invest 1980;66:962–970.

174. Frenckrier B, Freyschuss U. Pulmonary function after lobectomy for congenital lobar emphysema and congenital cystic adenomatoid malformation: A follow-up study. Scand J Thorac Cardiovasc Surg 1982;16:293–298.

175. Williams AJ, Schuster SR. Bronchial atresia associated with a bronchogenic cyst. Chest 1985;87:396–398.

176. Jones JC, Almond CH, Snyder HM, Meyer BW, Patrick JR. Lobar emphysema and congenital heart disease in infancy. J Thorac Cardiovasc Surg 1965;49:1–10.

177. Pierce WS, DeParedes CG, Friedman S, Waldhausen JA. Concomitant congenital heart disease and lobar emphysema in infants. Ann Surg 1970;172:951–956.

178. Roguin N, Peleg H, Lemer J, Naveh Y, Reis E. The value of cardiac catheterization and cineangiography in infantile lobar emphysema. Pediatr Radiol 1980;10:71–74.

179. Bolande RP, Schneider AF, Boggs JD. Infantile lobar emphysema: Etiologic concept. Arch Pathol Lab Pathol 1956;61:289–294.

180. Campbell PE. Congenital lobar emphysema: Etiological studies. Aust Paediatr J 1969;5:226–233.

181. Warner JO, Rubin S, Heard BE. Congenital lobar emphysema: A case with bronchial atresia and abnormal

bronchial cartilage. Br J Dis Chest 1982;76:177–184.

182. Hislop A, Reid L. New pathological findings in emphysema of childhood: I. Polyalveolar lobe with emphysema. Thorax 1970;25:682–690.

183. Munnell ER, Lambird PA, Austin RL. Polyalveolar lobe causing lobar emphysema of infancy. Ann Thorac Surg 1973;16:624–628.

184. Topper D, Schuster S, McBride J, et al. Polyalveolar lobe: Anatomic and physiologic parameters and their relationship to congenital lobar emphysema. J Pediatr Surg 1980;15:931–937.

185. Felman AH, Rhatigan RM, Pierson KK. Pulmonary lymphangiectasis: Observation in 17 patients and proposed classification. AJR 1972;116:548–558.

186. Noonan JA, Walters LR, Reeves JT. Congenital pulmonary lymphangiectasis. Am J Dis Child 1970;120:314–319.

187. Hunter WS, Becroft DMO. Congenital pulmonary lymphangiectasis associated with pleural effusions. Arch Dis Child 1984;59:278–279.

188. Gardner TW, Domm AC, Brock CE, Pruitt AW. Congenital pulmonary lymphangiectasis. Clin Pediatr (Phila) 1983;22:75–78.

189. Wilson RH, Duncan A, Hume R, Bain AD. Prenatal pleural effusion associated with congenital pulmonary lymphangiectasis. Prenat Diagn 1985;5:73–76.

190. Siegal A, Katsenstein M, Wolach B. Neonatal pneumothorax, a rare complication of pulmonary cystic lymphangiectasis. Eur J Respir Dis 1985;66:153–157.

191. Scott-Emuakpor AB, Warren ST, Kapur S, Quiachon EB, Higgins JV. Familial occurrence of congenital pulmonary lymphangiectasis: Genetic implications. Am J Dis Child 1981;135:532–534.

192. Pemot C, Bernard C, Hoeffel JG. Congenital pulmonary lymphangiectasis of late onset associated with congenital heart disease. Arch Fr Pediatr 1984;41:617–622.

193. Esterly JR, Oppenheimer EH. Lymphangiectasis and other pulmonary lesions in the asplenia syndrome. Arch Pathol Lab Med 1970;90:553–560.

194. France NE, Brown RJK. Congenital pulmonary lymphangiectasis; report of 11 examples with special reference to cardiovascular findings. Arch Dis Child 1971; 46:528–532.

195. Rhatigan RM, Hobin FP. Congenital pulmonary lymphangiectasis and ichthyosis congenita. Am J Clin Pathol 1970;53:95–99.

196. Chin KY, Tang MY. Congenital adenomatoid malformation of one lobe of a lung with general anasarca. Arch Pathol Lab Med 1949;48:221–229.

197. VanDijk C, Wagenvoort CA. The various type of congenital adenomatoid malformation of the lung. J Pathol 1973;110:131–134.

198. Madewell JE, Stocker JT, Korsower JM. Cystic adenomatoid malformation of the lung. AJR 1975;124:436–448.

199. Kwitten J, Reiner L. Congenital cystic adenomatoid malformation of the lung. Pediatrics 1962;30:759–768.

200. Avitabile AM, Hulnick DH, Greco A, Feiner HD. Congenital cystic adenomatoid malformation of the lung in adults. Am J Surg Pathol 1984;8:193–202.

201. Miller RK, Sieber WK, Yunis EJ. Congenital adenomatoid malformation of the lung: A report of 17 cases and review of the literature. Pathol Annu 1980;15(part 1):387–402.

202. Wexler HA, Valdes Dapena M. Congenital cystic adenomatoid malformation: A report of 3 unusual cases. Radiology 1978;126:737–741.

203. Alt B, Shikes RH, Stanford RE, Silverberg SG. Ultrastructure of congenital cystic adenomatoid malformation of the lung. Ultrastruct Pathol 1982;3:217–228.

204. Olson JL, Mendelsohn G. Congenital cystic adenomatoid malformation of the lung. Arch Pathol Lab Med 1978;102:248–251.

205. Glaves J, Baker JL. Spontaneous resolution of maternal hydramnios in congenital cystic adenomatoid malformation of the lung. Antenatal ultrasound features. Case report. Br J Obstet Gynaecol 1983;90:1065–1068.

206. Diwan RV, Brennan JN, Philipson EH, Jain S, Bellon EM. Ultrasonic prenatal diagnosis of type III congenital cystic adenomatoid malformation of lung. J Clin Ultrasound 1983;11:218–221.

207. Cohen RA, Moskowitz PS, McCallum WD. Sonographic diagnosis of cystic adenomatoid malformation in-utero. Prenat Diagn 1983;3:139–143.

208. Yadar K, Kataria S, Pathak IC. Congenital cystic lesion of the lung in a new-born. Int Surg 1982;67:430.

209. Benjavongkulchai S, Shuangshoti S. Congenital cystic adenomatoid malformation of the lung. J Med Assoc Thai 1982;65:333–339.

210. Bruno E. Congenital cystic adenomatoid malformation. IMJ 1982;162:485, 506–508.

211. Cachia R, Sobonya RE. Congenital cystic adenomatoid malformation of the lung with bronchial atresia. Hum Pathol 1981;12:947–950.

212. Donn SM, Martin JN, White SJ. Antenatal ultrasound findings in cystic adenomatoid malformation. Pediatr Radiol 1981;10:180–182.

213. Nishibayashi SW, Andrassy RJ, Woolley MM. Congenital cystic adenomatoid malformation: A 30-year experiment. J Pediatr Surg 1981;16:704–706.

214. Blane CE, Donn SM, Mori KW. Case report: Congenital cystic adenomatoid malformation of the lung. J Comput Assist Tomogr 1981;5:418–420.

215. Krous HF, Harper PE, Perlman M. Congenital cystic adenomatoid malformation in bilateral renal agenesis. Its mitigation of Potter's syndrome. Arch Pathol Lab Med 1980;104:368–370.

216. Stevenson DK, Silverman FN, Churg AM, Shochat SJ. Unusual roentgenographic presentation of a congenital cystic malformation of the lung. Eur J Pediatr 1979; 132:119–124.

217. Bale, PM. Congenital cystic malformation of the lung. Am J Clin Pathol 1979;71:411–420.

218. Weinberg AG, Zumwalt RE. Bilateral nephromegaly and multiple pulmonary cysts. Am J Clin Pathol 1977;67:284–288.

219. Chi JG, Shong YK. Diffuse striated muscle heteroplasia of the lung. Arch Pathol Lab Med 1982;106:641–644.

220. Vilanova JR, Burgos-Bretones J, Aguirre JM, Rivera-

Pomar JM. Rhabdomyomatous dysplasia of lung and congenital diaphragmatic hernia. J Pediatr Surg 1983; 18:201–203.

221. Ueda K, Gruppo R, Unger F, Martin L, Bove K. Rhabdomyosarcoma of lung arising in congenital cystic adenomatoid malformation. Cancer 1977;40:383–388.

222. Krous HF, Sexauer CL. Embryonal rhabdomyosarcoma arising within a congenital bronchogenic cyst in a child. J Pediatr Surg 1981;16:506–508.

223. Rutledge J, Jensen P. Acinar dysplasia: A new form of pulmonary maldevelopment. Hum Pathol 1986;17: 1290–1293.

224. Haller JO, Kauffman SL, Kassner EG. Congenital mesenchymal tumour of the lung. Br J Radiol 1977;50:217–219.

225. Fisher JE, Nelson SJ, Allen JE, Holzman RS. Congenital cystic adenomatoid malformation of the lung: a unique variant. Am J Dis Child 1982;136:1071–1074.

226. Janney CG, Askin FB, Kuhn C. Congenital alveolar capillary dysplasia; an unusual cause of respiratory distress in the newborn. Am J Clin Pathol 1981;76:722–727.

227. MacMahon HE. Congenital alveolar dysplasia of the lung. Am J Pathol 1984;24:919–930.

228. Kaufman N, Spiro RK. Congenital alveolar dysplasia of the lung. Arch Pathol Lab Med 1951;49:434–440.

229. Daentl DL, Passarge E. Familial agenesis of the diaphragm. Birth Defects 1972;8:24–26.

230. Benjamin HB. Agenesis of the left hemidiaphragm. J Thorac Cardiovasc Surg 1963;46:265–270.

231. Eichelberger MR, Kettrich RG, Hoelzer DJ, Swellow DB, Schnaufer L. Agenesis of the left diaphragm: surgical repair and physiologic consequences. J Pediatr Surg 1980;15:395–397.

232. Neville WE, Clowes GA. Congenital absence of hemidiaphragm and use of a lobe of liver in its surgical repair. Arch Surg 1954;69:282–290.

233. Ikeda T, Ishihara H, Yoshimatru H, et al. Accessory diaphragm associated with congenital posterolateral diaphragmatic hernia, aberrant systemic artery to the right lower lobe and anomalous pulmonary vein. J Thorac Cardiovasc Surg 1972;64:18–25.

234. Kenauoglu A, Tunchilek E. Accessory diaphragm on the left side. Pediatr Radiol 1978;7:172–174.

235. Hart JC, Cohen IT, Ballantine TVN, Varrano LF. Accessory diaphragm in an infant. J Pediatr Surg 1981;16:947–948.

236. Nazarian M, Currarino G, Webb WR, Willis K, Kiphart RJ, Wilson HE. Accessory diaphragm: report of a case with complete physiological evaluation and surgical correction. J Thorac Cardiovasc Surg 1971;61:293–299.

237. Hansen J, James S, Burrington J, Whitfield J. The decreasing incidence of pneumothorax and improving survival of infants with diaphragmatic hernia. J Pediatr Surg 1984;19:385–388.

238. Starrett RW, deLorimier AA. Congenital diaphragmatic hernia in lambs: hemodynamic and ventilatory changes with breathing. J Pediatr Surg 1975;10:575–582.

239. Levin DL. Morphologic analysis of the pulmonary vascular bed in congenital left-sided diaphragmatic hernia. J Pediatr 1978;92:805–809.

240. Dibbins AW, Wiener ES. Mortality from neonatal diaphragmatic hernia. J Pediatr Surg 1974;9:653–662.

241. Mishalany HG, Nakada K, Woolley MM. Congenital diaphragmatic hernias. Arch Surg 1979;114:1118–1123.

242. Bloss RS, Aranda JV, Beardmore HE. Congenital diaphragmatic hernia: Pathophysiology and pharmacologic support. Surgery 1981;89:518–524.

243. Campbell DN, Lilly JR. The clinical spectrum of right Bochdulek's hernia. Arch Surg 1982;117:341–344.

244. Banagale RC, Watters JH. Delayed right-sided diaphragmatic hernia following group B streptococcal infection. Hum Pathol 1983;14:67–69.

245. Greenwood RD, Rosenthal A, Nadas AS. Cardiovascular abnormalities associated with congenital diaphragmatic hernia. Pediatrics 1976;57:92–97.

246. Jewett TC, Thomson NB. Iatrogenic eventration of the diaphragm in infancy. J Thorac Cardiovasc Surg 1964;48:861–866.

247. Paris F, Blasco E, Canto A, Tarazona V, Casillas M. Diaphragmatic eventration in infants. Thorax 1973; 28:66–72.

248. Wayne ER, Campbell JB, Burrington JD, Davis WS. Eventration of the diaphragm. J Pediatr Surg 1974; 9:643–651.

249. Thomas TV. Congenital eventration of the diaphragm. Ann Thorac Surg 1970;10:180–192.

250. O'Shea PA. Chronic granulomatous disease of childhood. Perspect Pediatr Pathol 1981;6:237–258.

251. Schafer IA. Vascular and other genetic diseases affecting the lungs. In: Baum GL, Wolinsky E, eds. Textbook of pulmonary diseases. 3d Ed. Boston: Little, Brown, 1983:1261–1276.

CHAPTER 8

Acquired Neonatal and Pediatric Diseases

J. Thomas Stocker and Louis P. Dehner

If a chapter equivalent to this one had been available 35 or 45 years ago, we would have seen a number of familiar topics such as bacterial pneumonias, bronchiectasis, and some viral pneumonias, but many other clinicopathologic conditions and concepts would have been included. Children are still subject to pyogenic pneumonias from *Staphylococcus aureus* and *Streptococcus pneumoniae,* although effective antibiotic therapy has markedly diminished the fatal consequences in the nonimmunocompromised child. Today, the latter qualification in the immune status of the host is the critical factor in the type(s) of offending pathogens and the anticipated clinical syndrome.

Pediatric pulmonary surgical pathology today, in the experience of one of the authors (LPD), is dominated by sequential transbronchial biopsies in lung transplant recipients to monitor the presence of allograft rejection or an opportunistic infection like cytomegalovirus. The clinical indications for lung or bronchial biopsies in children are similar to those in adults except for the question of possible bronchogenic carcinoma in the older age groups. The nature and status of an undiagnosed or previously diagnosed interstitial-alveolar lung disease are the usual reasons for a transbronchial or open lung biopsy in a child. Exclusive of single or double lung explants, pulmonary resections are generally restricted to lobectomies for congenital lobar emphysema, congenital cystic adenomatoid malformation, and persistent interstitial emphysema. Abscess, mucoid impaction, inflammatory myofibroblastic tumor, pleuropulmonary blastoma, and carcinoid are various disorders of the lung in children that were diagnosed and treated by lobectomy and examined in our laboratory in the past 3 years.

There are other problems and questions unrelated to infections, which the pathologist may expect to encounter, that were either unrecognized or nonexistent earlier. New technology, drugs, and even pathogens (e.g., *Legionella pneumophilia*) are the major agents that have brought about these changes. For instance, pulmonary cysts in the newborn were generally regarded as congenital in most cases; however, persistent interstitial pulmonary emphysema in an infant with a history of bronchopulmonary dysplasia and/or vigorous ventilatory support is one of the more common indications for a segmental or total lobectomy in an infant with a "lung cyst."[1]

The *lung biopsy* is an established procedure to procure a pathologic diagnosis in a child who is usually immunocompromised and has developed pulmonic infiltrates suspicious for an opportunistic infection.[2–6] Improvements in pediatric anesthesia and surgery have reduced the operative complications to a minimum; however, many of these children are extremely ill and therefore are high-risk candidates for any invasive procedure. A biopsy can usually be taken through a small intercostal incision when localization is not especially important in a patient with diffuse changes[7] (see Chapter 1). The alternative method for tissue sampling is the endoscopic transbronchial biopsy.[8] There is less risk to the patient, but the specimen is smaller and crush artifacts from the instrument are more common. Transbronchical biopsies of multiple lobes are performed as a matter of routine follow-up to monitor for the presence of rejection or an infection in pulmonary allograft(s). An open lung biopsy is the exception in these particular patients.

Regardless of the biopsy technique, touch imprints from the moist surface of the fresh specimen should be taken immediately and fixed for cytologic examination. A methenamine silver stain is performed on the touch imprints for the identification of fungi and/or *Pneumocystis carinii*. Intranuclear inclusions and other cytologic aberrations are best appreciated with the Papanicolaou stain. Rapid tissue processing of the biopsy for routine histologic preparation is preferred to a frozen-section consultation because these specimens in children are often very small and may be exhausted in the preparation. If the clinician is mainly interested in knowing whether granulomas or recurrent tumor is present, however, a frozen section can serve that immediate purpose. Another function of the frozen section is to give the surgeon some indication whether lesional tissue has been sampled. A number of series have been published and should be consulted about the results of open lung and transbronchial biopsies in children.

Another procedure that has come into vogue recently is the *fine-needle aspiration biopsy*[9,10] in which the needle is guided by computed tomography (CT) or ultrasonography. The application of fine-needle aspiration biopsy is mainly confined to the presence of a discrete mass with the clinical prospects of recurrent or mestastatic tumor. A diagnosis by this biopsy technique has medical and economic advantages. If the changes in the lung(s) are diffuse in nature, rather than a single localized lesion, the positive yield in our experience has been quite low. A diagnosis of cytomegalovirus pneumonia was made in one case by fine-needle aspiration biopsy with the identification of the characteristic intranuclear inclusion in the aspirate. This case represents an exception rather than the rule.

Some of the disease entities presented in this chapter are also discussed elsewhere in this volume with more adult orientation, and the reader is referred to these chapters. Many other entities discussed here, however, do not have counterparts in adults. Rare examples of adult presentation of typically pediatric entities are included in this chapter.

Hyaline Membrane Disease

Hyaline membrane disease in the "classical" form as described by Lauweryns[11] in 1970 is seen only infrequently today, usually in the premature infant with mild respiratory distress who dies unexpectedly from intraventricular hemorrhage of the brain in the first day or two of life. Infants with more severe respiratory distress syndrome surviving longer than 2 or 3 days before death will usually display the changes of bronchopulmonary dysplasia described here. Hyaline membranes can also be seen in postmature infants. Seo and colleagues described the occurrence of hyaline membranes in 17 of 21 postterm infants dying within 10 days of birth. Amniotic and meconium aspiration was present in 95% of these cases.[12]

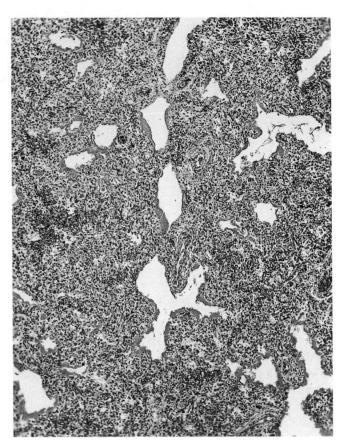

Fig. 8–1. Hyaline membrane disease. Autopsy section of lung with hyaline membrane disease displays diffuse atelectasis of alveolar sacs and alveoli with slight overdistension of alveolar ducts and terminal bronchioles. Smooth hyaline membranes are closely applied to walls of these airways. (AFIP Neg. 75–6696.) H and E, ×70.

"Uncomplicated" hyaline membrane disease, that is, those cases not requiring high oxygen tensions and ventilatory pressures, occurs in premature infants with idiopathic respiratory distress syndrome. This syndrome, characterized by tachypnea, intercostal retractions, and hypoxemia, is associated with a variety of clinical conditions, of which most involve deficiency of pulmonary surfactant leading to pulmonary atelectasis, anoxia, and alveolar cell necrosis. Radiographically, these infants display a typical ground-glass appearance of the lungs with an air bronchogram and diffusely scattered reticulogranular opacities.

On gross examination the lungs are firm, atelectatic, and typically sink when placed in water. The pleura is smooth and deep tan to red. The cut surface reveals a deep red parenchyma that oozes bloody fluid and resembles liver more than lung.

Microscopically there is a diffuse atelectasis that accentuates the bronchi and dilated bronchioles and alveolar ducts (Fig. 8–1). Smooth, homogeneous pink mem-

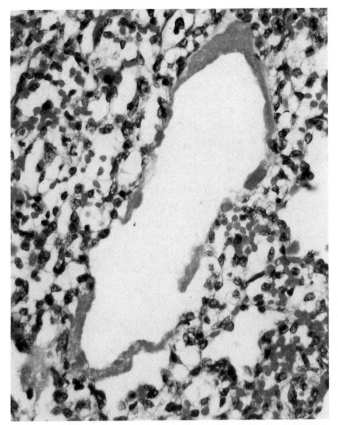

Fig. 8–2. Hyaline membrane disease. In this 1-day-old infant's lung, homogeneous membrane covers surface of alveolar duct. Note relatively smooth luminal surface. (AFIP Neg. 86–5551.) H and E, ×400.

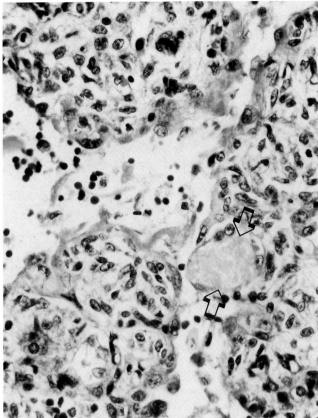

Fig. 8–3. Hyaline membrane disease in 4-day-old infant. Hyaline membranes are undergoing "organization" by macrophages and regenerating alveolar lining cells, which separate membranes from wall of alveolar duct. Note "rounded-up" membrane material (*arrows*). (AFIP Neg. 86–6762.) H and E, ×400.

branes, the "hyaline" membranes from which the disease derives its name, lie free in the lumen or are closely applied to surfaces of respiratory bronchioles and alveolar ducts (Fig. 8–2). The membranes are composed of necrotic alveolar lining cells, plasma transudate, inhaled amniotic fluid, and, if hemorrhage is present, fibrin. Homogeneously pink or finely granular transudate is often present in alveolar saccules, occasionally extending to bronchiolar and bronchial levels. Hemorrhagic material may be present focally throughout the lung. Pulmonary lymphatics are dilated particularly around pulmonary veins.[13]

Hyaline membranes may be seen in infants dying as early as 3–4 h after birth. Well-formed membranes are usually present by 12–24 h, and by 36–48 h, in cases of uncomplicated disease, organization of these membranes occurs with separation of the membrane from the underlying wall and engulfment of the material by macrophages (Fig. 8–3). Final repair of the bronchiolar and alveolar duct wall is accomplished by "resurfacing" of the wall by bronchiolar epithelial cells or type I and II alveolar lining cells.[14,15]

The appearance of the hyaline membranes may be altered by the presence of bacteria that find the membranes an ideal "culture media." Gram stains of membranes that are fragmented, granular, and faintly basophilic will often display the gram-positive cocci or gram-negative rods typical of streptococcal or *Escherichia coli* infections occasionally associated with this disease (Fig. 8–4). In infants with kernicterus, intraventricular hemorrhage, intrahepatic bile stasis, pulmonary hemorrhage, or disseminated intravascular coagulation who survive 3 or more days, yellow hyaline membranes may be present. The yellow pigment, visible in unstained paraffin sections, is an unconjugated bilirubin.[16,17]

Bronchopulmonary Dysplasia

The definition of bronchopulmonary dysplasia varies considerably depending on whether one is utilizing

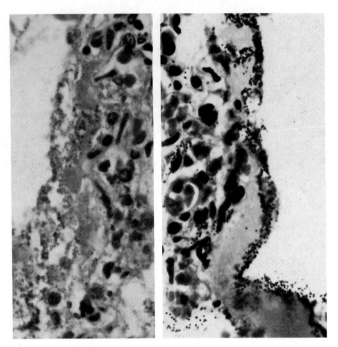

Fig. 8–4. Hyaline membrane disease with superimposed bacterial growth. On left, irregular, granular hyaline membrane lines alveolar duct. With special stains (right) cocci can be seen covering surface of membrane. (AFIP Neg. 75–6706.) Left, H and E, ×615; right, Humberstone stain, ×615.

clinical, radiographic, or pathologic characteristics.[18] Many neonatologists adopt a definition based on oxygen dependency and radiographic changes in the lung. Bancalari et al.,[19] for example, diagnosed bronchopulmonary dysplasia in all patients who are oxygen dependent for more than 28 days following mechanical ventilation during the first week of life and who have persistent increased densities in chest radiographs.[19,20] Pathologically, however, we are able to recognize the characteristic changes of bronchopulmonary dysplasia (bronchiolar epithelial dysplasia, necrotizing bronchiolitis, peribronchiolar edema, etc.) by the fifth day of life and often as early as 48–72 h of age. Because of this wide time discrepancy between the clinical and pathologic definition of bronchopulmonary dysplasia, we describe this disease primarily on the basis of its morphologic features, dividing those changes into (1) acute, (2) reparative or healing, and (3) long-standing "healed" bronchopulmonary dysplasia.

Clinically, bronchopulmonary dysplasia is noted in 2.5%–20% of infants with the respiratory distress syndrome who receive intermittent positive pressure ventilation.[20–23] In the United States, approximately 1,300 infants per year survive the more severe forms of this disease, with the numbers of infants surviving with milder forms of chronic lung damage being much

higher.[21] While most cases follow the treatment of the respiratory distress syndrome, others may occur following pneumonia, meconium aspiration syndrome, tracheoesophageal fistula, and congenital heart disease.[23,24]

The treatment of infants with bronchopulmonary dysplasia in its acute and reparative stages is primarily supportive. Mechanical ventilation using the lowest possible peak inspiratory pressure in conjunction with supplemental oxygen to maintain partial arterial oxygen pressure in the range of 50 to 80 torr constitute the major therapeutic approach in the early stages. The recent use of high-frequency ventilators of the jet ventilator, flow interrupter, or oscillator type may allow reduction of peak inspiratory pressure and help decrease the high incidence of interstitial pulmonary emphysema (as high as 40%) associated with bronchopulmonary dysplasia.[25–29] Fluid therapy, bronchodilator therapy, dexamethosome, Vitamin E, Vitamin A, and antihypertensive agents are also utilized in the treatment of bronchopulmonary dysplasia.[30–35] In recent years, surfactant replacement therapy has become widespread, and improvements in morbidity and mortality have been reported.[36–42] Davis and colleagues[41] reported an 89% survival rate in 28 infants with severe respiratory distress who initially deteriorated despite optimal conventional mechanical ventilation and exogenous surfactant therapy but responded to continued surfactant therapy and high-frequency jet ventilation.

Survival of infants who develop bronchopulmonary dysplasia is difficult to assess, again because of the difficulty in defining the entity. Severe bronchopulmonary dysplasia, however, using the radiographic criteria of Northway et al.[18] or the pathologic changes described by Edwards et al.,[43] is associated with a 54% mortality and significant morbidity even in long-term survivors.[44] Predictors of survival and outcome, not surprisingly, include degree of prematurity, duration of oxygen requirement, length of stay in the hospital, and severity of radiographic abnormalities.[44,45]

The pathogenesis of bronchopulmonary dysplasia is generally considered to be multifactorial.[24,46] The disease was first described in premature infants with severe respiratory distress syndrome who had been treated with high levels of oxygen (80%–100%) and intermittent positive-pressure respirators for longer than 6 days.[18,47,48] Subsequent experimental studies have clearly demonstrated the toxic effects of prolonged exposure to high oxygen levels on the lungs of animals.[49–53] Considered of equal importance by many is the role of barotrauma from artificial ventilation to the developing immature lung, contributing not only to the interstitial emphysema, pneumothorax, and pneumomediastinum seen in infants with bronchopulmo-

Table 8–1. Pathologic features of bronchopulmonary dysplasia

	Acute	Reparative	LSHBPD[a]
I. Trachea			
Mucosa	Dysplasia	Metaplasia	Normal or metaplasia
	Necrosis	Metaplasia	Metaplasia
Submucosa	Inflammation acute or chronic	Inflammation chronic	Inflammation chronic
	Necrosis and/or edema	Fibroplasia	Fibrosis (pseudopolyp)
Glands	Hypertrophy	Hyperplasia	Hyperplasia or normal
II. Bronchi			
Mucosa	Dysplasia	Metaplasia	Normal or metaplasia
Submucosa	Inflammation acute or chronic	Inflammation chronic	Normal
	Edema	Muscular hyperplasia	Normal
III. Bronchioles			
Mucosa	Luminal occlusion by hyaline membrane	Organization	Normal
	Dysplasia	Metaplasia	Normal
	Necrosis	Metaplasia	Normal
	Necrosis	Organization	Normal
Submucosa	Necrotizing "obstructive" bronchiolitis	Intrinsic fibroplasia	Partial or complete obliteration
	Edema	Muscular hyperplasia	Muscular hyperplasia
	Inflammation acute and chronic	Extrinsic fibroplasia	Fibrosis
IV. Alveolar Duct			
Mucosa	Hyaline membranes	Organization	Normal
	Dysplasia	Metaplasia	Normal
	Necrosis	Intrinsic fibroplasia	Fibrosis or obliteration
Submucosa	Necrosis and edema	Extrinsic fibroplasia	Fibrosis or obliteration
V. Alveolus			
Lining cells	Hyaline membranes	Organization	Normal
	Necrosis	Fibroplasia	Fibrosis or obliteration
Interstitium	Edema	Edema	Normal
	Necrosis	Fibroplasia	Fibrosis or obliteration
VI. Interlobular Septa			
	Edema	Edema	Normal
	Interstitial emphysema—acute	Organization	Normal
	Interstitial emphysema—persistent	Giant cell reaction	Fibrosis
VII. Pulmonary Arteries			
	Adventitial edema	Medial hyperplasia and adventitial edema	Medial hyperplasia and/or adventitial fibrosis

[a] LSHBPD, long-standing healed bronchopulmonary dysplasia.[53]

nary dysplasia but also directly injuring the acinus.[54,55] Other factors possibly involved in the development of bronchopulmonary dysplasia include pulmonary edema.[56,57] Vitamin E deficiency,[58] Vitamin A deficiency,[35] and ceruloplasmin deficiency.[46]

The pathology of the lungs of infants with bronchopulmonary dysplasia[59–65] varies considerably depending on (1) the gestational age of the infant, specifically, the degree of immaturity of the lung; (2) the type, duration, and peak pressures of artificial ventilation; (3) the duration and concentration of oxygen therapy; (4) the degree of pulmonary edema; and (5) the presence of intercurrent processes such as pneumonia, interstitial emphysema, or pneumothorax. Detailed description of all these variations is beyond the scope of this chapter, but the major changes in gross morphology and changes within the airways and acini are described and summarized (Table 8–1).

In the acute stages of the disease, following typical changes of hyaline membrane disease in the first 3 to 4 days of life, the lungs are bulky, firm, and heavy, and often two to four times expected weight (Fig. 8–5). The pink-to-tan pleura may be smooth or mildly irregular with areas of depressed or atelectatic parenchyma producing an uneven surface. Cut section displays a solid-appearing parenchyma that exudes fluid when compressed. By 1–2 weeks, the lungs begin to show a typical cobblestone surface with the development of an intricate sublobulation beneath the pleural representing alternating areas of atelectasis, interstitial fibroplasia, or hyperexpansion of acini (Fig. 8–6). As the disease progresses to the "healed" stage at 1–3 months, this sublobulation becomes more accentuated with shallow and deep depressions dividing the lung into irregular lobules (Fig. 8–7). Some of these depressions may be large enough to be confused with the fissures between lobes of the lung (Fig. 8–8). Hyperexpanded acini protrude from the surface of the lung with individual alveoli visible to the naked eye, implying an overexpansion of at least 5- to 10 fold.

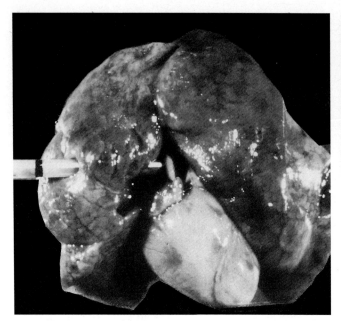

Fig. 8–5. Bronchopulmonary dysplasia at 8 days of age. Lungs are bulky and expanded with mildly irregular surface. Note chest tube perforating right lung. (AFIP Neg. 86–7729.)

Microscopically, the airways (trachea, bronchi, bronchioles) and gas-exchanging portions of the lung (alveolar ducts, saccules, and alveoli) undergo a series of acute changes followed by reparative processes that eventually lead to a "static" stage termed "long-standing 'healed' bronchopulmonary dysplasia." These changes will be considered in turn at each level of the lung.

The acute changes within the trachea range from

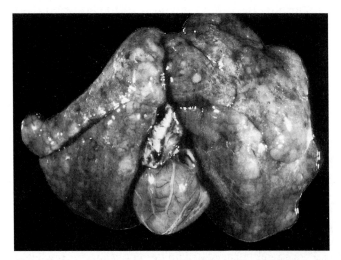

Fig. 8–6. Bronchopulmonary dysplasia at 21 days. Pleura of lung is markedly irregular with hyperexpanded acini bulging from surface. Discontinuous "pseudofissures" present in left-upper lobe. (AFIP Neg. 86–7731.)

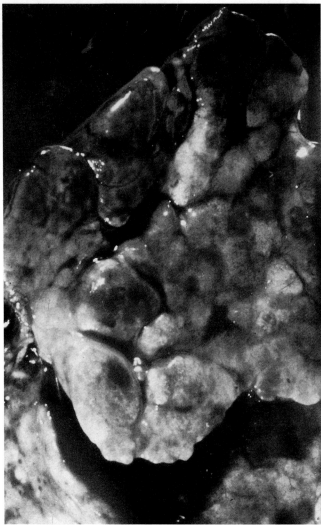

Fig. 8–7. Long-standing "healed" bronchopulmonary dysplasia at 3 months. Close-up view: Irregular depressions or fissures subdivide lung into multiple sublobules. Hyperexpanded acini protrude "above" pleura, further accentuating sublobules.

mild mucosal dysplasia to frank necrosis.[66,67] The earliest changes may consist only of loss of cilia and disruption of the pseudostratification typical of respiratory epithelium (Fig. 8–9). Epithelial cells may appear "dysplastic" with enlarged nuclei. Focal mucosal necrosis, which may extend through the submucosa to the level of the tracheal cartilage rings, may occur and is possibly related to excessive pressure from an endotracheal tube. Acute and chronic inflammation in the submucosal connective tissue is usually present in varying degrees, and submucosal glands may be hypertrophied with dilated acini and ducts. In the reparative stages, the mucosa may undergo significant metaplastic changes eventually resembling noncornified stratified squamous

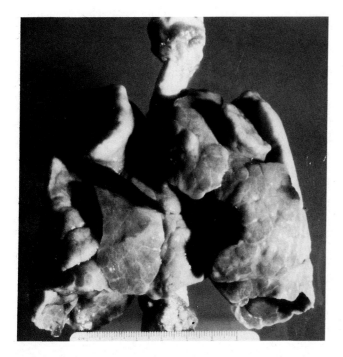

Fig. 8–8. Long-standing "healed" bronchopulmonary dysplasia at 10 months. With growth of new parenchyma, pleural surface becomes smoother (compare with Fig. 8–7), but large fissures remain, producing bizzare lobular configuration.

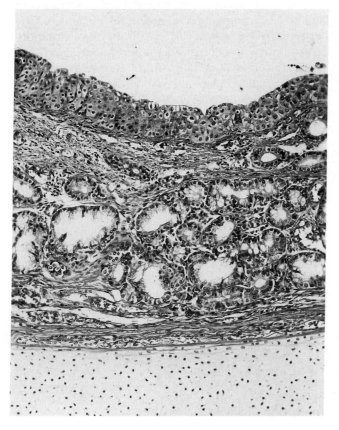

epithelium, which is usually focal and noted predominantly in the lower trachea but may line the entire trachea extending into the ducts of the submucosal glands (Fig. 8–10). Chronic inflammation persists in the submucosa, and glands may display hyperplasia producing a Reid index of 40%–60% that may persist into the healed stage. Focal fibrous and muscular hyperplasia in the lower trachea may produce epithelial-covered polyps that may narrow or rarely occlude the lumen (Fig. 8–11).

Bronchial changes in the acute, reparative, and healed stages are similar to those noted in the trachea. First- or second-division bronchi display mucosal dysplasia and, occasionally, necrosis. The submucosa is often edematous and mildly infiltrated by acute inflammatory cells. Submucosal glands may be hypertrophied in early stages, but hyperplasia infrequently occurs and is usually mild or nonexistent in the healed phase. Muscular hyperplasia may develop in the reparative stage and persist in distal bronchi in the healed phase.

The most striking changes of acute bronchopulmonary dysplasia occur at the level of the bronchioles and alveolar ducts, where several distinct lesions are observed. Total occlusion of a terminal or respiratory bronchiole by hyaline membranes and/or necrotic debris (Figs. 8–12 and 8–13) may effectively remove access to, and thus protect, the acinus distal to the occlusion from exposure to oxygen tensions and ventilatory pressures. The occluded bronchiole may display an intact epithelial lining, submucosa, and muscular wall, or the bronchiole may be recognizable only by remnants of the muscular wall with partial or total destruction of the epithelium. As the lesions resolve and most of the occluded bronchioles are cleared of debris or "recanalized." the epithelium may regenerate leaving a normal-appearing, cuboidal-to-columnar epithelium and unremarkable wall. Some of the severely involved bronchioles may remain permanently obliterated.

Bronchioles in the acute stage that remain free of hyaline membranes and necrotic debris, or are only partially occluded, may display striking epithelial cell dysplasia with large irregular cells containing hyperchromatic nuclei with densely clumped chromatin and prominent nucleoli (see Fig. 8–13). Focal necrosis may also be present. The submucosa is usually edematous and may be infiltrated by neutrophils and lymphocytes.

◁——————————————————

Fig. 8–9. Bronchopulmonary dysplasia at 16 days. Normal pseudostratified ciliated columnar epithelium of trachea is replaced by metaplastic squamous epithelium. Submucosal glands are hyperplastic and focally dilated, occupying nearly 75% of area between mucosa and cartilage (bottom). (AFIP Neg. 75–7020.) H and E, ×120.

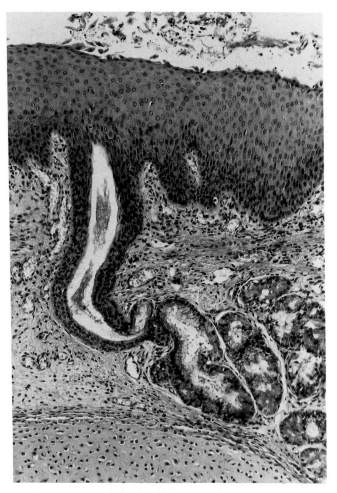

Fig. 8–10. Long-standing "healed" bronchopulmonary dysplasia at 8 months. Squamous epithelium covers surface and extends into duct of this segment of lower trachea. Note mild chronic inflammation. H and E, ×120.

As the lesion progresses, fibroblasts may proliferate within the submucosal connective tissue (intrinsic fibroplasia) or outside the muscular wall (extrinsic fibroplasia) (Fig. 8–14). With resolution of these injured bronchioles the epithelium also returns to normal, but muscular hyperplasia of the wall may persist.

The alveolar ducts not "protected" by an occluded bronchiole in the acute phase display striking epithelial cell dysplasia (for which the disease is named) and focal necrosis. Edema in the subepithelial region gives way to prominent fibroplasia, which may extend into adjacent alveolar septa. This fibroproliferative process and associated edema may expand the duct wall, leading to varying degrees of occlusion of the lumen and partially protecting the distal acinus in a manner similar to that provided by occluded bronchioles. With resolution, the ductular wall becomes thickened by fibrous connective tissue.

Alveoli in acini with occluded bronchioles remain unremarkable (Figs. 8–15 through 8–17). In acini exposed to the high oxygen tensions and ventilatory pressures, however, alveoli have increased numbers of macrophages with hyperplastic and bizarre nuclei. Alveolar lining cells may undergo necrosis or, more often, become hyperplastic, frequently forming a prominent cuboidal cell lining to the alveoli all the way to the periphery of the acinus (Fig. 8–18). In cases with more severe injury, interstitial edema is present along with plump fibroblasts that may proliferate and, in extreme cases, virtually replace an acinus. Resolution of this process may, depending on the degree of injury, lead to interstitial fibrosis (Fig. 8–19) or possibly total loss of the acinus. The degree of acinar injury seems to correlate with the long term survival of premature infants with bronchopulmonary dysplasia. Soboyna and colleagues[63] and Margrof and colleagues[68] noted a marked decrease in mean total alveolar number (less than 15% of expected) and internal surface area of the lung in long term survivors.

Interstitial fibrosis, the hallmark of longstanding "healed" bronchopulmonary dysplasia (Fig. 8–20A), is usually uniform within an acinus but may be extremely variable from one lobe of a lung to another or even from one acinus to another (Fig. 8–20B). The fibrous connective tissue within the alveolar wall separates the usually

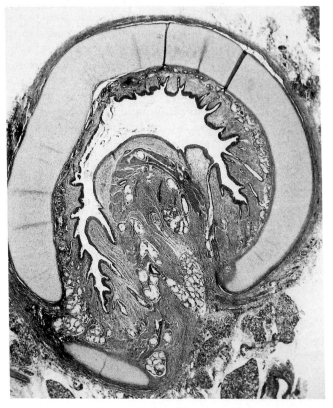

Fig. 8–11. Long-standing "healed" bronchopulmonary dysplasia at 6 months. Lumen of trachea is significantly narrowed by squamous epithelial-covered polyp with fibromuscular core. (AFIP Neg. 86–5362.) H and E, ×15.

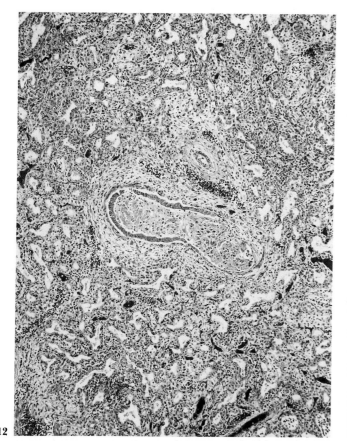

8-12

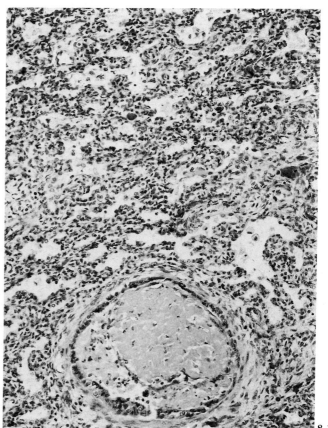

8-13

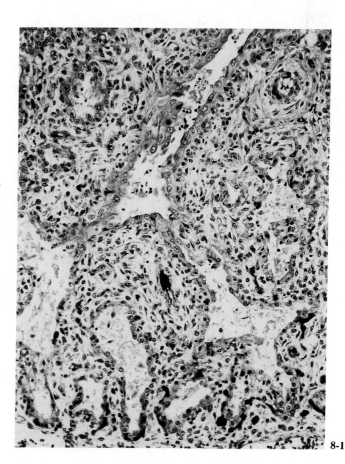

8-14

Fig. 8–12. Bronchopulmonary dysplasia at 8 days. Mixture of hyaline material and amorphous necrotic debris occludes bronchiole in 700-g infant, "protecting" surrounding acinus from venilatory pressure and high oxygen tension. (AFIP Neg. 86–6534.) H and E, ×60.

Fig. 8–13. Bronchopulmonary dysplasia at 8 days. In slightly more mature lung (820-g infant) than Fig. 8–12, protective effect of occluded bronchiole is readily seen in absence of acinar dysplasia or fibroplasia (see Fig. 8–14). (AFIP Neg. 86–7105.) H and E, ×160.

Fig. 8–14. Bronchopulmonary dysplasia at 8 days. In acinus in another area of same lung as in Fig. 8–13, open bronchiole/ alveolar duct displays marked dysplasia of cuboidal epithelium and prominent interstitial proliferation of fibroblasts. Note hyperplastic alveolar lining cells. (AFIP Neg. 86–6544.) H and E, ×160.

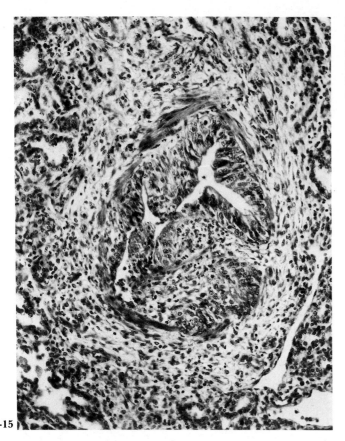

Fig. 8–15. Bronchopulmonary dysplasia at 23 days. Proliferating fibroblasts and regenerating columnar and metaplastic squamous epithelium partially occlude bronchiole. Fibroblasts are also prominent outside muscular wall. Surrounding alveoli, however, show only minimal change. (AFIP Neg. 86–7109.) H and E, ×160.

Fig. 8–16. Bronchopulmonary dysplasia at 8 days. Acinus (upper) in this immature lung from 700-g infant shows only mild atelectasis while adjacent acinus (lower) displays marked interstitial edema and early fibroplasia (see Fig. 8–17 for later stage). (AFIP Neg. 86–6541.) H and E, ×60.

Fig. 8–17. Bronchopulmonary dysplasia at 23 days. Interstitial emphysema extends along interlobular septa separating acini. Note prominent alveolar septal fibroplasia in acini below and to right, an accentuation of process seen in Fig. 8–16. (AFIP Neg. 86–7114.) H and E, ×25.

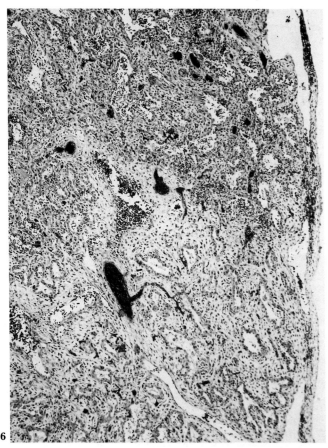

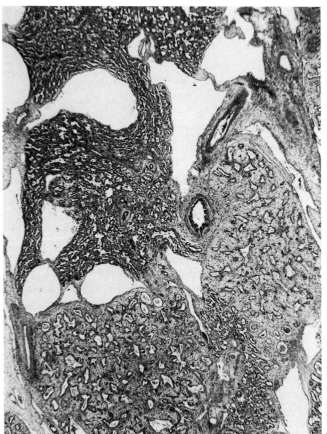

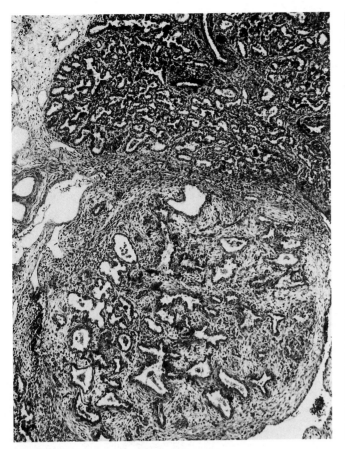

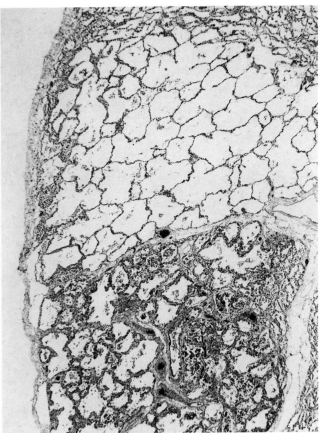

Fig. 8–18. Bronchopulmonary dysplasia at 23 days. Varying degrees of acinar damage are readily apparent; virtually normal acinus at top lies next to acinus displaying prominent alveolar septal fibrosis and alveolar cell dysplasia (below). (AFIP Neg. 86–7123.) H and E, ×60.

Fig. 8–19. Long-standing "healed" bronchopulmonary dysplasia at 6 months. Acinus below displays diffuse alveolar septal fibrosis while acinus at top, although hyperexpanded, shows little or no fibrosis (compare with Figs. 8–17 and 8–18). (AFIP Neg. 86–6089.) H and E, ×25.

intermeshed capillary beds supplying the alveoli on either side of the wall. In cases with severe fibrosis, a "third" capillary bed may be present within the connective tissue separating the two alveolar capillary beds.

Changes in the vessels within the lung, other than those in the alveolar capillary bed, are mild. Pulmonary arteries at the level of the bronchi display adventitial edema early in the course of the disease, and medial hypertrophy is present during the reparative and healed stages although changes beyond Heath and Edward grade I–II pulmonary hypertensive vascular disease are unusual.[69] Bronchial arteries and lymphatics show no significant changes. Changes within the interlobular septa and pleura are seen only in cases in which acute or persistent interstitial pulmonary emphysema develops.

Hyperexpansion of acini may be present following the early stages of the disease, accounting for the "cystic" changes noted radiographically and the accentuated sublobulation seen grossly. The enlarged alveoli are usually in acini with little or, more frequently, no interstitial fibrosis (see Figs. 8–19 and 8–20B). Alveoli

may be expanded to 5- to 10 fold or more normal size, and rupture of the highly elastic walls may be noted. As with the interstitial fibrosis, the emphysema may be patchy with an acinus containing normal-sized alveoli lying adjacent to one with markedly distended alveoli. The sequential changes of bronchopulmonary dysplasia are presented schematically in Fig. 8–21.

The changes of bronchopulmonary dysplasia just described are in many ways similar to those of diffuse alveolar damage seen in older children and adults following various types of injury. The immaturity of the lungs in these infants, however, along with the necrotizing "obstructive" bronchiolitis that is apparently a unique feature of bronchopulmonary dysplasia, probably accounts for the differences between these two types of lung injury.

Interstitial Pulmonary Emphysema

Interstitial pulmonary emphysema is the presence of air within the connective tissue, and possibly the lymphat-

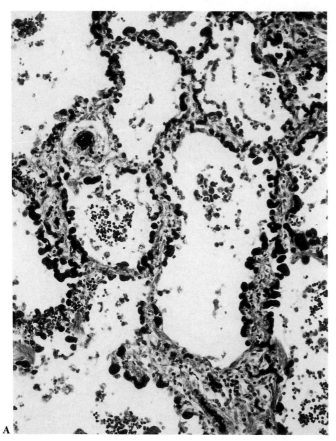
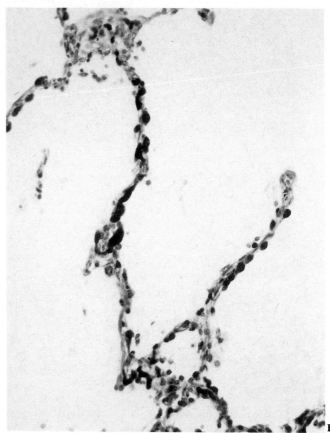

Fig. 8–20 A,B. Long-standing "healed" bronchopulmonary dysplasia at 6 months. **A.** Each alveolar wall is formed of distinct capillary beds separated by fibrous connective tissue. This alveolar septal fibrosis is the hallmark of "healed" bronchopulmonary dysplasia and is clearly delineated by the bulg-ing capillary plexuses. (AFIP Neg. 86–6104.) H and E, ×250. **B.** In acinus adjacent to that shown in **A** at same magnification, hyperexpanded or emphysematous alveoli are composed of septa with little or not fibrosis between capillary beds. (AFIP Neg. 86–6101.) H and E, ×250.

ics, of the perivascular and interlobular septa of the lungs.[70] Interstitial pulmonary emphysema develops along the interlobular septa of the lungs following the overdistension and rupture of the alveolar base, the segment of an alveolus directly contiguous to the fluid-rich tissue surrounding blood vessels. This allows air to leak into the septal connective tissue.[71,72] The air may remain localized to the septa, or dissect centrally along vessels to the mediastinum producing pneumomediastinum, or to the pericardium producing pneumopericardium, or peripherally to and through the pleura producing a pneumothorax.[73] The air of interstitial pulmonary emphysema may be rapidly reabsorbed with few sequelae, or it may persist, through continuous or repeated alveolar base rupture, for days or weeks to elicit a fibroblastic and foreign-body giant cell reaction called persistent interstitial pulmonary emphysema.[25,74] There is usually surprisingly little hemorrhage associated with this process.

Interstitial pulmonary emphysema is seen in as many as 20% of all preterm infants ventilated for the respiratory distress syndrome. Infants weighing less than 1,500 g show an incidence of nearly 33%, and infants less than 1,000 g, an incidence as high as 42%.[75,76] Mortality in these infants is higher (greater than 50%), again primarily (95%) in those infants with birth weights less than 1,500 g (64%) or who develop interstitial pulmonary emphysema in the first day of life (>75%). Preterm survivors of interstitial pulmonary emphysema also display significant morbidity with more than 50% developing bronchopulmonary dysplasia.[77]

Pneumothorax, pneumomediastinum, and pneumopericardium frequently accompany interstitial pulmonary emphysema (40%–77%) and contribute significantly to the mortality of preterm infants.[73,77] Pneumothorax and interstitial pulmonary emphysema are also seen in full-term infants, primarily in associa-

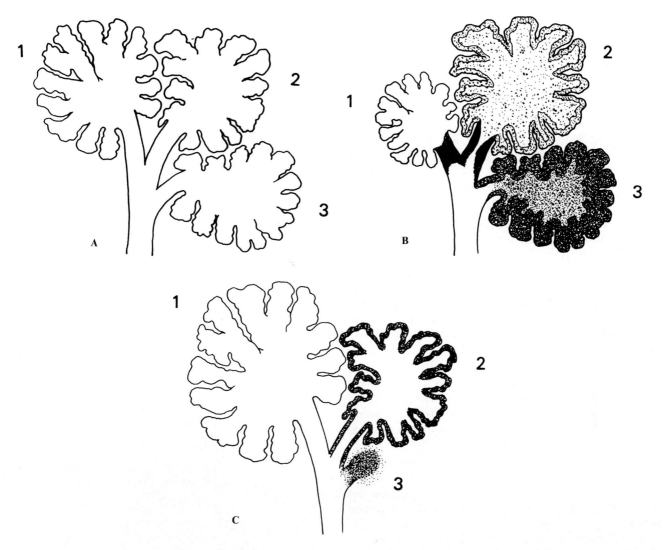

Fig. 8–21 A–C. Bronchopulmonary dysplasia. **A.** Three normal acini (1, 2, 3) arise from terminal bronchiole in this schematic drawing. **B.** In acute stages of bronchopulmonary dysplasia, bronchiole leading to acinus 1 is occluded by material (Hyaline membranes, necrotic debris, etc.) protecting acinus from ventilatory pressure and high oxygen tension Bronchiole to acinus 2 is only partially occluded, allowing some injury to alveolar saccules and alveoli. Acinus 3 receives full ventilatory pressure and oxygen tension through widely patent bronchiole, allowing extensive damage (dysplasia, inflammation, fibroplasia) to alveolar saccules and alveoli. **C.** With resolution and "healing," bronchiole in 1 is reopened allowing expansion (or overexpansion) of uninjured acinus. Acinus 2 displays interstitial fibrosis atypical of "healed" bronchopulmonary dysplasia; the most severely injured acinus 3 may partially or completely disappear, leading to contraction and fissuring of pleura. (Modified from Stocker JT. The pathology of long-standing "healed" bronchopulmonary dysplasia. Hum Pathol 1986;17:943–961,[65] with permission from W.B. Saunders Co.)

tion with aspiration or pulmonary hypoplasia. Pneumothorax has been observed in 60% of infants following repair of their congenital diaphragmatic hernia.[78]

Radiographically, interstitial pulmonary emphysema presents as lucent linear streaks with prominent interstitial markings and cystic spaces that tend to radiate from the hilum. Large subpleural lucent cystic spaces may be seen, being particularly noticeable if a pneumothorax is present. If interstitial pulmonary emphysema persists, radiographs may display an expanded multicystic pattern of one or more lobes. If it is localized to one lung, mediastinal shift and depression of the diaphragm may occur. Compression atelectasis of lung adjacent to the cysts will further accentuate the air-filled spaces.[79]

The treatment of infants with bilateral interstitial

Table 8–2. Comparison of forms of interstitial pulmonary emphysema[a]

Features	AIPE[b]	PIPE[c]	
		Localized	Diffuse
Patient's age (days)	<7	>7	>7
Mediastinal shift	+	++	−
Pneumothorax	++	+	++
Average size of interstitial air spaces (cm)	0.2	1.3	0.7
Shape of interstitial air spaces	Spherical cysts	Irregular cysts	Channels and cysts
Fibrosis of cyst wall	−	++	+
Giant cell reaction along wall	−	++	+
Parenchymal disease	+	+	++

[a] Reproduced with permission from Stocker JT, Drake RM, Madewell JE. Cystic and congenital lung disease in the newborn. In: Rosenberg HS, Bolande RP, eds. Perspectives in Pediatric Pathology, Volume 4. Copyright © 1978 by Year Book Medical Publishers, Inc., Chicago.
[b] AIPE, acute interstitial pulmonary emphysema.
[c] PIPE, persistent interstitial pulmonary emphysema.

pulmonary emphysema is difficult and varied. Reduction in ventilatory pressures is effective and alleviates the influx of air into interstitial tissues but may also prove inadequate to ventilate the infant. High-frequency ventilation has recently been shown to be helpful in these infants.[80,81] Many modes of therapy have been employed in the treatment of infants with persistent unilateral interstitial pulmonary emphysema, including selective bronchial intubation,[82–86] lateral decubitus positioning,[87,88] extracorporeal membrane oxygenation,[89] alveolar lavage during flexible bronchoscopy,[90] artifical pneumothorax and pneumonotomy,[91,92] and lobectomy.[83–95] Persistent interstitial pulmonary emphysema in recent years has become an indication for pulmonary resection in the newborn period.[96]

Interstitial pulmonary emphysema pathologically occurs in two forms (Table 8–2), an acute usually diffuse form noted in the first few days of life and a persistent form seen in either a localized or diffuse pattern in infants more than 1 week old.[25,97]

Acute interstitial pulmonary emphysema (AIPE) appears grossly as round-to-oval gas-filled spaces around bronchovascular bundles or along interlobular septa (Fig. 8–22). These spaces are usually visible beneath the pleura but are almost always limited to those areas in which the interlobular septa extend to the pleura. This is a major reason for establishing that the gas, for the most part, is within the connective tissue of the interlobular spaces rather than within lymphatics, which could lead to a lateral distribution of air within subpleural lymphatics.[25,98] The parenchyma adjacent to the interstitial pulmonary emphysema is often atelectatic and firmer than areas of uninvolved lung.

Microscopically, interstitial pulmonary emphysema is characterized by spherical "cysts" within the interlobular septa (Fig. 8–23). The walls of the cysts are com-

posed of thin fragments of connective tissue or, more frequently, the walls of collapsed alveoli of lobules adjacent to the interlobular septa. The cysts usually have no discernible lining, although rarely endothelial cells of interlobular septal lymphatics may be incorpo-

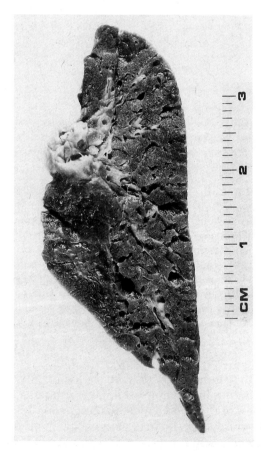

Fig. 8–22. Acute interstitial pulmonary emphysema. Air-filled cysts are present within interlobular septa extending radially from hilum (upper left) to subpleura. (AFIP Neg. 75–7068.)

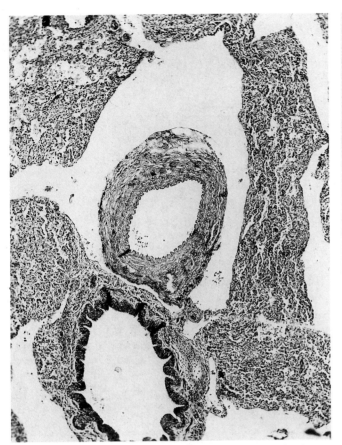

Fig. 8–23. Acute interstitial pulmonary emphysema. Bronchus (below) and pulmonary artery (above) are surrounded by clear spaces (grossly air-containing) that compress intervening pulmonary parenchyma. (AFIP Neg. 76–1114.) H and E, ×56.

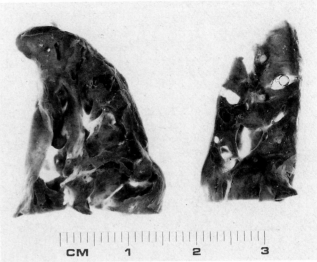

Fig. 8–24. Persistent interstitial pulmonary emphysema. Sections of lung are distorted by interconnecting irregular air-filled cysts varying from 0.2 to more than 1 cm in diameter. (AFIP Neg. 76–5618.)

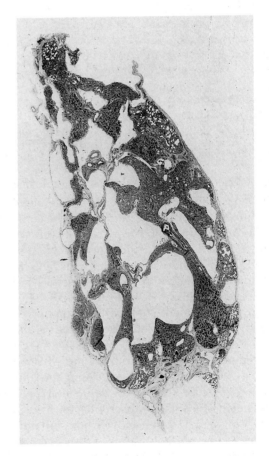

Fig. 8–25. Persistent interstitial pulmonary emphysema. Irregular air-filled spaces are limited to interlobular septa extending to but rarely laterally beneath pleura. (AFIP Neg. 76–1955.) H and E, ×4.

rated into some of the cysts. Other lymphatics, however, along with pulmonary veins, may be compressed by the interstitial cysts. Subpleural lymphatics, as previously mentioned, are rarely involved by this process. Adjacent parenchyma may display the changes of the hyaline membrane disease and bronchopulmonary dysplasia so frequently associated with interstitial pulmonary emphysema.

Persistent interstitial pulmonary emphysema (PIPE) in its localized form presents grossly with a picture of multiple intercommunicating cysts 0.2–2.0 cm in diameter, resembling, in some cases, congenital cystic adenomatoid malformation.[25,99,100] The cysts, again limited to interlobular septa, are often irregular and appear to be lined by a smooth membrane overlying atelectatic parenchyma (Fig. 8–24). Microscopically, the cysts display a thin to occasionally prominent fibrous connective tissue wall studded with multinucleated foreign-body giant cells (Figs. 8–25 and 8–26). These giant cells, the hallmark of persistent interstitial pulmonary

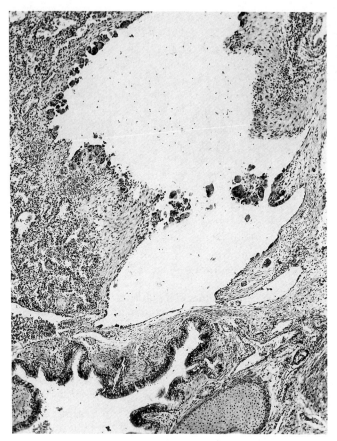

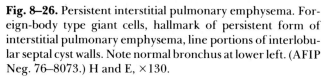

Fig. 8–26. Persistent interstitial pulmonary emphysema. Foreign-body type giant cells, hallmark of persistent form of interstitial pulmonary emphysema, line portions of interlobular septal cyst walls. Note normal bronchus at lower left. (AFIP Neg. 76–8073.) H and E, ×130.

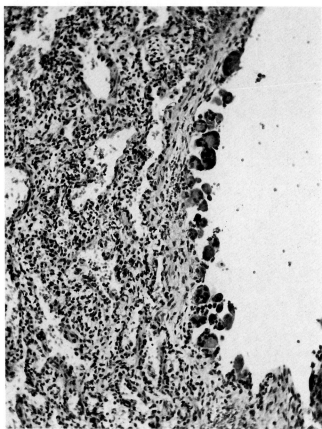

Fig. 8–27. Persistent interstitial pulmonary emphysema. Foreign-body giant cells are separated from underlying acinar parenchyma by fibrous connective tissue wall of variable thickness. (AFIP Neg. 76–8074.) H and E, ×250.

emphysema, may occur singly or in clusters along the surface of the cyst (Fig. 8–27) or within the connective tissue of the cyst wall, the latter probably reflecting an area of collapsed and "scarred" former cyst. The cells are 20–150 μm or more in diameter with 2–35 or more round-to-oval eccentrically placed nuclei, each with a prominent nucleolus (Figs. 8–28 and 8–29). The abundant cytoplasm is smooth to finely granular or vesicular and only rarely contains any identifiable or stainable material, as with hemosiderin.

The tissue in the walls of the cysts ranges from plump fibroblasts with prominent capillaries in young infants to dense collagenized connective tissue in older infants. Foci of hemosiderin-laden macrophages, probably reflecting old hemorrhage, and chronic inflammatory cells may also be present. Rarely, a direct communication between the interstitial cysts and a bronchiole or alveolar duct may be demonstrated with cuboidal epithelial lining cells extending from the bronchiole into the cyst. Adjacent lung parenchyma may be entirely

normal or display focal atelectasis, fibrosis, or pneumonia. Persistent interstitial pulmonary emphysema in its diffuse form with three or more lobes involved is closely associated with bronchopulmonary dysplasia. The lung is firm as in bronchopulmonary dysplasia but in addition small (0.1–0.4 cm in diameter), irregular gas-filled spaces are present as long thin channels around bronchovascular bundles and along interlobular septa. The channel walls are composed of loose fibrous connective tissue along which giant cells are seen. They occur, however, far less frequently than in the localized form of PIPE. The underlying pulmonary parenchyma usually displays the characteristic features of bronchopulmonary dysplasia.

The cyst walls of PIPE, particularly the localized form, are virtually identical to those seen in pneumotosis intestinalis and pneumotosis vaginalis.[25] The giant cells apparently reflect a reaction of the connective tissue to air, a "foreign" substance, which when present in the tissue for more than 7 days elicits this response.[74]

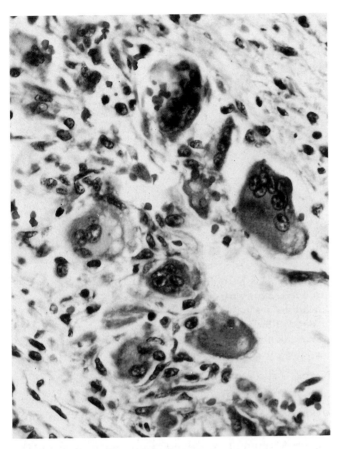

Fig. 8–28. Persistent interstitial pulmonary emphysema. Foreign-body giant cells contain 3–25 eccentrially placed nuclei and finely granular cytoplasm rarely displaying demonstrable foreign material. (AFIP Neg. 76–1959.) H and E, ×440.

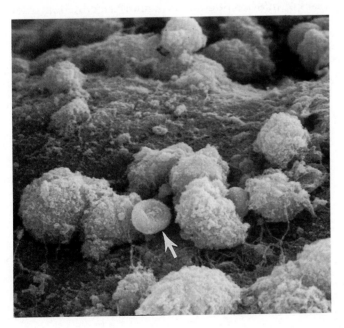

While lymphatics may be incorporated into the walls of the interstitial cysts through fibrosis or contribute to the "lining" of a small portion of the cysts, it is unlikely that the cysts represent only intralymphatic air. As previously mentioned, interstitial air is rarely seen in the subpleural region except for the area in direct continuity with the interlobular septum. In cases of bronchopulmonary dysplasia with AIPE or PIPE, the large subpleural lymphatic bed is uninvolved and in most cases appears virtually normal. Also, the air containing cysts of interstitial pulmonary emphysema are many times the size of normal lymphatics and the dilated lymphatics of congenital lymphangiectasis which, incidentally, does involve subpleural as well as interlobular lymphatics. Finally, an endothelial lining, as persent in lymphatics, cannot be identified with any consistency in the interstitial cysts.[25]

Tracheomalacia

While congenital tracheomalacia is a relatively rare disorder (see Chapter 7), "acquired" tracheomalacia has been seen with increasing frequency in premature infants requiring prolonged nasotracheal intubation as part of the treatment for the respiratory distress syndrome.[101] Damage to the lower trachea and mainstem bronchi has also been noted with aggressive airway suctioning through naso- or orotracheal tubes.[102,103] Tracheal perforation may, in fact, occur as a complication of vigorous nasotracheal intubation.[104]

Radiographically, tracheomalacia may be noted as a extremely mobile trachea that is more dilated and oval (or even collapsed) than normal.[103] Grossly the trachea is pliable and easily compressed and flattened. The internal diameter of the lumen may be enlarged with an increased width of the posterior fibromuscular membrane completing the cartilage ring.

Microscopically, squamous metaplasia of the epithelium is usually prominent, either focally or around the entire internal diameter of the trachea. Focal ulceration and necrosis may also be present.[101] The underlying fibromuscular connective tissue may display an acute or chronic inflammatory infiltrate, and mucous glands may be increased, occupying more than 50% of the area between the cartilage rings and epithelium. The cartilage rings (and plates in the bronchi) may be narrowed

◁—————————————————

Fig. 8–29. Persistent interstitial pulmonary emphysema. Cyst, scanning electromicroscopy. Foreign-body type giant cells are randomly scattered along surface. Thin strands of fibrous connective tissue crosscross wall. Note concave red blood cell (*arrow*). (AFIP Neg. 86–8050.) SEM, ×3,000.

or thinned, with rare foci of inflammation and necrosis, but in most cases are histologically unremarkable.

Pulmonary Changes in Extracorporeal Membrane Oxygenation

The development of extracorporeal membrane oxygenation and its use in the treatment of meconium aspiration, congenital heart malformations, and diaphragmatic hernia (among other causes of pulmonary hypoplasia) has produced a unique set of pathologic changes in the lung.[105] Chou and colleagues[106] described the autopsy finding in 17 patients receiving extracorporeal membrane oxygenation therapy and noted the presence of interstitial and intraalveolar hemorrhage with hyaline membrane formation during the first few days of therapy. Hyperplasia of type II alveolar cells and bronchial epithelial cells was noted after 2 days of extracorporeal membrane oxygenation therapy in some patients and by 7 days in all patients. Bronchial epithelium displayed squamous metaplasia in most cases with 1 case displaying mucinous metaplasia as well. Clusters of calcified material were noted in the alveoli of 5 of 18 cases. Interstitial fibrosis was a consistent finding after 7 days of extracorporeal membrane oxygenation therapy.

Pulmonary Hemorrhage

Hemorrhage into the alveoli and/or interstitium of the lung is a rather common histologic finding at autopsy or in tissue removed at surgery for various reasons. In the latter situation, one must keep in mind the possibility that intraoperative manipulation may have produced the hemorrhage. However, this section is concerned with the clinicopathologic entities of *massive pulmonary hemorrhage of the newborn* and the so-called *alveolar hemorrhage syndromes* (Fig. 8–30).[107,108] It is likely in some cases that these two disease categories may converge as pathogenetically identical processes. The alveolar hemorrhage syndromes include Goodpasture's syndrome, the collagen vascular diseases complicated by hemorrhage and idiopathic pulmonary hemosiderosis. The designation *pulmonary renal syndromes* has been applied as a collective appellation to this same basic group of diseases with the exception of idiopathic pulmonary hemosiderosis.[109,110] In the pediatric age population, the concerns are mainly focused on neonatal pulmonary hemorrhage and idiopathic pulmonary hemosiderosis.

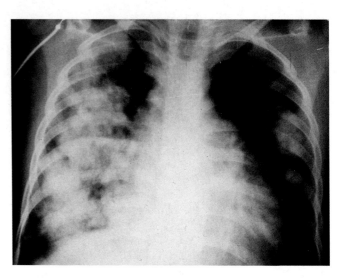

Fig. 8–30. Massive pulmonary hemorrhage in 7-year-old girl produced large fluffy radiodensities in left lung and peripheral infiltrates in right lung. Patient presented with cough and malaise of 3 days duration; kidney biopsy showed crescentic glomerulonephritis, and lung biopsy revealed small vessel vasculitis, alveolar damage, and hemorrhage.

If hyaline membrane disease or bronchopulmonary dysplasia is the most common cause of neonatal respiratory distress, massive pulmonary hemorrhage is one of the least frequent, as judged by our experience and the literature.[111] There is little to distinguish massive pulmonary hemorrhage from other etiologies of severe respiratory insufficiency in the early clinical stages until there is "bleeding" from the tracheobronchial tree. The changes on the chest radiograph are generally nonspecific. A study of the radiographic abnormalities in 46 cases of massive pulmonary hemorrhage by Bomsel et al.[112] identified two categories. One group (19 cases) only had massive pulmonary hemorrhage at autopsy, and their chest radiographs disclosed bilateral granular densities, indistinct pneumonic-like opacities, segmental opacification, or total "white-out" in a minority of cases. The second group (27 cases) of infants had a number of different pathologic findings in the lungs at autopsy in addition to massive pulmonary hemorrhage. Herein lies the problem of massive pulmonary hemorrhage and whether there is such a specific entity. An unmistakable impression from recent studies is that massive pulmonary hemorrhage is a diagnosis of exclusion, because there are other conditions such as disseminated intravascular coagulation, pneumonia, and congestive heart failure that produce a clinicopathologic picture of massive pulmonary hemorrhage.

The estimated frequency of massive pulmonary hemorrhage in neonates is 1 case per 1,000 live births, a figure derived from the British Perinatal Mortality survey.[113,114] As viewed from the perspective of an autopsy finding in neonates, the frequency of pulmonary hemorrhage is more difficult to access since the quantitative aspects are not explicitly addressed in each published study. For instance, Landing[115] examined the lung lesions in 125 infants who died within the first 7 days of life and found hemorrhage ("the presence of extravasated erythrocytes, in air spaces, in septa, or in both") in 68% of cases. Other than his conclusion that the hemorrhage was correlated with acute pneumonia, it was difficult to determine the degree or extent of hemorrhage. McAdams[116] studied "significant pulmonary hemorrhage" in the newborn and its relationship to other pathologic findings at autopsy, but he also only referred to the "diffuse" or "severe" nature of the hemorrhage. Both of these investigators, as well as others, were more intent upon the more basic issue of pathogenesis. A number of mechanisms and/or etiologies have been proposed including aspiration of maternal blood, viral or bacterial infections, hypothermia, coagulopathy, hemolytic disease of the newborn, early hyaline membrane disease, oxygen toxicity, birth asphyxia, and congenital hyperammonemia.[117–121] Yeung[122] examined 35 neonates who came to autopsy after culture-proven bacterial infections during life; massive pulmonary hemorrhage was found in the lungs in 19 cases. It may be fair to conclude that massive pulmonary hemorrhage is a tissue response to a variety of systemic and localized conditions. One suggestion is that massive pulmonary hemorrhage is a nonspecific terminal event, a viewpoint that is difficult to refute.

The infants who develop massive pulmonary hemorrhage may be premature or low weight for dates; others are full term or weigh in excess of 2,500 g at birth.[123–125] This variability in the clinical profile of neonates with massive pulmonary hemorrhage is best explained by the differences in etiology and pathogenesis. Since most studies are drawn from autopsy experiences, the conclusion is that massive pulmonary hemorrhage is universally fatal. However, there are individual reports of survivors, which is a testimonial to the fact that most infants succumb to this condition.[121,126]

Hemorrhage producing consolidation of at least two lobes of the lung is a definition of massive pulmonary hemorrhage that was proposed by Esterly and Oppenheimer[127] in their classic study. They emphasized the confluent nature of the hemorrhage, although focal areas of more normal-appearing parenchyma may be identified. The cut surface of the specimen releases a hemorrhagic and oftentimes frothy fluid.[128] This feature is interesting in light of the observation by Adamson and associates,[129] who examined the bloody liquid from the trachea of two neonates with massive pulmonary hemorrhage. They found that the hematocrit of

the fluid was very low and thus concluded that the "blood" was a plasma filtrate. Microscopically, the hemorrhage is typically found in the alveoli and interstitium; however, the alveolar extravasation is generally more apparent than the interstitial hemorrhage.[130] Many alveoli, in addition to the blood, contain palely staining fluid that is the predominant finding in some fields. The interlobar septa are often widened as the result of hemorrhage and edema. It is often difficult to be certain whether the changes in the alveolar septa are congestion or actual extravasation. When an area of lung is collapsed, there are further problems in the interpretation of the microscopic findings.

When the lungs are examined, it is important to evaluate them for the presence of other abnormalities that may be as important, if not more so, in explaining the cause of death. Focal bronchopneumonia, fibrin thrombi in arteriolar or capillary-sized vessels, and aspirated material should be carefully searched for in the sections.[131] Fibrin thrombi are an indication of disseminated intravascular coagulopathy; an examination of other organs such as the kidney, adrenal, and intestine will often disclose the presence of thrombi as well. Hyaline membrane formation is found in a minority of cases. It is important to recall that intraalveolar hemorrhage is one feature of bronchopulmonary dysplasia, but it is usually not "massive."

Idiopathic Pulmonary Hemosiderosis

Idiopathic pulmonary hemosiderosis shares many of the same diagnostic frustrations as massive pulmonary hemorrhage. The first and foremost of these is the fact that the diagnosis is established through a process of exclusion. Assuming that necrotizing glomerulonephritis and pulmonary collagen vascular disease with or without demonstrated vasculitis, congestive heart failure, mitral stenosis, venoocclusive disease, uremia, arteriovenous fistulas, pulmonary hypertension, thrombocytopenia, contusion, and viral pneumonitis have been satisfactorily eliminated, it is time to consider idiopathic pulmonary hemosiderosis. Cutz[132] thoroughly reviewed the topic of idiopathic pulmonary hemosiderosis and has devised a classification of diffuse pulmonary hemorrhage and hemosiderotic conditions in children.

Since idiopathic pulmonary hemosiderosis is a rare condition, other clinical possibilities are more likely in a given case. A review of the Swedish experience indicated that there were 0.24 cases of idiopathic pulmonary hemosiderosis per 1 million children.[133] For a period between 1962 and 1970, a cluster of cases occurred in village children in northern Greece; the authors suggested that a transient environmental toxin may have been responsible for these cases since there was a

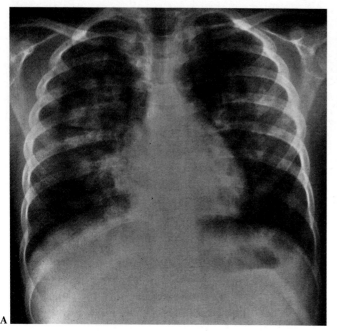
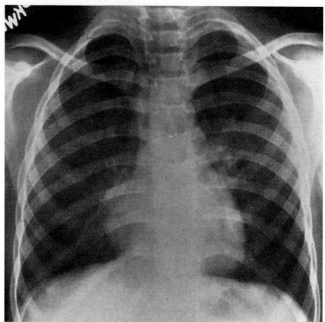

Fig. 8–31 A,B. Idiopathic pulmonary hemosiderosis in 4-year-old girl presented with shortness of breath, weakness, and iron-deficiency anemia. **A.** Admission chest radiograph shows multiple infiltrates and densities in both lung fields. **B.** Several weeks later, these abnormalities had almost completely resolved.

decline in numbers after 1974.[134] Children between the ages of 1 and 6 years are most affected, and the sex incidence is approximately equal. There are examples of idiopathic pulmonary hemosiderosis as young as 4–6 months of age; adolescents and young adults with idiopathic pulmonary hemosiderosis comprise 15%–20% of cases.[135]

Despite many vigorous attempts to elucidate its etiology and pathogenesis, idiopathic pulmonary hemosiderosis remains a veiled disease.[136,137] Some immunologic abnormalities have been demonstrated but their causative role is still uncertain.[138] There is the provocative association of idiopathic pulmonary hemosiderosis with gluten-sensitive enteropathy in some adults, with cow's milk hypersensitivity in a small subset of children (Heiner's syndrome) and with autoimmune hemolytic anemia in a young adult.[139,140] Some patients may have a peripheral eosinophilia. Autoantibodies and immune complexes have not been identified in idiopathic pulmonary hemosiderosis. When autoantibodies to alveolar basement membranes are found by immunofluorescence, the diagnosis of Goodpasture's syndrome is made. Pulmonary hemosiderosis has been reported in a child with cystic fibrosis.[141]

Cough, lethargy, dyspnea, and hemoptysis are the nonspecific, recurrent symptoms of idiopathic pulmonary hemosiderosis. Fever, in some children, may suggest an infection. Hepatosplenomegaly is reported in 20% of cases.[135] Hypochromic microcytic anemia is the characteristic laboratory abnormality in virtually all cases; eosinophilia is present in 12%–15% of patients. Reticulocytosis, elevated unconjugated bilirubin, and a low serum haptoglobin are the other abnormalities. The radiographic changes are quite variable, which may add to the delay in a diagnosis (Fig. 8–31). Serial scintographic scanning with radiolabeled erythrocytes was reported by Kurzweil et al.[142] to establish a diagnosis. Treatment to date is mainly supportive. The natural history is usually progressive respiratory insufficiency to death over a period of 2–5 years.[143]

The lung biopsy from a child with suspected or unsuspected idiopathic pulmonary hemosiderosis is useful in terms of excluding other causes of pulmonary hemorrhage but by itself is limited in providing a specific pathologic diagnosis. If at all possible, sufficient tissue should be provided to perform electron microscopy and immunofluorescence. Collections of hemosiderin-laden macrophages and fewer free erythrocytes are present in most if not all alveolar spaces and interstitium (Fig. 8–32). Fibrin deposition, hyaline membranes, and edema are usually not apparent. If these changes are noted in the presence of hyperplastic alveolar lining cells, alveolar damage secondary to a viral, immunologic, or chemical result may have occurred. Interstitial fibrous thickening is not apparent until later in the clinical course when it becomes a major finding

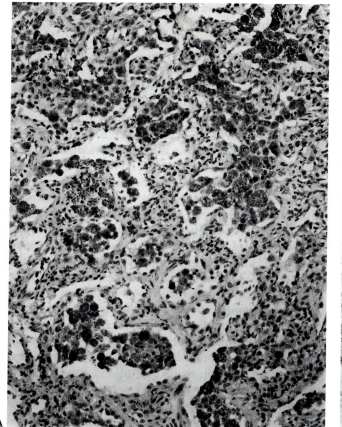

Fig. 8–32 A,B. Idiopathic pulmonary hemosiderosis (IPH). **A.** Lung biopsy shows collections of hemosiderin-laden maccophages in alveoli, moderate interstitial fibrosis, and hyperplastic alveolar lining cells. Changes are not specific for IPH, but this diagnosis is strongly suspected in presence of appropriate clinical and radiographic findings. H and E, ×160. **B.** Prussian blue stain for iron demonstrates hemosiderin-laden macrophages. Prussian blue, ×160.

on biopsy. Iron and calcium are found in the elastica of pulmonary vessels in the late stages. A number of changes have been described by electron microscopy, but these, like the features visible on light microscopy, are nonspecific and probably secondary to the hemorrhage.[144,145] However, Corrin and associates[146] observed ultrastructural abnormalities in the capillary endothelial cells and basement membrane. Swelling of the endothelial cells and platelet aggregates were seen. Immune deposits were not identified in the focally thickened capillary basement membranes. Cutz[147] noted reduplication of the capillary basement membrane in one case and focal thickening of the alveolar cell basement membrane. One interesting observation was the identification of mast cells by Dolan et al.[148] Progressive interstitial fibrosis is the cause of death in these patients, the lungs at autopsy have a brownish, indurated appearance.

There is a consensus that it is very difficult to differentiate Goodpasture's syndrome from other causes of pulmonary hemorrhage on the basis of routine histologic examination. However, we have been impressed with the presence of free alveolar hemorrhage and fewer pigment-laden macrophages in Goodpasture's syndrome as compared to other entities. Small vessel vasculitis excludes idiopathic pulmonary hemosiderosis and Goodpasture's syndrome. An accompanying infarct favors a vasculitic process such as Wegener's granulomatosis, an angio-invasive pathogen as with *Aspergillus* or *Mucor*, or pulmonary venoocclusive disease. Mitral stenosis and congestive heart failure are other causes of alveolar hemosiderosis.

Goodpasture's Syndrome

Whereas idiopathic pulmonary hemosiderosis is ordinarily regarded as a pediatric condition, Goodpasture's syndrome is usually diagnosed in young adult males. (See Chapters 20 and 22.) Levin and associates[149] reported three cases in children; one other pediatric case,

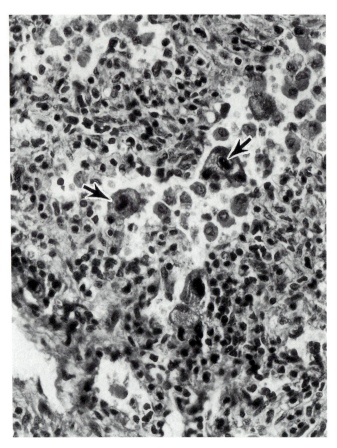

Fig. 8–34. Cytomegalovirus (CMV) pneumonia in neonate shows at least three virally infected cells with intranuclear and cytoplasmic inclusions (*arrows*). Prominent interstitial and alveolar cellular reaction is present. H and E, ×400.

sufficiently well preserved in an otherwise autolyzed background to make a diagnosis possible.[201,202] Although the CMV inclusion is easily recognized as such in most cases, an enlarged amphophilic nucleolus in a reactive alveolar lining cell or other types of inclusions may evoke uncertainty that can be resolved by immunohistochemistry. It is unnecessary in most cases to resort to the latter technique except to confirm the diagnosis. We have found immunohistochemistry especially helpful in the demonstration of the less apparent cytoplasmic inclusions.

Most experience with CMV pneumonitis is confined to lung biopsies from institutions with larger populations of immunocompromised children and adults. In addition to an interstitial inflammatory infiltrate, evidence of alveolar damage with plump lining cells, hyaline membranes, hemorrhage, and macrophages are common histologic features even in the neonate. However, these inflammatory and reactive changes are inconspicuous in the lungs of stillborn infants with CMV. Because the lungs have not inflated in the stillborn, we

have found it difficult to judge the presence of an interstitial inflammatory reaction. Focal lymphocytic collections in a peribronchiolar location or a minimal lymphocytic or plasmacellular infiltration in the interstitium is seen more frequently in the neonatal lung.

The pneumonitis in perinatal acquired CMV more closely resembles the infection of later childhood.[203] A flocculant alveolar exudate may be the clue to a coinfection by *Pneumocytis carinii*, but even in the absence of these changes, a methenamine silver stain is a justified routine. Necrosis in the lung should also alert one to the possibility of a coinfection since CMV pneumonitis alone is rarely accompanied by necrosis. Eventration of the diaphragm and hypoplasia of the lung are other less common intrathoracic complications of congenital-perinatal CMV.[204,205]

Herpes Simplex

Most neonates with herpes simplex virus (HSV) infection have clinical manifestations, unlike the majority of infants with the more common cytomegalovirus. A minority of cases of HSV are acquired in utero (congenital); exposure to genital secretions during the second stage of delivery accounts for the predominant HSV-2 infection (80% of cases).[206–208] The incidence is higher in the lower socioeconomic stratum, as has been noted in the Atlanta, Georgia (United States) area where 1 case of neonatal HSV occurs in every 3,500 births, whereas the range in other series is 1:2,500–1:30,000 live births.[209] Approximately 40–50% of infected infants are premature. After the neonate is infected with HSV, an incubation period of 2–12 days culminates in symptoms and signs in the first 2 weeks of life. The severity of the neonatal infection, as with cytomegalovirus, is determined to some degree by the type of maternal infection, whether primary or recurrent. Andiman[210] has reviewed other intrapartum factors that influence the prognosis of neonatal HSV. It is estimated that 40% of infants become infected during birth if there are active cervicovaginal lesions in the mother. However, there are any number of cases of neonatal HSV in which viral shedding was not apparent or recognized at birth. These are the unfortunate "de novo" cases.

Neonatal HSV is either generalized (40%–65% of cases) or localized to the brain, eyes, skin, or oral mucous membranes (35%–60% of cases).[211,212] The central nervous system is infected in approximately 80% of infants with disseminated HSV. Cutaneous vesicles are often the first sign, followed by the constitutional symptoms.[213] Only one organ may be the predominant site of clinical abnormalities or the infection may severely compromise several organs, resulting in multisystem failure. Pneumonia is reported as one of the less common presenting features of HSV; it is usually accompanied by other, often more serious extrapulmonary manifestations.[214,215] The spectrum of radiographic changes has been reviewed in a series of 16 cases by Dominguez et al.[216] If the infection is confined to the skin, the prognosis is excellent. The mortality ranges from 60% to 90% in the presence of disseminated HSV; somewhat better survival is reported for localized HSV encephalitis, but the long-term consequences are devastating in terms of psychomotor development.

The pathologic diagnosis of suspected HSV pneumonitis need not await a biopsy or autopsy; Drut and Drut[217] reported virus-containing multinucleated cells in a tracheobronchial aspiration from a 10-day-old infant. More often than not, unfortunately, the diagnosis is confirmed at autopsy. Singer[218] found intranuclear inclusions in the lungs of 8 of 23 (34%) infants who came to postmortem examination.

The lungs are heavier than normal, have petechiae on the pleural surfaces, and are variably hemorrhagic or consolidated on cut surface. Bloody fluid exudes from the surface. Necrosis is generally not apparent from the gross inspection, but diffuse parenchymal nodularity may indicate that secondary bronchopneumonia has occurred. The herpetic inclusions vary in appearance from a sharply delineated acidophilic structure surrounded by a halo and marginated chromatin to a smudged, amphophilic inclusion replacing the nucleoplasm.[219] Both mononuclear and multinucleated cells contain the inclusion(s). Cytomegaly is not a feature of the infected cells. If there are any questions about the type of viral inclusion, the issue can be settled by immunohistochemistry.[220]

Focal necrosis and a background of alveolar damage and hemorrhage should suggest the possibility of HSV pneumonitis even before the characteristic inclusions are found. The inclusions are present in alveolar macrophages and interstitial cells at or near the margins of necrosis. It may be necessary to examine several microscopic sections before the inclusions are identified. In a few cases, even in the presence of inclusions in other organs (adrenals, liver, brain, skin), the diagnostic cells may be difficult to find in the lungs because of extensive necrosis; careful search may be required.

If needed, immunohistochemistry for HSV can be performed.[221] The lung may also have features of massive pulmonary hemorrhage, diffuse alveolar damage with hyaline membranes, fibrin thrombi in small vessels, or nonspecific interstitial pneumonitis.[222] Neutrophils in the peripheral airspaces may indicate secondary bacterial pneumonia in an infant who has survived long enough to develop this complication.

Varicella-Zoster

The herpesvirus varicella-zoster is the cause of a very common contagious childhood infection; most individuals (95% or more) have been exposed to varicella-zoster by 15 years of age.[206] Only 1 case of varicella-zoster is reported in every 7,500 pregnancies. Varicella embryopathy (hypoplasia of extremities, cutaneous scarring, growth retardation, and neuroophthalmic damage) occurs in fetuses who are infected between the eighth and nineteenth week of gestation.[223,224] An infection in the last 4 days of gestation or within 2 days of birth results in severe generalized varicella with a very poor prognosis. Beyond this period, the infection is mild. Approximately 50 cases of varicella have been reported in the perinatal-neonatal period.[225]

The pathologic findings in the lungs are similar if not indistinguishable from herpes simplex pneumonitis, including the appearance of the intranuclear inclusions.[226] Diffuse alveolar damage, hyaline membranes, and interstitial inflammatory and focal necrosis are the principal microscopic features.

Rubella

Classic rubella embryopathy (cataracts, deafness, and congenital heart disease including patent ductus arteriosus, ventricular septal defect, and central and peripheral pulmonic stenosis) is the consequence of an in utero infection during the first two trimesters.[227,228] If the mother is seronegative in a nonepidemic period, 1 per 25,000 pregnancies is complicated by rubella embryopathy.[229] The "expanded" syndrome is manifested by thrombocytopenia purpura, neonatal hepatitis, encephalitis, and pneumonitis. Respiratory distress may be apparent soon after birth, or may be delayed for several weeks or months in infants with rubella pneumonitis. Gradual resolution of symptoms and signs is generally the case. Rosenberg and associates[230] indicated that pneumonitis with the late lesions of congenital rubella is probably a superimposed infection rather than rubella itself.

Interstitial pneumonitis with or without fibrosis is the less than specific finding in the lung.[231,232] Desquamative interstitial pneumonia was reported by Boner and associates,[233] but the specificity of this particular pattern is debated. It is safe to conclude that a diagnosis of rubella pneumonitis is only possible with appropriate supporting clinical and laboratory observations.

Listeria monocytogenes

Listeria monocytogenes, a gram-positive rod, is one of the three nonviral organisms (the others are Toxoplasma *gondii* and *Treponema pallidum*) that spread from an infected mother through the placenta resulting in fetal sepsis. However, the infant may be infected through the amniotic cavity, at the time of delivery through an infected birth canal, or in an infrequent nursery epidemic. Lallemand and associates[234] documented the presence of listeriosis in 3% of second-trimester abortions. A spontaneous abortion occurred shortly after the mother had become febrile. The clinical manifestations of fetal, perinatal, and neonatal listeriosis vary, but cutaneous pustules, respiratory distress, and hepatic dysfunction are among the more common features.[235] In the premature infant with respiratory symptoms, bronchopulmonary dysplasia and streptococcal pneumonia are plausible considerations. Later onset listeriosis at 2–3 weeks of age is characterized by meningitis.

Villitis and focal necrosis or abscess formation in the fetus are the hallmarks of intrauterine septicemia; chorioamnionitis and decidual abscesses are more typical of the ascending infection. Abscesses are present in multiple organs, including the lungs, in the septic fetus.[236] Aspiration of infected vaginal secretions produces bronchopneumonia with necrotizing and hemorrhagic features.

Treponema pallidum

Congenital syphilis is a complex disease with a host of clinical signs and symptoms.[172] The transmission of the spirochetes from an infected mother to the fetus may occur at any time during pregnancy. The resurgence of syphilis in the United States over the past decade (1981–1990) has also been manifested by an increase in the incidence of congenital syphilis.[237] Poor or nonexistent prenatal care and substance abuse by mothers have contributed significantly to the virtual epidemic of congenital syphilis.[238] The diagnosis of congenital syphilis may be unsuspected initially, but should be considered in a stillborn with evidence of nonimmune hydrops fetalis, hepatomegaly, and cutaneous lesions.[239]

So-called pneumonia alba is one of the classic pathologic features of congenital syphilis. There is delayed maturation of the lung and a severe fibrosing process with a zonal distribution.[240] The inflammatory reaction mainly consists of scattered lymphocytes and plasma cells in the interstitium (Fig. 8–35). These infiltrates may be confused with extramedullary hematopoiesis. A superimposed bacterial pneumonia is suggested by the presence of neutrophils. Spirochetes are often present in large numbers.

Toxoplasma gondii

Toxoplasmosis is the most common parasitic infection in the United States, according to some investiga-

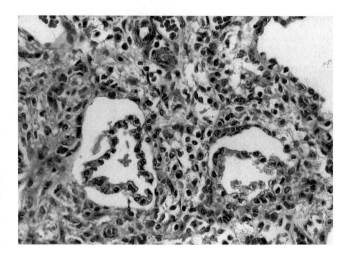

Fig. 8–35. Congenital syphilis shows moderately dense interstitial inflammatory infiltrate consisting in part of mature plasma cells. H and E, ×400.

tors.[241,242] The facultative intracellular coccidia, *Toxoplasma gondii*, produces a number of clinical syndromes, ranging from a flu-like illness to an overwhelming septic infection affecting multiple organs including the brain, heart, and eye. An infection during pregnancy is usually inconsequential to the mother but may have drastic effects on the fetus, depending on the time during gestation when the organisms pass through the placenta. The fetus of a seronegative primipara with an acute mononucleosis syndrome has a 25%–40% chance of being infected. Maternal toxoplasmosis between the third and sixth months of gestation is the most vulnerable period for a severe fetal infection.[243–245] Only 10%–20% of seropositive infants are clinically ill at birth. The complex of congenital toxoplasmosis (cerebral calcifications, chorioretinitis, thrombocytopenia) is similar to congenital cytomegalovirus. Pneumonitis is present in 35%–40% of neonates with generalized toxoplasmosis. These children have respiratory distress, which may constitute a significant problem in management.

Unless and until the encysted organisms are identified in the lung, the pulmonary changes are indistinguishable from other interstitial pneumonidites. There is widening of the alveolar septa by a mixed inflammatory infiltrate, and focal collections of alveolar macrophages are present in distal airspaces.[246] The cysts are found in macrophages, endothelium, smooth muscle, and epithelial cells.

Human Immunodeficiency Virus

Acquired immunodeficiency syndrome (AIDS) is the eventual consequence in most individuals of a human immunodeficiency virus (HIV-1; infrequently, HIV-2)

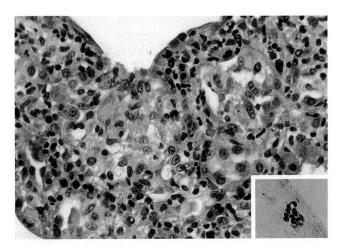

Fig. 8–36. *Pneumocystis carinii* pneumonia presenting in HIV-positive child. Numerous noncaseating epithelioid granulomas are present in widened interstitium. Mycobacterial infection was suspected, but clusters of cysts (*inset*) were identified in granulomas, and acid-fast stains were negative. H and E, ×400; Gomori methenamine silver, ×400.

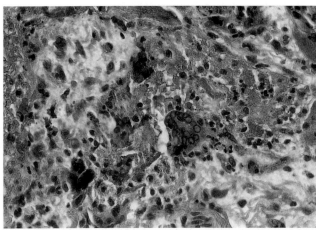

Fig. 8–37. Giant cell pneumonia in child with primary immunodeficiency disorder who had been inoculated with live attenuated measles vaccine. A similar pattern of lung injury is seen in respiratory syncytial virus and parainfluenza infections of the lung in immunocompromised patients regardless of etiology. H and E, ×400.

infection. Approximately 2% of all reported AIDS cases in the United States are diagnosed in individuals less than 13 years old.[247] The overwhelming majority of pediatric cases (80%–90%) are recognized in children 2 years old or less who have acquired HIV through vertical transmission from an infected mother. Some infants are seemingly infected in utero, but other neonates may acquire the virus intra- or peripartum. Even though the virus is transmitted across the placenta in some or most cases, neither villitis nor other pathologic evidence of infection, including pneumonia, has been documented in the fetus or neonate. The remaining HIV–AIDS cases in the pediatric age population are the results of an infected blood transfusion (uncommon in the United States) or sexual contact with a HIV-infected individual; these patients are more commonly older children or adolescents.[247]

Pulmonary complications of HIV–AIDS are manifested in 70% or more of infected children, especially among infants. Rather than opportunistic microorganisms, infants often have recurrent bacterial infections from *Hemophilus influenzae* type b, *Streptococcus pneumoniae*, and *Staphylococcus aureus*, or mucosal candidiasis.[248] Among the serious opportunistic infections, *Pneumocystis carinii* pneumonia is one of the most common in children and has been reported in almost 40% of pediatric cases.[249] Organisms are often identified in a bronchoalveolar lavage or transbronchial biopsy. A frothy alveolar exudate with abundant cysts is very often absent, and in its place is seen a pattern of diffuse alveolar injury and even granulomas of an epithelioid type without caseous necrosis (Fig. 8–36). Measles,

herpes simplex, varicella, and respiratory syncytial virus are known to cause severe, if not fatal, pneumonia in HIV-infected chldren just as these viruses are responsible for pneumonitis in children with one of the primary immunodeficiency syndromes[250] (Fig. 8–37).

Lymphoid hyperplasia-lymphoid interstitial pneumonia was initially recognized in HIV-infected infants and was considered sufficiently specific to qualify as a definitional lesion of pediatric AIDS.[251,252] However, Travis et al.[253] have reported similar changes in the lungs of adults. A dense infiltrate of mature lymphocytes, predominantly CD8-positive cells, and plasma cells infiltrate the interstitium and septa and around distal airways and vessels (Fig. 8–38). Small noncleaved cell lymphoma or Burkitt's lymphoma was documented in the lungs and other sites in a 2-year-old boy with AIDS who had been initially diagnosed with lymphoid interstitial pneumonia.[254]

Perinatal and Neonatal Infection

The infections in the previous sections are typically acquired at some point during gestation, even during the first stage of delivery. This section is concerned principally with those infections that are acquired perinatally and are manifested in the first days or weeks of life. Most of these infections are ultimately traced to the mother. Mothers can infect their children postnatally, but extramaternal sources (the nursery and its personnel, mechanical devices, and other family members) are important in the etiology of neonatal pneumonias.[255]

A prospective study of pneumonia developing in the

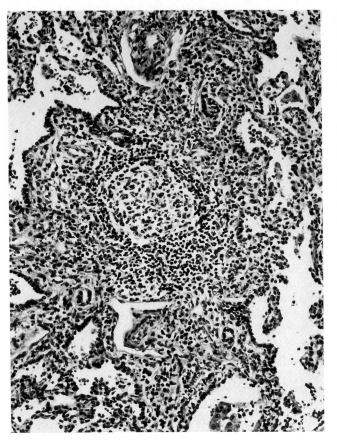

Fig. 8–38. Lymphocytic interstitial pneumonitis in infant with failure to thrive, fever, and chronic diarrhea provided clinical clues to diagnosis of acquired immune deficiency syndrome. A reactive follicular center is surrounded by concentric mantle of small lymphocytes that spilled into adjacent alveolar septa. H and E, ×160.

first 48 h of life revealed that 57% of cases were caused by group B beta-hemolytic *Streptococcus* and that approximately 50% of these neonates also had positive blood cultures.[256] Most of the neonates, regardless of the specific microorganism, were preterm and required mechanical ventilation. The overall mortality rate was 30%, which is comparable to the experience of others.[257]

Group B Beta-Hemolytic Streptococcus

Two bacteria, group B beta-hemolytic *Streptococcus* (GBS) and *Escherichia coli,* are together responsible for the majority of cases of neonatal sepsis, pneumonia, and meningitis.[172,173] It has only been in the past generation that group B beta-hemolytic *Streptococcus* has come to be recognized as one of the most important pathogens in the neonatal period.[258,269] The overall incidence of this disease is 2–3 cases per 1,000 live births; premature or low-weight-for-date infants have an even greater risk of infection.[259,260] There is a correlation between the degree of cervicovaginal colonization and the acquisition rate of GBS disease in the neonate.[261] Prolonged rupture of membranes and low birth weight enhance the risk for infection. Early-onset GBS disease in the first day of life is characterized by symptoms and signs of respiratory distress and radiographic changes resembling early bronchopulmonary dysplasia.[262–265] The infection evolves very rapidly and terminates in death in 50%–75% of cases. When GBS disease has a delayed onset, the prognosis is more favorable. A documented complication of GBS disease is the occurrence of a delayed right-sided diaphragmatic hernia.[266]

The pathologic findings of group B beta-hemolytic *Streptococcus* in the lungs have been carefully delineated by Craig.[267] In the early stages, the lungs both grossly and microscopically are similar to bronchopulmonary dysplasia with a hypoaerated appearance and widespread hyaline membranes in underexpanded air spaces (Fig. 8–39). Diffuse alveolar and interstitial hemorrhage simulates massive pulmonary hemorrhage of the newborn. There is a minimal neutrophilic infiltrate in the first few hours of the infection (Fig. 8–40); the Gram stain shows clumps of gram-positive cocci in the air spaces and within the hyaline membranes, and appropriate bacteriologic cultures establish the diagnosis. Antibiotic therapy may interfere with the results of culture and the demonstration of the bacteria. A focal or confluent neutrophilic exudate in the alveoli is present in the lungs of infants who survive 12–24 h. Abscesses are usually not found.

Chlamydia trachomatis

Chlamydia has long been known as the etiologic agent of neonatal inclusion conjunctivitis, but its role in genital tract infections in adults has been the subject of recent interest.[268–271] At the time of delivery, the cervix is infected by *Chlamydia* in approximately 10% of mothers. Conjunctivitis is the most typical form of *Chlamydia* infection (20%–25%); it is encountered in 1–4 infants per 1,000 live births.[272,273] Pneumonitis occurs in 3%–18% of cases and is preceded by conjunctivitis in a number of infants.[274,275] Approximately 30%–40% of all infectious pneumonidites in the first 6 months of life are caused by *Chlamydia*. Most of these cases are clinically mild; however, 25% of infants have moderate-to-severe respiratory distress.[276–279] Bilateral interstitial and/or reticulonodular infiltrates and hyperexpanded segments are the radiographic findings. The overall prognosis is excellent.[280]

The diagnosis of *Chlamydia* is based on the results of tissue culture and the detection of the specific IgM

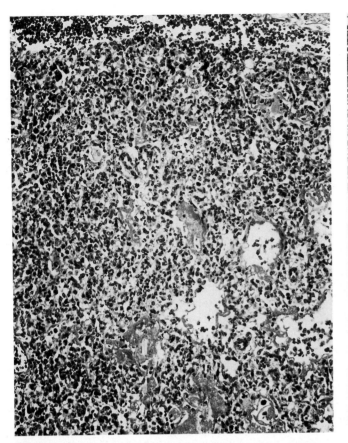

Fig. 8–39. Neonatal pneumonia in early state is characterized by presence of hyaline membranes, focal or diffuse interstitial and/or alveolar hemorrhage, and a predominantly interstitial inflammatory infiltrate. H and E, ×160.

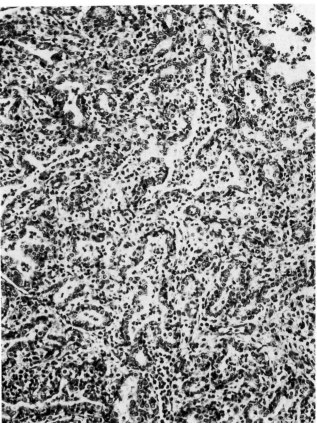

Fig. 8–40. Neonatal pneumonia in premature infant shows interstitial stromal cellularity that may obscure diagnosis until neutrophilic exudate is recognized in alveoli. Presence of squames within exudate may indicate that infected amniotic contents contributed to cause of pneumonia. H and E, ×160.

antibody. Infected cells contain an intracytoplasmic inclusion on Giemsa-stained material from the eye or nasopharynx. Fortunately, there are very few opportunities to examine lung tissue from these patients. An open lung biopsy was performed on the patient that was reported by Arth et al.[281] They described a necrotizing bronchiolitis and a mononuclear cell infiltrate. An interstitial pneumonia without specific histologic features was seen by Beem and Saxon[276] in open lung biopsies from two infants. Too few cases of chlamydia pneumonitis have been described to allow any definite characterization.

Mycoplasma pneumoniae

The presence of *Mycoplasma pneumoniae*, *Mycoplasma hominis*, and *ureaplasma urealyticum* in the lower genital tract explains the occasional neonatal pneumonia caused by one of these organisms.[272,282] *Ureaplasma* is a documented copathogen in cases of neonatal cytomeg-

alovirus pneumonitis. *Mycoplasma* pneumonia is generally uncommon in children less than 6 months old, but it occurs in 4 children per 1,000 between the ages of 5 and 9 years.[283]

There are a few descriptions in the literature of the pathologic findings of *Mycoplasma* pneumonia; most of these are in adults and a few prepubertal children.[284] Luminal exudate in the bronchioles, peribronchiolar lymphoplasmacytic infiltrate, interstitial mononuclear infiltrate, and alveolar damage are characteristic features.

Mycobacterium tuberculosis hominis

Tuberculosis has always been prevalent in the less developed countries of the world, where it is endemic. In the United States, tuberculosis was until recently regarded as a disease under control; however, the status quo has been altered substantially, in part because of the number of new cases in HIV-infected individuals.[285]

New cases of tuberculosis in children are most prevalent in those under 5 years of age;[286] most of these infections are airborne spread.

Infrequent examples of congenital tuberculosis have been documented and defined by active maternal disease and a primary complex in the liver of the infant.[287-294] Machin and associates[295] reported their experience with perinatally acquired tuberculosis and summarized the previous 13 cases in the literature. Infected secretions from mothers with pulmonary and genital tuberculosis are the source of the organisms. Although there is a miliary pattern of dissemination to the various organs including the lungs, caseous granulomas are uncommon. Collections of histiocytes are present in the terminal air spaces in a distribution like bronchopneumonia, but there is an absence of neutrophils, lymphocytes, and plasma cells. One potential misinterpretation is Langerhans' cell histiocytosis (histiocytosis X) and endogenous or exogenous lipid pneumonia.

Candida albicans

Candidiasis is the most common fungal infection of the neonatal period. Most of these infants have a localized infection in the oral cavity known as thrush. Approximately 4% of neonates develop thrush, which is probably acquired from organisms in the maternal cervicovaginal secretions. There are a few examples of intrauterine infections from organisms in the vagina gaining access to the amniotic cavity and producing chorioamnionitis.[296] In the past several years, candidiasis in premature infants has emerged as an important complication in neonatal intensive care units. These infants are extremely vulnerable to infections, and the parenteral route from intravascular catheters is well established both clinically and pathologically. Smith and Congdon,[297] among others, have reviewed their experiences with this infection. The postmortem findings in 34 small premature infants (birth weight of less than 1,500 g) revealed that 8 babies (23.5%) had candidiasis as a primary or a contributory cause of death. These infants have the expected early onset of respiratory distress, usually related to bronchopulmonary dysplasia. Symptoms and signs of sepsis ensue, and the radiographic findings are the combination of progressive bronchopulmonary dysplasia and focal or patchy parenchymal consolidation.[298] The latter may evolve into diffuse consolidation. Aggressive antibiotic therapy and other supportive measures are imperative to avoid the inevitable outcome.

The gross and microscopic changes in the lungs may vary by virtue of the mode of candidal spread via the bronchopulmonary, vascular emboli, or systemically disseminated routes. Among the 14 autopsy cases that Kassner et al.[299] examined, 50% of the infants had embolization of an infected thrombus from a major vein or right-sided heart valve to the lungs with one or several peripheral hemorrhagic infarcts. The lungs were diffusely consolidated and hemorrhagic in those cases of systemic candidiasis. Nodularity on palpation of the gross specimen may suggest the presence of abscesses or secondary bronchopneumonia. A shaggy, fibrinopurulent exudate alternating with denuded tracheobronchial mucosa in association with parenchymal consolidation was present in those cases of direct extension from the oropharynx.

Yeasts and pseudohyphae are easily identified in the mucosal exudate, but the invasive organisms may be obscured by the hemorrhage and necrosis. Occluded pulmonary vessels in the region of an infarct are often highlighted by a dense tangle of pseudohyphae invading the vessel wall in a similar manner as does *Aspergillus* or *Mucor*. Microabscesses with a minimal exudative component and rarely a granulomatous reaction are the features of capillary invasive candidiasis. An occasional case has more than one pattern of pulmonary involvement by *Candida*, or several simultaneous processes may be present as well, including bronchopulmonary dysplasia and/or secondary bacterial pneumonia. Separation of the various pathologic findings in the lung is a difficult and complicated problem that is best approached with a thorough knowledge of the clinical events.

Other Fungal Infections

Fungal infections other than candidiasis in the neonatal-early infancy period are extremely rare. Miller[300] found only six reported examples of cryptococcosis in the first month of life. Four cases of coccidioidomycosis in infants younger than 3 months old were reported by Child and associates.[301] Their review identified 17 cases, inclusive of their 4 cases of neonatal coccidioidomycosis. Occasional examples of histoplasmosis, aspergillosis, and phycomycosis can be found in the literature.

Pneumocystis carinii

Today, *Pneumocystis carinii* pneumonia is generally an opportunistic infection in children with primary or secondary immunodeficiency states. However, the earliest reports of this infection were nursery epidemics in poorly nourished, low-birth-weight infants who developed "plasma cell pneumonia." Very few epidemics of nursery pneumocystosis are reported in the developed countries of the world. However, sporadic cases in immunocompromised infants remain an ever-present clinical problem. It is the experience in many centers, especially in those located in large urban areas, that HIV-infected children are the source of most cases of pulmonary pneumocystosis.[302] Those infants and young children who are HIV infected and present with *Pneumocystis carinii* pneumonia have a shorter period of survival when compared to HIV-infected children with some other initial clinical presentation.[303] *Pneumocystis carinii* has been isolated as a copathogen in infants with cytomegalovirus pneumonia; Stagno and associates[304] documented this unicellular protozoa in 10 of 67 (14%) immunocompetent infants with pneumonitis in the first 12 weeks of life. Severe respiratory distress, tachypnea, apneic episodes, and small reticulonodular infiltrates on chest radiographs are the clinical manifestations. The organism is acquired from environmental exposure early in life; approximately one-third of children have antibodies to pneumocystis by 1 year of age and 75% by 4 years of age.

The interstitium of the lung is heavily infiltrated by mature plasma cells in classic infantile pneumocystosis. A flocculant, intraalveolar exudate containing the encysted organisms and a nonspecific, variably dense interstitial inflammatory infiltrate are the microscopic features usually associated with pneumocystis pneumonia. However, a number of other tissue reactions accompany the infection, including poorly formed granulomas, diffuse alveolar damage, and dystrophic calcification (see Fig. 8–36). Touch imprints from a positive lung biopsy or material from a bronchoalveolar and tracheal aspiration stained with methenamine silver demonstrate the 1- to 2-μm round to crescentric-shaped organisms in clustered or individual cysts[305] (see Chapter 14).

Respiratory Syncytial Virus

The respiratory syncytial virus, a RNA virus, is the single most important lower respiratory tract pathogen in childhood.[306,307] An epidemiologic study by Glezen and Denny[308] showed that the peak incidence of lower respiratory tract infections in children (240 per 1,000 children) occurs in the first year of life. Most of these cases are caused by respiratory syncytial virus or parainfluenza viruses type 1 or 3 (croup).[309] The symptomatology of classic respiratory syncytial virus-associated bronchiolitis is coughing and wheezing, except in infants under 4 weeks of age who are more likely to have an atypical pneumonia.[310] Respiratory syncytial virus has also been isolated in cases of sudden infant death syndrome, as a cause of giant cell pneumonitis in infants with primary immunodeficiency syndromes, and as severe bronchiolitis in young children with congenital

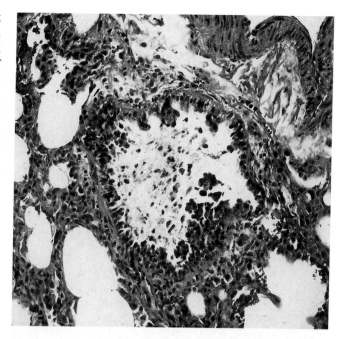

Fig. 8–41. Respiratory syncytial virus bronchiolitis accompanied by pneumonitis in infant with tachypnea and subcostal retractions. Biopsy disclosed papillary hyperplasia of bronchiolar epithelium, inspissated mucus, and interstitial inflammatory reaction. H and E, ×160.

heart disease.[311–313] For older children with underlying chronic disease or an HIV-infected child, the prognosis is poorer than for the immunologically intact child.[314,315]

The pathologic anatomy of respiratory syncytial virus is discussed at length in Chapter 12. Papillary hyperplasia of bronchiolar epithelium and distal mucous plugging are the principal microscopic features (Fig. 8–41).

Papillomavirus

Human papillomavirus is the general designation for a family of related DNA viruses with a number of distinct serotypes having a tropism for keratinizing epithelium. One subtype of human papillomavirus, type 6, is the etiologic agent for condyloma acuminatum and juvenile laryngeal papillomatosis.[316,317] Fewer than 0.1% of infants develop laryngeal papillomatosis, but in those with lesions, 50% or more of their mothers have documented genital tract involvement. There is a predilection for first-born infants. The initial lesions are found on the true vocal cords. The natural history is characterized by multiple local recurrences and even spread beyond the larynx into the hypopharynx, trachea, and even the lung. There are rare examples of spontaneous or induced malignant transformation.[318]

Pulmonary involvement by papillomatosis is the con-

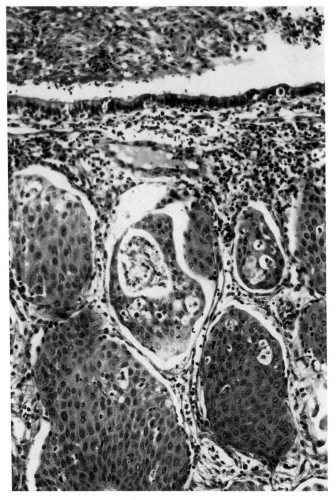

Fig. 8–42. Laryngeal papillomatosis disseminated to lung. Sheets of squamous cells fill alveoli, compressing alveolar septa between cell masses. Note bronchiole (above) filled with necrotic debris. (AFIP Neg. 82–7805.) H and E, ×160.

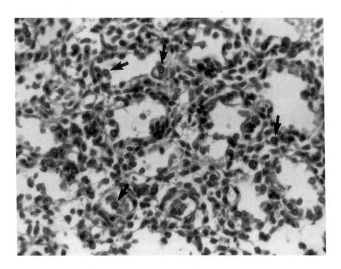

sequence of contiguous extension into the tracheobronchial tree (Fig. 8–42).[319–321] The proliferation of squamous epithelium retains its papillomatous configuration in the bronchus. Hyperplastic squamous epithelium with surface koilocytosis with accompanying cytologic atypia is the characteristic microscopic appearance.[322,323] In some cases, the cellular atypia is sufficiently disturbing as to suggest carcinoma in situ. It is best to reserve the diagnosis of carcinoma for those cases with unequivocal invasion.

Other Viral Infections

Many different types of major and minor viruses have been reported as etiologic agents of pneumonia in the neonatal period.[324] Somewhat surprising is the fact that adenovirus infection, a rather ubiquitous pathogen, is a rare cause of neonatal pneumonia. Sun and Duara[325] reported two such cases of necrotizing adenovirus bronchopneumonia in neonates, and only three other similar examples have been found in the literature. The enteroviruses, echo and coxsackie, are responsible for isolated cases of pneumonia in the newborn period. Epstein–Barr virus is an unimportant cause to date of congenital and neonatal infections.[326] Human parvovirus B19 is known to infect the fetus through placental transfer from the mother. A link with intrauterine fetal wastage has been established through mechanism of a cytopathic infection of erythroid precursors, resulting in anemia and fetal hydrops.[327] The characteristic glassy eosinophilic intranuclear inclusion is present in erythroid cells in vascular spaces in the lungs and other organs[328] (Fig. 8–43). Inflammation is minimal except in the liver.

Other Bacterial Infections

Virtually all the gram-negative enteric bacilli, particularly *Escherichia coli*, are causes of perinatal pneumonia.[329] *Streptococcus pneumoniae* sepsis is a rare infection of the neonatal period;[330] Bergqvist and Trovik[331] reported three cases that simulated group B beta-hemolytic streptococcal infection. Nursery epidemics of *Staphylococcus aureus* are manifested as necrotizing bronchopneumonia.[332,333] Hemophilus influenza, type B is one of the important causes of meningitis in infancy, but it is also the etiologic agent for a segmental pneumo-

◁————————————————

Fig. 8–43. Parvovirus B19 infection in stillborn fetus with severe hydrops fetalis. Virtually all capillaries of lung contained erythrocyte precursors with intranuclear inclusions (*arrows*). H and E, ×600,

nia in children between 3 and 12 months of age.[334–337] The pathologic appearance is one of necrotizing pneumonia. *Legionella pneumophilia* has been isolated in rare cases of sepsis and pneumonia in immunocompromised infants.[338–340]

Postinfarction and Down Syndrome-Associated "Peripheral Cysts"

The development of small subpleural cysts of the lung has been described in patients with Down syndrome and others with pulmonary artery thrombosis.[341–344] Gonzalez and colleagues[344] analyzed autopsies of 98 patients with Down syndrome and found small subpleural cysts in 19 patients. They suggested that the cysts result from reduced postnatal production of peripheral small air passages and alveoli, reflecting the slow rate of cell proliferation seen in Down syndrome. Stocker and colleagues[341] believed that the peripheral cysts develop through liquefaction necrosis of the lung secondary to hypoperfusion of that area, as the result of either pulmonary artery occlusion or possibly altered blood flow associated with a cardiovascular anomaly (Figs. 8–44 and 8–45).

Preservation of the central portion of the lung is accomplished through an intact bronchial artery circulation supplying both the bronchial tree and adjacent pulmonary parenchyma through direct bronchopulmonary arteries and anastomoses between pulmonary arteries and bronchial arteries (Table 8–3 and Fig. 8–46). The walls of the cysts represent preserved interlobular septa, which also receive their blood supply through the bronchial artery circulation. The cysts are 0.1–0.6 cm in diameter after reabsorption of the necrotic debris (Figs. 8–47 and 8–48), and are most prominent in the upper lobes, suggesting a possible relationship to the cysts of idiopathic spontaneous pneumothorax noted in other patients.[341] The air-filled cysts of older infants as well as adults with idiopathic spontaneous pneumothorax, are lined by low cuboidal to attenuated epithelial cells overlying a vascular connective tissue wall.

Intralobar Sequestration

An intralobar sequestration is a segment of pulmonary parenchyma invested along with the normal right or left lung by visceral pleura and supplied by a systemic artery. The segment is usually isolated from the tracheobronchial tree but may be partially air containing.[345]

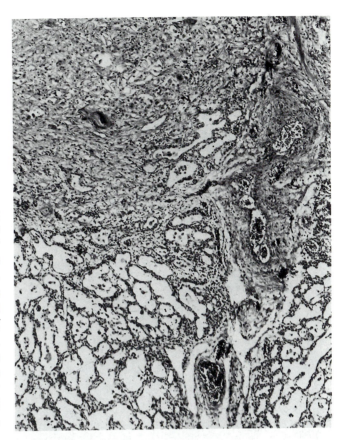

Fig. 8–44. Peripheral pulmonary infarction. Only amorphous debris (upper left) remains of acini after infarction of periphery of lung (intact pleura lies beyond top of field). Note preserved interlobular septa (right) with its intact blood supply from bronchial arteries. This 2-week-old infant had total occlusion of right pulmonary artery. H and E, ×50.

Intralobar sequestration is seen slightly more frequently in males than females (1.1:1).[346] Symptoms of cough, sputum production, and recurrent pneumonia are noted in 85% of patients, approximately 25% of whom present before the age of 10.[347] Intralobar sequestration, however, is rarely seen in infants. In a review of 42,000 autopsies of infants less than 2 months of age, not a single case of intralobar sequestration was noted, while 12 cases of extralobar sequestration were seen.[348] Intralobar sequestration has been described in 13 infants under 5 years of age,[349–358] 3 of whom had a bronchopulmonary foregut malformation with communication between the sequestration and the esophagus or stomach.[350,352,355] A 2-day-old infant, the youngest reported case of intralobar sequestration, had an unilobulated hypoplastic lung supplied exclusively by the abdominal aorta.[354] Two other patients with normal bronchial communication had a vascular malformation to their lower lobes[356] and thus were not truly sequestered. The remaining 7 had histories of chronic cough,

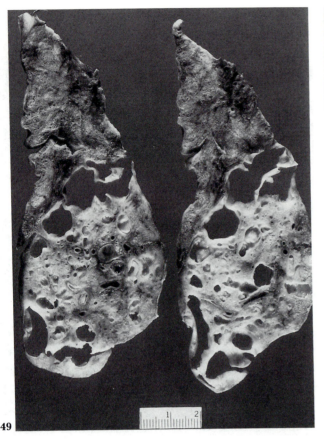

8-49

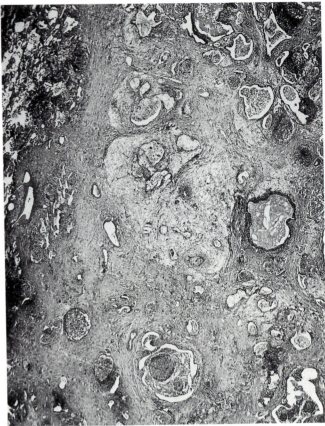

8-50

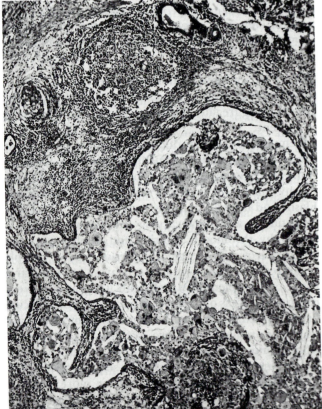

8-51

Fig. 8–49. Intralobar pulmonary sequestration. Cut sections of resected left-lower lobe reveal densely fibrotic and multi-cystic mass in lower portion that was isolated from tracheo-bronchial tree and supplied by large systemic artery that arose from thoracic aorta and passed through pulmonary ligament to enter lung. Similar smaller arteries are also noted within pulmonary ligament. Note normal lung in top third of each section.

Fig. 8–50. Intralobar pulmonary sequestration. Pulmonary parenchyma is distorted and largely replaced by dense fibrosis and chronic inflammation. Scattered bronchial-like structures lined by cuboidal-to-columnar epithelium are present. H and E, ×15.

Fig. 8–51. Intralobar pulmonary sequestration. Amorphous debris containing cholesterol clefts fills irregular bronchiole-like structure surrounded by fibrous connective tissue heavily infiltrated by chronic inflammatory cells. Note lymphoid follice at top. H and E, ×100.

(Table 8–4).[350,363–371] Gebauer and Mason[368] in 1959, however, suggested that intralobar sequestration resulted from "a destructive bronchial pulmonary disease." In 1984, Stocker and Malczak[371] described the presence of normally occurring pulmonary ligament arteries in 90% of infants and children, and postulated that these arteries could be parasitized in the formation of an intralobar sequestration. Under circumstances of bronchial obstruction and a chronic pneumonia with partial or complete interruption of the pulmonary artery supply to the infected portion, parasitization could occur through the development of a pleuritis and formation of a richly vascular granulation tissue deriving its blood supply from the hypertrophied pulmonary ligament arteries or, if the diaphragmatic surface of the lung is involved, the diaphragmatic vessels, that is, the phrenic arteries via the celiac axis (Fig. 8–52).

With progression and resolution of the pneumonia, accentuated by recurring bouts of pneumonia, one or more systemic arteries assume a substantial supply to the chronically infected segment of lung. The lack of systemic arteries other than the bronchial arteries available for parasitization by a chronic upper-lobe pneumonia accounts for the rare occurrence of intralobar sequestration in the upper lobes (less than 2%). Chronic pneumonia of the upper lobes, histologically similar to intralobar sequestration, is not, however, an unusual occurrence.

Intralobar sequestration is virtually absent in infants, with the notable exception of bronchopulmonary foregut malformations and the rare case of pulmonary vascular malformation producing congestive heart failure, both clearly congenital lesions. This absence supports the theory of an acquired origin of this lesion. So also does the relative infrequency of associated anomalies (6%–12%)[345] when compared with the anomalies seen in association with extralobar sequestration (49%–67%), congenital pulmonary lymphangiectasis (85%), infantile lobar emphysema (42%), and congenital cystic adenomatoid malformation (26%).[79] Finally, the fact that intralobar sequestrations drain via the normal pulmonary veins in 95% of cases, and may be partially air containing, again suggests a fluctuating inflammatory process superimposed on a developmentally normal lung. It is possible, however, that some intralobar sequestrations develop in other preexisting malformations, such as congenital cystic adenomatoid malformation of a lower lobe.

Interstitial and Alveolar Diseases

Acute lung injury with the resulting adult respiratory distress syndrome (ARDS) is well documented in the

Table 8–4. Theories of origin of intralobar sequestration[a]

Traction by anomalous branch of aorta on segment of developing lung results in separation from normal lung	Pryce, 1946[365]
Persistence of thoracic aortic arteries secondary to insufficient pulmonary arterial supply; systemic blood pressure causes cystic degeneration of the lung	Smith, 1956[366]
No causal relationship between nonfunctioning lung and systemic artery	Boyden, 1958[367]
Acquired disease secondary to localized infectious process	Gebauer and Mason, 1959[368]
Failure of normal embryonic organizer control	Blesovsky, 1967[369]
Accessory lung bud develops in embryo and either becomes incorporated into normally developing lung (intralobar) or remains separate (extralobar); suggested term "congenital bronchopulmonary foregut malformation"	Gerle et al., 1968[350]
Intralobar sequestration is collection of bronchogenic cysts associated with a systemic artery	Moscarella and Wylie, 1968[370]
Acquired disease utilizing normally occurring pulmonary ligament arteries	Stocker and Malczak, 1984[371]

[a] Modified from Stocker and Malczak. Chest 1984;86:611–615,[371] with permission.

pediatric age group despite its appellation.[372,373] Typically, ARDS presents in a previously healthy individual who has no known underlying pulmonary disease; however, a flu-like illness may precede the development of severe respiratory distress. The injury to the lungs may be direct, as in the case of an infection or inhalant, or indirect, as in the case of sepsis, shock, and trauma.[372] There are few data on the epidemiology of ARDS in children, but a viral infection is often suspected. The pediatric experience with ARDS is that the outcome is poor, with a mortality of 50%–60%.[373] In virtually all respects, the clinical and pathologic features are identical in children and adults. Histologically, the earliest changes are alveolar edema, which as an isolated finding is rarely seen in the initial lung biopsy. More often, the specimen is obtained during the phase of acute respiratory failure when hyaline membranes, interstitial edema, a mild acute inflammatory infiltrate, and necrosis of alveolar lining cells are the predominant microscopic findings (Fig. 8–53). The exudative phase is superseded by the proliferative phase with early fibrous ingrowth with fibromyxomatous cushions, type II cell hyperplasia and metaplasia, and more pronounced interstitial cellular infiltrates.[374]

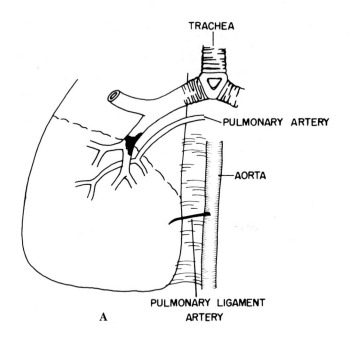

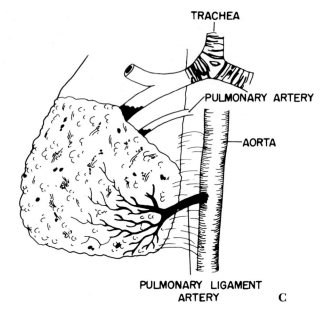

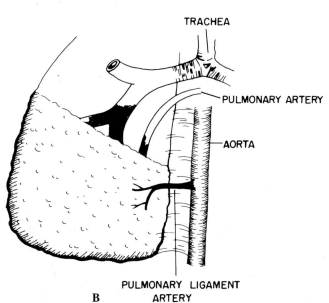

Fig. 8–52 A–C. Sequence of events leading to formation of intralobar sequestration. **A.** Bronchial occlusion (by aspiration, inflammatory debris, etc.) leads to development of pneumonia distal to obstruction. Note small pulmonary ligament artery that is normally present. **B.** As pneumonia progresses, obstruction of pulmonary artery may occur, promoting hypertrophy of pulmonary ligament artery as inflamed lung seeks oxygenated blood to aid in resolution of pneumonia. **C.** As pneumonia resolves, progresses, or recurs, involved segment of lung may derive its major arterial supply from single (or multiple) hypertrophied pulmonary ligament artery. (Modified from Stocker and Malczak. Chest 1984;86:611–615,[371] with permission.)

Interstitial lung disease is as well or poorly understood in children as it is in adults.[375,376] There are numerous etiologies and associated conditions and diseases of acquired and inherited types, but the fact remains that most cases are idiopathic or cryptogenic. Hypersensitivity pneumonitis or extrinsic allergic alveolitis is characterized by bronchiolitis, an inflammatory infiltrate of plasma cells, eosinophils, neutrophils, and macrophages. Noncaseating granulomas may be seen later in the evolution of the reaction. So-called desquamative interstitial pneumonitis is another pattern of lung response to injury with the filling of distal air-

spaces with macrophages and type II pneumocytes.[377] Usual interstitial pneumonitis is considered the morphologic end stage of any number of pulmonary insults, including ARDS, which has evolved into end-stage lung disease.[378] Dense fibrosis replaces the normal architectural landmarks of the lung with thickening of vessels leading to pulmonary hypertension (Fig. 8–54). It is uncommon for interstitial fibrosis in children to have a documented etiology, but it is associated with chronic aspiration, idiopathic pulmonary hemosiderosis, and Langerhans' cell histiocytosis.[379,380]

Bronchiolitis obliterans with or without organizing

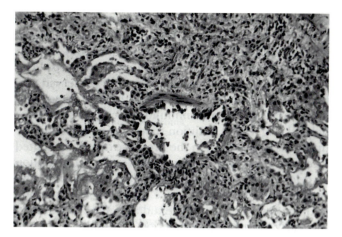

Fig. 8–53. Acute lung injury in young child who presented with rapidly progressive respiratory distress. Interstitial inflammatory infiltrate, edema, hyaline membranes, and occasional hyperplastic type II pneumocytes are present in this open lung biopsy. H and E, ×200.

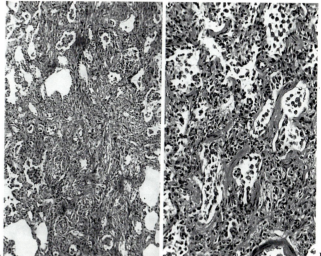

Fig. 8–54 A,B. Usual interstitial pneumonitis in explanted lung of 10-year-old boy with end-stage disease who received bilateral lung allografts. **A.** Fibrosis has replaced extensive areas of lung parenchyma. H and E, ×100. **B.** Residual foci of recognizable parenchyma show fibrosis of distal air spaces and mild chronic inflammation. H and E, ×200.

pneumonitis is known to occur in children, but its incidence is unknown.[381] Acute bronchiolitis is common in infancy, and most cases are caused by respiratory syncytial virus (60%–90% of cases).[382] Parainfluenza, influenza and adenovirus are the other offending pathogens. Of the various viruses, adenovirus is the more likely to produce obliterative bronchiolitis. The latter is also seen as a manifestation of graft-versus-host disease and chronic allograft rejection.[383,384] In the two clinicopathologic series on bronchiolotis obliterans organizing pneumonitis, the youngest patients were recognized in the third decade of life.[385,386]

Pulmonary alveolar proteinosis (PAP) is a clinicopathologic entity with several associations to suggest that more than one etiology may be responsible for a common pattern of lung injury.[387] In the case of PAP, the distal air spaces are filled with a pale-staining, flocculent, eosinophilic, lipoproteinaceous material that is rich in phospholipids, carbohydrates, and protein (Fig. 8–55). Interstitial fibrosis and hyperplasia of type II pneumocytes are other less constant histologic findings. Although PAP is uncommon, its occurrence in children is well documented, especially in the setting of a primary or secondary immunodeficiency disorder.[388–390] These children are also likely to have an infection caused by *Nocardia asteroides*, *Pneumocystis carinii*, or *Mycobacterium avium-intracellare*. PAP can also present in the neonatal period with respiratory distress that is not explained by hyaline membrane disease–bronchopulmonary dysplasia.[391] Bilateral air bronchograms and finely granular infiltrates are the roentgenographic findings. Reports of familial cases presenting

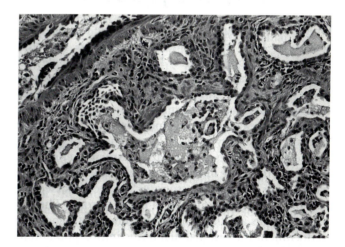

Fig. 8–55. Pulmonary alveolar proteinosis with thickened interstitium in full-term infant who developed respiratory distress shortly after birth. A sibling who died several years before in infancy and another sibling born after the death of this patient had similar pathologic findings in the lung on biopsy and subsequent autopsy. Flocculant eosinophilic material and macrophages are present in alveoli. Interstitial fibrosis is rather marked in this open lung biopsy. H and E, ×200.

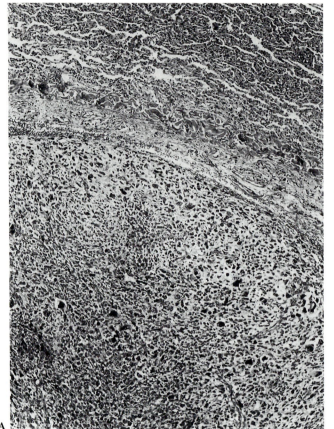

Fig. 8–64 A,B. Pleuropulmonary blastoma presenting as large pleural-based mass in 3-year-old boy. **A.** Tumor is demarcated from lung parenchyma by visceral pleura. Primitive mesenchyme, blastematous condensations, rhabdomyoblasts, and islands of cartilage are composite of findings. H and E, ×64.

B. Malignant cartilage is surrounded by anaplastic cells. Immunohistochemical profile of this neoplasm included focal staining for desmin, S-100 protein, alpha-1 antitrypsin, and vimentin. H and E, ×160.

not have accompanying solid nodule(s) or polypoid excrescences. The more common solid mass has a mutilobated appearance, weighs between 160 and 1100 g, and measures between 6 and 25 cm in diameter. A solid grey-white tumor with a glistening, mucoid appearance has alternating foci of necrosis, hemorrhage, and cystic degeneration. Variations occur in the gross and histologic features within a defined range. Blastematous foci of compact small cells, a loose-to-dense spindle cell stroma, foci of rhabdomyoblasts, collections of large anaplastic cells, and nodules of immature or overtly malignant-appearing cartilage are the histologic components of a typical pleuropulmonary blastoma (Fig. 8–64 A,B). Individual patterns may be absent or overly represented in a particular neoplasm. Among the purely cystic lesions, a cambium layer of small primitive or rhabdomyoblastic-appearing cells is situated beneath a lining of single or stratified cuboidal or ciliated columnar epithelium without atypical cytologic features (Fig.

8–65). Some have interpreted the cyst(s) as a congenital adenomatoid malformation, bronchogenic cyst, or simply a congenital cyst.[423,425] The relationship of pleuropulmonary blastoma to the cystic mesenchymal hamartoma of the lung and adult-type pulmonary blastoma is unsettled, but it is tempting to speculate about the existence of a histogenetic and morphological continuum.

The prognosis for the predominantly cystic pleuroplumonary blastoma without solid nodules is generally quite favorable, whereas the large, solid, multipatterned tumor generally has a dismal outcome.[419] Failure of local tumor control and metastasis to the brain are the major events responsible for the poor prognosis.

Malignant small cell tumor of the thoracopulmonary region (Askin tumor) presents in the soft tissues of the chest wall or as a mass involving both the lung and adjacent structures.[429] This tumor is diagnosed almost

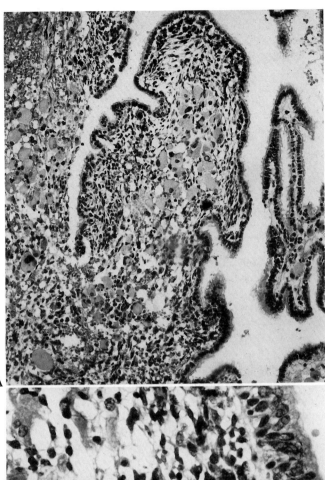

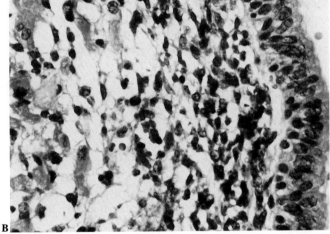

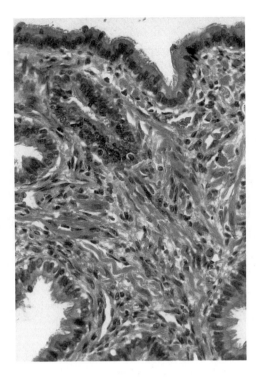

Fig. 8–66. Rhabdomyomatous dysplasia in extralobar sequestration. Immature rhabdomyoblasts in interstitium and other features of this sequestration resemble a type II adenomatoid malformation. H and E, ×400.

Fig. 8–65 A,B. Pleuropulmonary blastoma presenting in 30-month-old child with 3-month history of wheezing and cough. Large multioculated cyst partially replaced right-upper lobe. Electron microscopy confirmed impression that tumor cells had rhabomyoblastic differentiation. **A.** Solid and cystic areas are apparent in gross examination; respiratory type mucosa lines cysts and large rhabdomyoblastic cells occupy supporting stroma. H and E, ×160. **B.** Small hyperchromatic spindle cells beneath mucosal surface produce cambium-layer effect, a feature of botryoid embryonal rhabdomyosarcoma. H and E, ×460.

exclusively in the first two decades of life from infancy through late adolescence; most cases are seen between 10 and 19 years, and there is a female predilection. Nests and cords of uniform, cohesive small dark cells with focal rosette formation are the microscopic features. Both electron microscopy and immunohistochemistry support the conclusion that this neoplasm is a primitive neuroectodermal tumor or peripheral neuroepithelioma.[430,431]

Rhabdomyosarcoma as a primary neoplasm of the lung, exclusive of the setting of cystic pleuropulmonary blastoma, would appear to be quite rare; however, the lungs are one of the preferred sites for metastatic involvement by embryonal and alveolar rhabdomyosarcomas.[432,433] The metastases are usually multiple and have a bronchovascular distribution reflecting the hematogenous mode of spread to the lungs. Nonneoplastic skeletal muscle has been reported in the interstitium of fetal and neonatal lungs as rhabdomyomatous dysplasia, in extralobar sequestration, and type II adenomatoid malformation[434] (Fig. 8–66). The presence of skeletal muscle in these instances is an example of heterotopia, because straited muscle is not normally found in the lung.

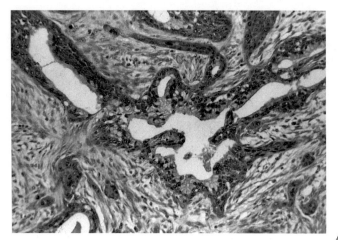

Fig. 8–67. Mucoepidermoid carcinoma of bronchus in 15-year-old female who presented with postobstructive pneumonia. Infiltrating neoplastic nests are composed mucinous and intermediate squamous cells in desmoplastic stroma. H and E, ×400.

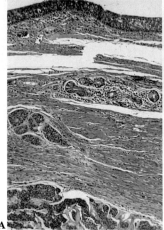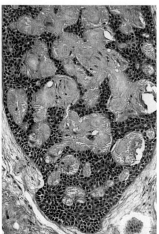

Fig. 8–68. Adenoid cystic carcinoma of trachea in 11-year-old girl. **A.** Submucosal sessile mass occluded approximately 50% of luminal area. H and E, ×100. **B.** Tumor had predominant cribiform pattern. Patient continues to do well almost 2 years after resection. H and E, ×400.

Epithelial Tumors

These are few benign epithelial neoplasms of the lung other than the rare true adenomas (see Chapter 29). Among the primary nonmesenchymal malignant tumors of the lung, the so-called bronchial adenomas or bronchial gland-derived neoplasms are the most common in children (see Table 8–5). Carcinoid, mucoepidermoid carcinoma, and adenoid cystic carcinoma, in descending order of frequency, are the three major tumor types of bronchial gland-derived tumors in children. Bronchial carcinoid in the pediatric age group typically presents between the ages of 12 and 19 years with symptoms and signs referable to the obstruction of a major bronchus.[435] A yellowish submucosal mass measuring 2–4 cm protrudes into the lumen of a bronchus. Microscopically, cords and nests of small uniform tumor cells with minor cytologic abnormalities infiltrate around and through the bronchial cartilage. Foci of necrosis, nuclear aberrations, and pleomorphism should be viewed as evidence of a higher grade neoplasm than the typical carcinoid, which has an excellent prognosis in 80%–90% of cases.[436] Mucoepidermoid carcinoma, although less common than carcinoid, has been well documented in the lung of children.[435] Like carcinoid, the tumor presents as a central obstructive lesion of the bronchus. A broad-based, endobronchial polypoid mass measuring 2–3 cm is the gross appearance. Microscopically, the tumor is compared of intermediate- to high-grade squamous cells forming nests and mucin-containing glands or luminal structures filled with mucin (Fig. 8–67). Adenoid cystic carcinoma

of the bronchus is a very uncommon neoplasm, but we have seen one example in the trachea in an 11-year-old girl (Fig. 8–68).

More conventional forms of bronchogenic carcinoma are infrequently reported in children and young adults.[437] Examples of invasive squamous cell carcinoma have been described as a de novo neoplasm in an adolescent with a history of smoking dating to early childhood or as malignant transformation in bronchopulmonary papillomatosis.[438] Travis and associates[439] reported the occurrence of single pulmonary nodules in the lung resembling bronchioloalveolar carcinoma (BAC) in adolescent patients who had received chemotherapy. Likewise, Benjamin and Cahill[440] described a BAC in a 19-year-old male with the history of a resected congenital cystic adenomatoid malformation as an infant.

Histiocytic and lymphoid infiltrates in the lung are not unique to children but at least one entity, Langerhans' cell histiocytosis (histiocytosis X) has a predilection to the pediatric age group. In the younger child, diffuse pulmonary involvement generally accompanies multisystem or generalized Langerhans' cell histiocytosis.[441,442] The adolescent or young adult is more likely to have eosinophilic granulomas restricted to the lung, but there are isolated cases of primary pulmonary histiocytosis in very young children (Fig. 8–69).[443–447] Aggregates of Langerhans' cells or a more subtle infiltration of the interstitium with or without a fibrous reaction are the variable histologic findings. A stellate scar may be the only remnant of an earlier active lesion.

One of several problems in histologic interpretation is

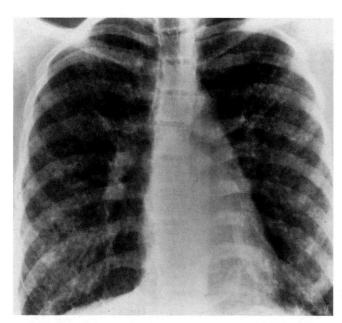

Fig. 8–69. Pulmonary histiocytosis X (Langerhans' cell histiocytosis) produces chest radiographic appearance of diffuse reticulonodular infiltrates in young female.

the distinction of pulmonary macrophages from Langerhans' cells. Also, the presence of some Langerhans' cells does not guarantee a diagnosis of eosinophilic granuloma because these cells occur in any number of inflammatory reactions in the lungs. Electron microscopy for cytoplasmic Birbeck granules, CD1 on the cell surface in frozen sections, and immunohistochemical demonstration of S-100 protein in the nucleus and cytoplasm are the means of confirming the diagnosis; however, Langerhans' cells have characteristic cytologic features (Fig. 8–70).[448–452]

The lung is also involved by malignant histiocytosis and acute monoblastic leukemia, but the original diagnosis is usually established by bone marrow or lymph node biopsy before the appearance of pulmonary manifestations.[453,454] Interstitial lymphoid infiltrates may represent acute lymphoblastic leukemia in a known case of lymphoid interstitial pneumonia in a child with acquired immune deficiency syndrome.[455–459] We and others have seen several examples of polymorphous B-cell hyperplasia and malignant lymphoma in children who had priumary immunodeficiency states or were bone marrow transplant recipients (Fig. 8–71). These tumors are either immunoblastic B-cell lymphomas or mixed small and large cell lymphomas. In addition to the obvious cytologic atypia, focal necrosis is a common finding in the lung biopsy. An angiocentric arrangement that should suggest a T-cell lymphoid neoplasm known as lymphomatoid granulomatosis has been recognized in childhood.[460–463]

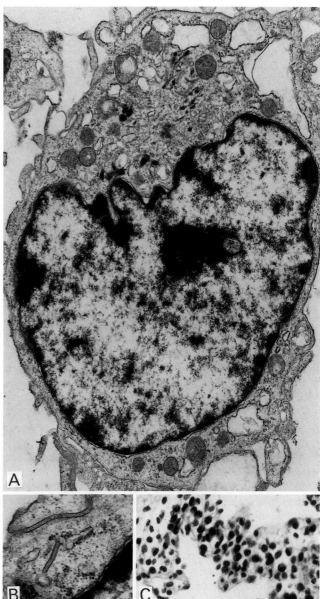

Fig. 8–70 A–C. A. Pulmonary histiocytosis X (Langerhans' cell histiocytosis) in infant shows numerous large cells of this type in lung biopsy by electron microscopy. Uranyl acetate and lead citrate, ×9,800. **B.** Cytoplasm contains pentalaminar Birbeck granules. Uranyl acetate and lead citrate, ×12,000. **C.** S-100 protein immunoreactivity in nucleus and cytoplasm are demonstrated in this collection of Langerhans' cells. Immunoperoxidase, ×400.

Metastatic tumor, as noted previously, is the type of pulmonary neoplasm from a child that is most frequently seen in our surgical pathology laboratory. Osteosarcoma to the lung is without question the malignancy that is most aggressively managed by surgical resection, since the lung is the site of metastatic disease

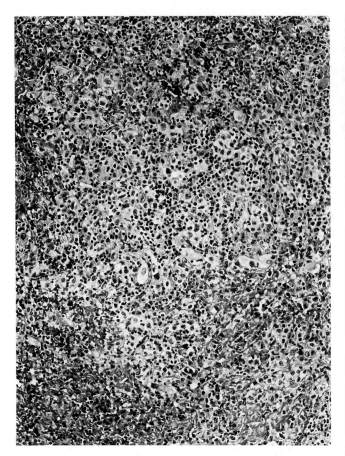

Fig. 8–71. Malignant lymphoma, predominantly large cell type, occurred in lung and liver of child who was bone marrow transplant recipient. Multiple nodules are present in chest radiograph; initially, patient was thought to have opportunistic infection. H and E, ×160.

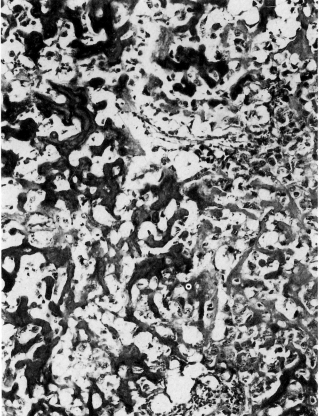

Fig. 8–72. Metastatic osteosarcoma presented this appearance in one of multiple nodules resected from lungs of 16-year-old boy. Histologic appearance of several lesions varies in terms of osteoid formation, cellularity, anaplasia, and extent of necrosis. On occasion, a nodule may consist only of mature trabecular bone or less mature woven bone. H and E, ×160.

in 75%–80% of cases.[464] In addition to chemotherapy, these patients may return to surgery several times for the resection of metastatic nodules through bilateral thoracotomies.[465] As many as 30–40 nodules measuring from 0.5 to 3 cm in diameter have been excised from the lung parenchyma. Some of the nodules are obviously calcified whereas others are firm to soft without mineralization. There is considerable microscopic diversity from one nodule to another from the same patient; bony trabeculae without an overtly neoplastic stroma to a purely anaplastic stroma constitute the range of findings (Fig. 8–72).[466] Between these extremes, the histologic appearance is clearly indicative of an osteosarcoma with dense strands of osteoid matrix situated among malignant-appearing mononuclear and multinucleated mesenchymal cells.

Wilms' tumor also has a predilection for metastasizing to the lungs. These metastases are often large and undergo cystic changes; pleural-based nodules are common as well (Fig. 8–73). Microscopically, the metastasis may recapitulate the primary tumor with a combination of blastoma and differentiated nephrogenic elements. On the other hand, the metastasis may show blastoma alone with or without cellular anaplasia or even a benign-appearing fibromatous mass.[467]

Clear cell sarcoma and the rhabdoid tumor are usually identifiable as such in the metastasis. Cellular mesoblastic nephroma with its uniform spindle cell features may rarely metastasize to the lungs.[468] Hepatoblastoma to the lungs resembles the primary tumor with its combined fetal and/or embryonal features.[469] Ewing's sarcoma and rhabdomyosarcoma may be difficult to differentiate on the basis of a small biopsy only since the crush artifacts affect virtually all small blue cell tumors in a similar manner. The tumor cells infiltrate along the alveolar septa and spill into the terminal air spaces with the formation of nodules that coalesce. Small vessels and capillaries may also contain collections of tumor

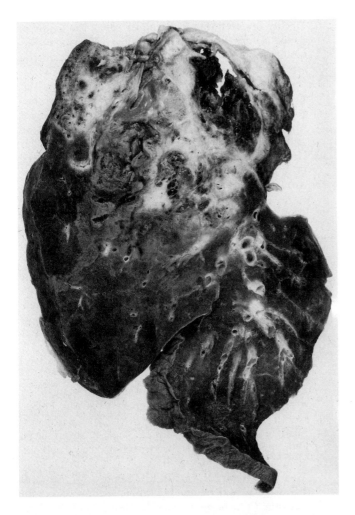

Fig. 8–73. Metastatic Wilms' tumor in lung resection shows large, partially cystic, solid mass occupying major portion of lobe. Metastasis often retains gross and microscopic features of primary tumor.

cells. Neuroblastoma generally does not metastasize to the pulmonary parenchyma until late in the clinical course. Only 20% of our autopsy cases of neuroblastoma had lung metastasis; pleural involvement was more common.

The malignant germ cell tumors, endodermal sinus tumor and mixed pattern germinal neoplasms, rather frequently produce pulmonary metastases in children with advanced clinical stage disease. Shortness of breath, chest pain, and multiple metastatic nodules in the lung of an adolescent male or female are the initial manifestations of a malignant germ cell tumor in a minority of patients. Other neoplasms in children that we have encountered as pulmonary metastases include nonkeratinizing squamous cell carcinoma, chordoma, various soft tissue sarcomas (angiosarcoma, synovial sarcoma, epithelioid sarcoma, fibrosarcoma, malignant schwannoma), and Hodgkin's disease.[470]

References

1. Schneider JR, St Cys JS, Thompson TR. The changing spectrum of cystic pulmonary lesions requiring surgical resection in infants. J Thorac Cardiovasc Surg 1985; 89:332–339.
2. Adeyemi SD, Ein SH, Simpson JS, Turner P. The value of emergency open lung biopsy in infants and children. J Pediatr Surg 1979;14:426–427.
3. Early GL, Williams TE, Kilman JW. Open lung biopsy. Its effects on therapy in the pediatric patient. Chest 1985;87:467–469.
4. Imoke E, Dudgeon DL, Colombani P, Leventhal B, Buck JR, Haller JA. Open lung biopsy in the immunocompromised pediatric patient. J Pediatr Surg 1983;18:816–820.
5. Prober CG, Whyte H, Smith CR. Open lung biopsy in immunocompromised children with pulmonary infiltrates. Am J Dis Child 1984;138:60–63.
6. Wolff LJ, Bartlett MS, Baehner RL, Grosfeld JL, Smith JW. The causes of interstitial pneumonitis in immunocompromised children: An aggressive systematic approach to diagnosis. Pediatrics 1977;60:41–45.
7. Leijala M, Louhimo I, Lindfors E-L. Open lung biopsy in children with diffuse pulmonary lesions. Acta Paediatr Scand 1982;71:717–720.
8. Fitzpatrick SB, Stokes, DC, Marsh B, Wang K-P. Transbronchial lung biopsy in pediatric and adolescent patients. Am J Dis Child 1985;139:46–49.
9. Diament MJ, Stanley P, Taylor S. Percutaneous fine needle biopsy in pediatrics. Pediatr Radiol 1985;15:409–411.
10. Towbin RB, Strife JL. Percutaneous aspiration, drainage and biopsies in children. Radiology 1985;157;81–85.
11. Lauweryns JM. "Hyaline membrane disease" in newborn infants. Hum Pathol 1970;1:175–204.
12. Seo IS, Gillim SE, Mirkin LD. Hyaline membranes in postmature infants. Pediatr Pathol 1990;10:539–548.
13. Lauweryns JM, Claessens S, Boussauw L. The pulmonary lymphatics in neonatal hyaline membrane disease. Pediatrics 1968;41:917–930.
14. Nakamura Y, Saitoh Y, Yamamoto I, Fukuda S, Hashimoto T. Regenerative process of hyaline membrane disease. Arch Pathol Lab Med 1988;112:821–824.
15. Fagan DG, Emery JL. A review and restatement of some problems in histological interpretation of the infant lung. Pediatr Pathol 1992;9:13–23.
16. Doshi N, Klionsky B, Fujikura T, MacDonald H. Pulmonary yellow hyaline membranes in neonates. Hum Pathol 1979;11:520–527.
17. Morgenstern B, Klionsky B, Doshi N. Yellow hyaline membrane disease. Lab Invest 1981;514–518.
18. Northway WH, Rosan RG, Porter DY. Pulmonary disease following therapy of hyaline membrane. N Engl J Med 1967;276:357–368.
19. Bancalari E, Abdenour GE, Feller R, Gannon J. Bronchopulmonary dysplasia: Clinical presentation. J Pediatr 1979;95:819–823.

20. Bancalari E. Pathogenesis of bronchopulmonary dysplasia: An overview. In: Bancalari E, Stocker JT, eds. Bronchopulmonary dysplasia. Washington, DC: Hemisphere, 1988:3–15.

21. Bancalari E, Gerhardt T. Bronchopulmonary dysplasia. Pediatr Clin North Am 1986;33:1–23.

22. Mayes L, Perkett E, Stahlman MT. Severe bronchopulmonary displasia: A retrospective review. Acta Pediatr Scand 1983;72:225–229.

23. Farrell PM. Bronchopulmonary dysplasia. In: Farrell PM, Taussig LM, eds. Bronchopulmonary dysplasia and related chronic respiratory disorders. Columbus: Ross Laboratories, 1986;1–6.

24. Bancalari E, Sosenko I. Pathogenesis and prevention of neonatal chronic lung disease: Recent developments. Pediatr Pulmonol 1990;8:109–116.

25. Stocker JT, Madewell JE. Persistent interstitial pulmonary emphysema. Another complication of the respiratory distress syndrome. Pediatrics 1977;59:847–857.

26. Fox WW, Spitzer AR. Treatment of lung injury in the early phases of bronchopulmonary dysplasia. In: Farrell PM, Taussig LM, eds. Bronchopulmonary dysplasia and related chronic disorders. Columbus: Ross Laboratories, 1986:115–120.

27. Frantz ID. Newer forms of ventilation for prevention or amelioration in bronchopulmonary dysplasia. In: Farrell PM, Taussig LM, eds. Bronchopulmonary dysplasia and related chronic respiratory disorders. Columbus: Ross Laboratories, 1986:135–144.

28. Moylan FMB, Walker AM, Kramer SS, Todres ID, Shannon DC. The relationship of bronchopulmonary dysplasia to the occurrence of alveolar rupture during positive pressure ventilation. Pediatrics 1975;55:783–787.

29. Boynton BR, Mannino FL, Davis RF, Kopotic RJ, Friederichsen G. Combined high-frequency oscillatory ventilation and intermittent mandatory ventilation in critically ill neonates. J Pediatr 1984;105:297–302.

30. Abman SH, Warady BA, Lum GM, Koops BL. Systemic hypertension in infants with bronchopulmonary dysplasia. J Pediatr 1984;104:928–931.

31. Ehrenkrantz RA, Bonta BW, Ablow RC, Warshaw JB. Amelioration of bronchopulmonary dysplasia after vitamin E administration. N Engl J Med 1978;299:564–569.

32. Moylan FMB, O'Connell KC, Todres ID, Shannon DC. Edema of the pulmonary interstitium in infants and children. Pediatrics 1975;55:783–787.

33. Logvinoff MM, Lumen RJ, Taussig LM, Lamont BA. Bronchodilators and diuretics in children with bronchopulmonary dysplasia. Pediatr Pulmonol 1985;1:198–203.

34. Mammel MC, Green TP, Johnson DE, Thompson TR. Controlled trial of dexamethasone therapy in infants with bronchopulmonary dysplasia. Lancet 1983;i:1356–1358.

35. Zachman RD. Vitamin A. In: Farrell PM, Taussig LM, eds. Bronchopulmonary dysplasia and related chronic respiratory disorders. Columbus: Ross Laboratories, 1986:86–96.

36. Liechty EA, Donovan E, Parohit D, et al. Reduction of neonatal mortality after multiple doses of bovine surfactant in low birth weight infants with respiratory distress syndrome. Pediatrics 1991;88:19–28.

37. Davis JM, Veness-Meehan K, Notter RH, Bhutani VK, Kendig JW, Shapiro DL. Changes in pulmonary mechanics after the administration of surfactant to infants with the respiratory distress syndrome. N Engl J Med 1988;319:476–479.

38. Hoekstra RE, Jackson JC, Myers TF, et al. Improved neonatal survival following multiple doses of bovine surfactant in very premature neonates at risk for respiratory distress syndrome. Pediatrics 1991;88:10–18.

39. Bose C, Corbet A, Bose G, et al. Improved outcome at 28 days of age for very low birthweight infants treated with a single dose of a synthetic surfactant. J Pediatr 1990;117:947–953.

40. Shapiro DC, Notter RH, eds. Surfactant replacement therapy. New York: Liss, 1989.

41. Davis JM, Richter SE, Kendig JW, Notter RH. High-frequency jet ventilation and surfactant treatment of newborns with severe respiratory failure. Pediatr Pulmonol 1992;13:108–112.

42. Merritt TA, Hallman M. Surfactant replacement. Am J Dis Child 1988;142:1333–1339.

43. Edwards DK, Dyer WM, Northway WH. Twelve years' experience with bronchopulmonary dysplasia. Pediatrics 1977;59:839–846.

44. Shankaran S, Szego E, Eizert D, Siegel P. Severe bronchopulmonary dysplasia: predictors of survival and outcome. Chest 1984;86:607–610.

45. Toce SS, Farrell PM, Leavitt LA, Samuels DP, Edwards DK. Clinical and roentgenographic scoring system for assessing bronchopulmonary dysplasia. Am J Dis Child 1984;138:581–585.

46. McCarthy K, Bhogal M, Nardi M, Hart D. Pathogenic factors in bronchopulmonary dysplasia. Pediatr Res 1984;18:483–487.

47. Nash G, Blennerhassett JB, Pantoppidan H. Pulmonary lesions associated with oxygen therapy and artificial respiration. N Engl J Med 1967;276:368–374.

48. Becker MJ, Koppe JG. Pulmonary structural changes in neonatal hyaline membrane disease treated with high pressure artificial respiration. Thorax 1969;24:689–694.

49. Northway WH, Rezeau L, Petriceks R, Bensch KG. Oxygen toxicity in the newborn lung: Reversal of inhibition of DNA synthesis in the mouse. Pediatrics 1976;57:41–46.

50. Bonikos DS, Bensch KG, Ludwin SK, Northway WH. Oxygen toxicity in the newborn. Lab Invest 1975;32:619–635.

51. Kapanci Y, Weibel ER, Kaplan HP, Robinson FR. Pathogenesis and reversibility of the pulmonary lesion of oxygen toxicity in monkeys. Lab Invest 1969;20:101–118.

52. Ludwin SK, Northway WH, Bensch KG. Oxygen toxicity in the newborn. Lab Invest 1974;31:425–435.

53. Pappas CTE, Obara H, Bensch KG, Northway WH.

Effect of prolonged exposure to 80% oxygen on the lung of the newborn mouse. Lab Invest 1983;48:735–748.

54. Taghizadeh A, Reynolds EOR. Pathogenesis of bronchopulmonary dysplasia following hyaline membrane disease. Am J Pathol 1976;82:241–258.

55. Rhodes PG, Graves GR, Patel DM, Campbell SB, Blumenthal BI. Minimizing pneumothorax and bronchopulmonary dysplasia in ventilated infants with hyaline membrane disease. J Pediatr 1983;103:634–637.

56. Brown ER, Stark A, Sosenko I, Lawson EE, Avery ME. Bronchopulmonary dysplasia: Possible relationship to pulmonary edema. J Pediatr 1978;92:982–984.

57. Pietra GG. New insights into mechanisms of pulmonary edema. Lab Invest 1984;51:489–494.

58. Ehrenkranz RA, Bonta BW, Ablow RC, Warshaw JB. Amelioration of bronchopulmonary dysplasia after vitamin E administration. N Engl J Med 1978;299:564–569.

59. Anderson WR, Strickland MB, Tsai SH, Haglin JJ. Light microscopic and ultrastructural study of the adverse effects of oxygen therapy on the neonate lung. Am J Pathol 1973;73:327–348.

60. Benerjee CK, Girling DJ, Wiggleworth JS. Pulmonary fibroplasia in newborn babies treated with oxygen and artificial ventilation. Arch Dis Child 1972;47:509–518.

61. Bonikos DS, Bensch KG, Northway WH, Edwards DK. Bronchopulmonary dysplasia: the pulmonary pathologic sequel of necrotizing bronchiolitis and fibrosis. Hum Pathol 1976;7:643–666.

62. Rosan CR. Hyaline membrane disease and a related spectrum of neonatal pneumopathies. Perspect Pediatr Pathol 1975;2:15–60.

63. Sobonya RA, Logvinoff MM, Taussig LM, Theriault A. Morphometric analysis of the lung in prolonged bronchopulmonary dysplasia. Pediatr Res 1982;16:969–972.

64. Anderson WR, Engel RR. Cardiopulmonary sequelae of reparative stages of bronchopulmonary dysplasia. Arch Pathol Lab Med 1983;107:603–608.

65. Stocker JT. The pathology of longstanding "healed" bronchopulmonary dysplasia. A study of 28 infants 3–40 months of age. Hum Pathol 1986;17:943–961.

66. Wiswell TE, Wiswell SH. The effect of 100% oxygen on the propagation of tracheobronchial injury during high-frequency and conventional mechanical ventilation. Am J Dis Child 1990;144:560–564.

67. Cordero L, Tallman RD, Qualman S, Gardner D. Necrotizing tracheobronchitis following high frequency ventilation: effect of hydrocortisone. Pediatr Pathol 1990; 10:663–670.

68. Margrof LR, Tomashefski JF, Bruce MC, Dahms BB. Morphometric analysis of the lung in bronchopulmonary dysplasia. Am Rev Respir Dis 1991;143:391–399.

69. Heath D, Edwards JE. The pathology of hypertensive pulmonary vascular disease. Circulation 1958;18:533–547.

70. Askin FB. Pulmonary interstitial air and pneumothorax in the neonate. In: Stocker JT, ed. Pediatric pulmonary disease. New York: Hemisphere, 1989:165–174.

71. Macklin MT, Macklin CC: Malignant interstitial emphysema of the lungs and mediastinum as an important occult complication in many respiratory diseases and other conditions. Medicine (Baltimore) 1944;23:281–358.

72. Caldwell EJ, Powell RD, Mullooly JP. Interstitial emphysema. A study of physiologic factors involved in experimental induction of the lesion. Am Rev Respir Dis 1970;102:516–525.

73. Thibeault DW, Lachman RS, Laul VR, Kwong MS. Pulmonary interstitial emphysema, pneumomediastinum and pneumothorax. Am J Dis Child 1973;126:611–614.

74. Wright AW. The local effect of the injection of gases into the subcutaneous tissues. Am J Pathol 1930;2:87–123.

75. Greenough A, Dixon AK, Robertson NRC. Pulmonary interstitial emphysema. Arch Dis Child 1984;59:1046–1051.

76. Hart SM, McNair M, Gdamsu HR, Price JF. Pulmonary interstitial emphysema in very low birth weight infants. Arch Dis Child 1983;58:612–615.

77. Gaylord MS, Thieme RE, Woodall DL, Quissell BJ. Predicting mortality in low-birth-weight infants with pulmonary interstitial emphysema. Pediatrics 1985;76:219–224.

78. Srouji MN, Buck B, Downes JJ. Congenital diaphragmatic hernia: deleterious effects of pulmonary interstitial emphysema and tension extrapulmonary air. J Pediatr Surg 1981;16:45–54.

79. Stocker JT, Drake RM, Madewell JE. Cystic and congenital lung disease in the newborn. Perspect Pediatr Pathol 1978;4:93–154.

80. Frantz ID, Warthammer J, Stark AR. High frequency ventilation in premature infants with lung disease: adequate gas exchange at low tracheal pressure. Pediatrics 1983;71:483–488.

81. Ng KPK, Easa D. Management of interstitial emphysema by high-frequency low positive-pressure hand ventilation in the neonate. J Pediatr 1979;95:117–118.

82. Campbell AN, Zarfin Y, Perlman M. Selective bronchial intubation for pulmonary emphysema. Arch Dis Child 1984;59:890–892.

83. Vahey TN, Pratt GB, Baum RS. Treatment of localized pulmonary interstitial emphysema with selective bronchial intubation. AJR 1983;140:1107–1109.

84. Mathew OP, Thach BT. Selective bronchial obstruction for treatment of bullous interstitial emphysema. J Pediatr 1980;86:475–477.

85. Seibert JJ, Dahlmann K, Hill DE. Selective left bronchial intubation for the treatment of pulmonary pseudocyst in the very premature infant. J Pediatr Surg 1984;19:198–199.

86. MacMahon P. Fleming PJ, Theaile MJ, Speidel BD. An improved selective bronchial intubation technique for managing severe localized interstitial emphysema. Acta Paediatr Scand 1982;71:151–153.

87. Cohen RS, Smith DW, Stevenson DK, Moskowitz PS, Graham CB. Lateral decubitus position as therapy for persistent focal pulmonary interstitial emphysema in neonates. A preliminary report. J Pediatr 1984;104:

441–442.

88. Swingle HM, Eggert LD, Bucciarelli RL. New approach to management of unilateal tension pulmonary interstitial emphysema in premature infants. Pediatrics 1984;74:354–357.

89. Bartlett RH, Andrews AF, Toomasian JM, Haiduc NJ, Gazzaniga AB. Extracorporeal membrane oxygenation for newborn respiratory failure: forty-five cases. Surgery 1982;92:425–433.

90. deBlio J, Scheinmann P, Paupe J. Successful treatment of persistent neonatal interstitial emphysema by flexible bronchoscopy. Lancet 1984;2:1389–1390.

91. Pear PRF, Conway SP. Treatment of severe bilateral interstitial emphysema in a baby by artificial pneumothorax and pneumonotomy. Lancet 1984;1:273–275.

92. Milligan DWA, Issler H, Masam M, Reynolds EOR. Treatment of neonatal pulmonary interstitial emphysema by lung puncture. Lancet 1984;1:1010–1011.

93. Reyes HM, Kagan RJ, Rowlatt UF, Vidyasagar D. Pulmonary interstitial emphysema—surgical management: report of three cases. J Pediatr Surg 1980;15:266–269.

94. Martinez-Frontanilla LA, Hernandez J, Haase GM, Burrington JD. Surgery of acquired lobar emphysema in the neonate. J Pediatr Surg 1984:19:375–379.

95. Levine DH, Trump DS, Waterkotti G. Unilateral pulmonary interstitial emphysema: a surgical approach to treatment. Pediatrics 1981;68:510–514.

96. Schneider JR, Cyr JA, Thompson TR, Johnson DE, Burke BA, Foker JE. The changing spectrums of cystic pulmonary lesions requiring surgical resection in infants. J Thorac Cardiovasc Surg 1985;89:332–339.

97. Brewer LL, Moskowitz PS, Carrington CB, Bursch KG. Pneumotosis pulmonalis: a complication of the idiopathic respiratory distress syndrome. Am J Pathol 1979;95:171–190.

98. Wood BP, Anderson VM, Mauk JE, Merritt TA. Pulmonary lymphatic air: locating "pulmonary interstitial emphysema" of the premature infant. AJR 1982;138:809–814.

99. Fletcher BD, Outerbridge EW, Youssef S, Bolande RP. Pulmonary interstitial emphysema in a newborn infant treated by lobectomy. Pediatrics 1974;54:808–811.

100. Magilner AD, Capitanio MA, Wertheimer I, Burke H. Persistent localized intrapulmonary interstitial emphysema: an observation in three infants. Radiology 1974;111:379–384.

101. Symchych PS, Cadotte M. Squamous metaplasia and necrosis of the trachea complicating prolonged nasotracheal intubation of small newborn infants. J Pediatr 1967;71:534–541.

102. Sackner MA, Landa JF, Greenletch N, Robinson MJ. Pathogenesis and prevention of tracheobronchial damage with suction procedures. Chest 1973;64:284–290.

103. Sotomayor JL, Godinez RI, Borden S, Wilmont RW. Large-airway collapse due to acquired tracheobronchomalacia in infancy. Am J Dis Child 1986;140:367–371.

104. Schild JP, Wuilloud A, Kollberg H, Bossi E. Trachael perforation as a complication of nasotracheal intubation

105. Scalzo AJ, Weber TR, Jaeger RW, Connors RH, Thompson MW. Extracorporeal membrane oxygenation for hydrocarbon aspiration. Am J Dis Child 1990;144:867–871.

106. Chou P, Shen-Schwarz S, Crawford SE, Blei ED, Crussi FG, Reynolds M. Pulmonary epithelial changes with extracorporeal membrane oxygenation (ECMO) therapy: Analysis of 17 autopsy cases. Mod Pathol 1991;4:2P.

107. Thomas HM, Irwin RS. Classification of diffuse intrapulmonary hemorrhage. Chest 1975;68:483–484.

108. Leatherman JW, Davies SF, Hoidal JR. Alveolar hemorrhage syndromes: Diffuse microvascular lung hemorrhage in immune and idiopathic disorders. Medicine (Baltimore) 1984;63:343–361.

109. Matthay RA, Bromberg SI, Putman CE. Pulmonary renal syndromes—a review. Yale J Biol Med 1980;53:497–533.

110. Rankin JA, Matthay RA. Pulmonary renal syndromes. II. Etiology and pathogenesis. Yale J Biol Med 1982;55:11–26.

111. Fedrick J, Butler NR. Certain causes of neonatal death. IV. Massive pulmonary haemorrhage. Biol Neonate 1971;18:243–261.

112. Bomsel F, Couchard M, Larroche J-Cl, Magder L. Diagnostic radiologique de l'hemorragie pulmonaire massive du nouveau-né. Ann Radiol (Paris) 1975;18:419–430.

113. Massive pulmonary haemorrhage in the newborn. (editorial). Br Med J 1973;3:553–554.

114. DeSa DJ, MacLean BS. An analysis of massive pulmonary haemorrhage in the newborn infant in Oxford, 1948–1968. Br J Obstet Gynecol 1970;77:158–163.

115. Landing BH. Pulmonary lesions of newborn infants. A statistical study. Pediatrics 1957;19:217–222.

116. McAdams AJ. Pulmonary hemorrhage in the newborn. Am J Dis Child 1967;113:255–262.

117. Roberts JT, Davies AJ, Bloom AL. Coagulation studies in massive pulmonary haemorrhage of the newborn. J Clin Pathol 1966;19:334–338.

118. Hurley R, Norman AP, Pryse-Davies J. Massive pulmonary haemorrhage in the newborn associated with coxsackie B virus infection. Br Med J 1969;3:636–637.

119. Ceballos R. Aspiration of maternal blood in the etiology of massive pulmonary hemorrhage in the newborn infant. J Pediatr 1968;72:390–393.

120. Sheffield LJ, Danks DM, Hammond JW, Hoogenraad NJ. Massive pulmonary hemorrhage as a presenting feature in congenital hyperammonemia. J Pediatr 1976;88:450–452.

121. Castile RG, Kleinberg F. The pathogenesis and management of massive pulmonary hemorrhage in the neonate. Case report of a normal survivor. Mayo Clin Proc 1976;51:155–158.

122. Yeung CY. Massive pulmonary hemorrhage in neonatal infection. Can Med Assoc J 1976;114:135–138.

123. Rowe S, Avery ME. Massive pulmonary hemorrhage in the newborn. II. Clinical considerations. J Pediatr 1966;69:12–20.

in a neonate. J Pediatr 1976;88:631–632.

124. Bhargava SK, Sharma BD, Saxena HMK, Ghosh S. Massive pulmonary hemorrhage in the newborn. Indian Pediatr 1970;7:46–48.

125. Trompeter R, Yu VYH, Aynsley-Green A, Roberton NRC. Massive pulmonary haemorrhage in the newborn infant. Arch Dis Child 1975;50:123–127.

126. Thomas DB. Survival after massive pulmonary haemorrhage in the neonatal period. Acta Paediatr Scand 1975;64:825–829.

127. Esterly JR, Oppenheimer EH. Massive pulmonary hemorrhage in the newborn. I. Pathologic considerations. J Pediatr 1966;69:3–11.

128. Keenan WJ, Altshuler G. Massive pulmonary hemorrhage in a neonate. J Pediatr 1975;86:466–471.

129. Adamson TM, Boyd RDH, Normand ICS, Reynolds EOR, Shaw JL. Haemorrhagic pulmonary oedema ("massive pulmonary haemorrhage") in the newborn. Lancet 1969;1:494–495.

130. Parker JC, Brown AL Jr, Harris LE. Pulmonary hemorrhages in the newborn. Mayo Clin Proc 1968;43:465–477.

131. Boothby CB, DeSa DJ. Massive pulmonary haemorrhage in the newborn. A changing pattern. Arch Dis Child 1973;48:21–30.

132. Cutz, E. Idiopathic pulmonary hemosiderosis and related disorders in infancy and childhood. Perspect Pediatr Pathol 1987;11:47–81.

133. Kjellman B, Elinder G, Garwicz S, Svan H. Idiopathic pulmonary hemosiderosis in Swedish children. Acta Paediatr Scand 1984;73:584–588.

134. Cassimos CD, Chryssanthopoulos C, Panagiotidou C. Epidemiologic observations in idiopathic pulmonary hemosiderosis. J Pediatr 1983;102:698–702.

135. Soergel KH, Sommers SC. Idiopathic pulmonary hemosiderosis and related syndromes. Am J Med 1962;32:499–511.

136. Beckerman RC, Taussig LM, Pinnas JI. Familial idiopathic pulmonary hemosiderosis. Am J Dis Child 1979;133:609–611.

137. Breckenridge RI, Jr., Ross JS. Idiopathic pulmonary hemosiderosis. A report of familial occurrence. Chest 1979;75:636–638.

138. O'Donohue WJ. Idiopathic pulmonary hemosiderosis with manifestations of multiple connective tissue and immune disorders. Am Rev Respir Dis 1984;109:473–479.

139. Rafferty JR, Cook MK. Idiopathic pulmonary hemosiderosis with autoimmune haemolytic anemia. Br J Dis Chest 1984;78:282–285.

140. Lee SK, Kniker WT, Cook CD, Heiner DC. Cow's milk-induced pulmonary disease in children. Adv Pediatr 1978;25:39–57.

141. Valletta EA, Cipolli M, Cazzola G, Mastella G. Pulmonary hemosiderosis in a child with cystic fibrosis. Helv Paediatr Acta 1988;43:487–490.

142. Kurzweil PR, Miller DR, Freeman JE, Reiman RE, Mayer K. Use of sodium chromate CR_{51} in diagnosing childhood idiopathic pulmonary hemosiderosis. Am J Dis Child 1984;138:746–748.

143. Chryssanthopoulos C, Cassimos C, Panagiotidou C. Prognostic criteria in idiopathic pulmonary hemosiderosis in children. Eur J Pediatr 1983;140:123–125.

144. Yaeger H, Jr., Powell D, Weinberg RM, Bauer H, Bellanti JA, Katz S. Idiopathic pulmonary hemosiderosis. Ultrastructural studies and response to azathioprine. Arch Intern Med 1976;136:1145–1149.

145. Gonzalez-Crussi F, Hull MT, Grosfeld JL. Idiopathic pulmonary hemosiderosis: Evidence of capillary basement membrane abnormality. Am Rev Respir Dis 1976;114:689–698.

146. Corrin B, Jagusch M, Dewar A, et al. Fine structural changes in idiopathic pulmonary haemosiderosis. J Pathol 1987;153:249–256.

147. Cutz E. Idiopathic pulmonary hemosiderosis and related disorders in infancy and childhood. Perspect Pediatr Pathol 1987;11:47–81.

148. Dolan J, McGuire S, Sweeney E, Bourke J, Ward OC. Mast cells in pulmonary hemosiderosis. Arch Dis Child 1984;59:276–278.

149. Levin M, Rigden SPA, Pincott JR, Lockwood CM, Barratt TM, Dillon MJ. Goodpasture's syndrome: Treatment with plasmapheresis, immunosuppression and anticoagulation. Arch Dis Child 1983;58:697–702.

150. Martini A, Binda S, Mariani G, Scotta MS, Ruberto G. Goodpasture's syndrome in a child: Natural history and effect of treatment. Acta Paediatr Scand 1981;70:435–439.

151. Harman EM. Immunologic lung disease. Med Clin North Am 1985;69:705–714.

152. Leatherman JW, Sibley RK, Davies SF. Diffuse intrapulmonary hemorrhage and glomerulonephritis unrelated to anti-glomerular basement membrane antibody. Am J Med 1982;72:401–410.

153. Walker RG, Scheinkestel C, Becker GJ, Owen JE, Dowling JP, Kincaid-Smith P. Clinical and morphologic aspects of the management of crescentic antiglomerular basement membrane antibody (anti-GBM) nephritis/Goodpasture's syndrome. Q J Med 1985;54:75–89.

154. Hoffman GS, Kerr GS, Leavitt RY, et al. Wegener's granulomatosis: An analysis of 158 patients. Ann Intern Med 1992;116:488–498.

155. Singer J, Suchet I, Horwitz T. Paediatric Wegener's granulomatosis: Two case histories and a review of the literature. Clin Radiol 1990;42:50–51.

156. Hunninghake CW, Fauli AS. Pulmonary involvement in the collagen vascular disease. Am Rev Respir Dis 1979;119:471–503.

157. DeRemee RA, Weiland LH, McDonald TJ. Respiratory vasculitis. Mayo Clin Proc 1980;55:492–498.

158. Mark EJ, Ramirez JF. Pulmonary capillaritis and hemorrhage in patients with systemic vasculitis. Arch Pathol Lab Med 1985;109:413–418.

159. Eagan JW, Memoli VA, Roberts JL, Matthew GR, Schwartz MM, Lewis EJ. Pulmonary hemorrhage in systemic lupus erythematosus. Medicine (Baltimore) 1978;57:545–560.

160. Miller LR, Greenberg SD, McLarty JW. Lupus lung. Chest 1985;88:265–269.

161. Carette S, Marcher AM, Nussbaum A, Plotz PH. Severe, acute pulmonary disease in patients with systemic lupus erythematosus: Ten years of experience at the National Institutes of Health. Semin Arthritis Rheum 1984;14: 52–59.

162. Miller RW, Salcedo JR, Fink RJ, Murphy TM, Magilavy DB. Pulmonary hemorrhage in pediatric patients with systemic lupus erythematosus. J Pediatr 1986;108:576–579.

163. Myers JL, Katzenstein A-LA. Microangiitis in lupus-induced pulmonary hemorrhage. Am J Clin Pathol 1986;85:552–556.

164. Fauci AS, Haynes BF, Katz P, Wolff SM. Wegener's granulomatosis: prosective clinical and therapeutic experience with 85 patients for 21 years. Ann Intern Med 1983;98:76–85.

165. Hall SL, Miller LC, Duggan E, Mauer SM, Beatty EC, Hellerstein S. Wegener granulomatosis in pediatric patients. J Pediatr 1985;106:739–744.

166. Chandler DB, Fulmer JD. Pulmonary vasculitis. Lung 1985;163:257–273.

167. Yoshikawa Y, Watanabe T. Pulmonary lesions in Wegener's granulomatosis: A clinicopathologic study of 22 autopsy cases. Hum Pathol 1986;17:401–410.

168. Fortoul TI, Cano-Valle F, Oliva E, Barrios R. Follicular bronchiolitis in association with connective tissue diseases. Lung 1985;163:305–314.

169. Lanham JG, Elkon KB, Pusey CD, Hughes GR. Systemic vasculitis with asthma and eosinophilia. A clinical approach to the Churg-Strauss syndrome. Medicine (Baltimore) 1984;63:65–81.

170. Avery MD, Fletcher BD, Williams RG. The lung and its disorders in the newborn infant. 4th Ed. Philadelphia: WB Saunders, 1981:203–221.

171. Klein JO, Remington JS, Marcy SM. Current concepts of infections of the fetus and newborn infant. In: Remington JS, Klein JO, eds. Infectious diseases of the fetus and newborn infant. 2nd Ed. Philadelphia: WB Saunders, 1983:1–26.

172. Ingall D, Musher D: Syphilis. In: Remington JS, Klein JO, eds. Infectious diseases of the fetus and newborn infant. 2d Ed. Philadelphia: WB Saunders, 1983:335–374.

173. Klein JO. Bacterial infections of the respiratory tract. In: Remington JS, Klein JO, eds. Infectious diseases of the fetus and newborn infant. 2d Ed. Philadelphia: WB Saunders, 1983:736–754.

174. Santos JI, Hill HR. Bacterial infections of the neonate. In: Wedgwood RJ, Davis SD, Ray CG, Kelley VC, eds. Infections in children. Philadelphia: Harper & Row, 1982;179–202.

175. Schachter J, Grossman M. Chlamydia. In: Remington JS, Klein JO, eds. Infectious diseases of the fetus and newborn infant. 2d Ed. Philadelphia: WB Saunders, 1983:450–463.

176. Wigglesworth JS. Perinatal infection. In: Bennington JL, ed. Perinatal pathology. Philadelphia: WB Saunders, 1984:137–167.

177. Potter EL, Craig JM. Pathology of the fetus and the infant. 3d Ed. Chicago: Year Book Medical, 1975;121–149.

178. Singer DB. Infections of fetuses and neonates. In: Wigglesworth JS, Singer DB, eds. Textbook of fetal and perinatal pathology. Boston: Blackwell, 1991:525–591.

179. Naeye RL, Dellinger WS, Blanc WA. Fetal and maternal features of antenatal bacterial infections. J Pediatr 1971;79:733–739.

180. Hammerschlag MR. Nonbacterial infections of the neonate. In: Wedgwood RJ, Davis SD, Ray CG, Kelley VC, eds. Infections in children. Philadelphia: Harper & Row, 1982:203–227.

181. Davies PA, Aherne W. Congenital pneumonia. Arch Dis Child 1962;37:598–602.

182. Dworsky ME, Stagno S. Newer agents causing pneumonitis in early infancy. Pediatr Infect Dis 1982;1:188–195.

183. Barter RA, Hudson JA. Bacteriological findings in perinatal pneumonia. Pathology 1974;6:223–230.

184. Langley FA, Smith JAM. Perinatal pneumonia: a retrospective study. J Obstet Gynaecol Br Empire 1959;66: 12–25.

185. Dworsky ME, Stagno S. Newer agents causing pneumonitis in early infancy. Pediatr Infect Dis 1982;1:188–195.

186. Barter R. The histopathology of congenital pneumonia: A clinical and experimental study. J Pathol 1983;66: 407–415.

187. Sherman MP, Goetzman BW, Ahlfors CE, Wennberg RP. Tracheal aspiration and its clinical correlation in the diagnosis of congenital pneumonia. Pediatrics 1980;65:258–263.

188. Bernstein J, Wang J. The pathology of neonatal pneumonia. Am J Dis Chld 1961;101:350–363.

189. Hanshaw JB, Dudgeon JA. Congenital cytomegalovirus. Maj Probl Clin Pediatr 1978;17:97–152.

190. Stagno S, Whitley RJ. Herpes virus infections of pregnancy. Part I: Cytomegalovirus and Epstein-Barr virus infections. N Engl J Med 1985;713:1270–1274.

191. Stagno S, Pass RF, Dworsky ME, Britt WJ, Alford CA. Congenital and perinatal cytomegalovirus infections: clinical characteristics and pathogenic factors. Birth Defects 1984;20:65–85.

192. Preece PM, Pearl KN, Peckham CS. Congenital cytomegalovirus infection. Arch Dis Child 1984;59:1120–1126.

193. Schopfer K, Lauber E, Krech U. Congenital cytomegalovirus infection in newborn infants of mothers infected before pregnancy. Arch Dis Child 1978;53:536–539.

194. McCracken GH, Shinefield HR, Cobb K, Rausen AR, Dische MR, Eichenwald HF. Congenital cytomegalic inclusion disease. A longitudinal study of 20 patients. Am J. Dis Child 1969;117:522–539.

195. Pass RF, Stagno S, Myers GJ, Alford CA. Outcome of symptomatic congenital cytomegalovirus infection: results of long-term longitudinal follow-up. Pediatrics 1980;66:758–762.

196. Stagno S, Brasfield DM, Brown MB, et al. Infant pneumonitis associated with cytomegalovirus, *Chalamydia*, *Pneumocystis* and *Ureaplasma*: a prospective study. Pedi-

atrics 1981;68:322–329.

197. Smith SD, Cho CT, Brahmacupta N, Lenahan MF. Pulmonary involvement with cytomegalovirus infections in children. Arch Dis Child 1977;52:441–446.

198. Kim YJ, Gururaj VJ, Mirkovic RR. Concomitant diffuse nodular pulmonary infiltration in an infant with cytomegalovirus infection. Pediatr Infect Dis 1982;1:173–176.

199. Whitley RJ, Brasfield D, Reynolds DW, Stagno S, Tiller RE, Alford CA. Protracted pneumonitis in young infants associated with perinatally acquired cytomegaloviral infection. J Pediatr 1976;89:16–22.

200. Becroft DMO. Prenatal cytomegalovirus infection: epidemiology, pathology and pathogenesis. Perspect Pediatr Pathol 1981;6:203–241.

201. Nakamura Y, Komatsu Y, Hosokawa Y, et al. Generalized cytomegalic inclusion disease in neonates and infants. Acta Pathol Jpn 1980;30:347–354.

202. Benirschke K, Mendoza GR, Bazeley PL. Placental and fetal manifestations of cytomegalovirus infection. Virchows Arch (Cell Pathol) 1974;16:121–139.

203. Hamazaki M. Histological study of congenital and acquired cytomegalovirus infection. Acts Pathol Jpn 1983;33:89–96.

204. Stocker JT: Congenital cytomegalovirus infection presenting as massive ascites with secondary pulmonary hypoplasia. Hum Pathol 1985;16:1173–1175.

205. Becroft DMO. Prenatal cytomegalovirus infection and muscular deficiency (eventration) of the diaphragm. J Pediatr 1979;94:74–75.

206. Stagno S, Whitley RJ. Herpes virus infections of pregnancy. Part II: Herpes simplex virus and varicella-zoster virus infections. N Engl J Med 1985;313:1327–1330.

207. Corey L, Spear PG. Infections with herpes simplex viruses. (First of two parts.) N Engl J Med 1986;314:686–691.

208. Corey L, Spear PG. Infections with herpes simplex viruses. (Second of two parts.) N Engl J Med 1986;314:749–756.

209. Nahmais AJ, Schwahn MG. Neonatal herpes simplex: a worldwide disease which is potentially preventable and treatable. Prog Clin Biol Res 1985;163B:355–362.

210. Andiman WA. Congenital herpes virus infections. Clin Perinatol 1979;6:331–346.

211. Committee on fetus and newborn. Perinatal herpes simplex virus infections. Pediatrics 1980;66:147–148.

212. Whitley RJ, Nahmias AJ, Visintine AM, Fleming CL, Alford CA. The natural history of herpes simplex virus infection of mother and newborn. Pediatrics 1980;66:489–494.

213. Honig PJ, Holzwanger J, Leyden JJ. Congenital herpes simplex virus infection. Report of three cases and review of the literature. Arch Dermatol 1979;115:1329–1333.

214. Lissauer TJ, Shaw PJ, Underhill G. Neonatal herpes simplex pneumonia. Arch Dis Child 1984;59:668–670.

215. Hull HF, Blumhagen JD, Benjamin D, Corey L. Herpes simplex viral pneumonitis in childhood. J Pediatr 1984;104:211–215.

216. Dominguez R, Rivero H, Gaisie G, Talmachoff P, Amortegvi A, Young LW: Neonatal herpes simplex pneu-

monia: radiographic findings. Radiology 1984;153:395–399.

217. Drut RM, Drut R. Congenital herpes simplex virus infections in diagnosed by cytology of aspirated tracheobronchial material. Acta Cytol (Baltimore) 1985;29:712–713.

218. Singer DB. Pathology of neonatal herpes simplex virus infection. Perspect Pediatr Pathol 1981;6:243–278.

219. Watanabe K, Tanaka J, Hatano M, et al. Generalized neonatal herpes virus infection (cytomegalovirus or herpes virus type 1). Comparative examination of loci attacked by two viruses. Acta Pathol Jpn 1984;34:847–858.

220. Nakamura Y, Yamamoto S, Tanaka S, et al. Herpes simplex viral infection in human neonates: an immunohistochemical and electron microscopic study. Hum Pathol 1985;16:1091–1097.

221. Anderson GH, Matisic JP, Thomas BA. Confirmation of genital herpes simplex viral infections by an immunoperoxidase technique. Acta Cytol (Baltimore) 1985;29:695–700.

222. Schaefer HE. Inflammatory disease of the human lung of definite or presumed viral origin. Cytologic and histologic topics. Curr Top Pathol 1983;73:153–205.

223. Paryani SG, Arvin AM. Intrauterine infection with varicella-zoster virus after maternal varicella. N Engl J Med 1986;314:1542–1546.

224. Brunell PA. Fetal and neonatal varicella-zoster infections. Semin Perinatol 1983;7:47–56.

225. Enders G. Varicella-zoster virus infection in pregnancy. Prog Med Virol 1984;29:166–196.

226. Brewer TF. Congenital varicella with primary varicella pneumonia. Calif Med 1980;92:350–353.

227. Cooper LZ. The history and medical consequences of rubella. Rev Infect Dis 1985;7(Suppl. 1):S2–S10.

228. Sever JL. Congenital rubella. Clin Perinatol 1979;6:347–352.

229. Bart KJ, Orenstein WA, Pueblud SR, Hinman AR, Lewis F Jr, Williams NM. Elimination of rubella and congenital rubella from the United States. Pediatr Infect Dis 1985;4:14–21.

230. Rosenberg HS, Oppenheimer Eh, Esterly JR. Congenital rubella syndrome: the late effects and their relation to early lesions. Perspect Pediatr Pathol 1981;6:183–202.

231. Menser MA, Reye RDK. The pathology of congenital rubella: A review written by request. Pathology 1974;6:215–222.

232. Phelan P, Campbell P. Pulmonary complications of rubella embryopathy. J Pediatr 1969;75:202–212.

233. Boner A, Wilmott RW, Dinwiddie R, et al. Desquamative interstitial pneumonia and antigen-antibody complexes in two infants with congenital rubella. Pediatrics 1983;72:835–839.

234. Lallemand AV, Gaillard DA, Paradis PH, Chippaux CG. Fetal listeriosis during the second trimester of gestation. Pediatr Pathol 1992;12:665–671.

235. Seeliger HPR, Finger H. Listeriosis. In: Remington JS, Klein JO, eds. Infectious diseases of the fetus and newborn infant. 2d Ed. Philadelphia: WB Saunders, 1983:

264–289.

236. Vawter GF. Perinatal listeriosis. Perspect Pediatr Pathol 1981;6:153–166.

237. Rolfs RT, Nakashima AK. Epidemiology of primary and secondary syphilis in the United States, 1981 through 1989. JAMA 1990;264:1432–1437.

238. Ricci JM, Fojaco RM, O'Sullivan MJ. Congenital syphilis: The University of Miami/Jackson Memorial Medical Center experience, 1986–1988. Obstet Gynecol 1989; 74:687–693.

239. Ikeda MK, Jenson HB. Evaluation and treatment of congenital syphilis. J Pediatr 1990;117:843–852.

240. Oppenheimer EH, Dahms BB. Congenital syphilis in the fetus and neonate. Perspect Pediatr Pathol 1981;6:115–138.

241. Feldman HA, Epidemiology of *Toxoplasma* infections. Epidemiol Rev 1982;4:204–213.

242. Remington JS, Desmonts G. Toxoplasmosis. In: Remington JS, Klein JO, eds. Infectious diseases of the fetus and newborn infant. 2d Ed. Philadelphia: WB Saunders, 1983:143–263.

243. Desmonts G, Couvreur J. Congenital toxoplasmosis. A prospective study of 378 pregnancies. N Engl J Med 1974;290:1110–1116.

244. Stray-Pederson B. Infants potentially at risk for congenital toxoplasmosis. A prospective study. Am J Dis Child 1980;134:638–642.

245. Stagno S. Congenital toxoplasmosis. Am J Dis Child 1980;134:635–637.

246. Dische MR, Gooch WM III. Congenital toxoplasmosis. Perspect Pediatr Pathol 1981;6:83–113.

247. Indacochea FJ, Scott GB. HIV-1 infection and the acquired immunodeficiency syndrome in children. Curr Probl Pediatr 1992;22:166–204.

248. Rubinstein A. Pulmonary disease in children infected by the human immunodeficiency virus. Semin Respir Med 1990;11:248–252.

249. Sanders-Laufer D, DeBruin W, Edelson PJ. *Pneumocystis carinii* infections in HIV-infected children. Pediatr Clin North Am 1991;38:69–88.

250. Nauseef WM. Pulmonary disease in other acquired and primary immunodeficiencies. Semin Respir Med 1989; 10:21–29.

251. Pitt, J. Lymphocytic interstitial pneumonia. Pediatr Clin North Am 1991;38:89–95.

252. Joshi VV. Pathology of acquired immunodeficiency syndrome (AIDS) in children. In: Joshi VV, ed. Pathology of AIDS and other manifestations of HIV infection. New York: Igaku-Shoin, 1990:239–270.

253. Travis WD, Fox CH, Devaney KO, et al. Lymphoid pneumonitis in 50 adult patients infected with the human immunodeficiency virus: Lymphocytic interstitial pneumonitis versus nonspecific interstitial pneumonitis. Hum Pathol 1992;23:529–541.

254. Young SA, Crocker DW. Burkitt's lymphoma in a child with AIDS. Pediatr Pathol 1991;11:115–121.

255. Krober MS, Bass JW, Powell JM, Smith FR, Seto DSY. Bacterial and viral pathogens causing fever in infants less than three months old. Am J Dis Child 1985;139: 889–892.

256. Webber S, Wilkinson AR, Lindsell D, Hope PL, Dobson SRM, Isaacs D. Neonatal pneumonia. Arch Dis Child 1990;65:207–211.

257. Klein JO. Bacterial infections of the respiratory tract. In: Remington JS, Klein JO, eds. Infectious diseases of the fetus and newborn infants. 3d Ed. Philadelphia: WB Saunders, 1990:656–673.

258. Baker CJ, Edwards MS. Group B streptococcal infections. In: Remington JS, Klein JO, eds. Infectious diseases of the fetus and newborn infant. 3d Ed. Philadelphia: WB Saunders, 1990:742–811.

259. Dillon HC, Jr., Gray BM. Infections caused by group B streptococci: Perinatal, neonatal and early infancy. In: Wedgwood RJ, Davis SD, Ray CG, Kelley VG, eds. Infections in children. Philadelphia: Harper & Row, 1982:567–579.

260. Ferrieri P. GBS infections in the newborn infant: diagnosis and treatment. Antibiot Chemother 1985;35:211–224.

261. Boyer KM, Gotoff SP. Prevention of early-onset neonatal group B streptococcal disease with selective intrapartum chemoprophylaxis. N Engl J Med 1986;314:1665–1669.

262. Christensen KK, Svenningsen N, Dahlander K, Ingemarsson E, Linden V, Christensen P. Relation between neonatal pneumonia and maternal carriage of group B streptococci. Scand J Infect Dis 1982;14:261–266.

263. Christensen KK, Christensen P, Dahlander K, Linden V, Lindroth M, Svenningsen N. The significance of group B streptococci in neonatal pneumonia. Eur J Pediatr 1983;140:118–122.

264. Ablow RC, Driscoll SG, Effmann EL, et al. A comparison of early-onset group B streptococcal neonatal infection and the respiratory-distress syndrome of the newborn. N Engl J Med 1976;294:65–70.

265. Katzenstein A-L, Davis C, Braude A. Pulmonary changes in neonatal sepsis due to group B β-hemolytic *Streptococcus:* Relation to hyaline membrane disease. J Infect Dis 1976;133:430–435.

266. Banagale RC, Watters JH. Delayed right-sided diaphragmatic hernia following group B streptococcal infection: A discussion of its pathogenesis, with a review of the literature. Hum Pathol 1983;14:67–69.

267. Craig JM. Group B beta hemolytic streptococcal sepsis in the newborn. Perspect Pediatr Pathol 1981;6:139–151.

268. Schachter J, Grossman M. Chlamydial infections. Annu Rev Med 1981;32:45–61.

269. Schachter J. Chlamydial infections (first of three parts). N Engl J Med 1978;298:428–435.

270. Schachter J. Chlamydial infections (second of three parts). N Engl J Med 1978;298:490–495.

271. Schachter J. Chlamydial infections (third of three parts). N Engl J Med 1978;298:540–549.

272. Bell TA. *Chlamydia trachomatis, Mycoplasma hominis,* and *Ureaplasma urealyticum* infections of infants. Semin Perinatal 1985;9:29–37.

273. Alexander ER, Harrison HR. Role of *Chlamydia trachomatis* in perinatal infection. Rev Infect Dis 1983;5:713–719.

274. Schaad UB, Rossi E. Infantile chlamydial pneumonia—A review based on 115 cases. Eur J Pediatr 1982;138:105–109.

275. Schachter J, Gross M, Sweet RL, Holt J, Jordan C, Bishop E. Prospective study of perinatal transmission of *Chlamydia trachomatis.* JAMA 1986;255:3374–3377.

276. Beem MO, Saxon EM. Respiratory-tract colonization and a distinctive pneumonia syndrome in infants infected with *Chlamydia trachomatis.* N Engl J Med 1977;296:306–310.

277. Harrison HR, English MG, Lee CK, Alexander ER. *Chlamydia trachomatis* infant pneumonitis. N Engl J Med 1978;298:702–708.

278. Attenburrow AA, Barker GM. Chlamydial pneumonia in the low birth-weight neonate. Arch Dis Child 1985;60;1169–1172.

279. Griffin M, Pushpanathan C, Andrews W. *Chlamydia trachomatis* pneumonitis: A case study and literature review. Pediatr Pathol 1990;10:843–852.

280. Schachter J, Sweet RL, Grossman M, Landers D, Robbie M, Bishop E. Experience with the routine use of erythromycin for chlamydia infections in pregnancy. N Engl J Med 1986;314:276–279.

281. Arth C, Von Schmidt B, Grossman M, Schachter J. Chlamydia pneumonitis. J Pediatr 1978;93:447–449.

282. Jennings LC, Dawson KP, Abbott GD, Allan J. Acute respiratory tract infections of children in hospital: A viral and *Mycoplasma pneumoniae* profile. NZ Med J 1985;98:582–585.

283. Broughton RA, Infections due to *Mycoplasma pneumoniae* in childhood. Pediatr Infect Dis 1986 1986;5:71–85.

284. Rollins S, Colby T, Clayton F. Open lung biopsy in *Mycoplasma pneumoniae* pneumonia. Arch Pathol Lab Med 1986;110:34–41.

285. Braun MM, Cauthen G. Relationship of the human immunodeficiency virus epidemic to pediatric tuberculosis and bacillus Calmette-Guerin immunization. Pediatr Infect Dis 1992;11:220–227.

286. Starke JR, Jacobs RF, Jereb J. Resurgence of tuberculosis in children. J Pediatr 1992;120:839–855.

287. Kendig EL Jr, Inselman LS. Tuberculosis in children. Adv Pediatr 1991;38:233–255.

288. Amodio J, Abramson S, Berdon W. Primary pulmonary tuberculosis in infancy: A resurgent disease in the urban United States. Pediatr Radiol 1986;16:185–189.

289. Powell K, Meador M, Farer L. Recent trends in tuberculosis in children. JAMA 1984;251:1289–1292.

290. Powell DA, Walker DH. Nontuberculous myobacterial endobronchitis in children. J Pediatr 1980;96:268–271.

291. Nemir RL, O'Hare D. Congenital tuberculosis. Review and diagnostic guidelines. Am J Dis Child 1985;139:284–287.

292. Lamont AC, Cremin BJ, Pelteret RM. Radiological patterns of pulmonary tuberculosis in the paediatric age group. Pediatr Radiol 1986;16:2–7.

293. Hageman J, Shulman S, Schreiber M, Luck S, Yogev R. Congenital tuberculosis: Critical reappraisal of clinical findings and diagnostic procedures. Pediatrics 1980;66:980–984.

294. Stallworth JR, Brasfield DM, Tiller RE. Congenital miliary tuberculosis proved by open lung biopsy specimen and successfully treated. Am J Dis Child 1980;134:320–321.

295. Machin GA, Honore' LH, Fanning EA, Molesky M. Perinatally acquired neonatal tuberculosis: Report of two cases. Pediatr Pathol 1992;12:707–716.

296. Delprado WJ, Baird PJ, Russell P. Placental candidiasis: Report of three cases with a review of the literature. Pathology 1982;14:191–195.

297. Smith H, Congdon P. Neonatal systemic candidiasis. Arch Dis Child 1985;60:365–369.

298. Patriquin H, Lebowitz R, Perreault G, Yousefzadeh D. Neonatal candidiasis: Renal and pulmonary manifestations. AJR 1980;135:1205–1210.

299. Kassner EG, Kauffman SL, Yoon JJ, Semiglia M, Kozinn PJ, Goldberg PL. Pulmonary candidiasis in infants: Clinical, radiologic and pathologic features. AJR 1981;137:707–716.

300. Miller MJ. Fungal infections. In: Remington JS, Klein JO, eds. Infectious diseases of the fetus and newborn infant. 3d Ed. Philadelphia: WB Saunders, 1990:475–515.

301. Child DD, Newell JD, Bjelland JC, Spark RP. Radiographic findings of pulmonary coccidioidomycosis in neonates and infants. AJR 1985;145:261–263.

302. Sanders-Laufer D, DeBruin W, Edelson PJ. *Pneumocystis carinii* infections in HIV-infected children. Pediatr Clin North Am 1991;38:69–88.

303. Bernstein LJ, Bye MR, Rubinstein A. Prognostic factors and life expectancy in children with acquired immunodeficiency syndrome and *Pneumocystis carinii* pneumonia. Am J Dis Child 1989;143:775–778.

304. Stagno S, Pifer LL, Hughes WT, Brasfield DM, Tiller RI. *Pneumocystis carinii* pneumonitis in young immunocompetent infants. Pediatrics 1980;66:56–62.

305. Leigh MW, Henshaw NG, Wood RE. Diagnosis of *Pneumocystis carinii* pneumonia in pediatric patients using bronchoscopic bronchoalveolar lavage. Pediatr Infect Dis 1985;4:408–410.

306. McIntosh K, Fishaut JM. Immunopathologic mechanisms in lower respiratory tract disease of infants due to respiratory syncytial virus. Prog Med Virol 1980;26:94–118.

307. Stott EJ, Taylor G. Respiratory syncytial virus. Brief review. Arch Virol 1985;84:1–52.

308. Glezen WP, Denny FW. Epidemiology of acute lower respiratory tract disease in children. N Engl J Med 1973;288:498–505.

309. Henderson FW, Collier AM, Clyde WA Jr, Denny FW. Respiratory-syncytial-virus infections, reinfections and immunity. A prospective, longitudinal study in young children. N Engl J Med 1979;300:530–534.

310. Ericksson J, Nordshus T, Carlsen K-H. Orstadvik I, Westvik J, Eng J. Radiological findings in children with respiratory syncytial virus infection: relationship to clinical and bacteriological findings. Pediatr Radiol 1986;16:120–122.

311. MacDonald NE, Hall CB, Suffin SC, Alexson C, Harris PJ, Manning JA Respiratory syncytial virus infection in infants with congenital heart disease. N Engl J Med 1982;307:397–400.

312. Delage G, Brochu P, Robillard L, Jasmin G, Joncas JH, Lapointe N. Giant cell pneumonia due to respiratory syncytial virus. Occurrence in severe combined immunodeficiency syndrome. Arch Pathol Lab Med 1983;108:623–625.

313. Hall CB, Powell KR, MacDonald NE, et al. Respiratory syncytial viral infection in children with compromised immune function. N Engl J Med 1986;315:77–80.

314. Groothuis JR, Salbenblatt CK, Lauer BA. Severe respiratory syncytial virus infection in older children. Am J Dis Child 1990;144:346–348.

315. Chandwani S, Borkowsky W, Krasinski K, Lawrence R, Welliver R. Respiratory syncytial virus infection in human immunodeficiency virus-infected children. J Pediatr 1990;117:251–254.

316. Mounts P, Shah KV. Respiratory papillomatosis: Etiologic relation to genital tract papillomavirus. Prog Med Virol 1984;29:90–114.

317. Mounts P, Wu TC, Leventhal B, et al. Analysis of human papillomarivus type 6 in respiratory and genital tracts during inferferon therapy. In: Howley PM, Broker TR, eds. Papillomaviruses: molecular and clinical aspects. New York: Alan R Liss, 1985:137–154.

318. Runckel D, Kessler S: Bronchogenic squamous carcinoma in nonirradiated juvenile laryngotracheal papillomatosis. Am J Surg Pathol 1980;4:293–296.

319. Kawanami T, Bowen A. Juvenile laryngeal papillomatosis with pulmonary parenchymal spread. Case report and review of the literature. Pediatr Radiol 1985;15:102–104.

320. Kramer SS, Wehunt WD, Stocker JT, Kashima H. Pulmonary manifestations of juvenile laryngotracheal papillomatosis. AJR 1985;144:687–694.

321. Borkowsky W, Martin D, Lawrence HS. Juvenile laryngeal papillomatosis with pulmonary spread. Regression following transfer factor therapy. Am J Dis Child 1984;138:667–669.

322. Nikolaidis ET, Trost DC, Buchholz CL, Wilkinson EJ. The relationship of histologic and clinical factors in laryngeal papillomatosis. Arch Pathol Lab Med 1985;109:24–29.

323. Quick CA, Foucar E, Dehner LP. Frequency and significance of epithelial atypia in laryngeal papillomatosis. Laryngoscope 1979;89:550–560.

324. Arvin AM, Yaeger AS. Other viral infections of the fetus and newborn infant. In: Remington JS, Klein JO, eds. Infectious diseases of the fetus and newborn infant. 3d Ed. Philadelphia: WB Saunders, 1990:516–527.

325. Sun C-C, Duara S. Fatal adenovirus pneumonia in two newborn infants, one case caused by adenovirus type 30. Pediatr Pathol 1985;4:247–255.

326. Le CT, Chang RS, Lipson MH. Epstein-Barr virus infections during pregnancy. A prospective study and review of the literature. Am J Dis Child 1983;137:466–468.

327. Anderson LJ, Hurwitz ES. Human parvovirus B19 and

328. Franciosi RA, Tattersall P. Fetal infection with human parvovirus B19. Hum Pathol 1988;19:489–491.

329. Brook I, Martin WJ, Finegold SM. Neonatal pneumonia caused by members of the *Bacteriodes fragilis* group. Clin Pediatr (Phila) 1980;19:541–544.

330. Moriartey RR, Finer NN. Pneumococcal sepsis and pneumonia in the neonate. Am J Dis Child 1979;133:601–602.

331. Bergqvist G, Trovik M. Neonatal infections with *Streptococcus pneumonia*. Scand J Infect Dis 1985;17:33–35.

332. Shinefield HR. Staphylococcal infections. In: Remington JS, Klein JO, eds. Infectious diseases of the fetus and newborn infant. 2d ed. Philadelphia: WB Saunders, 1983:882–916.

333. Sieber OF Jr, Handal GA. Staphylococcal infections. In: Wedgwood RJ, Davis SD, Ray CG, Kelley VC, eds. Infections in children. Philadelphia: Harper & Row, 1982;580–592.

334. Jacobs NM, Harris VS. Acute *Hemophilus* pneumonia in childhood. Am J Dis Child 1979;133:603–605.

335. Chitayat D, Diamant S, Lazevnick R, Spirer Z. *Hemophilus influenzae* type B pneumonia with pneumatocele formation. Clin Pediatr (Phila) 1980;19:151–152.

336. Asmar BI, Slovis TL, Reed JO, Dajani AS. *Hemophilus influenzae* type B pneumonia in 43 children. J Pediatr 1979;93:389–393.

337. Campognone P, Singer DB. Neonatal sepsis due to nontypable *Haemophilus influenzae*. Am J Dis Child 1986;140:117–121.

338. Cutz E, Thorner PS, Rao CP, Toma S, Gold R, Gelfand EW. Disseminated *Legionella pneumophilia* infection in an infant with severe combined immunodeficiency. J Pediatr 1982;100:760–762.

339. Davis GS, Winn WC Jr, Beaty NH. Legionnaires disease. Infections caused by *Legionella pneumophilia* and legionella-like organisms. Clin Chest Med 1981;2:145–166.

340. Sturm R, Staneck JL, Myers JP, Wilkinson HW, Cottrill CM, Towbin RB. Pediatric Legionnaire's disease: diagnosis by direct immunofluorescent staining of sputum. Pediatrics 1981;68:539–543.

341. Stocker JT, McGill LC, Orsini EN. Post-infarction peripheral cysts of the lung in pediatric patients: a possible cause of idiopathic spontaneous pneumothorax. Pediatr Pulmonol 1985;1:7–18.

342. Burrows PE, Leahy FA, Reed MH. Neonatal pulmonary infarction. Am J Dis Child 1983;137:61–64.

343. Joshi VV, Kasznica J, Khan MAA, Amato JJ, Levine DR. Cystic lung disease in Down's syndrome. Pediatr Pathol 1986;5:79–86.

344. Gonzalez OR, Gomez IG, Recalde AL, Landing BH. Postnatal development of the cystic lung lesion of Down syndrome: Suggestion that the cause is reduced formation of peripheral air spaces. Pediatr Pathol 1991;11:623–633.

345. Stocker JT, Sequestration of the lung. Semin Diagn Pathol 1986;3:106–121.

346. Savic B, Birtel FJ, Knoche R, Tholen W, Schild H.

pregnancy. Clin Perinatol 1988;15:273–286.

Pulmonary sequestration. In: Frick HP, Harnack GA, Martini GA, Prader A, Schoen R, Wolff HP, eds. Advances in internal medicine and pediatrics. Berlin: Springer-Verlag, 1979:58–92.

347. Carter R. Pulmonary sequestration. Ann Thorac Surg 1969;9:68–86.

348. Stocker JT, Kagan-Hallet K. Extralobar pulmonary sequestration: analysis of 15 cases. Am J Clin Pathol 1979;72:917–925.

349. Telander RL, Lennox C, Sieber W. Sequestration of the lung in children. Mayo Proc Clin 1976;51:578–584.

350. Gerle RD, Jaretski A, III, Ashley CA, Berne AS. Congenital bronchopulmonary-foregut malformation. Pulmonary sequestration communicating with the gastrointestinal tract. N Engl J Med 1968;278:1413–1419.

351. Pryce CM, Sellors TH, Blair LG. Intralobar sequestration of lung associated with an abnormal pulmonary artery. Br J Surg 1947;35:18–29.

352. Kafka V, Beco V. Simultaneous intra- and extralobar sequestration. Arch Dis Child 1960;35:51–65.

353. Witten DM, Clagett OT, Woolner LB. Intralobar bronchopulmonary sequestration involving the upper lobes. J Thorac Cardiovasc Surg 1962;43:523–529.

354. Jona JZ, Roffensperger JG. Total sequestration of the right lung. J Thorac Cardiovasc Surg 1975;69:361–364.

355. Johnson F, Laird T. Radionuclide evaluation of a communicating bronchopulmonary foregut malformation. Pediatr Radiol 1978;7:175–177.

356. Choplin RH, Siegel MG. Pulmonary sequestration: Six unusual presentations. AJR 1980;134:695–700.

357. Miller PA, Williamson BRJ, Minor GR, Buschi AJ. Pulmonary sequestration: Visualization of the feeding artery by CT. J Comput Assist Tomogr 1982;6:828–830.

358. Thilenius OG, Ruschhaupt DG, Replogle RL, Bharati S, Herman T, Arcilla RA. Spectrum of pulmonary sequestration: association with anomalous pulmonary venous drainage in infants. Pediatr Cardiol 1983;4:97–103.

359. Derkson OS. Scimitar syndrome and pulmonary sequestration. Radiologia Clin 1977;46:81–93.

360. Savic B, Birtel FJ, Tholen W, Funke HD, Kroche R. Lung sequestration: Report of seven cases and review of 540 published cases. Thorax 1979;34:96–101.

361. Hopkins RL, Levine SD, Waring WW. Intralobar sequestration. Chest 1982;82:192–193.

362. Ferris EJ, Smith PL, Mirza H, et al. Intralobar pulmonary sequestration: Value of aortography and pulmonary arteriorgraphy. Cardiovasc Intervent Radiol 1981; 4:17–23.

363. Roe JP, Mack JW, Shirley JH. Bilateral pulmonary sequestration. J Thorac Cardiovasc 1980;80:8–10.

364. Bell-Thompson J, Missier P, Sommers SC. Lung carcinoma arising in bronchopulmonary sequestration. Cancer (Philadelphia) 1979;44:334–339.

365. Pryce DM. Lower accessory pulmonary artery with intralobar sequestration of lung: A report of seven cases. J Pathol Bacteriol 1946;58:457–467.

366. Smith RA. A theory on the origin of intralobar sequestration of lung. Thorax 1956;11:10–24.

367. Boyden EA. Bronchogenic cysts and the theory of intra-

lobar sequestration: new embryologic data. J Thorac Surg 1958;35:604–616.

368. Gebauer PW, Mason CB. Intralobar pulmonary sequestration associated with anomalous pulmonary vessels: A nonentity. Dis Chest 1959;35:282–288.

369. Blesovsky A. Pulmonary sequestration: A report of an unusual case and a review of the literature. Thorax 1967;22:351–357.

370. Moscarella AA, Wylie RH. Congenital communication between the esophagus and isolated ectopic pulmonary tissue. J Thorac Cardiovasc Surg 1968;55:672–676.

371. Stocker JT, Malczak HT. A study of pulmonary ligament arteries. Relationship to intralobar pulmonary sequestration. Chest 1984;86:611–615.

372. Royall J, Levin DL. Adult respiratory distress syndrome in pediatric patients. 1. Clinical aspects, pathophysiology, pathology, and mechanisms of lung injury. J Pediatr 1988;112:169–180.

373. Royal JA. Adult respiratory distress syndrome in children. Semin Respir Med 1990;11:223–234.

374. Thurlbeck WM, Miller RR, Muller NL, Rosenow EC, III. Diffuse diseases of the lung. Philadelphia: BC Decker, 1991:46–49.

375. Laraya-Cuasay LR. The interstitial pneumonias. In: Laraya-Cuasay LR, Hughes WT, eds. Interstitial lung diseases in children. Vol. III. Boca Raton: CRC Press, 1988;122–150.

376. Henderson DW. The morphogenesis and classification of diffuse interstitial lung diseases: A clinicopathologic approach, based on tissue reaction patterns. Aust NZ J Med 1984;14:735–748.

377. Fleetham JA, Thurlbeck WM. Desquamative interstitial pneumonia and other variants of interstitial pneumonia. In: Chernick V, Kendig EL, eds. Kendig's disorders of the respiratory tract in children. 5th Ed. Philadelphia: WB Saunders, 1990:485–492.

378. Thurlbeck WM, Fleetham JA. Usual interstitial pneumonia (cryptogenic or idiopathic fibrosing alveolitis). In: Chernick V, Kendig EL, eds. Kendig's disorders of the respiratory tract in children. 5th Ed. Philadelphia: WB Saunders, 1990:480–485.

379. Diaz RP, Bowman CM. Childhood interstitial lung disease. Semin Respir Med 1990;11:253–268.

380. Platzker ACG, Lew CD. Childhood pulmonary aspiration. Semin Respir Med 1990;11:176–184.

381. Wohl MEB. Bronchiolitis. In: Chernick V, Kendig EL, eds. Kendig's disorders of the respiratory tract in children. 5th Ed. Philadelphia: WB Saunders, 1990:360–370.

382. Nicolai T, Pohl A. Acute viral bronchiolitis in infancy: Epidemiology and management. Lung 1990;168(Suppl): 396–405.

383. Snover DC. Biopsy interpretation in bone marrow transplantation. Pathol Annu 1989;24(Pt 2):63–101.

384. Yousem SA, Dauber JA, Keenan R, Paradis IL, Zeevi A, Griffith BP. Does histologic acute rejection in lung allografts predict the development of bronchiolitis obliterans? Transplantation 1991;52:306–309.

385. Epler GR, Colby TV, McLoud TC, Carrington CB,

lar lavage fluid. Am J Pathol 1984;115:225–232.

452. Soler P, Chollet S, Jacque C, Fukuda Y, Ferrans VJ, Basset F. Immunohistochemical characterization of pulmonary histiocytosis X cells in lung biopsies. Am J Pathol 1985;118:439–451.

453. Colby TV, Carrington CB, Mark GJ. Pulmonary involvement in malignant histiocytosis. A clinicopathologic spectrum. Am J Surg Pathol 1981;5:61–73.

454. Heitzman ER. Pulmonary neoplastic and lymphoproliferative disease in AIDS: A review. Radiology 1990; 177:347–351.

455. Kennedy JL, Nathwani BN, Burke JS, Hill LR, Rappaport H. Pulmonary lymphomas and other pulmonary lymphoid lesions. A clinicopathologic and immunologic study of 64 patients. Cancer (Philadelphia) 1985;56: 539–552.

456. Perreault C, Cousineau S, D'Angelo G, et al. Lymphoid interstitial pneumonia after allogenic bone marrow transplantation. A possible manifestation of chronic graft-versus-host disease. Cancer (Philadelphia) 1985; 55:1–9.

457. Colby TV, Yousem SA. Pulmonary lymphoid neoplasms. Semin Diagn Pathol 1985;2:183–196.

458. Kradin RL, Mark EJ. Benign lymphoid disorders of the lung, with a theory regarding their development. Hum Pathol 1983;14:857–867.

459. Hildebrand FL, Jr., Rosenow EC, III, Habermann TM, Tazelaar HD. Pulmonary complications of leukemia. Chest 1990;98:1233–1239.

460. Katzenstein A, Carrington CB, Liebow AA. Lymphomatoid granulomatosis: a clinicopathologic study of 152 cases. Cancer 1979;43:360–373.

461. Bekassy AN, Cameron R, Garwicz S, Laurin S, Wiebe T. Lymphomatoid granulomatosis during treatment of acute lymphoblastic leukemia in a 6-year-old girl. Am J Pediatr Hematol Oncol 1985;7:377–380.

462. Jaffe ES. Pathologic and clinical spectrum of post-thymic T-cell malignancies. Cancer Invest 1984;2:413–426.

463. Simrell CR, Margolick JB, Crabtree GR, Cossman J, Fauci AS, Jaffe ES. Lymphokine-induced phagocytosis in angiocentric immunoproliferative lesions (AIL) and malignant lymphoma arising in AIL. Blood 1985;65: 1469–1476.

464. Giuliano AE, Feig S, Eilber FR. Changing metastatic patterns of osteosarcoma. Cancer 1984;54:2160–2164.

465. Han MT, Telander RL, Pairolero PC, et al. Aggressive thoracotomy for pulmonary metastatic osteogenic sarcoma in children and young adolescents. J Pediatr Surg 1981;16:928–933.

466. Dunn D, Dehner LP. Metastatic osteosarcoma to lung. A clinicopathologic study of surgical biopsies and resections. Cancer 1977;40:3054–3064.

467. Alvarez Silván AM, Gonzalez del Castillo J, Martinez Caro A, et al. Maturation of Wilms' tumor pulmonary metastases to benign fibromas after therapy. Med Pediatr Oncol 1984;12:218–220.

468. Gonzalez-Crussi F, Sotelo-Avila C, Kidd JM. Malignant mesenchymal nephroma of infancy. Report of a case with pulmonary metastases. Am J Surg Pathol 1980;4: 185–190.

469. Stocker JT, Ishak KG. Heptoblastoma. In: Okuda K, Ishak KG, eds. Neoplasms of the liver. New York: Springer-Verlag (in press).

470. Grossman NJ, Luddy RE, Schwartz AD. Stage IVA Hodgkin's disease of the lung. Am J Pediatr Hematol Oncol 1984;6:332–334.

CHAPTER 9

Bacterial Infections

WASHINGTON C. WINN, JR. and FRANCIS W. CHANDLER

In Osler's time, bacterial pneumonia was a dreaded event, so important that he borrowed John Bunyan's characterization of tuberculosis and anointed the pneumococcus, as the prime pathogen, "Captain of the men of death"[1]. One hundred years later much has changed, but much remains the same. Pneumonia is now the sixth most common cause of death and the most common lethal infection in the United States. Hospital-acquired pneumonia is now the second most common nosocomial infection.[2] It was documented as a complication in 0.6% of patients in a national surveillance study,[3] and has been reported in as many as 20% of patients in critical care units.[4,5] Furthermore, it is the leading cause of death among nosocomial infections.[6] Leu and colleagues[7] were able to associate one-third of the mortality in patients with nosocomial pneumonia to the infection itself. The increase in hospital stay, which averaged 7 days, was statistically significant. It has been estimated that nosocomial pneumonia produces costs in excess of $500 million each year in the United States, largely related to the increased length of hospital stay.

For many years it appeared that the problem of infection in our society had been solved. The discovery and then commercialization of penicillin opened a new era of optimism, which was bolstered by discovery of the macrolides, such as erythromycin, and the aminoglycosides, such as streptomycin. It was not long, however, before the seemingly endless resilience and resourcefulness of bacterial pathogens became manifest. The Cold War between medicinal chemists and bacteria began in earnest in the 1960s with the emergence of *Staphylococcus aureus* that were resistant to penicillin and the increasing prominence of gram-negative bacilli as serious pathogens. The war has continued unabated in succeeding decades, shifting battlefields as immuno-suppressive therapies have been developed and patients survived previously fatal primary diseases, waxing and waning as new therapeutic strategies were developed and new mechanisms of resistance were elicited, and reaching virgin territory as new infectious agents were discovered. Legionnaires' disease taught us, in the mid-1970s, that we still had a lot to learn about the enemy. In the 1980s, gram-positive bacteria have reasserted their importance as methicillin-resistant staphylococci and enterococci joined their gram-negative counterparts.[8] In the 1990s the political and military Cold War has ended with the collapse of communism and the fall of the Berlin Wall, but we take one step backward for every two forward in our war against bacterial pneumonia. The "Men of Death" still stalk our hospital wards and lurk in our streets for the weak and the unprepared.

Definition and Classification

Pneumonia, (πνευμονια, of old, meant a disease of the lungs), *Peripneumo'nia,... Pleumo'nia,... Pneumoni'tis,... Pulmonitis, Pulmo'nia,... Lung-fever* (vulgarly).... The chief symptoms of pneumonia are: —pyrexia, accompanied by pain, sometimes obtuse, at others pungent, —in some part of the thorax; pulse more or less quick and hard, according to the violence and extent of the local disorder; pain, aggravated by the cough, which, with dyspnoea, exists throughout the disease.... When the inflammation, instead of going off by resolution, passes on to suppuration, rigors are experienced.... Pneumonia may, also, terminate by gangrene, —but this rarely happens, —by induration and by hepatization.

—Robley Dunglison, A Dictionary of Medical Science, 1874[9]

Table 9–1. Classification schemes for bacterial pneumonia

Category	Variables
Pathogenesis	Exogenous vs. endogenous
	Inhalation vs. aspiration vs. bacteremia
	Primary vs. Secondary
Epidemiology	Community acquired vs. nosocomial
Anatomic distribution	Focal (lobular) vs. lobar
	Diffuse vs. circumscribed (Round)
Time course	Acute vs. chronic
Etiologic agent	Various

Table 9–2. Characterization of bacterial pneumonia by infectious source

Endogenous	Exogenous
Streptococcus pneumoniae	Mycobacterium tuberculosis
Haemophilus influenzae	Mycobacterium spp.
Anaerobic bacteria	Legionella spp.
Staphylococcus aureus	Yersinia pestis
Enteric gram-negative bacilli	Francisella tularensis
Pseudomonas spp.	Bacillus anthracis
Acinetobacter spp.	
Yersinia pestis	
Francisella tularensis	
Miscellaneous	

Infections of the lower respiratory tract are defined by their anatomic location: larynx, trachea, bronchi, bronchioles, and distal air spaces. Infectious disease of the distal air spaces (respiratory bronchioles, alveolar ducts, and alveoli) is commonly described as pneumonia, but the usage is not always precise and occasionally the generic term pneumonitis is used synonymously. Some of the common etiologic agents are common to infections of the trachea, bronchi, and air spaces, but the infections may occur independently as well as concurrently.

This chapter discusses bacterial pneumonia in adult patients. Certain bacteria, such as *Mycobacterium* sp. (Chapter 10), *Chlamydia* sp., and *Mycoplasma* sp. (Chapter 13) are discussed elsewhere.

Pneumonia may be classified in many ways, as demonstrated in Table 9–1. Pathogenesis, epidemiology, macroscopic distribution, and inflammatory component/time course are discussed; the pathologic processes produced by individual bacteria or bacterial groups are then reviewed in detail.

Pathogenesis of Bacterial Pneumonia

The pathogenesis of bacterial pneumonia begins with the introduction of organisms into the airways. The relative sterility of the lower respiratory tract depends on the filtering action of the nasopharyngeal mucosa, the integrity of the epiglottic barrier, and, finally, the adequacy of pulmonary defense mechanisms. (See Chapter 3). The review of Green and colleagues[10] also remains a useful general reference.

Intrusions of bacteria into the lower respiratory tract may come from either exogenous or endogenous sources. The few instances in which the source of the inoculum is exogenous are paradoxically less challenging than the more common endogenous infections, because the external source can be identified and controlled. For example, many hospitals have been able to virtually banish *Legionella* pneumonia from their institutions by eliminating the bacteria from the aquatic environment, whether it be in potable water, in adjacent cooling towers, or both.[11–13] Immunization has been the primary stratagem for control of endogenous pathogens such as *Streptococcus pneumoniae*.[14,15] A classification of bacterial pneumonia by source of the inoculum is shown in Table 9–2.

Routes of Infection: Exogenous Pneumonia

The most important routes by which bacteria are delivered to the airspaces are by inhalation of an aerosol, by aspiration of respiratory or gastrointestinal secretions, and by bacteremic spread. Exogenous pneumonia is predominantly transmitted by inhalation of an infectious aerosol, as exemplified by *Mycobacterium tuberculosis*. *Bacillus anthracis* produces a variety of diseases, depending in part on the mechanism of bacterial transmission. Cutaneous anthrax, the most common manifestation of infection, results from direct inoculation of spores from contaminated soil or animal skins.[16,17] The infection remains localized to the skin. The most feared form of anthrax, however, is the overwhelming pneumonia that results from inhalation of aerosolized spores. Pneumonic anthrax is fortunately rare, because aerosols of large proportions are uncommon. Careful epidemiologic investigation may be necessary to establish the source of the aerosol, as occurred when workers in a woolen mill contracted inhalational anthrax.[18] Analogous situations are found in plague and tularemia, which usually infect the lungs as a by-product of bacteremic disease but may produce primary respiratory infection after inhalation of aerosolized bacteria.

The most recent example of an exogenous infection is *Legionella pneumophila* pneumonia, which as noted is almost exclusively associated with aquatic environments. Most investigators accept that an important source of infection is aerosolization of bacteria from cooling towers.[11,12,19,20] Much of the evidence is derived from epidemiologic studies, buttressed in many cases by molecular analysis of bacterial isolates. A particularly instructive incident ushered in a pair of epidemics in Burlington, Vermont, during the summer of 1980.[21] Two maintenance workers entered an inactive cooling tower on the roof of the building that houses the College of Medicine to prepare it for the summer season. During their work the fan in the tower was activated, producing a sudden blast of aerosolized water; the men then turned the fan off and continued their work. Within several days both men became sick and one developed a severe pneumonia that required prolonged hospitalization. Shortly thereafter a biphasic epidemic began that was associated epidemiologically with the cooling tower.[12] Further, strains of *Legionella pneumophila*, serogroup 1, which were isolated from the cooling tower water and from infected patients, displayed the same antigenic profile when tested with a panel of monoclonal antibodies.[22]

Cooling towers are not the only sources of *Legionella* aerosols, however. Small epidemics of legionnaires' disease have been traced to the use of drinking water that was contaminated with *Legionella* in nebulizers.[23] Hypothetically many other daily activities are associated with transient aerosols, such as turning on a faucet, flushing a toilet, or taking a shower. Despite the concentration of attention on cooling towers the source of most cases of sporadic legionnaires' disease is unknown, but probably includes transmission of bacteria from a source in potable water to the patient. It has not been determined whether the mechanism is inhalation of an aerosol, aspiration of potable water, or both. The role of drinking water has been further emphasized, however, by the dramatic demonstration that *Legionella dumoffii* produced sternal wound infections when tap water was used to bathe the incisions of patients who were recovering from cardiac surgery.[24]

Routes of Infection: Endogenous Pneumonia

The pathogenesis of most cases of endogenous pneumonia includes transmission of bacteria from the upper respiratory or gastrointestinal tracts into the lung. The mechanism is not always clear, but the most likely scenario is that oropharyngeal secretions are aspirated into the lower respiratory tract (Fig. 9–1). Experimental studies of humans have documented regular episodes of subclinical aspiration, which increase in magnitude as the level of consciousness decreases.[25] (Also see Chapter 5.) The interplay between volume of aspirated material, microbial composition of the inoculum, and adequacy of defense mechanisms then determines the outcome of the event.

Community-acquired and nosocomial pneumonias of endogenous origin are caused by different groups of bacteria, but in each case the bacterial inoculum originates in the upper airway. Factors that determine the

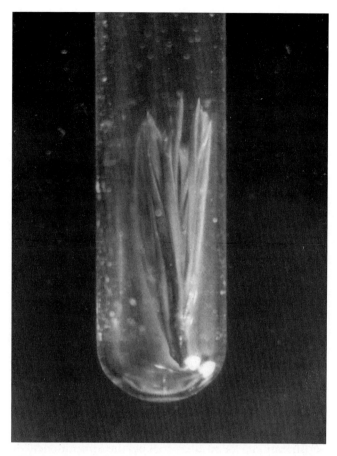

Fig. 9–1. Aspirated Christmas tree fragment removed from bronchus of young child. Specimen yielded pure growth of *Streptococcus pneumoniae*. Most episodes of aspiration are subtle and unrecognized by patient.

nature of the colonizing oropharyngeal flora also indirectly predict the etiologic agents of lower respiratory infection.

The oropharyngeal flora of normal individuals is predominantly gram positive.[26] The local environment with its narrow range of temperature and pH, flow of salivary secretions, and humoral factors such as IgA and lysozyme favor a plethora of streptococcal species.[26] *Streptococcus pneumoniae* colonizes the oropharynx in as many as 10%–15% of patients who do not have pneumococcal infections.[27] *Staphylococcus aureus* is a frequent inhabitant. *Haemophilus influenzae*, especially nontypable strains that lack capsular polysaccharide, *Neisseria* species, and *Moraxella (Branhamella) catarrhalis* are regular gram-negative members of the oropharyngeal flora. Even *Streptococcus pyogenes*, often considered a priori a pathogen when isolated from the oropharynx, may be recovered from asymptomatic individuals. Winther and colleagues[28] studied a group of healthy students five times during a single winter season. *Streptococcus pneumoniae* was isolated from 12.5%–25.6% of students, *Streptococcus pyogenes* from 3.5%–8.3%, and *Haemophilus* species from 1.2%–8.8% during a period of 8 months. Anaerobic bacteria, both gram positive and gram negative, make their home in the crevices of the gums and proliferate when dental hygiene is poor.

Colonization

Once patients are admitted to the hospital there is a dramatic shift in the colonizing flora of the upper airway from gram positive to gram negative. Enteric gram-negative bacilli and *Pseudomonas* species join or even replace gram-positive bacteria as colonizing flora of the upper airways. The alteration in flora does not occur in physiologically normal subjects who have been hospitalized and correlates best with severity of illness.[29] Gram-negative bacilli were isolated from pharyngeal cultures in 2% of normal subjects, whether hospitalized or not, from 16% of moderately ill patients, and from 57% of moribund individuals. This shift in colonizing flora is not related to duration of hospitalization and in fact frequently occurs within 24 h of admission to an intensive care unit.[30] Cigarette smokers and patients with chronic bronchitis also experience a change in the colonizing flora to gram-negative species.[31]

The importance of colonization in the pathogenesis of pneumonia is emphasized by the prominence of gram-positive bacteria, *Haemophilus influenzae*, and anaerobic bacteria in the etiology of community acquired pneumonia and by the prominence of gram-negative species in nosocomial pneumonia. The anaerobic bacteria most commonly isolated from pulmonary infections include anaerobic streptococci, *Fusobacterium nucleatum*, and black-pigmented genera such as *Porphyromonas* and *Prevotella* (formerly *Bacteroides melaninogenicus* group).[32–34] *Enterococcus* species, which heavily colonize the lower gastrointestinal tract and participate in abdominal infections, are notably infrequent in the oropharynx and infrequently produce bacterial pneumonia.

In one study of nosocomial pneumonia, Johanson and colleagues[30] noted that 22 of 26 patients in an intensive care unit who developed bacterial pneumonia had been colonized previously with gram-negative bacilli. Pneumonia resulted in 3.3% of patients who had not been colonized, but fully 23% of colonized patients developed infections of the air spaces.

Bacterial Adherence

The mechanism by which colonization occurs appears to involve adherence of bacteria to epithelial cells (Fig. 9–2). In a group of 34 patients who required intensive

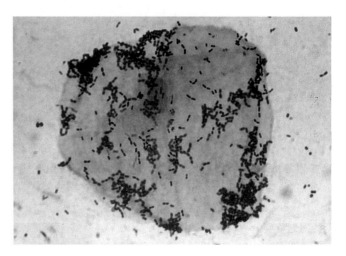

Fig. 9–2. Gram-positive cocci cover surface of desquamated squamous epithelial in expectorated sputum specimen. In many hospitalized patients, gram-positive organisms are replaced by gram-negative bacilli. Gram, ×1000.

care, 53% were colonized with gram-negative bacilli.[35] The buccal epithelial cells from colonized patients contained more adherent gram-negative bacilli and fewer adherent alpha-hemolytic streptococci than the cells of noncolonized individuals. Further, incubation of cells in vitro with one species of enteric bacillus inhibited adherence of a second species, suggesting that a specific receptor was responsible for the phenomenon. When buccal squamous epithelial cells from a group of 32 noncolonized patients who were undergoing cardiac surgery were studied in vitro, the frequency of adherence of *Pseudomonas aeruginosa* and three other gram-negative bacilli doubled in half the patients. Eleven of 16 (69%) patients whose buccal cells developed an affinity for gram-negative bacteria in vitro became colonized in vivo.[36] None of the patients who did not develop increased adherence in vitro in the perioperative period became colonized in vivo. Adherence to tracheal columnar epithelial cells may also be important. Todd and colleagues[37] studied the adhesion of *Pseudomonas aeruginosa* to tracheal cells in a group of 24 intensive care unit patients. Pneumonia was observed in 11 of 12 patients who had elevated bacterial adherence in contrast to only 1 of 12 patients with normal adherence. A prospective study was not performed, however.

The bacterial adhesive factors vary greatly, depending on the species.[38] As suggested by the epidemiologic studies, however, the critical factor appears to be changes in the epithelial cells that permit access to previously hidden receptors. Fibronectin is the prime candidate for the critical cellular factor. Woods and colleagues[39] studied 12 seriously ill patients, whose respiratory tract was colonized with *Pseudomonas aeruginosa*, and a group of noncolonized controls. The sialic

Fig. 9–3. "Clearance" of physical bacterial particles and viable organisms from lung in experimental pneumonia. After aerosol challenge, physical particles (represented by radioactive counts) are removed slowly over period of days. Effective clearance of viable bacteria combines physical removal with the antibacterial defenses of the lung.

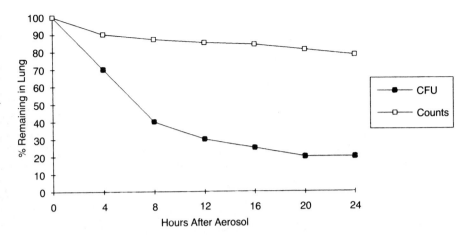

acid and fibronectin content of buccal epithelial cells from the seriously ill patients was less than that of controls. When normal cells were treated with neuraminidase to remove sialic acid, there was no change in bacterial adhesion, but trypsinization to remove fibronectin caused increased adherence of *Pseudomonas* to cells from the normal controls. The authors were able to demonstrate decreased cellular fibronectin by immunofluorescence and increased numbers of *Pseudomonas* by Gram's stain on the cells of colonized patients and on the trypsinized cells of controls. The factor that strips fibronectin from the surface of cells appears to be protease excreted into the saliva from the salivary glands of colonized patients.[40]

Bacterial Clearance

After inhalation or aspiration of bacteria and other particles into the lower respiratory tract, a congery of defense mechanisms attempt to eliminate ("clear") the particles from the lower respiratory tract. Many experimental studies have documented the variety of interactions that may take place, depending in part on the nature of the infecting organism, the bacterial inoculum, and the state of the infected host. Experimental systems that deliver bacteria to the lungs by aerosol utilize chambers that expose the whole animal[41] or only the snout.[42] These systems most closely simulate inhalation of nebulized or aerosolized bacteria from exogenous sources. Models that employ intranasal or intratracheal inoculation of bacterial suspensions resemble aspiration of endogenous or colonizing microflora.[43]

Bacteria are removed from the lung by two pathways, (1) retrograde up the respiratory tract on the "mucociliary escalator," to be expectorated or swallowed, and (2) into the interstitium.[44] Transport centripetally out of the lung occurs by both cellular and noncellular mechanisms. Free particles are swept along the surface of the

ciliated mucosa, following the flow of fluid being removed from the lung.[45] An additional and probably more important mechanism is the removal of cells, especially resident alveolar macrophages, that have phagocytized ingested bacteria.[46] Clearance of bacteria often follows a biphasic curve, and the ciliary mechanism accounts for the early phase, which occurs in a matter of minutes to hours. *Streptococcus pneumoniae* radiolabeled with technetium was cleared from the lung, but did not appear in the hepatic reticuloendothelial system within the first 6 hours after aerosol challenge.[47] Factors that reduce mucociliary clearance, such as influenza virus infection, also reduce the clearance of inhaled particles from the lower respiratory tract.[48] Ultrastructural examination of human upper-respiratory ciliated epithelium from children with respiratory viral infections demonstrated damaged cilia that persisted for 2 to 10 days after the infection.[49]

In contrast to the luminal mechanism, the interstitial transport pathways appear to be oriented radially along the terminal bronchiole and thence to the lymphatics and either the pleural surface or regional lymph nodes.[44] The familiar distribution of carbon in the pleura, peribronchial region, and lymph nodes at postmortem examination reflects this pathway. This second phase of clearance is considerably slower and may last days, weeks, or months.

When "clearance" is measured by titration of viable bacteria, a more rapid disappearance of the inoculum is usually observed (Fig. 9–3), representing cellular bactericidal activity as well as physical removal of the particles.[50] Experimental variations occur depending on design of the aerosol chamber, nature of the bacterial species, and placement of animals, but these factors can be controlled. Killing of bacteria by drying and shear forces while the aerosol is being generated cannot be completely eliminated.[51,52]

The interaction between the infecting bacteria and

the resident phagocytic cells is a critical factor in the outcome. When most respiratory pathogens are introduced into the air spaces, physical clearance occurs and bactericidal activity is expressed to varying degrees. In the initial encounter with an infectious agent, defense mechanisms are not immunologically specific, and the complement segment of the humoral immune system plays an important role. Some bacterial species, such as *Staphylococcus aureus*, are readily phagocytized by resident macrophages. In contrast encapsulated bacteria, such as *Streptococcus pneumoniae* and type b *Haemophilus influenzae*, are inherently resistant to phagocytosis in the absence of opsonins. Pneumococci are able to activate the complement cascade, either through the classical pathway in the presence of antibody or through the alternate pathway when antibody is absent.[53] Winkelstein and Tomasz[54] demonstrated that the teichoic acid component of the cell wall is responsible for the activation of the alternate pathway. Phagocytosis of pneumococci by neutrophils is enhanced by either complement or antibody through complement and Fc receptors on the cells. It appears that there are serotypic differences among pneumococci in their interaction with the complement system. Coonrod and colleagues[55] reported that type 1 strains were not opsonized by complement, type 3 strains were opsonized partly by the alternative pathway and partly by the classical pathway, and type 25 strains were readily opsonized by the alternate pathway.

The importance of complement is illustrated by the occurrence of overwhelming pneumococcal infection in patients with deficiencies in several complement components.[56] Experimentally, the effect of complement depletion on the clearance of bacteria from the lung depends on the in vitro interactions among complement, cells, and bacteria. Several groups have demonstrated impaired clearance of *Streptococcus pneumoniae* and *Pseudomonas aeruginosa* in animals rendered hypocomplementemic by cobra venom factor.[57,58] In contrast, clearance of *Staphylococcus aureus* and *Klebsiella pneumoniae* was unaffected by decomplementation.

Nonimmunologic humoral defenses may also be important in the early hours after bacteria are deposited in the lower airways. Coonrod and colleagues[55] demonstrated that encapsulated pneumococci were killed in vitro by incubation with a fraction of rat bronchoalveolar fluid that was rich in surfactant. In addition LaForce and associates[59] demonstrated that rat alveolar lining material enhanced the antibacterial activity of macrophages. Other investigators, using concentrated human alveolar fluid, have been unable to demonstrate any antibacterial activity.[60] Such nonimmunoglobulin factors as complement and alveolar lining material may explain the early observations in experimental pneumococcal pneumonia that limitation of the expanding

pneumonic lesion and phagocytosis of bacteria occurred so soon after infection that specific antibody could not be responsible for the effective host defense.[61]

Facultative intracellular pathogens, such as *Legionella pneumophila* or *Mycobacterium tuberculosis*, actually proliferate in the resident alveolar macrophages after phagocytosis so that only the relatively small component of physical clearance is operative.[62] In this situation the best strategy from the point of view of host defenses is to keep bacteria out of macrophages; opsonins may actually be undesirable. In vitro, at least, the addition of specific antibody opsonin to cultures of *Legionella pneumophila* and human alveolar macrophages promotes adherence of bacteria and does not inhibit intracellular multiplication.[63]

Inflammatory Responses

The resident alveolar macrophages are the critical first line of cellular defenses, but recruited polymorphonuclear neutrophils and circulating monocytes are essential backup forces (Fig. 9–4). Once the inflammatory process is initiated, a complex set of interactions among cells, bacteria, and plasma proteins sets in motion a series of events that is perpetuated by a continuing network of chemotactic stimuli.[64] The precise sequence of events depends in part on the virulence of the infecting bacterium and the quantity of organisms in the challenge. Onofrio and colleagues[65] studied the interactions of inflammatory cells and graded quantities of *Staphylococcus aureus* that had been introduced into the lungs of mice. If the inoculum is small and the resident macrophages are capable of engulfing and killing the bacteria, there is no need for additional cellular recruitment and chemotactic factors are not generated. With intermediate inocula an active recruitment of polymorphonuclear neutrophils ensues, after which bacterial growth is checked. If the inocula are sufficiently high, neutrophils are recruited but the combined cellular response is inadequate to control the growth of bacteria.

The inflammatory sequence of resident alveolar macrophage, recruited polymorphonuclear neutrophil, and recruited monocyte-macrophage can be generalized from several experimental models.[62,65–67] Although there may be variation in the propensity for recruitment of polymorphonuclear neutrophils, the standard response is an influx of neutrophils within a few to 24 h after infection. Pierce and associates[67] found that two enteric gram-negative bacilli, *Escherichia coli* and *Klebsiella pneumoniae*, elicited a greater neutrophilic response in the early hours after aerosol infection of mice than did *Staphylococcus aureus* or water. Vial and

Fig. 9–4. Cell populations in air spaces in bacterial pneumonia. Predominant cell in air spaces at onset of infection is alveolar macrophage (MAC). Recruited polymorphonuclear neutrophils (PMN) quickly become predominant cell type and are removed as the acute infection is contained. Recruited monocytes then increase numbers of macrophages and are cleared more slowly. Recruited lymphocytes (LYMPH), appearing approximately 5–7 days after infection represent cellular phase of immune response.

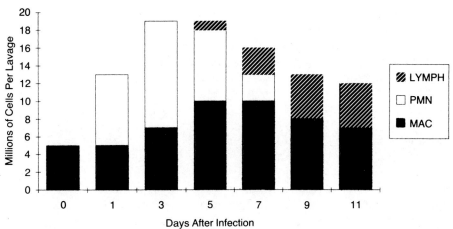

colleagues[68] demonstrated a dose dependence for *Streptococcus pneumoniae*. Both the recruitment of neutrophils into the air spaces and the chemoattractant ability of bronchoalveolar lavage fluid in vitro were directly related to the bacterial inoculum (log neutrophils recruited = 0.751 log *Pneumococcus* + 0.52; $r = .77$; $p < .005$).

The stimulus for the neutrophilic influx is multifactorial. An important mechanism is the activation of the complement cascade through either the classical or alternate pathway. Shaw and associates[69] instilled low molecular weight fragments of C5 into the trachea of rabbits and reproduced the full spectrum of the inflammatory response. Damage to endothelial and epithelial cells, extravasation of erythrocytes with fibrin clumps, and degranulating polymorphonuclear neutrophils were evident ultrastructurally. The process could be blocked by absorption of complement fragments with antibody to homogeneous human C5a. Larsen and colleagues[70] have suggested that C5a des arg, a metabolite of C5a produced in vivo, is actually responsible for the phlogistic responses in the lung. Coonrod and colleagues[71] have documented depressed levels of complement components that participate in the alternate pathway during the early phases of pneumococcal pneumonia, suggesting that complement activation is a part of the pathophysiologic response in human disease.

Chemotactic stimuli for neutrophils are also derived from resident alveolar macrophages. When particles such as Sepharose beads or bacteria are phagocytized by alveolar macrophages in vitro, the stimulated macrophages release a low molecular weight chemotactic factor that is distinct from C5a. Incubation of the particles with serum augments the chemotactic response and causes the fixation of C3b onto the particle surface.[72]

The appearance of polymorphonuclear neutrophils in the air spaces coincides with the development of leaky capillaries and transudation of immunoglobulin, albumin, and other serum factors.[62] Ultrastructurally, there is damage to endothelial cells and movement of neutrophils between the cells, through the basement membrane, and into the interstitium. Damage to epithelial lining cells and movement of neutrophils through the gaps into the alveoli ensues if the chemotactic response originates in the air space[69,73] (Fig. 9–5). Experimental damage to the pulmonary vascular endothelium is mediated by polymorphonuclear neutrophils and is blocked by depletion of circulating neutrophils, whether the process initiates within the vascular system[74,75] or within the alveoli.[69] In the trachea, neutrophils migrate through the mucosa serially, not randomly between epithelial cells.[76]

Accumulation of neutrophils in the air spaces begins within hours of infection and continues for as long as 3 days. The next phase in the inflammatory process is the recruitment of circulating peripheral blood monocytes, which begins within 1–2 days after infection and continues for days to weeks, depending on the nature of the stimulus. The origin of these cells in the bone marrow has been established by radiolabeling and by irradiation of bone marrow in experimental animals.[77] By the time the monocytes traverse the interstitium and reach the air spaces they are mature macrophages. These recruited macrophages differ immunochemically and functionally from the resident alveolar macrophages. They show evidence of having ingested neutrophilic enzymes, and their procoagulant and fibrinolytic activity is increased to maximize removal of fibrin.[78] Completing the cycle of inflammatory events, this recruitment of monocyte-macrophages is elicited by chemotactic factors produced by polymorphonuclear neutrophils. A complement stimulus for inflammatory cells does not result in macrophage recruitment if animals have been first rendered neutropenic.[79]

The final inflammatory cell component is the lymphocyte, which appears in the airspaces 5–7 days after

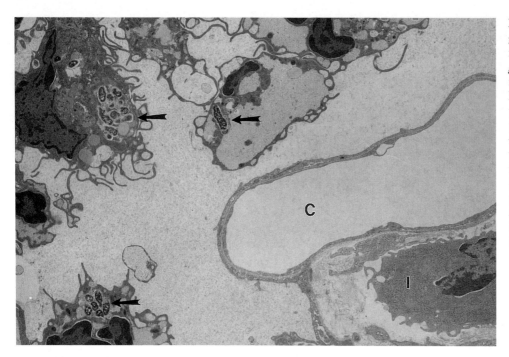

Fig. 9–5. Electron micrograph of guinea pig lung infected with serogroup 1 *Legionella pneumophila*. Inflammatory exudate has accumulated in edematous air space; phagocytized bacteria are present in phagosomes (*arrows*). Lungs were fixed by vascular perfusion so that capillary space has been cleared (C); note monocyte in expanded interstitium (I). Glutaraldehyde-fixed osmicated lung stained with uranyl acetate, ×2000.

infection.[62] There is experimental evidence that these immunologically specific cells may differ depending on the nature of the stimulus. Shennib and colleagues[80] noted that subsets of lymphocytes had distinctive characteristics when the injury was lung allotransplantation or *Pseudomonas aeruginosa* pneumonia in experimentally treated dogs.

Effect of Immunity on Defense Mechanisms

There are relatively few clinical or experimental data on the effectiveness of the immune response in preventing repeat episodes of pneumonia. Second episodes of serogroup 1 *Legionella pneumophila* pneumonia have not been documented definitively. Experimental studies with this pulmonary pathogen have documented solid protective immunity after a primary infection.[81] Protective immunity to *Legionella pneumophila* can be produced by immunization with the major secretory protein of the bacterium.[82] The immune response to *Legionella pneumophila* is both humoral and cellular. In vitro studies document the association of this pathogen with macrophages, the inability of specific antibody to prevent intracellular growth, and the ability of activated macrophages to inhibit growth within the cells.[83,84] These characteristics of the bacterium suggest that cellular immunity represents the primary defense in vivo also.

In contrast, *Haemophilus influenzae* pneumonia that is associated with subsequent bacteremia is usually caused by strains that possess the type B capsular polysaccha-

ride. The recent introduction of an immunogenic vaccine to the capsular polysaccharide has been associated with a dramatic reduction in the incidence of invasive *Haemophilus influenzae* type B disease.[85]

Similarly, a primary therapy for pneumococcal pneumonia before the development of effective antibiotics was immunotherapy with type-specific antibody. In classic studies performed by W. Barry Wood,[61] administration of antibody to experimental rats that had been infected with *Streptococcus pneumoniae* dramatically limited the spread of the inflammatory process, cleared the bloodstream of bacteria, and prevented the extension of early pleurisy. Musher and colleagues[86] demonstrated a quantitative relationship between the amount of anticapsular antibody to *Streptococcus pneumoniae* type 4 and protection from infection in experimental mice.

The large variety of immunotypes in many bacterial species makes assessment of protective immunity difficult. Recurrent infections with nonencapsulated strains of *Haemophilus influenzae* in patients with chronic obstructive pulmonary disease suggest, but do not prove, that immunity is incomplete.

Some of the effects of prior infection or immunization may be mediated by the mechanisms discussed. For example, mice that had been immunized with *Pseudomonas aeruginosa* cleared bacteria from the lung more effectively than their nonimmunized counterparts.[87] Some of the effects of immunization may be not immunologically specific but instead are caused by activation of the cellular phagocytic defenses of the lung. LaForce and colleagues[88] demonstrated enhanced intrapulmonary bactericidal activity against aerosolized *Serratia marcescens*, *Escherichia coli*, and *Staphylococcus aureus* in mice that had been experimentally immunized with the Re595 strain of *Salmonella minnesota* 2 weeks previously.

Secondary Pneumonia

In the scenarios outlined previously, pneumonia is the primary event. Bacteria may also reach the lung through the bloodstream after initiating a distant infection. The capillary bed of the lungs is one of the important filters in the circulatory system, providing an efficient trap for circulating bacteria or infected thromboemboli. The roster of microbes that produce secondary pneumonia includes important pathogens such as *Staphylococcus aureus*, enteric gram-negative bacilli, *Salmonella typhi*, *Francisella tularensis*, and *Yersinia pestis*.

When the bacterial inoculum is delivered to the lung through the bloodstream, the defense mechanisms are different and the interactions vary correspondingly. Harrow and colleagues[89] studied the effect of systemic inoculation of *Staphylococcus aureus* and *Proteus mirabilis* in mice. They found that larger quantities of *Staphylococcus aureus* lodged in the lung and that this bacterial species was killed by pulmonary defenses less efficiently than was the gram-negative organism. These experimental studies may have their counterpart in the frequency with which *Staphylococcus aureus* causes nosocomial pneumonia.

Epidemiology

Community-Acquired versus Nosocomial Pneumonia

The geographic site at which the pneumonia was acquired is of more than academic interest. As has been indicated, the colonizing oropharyngeal flora vary by age and hospitalization status. Knowledge of the most likely etiologic agents directs the selection of the most appropriate antibiotics. The patient-related risk factors also differ in community-acquired and nosocomial infections. A summary of etiologic agents for community-acquired and nosocomial pneumonia is presented in Tables 9–3 and 9–4. There is surprising agreement among these diverse studies, which were performed in various populations using nonstandardized methods. It is particularly important to note that the results will be influenced by the diagnostic methods used, by the types of agents sought, and by the criteria for documenting etiologic agents. As suggested by the data on normal flora and colonization of the upper airways, the predominant pathogens in community-acquired pneumonia are either members of the normal oropharyngeal flora or are exogenously acquired organisms such as *Legionella* species, *Mycoplasma pneumoniae*, and viruses. *Streptococcus pneumoniae* no longer occupies the overwhelmingly predominant position of earlier decades, but it still accounts for a substantial minority of infections. The switch to gram-negative pathogens, including *Pseudomonas aeruginosa*, and traditional hospital

Table 9–3. Etiology of community-acquired pneumonia

Reference	Holmberg[90]	Karalus et al.[91]	Woodhead et al.[92]	Lim et al.[93]	Fang et al.[94]	Marrie et al.[95]
Country	Sweden	Britain	Britain	Australia	United States	Canada
Number of cases	147	92	236	106	359	719
Age (years)	71[a]	56[b]	15–79[c]	60[b]	62[b]	63[b]
Streptococcus pneumoniae	46.9%	33%	36%	42%	15.3%	8.5%
Haemophilus influenzae	9.5%	2.1%	10%	9%	10.9%	
Legionella spp.	2.7%	4.2%	0.5%	3%	6.7%	2%
Mycoplasma pneumoniae	5.4%	18%	1%	8%	2.0%	5.6%
Moraxella (Branhamella) catarrhalis	2.0%					
Aerobic gram-negative bacilli		5%	1.5%	8%	5.9%	3.0%
Straphylococcus aureus		3.3%	1%	3%	3.3%	4%
Influenza A	9.5%	8%	6%	4%		5.6%
Chlamydia psittaci	1.4%	2%	1%	5%		
Chlamydia pneumoniae					6.1%	
Aspiration/postobstructive pneumonia					8.6%	7.2%
Mixed infections	10.3	11%	20%	18%	2.8%	10.3%
Unidentified/miscellaneous	22.6%	24.4%	43%	18%	49.8%	47%

[a] Median.
[b] Mean.
[c] Range.

Table 9–4. Etiology of nosocomial pneumonia

Reference	Torres et al.[96]	Fagon et al.[97]	Bartlett et al.[32]	Bryan and Reynolds[98]	Quoted in Scheld and Mandel[2]	Rello et al.[99]
Year	1989	1989	1986	1984	1984	1991
Country	Spain	France	United States[c]	United States[d]	United States	Spain[b]
Number of cases	78	52	159	172	—	68
Age (years)	54.5[e]	65[e]	68[f]	61–70[g]	—	—
Streptococcus pneumoniae		3%	44%	17%		4%
Straphylococcus aureus	3%	33%	10%	27%	12.9%	22%
Enteric gram-negative Bacilli	3%	16%	14%	33%	37.4%	8%
Pseudomonas spp.	6%	23%	3%	9%	16.9%	21%
Acinetobacter spp.	12%	11%				3%
Moraxella (Branhamella) catarrhalis		8%				2%
Haemophilus spp.		8%	3%			19%
Legionella spp.	3%	1%				
Mixed infections	16%	40%	—	12%	—	28%
Miscellaneous unidentified	76%	—	26%	14%	32.8%	21%

[a] Patients undergoing mechanical ventilation.

[b] Case definition required isolation of $>10^3$ colony-forming units of bacteria from protected catheter bronchoscopy.

[c] Etiology defined by isolation in pure culture.

[d] Etiology defined by positive blood culture.

[e] Mean.

[f] Median.

[g] Mode.

pathogens, such as *Staphylococcus aureus*, is evident in the causes of nosocomial pneumonia.[100]

It is important to document local conditions, because both pathogens and their susceptibilities to antimicrobial agents may vary greatly. The presence of potential pathogens in the local environment and existence of effective means for transmission of microbes to patients accounts for some variation, as demonstrated by epidemics of *Legionella*[101] and *Aspergillus*[102] infection. Methicillin-resistant *Staphylococcus aureus*, enteric gram-negative bacilli, and non-glucose-fermenting gram-negative bacilli such as species of *Pseudomonas* and *Acinetobacter* may cause local problems because of patterns of practice, including use of antibiotics, and because of susceptibility of particular patient populations.[103,104] Molecular diagnostic tools may be useful for dissecting the epidemiology of the infections.[105] Special epidemiologic intervention, such as isolation of patients, reinforcement of hand-washing technique, and restriction of antibiotic use, may be necessary to control the spread of drug-resistant pathogens.[106]

Risk Factors for Development of Bacterial Pneumonia

The risk factors for development of pneumonia are summarized in Table 9–5. The most rigorous studies are prospective, case-controlled epidemiologic analyses with sophisticated statistical evaluation. Those studies that utilize multivariate analysis and logistical regression are particularly instructive because they help to eliminate variables that are not independent risk factors. The quality of the information is, not surprisingly, considerably higher for nosocomial infection, because the population of patients at risk can be defined more precisely and appropriate controls identified more readily than can be done in community-acquired pneumonia. It is nevertheless obvious that many of the risk factors are similar.

In many instances the documented risk factors reflect variables that are operative in the pathogenesis of pneumonia. Conditions that predispose patients to aspiration, such as depressed consciousness from neurologic disease, anesthesia, or prolonged intubation, are prominent on the list. It is important to recognize that intubation does not prevent aspiration; in fact, the violation of laryngeal integrity by a foreign body may foster episodes of aspiration. It is well established that the tubing of modern ventilators with cascade humidification systems are contaminated by flora that originated in the patient.[112] These tubes do, however, provide a source for a bacterial inoculum that can be "dumped" back into the patient's lower respiratory tract as the patient is moved about. This mechanism may be responsible for the surprising finding that the increased manipulation of daily tubing changes actually increases the risk of pneumonia.[107] A recent development is the appreciation that bacterial colonization of the stomach may be an important source for aspirated bacterial inocula.[113] Gastric stress ulcers are a common complica-

Table 9–5. Risk factors for bacterial pneumonia

Reference	Craven et al.[107a]	Garibaldi et al.[108a]	Corensek et al.[109a]	Celis et al.[110a]	Torres et al.[96a]	England et al.[111]
Year	1986	1981	1988	1988	1990	1981
Number of patients	233	520	50	118	322	—
Setting	Intensive care with continuous mechanical ventilation	Postoperative pneumonia	Cardiac transplantation	Nonneutropenic hospitalized patients	Mechanically ventilated patients	Legionella pneumonia vs. U.S. population
Risk factors (p/odds ratio)	Intracranial pressure monitor ($p < .002$)	Low serum albumin ($p < .005$)	Posttransplant reintubation ($p = .009$)	Chronic lung disease ($p < .0003$)	More than one intubation ($p < .000012$)	End-stage renal disease (odds ratio = 340)
	Cimetidine therapy ($p < .01$)	High anesthesia risk ($p < .0001$)	High doses of steroids ($p = .02$)	Depressed consciousness ($p < .0002$)	Prior episode of gastric aspiration ($p < .00018$)	Immunosuppression (odds ratio = 26)
	Fall–winter hospitalization ($p < .04$)	History of smoking ($p < .001$)		Nasotracheal or orotracheal intubation ($p < .0001$)	Ventilation >3 days ($p < .015$)	Cancer (odds ratio = 11)
	Ventilator circuit changes q 24 h	Longer Preoperative stays ($p < .0001$)		Large-volume aspiration ($p < .003$)	Chronic lung disease ($p < .048$)	Chronic lung disease (odds ratio = 3.7)
		Longer operative procedures ($p < .0001$)		Thoracoabdominal surgery ($p < .0018$)		Smoking (odds ratio = 1.9)
		Thoracic or upper abdominal surgery ($p < .0001$)		Age >70 years ($p < .04$)		Diabetes mellitus (odds ratio = 1.3)

[a] Multivariate/logistical regression analysis performed.

tion of serious illness, but many common therapeutic approaches, such as administration of antacids or H2-antagonists, have the undesirable side effects of reducing gastric acidity and allowing bacterial proliferation. Several studies have documented that use of sucralfate, which does not increase the pH of the stomach, results in lower rates of nosocomial pneumonia.[114]

An additional group of risk factors includes conditions that reduce the effectiveness of pulmonary defense mechanisms, such as chronic obstructive lung disease and smoking. Alcohol intoxication and anesthesia may increase the risk of pneumonia by increasing the frequency of aspiration, but experimental intoxication of rabbits suggested many years ago that interference with migration of leukocytes into the air spaces may be an additional mechanism for enhanced susceptibility.[115] Although viral infections were not identified as a risk factor in these studies, bacterial superinfection has been a long recognized complication of influenza epidemics and also occurs in sporadic infection.[116] Exper-

imental studies in mice suggest that one mechanism for adverse effects of viral infection may be impairment of lung clearance of inhaled particles, presumably related to the destruction of ciliated epithelium.[117]

In addition to factors that compromise anatomic and epithelial defenses, diseases or therapy that compromise inflammatory and immunologic defense mechanisms are of critical importance. These diseases may be hereditary deficiencies in immunoglobulins[118–120] or in phagocytic function.[121] More commonly neoplastic disease is the cause of the immunosuppression, either directly or indirectly as a result of antitumor chemotherapy.[122,123] Patients who have received immunosuppressive therapy after organ transplantation represent another important risk group.[124–126] Although compromise in specific immunologic defenses is undoubtedly important, concomitant neutropenia is perhaps the most important risk factor.[127] The diminution in inflammation may cause atypical clinical presentations. Radiographic findings, the equivalent of gross pathologic examination, may be altered dramatically by the minimal inflammatory response.[128,129]

Human immunodeficiency virus (HIV) infection has now joined the ranks of important immunosuppressive conditions. Although attention has been focused on fungal, parasitic, and viral infections in patients with the acquired immunodeficiency syndrome, bacterial infections are also significantly increased.[130–133] The pathogens that infect patients with HIV infection are the same colonizing bacteria that cause community-acquired and nosocomial pneumonia in immunologically competent patients: *Staphylococcus aureus, Streptococcus pneumoniae, Haemophilus influenzae, Moraxella (Branhamella) catarrhalis*, etc.[133] The clinical and radiographic presentations of the disease may be atypical, however, perhaps because of the prophylactic use of trimethoprim-sulfamethoxazole for prevention of *Pneumocystis carinii* pneumonia.[130] The radiographic picture of bacterial pneumonia in patients with acquired immunodeficiency syndrome may actually mimic *Pneumocystis* infection.

A special risk group for severe pneumonia is the increasingly large elderly population.[134,135] The etiologic agents and specific risk factors are not distinctive, but they present ever-increasing challenges in this group of patients.

The concurrence of environmental and host risk factors is important. Arnow and associates[23] described a small epidemic of *Legionella pneumophila* pneumonia that was associated with nebulizers that had been filled with tap water. A statistically significant association of disease with risk factors required immunocompromised patients (corticosteroid therapy) and environmental exposure (water that was contaminated with *Legionella*). Many of the variables that are risk factors for development of pneumonia are also predictive of the prognosis in patients who have lower respiratory infection (Table 9–6).

Diagnosis of Bacterial Pneumonia

Difficulties in Diagnosing Pneumonia

Characterization of the etiology of bacterial pneumonia is complicated by the difficulty of making a definitive diagnosis in individual patients. Two factors complicate the laboratory diagnosis of bacterial pneumonia. First and foremost, the most common bacterial pathogens are also found in the upper airway. Thus, specimens that are collected through the upper airway can be contaminated with oral secretions. The presence of an endotracheal tube does not ensure the absence of contamination when specimens are obtained through the tube. In fact, the presence of the endotracheal tube may

lead to leakage of oropharyngeal secretions around the cuff of the tube.

The second complicating phenomenon is the presence of colonizing bacteria in the bronchial tree of patients who have chronic bronchitis and the presence of inflammatory cells elicited by irritation of the trachea from indwelling endotracheal tubes or tracheostomy tubes. The diagnosis of bacterial pneumonia, therefore, includes the documentation of lower tract disease clinically or radiographically if specimens cannot be obtained directly from the air spaces.

The most sensitive and specific means for an etiologic diagnosis of pneumonia is, of course, lung biopsy, but it is rarely necessary to resort to this extreme. The diagnostic approach to most pneumonias is graded, starting with the least invasive procedure. Common bacterial agents have usually been eliminated from consideration by the time the surgical stage is reached. If lung tissue is presented to the pathologist, however, it is important that a portion of the tissue be removed for bacterial culture if the surgeon has not submitted a separate biopsy to the microbiology laboratory. Any clinical considerations that might suggest special culture media, such as the possibility of legionnaires' disease, should be conveyed to the microbiologist so that special culture media can be inoculated. At the Medical Center Hospital or Vermont, uninoculated tissue from any source is frozen at −70°C so that additional microbiologic evaluations may be carried out if unsuspected histologic findings redirect diagnostic considerations.

The difficulty of making a specific etiologic diagnosis of pneumonia complicates analysis of other diagnostic methods, as well as clinical and epidemiologic investigations. There is no adequate gold standard in this area. Lung tissue is usually not available for culture. Isolation of an organism from blood or pleural fluid provides a solid diagnosis (100% specificity), so these cultures should be performed when appropriate in seriously ill patients. Reliance on culture of sterile body fluids is insufficient, however, because many pneumonias are not associated with infectious pleurisy or bacteremia. Bacterial pneumonia is accompanied by dissemination of bacteria through the bloodstream in only 20%–30% of cases.[138]

A variety of methods has been developed to diagnose bacterial pneumonia without surgical biopsy. Two percutaneous aspiration techniques avoid passage of the diagnostic instrument through the upper airways. Needle aspiration of pulmonary lesions that have been defined by chest radiograph has been employed primarily in children but also in adults.[139–141] The procedure may be fluoroscopically guided. Direct aspiration provides a specific diagnosis, the few false-positives being derived from the overlying skin. The sensitivity of

Table 9–6. Prognostic factors for bacterial pneumonia

Reference	Martin et al.[136]	Celis et al.[110a]	Torres et al.[96a]	Craven et al.[107a]	Torres et al.[137a]
Year	1984	1988	1990	1986	1991
Number of patients	136	118	322	233	92
Setting	Postoperative patients	Nonneutropenic hospitalized patients	Mechanically ventilated patients	Mechanically ventilated patients	Community-acquired pneumonia
Prognostic factors for mortality	Gram-negative pneumonia ($p < .001$)	"High-risk" microbe ($p < .0007$)	Ultimately or rapidly fatal disease ($p = .0018$)	Creatinine >1.5mg/dl (odds ratio = 3.3; $p < .0002$)	Spread of pneumonia (odds ratio = 181; $p < .0001$)
	Remote organ failure ($p < .001$)	Bilateral pneumonia ($p < .008$)	Septic shock ($p = .016$)	Admitted with pneumonia (odds ratio = 4.9; $p < .0002$)	Septic shock (odds ratio = 36; $p < .0002$)
	Bilateral pneumonia ($p < .001$)	Respiratory failure present ($p < .005$)	Inappropriate antibiotic treatment ($p < .02$)	No nebulized bronchodilator (odds ratio = 4.2; $p < .0004$)	Ultimately or rapidly fatal illness (odds ratio = 6.2; $p < .0185$)
	Pseudomonas-predominant ($p < .01$)	Inappropriate antibiotic therapy ($p < .02$)		Duration of ventilation (odds ratio = 1.2; $p < .005$)	
	Emergent operation ($p < .01$)	Age >60 years ($p < .02$)		No abdominal surgery (odds ratio = 3.2; $p < .03$)	
	Bacteremia ($p < .01$)	Underlying condition ultimately or rapidly fatal ($p < .02$)		Transferred from ward of other hospital (odds ratio = 2.9; $p < .003$)	
	Postoperative peritonitis ($p < .01$) Respiratory acquired pneumonia ($p < .05$)		Coma on admission (odds ratio = 2.6; $p < .009$)		

[a] Multivariate/logistical regression performed.

the technique is more difficult to gauge. Complications are most commonly pneumothorax, which is easily treated and not usually associated with infectious pleurisy. Serious morbidity is variously estimated to be rare[140] or frequent.[141] Alternatively, transtracheal aspiration has been employed to obtain uncontaminated lower respiratory secretions.[142] This technique has fallen from favor in many institutions because of occasional complications. Infrequent false-positive results were reported in studies of normal volunteers, but were as high as 21% in a clinical study.[142] The false-positives may result from aspiration of oral contents during the procedure or may represent colonizing tracheal flora in patients with chronic bronchitis.

The least invasive diagnostic technique is culture and Gram's stain examination of sputum obtained by expectoration or by endotracheal aspiration. Careful correlation of culture and smear with clinical and radiographic data is necessary to arrive at an informed clinical diagnosis. The problems with sputum as a diagnostic specimen have been emphasized,[143] but recent reports have been more optimistic.[144–146] In one prospective study of sputum, bronchial aspiration, and transtracheal aspiration, the authors recovered the predominant organism from all three types of specimen.[147] Homogenization of sputum and inoculation of mice did not improve the diagnostic yield.

In an attempt to select specimens that were enriched for lower respiratory secretions and relatively devoid of contaminating upper respiratory flora, Murray and Washington[148] studied several screening criteria using Gram's stain. The criteria most commonly employed in clinical microbiology laboratories at present are the presence of fewer than 10 squamous epithelial cells and more than 25 polymorphonuclear neutrophils per 100× microscopic field. The presence of macrophages documents the presence of alveolar contents, but does not increase the diagnostic usefulness of the screening criteria.[149,150] A careful comparison of expectorated sputum and transtracheal aspiration documented the usefulness of the criteria.[146] If more than 25 squamous epithelial cells were present in the expectorated sputum, there was agreement of bacterial isolates with transtracheal analysis in only 27% of cases. When fewer than 10 squamous cells and more than 25 neutrophils were present, a potential pathogen growing in the expectorated sputum was 92% predictive of growth in the transtracheal aspirate. When multiple potential pathogens are present in the sputum, careful correlation of the results with clinical data is necessary before the bacteria can be accepted as etiologic agents.

Assessment of bacteria in areas of the smear that are inflammatory and do not contain squamous epithelial cells provides useful information with which to interpret the results of culture. Assessment of pneumococci is particularly difficult because of the frequent presence of viridans streptococci in the specimens. Rein and colleagues[151] have assessed the effect of varying criteria on the sensitivity and specificity of the microscopic examination. The best balance of sensitivity and specificity occurred when at least 10 lancet-shaped diplococci per oil immersion field were present. While pneumococci may be confused with other streptococci, gram-negative bacteria, particularly *Haemophilus influenzae*, may be overlooked in the pink proteinaceous background. The myth that gram stain examination is a simple procedure is belied by studies such as the evaluation of sputum smears prepared by house staff.[152] Smears prepared by house staff were judged inadequate in 15% of cases compared to 3% for smears prepared by microbiology technologists. The sensitivity of interpretation of pneumococci by house staff was approximately 90% as judged by technologist interpretations or by culture, but there was a 50% false-positive rate. In contrast, the house staff underdiagnosed *Haemophilus* sp. on the smears.

In recent years more refined bronchoscopic techniques have been applied to diagnosis. Protected specimen brushes of distal bronchioles provide the most accurate specimens. Chastre and colleagues[153] compared the results of this technique with lung biopsy in patients immediately after death (a study made possible by a change in French law regarding postmortem examination). They found an excellent correlation between the techniques when more than 10^3 colony-forming units of a bacterium per milliliter were present. Subsequent studies from these investigators documented the predictive value of finding intracellular bacteria in

more than 25% of cells obtained by cytospin analysis of bronchoalveolar lavage fluid.[154]

The etiologic diagnosis of bacterial pneumonia is, therefore, difficult, but an informed analysis can be made when all possible means are employed. Isolation of pathogens that are not part of the normal respiratory flora is diagnostic. Unfortunately, with the exception of *Legionella pneumophila* and *Mycobacterium* sp., such instances are extremely rare.

Morphologic Detection and Identification of Bacteria

Gram's stain provides important information for the assessment of bacterial processes. Modifications of this procedure for histologic sections, most prominently the Brown and Brenn and Brown–Hopps procedures, have been developed, but these stains for histologic sections are much more difficult to evaluate than are gram-stained smears. The cut surface of lung tissue may be touched lightly to the surface of a flamed glass slide so that sterility of the tissue is maintained. Alternatively, a sterile scalpel blade may be drawn across the surface of the lung to collect exudate, which is then spread on a glass slide. The scrape technique is particularly effective when the exudate is fibrinous. Extra slides should be prepared to allow for a subsequent need for special examinations, such as calcofluor white staining for fungi, acid-fast stains, or immunofluorescence examination for selected pathogens. To wait for sections of paraffin-embedded tissue before doing special stains for microbial pathogens is analogous to waiting to examine postmortem lung tissue with the electron microscope when an open lung biopsy could have been fixed promptly in glutaraldehyde solution.

If the tissue has already been fixed in formaldehyde solution, several histologic stains can be used to demonstrate and characterize bacterial pathogens in tissue sections. The most useful stains and their diagnostic applications are listed in Table 9–7.

Modified Gram stains such as the Brown and Brenn, Brown–Hopps, and MacCallum–Goodpasture procedures are used to differentiate gram-positive and gram-negative bacteria in tissue, including the gram-positive agents of actinomycosis and nocardiosis. In our experience, the Brown–Hopps stain is superior for demonstrating gram-negative bacteria and is the best single choice for a tissue Gram stain. On the other hand, the Brown and Brenn procedure colors gram-positive bacteria somewhat better than the other methods.

Gomori's methenamine silver procedure, which is usually employed for the demonstration of fungi, will also stain *Actinomyces* and related organisms, *Nocardia*

Table 9–7. Special stains for bacteria in clinical specimens

Indication	Primary stain	Alternatives	Comments
General bacteria	Brown–Hopps	Brown and Brenn	Gram's stain of imprint preferred
Gram-positive bacteria	Brown and Brenn	Brown–Hopps	Gram's stain of imprint preferred
Gram-negative bacteria	Brown–Hopps	Brown and Brenn	Gram's stain of imprint preferred
Poorly staining bacteria	Steiner[a]	Warthin–Starry, Dieterle[a]	Distorts morphology; no gram reactivity
Acid-fast bacilli	Ziehl–Neelsen	Auramine, auramine-rhodamine	Should be used as general screen; Ziehl–Neelsen or Kinyoun on imprint preferred
Partially acid-fast organisms suspected	Fite–Farraco	Putt	Modifed Kinyoun on imprint preferred
Actinomyces	Brown and Brenn	Gormori's methenamine silver	
Nocardia	Brown and Brenn; Fite	Gomori's methenamine silver	
Legionella, Yersinia, Francisella, Brucella	Steiner, Warthin–Starry, or Dieterle	Brown–Hopps	Gram's stain on imprint useful

[a] The silver impregnation stains are essentially interchangeable. The preferred stain is the one for which the output of the local laboratory is most satisfactory.

spp., and nonfilamentous bacteria that have polysaccharide capsules such as *Streptococcus pneumoniae*, *Klebsiella pneumoniae*, *Haemophilus influenzae*, *Rhodococcus equi*, and certain strains of *Neisseria meningitidis*. If the incubation period is prolonged, mycobacteria, including *Mycobacterium tuberculosis*, may be stained by the Gomori method.

Silver impregnation stains such as the Steiner, Dieterle, and Warthin–Starry procedures are required to demonstrate *Calymmatobacterium granulomatis* and spirochetes such as *Treponema pallidum*, *Borrelia burgdorferi*, and *Leptospira* spp. The silver impregnation procedures stain all bacteria nonselectively and are excellent for demonstrating small, weakly gram-negative bacilli, such as *Legionella* spp., *Francisella tularensis* (tularemia), *Afipia felis* (proposed as an etiologic agent of cat-scratch disease), *Pseudomonas pseudomallei* (melioidosis), and *Rochalimaea henselae* (cat-scratch disease and bacillary angiomatosis).[155] The accretion of reduced silver on these bacteria greatly increases their visibility but also enlarges and distorts the form of the bacteria. When compared to Gram's stain, silver impregnation procedures provide much greater sensitivity for detecting small numbers of either gram-positive or gram-negative bacteria. Once bacteria are detected, a modification of Gram's stain can be applied to replicate tissue sections to determine gram reactivity of the organisms.

Most mycobacteria, particularly *Mycobacterium avium* complex, not only appear acid fast after staining with the Ziehl-Neelsen procedure, but are also weakly gram positive and stain positively with the periodic acid–Schiff[156] and Gomori's methenamine silver procedures in fixed paraffin-embedded tissue sections. (See also

Chapter 10.) Auramine or auramine-rhodamine may be used to screen sections efficiently for acid-fast bacilli if a fluorescence microscope is available. A mercury light source is not required as halogen lamps emit light efficiently in the exciting range for these dyes. The fluorescent methods are more sensitive than the Ziehl–Neelsen procedure and it is easier to screen sections quickly, but it is more difficult to assess the morphology of putative bacilli and to characterize correctly nonbacterial acid-fast material that may be abundant in sections. The routine acid-fast stain for most laboratories should be the Ziehl–Neelsen procedure, unless an observer is familiar with the fluorescent stains. A modified decolorization procedure should be employed only if a partially acid-fast bacterium is suspected. It should be noted that the fluorescent acid-fast stains operate on the same principles as the Ziehl–Neelsen stain; they are not immunologically specific procedures.

Nocardia spp., *Legionella micdadei*, and *Rhodococcus equi* are weakly acid fast and nonalcohol fast. In addition, the mycobacterial rapid growers such as *Mycobacterium fortuitum* or *Mycobacterium chelonii* may not be stained by the Ziehl–Neelsen procedure. Therefore, modified acid-fast procedures that use an aqueous solution of a weak acid, such as 1% sulfuric acid, as a decolorizer are required to stain these bacteria satisfactorily. The decolorization provided by the Putt modification of the acid-fast stain is more gentle than that provided by the Fite or Fite–Farraco procedures. Instances have been reported in which the Putt modification produced acid-fastness in *Actinomyces* spp., normally not considered acid-fast bacilli, whereas the Fite stain produced negative results.[157] For this reason the Fite modification is the preferred procedure. Rarely, *Legionella pneumophila* may appear acid fast in tissue (personal observation). It is important to recognize that *Legionella* spp. will be acid fast only in tissue and will not appear acid fast after isolation on agar media.

When immunologic reagents of adequate sensitivity and specificity are available, either immunofluorescence or immunoenzymatic staining of bacterial pathogens in smears or formalin-fixed deparaffinized tissue sections can be routinely used to extend the diagnostic capability of conventional histopathology. Immunohistologic staining is invaluable for confirming a presumptive diagnosis, especially when only fixed tissues are available, or for identifying a bacterium in a contaminated specimen. The limited commercial availability of many of the reagents limits the usefulness of this potentially important diagnostic approach.

Controls for histologic stains should be carefully selected to test the reliability of the reagents and the stain procedure. A section that is teeming with acid-fast bacilli is a very poor guarantor of adequate staining in a marginally positive specimen. On the other hand, it is not practical to include a positive control in which scant bacteria are present, because much time will be wasted in searching and there is a finite probability that bacteria will not be visualized even though the stain worked well. Therefore, a middle ground must be sought in which a moderate but not overwhelming number of organisms is present. It is not a good idea to use an "all-purpose" control, such as colonic material that contains mixed morphotypes. An appropriately screened control that contains gram-positive cocci and gram-negative bacilli may be useful, however. Jung[158] described a method for creating fibrin substrates into which cultured bacteria may be placed before fixation and embedding. If the stain is intended to detect a "difficult" organism, such as the Brown–Hopps stain for *Legionella*, it is important to use a control that matches the task; good coloration of *Escherichia coli* is no assurance that *Legionella* will be visualized similarly.

Macroscopic Distribution, Inflammatory Characteristics, and Time Course

Macroscopic Distribution

The classical pathologic characterization of pneumonia has been by macroscopic distribution. At the two poles are lobar and "broncho-" pneumonia.

Lobar Pneumonia

Lobar pneumonia was described as the manifestation of pneumococcal pneumonia. As the name implies, the

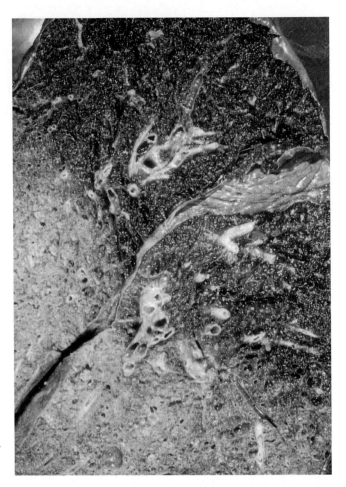

Fig. 9–6. Lobar pneumonia. Elderly man found by his family in unresponsive state died shortly after arriving at the Emergency Department. *Streptococcus pneumoniae* was isolated in pure culture from postmortem lung; extensively emphysematous air spaces are full of very cellular exudate (stage of grey hepatization). Exudate does not involve entire lobe but extends by contiguity to both pleural surface and lobar fissure. This case is unusual in that a major portion of two lobes is involved, but entire process is contiguous and additional foci are not present in other areas of lung.

inflammatory process consumes the greater part of a lobe of the lung and may involve the entire lobe. Typically, the consolidative process extends to and is sharply delimited by the pleura (Fig. 9–6) or by a major fissure (Fig. 9–7). Macroscopic consolidation occasionally may breach the boundary of the lobe. Osler considered[1] the involvement of a single lobe to be an important diagnostic criterion of lobar pneumonia. Microscopic inflammation often extends across the fissure and into the pleura, producing a roughened pleural surface or full-blown pleurisy (Fig. 9–8).

Although lobar pneumonia is classically associated with *Streptococcus pneumoniae*, other pathogens may produce a similar pathologic picture. A typical lobar inflammation caused by *Klebsiella pneumoniae*, type 1, is

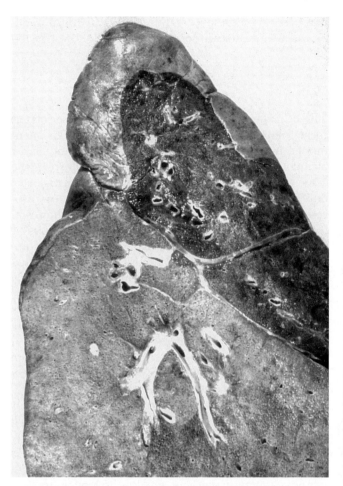

Fig. 9–7. Friedländer's lobar pneumonia. Elderly alcoholic was admitted to hospital with acute pneumonia that progressed rapidly. *Klebsiella pneumoniae*, type 1 was isolated in pure culture from antemortem sputum and postmortem lung tissue. Entire right-lower lobe is consolidated; inflammation extends both to pleural surfaces and lobar fissure. Volume of lung is expanded; some areas of lobe are beefy red while others are yellow-white (stages of red and grey hepatization).

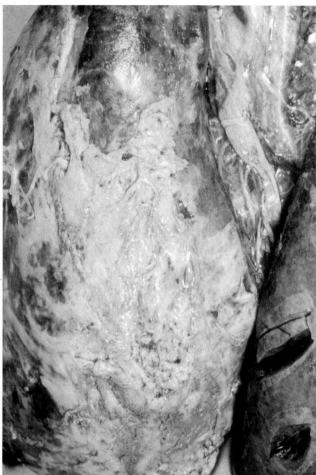

Fig. 9–8. Fibrinous pleurisy and empyema. Middle-aged woman developed influenza A pneumonia complicated by bacterial infection. *Haemophilus influenzae* was isolated from postmortem lung in pure culture. Note shaggy adherent yellow-white exudate on pleural surface.

Table 9–8. Pathologic features of lobar pneumonia in 400 autopsy cases[a]

Pathologic state	Number of cases
Red hepatization	212
Red and gray hepatization	225
Gray hepatization	317
Organizing pneumonia	2
Combination of above	44
Abscess or gangrene	19
Infarct	ˑ6

[a] Reference: 164.

demonstrated pathologically (see Figure 9–7). A minority of cases of *Legionella pneumophila* infection may also produce a typical lobar configuration. Individual cases of lobar pneumonia have been ascribed to *Staphylococcus aureus*,[159] *Neisseria gonorrhoeae*,[160] and *Mycoplasma pneumoniae*.[161]

The pathologic process of lobar pneumonia (primarily pneumococcal) was delineated as early as the first decades of the nineteenth century by Laennec who described the basic progression of the consolidative process (quoted in reference 162). The inflammatory process proceeds through stages of edema, red hepatization, gray hepatization, and resolution.[163] The frequency of various stages and manifestations of lobar pneumonia were tabulated in a series of 400 cases by Berry[164] (Table 9–8). It is noteworthy that two or more stages in the process of consolidation may coexist in the same lung (see Figure 9–7). The pneumonic process is dynamic, so that the inflammatory process is more advanced in the areas infected first than in recently infected areas.

Heffron described the sequence of inflammatory events in lobar pneumonia as follows:[162]

Engorgement

It is rare to find lungs that are totally in the stage of engorgement at autopsy. Rather one must examine the edges of older advancing lesions. The lung is heavy and doughy, but still crepitant. A frothy blood-tinged fluid exudes from the cut surface. Microscopically, the capillaries are engorged, the alveolar epithelium is "swollen," and the airspaces contain edema fluid, red blood cells, and desquamated epithelium. This stage probably lasts only a few hours in the usual case.

Red Hepatization

The lung is heavy, non-crepitant, and no longer floats on water. The surface is dark red or reddish-brown in color. In consistency it is dry and granular because of fibrin deposition in the airspaces. When the etiologic agent is heavily encapsulated, such as *Streptococcus pneumoniae* type 3 or *Klebsiella pneumoniae* type 1 may be, the exudate has been described as more viscid than usual. Microscopically, the air spaces are filled with a fibrin mesh containing erythrocytes, polymorphonuclear and mononuclear leukocytes, and desquamated epithelial cells. The cellular exudate is remarkably intact and well preserved.

Gray Hepatization

At this stage the lung is dense and friable, gray to white to yellow in color. The cut surface is somewhat more moist than in the previous stage and exuded fluid is turbid. Microscopically, the predominant cell in the alveolar exudate is the polymorphonuclear neutrophil. Most erythrocytes have lysed and the fibrin net is less obvious. At this stage the inflammatory exudate is undergoing lysis. Cells stain poorly, their outlines are indistinct, and hemosiderin pigment may be evident. The interstitial blood vessels are no longer engorged and occasionaly megakaryocytes, released from the bone marrow during the outpouring of leukocytes, may be trapped in the capillaries. In pneumococcal lobar pneumonia the bacteria stain well and are still viable during the stage of red hepatization, but are poorly stained and nonviable once the gray hepatization phase is reached.

The time course for the inflammatory process is variable, with the duration of the red and gray hepatization phases being estimated at two to three days each. The time of maximum consolidation has been variously estimated to be 2 days[165] or 3–6 days.[166] The physical effects of the extensive inflammatory consolidation are emphasized by the observation that an artificial pneumothorax produces little, if any, collapse of the affected lung.[167]

Focal Pneumonia

The other major anatomic pattern is best described as focal pneumonia, but has also been called lobular pneumonia, bronchopneumonia, bronchial pneumonia, or bronchiolar pneumonia. The latter names illustrate the association of the inflammation with the bronchial tree, but they are misnomers because the inflammatory process is essentially a disease of the air spaces—the respiratory bronchioles, alveolar ducts, and alveoli. Lobular pneumonia is an accurate description of the most common variant of focal pneumonia. A paper-mounted whole-lung section (Gough section) illustrates clearly the association of inflammation with the centrilobular portion of the pulmonary lobule (Fig. 9–9). The heavy carbon deposition in the patient, who was a cigarette smoker, clearly delineates the terminal bronchioles at the center of the lesions. It is usually difficult to see the distribution so clearly when an unfixed, untreated section of lung is examined macroscopically. The pathogenetic mechanisms are similar to those at work in lobar pneumonia. The stages of consolidation are not so well described as in lobar pneumonia, but undoubtedly follow a similar pattern. Spread of the infection is probably through the bronchial tree from lobule to lobule, segment to segment, and lobe to lobe. Extension from alveolus to alveolus through the pores of Kohn probably occurs also.

The differentiation of lobar from focal lobular pneumonia is not always clear and the processes probably represent a continuum rather than dichotomous entities. When focal pneumonia is extensive, differentiation from lobar pneumonia may be difficult or impossible,[168] a fact that has been recognized for many decades.[162] Such lesions are described as confluent lobular pneumonia (Fig. 9–10). Consolidation may appear lobar by radiographic analysis[169] but be characterized as confluent lobular pneumonia when examined at autopsy.[170]

Similarly, the etiologic associations are not precise. *Streptococcus pneumoniae* is the classic agent of lobar pneumonia, but frequently produces focal consolidation. Conversely, other agents may on occasion cause a lobar consolidation. Although *Staphylococcus aureus* pneumonia is usually described as a focal process, Chartrand and McCracken[159] described a radiographic picture of lobar pneumonia as the most frequent presenting manifestation of infection in 79 infants and children. A factor in characterizing the infections may be the relative imprecision of chest radiographs in

Fig. 9–9. Focal (lobular) pneumonia. Previously healthy young man, a cigarette smoker, developed acute *Legionella* pneumonia. *Legionella pneumophila*, serogroup 1 was isolated in pure culture from lung tissue. This paper-mounted whole-lung section (Gough technique) demonstrates well association of inflammatory exudate with pulmonary lobules because centrilobular regions are marked by intense carbon pigmentation.

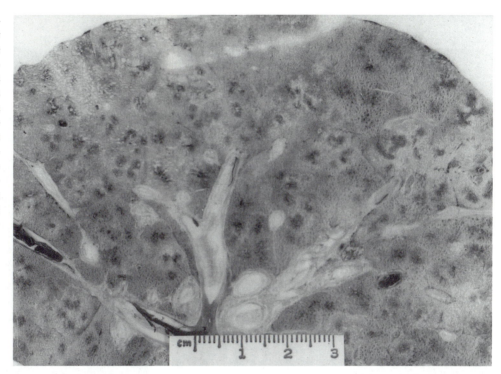

defining the exact anatomic distribution of infiltrates. The radiograph is the only tool that clinicians have to assess the distribution in most cases, however, so it is important to realize the limitations of the technique.

Round Pneumonia

A variant of focal pneumonia has been given the descriptive designation "round pneumonia" (Fig. 9–11). This distribution may be caused by a variety of infectious agents and is not distinctive in a pathogenetic sense. The lesions presumably result from centrifugal spread of the inflammatory process. They may become quite large (Fig. 9–12) and may be multiple (Fig. 9–13). Round pneumonia has been described primarily in children, but may also occur in adults.[171,172]

The radiographic differential diagnosis of round pneumonia is radiation pneumonitis, round atelectasis,

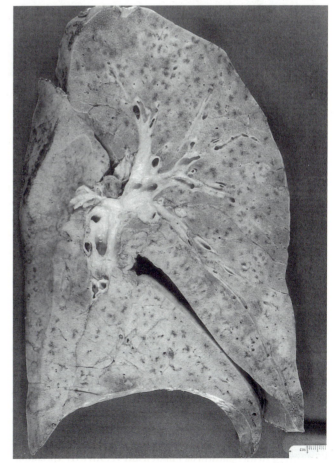

Fig. 9–10. Confluent focal (lobular) pneumonia is produced by coalescence of individual lobular lesions. In this section from lung of patient described in Fig. 9–9, lobular lesions are evident in upper lobe. Consolidation has become confluent in lower part of upper lobe and throughout lower lobe. Such extensive consolidation may be characterized as lobar or sublobar if focal nature of process is not recognized.

and *Peptostreptococcus* sp. are isolated. Although *Bacteroides fragilis* is not usually isolated from the upper airways, this important pathogen is present in a minority of lung abscesses.

Inflammatory Characteristics and Time Course

Acute Pneumonia

Most bacterial pneumonias, excepting mycobacterial infection, are an acute inflammatory process in which the polymorphonuclear neutrophil plays a prominent role. The preceding description of classical lobar pneumonia represents such a process. The development of the inflammatory process requires from 5 to 10 days, and acute symptoms persist a similar period in 70% of untreated cases.[162] Symptoms rarely last only 2–3 days, and occasionally symptoms persist for 2–3 weeks.

The characteristics of the inflammatory process are somewhat more variable. Cases of well-documented legionnaires' disease have been described in which the histologic reaction in biopsied lung resembled acute diffuse alveolar damage with prominent hyaline membranes and without a prominent accumulation of polymorphonuclear neutrophils in the air spaces.[185] Approximately one-third of *Legionella pneumophila* infections are characterized by an alveolar exudate exclusively of macrophages.[172] Walsh and Kelley[186] described an unusual case of legionnaires' disease in which the exudate was exclusively mature plasma cells. The clinical presentations and time course in these cases with atypical inflammatory cell populations did not differ from a typical case.

Chronic Pneumonia

Chronic pneumonias are most commonly caused by fungi and mycobacteria, but some bacterial species frequently produce a chronic process in which islands of acute inflammatory cells are mixed with chronic inflammation and fibrosis. *Actinomyces* spp. and related bacteria, *Nocardia* spp., and *Pseudomonas pseudomallei* typically produce such infections. It should be emphasized, however, that other pathogens typically associated with acute inflammation may on occasion produce a chronic process.

Organizing Pneumonia and Fibrosis

Most episodes of acute pneumonia resolve spontaneously or after antimicrobial chemotherapy by resorption of the inflammatory exudate with restitution of the normal underlying structure. In some cases, however, the stimulation of fibroblasts by the inflammatory response elicits a proliferation of connective tissue (Fig. 9–16). Kuhn[187] defined at least four pathologic processes that contribute to the remodeling of the lung: interstitial thickening, deposition of a connective tissue matrix within the air spaces, collapse of the air spaces, and contraction of the wound. The intraalveolar proliferation of fibroblasts produces nodular structures called Masson bodies (Fig. 9–17). (Also see Chapters 4 and 5 for the entity BOOP.) Pulmonary myofibroblasts participate in the contractile phase of pulmonary fibrosis,[188–190] producing a contracted residuum of mature fibroblasts.[191] The process of pulmonary fibrosis is discussed in detail in Chapter 20.

Specific Etiologic Agents of Pneumonia

Gram-Positive Cocci

Streptococcus pneumoniae

The pneumococcus is the king of pulmonary pathogens, although its relative position has been diminished by addition of new pathogens and new risk factors. The clinical,[192] epidemiologic, pathogenetic,[53,61,163,193] diagnostic,[194] and pathologic[162] aspects of pneumococcal pneumonia have been reviewed and discussed extensively. A variety of pneumococcal serotypes produce infection, but a select group of serotypes, which have been incorporated into pneumococcal vaccines, produces the majority of infections.[195] The recent development of pneumococcal strains resistant or relatively resistant to penicillin introduces a new therapeutic concern into the treatment of pneumococcal pneumonia.[196] Fortunately, fully resistant strains are still unusual in the United States and resistant isolates respond fully to therapy with third-generation cephalosporins. Pneumonia that is produced by relatively resistant pneumococcal strains may respond to penicillin therapy given in high doses.

The classical presentation of pneumococcal pneumonia is as a lobar consolidation (Figs. 9–6 and 9–18). It is important to recognize, however, that in a substantial proportion of cases the process is focal (Fig. 9–19). The inflammatory infiltrate consists of a mixture of polymorphonuclear neutrophils and macrophages (Fig. 9–20) surrounded by an edematous zone (Fig. 9–21). In the early stages of the infection pneumococci are easily demonstrated in the infiltrate (Fig. 9–22). An immunologically specific diagnosis can be made by reacting the bacteria with a polyvalent antiserum to capsular polysaccharide, the quellung reaction.[197] This procedure works better on sputum smears (Fig. 9–23) or tissue imprints than on isolated bacteria. Although the

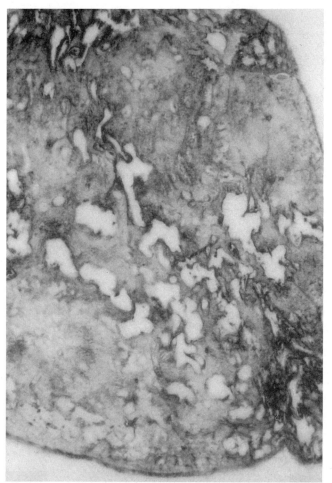

9-16

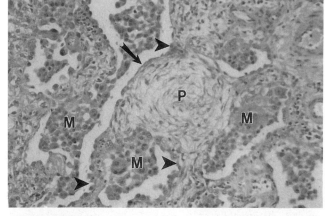

9-17

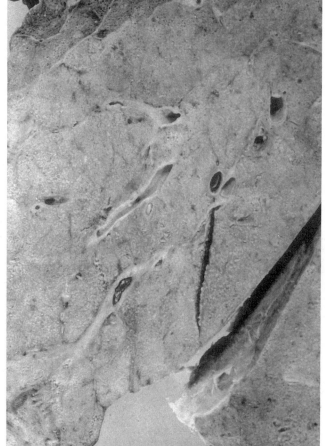

9-18

Fig. 9–16. Extensive area of fibrosis is evident in paper-mounted whole-lung section of patient who had had legionnaires' disease. Distal bronchioles are prominently outlined by fibrosis. *Legionella pneumophila* was isolated ante mortem.

Fig. 9–17. Masson polyp (P) composed of proliferating fibroblasts in air space. Epithelial cells cover surface (*arrow*), and attachments to cellular interstitium (arrowheads) represent route of fibroblastic ingrowth into air space. Macrophages (M) have accumulated in adjacent air spaces. H and E, ×250. (Courtesy of Kevin Leslie, M.D.)

Fig. 9–18. Pneumococcal lobar pneumonia. Major part of lobe is densely consolidated, primarily in stage of grey hepatization.

quellung reaction is useful for problem cases, the antiserum is very expensive and the information is not usually necessary.

Most nonfatal cases of pneumococcal pneumonia resolve without residua, but cavitary disease may occur, particularly in patients who have bacteremic disease.[173,198] In some cases concomitant infection with bacteria that typically produce necrotizing infection may be responsible.[199] Respiratory distress syndrome as defined clinically has been described as a complication in fatal pneumococcal pneumonia.[200] Pneumatoceles, typically associated with staphylococcal pneumonia, have been reported in childhood pneumococcal infection.[201]

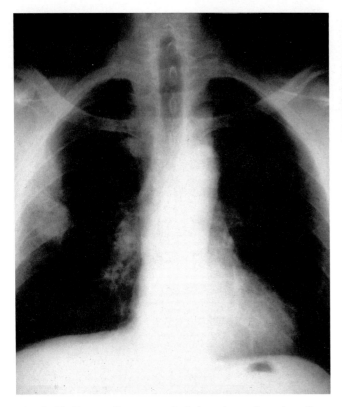

Fig. 9–19. Focus of pneumonia is based on pleural surface, suggesting differential diagnosis of pulmonary embolus and hemorrhage. Rounded nodular outline is discernible within larger infiltrate. *Streptococcus pneumoniae*, type 3 was isolated in pure culture from aspirate of lesion.

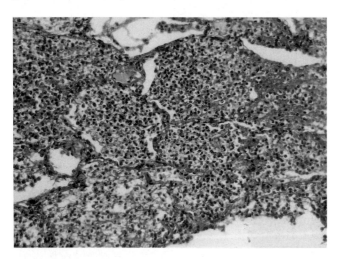

Fig. 9–20. Pneumococcal pneumonia. Air spaces are filled with intact inflammatory cells, fibrin, and edema fluid. Interstitium is distinctly outlined by congested vasculature in classical example of red hepatization. H and E, ×100.

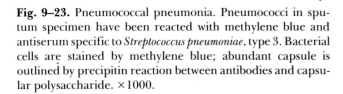

Fig. 9–23. Pneumococcal pneumonia. Pneumococci in sputum specimen have been reacted with methylene blue and antiserum specific to *Streptococcus pneumoniae*, type 3. Bacterial cells are stained by methylene blue; abundant capsule is outlined by precipitin reaction between antibodies and capsular polysaccharide. ×1000.

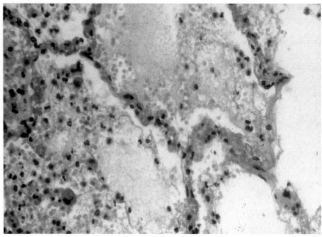

Fig. 9–21. Pneumococcal pneumonia. At edge of inflammatory focus is slight infiltrate of inflammatory cells in air spaces and surrounding acellular edema. Interstitial vasculature is congested. H and E, ×400.

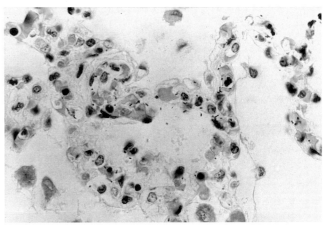

Fig. 9–22. Pneumococcal pneumonia. Gram-positive diplococci are well demonstrated in cellular exudate of child with pneumonia and Waterhouse-Friderichsen syndrome associated with *Streptococcus pneumoniae* bacteremia. Brown–Hopps procedure, ×580.

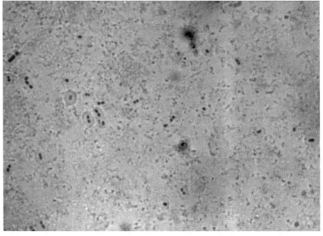

Beta-Hemolytic Streptococci

Streptococcus pyogenes (Group A beta-hemolytic streptococcus) pneumonia is exceedingly rare and was uncommon even in the preantibiotic era.[162] The pneumonia may be secondary to streptococcal sepsis. The recent resurgence of virulent streptococcal infection[202,203] may bode greater familiarity with this awesome pathogen, the cause of the death of Jim Henson, creator of the muppets. Primary pulmonary infection often follows viral illness, particularly influenza,[204–207] but primary streptococcal pneumonia also occurs without antecedent disease.[205,208] Mortality, which was as high as 54%,[162] decreased dramatically with the introduction of penicillin therapy. Bacteremia is uncommon in primary *Streptococcus pyogenes* pneumonia.[205,208] Keefer and colleagues[205] detected bacteremia in 12% of 55 patients with primary streptococcal pneumonia; in those patients the mortality rate was 57% compared to 9% in the nonbacteremic patients. Although penicillin-resistant isolates have not yet been recognized, some of the virulent strains produce such rapidly fatal disease that antibiotics do not have a chance to kill the organisms.

The distribution of the lesions ranges from focal, lobular infiltrates, often confluent and extensive,[209,210] to lobar pneumonia. An interstitial pattern has also been described radiographically[204] and pathologically,[210] perhaps analogous to the familiar streptococcal cellulitis in the skin, but Goodpasture commented that the interstitial bronchopneumonia described by MacCallum as a sequel to measles was not present in his cases.[211] Macroscopically, Goodpasture[211] described the gray-purple color of the cut lung surface and the dry nature of the exudate in the bronchioles.

Early in the infection bacteria and inflammatory cells are scarce and hyaline membranes may be prominent.[211] At this early stage it may be difficult to distinguish between cases that were preceded clinically by a viral infection and those that were not, an observation that was later made by those who studied staphylococcal pneumonia in the influenza pandemic of 1957. Later, the infiltrate is rich in polymorphonuclear neutrophils, which may be extensively lysed by the bacterial enzymes, leaving a battlefield strewn with nuclear fragments and dead bacteria (Fig. 9–24). The result may be a very "dusty"-looking microscopic field at low power. Abscess formation is well described,[212] as is empyema.[204] Kevy and Lowe[213] described empyema as a complication in 100% of their cases of Group A streptococcal pneumonia.

Streptococcus agalactiae (Group B beta-hemolytic streptococcus) is best known as an important cause of neonatal pneumonia (see Chapter 8). There is a second peak of group B infections in the elderly, however,[214] and

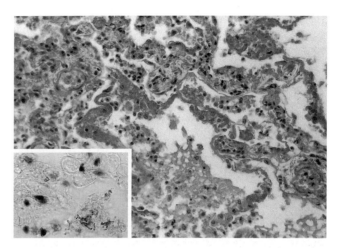

Fig. 9–24. *Streptococcus pyogenes* pneumonia. Interstitial infiltrate and alveolar exudate of edema and fibrin with hyaline membranes characterize this case of streptococcal pneumonia. Other areas of the lung contained intense neutrophilic alveolar exudates with microabscesses. *Streptococcus pyogenes* (Group A beta hemolytic streptococcus) was isolated in pure culture from lung. H and E, ×250. Inset: Small gram-positive cocci chains in various planes of focus. Brown–Hopps procedure, ×1000.

occasional cases of pneumonia have been reported. Verghese and colleagues reported seven cases, two of whom had diabetes mellitus.[215] All seven patients died, but five of the seven cases were polymicrobial.

Group C beta-hemolytic streptococci commonly produce disease in animals, including strangles in horses. They are generally recognized as etiologic agents of streptococcal pharyngitis and peritonsillar abscess[216,217] and may cause serious systemic disease.[218] Group C streptococci also may rarely produce serious pneumonia that resembles *Streptococcus pyogenes* infection in most parameters.[217–220] As in group A infections an interstitial pattern of infiltrates is often seen radiographically and empyema is a common complication.

Group C streptococci have been identified as *Streptococcus zooepidemicus* and *Streptococcus equisimilis* when appropriate biochemical studies are performed. These organisms are beta hemolytic on sheep blood agar, but may be gamma hemolytic on horse blood agar. Many strains are very susceptible to bacitracin and may be identified as group A streptococci if the taxonomic bacitracin disk is used for presumptive identification.[218]

These species rarely cause pneumonia and are more frequently found in the oropharynx of healthy individuals than are group A beta-hemolytic streptococci, so that isolation from normally sterile sites, seroconversion, or critical analysis of laboratory and clinical data is necessary to document the isolate as an etiologic agent of the infection. Group C streptococci are susceptible to the action of penicillin, and resistant strains have not been described.

Other beta-hemolytic streptococci rarely cause infection. A possible case of group G beta-hemolytic streptococcal pneumonia in a newborn infant has been described.[221] Group D and F streptococci usually have an alpha or gamma hemolytic reaction on blood agar and are discussed below.

Viridans Streptococci

Lancefield group F streptococci that are not beta hemolytic (α or γ hemolysis) have been recovered from serious lower respiratory infections.[181] These organisms are physiologically characterized variously as *Streptococcus milleri* in the British literature (not a taxonomically valid name) and *Streptococcus anginosus* in the American literature. They cause abscesses in many organs, including lung, liver, and brain. In the lung they have been described as a component of polymicrobial lung abscess and as the sole cause of lung abscess. In one case the abscess was described as "foul smelling," a feature of anaerobic infection, but gram-positive cocci in chains were seen in smears and only *Streptococcus anginosus* was isolated. The possibility that *Peptostreptococcus* sp. was also present, but not isolated, cannot be eliminated. A case of empyema secondary to liver abscess without primary pneumonia has also been described.[222]

Sarkar and colleagues[223] described three cases of bacteremic pneumonia caused by *Streptococcus uberis*. The clinical course was uncomplicated, abscesses were not present, and the patients responded to penicillin therapy. Pratter and Irwin[224] reported a case of lung abscess and empyema caused by viridans streptococcus. The isolate was not completely identified, and the case may represent another example of *Streptococcus anginosus* infection.

Enterococcus spp.

Enterococci (formerly classified as streptococci) are rarely isolated from the oropharynx and the lower respiratory tract. Berk and colleagues[225] described a case of enterococcal pneumonia that developed after therapy with cephalosporins. The inflammatory response as observed in transtracheal aspirates consisted of polymorphonuclear neutrophils. One isolate was completely identified as *Enterococcus faecalis*, the most common enterococcal species. Enterococci are naturally resistant to cephalosporins and are recognized as potential problems in abdominal infections that are treated with these commonly used antibiotics. Optimal therapy is provided by the combination of a beta-lactam antibiotic and an aminoglycoside (usually ampicillin and gentamicin). Strains that are intrinsically resistant to aminoglycosides and do not respond to combination therapy have been described with increasing frequency[226]; vancomycin alone or vancomycin and an aminoglycoside must then be used. Vancomycin-resistant strains have also been identified, leaving infectious disease physicians anxiously searching for alternatives.[227]

Staphylococcus aureus (Coagulase-Positive Staphylococcus)

Staphylococcus aureus is an uncommon but life-threatening cause of pneumonia both in the community and in hospitals; its incidence may be increasing.[99] Most patients who develop staphylococcal pneumonia have some underlying disease. Influenza virus infection is a frequent antecedent event when disease is community acquired. In a recent study of staphylococcal pneumonia, 52% of patients who were also tested for viral infection had either influenza A or B.[228] Staphylococcal pneumonia was a very frequent cause of secondary pneumonia in the 1957 influenza pandemic,[229] but has been less prominent in subsequent epidemics. Staphylococcal pneumonia also occurs in sporadic forms without regard to outbreaks of influenza virus, usually as a nosocomial infection.[174,230] In such cases the pneumonia may be primary, contracted through a respiratory route,[230] or may be secondary to infected foci in the viscera or soft tissues.[175]

Staphylococcal infections occur at the extremes of life.[159,174] Patients with coma[99] or on neurosurgical nursing units[231] are more likely to develop staphylococcal pneumonia. Patients infected with human immunodeficiency virus are also at increased risk. Levine and colleagues[132] identified *Staphylococcus aureus* as the etiologic agent in 7 of 102 patients who developed respiratory illness. It is noteworthy that *Staphylococcus aureus* was isolated from respiratory secretions in 30 clinical episodes, but the bacteria were believed to be the etiologic agent in only 8 instances. Even in severely immunosuppressed patients the isolation of most bacteria from potentially contaminated secretions does not establish an etiologic diagnosis. Finally, patients with cystic fibrosis are often colonized with *Staphylococcus aureus* and may develop symptomatic infection of the lower respiratory tract. *Staphylococcus* usually is found in the early stages of disease, to be supplanted later by *Pseudomonas aeruginosa*.[232]

The clinical presentation is quite variable. Patients are usually acutely ill; septicemic signs and symptoms may be dominant in disseminated infection. The radiographic distribution of the lesions may take any pattern, including lobar.[159] When the lungs are seeded from

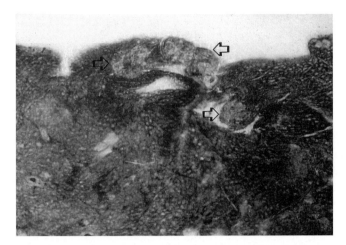

Fig. 9–25. Mixed pneumonia caused by *Legionella pneumophila* and *Staphylococcus aureus*. Staphylococcal lesions in paper-mounted whole-lung section are discrete, focal rounded densities that were microabscesses histologically (*arrows*). *Legionella pneumophila* and *Staphylococcus aureus*, isolated from postmortem lung.

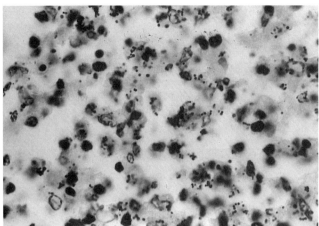

Fig. 9–26. *Staphylococcus aureus* pneumonia. Numerous gram-positive rounded cocci in pairs and small clusters both within phagocytic cells and free in air space. Contrast these forms with chains seen in streptococcal pneumonia and elongated pairs and short chains of cocci in pneumococcal pneumonia. *Staphylococcus aureus* isolated in pure culture from the lung. Brown–Hopps procedure, ×1000.

distant foci of infection, a metastatic pattern of multiple rounded densities may occur (Fig. 9–25).[175]

The inflammatory reaction is usually rich in polymorphonuclear leukocytes and bacteria are easily visualized with Gram's stain (Fig. 9–26). Abscesses occur in 15% to 20% of patients,[174,228] but have been described in as many as 70% of primary pneumonias[230] and 80% of hematogenously derived infections.[175] Pneumatoceles, thin-walled "abscesses" visualized on chest radiographs, are classically described in children with staphylococcal pneumonia[159] but may occur after other bacterial infections as well.[233] Chartrand and McCracken[159] described pneumatoceles in 33 of 79 children (41%), usually by the fifth to the seventh day after admission (also see Chapter 8). Likewise, empyema is a recognized complication of staphylococcal pneumonia, occurring in 20% of adult cases[174] and as many as 75% of pediatric infections.[159,234] Atypical cases have been described in which a mixture of acute and chronic inflammation with fibrosis was present, perhaps influenced by partially effective antimicrobial chemotherapy.[235]

The mortality from staphylococcal pneumonia may be considerable. Bacteremia after primary infection develops in 25%–40% of patients.[230,236] A rate of bacteremia as high as 89% has been reported when disseminated staphylococcal lesions are present; in this situation the bacteremia may persist even in the face of appropriate antimicrobial chemotherapy.[159] The death rate is commonly in the range of 25%–30%,[159,174,228] but may be as high as 84% when bacteremia is present.[237] Therapy of the infections is complicated by the existence in many hospitals of bacterial strains that are resistant to multiple antibiotics, including the penicillinase-resistant penicillins and cephalosporins that are usually selected as therapy.[238] In these cases vancomycin is the only readily available alternative.

Other Gram-Positive Cocci

Souhami et al.[239] described a case of pneumonia in which *Micrococcus luteus* was isolated in heavy quantities and pure culture from a bronchial brush specimen. The patient, who had acute myelogenous leukemia and was leukopenic, developed cavitary disease but was successfully treated. The sputum was described as purulent, but the inflammatory nature of the material from the brushings was not mentioned. This organism is usually a saprophyte and is pathogenic in only rare instances.

Gram-Positive Bacilli

Nocardia spp.

Nocardiosis is an acute progressive or chronic bacterial infection caused by aerobic, exogenous, filamentous actinomycetes in the genus *Nocardia* and the order Actinomycetales.[240,241] The disease occurs worldwide and is often seen in persons who are immunocompromised or who have underlying medical conditions,[242–244] especially lymphoreticular malignancies,[245] granulocytopenia, chronic granulomatous dis-

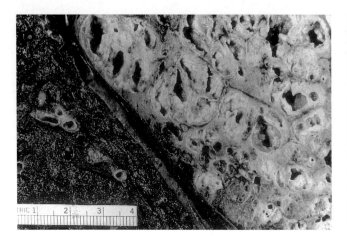

Fig. 9–27. Pulmonary nocardiosis. Sectioned surface of lung reveals multiple abscesses with fibrotic walls.

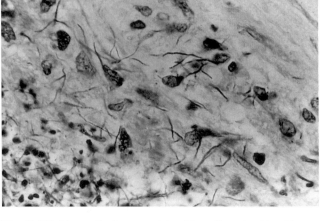

Fig. 9–28. Nocardiosis caused by *Nocardia asteroides*. Gram-positive filaments branching at predominantly right angles are embedded in fibrogranulomatous wall of pulmonary abscess. Brown and Brenn procedure, ×750.

ease of childhood,[246,247] and pulmonary alveolar proteinosis.[248–250] Most primary infections are pulmonary and result from inhalation of nocardiae that live as saprophytes in soil. Hematogenous dissemination from a primary pulmonary focus can involve almost any organ, but the brain, subcutaneous tissue, bones, joints, heart, and peritoneum are most often affected. Primary cutaneous lesions are rare and result from the accidental percutaneous inoculation of nocardiae in the environment.[251–253] The term nocardiosis refers to the disseminated disease in which nocardial filaments are randomly scattered within the invaded tissue. When nocardiae develop in the form of grains or granules in tissue, this rare localized form of the disease, usually seen in noncompromised patients, is classified as an actinomycotic mycetoma.

The three principal species that cause nocardiosis are *Nocardia asteroides*, *Nocardia brasiliensis*, and *Nocardia otitidiscaviarum*. Rarely, other species, such as *Nocardia transvalensis*, may produce similar disease.[254] Approximately 85% of nocardial infections are caused by *Nocardia asteroides*, and this species is most often implicated in pulmonary infections. All three species are aerobic and easily cultured on Lowenstein–Jensen medium at 30°C to 37°C. They will also grow, however, on blood agar and Sabouraud's agar that are antibiotic free. Colonies usually develop within 3–7 days, are heaped and folded, cream to yellowish-orange, and have a surface that is either moist and glabrous or covered with a powdery white aerial mycelium. The nocardiae are morphologically similar in cultures and clinical materials, appearing as delicate, branched filaments ≤1 μm in diameter. The filaments are often beaded, and fragmented bacillary and coccoid forms are occasionally seen. Isolates can be

identified in culture by studying their physiologic and biochemical properties.[240,255,256]

Nocardiosis occurs three times as often in males as in females. It usually presents as either a chronic pneumonia in apparently immunocompetent individuals or as an acute, progressive pneumonia in immunodeficient patients.[257–264] Symptoms of pulmonary infection mimic those of tuberculosis and include fever, chills, dyspnea, cough, hemoptysis, chest pain, night sweats, and weight loss. Chest radiographs, which are nonspecific, usually reveal bilateral infiltrates and thin-walled cavities. Therapy consists of surgical drainage combined with high doses of trimethoprim-sulfamethoxazole or penicillins.[240,255,256,266]

The inflammatory response in nocardiosis is typically suppurative and necrotizing, leading to sinus tracts and encapsulated abscesses.[241] In chronic infections, multiple abscesses filled with thick, greenish-yellow, odorless pus are separated by areas of fibrosis (Fig. 9–27). The abscesses, which vary from 1 to 10 mm or more in diameter, are filled with neutrophils and macrophages. In chronic infections, epithelioid histiocytes and multinucleated giant cells are usually present at the periphery of the abscesses. The overall appearance of nocardiosis differs somewhat from actinomycosis in that the abscess cavities are less well defined and the fibrosis is less pronounced. Cavitation and pleuritis with empyema are frequent complications of pulmonary nocardiosis.[243,245,259,262]

In both acute and chronic lesions, individual nocardiae are diffusely distributed in the inflammatory exudate. The organisms appear as delicate, beaded filaments, ≤1 μm in width, that branch at predominantly right angles (Fig. 9–28).[241,267,268] Frequently individual filaments are so highly branched that they have been described as resembling "Chinese characters." In tissue sections the nocardiae are readily demonstrated with Gomori's methenamine silver stain and by a modified Gram's stain, such as Brown and Brenn and Brown–Hopps. They are not reliably stained, however, with hematoxylin and eosin, periodic acid–Schiff, and Gridley fungus procedures. *Nocardia* spp. are weakly acid fast and nonalcohol fast when stained with modified acid-fast procedures that use an aqueous solution of a weak acid for decolorization (Fig. 9–29).[241,267]

Patients with pulmonary nocardiosis who are severely immunocompromised often present with progressive disease that appears as lobar, lobular, or fulminant necrotizing pneumonia.[241,243,257,264] Pulmonary fibrosis is minimal in these patients. The pneumonia is histologically similar to that caused by more commonly encountered bacteria. In the fulminant form of the disease, myriad nocardiae are often present and appear as faintly basophilic filaments and fragmented bacillary forms in hematoxylin and eosin stained sections. Large numbers of entangled nocardial filaments can form loose aggregates, but these aggregates do not resemble "sulfur granules" as seen in actinomycosis. Nor are they surrounded by clublike Splendore–Hoeppli material.

An unusual association of nocardiosis is that with pulmonary alveolar proteinosis (see Chapter 22). The pathogenic relationship between these two entities is not completely understood.[248,249] *Nocardia* spp. have a predilection for causing pulmonary infection, and it is likely that alveolar proteinosis provides a favorable condition for growth of these actinomycetes. In addition to pulmonary nocardiosis, cerebral nocardiosis has also been reported in association with pulmonary alveolar proteinosis.[249]

Bacillus anthracis

Anthrax, historically referred to as "woolsorters' disease" in England,[269–271] is a highly lethal form of pneumonia and septicemia. Anthrax is caused by inhalation of spores of the large (1 μm in width by 3 μm to 10 μm in length) gram-positive, nonmotile, toxin-producing rod *Bacillus anthracis*. This rare zoonotic disease is endemic in goats, sheep, cattle, horses, and pigs. It is usually spread to humans through the handling of contaminated hides, wool, hair, bone meal, or other animal products.[272] Those in close contact with these products or with animal tissues and fluids are at greatest risk. Infection occurs when spores of *Bacillus anthracis* enter the body via percutaneous implantation, inhalation, or ingestion. The four major clinical forms of anthrax are cutaneous (malignant pustule), septicemic, pulmonary, and gastrointestinal. The malignant pus-

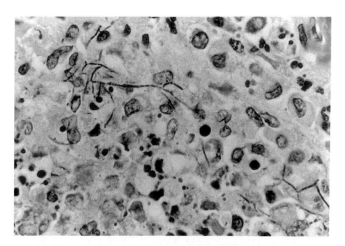

Fig. 9–29. Pulmonary nocardiosis. Delicate beaded and branched acid-fast filaments of *Nocardia asteroides* embedded in pulmonary abscess. Modified Ziehl–Neelsen stain, ×750.

tule is the most common form and accounts for 95% of all infections.[273] Patients with pulmonary anthrax typically have no predisposing underlying illness, and the disease has a rapid onset characterized by fever, extreme weakness, nonproductive cough, severe dyspnea, tachycardia, and cyanosis. Anthrax is usually fatal within 4 days after the onset of symptoms. The diagnosis is seldom suspected, and the clinical course is usually very short.[274,275]

Experimental animal models of anthrax have shown that, after inhalation of spores, germination and multiplication of organisms occur in the tracheobronchial lymph nodes rather than in the lungs. A generalized septicemia follows germination. The lungs and other body sites are then involved by secondary spread. Vascular injury results from sepsis and individual toxin components.[18,276–279]

The most characteristic lesion of pulmonary anthrax is hemorrhagic edema (Fig. 9–30).[18,274,276] The lungs are heavy and have decreased crepitance. The pleural surfaces are smooth and there is usually a serosanguinous pleural effusion. The cut surfaces of the lungs are wet, and bloody fluid can easily be expressed from both bronchi and alveoli. Microscopically the lungs show massive hemorrhage and edema of all air spaces (see Fig. 9–30). The most significant feature is the presence of a serofibrinous exudate and many large gram-positive bacilli in the absence of neutrophilic inflammatory exudate (Fig. 9–31). In the few patients who have a prolonged survival, septal necrosis may evolve and fibrin thrombi are present in alveolar capillaries.

Patients who are diagnosed as having anthrax before death should be autopsied only with extreme care, because of the extreme hazards associated with han-

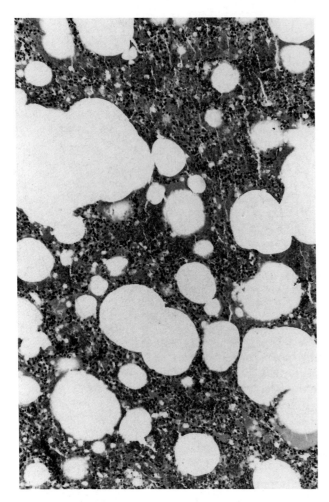

Fig. 9–30. Pulmonary anthrax characterized by diffuse intraalveolar hemorrhage and edema. H and E, ×100.

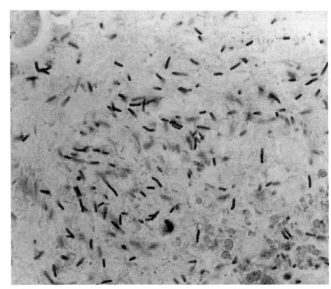

Fig. 9–31. Pulmonary anthrax. Numerous large, elongated bacilli of *Bacillus anthracis* occupy a bronchiole and contiguous alveolar spaces. Note absence of neutrophilic inflammatory exudate. Steiner silver impregnation method, ×750.

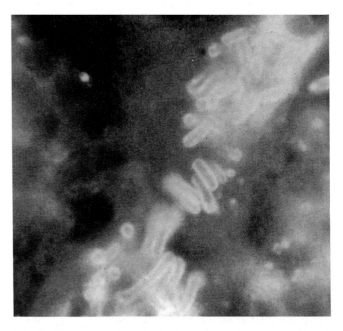

Fig. 9–32. Immunohistologic detection of *Bacillus anthracis* uses fluorescein-labeled antiglobulins specific for this bacterium. Large, brightly fluorescent bacilli with rounded ends in terminal bronchiole. ×1,500.

dling *Bacillus anthracis.* If tissue from suspected cases is available, the organism can be identified in impression smears or in fixed deparaffinized tissue sections by direct immunofluorescence (Fig. 9–32).[280]

Rhodococcus equi (Corynebacterium equi)

Infection with the aerobic gram-positive opportunistic bacterium *Rhodococcus equi* (formerly *Corynebacterium equi*) is being reported with increased frequency in immunocompromised humans, particularly those with defective cell-mediated immunity.[281–288] Since *Rhodococcus equi* was first reported to cause human infection in 1967,[289] more than 35 cases have appeared in the refereed literature.[285] Approximately one-third of the infections have occurred in patients with AIDS or HIV infection. (See also Chapter 6). This bacterium has now been added to the list of opportunistic pathogens that define the acquired immunodeficiency syndrome.[285,290–292]

Rhodococcus equi is a well-recognized agent of respiratory and other infections in domestic animals, including horses, cattle, sheep, and swine. Foals are especially susceptible to infection and often develop suppurative pneumonia.[281,283,293,294] The bacterium is a common saprophyte of soil, which is believed to be the source for infections in animals.[293,294] Humans with *Rhodococcus equi* infections usually have a history of contact with farm animals or manure.[286,295] In patients who cannot recall animal contact, soil is believed to be the natural reservoir and source of the bacterium. In most instances, *Rhodococcus equi* is probably acquired by inhalation of animal secretions or contaminated soil, after which there is a primary pulmonary infection.

The most common clinical manifestation of *Rhodococcus equi* infection in humans is pneumonia, occurring in about 75% of all cases.[285] The onset is typically insidious with fever, cough, dyspnea, and fatigue. Chest radiographs often reveal a unilobar pulmonary infiltrate with no predilection for involvement of a particular lobe. After 2–3 weeks, the infiltrate may progress to involve several lobes or cavitate.[282,286,291,292] Pulmonary infections tend to be chronic, may mimic tuberculosis or other slowly progressive infections, may cavitate, and may produce pleural effusion or frank empyema.[296] The spectrum of pathologic findings includes acute suppurative bronchopneumonia, necrotizing pneumonia with abscess formation and cavitation, and mixed suppurative and granulomatous pneumonia involving one or more lobes.[282,285,288–290] *Rhodococcus equi* has also been reported to cause osteomyelitis, endophthalmitis, wound infection in a noncompromised individual,[297] and recurring bacteremia.[282,283,285]

Hematogenous dissemination from a primary pulmonary focus has been reported and *Rhodococcus equi* has been isolated from several distant infected sites.[285,292] The mortality of disseminated *Rhodococcus equi* infection is higher for patients who are infected with human immunodeficiency virus than for those who are not (55% versus 20%).[285]

In tissue sections there are foci of suppurative and granulomatous inflammation. *Rhodococcus equi* appears as numerous pleomorphic, gram-positive coccobacilli within macrophages and, less often, polymorphonuclear leukocytes (Fig. 9–33). The bacterium is easily delineated with modified gram stains such as Brown and Brenn, and Gomori's methenamine silver stain (Fig. 9–34). Most strains of *Rhodococcus equi* are partially acid-fast with the Fite or Fite–Farraco stains, but they do not retain their acid-fastness when stained with the standard Ziehl–Neelsen procedure for mycobacteria. Partial acid-fastness can be an important clue to the identity of *Rhodococcus* spp. in tissue sections.[281,292]

In culture, most *Rhodococcus equi* isolates of human origin are resistant to penicillins and cephalosporins. In vitro studies have shown that virulent strains of *Rhodococcus equi* are resistant to phagocytosis and intracellular killing by macrophages.[298] It has been suggested therefore that antibiotics with two distinct characteristics, activitiy against *Rhodococcus equi* in vitro and the ability

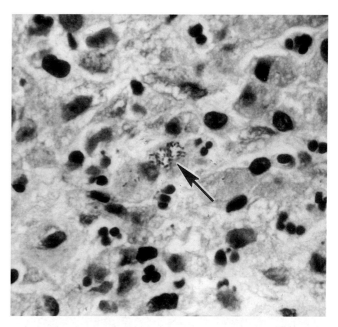

Fig. 9–33. Wound infection caused by *Rhodococcus equi*. Occasional macrophages contain gram-positive, pleomorphic coccobacilli (*arrow*). Brown–Hopps procedure, ×750.

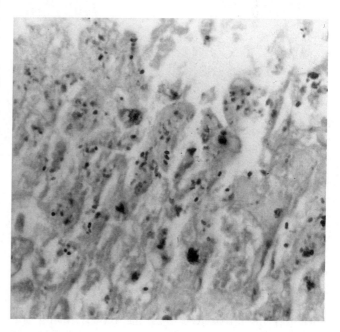

Fig. 9–34. *Rhodococcus equi* infection. Pleomorphic, argyrophilic coccobacilli within epithelioid histiocytes at periphery of abscess. Gomori methenamine silver, ×750.

to penetrate macrophages, should be selected for treatment.[285,296] Erythromycin and rifampin are two commonly used antibiotics that share these characteristics. Similar reasoning has been used to justify the efficacy of these two antibiotics against *Legionella* spp. in vivo. A prolonged course of antibiotics has been recommended

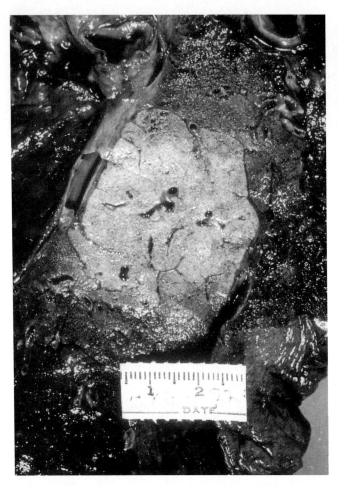

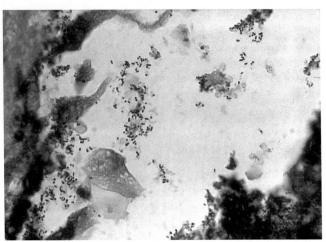

Fig. 9–36. *Corynebacterium jeikeium* pneumonia. Tissue Gram stain from case shown in Fig. 9–35 demonstrates numerous small gram-positive coccobacilli, primarily extracellular. Differential diagnosis includes other "diptheroids" and elongated streptococci. Brown–Hopps procedure, ×1000.

◁

Fig. 9–35. *Corynebacterium jeikeium* pneumonia. Large consolidated necrotic grey nodule is surrounded by hemorrhagic lung. Note lobular demarcation of lesion. (Courtesy of B. Waters, M.D.)

because of frequent relapses. In addition to antibiotics, surgical extirpation or drainage of persistent, isolated lesions may also be beneficial.

Corynebacterium spp.

Several *Corynebacterium* species may produce pneumonia in immunosuppressed patients.

Corynebacterium jeikeium (formerly *Corynebacterium* Group JK) is a species that produces septicemia in immunosuppressed patients, usually in the terminal stages of their illness. This species is found on the skin and may be introduced into the blood during the process of collection, so that routine identification of isolates is not useful. If multiple cultures from an immunosuppressed patient are positive, however, the isolate should be identified and tested for antimicrobial susceptibility, because this species is resistant to the commonly used beta lactam antibiotics. Pneumonia may result as a part of the septicemic process. Waters[299] described a case of *Corynebacterium jeikeium* pneumonia in a neutropenic patient. The lung was edematous and hemorrhagic. Alveolar septa were focally necrotic and contained masses of proliferating bacteria (Figs. 9–35 and 9–36). Abscess cavities have been documented radiographically in pneumonia produced by this species.[300] Cases of pneumonia caused by *Corynebacterium pseudodiphtheriticum* and *Corynebacterium* Group D2 have been reported in immunocompetent individuals.[301,302] A case of pneumonia attributed to *Corynebacterium pseudotuberculosis*, ordinarily an animal pathogen, has been described in a veterinary medical student.[303] A transtracheal aspirate from which the bacterium was isolated contained polymorphonuclear neutrophils, but a transbronchial biopsy demonstrated interstitial fibrosis and intraalveolar eosinophils.

Miscellaneous Gram-Positive Bacilli

Listeria monocytogenes is a well-recognized cause of intrauterine and neonatal infection, as well as meningitis in adults. In patients who are infected with HIV this bacterium produces a greater variety of infections, including brain abscess.[304] Pneumonia is a rare manifestation of *Listeria* infection. Whitelock-Jones and colleagues[305] reported an unusual case of cavitating pneumonia in a previously healthy man. *Listeria monocytogenes* was isolated from blood.

Bacillus cereus may cause serious infections, including pneumonia, especially in patients who are immunosuppressed.[306] Bekemeyer and Zimmerman[307] reported an 18-year-old, previously healthy, man who developed massive hemoptysis, bronchopleural fistula, and empyema. *Bacillus cereus* was isolated from sputum and in pure culture from pleural fluid.

Lactobacillus spp. are common commensals in the vagina and in the upper respiratory tract. This genus is difficult to identify, and differentiation from streptococci may even be a problem occasionally. Rarely *Lactobacillus* spp. may produce serious infection, including pneumonia. Querol and colleagues[308] reported a cavitating lesion in a 40-year-old heavy smoker and drinker who developed foul smelling sputum, usually associated with anaerobic infection. *Lactobacillus* sp. was isolated from blood and from the lung in pure culture by a needle aspirate that also contained many neutrophils. We have observed a similar patient at the Medical Center Hospital of Vermont who was infected with a strain of *Lactobacillus* sp. that was resistant to vancomycin, an antibiotic that is very effective against most gram-positive organisms.[227]

Rothia dentocariosa is a gram-positive coccobacillus that resembles *Corynebacterium* and normally inhabits the oral cavity. On rare occasion this bacterium may produce severe infection, such as endocarditis. Schiff and Kaplan have described an acute upper lobe pneumonia in an 84-year-old woman with acute myelocytic leukemia. *Rothia* was isolated in pure culture from a lung aspirate, but the inflammatory reaction was not described.[309] This organism can also produce a pathologic process that resembles actinomycosis (see p. 308).

Gram-Negative Cocci

Neisseria meningitidis

Neisseria meningitidis is a well-established pathogen that usually causes meningitis or septicemia, but also colonizes the upper respiratory tract of many individuals. Colonization is not a risk factor for subsequent disease in nonepidemic situations. Pneumonia is an uncommon manifestation of *Neisseria meningitidis* infection, although the true incidence is difficult to determine.[310] This infection is frequently preceded by a viral upper respiratory infection, but may also be one of the bacterial complications of measles.[311] The source of the bacterial inoculum is presumably the upper respiratory tract. Most infections are community acquired, but nosocomial meningococcal pneumonia has also been described.[312] The pathogenesis of meningococcal pneumonia may be aspiration of indigenous flora, even in the hospital setting, but Rose and colleagues[313] have reported two cases of pneumonia caused by *Neisseria meningitidis* serogroup B in which transmission of bacteria from one patient to another may have been accomplished by hospital staff.

Most cases of meningococcal pneumonia, in which typing of the bacterial isolates has been done, are caused by serogroup Y,[311,314–316] but serogroup W-135[317,318] and serogroup B[313] have also been reported. Meningococci may be isolated from sputum in the absence of lower respiratory tract disease. If the isolate is typed as serogroup Y, there is a greater association with pneumonia, but careful correlation with clinical data must be done before accepting the isolate as the etiologic agent of the infection.

Most cases of meningococcal pneumonia appear to be focally distributed. A lobar radiographic pattern has been described in one case.[316] The clinical course is usually uncomplicated, although bacteremia may occur,[318] and empyema may rarely ensue.[319]

Other *Neisseria* spp.

Neisseria gonorrhoeae ordinarily is found in the respiratory tract only in the pharynx, where it can produce acute pharyngitis.[320] An unusual case of pneumonia complicated by empyema has been attributed to *Neisseria gonorrhoeae*.[160]

Other *Neisseria* species are common members of the indigenous upper respiratory tract flora. They may be isolated from polymicrobial infections, but are unusual sole isolates from cases of pneumonia. *Neisseria cinerea* has been reported as the etiologic agent of a case of nosocomial pneumonia.[321] *Neisseria sicca*, frequently present in the upper airway, has caused pneumonia in patients who had bronchiectasis,[322] were pregnant, or had bullous pemphigoid that was treated with steroids.[323] *Neisseria catarrhalis*, which has been reclassified as *Moraxella catarrhalis*, is discussed with the gram-negative bacilli.

Gram-Negative Bacilli

Enteric Gram-Negative Bacilli

The enteric gram-negative bacilli constitute a large group of organisms in the family Enterobacteriaceae. They are genetically related and share phenotypic characteristics that allow microbiologists to classify them. They are relatively plump bacilli, which may sometimes be coccobacillary but without the pleomorphism of

Serratia spp.

Serratia marcescens is the most important pathogen in the genus. This bacterium has a venerable and colorful history, often related to the bright red pigment that many isolates produce. Raphael's fresco "The Mass of Bolsensa" commemorates the miraculous appearance of "blood" on the Eucharistic wafer, now interpreted as contamination of the bread by *Serratia marcescens*. This organism was once considered a harmless commensal, to be swabbed on the hands of medical students in epidemiology demonstrations or released into the environment as experiments in biological warfare.[347] Outbreaks of nosocomial infection were associated with some of the military aerosol experiments, but retrospective analysis has suggested that the associations were fortuitous. Rather, the outbreaks called attention to nosocomial infections that had not been recognized previously. *Serratia marcescens* may cause infections as a member of the patient's indigenous flora, after transfer on the hands of medical personnel or through contamination of therapeutic or diagnostic reagents.[348] Most patients have serious underlying disease. The etiologic agent is usually isolated from sputum, where it must be differentiated from colonizing flora. A minority of patients develop bacteremia. *Serratia marcescens* was recovered only at postmortem examination in 7 of 40 patients reported by Goldstein and colleagues.[176]

The radiographic[349] and pathologic[176] features of nosocomial *Serratia* pneumonia at one institution have been described. Goldstein and associates[176] reviewed the pathologic findings in 40 cases of pneumonia in which *Serratia marcescens* was isolated, including 16 cases in which the bacterium was isolated in pure culture. The pathologic response differed in patients who were neutropenic and those in whom the circulating neutrophils were intact. The most common macroscopic appearance was focal consolidation and focal hemorrhage, which occasionally became confluent. The radiographic analysis of cases from this institution included 2 cases in which the distribution was described as lobar, perhaps reflecting the difficulty of differentiating confluent focal pneumonia from lobar consolidation radiographically.[349] In the neutropenic patients the lungs were diffusely edematous and hemorrhagic.

Microscopically, the inflammatory exudate in nonneutropenic patients consisted of polymorphonuclear neutrophils, macrophages, fibrin, and hemorrhage. Necrotizing inflammation was common, as were microabscesses or macroscopically and radiographically visible cavities. Gram-negative bacilli were readily demonstrable in the exudate. In seven of nine cases there was a distinctive vasculitis of arteries and veins. Polymorphonuclear neutrophils infiltrated the intima and media, and gram-negative bacilli were demonstrated intramu-

rally in two cases. Vascular thrombosis and necrosis were not observed. The authors noted the similarity of this "vasculitis" to that found in *Legionella* pneumonia and the differences from the lesions found in *Pseudomonas* infections.[176]

The inflammatory exudate in the neutropenic patients included fibrin, hemorrhage, and hyaline membranes. In some cases bacteria were present without cellular reaction; in others macrophages were increased in number.

The lungs of four patients with *Serratia marcescens* pneumonia contained intraalveolar inflammatory organization or bronchiolitis obliterans in addition to necrotizing or neutrophilic pneumonia.[176] Carlon and associates[350] reported a patient who developed interstitial fibrosis, as demonstrated by chest radiographs, after an acute *Serratia* pneumonia.

Proteus spp. and Related Organisms

The tribe Proteeae consists of the genera *Proteus*, *Providencia*, and *Morganella*, which are infrequent causes of pneumonia. Walter Reed reported an early case in which *Proteus vulgaris* was isolated from lung and from sputum by inoculation of rabbits.[351] Lancet-shaped diplococci were also present, although not isolated in either culture, so the role of *Proteus* in the infection is unclear. Tillotson and Lerner[352] described six cases caused by *Proteus mirabilis*, *Proteus vulgaris*, and *Proteus morganii* (currently classified as *Morganella morganii*). All patients had chronic lung disease and five were alcoholic. The episodes of pneumonia were preceded by episodes of decreased consciousness, and the resultant pneumonia had a lobar appearance radiographically. Microscopically, there was a mixed mononuclear and polymorphonuclear inflammatory cell infiltrate. Abscesses were present in five of six cases. Empyema was not observed in this series, but has been reported. Lysy and colleagues[353] described pneumatoceles, large airfilled spaces usually associated with staphylococcal pneumonia, in an infection produced by *Proteus mirabilis*. Pneumatoceles are produced by destruction of lung tissue, but are thin walled in comparison to chronic abscesses, are usually visualized radiographically, and ordinarily resolve without clinically evident residua. *Proteus* lobar pneumonia has also been reported in a previously healthy adult.[354] Focal pneumonia with abscess formation has also been associated with infection by *Providencia* species, but detailed descriptions of the pathology are not available.[355]

Salmonella spp.

Cough and pulmonary infiltrates are a regular part of the typhoid fever syndrome,[356–358] but *Salmonella* species are not usually considered primary pulmonary pathogens. Aguado and colleagues[359] described 8 patients with pleuropulmonary infections caused by nontyphoidal *Salmonella* species; *Salmonella* was isolated from the stool of only 2 patients. Serious underlying disease was present in all patients, and 7 of 11 were immunosuppressed. Eight patients had focal pneumonia, 2 had discrete lung abscesses, and 1 had an empyema. *Salmonella* pneumonia has been described as a complication of neoplastic disease, including carcinoma[360] and lymphoma.[361]

Yersinia pestis

Plague is caused by the small, gram-negative, nonmotile, and non-spore-forming coccobacillus, *Yersinia pestis*. This organism, which was formerly named *Pasteurella pestis*, was transferred into the newly created genus *Yersinia*, a member of the family Enterobacteriaceae, on the basis of biochemical and genetic relatedness.[34] At the same time, *Pasteurella tularensis* was placed in the newly created genus *Francisella*.

Plague, which is a disease of both historic and current interest, can exist in either the bubonic, primary septicemic, or pneumonic forms. Clinical disease results from the rapid, uncontrolled multiplication of plague bacilli in infected tissues and the subsequent production of two major toxins—endotoxin and murine toxin.[362-364] The gross and microscopic appearances of the lungs are similar in all forms of the disease.

Bubonic plague, which decimated the population of Western Europe during the Middle Ages, has been referred to as the "black death." The environmental disease reservoirs are wild rodents, especially rats and mice in urban environments, and ground squirrels, chipmunks, and prairie dogs in the southwestern United States. The disease is transmitted to humans either by direct contact or by the bite of a rodent flea.[365,366] Following entry of the organism, the regional lymph nodes become infected. After a few days the lymph nodes may enlarge to form the characteristic painful, fluctuant buboes of bubonic plague.[367] If bacteremia develops by release of bacteria from the buboes, the lungs as well as the spleen, liver, meninges, and other body sites may become secondarily infected via hematogenous dissemination. In primary septicemic plague, patients have minimal or no lymphadenopathy, and organisms pass rapidly through regional lymph nodes to the vascular system. In either bubonic or primary septicemic plague, patients with pulmonary infection typically produce large amounts of bloody or frothy sputum containing myriad bacilli. They readily disseminate bacteria into their environment by the aerosol route.

Pneumonic plague, or primary plague pneumonia, is the most rapidly lethal form and results from the inhalation of aerosolized droplets of infected secretions. Historically, pneumonic plague has been much less common than bubonic or septicemic plague, although occasional cases have been seen during outbreaks of bubonic disease. The only well-investigated epidemic of primary pneumonic plague occurred in Manchuria during the early twentieth century.[368] In this outbreak the disease apparently spread rapidly from person to person among those living in poorly developed, cold, crowded areas. Although the disease probably originated in rodents, rapid and efficient transmission no longer required an insect vector after the airborne route of spread evolved.

Sporadic cases of pneumonic plague also occur. In the western part of the United States these cases are usually associated directly or indirectly with endemic foci of disease in wildlife. Werner and colleagues[369] reported a fatal case of primary plague pneumonia in a woman who contracted the disease from a cat that also had pneumonic disease. A recent case illustrates the transient nature of the contact necessary to produce fatal pneumonic infection. A 31-year-old man died of primary *Yersinia pestis* pneumonia after he removed an infected domesticated cat from the crawlspace under a house in Colorado.[370] The cat, which had oral and submandibular lesions compatible with feline plague, probably was infected after contact with endemically infected chipmunks in the area. In this case the correct diagnosis was delayed because a packaged microbiology system, which did not contain *Yersinia pestis* in its database, incorrectly identified the sputum isolates as *Yersinia pseudotuberculosis*.

Primary plague pneumonia is characterized by widespread hemorrhagic lobular lesions that may become confluent over large areas of the lung to produce a lobar and then multilobar pneumonia.[371] Fluid can be expressed readily from cut surfaces. Peribronchial and mediastinal lymph nodes are enlarged and may be edematous and hemorrhagic.

Microscopically, the inflammatory exudate is characterized by hemorrhage and edema; fibrin is almost always absent (Fig. 9–40). Macrophages and scant neutrophils are present within the alveoli, and there is extensive parenchymal necrosis. Massive numbers of gram-negative, bipolar-staining coccobacilli that measure 0.5 μm–1.0 μm × 1.0 μm–2.0 μm are present in bronchi, bronchioles, and alveoli (Fig. 9–41). The organisms are best demonstrated with Gram's stain of impression smears. In tissue, the Brown–Hopps tissue gram stain and silver impregnation stains, such as the Steiner, Warthin–Starry, or Dieterle procedures, are preferred. Because bipolar staining is typically present, *Yersinia pestis* has been described as having a safety-pin appearance. This bipolar staining is best demonstrated

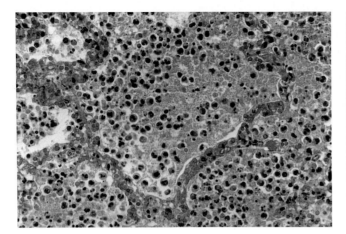

Fig. 9–40. Pneumonic plague. Alveolar spaces contain compact masses of poorly stained coccobacilli mixed with fewer neutrophils and macrophages; fibrin is absent. H and E, ×300.

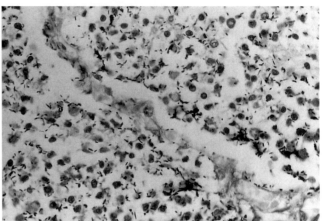

Fig. 9–41. Pneumonic plague. Inflammatory cells and numerous argyrophilic coccobacilli of *Yersinia pestis* fill alveolar spaces. Steiner silver impregnation method, ×480.

in methylene blue or gram-stained impression smears; such structural detail is lost when the silver impregnation stains are employed. In pneumonic plague secondary to septicemia, the inflammatory response is similar to that seen in primary plague pneumonia. In septicemic disease, however, plague bacilli associated with parenchymal necrosis are often more numerous in the interstitium than in the alveoli.[372] Extreme caution should be taken when caring for plague patients, when handling autopsy and surgical specimens, and when handling the organism in the laboratory. The disease can be acquired by the respiratory route, and laboratory-acquired cases have been reported.[371] It is frequently desirable to identify *Yersinia pestis* in smears of respiratory secretions or in formalin-fixed deparaffinized tissue sections by direct immunofluorescence (Fig. 9–42), because of the risks associated with handling cultures of the organism.[280]

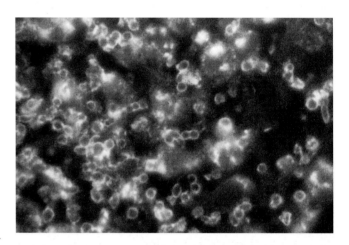

Fig. 9–42. Compact intraalveolar aggregates of *Yersinia pestis* in formalin-fixed deparaffinized lung section are brightly fluorescent when stained with fluorescein-labeled immunoglobulins specific for this bacterium. ×800.

Yersinia enterocolitica

Yersinia enterocolitica most frequently causes gastroenteritis and mesenteric adenitis, but may also cause septic arthritis[373] and overwhelming sepsis, particularly in patients with hemochromatosis.[374] Focal pneumonia is an uncommon manifestation of the infection.[375–377] Nodular infiltrates,[378] abscess formation,[379,380] and empyema[381] have also been described.

Miscellaneous Enteric Bacilli

A case of pneumonia has been attributed to CDC Enteric Group 15 (currently classified as *Cedecea* species).[382]

Haemophilus influenzae

Haemophilus influenzae was isolated with such high frequency from patients with influenza that early investigators attributed causality to the bacterium, not yet recognizing the existence of viruses.[383] The "Pfeiffer bacillus" was accepted by Opie and colleagues[207] as the cause of the underlying pneumonia when he described the bacterial complications of influenza after World War I. Opie described the association of the gram-negative bacillus with purulent bronchitis in his patients, as opposed to the isolation of the gram-positive cocci more commonly from lung parenchyma. That association has been noted also by modern investigators, who were unable to distinguish clinically acute febrile tracheobronchitis from pneumonia except for the absence of radiographic infiltrates in the former.[384] MacCallum[385] also emphasized the bronchial association of the lesions in *Haemophilus influenzae* pneumonia, but challenged the etiologic association with the influenza syndrome. Some years later Pittman[386] defined the existence of strains that had polysaccharide capsules and others that were unencapsulated. Pittman noted the antigenic differences among the encapsulated isolates and first suggested that the type B strains were associated with severe bacteremic disease. The matter was finally settled when Smith and colleagues[387] isolated influenza virus by inoculation of ferrets in 1933.

MacCallum[385] noted a purulent exudate in the bronchi where the gram-negative bacilli could be demonstrated readily. The corresponding macroscopic appearance was of multiple nodular yellowish lesions and relatively intact lung parenchyma. In the air spaces, the infiltrate was either neutrophilic or mononuclear, and bacteria were difficult to demonstrate.

MacCallum described a fibrinous exudate frequently, but noted the rarity of empyema. This observation has been confirmed by others,[388] but empyema does occur in *Haemophilus influenzae* infection (see Fig. 9–8).[389,390] Likewise, suppuration and abscess formation are uncommon, but have been described.[390–392] Pneumatoceles similar to those found in staphylococcal pneumonia have also been described radiographically in children with *Haemophilus influenzae* infection.[393]

The pathogenesis of *Haemophilus* pneumonia has been reviewed by Moxon and Wilson.[394] Traditionally serious systemic infections were thought to be caused by encapsulated type B strains, usually in young children.[388,395,396] The first cases in adults were described by Keefer and Rammelkamp in 1942,[397] and this association has been emphasized increasingly in recent years.[398] Bacteremic pneumonia is usually caused by encapsulated type B strains,[399] but type C,[400] type D,[401] type E,[391] and type F strains[402] have also produced bacteremic disease and fatal infections. Type F encapsulated strains are next most common after type B in bacteremic pneumonia.[399] Encapsulated *Haemophilus* produces a variety of diseases in adults that is similar to the spectrum of serious disease in children, including meningitis, arthritis, and epiglottitis as well as pneumonia.[403]

The importance of nonencapsulated (nontypable) strains has recently become recognized both in children[404] and in adults.[384,398] Nontypable strains have been recorded as important pathogens in community and hospital-acquired pneumonia in the elderly, accounting for 11% of episodes of pneumonia documented by transtracheal aspirates.[405] Nosocomial *Haemophilus* pneumonia has increasingly been recognized as a problem in younger patients also.[406] Bacteremia also occurs with nontypable strains but less frequently than with type B *Haemophilus influenzae*.

Patients with *Haemophilus influenzae* pneumonia usually survive the acute episodes, so there has been very little recent description of the histopathology. Most reports emphasize the occurrence of both focal pneumonia (see Fig. 9–11) and lobar or segmental infiltrates, as defined by chest radiographs.* It has been suggested that type F *Haemophilus influenzae* is particularly prone to cause lobar pneumonia.[408] Henry and colleagues[409] described an unusual case of *Haemophilus influenzae* pneumonia in which the clinical course was prolonged. Polymorphonuclear neutrophilic leukocytes, partial destruction of the bronchial walls, and fibroblastic proliferation were demonstrated in a lung biopsy.

The challenge of managing serious infections caused by *Haemophilus influenzae* has increased during the past 15 years as bacterial resistance has developed to the two first-line chemotherapeutic agents, ampicillin and chloramphenicol.[410] The third-generation cephalosporin antibiotics now serve as the major therapeutic agents for serious systemic infection. The importance of interpretation of Gram's stains of sputum by skilled observers has been emphasized by the frequency with which the thin, pleomorphic gram-negative *Haemophilus* in smears have been overlooked or misinterpreted by medical house officers and other observers.[391,398,411]

Other *Haemophilus* Species

Haemophilus parainfluenzae, a frequent component of the oropharyngeal flora, is not considered a pulmonary pathogen but a case of thoracic empyema has been described.[412] A single case of *Haemophilus aphrophilus* pneumonia in a previously normal child has been reported.[413] Pneumatoceles and a single abscess developed radiographically in the setting of diffuse air space infiltrates.

Legionella Species

The newest addition to the list of major pulmonary pathogens is the genus *Legionella*.[414] As has been true of most recently "discovered" pathogens, the bacteria had been recognized for many years but their true role in human disease had not been appreciated. It took the combined effects of a point-source outbreak and intense scrutiny from the media to generate the concerted investigations required to unravel the mystery.[101] After 15 years of study, there are now 36 accepted or pro-

---

*References: 384, 391, 398, 405, 407.

posed species within the genus, several of which have multiple serotypes.[34] By far the most important human pathogen is *Legionella pneumophila*, which accounts for 75% or more of human infections.[415] Within the species *Legionella pneumophila*, serogroup 1 strains account for the majority of infections and serogroup 6 strains for most of the rest. The other pathogenic species of note is *Legionella micdadei*, named for Joseph McDade, who isolated the strains from the original epidemic of pneumonia at the American Legion convention in Philadelphia during the bicentennial celebration.

Two clinically and epidemiologically distinct respiratory syndromes are caused by *Legionella* spp. The first, known as Pontiac fever, is an acute, self-limited flu-like syndrome that includes cough but not radiographic evidence of pulmonary infiltrates. The incubation period is very short, and the attack rate is very high. This syndrome has been caused by *Legionella pneumophila*,[416] *Legionella feeleii*,[417] *Legionella micdadei*,[418,419] and *Legionella anisa*.[420]

The second and most common manifestation of *Legionella* infection is acute pneumonia.[421] The original epidemic was known as legionnaires' disease, but the etiologic designation *Legionella* pneumonia is more generic. Much of the epidemiology and pathogenesis has been described in the introductory sections of this chapter, and the history of the disease has been reviewed.[101] The epidemic of mysterious respiratory disease at the Pennsylvania American Legion convention during the bicentennial celebration in 1976 caused a great furor, because the country was ready for an outbreak of swine influenza, a strain with the antigenic characteristics of the swine virus having been isolated the previous year in Fort Dix, New Jersey. Influenza virus was not isolated until 1933,[387] so that strains from the great pandemic of 1981–1919 were not available, but serologic analysis had suggested that the epidemic was caused by a virus that resembled the swine strains isolated by Shope the next year.[422]

Epidemiologists pointed out that the great fall pandemic was preceded by a first wave of disease in the spring and summer. Epidemic pneumonia is unusual in the summertime, and the sudden appearance of a mysterious epidemic caught the attention of the media and put great pressure on the epidemic investigators. Initial investigations of the tissues from Philadelphia failed to identify an etiologic agent, and speculations about chemical intoxication began to emerge. During the pathologic analysis bacteria were seen in the tissues, but they were dismissed as secondary invaders. An expert panel was convened to review the pathologic evidence, which consisted of tissue blocks and sections retrieved from the hospitals where convention attendees had died. After reviewing the macroscopic pathol-

ogy from the first Burlington epidemic of *Legionella* pneumonia the next year, one of the members of this panel commented that he thought they would not have been sidetracked if they had had the benefit of seeing the whole lungs (Charles Carrington, personal communication).

The experience with legionnaires' disease had a major impact on microbiologists and infectious disease clinicians, who were beginning to realize emphatically that the age of infectious diseases was still with us. A few years later astute investigators in Charlottesville, Virginia,[423] and Pittsburgh, Pennsylvania,[424] recognized an unusual combination of events: acute purulent pneumonia in immunosuppressed patients, the presence of acid-fast bacilli in sections, and cultures negative for bacteria and mycobacteria. Using techniques that had been employed in the investigation of the American Legion epidemic, the Pittsburgh investigators isolated a gram-negative bacillus that was originally called the Pittsburgh Pneumonia Agent and later classified as *Legionella micdadei*. This species has the unusual characteristic of partial acid-fastness in tissues and secretions but not after growth on agar. The bacterium also undergoes morphologic transformation ultrastructurally, which may correlate with the changes in acid-fastness.[425] Surgical pathologists can learn a lesson from this experience: When the population of patients is sufficiently immunosuppressed and *either* clinical or pathologic markers of infection are present, use of a battery of special stains should be encouraged. The rules that define which organism should be sought as an etiologic agent for a certain type of inflammation must be thrown out the window. Appropriate special stains are discussed in the section on **Morphologic Detection and Identification of Bacteria**.

Most of our information about the pathology of *Legionella* infections has come from study of *Legionella micdadei* and serogroups 1 and 6 *Legionella pneumophila* infections. The pathologic information on these recently recognized pathogens is, in fact, far more complete than the data we have on such venerable bacteria as *Streptococcus*, *Staphylococcus*, *Haemophilus*, and enteric gram-negative bacilli.

Most of the pathologic features of *Legionella pneumophila* pneumonia were defined during the study of the 1976 epidemic in Philadelphia[426] and the 1977 epidemics in Los Angeles[427] and in Burlington, Vermont.[168,170] The review of the pathology of *Legionella* pneumonia by Winn and Myerowitz remains current.[172] The macroscopic distribution of lesions is most frequently focal and lobular, as has been illustrated in Figs. 9–9 and 9–10.[168] Multilobar involvement is common, however, and extensive confluence of the focal consolidation may produce the familiar difficulty in

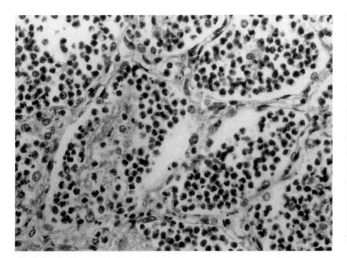

Fig. 9–43. *Legionella pneumophila* pneumonia. Air spaces are infiltrated with intact polymorphonuclear leukocytes. Legionella pneumophila, serogroup 1 demonstrated in lung tissue by direct immunofluorescence. H and E, ×400.

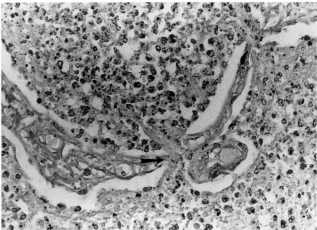

Fig. 9–44. *Legionella pneumophila* pneumonia. Air space is filled with macrophages, some of which are undergoing disintegration. Note extension of inflammatory exudate from one air space to another through pore of Kohn. H and E, ×400.

deciding whether extensive lesions are lobar or confluent lobular in nature. Cases of lobar pneumonia caused by *Legionella* spp. have been described by several investigators.[172,426–428] A careful study of serial macroscopic sections and paper-mounted whole-lung sections suggested that most cases were best described as confluent lobular pneumonia.[168] It should be noted that the infiltrates from patients in that same epidemic were frequently described as lobar radiographically.[169]

A prominent subset of *Legionella* pneumonias present as poorly marginated rounded opacities that may suggest neoplastic disease (see Figs. 9–12, 9–13, and 9–14). Localized, poorly marginated opacities have been described in chest radiographs of both patients with *Legionella pneumophila*[169,429–431] and those with *Legionella micdadei*[432] pneumonia. Winn and Myerowitz[172] noted that distinct round lesions were present in 12 of 42 cases that could be analyzed. The macroscopic lesions have a tan-white appearance and a very friable texture because of the high fibrin content.

Initial reports did not emphasize abscess formation, but subsequent studies documented the potential for destructive pneumonia.[179,180,433–437] In a large series macroscopic abscesses were documented in 10 of 42 cases of *Legionella pneumophila* pneumonia and in 5 of 9 cases caused by *Legionella micdadei*.[172] Most abscesses are small and are not demonstrable radiographically. The presence of cavitary lesions, however, is entirely compatible with *Legionella* pneumonia.[430,438] Small pleural effusions are common in *Legionella* pneumonia. Large effusions and empyema have been reported only rarely in cases caused by *Legionella pneumophila*,[172,439] *Legionella micdadei*,[440] and *Legionella bozemanii*.[441,442]

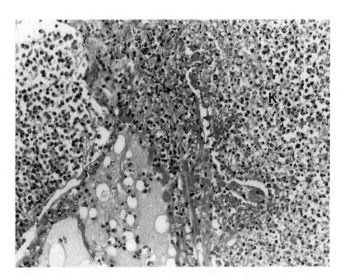

Fig. 9–45. *Legionella pneumophila* pneumonia. Fibrin and edema fill air spaces; cellular exudate is undergoing extensive lysis, leaving karyorrhectic debris. H and E, ×250.

Microscopically, the inflammatory infiltrate in *Legionella* pneumonia is variable. In approximately one-third of cases the infiltrate is composed predominantly of polymorphonuclear neutrophils (Fig. 9–43); in one-third, monocytes/macrophages predominate (Fig. 9–44); in the final third there is a mixture of macrophages and neutrophilic leukocytes. Fibrin is a prominent part of the exudate (Fig. 9–45), and hemorrhage in the air spaces is common. Edema and a sparse cellular infiltrate are seen around the periphery of active lesions. The interstitium is also frequently cellular but always considerably less so than the adjacent air spaces.

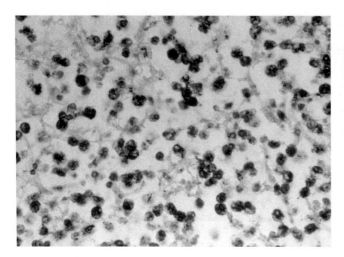

Fig. 9–46. *Legionella pneumophila* pneumonia. Leder stain colors the granules of polymorphonuclear neutrophils and highlights these cells in inflammatory exudate. *Legionella pneumophila* isolated in pure culture from postmortem lung. Leder procedure, ×800.

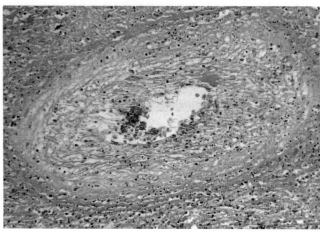

Fig. 9–47. *Legionella pneumophila* pneumonia. Necrosis of pulmonary blood vessel, possibly pulmonary vein, with inflammatory cell infiltration of wall. *Legionella pneumophila* isolated in pure culture from postmortem lung. H and E, ×160.

One of the distinctive features of *Legionella* pneumonia is an intense lytic process in the inflammatory exudate, leaving many nuclear fragments and a "dusty" appearance, dubbed leukocytoclastic by analogy to the dermal vasculitis (Fig. 9–45). In its extreme form the lysis of the infiltrate may be so complete that the hematoxylin and eosin-stained exudate has a bluish homogeneous appearance. Weisenburger and colleagues[443] have described an acellular fibrinoserous exudate in the air spaces of neutropenic patients. Some of the confusion about the nature of the cellular exudate in *Legionella* infection derives from the difficulty of distinguishing cell types when the exudate is undergoing lysis. In such cases application of the Leder stain[444] for neutrophils may resolve the issue (Fig. 9–46).

Diffuse alveolar damage, including hyaline membranes remote from the primary inflammatory foci, were found in 13 of 53 cases of *Legionella pneumophila* pneumonia and in 1 of 7 autopsied cases of *Legionella micdadei* pneumonia.[172] An expected etiology for diffuse alveolar damage was usually present, but some cases could not be explained by factors other than *Legionella*, and a lung biopsy was reported in which diffuse alveolar damage was the only pathologic finding.[185]

Coagulative necrosis, which is present in a minority of cases and may mimic pulmonary infarcts, may be associated with vasculitis.[172,427] Small pulmonary vessels are infiltrated with inflammatory cells and often contain thrombi (Fig. 9–47). In contrast to *Pseudomonas* vasculitis, bacteria are infrequent in the damaged blood vessels. Vasculitis may occur without coagulative necrosis,

however. In one series vasculitis was seen in 16 of 53 cases of *Legionella pneumophila* pneumonia (30%), but coagulative necrosis was found in only 6 cases, all of which contained inflamed blood vessels.[172]

Ultrastructural examination of tissues has expanded our knowledge of the cellular interactions with *Legionella* and provided some useful pathogenetic clues.[425,445] The initial ultrastructural examinations documented the gram-negative cell wall structure of the bacteria and the close association of the bacteria with macrophages in the air space infiltrate (Fig. 9–48). Most of the specimens were obtained at autopsy, however, and cells were insufficiently preserved to make definitive observations of subcellular structure. Glavin and colleagues[446] examined three lung biopsies that had been freshly fixed in glutaraldehyde solution. They noted the association of phagocytized *Legionella* with alveolar macrophages (Fig. 9–49) but also described phagocytized organisms in polymorphonuclear neutrophils. They further noted that the intracellular bacteria were in vacuoles that had closely apposed, ribosome-like structures (Fig. 9–50). This association of bacteria with ribosome-studded phagosomes has been noted experimentally also.[447] The association appears related to intracellular parasitism, but the precise function associated with the physical relationship is not known.[448]

Legionella sp. can be demonstrated in tissue readily, a considerable irony because the failure to visualize them delayed the recognition of the cause of the Philadelphia outbreak. As usual, the task is easy once the ground has been broken. A monoclonal fluorescent reagent that

Fig. 9–48. *Legionella pneumophila*, serogroup 1 pneumonia. Multiple bacteria have been engulfed by or multiplied in alveolar macrophage in air space. Phagocytized debris and bacteria present in adjacent macrophage. Formalin-fixed lung tissue with uranyl acetate stain, ×10,000.

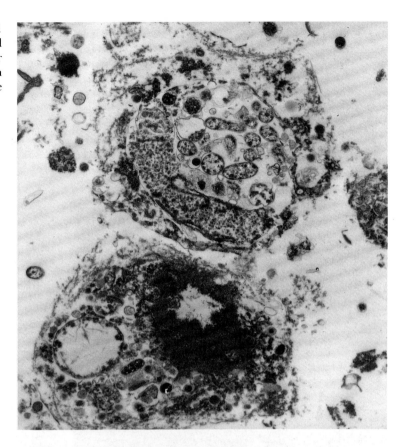

Fig. 9–49. *Legionella pneumophila*, serogroup 1 pneumonia. Bacteria phagocytized by inflammatory cells, probably polymorphonuclear neutrophils, that are undergoing extensive degeneration. One bacterium is undergoing binary fission, suggesting intracellular multiplication. Glutaraldehyde-fixed, osmicated lung biopsy, uranyl acetate stain, ×15,000.

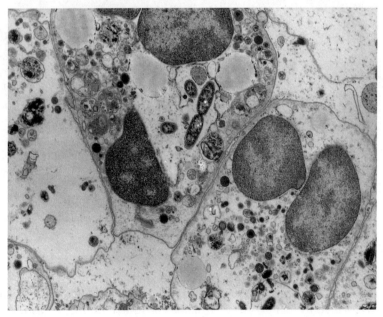

reacts with all serogroups of *Legionella pneumophila* is commercially available. This reagent has the advantage of good specificity, but does not detect other species.[449,450] Even the monoclonal reagent, however, may cross-react with other bacteria, such as spores of *Bacillus cereus*[451] and *Bordetella pertussis*.[452] Polyclonal fluores-

cent reagents that react with many species have also been evaluated and are commercially available,[450,453] but it is important to remember that cross-reactions with other bacterial species will occur.

Legionella antigen survives prolonged formalin fixation and processing for paraffin-embedded sections, so

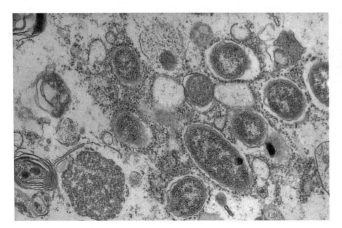

Fig. 9–50. *Legionella pneumophila*, serogroup 1 pneumonia. Bacteria have been taken up by macrophage into phagosomes that are lined by ribosome-like structures. Glutaraldehyde-fixed lung biopsy, uranyl acetate stain, ×20,000. (Photograph courtesy of Frederick Glavin, M.D.).

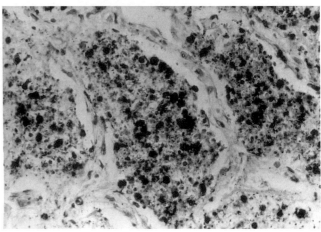

Fig. 9–52. *Legionella pneumophila* pneumonia. Airspaces are filled with inflammatory exudate that is heavily stained by antibody to *Legionella pneumophila* which has been conjugated to immunoperoxidase. ×250.

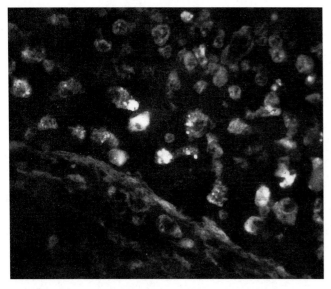

Fig. 9–51. *Legionella pneumophila* pneumonia. Phagocytic cells in air spaces contain fluorescent bacteria and antigenic debris. Formalin-fixed, paraffin-embedded lung tissue has been reacted with fluorescein-conjugated antiserum to *Legionella pneumophila*. ×400.

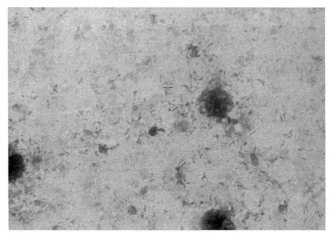

Fig. 9–53. *Legionella pneumophila* pneumonia. Gram's stain of lung imprint shows multiple thin, somewhat pleomorphic gram-negative bacilli. *Legionella pneumophila*, serogroup 1 isolated in pure culture from lung. ×1000.

that special manipulations are not needed to visualize the bacteria in archival material (Figs. 9–51 and 9–52). If formalin-fixed tissue is available, a much simpler method for preparation of smears is to scrape the surface of fibrinous lesions with a scalpel blade and transfer the exudate to clean glass slides.

The traditional adaptations of Gram's stain for tissue, such as the Brown–Hopps and Brown and Brenn versions, do not color *Legionella* and some other fastidious gram-negative bacilli well. Unfortunately our experi-

ence is that considerable variation still occurs from laboratory to laboratory.

With some forethought the problem may be avoided, because scrapings from the surface of the lung or impression smears may be prepared and stained with the traditional Gram's stain (Fig. 9–53). The staining of fastidious gram-negative bacilli can be enhanced greatly by addition of basic fuchsin (0.5 g/liter) to the safranin counterstain. The successful demonstration of *Legionella pneumophila* in tissue was first accomplished reliably by use of the Dieterle silver impregnation stain, first intended for demonstration of spirochetes.[454,455] Other silver stains, such as the Steiner (Fig. 9–54)[456] or Warthin–Starry[457] modifications, also stain the bacteria

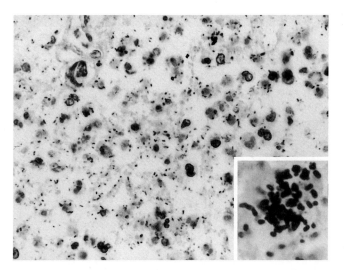

Fig. 9–54. *Legionella pneumophila* pneumonia. Innumerable bacilli are demonstrated by silver impregnation stain of air space exudate. Many bacteria are cell associated. Diffuse bacterial antigen revealed by immunologic procedures is not revealed by this stain. ×250. Inset: bacilli at high power. Fine morphology discernible with Gram's stain is obscured by heavy deposition of silver salts. Steiner silver impregnation method, ×1000.

well. The silver-stained bacteria appear larger and more regular than do gram-stained organisms because of the deposition of silver on the surface of the bacteria (see Fig. 9–54, inset). The information on gram reactivity is, of course, lost when the silver impregnation stains are employed. Other stains such as the Giemsa[458] or Gimenez[459] procedures may also be used but offer little additional advantage. All these chemical stains are immunologically nonspecific. They have the advantage of not being limited by serologic specificity, but they provide little or no information as to the nature of the bacterium. The temptation to ascribe a genus and species designation to bacteria in tissue should be resolutely resisted.

The radiographic abnormalities in *Legionella* pneumonia resolve slowly, and patients may have a prolonged convalescence.[438,460] Focal organization of infiltrate has been noted occasionally in fatal acute cases,[427] not surprising in view of the accompanying necrosis. A few cases of chronic organizing pneumonia have been attributed to *Legionella*.[461–463] In most of these cases the diagnosis was made serologically and the patients experienced a prolonged, complicated clinical course. Chastre and colleagues[464] have described five well-documented cases of pulmonary fibrosis following acute *Legionella pneumophila* infection. Two patterns of fibrosis were observed: one in which the interstitium was primarily involved, and a second in which the air spaces

were the principal site of fibrosis. In both patterns there was ultrastructural damage to the alveolar epithelial lining and basement membrane. Types one and three collagen were demonstrated in the areas of interstitial and intraalveolar fibrosis.

Walsh and Kelley[186] described a patient with acute pneumonia and a plasma cell infiltrate in the lung. Serogroup 1 *Legionella pneumophila* was isolated in pure culture from the lung of this case, but the significance of the unusual infiltrate is hard to assess.

Control of *Legionella* pneumonia consists of preventive measures to eradicate environmental bacteria and antimicrobial chemotherapy of patients using erythromycin. Some antibiotics that are effective against *Legionella* in vitro, such as aminoglycosides, are not active in vivo, probably because the antimicrobial agents do not accumulate intracellularly in macrophages.[465]

Other Legionella spp.

Many of the other defined species of *Legionella* have been isolated from cases of pneumonia: these include *Legionella bozemanii*,[466] *Legionella dumoffii*,[467] *Legionella gormanii*,[468] *Legionella feeleii*,[469–471] *Legionella longbeachae*,[472,473] *Legionella oakridgensis*,[474] *Legionella jordanis*,[475] *Legionella anisa*,[476] *Legionella cincinnatiensis*,[477] *Legionella wadsworthii*,[478] *Legionella hackeliae*,[479,480] *Legionella tucsonensis*,[481] *Legionella maceachernii*,[482] and *Legionella birminghamensis*.[483] The limited information from the few cases of each species described suggest that the pathologic response to infection is similar to that found in *Legionella pneumophila* and *Legionella micdadei* infections.[172] Some of the recently characterized strains have only been isolated from the environment, but from past experience it can be expected that any species may cause human disease in a sufficiently immunosuppressed patient.

Pseudomonas aeruginosa

Pseudomonas aeruginosa is the most virulent species of the genus and the predominant isolate in clinical microbiology laboratories. In contrast to the Enterobacteriaceae this species of *Pseudomonas* produces indophenol oxidase, providing an easy differentiation for the microbiologist. *Pseudomonas* spp. are gram-negative bacilli, but tend to be thin and long compared to the shorter, fatter enteric bacilli. *Pseudomonas aeruginosa* produces powerful exoenzymes, such as proteases and elastases, that contribute to tissue destruction. Consequently the hallmarks of *Pseudomonas* infections are hemorrhage, necrosis, and abscess formation.

There are two pathogenic mechanisms for *Pseudomonas aeruginosa* pneumonia. The first is aspiration of oral contents, usually in a nosocomial setting after shifting of the oral flora to gram-negative species.[29] Patients who are at risk usually have a serious underlying disease that is immunosuppressive, particularly acute leukemia.* Bodey and colleagues[486] reported that *Pseudomonas* bacteremia was 19 times more frequent in patients with acute leukemia than in those with solid tumors. In recent years AIDS has joined the list of predisposing conditions. Patients with HIV infection may develop *Pseudomonas aeruginosa* pneumonia as a nosocomial infection, but traditional causes of community-acquired bacterial pneumonia appear to be more common etiologic agents.[130,131] Neutropenia is a particularly important risk factor. In their series of patients with *Pseudomonas aeruginosa* bacteremia, Bodey and colleagues[486] noted that 69% of patients had absolute initial neutrophil counts less than 1,000/mm^3 and 46% had initial neutrophil counts less than 100/mm^3.[486] Recovery from the infectious episode is often as dependent on recovery of neutrophils as on antimicrobial therapy.[127] In some series chronic cardiopulmonary disease was a common underlying condition,[488,489] but in other series these diseases have not been represented,[127,484] perhaps because of the nature of the patient populations served. Bacteremic infection appears to be more common when the patient populations are severely immunosuppressed or leukopenic.

Bacteremia is common in *Pseudomonas* pneumonia. Unger and colleagues[336] noted positive blood cultures in 8 of 19 cases, in all of which the pneumonia was the initial event.[336] Metastatic infection, such as vertebral osteomyelitis[490] and ecthyma gangrenosum, are frequent complications of the bacteremia.[491] The mortality in patients who are bacteremic is very high.

Pseudomonas aeruginosa pneumonia is rarely acquired in the community and in the absence of immunosuppression, but has been described in patients with status asthmaticus[492] and in previously healthy individuals.[491,493–495]

The second pathogenetic mechanism for *Pseudomonas aeruginosa* pneumonia is secondary spread to the lungs from distant foci through the bloodstream.[496,497] The early radiographic appearance of the lungs may suggest congestion[484] or even unilateral pulmonary edema,[498] but by the time the patient dies necrotizing or hemorrhagic inflammatory lesions predominate.

Tillotson and Lerner[488] described the pathology of eight fatal cases of *Pseudomonas aeruginosa* pneumonia at autopsy. Criteria for inclusion in the study were either (1) isolation of the bacterium from two or more successive sputa, (2) isolation of the bacterium from one

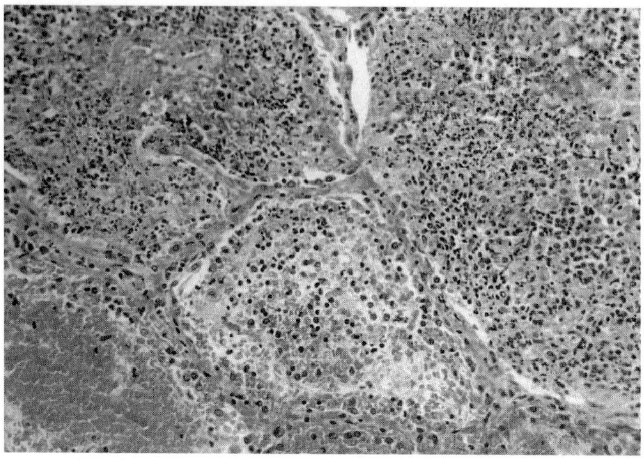

Fig. 9–55. *Pseudomonas aeruginosa* pneumonia. Intense neutrophilic inflammation has produced microabscess with destruction of alveolar septa. Surrounding lung contains macrophages and fibrin. Pseudomonas aeruginosa was isolated from lung in pure culture. H and E, ×100.

sputum and blood, or (3) isolation of the bacterium from pleural fluid. It is likely that most of these cases represented primary *Pseudomonas* pneumonia. Macroscopically there were extensive confluent focal pneumonia and pleural adhesions. There was a variable histopathologic picture within each case. Some areas that contained intense inflammatory exudates were associated with microabscesses and destruction of alveolar septa (Fig. 9–55). In other sites the lesions were hemorrhagic, but deficient in leukocytes, while still other sites contained edema and a moderate mixed inflammatory exudate in the air spaces. Thrombosis and necrosis of vascular walls were not observed.

Rose and colleagues,[489] who used diagnostic criteria similar to those employed by Tillotson and Lerner, described air space infiltrates as the predominant radiographic appearance and a polymorphonuclear neutrophilic exudate as the microscopic appearance of all 19 patients. Necrosis of alveolar septa occurred in 16 patients, and 14 patients had abscesses that exceeded 1.0 cm in diameter.

Fetzer and colleagues[178] described two types of macroscopic pathology in *Pseudomonas* pneumonia in seven patients. Criteria for inclusion in the study were (1) a positive antemortem culture from blood, (2) a positive postmortem culture from lung, and (3) a postmortem diagnosis of pneumonia. Extrapulmonary inflammatory lesions were described, but the number of patients affected was not stated.

The first macroscopic pattern was characterized by focal nodular, poorly delimited, hemorrhagic lesions that were often located in a subpleural location and resembled noninfectious pulmonary hemorrhages (Fig.

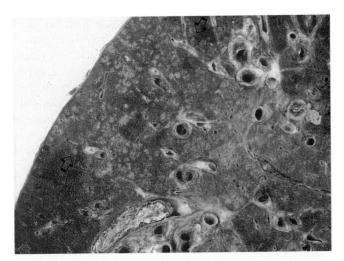

Fig. 9–56. *Pseudomonas aeruginosa* pneumonia. Pleural-based peripheral focus is hemorrhagic, suggesting embolic event.

9–56). Microscopically these lesions were hemorrhagic, noninflammatory, and contained many gram-negative bacteria. The lesions were centered around small pulmonary blood vessels. Necrosis of alveolar septa was variably present.

The second macroscopic pattern was characterized by firm, yellow-brown or tan necrotic nodules that were elevated above the cut surface and sharply delimited from the surrounding lung tissue.[178] Microscopically these lesions had two slightly different appearances. In one subset there was a mixed inflammatory infiltrate that consisted of lymphocytes, macrophages, and polymorphonuclear neutrophils that had undergone extensive lysis. Liquefactive necrosis and abscess formation were common. Bacteria, which were sparse, lined the walls of septal capillaries at the periphery of the lesion. Thrombosis was uncommon and bacterial invasion of muscular arteries was minimal.

The more common histopathological pattern in these yellow, necrotic nodules was distinctive and suggested a diagnosis of *Pseudomonas aeruginosa* infection. This pattern was characterized by "vasculitis" and coagulative necrosis. Small muscular arteries and veins were necrotic, hyalinized, and infiltrated with leukocytes, which often lined the endothelial surface. Thrombi were uncommonly present. Large numbers of gram-negative bacilli, however, were present in the blood vessels, concentrated on the adventitial surfaces. The bacterial aggregates were never as prominent as those seen in other organs. Coagulative necrosis was accompanied by large numbers of bacteria and few inflammatory cells.

The vasculitic lesions may resemble pulmonary infarcts. Soave and colleagues[496] described a woman with rheumatic heart disease and systemic lupus erythematosus who developed a rapidly progressing pneumonia

accompanied by bacteremia and metastatic necrotic lesions in the skin and other organs. Scant *Pseudomonas aeruginosa* had been isolated from the sputum 2 days earlier. An extrapulmonary source for the infection was not evident. At autopsy there was patchy consolidation throughout the lungs, and numerous 2- to 4-mm, gray-yellow nodules were present. Microscopically there was extensive focal pneumonia with microabscess formation and diffuse hemorrhagic necrosis. Vascular necrosis and infiltration by bacteria occurred, but intraluminal organisms were not seen. Similar lesions were present in other organs.

Swartz and Castleman[497] discussed a patient in the case records of the Massachusetts General Hospital who was similar to the patient reported by Soave, except that extensive burn wounds with suppurative infection were present. Septic infarcts of the lung and focal pneumonia developed in close temporal proximity to *Pseudomonas* bacteremia, and multifocal abscesses were present in the kidneys. At autopsy the pulmonary vasculature was focally necrotic, and bacteria were seen in the walls of the blood vessels.

The pulmonary vasculitis has been reproduced by Teplitz.[499] He produced a fatal wound sepsis in rats by inducing an extensive full-thickness burn of the skin followed by infection with clinical strains of *Pseudomonas aeruginosa*. Hemorrhagic subpleural pulmonary lesions resulted. Of the animals that developed metastatic infection, 30% also developed vascular lesions that were very similar to the vasculitis in humans. Although the bacteria had clearly reached the lungs through the bloodstream, large numbers of bacilli were densely packed in the medial and adventitial layers or concentrated as partial or circumferential perivascular bacterial cuffs without appreciable invasion of the media.

In summary, the most common macroscopic manifestations of *Pseudomonas* pneumonia are confluent focal pneumonia with abscess formation, focal pulmonary hemorrhage, focal nodular necrotic lesions, or septic infarcts. Microscopically a similar spectrum included necrotizing acute inflammation, relatively noninflammatory hemorrhage into the air spaces with focal acellular necrosis, and coagulation necrosis with necrotic pulmonary muscular veins and arteries. It is difficult to distinguish between aspiration and bacteremic pathogenetic mechanisms in the reports of human disease. Several lines of evidence suggest, however, that the vasculitis and septic infarcts occur predominantly in pneumonia that is secondary to bacteremia. Although the bacteria are concentrated in the external layers of the blood vessels, identical lesions can be produced experimentally when bacteremia originates in a septic burn wound. The same sequence of events has been described in humans. The concentration of the pulmonary lesions around small arteries and veins, rather than around terminal and respiratory bronchioles, also suggests a vascular focus. It appears that this very characteristic *Pseudomonas* vasculitis may be decreasing in frequency as the antimicrobial therapy for *Pseudomonas aeruginosa* has become more effective.

The course of *Pseudomonas* pneumonia is acute, but a protracted clinical course has been described in occasional cases.[489] Patients with cystic fibrosis are commonly colonized with *Pseudomonas aeruginosa* late in the course of their disease, often after initial colonization with *Staphylococcus aureus* or *Haemophilus influenzae*.[232] The characteristic pulmonary lesion in cystic fibrosis is bronchiectasis. The colonizing bacteria often produce chronic infection with periodic acute exacerbations of symptoms. A close association has been documented between very mucoid strains of *Pseudomonas aeruginosa* and cystic fibrosis.[232] Rivera and Nicotra[500] suggested that the association may be with bronchiectasis rather than with cystic fibrosis per se. The presence of a mononuclear infiltrate in some lesions of *Pseudomonas aeruginosa* pneumonia has been noted. Tillotson and Lerner[488] also emphasized the coexistence of predominantly mononuclear infiltrates with liquefactive neutrophilic lesions.

The sputum contains *Pseudomonas aeruginosa* in approximately 80% of cases, but as it often also contains other pathogens careful clinical correlation or additional diagnostic studies must be performed. In various reports, 20%–50% of patients with primary pneumonia had an accompanying bacteremia.[127,488,489]

Other *Pseudomonas* Species and Non-Glucose-Fermenting Bacteria

Pseudomonas cepacia

Pseudomonas cepacia has recently been recognized as an important pathogen in patients with cystic fibrosis, associated with a significant worsening of the clinical condition. Reliable recovery of this bacterium from sputum may require selective media to inhibit overgrowth by *Pseudomonas aeruginosa*. This species is usually resistant to aminoglycoside antibiotics.

Tomashefski and colleagues[501] have described the pathologic patterns of *Pseudomonas cepacia* pneumonia at autopsy in 40 patients. Lobular or peribronchial pneumonia was the most common pathologic manifestation of infection. Well-delineated yellow peribronchial nodules were present. Diffuse alveolar damage was uncommon, and vasculitis was not observed. The first group of patients had a rapidly progressing clinical course; purulent focal pneumonia occurred most frequently in this group. Polymorphonuclear neutrophils were prominent and abscesses were a regular feature. The second group experienced slow clinical deterioration after colonization with *Pseudomonas cepacia*. Chronic inflammatory lesions, including macrophages, lymphocytes, and plasma cells, were more commonly found in this group. Chronic interstitial pneumonia with or without an organizing alveolar component was found almost exclusively in this group. Lesions of varying types occurred in each clinical category, however.

A case of chronic progressive pneumonia caused by *Pseudomonas cepacia* was reported in a patient with chronic granulomatous disease.[121] This group of patients develops atypical granulomatous lesions in response to bacterial pathogens that usually elicit an acute inflammatory reaction.[121] Dailey and Benner,[502] however, reported a case of chronic, necrotizing pneumonia that was caused by *Pseudomonas cepacia*, then classified as "Eugonic oxidizer—Group 1 (EO-1)."

Pseudomonas pseudomallei

Melioidosis is a geographically limited bacterial disease of protean clinical manifestations first described by Whitmore and Krishnaswami in 1912.[503] It is caused by *Pseudomonas pseudomallei* (Whitmore's bacillus), a small, motile, gram-negative, aerobic bacillus that is a ubiquitous saprophyte of soil, ponds, stagnant water, and rice paddies in tropical regions between 20° north and south latitudes.[504] The disease is endemic in Southeast Asia. Humans as well as wild and domestic animals are susceptible to infection, but it is thought that animals do not serve as a reservoir for human disease. Serologic data indicate that approximately 9% of U.S. soldiers had subclinical infection with *Pseudomonas pseudomallei* while in Southeast Asia during the Vietnam War.[505] More than 300 cases have been encountered in military personnel months to years after their return from Vietnam, because melioidosis often has a long latent period.[506,507]

The usual portals of entry for *Pseudomonas pseudomallei* are the alimentary tract and abraded or traumatized skin. In addition primary pulmonary infection can follow inhalation of aerosolized water droplets or dust particles contaminated with the organism.[504] The incubation period is extremely variable, ranging from a few days in the acute pulmonary form of melioidosis up to months and even years in the localized subacute and chronic forms. Human-to-human transmission of infection has been suggested on the basis of serologic data.[508]

Clinically patients with melioidosis can present with an acute localized suppurative infection, acute pulmonary disease, acute septicemia, or a chronic suppurative

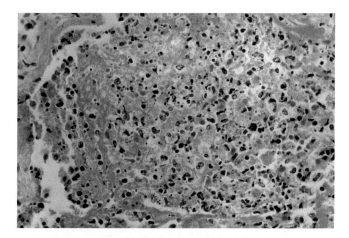

Fig. 9–57. Pulmonary melioidosis caused by *Pseudomonas pseudomallei*. Masses of fibrin, polymorphonuclear leukocytes, and fewer macrophages fill alveolar spaces at periphery of abscess. Exudate is undergoing lysis similar to that seen in *Legionella* pneumonia. Vasculitis, as seen in *Pseudomonas aeruginosa* infections, is absent. H and E, ×300.

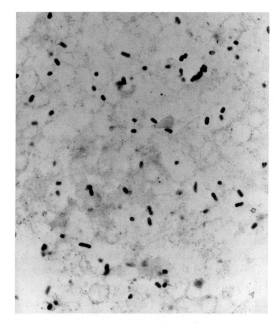

Fig. 9–58. Small pleomorphic bacilli of *Pseudomonas pseudomallei* within necrotic center of pulmonary granuloma. Few bacilli show bipolar staining. Steiner silver impregnation method, ×750.

infection.[504,509–511] The most common clinical form is pulmonary infection, which can be either primary from direct inhalation of the organism or secondary after hematogenous dissemination in the septicemic form. Chest radiographs usually reveal consolidation or nodular densities of the upper lobes. Cavitation, which occurs frequently, can mimic tuberculosis.[504,512] Pleural effusions are uncommon, but a localized pleural mass caused by *Pseudomonas pseudomallei* has been reported.[513] In chronic suppurative infections, localized lesions occur in the skin, lungs, liver, spleen, lymph nodes, brain, myocardium, bones, and joints.[514–517]

Microscopically the acute form of melioidosis is characterized by multiple discrete abscesses that measure 1 to several millimeters in diameter and are most often found in the lungs, liver, and spleen (Fig. 9–57).[510,511] The abscesses contain neutrophils, macrophages, fibrin, and giant cells that superficially resemble megakaryocytes. If a patient survives the acute infection, epithelioid histiocytes, lymphocytes, and multinucleated giant cells of both the Langhans' and foreign-body types surround the abscess as the lesion becomes granulomatous.[504,511,512] In long-standing infections granulomas are often encapsulated by dense fibrous connective tissue. The centers of granulomas consist of either stellate abscesses or caseous necrosis that resembles the lesions of tuberculosis. In the lymph nodes stellate abscesses are similar to those seen in tularemia, cat scratch disease, and lymphogranuloma venereum. Numerous bacilli of *Pseudomonas pseudomallei* that measure 0.8 × 2.0 μm are readily demonstrated within macrophages in acute lesions. The bacilli, however, are very sparse and difficult to detect in the suppurative or caseous centers of the granulomas in chronic lesions (Fig. 9–58). Although the Brown–Hopps and Giemsa stains have been recommended for demonstrating *Pseudomonas pseudomallei* in tissue sections,[511] organisms are much more easily seen with silver impregnation stains such as the Steiner and Dieterle procedures (see Fig. 9–58).

A diagnosis of melioidosis can be made by microbiologic culture, by serologic testing, or by immunofluorescence staining of *Pseudomonas pseudomallei* in smears and formalin-fixed deparaffinized tissue sections (see Fig. 9–58, inset).[280,504,518] Laboratory-acquired infection with *Pseudomonas pseudomallei* has been described.[519]

Miscellaneous Pseudomonads

Rosenthal and associates[520] have described a case of pneumonia in a patient who experienced near-drowning. *Pseudomonas putrefaciens* was recovered repeatedly from sputum and from water at the site of the accident. It is the likely cause of the pneumonia, but was not isolated from sterile sites. *Xanthomonas maltophilia* (formerly *Pseudomonas maltophilia*) has been isolated from aspirated bronchial secretions of a patient with pneumonia, whose disease responded to therapy only when an effective antibiotic was employed for this multiply resistant bacterium.[521] This species has been recognized as a cause of nosocomial pneumonia,[522,523] but geographic and environmental factors determine its importance. The respiratory tracts of many patients are colonized without resultant infection. Recently Trotter and associates[524] reported a case of pneumonia caused by an unclassified pseudomonad that phenotypically resembled *Pseudomonas cepacia*.

Moraxella spp.

Moraxella species are gram-negative coccobacilli that may resemble *Neisseria* species morphologically. The most important human pathogen, *Moraxella catarrhalis*, has the appearance of a diplococcus and was previously classified as *Neisseria catarrhalis*, then as *Branhamella catarrhalis*. *Moraxella catarrhalis* was recognized only recently as a cause of pneumonia because it is frequently a part of the resident oropharyngeal flora. The clinical illness is rarely life threatening, and bacteremic infection is rare.[525] Wright and colleagues[526] summarized the characteristics of *Moraxella catarrhalis* pneumonia. Most patients have a serious underlying disease, including immunoglobulin deficiencies.[119,120] Many patients are elderly and have chronic obstructive lung disease, but infection in neonates has also been described.[527] The radiographic infiltrates are typically described as patchy with focal consolidation. In as many as half the patients, the infiltrates have an interstitial appearance that suggests pulmonary edema. Bacteremia occurs rarely,[528,529] but abscess formation and empyema have not been described. Most *Moraxella* species are susceptible to the action of penicillin and other beta-lactam antibiotics. *Moraxella catarrhalis*, however, frequently produces beta lactamase and may not respond to therapy with beta-lactam antibiotics even if standard tests indicate susceptibility.

Rosett and colleagues[530] described the case of a 78-year-old man with an indolent pneumonia, productive of purulent sputum. Chest radiographs demonstrated a patchy pneumonia in the left-lower lobe and consolidation of the superior segment. Infiltrates later appeared in the right lung, and an abscess was noted in the consolidated segment of the left lung. *Moraxella non-liquefaciens* was recovered from sputum and a transtracheal aspirate. A case of pneumonia in a renal transplant patient has been attributed to a *Moraxella*-like bacterium that most closely resembled CDC Group M-5, which is usually associated with dog bites.[531]

Flavobacteria spp. and Related Organisms

Flavobacteria are yellow-pigmented gram-negative bacilli that are frequently found in the environment. Most infections have occurred in neonates, in whom *Flavobacterium meningosepticum* may produce a devastating meningitis,[532] but meningitis may occur in adults also.[533]

Only a few cases of pneumonia have been attributed to *Flavobacterium meningosepticum*. Ashdown and Previtera[534] reported a community-acquired pneumonia in a 76-year-old man who had a *Flavobacterium meningosepticum* septicemia. The authors commented on the similarity of the clinical presentation to melioidosis. Sundin and colleagues[535] described a previously healthy 5-year-old girl in whom pneumonia developed as part of a disseminated infection. At autopsy there were bilateral bronchopneumonia, bronchiolitis, and focal hyaline membranes; further details were not given. Tam and colleagues[536] described a 2-week-old infant with primary nosocomial pneumonia. At autopsy there were diffuse consolidation and focal hemorrhage. Microscopically extensive denuding of the bronchiolar and bronchial epithelium occurred. Polymorphonuclear neutrophilic leukocytes accompanied hemorrhage and hyaline membranes in the air spaces. A mixed inflammatory infiltrate was present in the interstitium. Nosocomial pneumonia has also been reported in adults,[537] including an outbreak associated with aerosolized polymyxin B.[538]

One of the peculiarities of *Flavobacterium meningosepticum* is resistance to antibiotics that are usually employed for gram-negative infections and susceptibility to certain antibiotics that are ordinarily reserved for gram-positive bacteria, such as rifampin and vancomycin.[539]

Casalta and colleagues[540] described an unidentified gram-negative bacterium that resembled *Flavobacterium* sp. The pulmonary process was described as lobar radiographically, but no further details were given.

Vibrionaceae

The family Vibrionaceae includes the genera *Aeromonas* and *Vibrio*. Both these genera consist of fermentative gram-negative bacilli that contain indophenol oxidase. They are environmental aquatic organisms that most commonly produce gastroenteritis or wound infection, depending on the species.

Several cases of *Aeromonas hydrophila* pneumonia have been reported. Reines and Cook[541] described three patients with pneumonia and sepsis. One patient was immunocompromised, and the two normal individuals had experienced near-drowning. At autopsy of the one fatal case there was a necrotizing pneumonia with abscesses. Baddour and Baselski[542] reported eight cases of *Aeromonas* pneumonia and reviewed other cases from the literature. All patients had serious underlying diseases, and an episode of aspiration was documented in six individuals. Once again, the two healthy patients had experienced near-drowning episodes.

Kelly and Avery[543] reported a case of pneumonia and septicemia caused by *Vibrio vulnificus* (formerly lactose-positive *Vibrio*) in a previously healthy man who was found floating face down in the sea. This species has been responsible for serious wound infections with a high mortality rate.[544]

Acinetobacter species

Acinetobacter includes five species of which the most important is *Acinetobacter baumanii*. The taxonomy and nomenclature of this genus have been a kaleidoscopic tapestry rivaling that of non-Hodgkins lymphoma. Previous names include *Acinetobacter anitratum*, *Acinetobacter calcoaceticus* var. *anitratus*, and *Herrelea vaginicola*.[34]

Acinetobacter baumannii has been described as a cause of community-acquired pneumonia in patients with serious underlying disease,[545–547] of epidemic pneumonia in an industrial setting,[548] and of epidemic nosocomial pneumonia associated with contaminated respirometers.[549] All patients have been immunocompromised or afflicted with serious underlying diseases. The pneumonia has been described as focal, occasionally with confluence. Microscopically there is an air space exudate of polymorphonuclear neutrophils and macrophages. Abscesses may develop. Bacteria are usually demonstrable in the lesions, but this very short gram-negative bacillus may be misidentified as a gram-negative coccus.[547]

Pasteurella spp.

All the major pathogens have been transferred from the genus *Pasteurella* to other genera, such as *Yersinia* and *Francisella*. The species most commonly isolated from human specimens is *Pasteurella multocida*. This species is commonly found in animals and often causes wound infections after dog or cat bites, but colonization and infection of the respiratory tract occur in the absence of exposure to animals.[34] Most cases of *Pasteurella multocida* pneumonia have occurred in patients with chronic bronchitis or a history of aspiration.[550–552] The pneumonia is usually described as patchy and focal. The bacteria may be pleomorphic, resembling *Haemophilus*, or coccobacillary, even resembling *Neisseria* spp. Necrotizing infection with abscess formation and empyema may occur rarely.[553–555]

A case of focal pneumonia attributed to *Pasteurella ureae* has been described. The infection was acquired in the hospital and was documented by culture and Gram stain of tracheal aspirates.[556]

Francisella tularensis

Tularemia is a systemic bacterial infection caused by the small, gram-negative, pleomorphic bacterium *Francisella tularensis*. The disease, which is endemic in

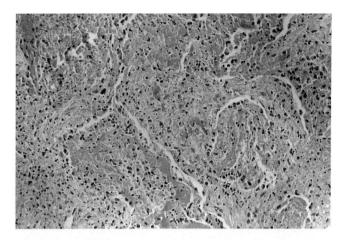

Fig. 9–59. Tularemic pneumonia. Abundant fibrin and macrophages fill alveoli and bronchioles. Note necrosis of alveolar septa. H and E, ×150.

ground animals, particularly rabbits, rodents, squirrels, cats and raccoons, is sometimes transmitted to humans through handling these animals.[557,558] Insect vectors, especially ticks, can also be the source of infection.[557–559] Most cases of tularemia therefore occur in rural areas, but suburban residents are also at risk.[560]

The principal clinical forms of tularemia are ulceroglandular, pneumonic, oculoglandular, and typhoidal.[561] Pulmonary involvement is present in most fatal cases of tularemia and may represent either the primary or secondary form of the disease.[562–564] Pneumonia may result from septicemia or from inhalation of aerosolized infectious droplets. Although most patients with tularemia survive the disease, pulmonary involvement usually portends a poor prognosis.[562–564] Sunderrajan and colleagues[565] reported three patients who developed the clinical picture of adult respiratory distress syndrome with diffuse parenchymal infiltrates as a part of *Francisella tularensis* pneumonia.

Macroscopically the lungs from patients who die of tularemia with pulmonary involvement exhibit a multifocal pneumonia. The areas of pneumonia may be confluent, resulting in a lobar pattern of consolidation. Multiple small abscesses also may be present. Microscopically abundant fibrin is present in alveoli, and the cellular component of the exudate consists primarily of mononuclear cells (Fig. 9–59). As the disease progresses, parenchymal necrosis develops. The necrotic areas may resemble infarcts or geographic foci of caseation.[566,567]

The vascular changes in acute tularemic pneumonia may be quite pronounced, including extensive thrombosis and necrosis of small and medium-sized arteries and veins (Fig. 9–60). Although small foci of granulomatous inflammation may be seen in tularemia, giant cells are usually absent. *Francisella tularensis* stains

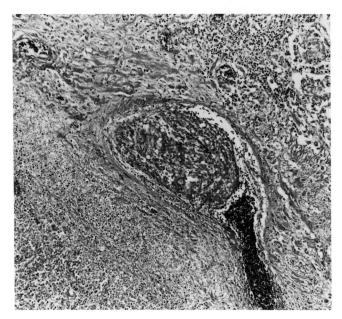

Fig. 9–60. Vascular thrombosis in tularemic pneumonia. H and E, ×100.

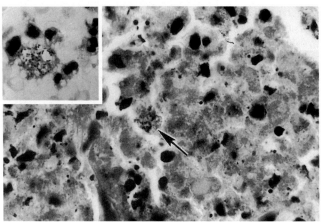

Fig. 9–61. Tularemic pneumonia. Alveolar macrophages contain rare, minute, weakly gram-negative coccobacilli (*arrow*). Brown–Hopps procedure, ×750. Inset: Macrophage contains numerous pleomorphic coccobacilli of *Francisella tularensis* in touch preparation of fresh lung. Giemsa stain, ×750.

poorly with tissue gram stains and is very difficult to demonstrate in histologic sections (Fig. 9–61). When present, the bacilli are usually within macrophages and epithelioid histiocytes. Although only faintly gram negative, the bacterium is intensely argyrophilic when stained with the Steiner, Dieterle, or Warthin–Starry silver impregnation procedures. Diagnosis of the disease requires either the bacteriologic isolation of the causative organism, demonstration of a specific immunologic response, or demonstration of the organism by direct immunofluorescence in smears of lesional exudate or in formalin-fixed, deparaffinized tissue sections (Fig. 9–62).[280,568] Roy and colleagues[569] reported cross-reactions between *Legionella pneumophila* and *Francisella tularensis* in the direct immunofluorescence test. Further, *Francisella tularensis* may be isolated on buffered charcoal yeast extract agar, the medium normally used for culture of *Legionella* spp.[570] Both genera require cysteine in the medium for optimal isolation. *Legionella* spp. do not present a biohazard in the laboratory under normal conditions, but *Francisella tularensis* must be handled with great care.

Brucella spp.

Brucellosis is a zoonotic disease caused by six species of small, gram-negative, nonmotile, and non-spore-forming coccobacilli in the genus *Brucella*.[571,572] Humans are infected by direct contact with tissues and body fluids of chronically infected animals, especially cattle, goats, sheep, and swine, or by ingestion of raw milk, milk

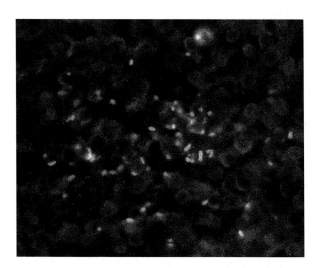

Fig. 9–62. Tularemic lymphadenitis. Minute, brightly fluorescent coccobacilli in center of abscess. Formalin-fixed deparaffinized section was stained with fluorescein-conjugated antiglobulins specific for *Francisella tularensis*. ×1000.

products, and tissues contaminated with the bacterium.[573–575] *Brucella* spp. gain entrance into the body via the skin, mucous membranes, alimentary tract, and lungs. Individuals who have close, continuous contact with domestic animals are at increased risk of infection. Most human infections are caused by four species: *Brucella abortus*, from cattle; *Brucella melitensis*, from goats and sheep; *Brucella suis*, from swine; and *Brucella canis*, from dogs.[574,576] In the United States and Canada, most human infections are caused by *Brucella abortus*, whereas *Brucella melitensis* and *Brucella suis* are the most common etiologic agents in other countries.

The three major clinical forms of brucellosis are acute malignant infection, relapsing or "undulant" fever, and intermittent or chronic disease.[571–573]

Following entry into the body, the *Brucella* spp. disseminate via the mononuclear phagocyte system. As facultative intracellular pathogens, they multiply predominantly within monocytes and macrophages.[571,577] Generalized hyperplasia of the mononuclear phagocyte system usually results in lymphadenopathy and hepatosplenomegaly in about half of infected patients. In the subacute stage of infection patients may also develop noncaseating epithelioid cell granulomas and lymphocytic infiltrates in the lymph nodes, spleen, liver, bone marrow, synovial membranes, meninges, genitourinary tract, and lungs.[577–582] Acute bacterial endocarditis has also been described, as have multifocal abscesses in the myocardium.[577,583] Intracellular gram-negative coccobacilli are more easily demonstrated in the acute and subacute lesions than in the more chronic stages. The organism can usually be isolated from the blood and infected tissues in all forms of brucellosis, however. In our experience, silver impregnation stains (Steiner, Dieterle or Warthin–Starry) have been superior to the Brown–Hopps or other tissue Gram stains for demonstrating sparse intracellular organisms in histologic sections (Fig. 9–63).

In chronic brucellosis, the organs mentioned previously often contain solitary or multiple, sharply outlined, caseous or suppurative granulomas that resemble those seen in tuberculosis.[577,584] Residual fibrocaseous nodules or "coin" lesions that resemble tuberculomas, histoplasmomas, or coccidioidomas in hematoxylin and eosin-stained sections have been described in the lungs.[584]

A diagnosis of brucellosis can be confirmed by microbiologic culture of blood and tissue specimens, by serologic procedures, or by immunofluorescence staining of the bacterium in smears or formalin-fixed deparaffinized tissue sections (see Fig. 9–63, inset).[280,585–587]

Bordetella spp.

Whooping cough was one of the diseases that effective immunization practices had virtually eliminated, but changes in those practices have led to a resurgence of disease in the past decade.[588] The pertussis syndrome is most commonly caused by *Bordetella pertussis*, a tiny gram-negative coccobacillus.[589,590] *Bordetella parapertussis* may cause a milder syndrome.[591] The clinical syndrome includes an early catarrhal phase, followed by a period of laryngotracheobronchitis, a phase of characteristic paroxysmal cough, and finally a recovery phase. Atypical lymphocytosis may occur, but is inconstant. The differential diagnosis includes viral infection of the

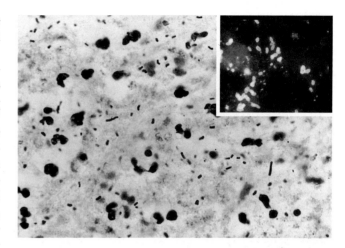

Fig. 9–63. Chronic pulmonary brucellosis. Small bacilli and coccobacilli seen at the margin of a caseous granuloma. H and E, ×800. Inset: In replicate deparaffinized section, bacilli are intensely decorated with immunofluorescence conjugate specific for *Brucella* spp. (to genus level only). ×1000.

lower respiratory tract.[592] In fact, whooping cough and viral infection may coexist in young children.[593]

Most cases of whooping cough occur in nonvaccinated infants, but cases have been reported in adults,[594] including those with waning immunization.[595] Infections in adults and immunized patients tend to be mild. *Bordetella pertussis*, which is found only in humans, is maintained in nature by person-to-person spread, usually with mild or subclinical infection resulting.[596] *Bordetella pertussis* has been isolated from patients with AIDS and respiratory infections.[597]

The clinical diagnosis of pertussis is imprecise,[598] and laboratory support is important. The primary diagnostic modality is bacterial culture,[599] but the bacterial colonies require several days to develop. Bordet–Gengou medium, the traditional choice, has been replaced or supplemented by a charcoal-based medium.[600] Direct immunofluorescence of the bacteria in clinical specimens provides a more rapid diagnosis,[601,602] but this method is plagued by insensitivity and nonspecificity.[452,599,603] Serologic diagnosis is particularly useful for mild cases[596,604] but is perforce retrospective and is not readily available in this country.

Most cases of whooping cough are not fatal, and there is little published information on the pathology of the infection. As suggested by the clinical symptoms, the site of injury is primarily in the airways rather than in the alveoli themselves. The lymphocytic inflammatory exudate infiltrates the submucosa of the large airways (Fig. 9–64) and all layers of distal bronchioles (Fig. 9–65). Toxic effects on the epithelial cells are difficult to differentiate from postmortem effects. *Bordetella pertussis* is most readily cultured during the early, unfortu-

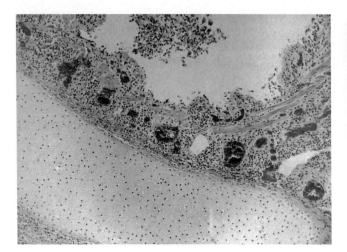

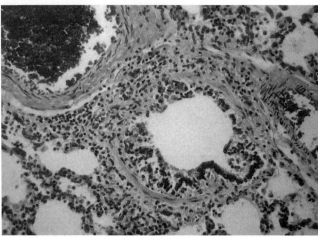

Fig. 9–64. *Bordetella pertussis* bronchitis. Infant girl, who had not been immunized for religious reasons, died of whooping cough. Bronchial mucosa is extensively infiltrated with mononuclear cells; epithelial cells are largely sloughed. *Bordetella pertussis* was isolated in pure culture from lung post mortem. H and E, ×100. (Case contributed by Paul Morrow, M.D.)

Fig. 9–65. *Bordetella pertussis* bronchiolitis. Bronchiolar mucosa and submucosa and pulmonary interstitium from case shown in Fig. 9–64 is infiltrated with mononuclear cells. Mucosa is focally sloughed. H and E, ×400.

nately nonspecific, catarrhal phase of the illness. Recovery of the bacteria is increasingly difficult as the infection progresses and demonstration of the organism in tissue is usually not accomplished. The differential diagnosis of the pathologic lesions, as well as the clinical symptoms, is viral infection, particularly respiratory syncytial virus, adenoviruses, and parainfluenza viruses.

Bordetella bronchiseptica is a pathogen of animals.[605] This easily cultivated species may also cause chronic bronchitis and has been suggested as a cause of pneumonia in a patient who may have acquired the infection from his dog.[606]

Miscellaneous Gram-Negative Bacilli

Several cases of bacteremic pneumonia caused by *Alcaligenes xylosoxidans* (formerly *Achromobacter xylosoxidans*) have been described.[607,608] In each case there was a serious underlying disease. Details of the pathologic processes were not given.

Eikenella corrodens is a facultatively anaerobic, gram-negative bacterium that is commonly a part of the microflora of the oropharynx. The bacterium gets its name from the distinctive manner in which the colonies "pit" the agar medium, producing a dewdrop or fried egg appearance.[34] Goldstein and colleagues[609] described the recovery of this organism from respiratory secretions of 16 patients, 7 of whom had pneumonia or lung abscess. All 7 patients had serious underlying disease and 4 had carcinomas. In all 7 cases *Eikenella* was

isolated as part of a polymicrobial infection. The nature of the pulmonary lesions was not detailed.

Obligately Anaerobic Bacteria

Most anaerobic infections of the lung are polymicrobial and follow aspiration of oropharyngeal contents, where anaerobes constitute a majority of the normal flora. The most distinctive manifestations of anaerobic pleuropulmonary infections are thoracic actinomycosis, putrid lung abscess, and empyema. A foul or "fecal" odor in a clinical specimen suggests an anaerobic component to the infection. Certain anaerobes, such as *Peptostreptococcus anaerobius* and some *Bacteroides* species, have a very disagreeable odor even on agar plates. One suggested criterion for the identification of *Clostridium difficile* at the Medical Center Hospital of Vermont has been complaints about air pollution from the hematology laboratory next door. Not all anaerobic bacteria produce odoriferous end products, however. Actinomycotic infections should not be expected to smell bad.

Actinomyces spp. and Related Bacteria

Actinomycosis is a sporadic localized infection of worldwide distribution caused by anaerobic or microaerophilic filamentous bacteria in the order Actinomycetales.[241,610–612] The disease is not contagious, and its causative agents have never been isolated from any natural habitats outside the body. The agents of actinomycosis occur as commensals of the mouth, throat, gastrointestinal tract, and vagina of healthy individuals.[241,611–613] These endogenous microorganisms are opportunists that have the capacity to invade injured tissues and intraabdominal mucosal breaks. Unlike nocardiosis, actinomycosis does not occur preferentially in immunocompromised patients. Because actinomycosis is an endogenous disease, it is not included under mycetoma, despite the fact that its etiologic agents commonly form granules in tissue. The principal agent of actinomycosis in humans is *Actinomyces israelii*. Other causes of the disease are *Actinomyces naeslundii*,[614–616] *Actinomyces viscosus*,[616–620] *Arachnia propionica*,[621,622] and, rarely, *Actinomyces odontolyticus*,[623–625] *Actinomyces meyeri*,[626,627] *Eubacterium nodatum*,[628] and *Rothia dentocariosa*. *Actinomyces* spp. and related bacteria may be part of a mixed anaerobic infection, and there is experimental evidence that other bacteria may enhance the pathogenicity of the actinomycetes.[629]

Based on the anatomic site of infection, most cases of actinomycosis are classified as either cervicofacial, thoracic, abdominal, or pelvic. Cervicofacial infection or "lumpy jaw" is the most common clinical form. It may develop without any known antecedent injury to the oral mucosa.[610,630] Frequently, however, cervicofacial actinomycosis follows a dental extraction. Less commonly it is a sequel to dental caries, periodontal disease,[616] or an accidental injury to the oral mucosa. Infected tissues are swollen, firm, and elastic. As the disease progresses, abscesses form and draining sinus tracts emerge. If untreated, the infection may extend upward to involve the sinuses, the orbit, or the cranial bones.

Thoracic actinomycosis usually results from aspiration of infectious materials, but it may also develop by direct extension of a cervicofacial infection.[612,626,631–633] Patients have either isolated lung disease or a combination of lung and chest wall involvement. Clinically, symptoms of thoracic actinomycosis often suggest a malignancy.[634,635] Abdominal actinomycosis can develop by direct extension of a thoracic infection but more commonly results from a ruptured appendix or penetration of the etiologic agent through the wall of the stomach or intestines.[610,636] Pelvic or genital actinomycosis is a well-documented complication of intrauterine contraceptive devices.[637–639] Primary actinomycotic infections have also been reported in other sites such as the extremities, following human bites, and in the lacrimal glands.[610,611]

Thoracic actinomycosis represents approximately one-fifth of all cases and is characterized by chest pain, fever, chills, night sweats, and weight loss.[640] Chest radiographs usually reveal pulmonary consolidation, numerous small opacities with cavitation, and pleural thickening. Osteomyelitis of adjacent ribs may also be

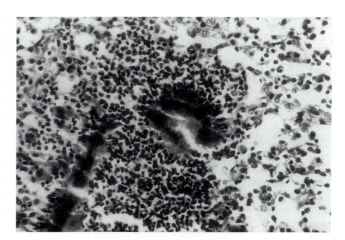

Fig. 9–66. Pulmonary actinomycosis caused by *Arachnia propionica*. Two irregular granules are embedded in abscess and surrounded by deeply eosinophilic, radiating clubs of Splendore–Hoeppli material. Individual actinomycetes within granules are unstained. H and E, ×480.

present.[641–644] Macroscopically lungs infected with the agents of actinomycosis exhibit scarring and multiple abscesses 0.1 cm to several centimeters in diameter. The lung is often adherent to the parietal pleura, and there may be inflammation in the soft tissues of the chest wall. Sinus tracts discharging to the skin are occasionally seen, and sinus exudates may contain "sulfur granules".[645,646] The diagnosis is generally made by histologic examination of surgical specimens because the responsible agents are anaerobic and difficult to culture from lung. Actinomycosis is usually not suspected before surgery.[647]

The drugs of choice for treating actinomycosis are penicillins given in high doses.[611,640,648] Prolonged treatment (6 weeks) followed by tetracycline for 6–12 months is generally required because relapse is common with short courses of therapy. Surgical drainage and excision of diseased tissues are also important in the treatment of this disease.[647]

The suppurative reaction to the agents of actinomycosis is characterized by the formation of abscesses that contain one or more actinomycotic granules and are encapsulated by fibrosing granulation tissue.[241] In most cases the granules are bordered by intensely eosinophilic, club-like projections of Splendore–Hoeppli material (Fig. 9–66). Granules range from 30 to 3000 μm in diameter and can sometimes be seen with the naked eye when a stained tissue section is held up to the light.[241,610,645] Abscesses vary in size, may be solitary or multiple, and are characteristically surrounded by numerous histiocytes that have foamy cytoplasm because of their lipid content.

A modified Gram's stain, such as the Brown and

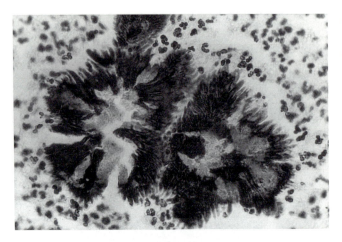

Fig. 9–70. Pulmonary botryomycosis caused by *Pseudomonas aeruginosa*. Bacteria in center of two granules are poorly stained. Prominent radiating clubs of intensely eosinophilic Splendore–Hoeppli material surround granules, which are embedded in abscess. H and E, ×480.

agent of botryomycosis is *Staphylococcus aureus*. Agents less frequently encountered include *Pseudomonas aeruginosa*, *Escherichia coli*, *Actinobacillus lignieresi*, *Neisseria mucosa*, and species belonging to the genera *Bacillus*, *Bacteroides*, *Proteus*, and *Streptococcus*.[659–662,666,669]

In lesions and purulent exudates that drain from sinus tracts, botryomycotic granules appear as soft, yellow or white, organized bacterial aggregates (microcolonies) that range from 0.2 to 2.0 mm in diameter. One or more granules are embedded in an abscess that is usually surrounded by epithelioid histiocytes, multinucleated giant cells, and fibrous connective tissue. The bacteria within botryomycotic granules are usually hematoxylinophilic, are embedded in an amorphous eosinophilic matrix or ground substance, and are intimately surrounded by brightly eosinophilic, radiating clubs of Splendore–Hoeppli material (Fig. 9–70). The bacterial cocci or bacilli that form the granules are best demonstrated with modified gram stains, such as Brown–Hopps (best for gram-negative bacteria) or Brown and Brenn (best for gram-positive bacteria). The peripheral Splendore–Hoeppli material is gram negative. A presumptive histopathologic diagnosis can be confirmed by culture.

The pathogenesis of granule formation in botryomycosis is poorly understood. Brunken et al.[670] postulated that either defective host resistance or infection by bacteria with attenuated virulence may be important factors in this localized disease. There have been several recent reports of immunodeficiency states, including chronic granulomatous disease, immunoglobulin deficiencies, steroid therapy, and AIDS associated with botryomycosis.[666,668,669,671] Botryomycosis has also been reported to be a complication of cystic fibrosis,[672]

diabetes mellitus,[667] and extensive follicular mucinosis.[673] Of the 10 reported cases of pulmonary botryomycosis, 7 have been in children with cystic fibrosis.[667,672]

References

1. Osler W. Practice of medicine. 5th Ed. New York: Appleton, 1904:108.
2. Scheld WM, Mandell GL. Nosocomial pneumonia: Pathogenesis and recent advances in diagnosis and therapy. Rev Infect Dis 1991;13:S743–S751.
3. Horan TC, White JW, Jarvis WR, et al. Nosocomial infection surveillance 1984. MMWR CDC Surveill Summ 1986;35:17SS–29SS.
4. Haley RW, Hooten TM, Culver DH, et al. Nosocomial infections in U.S. hospitals, 1975–1976; estimated frequency by selected characteristics of patients. Am J Med 1981;70:947–959.
5. Pugliese G, Lichtenberg DA. Nosocomial bacterial pneumonia: An overview. Am J Infect Control 1987;15:249–265.
6. Gross PA, Neu HC, Aswapokee P, van Antwerpen C, Aswapokee N. Deaths from nosocomial infections: Experience in a university hospital and a community hospital. Am J Med 1980;68:219–223.
7. Leu HS, Kaiser DL, Mori M, Woolson RF, Wenzel RP. Hospital-acquired pneumonia. Attributable mortality and morbidity. Am J Epidemiol 1989;129:1258–1267.
8. McGowan JE, Jr. Changing etiology of nosocomial bacteremia and fungemia and other hospital-acquired infections. Rev Infect Dis 1985;73:S357–S370.
9. Dunglison R. Medical lexicon. A dictionary of medical science. Philadelphia: Henry C. Lea, 1874:817–818.
10. Green GM, Jakab GJ, Low RB, Davis GS. Defense mechanisms of the respiratory membrane. Am Rev Respir Dis 1977;115:479–514.
11. Dondero TJ, Jr., Rendtorff RC, Mallison GF, et al. An outbreak of legionnaires' disease associated with a contaminated air-conditioning cooling tower. N Engl J Med 1980;302:365–370.
12. Klaucke DN, Vogt RL, LaRue D, et al. Legionnaires' disease: The epidemiology of two outbreaks in Burlington, Vermont, 1980. Am J Epidemiol 1984;119:382–391.
13. Helms CM, Massanari RM, Zeitler R, et al. Legionnaires' disease associated with a hospital water system: A cluster of 24 nosocomial cases. Ann Intern Med 1983;99:172–178.
14. Shapiro ED, Berg AT, Austrian R, et al. The protective efficacy of polyvalent pneumococcal polysaccharide vaccine. N Engl J Med 1991;325:1453–1460.
15. Sims RV, Steinmann WC, McConville JH, King LR, Zwick WC, Schwartz JS. The clinical effectiveness of pneumococcal vaccine in the elderly. Ann Intern Med 1988;108:653–657.
16. Anthrax contamination of Haitian goatskin products. MMWR 1977;26:31.
17. Human anthrax—Colorado. MMWR 1980;29:469–470.

18. Albrink WS, Brooks SM, Biron RE, Kopel M. Human inhalation anthrax. A report of three fatal cases. Am J Pathol 1960;36:457–471.

19. Muder RR, Yu VL, Woo AH. Mode of transmission of *Legionella pneumophila*. A critical review. Arch Intern Med 1986;146:1607–1612.

20. Addiss DG, Davis JP, Wand PJ, McKinney RM, Gradus MS, Martins RR. Two cases of community-acquired legionnaires' disease: Evidence for association with a cooling tower. J Infect Dis 1989;159:572–575.

21. Girod JC, Reichman RC, Winn WC, Jr., Klaucke DN, Vogt RL, Dolin R. Pneumonic and nonpneumonic forms of legionellosis. The result of a common-source exposure to *Legionella pneumophila*. Arch Intern Med 1982;142:545–547.

22. Joly JR, Winn WC. Correlation of subtypes of *Legionella pneumophila* defined by monoclonal antibodies with epidemiological classification of cases and environmental sources. J Infect Dis 1984;150:667–671.

23. Arnow PM, Chou T, Weil D, Shapiro EN, Kretzschmar C. Nosocomial legionnaires' disease caused by aerosolized tap water from respiratory devices. J Infect Dis 1982;146:460–467.

24. Lowry PW, Blankenship RJ, Gridley W, Troup NJ, Tompkins LS. A cluster of *Legionella* sternal-wound infections due to postoperative topical exposure to contaminated tap water. N Engl J Med 1991;324:109–113.

25. Huxley EJ, Viroslav J, Gray WR, et al. Pharyngeal aspiration in normal adults and patients with depressed consciousness. Am J Med 1978;64:564–568.

26. Mackowiak PA. The normal microbial flora. N Engl J Med 1982;307:83–93.

27. Foy HM, Wentworth B, Kenny GE, Kloeck JM, Grayston JT. Pneumococcal isolations from patients with pneumonia and control subjects in a prepaid medical care group. Am Rev Respir Dis 1975;111:595–603.

28. Winther FO, Horthe K, Lystad A, Vellar OD. Pathogenic bacterial flora in the upper respiratory tract of healthy students. Prevalence and relationship to nasopharyngeal inflammatory symptoms. J Laryngol Otol 1974;88:407–412.

29. Johanson WG, Jr., Pierce AK, Sanford JP. Changing pharyngeal bacterial flora of hospitalized patients. Emergence of gram-negative bacilli. N Engl J Med 1969;281:1137–1140.

30. Johanson WG, Jr., Pierce AK, Sanford JP, Thomas GD. Nosocomial respiratory infections with gram negative bacilli. The significance of colonization of the respiratory tract. Ann Intern Med 1972;77:701–706.

31. Fainstein V, Musher D. Bacterial adherence to pharyngeal cells in smokers, nonsmokers, and chronic bronchitics. Infect Immun 1979;26(1):178–182.

32. Bartlett JG, O'Keefe P, Tally FP, Louie TJ, Gorbach SL. Bacteriology of hospital-acquired pneumonia. Arch Intern Med 1986;146:868–871.

33. Lorber B, Swenson RM. Bacteriology of aspiration pneumonia. A prospective study of community- and hospital-acquired cases. Ann Intern Med 1974;81:329–331.

34. Koneman EW, Allen SD, Janda WM, Schreckenberger PC, Winn WC, Jr. Color atlas and textbook of diagnostic microbiology. 4th Ed. Philadelphia: Lippincott, 1992.

35. Johanson WG, Jr., Woods DE, Chaudhuri T. Association of respiratory tract colonization with adherence of gram-negative bacilli to epithelial cells. J Infect Dis 1979;139:667–673.

36. Johanson WG, Jr., Higuchi JH, Chaudhuri TR, Woods DE. Bacterial adherence to epithelial cells in bacillary colonization of the respiratory tract. Am Rev Respir Dis 1980;121:55–63.

37. Todd TR, Franklin A, Mankinen-Irvin P, Gurman G, Irvin RT. Augmented bacterial adherence to tracheal epithelial cells is associated with gram-negative pneumonia in an intensive care unit population. Am Rev Respir Dis 1989;140:1585–1589.

38. Conway B, Ronald A. An overview of some mechanisms of bacterial pathogenesis. Can J Microbiol 1988;34:281–286.

39. Woods DE, Strauss DC, Johanson WG, Jr., Bass JA. Role of fibronectin in the prevention of adherence of *Pseudomonas aeruginosa* to mammalian buccal epithelial cells. J Infect Dis 1981;143:784–790.

40. Woods DE, Strauss DC, Johanson WG, Jr., Bass JA. Role of salivary protease activity in adherence of gram-negative bacilli to mammalian buccal epithelial cells in vivo. J Clin Invest 1981;68:1435–1440.

41. Baskerville A, Fitzgeorge RB, Broster M, Hambleton P, Dennis PJ. Experimental transmission of legionnaires' disease by exposure to aerosols of *Legionella pneumophila*. Lancet 1981;ii:1389–1390.

42. Davis GS, Winn WG, Jr., Gump DW, Craighead JE, Beaty HN. Legionnaires' pneumonia after aerosol exposure in guinea pigs and rats. Am Rev Respir Dis 1982;126:1050–1057.

43. Winn WC, Jr., Davis GS, Gump DW, Craighead JE, Beaty HN. Legionnaires' pneumonia after intratracheal inoculation of guinea pigs and rats. Lab Invest 1982;47:568–578.

44. Green GM. Alveolobronchiolar transport mechanisms. Arch Intern Med 1973;131:109–114.

45. Sorokin SP, Brain JD. Pathways of clearance in mouse lungs exposed to iron oxide aerosols. Anat Rec 1975;181:581–626.

46. Green GM, Kass EH. The role of the alveolar macrophage in the clearance of bacteria from the lung. J Exp Med 1964;119:167–175.

47. Johanson WG, Jr., Kennedy MG, Bonte FJ. Use of technetium (^{99m}Tc) as a bacterial label in lung clearance studies. Appl Microbiol 1973;25:592–594.

48. Creasia DA, Nettesheim P, Hammons AS. Impairment of deep lung clearance by influenza virus infection. Arch Environ Health 1973;26:197–201.

49. Carson JL, Collier AM, Hu SS. Acquired ciliary defects in nasal epithelium of children with acute viral upper respiratory infections. N Engl J Med 1985;312:463–468.

50. Ruppert D, Jakab GJ, Sylwester DL, Green GM. Sources of variance in the measurement of intrapulmonary kill-

ing of bacteria. J Lab Clin Med 1976;87:544–558.

51. Berendt RF. Survival of Legionella pneumophila in aerosols: Effect of relative humidity. J Infect Dis 1980; 141:689.

52. Hambleton P, Broster MG, Dennis PJ, Henstridge R, Fitzgeorge R, Conlan JW. Survival of virulent Legionella pneumophila in aerosols. J Hyg (Lond) 1983;90:451–460.

53. Johnston RB, Jr. The host response to invasion by Streptococcus pneumoniae: Protection and the pathogenesis of tissue damage. Rev Infect Dis 1981;3:282–288.

54. Winkelstein JA, Tomasz A. Activation of the alternative complement pathway by pneumococcal cell wall teichoic acid. J Immunol 1978;120:174–178.

55. Coonrod JD, Rehm SR, Yoneda MD. Pneumococcal killing in the alveolus. Evidence for a non-phagocytic mechanism for early clearance. Chest 1983;83:S89.

56. Winkelstein JA. The role of complement in the host's defense against Streptococcus pneumoniae. Rev Infect Dis 1981;3:289–298.

57. Gross GN, Rehm SR, Pierce AK. The effect of complement depletion on lung clearance of bacteria. J Clin Invest 1978;62:373–378.

58. Heidbrink PJ, Toews GB, Gross GN, et al. Mechanisms of complement-mediated clearance of bacteria from the murine lung. Am Rev Respir Dis 1982;125:517–520.

59. LaForce FM, Kelley WJ, Huber GL. Inactivation of staphylococci by alveolar macrophages with preliminary observations on the importance of alveolar lining material. Am Rev Respir Dis 1977;108:784–790.

60. Jonsson S, Musher DM, Goree A, Lawrence EC. Human alveolar lining material and antibacterial defenses. Am Rev Respir Dis 1986;133:136–140.

61. Wood WB. Studies on the mechanism of recovery in pneumococcal pneumonia. I. The action of type specific antibody upon the pulmonary lesion in experimental pneumonia. J Exp Med 1941;73:201–222.

62. Davis GS, Winn WC, Jr., Gump DW, Beaty HN. The kinetics of early inflammatory events during experimental pneumonia due to Legionella pneumophila in guinea pigs. J Infect Dis 1983;148:823–835.

63. Horwitz MA, Silverstein SC. Interaction of the legionnaires' disease bacterium (Legionella pneumophila) with human phagocytes. II. Antibody promotes binding of L. pneumophila to monocytes but does not inhibit intracellular multiplication. J Exp Med 1981;153:398–406.

64. Kunkel SL, Strieter RM. Cytokine networking in lung inflammation. Hosp Pract 1990;25:63–69.

65. Onofrio JM, Toews GB, Lipscomb MF, Pierce AK. Granulocyte-alveolar-macrophage interaction in the pulmonary clearance of Staphylococcus aureus. Am Rev. Respir Dis 1983;127:335–341.

66. Pine JH, Richter WR, Esterly JR. Experimental lung injury. I. Bacterial pneumonia: Ultrastructural, autoradiographic and histochemical observations. Am J Pathol 1973;73:115–130.

67. Pierce AK, Reynolds RC, Harris GD. Leukocytic response to inhaled bacteria. Am Rev Respir Dis 1977; 116:679–684.

68. Vial WC, Toews GB, Pierce AK. Early pulmonary granulocyte recruitment in response to Streptococcus pneumoniae. Am Rev Respir Dis 1984;129:87–91.

69. Shaw JO, Henson PM, Henson JE, et al. Lung inflammation induced by complement-derived chemotactic fragments in the alveolus. Lab Invest 1980;42:547–558.

70. Larsen GL, McCarthy K, Webster RO, Henson J, Henson PM. A differential effect of C5a and C5a des arg in the induction of pulmonary inflammation. Am J Pathol 1980;100:179–192.

71. Coonrod JD, Rylko-Bauer B. Complement levels in pneumococcal pneumonia. Infect Immun 1977;18:14–22.

72. Gadek JE, Hunninghake GW, Zimmerman RL, Crystal RG. Regulation of the release of alveolar macrophage-derived neutrophil chemotactic factor. Am Rev Respir Dis 1980;121:723–733.

73. Loosli CG, Baker RF. Acute experimental pneumococcal (type 1) pneumonia in the mouse: The migration of leukocytes from the pulmonary capillaries into the alveolar spaces as revealed by the electron microscope. Trans Am Clin Climatol Assoc 1962;74:15–28.

74. Till GO, Morganroth ML, Kunkel R, Ward PA. Activation of C5 by cobra venom factor is required in neutrophil-mediated lung injury in the rat. Am J Pathol 1987;129:44–53.

75. Morganroth ML, Till GO, Kunkel RG, Ward PA. Complement and neutrophil-mediated injury of perfused rat lungs. Lab Invest 1986;54:507–514.

76. Hulbert WC, Walker DC, Hogg JC. The site of leukocyte migration through the tracheal mucosa in the guinea pig. Am Rev Respir Dis 1981;124:310–316.

77. Velo GP, Spector WG. The origin and turnover of alveolar macrophages in experimental pneumonia. J Pathol 1973;109:7–19.

78. Dal Nogare AR, Toews GB. Characteristics of alveolar macrophages in an animal model of resolving pulmonary inflammation. Am Rev Respir Dis 1990;142:660–667.

79. Doherty DE, Downey GP, Worthen GS, Haslett C, Henson PM. Monocyte retention and migration in pulmonary inflammation. Requirement for neutrophils. Lab Invest 1988;59:200–213.

80. Shennib H, Nguyen D, Guttmann RD, Mulder DS. Phenotypic expression of bronchoalveolar lavage cells in lung rejection and infection. Ann Thorac Surg 1991; 51:630–635.

81. Breiman RF, Horwitz MA. Guinea pigs sublethally infected with aerosolized Legionella pneumophila develop humoral and cell-mediated immune responses and are protected against lethal aerosol challenge. A model for studying host defense against lung infections caused by intracellular pathogens. J Exp Med 1987; 165:799–811.

82. Blander SJ, Horwitz MA. Vaccination with the major secretory protein of Legionella pneumophila induces cell-mediated and protective immunity in a guinea pig model of Legionnaires' disease. J Exp Med 1989;

169:691–705.

83. Nash TW, Libby DM, Horwitz MA. Interaction between the legionnaires' disease bacterium (Legionella pneumophila) and human alveolar macrophages. Influence of antibody, lymphokines, and hydrocortisone. J Clin Invest 1984;74:771–782.

84. Nash TW, Libby DM, Horwitz MA. IFN-gamma-activated human alveolar macrophages inhibit the intracellular multiplication Legionella pneumophila. J Immunol 1988;140:3978–3981.

85. Black SB, Shinefield HR. Immunization with oligosaccharide conjugate Haemophilus influenzae type b (HbOC) vaccine on a large health maintenance organization population: extended follow-up and impact on Haemophilus influenzae disease epidemiology. The Kaiser Permanente Pediatric Vaccine Study Group. Pediatr Infect Dis J 1992;11:610–613.

86. Musher DM, Johnson B, Jr., Watson DA. Quantitative relationship between anticapsular antibody measured by enzyme-linked immunosorbent assay or radioimmunoassay and protection of mice against challenge with Streptococcus pneumoniae serotype 4. Infect Immun 1990;58:3871–3876.

87. Dunn MM, Toews GB, Hart D, Pierce AK. The effects of systemic immunization on pulmonary clearance of Pseudomonas aeruginosa. Am Rev Respir Dis 1985; 131:426–431.

88. LaForce FM, Boose DS, Mills DM. Heightened lung bactericidal activity in mice after aerosol immunization with Re 595 Salmonella minnesota: Importance of cellular rather than humoral factors. J Infect Dis 1980; 142:421–431.

89. Harrow EM, Jakab GJ, Brody AR, Green GM. The pulmonary response to a bacteremic challenge. Am Rev Respir Dis 1975;112:7–16.

90. Holmberg H. Aetiology of community-acquired pneumonia in hospital-treated patients. Scand J Infect Dis 1987;19:491–501.

91. Karalus NC, Cursons RT, Leng RA, et al. Community-acquired pneumonia: Aetiology and prognostic index evaluation. Thorax 1991;46:413–418.

92. Woodhead MA, Macfarlane JT, McCracken JS, Rose DH, Finch RG. Prospective study of the aetiology and outcome of pneumonia in the community. Lancet 1987;i:671–674.

93. Lim I, Shaw DR, Stanley DP, Lumb R, McLennan G. A prospective hospital study of the aetiology of community-acquired pneumonia. Med J Aust 1989;151:87–91.

94. Fang GD, Fine M, Orloff J, et al. New and emerging etiologies for community-acquired pneumonia with implications for therapy. A prospective multicenter study of 359 cases. Medicine (Baltimore) 1990;69:307–316.

95. Marrie TJ, Haldane EV, Noble MA, Faulkner RS, Martin RS, Lee SH. Causes of atypical pneumonia: results of a 1-year prospective study. Can Med Assoc J 1981; 125:1118–1123.

96. Torres A, Aznar R, Gatell JM, et al. Incidence, risk, and prognosis factors of nosocomial pneumonia in mechanically ventilated patients. Am Rev Respir Dis 1990;

142:523–528.

97. Fagon JY, Chastre J, Domart Y, et al. Nosocomial pneumonia in patients receiving continuous mechanical ventilation. Prospective analysis of 52 episodes with use of a protected specimen brush and quantitative culture techniques. Am Rev Respir Dis 1989;139:877–884.

98. Bryan CS, Reynolds KL. Bacteremic nosocomial pneumonia. Analysis of 172 episodes from a single metropolitan area. Am Rev Respir Dis 1984;129:668–671.

99. Rello J, Quintana E, Ausina V, Puzo C, Net A, Prats G. Risk factors for Staphylococcus aureus nosocomial pneumonia in critically ill patients. Am Rev Respir Dis 1990;142:1320–1324.

100. Mayer KH, Zinner SH. Bacterial pathogens of increasing significance in hospital-acquired infections. Rev Infect Dis 1985;73:S371–S379.

101. Winn WC, Jr. Legionnaires disease: Historical perspective. Clin Microbiol Rev 1988;1:60–81.

102. Rhame FS, Streifel AJ, Kersey JH, Jr., McGlave PB. Extrinsic risk factors for pneumonia in the patient at high risk of infection. Am J Med 1984;76:42–52.

103. Shlaes DM, Currie CA, Rotter G, Eanes M, Floyd R. Epidemiology of gentamicin-resistant, gram-negative bacillary colonization in a spinal cord injury unit. J Clin Microbiol 1983;18:227–235.

104. Thompson RL, Wenzel RP. International recognition of methicillin-resistant strains of Staphylococcus aureus. Ann Intern Med 1982;97:925–926.

105. John JF, Jr., Twitty JA. Plasmids as epidemiologic markers in nosocomial gram-negative bacilli: Experience at a university and review of the literature. Rev Infect Dis 1986;8:693–704.

106. Doebbeling BN, Stanley GL, Sheetz CT, et al. Comparative efficacy of alternative hand-washing agents in reducing nosocomial infections in intensive care units. N Engl J Med 1992;327:88–93.

107. Craven DE, Kunches LM, Kilinsky V, Lichtenberg DA, Make BJ, McCabe WR. Risk factors for pneumonia and fatality in patients receiving continuous mechanical ventilation. Am Rev Respir Dis 1986;133:792–796.

108. Garibaldi RA, Britt MR, Coleman ML, Reading JC, Pace NL. Risk factors for postoperative pneumonia. Am J Med 1981;70:677–680.

109. Corensek MJ, Stewart RW, Keys TF, Mehta AC, McHenry MC, Goormastic M. A multivariate analysis of risk factors for pneumonia following cardiac transplantation. Transplantation 1988;46:860–865.

110. Celis R, Torres A, Gatell JM, Almela M, Rodriguez-Roisin R, Agusti-Vidal A. Nosocomial pneumonia. A multivariate analysis of risk and prognosis. Chest 1988; 93:318–324.

111. England AC, III, Fraser DW. Sporadic and epidemic nosocomial legionellosis in the United States. Epidemiologic features. Am J Med 1981;70:707–711.

112. Craven DE, Goularte TA, Make BJ. Contaminated condensate in mechanical ventilator circuits. A risk factor for nosocomial pneumonia? Am Rev Respir Dis 1984; 129:625–628.

113. du Moulin GC, Paterson DG, Hedley-Whyte J, Lisbon A.

Aspiration of gastric bacteria in antacid-treated patients: A frequent cause of postoperative colonisation of the airway. Lancet 1982;i:242–245.

114. Tryba M. Sucralfate versus antacids or H2-antagonists for stress ulcer prophylaxis: A meta-analysis on efficacy and pneumonia rate. Crit Care Med 1991;19:942–949.

115. Pickrell KL. The effect of alcohol intoxication and ether anesthesia on resistance to pneumococcal infection. Bull Johns Hopkins Hosp 1938;63:238–260.

116. Klimek JJ, Lindenberg LB, Cole S, Ellison LH, Quintiliani R. Fatal case of influenza pneumonia with suprainfection by multiple bacteria and Herpes simplex virus. Am Rev Respir Dis 1976;113:683–688.

117. Creasia DA, Nettesheim P, Hammons AS. Impairment of the lung clearance mechanism by respiratory infection. Health Phys 1972;23:865–867.

118. Umetsu DT, Ambrosino DM, Quinti I, Siber GR, Geha RS. Recurrent sinopulmonary infection and impaired antibody response to bacterial capsular polysaccharide antigen in children with selective IgG-subclass deficiency. N Engl J Med 1985;313:1247–1251.

119. Diamond LA, Lorber B. Branhamella catarrhalis pneumonia and immunoglobulin abnormalities: A new association. Am Rev Respir Dis 1984;129:876–878.

120. Karnad A, Alvarez S, Berk SL. Branhamella catarrhalis pneumonia in patients with immunoglobulin abnormalities. South Med J 1986;79:1360–1362.

121. Sieber OF, Jr., Fulginiti VA. Pseudomonas cepacia pneumonia in a child with chronic granulomatous disease and selective IgA deficiency. Acta Paediatr Scand 1976;65:519–520.

122. Polsky B, Armstrong D. Infectious complications of neoplastic disease. Am J Infect Control 1985;13:199–209.

123. Valdivieso M, Gil-Extremera B, Zornoza J, Rodriquez V, Bodey GP. Gram-negative bacillary pneumonia in the compromised host. Medicine (Baltimore) 1977;56:241–254.

124. Huertas VE, Port FK, Rozas VV, Niederhuber JE. Pneumonia in recipients of renal allografts. Arch Surg 1976;111:162–166.

125. Mermel LA, Maki DG. Bacterial pneumonia in solid organ transplantation. Semin Respir Infect 1990;5:10–29.

126. Rand KH, Pollard RB, Merigan TC. Increased pulmonary superinfections in cardiac-transplant patients undergoing primary cytomegalovirus infection. N Engl J Med 1978;298:951–953.

127. Pennington JE, Reynolds HY, Carbone PP. Pseudomonas pneumonia. A retrospective study of 36 cases. Am J Med 1973;55:155–160.

128. Zornoza J, Goldman AM, Wallace S, Valdivieso M, Body GP. Radiologic features of gram-negative pneumonias in the neutropenic patient. AJR 1976;127:989–996.

129. Donowitz GR, Harman C, Pope T, Stewart FM. The role of the chest roentgenogram in febrile neutropenic patients. Arch Intern Med 1991;151:701–704.

130. Magnenat JL, Nicod LP, Auckenthaler R, Junod AF. Mode of presentation and diagnosis of bacterial pneumonia in human immunodeficiency virus-infected patients. Am Rev Respir Dis 1991;144:917–922.

131. Polsky B, Gold JW, Whimbey E, et al. Bacterial pneumonia in patients with the acquired immunodeficiency syndrome. Ann Intern Med 1986;104:38–41.

132. Levine SJ, White DA, Fels AO. The incidence and significance of Staphylococcus aureus in respiratory cultures from patients infected with the human immunodeficiency virus. Am Rev Respir Dis 1990;141:89–93.

133. Witt DJ, Craven DE, McCabe WR. Bacterial infections in adult patients with the acquired immune deficiency syndrome (AIDS) and AIDS-related complex. Am J Med 1987;82:900–906.

134. Harkness GA, Bentley DW, Roghmann KJ. Risk factors for nosocomial pneumonia in the elderly. Am J Med 1990;89:457–463.

135. Verghese A, Berk SL. Bacterial pneumonia in the elderly. Medicine (Baltimore) 1983;62:271–285.

136. Martin LF, Asher EF, Casey JM, Fry DE. Postoperative pneumonia. Determinants of mortality. Arch Surg 1984;119:379–383.

137. Torres A, Serra-Batlles J, Ferrer A, et al. Severe community-acquired pneumonia. Epidemiology and prognostic factors. Am Rev Respir Dis 1991;144:312–318.

138. Donowitz GR, Mandell GL. Acute pneumonia. In: Mandell GL, Douglas RG, Jr., Bennett JE, eds. Principles and practice of infectious diseases. 3d Ed. New York: Churchill Livingstone, 1990:540–555.

139. Torres A, Jimenez P, Puig de la Bellacasa J, Celis R, Gonzalez J, Gea J. Diagnostic value of nonfluoroscopic percutaneous lung needle aspiration in patients with pneumonia. Chest 1990;98:840–844.

140. Barnes DJ, Naraqi S, Igo JD. The role of percutaneous lung aspiration in the bacteriological diagnosis of pneumonia in adults. Aust NZ J Med 1988;18:754–757.

141. Palmer DL, Davidson M, Lusk R. Needle aspiration of the lung in complex pneumonias. Chest 1980;78:16–21.

142. Bartlett JG. Diagnostic accuracy of transtracheal aspiration. Bacteriologic studies. Am Rev Respir Dis 1977; 115:777–782.

143. Barrett-Connor E. The nonvalue of sputum culture in the diagnosis of pneumococcal pneumonia. Am Rev Respir Dis 1971;103:845–848.

144. Drew WL. Value of sputum culture in diagnosis of pneumococcal pneumonia. J Clin Microbiol 1977;6:52–55.

145. Gleckman R, DeVita J, Hibert D, Pelletier C, Martin R. Sputum gram stain assessment in community-acquired bacteremic pneumonia. J Clin Microbiol 1988;26:846–849.

146. Geckler RW, Gremillion DH, McAllister CK, Ellenbogen C. Microscopic and bacteriological comparison of paired sputa and transtracheal aspirates. J Clin Microbiol 1977;6:396–399.

147. Thorsteinsson SB, Musher DM, Fagan T. The diagnostic value of sputum culture in acute pneumonia. JAMA 1975;233:894–895.

148. Murray PR, Washington JA, II. Microscopic and bacteriologic analysis of expectorated sputum. Mayo Clin

Proc 1975;50:339–344.

149. Kalin M, Lindberg AA, Tunevall G. Etiological diagnosis of bacterial pneumonia by gram stain and quantitative culture of expectorates. Leukocytes or alveolar macrophages as indicators of sample representativity. Scand J Infect Dis 1983;15:153–160.

150. Salata RA, Lederman MM, Shlaes DM, et al. Diagnosis of nosocomial pneumonia in intubated, intensive care unit patients. Am Rev Respir Dis 1987;135:426–432.

151. Rein MF, Gwaltney JM, Jr., O'Brien WM, Jennings RH, Mandell GL. Accuracy of Gram's stain in identifying pneumococci in sputum. JAMA 1978;239:2671–2673.

152. Fine MJ, Orloff JJ, Rihs JD, et al. Evaluation of housestaff physicians' preparation and interpretation of sputum Gram stains for community-acquired pneumonia. J Gen Intern Med 1991;6:189–198.

153. Chastre J, Viau F, Brun P, et al. Prospective evaluation of the protected specimen brush for the diagnosis of pulmonary infections in ventilated patients. Am Rev Respir Dis 1984;130:924–929.

154. Chastre J, Fagon JY, Soler P, et al. Diagnosis of nosocomial bacterial pneumonia in intubated patients undergoing ventilation: Comparison of the usefulness of bronchoalveolar lavage and the protected specimen brush. Am J Med 1988;85:499–506.

155. Schwartzman WA. Infections due to Rochalimaea: The expanding clinical spectrum. Clin Infect Dis 1992; 15:893–902.

156. Wear DJ, Hadfield TL, Connor DH, et al. Periodic acid–Schiff reaction stains Mycobacterium tuberculosis, Mycobacterium leprae, Mycobacterium ulcerans, Mycobacterium chelonei (abscessus), and Mycobacterium kansasii. Arch Pathol Lab Med 1985;109:701–703.

157. Lowe RN, Azimi PH, McQuitty J. Acid-fast Actinomyces in a child with pulmonary actinomycosis. J Clin Microbiol 1980;12:124–126.

158. Jung WK. In vitro positive controls for histochemical stains of bacteria and fungi. Am J Clin Pathol 1985; 84:342–345.

159. Chartrand SA, McCracken GH, Jr. Staphylococcal pneumonia in infants and children. Pediatr Infect Dis 1982;1:19–23.

160. Enos WF, Beyer JC, Zimmet SM, Kiesel JA. Unilateral lobar pneumonia with empyema caused by Neisseria gonorrhoeae. South Med J 1980;73:266–267.

161. Cockcroft DW, Stilwell GA. Lobar pneumonia caused by Mycoplasma pneumoniae. Can Med Assoc J 1981;124: 1463–1468.

162. Heffron R. Pneumonia. Cambridge: Harvard University Press, 1939.

163. Loosli CG. Pathogenesis and pathology of lobar pneumonia. J Lancet 1940;60:49–54.

164. Berry FB. Lobar pneumonia: analysis of 400 autopsies. Med Clin N Am 1920;4:571.

165. Loeschcke H. Untersuchungen über die kruppöse Pneumonie. Beitr Pathol Anat Allg Pathol 1931;86:201.

166. Graeser JB, Wu C, Robertson OH. Physical signs and roentgenographic findings in lobar pneumonia in adults. Arch Intern Med 1934;53:249.

167. Blake FG, Howard ME, Hull WS. Artificial pneumothorax in the treatment of lobar pneumonia. JAMA 1935;105:1489.

168. Winn WC, Jr., Glavin FL, Perl DP, Craighead JE. Macroscopic pathology of the lungs in legionnaires' disease. Ann Intern Med 1979;90:548–551.

169. Dietrich PA, Johnson RD, Fairbank JT, Walke JS. The chest radiograph in legionnaires' disease. Radiology 1978;127:577–582.

170. Winn WC, Jr., Glavin FL, Perl DP, et al. The pathology of legionnaires' disease. Fourteen fatal cases from the 1977 outbreak in Vermont. Arch Pathol Lab Med 1978;102:344–350.

171. Hershey CO, Panaro V. Round pneumonia in adults. Arch Intern Med 1988;148:1155–1157.

172. Winn WC, Jr., Myerowitz RL. The pathology of the Legionella pneumonias. A review of 74 cases and the literature. Hum Pathol 1981;12:401–422.

173. Yangco BG, Deresinski SC. Necrotizing or cavitating pneumonia due to Streptococcus pneumoniae: Report of four cases and review of the literature. Medicine (Baltimore) 1980;59:449–457.

174. Kaye MG, Fox MJ, Bartlett JG, Braman SS, Glassroth J. The clinical spectrum of Staphylococcus aureus pulmonary infection. Chest 1990;97:788–792.

175. Naraqi S, McDonnell G. Hematogenous staphylococcal pneumonia secondary to soft tissue infection. Chest 1981;79:173–175.

176. Goldstein JD, Godleski JJ, Balikian JP, Herman PG. Pathologic patterns of Serratia marcescens pneumonia. Hum Pathol 1982;13:479–484.

177. Knight L, Fraser RG, Robson HG. Massive pulmonary gangrene: A severe complication of Klebsiella pneumonia. Can Med Assoc J 1975;112:196–198.

178. Fetzer AE, Werner AS, Hagstrom JW. Pathologic features of pseudomonal pneumonia. Am Rev Respir Dis 1967;96:1121–1130.

179. Lewin S, Brettman LR, Goldstein EJ, et al. Legionnaires' disease. A cause of severe abscess-forming pneumonia. Am J Med 1979;67:339–342.

180. Dowling JN, Kroboth FJ, Karpf M, Yee RB, Pasculle AW. Pneumonia and multiple lung abscesses caused by dual infection with Legionella micdadei and Legionella pneumophila. Am Rev Respir Dis 1983;127:121–125.

181. Shlaes DM, Lerner PI, Wolinsky E, Gopalakrishna KV. Infections due to Lancefield group F and related streptococci (S. milleri, S. anginosus). Medicine (Baltimore) 1981;60:197–207.

182. Singh KP, Morris A, Lang SD, MacCulloch DM, Bremmer DA. Clinically significant Streptococcus anginosus (Streptococcus milleri) infections: A review of 186 cases. NZ Med J 1988;101:813–816.

183. Shales DM, Lederman MM, Chmielewski R, Tweardy D, Krause G, Saffai C. Sputum elastin fibers and the diagnosis of necrotizing pneumonia. Chest 1984;85:763–766.

184. Bartlett JG, Gorbach SL, Finegold SM. The bacteriology of aspiration pneumonia. Am J Med 1974;56:202–207.

185. Nusser RA, Tarkoff MP. Legionnaires disease causing

adult respiratory distress syndrome. Survival and report of open lung biopsy. West J Med 1978;128:443–448.

186. Walsh JJ, Kelley J. Plasma cell pneumonia induced by Legionella pneumophila. Chest 1991;100:1170–1172.

187. Kuhn C. Patterns of lung repair. A morphologist's view. Chest 1991;99:11S–14S.

188. Kuhn C, McDonald JA. The roles of the myofibroblast in idiopathic pulmonary fibrosis. Ultrastructural and immunohistochemical features of sites of active extracellular matrix synthesis. Am J Pathol 1991;138:1257–1265.

189. Leslie KO, Mitchell J, Low R. Lung myofibroblasts. Cell Motil Cytoskeleton 1992;22:92–98.

190. Adler KB, Low RB, Leslie KO, Mitchell J, Evans JN. Biology of disease. Contractile cells in normal and fibrotic lung. Lab Invest 1989;60:473–485.

191. Auerbach SH, Mims OM, Goodpasture EW. Pulmonary fibrosis secondary to pneumonia. Am J Pathol 1951;69–81.

192. Ort S, Ryan JL, Barden G, D'Esopo N. Pneumococcal pneumonia in hospitalized patients. Clinical and radiological presentations. JAMA 1983;249:214–218.

193. Loosli CG. The pathogenesis and pathology of experimental pneumonia in the monkey. J Exp Med 1942;76:79–95.

194. Perlino CA. Laboratory diagnosis of pneumonia due to Streptococcus pneumoniae. J Infect Dis 1984;150:139–144.

195. Valenti WM, Jenzer M, Bentley DW. Type-specific pneumococcal respiratory disease in the elderly and chronically ill. Am Rev Respir Dis 1978;117:233–238.

196. Perlino CA, Burleigh P. Penicillin-insensitive pneumococci: Isolation from patients with pneumonia. South Med J 1979;72:20–22.

197. Merrill CW, Gwaltney JM, Jr., Hendley JW, Sande MA. Rapid identification of pneumococci. Gram stain vs. the quellung reaction. N Engl J Med 1973;288:510–512.

198. Isaacs RD. Necrotizing pneumonia in bacteraemic pneumococcal infection. Br J Dis Chest 1986;80:295–296.

199. Leatherman JW, Iber C, Davies SF. Cavitation in bacteremic pneumococcal pneumonia. Causal role of mixed infection with anaerobic bacteria. Am Rev Respir Dis 1984;129:317–321.

200. Fruchtman SM, Gombert ME, Lyons HA. Adult respiratory distress syndrome as a cause of death in pneumococcal pneumonia. Report of ten cases. Chest 1983;83:598–601.

201. Asmar BI, Thirumoorthi MC, Dajani AS. Pneumococcal pneumonia with pneumatocele formation. Am J Dis Child 1978;132:1091–1093.

202. Stevens DL, Tanner MH, Winship J, et al. Severe group A streptococcal infections associated with a toxic shock-like syndrome and scarlet fever toxin A. N Engl J Med 1989;321:1–7.

203. Gray GC, Escamilla J, Hyams KC, Struewing JP, Kaplan EL, Tupponce AK. Hyperendemic Streptococcus pyogenes infection despite prophylaxis with penicillin G benzathine. N Engl J Med 1991;325:92–97.

204. Molteni RA. Group A beta-hemolytic streptococcal pneumonia: Clinical course and complications of management. Am J Dis Child 1977;131:1366–1371.

205. Keefer CS, Rantz LA, Rammelkamp CH. Hemolytic streptococcal pneumonia and empyema; a study of 55 cases with special reference to treatment. Ann Intern Med 1941;14:1533–1550.

206. Gerber GJ, Farmer WC, Fulkerson LL. β-hemolytic streptococcal pneumonia following influenza. JAMA 1978;240:242–243.

207. Opie EL, Freeman AW, Blake FG, Small JC, Rivers TM. Pneumonia following influenza (at Camp Pike, Ark.). JAMA 1919;72:556–565.

208. Basiliere JL, Bistrong HW, Spence WF. Streptococcal pneumonia. Recent outbreaks in military recruit populations. Am J Med 1968;44:580–589.

209. Cecil RL. Pneumonia and empyema at Camp Upton, N.Y. Med Clin North Am 1918;2:567.

210. MacCallum WG. Pathology of epidemic streptococcal bronchopneumonia in army camps. JAMA 1981;71:704.

211. Goodpasture EW. Bronchopneumonia due to hemolytic streptococci following influenza. JAMA 1919;72:724–725.

212. McIntyre HD, Armstrong JG, Mitchell CA. Streptococcus pyogenes pneumonia with abscess formation. Aust NZ J Med 1989;19:248–249.

213. Kevy SV, Lowe BA. Streptococcal pneumonia and empyema in childhood. N Engl J Med 1961;264:738.

214. Lerner PI, Gopalakrishna KV, Wolinsky E, et al. Group B Streptococcus bacteremia in adults: Analysis of 32 cases and review of the literature. Medicine (Baltimore) 1977;56:457–473.

215. Verghese A, Berk SL, Boelen LJ, Smith JK. Group B streptococcal pneumonia in the elderly. Arch Intern Med 1982;142:1642–1645.

216. Schwartz RH, Shulman ST. Group C and group G streptococci. In-office isolation from children and adolescents with pharyngitis. Clin Pediatr (Philadelphia) 1986;25:496–502.

217. Stamm AM, Cobbs CG. Group C streptococcal pneumonia: Report of a fatal case and review of the literature. Rev Infect Dis 1980;2:889–898.

218. Mohr DN, Feist DJ, Washington JA, Hermans PE. Infections due to group C streptococci in man. Am J Med 1979;66:450–456.

219. Siefkin AD, Peterson DL, Hansen B. Streptococcus equisimilis pneumonia in a compromised host. J Clin Microbiol 1983;17:386–388.

220. Rose HD, Allen JR, Witte G. Streptococcus zooepidemicus (group C) pneumonia in a human. J Clin Microbiol 1980;11:76–78.

221. Ancona RJ, Thompson TR, Ferrieri P. Group G streptococcal pneumonia and sepsis in a newborn infant. J Clin Microbiol 1979;10:758–759.

222. Koshi G, John L. Lancefield group F streptococci causing liver abscess and empyema. Indian J Med Res 1971;59:45–49.

223. Sarkar TK, Murarka RS, Gilardi GL. Primary Streptococcus viridans pneumonia. Chest 1989;96:831–834.

224. Pratter MR, Irwin RS. Viridans streptococcal pulmonary parenchymal infections. JAMA 1980;243:2515–2517.

225. Berk SL, Verghese A, Holtsclaw SA, Smith JK. Enterococcal pneumonia. Occurrence in patients receiving broad-spectrum antibiotic regimens and enteral feeding. Am J Med 1983;74:153–154.

226. Eliopoulos GM, Wennersten C, Reiszner E, Goldmann D, Moellering RC, Jr. High-level resistance to gentamicin in clinical isolates of Streptococcus (Enterococcus) faecium. Antimicrob Agents Chemother 1988;32,10:1528–1532.

227. Johnson AP, Uttley AHC, Woodford N, George RC. Resistance to vancomycin and teicoplanin: An emerging clinical problem. Clin Microbiol Rev 1990;3:280–291.

228. Woodhead MA, Radvan J, Macfarlane JT. Adult community-acquired staphylococcal pneumonia in the antibiotic era: A review of 61 cases. Q J Med 1987;64:783–790.

229. Robertson L, Caley JP, Moore J. Importance of Staphylococcus aureus in pneumonia in the 1957 epidemic of influenza A. Lancet 1958;ii:233–236.

230. Fisher AM, Trever RW, Curtin JA, Schultze G, Miller DF. Staphylococcal pneumonia. A review of 21 cases in adults. N Engl J Med 1958;258:919–928.

231. Espersen F, Gabrielsen J. Pneumonia due to Staphylococcus aureus during mechanical ventilation. J Infect Dis 1981;144:19–23.

232. Stutman HR, Marks MI. Pulmonary infections in children with cystic fibrosis. Semin Respir Infect 1987;2:166–176.

233. McGarry T, Giosa R, Rohman M, Huang CT. Pneumatocele formation in adult pneumonia. Chest 1987;92:717–720.

234. Chonmaitree T, Powell KR. Parapneumonic pleural effusion and empyema in children. Review of a 19-year experience, 1962–1980. Clin Pediatr 1983;22:414–419.

235. Gallis HA. Subacute staphylococcal pneumonia in a renal transplant recipient. Am Rev Respir Dis 1975;112:109–112.

236. Musher DM, McKenzie SO. Infections due to Staphylococcus aureus. Medicine (Baltimore) 1977;56:383–409.

237. Watanakunakorn C. Bacteremic Staphylococcus aureus pneumonia. Scand J Infect Dis 1987;19:623–627.

238. Massanari RM, Pfaller MA, Wakefield DS, et al. Implications of acquired oxacillin resistance in the management and control of Staphylococcus aureus infections. J Infect Dis 1988;158:702–709.

239. Souhami L, Feld R, Tuffnell PG, Feller T. Micrococcus luteus pneumonia: A case report and review of the literature. Med Pediatr Oncol 1979;7:309–314.

240. Causey WA, Lee R. Nocardiosis: In: Vinken PJ, Bruyn GW. eds. Handbook of clinical neurology, Vol. 35. Infections of the nervous system, Part III. Amsterdam: North Holland, 1978:517–530.

241. Chandler FW, Watts JC. Pathologic diagnosis of fungal infections. Chicago: American Society of Clinical Pathologists, 1987:265–271.

242. Krick JA, Stinson EB, Remington JS. Nocardia infection in heart transplant patients. Ann Intern Med 1975;82:18–26.

243. Simpson GL, Stinson EB, Egger MJ, et al. Nocardial infections in the immunocompromised host: A detailed study in a defined population. Rev Infect Dis 1981;3:492–507.

244. Smego RAJ, Gallis HA. The clinical spectrum of Nocardia brasiliensis infection in the United States. Rev Infect Dis 1984;6:164–180.

245. Young LS, Armstrong D, Blevins A, Lieberman P. Nocardia asteroid infection complicating neoplastic disease. Am J Med 1971;50:356–367.

246. Casale TB, Macher AM, Fauci AS. Concomitant pulmonary aspergillosis and nocardiosis in a patient with chronic granulomatous disease of childhood. South Med J 1984;77:274–275.

247. Jonsson S, Wallace RJ, Jr., Hull SI. Recurrent Nocardia pneumonia in an adult with chronic granulomatous disease. Am Rev Respir Dis 1986;133:932–934.

248. Burbank B, Morrione TG, Cutler SS. Pulmonary alveolar proteinosis and nocardiosis. Am J Med 1960;28:1002–1007.

249. Carlsen ET, Hill RB, Rowlands DT. Nocardiosis and pulmonary alveolar proteinosis. Ann Intern Med 1964;60:275–281.

250. Clague HW, Harth M, Hellyer D, et al. Septic arthritis due to Nocardia asteroides in association with pulmonary alveolar proteinosis. J Rheumatol 1982;9:469–472.

251. Kahn FW, Gornick CC, Tofte RW. Primary cutaneous Nocardia asteroides infection with dissemination. Am J Med 1981;70:859–863.

252. Kalb RE, Kaplan MH, Grossman ME. Cutaneous nocardiosis: Case reports and review. J Am Acad Dermatol 1985;13:125–133.

253. Tsuboi R, Takamori K, Ogawa H. Lymphocutaneous nocardiosis caused by Nocardia asteroides. Arch Dermatol 1986;122:1183–1185.

254. McNeil MM, Brown JM, Georghiou PR, Allworth AM, Blacklock ZM. Infections due to Nocardia transvalensis: Clinical spectrum and antimicrobial therapy. Clin Infect Dis 1992;15:453–463.

255. Palmer DL, Harvey RL, Wheeler JK. Diagnostic and therapeutic considerations in Nocardia asteroides infection. Medicine (Baltimore) 1974;53:391–401.

256. Stevens DA. Clinical and clinical laboratory aspects of nocardial infection. J Hyg 1983;91:377–384.

257. Neu HC, Silva M, Hazen E. Necrotizing nocardial pneumonitis. Ann Intern Med 1967;66:274–284.

258. Berd D. Nocardia brasiliensis infection in the United States: A report of nine cases and a review of the literature. Am J Clin Pathol 1973;60:254–258.

259. Frazier AR, Rosenow EC, Roberts GD. Nocardiosis: A review of 25 cases occurring during 24 months. Mayo Clin Proc 1975;50:657–663.

260. Beaman BL, Burnside J, Edward B, et al. Nocardia infections in the United States, 1972–1974. J Infect Dis 1976;134:286–289.

261. Stropes L, Bartlett M, White A. Multiple recurrences of Nocardia pneumonia. Am J Med Sci 1980;280:119–122.

262. Curry WA. Human nocardiosis: A clinical review with selected case reports. Arch Intern Med 1980;140:818–826.

Med 1982;72:899–902.

345. Broughton WA, Kirkpatrick MB. Acute necrotizing pneumonia caused by Enterobacter cloacae. South Med J 1988;81:1061–1062.

346. Svarva PL, Lyng RV, Maeland JA. Emergence of beta-lactam multiresistant variants of gram-negative bacilli in the presence of cefotaxime. Scand J Infect Dis 1985;17:387–391.

347. Yu VL. Serratia marcescens. Historical perspective and clinical review. N Engl J Med 1979;300:887–893.

348. Sanders CV, Jr., Luby JP, Johanson WG, Barnett JA, Sanford JP. Serratia marcescens infections from inhalation therapy medications: Nosocomial outbreak. Ann Intern Med 1970;73:15–21.

349. Balikian JP, Herman PG, Godleski JJ. Serratia pneumonia. Radiology 1980;137:309–311.

350. Carlon GC, Dickinson PC, Goldiner PL, Turnbull AD, Howland WS. Serratia marcescens pneumonia. Arch Surg 1977;112:1220–1224.

351. Reed W. Association of Proteus vulgaris and Diplococcus lanceolatus in a case of croupous pneumonia. Hopkins Hosp Bull 1894;5:24.

352. Tillotson JR, Lerner AM. Characteristics of pneumonias caused by Bacillus proteus. Ann Intern Med 1968;68:287–294.

353. Lysy J, Werczberger A, Globus M, Chowers I. Pneumatocele formation in a patient with Proteus Mirabilis pneumonia. Postgrad Med J 1985;61:255–257.

354. Seriff NS. Lobar pneumonia due to Proteus infection in a previously healthy adult. Am J Med 1969;46:480–488.

355. Solberg CO, Matsen JM. Infections with providence bacilli. A clinical and bacteriologic study. Am J Med 1971;50:241–246.

356. Neva F. Pulmonary involvement in typhoid and paratyphoid fevers. Ann Intern Med 1950;33:83–89.

357. Stuart BM, Pullen RL. Typhoid: Clinical analysis of three hundred and sixty cases. Arch Intern Med 1946;8:629–661.

358. Cohen JI, Bartlett JA, Corey GR. Extra-intestinal manifestations of Salmonella infections. Medicine (Baltimore) 1987;66:349–388.

359. Aguado JM, Obeso G, Cabanillas JJ, Fernandez-Guerrero M, Ales J. Pleuropulmonary infections due to nontyphoid strains of Salmonella. Arch Intern Med 1990;150:54–56.

360. Berkeley D, Mangels J. Salmonella pneumonia in a patient with carcinoma of the lung. Am J Clin Pathol 1980;74:476–478.

361. Canney PA, Larsson SN, Hay JH, Yussuf MA. Case report: Salmonella pneumonia associated with chemotherapy for non-Hodgkin's lymphoma. Clin Radiol 1985;36:459–460.

362. Finegold MJ. Pneumonic plague in monkeys. An electron microscopic study. Am J Pathol 1969;54:167–185.

363. Cavanaugh DC, Randall R. The role of multiplication of Pasteurella pestis in mononuclear phagocytes. J Immunol 1959;83:348–363.

364. Monte TC. Properties and pharmacological action of plague murine toxin. Pharmacol Ther 1981;12:491–499.

365. World Health Organization Technical Report Series (No. 165). Expert committee on plague. Geneva: World Health Organization, 1959.

366. Meyer KF. The ecology of plague. Medicine (Baltimore) 1942;21:143–174.

367. Morris JT, McAllister CK. Bubonic plague. South Med J 1992;85:326–327.

368. Wu L-T, Woodhead GS. Notes on the histology of some of the lesions present in pneumonic plague. J Pathol Bacteriol 1914;19:1–32.

369. Werner SB, Weidmer CE, Nelson BC, Nygaard GS, Goethals RM, Poland JD. Primary plague pneumonia contracted from a domestic cat at South Lake Tahoe, Calif. JAMA 1984;251:929–931.

370. Centers for Disease Control. Pneumonic plague—Arizona, 1992. MMWR 1992;41:737–739.

371. Burmeister RW, Tigertt WD, Overholt EL. Laboratory-acquired pneumonic plague. Report of a case and review of previous cases. Ann Intern Med 1962;56:789–800.

372. Smith JH. Plague. In: Binford CH, Connor DH, eds. Pathology of tropical and extraordinary diseases. Washington, D.C.: Armed Forces Institute of Pathology, 1976;130–134.

373. Ostroff SM, Kapperud G, Lassen J, Aasen S, Tauxe RV. Clinical features of sporadic Yersinia enterocolitica infections in Norway. J Infect Dis 1992;166:812–817.

374. Bottone EJ. Yersinia enterocolitica: A panoramic view of a charismatic microorganism. CRC Crit Rev Clin Lab Sci 1977;5:211–241.

375. Portnoy D, Martinez LA. Yersinia enterocolitica septicemia with pneumonia. Can Med Assoc J 1979;120:61–62.

376. Ettensohn DB, Roberts NJ, Jr. Yersinia enterocolitica pneumonia. NY State J Med 1981;81:791–794.

377. Bigler RD, Atkins RR, Wing EJ. Yersinia enterocolitica lung infection. Arch Intern Med 1981;141:1529–1530.

378. Taylor BG, Zafarzai MZ, Humphreys DW, et al. Nodular pulmonary infiltrates and septic arthritis associated with Yersinia enterocolitica bacteremia. Am Rev Respir Dis 1977;116:525–529.

379. Sebes JI, Mabry EH, Jr., Rabinowitz JG. Lung abscess and osteomyelitis of rib due to Yersinia enterocolitica. Chest 1976;69:546–548.

380. Cropp AJ, Gaylord SF, Watanakunakorn C. Cavitary pneumonia due to Yersinia enterocolitica in a healthy man. Am J Med Sci 1984;288:130–132.

381. Kane DR, Reuman DD. Yersinia enterocolitica causing pneumonia and empyema in a child and a review of the literature. Pediatr Infect Dis J 1992;11:591–593.

382. Bae BH, Sureka SB, Ajamy JA. Enteric group 15 (Enterobacteriaceae) associated with pneumonia. J Clin Microbiol 1981;14:596–597.

383. Pfeiffer R. Vorläufige Mitteilungen über die Erreger der Influenza. Dtsch Med Wochenschr 1892;18:28.

384. Musher DM, Kubitschek KR, Crennan J, Baughn RE. Pneumonia and acute febrile tracheobronchitis due to Haemophilus influenzae. Ann Intern Med 1983;99:444–450.

385. MacCallum WG. Pathology of the pneumonia following

influenza. JAMA 1919;72:720–723.

386. Pittman M. Variation and type specificity in the bacterial species Haemophilus influenzae. J Exp Med 1931;53:471.

387. Smith W, Andrews CH, Laidlaw PP. A virus obtained from influenza patients. Lancet 1933;ii:66.

388. Ginsburg CM, Howard JB, Nelson JD. Report of 65 cases of Haemophilus influenzae b pneumonia. Pediatrics 1979;64:283–286.

389. Alsever RN, Stiver HG, Dinerman N, Dahl CR, Eickhoff TC. Haemophilus influenzae pericarditis and empyema with thyroiditis in an adult. JAMA 1974;230:1426–1427.

390. Levin DC, Schwarz MI, Matthay RA, LaForce FM. Bacteremic Haemophilus influenzae pneumonia in adults. A report of 24 cases and a review of the literature. Am J Med 1977;62:219–224.

391. Wallace RJ Jr., Musher DM, Martin RR. Hemophilus influenzae pneumonia in adults. Am J Med 1978;64:87–93.

392. Kaplan NM, Braude AI. Hemophilus influenzae infection in adults. Arch Intern Med 1958;101:515.

393. Warner JO, Gordon I. Pneumatocoeles following Haemophilus influenzae pneumonia. Clin Radiol 1981;32:99–105.

394. Moxon ER, Wilson R. The role of Haemophilus influenzae in the pathogenesis of pneumonia. Rev Infect Dis 1991;13:S518–S527.

395. Asmar BI, Slovis TL, Reed JO, Dajani AS. Hemophilus influenzae type b pneumonia in 43 children. J Pediatr 1978;93:389–393.

396. Jacobs NM, Harris VJ. Acute Haemophilus pneumonia in childhood. Am J Dis Child 1979;133:603–605.

397. Keefer CS, Rammelkamp CH. Hemophilus influenzae bacteremia: Report of two cases recovering following sulfathiazole and sulfapyridine. Ann Intern Med 1942;16:1221–1227.

398. Everett ED, Rham AE, Jr., Adaniya R, Stevens DL, McNitt TR. Haemophilus influenzae pneumonia in adults. JAMA 1977;238:319–321.

399. Quintiliani R, Hymans PJ. The association of bacteremic Haemophilus influenzae pneumonia in adults with typable strains. Am J Med 1971;50:781–786.

400. Lowe MB. Haemophilus influenzae type c bronchopneumonia. J Pathol Bacteriol 1964;88:315.

401. Holmes RL, Kozinn WP. Pneumonia and bacteremia associated with Haemophilus influenzae serotype d. J Clin Microbiol 1983;18:730–732.

402. Dworzack DL, Blessing LD, Hodges GR, Barnes WG. Hemophilus influenzae type F pneumonia in adults. Am J Med Sci 1978;275:87–91.

403. Takala AK, Eskola J, van Alphen L. Spectrum of invasive Haemophilus influenzae type b disease in adults. Arch Intern Med 1990;150:2573–2576.

404. Liston TE, Foshee WS. Invasive disease due to nontypable Haemophilus influenzae in children. South Med J 1982;75:753–754.

405. Berk SL, Holtsclaw SA, Wiener SL, Smith JK. Nontypeable Haemophilus influenzae in the elderly. Arch Intern Med 1982;142:537–539.

406. Miller EH, Jr., Caplan ES. Nosocomial Hemophilus pneumonia in patients with severe trauma. Surg Gynecol Obstet 1984;159:153–156.

407. Pearlberg J, Haggar AM, Saravolatz L, Beute GH, Popovich J. Hemophilus influenzae pneumonia in the adult. Radiographic appearance with clinical correlation. Radiology 1984;151:23–26.

408. Tillotson JR, Lerner AM. Hemophilus influenzae bronchopneumonia in adults. Arch Intern Med 1968;121:428–432.

409. Henry SA, Gold JW, Freiman AH, Armstrong D. Chronic pneumonitis caused by Hemophilus influenzae in an adult. Arch Intern Med 1983;143:1461–1462.

410. Doern GV, Jorgensen JH, Thornsberry C, et al. National collaborative study of the prevalence of antimicrobial resistance among clinical isolates of Haemophilus influenzae. Antimicrob Agents Chemother 1988;32:180–185.

411. Johnson WD, Kaye D, Hook EW. Haemophilus influenzae pneumonia in adults. Am Rev Respir Dis 1968;97:1112–1117.

412. Cooney TG, Harwood BR, Meisner DJ. Haemophilus parainfluenzae thoracic empyema. Arch Intern Med 1981;141:940–941.

413. Arneborn P, Lindquist BL, Sjöberg L. Severe pulmonary infection by Haemophilus aphrophilus in a noncompromised child. Scand J Infect Dis 1985;17:327–329.

414. McDade JE, Shepard CC, Fraser DW, Tsai TR, Redus MA, Dowdle WR. Legionnaires' disease: isolation of a bacterium and demonstration of its role in other respiratory disease. N Engl J Med 1977;297:1197–1203.

415. Reingold AL, Thomason BM, Brake BJ, Thacker L, Wilkinson HW, Kuritsky JN. Legionella pneumonia in the United States: The distribution of serogroups and species causing human illness. J Infect Dis 1984;149:819.

416. Glick TH, Gregg MB, Berman B, Mallison G, Rhodes WW, Jr., Kassanoff I. Pontiac fever. An epidemic of unknown etiology in a health department: I. Clinical and epidemiologic aspects. Am J Epidemiol 1978;107:149–160.

417. Herwaldt LA, Gorman GW, McGrath T, et al. A new Legionella species, Legionella feeleii species nova, causes Pontiac fever in an automobile plant. Ann Intern Med 1984;100:333–338.

418. Knudsen F, Nielsen AH, Hansen KB. Legionella micdadei (Pittsburgh pneumonia agent) may cause non-pneumonic legionellosis. Lancet 1983;i:708.

419. Goldberg DJ, Wrench JG, Collier PW, et al. Lochgoilhead fever: Outbreak of non-pneumonic legionellosis due to Legionella micdadei. Lancet 1989;i:316–318.

420. Fenstersheib MD, Miller M, Diggins C, et al. Outbreak of Pontiac fever due to Legionella anisa. Lancet 1990;336:35–37.

421. Fraser DW, Tsai TR, Orenstein W, et al. Legionnaires' disease: Description of an epidemic of pneumonia. N Engl J Med 1977;297:1189–1197.

422. Shope RE. The infection of ferrets with swine influenza virus. J Exp Med 1934;60:49–61.

423. Rogers BH, Donowitz GR, Walker GK, Harding SA, Sande MA. Opportunistic pneumonia: A clinicopathological study of five cases caused by an unidentified acid-fast bacterium. N Engl J Med 1979;301:959–961.

424. Myerowitz RL, Pasculle AW, Dowling JN, et al. Opportunistic lung infection due to "Pittsburgh Pneumonia Agent." N Engl J Med 1979;301:953–958.

425. Gress FM, Myerowitz RL. The ultrastructural morphologic features of Pittsburgh pneumonia agent. Am J Pathol 1980;101:63–78.

426. Blackmon JA, Hicklin MD, Chandler FW. Legionnaires' disease. Pathological and historical aspects of a 'new' disease. Arch Pathol Lab Med 1978;102:337–343.

427. Hernandez FJ, Kirby BD, Stanley TM, Edelstein PH. Legionnaires' disease. Postmortem pathologic findings of 20 cases. Am J Clin Pathol 1980;73:488–495.

428. Boyd JF, Buchanan WM, MacLeod TI, Dunn RI, Weir WP. Pathology of five Scottish deaths from pneumonic illnesses acquired in Spain due to legionnaires' disease agent. J Clin Pathol 1978;31:809–816.

429. Carter JB, Wolter RK, Angres G, Saltzman P. Nodular legionnaire's disease. AJR 1981;137:612–613.

430. Muder RR, Yu VL, Parry MF. The radiologic manifestations of Legionella pneumonia. Semin Respir Infect 1987;2:242–254.

431. Wade JS, Griffin FM, Jr. Multinodular pneumonia caused by Legionella. Am J Med 1987;83:603.

432. Pope TI, Jr., Armstrong P, Thompson R, Donowitz GR. Pittsburgh pneumonia agent: Chest film manifestations. AJR 1982;138:237–241.

433. Venkatachalam KK, Saravolatz LD, Christopher KL. Legionnaires' disease. A cause of lung abscess. JAMA 1979;241:597–598.

434. Lake KB, van Dyke JJ, Gerberg E, Browne PM. Legionnaires' disease and pulmonary cavitation. Arch Intern Med 1979;139:485–486.

435. Edwards D, Finlayson DM. Legionnaires' disease causing severe lung abscesses. Can Med Assoc J 1980;123:524–527.

436. Gibney RT, Herbert FA, King EG, Elliot JF. Prolonged cavitating pneumonia in a patient with serologic evidence of legionnaires' disease. Chest 1980;78:671–672.

437. Magnussen CR, Israel RH. Legionnaires' lung abscess. Am J Med Sci 1980;279:117–120.

438. Fairbank JT, Mamourian AC, Dietrich PA, Girod JC. The chest radiograph in legionnaires' disease. Further observations. Radiology 1983;147:33–34.

439. Randolph KA, Beekman JF. Legionnaires' disease presenting with empyema. Chest 1979;75:404–406.

440. Halberstam M, Isenberg HD, Hilton E. Abscess and empyema caused by Legionella micdadei. J Clin Microbiol 1992;30:512–513.

441. Strampfer MJ, Schoch PE, Scoma S, Cunha BA. Empyema and Legionella bozemanii. Ann Intern Med 1986;105:626.

442. Brettman LR, DeHertogh D, Rank EL, Mandour MA. Legionella bozemanii and empyema. Ann Intern Med 1986;105:146–147.

443. Weisenburger DD, Helms CM, Renner ED. Sporadic legionnaires' disease. A pathologic study of 23 fatal cases. Arch Pathol Lab Med 1981;105:130–137.

444. Leder LD. Uber die selektive fermentcytochemische Darstellung von neutrophilen myeloischen Zellen und Gewabsmastzellen im Paraffinschnitt. Klin Wochenschr 1964;42:553.

445. Chandler FW, Cole RM, Hicklin MD, Blackmon JA, Callaway CS. Ultrastructure of the legionnaires' disease bacterium. A study using transmission electron microscopy. Ann Intern Med 1979;90:642–647.

446. Glavin FL, Winn WC, Jr., Craighead JE. Ultrastructure of lung in legionnaires' disease. Observations of three biopsies done during the Vermont epidemic. Ann Intern Med 1979;90:555–559.

447. Horwitz MA, Silverstein SC. Legionnaires' disease bacterium (Legionella pneumophila) multiples intracellularly in human monocytes. J Clin Invest 1980;66:441–450.

448. Silverman DJ, Wisseman CC, Jr., Waddell AD, Jones M. External slime layers of Rickettsia prowazekii and Rickettsia rickettsii: Occurrence of a slime layer. Infect Immun 1978;22:233–246.

449. Tenover FC, Edelstein PH, Goldstein LC, Sturge JC, Plorde JJ. Comparison of cross-staining reactions by Pseudomonas spp. and fluorescein-labeled polyclonal and monoclonal antibodies directed against Legionella pneumophila. J Clin Microbiol 1986;23:647–649.

450. Edelstein PH, Beer KB, Sturge JC, Watson AJ, Goldstein LC. Clinical utility of a monoclonal direct fluorescent reagent specific for Legionella pneumophila: Comparative study with other reagents. J Clin Microbiol 1985;22:419–421.

451. Flournoy DJ, Belobraydic KA, Silberg SL, Lawrence CH, Guthrie PJ. False positive Legionella pneumophila direct immunofluorescent monoclonal antibody test caused by Bacillus cereus spores. Diagn Microbiol Infect Dis 1988;9:123–125.

452. Benson RF, Thacker WL, Plikaytis BB, Wilkinson HW. Cross-reactions in Legionella antisera with Bordetella pertussis strains. J Clin Microbiol 1987;25:594–596.

453. Edelstein PH, Edelstein MAC. Evaluation of the Merifluor-Legionella immunofluorescent reagent for identifying and detecting 21 Legionella species. J Clin Microbiol 1989;27:2455–2458.

454. Chandler FW, Hicklin MD, Blackmon JA. Demonstration of the agent of legionnaires' disease in tissue. N Engl J Med 1977;297:1218–1220.

455. Van Orden AE, Greer PW. Modification of the Dieterle spirochete stain. Histotechnology 1977;1:51–53.

456. Elias JM, Greene C. Modified Steiner method for the demonstration of spirochetes in tissue. Am J Clin Pathol 1979;71:109–111.

457. Pounder DJ. Warthin-Starry for Legionella. Am J Clin Pathol 1983;80:276.

458. Frenkel JK, Baker LH, Chonko AM. Autopsy diagnosis of legionnaires' disease in immunosuppressed patients. A paleodiagnosis using Giemsa stain (Wohlbach modifi-

cation). Ann Intern Med 1979;90:559–562.

459. Greer PW, Chandler FW, Hicklin MD. Rapid demonstration of Legionella pneumophila in unembedded tissue. An adaptation of the Gimenez stain. Am J Clin Pathol 1980;73:788–790.

460. Edelstein PH, Meyer RD, Finegold SM. Long-term followup of two patients with pulmonary cavitation caused by Legionella pneumophila. Am Rev Respir Dis 1981; 124:90–93.

461. Kariman K, Shelburne JD, Gough W, Zacheck MJ, Blackmon JA. Pathologic findings and long-term sequelae in legionnaires' disease. Chest 1979;75:736–739.

462. Blackmon JA, Harley RA, Hicklin MD, Chandler FW. Pulmonary sequelae of acute legionnaires' disease pneumonia. Ann Intern Med 1979;90:552–554.

463. Case records of the Massachusetts General Hospital. Case 32-1978. N Engl J Med 1978;299:347–354.

464. Chastre J, Raghu G, Soler P, Brun P, Basset F, Gibert C. Pulmonary fibrosis following pneumonia due to acute legionnaires' disease. Clinical, ultrastructural, and immunofluorescent study. Chest 1987;91:57–62.

465. Fraser DW, Wachsmuth I, Bopp C, Feeley JC, Tsai TF. Antibiotic treatment of guinea-pigs infected with agent of legionnaires' disease. Lancet 1978;i:175–178.

466. Parry MF, Stampleman L, Hutchinson JH, Folta D, Steinberg MG, Krasnogor LJ. Waterborne Legionella bozemanii and nosocomial pneumonia in immunosuppressed patients. Ann Intern Med 1985;103:205–210.

467. Brenner DJ, Steigerwalt AG, Gorman GW, et al. Legionella bozemanii sp. nov. and Legionella dumoffii sp. nov.: Classification of two additional species of Legionella associated with human pneumonia. Curr Microbiol 1980;4:111–116.

468. Griffith ME, Lindquist DS, Benson RF, Thacker WL, Brenner DJ, Wilkinson HW. First isolation of Legionella gormanii from human disease. J Clin Microbiol 1988; 26:380–381.

469. Thacker WL, Wilkinson HW, Plikaytis BB, et al. Second serogroup of Legionella feeleii strains isolated from humans. J Clin Microbiol 1985;22:1–4.

470. Misra DP, Harris LF, Shasteen WJ. Legionella feeleii pneumonia. South Med J 1987;80:1063–1064.

471. Palutke WA, Crane LR, Wentworth BB, et al. Legionella feeleii-associated pneumonia in humans. Am J Clin Pathol 1986;86:348–351.

472. McKinney RM, Porschen RK, Edelstein PH, et al. Legionella longbeachae species nova, another etiologic agent of human pneumonia. Ann Intern Med 1981; 94:739–743.

473. Bibb WF, Sorg RJ, Thomason BM, et al. Recognition of a second serogroup of Legionella longbeachae. J Clin Microbiol 1981;14:674–677.

474. Tang PW, Toma S, MacMillan LG. Legionella oakridgensis: Laboratory diagnosis of a human infection. J Clin Microbiol 1985;21:462–463.

475. Thacker WL, Wilkinson HW, Benson RF, Edberg SC, Brenner DJ. Legionella jordanis isolated from a patient with fatal pneumonia. J Clin Microbiol 1988;26:1400–1401.

476. Thacker WL, Benson RF, Hawes L, Mayberry WR, Brenner DJ. Characterization of a Legionella anisa strain isolated from a patient with pneumonia. J Clin Microbiol 1990;28:122–123.

477. Thacker WL, Benson RF, Staneck JL, et al. Legionella cincinnatiensis sp. nov. isolated from a patient with pneumonia. J Clin Microbiol 1988;26:418–420.

478. Edelstein PH, Brenner DJ, Moss CW, Steigerwalt AG, Francis EM, George WL. Legionella wadsworthii species nova: A cause of human pneumonia. Ann Intern Med 1982;97:809–813.

479. Wilkinson HW, Thacker WL, Steigerwalt AG, Brenner DJ, Ampel NM, Wing EJ. Second serogroup of Legionella hackeliae isolated from a patient with pneumonia. J Clin Microbiol 1985;22:488–489.

480. Brenner DJ, Steigerwalt AG, Gorman GW, et al. Ten new species of Legionella. Int J Syst Bacteriol 1985; 35:50–59.

481. Thacker WL, Benson RF, Schifman RB, et al. Legionella tucsonensis sp. nov. isolated from a renal transplant recipient. J Clin Microbiol 1989;27:1831–1834.

482. Wilkinson HW, Thacker WL, Brenner DJ, Ryan KJ. Fatal Legionella maceachernii pneumonia. J Clin Microbiol 1985;22:1055.

483. Wilkinson HW, Thacker WL, Benson RF, et al. Legionella birminghamensis sp. nov. isolated from a cardiac transplant recipient. J Clin Microbiol 1987;25: 2120–2122.

484. Iannini PB, Claffey T, Quintiliani R. Bacteremic Pseudomonas pneumonia. JAMA 1974;230:558–561.

485. Hoogwerf BJ, Khan MY. Community-acquired bacteremic Pseudomonas pneumonia in a health adult. Am Rev Respir Dis 1981;123:132–134.

486. Bodey GP, Jadeja L, Elting L. Pseudomonas bacteremia. Retrospective analysis of 410 episodes. Arch Intern Med 1985;145:1621–1629.

487. Bodey GP, Bolivar R, Fainstein V, Jadeja L. Infections caused by Pseudomonas aeruginosa. Rev Infect Dis 1983;5:279–313.

488. Tillotson JR, Lerner AM. Characteristics of nonbacteremic Pseudomonas pneumonia. Ann Intern Med 1968; 68:295–307.

489. Rose HD, Heckman MG, Unger JD. Pseudomonas aeruginosa pneumonia in adults. Am Rev Respir Dis 1973;107:416–422.

490. Watanakunakorn C. Vertebral osteomyelitis as a complication of Pseudomonas aeruginosa pneumonia. South Med J 1975;68:173–176.

491. Quirk JA, Beaman MH, Blake M. Community-acquired Pseudomonas pneumonia in a normal host complicated by metastatic panophthalmitis and cutaneous pustules. Aust NZ J Med 1990;20:254–256.

492. Mungall IP, Jackson EW, Dibble JB. Pseudomonas pneumonia in status asthmaticus. Postgrad Med J 1977;53:764–765.

493. Fishman H, Eaton B, Lipson A, Delaney MD. Primary Pseudomonas pneumonia in a previously healthy man. South Med J 1983;76:260–262.

494. Govan J, Reiss-Levy E, Bader L, Schonell M. Pseudomo-

nas pneumonia with bacteraemia. Med J Aust 1977; 1:627–628.

495. Siebert WT, Williams TW, Jr. Primary Pseudomonas pneumonia. South Med J 1980;73:75–77.

496. Soave R, Murray HW, Litrenta MM. Bacterial invasion of pulmonary vessels. Pseudomonas bacteremia mimicking pulmonary thromboembolism with infarction. Am J Med 1978;65:864–867.

497. Case Records of the Massachusetts General Hospital. Case 15-1966. N Engl J Med 1966;274:736–744.

498. Uppington J, Penney MD. Unilateral pulmonary oedema and Pseudomonas pneumonia. Postgrad Med J 1980;56:677–678.

499. Teplitz C. Pathogenesis of Pseudomonas vasculitis and septic lesions. Arch Pathol 1965;80:297–307.

500. Rivera M, Nicotra MB. Pseudomonas aeruginosa mucoid strain. Its significance in adult chest diseases. Am Rev Respir Dis 1982;126:833–836.

501. Tomashefski JF, Thomassen MJ, Bruce MC, Goldberg HI, Konstan MW, Stern RC. Pseudomonas cepacia-associated pneumonia in cystic fibrosis. Relation of clinical features to histopathologic patterns of pneumonia. Arch Pathol Lab Med 1988;112:166–172.

502. Dailey RH, Benner EJ. Necrotizing pneumonitis due to the pseudomonad "Eugonic Oxidizer—Group I". N Engl J Med 1968;279:361–362.

503. Whitmore A, Krishnaswami CS. An account of the discovery of a hitherto undescribed infective disease occurring among the population of Rangoon. Indian Med Gaz 1912;47:262.

504. Sanford JP. Pseudomonas species. In: Mandell GL, Douglas RG, Jr., Bennett JE, eds. Principles and practice of infectious diseases. 3d Ed. New York: Churchill Livingstone, 1990;1692–1696.

505. Clayton AJ, Lisella RS, Martin DG. Melioidosis: A serological survey in military personnel. Milit Med 1973; 138:24.

506. Weber DR, Douglass LE, Brundage WG, Stallkamp TC. Acute varieties of melioidosis occurring in US soldiers in Vietnam. Am J Med 1969;46:234–244.

507. Mackowiak PA, Smith JW. Septicemic melioidosis. Occurrence following acute influenza A six years after exposure in Vietnam. JAMA 1978;240:764–766.

508. McCormick JB, Sexton DJ, McMurray JG, Carey E, Hayes P, Feldman RA. Human-to-human transmission of Pseudomonas pseudomallei. Ann Intern Med 1975; 83:512–513.

509. James AE, Dixon GD, Johnson HG. Melioidosis: a correlation of the radiologic and pathologic findings. Radiology 1967;89:230–235.

510. Greenwald KA, Nash G, Foley FD. Acute systemic melioidosis: Autopsy findings in four patients. Am J Clin Pathol 1969;52:188–198.

511. Piggott JA, Hochholzer L. Human melioidosis. A histopathologic study of acute and chronic melioidosis. Arch Pathol 1970;90:101–111.

512. Everett ED, Nelson RA. Pulmonary melioidosis. Observations in thirty-nine cases. Am Rev Respir Dis 1975; 112:331–340.

513. Girard DE, Nardone DA, Jones SR. Pleural melioidosis. Am Rev Respir Dis 1976;114:1175–1178.

514. Buchman RJ, Kmiecik JE, LaNoue AM. Extrapulmonary melioidosis. Am J Surg 1973;125:324–327.

515. Saengnipanthkul S, Laupattarakasem W, Kowsuwon W, Mahaisavariya B. Isolated articular melioidosis. Clin Orthop 1991;267:182–185.

516. Baumann BB, Morita ET. Systemic melioidosis presenting as myocardial infarct. Ann Intern Med 1967; 67:836–842.

517. Jackson AE, Moore WL, Jr., Sanford JP. Recrudescent melioidosis associated with diabetic ketoacidosis. Arch Intern Med 1972;130:268–271.

518. Kunakorn M, Petchclai B, Khupulsup K, Naigowit P. Gold blot for detection of immunoglobulin M (IgM)- and IgG-specific antibodies for rapid serodiagnosis of melioidosis. J Clin Microbiol 1991;29:2065–2067.

519. Green RN, Tuffnell PG. Laboratory acquired melioidosis. Am J Med 1968;44:599–605.

520. Rosenthal SL, Zuger JH, Apollo E. Respiratory colonization with Pseudomonas putrefaciens after near-drowning in salt water. Am J Clin Pathol 1975;64:382–384.

521. Sarkar TK, Gilardi G, Aguam AS, Josephson J, Leventhal GL. Primary Pseudomonas maltophilia infection of the lung. Postgrad Med 1979;65:253–256, 260.

522. Zuravleff JJ, Yu VL. Infections caused by Pseudomonas maltophilia with emphasis on bacteremia: Case reports and a review of the literature. Rev Infect Dis 1982; 4:1236–1246.

523. Khardori N, Elting L, Wong E, Schable B, Bodey GP. Nosocomial infections due to Xanthomonas maltophilia (Pseudomonas maltophilia) in patients with cancer. Rev Infect Dis 1990;12:997–1003.

524. Trotter JA, Kuhls TL, Pickett DA, Reyes de la Rocha S, Welch DF. Pneumonia caused by a newly recognized pseudomonad in a child with chronic granulomatous disease. J Clin Microbiol 1990;28:1120–1124.

525. Srinivasan G, Raff MJ, Templeton WC, Givens SJ, Graves RC, Melo JC. Branhamella catarrhalis pneumonia: Report of two cases and review of the literature. Am Rev Respir Dis 1981;123:553–555.

526. Wright PW, Wallace RJ, Jr., Shepherd JR. A descriptive study of 42 cases of Branhamella catarrhalis pneumonia. Am J Med 1990;88:2S–8S.

527. Ohlsson A, Bailey T. Neonatal pneumonia caused by Branhamella catarrhalis. Scand J Infect Dis 1985;17: 225–228.

528. Malkamaki M, Honkanen E, Leinonen M, Makela PH. Branhamella catarrhalis as a cause of bacteremic pneumonia. Scand J Infect Dis 1983;15:125–126.

529. Choo PW, Gantz NM. Branhamella catarrhalis pneumonia with bacteremia. South Med J 1989;82:1317–1318.

530. Rosett W, Heck DM, Hodges GR. Pneumonitis and pulmonary abscess associated with Moraxella nonliquefaciens. Chest 1976;70:664–665.

531. Goetz MB, Jones J. Pneumonia and bacteremia caused by a previously undescribed Moraxella-like bacterium. J Clin Microbiol 1982;15:720–722.

532. Abrahamsen TG, Finne PH, Lingaas E. Flavobacterium meningosepticum infections in a neonatal intensive care unit. Acta Paediatr Scand 1989;78:51–55.

533. Uchihara T, Yokota T, Watabiki S, Ueki M, Miyake S, Tsukagoshi H. Flavobacterium meningosepticum meningitis in an adult. Am J Med 1988;85:738–739.

534. Ashdown LR, Previtera S. Community-acquired Flavobacterium meningosepticum pneumonia and septicaemia. Med J Aust 1992;156:69–70.

535. Sundin D, Gold BD, Berkowitz FE, Schwartz DA, Goo D. Community-acquired Flavobacterium meningosepticum meningitis, pneumonia and septicemia in a normal infant. Pediatr Infect Dis J 1991;10:73–76.

536. Tam AY, Yung RW, Fu KH. Fatal pneumonia caused by Flavobacterium meningosepticum. Pediatr Infect Dis J 1989;8:252–254.

537. Teres D. ICU-acquired pneumonia due to Flavobacterium meningosepticum. JAMA 1974;228:732.

538. Brown RB, Phillips D, Barker MJ, Pieczarka R, Sands M, Teres D. Outbreak of nosocomial Flavobacterium meningosepticum respiratory infections associated with use of aerosolized polymyxin B. Am J Infect Control 1989;17:121–125.

539. Raimondi A, Moosdeen F, Williams JD. Antibiotic resistance pattern of Flavobacterium meningosepticum. Eur J Clin Microbiol 1986;5:461–463.

540. Casalta JP, Peloux Y, Raoult D, Brunet P, Gallais H. Pneumonia and meningitis caused by a new nonfermentative unknown gram-negative bacterium. J Clin Microbiol 1989;27:1446–1448.

541. Reines HD, Cook FV. Pneumonia and bacteremia due to Aeromonas hydrophila. Chest 1981;80:264–267.

542. Baddour LM, Baselski VS. Pneumonia due to Aeromonas hydrophila-complex: Epidemiologic, clinical, and microbiologic features. South Med J 1988;81:461–463.

543. Kelley MT, Avery DM. Lactose-positive Vibrio in seawater: A cause of pneumonia and septicemia in a drowning victim. J Clin Microbiol 1980;11:278–280.

544. Janda JM, Powers C, Bryant RG, et al. Current perspectives on the epidemiology and pathogenesis of clinically significant Vibrio spp. Clin Microbiol Rev 1988;1:245–267.

545. Gottlieb T, Barnes DJ. Community-acquired Acinetobacter pneumonia. Aust NZ J Med 1989;19:259–260.

546. Goodhart GL, Abrutyn E, Watson R, Root RK, Egert J. Community-acquired Acinetobacter calcoaceticus var anitratus pneumonia. JAMA 1977;238:1516–1518.

547. Wallace RJ, Jr., Awe RJ, Martin RR. Bacteremic Acinetobacter (Herellea) pneumonia with survival: Case report. Am Rev Respir Dis 1976;113:695–699.

548. Cordes LG, Brink EW, Checko PJ, et al. A cluster of Acinetobacter pneumonia in foundry workers. Ann Intern Med 1981;95:688–693.

549. Cunha BA, Klimek JJ, Gracewski J, McLaughlin JC, Quintiliani R. A common source outbreak of Acinetobacter pulmonary infections traced to Wright respirometers. Postgrad Med J 1980;56:169–172.

550. Milder JE, Hall NK, Finley RA. Pasteurella multocida pneumonia and bacteremia. South Med J 1977;70: 1123–1124.

551. Rose HD, Mathai G. Acute Pasteurella multocida pneumonia. Br J Dis Chest 1977;71:123–126.

552. Ruiz-Santana S, Antunez IA, Armas M, Rodriguez de Castro F, Manzano JL. Telescoping plugged catheter. An unusual way of diagnosing Pasteurella multocida pneumonia. Chest 1991;99:1517.

553. Olsen AM, Needham GM. Pasteurella multocida in suppurative diseases of the respiratory tract. Am J Med Sci 1952;224:77–81.

554. Maneche HC, Toll HW. Pulmonary cavitation and massive hemorrhage caused by Pasteurella multocida. N Engl J Med 1964;271:491–494.

555. Schmidt EC, Truitt LV, Koch ML. Pulmonary abscess with empyema caused by Pasteurella multocida. Am J Clin Pathol 1970;54:733–736.

556. Starkebaum GA, Plorde JJ. Pasteurella pneumonia: Report of a case and review of the literature. J Clin Microbiol 1977;5:332–335.

557. Taylor JP, Istre GR, McChesney TC, et al. Epidemiologic characteristics of human tularemia in the southwest-central states, 1981–1987. Am J Epidemiol 1991;133:1032–1038.

558. Boyce JM. Recent trends in the epidemiology of tularemia in the United States. J Infect Dis 1975;131:197–199.

559. Rohrbach BW, Westerman E, Istre GR. Epidemiology and clinical characteristics of tularemia in Oklahoma, 1979 to 1985. South Med J 1991;84:1091–1096.

560. Martone WJ, Marshall LW, Kaufmann AF, Hobbs JH, Levy ME. Tularemia pneumonia in Washington, DC. A report of three cases with possible common-source exposures. JAMA 1979;242:2315–2317.

561. Pullen RL, Stuart BM. Tularemia analysis of 225 cases. JAMA 1945;129:495–500.

562. Stuart BM, Pullen RL. Tularemic pneumonia. Review of American literature and report of 15 additional cases. Am J Med Sci 1945;210:223–236.

563. Mille RP, Bates JH. Pleuropulmonary tularemia. A review of 29 patients. Am Rev Respir Dis 1969;99: 31–41.

564. Avery FW, Barnett TB. Pulmonary tularemia. A report of five cases and consideration of pathogenesis and terminology. Am Rev Respir Dis 1967;95:584–591.

565. Sunderrajan EV, Hutton J, Marienfeld RD. Adult respiratory distress syndrome secondary to tularemia pneumonia. Arch Intern Med 1985;145:1435–1437.

566. Verbrycke JR. Tularemia. With report of fatal case simulating cholangeitis, with postmortem report. JAMA 1924;82:1577–1581.

567. Permar HH, MacLachlan WWG. Tularemic pneumonia. Ann Intern Med 1931;5:687–698.

568. Sato T, Fujita H, Ohara Y, Homma M. Microagglutination test for early and specific serodiagnosis of tularemia. J Clin Microbiol 1990;28:2372–2374.

569. Roy TM, Fleming D, Anderson WH. Tularemic pneumonia mimicking legionnaires' disease with false-positive direct fluorescent antibody stains for Legionella. South Med J 1989;82:1429–1431.

570. Westerman EL, McDonald J. Tularemia pneumonia

mimicking legionnaires' disease: Isolation of organism on CYE agar and successful treatment with erythromycin. South Med J 1983;76:1169–1170.

571. Young EJ. Human brucellosis. Rev Infect Dis 1983; 5:821–842.

572. Joint FAO/WHO Expert Committee on Brucellosis. Geneva: World Health Organization, 1986.

573. Buchanan TM, Faber LC, Feldman RA. Brucellosis in the United States 1960–1972. An abbatoir-associated disease. Part 1. Clinical features and therapy. Medicine (Baltimore) 1974;53:403–413.

574. Schirger A, Nichols DR, Martin WJ, Wellman WE, Weed LA. Brucellosis. Experiences with 224 patients. Ann Intern Med 1960;52:827–837.

575. Pfischner WCE, Tshak KG, Neptume EM, et al. Brucellosis in Egypt. A review of experience with 228 patients. Am J Med 1957;22:915–929.

576. Blankenship RM, Sanford JP. Brucella canis: A cause of undulant fever. Am J Med 1975;59:424–426.

577. Hunt AC, Bothwell PW. Histologic findings in human brucellosis. J Clin Pathol 1967;20:267–272.

578. Haden RL, Kyger ER. Pulmonary manifestations of brucellosis. Cleve Clin Q 1946;13:220–227.

579. Harvey WA. Pulmonary brucellosis. Ann Intern Med 1948;28:768–781.

580. Greer AE. Pulmonary brucellosis. Dis Chest 1956;29: 508–519.

581. Walus MA, Young EJ. Concomitant neurocysticercosis and brucellosis. Am J Clin Pathol 1990;94:790–792.

582. Agarwal S, Kadhi SK, Rooney RJ. Brucellosis complicating bilateral total knee arthroplasty. Clin Orthop 1991;267:179–181.

583. Peery TM, Belter LF. Brucellosis and heart disease. II. Fatal brucellosis: A review of the literature and report of new cases. Am J Pathol 1960;36:673–697.

584. Weed LA, Sloss PT, Clagett OT. Chronic localized pulmonary brucellosis. JAMA 1956;161:1044–1047.

585. Hunter SB, Bibb WF, Shih CN, et al. Enzyme-linked immunosorbent assay with outer membrane proteins of Brucella melitensis to measure immune response to Brucella species. J Clin Microbiol 1986;24:566–572.

586. Goldbaum FA, Rubbi CP, Wallach JC, et al. Differentiation between active and inactive human brucellosis by measuring antiprotein humoral immune responses. J Clin Microbiol 1992;30:604–607.

587. Castaneda MR. Laboratory diagnosis of brucellosis in man. Bull WHO 1961;24:73–84.

588. Geller RJ. The pertussis syndrome: A persistent problem. Pediatr Infect Dis 1984;3:182–186.

589. Field LH, Parker CD. Pertussis outbreak in Austin and Travis County, Texas, 1975. J Clin Microbiol 1977;6: 154–160.

590. Brooksaler F, Nelson JD. Pertussis. A reappraisal and report of 190 confirmed cases. Am J Dis Child 1967; 114:389–396.

591. Granstrom M, Askelof P. Parapertussis: An abortive pertussis infection? Lancet 1982;ii:1249–1250.

592. Feldmann GV, Macaulay D, Abott JD, Cradock Watson JE, Tobin JO. Viruses and whooping-cough. Lancet 1972;i:379.

593. Nelson WL, Hopkins RS, Roe MH, Glode MP. Simultaneous infection with Bordetella pertussis and respiratory syncytial virus in hospitalized children. Pediatr Infect Dis 1986;5:540–544.

594. MacLean DW. Adults with pertussis. J R Coll Gen Pract 1982;32:298–300.

595. Sheps S. Pertussis in a vaccinated 12-year-old girl. Can Med Assoc J 1984;131:1467–1468.

596. Mertsola J, Ruuskanen O, Eerola E, Viljanen MK. Intrafamilial spread of pertussis. J Pediatr 1983;103:359–363.

597. Ng VL, York M, Hadley WK. Unexpected isolation of Bordetella pertussis from patients with acquired immunodeficiency syndrome. J Clin Microbiol 1989;27:337–338.

598. Sotomayor J, Weiner LB, McMillan JA. Inaccurate diagnosis in infants with pertussis. An eight-year experience. Am J Dis Child 1985;139:724–727.

599. Gilligan PH, Fisher MC. Importance of culture in laboratory diagnosis of Bordetella pertussis infections. J Clin Microbiol 1984;20:891–893.

600. Regan J, Lowe F. Enrichment medium for the isolation of Bordetella. J Clin Microbiol 1977;6:303–309.

601. Donaldson P, Whitaker JA. Diagnosis of pertussis by fluorescent antibody staining of nasopharyngeal smears. Am J Dis Child 1960;99:423–427.

602. Whitaker JA, Donaldson P, Nelson JD. Diagnosis of pertussis by the fluorescent-antibody method. N Engl J Med 1960;263:850–851.

603. Broome CV, Fraser DW, English WJ, Jr. International Symposium on Pertussis. U.S. Department of Health, Education, and Welfare, DHEW Publ. No. (NIH)79-1830. Bethesda, 1978:19–22.

604. Hakansson S, Sundin CG, Granstrom M, Gastrin B. Diagnosis of whooping cough—a comparison of culture, immunofluorescence and serology with ELISA. Scand J Infect Dis 1984;16:281–284.

605. Duncan JR, Ramsey RK, Switzer WP. Pathology of experimental Bordetella bronchiseptica infection in swine: Pneumonia. Am J Vet Res 1966;27:467–472.

606. Reina J, Bassa A, Llompart I, Borrell N, Gomez J, Serra A. Pneumonia caused by Bordetella bronchiseptica in a patient with a thoracic trauma. Infect 1991;19:46–48.

607. Dworzack DL, Murray CM, Hodges GR, Barnes WG. Community-acquired bacteremic Achromobacter xylosoxidans type IIIa pneumonia in a patient with idiopathic IgM deficiency. Am J Clin Pathol 1978;70:712–717.

608. Mandell WF, Garvey GJ, Neu HC. Achromobacter xylosoxidans bacteremia. Rev Infect Dis 1987;9:1001–1005.

609. Goldstein EJ, Kirby BD, Finegold SM. Isolation of Eikenella corrodens from pulmonary infections. Am Rev Respir Dis 1979;119:55–58.

610. Brown JR. Human actinomycosis: A study of 181 subjects. Hum Pathol 1973;4:319–330.

611. Causey WA. Actinomycosis. In: Vinken PJ, Bruyn GW, eds. Handbook of clinical neurology, Vol. 35. Infections

of the nervous system, Part III. Amsterdam: North Holland, 1978;383–394.

612. Peabody JW, Seabury JH. Actinomycosis and nocardiosis. J Chron Dis 1975;5:374–403.

613. Gruner OPN. Actinomyces in tonsillar tissue. A histological study of a tonsillectomy material. Acta Pathol Microbiol Scand 1969;76:239–244.

614. Coleman RM, Georg LK, Rozzell AR. Actinomyces naeslundii as an agent of human actinomycosis. Appl Microbiol 1969;18:420–426.

615. Dobson SR, Edwards MS. Extensive Actinomyces naeslundii infection in a child. J Clin Microbiol 1987;25:1327–1329.

616. Suzuki JB, Delisle AL. Pulmonary actinomycosis of periodontal origin. J Periodontol 1984;55:581–584.

617. Lewis R, Gorbach SL. Actinomyces viscosus in man. Lancet 1972;i:641–642.

618. Spiegel CA, Telford G. Isolation of Wolinella recta and Actinomyces viscosus from an actinomycotic chest wall mass. J Clin Microbiol 1984;20:1187–1189.

619. Eng RH, Corrado ML, Cleri D, Cherubin C, Goldstein EJ. Infections caused by Actinomyces viscosus. Am J Clin Pathol 1981;75:113–116.

620. Brown JR, Von Lichtenberg F. Experimental actinomycosis in mice. Arch Pathol Lab Med 1970;90:391–402.

621. Brock DW, Georg LK, Brown JM, Hicklin MD. Actinomycosis caused by Arachnia propionica: Report of 11 cases. Am J Clin Pathol 1973;59:66–77.

622. Albright L, Toczek S, Brenner VJ, Ommaya AK. Osteomyelitis and epidural abscess caused by Arachnia propionica. Case report. J Neurosurg 1974;40:115–119.

623. Klaaborg KE, Kronborg O, Olsen H. Enterocutaneous fistulization due to Actinomyces odontolyticus. Report of a case. Dis Colon Rectum 1985;28:526–527.

624. Baron EJ, Angevine JM, Sundstrom W. Actinomycotic pulmonary abscess in an immunosuppressed patient. Am J Clin Pathol 1979;72:637–639.

625. Ruutu P, Pentikainen PJ, Larinkari U, Lempinen M. Hepatic actinomycosis presenting as repeated cholestatic reactions. Scand J Infect Dis 1982;14:235–238.

626. Rippon JW, Kathuria SK. Actinomyces meyeri presenting as an asymptomatic lung mass. Mycopathology 1984;84:187–192.

627. Allworth AM, Ghosh HK, Saltos N. A case of Actinomyces meyeri pneumonia in a child. Med J Aust 1986;145:33.

628. Hill GB. Eubacterium nodatum mimics Actinomyces in intrauterine device-associated infections and other settings within the female genital tract. Obstet Gynecol 1992;79:534–538.

629. Jordan HV, Kelly DM, Heeley JD. Enhancement of experimental actinomycosis in mice by Eikenella corrodens. Infect Immun 1984;46:367–371.

630. Kanya KJ. Cervico-facila actinomycosis (a case report). J Oral Med 1985;40:166–167.

631. Spinola SM, Bell RA, Henderson FW. Actinomycosis: A cause of pulmonary and mediastinal mass lesions in children. Am J Dis Child 1981;135:336–339.

632. Golden N, Cohen H, Weissbrot J, Silverman S. Thoracic actinomycosis in childhood. Clin Pediatr 1985;24:646–650.

633. Dicpinigaitis PV, Bleiwelss U, Krellenstein DJ, Halton KP, Teirstein AS. Primary endobronchial actinomycosis in association with foreign body aspiration. Chest 1992;101:283–285.

634. Wright EP, Holmberg K, Houston J. Pulmonary actinomycosis simulating a bronchial neoplasm. J Infect Dis 1983;6:179–181.

635. Ariel I, Breuer R, Kamal NS. Endobronchial actinomycosis simulating bronchogenic carcinoma. Diagnosis by bronchial biopsy. Chest 1991;99:493–495.

636. Berardi RS. Abdominal actinomycosis. Surg Gynecol Obstet 1979;149:257–266.

637. Bhagavan BS, Gupta PK. Genital actinomycosis and intrauterine contraceptive devices. Hum Pathol 1978;9:567–578.

638. Gupta PK. Intrauterine contraceptive devices: Vaginal cytology, pathologic changes and clinical implications. Acta Cytol 1982;26:571–613.

639. Nayar M, Chandra M, Chitraratha K, Das SK, Chowdhary GR. Incidence of actinomycetes infection in women using intrauterine contraceptive devices. Acta Cytol 1985;29:111–116.

640. Weese WC, Smith IM. A study of 57 cases of actinomycosis over a 36-year period. A diagnostic "failure" with good prognosis after treatment. Arch Intern Med 1975;135:1562–1568.

641. Frank P, Strickland B. Pulmonary actinomycosis. Br J Radiol 1974;47:373–378.

642. Balikian JP, Cheng TH, Costello P, Herman PG. Pulmonary actinomycosis. A report of three cases. Radiology 1978;128:613–616.

643. Webb WR, Sagel SS. Actinomycosis involving the chest wall: CT findings. Am J Radiol 1982;139:1007–1009.

644. Kwong JS, Muller NL, Godwin JD, Aberle D, Grymaloski MR. Thoracic actinomycosis: CT findings in eight patients. Radiology 1992;183:189–192.

645. Hotchi M, Schwarz J. Characterization of actinomycotic granules by architecture and staining methods. Arch Pathol 1972;93:392–400.

646. Oddó D, González S. Actinomycosis and nocardiosis: A morphologic study of 17 cases. Pathol Res Pract 1986;181:320–326.

647. Harris LF, Kakani PR, Selah CE. Actinomycosis. Surgical aspects. Am Surg 1985;51:262–264.

648. Bennhoff DF. Actinomycosis: Diagnostic and therapeutic considerations and a review of 32 cases. Laryngoscope 1984;94:1198–1217.

649. Behbehani MJ, Heeley JD, Jordan HV. Comparative histopathology of lesions produced by Actinomyces israelii, Actinomyces naeslundii, and Actinomyces viscosus in mice. Am J Pathol 1983;110:267–274.

650. Holmberg K, Forsum U. Identification of Actinomyces, Arachnia, Bacterionema, Rothia and Propionibacterium species by defined immunofluorescence. Appl Microbiol 1973;25:834–843.

651. Happonen RP, Viander M. Comparison of fluorescent antibody technique and conventional staining methods

in diagnosis of cervicofacial actinomycosis. J Oral Med 1982;11:417–425.

652. Kleinman PK, Flowers RA. Necrotizing pneumonia after pharyngitis due to Fusobacterium necrophorum. Pediatr Radiol 1984;14:49–51.

653. Bartlett JG, Gorbach SL, Thadepalli H, Finegold SM. Bacteriology of empyema. Lancet 1974;i:338–340.

654. Morgenstein AA, Citron DM, Orisek B, Finegold SM. Serious infection with Leptotrichia buccalis. Report of a case and review of the literature. Am J Med 1980; 69:782–785.

655. Bartlett JG. Anaerobic bacterial pneumonitis. Am Rev Respir Dis 1979;119:19–23.

656. Brook I, Martin WJ, Finegold SM. Neonatal pneumonia caused by members of the Bacteroides fragilis group. Clin Pediatr 1980;19:541–544.

657. Bayer AS, Nelson SC, Galpin JE, Chow AW, Guze LB. Necrotizing pneumonia and empyema due to Clostridium perfringens. Report of a case and review of the literature. Am J Med 1975;59:851–856.

658. File TM, Jr., Fass RJ, Perkins RL. Pneumonia and empyema caused by Clostridium sordellii. Am J Med Sci 1977;274:211–212.

659. Winslow DJ. Botryomycosis. Am J Pathol 1959;35:153–167.

660. Greenblatt M, Heredia R, Rubenstein L, Alpert S. Bacterial pseudomycosis ("botryomycosis"). Am J Clin Pathol 1964;41:188–193.

661. Martin-Pasqual A, Perez AG. Botryomycosis. Dermatologica (Basel) 1975;51:302–308.

662. Hacker P. Botryomycosis review. Int J Dermatol 1983; 22:455–458.

663. Picou K, Batres E, Jarratt M. Botryomycosis. A bacterial cause of mycetoma. Arch Dermatol 1979;115:609–610.

664. Winslow DJ, Chamblin SA. Disseminated visceral botryomycosis. Report of a fatal case probably caused by Pseudomonas aeruginosa. Am J Clin Pathol 1960;33: 43–47.

665. Leibowitz MR, Asvat MS, Kalla AA, Wing G. Extensive botryomycosis in a patient with diabetes and chronic active hepatitis. Arch Dermatol 1981;117:739–742.

666. Washburn RG, Bryan CS, DiSalvo AF, Macher AM, Gallin JI. Visceral botryomycosis caused by Neisseria mucosa in a patient with chronic granulomatous disease. J Infect Dis 1985;151:563–564.

667. Speir WA, Mitchener JW, Galloway RF. Primary pulmonary botryomycosis. Chest 1971;60:92–93.

668. Paz HL, Little BJ, Winkelstein JA. Primary pulmonary botryomycosis. A manifestation of chronic granulomatous disease. Chest 1992;101:1160–1162.

669. Bishop GF, Greer KE, Horwitz DA. Pseudomonas botryomycosis. Arch Dermatol 1976;112:1568–1570.

670. Brunken RC, Lichon-Chao N, van den Broeck H. Immunologic abnormalities in botryomycosis. J Am Acad Dermatol 1983;9:428–434.

671. Toth IR, Kazal HL. Botryomycosis in acquired immunodeficiency syndrome. Arch Pathol Lab Med 1987; 111:246–249.

672. Katznelson D, Vawwter GF, Foley GE, Shwachman H. Botryomycosis: A complication of cystic fibrosis. J Pediatr 1964;65:525–539.

673. Harman RRM, English MP, Halford M, Saihan EM, Greenham LW. Botryomycosis. A complication of extensive follicular mucinosis. Br J Dermatol 1980; 102:215–222.

CHAPTER 10

Mycobacterial Infections

RALPH H. HRUBAN and GROVER M. HUTCHINS

Mycobacteria cause a variety of diseases in man. Diseases caused by *Mycobacterium tuberculosis* are among the oldest of the life-threatening infectious diseases known, but it was only in the 1950s that the nontuberculous mycobacteria were recognized to be pathogenic in humans. Although tuberculous and nontuberculous mycobacterial diseases differ in many important respects, both are undergoing an unprecedented resurgence in their numbers, in large part as a result of the current epidemic of human immunodeficiency virus (HIV).

This chapter begins with a discussion of diseases caused by *Mycobacterium tuberculosis*. This section is followed by a consideration of diseases caused by nontuberculous mycobacteria. Finally, the dramatic impact that HIV infection has had on both tuberculous and nontuberculous mycobacterial infections is examined.

Mycobacterium Tuberculosis

Tuberculosis and History

Tuberculosis has played an important role in history.[1] Examination of literature, art representations, and human remains of ancient Egypt has revealed that tuberculosis has been present in the Old World for thousands of years.[2] The organism has even been identified in an Incan mummy from 700 A.D. in the Americas.[3] More recently, its victims have included the poet John Keats, President Andrew Jackson, First Lady Eleanor Roosevelt, and the composer Frederic Chopin. Tuberculosis has been called "consumption" and "the white plague," and in the nineteenth century it was a major cause of death in the Western world.[1] Also, it was in the nineteenth century that the role of bacteria in the etiology of tuberculosis was established by Robert Koch.[4]

Epidemiology

Tuberculosis is a disease not only of the individual but of the community as well.[5] In the community, tuberculosis, like measles, has been shown to follow an epidemic curve with a short ascent, a peak, and a gradual descent.[6] When tuberculosis is first introduced into a population of susceptible individuals, its mortality rates rise sharply, peak, and then very gradually decline until only a small portion of the population develops clinical disease when infected with the organism.[7] This epidemic wave of tuberculosis takes not weeks or months, but hundreds of years, to resolve.[6] Grigg, in his classic study of the epidemiology of tuberculosis,[6] demonstrated that the peak of mortality for tuberculosis in the United States occurred before the end of the nineteenth century and that since then tuberculosis has declined in an almost linear fashion. The fact that the slope of this decline has not been altered appreciably by the discovery of the agent that causes tuberculosis, the development of the bacille Calmette-Guérin (BCG) vaccine, or the discovery of streptomycin suggests that natural factors such as the selection of susceptible individuals and the development of host resistance have played a greater role in the decline of tuberculosis than has the intervention of modern medicine.[8,8a]

Within a given society, factors such as poverty, overcrowded housing, and undernourishment can increase the rates of tuberculosis.[9] It is therefore not surprising that in the United States the highest rates of tuberculosis infection are found in minorities living in inner city slums where there is crowding of the poor and elderly.[10]

A variety of diseases have been identified that may predispose a given member of society to the development of tuberculosis. For example, silicosis, diabetes mellitus, malignancy, and human immunodeficiency virus infection have all been shown to predispose to infection by *Mycobacterium tuberculosis*.[7,11–15] Recently tuberculosis has also been linked to crack cocaine use.[16] In Contra Costa County, California, 16% of the tuberculosis cases reported between January 1987 and June 1990 occurred in patients using crack cocaine. This high prevalence of tuberculosis in crack cocaine users was probably caused by several factors. For example, not only is crack cocaine use associated with an increased risk of human immunodeficiency virus infection, but also (in Contra Costa County) crack use in patients with tuberculosis occurred predominantly among African-American males from an economically depressed area who frequented poorly ventilated crack houses.[16]

Microbiology of Tuberculosis

Mycobacteria are nonmotile, nonsporulating, weakly gram-positive rods of the order Actinomycetales.[17] The genus *Mycobacterium* is largely defined by the property of acid-fastness, which means that when the bacilli are stained with certain dyes and then washed with acid alcohol, they retain the dyes.[18–20] This acid-fast staining characteristic of organisms in the genus *Mycobacterium* is due to their high lipid content.

Mycobacterium tuberculosis is an obligate aerobe. It can be recognized by the characteristic morphology of clones of the bacilli grown in culture. Clones of *M. tuberculosis* lack pigmentation and have slow or delayed catalase activity and a positive niacin test.[17] In tissue sections, the microscopic appearance of *M. tuberculosis* is not specific enough to permit the definite classification of the organism.[18] In general, bacilli of *M. tuberculosis* are slim rods averaging 4 μm in length. A variety of stains can be used to detect the organism in tissue sections. The Ziehl–Neelsen is the stain most commonly used; however, it must be emphasized that it may take as many as 10^6 organisms per milliliter of tissue to detect the organism using this stain.[19,20] Fluorescent dyes such as auramine and rhodamine, silver stains, and DNA amplification and hybridization techniques have also been used.[21–24c]

Transmission of Tuberculosis

Mycobacterium tuberculosis is transmitted person to person by small (1–5 μm) airborne droplet nuclei.[25–27] These nuclei are so small that they remain airborne for extended periods of time and disperse uniformly throughout enclosed spaces.[27] In contrast, particles larger than 10 μm do not remain airborne, and when inhaled impact on the proximal portions of the airways and therefore do not cause disease. The infectiousness of airborne droplet nuclei was established by Riley et al.[28] in a study from the Veterans Administration Hospital in Baltimore, Maryland. In their classic study, they funneled air from a tuberculosis ward into rooms that housed caged guinea pigs. Half the guinea pigs received irradiated ward air and half received nonirradiated ward air. Sixty-three of the guinea pigs contracted tuberculosis during their study, and all 63 were from the group that received nonirradiated ward air. Further, there was no pattern to the distribution of the cages in which the infected guinea pigs were housed, suggesting that the infectious airborne particles were randomly distributed throughout the ward air.[28] These observations not only explain the transmission of tuberculosis but also have important implications for the prevention of its transmission. Regular surgical masks, while they effectively block large particles, allow the passage of air and of minute airborne droplet nuclei around their periphery.[29] This passage of air around the periphery of regular surgical face masks suggests that they do not effectively screen airborne contaminants such as tuberculous bacteria;[29] masks that fit tightly around the face are needed.

Primary Infection with Tuberculosis

Inhaled droplet nuclei measuring 1–5 μm in size containing *M. tuberculosis* may implant on respiratory bronchioles or alveoli beyond the mucocilliary system.[25] On the basis of the volume distribution of inhaled air in the lung, these droplet nuclei usually implant in the middle or lower lung fields.[17]

Once implanted in the alveoli, the bacilli elicit a nonspecific polymorphonuclear leukocyte reaction.[30] These polymorphonuclear leukocytes are then gradually replaced by alveolar macrophages. The mycobacteria are engulfed by the macrophages, but the bacilli may remain viable and multiply within these cells.[25] Some of the infected macrophages remain at the site of implantation while others enter the lymphatic system. Those that enter the lymphatic system transport bacilli to regional lymph nodes, from which they can carry them lymphohematogenously throughout the body.[17,30–32] These hematogenously distributed bacilli often lodge and multiply in the posterior half of the upper lobes of the lungs. Such apical foci of tuberculous infection, termed "Simon" foci, probably develop in the lung apices because of the high oxygen tension and the relative lymphostasis in the upper lobes.[31,33] The lesion produced where the first infection with the tuberculosis bacilli occurred is called a "primary" or "Ghon" focus, and the primary focus and the involved regional lymph nodes together are called a "primary" or "Ghon" complex.[32]

Some of the macrophages do succeed in killing the bacteria. These macrophages then process and present mycobacterial antigens to specific CD-4-positive T-helper lymphocytes.[7,34–36] These lymphocytes then synthesize and release a variety of lymphokines that cause bloodborne monocytes to enter the lesion and which activate macrophages within the lesion.[34–36] Activated macrophages tend to fuse and form typical granulomas, and they are more efficient at phagocytizing mycobacteria and killing the mycobacteria after the bacilli are phagocytized.[30] The activated macrophages have the appearance of epithelioid histiocytes, and when they fuse they form Langerhans'-type giant cells. Thus, cellular immunity becomes the major host defense against tuberculosis infection. Needless to say, humoral immunity does not appear to play a major role in this process. Once the cellular immune system has been activated, the host develops delayed hypersensitivity to tuberculin antigens.[37] As the inflammatory response develops in hypersensitive hosts, it can cause cell death and tissue destruction resulting in the development of caseous necrosis at the site of infection (Fig. 10–1).[35] Cell lysis by activated cytolytic T-cells may also play a role in the development of specific resistance to mycobacterial infections.[37a] The infection may then either heal or progress, depending on the ability of the activated macrophages to inhibit the growth of bacilli.[35]

The primary tuberculous infection (Fig. 10–2 and 10–3) heals without progression of disease in more than 90% of cases. In these cases the patients are often asymptomatic, and the only clue to their infection is a positive tuberculin skin test. Healed tuberculous lesions may resolve completely with restitution of the involved tissue to normal; they can undergo fibrosis and form a fibrotic scarred nodule, or they may calcify.[30] Despite the healing of these tuberculous lesions, viable tubercle bacilli may persist for years, and infected individuals therefore remain indefinitely at risk for the development of recurrent disease.[30,38]

In a minority of patients, primarily those with lowered immunity, the primary infection does not heal, but instead progresses (Figs. 10–4 and 10–5). Such cases, termed progressive primary tuberculosis, are characterized by rapid enlargement of the primary complex.[32,39] These enlarging lesions may erode into a blood vessel, bronchus, or the pleura.[32] If the lesions erode into a blood vessel, bacilli can then embolize in large numbers into the capillary beds of the organs supplied by the eroded vessel.[39–43] If the vessel is a

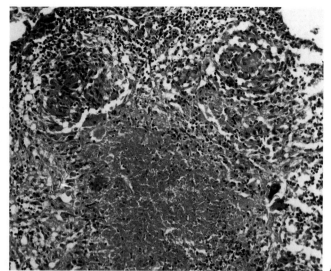

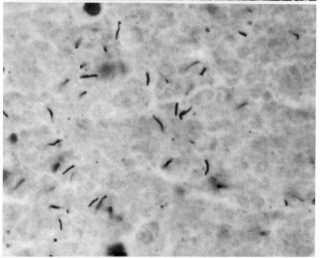

Fig. 10–1A,B. Epithelioid granulomas (**A**) and caseous necrosis with palisading epithelioid cells and occasional multinucleated giant cells in patient with tuberculosis. Ziehl–Neelsen stain (**B**) reveals multiple acid-fast organisms with caseum. **A**, H and E, ×180; **B**, Ziehl–Neelsen stain, ×1500.

pulmonary artery, then only the lung supplied by that artery will be affected; however, if the vessel is a vein, sepsis will result and bacilli will gain access to all organs. The simultaneous embolization of numerous bacilli will produce numerous tiny lesions of the same size and age in the organs infected (Fig. 10–6). These 2- to 3-mm lesions tend to be discrete and resemble millet seeds; thus, this disorder has been named "miliary tuberculosis" from the Latin *miliarius*, meaning "of the millet seed."[41]

If, on the other hand, the tuberculous lesion erodes into a bronchus, then a large number of bacilli will be discharged into the airways and numerous bacilli will be spread into other areas of the lung.[30] The resulting

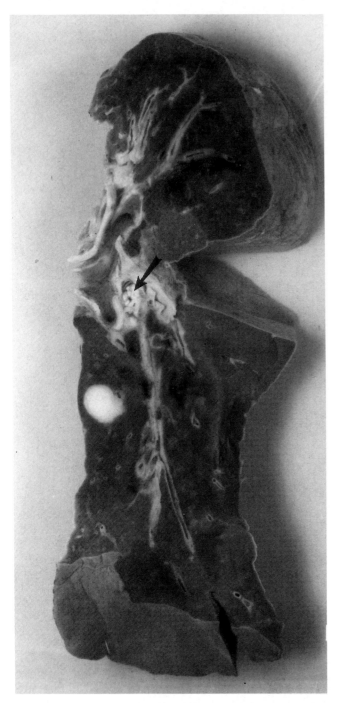

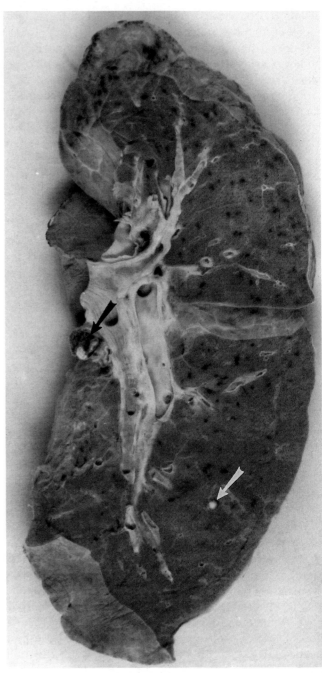

Fig. 10–2. Healing primary complex in a 16-year-old white female. Caseous primary focus in lower lobe shows early encapsulation; draining lymph node in hilum (*arrow*) has multiple confluent caseous foci that are also undergoing healing.

Fig. 10–3. A 32-year-old white male with healed primary parenchymal lesion in lower lobe (*white arrow*) and healed hilar lymph node lesion (*black arrow*). Primary lesion and involved regional lymph nodes together are called a "Ghon" complex.

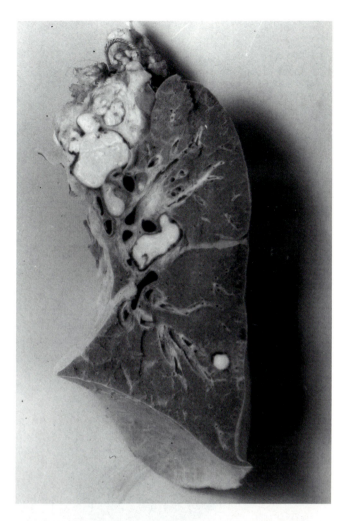

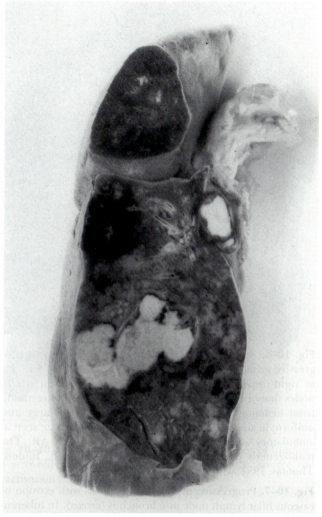

Fig. 10–4. Progressive primary tuberculosis in 21-month-old white girl. Primary focus in lower lobe is small but hilar and peritracheal lymph nodes show massive enlargement with caseous necrosis. (From Rich AR. The pathogenesis of tuberulosis. 2d Ed. Springfield, Illinois: Charles C. Thomas, 1951, with permission.)

Fig. 10–5. Progressive primary tuberculosis in 14-month-old African-American boy. Primary parenchymal focus in the lower lobe is quite large, and the associated hilar lymph node, although not massively enlarged, is replaced by caseous necrosis.

tuberculous bronchopneumonia (Figs. 10–7 and 10–8) will differ from miliary tuberculosis in that the nodules will cluster and vary in size.[30] In some cases the tuberculous lesions may erode into the pleura, resulting in tuberculous pleurisy or empyema (Fig. 10–9).[44–47]

Although traditionally considered a complication of cavitary tuberculosis, some adults with progressive primary tuberculosis develop endobronchial tuberculosis.[48–50] Endobronchial tuberculosis is believed to be caused either by lymphatic spread of tubercle bacilli from parenchymal lesions to the bronchial submucosa or by direct surface implantation from cavitary tuberculosis.[48–50] Fiberoptic bronchoscopy has revealed a progression in the lesions of endobronchial tuberculosis from mucosal ulceration to hyperplastic polyp to healing with bronchostenosis. This bronchostenosis can

mimic bronchogenic carcinoma both grossly and radiographically, and may result in lobar atelectasis.[48–50]

Postprimary Tuberculosis

Postprimary tuberculosis, also known as "reactivation" or "secondary" tuberculosis, refers to those infections that develop in individuals with immunity to the bacillus.[42,51] Postprimary tuberculosis may develop either from reactivation of a previously healed tuberculosis infection or from reinfection of a previously infected individual.[38,52–57]

Reactivation of a previously healed tuberculous infection can occur, because, as was noted earlier, residual

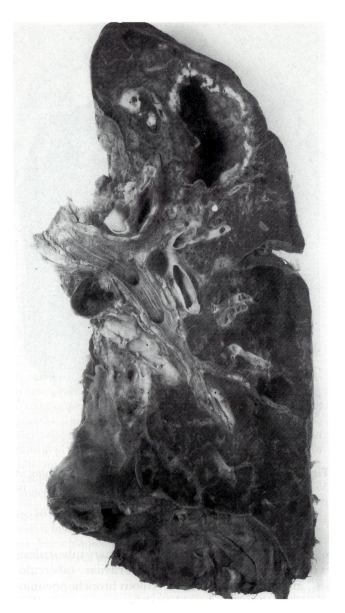

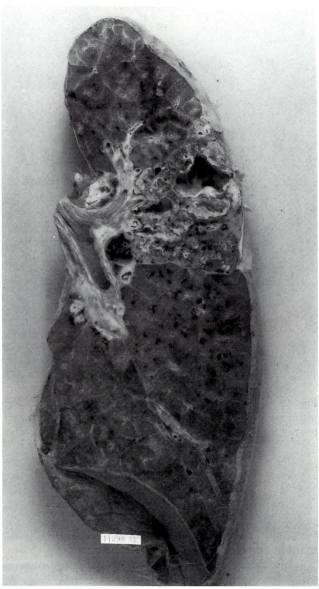

Fig. 10–11. Cavitation of postprimary tuberculosis in upper lobe of lung from 44-year-old African-American female. (From Rich AR. The pathogenesis of tuberculosis. 2d Ed. Springfield, Illinois: Charles C. Thomas, 1951, with permission.)

Fig. 10–12. Cavitation in postprimary tuberculosis. In contrast to Fig. 10–11, there is also local endobronchial dissemination.

lymph nodes, the adrenal glands, kidneys, brain, and bone.[39] Slavin et al. also found that once hematogenous dissemination was established, the spleen was involved in 100% of cases, the liver in 97%, the lungs in 86%, and the bone marrow in 77%.[39] These findings therefore suggest that biopsies of liver, lung, or bone marrow may help make the diagnosis of miliary tuberculosis.

Finally, carcinomas may occasionally arise in healed or active tuberculous lesions (Fig. 10–24). Although the role of the tuberculous scar in the development of these carcinomas has been questioned, it is clear that patients

with malignancies are at increased risk for developing reactivation of their tuberculosis.[13–15]

Summary of Mycobacterium Tuberculosis Infection

In summary, tuberculosis is spread person to person by airborne droplet nuclei. When infected, persons not previously exposed to the organism develop "primary tuberculosis." Primary tuberculosis is characterized by the development of a lesion, called a Ghon focus, at the

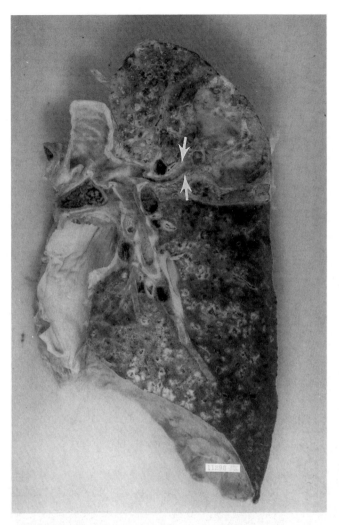

Fig. 10–13. Postprimary tuberculosis with cavitation and extensive endobronchial dissemination of bacilli resulting in tuberculous bronchopneumonia. Note connection between cavity and bronchus (*arrows*). (From MacCallum WG, A textbook of pathology. Philadelphia: Saunders, 1940, with permission.)

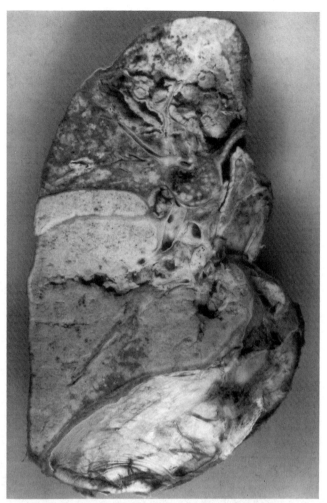

Fig. 10–14. Tuberculous lobar pneumonia caused by endobronchial dissemination of caseous material from cavitation of postprimary tuberculous infection in upper lobe. Lower lobe is uniformly consolidated by massive caseous material.

site of implantation of the bacilli. Macrophages carry the bacilli to regional lymph nodes, which may enlarge, and from there the bacilli disseminate hematogenously in small numbers throughout the body, including the apices of the lungs. In most individuals the infection heals and the infected individuals remain asymptomatic. In a small percentage of people, the disease progresses. If the disease progresses during the initial infection it is called progressive primary tuberculosis; if it progresses following a period of latency it is termed progressive postprimary tuberculosis. Progressive tuberculosis is usually symptomatic and may be complicated by the development of tuberculous bronchopneumonia, miliary tuberculosis, or tuberculous empyema.

The impact of the current epidemic of human immunodeficiency virus infection on tuberculosis is discussed later in this chapter.

The Nontuberculous Mycobacteria

Mycobacteria other than *Mycobacterium tuberculosis* have been called by a variety of names, including nontuberculous mycobacteria, atypical mycobacteria, anonymous mycobacteria, and pseudotubercle bacilli. We prefer the term nontuberculous mycobacteria because this term highlights their distinction from *Mycobacterium*

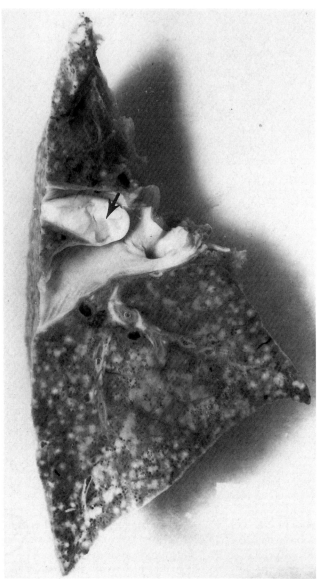

10-15

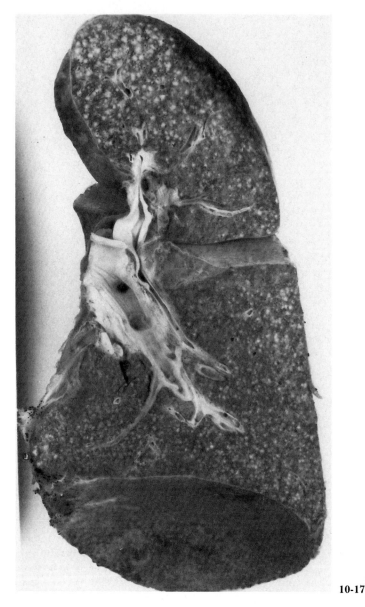

10-17

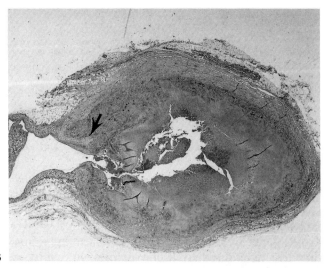

10-16

Fig. 10–15. Postprimary miliary tuberculosis in 28-year-old African-American female. A lymph node (*arrow*) in hilum of lung has eroded into a pulmonary vein, resulting in simultaneous hematogenous dissemination of numerous bacilli and the development of miliary tuberculosis.

Fig. 10–16. Fistulous communication (*arrow*) between a pelvic lymph node with tuberculosis and a vein. Drainage of the caseous material into the circulation produced miliary tuberculosis. H and E, ×10.

Fig. 10–17. Miliary tuberculosis in 8-year-old African-American female. Note decreasing size of tubercles from apex to base of lung. This pattern of miliary tuberculosis contrasts with that seen in infant lung in Fig. 10–6. (From Rich AR. The pathogenesis of tuberculosis, 2d. Ed. Springfield, Illinois: Charles C. Thomas, 1951, with permission.)

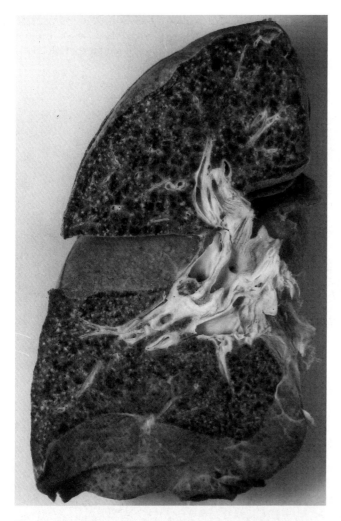

Fig. 10–18. Miliary tuberculosis in 40-year-old African-American female. Nodules of miliary tuberculosis in this case are smaller and less numerous, and presumably earlier, than those seen in Figs. 10–6 and 10–17.

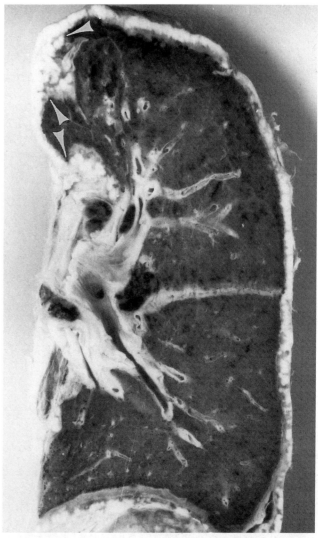

Fig. 10–19. Postprimary tuberculosis with erosion of lesions (*arrowheads*) in upper lobe into pleural space. Entire lung is encased in tuberculous pleuritis. (From MacCallum WG. A textbook of pathology. Philadelphia: Saunders, 1940, with permission.)

tuberculosis without carrying the connotations of the other terms.[60]

Although nontuberculous mycobacteria were identified in the nineteenth century, they were initially not believed to be pathogenic in man because they lacked virulence in guinea pigs. It was not until the publication of Timpe and Runyon's classical work in 1954 that the nontuberculous mycobacteria were accepted as a cause of human disease.[61–63] Timpe and Runyon[62] conducted a survey of mycobacterial diseases in man through the Veterans Administration and identified 88 patients with nontuberculous mycobacterial infections. They noted that a wide variety of nontuberculous my-

cobacteria can cause disease in man and that these organisms occur throughout the United States.[61] Based on their observations they proposed a classification system for nontuberculous mycobacteria.[61,64]

Runyon and Timpe classified the nontuberculous mycobacteria into four groups based on colony pigmentation, colony growth rate, colony morphology, catalase activity, drug susceptibilities, and pathogenicity for animals.[61,64] The colonies of Group I nontuberculous mycobacteria, the photochromogens, lack color if grown in the dark but are bright yellow to red if grown in the light.[60,61,63] The bright yellow color of the organisms in this group is derived from their ability to

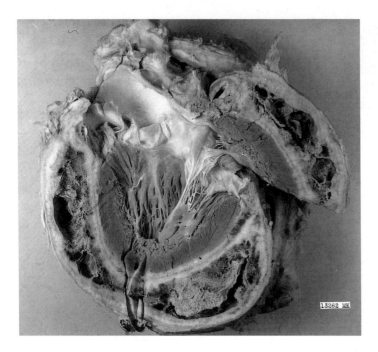

Fig. 10–20. Tuberculous pericarditis in 32-year-old African-American male. Lesion arose when caseous material from a tuberculous carinal lymph node drained into the pericardial space.

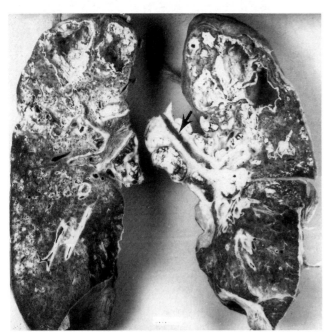

Fig. 10–21. Severe bilateral postprimary tuberculosis with extensive cavitation of upper-lobe lesions. In this posterior view, right mainstem bronchus shows endobronchial tuberculosis (*arrow*) as well as tuberculous bronchopneumonia. (From MacCallum WG. A textbook of Pathology. Philadelphia: Saunders, 1940, with permission.)

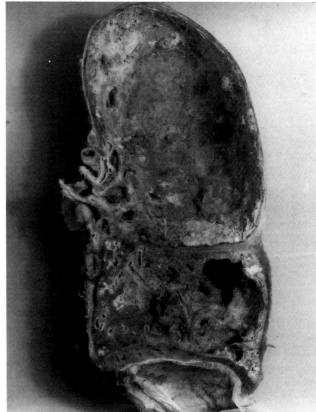

Fig. 10–22. End-stage, upper-lobe cavitation of postprimary tuberculosis. Note cavitation of lower lobe produced by endobronchial dissemination of bacilli.

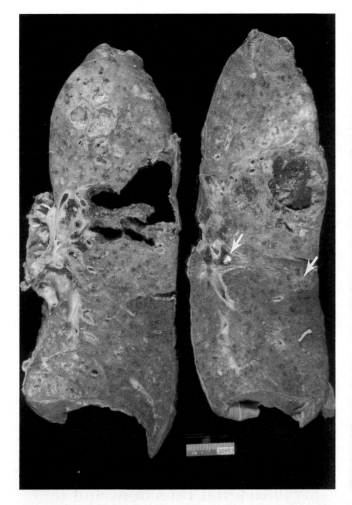

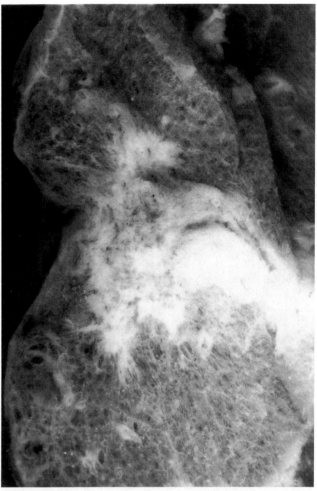

Fig. 10–23. Postprimary cavitary tuberculosis complicated by endobronchial dissemination and massive hemorrhage into emptied cavity. Note poorly defined, healed parenchymal (*right arrow*) and lymph node (*left arrow*) lesions of Ghon complex.

Fig. 10–24. Adenocarcinoma arising in fibrotic Simon focus. Tuberculous process is inactive in this case.

synthesize a carotene pigment on exposure to light. *Mycobacterium kansasii* belongs to group I. The colonies of group II nontuberculous mycobacteria, the scotochromogens, are yellow-orange in the dark and red when grown in the light. *Mycobacterium scrofulaceum* and *M. gordonae* belong to this group. The colonies of Group III mycobacteria are small, smooth, circular, and generally weakly pigmented; *M. intracellulare*, *M. avium*, and *M. xenopi* belong to this group, the nonphotochromogens. Finally, Group IV mycobacteria are the rapid growers, forming rough or smooth colonies that usually lack color. *M. fortuitum*, *M. abscessus*, and *M. flavescens* belong to Group IV.[60,61,64] While this classification system for mycobacteria has proven useful, modern molecular biology techniques will undoubtedly expand our understanding of the microbiology of these organ-

isms, and it is reasonable to expect that this classification scheme will be revised in the future.[65]

The nontuberculous mycobacteria are generally acquired directly from the environment, and in contrast to *M. tuberculosis*, person-to-person transmission generally does not occur.[60,64,66] Natural habitats for the nontuberculous mycobacteria include the soil, water, plants, and animals.[60] They also differ from the tuberculous mycobacteria in that they generally infect individuals with underlying lung diseases or decreased immunity.[60,66–68] Contreras et al.[68] reviewed the clinical findings in 89 patients with nontuberculous mycobacterial infections and found that 82% of these patients had preexisting lung disease. The lung diseases that appear to predispose to the development of nontuberculous mycobacterial infections include chronic ob-

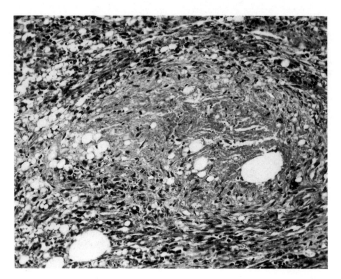

Fig. 10–25. Mineral oil pneumonia complicated by *Mycobacterium fortuitum* infection. Focus of caseous necrosis contains numerous droplets of lipid. H and E, ×180.

structive pulmonary disease (COPD), previous tuberculosis, pulmonary fibrosis (such as silicosis), carcinoma of the lung, and mineral oil pneumonia (Fig. 10–25).[67–69] Alcoholism, acquired immunodeficiency syndrome (AIDS), and diabetes mellitus, all disorders that decrease an individual's immunity, have also been associated with the development of these infections.[67,68]

Mycobacterium avium and *M. intracellulare* are two closely related mycobacteria that are often grouped together as the "Mycobacterium avium-intracellulare complex" (MAI).[70,71] These mycobacteria are generally resistant to currently available antibiotic therapy, and they probably gain entry into the human body via the oropharynx, intestine, or respiratory tract.[72] Infection with these organisms can cause a wide variety of diseases including asymptomatic lesions, cavitary lung disease, and severe disseminated infection.[60] Cavitary lung disease caused by MAI often involves the upper lobes of the lungs.[64,73,74] These cavities are frequently thin walled, but otherwise may grossly resemble those caused by *M. tuberculosis*.[68,75] Like tuberculosis, the organisms in these lesions in non-AIDS patients often elicit a granulomatous response, but unlike tuberculosis these granulomas usually do not caseate.[73,75] Despite these differences, lung diseases caused by MAI can be difficult to distinguish from those caused by *M. tuberculosis*.[73] Patients with the cavitary form of MAI infection often have an indolent course, but the organism can be difficult to eradicate.[67] More severe disseminated forms of MAI occur in severely immunosuppressed individuals; these infections are discussed later in this chapter. discussed later in this chapter.

Mycobacterium kansasii may also cause pulmonary disease. These organisms are slightly larger and more coarsely beaded than most of the other mycobacteria.[75–80] *M. kansasii* generally causes a milder disease than *M. tuberculosis*, but otherwise the gross and microscopic findings may be similar to those seen in MAI infection.[64] The disease usually involves the posterior portion of the upper lobes, and cavitation and endobronchial spread are common.[78] Like MAI, *M. kansasii* infection may disseminate in hosts with severely compromised immune systems.

A variety of the other nontuberculosis mycobacteria have been reported to cause lung disease in man, including *M. africanum*, *M. asiaticum*, *M. ulcerans*, *M. scrofulaceum*, *M. xenopi*, *M. szulgai*, *M. simiae*, *M. fortuitum*, *M. genavense*, *M. bovis*, and *M. chelonei*.[65,81,81a,81b] These organisms generally produce diseases similar to those caused by the other nontuberculous mycobacteria discussed previously.

In summary, the nontuberculous mycobacteria are now clearly recognized pulmonary pathogens in man. They usually infect persons with an underlying lung disease or with severe immune deficiency. In individuals with an intact immune response, they can cause cavitary lung disease that may mimic tuberculosis, while persons with severe immunodeficiency may develop disseminated disease. The dramatic effect of immunodeficiency on mycobacterial disease is most apparent in patients with AIDS, as is discussed in the next section.

Mycobacterial Infections and the HIV Epidemic

The epidemic of human immunodeficiency virus (HIV) infection has had a dramatic impact on diseases caused by mycobacteria. The HIV epidemic has not only led to a significant rise in the number of reported cases of mycobacterial infection in the United States, but it has also significantly changed the patterns of disease caused by these infections.[39,82]

HIV and Tuberculosis

The number of tuberculosis cases reported in the United States had fallen at a relatively constant rate from 84,304 cases in 1953 to 22,255 cases in 1984.[82–85] This steady downward trend dramatically came to an end in 1985, and in 1986 the number of tuberculosis cases reported in the United States rose to 22,768.[85] The number of cases has continued to rise since then, and in 1989 23,495 cases were reported.[82] This reversal of the downward trend in the number of reported cases of tuberculosis means that there have been 14,768 more cases of tuberculosis in the United States than expected had the downward trend continued for the years 1985 through 1988.[85]

It is widely believed that this resurgence in tuberculosis results, in large part, from the HIV epidemic.[12,82,86] Several lines of evidence support this belief. First, those populations with the greatest numbers of acquired immunodeficiency disease syndrome (AIDS) cases have had the largest rise in the number of reported cases of tuberculosis.* For example, in New York City, where there is a high incidence of HIV infection, the number of tuberculosis cases reported rose by a remarkable 36% from 1984 to 1986.[89]

Second, the incidence of tuberculosis is much higher in individuals with HIV infection than it is in the general population.† In Florida, of 1,094 people diagnosed with AIDS between 1981 and 1985, 109 (or 10%) were also diagnosed as having tuberculosis between the years 1978 and 1985.[88] The same is true in New York City where nearly 5% of the AIDS patients were found to have tuberculosis.[89] These numbers are approximately 100 to 500 times the prevalence of tuberculosis in the general population.[36,82,90]

Third, within a population of HIV-infected patients, those who have a positive tuberculin skin test have an extremely high risk of developing active tuberculosis.‡ Thus, in Dade County, Florida, where there is a very high prevalence of positive tuberculin skin tests among Haitian immigrants, nearly 60% of Haitians with AIDS had active tuberculosis, while only 2.7% of non-Haitians with AIDS developed tuberculosis.[87] While the extremely high prevalence of active tuberculosis in AIDS patients with positive tuberculin skin tests supports the association between HIV infection and tuberculosis, it also suggests that the active disease which develops in HIV-infected patients might be the result of reactivation of old healed tuberculosis.

From these epidemiologic studies one can conclude that HIV infection has played a major role in the resurgence of tuberculosis and that some cases of tuberculosis in HIV-infected patients are the result of reactivation of old healed tuberculosis.[12,82,91] Restriction-fragment-length polymorphism analyses of outbreaks of tuberculosis has revealed that HIV-infected individuals are also highly susceptible to new primary infections.[91a] The impact of HIV infection on the diseases caused by tuberculosis should not be surprising; HIV infection not only depletes the body of CD-4-positive T-helper lymphocytes, but it also results in defective monocyte and macrophage function.[92] As discussed previously, these are the very same cells responsible for controlling the progression of mycobacterial infections.[34,35] The quantitative and qualitative defect in T-helper lymphocytes produced by HIV infection results in decreased lymphokine production, which in turn reduces macrophage activation and mycobacterial killing.[36]

Several interesting observations highlight the impact of HIV infection on tuberculosis. For example, among HIV-infected individuals, most cases of tuberculosis are diagnosed within 6 months of their AIDS diagnosis.[36,87,90] Pitchenik et al.[87] followed 45 Haitian patients with AIDS and found that among the 27 with both AIDS and tuberculosis, the diagnosis of tuberculosis preceded the diagnosis of AIDS in 22 (81%) and that the diagnosis of tuberculosis preceded the symptoms of AIDS by an average of 6 months. This suggests that tuberculosis, because it is more virulent, may cause disease at an earlier state of immunodeficiency than do opportunistic infections.[93]

The immunodeficiency caused by HIV infection not only affects the timing of tuberculosis infections in these patients but has also dramatically impacted on the patterns of diseases seen. For example, there is a high frequency of extrapulmonary tuberculosis in HIV-infected patients.* Pitchenik et al.[87] found that among Haitian immigrants with tuberculosis those with AIDS had extrapulmonary tuberculosis 70% of the time. This incidence was much higher than the 20% found in patients without AIDS.

Several other aspects of the clinical features of tuberculosis infections in HIV infected patients are somewhat unusual, and these deserve further discussion. Not only is extrapulmonary disease common, but when the lungs are involved they are often involved in an unusual pattern.[36,95] Pitchenik et al.[95] reviewed the radiographic appearance of tuberculosis in 17 patients with tuberculosis and HIV infection. Ten (59%) of the 17 patients had hilar or mediastinal adenopathy, 5 (29%) had localized pulmonary infiltrates limited to the middle or lower lung fields, 3 (18%) had localized pulmonary infiltrates limited to the upper lung fields, 3 (18%) had diffuse miliary infiltrates, and 6 (35%) had no infiltrates whatsoever.[95] In a similar manner, the gross and microscopic pathologic appearance of tuberculosis in HIV-infected patients can be unusual. The lesions are often nonapical and noncavitary, and microscopically they may form poorly developed granulomas or even no granulomas at all.[36,93,94,96] Sunderam et al.[94] reviewed 17 biopsies obtained from HIV infected patients with tuberculosis. They found necrotizing granu-

---

*References: 10, 36, 82, 83, 86–89.
†References: 36, 82, 88, 89, 89a.
‡References: 70, 82, 87, 90, 91.

---

*References: 36, 70, 82, 87, 93, 94, 94a.

lomas in 8 of the 17 cases, nonnecrotizing granulomas in 6, and no granulomas in 3. Similarly, caseation is often not seen. This failure to develop well-formed granulomas and caseous necrosis is most likely the result of viral-induced immunodeficiency.

One of the most concerning aspects of tuberculosis in HIV-infected patients is the recent appearance of drug-resistant strains of tuberculosis.[96a–96e] In the past several years over 200 cases of drug resistant tuberculosis have been reported and most strains isolated have been found to be resistant to both isoniazid and rifampin.[96b] Although most of these cases of drug-resistant tuberculosis have occurred in HIV-infected individuals, there is no reason to believe that drug-resistant tuberculosis will not spread into the general population.[96b]

In summary, tuberculosis is common in HIV-infected patients. Tuberculosis in HIV-infected patients differs from tuberculosis in immunocompetent patients in many important respects. In the HIV-infected patient, tuberculosis is more often extrapulmonary. When the lungs are involved, well-formed granulomas are often not present, and the radiographic presentation is unusual. Recently, drug-resistant tuberculosis has appeared in HIV-infected patients and pulmonary tuberculosis has been added to the Center for Disease Control's list of AIDS defining illnesses in HIV-infected patients.[96f] Pathologists and clinicians need to be aware of these changes.

HIV and Nontuberculous Mycobacterial Infections

As is true with tuberculosis, there are differences between nontuberculous mycobacterial infections in patients with AIDS and nontuberculous mycobacterial infection in patients without AIDS.[97,98]

Nontuberculous mycobacterial infections are common in AIDS patients, and the *Mycobacterium avium-intracellulare* complex (MAI) is perhaps the most common group of mycobacteria isolated from patients with AIDS.* Hawkins et al.,[102] in a review of MAI infections in AIDS patients treated at Memorial Sloan-Kettering Cancer Center, found that 18.3% of the AIDS patients were clinically recognized to have MAI infections. An even larger percentage of patients must have had an MAI infection that was clinically silent, because more than half (53%) of the autopsied patients with AIDS at that institution were found to have MAI infections.[102]

Unlike tuberculosis which occurs early in HIV infection, infections with the nontuberculous mycobacteria occur late in the course of the patient's HIV infec-

---

*References: 70, 96, 97, 99–102.

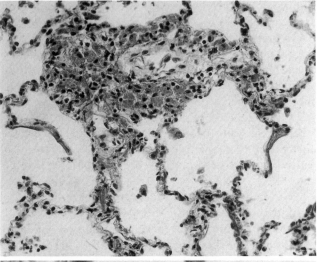

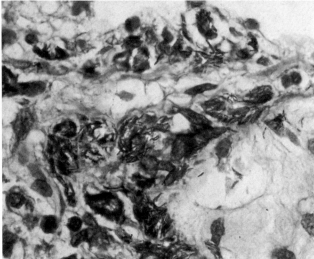

Fig. 10–26. *Mycobacterium avium-intracellulare* involving lung of man with AIDS. Note perivascular accumulation of striated histiocytes (top half). These histiocytes are packed with mycobacteria, as shown in Ziehl–Neelsen stain (bottom half). Numerous extracellular organisms are present. Top, H and E, ×200; bottom, Ziehl–Neelsen, ×1,000.

tion.[100,102] Horsburgh et al.,[100] in a review of MAI infections in AIDS patients, found that MAI infections occurred 7 to 15 months after the diagnosis of AIDS and that the major risk factor for this infection was the severity of the immunodeficiency as measured by the CD-4-positive cell count.

These infections are usually primary infections, and the gastrointestinal tract appears to be the most common portal of entry.[100] Once AIDS patients are infected, disseminated disease is common, and it is usually manifested clinically by the development of fever, weight loss, diarrhea, abdominal pain, and anuria.[100] Although the lungs are often spared, when they are involved they will show a mild mixed chronic inflammatory cell infiltrate with numerous histiocytes packed with bacilli.**

These histiocytes do not form well-defined granulomas (Figure 10–26).[97,100,103,104] In hematoxylin and eosin-H and E-stained tissue sections, the histiocytes have a characteristic light-steel-blue, "globoid," or pseudo-Gaucher appearance, while Ziehl–Neelsen and periodic acid-Schiff (PAS) stains show them to be distended with innumerable bacilli.[97,105,106] Recognition of these unusual light-steel-blue-tinged histiocytes is often the first clue in establishing the diagnosis in tissue sections.

In summary, the HIV epidemic has had an enormous impact on mycobacterial infections. Tuberculosis tends to occur relatively early in the infection and it may have an atypical presentation. The nontuberculous mycobacterial infections in AIDS patients are usually disseminated and the bacilli are numerous, producing characteristic light-steel-blue histiocytes. Pathologists and clinicians must not only be aware of the new patterns of mycobacterial diseases caused by the HIV epidemic, but they must also be prepared to face the new diagnostic and therapeutic challenges that this epidemic surely will bring.

References

1. Dubos RJ, Dubos J, Rosenkrantz BG. The white plague: Tuberculosis, man, and society. New Brunswick: Rutgers University Press, 1987.
2. Morse D, Brothwell DR, Ucko PJ. Tuberculosis in ancient Egypt. Am Rev Respir Dis 1964;90:524–541.
3. Stead WW, Bates JH. Epidemiology and prevention of tuberculosis. In: Fishman AP, ed. Pulmonary diseases and disorders. 2d Ed. New York: McGraw-Hill, 1988:1795–1810.
4. Koch R. Die Aetiologie der Tuberculose. Berlin Klin Wochenschr 1882;19:221–230.
5. Sbarbaro JA. Tuberculosis: A portal through which to view the future. Am Rev Respir Dis 1982;125(Suppl): 127–132.
6. Grigg ERN. The arcana of tuberculosis. Am Rev Tuberc Pulm Dis 1958;78:151–172.
7. Bates JH. Tuberculosis: Susceptibility and resistance. Am Rev Respir Dis 1982;125(Suppl):20–23.
8. Kass EH. Infectious diseases and social change. J Infect Dis 1971;123:110–114.
8a. Stead WW. Genetics and resistance to tuberculosis. Could resistance be enhanced by genetic engineering? Ann Int Med 1992;116:937–941.
9. Grzybowski S. Impact of tuberculosis on human health in the world. Am Rev Respir Dis 1982;125(Suppl):125.
10. Tuberculosis in minorities—United States. MMWR 1987;36:77–80.
11. Morgan EJ. Silicosis and tuberculosis. Chest 1979; 75:202–203.
12. Rieder HL, Cauthen GM, Comstock GW, Snider DE, Jr. Epidemiology of tuberculosis in the United States. Epidemiol Rev 1989;11:79–98.
13. Browne M, Healy TM. Coexisting carcinoma and active tuberculosis of the lung: 24 patients. Ir J Med Sci 1982;151:75–78.
14. Ortbals DW, Marr JJ. A comparative study of tuberculous and other mycobacterial infections and their associations with malignancy. Am Rev Respir Dis 1978; 117:39–45.
15. Kaplan MH, Armstrong D, Rosen P. Tuberculosis complicating neoplastic disease. A review of 201 cases. Cancer 1974;33:850–858.
16. Crack cocaine use among persons with tuberculosis—Contra Costa County, California, 1987–1990. MMWR 1991;40:485–489.
17. Sbarbaro JA. Tuberculosis. Med Clin N Am 1980; 64:417–431.
18. Wayne LG, Hawkins JE. Microbiology of tuberculosis. In: Fishman AP, ed. Pulmonary diseases and disorders. 2d Ed. New York: McGraw-Hill, 1988:1811–1820.
19. Ziehl F. Zur Färbung des Tuberkelbacillus. Dtsch Med Wochenschr 1882;8:451.
20. Wayne LG. Microbiology of tubercle bacilli. Am Rev Respir Dis 1982;125(Suppl):31–41.
21. Nyka W. Studies on mycobacterium tuberculosis in lesions of the human lung. A new method of staining tubercle bacilli in tissue sections. Am Rev Respir Dis 1963;88:670–679.
22. Truant JP, Brett WA, Thomas W, Jr. Fluorescence microscopy of tubercle bacilli stained with auramine and rhodamine. Henry Ford Hosp Med Bull 1962;10:287–296.
23. Shoemaker SA, Fisher JH, Scoggin CH. Techniques of DNA hybridization detect small numbers of mycobacteria with no cross-hybridization with nonmycobacterial respiratory organisms. Am Rev Respir Dis 1985;131: 760–763.
24. Brisson-Noel AN, Lecossier D, Nassif X, Gicquel B, Levy-Frebault V, Hance AJ. Rapid diagnosis of tuberculosis by amplification of mycobacterial DNA in clinical samples. Lancet 1989; ii:1069–1071.
24a. Walker GT, Little MC, Nadeau JG, Shank DD. Isothermal in vitro amplification of DNA by a restriction enzyme/DNA polymerase system. Proc Natl Acad Sci USA 1992;89:392–396.
24b. Lim SD, Todd J, Lopez J, Ford E, Janda JM. Genotypic identification of pathogenic mycobacterium species by using a nonradioactive oligonucleotide probe. J Clin Microbiol 1991;29:1276–1278.
24c. Otal I, Martin C, Vincent-Lévy-Frebault V, Thierry D, Gicquel B. Restriction fragment length polymorphism analysis using IS6110 as an epidemiological marker in tuberculosis. J Clin Microbiol 1991;29:1252–1254.
25. American Thoracic Society. Diagnostic standards and classification of tuberculosis. Am Rev Respir Dis 1990; 142:725–735.

**References: 97, 98, 100, 103, 104.

26. Ratcliffe HL, Palladino VS. Tuberculosis induced by droplet nuclei infection. J Exp Med 1953;97:61–97.

27. Riley RL. Disease transmission and contagion control. Am Rev Respir Dis 1982;125(Suppl):16–19.

28. Riley RL, Mills CC, O'Grady F, Sultan LU, Wittstadt F, Shivpuri DN. Infectiousness of air from a tuberculosis ward. Ultraviolet irradiation of infected air: Comparative infectiousness of different patients. Am Rev Respir Dis 1962;85:511–525.

29. Pippin DJ, Verderame RA, Weber KK. Efficacy of face masks in preventing inhalation of airborne contaminants. J Oral Maxillofac Surg 1987;45:319–323.

30. Pratt PC. Pathology of tuberculosis. Semin Roentgenol 1979;14:196–203.

31. Goodwin RA, Des Prez RM. Apical localization of pulmonary tuberculosis, chronic pulmonary histoplasmosis, and progressive massive fibrosis of the lung. Chest 1983;83:801–805.

32. Nice CM Jr. The pathogenesis of tuberculosis. Dis Chest 1950;17:550–560.

33. Simon G. Die Tuberkulose der Lungenspitzen. Beitr Klin Tuberk 1927;67:467–479.

34. Collins FM. The immunology of tuberculosis. Am Rev Respir Dis 1982;125(Suppl):42–49.

35. Dannenberg AM, Jr. Pathogenesis of pulmonary tuberculosis. Am Rev Respir Dis 1982;125(Suppl):25–29.

36. Pitchenik AE, Fertel D, Bloch AB. Mycobacterial disease: Epidemiology, diagnosis, treatment and prevention. Clin Chest Med 1988;9:425–441.

37. Salvin SB, Neta R. A possible relationship between delayed hypersensitivity and cell-mediated immunity. Am Rev Respir Dis 1975;111:373–377.

37a. Orme IM, Miller ES, Roberts AD, Furney SK, Griffin JP, Dobos KM, Chi D, Rivoire B, Brennan PJ. T lymphocytes mediating protection and cellular cytolysis during the course of mycobacterium tuberculosis infection. Evidence for different kinetics and recognition of a wide spectrum of protein antigens. J Immunol 1992;148:189–196.

38. Opie EL, Aronson JD. Tubercle bacilli in latent tuberculous lesions and in lung tissue without tuberculous lesions. Arch Pathol Lab Med 1927;4:1–21.

39. Slavin RE, Walsh TJ, Pollack AD. Late generalized tuberculosis: A clinical pathologic analysis and comparison of 100 cases in the preantibiotic and antibiotic eras. Medicine (Baltimore) 1980;59:352–366.

40. Gelb AF, Leffler C, Brewin A, Mascatello V, Lyons HA. Miliary tuberculosis. Am Rev Respir Dis 1973;108:1327–1333.

41. Sahn SA, Neff TA. Miliary tuberculosis. Am J Med 1974;56:495–505.

42. Auerbach O. The natural history of the tuberculous pulmonary lesion. Med Clin N Am 1959;43:239–251.

43. Biehl JP. Miliary tuberculosis: A review of sixty-eight adult patients admitted to a municipal general hospital. Am Rev Tuberc Pulm Dis 1958;77:605–622.

44. Epstein DM, Kline LR, Albelda SM, Miller WT. Tuberculous pleural effusions. Chest 1987;91:106–109.

45. Hulnick DH, Naidich DP, McCauley DI. Pleural tuberculosis evaluated by computed tomography. Radiology 1983;149:759–765.

46. Enarson DA, Dorken E, Grzybowski S. Tuberculous pleurisy. Can Med Assoc J 1982;126:493–495.

47. Donath J, Khan FA. Tuberculous and posttuberculous bronchopleural fistula. Ten-year clinical experience. Chest 1984;86:697–703.

48. Smith LS, Schillaci RF, Sarlin RF. Endobronchial tuberculosis. Serial fiberoptic bronchoscopy and natural history. Chest 1987;91:644–647.

49. Thompson JR, Kent G. Occult tuberculous endobronchitis in surgically resected lung specimens. Am Rev Tuberc Pulm Dis 1958;77:931–939.

50. Volckaert A, Roels P, Van Der Niepen P, Schandevyl W. Endobronchial tuberculosis: Report of three cases. Eur J Respir Dis 1987;70:99–101.

51. Rich AR. The pathogenesis of tuberculosis. 2nd Ed. Springfield: Thomas, 1951.

52. Stead WW. Pathogenesis of a first episode of chronic pulmonary tuberculosis in man: Recrudescence of residuals of the primary infection or exogenous reinfection? Am Rev Respir Dis 1967;95:729–745.

53. Bates JH, Stead WW, Rado TA. Phage type of tubercle bacilli isolated from patients with two or more sites of organ involvement. Am Rev Respir Dis 1976;114:353–358.

54. Mankiewicz E, Liivak M. Phage types of mycobacterium tuberculosis in cultures isolated from Eskimo patients. Am Rev Respir Dis 1975;111:307–312.

55. Ormerod P, Skinner C. Reinfection tuberculosis: Two cases in the family of a patient with drug-resistant disease. Thorax 1980;35:56–59.

56. Raleigh JW, Wichelhausen RH, Rado TA, Bates JH. Evidence for infection by two distinct strains of *Mycobacterium tuberculosis* in pulmonary tuberculosis: Report of 9 cases. Am Rev Respir Dis 1975;112:497–503.

57. Raliegh JW, Wichelhausen R. Exogenous reinfection with mycobacterium tuberculosis confirmed by phage typing. Am Rev Respir Dis 1973;108:639–642.

58. Khan MA, Kovnat DM, Bachus B, Whitcomb ME, Brody JS, Snider GL. Clinical and roentgenographic spectrum of pulmonary tuberculosis in the adult. Am J Med 1977;62:31–38.

59. Kuhlman JE, Deutsch JH, Fishman EK, Siegelman SS. CT features of thoracic mycobacterial disease. RadioGraphics 1990;10:413–431.

60. Wolinsky E. Nontuberculous mycobacteria and associated diseases. Am Rev Respir Dis 1979;119:107–159.

61. Runyon EH. Anonymous mycobacteria in pulmonary disease. Med Clin N Am 1959;43:273–290.

62. Timpe A, Runyon EH. The relationship of "atypical" acid-fast bacteria to human disease. J Lab Clin Med 1954;44:202–209.

63. Clark M, Hall WH, Pollak A, et al. Veterans Administration—National Tuberculosis Association Cooperative Study of Mycobacteria. Am Rev Tuberc Pulm Dis 1955;72:866–869.

64. Tellis CJ, Putnam JS. Pulmonary disease caused by nontuberculous mycobacteria. Med Clin N Am 1980;

64:433–446.

65. Sommers HM. The identification of mycobacteria. Lab Med 1978;9:34–43.

66. Chapman JS. The atypical mycobacteria. Am Rev Respir Dis 1982;125(Suppl):119–124.

67. Rosenzweig DY. Pulmonary mycobacterial infections due to mycobacterium intracellulare-avium complex. Chest 1979;75:115–119.

68. Contreras MA, Cheung OT, Sanders DE, Goldstein RS. Pulmonary infection with nontuberculous mycobacteria. Am Rev Respir Dis 1988;137:149–152.

69. Hutchins GM, Boitnott JK. Atypical mycobacterial infection complicating mineral oil pneumonia. JAMA 1978;240:539–541.

70. American Thoracic Society. Mycobacterioses and the acquired immunodeficiency syndrome. Am Rev Respir Dis 1987;136:492–496.

71. Iseman MD, Corpe RF, O'Brien RJ, Rosenzweig DY, Wolinsky E. Disease due to mycobacterium avium-intracellulare. Chest 1985;87:139S–149S.

72. Horsburgh CR, Jr. Mason UG III, Farhi DC, Iseman MD. Disseminated infection with mycobacterium avium-intracellulare. Medicine (Baltimore) 1985;64:36–48.

73. Marchevsky A, Damsker B, Gribetz A, Tepper S, Geller SA. The spectrum of pathology of nontuberculous mycobacterial infections in open-lung biopsy specimens. Am J Clin Pathol 1982;78:695–700.

74. Albelda SM, Kern JA, Marinelli DL, Miller WT. Expanding spectrum of pulmonary disease caused by nontuberculous mycobacteria. Radiology 1985;157:289–296.

75. Snijder J. Histopathology of pulmonary lesions caused by atypical mycobacteria. J Pathol Bacteriol 1965;90:65–73.

76. Smith ER, Penman HG. Histological diagnosis of *M. kansasii* lung infection: A case report. Pathology 1971;3:93–98.

77. Francis PB, Jay SJ, Johanson WG, Jr. The course of untreated *Mycobacterium kansasii* disease. Am Rev Respir Dis 1975;111:477–487.

78. Christensen EE, Dietz GW, Ahn CH, Chapman JS, Murry RC, Hurst GA. Radiographic manifestations of pulmonary *Mycobacterium kansasii* infections. AJR 1978;131:985–993.

79. Bialkin G, Pollak A, Weil AJ. Pulmonary infection with *Mycobacterium kansasii*. Am J Dis Child 1961;101:95–104.

80. Ahn CH, McLarty JW, Ahn SS, Ahn SI, Hurst GA. Diagnostic criteria for pulmonary disease caused by *Mycobacterium kansasii* and *Mycobacterium intracellulare*. Am Rev Respir Dis 1982;125:388–391.

81. Dannenberg AM, Jr., Tomashefski JF, Jr. Pathogenesis of tuberculosis. In: Fishman AP, ed. Pulmonary diseases and disorders. 2d Ed. New York: McGraw-Hill, 1988:1821–1842.

81a. Böttger EC, Teske A, Kirschner P, Bost S, Chang HR, Beer V, Hirschel B. Disseminated "Mycobacterium genavense" infection in patients with AIDS. The Lancet 1992;340:76–80.

81b. Fanning A, Edwards S. Mycobacterium bovis infection in human beings in contact with elk (Cervus elaphus) in Alberta, Canada. The Lancet 1991;338:1253–1255.

82. Barnes PF, Bloch AB, Davidson PT, Snider DE, Jr. Tuberculosis in patients with human immunodeficiency virus infection. N Engl J Med 1991;324:1644–1650.

83. Tuberculosis—United States, 1985. MMWR 1986;35:699–703.

84. Tuberculosis, Final Data—United States, 1986. MMWR 1988;36:817–820.

85. Update: Tuberculosis elimination—United States. MMWR 1990;39:153–156.

86. Tuberculosis—United States, 1985—and the possible impact of human T-lymphotrophic virus type III/lymphadenopathy-associated virus infection. MMWR 1986;35:74–76.

87. Pitchenik AE, Cole C, Russell BW, Fischl MA, Spira TJ, Snider DE, Jr. Tuberculosis, atypical mycobacteriosis, and the acquired immunodeficiency syndrome among Haitian and non-Haitian patients in South Florida. Ann Intern Med 1984;101:641–645.

88. Tuberculosis and acquired immunodeficiency syndrome—Florida. MMWR 1986;35:587–590.

89. Tuberculosis and acquired immunodeficiency syndrome—New York City. MMWR 1987;36:785–795.

89a. De Cock KM, Soro B, Coulibaly IM, Lucas SB. Tuberculosis and HIV infection in sub-saharan Africa. JAMA 1992;268:1581–1587.

90. Tuberculosis and AIDS—Connecticut. MMWR 1987;36:133–135.

91. Selwyn PA, Hartel D, Lewis VA, et al. A prospective study of the risk of tuberculosis among intravenous drug users with human immunodeficiency virus infection. N Engl J Med 1989;320:545–550.

91a. Daley CL, Small PM, Schecter GF, Schoolnik GK, McAdam RA, Jacobs WR Jr., Hopewell PC. An outbreak of tuberculosis with accelerated progression among persons infected with the human immunodeficiency virus. An analysis using restriction-fragment-length polymorphisms. N Engl J Med 1992;326:231–235.

92. Bender BS, Davidson BL, Kline R, Brown C, Quinn TC. Role of the mononuclear phagocyte system in the immunopathogenesis of human immunodeficiency virus infection and the acquired immunodeficiency syndrome. Rev Infect Dis 1988;10:1142–1154.

93. Duncanson FP, Hewlett D, Jr., Maayan S, et al. Mycobacterium tuberculosis infection in the acquired immunodeficiency syndrome. A review of 14 patients. Tubercle 1986;67:295–302.

94. Sunderam G, McDonald RJ, Maniatis T, Oleske J, Kapila R, Reichman LB. Tuberculosis as a manifestation of the acquired immunodeficiency syndrome (AIDS). JAMA 1986;362–366.

94a. Berenguer J, Moreno S, Laguna F, Vicente T, Adrados M, Ortega A, González-LaHoz J, Bouza E. Tuberculous meningitis in patients infected with the human immunodeficiency virus. N Engl J Med 1992;326:668–672.

95. Pitchenik AE, Rubinson HA. The radiographic appearance of tuberculosis in patients with the acquired immune deficiency syndrome (AIDS) and pre-AIDS. Am Rev Respir Dis 1985;131:393–396.

96. Centers for Disease Control. Diagnosis and management of mycobacterial infection and disease in persons with human immunodeficiency virus infection. Ann Intern Med 1987;106:254–256.

96a. Weiss R. On the track of "killer" TB. Science 1992; 255:148–150.

96b. Snider DE Jr., Roper WL. The new tuberculosis. N Engl J Med 1992;326:703–705.

96c. Zhang Y, Heym B, Allen B, Young D, Cole S. The catalase-peroxidase gene and isoniazid resistance of Mycobacterium tuberculosis. Nature 1992;358:591–593.

96d. Glassroth J. Tuberculosis in the United States. Looking for a silver lining among the clouds. Am Rev Respir Dis 1992;146:278–279.

96e. Chawla PK, Klapper PJ, Kamholz SL, Pollack AH, Heurich AE. Drug-resistant Tuberculosis in an urban population including patients at risk for human immunodeficiency virus infection. Am Rev Respir Dis 1992;146:280–284.

96f. MMWR, 1992 Revised classification system for Human Immunodeficiency Virus infection and expanded AIDS surveillance case definition for adolescents and adults. In Press.

97. Klatt EC, Jensen DF, Meyer PR. Pathology of Mycobacterium avium-intracellulare infection in acquired immunodeficiency syndrome. Hum Pathol 1987;18:709–714.

98. Marinelli DL, Albelda SM, Williams TM, Kern JA, Iozzo RV, Miller WT. Nontuberculous mycobacterial infection in AIDS: Clinical, pathologic and radiographic features. Radiology 1986;160:77–82.

99. Greene JB, Sidhu GS, Lewin S, et al. Mycobacterium avium-intracellulare: A cause of disseminated life-threatening infection in homosexuals and drug abusers. Ann Intern Med 1982;97:539–546.

100. Horsburgh CR, Jr. Mycobacterium avium complex infection in the acquired immunodeficiency syndrome. N Engl J Med 1991;324:1332–1338.

101. Kiehn TE, Cammarata R. Laboratory diagnosis of mycobacterial infections in patients with acquired immunodeficiency syndrome. J Clin Microbiol 1986;24:708–711.

102. Hawkins CC, Gold JWM, Whimbey E, et al. Mycobacterium avium complex infections in patients with the acquired immunodeficiency syndrome. Ann Intern Med 1986;105:184–188.

103. Farhi DC, Mason UG, III, Horsburgh CR, Jr. Pathologic findings in disseminated Mycobacterium avium-intracellulare infection: A report of all 11 cases. Am J Clin Pathol 1986;85:67–72.

104. Nash G, Fligiel S. Pathologic features of the lung in the acquired immune deficiency syndrome (AIDS): An autopsy study of seventeen homosexual males. Am J Clin Pathol 1984;81:6–12.

105. Wear DJ, Hadfield TL, Connor DH, et al. Periodic acid-Schiff reaction stains *Mycobacterium tuberculosis*, *Mycobacterium leprae*, *Mycobacterium ulcerans*, *Mycobacterium chelonei (abscessus)*, and *Mycobacterium kansasii*. Arch Pathol Lab Med 1985;109:701–702.

106. Solis OG, Belmonte AH, Ramaswamy G, Tchertkoff V. Pseudogaucher cells in Mycobacterium avium-intracellulare infections in acquired immune deficiency syndrome (AIDS). Am J Clin Pathol 1986;85:233–235.

CHAPTER 11

Fungal Infections

FRANCIS W. CHANDLER and JOHN C. WATTS

Fungi are eukaryotic, unicellular, or filamentous organisms that lack chlorophyll, have chitinous cell walls, and reproduce asexually, sexually, or both ways. All available evidence indicates that humans and animals contract most fungal infections by exposure to infectious particles originating from saprophytic moulds and yeasts growing in nature. Of more than 100,000 fungal species in our environment, only about 150 are known to be pathogenic. Their ability to invade body tissues and to produce disease depends on the virulence of the infectious particle, the infecting dose, the route of infection, the resistance or immune status of the host, the organs affected, and the coexistence of infections and other underlying medical conditions. A few fungi, such as the *Candida* spp., are endogenous, occurring as commensals on the skin and mucous membranes and in the gastrointestinal tract.[1,2] These fungi, which are part of the normal body flora, are opportunists that only rarely infect the noncompromised, healthy individual. The *Prototheca* spp. are not fungi, but are considered by most taxonomists to be achloric mutants of green algae of the genus *Chlorella*.[3] Nevertheless, diseases caused by the prototothecae have traditionally fallen within the province of medical mycology and are therefore included in this chapter. For detailed information on the taxonomy of the fungi, several texts are recommended.[2–5]

No clear-cut evidence exists that fungal infections—other than tinea versicolor, the dermatophytoses, and candidiasis of the newborn—are contagious. However, infections can be transmitted by accidental inoculation or by direct contamination of an open wound,[6,7] and one should therefore take care when handling contaminated body discharges and tissues. There is no justification for isolating a patient solely because he or she has a systemic mycosis.

Classification of Fungal Infections

Based on the principal location of lesions on or within the body, fungal infections (mycoses) can be grouped arbitrarily into three broad categories: (1) superficial and cutaneous; (2) subcutaneous; and (3) systemic. Most of the systemic mycoses, such as blastomycosis and coccidioidomycosis, begin in the lungs following inhalation of aerosolized fungal elements from environmental sources.[2,5,8] Having reached the lungs, infection can remain localized or it can disseminate via hematogenous, lymphatic, and bronchial routes to produce severe disease that is often fatal if not promptly diagnosed and treated. Rarely, the gastrointestinal tract and skin are primary foci of systemic infection as a result of direct inoculation of a fungus following injury. The subcutaneous mycoses, such as some forms of phaeohyphomycosis and sporotrichosis, are usually localized infections that result from the traumatic implantation of fungal elements. Dissemination from these sites sometimes involves the lung and other organs, and these same infections occasionally have a primary pulmonary focus following inhalation of infectious fungal elements. The superficial and cutaneous mycoses, such as tinea versicolor and the dermatophytoses, are usually confined to the keratinized layer of the skin and its appendages. Invasive cutaneous infections are very rare and do not ordinarily involve the lungs.

Opportunistic Fungal Infections

Fungi that cause invasive pulmonary infection can be divided into (1) the primary or true pathogens and (2) the opportunistic pathogens.[9–11] Primary pathogens infect healthy, immunologically competent people. In contrast, opportunistic fungi, which are normally innocuous saprophytes, become pathogenic only under conditions that increase the host's susceptibility to infection. With the exception of the endogenous *Candida* spp., these fungi usually gain entry through the lungs. The more common opportunistic mycoses include, in order of decreasing frequency: candidiasis, aspergillosis, cryptococcosis, zygomycosis, torulopsosis, pseudallescheriasis, fusariosis, and trichosporonosis. Those fungi that are primarily pathogens in healthy people can also be aggressive opportunists, and cause severe disseminated and often fatal infections in compromised individuals.

Since the early 1960s, the incidence of opportunistic fungal infections has risen dramatically; new ones are described with increasing frequency.[9–14] Important factors contributing to this increase have been immunosuppressive therapy of allograft rejection, chemotherapy of neoplasia, broad-spectrum antibiotic therapy of bacterial infections, and the long-term placement of vascular catheters. Other conditions that predispose to opportunistic infections are malignancies, especially leukemia and lymphoma, chronic lung disease, severe burns, abdominal surgery, cardiac valve replacement surgery, diabetes mellitus, Cushing's syndrome, uremia, malnutrition, alcohol abuse, drug abuse, genetic immune defects, and the acquired immunodeficiency syndrome (AIDS).[9–18] Epidemiologic factors include aging of the population, migration of susceptible persons into highly endemic areas, and greater awareness of fungal and other opportunistic infections in compromised patients.[3,6,18]

The subject of host resistance to fungi has been discussed extensively by Grieco[19] and others.[8,11,18] Immunologic defects thought to be responsible for increased susceptibility to fungal infections include: (1) a decrease in number or functional impairment of mature granulocytes and mononuclear phagocytes; (2) depressed B-lymphocyte (humoral) immunity with decreased production of immunoglobulins and impaired opsonization; (3) depressed T-lymphocyte (cell-mediated) immunity; and (4) abnormalities in immunoregulatory mechanisms. Disruption of mucosal and cutaneous barriers, disorders of the complement system, and hereditary enzyme deficiencies specifically associated with immunologic dysfunction are other factors responsible for increased susceptibility.[18–21]

Clinical features in severely immunosuppressed patients often differ from those seen in normal, immunocompetent hosts. Further, there may be little or no inflammatory response to enormous numbers of invasive fungi in tissue specimens; granulomas may not be formed, regardless of the causative agent. Because of these quantitative and qualitative differences in host response, special histologic stains for demonstrating fungi and other microorganisms should be routinely ordered along with hematoxylin and eosin (H and E). Certain coexisting infections occur with a surprising degree of regularity in the profoundly immunodeficient patient, and the possibility of multiple infectious agents in a single specimen should never be overlooked. Beause of the greater tendency for dissemination of fungal infections in such patients, timely and accurate diagnoses followed by aggressive treatment are of paramount importance in reducing morbidity and mortality.

Approach to the Histologic Diagnosis of Fungal Infections

Because the symptoms and radiographic findings of the pulmonary mycoses are not specific, diagnosis relies heavily on three basic laboratory procedures: (1) serologic; (2) mycologic; and (3) histologic.[22,23] A combination of these approaches is always recommended but is not always possible. Serologic tests on acute- and convalescent-phase sera have prognostic as well as diagnostic value, since changes in titer often indicate progression or regression of disease during therapy.[24,25] However, serologic tests have not been developed for some fungal diseases. When tests are available, one must be cautious in their interpretation, because both false-positive and false-negative results can occur.[25] The latter are particularly prevalent in patients with profound immunodeficiencies.

Most of the fungi that cause invasive pulmonary infection can be cultured on standard synthetic media.[2,4,5] However, cultivation and characterization of some isolates can take as long as 6 weeks. When a fungus is isolated, the question remains whether the isolate is an invasive pathogen or an environmental contaminant. In other instances, cultural studies are not possible because a mycosis is not suspected, and entire tissue specimens are fixed for histopathological evaluation. In all these situations, pathologists must rely on their ability to recognize and identify fungi in smears and fixed, paraffin-embedded tissue sections.[3,26] The presence of a fungus in tissue sections provides indisputable evidence of invasive infection. Histologic studies can also confirm the presence of coexisting infections by other fungi, viruses, bacteria, protozoans, and helminths. Finally, no other diagnostic approach can determine whether the host response signifies tissue invasion or a purely allergic reaction, for example, invasive versus allergic pulmonary aspergillosis. Although certain patterns of host reaction suggest that a mycosis exists, no absolute histologic criteria are available that permit an etiologic diagnosis unless a fungus is detected and identified.

Becuase of their size, chemical composition, and morphologic diversity, many fungi can be identified in tissue sections by conventional light microscopy. In tissue, fungi are either hyaline or dematiaceous, and usually occur as either hyphae, budding yeast-like cells, endosporulating spherules, granules, or a combination of these forms. Certain mycoses are caused by fungi that can be specifically identifed because they have a distinctive morphology in tissue. When classic forms are observed, an etiologic diagnosis can be made: for example, adiaspiromycosis, blastomycosis, coccidioidomycosis, cryptococcosis, histoplasmosis capsulati, histoplasmosis duboisii, paracoccidioidomycosis, penicilliosis marneffei, protothecosis, rhinosporidiosis, and sporotrichosis. In this group, only one species or variety of fungus is the cause of each particular mycosis. Other mycoses are caused by any of several species of a genus, all of which appear morphologically similar in tissue sections. Although these agents cannot be identified as to species by conventional histologic methods, the diseases that they cause can be diagnosed generically; for example, aspergillosis, candidiasis, and trichosporonosis. Still other mycoses are caused by any of a number of fungi belonging to different genera. These fungi appear similar if not identical to one another in tissue, and, although it is not possible to identify the etiologic agent, the mycosis can be named. This group includes diseases such a phaeohyphomycosis and zygomycosis.

Histologic Stains for Demonstrating Fungi

Several special stains can be used to demonstrate fungi in histologic sections. Detailed descriptions of these staining procedures, which are given in many excellent texts[27-30] and manuals,[31,32] are not included here.

Hematoxylin and eosin (H and E) is a versatile stain that enables the pathologist to evaluate the host response, including the Splendore–Hoeppli phenomenon,[33] and to detect some fungi and other microorganisms. It is the stain of choice to confirm the presence of naturally pigmented fungi and to demonstrate the nuclei of yeast-like cells. With H and E, however, it is often difficult to distinguish poorly stained fungi from tissue components, even at higher magnifications. When sparse, fungi are easily overlooked. Special stains for fungi and other microbes are therefore essential for the histopathological evaluation of unexplained inflammatory processes.

Most fungi can be readily demonstrated with any of the special fungal stains, the most common of which are Gomori's methenamine silver (GMS), Gridley's fungus (GF), and the periodic acid–Schiff (PAS) reaction procedures. However, GMS is preferred for screening; it gives better contrast and can stain degenerated and nonviable fungal elements that are sometimes refractory to the other two stains. GMS will also stain algae (*Prototheca* and *Chlorella* spp.), cyst walls of *Pneumocystis carinii* and pathogenic free-living soil amebas, the spore coat of most microsporidian parasites, intracytoplasmic granular inclusions of cytomegalovirus, *Actinomyces israelii* and related-species, *Nocardia* spp., most *Mycobacterium* spp., and nonfilamentous bacteria with polysaccharide capsules such as *Klebsiella pneumoniae* and *Streptococcus pneumoniae*. Prolonged staining in the silver nitrate solution may be required to adequately demonstrate degenerated fungal elements such as the yeast-like cells of *Histoplasma capsulatum* var. *capsulatum* in residual pulmonary granulomas.

The main disadvantage of special fungal stains is that they mask the natural color of pigmented fungi, making it impossible to determine whether a fungus is hyaline (colorless) or dematiaceous (pigmented). Such a determination is crucial in the histologic diagnosis of mycoses caused by dematiaceous fungi, such as phaeohyphomycosis.[3] Except for the PAS reaction, special fungal stains do not adequately demonstrate the inflammatory response to fungal invasion. To accomplish this, a GMS-stained section can be counterstained with H and E for simultaneous study of the fungus and the host response. Calcific bodies that are sometimes found in caseated granulomas are readily stained with H and E and the PAS reaction, and they can be mistaken for yeast-like fungi. This is especially true when calcific bodies are apposed to give the false impression of budding yeasts, or when the bodies are laminated to give the appearance of a capsule or thick cell wall. GMS and GF stains preclude this misinterpretation because the chromic acid used as an oxidizer in these procedures dissolves calcium, leaving calcific bodies unstained.

Mucin stains such as alcian blue and Mayer's or Southgate's mucicarmine procedures readily demonstrate the mucoid capsule of *Cryptococcus neoformans*. This staining reaction usually differentiates this pathogenic yeast from others of similar morphology. In some cases, however, poorly encapsulated cryptococci in tissue sections may not be carminophilic.[3] Further, mucin stains are not specific for *C. neoformans;* the cell walls of *Blastomyces dermatitidis* and *Rhinosporidium seeberi* are often colored to varying degrees. Because the latter two fungi are nonencapsulated and morphologically distinct, they are not ordinarily mistaken for cryptococci.

The cell wall of *C. neoformans* contains silver-reducing substances (melanin-like substances derived from dihydroxyphenylalanine) and can be stained with Fontana–Masson's silver procedure for melanin.[34-37] This stain is especially useful in those cases of cryptococcosis where the invasive yeast forms do not have readily detectable capsules (poorly encapsulated or so-called dry variants). Such forms could possibly be confused with nonencapsulated yeasts of similar morphology. Fontana–Masson's and Lillie's ferrous iron stains for melanin can also be used to confirm and accentuate the presence of melanin or melanin-like pigments in the cell walls of poorly pigmented agents of phaeohyphomycosis in tissue sections.[38]

The cytoplasm of certain fungi in tissue sections, especially the yeast-like cells of *Blastomyces dermatitidis* and *Histoplasma capsulatum* var. *capsulatum*, is variably acid fast.[39] However, this staining property is inconsistent and should not be used routinely for diagnosis. In our experience, the cell walls of fungi are not acid fast.

When examined under ultraviolet light, some fungi or fungal components in H and E-stained tissue sections are autofluorescent. Graham[40] reported bright green to yellow-green autofluorescence of *Aspergillus* spp., *Candida* spp. and *Coccidioides immitis*. Bright yellow fungal autofluorescence against a deep red-orange background was observed when sections were stained with the PAS reaction. Autofluorescence may help delineate sparse or poorly stained fungi in H and E-stained sections, but, in our experience, this property is inconsistent and should not be used for definitive diagnosis or to replace special histologic and immunohistologic procedures. Most fungi in frozen or paraffin-embedded tissue sections also stain nonspecifically with calcofluor white, a cotton whitener that fluoresces under ultraviolet light.[41] This rapid and simple fluorescence procedure can be routinely used in the intraoperative examination of fresh-frozen tissues for fungi.

Diagnostic Applications of Immunofluorescence

Direct immunofluorescence (IF) can extend the diagnostic capability of conventional histopathology in the diagnosis of mycotic diseases.[3,42,43] The IF procedure, which can be performed on smears and on formalin-fixed, paraffin-embedded tissue sections, is very helpful in confirming a presumptive histologic diagnosis, especially when fresh tissues are not available for culture or when only atypical forms of a fungus are seen. The Centers for Disease Control, Atlanta (United States), and others have developed a broad battery of sensitive and specific reagents for detecting and identifying the more common pathogenic fungi.

The IF procedure has several advantages. Final identification of an unknown fungus in replicate (sectioned from the same block) deparaffinized tissue sections is possible within hours after H and E- and GMS-stained sections are initially examined. The need for time-consuming and costly culture procedures is often obviated by IF, and the hazards of handling potentially infectious materials are reduced when microorganisms are inactivated by formalin before IF staining. Prolonged storage of formalin-fixed tissues, either "wet" or paraffin-embedded, does not appear to affect the antigenicity of fungi. This antigenic stability makes possible retrospective studies of paraffinized tissue blocks and the shipment of specimens to distant reference laboratories for confirmatory identification. Details of the IF technique are given in several references.[24,42,43] Immunoperoxidase labeling can also be used to identify certain fungi in smears and formalin-fixed, paraffin-embedded tissue sections.[44–48] At present, however, this technique has had limited diagnostic use.

Terminology

Because medical mycology is highly specialized, the following terms used to describe fungi and algae in tissue are defined:

adiaconidium: asexual conidium (spore) that enlarges after formation in vitro or implantation in vivo. Such conidia do not reproduce in vivo

alga (plural, algae): eukaryotic, photoautotrophic, unicellular or multicellular organisms of the kingdom Protista

arthroconidium: asexual conidium (spore) formed by mycelial disarticulation

bud (blastoconidium): a variety of conidium produced by lateral outgrowth from a parent cell; buds may be single or multiple

capsule: hyaline (colorless) mucopolysaccharide coat external to the wall of a fungal cell or conidium

chlamydoconidium: thick-walled, rounded, resistant conidium formed by direct differentiation of the mycelium

conidiophore: specialized hypha that produces and bears conidia

conidium: asexual spore formed on, but easily detached from, a hypha or conidiophore

dematiaceous: naturally pigmented, usually brown or black

dichotomous: equal branching of hyphae

dimorphic: growth as hyphae in vitro at 25°C and as budding yeasts or spherules in infected tissues or in vitro at 37°C on special media

endospore: asexual spore formed within a closed structure such as a spherule

endosporulation: process of producing endospores

"fruiting body": imprecise term for conidia-bearing organs produced by fungi germ tube: tube-like process, produced by a germinating conidium, that eventually develops into a hypha

hyaline: colorless

hypha: filament that forms the thallus or body of most fungi

intercalary: between two fungal cells

mycelium (plural, mycelia): mass of intertwined and branched hyphae

perfect state: developmental state of a fungus when sexual reproduction takes place and sexual spores are produced

phialide: a conidiogenous cell that successively produces conidia from within

pseudohypha: short hyphal-like filament produced by successive yeast buds that elongate and fail to separate

septate: having cross walls

septum (plural, septa): cross wall of a mycelial filament or conidium

spherule: closed, thick-walled, spherical structure within which asexual endospores are produced by progressive cytoplasmic cleavage

Splendore–Hoeppli phenomenon: eosinophilic, refractile, homogeneous, and often radially oriented material found around some fungi in tissue sections; represents a localized antigen–antibody reaction in the hypersensitized host

sporangium (plural, sporangia): a closed structure within which asexual spores (sporangiospores) are produced by cytoplasmic cleavage

sterigma (plural, sterigmata): short or elongate specialized projection of a sporophore on which spores are developed (see phialide)

yeast: round-to-oval unicellular fungus that reproduces by budding or fission

To facilitate differential diagnosis, fungal infections in this chapter are grouped according to the morphologic similarities of their etiologic agents in tissue. For further reading, several texts are recommended.* Numerous cases have been reported of allergic pulmonary disease in patients exposed to saprophytic moulds and yeasts in modern living and working environments. These allergic reactions to fungi are covered in Chapter 12.

Specific Fungal Diseases

Histoplasmosis Capsulati

Histoplasmosis capsulati is a respiratory infection contracted by inhalation of the airborne infectious conidia

---

*References: 2–5, 23, 49–51.

of *Histoplasma capsulatum* var. *capsulatum*.[52–54] There is marked proclivity for dissemination via the mononuclear phagocyte system from the primary pulmonary focus, which may not be clinically apparent. The mycosis occurs worldwide in both rural and urban settings where avian and chiropteran habitats such as chicken coops, roosting shelters, caves, and attics favor growth and multiplication of the fungus in soil enriched with fecal material. In the United States, the Mississippi and Ohio River valleys are highly endemic areas for histoplasmosis capsulati. Other endemic areas in the Western Hemisphere include Guatemala, Mexico, Peru, and Venezuela.

In this chapter, the term histoplasmosis capsulati refers to infection by the classic, small-celled, or *capsulatum* variety of *H. capsulatum*. Disease caused by the African, large-celled, or *duboisii* variety of this fungus is discussed separately because it is a distinct clinical and pathologic entity. Histoplasmosis duboisii is seen only in humans and nonhuman primates on the African continent, where both varieties of *H. capsulatum* exist. The two varieties are indistinguishable in culture and can be identified only by the difference in size of their yeast forms in tissue.[53] No evidence is available that either mycosis is contagious.

H. capsulatum var. *capsulatum* is a dimorphic pathogen. It grows as a mould in soil and in culture at 25°C, and as budding yeast-like cells 2–4 μm in diameter in human tissues and in culture at 37°C on enriched media. On Sabouraud's agar, mycelial-form colonies are downy, white to golden brown, and produce two types of asexual conidia: large (8–14 μm), thick-walled, tuberculate macroconidia with digitate protuberances; and small (2–4 μm), smooth-surfaced microconidia.[52–54]

The pathogenesis of histoplasmosis capsulati has been clearly established.[52,54–56] When soil or other contaminated matter is disturbed, aerosolized conidia are inhaled and germinate in alveolar ducts and alveoli. The yeast-like cells of the fungus proliferate, enter lymphatics, and are carried to the hilar lymph nodes, which in turn drain into the circulation. Bloodborne fungal elements are then disseminated to many organs and are sequestered in mononuclear phagocytes in the spleen, liver, lymph nodes, and bone marrow, where organisms are phagocytosed and removed from the circulation. Despite the fact that hematogenous dissemination occurs in most primary pulmonary infections, the disease is usually self limited and should not be confused with the progressive disseminated form of histoplasmosis capsulati.[57,58] Within days to a few weeks, a cell-mediated immune response develops in the normal host at sites of primary and metastatic infection; granuloma formation, caseation, and fibrotic encapsulation follow. Calcification of necrotic foci may occur months to years later in the lung as well as in other organs, especially in the hilar lymph nodes and spleen. If an effective cell-mediated immune response does not develop, progressive disseminated infection occurs. Endogenous reinfection also results in disseminated infection in many immunosuppressed patients.[59,60]

It has been estimated that about 500,000 new cases of histoplasmosis capsulati occur each year in the United States.[52,54] However, data from epidemiologic surveys indicate that 90%–95% of these cases represent asymptomatic, self-limited pulmonary infections. Localized lesions usually heal without antifungal therapy, but they may calcify and be discovered inadvertently in chest radiographs or at autopsy. The remaining 5%–10% of patients have symptomatic infections that fall into three broad clinical categories: (1) acute pulmonary form; (2) disseminated form; and (3) chronic pulmonary form.[56,61–65]

Three to 14 days after exposure, patients with the acute pulmonary form develop mild influenza-like symptoms such as fever, cough, malaise, myalgia, and arthralgia. A primary complex of hilar lymphadenopathy and a single small area of pulmonary infiltration is usually seen in chest radiographs (Fig. 11–1A); cavitation is very rare.[66] The severity and duration of infection depend on host resistance and the quantity of fungal conidia inhaled, and symptoms usually last for a few days to 2 weeks before recovery. A few patients may have a rapidly progressive pulmonary infection in which bilateral and often miliary reticulonodular infiltrates are seen on chest radiographs[58,67] (Figs. 11–1B and 11–2).

Disseminated histoplasmosis capsulati is a frequent complication of hematologic malignancies and cytotoxic chemotherapy,[57–59] aggressive immunosuppressive therapy in organ transplant recipients,[68,69] and the acquired immunodeficiency syndrome,[70–74] all of which compromise cell-mediated immunity.[60,75,76] Disseminated infection also occurs in very young children in the "infantile" form, and occurs in apparently healthy persons with no detectable immunologic defect in the "adult" form of histoplasmosis capsulati.[56,58,62] Some investigators believe that patients with the adult form may have transient immunosuppression resulting from a coexisting viral infection.[56] Hematogenous dissemination is characterized either by slowly progressive spread of infection to various organs or by fulminating infection with rapid clinical deterioration and death. The mortality rate can be as high as 80% without antifungal therapy.[54,56,58] Patients are often found to have fever, chills, productive cough, hemoptysis, dyspnea, weight loss, malaise, headache, drowsiness, diarrhea, generalized lymphadenopathy, hepatospleno-

megaly, purpura, and ulcerations of the oropharynx and intestines. Symptoms may mimic those of rapidly progressive lymphoma.[77,78] The most common pulmonary radiologic pattern is a diffuse interstitial infiltrate resulting from hematogenous dissemination.[56,58,62] Occasionally, however, chest radiographs are normal, despite other evidence of dissemination. Because of extensive parasitization of the mononuclear phagocyte system, bone marrow suppression occurs and results in one or more cytopenias.[79] Some patients may have symptoms of Addison's disease because of diffuse involvement of both adrenal glands.[80] Histoplasma endocarditis is a rare but serious manifestation of disseminated infection, which may occur without predisposing valvular disease or deformity.[81,82]

The chronic pulmonary form of histoplasmosis capsulati is primarily a disease of adults, and symptoms are indistinguishable from those of other chronic progressive pulmonary infections such as reinfection tuberculosis.[56,62,83–85] Four radiographic patterns have been described: infiltration, cavitation, fibrosis with emphysema, and the residual solitary nodule or histoplasmoma[84–87] (Figs. 11–1C,D and 11–3). The infiltrative pattern is frequently apical and appears as unilateral mottled densities that occasionally extend to the opposite lung. Thin-walled unilateral or bilateral cavities are seen in about 50% of these patients. Cavitary lesions may result from slow but progressive destruction of pulmonary parenchyma from unresolved primary infection occurring months to years earlier. However, cavitary lesions represent endogenous reinfection similar to that seen in tuberculosis. Fibrosis may be severe, and is sometimes associated with extensive irregular emphysema and bronchiectasis. Solitary residual nodules (histoplasmomas or "coin" lesions) often resemble carcinoma, especially when they are noncalcified and enlarge progressively on sequential chest radiographs.[86–88] Histoplasmomas are discretely rounded and vary from 0.5 to several centimeters in diameter; usually subpleural, they often contain stippled or concentric calcifications, and may be accompanied by enlarged and calcified hilar lymph nodes (Fig. 11–3). Granulomatous and sclerosing mediastinitis can result from direct extension of infection from hilar lymph nodes into the mediastinum.[56,61,83,84]

Radiographic abnormalities, when combined with clinical and laboratory findings, often allow for a presumptive diagnosis of histoplasmosis capsulati.[67,85–87] Silverman[89] studied the radiographic findings of the primary complex in histoplasmosis capsulati and concluded that larger and more numerous calcifications (primary foci of infection) in the lung and hilar lymph nodes strongly suggested histoplasmosis rather than tuberculosis, in which the primary pulmonary focus is

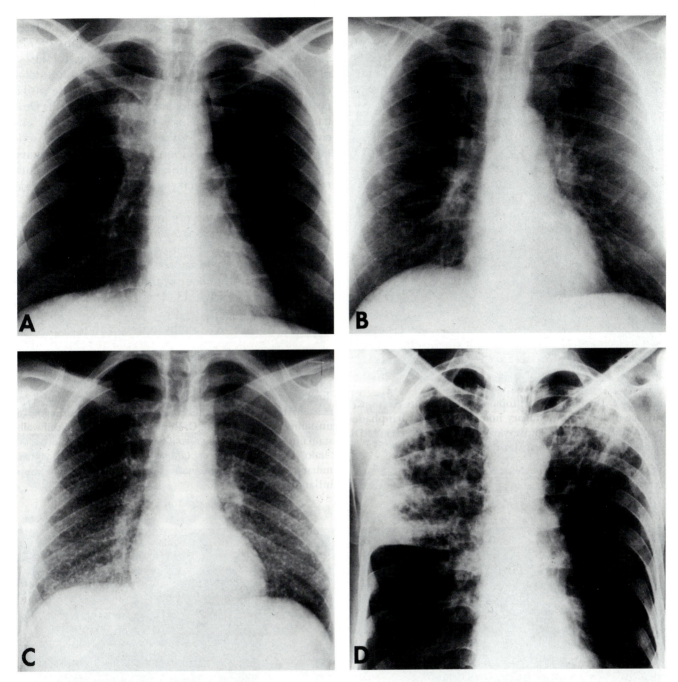

Fig. 11–1 A–D. Histoplasmosis capsulati. **A.** Acute pneumonic form with bulky mediastinal lymphadenopathy and infiltrates in periphery of right-upper lobe. **B.** Active miliary form characterized by poorly defined, noncalcified, 3- to 5-mm nodules in both lung fields. **C.** Chronic miliary form with calcified nodules throughout both lung fields. (Radiographs A–C courtesy of Harry D. Tabor, M.D., Department of Diagnostic Radiology, William Beaumont Hospital, Royal Oak, Michigan.) **D.** Chronic fibrocavitary form with bilateral involvement of upper lung fields. (Radiograph courtesy of Karlhanns Salfelder, M.D., Universidad de los Andes, Merida, Venezuela.)

usually solitary. Miliary calcifications throughout both lungs were found in some patients with histoplasmosis. In others, enlarged hilar lymph nodes obscured the smaller primary pulmonary lesion of the complex and were the only apparent radiographic abnormality. Pleu-ral thickening was often seen, but effusion was rare. Uncommon chest radiographic findings in patients with progressive pulmonary infection included bron-cholithiasis (see Chapter 5), vena caval obstruction, esophageal compression, pericardial calcification, and

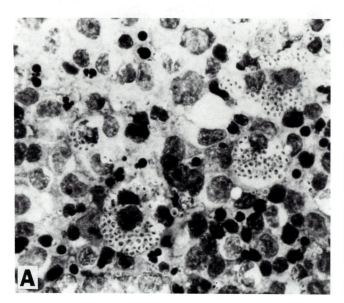

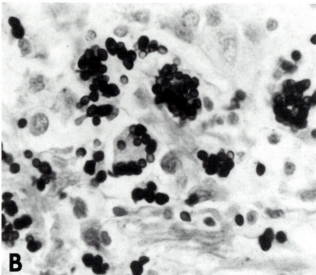

Fig. 11–5 A,B. Disseminated histoplasmosis capsulati. **A.** Yeast-laden histiocytes in bone marrow smear. Wright–Giemsa, ×480. **B.** Granulomatous adrenalitis with aggregates of yeast-like cells within histiocytes and multinucleated giant cells. GMS/H and E, ×600.

stained sections, the basophilic cytoplasm is retracted from the thin, poorly stained cell wall, creating a clear space or "halo" that gives the false impression of an unstained capsule (Fig. 11–4B). This "halo" effect is eliminated in sections stained with the special fungal stains, all of which stain the fungal cells entirely (Figs. 11–4C and 11–5B). Germ tubes and pseudohyphae are occasionally seen in active lesions that contain abundant fungal cells, and both hyphae and huge, bizarre, thick-walled yeast forms have been described on or near the surface of valvular vegetations in histoplasma endocarditis.[93]

The host response to *H. capsulatum* var. *capsulatum* varies with the dose of inoculum and the age and immunologic status of the host.[54,56,58,91] When many conidia have been inhaled, pulmonary lesions may be rapidly progressive even in the immunocompetent host, and may contain enormous numbers of proliferating intraalveolar and interstitial yeast forms associated with necrosis and mononuclear interstitial infiltrates (See Fig. 11–4). In contrast, fungal cells are relatively sparse in mild, self-limited and chronic, progressive pulmonary infections. In the very young and in persons who are immunosuppressed, the host response is predominantly histiocytic and characterized by intracellular multiplication of fungal cells. Dispersed infiltrates of yeast-laden histiocytes often efface the normal architecture of an organ, and widespread involvement of the mononuclear phagocyte system occurs (Fig. 11–5). In patients with profound cell-mediated immunodeficiency, for example, AIDS, yeast forms multiply pro-

fusely and sometimes form extracellular "yeast lakes" associated with bland necrosis. In immunocompetent hosts and patients with the "adult" form of disseminated disease, the fungus usually elicits an epithelioid and giant-cell granulomatous response with or without caseation (Fig. 11–6). Slowly evolving pulmonary granulomas may be followed by cavitation, fibrosis, emphysema, and at times calcification.

The residual pulmonary nodule (histoplasmoma) consists of a large central zone of caseous necrosis surrounded by a thick fibrotic capsule that contains peripheral lymphoid aggregates and rare epithelioid and multinucleated giant cells[61,94,95] (Fig. 11–7A). The central caseous material may be irregularly calcified and may rarely undergo osseous and myeloid metaplasia.[54] If present, fungal cells are scattered in the caseous material but are almost impossible to detect in H and E-stained sections. With GMS, they are often poorly stained ("ghost" forms), distorted, fragmented, and most abundant in the caseous center of the nodule (Fig. 11–7B). Attempts to culture the fungus from these residual lesions are usually unsuccessful, but a diagnosis can be made by demonstrating typical yeast forms of *H. capsulatum* var. *capsulatum* in tissue sections.

Definitive diagnosis of histoplasmosis capsulati rests on the isolation of the etiologic agent from clinical specimens or its demonstration in smears and tissue sections. Examination of Wright's-stained peripheral blood smears for yeast-like cells in monocytes and occasionally in neutrophils is a procedure often overlooked, but blood smears are positive in up to 50% of patients

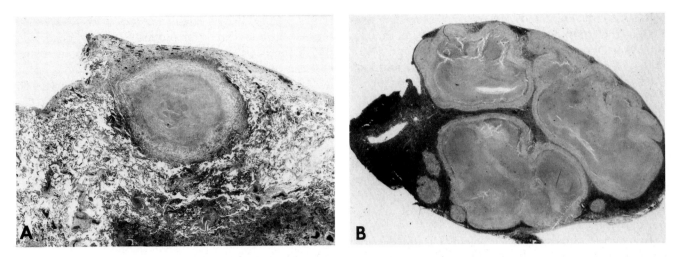

Fig. 11–6 A,B. Primary complex in histoplasmosis capsulati. **A.** Subpleural caseated granuloma. ×10. **B.** Fibrocaseous nodules in mediastinal lymph node. ×8.

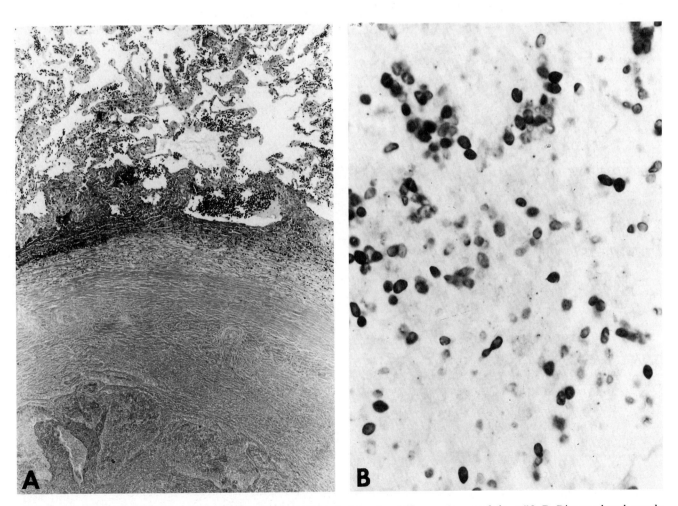

Fig. 11–7 A,B. Residual pulmonary histoplasmosis capsulati. **A.** Margin of fibrocaseous nodule. ×50. **B.** Distorted and poorly stained yeast-like cells in caseous center of nodule. GMS, ×760.

with severe disseminated infection.[96,97] Serologic tests such as the complement fixation and agar gel double-diffusion methods may also provide presumptive evidence of infection. However, a single high antibody titer has no diagnostic or prognostic significance.[56] Although the histoplasmin skin test is useful for mapping endemic regions and for epidemiologic investigations of acute histoplasmosis capsulati, it is not recommended for definitive diagnosis.[54,56] Measurement of H. capsulatum var. capsulatum polysaccharide antigen levels by radioimmunoassay has been shown to assist in the identification of histoplasmosis relapse in patients with AIDS, and is useful for management of maintenance therapy.[98]

In tissue sections, capsule-deficient cells of *Cryptococcus neoformans* and microforms of *Blastomyces dermatitidis* can resemble yeast forms of *H. capsulatum* var. *capsulatum*. However, a minority of these cryptococci will usually have some capsular material detectable with mucin stains; *B. dermatitidis* cells are multinucleated, have thick "doubly contoured" walls, and bud by a broad base. Yeast forms of *Torulopsis glabrata* may also resemble those of *H. capsulatum* var. *capsulatum*, but the former are amphophilic and stain entirely with H and E. When these differentiating features are equivocal, direct immunofluorescence using a screening conjugate directed against cell wall polysaccharide antigens of all known serotypes of *H. capsulatum* is invaluable for confirming a presumptive histologic diagnosis.[42,43]

The acute pulmonary form of histoplasmosis capsulati is usually a benign, self-limited illness that heals without antifungal therapy. However, progressive pulmonary and disseminated infections require prompt treatment with amphotericin B.[54,56] Ketoconazole has also been used with success in indolent chronic infections and as prophylactic treatment for patients who have a positive histoplasmin skin test and are receiving corticosteroids.[99,100] Surgical resection of cavities may be a valuable adjunct to antifungal therapy in patients with chronic cavitary pulmonary lesions.[56]

Histoplasmosis Duboisii

Histoplasmosis duboisii (African histoplasmosis) is a chronic progressive pulmonary mycosis with a marked tropism for the skin and bones. It is caused by the large-celled form or *duboisii* variety of *Histoplasma capsulatum*, first described and validated as a separate entity by Vanbreuseghem[101] in 1952. Infection by this dimorphic fungus results from inhalation of microconidia 2–4 μm in diameter that are produced by the saprophytic mycelial form in soil.

In culture, the mycelial and yeast forms of *H. capsulatum* var. *duboisii* are indistinguishable from those of the classic, small-celled or *capsulatum* variety of this species; the two varieties can be distinguished only by observing the differences in size of their yeast forms in tissue. Diseases caused by both varieties of *H. capsulatum* occur in Africa, but they are discussed separately because each is clinically and pathologically distinct.[102] With the exception of two cases, one from Japan[103] and the other from Madagascar,[104] natural infection with *H. capsulatum* var. *duboisii* is known to occur only in humans and in nonhuman primates on the African continent.[105,106] Most cases are further confined to the region that extends from 15° latitude in the north to 10° latitude in the south. Nevertheless, it is important to be aware of this mycosis because it is occasionally seen in the United States and elsewhere in individuals who previously lived or traveled in Africa.[107–110]

Unlike classic histoplasmosis, pulmonary lesions in histoplasmosis duboisii are exceptional, and when detected are often subtle. However, epidemiologic and clinical data support the concept of a pulmonary origin. Clark and Greenwood[111] strengthened this concept when they reported 2 cases with pulmonary involvement and reviewed 10 others from the literature with evidence of lung lesions. Chest radiographs of their two patients revealed diffuse infiltrates in both lung fields, and multiple granulomas with caseous centers were described at autopsy. Lanceley et al.[112] reported miliary opacities throughout both lung fields and enlarged hilar shadows in roentgenograms of an East African child with histoplasmosis duboisii. This was the first reported case that was culture proven and the first with radiologic evidence of pulmonary involvement in which typical cells of *H. capsulatum* var. *duboisii* were demonstrated in disseminated lesions. Quere et al.[113] described "tumor-like pulmonary infiltrates" in a young man with orbital and osseous involvement. In general, pulmonary radiographic findings vary from no detectable abnormalities to mild nonspecific infiltrates or small, miliary, nodular opacities.[102,111,114] Hilar adenopathy may also be present,[112,115] but cavitation and pleural effusion are seldom observed. Self-limited asymptomatic infection is thought to result in calcified foci occasionally detected in chest radiographs, at surgery, or at autopsy.[102]

There are two clinical forms of histoplasmosis duboisii: localized and disseminated. Patients with the localized form usually have lymphadenopathy, mucocutaneous ulcers, and insidious osteolytic lesions, particularly involving the cranium, ribs, sternum, scapula, vertebrae, and long bones.[102,113,115] Multiple skin ulcers frequently communicate with subcutaneous abscesses that are secondary to osteitis and osteomyelitis. Osteoarthritis and the formation of fistulas and draining sinuses may also occur. Hematogenous or lymphatic

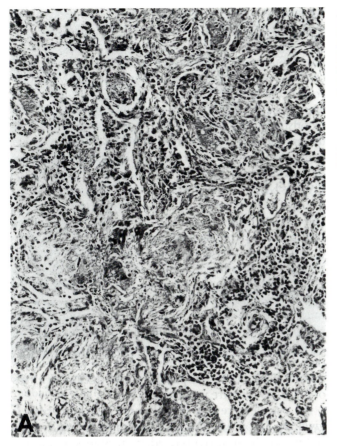

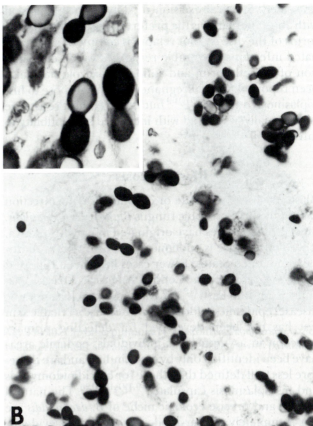

Fig. 11–8 A,B. Pulmonary histoplasmosis duboisii. **A.** Dispersed granulomatous inflammation and interstitial fibrosis. ×120. **B.** Single and budding yeast-like cells of *Histoplasma capsulatum* var. *duboisii* within macrophages and multinucle- ated giant cells. GM$_S$, ×480. *Inset:* Detail of three "double-cell" forms created when budding daughter cells enlarge until they are equal in size to the parent cells, to which they remain attached. GMS/H and E, ×760.

dissemination from pulmonary or localized foci is often fatal and can involve virtually any organ, particularly those previously mentioned and the spleen, liver, lung, and intestine.[102,105,116] Patients often have hepatosplenomegaly and prominent lymphadenopathy.

In all organs, lesions are microscopically similar. They consist typically of a dispersed granulomatous inflammatory reaction in which enormous numbers of yeast-like cells, 8–15 μm in diameter, are seen within histiocytes and huge multinucleated giant cells of both the foreign body and Langhans' types (Fig. 11–8). Irregular foci of caseous necrosis that contain extracellular yeast forms may also be present. In the lung, slowly evolving granulomas may be accompanied by fibrosis, cavitation, and rarely calcification (Fig. 11–8A). Involvement of thoracic lymph nodes, pleura, and contiguous bone may also occur. Cells of *H. capsulatum* var. *duboisii* are uninucleate, have thick walls, and bud by a relatively narrow base to create "double-cell" forms when daughter cells enlarge until they are equal in size

to the parent cells to which they remain attached (Fig. 11–8B). "Hour-glass" cells refer to those "double-cell" forms that share a centrally constricted cytoplasm. The yeast-like cells are usually abundant and easily demonstrated in smears of lesion exudate.

Tissue forms of *H. capsulatum* var. *duboisii* and *Blastomyces dermatitidis* can be mistaken for each other because both have thick cell walls and are similar in size. Blastomycosis is common in North America, and the problem of differential diagnosis is compounded because indigenous cases of this mycosis occur in Africa as well.[117] However, *B. dermatitidis* is multinucleated (best seen with H and E) and buds by a broader base. Tissue forms of *H. capsulatum* var. *capsulatum*, the agent of classic histoplasmosis, are much smaller (2–4 μm) than those of the large-celled *duboisii* variety.

The localized chronic form of histoplasmosis duboisii can sometimes persist for several decades with periods of quiescence and recrudescence, whereas the disseminated form can be rapidly progressive and fatal if

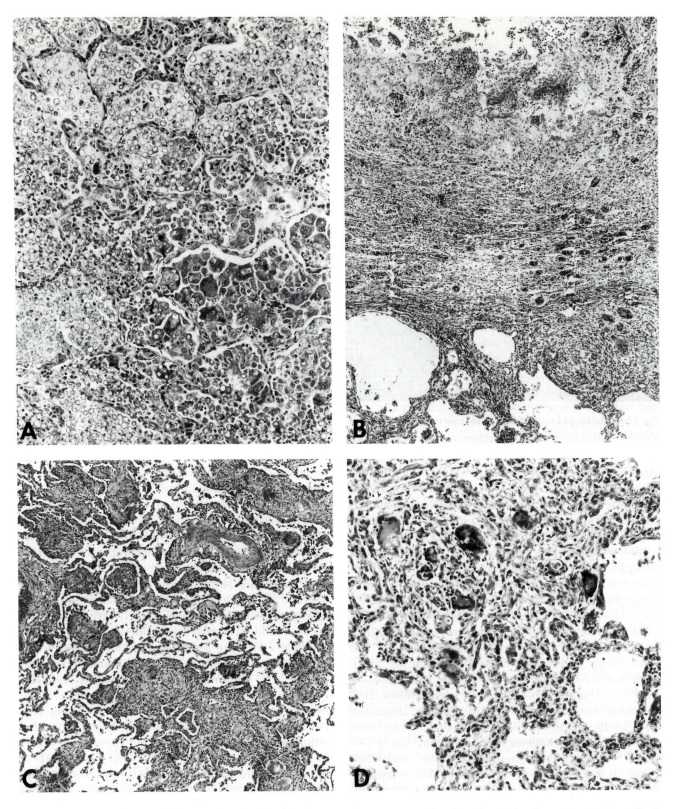

Fig. 11–11 A–D. Pulmonary blastomycosis. **A.** Alveolar spaces contain neutrophils, multinucleated giant cells, and enormous numbers of intra- and extracellular yeast forms of *Blastomyces dermatitidis*. ×120. **B.** Chronic suppurative and granuloma- tous pneumonitis with pleural involvement at top. ×48. **C.** Interstitial granulomatous pattern. ×48. **D.** Interstitial fibro- sis with mixed suppurative and granulomatous inflammation. ×120.

Fig. 11–12 A–D. Blastomycosis. **A.** Numerous thick-walled, multinucleated yeast forms of *Blastomyces dermatitidis* within a pulmonary granuloma. Broad-based budding (*arrow*) is diag- nostic. ×760. **B.** Single and budding yeast forms within alveolar space. The thick "doubly contoured" walls of the fungal cells are not readily apparent when special fungal stains are used. GMS, ×480. **C.** Microforms of *B. dermatitidis* in cerebellar granuloma of patient with chronic systemic infec- tion. GMS/H and E, ×480. **D.** Single and budding yeast forms with brightly fluorescent cell walls in section of lung. Direct immunofluorescence, ×600.

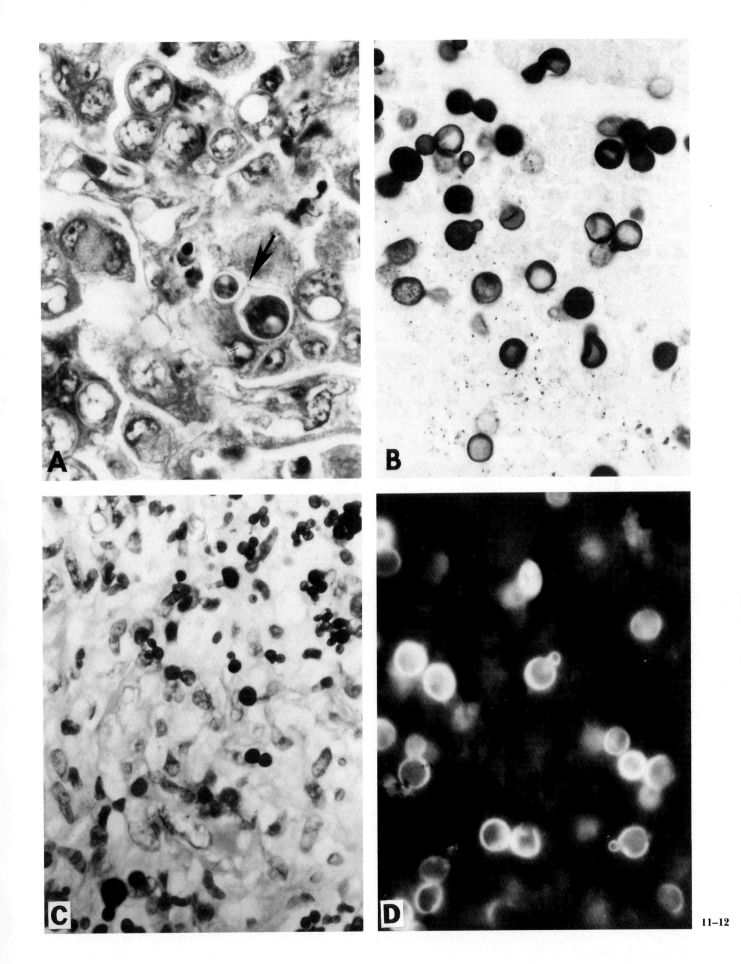

seen in cryptococcosis.[146,147] Within days to weeks, a granulomatous response develops; epithelioid cells, lymphocytes, plasma cells, and multinucleated giant cells of both the Langhans' and foreign body types surround foci of suppurative necrosis and caseation (Fig. 11–11). A primary pulmonary-lymph node complex is sometimes found, but it occurs much less frequently than in histoplasmosis capsulati.[146] In chronic pulmonary blastomycosis, fibrosis is common and is often accompanied by cavitation. Solitary residual fibrocaseous nodules or "coin lesions" are rare, and calcification of such lesions is even rarer.[126,146]

B. dermatitidis is found in both suppurative and granulomatous foci as intra- and extracellular, spherical to oval, multinucleated yeast-like cells 8–15 μm in diameter with thick, refractile, "doubly contoured" walls and single, broad-based buds (Fig. 11–12). The broad basal attachment of buds to their parent cells is diagnostic and aids in differentiating *B. dermatitidis* from yeast forms of similar size, especially *H. capsulatum* var. *duboisii*. Occasionally, very small (2–4 μm) but morphologically typical cells of *B. dermatitidis* are found in tissue[148] (Fig. 11–12C). These so-called microforms are almost always present as part of a continuous series of sizes ranging from the very small to the larger yeast forms typical of this fungus. Giant forms of *B. dermatitidis* are also rarely encountered.[149] These abnormally large yeast forms usually lack blastoconidia and measure up to 40 μm in diameter. Their morphology is otherwise similar to that of adjacent, typical blastomyces cells. Germ tubes and hyphae are rarely formed in tissue.[142,146]

Because acute pulmonary blastomycosis is often mild and self-limited, antifungal therapy is not always required.[126,150,151] However, long-term follow-up is necessary because patients may present with extrapulmonary lesions months to years after resolution of the primary infection. The chemotherapeutic agents of choice for patients with noncavitary pulmonary disease or disseminated lesions confined to the skin are amphotericin B or 2-hydroxystilbamidine, either alone or in combination.[150–152] Both of these antifungals are reported to be effective, but when cavitary lung disease or extracutaneous dissemination occurs, high-dose amphotericin B alone gives better results.[153] Another course of amphotericin B should be given if relapse occurs. Ketoconazole has been effective in patients who are not seriously ill, and this drug is recommended as a second choice.[154] Surgical excision of cavitary lung lesions may be a valuable adjunct to antifungal chemotherapy.

The mycelial form of *B. dermatitidis* can be isolated from clinical specimens on standard mycologic media at 25°C, but growth is very slow and often requires 4 weeks or more. Once isolated, subculture on blood agar at 37°C is required to convert this dimorphic fungus to the yeast form. Because *B. dermatitidis* is sensitive to cycloheximide, only culture media that are free of this antibiotic should be used. More rapid diagnosis is achieved by demonstrating classical yeast forms with broad-based buds in clinical specimens from patients with either acute or chronic infection. Diagnosis of blastomycosis by direct microscopic examination of Papanicolaou-stained smears of respiratory secretions is well documented.[155,156] When fungal elements are atypical or sparse, direct immunofluorescence using a specific conjugate directed against fungal cell wall polysaccharide antigens is invaluable for identifying *B. dermatitidis* in smears or tissue sections[42,43] (Fig. 11–12D). Serologic tests using the purified *B. dermatitidis* "A" antigen are rapid, specific, and provide presumptive evidence of infection.[157]

Cryptococcosis

Cryptococcosis is a systemic infection caused by the basidiomycetous, yeast-like fungus *Cryptococcus neoformans*.[158] This fungus is found worldwide as a ubiquitous saprophyte of soil, and it is most abundant in avian habitats, particularly those heavily contaminated with pigeon excreta.[159] Pigeons and other birds harbor the fungus in their gastrointestinal tracts, but they do not develop invasive infection.[160] The respiratory tract serves as the portal of entry for aerosolized cryptococci in almost all human infections, and there is a marked predilection for cerebromeningeal dissemination from the primary pulmonary focus, which may not be clinically apparent.[160–163] Primary cutaneous infection is rare and results from direct percutaneous inoculation.[164]

Although cryptococcosis is a cosmopolitan disease, the prevalence of clinically apparent infection appears to be highest in the United States and Australia.[158] Epidemiologic studies have shown that most infections are sporadic and occur in young and middle-aged adults; clustered outbreaks seldom occur. Although *C. neoformans* is pathogenic in apparently healthy individuals, it is more often encountered as an opportunist. Surveys indicate that between 40% and 85% of patients with this mycosis have defective cellular immunity or severe underlying disease.[160,165,166] Disseminated cryptococcosis is almost never seen in the immunocompetent host. Factors that predispose to opportunistic cryptococcosis include hematologic malignancies (especially Hodgkin's disease), long-term corticosteroid therapy, sarcoidosis, diabetes mellitus, the acquired immunodeficiency syndrome, and other conditions that are known to impair cell-mediated immunity.[160,165–169]

Unlike most invasive yeast-like fungi, *C. neoformans* is

not dimorphic. On Sabouraud's agar, typical isolates grow rapidly at 37°C or at room temperature to form moist, smooth, mucoid, convex, white to pale-yellow colonies. Microscopically, the colonies are composed of pleomorphic, spherical, thin-walled, yeast-like cells that are 2–20 μm in diameter, encapsulated, and have single buds attached to the parent cells by narrow necks. Chains of budding cells and pseudohyphae are also occasionally formed. The capsule varies in thickness from isolate to isolate, and it is best demonstrated by negative staining with India ink or by mucin stains such as mucicarmine or alcian blue. Although *C. neoformans* is the organism that usually causes cryptococcosis, two other saprophytic species—*C. albidus*[170] and *C. laurentii*[171]—have occasionally been implicated in human infections. The colonies and cells of *C. neoformans* cannot be distinguished morphologically from these ordinarily nonpathogenic species, but the latter usually do not grow at 37°C. Specific identification is based on appropriate biochemical and physiologic tests or on immunofluorescence studies.[42,43,160] The routine use of *Guizotia abyssinica* seed extract (birdseed) agar as the primary culture medium for sputum and urine specimens from patients with AIDS increases sensitivity and facilitates the isolation of *C. neoformans*.[172]

Clinically, two forms of cryptococcosis predominate: pulmonary and, via hematogenous spread from the lungs, cerebromeningeal.[160,163] Other organs less commonly involved by dissemination from a primary pulmonary focus include the skin, bones and joints, lymph nodes, kidneys, prostate, spleen, liver, and other internal organs. Skin lesions are encountered in 10%–20% of cases,[173–177] and osteolytic lesions, particularly of the pelvis, ribs, vertebrae, and long bones, occur in about 10% of cases of disseminated cryptococcosis.[160,163,165] Approximately 10% of patients with AIDS develop cryptococcal meningitis, and nearly 60% of these patients die from the infection.[178,179]

The spectrum of pulmonary involvement by *C. neoformans* includes: (1) transient, asymptomatic colonization of the tracheobronchial tree without tissue invasion; (2) self-limited or progressive pulmonary disease with or without extrapulmonary dissemination; and (3) the residual pulmonary nodule or cryptococcoma.[160,180–182] Saprophytic colonization of the respiratory tract by *C. neoformans* has been reported to occur in about 1% of patients with preexisting bronchopulmonary disease such as neoplasms, tuberculosis, chronic bronchitis, asthma, chronic obstructive pulmonary disease, and allergic bronchopulmonary aspergillosis.[182,183] Thus, a positive sputum culture alone cannot be considered diagnostic of cryptococcosis. These patients are at little or no risk of developing

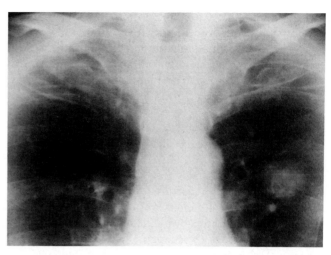

Fig. 11–13. Residual pulmonary cryptococcosis. Nodule (cryptococcoma) in left-upper lobe.

invasive cryptococcal infection, and antifungal chemotherapy is not indicated.

The majority of immunocompetent, apparently healthy patients with cryptococcosis are thought to have asymptomatic or mildly symptomatic but self-limited pulmonary infections for which antifungal therapy is not usually required.[160,182] These localized infections either resolve spontaneously or encapsulate, to be detected months to years later in chest radiographs or incidentally at autopsy as residual fibrocaseous nodules (cryptococcomas) (Fig. 11–13). These nodules are usually subpleural, discretely rounded, 0.2 to several centimeters in diameter, and noncalcified.[160,184,185] A primary pulmonary–lymph node complex develops in about 1% of patients with first-infection cryptococcosis.[186,187]

Progressive pulmonary cryptococcosis usually has a subacute or chronic course and may be associated with concomitant extrapulmonary infection. In one autopsy series, 45% of patients with cerebromeningeal cryptococcosis had active pulmonary lesions.[163] About one-third of patients with progressive pulmonary infection are asymptomatic.[160,166] The remainder usually present with chronic cough, low-grade fever, pleuritic or nonpleuritic chest pain, mucoid sputum, malaise, and weight loss. Chest radiographs may reveal alveolar and interstitial infiltrates, single or multiple nodules that resemble neoplasms, segmental or lobar consolidation, and, less commonly, hilar adenopathy and pleural effusion.[160,185,188–191] The upper lobes are reported to be more frequently involved.[190] Fibrosis and calcification are uncommon, and cavitation occurs in 10% or less of cases.[162,190] Diffuse interstitial, peribronchial, or miliary pneumonic infiltrates develop in profoundly immunodeficient patients who are exposed to a sufficiently large dose of inoculum.[162,169,190,192] Chest radiographs often reveal a diffuse interstitial or perivascular pattern that suggests hematogenous dissemination.[193] Massive pulmonary infection with rapid clinical deterioration, cerebromeningeal dissemination, and death may occur.[194] In one series, 24 of 25 immunosuppressed patients with progressive pulmonary cryptococcosis developed metastatic cerebromeningeal infection 2–20 weeks after radiographic documentation of pulmonary infection.[166]

Because the symptoms and radiographic findings in pulmonary cryptococcosis are not specific, the diagnosis must be based on the microscopic demonstration of *C. neoformans* in sputum, bronchial brushings and washings, or lung biopsy specimens (Figs. 11–14 through 11–18). Direct immunofluorescence can be used to specifically identify the fungus in smears and conventional tissue sections,[42,43] but whenever possible the diagnosis should be confirmed by isolating and identifying *C. neoformans* in culture. The latex agglutination test for capsular polysaccharide antigen is the best method available for serologic diagnosis.[195] However, sera with high titers of rheumatoid factor can give a false-positive reaction unless they are pretreated with dithiothreitol to inactivate IgM.[160]

The most common clinical presentation of cryptococcosis is cerebromeningeal. For reasons that are poorly understood, *C. neoformans* is extremely neurotropic, involving the central nervous system via hematogenous spread from a primary pulmonary focus that may not be clinically apparent. The leptomeninges are involved most often, and infection may extend into contiguous brain parenchyma to form cryptococcal "mucoid cysts" and intracerebral mass lesions. The onset of symptoms is usually insidious, and the clinical course varies from a few days to 20 years or more. In most patients, however, the course is fulminant and is almost always fatal unless promptly treated.[162,163] Presenting symptoms include fever, headache, altered consciousness, nausea, and vomiting. About 25% of patients undergo exploratory craniotomy because they have symptoms of an expanding intracranial lesion that mimic those of a neoplasm. The diagnosis of cerebromeningeal cryptococcosis is made by isolating and identifying the fungus in culture, by demonstrating typical fungal cells in an India-ink preparation of cerebrospinal fluid (CSF) or in tissue, or by detecting capsular polysaccharide antigen in the CSF by the latex agglutination test.[160,195,196] In addition to CSF, the blood, urine, and sputum should be cultured for *C. neoformans*. Only about 50% of patients with culture-proven cerebromeningeal cryptococcosis have a positive India-ink preparation.[196]

The combination of amphotericin B and 5-fluorocytosine is synergistic against *C. neoformans* in vitro, and this is the treatment of choice for the cerebromeningeal and progressive pulmonary forms of cryptococcosis.[160,182,196–198] Miconazole and ketoconazole have sometimes been effective in patients who are not seriously ill, and these chemotherapeutic agents are recommended as substitutes for amphotericin B when toxicity precludes its use.[160] Oral fluconazole, a new triazole antifungal agent, has been effective as suppressive therapy of disseminated cryptococcosis in patients with AIDS.[199] Surgical excision of chronic, localized, pulmonary lesions may be a valuable adjunct to antifungal chemotherapy.[200]

In H and E-stained tissue sections, typical cryptococci appear as pleomorphic, lightly eosinophilic, uninucleate, thin-walled, spherical, oval, and elliptical yeast forms that are 2–20 μm in diameter and surrounded by wide, clear spaces that represent unstained capsules[201,202] (see Figs. 11–14 and 11–15). Single buds attached to parent cells by narrow necks are common. In active lesions that contain myriad, rapidly dividing cryptococci, however, chains of budding cells and short hyphae may be seen (see Fig. 11–17). *C. neoformans* cells are easily demonstrated with any of the special stains for fungi. When the capsules of morphologically typical yeast forms react positively with mucin stains such as mucicarmine and alcian blue, a histologic diagnosis is established, because *Cryptococcus* spp. are the only pathogenic fungi that produce capsular material. The mucin-positive capsule often has a spinous appearance because of irregular shrinkage during tissue processing (see Fig. 11–15B).

The host response to *C. neoformans* is variable and usually depends on the degree of cell-mediated immunodeficiency, the severity of underlying disease, and whether or not the fungus is encapsulated.[160,196,203] T-cell-activated macrophages probably play a major role in preventing progressive infection.[167] In profoundly immunodeficient patients with progressive pulmonary or disseminated cryptococcosis, there is often a paucireactive pattern with little or no inflammation regardless of the organ involved (Fig. 11–15B). Cryptococci multiply profusely, displace normal tissues, and form "cystic" lesions composed of densely packed, heavily encapsulated organisms that elicit little surrounding reaction and impart a glistening appearance and slimy consistency on gross examination.[201] In the lungs, cryptococci partially or completely fill alveolar spaces, and individual and clustered organisms may be seen in thickened alveolar septa and within the lumens of septal capillaries, accompanied by a lymphocytic and histiocytic infiltrate (See Fig. 11–14).[202]

The initial pulmonary lesion in persons who do not have underlying immunodeficiency or other predisposing conditions consists of an intense, focal inflammatory

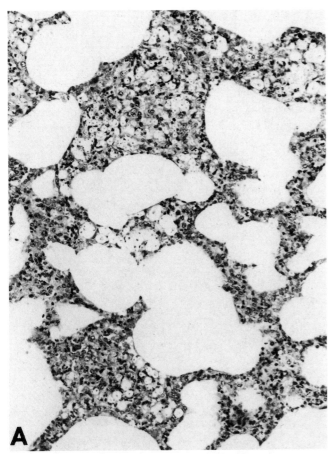

Fig. 11–14 A,B. Pulmonary cryptococcosis. **A.** Chronic interstitial inflammation and numerous interstitial *Cryptococcus neoformans* cells. ×120. **B.** Cryptococci with wide unstained capsules (*arrow*) in thickened alveolar septa of patient with acquired immunodeficiency syndrome and *Pneumocystis carinii* pneumonia (PCP). ×300.

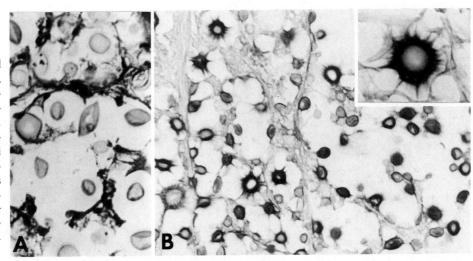

Fig. 11–15 A,B. Cryptococcal meningitis. **A.** Spherical, elliptical, and cup-shaped cryptococci surrounded by wide clear spaces representing unstained capsules. ×600. **B.** Distension of leptomeninges by myriad cryptococci with carminophilic capsules. Inflammation is minimal. Mayer's mucicarmine, ×300. *Inset:* Carminophilic capsule with radiate or spiny appearance caused by shrinkage during tissue processing. Mayer's mucicarmine, ×600.

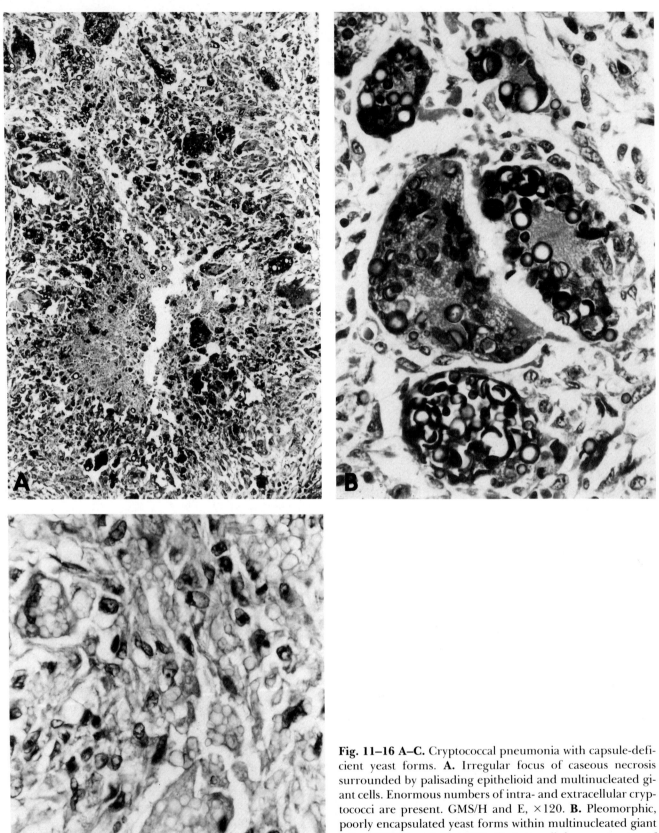

Fig. 11–16 A–C. Cryptococcal pneumonia with capsule-deficient yeast forms. **A.** Irregular focus of caseous necrosis surrounded by palisading epithelioid and multinucleated giant cells. Enormous numbers of intra- and extracellular cryptococci are present. GMS/H and E, ×120. **B.** Pleomorphic, poorly encapsulated yeast forms within multinucleated giant cells. GMS/H and E, ×480. **C.** Intracellular aggregates of cryptococci are unstained or only faintly stained with Mayer's mucicarmine procedure. ×480.

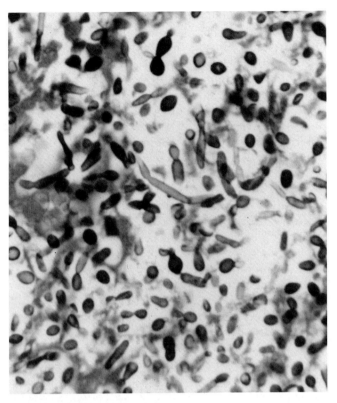

Fig. 11–17. Cryptococcal pneumonia in immunosuppressed patient. Proliferating yeast-like cells, chains of cells, germ tubes, and short hyphae elicit little or no inflammatory reaction. GMS, ×300.

reaction with suppuration and necrosis.[160] The lesion usually remains localized, and either resolves or becomes granulomatous and, in time, nodular and fibrocaseous (see Fig. 11–18A). These firm, grayish-white fibrotic nodules (cryptococcomas) with central necrosis and cavitation are similar to those that develop in residual pulmonary histoplasmosis capsulati and coccidioidomycosis, but they rarely calcify.[160,204] Smaller satellite nodules may also be present, but they are usually not connected to the bronchial tree. Cryptococci are not easily seen in these lesions with the H and E stain. However, with GMS, varying numbers of organisms are readily demonstrated within the central caseous material and at the nodule's margin within epithelioid histiocytes and multinucleated giant cells (see Fig. 11–18B,C). The cryptococci are usually capsule deficient, distorted, fragmented, unevenly stained, and small (2–4 μm in diameter); in this setting, they can be easily confused with *Histoplasma capsulatum* var. *capsulatum*.[205] Attempts to culture the fungus from residual nodules are often unsuccessful, but a presumptive histologic diagnosis can be confirmed by direct immunofluorescence.[42,43]

Pulmonary infections caused by capsule-deficient strains of cryptococci almost always occur in immunocompetent, apparently healthy subjects, and extrapulmonary dissemination has not been reported.[203,206] The host response to poorly encapsulated cryptococci is characterized by a dispersed granulomatous inflammatory reaction with suppuration, caseation, and fibrosis (see Fig. 11–16). Varying numbers of small, pleomorphic yeast forms are located within the cytoplasm of epithelioid and multinucleated giant cells. The majority of cryptococci in these lesions lack detectable capsular material with mucin stains, but a few fungal cells with attenuated and faintly mucin-positive capsules can usually be demonstrated (see Fig. 11–16C). As mentioned in the introduction, a modified Fontana–Masson stain

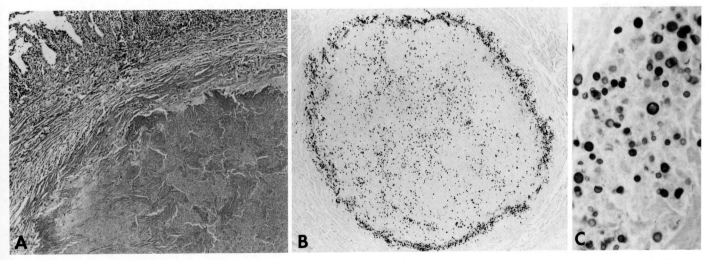

Fig. 11–18 A–C. Residual pulmonary cryptococcosis (cryptococcoma). **A.** Margin of solitary fibrocaseous nodule. ×120. **B.** Myriad yeast forms in central caseous material of nodule. Note peripheral concentration of organisms. GMS, ×48. **C.** Details of pleomorphic, poorly encapsulated cryptococci near margin of nodule. GMS, ×480.

can be used to identify poorly encapsulated cryptococci, because a positive reaction does not depend on the presence of capsular material.[34] However, the histologic diagnosis is best confirmed by isolating and identifying *C. neoformans* in culture.

Paracoccidioidomycosis

Paracoccidioidomycosis (South American blastomycosis) is a chronic progressive fungal infection that is largely confined to Latin America. The disease is caused by a single species, *Paracoccidioides brasiliensis*. Primary infection begins in the lungs; dissemination occurs eventually in most patients and may involve the mucosa of the oral cavity and upper respiratory tract and the skin, lymph nodes, liver, spleen, adrenal glands, intestines, and other organs.[207–209]

Although cases occur in Mexico and much of Central America, paracoccidioidomycosis is found more often in South America, particularly in tropical and subtropical regions of Brazil, Colombia, and Venezuela.[207] Cases diagnosed in the United States have been acquired in endemic regions of Latin America, and most of these cases represent reactivation of quiescent pulmonary disease following clinical latency of 3–20 years.[210–213] The disease occurs almost exclusively in adult males over the age of 30 years, most of whom are rural dwellers and have occupational contact with the soil.[208,214,215] Despite these epidemiologic observations, the natural habitat of *P. brasiliensis* remains largely undefined, although the fungus has been isolated from soil.[216]

P. brasiliensis is a dimorphic pathogen. In culture, the mycelial form grows slowly at 30°C to produce a white mould, whereas the yeast form grows as cerebriform colonies after 5–10 days of incubation at 35°–37°C.[207] The yeast-form colonies are composed of round or oval yeast-like cells 3–30 μm or more in diameter that produce one or more blastoconidia (buds) attached to the parent cells by narrow necks. Cells covered with multiple blastoconidia resemble "mariner's wheels" and are considered characteristic of *P. brasiliensis* in culture and in tissue.

Three clinical forms of paracoccidioidomycosis occur.[208,209] The acute (or subacute) progressive form is uncommon and occurs almost exclusively in young patients, in whom initial pulmonary infection is followed rapidly by dissemination to lymph nodes, liver, and spleen, in some cases with detectable fungemia. The chronic progressive form, occurring predominantly in older patients, follows initial infection by a latent period of many years. This is the most frequent clinical form of infection, accounting for 90% of cases in some series.[208] The disease remains clinically confined to the lungs in about 40% of these patients, whereas limited or widespread dissemination, most often to the oropharyngeal mucous membranes, occurs in the remaining 60%. The inactive or residual form follows successful treatment or natural resolution of the disease. Clinically overt pulmonary disease is present at some time during the course of infection in 85% or more of all patients.[208,214] Paracoccidioidomycosis is not considered to be an opportunistic infection, although reactivation of quiescent disease with delayed response to therapy may occur following immunosuppression.[217]

Patients usually present with symptoms referable to the respiratory tract that include cough, dyspnea, and fever.[214,218] Hemoptysis occurs in about 25% of patients, and constitutional symptoms such as fatigue, malaise, and weight loss in 40–50%. Pleuritic chest pain and pleural effusions are infrequent. Lesions of mucous membranes, found in half the patients, consist of painful ulcers involving the gingiva, palate, tongue, tonsils, nasal cavity, nasopharynx, and larynx,[211,214] often with regional lymphadenopathy. About 10% of patients present with lesions clinically restricted to the mucous membranes, and less than 5% of patients present with disseminated lymphadenopathy resembling malignant lymphoma.[214]

Chest radiographic abnormalities in paracoccidioidomycosis are protean, and none is considered pathognomonic of the disease.[219] Bilateral, symmetrical interstitial or micronodular infiltrates, often involving basal and central lung fields (Fig. 11–19), are found in 80% of patients, whereas areas of consolidation or fibrosis are found in about 50%.[214] Cavities develop in 20%–30% of patients, and residual nodules similar to those seen in histoplasmosis or coccidioidomycosis are found in about 15%,[214,218] usually without calcification. Radiographic patterns that can be confused with those of other diseases include tumorous masses or multiple nodules resembling metastatic carcinoma, bilateral juxtahilar consolidation with mediastinal adenopathy in young patients resembling lymphoma, consolidation with central cavitation resembling bacterial lung abscess, and a diffuse bilateral interstitial pattern resembling idiopathic interstitial fibrosis.[207,218–220] Late changes include fibrosis and emphysema. Radiographic changes are most often confused with those of tuberculosis[218,219] which may coexist in as many as 30% of patients with paracoccidioidomycosis.[207,215]

Pulmonary lesions are found at autopsy in 94%–100% of cases.[207,215] Most of these patients have had chronic progressive pulmonary disease of many years' duration. Externally, the lungs have a cobblestoned appearance resulting from advanced fibrosis and emphysema. Sectioned surfaces show a variety of changes

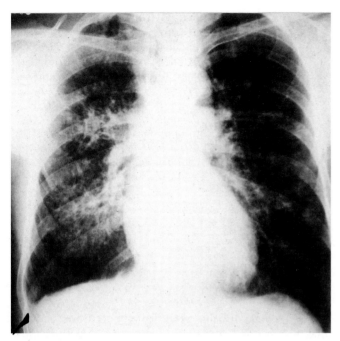

Fig. 11–19. Paracoccidioidomycosis. Bilateral diffuse reticulonodular infiltrates with parahilar accentuation. (Radiograph courtesy of Samir E. Noujaim, M.D., Department of Diagnostic Radiology, William Beaumont Hospital, Royal Oak, Michigan.)

that correlate with the patterns observed in chest radiographs. In the interstitial form, linear streaks of fibrosis radiate peripherally from the hilum.[221] This form is usually accompanied by emphysema. Microscopically, fibrosis of interalveolar and interlobular septa occurs, and remnant granulomas or multinucleated giant cells may be found in areas of fibrosis. Pulmonary blood vessels show marked intimal proliferation that is often

associated with right-ventricular enlargement. Cor pulmonale was found at autopsy in 70% of patients in Salfelder's series.[215]

Nodular lesions consist of miliary interstitial tuberculoid granulomas or larger granulomas with central caseous or suppurative necrosis and peripheral fibrosis[207] (Fig. 11–20). Cavitary lesions consist of large, centrally necrotic granulomas. Infrequently, an acute bronchopneumonic form (Fig. 11–21A) is found in patients with an acute or subacute clinical course, most often juveniles or patients treated with corticosteroids. The residual lesion consists of a solitary, circumscribed granuloma. This lesion, rarely encountered at autopsy, is similar to the residual pulmonary lesion of histoplasmosis,[222] except that calcification is uncommon. Hilar and mediastinal lymphadenopathy is found at autopsy in about 70% of patients who have pulmonary lesions.[215]

Extrathoracic lesions, manifestations of hematogenous or lymphatic dissemination, are found in the majority of patients at autopsy. Although any organ can be involved, lesions are typically found in the oropharyngeal mucosa (60% of cases), larynx (20%–40%), trachea (10%–20%), skin (50%; often contiguous with mucosal lesions), lymph nodes (90%), spleen (60%), liver (45%–65%), adrenal glands (50%), intestines (20%–30%), and kidneys (10%–15%).[207,215] Extrathoracic lesions are granulomatous, or suppurative and granulomatous, and the cutaneous and mucosal lesions are further characterized by pseudoepitheliomatous hyperplasia.

The yeast-like cells of *P. brasiliensis* are optimally identified in histologic sections with GMS, although they can often be seen in H and E-stained sections. The cells vary in diameter from 3 to 30 μm and occasionally

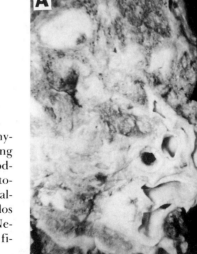
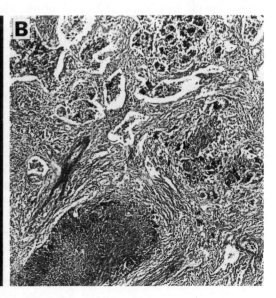

Fig. 11–20 A,B. Paracoccidioidomycosis. **A.** Sectioned surface of lung shows caseated granulomatous nodules and parahilar fibrosis. (Photograph courtesy of Karlhanns Salfelder, M.D., Universidad de los Andes, Merida, Venezuela.) **B.** Necrotic granulomas and interstitial fibrosis. GMS/H and E, ×50.

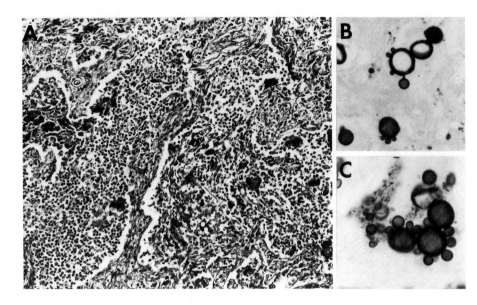

Fig. 11–21 A–C. Paracoccidioido-mycosis. **A.** Acute paracoccidioidal pneumonia. Suppurative alveolar exudate contains multinucleated giant cells and yeast forms of *Paracoccidioides brasiliensis*. GMS/H and E, ×120. **B.** Multiple-budding cells of *P. brasiliensis*. Note "teardrop" blastoconidium. GMS, ×480. **C.** Yeast forms of *P. brasiliensis* covered with round and oval blastoconidia. GMS, ×760.

attain a diameter as great as 60 μm. Larger cells have walls up to 1 μm thick. Most of the yeast-like cells in pulmonary and extrathoracic lesions are aconidiogenous or have single blastoconidia. However, unless confirmed by direct immunofluorescence, a specific histologic diagnosis of paracoccidioidomycosis is warranted only when typical multiple-budding cells are identified. Two patterns of budding are found: large "teardrop" blastoconidia attached to parent cells by narrow necks (Fig. 11–21B), and smaller, oval or tubular blastoconidia (Fig. 11–21C). Hyphae and pseudohyphae are rarely produced. "Mosaic" forms, effete cells with fractured walls, are almost constantly present in chronic pulmonary lesions; although characteristic, they are not specific for this disease. Small yeast-like cells 2–4 μm in diameter occasionally predominate in the lesions and can be mistaken for the cells of *Histoplasma capsulatum* var. *capsulatum*.[223] Confusion with *H. capsulatum* and other yeast-like fungi in tissue sections can be resolved by direct immunofluorescence or by the identification of typical multiple-budding cells and wide variation in cell size in the lesions of paracoccidioidomycosis. In active granulomatous lesions, the cells of *P. brasiliensis* are found within the cytoplasm of histiocytes and multinucleated giant cells. In necrotic granulomas, the yeast-like cells are found within necrotic material and are concentrated circumferentially at the interface between necrosis and granuloma.

The clinical diagnosis of paracoccidioidomycosis in endemic areas is strongly suggested by the combination of chronic pulmonary symptoms, chest radiographic abnormalities, and mucosal lesions of the oral cavity and upper respiratory tract.[214] Clinical confusion with Wegener's granulomatosis has been reported,[213] however, and cases with disease clinically confined to the lungs are usually mistaken for tuberculosis.[218] The clinical diagnosis can be confirmed serologically in most cases by complement fixation and immunodiffusion tests, which are sensitive to disease activity and can be used to monitor success of therapy. Direct microscopy and culture of respiratory secretions yield a positive diagnosis in up to 95% of patients.[214,224] The diagnosis is also confirmed by culture or biopsy of accessible lesions such as those of the oral mucosa, skin, and lymph nodes.

Ketoconazole is the drug of choice for treatment of most patients who have paracoccidioidomycosis.[225,226] Amphotericin B is also effective. Sulfonamides can be used alone in less advanced cases, but relapse following treatment with this drug is seen in as many as 40% of patients.[214] Initial experience with itraconazole has been promising, and this orally administered drug may soon become the treatment of choice for paracoccidioidomycosis.[227]

Sporotrichosis

Sporotrichosis is a chronic, localized or disseminated infection caused by the dimorphic fungus *Sporothrix schenckii*.[228,229] This organism is found in nature as a saprophyte of soil, wild and domesticated plants, trees, wood timbers, sphagnum moss, and other plant materials. Sporotrichosis occurs worldwide in temperate as well as tropical zones, but most documented cases have originated from the United States, South Africa, Mexico, and South America. Most infections are nonpulmonary and result from accidental percutaneous inoculation of the fungus growing on plant materials such as thorns and barbs.[228–230] The mycosis is considered to be an occupational disease, occurring most often in farmers, gardeners, forestry workers, florists, and others who are frequently exposed to plants and soil. Primary pulmonary infections are rare and result from inhalation of infectious conidia.[231–236] Cutaneous or, rarely, primary pulmonary infection can disseminate to involve the bones, joints, lungs, meninges, and other internal organs.[237–241] Patients who have serious underlying diseases or who are profoundly immunosuppressed or are alcoholics are at greatest risk of disseminated disease.[234–238]

Sporotrichosis is not contagious, but infections can result from contamination or inoculation of the broken skin with lesional exudate from humans or animals with the disease. Care should therefore be taken when handling infectious materials to prevent accidental infection.

S. schenckii grows as a yeast form in culture at 37°C and in the tissues of a living host, and as a mycelial form when cultivated at room temperature. Yeast-form colonies are moist, creamy, white, and composed of spherical, oval and elongated, single and budding yeast-like cells, 2–6 μm or more in diameter. In culture, the mycelial form develops as rapidly growing, whitish, and, in time, brownish-black moulds that have a wrinkled or folded membranous surface. Microscopically, the mycelium is composed of narrow, branched, septate, hyaline hyphae and abundant conidia formed on delicate sterigmata along the hyphae and terminally on conidiophores.

The classic clinical form of sporotrichosis, termed lymphocutaneous,[228–230] consists of a series of chronic subcutaneous nodules along the course of lymphatic drainage from a primary nodular-ulcerative skin lesion. These lesions may develop within 7–90 days or longer after a penetrating injury. In time, the lymphatic nodules ulcerate and discharge pus, but regional lymphadenopathy is usually absent. In addition to the classic lymphocutaneous form, primary cutaneous lesions without lymphatic involvement are common.

The pulmonary lesions seen in sporotrichosis sometimes develop during the course of dissemination from a primary cutaneous infection, where articular, osseous, and widespread cutaneous lesions predominate;[237,238,242] the lungs are involved secondarily in less than 20% of these cases.[238] Lesions are insidious but progressive if left untreated; even when these are treated, the prognosis is poor. Clinical findings in patients with pulmonary involvement are indistinguishable from those of other pulmonary infections causing chronic progressive granulomatous and cavitating lesions.* Radiographic findings are nonspecific and include linear streaks, patchy and fibronodular infiltrates, cavitary lesions, and rarely pleural effusions.[228,244,245]

The true prevalence of primary pulmonary sporotrichosis is unknown.[236] England and Hochholzer[234] described the histopathological findings of primary pulmonary sporotrichosis in 8 cases identified from the files of the Armed Forces Institute of Pathology (Washington, D.C.). An additional 23 cases reported in the literature during the 10-year period 1974–1983 were also reviewed. They found that primary pulmonary sporotrichosis is usually a bilateral, apical, cavitary, progressive, destructive, and debilitating infection that most often occurs in middle-aged men with a history of chronic obstructive pulmonary disease and alcoholism. Clinically, radiologically, and pathologically, the pulmonary lesions closely resemble tuberculosis and histoplasmosis capsulati. Patients usually presented with nonspecific symptoms including fever, chills, chest pain, dyspnea, hemoptysis, cough, malaise, and weight loss. Pulmonary lesions usually consisted of large, often confluent, necrotizing and nonnecrotizing granulomas that contained scattered or clustered yeast-like cells of *S. schenckii*. Granulomas were sometimes fibrotic, and two patients had solitary, peripheral, necrotizing, pulmonary nodules similar to those seen in residual pulmonary histoplasmosis capsulati. However, unlike the latter, calcification was not observed.

In a few patients with disseminated infection, a primary cutaneous or pulmonary lesion may not be evident, and the predominant manifestations are those of a suppurative arthritis, osteomyelitis, periostitis, or tenosynovitis, often involving the elbows and knees.[234–238] Without preexisting cutaneous involvement, these lesions may result from hematogenous spread of inapparent pulmonary infection. It has been speculated that many asymptomatic, immunocompetent individuals who have high antibody titers to *S. schenckii* may have had previous pulmonary exposure with infection limited to hilar lymph nodes, similar to that seen in asymptomatic histoplasmosis capsulati.[234]

The patterns of host response in localized and disseminated sporotrichosis are similar.[228–230] Skin lesions show pseudoepitheliomatous hyperplasia and epidermal ulceration, and a mixed suppurative and granulomatous inflammatory reaction in the dermis and subcutaneous tissue. In the lung, caseating granulomas may develop peripheral fibrosis and subsequently cavitate (Fig. 11–22A), but calcification has not been reported.

Because of their scarcity, *S. schenckii* cells are difficult to detect in H and E-stained tissue sections. They can usually be demonstrated in replicate sections stained with GMS, however, in which they appear as spherical, oval, or elongated (cigar-shaped) single or budding

---

*References: 231, 232, 237, 238, 243.

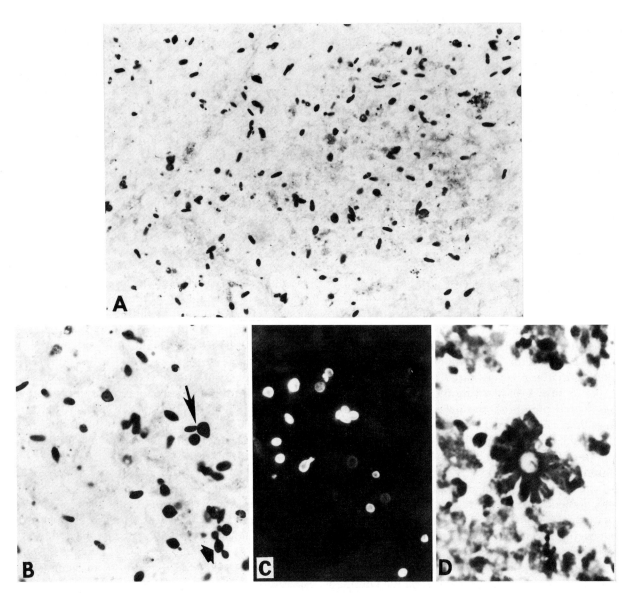

Fig. 11–22 A–D. Pulmonary sporotrichosis. **A.** Spherical, oval, and elongated (cigar-shaped) yeast-like cells in caseated granuloma. GMS, ×480. **B.** *Sporothrix schenckii* cells with elongated (*arrow*) and multiple (*blunt arrow*) buds attached to parent cells by narrow bases. GMS, ×760. **C.** Individual and clustered yeast forms in fibrotic granuloma. Direct immunofluorescence, ×680. **D.** Asteroid body in suppurative center of granuloma. ×700.

yeast-like cells 2–6 μm or more in diameter (Figs. 11–22A,B). Some of the yeast-like cells produce elongated "teardrop" or "pipestem" buds, and multiple budding is occasionally seen. The yeast-like cells may be coated with eosinophilic, refractile, radially oriented Splendore–Hoeppli material to form asteroid bodies that are usually located in microabscesses or suppurative centers of granulomas[228,230,246] (Fig. 11–22D). Asteroid bodies are not often found in the lesions of sporotrichosis, and when present are not pathognomonic for this disease, since Splendore–Hoeppli material may be seen surrounding parasite ova, foreign objects such as silk sutures, other species of fungi, and

actinomycotic and botryomycotic granules.[3,23,33,51] *S. schenckii* rarely forms hyphae in tissue, and intracavitary pulmonary fungus balls are also unusual.[233,247,248]

Diagnosis is established by isolating the fungus from clinical specimens or by direct immunofluorescence of *S. schenckii* in smears and tissue sections[249] (Fig. 11–22C). Serology is also a useful adjunct to diagnosis. The tube agglutination and latex agglutination tests are considered to be the most reliable and are of particular value for the diagnosis of extracutaneous infections.[24,25] However, low titers do not exclude invasive infection.

The prognosis is good in the cutaneous and lymphocutaneous forms of sporotrichosis, where oral saturated potassium iodide is the treatment of choice. This drug has also been given to patients with disseminated infection, but relapses may occur following initial clinical improvement.[237,238,250] Oral itraconazole has been shown to be an adequate alternative to iodide treatment in cutaneous and lymphocutaneous infections.[251] Amphotericin B is the preferred treatment for disseminated sporotrichosis, although favorable responses have sometimes been attained with miconazole, ketoconazole, and itraconazole.[234–238,250–254] However, the prognosis of disseminated infection is poor even when treated; in one series, 11 of 37 patients with disseminated sporotrichosis died despite treatment.[238] Chronic cavitary pulmonary sporotrichosis is usually refractory to antifungal chemotherapy, but can be cured when chemotherapy is combined with surgical resection.[255]

Torulopsosis

Torulopsosis is a rare opportunistic infection caused by *Torulopsis glabrata*, a small yeast-like fungus of the family Cryptococcaceae that has very low virulence.[256,257] This organism occurs as a saprophyte in nature, but it is also part of the normal microflora of the oropharynx, the skin, and the respiratory, urogenital, and gastrointestinal tracts. The recently proposed merger of the genera *Torulopsis* and *Candida* has now been rejected because members of these two groups are taxonomically distinct.[258,259] Unlike *Candida* spp., *T. glabrata* reproduces only by budding and does not form hyphae and pseudohyphae in culture or in tissue. On standard media, colonies are creamy white, smooth, soft, and glistening, and may become grayish-brown with age. Microscopically, they are composed entirely of yeast-like cells 2–5 μm in diameter with single buds. *T. glabrata* can be further differentiated from the *Candida* spp. by its failure to utilize potassium nitrate and by its pattern of fermentation and assimilation reactions against a battery of sugars.[260]

T. glabrata is responsible for a wide spectrum of disease in humans, including fungemia,[261–267] funguria,[268,269] pyelonephritis,[268,270] pneumonitis,[271–273] osteomyelitis,[274–276] endocarditis,[277,278] cholecystitis,[279] enterocolitis,[280] endophthalmitis,[280] meningoencephalitis,[281] wound infection,[282] ulcerative vaginitis,[283] and ulcerative esophagitis.[284] Surveys indicate that 40%–50% of *T. glabrata* infections are transient, asymptomatic, self-limited fungemias and fungurias without tissue invasion.[256,257,265,267] Most of these are nosocomial, and underlying disease, particularly neoplasia and bacterial sepsis, are the most important causes of death. Common predisposing factors in patients who develop *T. glabrata* fungemia or funguria include intravenous catheters, indwelling urethral catheters, prolonged antibiotic therapy, abdominal or urologic surgery, appendiceal abscesses, poorly controlled diabetes mellitus, malnutrition, drug abuse, and systemic therapy with corticosteroids and cytostatic drugs. Hematogenous seeding of *T. glabrata* occurs via contaminated catheter tips and intravenous lines, open wounds, and sites of endogenous colonization. The source of fungemia is often unexplained, but patients usually improve clinically once predisposing factors are eliminated.

Autopsy surveys indicate that lesions in disseminated torulopsosis are most often found in the kidneys, gastrointestinal tract, peritoneum, and heart. Although pulmonary lesions are rare, several case reports have documented the occurrence of *T. glabrata* pneumonitis in patients with severe myelosuppression and hematologic neoplasia.[271,272] In these cases, the pneumonitis was considered to be either primary or secondary to fungemia. Symptoms usually included a nonproductive cough, fever to 103°F, dyspnea, fatigue, and rales. Chest radiographs often revealed patchy or nodular infiltrates, and *T. glabrata* was demonstrated in and cultured from either transtracheal aspirates, endobronchial brushings, or lung biopsies. The pulmonary infiltrates usually resolved without antifungal therapy within 2–4 weeks after bone marrow recovery, but if severe myelosuppression persisted, rapidly progressive pulmonary infection with fungemia and widespread dissemination was the rule. Transfusions of granulocytes were usually ineffective in this setting, and infection was almost always fatal despite aggressive treatment with amphotericin B. In one case,[272] abundant fungal cells were present in the lungs at autopsy.

T. glabrata pneumonitis was also described in a malnourished woman who was neither leukopenic nor diabetic.[273] Chest radiographs revealed a dense infiltrate in the right-upper lobe. When she was given frequent feedings of a high-calorie isotonic diet, the pneumonitis resolved without antifungal therapy. In this case, the respiratory tract was apparently the primary focus of infection, which was confined to the lungs; repeated blood cultures during her illness were negative.

The host response in *T. glabrata* pneumonitis varies from little or no inflammation to suppurative and necrotizing bronchopneumonia with abscess formation[256,257,271,272] (Fig. 11–23A). Scattered yeast-like cells can be seen in alveolar spaces, bronchial lumens, and preexisting cavities; in most instances, the fungus does not invade the pulmonary parenchyma. In smears and tissue sections, *T. glabrata* appears as spherical to oval, nonencapsulated, intra- and extracellular yeast-like cells 2–5 μm in diameter with single buds (Fig.

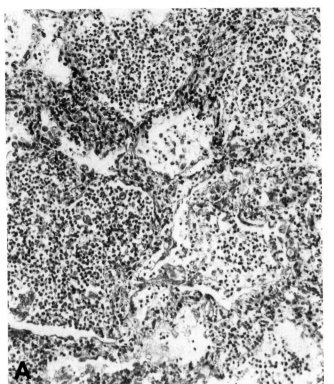

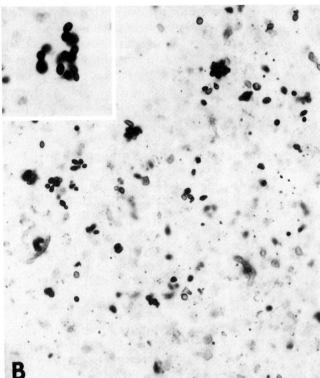

Fig. 11–23 A,B. Torulopsosis. **A.** Acute bronchopneumonia with suppurative alveolar exudate. ×120. **B.** Individual and clustered yeast forms of *Torulopsis glabrata* that closely resemble those of *Histoplasma capsulatum* var. *capsulatum*. GMS, ×480. *Inset:* Details of single and budding yeast forms. GMS, ×760.

11–23B). The cells of this fungus resemble those of *Histoplasma capsulatum* var. *capsulatum*, especially when they are clustered within macrophages. However, *T. glabrata* is more pleomorphic, slightly larger, and entire fungal cells are amphophilic with H and E. Budding is more frequent, and buds are sometimes attached to parent cells by a broader base. Definitive identification is accomplished by direct immunofluorescence of *T. glabrata* in smears and tissue sections and by culture.[257,285]

The treatment of choice in severe pulmonary and disseminated infections is amphotericin B.[257,272,286] Favorable responses have also been achieved with 5-fluorocytosine, miconazole, ketoconazole, and fluconazole.[281,282,287] Elimination of predisposing factors sometimes results in rapid improvement without specific treatment.

Candidiasis

Candidiasis comprises a group of superficial, mucocutaneous, and systemic opportunistic mycoses of cosmopolitan distribution caused by yeast-like fungi of the genus *Candida*. Candidiasis, the most frequently encountered human opportunistic mycosis, accounts for about 50% of fungal infections among immunocompromised patients[14,288,289] and up to 75% or more of such infections in patients with acute leukemia, lymphoma, or solid tumors.[290,291] Although the genus *Candida* contains more than 100 different species, only 7 have been isolated from human tissues or fluids with sufficient frequency to be considered pathogenic.[292] *C. albicans*, by far the most common isolant, is implicated in 70%–80% of cases of systemic candidiasis. *C. tropicalis* is the next most common pathogen, and the remaining occasional isolants include *C. parapsilosis*, *C. krusei*, *C. pseudotropicalis*, *C. guilliermondii*, *C. lusitaniae*, and *C. stellatoidea*.[290,293–298] *Torulopsis glabrata*, tentatively merged into the genus *Candida* as *C. glabrata*, is now considered taxonomically distinct[259] and is not included in the present discussion. *Candida* spp. and *T. glabrata* together account for 98% of all yeasts isolated from clinical specimens of cancer patients.[295]

C. albicans constitutes part of the normal microflora of the mouth and oropharynx, upper respiratory tract, digestive tract, and vagina, but is seldom isolated from environmental sources;[299,300] it is therefore considered a true endogenous pathogen. The other *Candida* spp. can be isolated from both human and environmental sources. The *Candida* spp. grow rapidly on standard mycologic media at room temperature or at 37°C, producing smooth or wrinkled, creamy white, yeast-like colonies. Although *C. albicans* forms germ tubes and terminal chlamydoconidia under certain conditions of growth, the other *Candida* spp. do not. However, occasional strains of *C. stellatoidea* (considered by some to be a variety of *C. albicans*) and *C. tropicalis* also produce chlamydoconidia.[300] Colonies of *C. albicans* are composed of spheroidal to oval yeast-like cells 5–7 μm in diameter, pseudohyphae (chains of elongated yeast-like cells), and septate hyphae 3–5 μm in width. The thick-walled chlamydoconidia, 8–12 μm in diameter, are spheroidal. *Candida* spp. can be further identified by their patterns of carbohydrate fermentation and assimilation.[300]

Normal skin and mucosal surfaces are an effective barrier against invasive candidiasis, and phagocytic leukocytes, particularly neutrophils, are the most important line of defense once mucosal penetration has occurred.[9,301,302] Humoral factors play a less important role in host defense, although IgG and complement components enhance phagocytosis of *Candida* spp. Defective cell-mediated immunity may result in severe, progressive, but localized mucocutaneous infection as seen in chronic mucocutaneous candidiasis, or in invasive bronchopulmonary candidiasis as seen in some patients with the acquired immunodeficiency syndrome.[303]

Factors that impair these host defense mechanisms predispose to invasive candidiasis. Thus, "barrier breaks" such as trauma, burns, peritoneal dialysis,[300] gastrointestinal surgery,[288,293,294,297] mucosal ulcers,[9,304] and indwelling venous catheters* permit submucosal invasion or provide direct access to the vascular system. Neutropenia induced by acute leukemia and cytotoxic chemotherapy,[291,296,307] and defective leukocyte function caused by corticosteroid therapy,[293,307] impair phagocytosis and killing of the *Candida* spp. Broad-spectrum antibiotic therapy promotes local overgrowth and mucosal colonization by *C. albicans*.[296,297] Broad-spectrum antibiotics, corticosteroids, and neutropenia are a potent predisposing combination[308] and account in part for the high incidence of candidiasis in patients treated for acute leukemia and lymphoma. Other predisposing factors include parenteral hyperalimentation,[288,300] prematurity,[305] diabetes mellitus,[300,304] and associated bacterial infection.[290] Pulmonary candidiasis occurs rarely in patients who have no recognized underlying illness or predisposition to infection.[309–311]

The clinical features of pulmonary candidiasis are nonspecific and resemble those of other opportunistic

*References: 288, 290, 293, 297, 304, 305, 306.

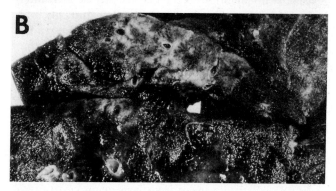

Fig. 11–24 A,B. Endobronchial pulmonary candidiasis. **A.** Diffuse bilateral alveolar infiltrates, predominantly perihilar. (Radiograph courtesy of Harry D. Tabor, M.D., Department of Diagnostic Radiology, William Beaumont Hospital, Royal Oak, Michigan.) **B.** Sectioned surface of lung shows bronchocentric foci of consolidation.

pulmonary infections. Typically, patients who are being treated for severe underlying disease develop persistent fever unresponsive to broad-spectrum antibiotic therapy, and exhibit new or changing pulmonary infiltrates on chest radiographs.[289,296,308] Some patients may develop cough and dyspnea.[290,300]

Radiographic abnormalities are correspondingly nonspecific[305,312,313] and can often be attributed to concurrent infection, hemorrhage, or underlying disease and its treatment.[307,314] Patterns of radiographic abnormality correlate with the route of pulmonary infection. Thus, patients with endobronchial pulmonary candidiasis develop patchy or diffuse bilateral areas of airspace consolidation (Fig. 11–24A) that are indistinguishable from bronchopneumonia resulting from other causes.* Patients with hematogenous pul-

*References: 305, 312, 313, 315, 316.

monary candidiasis develop bilateral miliary nodules several millimeters to 1 cm in size.[312,313] Embolic pulmonary candidiasis, virtually restricted to children, produces a pattern consistent with pulmonary infarction.[305] Abnormalities that can almost always be attributed to concurrent disease rather than to candidiasis include hilar or mediastinal lymphadenopathy, pleural effusion, large mass-like opacities, infarct patterns in adults, and cavities.[312–314,316,317] Patients with pulmonary candidiasis often have concurrent bacterial or fungal infections, pulmonary edema, hemorrhage, infarcts, aspiration pneumonia, or diffuse alveolar damage, which could also account for many of the observed radiographic abnormalities.[305,307,314,318] As many as 50% of patients with histologically documented pulmonary candidiasis have no demonstrable radiographic abnormalities, which can usually be attributed to agranulocytosis, small lesion size, or technically inferior (portable) films.[296,312,313,318] Thus, the radiographic diagnosis of pulmonary candidiasis is neither specific nor very sensitive.

The laboratory diagnosis of pulmonary and disseminated candidiasis is likewise fraught with difficulties. Because the *Candida* spp. constitute part of the normal human microflora and readily colonize mucosal surfaces, positive cultures of sputum, bronchoscopy specimens, urine, and feces are usually diagnostically inconclusive.[299,307,314,319] Blood cultures, widely considered to be diagnostically insensitive, are negative in 50%–60% of patients with disseminated candidiasis.[290,319,320] A positive blood culture may indicate only transient catheter-associated candidemia and does not prove that invasive infection is present. Problems with both false-positive and false-negative results limit the usefulness of serologic tests for antibodies against *Candida* spp.,[290,301,319,321] and serologic tests for candidal antigens are highly specific but insensitive.[290,319,322] Therefore, conclusive evidence of pulmonary candidiasis requires histologic demonstration of pulmonary parenchymal invasion[301,308,318] or isolation in culture of a *Candida* sp. from material obtained by transthoracic needle aspiration of a pulmonary lesion.[307,311]

The antifungal chemotherapeutic agent of choice for immunocompromised patients with systemic candidiasis is amphotericin B, alone or in combination with the synergistic drug flucytosine.[301,323] Survival depends on early diagnosis, removal of indwelling catheters, and control or reversal of the underlying disease, particularly granulocytopenia.[290,301] Antifungal chemotherapy has had little impact on survival in some series, because the lesions of candidiasis alone rarely involve enough parenchyma to compromise pulmonary function.[296,307]

The macroscopic features of pulmonary candidiasis at autopsy are largely determined by the route of infection.[304–307,314] Endobronchial infection caused by aspiration of *Candida* spp. from a focus of infection in the oropharynx or upper respiratory tract produces patchy, asymmetric areas of consolidation with a predilection for the lower lobes (Fig. 11–24B). Extensive pulmonary hemorrhage is associated with this form of infection in about 50% of cases,[307] but extrapulmonary candidal lesions are infrequent. When aspiration occurs as a preterminal event, the lesions are grossly inconspicuous and clinically insignificant. Hematogenous seeding of the lungs produces random, bilateral, more or less symmetrically distributed miliary or nodular lesions. This form of infection, a manifestation of dissemination, is frequently associated with extrapulmonary candidal lesions in the kidneys, liver, spleen, and myocardium; the gastrointestinal tract and indwelling venous catheters are the usual portals of entry. The hematogenous nodules, termed "target lesions" by Myerowitz and coworkers[304,314] are round and well circumscribed, 2–4 mm in diameter, and have yellow or gray granular centers with peripheral hemorrhagic rims. Abscesses several centimeters in diameter are occasionally found. Gross embolic spread to the lungs in about 50% of infants with fatal pulmonary candidiasis was reported in one series.[305] In this form of infection, the pulmonary arterial tree is seeded with emboli originating in central or peripheral veins or the right atrium; all such patients have indwelling venous catheters. Embolic pulmonary candidiasis produces peripheral hemorrhagic infarcts that may undergo cavitation. Pulmonary infarcts are distinctly unusual in adult patients with disseminated candidiasis, whereas they are the pathologic hallmark of pulmonary infection caused by *Aspergillus* spp. and the zygomycetes.

Microscopically, the lesions of invasive and disseminated candidiasis contain budding yeast-like cells, pseudohyphae, and occasional true hyphae. All the pathogenic *Candida* spp. have a similar appearance in histologic sections and therefore cannot be identified as to species by their morphology. The yeast-like cells are 2–6 μm in diameter, spheroidal to oval, rather uniform, and may produce oval blastoconidia. Pseudohyphae are composed of chains of elongated yeast-like cells attached end to end, whereas true hyphae, which are 3–5 μm in width, are septate and tubular or filamentous. Pseudohyphae can usually be distinguished from true hyphae by the presence (in the former) of constrictions at points of attachment between adjacent cells that give the pseudohyphal segments an elliptical contour (Fig. 11–25A). True hyphae are narrower than pseudohyphae and have parallel contours without constrictions at sites of septation (Fig. 11–25B). The distinction is at times difficult and somewhat arbitrary, but it has little

Fig. 11–25 A,B. Pulmonary candidiasis. **A.** Blastoconidia and pseudohyphae of *Candida albicans*. GMS, ×480. **B.** Septate hyphae and blastoconidia of *C. albicans*. GMS, ×480.

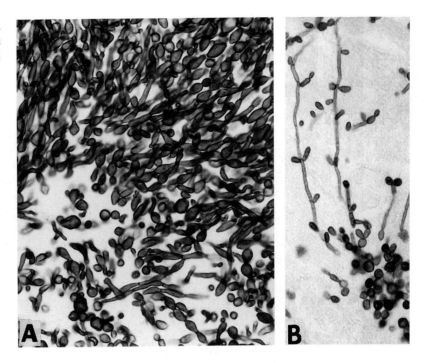

practical significance. Germinating cells are rarely found in histologic sections, but chlamydoconidia are either not produced in tissue or cannot be recognized as such. The various developmental forms of the *Candida* spp. are hyaline or weakly basophilic and, while often visible in sections stained with H and E, are demonstrated best with special stains such as GMS or PAS.

The cellular reaction to invasive infection by the *Candidia* spp. in the nongranulocytopenic host is characteristically neutrophilic. Yeast-like cells and mycelial elements may be diffusely distributed throughout areas of acute suppurative inflammation or may form compact radiating microcolonies similar to those seen in invasive pulmonary aspergillosis. In the granulocytopenic host, cellular reaction is minimal, and the lesions are mainly characterized by bland coagulative necrosis and hemorrhage.[304,307,324,325] A component of granulomatous inflammation may be seen in patients with chronic, indolent infections or in those who have been treated with antifungal chemotherapy.[304,315]

The microscopic pattern and distribution of the pulmonary lesions are also largely determined by the route of infection.[304–307,314,318] By the endobronchial route, yeast-like cells and mycelial elements proliferate within the conducting airways and extend out of bronchiolar lumens and through the walls of distal bronchi into peripheral and peribronchial alveolar spaces (Fig. 11–26A). Foreign material in these lesions, particularly food particles, provides additional evidence of aspiration. Because endobronchial candidiasis is frequently a preterminal infection, invasion of small veins and lym-

phatics by mycelial elements is unusual. Occasionally, however, such lesions may serve as a primary site for hematogenous dissemination, in which case microscopic vascular invasion is conspicuous.[318]

The "target lesions" of hematogenous pulmonary candidiasis, angiocentric rather than bronchocentric, are nodular infarcts composed of a central core of necrotic pulmonary parenchyma, yeast-like cells, and mycelial elements surrounded by an intermediate zone of polymorphonuclear neutrophils and a peripheral ring of parenchymal hemorrhage (Fig. 11–26B). A necrotic arteriole or small artery can usually be found within or at the edge of such lesions. With time, these lesions may enlarge and coalesce to produce necrotic abscesses, which may then be indistinguishable from the lesions produced by endobronchial infection. The embolic lesions in infants are characterized by thromboembolic occlusion of medium-sized or small pulmonary arteries (Fig. 11–26C) and hemorrhagic infarction of distal pulmonary parenchyma. The thromboemboli contain yeast-like cells and mycelial elements that penetrate through arterial walls into the infarcts and adjacent alveolar spaces. Acute suppurative inflammation may then produce liquefaction and cavitation of the infarcts. As a rule, the *Candida* spp. do not invade large arteries and veins in adults.

The results of a recent immunohistochemical study, applicable to biopsy specimens, suggested that invasive candidal pneumonia can be distinguished from noninvasive aspiration, colonization, or specimen contamination by *C. albicans* on the basis of the character, extent,

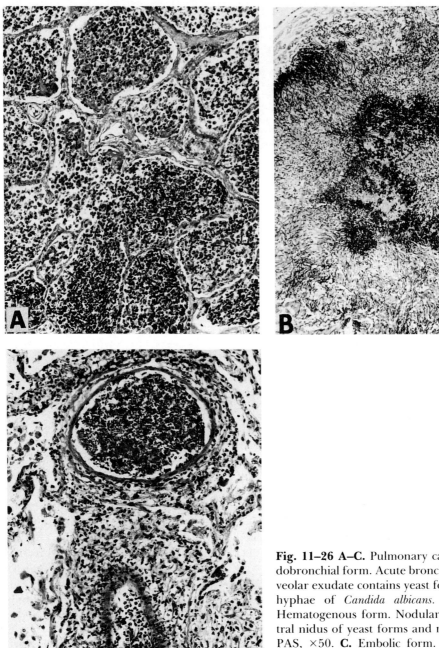

Fig. 11–26 A–C. Pulmonary candidiasis. A. Endobronchial form. Acute bronchopneumonia; alveolar exudate contains yeast forms and pseudohyphae of *Candida albicans*. PAS, ×120. B. Hematogenous form. Nodular infarct with central nidus of yeast forms and mycelial elements. PAS, ×50. C. Embolic form. Candidal thromboembolus with secondary necrotizing vasculitis, ×120.

and distribution of candidal antigens in histologic sections.[46] While intriguing, this conclusion needs confirmation. At present, the demonstration of typical budding yeast-like cells and mycelial elements in a lung biopsy specimen from a compromised patient with clinical and cultural evidence of candidiasis must be regarded as diagnostic of invasive infection.

The *Candida* spp. as a group can easily be distinguished from most other pathogens in histologic sections if both budding yeast-like cells of the appropriate

size and mycelial elements (pseudohyphae and hyphae) are present. Other pathogens such as *Sporothrix schenckii, Blastomyces dermatitidis, Cryptococcus neoformans,* and *Histoplasma capsulatum,* the tissue forms of which are yeast-like, rarely produce pseudohyphae or hyphae in tissues. *Torulopsis glabrata,* a yeast-like fungus closely related to *Candida* spp., never produces mycelial elements. Conversely, mycelial pathogens belonging to the genera *Aspergillus, Fusarium,* and *Pseudallescheria* do not produce yeast forms in tissues. The *Trichosporon* spp.

may be difficult to distinguish from the *Candida* spp. because both produce yeast-like cells and mycelial elements. However, the yeast forms of *Trichosporon* spp. are slightly larger and more pleomorphic than those of *Candida* spp. and are often accompanied by rectangular arthroconidia that facilitate the morphologic distinction. Poorly pigmented strains of the dematiaceous fungi that cause phaeohyphomycosis can also be mistaken for *Candida* spp. in some circumstances. Therefore, it is imperative to submit fresh tissue, if available, for cultural confirmation of the histologic diagnosis. *Candida* spp. can be identified generically in deparaffinized sections of formalin-fixed tissue by direct immunofluorescence[326] or by immunoperoxidase staining.[46]

Aspergillosis

The spectrum of pulmonary aspergillosis includes (1) a variety of allergic reactions in hypersensitized hosts; (2) saprophytic colonization of preexisting cavities in patients with normal immunity; (3) noninvasive or superficially invasive necrotizing tracheobronchitis; (4) chronic progressive and destructive pulmonary infection in mildly compromised patients, clinically resembling chronic tuberculosis or histoplasmosis; and (5) rapidly progressive, invasive infection in severely immunosuppressed patients, particularly those with acute leukemia.

Although these various forms of disease are often compartmentalized as discrete clinicopathologic entities, a degree of overlap actually exists among them.[327,328] Allergic aspergillosis, which includes the syndrome of allergic bronchopulmonary aspergillosis, eosinophilic pneumonia, mucoid impaction of proximal bronchi, bronchocentric granulomatosis with asthma,[329] and perhaps some cases designated as necrotizing sarcoid granulomatosis,[330] is discussed in Chapter 16; microgranulomatous hypersensitivity pneumonitis, caused by *Aspergillus clavatus* (malt workers' lung), is discussed in Chapter 18. The present discussion covers the colonizing and invasive forms of pulmonary aspergillosis.

The aspergilli are second only to *Candida* spp. as agents of opportunistic fungal infection, accounting for about 15%–30% of such infections in patients with malignant diseases.[13,14,288] However, the aspergilli are the most common etiologic agents of clinically significant pulmonary mycotic disease.[331,332] *Aspergillus* spp. are cosmopolitan moulds and are ubiquitous within the environment. They can be isolated from soil, decaying vegetation, and organic debris, and their conidia are constantly present in ambient air.[333] Although hundreds of *Aspergillus* spp. are recognized, only about 10 are authentic agents of human disease. *Aspergillus fumi-*

gatus, *A. flavus*, and *A. niger* are the most frequently isolated pathogens, and *A. clavatus*, *A. glaucus*, *A. nidulans*, *A. niveus*, *A. restrictus*, and *A. terreus* are occasional pathogens.[333–341] *A. fumigatus* is by far the most common agent of invasive pulmonary aspergillosis and, together with *A. niger*, accounts for most cases of intracavitary aspergilloma. The pathogenic aspergilli are thermotolerant and grow rapidly on standard mycologic media free of cycloheximide. Species identification is based on colony morphology, pigmentation, and the morphology of the conidial heads and conidia.[333,342] The common pathogenic species can be accurately identified in most clinical laboratories.

The aspergilli readily colonize the obstructed bronchial tree, where they proliferate as harmless saprophytes. Obstructive bronchial colonization occurs most frequently in patients with cystic fibrosis and occasionally in patients with bronchial asthma, chronic bronchitis, bronchiectasis, or neoplasm.[343] Colonization produces no symptoms, and patients are recognized incidentally by isolation of an *Aspergillus* sp. from sputum cultures. Specific antifungal therapy is unnecessary. Such patients may rarely develop specific antibodies and symptoms of allergic bronchopulmonary aspergillosis.

An aspergilloma, or fungus ball, develops when aspergilli colonize a preformed pulmonary cavity. Aspergillomas complicate a variety of chronic cavitary lung diseases, most frequently tuberculosis and sarcoidosis (see Chapter 10). In one survey, 11% of patients with residual tuberculous cavities at least 2.5 cm in diameter had radiographic evidence of aspergilloma.[344] Other diseases that predispose to the formation of aspergilloma include histoplasmosis, asbestosis, lung abscess, pulmonary infarct, bronchial cyst, ankylosing spondylitis, bullous emphysema, bronchiectasis, and necrotic neoplasms.[343,345–349] Fungus balls may also develop in the cavitary infarcts of invasive aspergillosis,[350,351] and they occur in about 40% of cases of chronic necrotizing pulmonary aspergillosis.[337] Although sometimes asymptomatic for years, about 75% of patients eventually develop hemoptysis,[346,348] and about 5% of patients die of uncontrollable hemorrhage.[343]

The clinical diagnosis of aspergilloma is based on the triad of hemoptysis, positive serology, and radiographic demonstration of an intracavitary mass. Serum precipitins are present in 92%–100% of patients, but culture of respiratory secretions yields an *Aspergillus* sp. in only about half.[343,348,352] Radiographs typically disclose a thick-walled cavity 3–5 cm in diameter, usually in an upper lobe or apex, that contains an opaque, rounded mass surrounded by a crescent of air (Monod's sign)[348,353] (Fig. 11–27). The adjacent pleura is usually

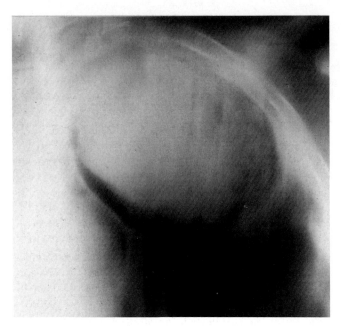

Fig. 11–27. Aspergilloma. Tomogram shows large intracavitary mass separated from cavity wall along inferior margin by crescent of air. (Radiograph courtesy of Harry D. Tabor, M.D., Department of Diagnostic Radiology, William Beaumont Hospital, Royal Oak, Michigan.)

thickened, and positional movement of the fungus ball can be demonstrated with decubitus films. Severe or recurrent hemoptysis is an indication for surgical resection. Direct instillation of amphotericin B into the cavity may benefit some symptomatic patients who are not surgical candidates, but the effectiveness of this form of therapy remains unproven. About 10% of fungus balls disappear spontaneously.

Necrotizing pseudomembranous bronchial aspergillosis and chronic necrotizing pulmonary aspergillosis are transitional diseases that occupy an intermediate position in the spectrum between colonizing and invasive forms of aspergillosis. Both occur in mildly compromised patients and are characterized by limited invasiveness. Bronchial aspergillosis develops in patients with mild leukopenia, some of whom have been treated with corticosteroids or antineoplastic drugs.[334,354] A case rapidly terminating in respiratory failure has been reported recently in a hemophiliac with the acquired immunodeficiency syndrome.[355] However, recovery from this superficially invasive infection following antifungal chemotherapy has also been reported.[356] Symptoms include dyspnea, wheezing, and nonproductive cough. Mycelium proliferates extensively throughout the bronchial tree and causes mucosal erosion or ulceration. Denuded mucosal surfaces are covered by pseudomembrane, and bronchial lumens may become plugged by casts composed of mucus and compacted mycelium.[357] Sputum cultures are rarely positive.[334]

Chronic necrotizing pulmonary aspergillosis (CNPA) is a progressive, locally destructive form of aspergillosis that occurs in mildly compromised patients, most of whom have underlying noncavitary structural lung disease.[337] It is closely related if not identical to "semi-invasive" pulmonary aspergillosis described by Gefter et al.[358] and clinically resembles chronic tuberculosis or histoplasmosis capsulati. Underlying diseases or conditions associated with CNPA include chronic obstructive pulmonary disease, inactive mycobacterial infection, sarcoidosis, pneumoconiosis, rheumatoid arthritis, ankylosing spondylitis, postradiation fibrosis, diabetes mellitus, alcoholism, anergy, and previous pulmonary resection, but about 25% of patients have no recognized predisposition. Most patients are middle aged, and about 25% have recently been treated with low-dose corticosteroids.[359] Fever, productive cough, weight loss, and malaise are the predominant symptoms. More than 90% of patients have serum precipitins against *Aspergillus* antigens and a positive culture of respiratory secretions for an *Aspergillus* sp., and most have a normal leukocyte count. Chest radiographs disclose parenchymal infiltrates and thick-walled cavities involving the upper lobes or superior segments of the lower lobes, often associated with pleural thickening. About 40% of patients develop fungus balls in these newly formed cavities. Therapy consists of surgical resection or antifungal chemotherapy with external drainage of cavities. The duration of the disease ranges from several months to several years. About 80% of patients survive the chronic necrotizing pulmonary form, although many are left with residual fibrocavitary disease. Systemic dissemination does not occur in this form.

Invasive pulmonary aspergillosis (IPA) is the most familiar and most devastating form of aspergillosis. With rare exception, it is a fulminant and highly lethal opportunistic infection of severely compromised patients. Experimental studies indicate that phagocytic leukocytes are the single most important line of host defense against invasive aspergillosis. Mononuclear phagocytes ingest and kill the conidia of *Aspergillus*, whereas polymorphonuclear neutrophils damage the hyphal forms, probably by nonphagocytic microbicidal mechanisms.[360,361] Thus, it is not surprising that profound granulocytopenia (<500/mm^3) and treatment for hematologic malignancy, particularly acute leukemia, are major risk factors for the development of IPA.[334,362–366] Both experimental evidence[360,361,367] and clinical observations[334,362–364] implicate corticosteroid therapy as another major predisposing factor. Other factors that are frequently associated with IPA include cytotoxic chemotherapy, broad-spectrum antibiotic therapy, concurrent or recent bacterial infection, immunosuppression following organ transplantation, and exposure to large doses of aerosolized conidia.* Some, such as antibiotic therapy, are undoubtedly epiphenomena related to treatment of underlying or concurrent disease rather than independent risk factors. In a case-control study, Gerson et al.[366] demonstrated that persistent granulocytopenia is the only independent risk factor that predisposes to IPA in patients with acute leukemia. Humoral and cellular immune mechanisms appear to play a minor role in host defense against invasive aspergillosis,[334,361] and the disease occurs rarely in the absence of identifiable predisposing factors.[369,370]

The symptoms of IPA, like those of many other opportunistic pneumonias, are nonspecific. Patients typically develop fever unresponsive to broad-spectrum antibiotics and new or changing pulmonary infiltrates in the setting of neutropenia and corticosteroid therapy.[289,327,362] Nonproductive cough and dyspnea occur less often. The sudden onset of pleuritic chest pain and hemoptysis, symptoms suggesting acute pulmonary infarction, should raise suspicion of IPA or other angioinvasive fungal infection in compromised patients.[350,362] Sputum cultures yield an *Aspergillus* sp. in less than one-third of cases,† and false-positive culture results are common.[338,362,365] Nevertheless, isolation of an *Aspergillus* sp. from respiratory secretions must be regarded as strong presumptive evidence of IPA in the appropriate clinical setting, and confirmation by other means should be aggressively pursued. Blood cultures are almost always negative‡, and serodiagnosis is notoriously unreliable.[327,333,362,365] However, recent evidence suggests that the detection of aspergillus antigens in the sera of neutropenic patients by ELISA is a sensitive and specific indicator of early invasive aspergillosis.[371] Chest radiographs disclose a variety of abnormalities: patchy, multifocal or diffuse, bilateral areas of consolidation; nodules; peripheral wedge-shaped, pleural-based infiltrates (infarct pattern); and, rarely, bilateral miliary nodules.§ Nodules and infarcts may cavitate, particularly following recovery from granulocytopenia,[339] and fungus balls may then develop within the cavities.[350,351,362] Chest radiographs are negative at clinical onset of disease in up to one-third of patients,[328] and about 10% or more of patients never develop recognizable radiographic abnormalities.[362,365] In a recent pathoradiologic correlative study,[363] about 50% of patients had concurrent pulmo-

nary infection that obscured or mimicked the radiographic lesions of IPA; only 60% of radiographic abnormalities were actually produced by the lesions of IPA.

The clinical diagnosis of IPA is exceedingly difficult because of the nonspecific nature of symptoms, the frequency of concurrent infection, and the lack of reliability of microbiologic, serologic, and radiographic findings. Less than 30% of patients survive the infection.[327,365] Survival is crucially dependent on early diagnosis, aggressive therapy, and remission of underlying disease. Amphotericin B is the chemotherapeutic agent of choice[327,343,347,368] and may have a role in prophylaxis against invasive aspergillosis in neutropenic patients.[374] Flucytosine can be given with amphotericin B, but its efficacy is unproven and it may exacerbate myelosuppression. Recent experience with the new oral triazole drug, itraconazole, in the treatment of invasive aspergillosis has been promising.[375] Surgical excision is reserved for localized infection and for aspergillomas developing within cavitary lesions of IPA.

Aspergillosis does not occur frequently among patients with AIDS, nor is it a sentinel opportunistic infection in these patients. When it does occur as a late complication of AIDS, invasive infection and colonization of obstructed bronchi are the two forms observed most frequently.[376]

Well-preserved hyphae of *Aspergillus* spp. have a characteristic appearance in histologic sections (Fig. 11–28A). The hyphae, 3–6 μm in width, are uniform, regularly septate, and have parallel contours. Branches arise at acute angles from parent hyphae, and the pattern of branching is progressive and dichotomous. Viable hyphae are basophilic, whereas necrotic hyphae are hyaline or eosinophilic. Although visible with H and E, hyphal morphology is demonstrated much better with special stains such as GMS. Under certain circumstances, the hyphae exhibit atypical or degenerative features. For instance, the mycelium composing an aspergilloma may contain bizarre, swollen, varicose, or globose hyphal segments up to 15 μm in diameter with irregular contours, inconspicuous septa, and abortive branches (Fig. 11–28B). Fan-shaped crystals of calcium oxalate, recognizable by polarization, are occasionally deposited within aspergillomas, particularly those formed of *A. niger*.[377,378]

The hyphae in chronic granulomatous lesions may be surrounded by a radiating, eosinophilic corona of Splendore–Hoeppli material, and intravascular hyphae are sometimes vacuolated and coated with a layer of amorphous, eosinophilic plasma protein (Fig. 11–28C). Species in the *A. flavipes-terreus* group produce pyriform or globose aleurioconidia (Fig. 11–29A), 3–6 μm in diameter, on short conidiophores that arise laterally

---

*References: 9, 13, 334, 335, 343, 347, 362–364, 368.
†References: 327, 334, 343, 362, 365.
‡References: 320, 327, 334, 343, 347, 362, 368.
§References: 312, 328, 331, 332, 362–364, 372, 373.

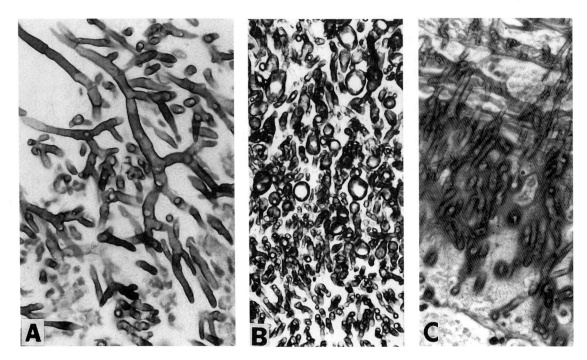

Fig. 11–28 A–C. Aspergillosis. **A.** Typical hyphae are septate, and branching is progressive and dichotomous. GMS, ×480. **B.** Bizarre, thick-walled, globose hyphae in aspergilloma.

GMS, ×300. **C.** Sheath of coagulated plasma protein surrounds intravascular hyphae. PAS, ×480.

from the hyphae.[379] Finally, conidial heads, produced occasionally by *Aspergillus* spp. in lesions exposed to ambient air, may be found in aspergillomas and in the lesions of necrotizing tracheobronchitis. The conidial heads, which are specialized for asexual reproduction, are borne upon conidiophores that arise directly from

thick-walled foot cells in the vegetative mycelium. The heads are composed of a vesicle, which is the terminal bulbous dilatation of a conidiophore, upon which are borne one or two layers of phialides (sterigmata) (Fig. 11–29B). Conidia arise in chains from the distal ends of the phialides. A definitive histologic diagnosis of as-

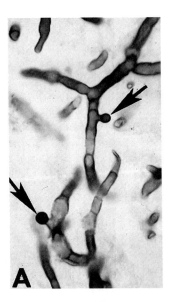
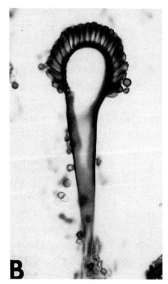
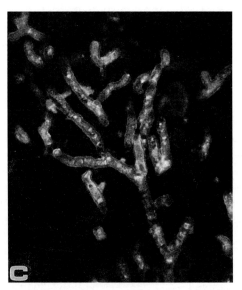

Fig. 11–29 A–C. Aspergillosis. **A.** Hyphae of *Aspergillus terreus* bear lateral aleurioconidia (*arrows*). GMS, ×760. **B.** Conidial head of *A. fumigatus* in intracavitary aspergilloma. Single row of phialides covers much of vesicle. Only a few globose conidia

remain attached to tips of some phialides. GMS, ×760. **C.** Hyphae of *A. fumigatus* in section of lung from patient with invasive aspergillosis. Direct immunofluorescence, ×750.

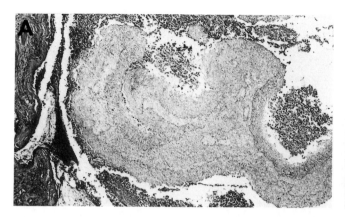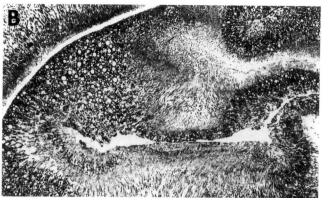

Fig. 11–30 A,B. Intracavitary aspergilloma. **A.** Inflammatory exudate surrounds portion of *Aspergillus niger* fungus ball in bronchiectatic cavity. Fungus ball is not attached to wall of cavity (left). ×50. **B.** Fungus ball consists of convoluted mycelium containing both typical and varicose hyphae. GMS, ×50.

pergillosis can be made when conidial heads are present, and their distinctive morphology often suggests the species designation. Because the hyphae of some other opportunistic pathogens closely resemble those of the aspergilli, a specific histologic diagnosis of aspergillosis on the basis of hyphal morphology alone is not justified unless confirmed by culture, direct immunofluorescence (Fig. 11–29C), or peroxidase immunohistochemical techniques.[380]

The intracavitary aspergilloma, sometimes erroneously referred to as "mycetoma," is a compact, spherical conglomerate of hyphae that develops within a preformed cavity.[335,381,382] Most such cavities are round or oval and sharply circumscribed, 1–7 cm or more in diameter, and communicate with the bronchial tree. Aspergillomas are occasionally multiple or bilateral. The walls of the cavities, 1–5 mm thick, are grayish white and fibrous with smooth or shaggy inner surfaces. The adjacent pleura is thickened and fibrotic. Microscopically, the walls of the cavities are composed of vascularized fibrous connective tissue infiltrated by lymphocytes, plasma cells, histiocytes, and occasional neutrophils and eosinophils. Granulomas are found occasionally, particularly in the walls of tuberculous cavities. The internal surfaces may be lined by respiratory or metaplastic epithelium that is often extensively eroded, which may account for the frequency of hemoptysis. The fungus ball, which may fill most of the cavity but is usually unattached to the wall, is smooth or lobulated, yellowish brown, and friable. Sectioned surfaces often appear laminated.

Microscopically, the fungus ball is composed of concentric or convoluted layers of radially arranged and intertwined hyphae (Fig. 11–30). Variation in the density of hyphae in adjacent layers, produced by alternation of rapid and slow phases of hyphal growth, resembles the zonation that may be observed in colonies cultured on solid media.[381] Hyphae in the center of the fungus ball are often nonviable and eosinophilic, whereas those at the periphery are basophilic. As noted previously, the morphology of degenerated hyphae can be quite atypical, and such hyphae can be mistaken for other pathogens, such as the zygomycetes. Conidial heads, produced in some cases, emerge from the surfaces of the fungus ball and cavity wall and are shed into the cavity. Although hyphae can be found along the surface and within the fibrous wall of the cavity, invasion into adjacent lung parenchyma does not occur unless host defense mechanisms are otherwise compromised. Most examples of "invasive aspergilloma" previously reported in the literature represent CNPA or aspergilloma developing in IPA. Fungus balls that develop within the lesions of IPA following recovery of patients from granulocytopenia differ in their histogenesis from those that develop in preformed cavities; the former are autoamputated spheres of necrotic lung tissue that contain invasive hyphae.[351,383] The margins of these sequestra and of lung tissue forming the cavity walls contain an unusually large number of degenerated polymorphonuclear neutrophils, which are thought to produce these lesions by enzymatic digestion of necrotic lung tissue.

Necrotizing bronchial aspergillosis accounts for 6%–9% of cases of bronchopulmonary aspergillosis in some series.[334,362,363] Patients in whom the infection remains confined to the airways are less severely compromised than those with IPA.[334] Bronchial aspergillosis may involve much of the tracheobronchial tree or remain confined to localized segments.[335,355,381] The eroded respiratory mucosa is replaced by a granular, brown, adherent pseudomembrane composed of inflammatory exudate, mucus, and hyphae that may occlude subsegmental bronchi.[357] Conidial heads are found in about 40% of cases.[355,362] Although the infec-

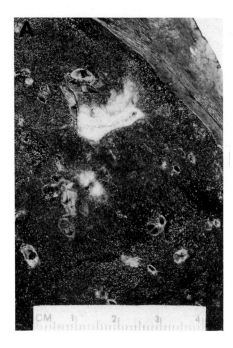 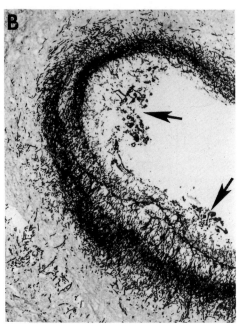

Fig. 11–31 A,B. Necrotizing bronchial aspergillosis. **A.** Thickening of bronchial wall with peribronchial consolidation. Bronchial mucosa is replaced by granular pseudomembrane. **B.** Pseudomembrane is composed of mycelial meshwork. Two clusters of conidial heads (*arrows*) emerge from pseudomembrane into bronchial lumen. Note limited peribronchial invasion. GMS, ×50.

tion is often confined to airways, limited invasion of hyphae into peribronchial lung tissue sometimes occurs. Sectioned surfaces of such lungs disclose zones of grayish-tan consolidation, 1–2 mm thick, distributed circumferentially around bronchi and bronchioles with sparing of intervening lung tissue (Fig. 11–31A). Microscopically, there is invasion and destruction of bronchial walls, and hyphae extend into peribronchial blood vessels and parenchyma[357] (Fig. 11–31B).

The pathologic features of CNPA have not yet been thoroughly delineated. As might be expected from its intermediate position in the clinical spectrum of pulmonary aspergillosis, CNPA incorporates some pathologic features of both aspergilloma and IPA. The major findings include large cavities that contain amorphous hyphal aggregates or well-formed fungus balls and some degree of invasion and destruction of surrounding lung tissue.[337,358,359] Parenchyma adjacent to the cavities usually shows chronic inflammation and fibrosis, which seems often to result from preexisting lung disease, but abscesses that contain hyphae have also been described.[337] Fungus balls develop dynamically in CNPA concurrent with and as a direct result of cavitation produced by invasive *Aspergillus* infection, apparently by a process similar to that described by Pryjemski and Mattii,[351] whereas fungus balls develop in preformed cavities by a passive process of colonization and progressive, noninvasive mycelial growth. Thus, the pathologic diagnosis of CNPA requires demonstration of invasion and destruction of noncavitary lung tissue in an appropriate clinical and roentgenographic setting. CNPA is distinguished from IPA by the limited extent

of parenchymal invasion and absence of vascular invasion and infarction.

Bardana[343] has coherently outlined the pathogenesis of IPA. The infection is initiated by colonization of the tracheobronchial tree with an *Aspergillus* sp. Endobronchial mycelial proliferation then results in necrotizing bronchial aspergillosis ("aspergillary bronchitis"), followed by transbronchial hyphal invasion. Invasion that occurs distally in the bronchial tree into adjacent small pulmonary blood vessels produces focal parenchymal lesions, whereas more proximal invasion into lobar or segmental blood vessels produces large hemorrhagic infarcts.[343,363] Hyphal invasion of arteries and veins is the pathologic hallmark of IPA and accounts for most of the observed parenchymal lesions. Secondary infection by an *Aspergillus* sp. of the necrotic lesions produced by coexistent pathogens, most often *Pseudomonas aeruginosa* or a *Candida* sp.,[334,362,363,365] may account for some of the focal parenchymal lesions of IPA. Hematogenous dissemination of an *Aspergillus* sp. to the lungs from an extrapulmonary focus seldom occurs.

Myerowitz and coworkers[332,363] have critically reappraised the histogenesis of the lesions of IPA, and the results of their studies have helped clarify much of the terminologic confusion surrounding its pathologic features. The characteristic lesion of IPA, occurring in about 60% of patients, is a nodular pulmonary infarct ("target lesion") that results from hyphal invasion of a small, peripheral pulmonary artery. Target lesions, several millimeters to 3 cm or more in diameter, are yellowish gray, necrotic nodules surrounded by hemorrhagic rims (Fig. 11–32). Microscopically, they are com-

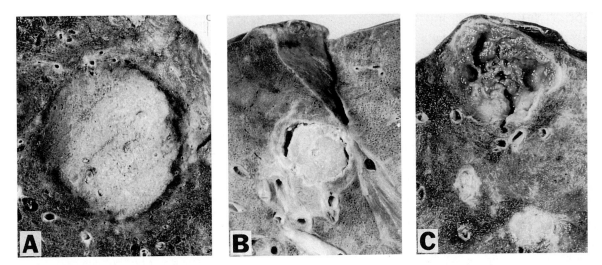

Fig. 11–32 A–C. Invasive pulmonary aspergillosis (IPA). **A.** Nodular infarct ("target lesion") with hemorrhagic rum. **B.** Early cavitation in nodular infarct. **C.** Advanced cavitation. Cavity contains amorphous mycelial aggregates.

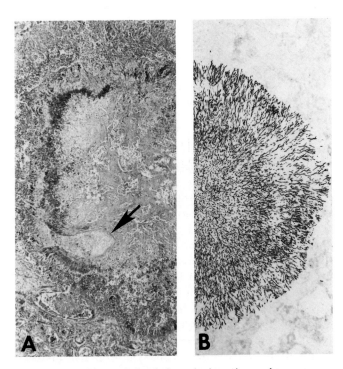

Fig. 11–33 A,B. Nodular infarct in invasive pulmonary aspergillosis (IPA). **A.** Central zone of ischemic necrosis with peripheral rim of inflammatory exudate. Artery near margin of infarct (*arrow*) is occluded by thrombus. ×30. **B.** Radial growth pattern typical of *Aspergillus* hyphae in nodular infarct. GMS, ×50.

posed of a central zone of ischemic necrosis, an intermediate zone of fibrinous exudate that may contain degenerated neutrophils, and a peripheral zone of parenchymal hemorrhage (Fig. 11–33A). An occluded, necrotic artery can often be identified within or at the edge of this lesion. Hyphae extend through the vascular wall and invade by radial growth throughout the surrounding necrotic parenchyma (Fig. 11–33B). Target lesions are usually multiple, and about half of the larger nodules undergo cavitation (Fig. 11–32B). A variety of terms, some histogenetically inaccurate, have been used to describe lesions of IPA that appear to correspond to the target lesions described by Myerowitz; patchy necrotizing (broncho-)pneumonia,[13,334,362,381] focal pulmonary necrosis,[362] nodular consolidation,[335] and rounded bronchopneumonia.[372] Intrapulmonary hematogenous dissemination, occurring in less than 10% of cases, produces myriads of small target lesions that are referred to by some investigators as miliary microabscesses.[334,362] The target lesion is not specific for IPA, and is found in other opportunistic angioinvasive mycotic infections, such as candidiasis.

Large, wedge-shaped, pleural-based hemorrhagic infarcts, often involving most of a lobe, are invariably associated with thrombosis of a major pulmonary arterial branch caused by hyphal invasion from an adjacent bronchus. Such infarcts, which are often multiple and bilateral, are found in about one-third of cases.[334,362,363] Suppurative basal bronchopneumonia may occur in nongranulocytopenic patients,[363] and necrotizing bronchial aspergillosis without extensive vascular or parenchymal invasion is found in about 10% of IPA cases.[334,362,363] Fungus balls develop within the necrotic lesions of IPA (Fig. 11–32C) in 1–6% of patients,[334,362] more commonly in those diagnosed early and treated aggressively.[350]

Typical hyphae are abundant in the bronchial, vascular, and parenchymal lesions of IPA. They often radiate outward from the center of target lesions and extend through tissue planes in parallel waves. A granulomatous inflammatory reaction sometimes occurs in noncompromised patients[370] and in patients treated with antifungal chemotherapy[13,332,363,382] but is not otherwise usually encountered. Hematogenous dissemination occurs in 25%–35% of severely compromised patients with aspergillosis. The respiratory tract is almost always the portal of entry, and pulmonary lesions can be demonstrated in 90%–97% of cases. Other organs frequently involved in systemic aspergillosis include the brain, heart, kidneys, gastrointestinal tract, liver, spleen, and thyroid gland.*

Difficulties may be encountered in the histopathologic diagnosis of pulmonary aspergillosis, particularly in biopsy specimens of limited size. Atypical hyphal forms, which occur in aspergillomas and in some chronic granulomatous lesions, may be difficult to distinguish from the hyphae of the zygomycetes. Angioinvasive opportunistic pathogens in the genera *Fusarium* and *Pseudallescheria* form branched, septate hyphae that closely resemble those of the *Aspergillus* spp. Like the aspergilli, *Pseudallescheria boydii* causes invasive pulmonary infection and forms intracavitary fungus balls. The hyphal forms of the *Candida* and *Trichosporon* spp. are easily distinguished histologically from the aspergilli, because they are accompanied by yeast-like cells and either pseudohyphae or arthroconidia, respectively. Fluorescent antibody[326] and immunoperoxidase[45,380] conjugates can help confirm a generic histologic diagnosis of aspergillosis when conidial heads are not present and fresh tissue is not available for culture.

Mucormycosis (Zygomycosis)

The term "mucormycosis" refers to a variety of opportunistic infections caused by fungi in the Order Mucorales, Class Zygomycetes (formerly Phycomycetes). The more general term "zygomycosis" ("phycomycosis" in the older literature) is often used synonymously. However, this designation also includes localized, nonopportunistic infections of subcutaneous tissue and rhinofacial structures, prevalent in the tropics, that are caused by zygomycetes in the Order Entomophthorales.[386] Because the two forms of zygomycosis are clinically and pathologically distinct, they are best designated respectively as "mucormycosis" and "entomophthoromycosis" to avoid confusion.

The clinicopathologic spectrum of mucormycosis has been the subject of several detailed reviews.[387–394] The rhinocerebral form is a fulminant, invasive infection of the nasal cavity, paranasal sinuses, palate, face, and

orbit that extends to the central nervous system.[395] This form of infection occurs most often in acidotic diabetics but is also seen in patients with leukemia. Gastrointestinal mycormycosis occurs in malnourished patients or patients with preexisting ulcerative lesions such as amebic colitis and produces ulcers or segmental areas of necrosis, most commonly in the stomach or colon.[396,397] Cutaneous infections occur in burned patients, diabetics, and patients whose surgical bandages have been contaminated with *Rhizopus* spp. Pulmonary and disseminated mucormycosis are particularly prone to occur in patients with acute leukemia or lymphoma.

Authenticated agents of mucormycosis include species within the genera *Rhizopus, Absidia, Mucor, Rhizomucor, Saksenaea, Cunninghamella, Mortierella, Syncephalastrum,* and *Apophysomyces*. The *Rhizopus* spp., particularly *R. oryzae (=R. arrhizus)*, are the most frequently implicated agents of human infection.[389,393,395] Most of the pathogenic zygomycetes grow rapidly in culture on enriched media, producing cottony mould-like colonies composed of sparsely septate mycelium. Asexual reproduction occurs by formation of sporangiospores or conidia, and sexual reproduction by formation of zygospores. Some genera produce rhizoids or anchoring rootlets. Species identification, both complex and difficult, is based on the morphology of the asexual cycle, physiologic characteristics such as thermotolerance, and mating behavior and the morphology of the sexual cycle.[392] The zygomycetes are widely distributed in nature and can be isolated from soil and decaying organic material.[389] The sporadic occurrence of mucormycosis throughout the world relates more to host susceptibility than to geographic or environmental factors.[391]

Mucormycosis is the third most common opportunistic mycosis among patients with neoplastic diseases, yet accounts for less than 5% of such infections in most series.[13,14,289] The incidence of mucormycosis appears to be increasing,[390,393] however, largely because of advances in the treatment of hematologic malignancy. Pulmonary mucormycosis occurs most frequently in patients with acute leukemia or lymphoma and is associated with leukopenia, corticosteroid and cytotoxic drug therapy, antibiotic therapy, concurrent bacterial infection, and relapse or lack of sustained remission of the underlying disease. Other underlying diseases or factors that can predispose to pulmonary mucormycosis include poorly controlled or acidotic diabetes mellitus, renal failure with acidosis, deferoxamine therapy for patients on hemodialysis,[398] severe burns, and therapy for nonhematologic neoplasms.[387–392,399,400] Pulmonary infection rarely occurs in patients without an identifiable predisposing illness.

The clinical features of pulmonary mucormycosis are

---

*References: 332, 334, 335, 362, 365, 382, 384, 385.

similar to those of invasive aspergillosis. Patients typically have persistent fever and new or progressive pulmonary infiltrates that are unresponsive to antibacterial therapy.[390,391,399] Signs and symptoms of pulmonary infarction may develop because of the propensity of these fungi to invade the pulmonary vascular tree and cause pulmonary arterial thrombosis. Rarely, patients die abruptly of massive, exsanguinating hemoptysis from mycotic erosion and rupture of a lobar or segmental pulmonary artery.[393,401,402] Chest radiographic abnormalities include patchy or nonhomogeneous infiltrates and solitary or multiple areas of consolidation.[331,390,403] Cavitation and pleural effusion are infrequent, and occasionally no abnormalities can be detected. Similar radiographic changes occur in some other opportunistic pneumonias such as aspergillosis and nocardiosis. The sequence of radiographic changes beginning with "rounded pneumonia," which progresses to a pulmonary infarction pattern or to large areas with the appearance of bronchopneumonia, is considered by some to be highly indicative of an opportunistic pulmonary mycosis in the appropriate clinical setting.[312,372] A miliary or nodular pattern may be found in patients with hematogenous pulmonary dissemination from another primary site.

The clinical diagnosis of pulmonary mucormycosis is exceedingly difficult to establish. Cultures of material derived from the respiratory tract or other sites in patients with pulmonary mucormycosis are usually negative,[390,399] and no reliable serologic tests to confirm the diagnosis are available. Therefore, definitive diagnosis usually depends on the identification of mucoraceous hyphae in biopsy specimens obtained from the respiratory tract.

The pathogenesis of pulmonary mucormycosis was described initially by Baker.[400] Following germination of inhaled sporangiospores or aspiration of hyphae from a focus of infection in the upper respiratory tract, the mycelium proliferates within the proximal bronchial tree. Aggressively invasive, the hyphae penetrate through bronchial walls and grow into adjacent blood vessels, particularly arteries, where thrombosis ensues. This results in pulmonary infarction, usually hemorrhagic, which is often parahilar as well as more peripheral in location (Fig. 11–34). Proximal infarcts are rounded or irregular in configuration, whereas peripheral infarcts are more often typically wedge shaped and accompanied by pleural invasion. Acute exudative bronchopneumonia results from spread of hyphae into adjacent parenchyma in the nongranulocytopenic host. Cavities develop in some of the infarcts and may contain necrotic tissue fragments admixed with hyphae.[390] Abscesses are uncommon and often signify secondary bacterial infection. Subsequent reports have confirmed

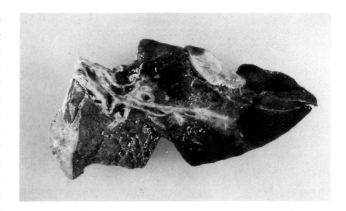

Fig. 11–34. Pulmonary mucormycosis. Sectioned surface of pulmonary lobe shows large hemorrhagic infarct (right).

Baker's observations and emphasized the frequency of hyphal vascular invasion and pulmonary infarction.* Rupture of a proximal pulmonary artery secondary to hyphal invasion is found in patients who die abruptly of massive hemoptysis,[393,401,402] and granulomatous mediastinitis may result from extension of the infection into the mediastinum.[405] Pulmonary involvement is found in 80%–100% of patients who die of disseminated mucormycosis;[13,389] also frequently involved are the central nervous system, kidneys, spleen, liver, heart, and gastrointestinal tract.[13,388–390,394]

Microscopically, the lesions of pulmonary mucormycosis consist of hemorrhagic infarcts (Fig. 11–35), nodular infarcts, and suppurative pneumonitis. Chronic, indolent, and partially treated infections may have a granulomatous component.[388,393] Mucoraceous hyphae are distributed haphazardly throughout these lesions and are conspicuous within the walls of blood vessels and in thrombi. The pleomorphic hyphae are broad (10–25 μm or more in width), delicate, thin walled, and pauciseptate (Fig. 11–36A). They are often twisted, folded, or wrinkled. Variation in hyphal caliber produces uneven contours in longitudinally sectioned hyphae. The pattern of branching is irregular, and branches are often oriented at right angles to parent hyphae. The hyphae are demonstrated as well with H and E as with the special stains for fungi. Thick-walled, densely stained, spherical, or ovoid chlamydoconidia (Fig. 11–36B) are occasionally found in tissue sections,[406] and sporangia have been described rarely in lesions exposed to the air.[387,389] However, some reports of sporangia in tissue sections are unconvincing;[387,407] the illustrated structures lack sporangiospores and appear to represent swollen, transected hyphae or chlamydoconidia.

---

*References: 387–390, 393, 403, 404.

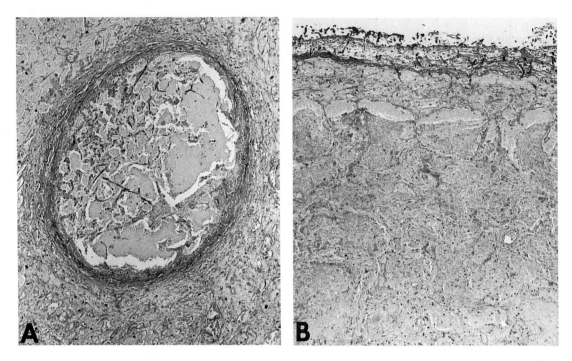

Fig. 11–35 A,B. Hemorrhagic infarct pictured in Fig. 11–34. **A.** Thrombotic vascular occlusion. Thrombus contains mucoraceous hyphae. PAS, ×50, **B.** Periphery of infarct. Note proliferation of hyphae on pleural surface (top). PAS, ×50.

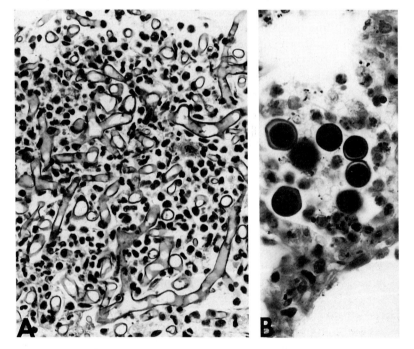

Fig. 11–36 A,B. Mucormycosis. **A.** Broad, pleomorphic, thin-walled hyphae in area of acute suppurative inflammation. Transected hyphae appear oval or round. GMS/H and E, ×300. **B.** Thick-walled chlamydoconidia of *Rhizopus* sp. ×480.

Although mucoraceous hyphae are occasionally confused with those of the *Aspergillus* spp. in tissue sections, typical hyphae of the aspergilli are narrower, more uniform, regularly septate, and have an orderly, progressive, dichotomous pattern of branching. The hyphae of *Rhizopus* and *Absidia* spp. can be identified in deparaffinized sections of formalin-fixed tissue by direct immunofluorescence with a screening conjugate.

Successful treatment of mucormycosis is predicated on the following principles: early diagnosis, control or remission of underlying disease, aggressive debridement or resection of localized foci of infection, and systemic antifungal chemotherapy.* Pulmonary mucormycosis is an almost uniformly fatal infection for several reasons: the patients are debilitated; the underlying disease, most often acute leukemia, may not be controllable; the clinical diagnosis is difficult to establish; and invasive diagnostic procedures may be delayed until the infection has progressed beyond a localized stage. The antifungal agent of choice is amphotericin B, but its effectiveness may be limited by poor penetration of infarcted tissue.[391,399,408] In the appropriate clinical setting, a positive culture result justifies empirical therapy with amphotericin B while efforts to confirm the diagnosis are pursued. Patients with the best chance of surviving pulmonary mucormycosis are those with a localized focus of infection amenable to segmental resection or lobectomy who have a controllable underlying disease such as diabetes mellitus.[399,410]

Coccidioidomycosis

Coccidioidomycosis is a pulmonary mycosis that is endemic in the Western Hemisphere. The majority of cases are clinically inapparent and resolve spontaneously. Symptomatic primary infection usually resolves as well but may lead to benign residual nodules or cavities, persistent pneumonia, or chronic progressive pneumonia. Extrapulmonary dissemination is rare except in certain high-risk groups. Acquisition of coccidioidomycosis is related primarily to environmental factors, whereas the course of the disease is largely determined by host factors.[411] Approximately 100,000 new cases occur annually in the United States, and about 70 cases per year are fatal.[412]

The disease is caused by a single dimorphic species, *Coccidioides immitis*. This fungus is widely distributed in soil throughout the Lower Sonoran Life Zone, which is characterized by a semiarid climate with a short, intense rainy season. Coccidioidomycosis is highly endemic within this life zone in parts of southern California, Arizona, New Mexico, Nevada, Utah, and Texas. The infection also occurs in northern and central Mexico, Baja California, Guatemala, Honduras, Nicaragua, Venezuela, Argentina, Colombia, Bolivia, and Paraguay.[412,413] *C. immitis* exists in nature and in culture at room temperature as a mould composed of septate, branched hyphae 2–4 μm wide. Arthroconidia, often barrel shaped and alternating with empty cells (disjunctors), are produced from aerial mycelium. Although racquet hyphae and arthroconidia typify the mycelium of *C. immitis* in culture, definitive identification requires conversion of the isolant to the spherule form, either in

special liquid media or by animal inoculation.[412,413] Alternatively, an extract of the mycelial form culture can be identified immunologically (exoantigen test). Because the airborne arthroconidia are highly infectious, mycelial form cultures of *C. immitis* must be handled with extreme caution in the laboratory.

In mammalian tissues, *C. immitis* exists in the form of spherules that replicate asexually by endosporulation. Immature spherules 5–30 μm in diameter develop directly from inhaled arthroconidia. These spherules endosporulate by a process of progressive cytoplasmic cleavage to become mature spherules 30–100 μm or more in diameter with refractile walls 1–2 μm thick. The uninucleate endospores, 2–5 μm in diameter, are released in packets following rupture of the spherule wall; they then enlarge to become immature spherules and repeat the sporangial cycle.[414,415] Under certain circumstances, endospores can germinate within host tissues to produce hyphae and arthroconidia.[416]

The varied clinical forms of coccidioidomycosis, recorded in detail by Fiese,[417] have been the subject of several recent reviews.[411,413,418–420] About 60% of cases of primary pulmonary coccidioidomycosis are clinically inapparent; these asymptomatic individuals can be recognized retrospectively by a positive skin test reaction to coccidioidin. The remaining 40% of patients develop a spectrum of symptoms ranging from a flu-like syndrome to frank pneumonia following an incubation period of 1–4 weeks. Symptoms most often include cough, fever, headache, chest pain, dyspnea, and malaise. About 10% of symptomatic patients develop allergic manifestations such as erythema nodosum, erythema multiforme, and arthralgias, which signify the development of hypersensitivity to *C. immitis* and usually portend a benign clinical course. Chest radiographs, normal in up to 20% of symptomatic patients, may show soft, hazy, patchy or segmental pneumonic infiltrates (75%), solitary or multiple nodules (15%), cavities (15%), hilar lymphadenopathy (20%), and pleural effusion (6%–20%).[421–423] The clinical diagnosis can be confirmed by isolation of *C. immitis* from respiratory secretions, skin test conversion, or positive serology (tube precipitin, immunodiffusion, and complement fixation tests). The illness is self limited in most patients, and symptoms generally resolve within several weeks. Persistent coccidioidal pneumonia is diagnosed when symptoms or radiographic abnormalities persist beyond 6–8 weeks. These patients are usually treated with amphotericin B, because some will develop progressive pneumonia or disseminated infection if untreated.

Chronic progressive coccidioidal pneumonia (CPCP) develops in less than 1% of patients hospitalized for primary pulmonary coccidioidomycosis. This indolent form of chronic infection mimics chronic tuberculosis

---

*References: 390–392, 399, 408–410.

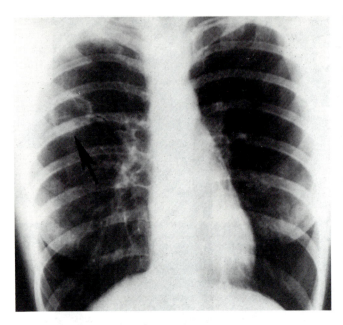

Fig. 11–41. Colonizing form of pulmonary pseudallescheriasis. Thin-walled cavity in right-upper lung field contains fungus ball (*arrow*) that is partially obscured by rib shadow.

hyphae.[453–456,459] The hyphae are not invasive unless the patient is otherwise immunosuppressed.[468] In one such patient, the intracavitary fungus ball was shown to develop from an infected lung sequestrum by a process similar to that which occurs in aspergillosis.[469] Invasive pulmonary pseudallescheriasis (Fig. 11–42A) is a destructive, necrotizing pneumonia with abscess formation,[449,464,467,468] mycelial vascular invasion,[449,455,463–466] and hemorrhagic infarction.[463] The hyphae in this form of the disease are scattered throughout areas of pneumonia or infarction. At autopsy, disseminated abscesses may be found in the brain and thyroid gland; they are less often found in the heart, kidneys, and other organs.* The pathogenesis of invasive pseudallescheriasis is presumed to be similar to that of invasive aspergillosis.

In tissue sections, the hyaline hyphae of *P. boydii* are septate, branched, and narrow, 2–5 μm wide (Fig. 11–42B). Although their pattern of branching is not progressive and dichotomous, they may be exceedingly difficult to distinguish from the hyphae of *Aspergillus* spp. The hyphae of *P. boydii* may produce thin-walled vesicles (swollen hyphal cells)[449,463,464,466] and terminal conidia of the *Scedosporium* type.† Only the latter are helpful in distinguishing *P. boydii* from an *Aspergillus* sp. in tissue sections. Morphology is unreliable in this regard, however, and definitive diagnosis requires isolation and identification of the fungus in culture. Direct

the bronchial tree. The walls of these cavities are formed of granulation tissue with suppurative or granulomatous inflammation. Bronchiectatic cavities and bronchogenic cysts may be lined partially by respiratory epithelium with squamous metaplasia. The intracavitary mycelium consists of either soft, amorphous yellow-brown hyphal aggregates[452,461,462] or true fungus balls formed of concentric rings of compact, tangled

---

*References: 448, 449, 455, 463–466.
†References: 453, 455, 458, 463–465.

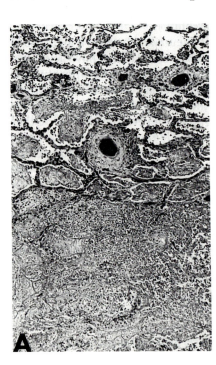
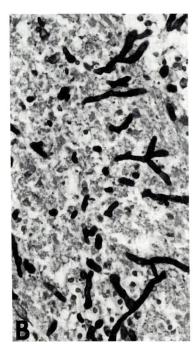

Fig. 11–42 A,B. Invasive pulmonary pseudallescheriasis. **A.** Margin of nodular pulmonary infarct. ×50. **B.** Branched, septate hyphae of *Pseudallescheria boydii*. GMS, ×300.

immunofluorescence may be helpful in diagnosis,[466] particularly if fresh tissue is not available for culture.

Although *P. boydii* can be isolated from sputum in up to 75% of patients with pulmonary pseudallescheriasis,[447] most isolants from the respiratory tract are environmental contaminants or colonizers of no clinical significance.[470] Surgical resection is the treatment of choice for noninvasive pseudallescheriasis,[447,452,458] and is usually reserved for patients with recurrent or uncontrolled hemoptysis. *P. boydii* is generally resistant to amphotericin B and flucytosine,[448,452,458,463,465] but may be susceptible to miconazole and ketoconazole.[463] Therapy with amphotericin B in patients with invasive pneumonia is ineffective, but survival following treatment with miconazole has been reported.[448,454]

Fusariosis

Infectious diseases caused by the *Fusarium* spp. include mycotic keratitis, endophthalmitis, onychomycosis, mycetoma, and cutaneous or disseminated infections in immunocompromised and burned patients.[471–473] The three major human pathogens within the genus *Fusarium* are *F. oxysporum*, *F. moniliforme*, and *F. solani*,[472] although *F. proliferatum* has emerged recently as an opportunistic human pathogen.[474] These species are widely distributed in nature as soil saprophytes and plant pathogens, and are occasionally isolated as laboratory contaminants.[475,476] They grow rapidly in culture at 25° or 37°C, producing mycelium composed of hyaline septate hyphae, often with intercalated or terminal chlamydoconidia.[471,472] Their characteristic septate macroconidia are fusoid or sickle shaped.

Localized and disseminated infections with these fungi have been reported in burned patients;[472,475] in patients treated for malignant lymphoma[471] and acute leukemia,[476–479] especially following bone marrow transplantation;[473,480] in a renal transplant recipient,[481] and in a patient with aplastic anemia.[482] Disruption of cutaneous or mucosal barriers appears to be a major factor in the pathogenesis of invasive fusariosis, and the paranasal sinuses, lungs, and skin are the usual portals of entry for the infection.[478] Patients usually have coexisting infections with bacteria, herpesviruses, or fungi, most often *Candida* or *Aspergillus* spp. Other factors predisposing to opportunistic infection among these patients include neutropenia and therapy with cytotoxic drugs, corticosteroids, and multiple antibiotics.[478,479]

Several immunosuppressed patients developed painful erythematous cutaneous nodules that progressed to necrotic ulcers, biopsy and culture of which helped to establish the diagnosis.[473,476,478,481] Chest radiographic abnormalities included nodular or fluffy densities or progressive pulmonary infiltrates.[471–473] However, some of these patients had coexisting pulmonary infection with herpesviruses and *Candida* spp. that could have produced or contributed to the radiographic findings. Unlike many other hyphomycoses, such as aspergillosis and mucormycosis, the diagnosis of disseminated fusariosis can be confirmed reliably by blood culture.[478]

Invasive and disseminated lesions produced by the *Fusarium* spp. consist of abscesses,[475] infarcts secondary to vascular invasion and thrombosis[472] (Fig. 11–43A), and granulomas.[482] The hyaline septate hyphae of *Fusarium* spp. measure 3–7 μm in width and are sparsely branched, the branches often arising perpendicular to parent hyphae (Fig. 11–43B). Intercalated chlamydoconidia are occasionally found, but the characteristic macroconidia are not produced in tissue. Hyphal angioinvasion is typical of disseminated infection with these fungi. In histologic sections, the hyphae of *Fusarium* spp. are most frequently mistaken for those of *Aspergillus* spp. and *Pseudallescheria boydii*. Although the *Fusarium* spp. do not show the regular pattern of progressive dichotomous branching so characteristic of the aspergilli, definitive diagnosis requires isolation and identification of the fungus in culture. The drug of choice for the treatment of invasive fusariosis is amphotericin B,[473,478] although in vitro resistance to this drug has been reported.[472,473,476] Most *Fusarium* isolants are resistant to flucytosine.[477,479]

Trichosporonosis

Trichosporonosis is a disseminated opportunistic mycosis caused by *Trichosporon* spp., yeast-like fungi within the Family Cryptococcaceae. *Trichosporon beigelii* (= *T. cutaneum*), the agent of white piedra, is the usual etiologic agent of disseminated trichosporonosis, although occasional cases have been caused by *T. capitatum*. These soil saprophytes are widely distributed in nature, form a minor component of normal skin flora, and are occasionally isolated as presumed contaminants from urine and throat cultures.[483,484]

The *Trichosporon* spp. grow rapidly in culture and produce cream-colored colonies that consist of hyaline yeast-like cells, mycelium, and arthroconidia, the last being characteristic of the genus. The two pathogenic species, *T. beigelii* and *T. capitatum*, are differentiated from each other by their urease activity and patterns of carbohydrate and nitrate assimilation.[483–489] *T. capitatum* has been reclassified recently into the genus *Blastoschizomyces* as *B. capitatus*.[490]

Most reported cases of disseminated trichosporonosis have been published since 1980.[483–504] This recently recognized disease occurs principally in patients treated

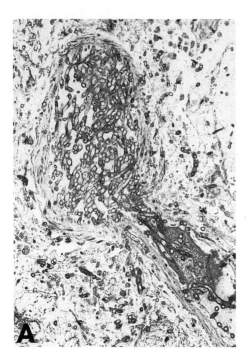
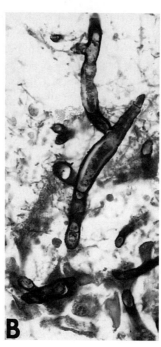

Fig. 11–43 A,B. Fusariosis. **A.** Vascular occlusion by hyphae of a *Fusarium* sp. at edge of nodular pulmonary infarct GMS/H and E, ×120. **B.** Branched, septate hyphae of *Fusarium* sp. are difficult to distinguish from those of *Aspergillus* sp. GMS/H and E, ×480.

for acute leukemia or lymphoma but has been reported also in renal transplant,[486,488] liver transplant,[502] and bone marrow transplant[487,489] recipients, in a patient following mitral valve replacement,[488] and in a heroin addict with mycotic endocarditis.[495] All the patients were immunosuppressed, either from underlying diseases such as acute leukemia or from therapy with cytotoxic drugs, corticosteroids, or azathioprine. About 50% of patients were neutropenic, and all had received multiple or broad-spectrum antibiotics for documented or presumed bacterial infections. Clinical findings were those of sepsis, most often fever unresponsive to antibiotic therapy. About one-third of patients developed purpuric papular or nodular skin lesions with vesiculation or ulceration.* Chest radiographic findings in patients with pulmonary involvement included localized[496] or bilateral[485,486] pulmonary infiltrates. Most patients had one or more positive blood cultures for a *Trichosporon* sp., and many had positive cultures from multiple sites, including urine, stool, respiratory secretions, throat, and skin lesions.

The mortality rate from disseminated trichosporonosis approaches 75%.[502] At autopsy, pulmonary lesions are found in about 75% of patients. Other organs frequently involved at autopsy include the kidneys, myocardium, liver and spleen, and less frequently the bone marrow, gastrointestinal tract, thyroid, lymph nodes, skin, and brain. Pulmonary lesions include hem-

orrhagic, necrotizing bronchopneumonia,[486,491] nodular infarcts containing radiating fungal colonies with little inflammatory response,[492,496] and widespread mycotic emboli with hemorrhagic infarcts.[489] Mycotic vascular invasion is found in more than 50% of the patients. Extrapulmonary lesions usually consist of abscesses, occasionally of necrotic granulomas.[491,498]

Trichosporon beigelii exists in tissue lesions in the form of pleomorphic hyaline yeast-like cells 3–8 μm in diameter, septate hyphae, and arthroconidia, the last produced by segmentation and fragmentation of hyphae (Fig. 11–44). However, the arthroconidia or yeast forms may be inconspicuous, in which case the fungi can be mistaken for a *Candida* sp. or an *Aspergillus* sp., respectively. Although the yeast-like cells of *Trichosporon* are typically more pleomorphic than those of *Candida* spp., definitive diagnosis requires confirmation by culture.

Immunohistologic identification of *T. beigelii* by immunoperoxidase methods in deparaffinized tissue sections has been reported recently.[503,505,506] Cross-reactivity with *Cryptococcus neoformans* (but not the *Candida* spp.) is a problem with the polyclonal antibody, but this can be removed by adsorption with *C. neoformans* cells.[505] The monoclonal antibody does not cross react with either *C. neoformans* or the *Candida* spp.[506]

In vitro susceptibility tests indicate that most isolants of *T. beigelii* are sensitive to amphotericin B and flucytosine, although strains resistant to one or the other drug have been reported.[493,494] Survival from trichosporonosis depends on prompt diagnosis, an adequate course of antifungal chemotherapy, and, most impor-

_____

*References: 484, 485, 489, 493, 494.

Fig. 11–44 A,B. Trichosporonosis. **A.** Yeast forms, hyphae, and arthroconidia of *Trichosporon beigelii*. GMS, ×480. **B.** Arthroconidia produced by septal disarticulation of hyphal segments. GMS, ×480.

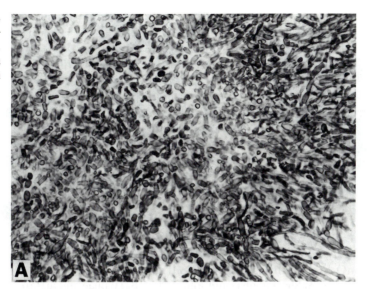
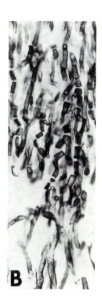

tantly, remission of underlying immunosuppression.* The diagnosis should be considered in any immunosuppressed patient with unremitting fever, neutropenia, skin lesions, and repeated cultural isolation of a *Trichosporon* sp. from blood, urine, skin lesions, or other sites. The portal of entry of infection in immunosuppressed patients is unknown, although respiratory, transcutaneous, and enteric routes have been proposed.[490,494,497]

Geotrichosis

Geotrichosis is an uncommon opportunistic fungal infection caused by *Geotrichum candidum*, a ubiquitous saprophyte found in soil, decomposing organic matter, and contaminated food.[507] The organism is also a transient commensal of the oropharynx, tracheobronchial tree, and gastrointestinal tract—sites that have been implicated as potential endogenous sources of infection. *G. candidum* is frequently isolated from sputum and stool specimens of normal persons, but, unlike *Candida albicans*, it is not an aggressive opportunist and rarely causes invasive infection. The clinical spectrum of geotrichosis includes transient fungemia,[507,508] colonization of bronchi and cavitary lung lesions,[509–512] and, rarely, oropharyngeal, gastrointestinal, cutaneous, and invasive disseminated infection.[507,513,514] Infections almost always occur in debilitated patients with preexisting pulmonary or other serious underlying disease, or as a complication of immunosuppressive therapy, parenteral alimentation, and prolonged treatment with broad-spectrum antibiotics.[515]

Transient or prolonged colonization of the respiratory tract, especially the bronchial tree and preexisting pulmonary cavities, is the most common clinical form of geotrichosis. Important predisposing factors are tuberculosis, chronic obstructive lung disease, chronic bronchitis, bronchogenic carcinoma, and certain other mycoses. About 26 cases have been reported.[507,509,512] Clinical signs, usually nonspecific, may include persistent cough; thick, grayish, mucoid or purulent, and rarely blood-tinged sputum; low-grade fever; and medium-to-coarse rales. Occasional patients with endobronchial geotrichosis may also have symptoms of severe asthma.[510] Chest radiographs may be normal or show peribronchial thickening and patchy infiltrates with cavitation, especially in apical and hilar regions. Bronchoscopy sometimes reveals white, thrush-like patches on the bronchial mucosa, and abundant fungal elements can be demonstrated in or isolated from the sputum. Endobronchial and intracavitary infections persist if predisposing factors are not eliminated, and fulminating fatal infections with fungemia have been reported rarely in patients who are profoundly immunosuppressed, neutropenic, or have malignant hematopoietic neoplasia.[507,511,512]

To our knowledge, only two cases of geotrichosis have been reported in which tissue invasion has been adequately documented.[513,514] In both, the gastrointestinal tract was the primary site of infection. In one patient with severe neutropenia and obstructing colonic adenocarcinoma, disseminated geotrichosis involved the lungs, heart, and spleen.[513] In the second patient, who had hairy-cell leukemia, invasion of *G. candidum* was confined to "plaque-like lesions" in the terminal ileum.[514] Lesions in these cases were suppurative and necrotizing or granulomatous, and were regarded as similar to those caused by *Candida* and *Aspergillus* spp.

*References: 484, 485, 490, 498–500.

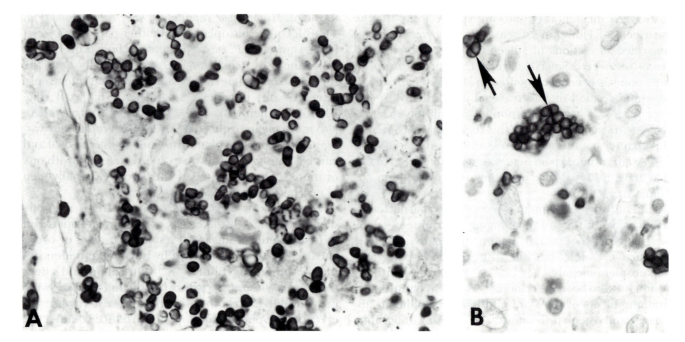

Fig. 11–46 A,B. Disseminated penicilliosis marneffei. **A.** Spherical, oval, and elongated intra- and extracellular yeast-like cells of *Penicillium marneffei* in hepatic abscess. GMS, ×760. **B.** Splenic granuloma contains pleomorphic intracellu-lar yeast forms, some of which have transverse septa and rounded ends (*arrows*). Unlike *Histoplasma capsulatum* var. *capsulatum, P. marneffei* does not bud. GMS, ×760.

Most disseminated infections have been reported in premature infants and, less often, in immunosup-pressed adults with severe, chronic gastrointestinal dis-ease who received lipid-supplemented total parenteral nutrition.[533,534] Although adults with *M. furfur* fun-gemia may be asymptomatic except for low-grade fever, neonates usually present with signs and symptoms of sepsis and thrombocytopenia. To date, approximately 55 cases of *M. furfur* fungemia in neonates have been reported.[528,536]

In disseminated malasseziasis, the lungs are most frequently involved, apparently because of increased lipid deposits in the walls of pulmonary blood ves-sels.[533,535] Histopathological findings within the lung range from numerous mycotic emboli without associ-ated vasculitis to massive consolidation, granulomatous inflammation, vasculitis, mycotic thrombosis, and my-cotic infarction of the pulmonary parenchyma. Organs less often involved include heart, liver, kidney, spleen, adrenal gland, colon, and brain.[535] In deep lesions, fungal elements are usually numerous and they appear as clusters of spherical or oval, thick-walled, single or budding yeast-like cells, 3–8 μm in diameter, that are considered to be phialoconidia (Fig. 11–47). A morpho-logically distinct, unipolar, phialidic collarette can sometimes be seen at the point where a bud was ex-truded from a parent cell. The yeast-like cells of

M. furfur are usually hematoxylinophilic in H and E-stained tissue sections, but are best demonstrated with the special stains for fungi.

M. furfur can be easily cultured on standard myco-logic media overlaid with a thin layer of sterile olive oil. Within 5–7 days, small, cream-to-tan, yeast-like colonies develop when incubated at 30°C. Microscopically, the colonies consist of budding yeast-like cells; however, under certain conditions, short curved hyphae are also formed.

Prompt removal of central venous catheters colo-nized with *M. furfur* is sometimes the only treatment necessary for fungemia. Severe disseminated infections have been treated successfully with amphotericin B and miconazole after discontinuation of intravenous lipid emulsion alimentation.[533,534]

Phaeohyphomycosis

The term "phaeohyphomycosis" refers to those subcu-taneous and systemic infections caused by a wide variety of dematiaceous (naturally pigmented) opportunistic fungi that develop as black moulds in culture and as dark-walled (brown) septate hyphae in tissue.[537–540] Because these soil and wood saprophytes are ubiquitous in many environments, proof of their etiologic role in disease usually requires direct microscopic demonstra-

Fig. 11–47. Disseminated malasseziasis in neonate. Myriad yeast-like cells of *Malassezia furfur*, 3–8 μm in diameter, with single buds (phialoconidia), are located within a pulmonary thromboembolus. GMS, ×560.

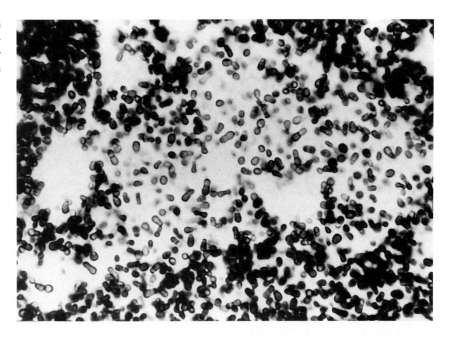

tion of characteristic fungal elements in tissue; a positive culture in the absence of compatible lesions is insufficient for diagnosis. Although infections have been reported in healthy persons, those who are immunocompromised or severely debilitated are more susceptible.

Two clinical forms of phaeohyphomycosis are recognized in humans: subcutaneous (phaeomycotic cyst) and systemic (cerebral phaeohyphomycosis). Subcutaneous infections are most common.[541–545] They occur when fungi enter the body through a skin wound or by traumatic implantation of a wood splinter or other foreign object that serves as a vehicle of infection.[542,545] Patients are typically found to have solitary, firm-to-fluctuant, painless, subcutaneous abscesses up to 7 cm in diameter on exposed parts of the body; lymphangitis and regional lymphadenopathy are uncommon. The etiologic agents of subcutaneous phaeohyphomycosis include more than 70 recognized genera and species of dematiaceous fungi, the more common being *Exophiala (Phialophora) jeanselmei*, *Phialophora parasitica*, *P. richardsiae*, and *Wangiella dermatitidis*.[537,539,540]

Systemic phaeohyphomycosis usually has a pulmonary inception with a marked but unexplained tropism for the brain, particularly the cerebral hemispheres.[546–550] Involvement of other organs is extremely rare. *Xylohypha bantiana (Cladosporium bantianum)*, the most commonly encountered agent, reaches the brain via hematogenous dissemination from a primary but usually clinically inapparent pulmonary lesion acquired by inhalation of fungal particles from the environment.[551] Some patients may have pulmonary symptoms such as cough, chest pain, dysp-

nea, and hemoptysis. Symptoms of cerebral phaeohyphomycosis include headache, nausea, vomiting, fever, and nuchal pain and rigidity. Cerebral lesions are solitary or multiple, up to 5 cm in diameter, and consist of encapsulated abscesses or generalized inflammatory infiltrates.[546–549] Recent findings in an animal model suggest that immunosuppression may be the most important predisposing factor in cerebral phaeohyphomycosis caused by *Xylohypha bantiana*.[552]

Certain agents of phaeohyphomycosis have been implicated as noninvasive stimuli for allergic bronchopulmonary disease.[553,554] Few descriptions of invasive pulmonary infection in systemic phaeohyphomycosis, however, have been published. Limsila et al.[555] described an indurated mass 6 cm in diameter that developed in the apex of the left-lower lobe of a patient who was infected with *Xylohypha bantiana* but did not have cerebral involvement. After lobectomy, the pulmonary "cladosporoma" was found to be confined to a bronchiectatic cavity that contained septate hyphae embedded in grayish-white necrotic material. In another report, pulmonary and cerebral "mycetomas" caused by *Curvularia pallescens* were discovered following inhalation of dirt by a retarded child who was otherwise apparently healthy.[556] Chest radiographs showed a large right perihilar mass that displaced the right mainstem bronchus and extended almost to the anterior axillary line. Biopsy of the mass revealed hyalinized fibrous tissue with numerous noncaseating granulomas that contained pigmented fungal elements; cultures of this lesion yielded *Curvularia pallescens*. Excision of a 3 × 5 cm mass in the frontoparietal cerebrum of this child revealed cystic granulomas containing fungi that

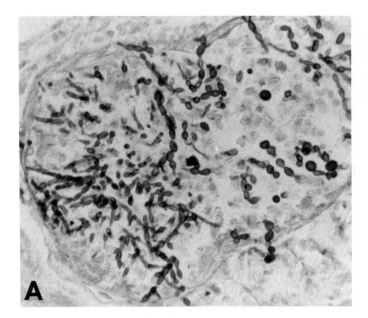

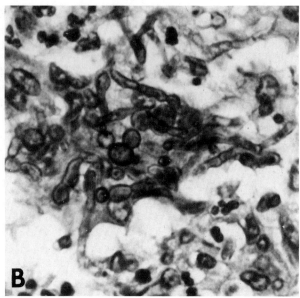

Fig. 11–48 A,B. Systemic phaeohyphomycosis. **A.** Acute pneumonia. Suppurative alveolar exudate contains yeast-like cells, chains of cells, and closely septate hyphae of *Xylohypha* *bantiana.* Gridley, ×300. **B.** Dematiaceous hyphae and budding yeast-like cells of *X. bantiana* in cerebral abscess. ×600.

were histologically and mycologically identical to those in the lung biopsy. More recently, primary pulmonary infection by *Curvularia lunata* with dissemination to the brain was reported in a man with chronic obstructive pulmonary disease and a history of alcohol abuse.[557] Clinically, this patient was thought to have a primary bronchogenic carcinoma with cerebral metastases. However, open lung biopsy revealed a 9 × 9 cm fibrogranulomatous mass; *Curvularia lunata* was demonstrated in and cultured from this lesion. Lobritz et al.[558] reported pulmonary granulomas caused by an *Alternaria* sp. in a patient who had no evidence of immunodeficiency or underlying disease. Open lung biopsy revealed a right-upper-lobe lesion composed of discrete peribronchial granulomas that contained pigmented fungi; an *Alternaria* sp. was recovered in pure culture. Finally, Borges et al.[559] reported a localized pulmonary nodule that contained pigmented hyphal fragments of culture-proven *Xylohypha bantiana* in a woman with a history of steroid-treated inflammatory bowel disease. In this case, surgical excision of the granulomatous lesion was both diagnostic and curative.

Progressive disseminated infection following cutaneous inoculation is rare. Rohwedder et al.[560] reported disseminated infection with *Curvularia lunata* in an immunocompetent man following presumed cutaneous inoculation of the saprophytic soil fungus while the man was playing football. Lymphadenopathy, empyema, and subcutaneous, pulmonary, paravertebral, and cerebral abscesses all resulted from infected leg ulcers

that developed from neglected abrasions. Chest radiographs revealed pleural effusion and a paraspinous abscess that communicated with the mediastinum and with a pleurocutaneous fistula. Sections of the fistulous tract showed necrotizing and suppurative granulomas that contained numerous pigmented hyphae; cultures yielded *C. lunata.* Ferraro and Morgan[561] reported a case of disseminated *Phialophora parasitica* infection in an elderly woman known to have a chronic subcutaneous infection with this fungus. At autopsy, *P. parasitica* was isolated from a thrombus within an abdominal aortic aneurysm and was directly demonstrated in sections obtained from the aneurysm wall.

Regardless of the anatomic site of involvement, the agents of phaeohyphomycosis almost always elicit the formation of cystic or dispersed granulomas that are usually solitary, encapsulated by dense collagenous connective tissue, and have suppurative or liquefied centers. The fungi appear as either individual or small but loose aggregates of closely septate and branched hyphae 2–6 μm wide, budding yeast-like cells, and large, thick-walled, chlamydoconidium-like cells within the walls and necrotic centers of the granulomas (Fig. 11–48). The brown cell walls of these moniliform fungi are easily detected in H and E-stained sections (Fig. 11–48B), but special fungal stains such as GMS and PAS are usually needed for detailed morphologic studies; the distribution and actual number of fungal elements are much more evident when these special stains are used.

Because most of the agents of phaeohyphomycosis

are morphologically and tinctorially similar in tissue, an etiologic diagnosis can be made only by isolating and identifying the organism in culture. Nevertheless, a disease diagnosis can be based on the natural brown color of morphologically typical fungal elements in clinical or biopsy specimens. In tissue sections, the dematiaceous agents of chromoblastomycosis appear as muriform cells that characteristically have thick walls, divide by septation in two planes, and do not form chains.[3,23,539] Because the typical forms of these fungi are morphologically distinctive, they are not ordinarily mistaken for the agents of phaeohyphomycosis.

Because most phaeomycotic cysts are solitary and encapsulated, surgical extirpation is usually sufficient for cure. Excision of localized lesions and prompt aggressive use of amphotericin B are the treatments of choice in systemic phaeohyphomycosis.[557,560] Initial experience with itraconazole in the management of mycoses caused by pigmented fungi has been promising, and this orally administered triazole compound may soon become the treatment of choice in systemic phaeohyphomycosis.[562]

Adiaspiromycosis

Adiaspiromycosis is a pulmonary mycosis caused by the dimorphic fungus *Chrysosporium parvum* var. *crescens* (*Emmonsia crescens*). This soil saprophyte is widely distributed throughout the world in temperate climates and frequently infects rodents and other small mammals. Human infection is uncommon, self limited, and confined to the lungs.[563,564]

In culture at room temperature, *C. parvum* var. *crescens* produces white, glabrous-to-floccose colonies composed of branching, septate mycelium with aleurioconidia 2–4 μm in diameter. When incubated at 37°C, the aleurioconidia progressively enlarge to become thick walled, spherical adiaconidia 400–700 μm in diameter.[563–565] The other variety of this species, *C. parvum* var. *parvum*, is not known to infect humans.

Human adiaspiromycosis has been reported from France, Czechoslovakia, the Soviet Union, Honduras, Guatemala, Venezuela, and Brazil.[563,564,566] Many of these patients had solitary adiaspiromycotic granulomas, clinically and radiographically inapparent, which were detected incidentally in lung tissue examined at autopsy or excised surgically for other reasons. The remaining patients had localized or diffuse bilateral lung disease that produced a finely nodular pattern in chest radiographs.[563,564,567–569] Only those patients with widespread, severe bilateral disease manifest symptoms, which include cough and slowly progressive dyspnea.[568] In its severest form, adiaspiromycosis can result in transient respiratory failure.[566]

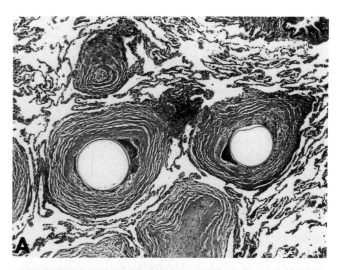
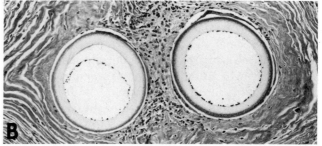

Fig. 11–49 A,B. Adiaspiromycosis. **A.** Large, thick-walled adiaconidia of *Chrysosporium parvum* var. *crescens* within fibrotic granulomas. ×50. **B.** Detail of adiaconidial walls. Note outer eosinophilic and inner hyaline layers. ×120.

The pulmonary lesions consist of discrete or confluent fibrotic granulomas 1–2 mm in size (Fig. 11–49A). Each granuloma contains one or more spherical adiaconidia, the only developmental form of this fungus thus far detected in humans. The largest conidia measure 200–300 μm in diameter, occasionally up to 500 μm. The conidial walls, 20–70 μm thick, have an eosinophilic outer layer and a broad hyaline inner layer (Fig. 11–49B). The Gridley stain defines three wall layers, which correspond to the trilaminar appearance demonstrated by electron microscopy.[569] Fenestrations can be seen in conidial walls sectioned laterally or tangentially and in those examined by electron microscopy. The interior of the adiaconidia is empty or contains small eosinophilic globules 1–3 μm in size. Some adiaconidia may contain an internal honeycombed cytoplasmic meshwork of unknown composition.[564–567] Reports of budding and endosporulation in human lesions[563,568] are not convincing; the adiaconidia seem to be incapable of replication or dissemination in the human host.[564–567] Symptoms, when present, can be attributed to mechanical displacement of tissue by the progressively enlarging adiaconidia.

Rhinosporidiosis

Rhinosporidiosis is primarily an infection of mucosal surfaces caused by *Rhinosporidium seeberi*. The disease is hyperendemic in India and Sri Lanka, but sporadic autochthonous cases have been reported from all over the world, including the United States.[570,571] The distribution of *R. seeberi* in nature is unknown, although infection is associated epidemiologically with rural and aquatic environments. Because the fungus cannot be isolated on synthetic media or transmitted experimentally to animals, diagnosis depends on identification of the characteristic endosporulating sporangia in smears or tissue sections. *R. seeberi* can propagate in tissue culture, but this is not used currently for diagnosis.[572]

Clinically, rhinosporidiosis produces bulky, friable mucosal polyps involving the nasal cavity, nasopharynx, palate, and upper respiratory tract. Other mucosal surfaces less commonly involved include the conjunctiva and lacrimal sac and the external genitalia.[570] Cutaneous lesions arise directly from adjacent mucosae or secondarily by autoinoculation. Authentic examples of disseminated infection are rare.[573,574] In one such case, small granulomas that contained the characteristic sporangia of *R. seeberi* were found throughout both lungs at autopsy.[574]

Two developmental forms of *R. seeberi* are recognized in tissue sections.[575–578] The vegetative (nonendosporulating) form, or trophocyte, is 10–100 μm in diameter and has a single, large, central karyosome (nucleus) with a prominent nucleolus. The cytoplasm is granular or lacy, and the refractile eosinophilic cell wall is 1–3 μm thick. The larger trophocytes endosporulate by a process of nuclear division and progressive cytoplasmic cleavage to produce mature sporangia 100–300 μm in diameter. The walls of mature sporangia, which are as thick as 5 μm, have a thin, eosinophilic outer layer and a broad, hyaline inner layer. The distinctive morphology and zonation of endospores within the sporangia are characteristic of this fungus (Fig. 11–50). Immature, uninucleate endospores 1–2 μm in size are flattened or oval and are distributed around the periphery of the sporangia in a germinative layer. As they mature, the endospores enlarge and move centrally within the sporangia. Fully mature endospores are 8–10 μm in diameter and contain multiple eosinophilic globules. Following sporangial rupture, the endospores are released into the surrounding tissues and enlarge to become trophocytes.

Rhinosporidial polyps involving mucosal surfaces are best treated by surgical excision. Recurrence rates are high if excision is incomplete. Antifungal chemotherapy alone is ineffective in eradicating the infection.

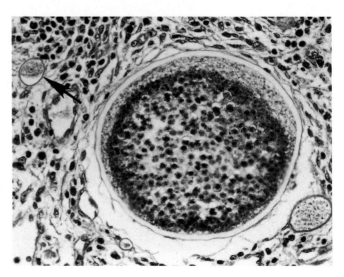

Fig. 11–50. Rhinosporidiosis. Zonation of endospores within sporangium of *Rhinosporidium seeberi*. Larger, mature endospores contain globular inclusions. Trophocyte (*arrow*) contains a small nucleus with prominent nucleolus. ×300.

Protothecosis

Protothecosis is an uncommon infectious disease caused by achlorophyllous algae of the genus *Prototheca*. Two of the three species in this genus, *P. wickerhamii* and *P. zopfii*, are pathogenic for animals and humans.[579] They are widely distributed in nature and can be isolated from soil, sewage, stream water, and other sites.[579,580] In culture at 25° or 37°C, the protothecae produce smooth, white-to-cream-colored yeast-like colonies that are composed of endosporulating sporangia. The two pathogenic species can be identified in culture by their patterns of sugar and alcohol assimilation and by direct immunofluorescence.[581]

About 30 cases of human protothecosis have been reported; most were from the United States and caused by *P. wickerhamii*.[582] Only rarely is *P. zopfii* implicated in human infection.[583] Cutaneous infection, accounting for almost two-thirds of cases, produces a localized or slowly progressive papular or eczematous dermatitis, usually on an extremity. This form of infection occurs in patients with underlying debilitating diseases such as malnutrition, diabetes mellitus, and alcoholism, in patients treated with immunosuppressive drugs, and in patients with intrinsic defects in cell-mediated immunity or neutrophil function.[582] Olecranon bursitis, the other major form of protothecosis, occurs in otherwise healthy people and is often associated with local injury to the elbow.

Regional lymphatic[584] and distant hematogenous[585] dissemination occur rarely in patients with cutaneous

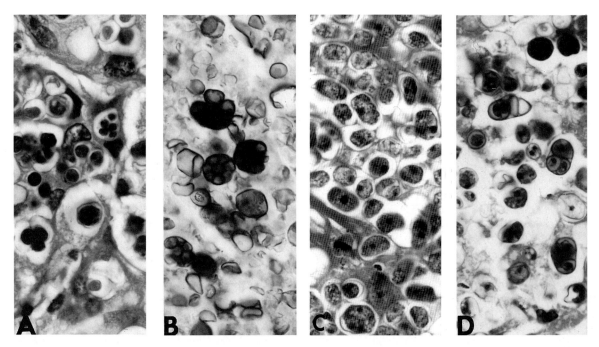

Fig. 11–51 A–D. Prototothecosis. **A.** Endosporulating sporangia of *Prototheca wickerhamii*, ×760. **B.** Distinctive "morula" form of *P. wickerhamii*. Gridley, ×760. **C.** Oval cells of *P. zopfii*. Note vacuolated cytoplasm and small, dense nuclei. ×760. **D.** Endosporulating sporangia of *P. zopfii*. Gridley, ×760.

prototothecosis. One such patient with chronic progressive cutaneous infection had multiple episodes of pneumonia of undetermined etiology.[586] *P. wickerhamii* was repeatedly isolated in culture from her skin lesions, stool, and sputum. This patient's neutrophils were specifically defective in their ability to kill *P. wickerhamii* in vitro. She recovered following treatment with tetracycline and amphotericin B despite persistence of the neutrophil defect. Dissemination from an enteric portal of entry can lead to biliary, hepatic, and intestinal infection.[587]

The prototothecae appear in culture and tissue sections as spherical-to-ovoid cells (sporangia) that replicate asexually by nuclear division and cytoplasmic cleavage, producing 2–20 uninucleate endospores (Fig. 11–51). In tissue sections, the sporangia of *P. wickerhamii* are 2–12 μm in diameter whereas those of *P. zopfii* are 10–25 μm or more. Each endospore produces its own cell wall while still inside the sporangium,[579] and molding of adjacent endospores creates the illusion of sporangial septation. The sporangia of *P. wickerhamii* sometimes occur as distinctive "morula" forms in which a central endospore is surrounded by a corona of polygonal or wedge-shaped molded endospores (Fig. 11–51B). Morula forms are only rarely found in infections caused by *P. zopfii*. The hyaline walls of the sporangia and endospores stain well with GMS, PAS, and Gridley stains, all of which highlight the distinctive morula cells.

The cutaneous lesions may show either little cellular reaction or a mixed cellular infiltrate with multinucleated giant cells and focal necrosis. The lesions of olecranon bursitis consist of geographic necrotizing or suppurative granulomas[588] that can be confused with rheumatoid nodules. Disseminated lesions, described histopathologically in only two cases, were granulomatous.[585,587]

Although the sporangia of *P. wickerhamii* and *P. zopfii* can often be distinguished from each other in tissue sections on the basis of size, shape, and frequency of morula forms, definitive diagnosis requires confirmation by culture or direct immunofluorescence.[579,581] Olecranon bursitis is cured by surgical excision. Antifungal chemotherapy of cutaneous and disseminated infections is usually ineffective.[579,580,582]

References

Introduction

1. Mackowiak PA. The normal microbial flora. N Engl J Med 1982;307:83–93.
2. Emmons CW, Binford CH, Utz JP, Kwon-Chung KJ. Medical mycology. 3d Ed. Philadelphia: Lea and Fe-

biger, 1977.

3. Chandler FW, Kaplan W, Ajello L. Color atlas and text of the histopathology of mycotic diseases. Chicago: Year Book Medical, 1980.

4. McGinnis MR. Laboratory handbook of medical mycology. New York: Academic Press, 1980.

5. Rippon JW. Medical mycology: The pathogenic fungi and the pathogenic actinomycetes. 3rd Ed. Philadelphia: W.B. Saunders, 1988.

6. Shaffer PJ, Medoff G, Kobayashi GS. New directions in diagnosis and treatment of fungus infections. Semin Infect Dis 1979;2:193–216.

7. Larson DM, Eckman Mr, Alber RL, Goldschmidt VG. Primary cutaneous (inoculation) blastomycosis: An occupational hazard to pathologists. Am J Clin Pathol 1983;79:253–255.

8. Newhouse M, Sanchis J, Bienenstock J. Lung defense mechanisms (Part 1). N Engl J Med 1976;295:990–998.

9. Williams DM, Krick JA, Remington JA. Pulmonary infection in the compromised host, part I. Am Rev Respir Dis 1976:114:359–394.

10. Ray TL. Fungal infections in the immunocompromised host. Med Clin North Am 1980;64:955–966.

11. Hawkins C, Armstrong D. Fungal infections in the immunocompromised host. Clin Haematol 1984;13: 599–630.

12. Krick Ja, Remington JS. Opportunistic invasive fungal infections in patients with leukemia and lymphoma. Clin Haematol 1976;5:249–310.

13. Rosen PP. Opportunistic fungal infections in patients with neoplastic diseases. Pathol Annu 1976;11:255–315.

14. Cho SY, Choi HY. Opportunistic fungal infection among cancer patients: A ten-year autopsy study. Am J Clin Pathol 1979;72:617–621.

15. Nash G. Pathologic features of the lung in the immunocompromised host. Hum Pathol 1982;13:841–858.

16. Nash G, Fligiel S. Pathologic features of the lung in the acquired immune deficiency syndrome (AIDS): An autopsy study of seventeen homosexual males. Am J Clin Pathol 1984;81:6–12.

17. Chandler FW. Pathology of the mycoses in patients with the acquired immunodeficiency syndrome (AIDS). Curr Top Med Mycol 1985;1:1–23.

18. Warnock DW, Richardson MD, eds. Fungal infection in the compromised patient. New York: Wiley, 1982.

19. Grieco MH. Humoral and cellular responses to infection. In: Grieco MH, ed. Infections in the abnormal host. New York: Yorke Medical, 1980:131–304.

20. Chandra RK, ed. Primary and secondary immunodeficiency disorders. New York: Churchill Livingstone, 1983.

21. Elliott K, Whelan J, eds. Enzyme defects and immune dysfunction. Ciba Foundation Symposium No. 68. Amsterdam: Excerpta Medica, 1979.

22. Thomson RB, Jr., Roberts DG. A practical approach to the diagnosis of fungal infections of the respiratory tract. Clin Lab Med 1982;2:321–342.

23. Chandler FW, Watts JC. Pathologic diagnosis of fungal infections. Chicago: ASCP Press, 1987.

24. Palmer DF, Kaufman L, Kaplan W, Cavallaro JJ. Serodiagnosis of mycotic diseases. Springfield: Thomas, 1977.

25. Kaufman L, Reiss E. Serodiagnosis of fungal diseases. In: Lennett EH, ed. Manual of clinical microbiology. 4th Ed. Washington DC: American Society for Microbiology, 1985:924–944.

26. Schwarz J. The diagnosis of deep mycoses by morphologic methods. Hum Pathol 1982;13:519–533.

27. Bancroft JD, Stevens A, eds. Theory and practice of histological techniques. London: Churchill Livingstone, 1977.

28. Kennedy A. Basic techniques in diagnostic histopathology. London: Churchill Livingstone, 1977.

29. Sheehan DC, Hnapchak BB. Theory and practice of histotechnology. 3d Ed. St. Louis: CV Mosby, 1980.

30. Elias JM. Principles and techniques in diagnostic histopathology. Park Ridge: Noyes, 1982.

31. Prophet EB, Mills B, Arrington JB, Sobin LH, eds. Laboratory Methods in Histotechnology. Washington, D.C.: American Registry of Pathology, 1992.

32. Vacca LL. Laboratory manual of histochemistry. New York: Raven, 1985.

33. Liber AF, Choi HS. Splendore-Hoeppli phenomenon about silk sutures in tissue. Arch Pathol Lab Med 1973;95:217–220.

34. Kwon-Chung KJ, Hill WB, Bennett JE. New, special stain for histopathological diagnosis of cryptococcosis. J Clin Microbiol 1981;13:383–387.

35. Ro JY, Lee SS, Ayala AG. Advantage of Fontana-Masson stain in capsule-deficient cryptococcal infection. Arch Pathol Lab Med 1987;111:53–57.

36. Wheeler MH, Bell AA. Melanins and their importance in pathogenic fungi. Curr Topics Med Mycol 1987; 2:338–387.

37. Dixon DM, Polak A. The medically important dematiaceous fungi and their identification. Mycoses 1991; 34:1–18.

38. Wood C, Russel-Bell B. Characterization of pigmented fungi by melanin staining. Am J Dermatopathol 1983; 5:77–81.

39. Wages DS, Wear DJ. Acid-fastness of fungi in blastomycosis and histoplasmosis. Arch Pathol Lab Med 1982; 106:440–441.

40. Graham AR. Fungal autofluorescence with ultraviolet illumination. Am J Clin Pathol 1983;79:231–234.

41. Monheit JE, Cowan DF, Moore DG. Rapid detection of fungi in tissues using calcofluor white and fluorescence microscopy. Arch Pathol Lab Med 1984;108:616–618.

42. Kaplan W, Kraft DE. Demonstration of pathogenic fungi in formalin-fixed tissues by immunofluorescence. Am J Clin Pathol 1969;52:420–432.

43. Kaplan W. Practical application of fluorescent antibody procedures in medical mycology. In: Mycoses. Sci Pub No 304. Washington DC: Pan American Health Organization, 1975:178–185.

44. Russell B, Beckett JH, Jacobs PH. Immunoperoxidase localization of *Sporothrix schenkii* and *Cryptococcus neoformans*. Staining of tissue sections fixed in 4% formaldehyde solution and embedded in paraffin. Arch Derma-

tol 1979;115:433–435.

45. El Nageeb S, Hay RJ. Immunoperoxidase staining in the recognition of *Aspergillus* infections. Histopathology 1981;5:437–444.

46. Humphrey DM, Weiner MH. Candidal antigen detection in pulmonary candidiasis. Am J Med 1983;74:630–640.

47. Klatt EC, Cosgrove M, Meyer RR. Rapid diagnosis of disseminated histoplasmosis in tissues. Arch Pathol Lab Med 1986;110:1173–1175.

48. Moskowitz LB, Ganjei P, Ziegels-Weissman J, et al. Immunohistologic identification of fungi in systemic and cutaneous mycoses. Arch Pathol Lab Med 1986; 110:433–436.

49. Baker RD, ed. The pathologic anatomy of mycoses: Human infection with fungi, actinomycetes and algae. Berlin: Springer-Verlag, 1971.

50. Conant NF, Smith DT, Baker RD, Callaway JL. Manual of clinical mycology. 3d Ed. Philadelphia: WB Saunders, 1971.

51. Binford CH, Dooley JR. Diseases caused by fungi and actinomycetes. In: Binford CH, Connor DH, eds. Pathology of tropical and extraordinary diseases. Washington DC: Armed Forces Institute of Pathology, 1976: 551–609.

Histoplasmosis Capsulati

52. Ajello L, Chick EW, Furcolow ML, eds. Histoplasmosis. Proceedings of the second national conference. Springfield: Thomas, 1971.

53. Domer JE, Moser SA. Histoplasmosis—a review. Rev Med Vet Mycol 1980;15:159–182.

54. Schwarz J. Histoplasmosis. New York: Praeger, 1981.

55. Schwarz J, Baum GL, Floyd H. The pathogenesis of "epidemic" histoplasmosis. Ann NY Acad Sci 1960; 89:47–58.

56. Goodwin RA, Jr., Des Prez RM. Histoplasmosis. State of the art. Am Rev. Respir Dis 1978;117:929–956.

57. Davies SF, Khan M, Sarosi GA. Disseminated histoplasmosis in immunologically suppressed patients. Occurrence in a non-endemic area. Am J Med 1978;64:94–100.

58. Goodwin RA, Jr., Shapiro JL, Thurman GH, Thurman SS, Des Prez RM. Disseminated histoplasmosis: Clinical and pathologic correlations. Medicine (Baltimore) 1980;59:1–33.

59. Kauffman CA, Israel KS, Smith JW, White AC, Schwarz J, Brooks GF. Histoplasmosis in immunosuppressed patients. Am J Med 1978;64:923–932.

60. Wheat LJ, Slama TG, Norton JA, et al. Risk factors for disseminated or fatal histoplasmosis. Ann Intern Med 1982;96:159–163.

61. Baker RD. Histoplasmosis in routine autopsies. Am J Clin Pathol 1964;41:457–470.

62. Vanek J, Schwarz J. The gamut of histoplasmosis. Am J Med 1971;50:89–104.

63. Straus SE, Jacobson ES. The spectrum of histoplasmosis in a general hospital: A review of 55 cases diagnosed at Barnes Hospital between 1966 and 1977. Am J Med Sci 1980;279:147–158.

64. Sarosi GA, Davies SF. *Histoplasma capsulatum* pneumonia. In: Pennington JE, ed. Respiratory infections: Diagnosis and management. New York: Raven, 1983:375–379.

65. Sutliff WD. Histoplasmosis in Veterans Administration hospitals in middle America. Mycopathologia 1983; 83:57–62.

66. Bennish M, Radkowski MA, Rippon JW. Cavitation in acute histoplasmosis. Chest 1983;84:496–497.

67. Sathapatavavongs B, Batteiger BE, Wheat J, Slama TG, Wass JL. Clinical and laboratory features of disseminated histoplasmosis during two large urban outbreaks. Medicine (Baltimore) 1983;62:263–270.

68. Walsh TJ, Catchatourian R, Cohen H. Disseminated histoplasmosis complicating bone marrow transplantation. Am J Clin Pathol 1983;79:509–511.

69. Wheat LJ, Smith EJ, Sathapatayavongs B, et al. Histoplasmosis in renal allograft recipients. Two large urban outbreaks. Arch Intern Med 1983;143:703–707.

70. Bonner JR, Alexander WJ, Dismukes WE, et al. Disseminated histoplasmosis in patients with the acquired immune deficiency syndrome. Arch Intern Med 1984; 144:2178–2181.

71. Wheat LJ, Small CB. Disseminated histoplasmosis in the acquired immune deficiency syndrome. Arch Intern Med 1984;144:2147–2149.

72. Wheat LJ, Slama TG, Zeckel ML. Histoplasmosis in the acquired immune deficiency syndrome. Am J Med 1985;78:203–210.

73. Minamoto G, Armstrong D. Fungal infections in AIDS: Histoplasmosis and coccidioidomycosis. Infect Dis Clin North Am 1988;2:447–456.

74. Case records of the Massachusetts General Hospital. Weekly clinicopathological exercises. Case 43-1991. A 27-year-old man with AIDS, a cough, fever, and pulmonary infiltrates. N Engl J Med 1991;325:1228–1239.

75. Kaur J, Myers AM. Homosexuality, steroid therapy, and histoplasmosis (letter). Ann Intern Med 1983;99:567.

76. Lehmann PF, Gibbons J, Senitzer D, Ribner BS, Freimer EH. T-lymphocyte abnormalities in disseminated histoplasmosis. Am J Med 1983;75:790–794.

77. Zeanah CH, Zusman J. Mediastinal and cervical histoplasmosis simulating malignancy. Am J Dis Child 1979;133:47–49.

78. Gaebler JW, Kleiman MB, Cohen M, et al. Differentiation of lymphoma from histoplasmosis in children with mediastinal masses. J Pediatr 1984;104:706–709.

79. Kurtin PL, McKinsey DS, Gupta MR, Driks M. Histoplasmosis in patients with the acquired immunodeficiency syndrome: Hematologic and bone marrow manifestations. Am J Clin Pathol 1990;93:367–372.

80. Crispell KR, Parson W, Hamlin J, Hollifield G. Addison's disease associated with histoplasmosis: Report of four cases and review of the literature. Am J Med 1956;20:23–29.

81. Canlas MS, Dillon ML Jr. *Histoplasma capsulatum* en-

docarditis: Report of a case following heart surgery. Angiology 1977;28:454–463.

82. Gaynes RP, Gardner P, Causey W. Prosthetic valve endocarditis caused by *Histoplasma capsulatum*. Arch Intern Med 1981;141:1533–1537.

83. Strimlan CV, Dines DE, Payne WS. Mediastinal granuloma. Mayo Clin Proc 1975;50:702–705.

84. Goodwin RA, Jr., Owens FT, Snell JD, et al. Chronic pulmonary histoplasmosis. Medicine (Baltimore) 1976; 55:413–452.

85. Wheat LJ, Wass J, Norton J, Kohler RB, French ML. Cavitary histoplasmosis occurring during two large urban outbreaks. Analysis of clinical, epidemiologic, roentgenographic, and laboratory features. Medicine (Baltimore) 1984;63:201–209.

86. Schwarz J, Baum GL. Fungus diseases of the lungs. Pulmonary histoplasmosis. Semin Roentgenol 1970;5: 13–28.

87. Connell JW, Muhm JR. Radiographic manifestations of pulmonary histoplasmosis: A 10-year review. Radiology 1976;121:281–285.

88. Goodwin RA, Jr., Snell JD. The enlarging histoplasmoma. Am Rev Respir Dis 1969;100:1–12.

89. Silverman FN. Roentgenographic aspects of histoplasmosis. In: Sweeny HC, ed. Histoplasmosis. Springfield: Thomas, 1960:337–381.

90. Whitehouse WM, Davey WM, Engelke OK, Holt JF. Roentgen findings in histoplasmin-positive school children. J Mich Med Soc 1959;58:1266–1269.

91. Binford CH. Histoplasmosis: tissue reactions and morphologic variations of the fungus. Am J Clin Pathol 1955;25:25–36.

92. Reynolds RJ, III, Penn RL, Grafton WD, George RB. Tissue morphology of *Histoplasma capsulatum* in acute histoplasmosis. Am Rev Respir Dis 1984;130:317–320.

93. Hutton JP, Durham JB, Miller DP, Everett ED. Hyphal forms of *Histoplasma capsulatum*. A common manifestation of intravascular infections. Arch Pathol Lab Med 1985;109:330–332.

94. Puckett TK. Pulmonary histoplasmosis: A study of twenty-two cases with the identification of *Histoplasma capsulatum* in resected tissues. Am Rev Tuberc 1963;67:453–476.

95. Ulbright TM, Katzenstein ALA. Solitary necrotizing granulomas of the lung. Am J Surg Pathol 1980;4: 13–28.

96. Girard DE, Fred HL, Bradshaw MW, Blakely RW, Ettlinger R. Disseminated histoplasmosis diagnosed from peripheral blood film. South Med J 1977;70:65–66.

97. Henochowicz S, Sahovic E, Pistole M, Rodrigues M, Macher A. Histoplasmosis diagnosed on peripheral blood smear from a patient with AIDS. JAMA 1985; 253:3148.

98. Wheat LJ, Connolly-Stringfield P, Blair R, et al. Histoplasmosis relapse in patients with AIDS: Detection using *Histoplasma capsulatum* var. *capsulatum* antigen levels. Ann Intern Med 1991;115:936–941.

99. Hawkins SS, Gregory DW, Alford RH. Progressive disseminated histoplasmosis: favorable response to ketoconazole. Ann Intern Med 1981;95:446–449.

100. Slama TG. Treatment of disseminated and progressive cavitary histoplasmosis with ketoconazole. Proceedings of a symposium on new developments in therapy for the mycoses. Am J Med 1983;74:70–73.

Histoplasmosis Duboisii

101. Vanbreuseghem R. L'histoplasmose africaine un histoplasmose causes pour *Histoplasma duboisii* Vanbreuseghem 1952. Bull Acad R Med Belg 1964;4:543–585.

102. Schwarz J. African histoplasmosis (part 2). In: Baker RD, ed. The pathologic anatomy of mycoses: Human infection with fungi, actinomycetes and algae. Berlin: Springer-Verlag, 1971:139–146.

103. Yamato H, Hitomi H, Maekawa S, Mimura K. A case of histoplasmosis. Acta Med Okayama 1957;11:347–364.

104. Coulanges P, Raveloarison G, Ravisse P. Existence of histoplasmosis with *Histoplasma duboisii* outside Continental Africa (on the first Malagash case). Bull Soc Pathol Exot Filiales 1982;75:400–403.

105. Cockshott WP, Lucas AO. *Histoplasma duboisii*. Q J Med 1964;33:223–238.

106. Walker J, Spooner ETC. Natural infection of the African baboon (*Papio papio*) with the large cell form of histoplasmosis. J Pathol Bacteriol 1960;8:436–439.

107. Williams AO, Lawson EA, Lucas AO. African histoplasmosis due to *Histoplasma duboisii*. Arch Pathol 1971; 92:306–318.

108. Nethercott JR, Schachter RK, Givan KF, Ryder DE. Histoplasmosis due to *Histoplasma capsulatum* var. *duboisii* in a Canadian immigrant. Arch Dermatol 1978;114: 595–598.

109. Shore RN, Waltersdorff RL, Edelstein MV, Teske JH. African histoplasmosis in the United States. JAMA 1981;245:734.

110. Lobdell DH, Cappiello MA, Riccio FJ. African histoplasmosis in Connecticut. Conn Med 1982;46:187.

111. Clark BM, Greenwood BB. Pulmonary lesions in African histoplasmosis. J Trop Med Hyg 1968;71:4–10.

112. Lanceley LJ, Lunn HF, Wilson AMM. Histoplasmosis in an African child. J Pediatr 1961;59:756–764.

113. Quere MA, Basset A, Basset M, Cave L. Histoplasmose generalisee avec localisation orbitopalpebrale et lacunes craniennes. Ann Oculist 1065;198:105–114.

114. Cockshott WP, Lucas AO. Radiological findings in *Histoplasma duboisii* infections. Br J Radiol 1964;37:653–660.

115. Lunn HF. A case of histoplasmosis of bone in East Africa. J Trop Med Hyg 1960;63:175–180.

116. Adekunle OO, Sudhakaran P, Timeyin ED. African histoplasmosis of the jejunum. Report of a case. J Trop Med Hyg 1978;81:88–90.

117. Young CN. North American blastomycosis in South Africa. S Afr Med J 1977;51:865.

118. Brown KGE, Molesworth BD, Boerrigter FGG, et al. Disseminated histoplasmosis duboisii in Malawi. Partial

response to sulphonamide/trimethoprim combination. East Afr Med J 1974;51:584–590.

Blastomycosis

119. McDonough ES. Blastomycosis: Epidemiology and biology of its etiologic agent, *Ajellomyces dermatitidis.* Mycopathologia 1970;41:195–201.

120. Sekhon AS, Jackson FL, Jacobs HJ. Blastomycosis: Report of the first case from Alberta, Canada. Mycopathologia 1982;79:65–69.

121. Tenenbaum MJ, Greenspan J, Kerkering TM. Blastomycosis. CRC Crit Rev Microbiol 1982;9:139–163.

122. Kane J, Righter J, Krajden S, Lester RS. Blastomycosis: A new endemic focus in Canada. Can Med Assoc J 1983;129:728–731.

123. Schwarz J. Epidemiology and epidemics of blastomycosis. Mykosen 1983;16:7–14.

124. Emerson PA, Higgins E, Branfoot A. North American blastomycosis in Africans. Br J Dis Chest 1984;78:286–291.

125. Randhawa HS, Khan Z, Gaur S. *Blastomyces dermatitidis* in India: First report of its isolation from clinical material. Sabouraudia 1983;21:215–221.

126. Sarosi GA, Davies, SF. Blastomycosis. Am Rev Respir Dis 1979;120:911–938.

127. Denton JF, McDonough ES, Ajello L, Ausherman RJ. Isolation of *Blastomyces dermatitidis* from soil. Science 1961;133:1126–1127.

128. Baum GL, Lerner PI. Primary pulmonary blastomycosis: A laboratory acquired infection. Ann Intern Med 1970;73:263–265.

129. Busey JP, ed. Blastomycosis: I. A review of 198 collected cases in the Veterans Administration hospitals. Am Rev Respir Dis 1964;89:659–672.

130. Witorsch P, Utz JP. North American blastomycosis: A study of 40 patients. Medicine (Baltimore) 1968;47:169–200.

131. Vanek J, Schwarz J, Haken S. North Ameirican blastomycosis. Am J Clin Pathol 1970;54:384–400.

132. Schwarz J, Baum GL. Fungus diseases of the lungs. North American blastomycosis. Semin Roentgenol 1970;5:40–48.

133. Cush R, Light RW, George RB. Clinical and roentgenographic manifestations of acute and chronic blastomycosis. Chest 1976;69:345–349.

134. Halvorsen RA, Duncan JD, Merten DJ, Gallis HA, Putman CE. Pulmonary blastomycosis: radiologic manifestations. Radiology 1984;150:1–5.

135. Laskey W, Sarosi GA. The radiologic appearance of pulmonary blastomycosis. Radiology 1978;126:351–357.

136. Abernathy RS. Clinical manifestations of pulmonary blastomycosis. Ann Intern Med 1959;51:707–727.

137. Inoshita T, Youngberg GA, Boelen LJ, Langston J. Blastomycosis presenting with prostatic involvement: Report of 2 cases and review of the literature. J Urol 1983;130:160–162.

138. Stelling CB, Woodring JH, Rehm SR, Hopper DW, Noble RC. Miliary pulmonary blastomycosis. Radiology 1984;150:7–13.

139. Poe RH, Vassalo CL, Plessingar VA, Pulmonary blastomycosis versus carcinoma: A challenging differential. Am J Med Sci 1972;263:145–155.

140. Kinasewitz GT, Penn RL, George RB. The spectrum and significance of pleural disease in blastomycosis. Chest 1984;86:580–584.

141. Onal E, Lopata M, Lourence RV. Disseminated pulmonary blastomycosis in an immunosuppressed patient: Diagnosis by fiberoptic bronchoscopy. Am Rev Respir Dis 1976;113:83–86.

142. Atkinson JB, McCurley TL. Pulmonary blastomycosis: filamentous forms in an immunocompromised patient with fulminating respiratory failure. Hum Pathol 1983;14:186–188.

143. Laskey WL, Sarosi GA. Endogenous reactivation in blastomycosis. Ann Intern Med 1978;88:50–52.

144. Harding CV. Blastomycosis and opportunistic infections in patients with acquired immunodeficiency syndrome. Arch Pathol Lab Med 1991;115:1133–1136.

145. Butka BJ, Bennett SR, Johnson AC. Disseminated inoculation blastomycosis in a renal transplant recipient. Am Rev Respir Dis 1984;130:1180–1183.

146. Schwarz J, Salfelder K. Blastomycosis: a review of 152 cases. In: Grundmann E, Kirsten WH, eds. Current topics in pathology. Berlin: Springer-Verlag, 1977;65:165–200.

147. Chandler FW, Watts JC. Pathologic features of blastomycosis. In: Al-Doory Y, DiSalvo AF, eds. Blastomycosis. New York: Plenum Press, 1992:189–220.

148. Tuttle JG, Lichtwardt HE, Altshuler CH. Systemic North American blastomycosis. Report of a case with small forms of blastomycetes. Am J Clin Pathol 1953;23:890–897.

149. Watts JC, Chandler FW, Mihalov ML, Kammeyer PL, Armin AR. Giant forms of *Blastomyces dermatitidis* in the pulmonary lesions of blastomycosis. Potential confusion with *Coccidioides immitis.* Am J Clin Pathol 1990;93:119–122.

150. Lockwood WR, Allison F, Blair BE, Busey JF. The treatment of North American blastomycosis. Ten years' experience. Am Rev Respir Dis 1969;100:314–320.

151. Parker JD, Doto IL, Tosh FE. A decade of experience with blastomycosis and its treatment with amphotericin B. Am Rev Respir Dis 1969;99:895–902.

152. Busey JF. Blastomycosis. III. A comparative study of 2-hydroxystilbamidine and amphotericin B therapy. Am Rev Respir Dis 1972;105:812–818.

153. Bradsher RW. Prognosis and therapy of blastomycosis. In: Al-Doory Y, DiSalvo AF, eds. Blastomycosis. New York: Plenum Press, 1992:237–247.

154. Short KL, Harty JI, Amin M, Short LF. The use of ketoconazole to treat systemic blastomycosis presenting as acute epididymitis. J Urol 1983;129:382–384.

155. Sanders JS, Sarosi GA, Nollet DJ, Thompson JI. Exfoliative cytology in the rapid diagnosis of pulmonary blastomycosis. Chest 1977;72:193–196.

156. Trumbull ML, Chesney TM. The cytological diagnosis of pulmonary blastomycosis. JAMA 1981;245:836–838.

157. Kaufman L. Immunodiagnosis of blastomycosis. In: Al-Doory Y, DiSalvo AF, eds. Blastomycosis. New York: Plenum Press, 1992:123–132.

Cryptococcosis

158. Kaufman L, Blumer S. Cryptococcosis: The awakening giant. In: The black and white yeasts. Sci Pub 356. Washington DC: Pan American Health Organization, 1978:176–182.

159. Powell KE, Dahl BA, Weeks RJ, Tosh FE. Airborne *Cryptococcus neoformans:* Particles from pigeon excreta compatible with alveolar deposition. J Infect Dis 1972;125:412–415.

160. Diamond RD. *Cryptococcus neoformans* pneumonia. In: Pennington JE, ed. Respiratory infections: Diagnosis and management. New York: Raven, 1983:341–351.

161. Nielson JB, Fromtling RA, Bulmer GS. *Cryptococcus neoformans:* Size range of infectious particles from aerosolized soil. Infect Immun 1977;17:634–638.

162. Littman ML, Walter JE. Cryptococcosis: current status. Am J Med 1968;45:922–932.

163. Lewis RL, Rabinovich S. The wide spectrum of cryptococcal infections. Am J Med 1972;53:315–322.

164. Noble RC, Fajardo LF. Primary cutaneous cryptococcosis: Review and morphologic study. Am J Clin Pathol 1972;57:13–22.

165. Kaplan MH, Rosen PP, Armstrong D. Cryptococcosis in a cancer hospital. Clinical and pathological correlates in forty-six patients. Cancer 1977;39:2265–2274.

166. Kerkering TM, Duma RJ, Shadomy S. The evolution of pulmonary cryptococcosis: Clinical implications from a study of 41 patients with and without compromising host factors. Ann Intern Med 1981;94:611–616.

167. Schimpff SC, Bennett JE. Abnormalities in cell-mediated immunity in patients with *Cryptococcus neoformans* infections. J Allergy Clin Immunol 1975;55:430–441.

168. Clark RA, Greer D, Atkinson W, Valainis GT, Hyslop N. Spectrum of *Cryptococcus neoformans* infection in 68 patients infected with human immunodeficiency virus. Rev Infect Dis 1990;12:768–777.

169. Chechani V, Kamholz SL. Pulmonary manifestations of disseminated cryptococcosis in patients with AIDS. Chest 1990;98:1060–1066.

170. Krumholz RA. Pulmonary cryptococcosis: a case due to *Cryptococcus albidus.* Am Rev Respir Dis 1972;105:421–424.

171. Lynch JP, III, Schaberg DR, Kissner DG, Kauffman CA. *Cryptococcus laurentii* lung abscess. Am Rev Respir Dis 1981;123:135–138.

172. Denning DW, Stevens DA, Hamilton JR. Comparison of *Guizotia abyssinica* seed extract (birdseed) agar with conventional media for selective identification of *Cryptococcus neoformans* in patients with acquired immunodeficiency syndrome. J Clin Microbiol 1990;28:2565–2567.

173. Sarosi GA, Silberfarb PM, Tosh FE. Cutaneous cryptococcosis: A sentinel of disseminated disease. Arch Dermatol 1971;104:1–3.

174. Schupbach CW, Wheeler CE, Briggaman RA, Warner NA, Kanof EP. Cutaneous manifestations of disseminated cryptococcosis. Arch Dermatol 1976;112:1734–1740.

175. Massa MG, Doyle JA. Cutaneous cryptococcosis simulating pyoderma gangrenosum. J Am Acad Dermatol 1981;5:32–36.

176. Borton LK, Wintroub BU. Disseminated cryptococcosis presenting as herpetiform lesions in a homosexual man with acquired immunodeficiency syndrome. J Am Acad Dermatol 1984;10:387–390.

177. Rico MJ, Penneys NS. Cutaneous cryptococcosis resembling molluscum contagiosum in a patient with AIDS. Arch Dermatol 1985;121:901–902.

178. Eng RH, Bishburg E, Smith SM, Kapila R. Cryptococcal infections in patients with acquired immune deficiency syndrome. Am J Med 1986;81:19–23.

179. Zuger A, Louie E, Holzman RS, Simberkoff MS, Rahal JJ. Cryptococcal disease in patients with the acquired immunodeficiency syndrome. Ann Intern Med 1986; 104:234–240.

180. Campbell GD. Primary pulmonary cryptococcosis. Am Rev Respir Dis1966;94:236–243.

181. Warr W, Bates JH, Stone A. The spectrum of pulmonary cryptococcosis. Ann Intern Med 1968;69:1109–1116.

182. Hammerman KJ, Powell KE, Christianson CS, et al. Pulmonary cryptococcosis: Clinical forms and treatment. A Center for Disease Control cooperative mycoses study. Am Rev Respir Dis 1973;108:1116–1123.

183. Tynes B, Mason KN, Jennings AE, Bennett JE. Variant forms of pulmonary cryptococcosis. Ann Intern Med 1968;69:1117–1125.

184. Cohen AA, Davis W, Finegold SM. Chronic pulmonary cryptococcosis. Am Rev Respir Dis 1965;91:414–423.

185. Feigin DS. Pulmonary cryptococcosis: Radiologic–pathologic correlates of its three forms. AJR 1983; 141:1262–1272.

186. Salyer WR. Primary complex of *Cryptococcus* and pulmonary lymph nodes. J Infect Dis 1974;130:74–77.

187. Baker RD. The primary pulmonary lymph node complex of cryptococcosis. Am J Clin Pathol 1976;65:83–92.

188. Schwarz J, Baum GL. Fungus diseases of the lungs. Cryptococcosis. Semin Roentgenol 1970;5:49–54.

189. Khoury MB, Godwin JD, Ravin CE, Gallis HA, Halvorsen RA, Putman CE. Thoracic cryptococcosis: Immunologic competence and radiologic appearance. AJR 1984;142:893–896.

190. Gordonson J, Birnbaum W, Jacobson G, Sargent EN. Pulmonary cryptococcosis. Radiology 1974;112:557–561.

191. Young EJ, Hirsh DD, Fainstein V, Williams TW. Pleural effusions due to *Cryptococcus neoformans:* A review of the literature and report of two cases with cryptococcal antigen determinations. Am Rev Respir Dis 1980;121:743–747.

192. Fisher BD, Armstrong D. Cryptococcal interstitial pneumonia: Value of antigen determination. N Engl J Med 1977;297:1440–1441.

193. Stansell JD. Fungal disease in HIV-infected persons: Cryptococcosis, histoplasmosis, and coccidioidomycosis. J Thorac Imaging 1991;66:153–156.

194. Kent TH, Layton JM. Massive pulmonary cryptococcosis. Am J Clin Pathol 1962;38:596–604.

195. Bloomfield N, Gordon MA, Elmendorf DF, Jr. Detection of *Cryptococcus neoformans* antigen in body fluids by latex particle agglutination. Proc Soc Exp Biol Med 1963;114:64–67.

196. Diamond RD. *Cryptococcus neoformans.* In: Mandell GL, Douglas RG, Bennett JE, eds. Principles and practice of infectious diseases. 2d Ed. New York: Wiley, 1985: 1460–1468.

197. Perkins W. Pulmonary cryptococcosis: Report on the treatment of nine cases. Chest 1969;56:389–394.

198. Larsen RA, Leal MAE, Chan LS. Fluconazole compared with amphotericin B plus flucytosine for cryptococcal meningitis in AIDS. A randomized trial. Ann Intern Med 1990;113:183–187.

199. Sugar AM, Saunders C. Oral fluconazole as suppressive therapy of disseminated cryptococcosis in patients with acquired immunodeficiency syndrome. Am J Med 1988; 85:481–489.

200. Smith FS, Gibson P, Nicholls TT, Simpson JA. Pulmonary resection for localized lesions of cryptococcosis (torulosis): A review of eight cases. Thorax 1976;31: 121–126.

201. Baker RD, Haugh RK. Tissue changes and tissue diagnosis in cryptococcosis. A study of twenty-six cases. Am J Clin Pathol 1955;25:14–24.

202. McDonnell JM, Hutchins GM. Pulmonary cryptococcosis. Hum Pathol 1985;16:121–128.

203. Farmer SG, Komorowski RA. Histologic response to capsule-deficient *Cryptococcus neoformans.* Arch Pathol 1973;96:383–387.

204. Rosenheim SH, Schwarz J. Cavitary pulmonary cryptococcosis complicated by aspergilloma. Am Rev Respir Dis 1975;111:549–553.

205. Gutierrez F, Fu YS, Lurie HI. Cryptococcosis histologically resembling histoplasmosis. A light and electron microscopical study. Arch Pathol 1975;99:347–352.

206. Harding SA, Scheld WM, Feldman PS, Sande MA. Pulmonary infection with capsule-deficient *Cryptococcus neoformans.* Virchows Arch [A] 1979;382:113–118.

Paracoccidioidomycosis

207. Angulo-Ortega A, Pollak L. Paracoccidioidomycosis. In: Baker RD, ed. The pathologic anatomy of mycoses: Human infection with fungi, actinomycetes and algae. Berlin: Springer-Verlag, 1971:507–576.

208. Giraldo R, Restrepo A, Gutierrez F, et al. Pathogenesis of paracoccidioidomycosis: A model based on the study of 46 patients. Mycopathologia 1976;58:63–70.

209. Restrepo A, Robledo M, Giraldo R, et al. The gamut of paracoccidioidomycosis. Am J Med 1976;61:33–42.

210. Fountain FF, Sutliff WD. Paracoccidioidomycosis in the United States. Am Rev Respir Dis 1969;99:89–93.

211. Kroll JJ, Walzer RA. Paracoccidioidomycosis in the United States. Arch Dermatol 1972;106:543–546.

212. Murray HW, Littman ML, Roberts RB. Disseminated paracoccidioidomycosis (South American blastomycosis) in the United States. Am J Med 1974;56:209–220.

213. Bouza E, Winston DJ, Rhodes J, Hewitt WL. Paracoccidioidomycosis (South American blastomycosis) in the United States. Chest 1977;72:100–102.

214. Restrepo A, Robledo M, Gutierrez F, Sanclemente M, Castaneda E, Calle G. Paracoccidioidomycosis (South American blastomycosis): A study of 39 cases observed in Medellin, Colombia. Am J Trop Med Hyg 1970; 19:68–76.

215. Salfelder K, Doehnert G, Doehnert HR. Paracoccidioidomycosis: Anatomic study with complete autopsies. Virchows Arch [A] 1969;348:51–76.

216. Restrepo A. The ecology of *Paracoccidioides brasiliensis:* A puzzle still unsolved. Sabouraudia 1985;23:323–334.

217. Sugar AM, Restrepo A, Stevens DA. Paracoccidioidomycosis in the immunosuppressed host: Report of a case and review of the literature. Am Rev Respir Dis 1984;129:340–342.

218. Londero AT, Ramos CD, Lopes JOS. Progressive pulmonary paracoccidioidomycosis: A study of 34 cases observed in Rio Grande do Sul (Brazil). Mycopathologia 1978;63:53–56.

219. Londero AT, Severo LC. The gamut of progressive pulmonary paracoccidioidomycosis. Mycopathologia 1981;75:65–74.

220. Schwarz J, Baum GL. Paracoccidioidomycosis (South American blastomycosis). Semin Roentgenol 1970; 5:69–72.

221. Tuder RM, El Ibrahim R, Godoy CE, DeBrito T. Pathology of the human pulmonary paracoccidioidomycosis. Mycopathologia 1985;92:179–188.

222. Severo LC, Geyer GR, Londero AT, Porto NS, Rizzon CFC. The primary pulmonary lymph node complex in paracoccidioidomycosis. Mycopathologia 1979;67:115–118.

223. Londero AT, Severo LC, Ramos CD. Small forms and hyphae of *Paracoccidioides brasiliensis* in human tissue. Mycopathologia 1980;72:17–19.

224. Tani EM, Franco M. Pulmonary cytology in paracoccidioidomycosis. Acta Cytol 1984;28:571–575.

225. Cohen J. Antifungal chemotherapy. Lancet 1982;ii: 532–537.

226. Hermans PE, Key TF. Antifungal agents used for deep-seated mycotic infections. Mayo Clin Proc 1983;58:223–231.

227. Restrepo A, Gomez I, Robledo J, Patiño MM, Cano LE. Itraconazole in the treatment of paracoccidioidomycosis. A preliminary report. Rev Infect Dis 1987;9(Suppl. 1):S51–S56.

Sporotrichosis

228. Lurie HI. Sporotrichosis. In: Baker RD, ed. The pathologic anatomy of mycoses: Human infection with fungi, actinomycetes and algae. Berlin: Springer-Verlag, 1971:

614–675.

229. Bullpitt P, Weedon D. Sporotrichosis: A review of 39 cases. Pathology 1978;10:249–256.

230. Lurie HI. Histopathology of sporotrichosis. Arch Pathol 1963;75:92–109.

231. Scott SM, Peasley ED, Crymes TP. Pulmonary sporotrichosis. Report of two cases with cavitation. N Engl J Med 1961;265:453–457.

232. Baum GL, Donnerberg RL, Steward D, Mulligan WJ, Putnam LR. Pulmonary sporotrichosis. N Engl J Med 1969;280:410–413.

233. Berson SD, Brandt FA. Primary pulmonary sporotrichosis with unusual fungal morphology. Thorax 1977;32:505–508.

234. England DM, Hochholzer L. Primary pulmonary sporotrichosis. Report of eight cases with clinicopathologic review. Am J Surg Pathol 1985;9:193–204.

235. England DM, Hochholzer L. *Sporothrix* infection of the lung without cutaneous disease: Primary pulmonary sporotrichosis. Arch Pathol Lab Med 1987;111:298–300.

236. Watts JC, Chandler FW. Primary pulmonary sporotrichosis. Arch Pathol Lab Med 1987;111:215–217.

237. Wilson DE, Mann JJ, Bennett JE, Utz JP. Clinical features of extracutaneous sporotrichosis. Medicine (Baltimore) 1967;46:265–279.

238. Lynch PJ, Voorhees JJ, Harrell ER. Systemic sporotrichosis. Ann Intern Med 1970;73:23–30.

239. Font RI,Jakobiec FA. Granulomatous necrotizing retinochoroiditis caused by *Sporotrichum schenckii*. Report of a case including immunofluorescence and electron microscopical studies. Arch Ophthalmol 1976;94:1513–1519.

240. Brook CJ, Ravikrishnan KP, Weg JG. Pulmonary and articular sporotrichosis. Am Rev Respir Dis 1977;116:141–143.

241. Friedman SJ, Doyle JA. Extracutaneous sporotrichosis. Int J Dermatol 1983;22:171–176.

242. Smith PW, Loomis GW, Luckasen JL, Osterholm RK. Disseminated cutaneous sporotrichosis. Three illustrative cases. Arch Dermatol 1981;117:143–144.

243. Smith AG, Morgan WKC, Hornick RB, Funk AM, Chronic pulmonary sporotrichosis: report of a case, including morphologic and mycologic studies. Am J Clin Pathol 1970;54:401–409.

244. Schwarz J, Baum GL. Fungus diseases of the lungs. Sporotrichosis. Semin Roentgenol 1970;5:55–57.

245. Comstock C, Wolson AH. Roentgenology of sporotrichosis. Am J Roentgenol Radium Ther Nucl Med 1975;125:651–655.

246. Lurie HI, Still WJS. The "capsule" of *Sporotrichum schenckii* and the evolution of the asteroid body. A light and electron microscopic study. Sabouraudia 1969;7:64–70.

247. Maberry JD, Mullins JF, Stone OJ. Sporotrichosis with demonstration of hyphae in human tissue. Arch Dermatol 1966;93:65–67.

248. Mohr JA, Patterson CD,Eaton BG, Rhoades ER, Nichols NB. Primary pulmonary sporotrichosis. Am Rev Respir Dis 1972;106:260–264.

249. Kaplan W, Gonzalez-Ochoa A. Application of the fluorescent antibody technique to the rapid diagnosis of sporotrichosis. J Lab Clin Med 1963;62:835–841.

250. Parker JD, Sarosi GA, Tosh FE. Treatment of extracutaneous sporotrichosis. Arch Intern Med 1970;125:858–863.

251. Restrepo A, Robledo J, Gomez I, Tabares AM, Gutierrez R. Itraconazole therapy in lymphangitic and cutaneous sporotrichosis. Arch Dermatol 1986;122:413–417.

252. Rohwedder JJ, Archer G. Pulmonary sporotrichosis: Treatment with miconazole. Am Rev Respir Dis 1976;114:403–406.

253. Baker JH, Goodpasture HC, Kuhns HR, Rinaldi MG. Fungemia caused by an amphotericin B-resistant isolate of *Sporothrix schenckii*. Successful treatment with itraconazole. Arch Pathol Lab Med 1989;113:1279–1281.

254. Gullberg RM, Quintanilla A, Levin ML, Williams J, Phair JP. Sporotrichosis: Recurrent cutaneous, articular, and central nervous system infection in a renal transplant recipient. Rev Infect Dis 1987;9:369–375.

255. Jung JY, Almond CH, Campbell DC, Elkadi A, Tenorio A. Role of surgery in the management of pulmonary sporotrichosis. J Thorac Cardioavasc Surg 1979;77:234–239.

Torulopsosis

256. Grimley PM, Wright LD, Jennings AE. *Torulopsis glabrata* infection in man. Am J Clin Pathol 1965;43:216–223.

257. Marks MI, Langston C, Eickhoff TC. *Torulopsis glabrata*—an opportunistic pathogen of man. N Engl J Med 1970;283:1131–1135.

258. Yarrow D, Meyer SA. Proposal for amendment of the diagnosis of the genus *Candida* Berkhout *nom. cons.* Int J Syst Bacteriol 1978;28:611–615.

259. McGinnis MR, Ajello L, Beneke ES, et al. Taxonomic and nomenclatural evaluation of the genera *Candida* and *Torulopsis*. J Clin Microbiol 1984;20:813–814.

260. Lodder J. The yeasts. A taxonomic study. 2d Ed. Amsterdam: North-Holland, 1970.

261. Katz D, Pickard RE. Systemic *Torulopsis glabrata* infection causing shock, fever and coma. Am J Med 1967;42:151–152.

262. Louria DB, Belvins A, Armstrong D, Burdick R. Lieberman P. Fungemia caused by "nonpathogenic" yeasts. Arch Intern Med 1967;119:247–252.

263. Rodrigues RJ, Shinya H, Wolff WI, Puttlitz D. *Torulopsis glabrata* fungemia during prolonged intravenous alimentation therapy. N Engl J Med 1971;284:540–541.

264. Pankey GA, Daloviso JR. Fungemia caused by *Torulopsis glabrata*. Medicine (Baltimore) 1973;52:395–403.

265. Young RC, Bennett JE, Geelhoed GW, Levine AS. Fungemia with compromised host resistance. A study of 70 cases. Ann Intern Med 1974;80:605–612.

266. Valdivieso M, Luna M, Bodey GP, Rodriguez V, Groschel D. Fungemia due to *Torulopsis glabrata* in the

compromised host. Cancer 1976;38:1750–1756.

267. Berkowitz ID, Robboy SJ, Karchmer AW, Kunz LJ. *Torulopsis glabrata* fungemia—a clinical pathological study. Medicine (Baltimore) 1979;58:430–440.

268. Kauffman CA, Tan JS. *Torulopsis glabrata* renal infection. Am J Med 1974;57:217–224.

269. Takeuchi H, Tomoyoshi T. Torulopsis infection extensively involving urinary tract. Urology 1983;22:173–175.

270. Vordermark JS, II, Modarelli RO, Buck AS. Torulopsis pyelonephritis associated with papillary necrosis. A case report. J Urol 1980;123:96–97.

271. Oldfield FS, Kapica L, Pirozynski WJ. Pulmonary infection due to *Torulopsis glabrata*. Can Med Assoc J 1968;98:165–168.

272. Aisner J, Sickles EA, Schimpff SC, Young VM, Greene WH, Wiernik PH. *Torulopsis glabrata* pneumonitis in patients with cancer: Report of three cases. JAMA 1974;230:584–585.

273. Sander LA, Young EJ, Musher DM, Clarridge JE. *Torulopsis glabrata* pneumonia in a malnourished woman. South Med J 1979;72:1477–1479.

274. Gustke KA, Wu KK. *Torulopsis glabrata* osteomyelitis: Report of a case. Clin Orthop 1981;154:197–200.

275. Thurston AJ, Gillespie WJ. *Torulopsis glabrata* osteomyelitis of the spine: A case report and review of the literature. Aust NZ J Surg 1981;51:374–376.

276. Rubin MM, Sanfilippo RJ. Osteomyelitis of the hyoid caused by *Torulopsis glabrata* in a patient with acquired immunodeficiency syndrome. J Oral Maxillofac Surg 1990;48:1217–1219.

277. Heffner DK, Franklin WA. Endocarditis caused by *Torulopsis glabrata*. Am J Clin Pathol 1978;70:420–423.

278. Holliday HD, Keipper V, Kaiser AB. *Torulopsis glabrata* endocarditis. JAMA 1980;244:2088–2089.

279. Miller DD. Postoperative acalculous cholecystitis due to *Torulopsis glabrata*. Arch Surg 1976;111:1404–1405.

280. Baley JE, Dliegman RM, Annable WL, Dahms BB, Fanaroff AA. *Torulopsis glabrata* sepsis appearing as necrotizing enterocolitis and endophthalmitis. Am J Dis Child 1984;138:965–966.

281. Wurzel B, Goldberg P, Caroline L, Bozza AT, Kozinn PJ. *Torulopsis glabrata* meningoencephalitis treated with 5-flucytosine. Ann Intern Med 1972;77:814–815.

282. Fitzsimons RB, Nicholls MD, Billson FA, Robertson TI, Hersey P. Fungal retinitis: A case of *Torulopsis glabrata* infection treated with miconazole. Br J Ophthalmol 1980;64:672–675.

283. Clark JFJ, Faggett T, Peters B, et al. Ulcerative vaginitis due to *Torulopsis glabrata:* A case report. J Natl Med Assoc 1978;70:913–914.

284. Tom W, Aaron JS. Esophageal ulcers caused by *Torulopsis glabrata* in a patient with acquired immune deficiency syndrome. Am J Gastroenterol 1987;82:766–768.

285. Hahn H, Condie F, Bulger RF. Diagnosis of *Torulopsis glabrata* infection. JAMA 1968;203:835–837.

286. Rose HD, Heckman MG. Persistent fungemia caused by *Torulopsis glabrata:* Treatment with amphotericin B. Am J Clin Pathol 1970;54:205–208.

287. Corbella X, Carratala J, Castells M, Berlanga B. Fluconazole treatment in *Torulopsis glabrata* upper urinary tract infection causing ureteral obstruction. J Urol 1992; 147:1112–1114.

Candidiasis

288. Rose HD, Varkey B. Deep mycotic infection in the hospitalized adult: A study of 123 patients. Medicine (Baltimore) 1975;54:499–507.

289. DeGregorio MW, Lee WMF, Linker CA, Jacobs RA, Ries CA. Fungal infections in patients with acute leukemia. Am J Med 1982;73:543–548.

290. Maksymiuk AW, Thongprasert S, Hopfer R, Luna M, Fainstein V. Bodey GP. Systemic candidiasis in cancer patients. Am J Med 1984;77(4D):20–27.

291. Schwartz RS, Mackintosh FR, Schrier SL, Greenberg PL. Multivariate analysis of factors associated with invasive fungal disease during remission induction therapy for acute myelogenous leukemia. Cancer 1984;53:411–419.

292. Hopfer RL. Mycology of candida infections. In: Bodey GP, Fainstein V, eds. Candidiasis. New York: Raven, 1985:1–12.

293. Parker JC, McCloskey JJ, Knauer KA. Pathobiologic features of human candidiasis: a common deep mycosis of the brain, heart and kidney in the altered host. Am J Clin Pathol 1976;65:991–1000.

294. Myerowitz RL, Pazin GJ, Allen CM. Disseminated candidiasis: changes in incidence, underlying diseases, and pathology. Am J Clin Pathol 1977;68:29–38.

295. Kiehn TE, Edwards FF, Armstrong D. The prevalence of yeasts in clinical specimens from cancer patients. Am J Clin Pathol 1980;73:518–521.

296. Hughes WT. Systemic candidiasis: A study of 109 fatal cases. Pediatr Infect Dis 1982;1:11–18.

297. Marsh PK, Tally FP, Kellum J, Callow A, Gorbach SL. Candida infections in surgical patients. Ann Surg 1983;198:42–47.

298. Blinkhorn RJ, Adelstein D, Spagnuolo PJ. Emergence of a new opportunistic pathogen, *Candida lusitaniae*. J Clin Microbiol 1989;27:236–240.

299. Kozinn PJ, Taschdjian CL. *Candida albicans:* Saprophyte or pathogen? JAMA 1966;198:170–172.

300. Rippon JW. Medical mycology: The pathogenic fungi and the pathogenic actinomycetes. 3rd Ed. Philadelphia: W.B. Saunders, 1988:536–581.

301. Edwards JW, moderator. Severe candidal infections: Clinical perspective, immune defense mechanisms, and current concepts of therapy. Ann Intern Med 1978; 89:91–106.

302. Smith CB. Candidiasis: Pathogenesis, host resistance, and predisposing factors. In: Bodey GP, Fainstein V. eds. Candidiasis. New York: Raven, 1985:53–70.

303. Marchevsky A, Rosen MJ, Chrystal G, Kleinerman J. Pulmonary complications of the acquired immunodeficiency syndrome: A clinicopathologic study of 70 cases. Hum Pathol 1985;16:659–670.

304. Myerowitz RL. The pathology of opportunistic infec-

tions with pathogenetic, diagnostic, and clinical correlations. New York: Raven, 1983:95–114.

305. Kassner EG, Kauffman SL, Yoon JJ, Semiglia M, Kozinn PJ, Goldberg PL. Pulmonary candidiasis in infants: Clinical, radiologic, and pathologic features. AJR 1981; 137:707–716.

306. Bross J, Talbot GH, Maislin G, Hurwitz S, Strom BL. Risk factors for nosocomial candidemia: A case-control study in adults without leukemia. Am J Med 1989; 87:614–620.

307. Masur H, Rosen PP, Armstrong D. Pulmonary disease caused by *Candida* species. Am J Med 1977;63:914–925.

308. Bodey GP, Fainstein V. Systemic candidiasis. In: Bodey GP, Fainstein V, eds. Candidiasis. New York: Raven, 1985:135–168.

309. Ramirez G, Shuster M, Kozub W, Pribor HC. Fatal acute *Candida albicans* bronchopneumonia: Report of a case. JAMA 1967;199:340–342.

310. Steven PJ, Jameson JW, Philpott CM. Fatal pulmonary candidiasis. Lancet 1972;i:962–963.

311. Rosenbaum RB, Barber JV, Stevens DA. *Candida albicans* pneumonia: Diagnosis by pulmonary aspiration, recovery without treatment. Am Rev Respir Dis 1974; 109:373–378.

312. Pagani JJ, Libshitz HI. Opportunistic fungal pneumonias in cancer patients. AJR 1981;137:1033–1039.

313. Pagani JJ, Libshitz HI. Radiology of *Candida* infections. In: Bodey GP, Fainstein V, eds. Candidiasis. New York: Raven, 1985:71–84.

314. Dubois PJ, Myerowitz RL, Allen CM. Pathoradiologic correlation of pulmonary candidiasis in immunosuppressed patients. Cancer 1977;40:1026–1036.

315. Bode FR, Paré JAP, Fraser RG. Pulmonary diseases in the compromised host: A review of clinical and roentgenographic manifestations in patients with impaired host defense mechanisms. Medicine (Baltimore) 1974; 53:255–293.

316. Buff SJ, McLelland R, Gallis HA, Matthay R, Putman CE. *Candida albicans* pneumonia: radiographic appearance. AJR 1982;138:645–648.

317. Hietala SO, Jonsson M, Burman LA. *Candida albicans* pneumonia. Acta Radiol [Diagn] (Stockh) 1982;23:507–511.

318. Rose HS, Sheth NK. Pulmonary candidiasis: A clinical and pathologic correlation. Arch Intern Med 1978; 138:964–965.

319. Kozinn PJ, Taschdjian CL. Laboratory diagnosis of candidiasis. In: Bodey GP, Fainstein V, eds. Candidiasis. New York: Raven, 1985:85–110.

320. Gold, JWM. Opportunistic fungal infections in patients with neoplastic disease. Am J Med 1984;76:458–463.

321. Goldstein E, Hoeprich PD. Problems in the diagnosis and treatment of systemic candidiasis. J Infect Dis 1972;125:190–193.

322. Walsh TJ, Hathorn JW, Sobel JD, et al. Detection of circulating Candida enolase by immunoassay in patients with cancer and invasive candidiasis. N Engl J Med 1991;324:1026–1031.

323. Utz JP, Drouhet E. Treatment of *Candida* infections. In:

Bodey GP, Fainstein V, eds. Candidiasis. New York: Raven, 1985:253–269.

324. Nakamura T. Experimental pulmonary candidiasis in modified rabbits. Mycopathologia 1984;85:129–144.

325. Luna MA, Tortoledo ME. Histologic identification and pathologic patterns of disease due to *Candida*. In: Bodey GP, Fainstein V, eds. Candidiasis. New York: Raven, 1985:13–27.

326. Kaplan W. Direct fluorescent antibody tests for the diagnosis of mycotic diseases. Ann Clin Lab Sci 1973; 3:25–29.

Aspergillosis

327. Pennington JE. *Aspergillus* lung disease. Med Clin North Am 1980;64:475–490.

328. Greene R. The pulmonary aspergilloses: Three distinct entities or a spectrum of disease. Radiology 1981; 140:527–530.

329. Katzenstein AL, Liebow AA, Friedman PJ. Bronchocentric granulomatosis, mucoid impaction, and hypersensitivity reactions to fungi. Am Rev Respir Dis 1975; 111:497–537.

330. Koss MN, Hochholzer L., Feigin DS, Garancis JC, Ward PA. Necrotizing sarcoid-like granulomatosis: Clinical, pathologic, and immunopathologic findings. Hum Pathol 1980;11:510–519.

331. Greene R. Opportunistic pneumonias. Semin Roentgenol 1980;15:50–72.

332. Myerowitz RL. The pathology of opportunistic infections with pathogenetic, diagnostic, and clinical correlations. New York: Raven, 1983:115–128.

333. Rippon JW. Medical mycology: The pathogenic fungi and the pathogenic actinomycetes. 3rd Ed. Philadelphia: WB Saunders, 1988:618–650.

334. Young RC, Bennett JE, Vogel CL, Carbone PP, DeVita VT. Aspergillosis: The spectrum of the disease in 98 patients. Medicine (Baltimore) 1970;49:147–173.

335. Peña CE. Aspergillosis. In: Baker RD, ed. The pathologic anatomy of mycoses: Human infection with fungi, actinomycetes and algae. Berlin: Springer-Verlag, 1971: 762–831.

336. Young RC, Jennings A, Bennett JE. Species identification of invasive aspergillosis in man. Am J Clin Pathol 1972;58:554–557.

337. Binder RE, Faling LJ, Pugatch RD, Mahasaen C, Snider GL. Chronic necrotizing pulmonary aspergillosis: A discrete clinical entity. Medicine (Baltimore) 1982; 61:109–124.

338. Weiland D, Ferguson RM, Peterson PK, Snover DC, Simmons RL, Najarian JS. Aspergillosis in 25 renal transplant patients: Epidemiology, clinical presentation, diagnosis, and management. Ann Surg 1983;198:622–629.

339. Albelda SM, Talbot GH, Gerson SL, Miller WT, Cassileth PA. Pulmonary cavitation and massive hemoptysis in invasive pulmonary aspergillosis: Influence of bone marrow recovery in patients with acute leukemia. Am Rev Respir Dis 1985;131:115–120.

340. White CJ, Kwon-Chung KJ, Gallin JI. Chronic granulomatous disease of childhood: An unusual case of infection with *Aspergillus nidulans* var. *echinulatus*. Am J Clin Pathol 1988;90:312–316.

341. Hara KS, Ryu JH, Lie JT, Roberts GD. Disseminated *Aspergillus terreus* infection in immunocompromised hosts. Mayo Clin Proc 1989;64:770–775.

342. Raper KB, Fennell DI. The genus *Aspergillus*. Baltimore: Williams & Wilkins, 1965.

343. Bardana EJ. Pulmonary aspergillosis. In: Al-Doory Y, Wagner GE, eds. Aspergillosis. Springfield: Thomas, 1985:43–78.

344. British Thoracic and Tuberculosis Association. Aspergilloma and residual tuberculous cavities: The results of a resurvey. Tubercle 1970;51:227–245.

345. Aslam PA, Eastridge CE, Hughes FA. Aspergillosis of the lung—an eighteen-year experience. Chest 1971; 59:28–32.

346. Freundlich IM, Israel HL. Pulmonary aspergillosis. Clin Radiol 1973;24:248–253.

347. Pennington JE. Opportunistic fungal pneumonias: *Aspergillus, Mucor, Candida, Torulopsis*. In: Pennington JE, ed. Respiratory infections: Diagnosis and management. New York: Raven, 1983:329–339.

348. Glimp RA, Bayer AS. Pulmonary aspergilloma: Diagnostic and therapeutic considerations. Arch Intern Med 1983;143:303–308.

349. McGregor DH, Papasian CJ, Pierce PD. Aspergilloma within cavitating pulmonary adenocarcinoma. Am J Clin Pathol 1989;91:100–103.

350. Sinclair AJ, Rossof AH, Coltman CA. Recognition and successful management in pulmonary aspergillosis in leukemia. Cancer 1978;42:2019–2024.

351. Przyjemski C, Mattii R. The formation of pulmonary mycetomata. Cancer 1980;46:1701–1704.

352. Henderson AH, English MP, Vecht RJ. Pulmonary aspergillosis: A survey of its occurrence in patients with chronic lung disease and a discussion of the significance of diagnostic tests Thorax 1968;23:513–518.

353. Klein DL, Gamsu G. Thoracic manifestations of aspergillosis. AJR 1980;134:543–552.

354. Niimi T, Kajita M, Saito H. Necrotizing bronchial aspergillosis in a patient receiving neoadjuvant chemotherapy for non-small cell lung cancer. Chest 1991; 100:277–279.

355. Pervez NK, Kleinerman J, Kattan M, et al. Pseudomembranous necrotizing bronchial aspergillosis: A variant of invasive aspergillosis in a patient with hemophilia and acquired immune deficiency syndrome. Am Rev Respir Dis 1985;131:961–963.

356. Kramer Mr, Denning DW, Marshall SE, et al. Ulcerative tracheobronchitis after lung transplantation. A new form of invasive aspergillosis. Am Rev Respir Dis 1991;144:552–556.

357. Clarke A, Skelton J, Fraser RS. Fungal tracheobronchitis. Report of 9 cases and review of the literature. Medicine (Baltimore) 1991;70:1–14.

358. Gefter WB, Weingrad TR, Epstein DM, Ochs RH, Miller WT."Semi-invasive" pulmonary aspergillosis: A new

look at the spectrum of *Aspergillus* infections of the lung. Radiology 1981;140:313–321.

359. Palmer LB, Greenberg HE, Schiff MJ. Corticosteroid treatment as a risk factor for invasive aspergillosis in patients with lung disease. Thorax 1991;46:15–20.

360. Diamond RD, Krzesicki R, Epstein B, Jao W. Damage to hyphal forms of fungi by human leukocytes in vitro: A possible host defense mechanism in aspergillosis and mucormycosis. Am J Pathol 1978;91:313–328.

361. Schaffner A, Douglas H, Braude A. Selective protection against conìda by mononuclear and against mycelia by polymorphonuclear phagocytes in resistance to *Aspergillus:* Observations on these two lines of defense in vivo and in vitro with human and mouse phagocytes. J Clin Invest 1982;69:617–631.

362. Meyer RD, Young LS, Armstrong D, Yu B. Aspergillosis complicating neoplastic disease. Am J Med 1973;54: 6–15.

363. Orr DP, Myerowitz RL, Dubois PJ. Patho-radiologic correlation of invasive pulmonary aspergillosis in the compromised host. Cancer 1978;41:2028–2039.

364. Herbert PA, Bayer AS. Fungal pneumonia (part 4): Invasive pulmonary aspergillosis. Chest 1981;80:220–225.

365. Fisher BD, Armstrong D, Yu B, Gold JWM. Invasive aspergillosis: progress in early diagnosis and treatment. Am J Med 1981;71:571–577.

366. Gerson SL, Talbot GH, Hurwitz S, Strom BL, Lusk EJ, Cassileth PA. Prolonged granulocytopenia: The major risk factor for invasive pulmonary aspergillosis in patients with acute leukemia. Ann Intern Med 1984; 100:345–351.

367. Sidransky H, Friedman L. The effect of cortisone and antibiotic agents on experimental pulmonary aspergillosis. Am J Pathol 1959;35:169–183.

368. Davies SF, Sarosi GA. Aspergillosis in the immunosuppressed patient. In: Al-Doory Y, Wagner GE, eds. Aspergillosis. Springfield: Thomas, 1985:96–114.

369. Brown E, Freedman S, Arbeit R, Come S. Invasive pulmonary aspergillosis in an apparently nonimmunocompromised host. Am J Med 1980;69:624–627.

370. Cooper JAD, Weinbaum DL, Aldrich TK, Mandell GL. Invasive aspergillosis of the lung and pericardium in a nonimmunocompromised 33-year-old man. Am J Med 1981;71:903–907.

371. Rogers TR, Haynes KA, Barnes RA. Value of antigen detection in predicting invasive pulmonary aspergillosis. Lancet 1990;ii:1210–1213.

372. Libshitz HI, Pagani JJ. Aspergillosis and mucormycosis: Two types of opportunistic fungal pneumonia. Radiology 1981;140:301–306.

373. Kuhlman JE, Fishman EK, Burch PA, Karp JE, Zerhouni EA, Siegelman SS. CT of invasive pulmonary aspergillosis. AJR 1988;150:1015–1020.

374. Rousey SR, Russler S, Gottlieb M, Ash RC. Low-dose amphotericin B prophylaxis against invasive *Aspergillus* infections in allogeneic marrow transplantation. Am J Med 1991;91:484–492.

375. Denning DW, Tucker RM, Hanson LH, Stevens DA.

Treatment of invasive aspergillosis with itraconazole. Am J Med 1989;86:791–800.

376. Denning DW, Follansbee SE, Scolaro M, Norris S, Edelstein H, Stevens DA. Pulmonary aspergillosis in the acquired immunodeficiency syndrome. N Engl J Med 1991;324:654–662.

377. Nime FA, Hutchins GM. Oxalosis caused by *Aspergillus* infection. Johns Hopkins Med J 1973;133:183–194.

378. Kurrein F, Green GH, Rowles SL. Localized deposition of calcium oxalate around a pulmonary *Aspergillus niger* fungus ball. Am J Clin Pathol 1975;64:556–563.

379. Pore RS, Larsh HW. Aleuriospore formation in four related *Aspergillus* species. Mycologia 1967;59:318–325.

380. Phillips P, Weiner MH. Invasive aspergillosis diagnosed by immunohistochemistry with monoclonal and polyclonal reagents. Hum Pathol 1987;18:1015–1024.

381. Schwarz J. Aspergillosis. Pathol Annu 1973;8:81–107.

382. Lemos LB, Jensen AB. Pathology of aspergillosis. In: Al-Doory Y, Wagner GE, eds. Aspergillosis. Springfield: Thomas, 1985:156–195.

383. Kibbler CC, Milkins SR, Bhamra A, Spiteri MA, Noone P, Prentice HG. Apparent pulmonary mycetoma following invasive aspergillosis in neutropenic patients. Thorax 1988;43:108–112.

384. Khoo TK, Sugai K, Leong TK. Disseminated aspergillosis: Case report and review of the world literature. Am J Clin Pathol 1966;45:697–703.

385. Boon AP, O'Brien D, Adams DH. Ten year review of invasive aspergillosis detected at necropsy. J Clin Pathol 1991;44:452–454.

Mucormycosis

386. Baker RD. The phycomycoses. Ann NY Acad Sci 1970;174:592–605.

387. Hutter RVP. Phycomycetous infection (mucormycosis) in cancer patients: A complication of therapy. Cancer 1959;12:330–350.

388. Straatsma BR, Zimmerman LE, Gass JDM. Phycomycosis: A clinicopathologic study of fifty-one cases. Lab Invest 1962;11:963–985.

389. Baker RD. Mucormycosis (opportunistic phycomycosis). In: Baker RD, ed. The pathologic anatomy of mycoses: Human infection with fungi, actinomycetes and algae. Berlin: Springer-Verlag, 1971:832–918.

390. Meyer RD, Rosen P, Armstrong D. Phycomycosis complicating leukemia and lymphoma. Ann Intern Med 1972;77:871–879.

391. Meyer RD, Armstrong D. Mucormycosis—changing status. CRC Crit Rev Clin Lab Sci 1973;4:421–451.

392. Lehrer RI, moderator. Mucormycosis. Ann Intern Med 1980;93(Part 1):93–108.

393. Marchevsky AM, Bottone EJ, Geller SA, Giger DK. The changing spectrum of disease, etiology, and diagnosis of mucormycosis. Hum Pathol 1980;11:457–464.

394. Ingram CW, Sennesh J, Cooper JN, Perfect JR. Disseminated zygomycosis: Report of four cases and review. Rev Infect Dis 1989;11:741–754.

395. Ferry AP, Abedi S. Diagnosis and management of rhinoorbitocerebral mucormycosis (phycomycosis): A report of 16 personally observed cases. Ophthalmology 1983;90:1096–1104.

396. Neame P, Rayner D. Mucormycosis: A report on twenty-two cases. Arch Pathol 1960;70:261–268.

397. Lyon DT, Schubert TT, Mantia AG. Phycomycosis of the gastrointestinal tract. Am J Gastroenterol 1979;72:379–394.

398. Windus DW, Stokes TJ, Julian BA, Fenves AZ. Fatal Rhizopus infections in hemodialysis patients receiving deferoxamine. Ann Intern Med 1987;107:678–680.

399. Murray HW. Pulmonary mucormycosis: One hundred years later. Chest 1977;72:1–2.

400. Baker RD. Pulmonary mucormycosis. Am J Pathol 1956;32:287–313.

401. Murray HW. Pulmonary mucormycosis with massive fatal hemoptysis. Chest 1975;68:65–68.

402. Passamonte PM, Dix JD. Nosocomial pulmonary mucormycosis with fatal massive hemoptysis. Am J Med Sci 1985;289:65–67.

403. Bartrum RJ, Watnick M, Herman PG. Roentgenographic findings in pulmonary mucormycosis. Am J Roentgenol Radium Ther Nucl Med 1973;117:810–815.

404. Myerowitz RL. The pathology of opportunistic infections with pathogenetic, diagnostic, and clinical correlations. New York: Raven, 1983:129–135.

405. Leong ASY. Granulomatous mediastinitis due to *Rhizopus* species. Am J Clin Pathol 1978;70:103–107.

406. Chandler FW, Watts JC, Kaplan W, Hendry AT, McGinnis MR, Ajello L. Zygomycosis: Report of four cases with formation of chlamydoconidia in tissue. Am J Clin Pathol 1985;84:99–103.

407. Espinoza CG, Halkias DG. Pulmonary mucormycosis as a complication of chronic salicylate poisoning. Am J Clin Pathol 1983;80:508–511.

408. Medoff G, Kobayashi GS. Pulmonary mucormycosis. N Engl J Med 1972;286:86–87.

409. Brown JF, Gottlieb LS, McCormick RA. Pulmonary and rhinocerebral mucormycosis: Successful outcome with amphotericin B and griseofulvin therapy. Arch Intern Med 1977;137:936–938.

410. DeSouza R, MacKinnon S, Spagnolo SV, Fossieck BE. Treatment of localized pulmonary phycomycosis. South Med J 1979;72:609–612.

Coccidioidomycosis

411. Drutz DJ. Coccidioidal pneumonia. In: Pennington JE, ed. Respiratory infections: Diagnosis and management. New York: Raven, 1983:353–373.

412. Drutz DJ, Catanzaro A. Coccidioidomycosis: part I. Am Rev Respir Dis 1978;117:559–585.

413. Rippon JW. Medical mycology: The pathogenic fungi and the pathogenic actinomycetes. 3rd Ed. Philadelphia: W.B. Saunders, 1988:433–469.

414. Drutz DJ, Huppert M. Coccidioidomycosis: Factors af-

fecting the host–parasite interaction. J Infect Dis 1983;147:372–390.

415. Sun SH, Cole GT, Drutz DJ, Harrison JL. Electron-microscopic observations of the *Coccidioides immitis* parasitic cycle *in vivo*. J Med Vet Mycol 1986;24:183–192.

416. Meyer PR, Hui AN, Biddle M. *Coccidioides immitis* meningitis with arthroconidia in cerebrospinal fluid: Report of the first case and review of the arthroconidia literature. Hum Pathol 1982;13:1136–1138.

417. Fiese MJ. Coccidioidomycosis. Springfield: Thomas, 1958.

418. Drutz DJ, Catanzaro A. Coccidioidomycosis: Part II. Am Rev Respir Dis 1978;117:727–771.

419. Bayer AS. Fungal pneumonias; pulmonary coccidioidal syndromes (part I): Primary and progressive primary coccidioidal pneumonias—diagnostic, therapeutic, and prognostic considerations. Chest 1981;79:575–583.

420. Bayer AS. Fungal pneumonias: pulmonary coccidioidal syndromes (part 2): Miliary, nodular, and cavitary pulmonary coccidioidomycosis; chemotherapeutic and surgical considerations. Chest 1981;79:686–691.

421. Birsner JW. The roentgen aspects of five hundred cases of pulmonary coccidioidomycosis. Am J Roentgenol Radium Ther Nucl Med 1954;72:556–573.

422. Greendyke WH, Resnick DL, Harvey WC. The varied roentgen manifestations of primary coccidioidomycosis. Am J Roentgenol Radium Ther Nucl Med 1970; 109:491–499.

423. McGahan JP, Graves DS, Palmer PES, Stadalnik RC, Dublin AB. Classic and contemporary imaging of coccidioidomycosis. AJR 1981;136:393–404.

424. Deresinsky SC, Stevens DA. Coccidioidomycosis in compromised hosts. Medicine (Baltimore) 1974;54:377–395.

425. Wack EE, Ampel NM, Galgiani JN, Bronnimann DA. Coccidioidomycosis during pregnancy: An analysis of ten cases among 47,120 pregnancies. Chest 1988; 94:376–379.

426. MacDonald N, Steinhoff MC, Powell KR. Review of coccidioidomycosis in immunocompromised children. Am J Dis Child 1981;135:553–556.

427. Forbus WD, Bestebreurtje AM. Coccidioidomycosis: A study of 95 cases of the disseminated type with special reference to the pathogenesis of the disease. Mil Surg 1946;99:653–719.

428. Huntington RW. Coccidioidomycosis. In: Baker RD, ed. The pathology anatomy of mycoses: Human infection with fungi, actinomycetes, and algae. Berlin: Springer-Verlag, 1971:147–210.

429. Winn WR, Finegold SM, Huntington RW. Coccidioidomycosis with fungemia. In: Ajello L. ed. Coccidioidomycosis: The second symposium on coccidioidomycosis. Tucson: Univ. Arizona Press, 1967:93–109.

430. Ampel NM, Ryan KJ, Carry PJ, Wieden MA, Schifman RB. Fungemia due to *Coccidioides immitis:* An analysis of 16 episodes in 15 patients and a review of the literature. Medicine (Baltimore) 1986;65:312–321.

431. Galgiani JN, Ampel NM. Coccidioidomycosis in human immunodeficiency virus-infected patients. J Infect Dis 1990;162:1165–1169.

432. Huntington RW, Waldmann WJ, Sargent JA, O'Connell H, Wybel R, Croll D. Pathologic and clinical observations on 142 cases of fatal coccidioidomycosis with necropsy. In: Ajello L, ed. Coccidioidomycosis: The second symposium on coccidioidomycosis. Tucson: Univ. Arizona Press, 1967:143–167.

433. Putnam JS, Harper WK, Greene JF, Nelson KG, Zurek RC. *Coccidioides immitis:* A rare cause of pulmonary mycetoma. Am Rev Respir Dis 1975;112:733–738.

434. Fee HJ, McAvoy JM, Michals AA, Gold PM. Unusual manifestation of *Coccidioides immitis* infection. J Thorac Cardiovasc Surg 1977;74:548–550.

435. Thadepalli H, Salem FA, Mandal AK, Rambhatla K, Einstein HE. Pulmonary mycetoma due to *Coccidioides immitis*. Chest 1977;71:429–430.

436. Rohatgi PK, Schmitt RG. Pulmonary coccidioidal mycetoma. Am J Med Sci 1984;287:27–30.

437. Graham AR, Sobonya RE, Bronnimann DA, Galgiani JN. Quantitative pathology of coccidioidomycosis in acquired immunodeficiency syndrome. Hum Pathol 1988;19:800–806.

438. Deppisch LM, Donowho EM. Pulmonary coccidioidomycosis. Am J Clin Pathol 1972;58:489–500.

439. Lombard CM, Tazelaar HD, Krasne DL. Pulmonary eosinophilia in coccidioidal infections. Chest 1987; 91:734–736.

440. Freedman SI, Ang EP, Haley RS. Identification of coccidioidomycosis of the lung by fine needle aspiration biopsy. Acta Cytol 1986;30:420–424.

441. Howard PF, Smith JW. Diagnosis of disseminated coccidioidomycosis by liver biopsy. Arch Intern Med 1983; 143:1335–1338.

442. Bayer AS, Yoshikawa TT, Galpin JE, Guze LB. Unusual syndromes of coccidioidomycosis: Diagnostic and therapeutic considerations. Medicine (Baltimore) 1976; 55:131–152.

443. McClatchie S, Warambo MW, Bremner AD. Myospherulosis: A previously unreported disease? Am J Clin Pathol 1969;51:699–704.

444. Kyriakos M. Myospherulosis of the paranasal sinuses, nose and middle ear: A possible iatrogenic disease. Am J Clin Pathol 1977;67:118–130.

445. Rosai J. The nature of myospherulosis of the upper respiratory tract. Am J Clin Pathol 1978;69:475–481.

446. Travis WD, Li CY, Weiland LH. Immunostaining for hemoglobin in two cases of myospherulosis. Arch Pathol Lab Med 1986;110:763–765.

Pseudallescheriasis

447. Jung JY, Salas R, Almond CH, Saab S, Reyna R. The role of surgery in the management of pulmonary monosporiosis: A collective review. J Thorac Cardiovasc Surg 1977;73:139–144.

448. Lutwick LI, Galgiani JN, Johnson RH, Stevens DA. Visceral fungal infections due to *Petriellidium boydii (Allescheria boydii):* In vitro drug sensitivity studies. Am J

Med 1976;61:632–640.

449. Winston DJ, Jordan MC, Rhodes J. *Allescheria boydii* infections in the immunosuppressed host. Am J Med 1977;63:830–835.

450. Lake FR, Tribe AE, McAleer R, Froudist J, Thompson PJ. Mixed allergic bronchopulmonary fungal disease due to *Pseudallescheria boydii* and *Aspergillus*. Thorax 1990;45:489–492.

451. McGinnis MR, Padhye AA, Ajello L. *Pseudallescheria* Negroni et Fischer, 1943 and its later synonym *Petriellidium* Malloch, 1970. Mycotaxon 1982;14:94–102.

452. Arnett JC, Hatch HB. Pulmonary allescheriasis: Report of a case and review of the literature. Arch Intern Med 1975;135:1250–1253.

453. Rippon JW, Carmichael JW. Petriellidiosis (Allescheriosis): Four unusual cases and review of literature. Mycopathologia 1976;58:117–124.

454. Dworzack DL, Clark RB, Borkowski WJ, et al. *Pseudallescheria boydii* brain abscess: Association with near-drowning and efficacy of high dose, prolonged miconazole therapy in patients with multiple abscesses. Medicine (Baltimore) 1989;68:218–224.

455. Shih LY, Lee N. Disseminated petriellidiosis (allescheriasis) in a patient with refractory acute lymphoblastic leukaemia. J Clin Pathol 1984;37:78–82.

456. Reddy PC, Christianson CS, Gorelick DF, Larsh HW. Pulmonary monosporiosis: An uncommon pulmonary mycotic infection. Thorax 1969;24:722–728.

457. Hainer JW, Ostrow JH, Mackenzie DWR. Pulmonary monosporiosis: Report of a case with precipitating antibody. Chest 1974;66:601–603.

458. Bakerspigel A, Wood T, Burke S. Pulmonary allescheriasis: Report of a case from Ontario, Canada. Am J Clin Pathol 1977;68:299–303.

459. Kathuria SK, Rippon J. Non-aspergillus aspergilloma. Am J Clin Pathol 1982;78:870–873.

460. Louria DB, Lieberman PH, Collins HS, Blevins A. Pulmonary mycetoma due to *Allescheria boydii*. Arch Intern Med 1966;117:748–751.

461. Travis RE, Ulrich EW, Phillips S. Pulmonary allescheriasis. Ann Intern Med 1961;54:141–152.

462. McCarthy DS, Longbottom JL, Riddell RW, Batten JC. Pulmonary mycetoma due to *Allescheria boydii*. Am Rev Respir Dis 1969;100:213–216.

463. DeMent SH, Smith RRL, Karp JE, Merz WG. Pulmonary, cardiac, and thyroid involvement in disseminated *Pseudallescheria boydii* (letter). Arch Pathol Lab Med 1984;108:859–861.

464. Enggano IL, Hughes WT, Kalwinsky DK, Pearson TA, Parham DM, Stass SA. *Pseudallescheria boydii* in a patient with acute lymphoblastic leukemia. Arch Pathol Lab Med 1984;198:619–622.

465. Smith AG, Crain SM, Dejongh C, Thomas GM, Vigorito RD. Systemic pseudallescheriasis in a patient with acute myelocytic leukemia. Mycopathologia 1985;90:85–89.

466. Walker DH, Adamec T, Krigman M. Disseminated petriellidiosis (allescheriosis). Arch Pathol Lab Med 1978; 102:158–160.

467. Saadah HA, Dixon T. *Petriellidium boydii (Allescheria boy-*

dii): necrotizing pneumonia in a normal host. JAMA 1981;245:605–606.

468. Alture-Werber E, Edberg SC, Singer JM. Pulmonary infection with *Allescheria boydii*. Am J Clin Pathol 1976; 66:1019–1024.

469. Schwartz DA. Organ-specific variation in the morphology of the fungomas (fungus balls) of *Pseudallescheria boydii*. Arch Pathol Lab Med 1989;113:476–480.

470. Travis LB, Roberts GD, Wilson WR. Clinical significance of *Pseudallescheria boydii:* A review of 10 years' experience. Mayo Clin Proc 1985;60:531–537.

Fusariosis

471. Young NA, Kwon-Chung KJ, Kubota TT, Jennings AE, Fisher RI. Disseminated infection by *Fusarium moniliforme* during treatment for malignant lymphoma. J Clin Microbiol 1978;7:589–594.

472. Wheeler MS, McGinnis MR, Schell WA, Walker DH. *Fusarium* infection in burned patients. Am J Clin Pathol 1981;75:304–311.

473. Blazar BR, Hurd DD, Snover DC, Alexander JW, McGlave PB. Invasive *Fusarium* infections in bone marrow transplant recipients. Am J Med 1984;77:645–651.

474. Summerbell RC, Richardson SE, Kane J. *Fusarium proliferatum* as an agent of disseminated infection in an immunosuppressed patient. J Clin Microbiol 1988;26: 82–87.

475. Abramowsky CR, Quinn D, Bradford WD, Conant NF. Systemic infection by *Fusarium* in a burned child: The emergence of a saprophytic strain. J Pediatr 1974; 84:561–564.

476. Cho CT, Vats Ts, Lowman JT, Brandsberg JW, Tosh FE. *Fusarium solani* infection during treatment for acute leukemia. J Pediatr 1973;83:1028–1031.

477. Venditti M, Micozzi A, Gentile G, et al. Invasive *Fusarium solani* infections in patients with acute leukemia. Rev Infect Dis 1988;10:653–660.

478. Anaissie E, Kantarjian H, Ro J, et al. The emerging role of *Fusarium* infections in patients with cancer. Medicine (Baltimore) 1988;67:77–83.

479. Richardson SE, Bannatyne RM, Summerbell RC, Milliken J, Gold R, Weitzman SS. Disseminated fusarial infection in the immunocompromised host. Rev Infect Dis 1988;10:1171–1181.

480. Mutton KJ, Lucas TJ, Harkness JL. Disseminated *Fusarium* infection. Med J Aust 1980;2:624–625.

481. Young CN, Meyers AM. Opportunistic fungal infection by *Fusarium oxysporum* in a renal transplant patient. Sabouraudia 1979;17:219–223.

482. Gutmann L, Chou SM, Pore RS. Fusariosis, myasthenic syndrome, and aplastic anemia. Neurology 1975;25: 922–926.

Trichosporonosis

483. Rivera R, Cangir A. *Trichosporon* sepsis and leukemia. Cancer 1975;36:1106–1110.

484. Evans HL, Kletzel M, Lawson RD, Frankel LS, Hopfer RL. Systemic mycosis due to *Trichosporon cutaneum*: A report of two additional cases. Cancer 1980;45:367–371.

485. Yung CW, Hanauer SB, Fretzin D, Rippon JW, Shapiro C, Gonzalez M. Disseminated *Trichosporon beigelii (cutaneum)*. Cancer 1981;48:2107–2111.

486. Saul SH, Khachatoorian T, Poorsattar A, et al. Opportunistic *Trichosporon* pneumonia: association with invasive aspergillosis. Arch Pathol Lab Med 1981;105:456–459.

487. Gardella S, Nomdedeu B, Bombi JA, et al. Fatal fungemia with arthritic involvement caused by *Trichosporon beigelii* in a bone marrow transplant recipient (letter). J Infect Dis 1985;151:566.

488. Madhaven T, Eisses J. Systemic infections due to *Trichosporon cutaneum*, an uncommon pathogen (abstr). Am J Clin Pathol 1975;63:598.

489. Winston DJ, Balsley GE, Rhodes J, Linne SR. Disseminated *Trichosporon capitatum* infection in an immunosuppressed host. Arch Intern Med 1977;137:1192–1195.

490. Martino P, Venditti M, Micozzi A, et al. *Blastoschizomyces capitatus*: An emerging cause of invasive fungal disease in leukemia patients. Rev Infect Dis 1990;12:570–582.

491. Kirmani N, Tuazon CU, Geelhoed GW. Disseminated *Trichosporon* infection: occurrence in an immunosuppressed patient with chronic active hepatitis. Arch Intern Med 1980;140:277–278.

492. Jameson B, Carter RL, Watson JG, Hay RJ. An unexpected fungal infection in a patient with leukaemia. J Clin Pathol 1981;34:267–270.

493. Gold JWM, Poston W, Mertelsmann R, et al. Systemic infection with *Trichosporon cutaneum* in a patient with acute leukemia. Cancer (Phila) 1981;48:2163–2167.

494. Manzella JP, Berman IJ, Kukrika MD. *Trichosporon beigelii* fungemia and cutaneous dissemination. Arch Dermatol 1982;118:343–345.

495. Brahn E, Leonard Pa. *Trichosporon cutaneum* endocarditis: A sequela of intravenous drug abuse. Am J Clin Pathol 1982;78:792–794.

496. Libertin CR, Davies NJ, Halper J, Edson RS, Roberts GD. Invasive disease caused by *Trichosporon beigelii*. Mayo Clin Proc 1983;58:684–686.

497. Haupt HM, Merz WG, Beschorner WE, Vaughan WP, Saral R. Colonization and infection with *Trichosporon* species in the immunosuppressed host. J Infect Dis 1983;147:199–203.

498. Bhansali S, Karanes C, Palutke W, Crane L, Kiel R, Ratanatharathorn V. Successful treatment of disseminated *Trichosporon beigelii (cutaneum)* infection with associated splenic involvement. Cancer (Phila) 1986; 58:1630–1632.

499. Leblond V, Saint-Jean O, Datry A, et al. Systemic infections with *Trichosporon beigelii (cutaneum)*. Cancer (Phila) 1986;58:2399–2405.

500. Walling DM, McGraw DJ, Merz WG, Karp JE, Hutchins GM. Disseminated infection with *Trichosporon beigelii*. Rev Infect Dis 1987;9:1013–1019.

501. Ito T, Ishikawa Y, Fujii R, et al. Disseminated *Trichosporon capitatum*. Cancer (Phila) 1988;61:585–588.

502. Ness MJ, Markin RS, Wood RP, Shaw BW, Woods GL. Disseminated *Trichosporon beigelii* infection after orthotopic liver transplantation. Am J Clin Pathol 1989; 92:119–123.

503. Kimura M, Takahashi H, Satou T, Hashimoto S. An autopsy case of disseminated trichosporonosis with candidiasis of the urinary bladder. Virchows Arch A [Pathol Anal] 1989;416:159–162.

504. Ogata K, Tanabe Y, Iwakiri K, et al. Two cases of disseminated *Trichosporon beigelii* infection treated with combination antifungal therapy. Cancer (Phila) 1990; 65:2793–2795.

505. Kobayashi M, Kotani S, Fujishita M, et al. Immunohistochemical identification of *Trichosporon beigelii* in histologic section by immunoperoxidase method. Am J Clin Pathol 1988;89:100–105.

506. Takeuchi T, Kobayashi M, Moriki T, Miyoshi I. Application of a monoclonal antibody for the detection of *Trichosporon beigelii* in paraffin-embedded tissue sections. J Pathol 1988;156:23–27.

Geotrichosis

507. Morenz J. Geotrichosis. In: Baker RD, ed. The pathologic anatomy of mycoses: Human infection with fungi, actinomycetes and algae. Berlin: Springer-Verlag, 1971: 919–952.

508. Sheehy TW, Honeycutt BK, Spency JT. *Geotrichum* septicemia. JAMA 1976;235:1035–1037.

509. Webster BH. Bronchopulmonary geotrichosis. Dis Chest 1959;35:273–281.

510. Ross JD, Reid KDG, Speirs CF. Bronchopulmonary geotrichosis with severe asthma. Br Med J 1962;1:1400–1402.

511. Ghamande AR, Landis FB, Snider GL. Bronchial geotrichosis with fungemia complicating bronchial carcinoma. Chest 1971;59:98–101.

512. Fishbach RS, White ML, Finegold SM. Bronchopulmonary geotrichosis. Am Rev Respir Dis 1973;108:1388–1392.

513. Chang WWL, Buerger L. Disseminated geotrichosis. Arch Intern Med 1964;113:356–360.

514. Jagirdar J, Geller SA, Bottone EJ. *Geotrichum candidum* as a tissue invasive human pathogen. Hum Pathol 1981;12:668–671.

515. Winer-Muram HT. Geotrichosis: Who is susceptible? (letter). Chest 1988;94:1315–1316.

516. Hamilton-Miller JMT. A comparative in vitro study of amphotericin B, clotrimazole and 5-fluorocytosine against clinically isolated yeasts. Sabouraudia 1972; 10:276–283.

Penicilliosis Marneffei

517. Pitt JI. The genus *Penicillium* and its teleomorphic states *Eupenicillium* and *Talaromyces*. New York: Academic Press, 1979.

518. Tsang DNC, Chan JKC, Lau YT, et al. *Penicillium marn-*

effei infection: An underdiagnosed disease? Histopathology 1988;13:311–318.

519. Deng Z, Connor DH. Progressive disseminated penicilliosis caused by *Penicillium marneffei*. Report of eight cases and differentiation of the causative organism from *Histoplasma capsulatum*. Am J Clin Pathol 1985;84:323–327.

520. Tsang DNC, Li PCK, Tsui MS, et al. *Penicillium marneffei:* Another pathogen to consider in patients infected with human immunodeficiency virus. Rev Infect Dis 1991;13:766–767.

521. Deng Z, Ribas JL, Gibson DW, Connor DH. Infections caused by *Penicillium marneffei* in China and Southeast Asia. Review of eighteen published cases and report of four more Chinese cases. Rev Infect Dis 1988;10:640–652.

522. Segretain G. Description d'une nouvelle espece de penicillium: *Penicillium marneffei*, n. sp. Bull Soc Mycol Fr 1959;75:412–416.

523. DiSalvo AF, Fickling AM, Ajello L. Infection caused by *Penicillium marneffei:* Description of first natural infection in man. Am J Clin Pathol 1973;60:259–263.

524. Pautler KB, Padhye AA, Ajello L. Imported penicilliosis marneffei in the United States: Report of a second human infection. Sabouraudia 1984;22:433–438.

525. Jayanetra P, Nitiyanant P, Ajello L, et al. Penicilliosis marneffei in Thailand: Report of five human cases. Am J Trop Med Hyg 1984;33:637–644.

526. So SY, Chau PY, Jones BM, et al. A case of invasive penicilliosis in Hong Kong with immunologic evaluation. Am Rev Respir Dis 1984;131:662–665.

527. Chan JKC, Tsang DNC, Wong DKK. *Penicillium marneffei* in bronchoalveolar lavage fluid. Acta Cytol 1989;33:533–536.

Malasseziasis

528. Marcon MJ, Powell DA. Human infections due to *Malassezia* spp. Clin Microbiol Rev 1992;5:101–119.

529. Bertini B, Kuttin ES, Beemer AM. Cytopathology of nipple discharge due to *Pityrosporum orbiculare* and cocci in an elderly woman. Acta Cytol 1975;19:38–42.

530. Oberle AD, Fowler M, Grafton WD. *Pityrosporum* isolate from the upper respiratory tract. Am J Clin Pathol 1981;76:112–116.

531. Wallace M, Bagnall H, Glen D. Isolation of lipophilic yeast in "sterile" peritonitis. Lancet 1979;ii:956.

532. Redline RW, Redline SS, Boxerbaum B, Dahms BB. Systemic *Malassezia furfur* infections in patients receiving intralipid therapy. Hum Pathol 1985;16:815–822.

533. Dankner WM, Spector SA, Fierer J, Davis CE. Malassezia fungemia in neonates and adults: Complication of hyperalimentation. Rev Infect Dis 1987;9:743–753.

534. Marcon MJ, Powell DA. Epidemiology, diagnosis and management of *Malassezia furfur* systemic infection. Diagn Microbiol Infect Dis 1987;7:161–175.

535. Shek YH, Tucker MC, Viciana AL, Manz HJ, Connor DH. *Malassëzia furfur*—Disseminated infection in premature infants. Am J Clin Pathol 1989;92:595–603.

536. Weiss SJ, Schoch PE, Cunha BA. *Malassezia furfur* fungemia associated with central venous catheter lipid emulsion infusion. Heart Lung 1991;20:87–90.

Phaeohyphomycosis

537. Ajello L. Phaeohyphomycosis: definition and etiology. In: Mycoses. Sci Pub 304. Washington DC: Pan American Health Organization, 1975:126–133.

538. McGinnis MR. Human pathogenic species of *Exophiala*, *Phialophora* and *Wangiella*. In: The black and white yeasts. Sci Pub 356. Washington, DC: Pan American Health Organization, 1978:37–59.

539. McGinnis MR. Chromoblastomycosis and phaeohyphomycosis: New concepts, diagnosis, and mycology. J Am Acad Dermatol 1983;8:1–16.

540. Fader RC, McGinnis MR. Infections caused by dematiaceous fungi: Chromoblastomycosis and phaeohyphomycosis. Infect Dis Clin North Am 1988;2:925–938.

541. Ichinose H. Subcutaneous abscesses due to brown fungi. In: Baker RD, ed. The pathologic anatomy of mycoses: Human infection with fungi, actinomycetes and algae. Berlin: Springer-Verlag, 1971:719–730.

542. Ziefer A, Connor DH. Phaeomycotic cyst. A clinicopathologic study of twenty-five patients. Am J Trop Med Hyg 1980;29:901–911.

543. Bambirra EA, Miranda D, Nogueira AMF, Barbosa CSP. Phaeohyphomycotic cyst: A clinicopathologic study of the first four cases described from Brazil. Am J Trop Med Hyg 1983;32:794–798.

544. Moskowitz LB, Cleary TJ, McGinnis Mr, Thomson CB. *Phialophora richardsiae* in a lesion appearing as a giant cell tumor in the tendon sheath. Arch Pathol Lab Med 1983;107:374–376.

545. Tschen JA, Knox JM, McGavran MH, Duncan WC. Chromomycosis, the association of fungal elements and wood splinters. Arch Dermatol 1984;120:107–108.

546. Riley O Jr, Mann SH. Brain abscess caused by *Cladosporium trichoides:* Review of 3 cases and report of fourth case. Am J Clin Pathol 1960;33:525–531.

547. Crichlow DK, Enrile FT, Memon MY. Cerebellar abscess due to *Cladosporium trichoides (bantianum):* case report. Am J Clin Pathol 1973;60:416–421.

548. Chandramukki A, Ramadevi MG, Shankar SK. Cerebral cladosporiosis—a neuropathological and microbiological study. Clin Neurol Neurosurg 1983;85:245–253.

549. Seaworth BJ, Kwon-Chung KJ, Hamilton JD, Perfect JR. Brain abscess caused by a variety of *Cladosporium trichoides*. Am J Clin Pathol 1983;79:747–752.

550. Dixon DM, Walsh TJ, Merz WG, McGinnis MR. Infections due to *Xylohypha bantiana (Cladosporium trichoides)*. Rev Infect Dis 1989;11:515–525.

551. McGinnis MR, Borelli D, Padhye AA, Ajello L. Reclassification of *Cladosporium bantianum* in the genus *Xylohypha*. J Clin Microbiol 1986;23:1148–1151.

552. Dixon DM, Merz WG, Elliot HL, Macleay S. Experimental central nervous system phaeohyphomycosis following intranasal inoculation of *Xylohypha bantiana* in cortisone-treated mice. Mycopathologia 1987;100:145–153.

553. Fink JN, Schlueter DP, Barboriak JJ. Hypersensitivity pneumonitis due to exposure to *Alternaria*. Chest 1973;63:49S.

554. McAleer R, Kroenert DB, Elder JL, Froudist JH. Allergic bronchopulmonary disease caused by *Curvularia lunata* and *Drechslera hawaiiensis*. Thorax 1981;36:338–344.

555. Limsila T, Stituimankaru T, Thasnakorn P. Pulmonary cladosporoma. Report of a case. J Med Assoc Thailand 1970;53:586–590.

556. Lampert RP, Hutto JH, Donnelly WH, Shulman ST. Pulmonary and cerebral mycetoma caused by *Curvularia pallescens*. J Pediatr 1977;91:603–605.

557. de la Monte SM, Hutchins GM. Disseminated *Curvularia* infection. Arch Pathol Lab Med 1985;109:872–874.

558. Lobritz RW, Roberts TH, Marraro RV, Carlton PK, Thorp DJ. Granulomatous pulmonary disease secondary to *Alternaria*. JAMA 1979;241:596–597.

559. Borges MC, Jr., Warren S, White W, Pellettiere EV. Pulmonary phaeohyphomycosis due to *Xylohypha bantiana*. Arch Pathol Lab Med 1991;115:627–629.

560. Rohwedder JJ, Simmons JL, Colfer H, Gatmaitan B. Disseminated *Curvularia lunata* infection in a football player. Arch Intern Med 1979;139:940–941.

561. Ferraro FA, Morgan MA. A case of disseminated *Phialophora parasitica* infection. Arch Pathol Lab Med 1989;113:1379–1381.

562. Hay RJ, Dupont B, Graybill JR, eds. First international symposium on itraconazole. Rev Infect Dis 1987;9 (Suppl.):S1–152.

Adiaspiromycosis

563. Kodousek R. Adiaspiromycosis. Acta Univ Palacki Olomuc Fac Med 1974;70:5–68.

564. Schwarz J. Adiaspiromycosis. Pathol Annu 1978;13:41–53.

565. Emmons CW, Binford CH, Utz JP, Kwon-Chung KJ. Medical mycology. 3d Ed. Philadelphia: Lea & Febiger, 1977:493–505.

566. Barbas Filho JV, Amato MBP, Deheinzelin D, Saldiva RHN, de Carvalho CRR. Respiratory failure caused by adiaspiromycosis. Chest 1990;97:1171–1175.

567. Cueva JA, Little MD. *Emmonsia crescens* infection (adiaspiromycosis) in man in Honduras. Am J Trop Med Hyg 1971;20:282–287.

568. Kodousek R, Vortel V, Fingerland A, et al. Pulmonary adiaspiromycosis in man caused by *Emmonsia crescens*: Report of a unique case. Am J Clin Pathol 1971;56:394–399.

569. Watts JC, Callaway CS, Chandler FW, Kaplan W. Human pulmonary adiaspiromycosis. Arch Pathol 1975;99:11–15.

Rhinosporidiosis

570. Karunaratne WAE. Rhinosporidiosis in man. London: Athlone, 1964.

571. Rippon JW. Medical mycology: The pathogenic fungi and the pathogenic actinomycetes. 3rd Ed. Philadelphia: W.B. Saunders, 1988:718–721.

572. Levy MG, Meuten DJ, Breitschwerdt EB. Cultivation of *Rhinosporidium seeberi* in vitro: Interaction with epithelial cells. Science 1986;234:474–476.

573. Rajam RV, Viswanathan GS, Rao AR, Rangiah PN, Anguli VS. Rhinosporidiosis: A study with report of a fatal case of systemic dissemination. Indian J Surg 1955;17:269–298.

574. Agrawal S, Sharma KD, Shrivastava JB. Generalized rhinosporidiosis with visceral involvement: Report of a case. Arch Dermatol 1959;80:22–26.

575. Bader G, Grueber HLE. Histochemical studies of *Rhinosporidium seeberi*. Virchows Arch [Pathol Anat] 1970;350:76–86.

576. Kannan-Kutty M, Teh EC. *Rhinosporidium seeberi*: An electron microscopy study of its life cycle. Pathology 1974;6:63–70.

577. Kannan-Kutty M, Teh EC. *Rhinosporidium seeberi*: An ultrastructural study of its endosporulation phase and trophocyte phase. Arch Pathol 1975;99:51–54.

578. Savino DF, Margo CE. Conjunctival rhinosporidiosis: Light and electron microscopic study. Ophthalmology 1983;90:1482–1489.

Prototothecosis

579. Kaplan W. Protothecosis and infections caused by morphologically similar green algae. In: The black and white yeasts. Sci Pub 356. Washington DC: Pan American Health Association, 1978:218–232.

580. Sudman MS. Protothecosis: A critical review. Am J Clin Pathol 1974;61:10–19.

581. Sudman MS, Kaplan W. Identification of the *Prototheca* species by immunofluorescence. Appl Microbiol 1973;25:981–990.

582. Conner DH, Gibson DW, Ziefer A. Diagnostic features of three unusual infections: micronemiasis, pheomycotic cyst, and protothecosis. In: Majno G, Cotran RS, Kaufman N, eds. Current topics in inflammation and infection. International Academy of Pathology monograph no. 23. Baltimore: Williams & Wilkins, 1982:205–239.

583. Naryshkin S, Frank I, Nachamkin I. *Prototheca zopfii* isolated from a patient with olecranon bursitis. Diagn Microbiol Infect Dis 1987;6:171–174.

584. Davies RR, Wilkinson JL. Human protothecosis: supplementary studies. Ann Trop Med Parasitol 1967;61:112–115.

585. Cox GE, Wilson JD, Brown P. Protothecosis: a case of disseminated algal infection. Lancet 1974;ii:379–382.

586. Venezio FR, Lavoo E, Williams JW, et al. Progressive cutaneous protothecosis. Am J Clin Pathol 1982;77:485–493.

587. Chan JC, Jeffers LJ, Gould EW, et al. Visceral protothecosis mimicking sclerosing cholangitis in an immunocompetent host: Successful antifungal therapy. Rev Infect Dis 1990;12:802–807.

588. Nosanchuk JS, Greenberg RD. Protothecosis of the olecranon bursa caused by achloric algae. Am J Clin Pathol 1973;59:567–573.

CHAPTER 12

Viral Infections

WASHINGTON C. WINN, JR. and DAVID H. WALKER

Viral infections are among the most common afflictions of man. It has been estimated that children experience two to seven respiratory infections each year; adults are afflicted with one to three such episodes.[1]

Many viral infections, such as chickenpox and measles, are contracted through the respiratory tract but usually manifest themselves in other organ systems. Despite the frequency with which viruses infect respiratory epithelium, very few viral pneumonias come to the attention of the anatomic pathologist. The reasons for this paradox are multiple. Most viral respiratory infections, excluding epidemic influenza, produce acute morbidity but little mortality in healthy individuals. The specific etiologic agent may not be known, but the likely identity of the culprit as viral is often suspected from clinical or epidemiologic data. Invasive procedures to procure tissues are unlikely under these conditions, except in those few cases that have unusual or severe clinical presentations.

With rare exceptions the specific identification of a viral infection must come from the clinical virology laboratory. The cytopathic effect of cytomegalovirus in tissue is pathognomonic, and the cytopathic effect of certain other viruses, such as adenovirus and herpes simplex virus, strongly suggests the specific diagnosis. However, definitive identification must come from virologic and/or immunologic investigations. What, then, is the role of the anatomic pathologist? First and most importantly, he or she should be at the center of the diagnostic action once a specimen of tissue has been obtained. If the clinician has suspected a viral etiology, the pathologist must ensure that specimens are preserved for culture and immunologic studies. If the correct diagnosis has not been suspected and if fresh tissue in sufficient volume has been submitted to the laboratory, the pathologist has a chance to salvage an etiologically specific diagnosis before the tissue is irreversibly immersed in fixative. If, as happens all too often, tissue has been immersed in chemical fixatives, the anatomic pathologist may be able to provide a specific diagnosis by molecular or immunologic means. It should be emphasized, however, that the optimal approach to diagnosis of viral infections includes attempts to recover the infectious agent in culture.

General Features

Viruses Causing Lower Respiratory Tract Infection

The number of viral immunotypes that produce upper respiratory tract infection is large, primarily because more than 100 types of rhinovirus can produce the common cold. A relatively restricted number of viruses account for almost all infections below the level of the larynx. With few exceptions, serious viral infections of the trachea, bronchi, and lung are diseases of infants, children, and immunocompromised adults. To a considerable extent, discrete clinical syndromes in defined age groups can be associated with specific viruses. These syndromes and associated viruses are detailed below and summarized in Table 12–1.

Clinical Syndromes

In neonates and infants less than 2 years old, respiratory syncytial virus (RSV) is the most important cause of viral bronchiolitis and pneumonia[1] (see Chapter 8). Parainfluenzavirus 3 is second only to RSV as a cause of

429

Table 12–1. Viral causes of respiratory disease syndromes[a]

Syndrome	Common agents	Less common agents
Coryza: "cold"	Rhinovirus	Influenza A and B
	Coronavirus	Parainfluenza 1 or 2
	Adenovirus	RSV
	Parainfluenza 3	Enterovirus
Pharyngitis	Adenovirus	Influenza A or B
	EBV	RSV
	Enterovirus	Parainfluenza 1 or 2
	Herpes simplex	Rhinovirus
		Coronavirus
Group	Parainfluenza 1–3	Influenza A
		RSV
Bronchiolitis	RSV	Adenovirus
	Parainfluenza 3	Parainfluenza 1 or 2
		Influenza A or B
		Rhinovirus
Pneumonia	RSV	Parainfluenza 1 or 2
	Parainfluenza 3	Rhinovirus
	Adenovirus	EBV
	Influenza A or B	Varicella-zoster virus
	CMV (compromised host)	HSV (compromised hosts)
		Adenovirus

[a] Adapted from McIntosh.[28]

bronchiolitis in this age group. Although much less common, adenoviruses may also produce severe bronchiolitis and fatal pneumonia in very young children.[2,3] The bronchiolitis may be obstructive, and apnea may occur. Viruses have been established as etiologic agents in some cases of sudden infant death syndrome,[4] particularly those associated with a lymphocytic bronchiolar infiltrate.

Parainfluenza viruses 1 and 2 are important causes of croup (infectious laryngotracheobronchitis) and pneumonia in older children (aged 2–6 years). These infections occur primarily in epidemics, and most children have been infected by the time they are 5 years old.

Immunity to these pediatric respiratory viruses is incomplete. Infections recur throughout life, usually as mild upper respiratory disease. It is now recognized, however, that severe lower respiratory tract disease is more common in adults than was previously appreciated.[5,6]

A common manifestation of severe respiratory infection in children and adults is the influenza syndrome—the abrupt onset of fever, headache, malaise, severe myalgias, and prostration in addition to cough, nasal congestion, and sore throat. The etiology of approximately half of these infections is unknown. Influenzaviruses A and B are responsible for one-third of cases; the remainder of the influenza syndromes are produced by a variety of agents, including coronaviruses, which usually cause upper respiratory tract disease.[1] Adenoviruses are particularly likely to infect military recruits.

Infection of the lower respiratory tract may occur as a complication of disseminated infection by viruses that usually cause disease in other organs. The most common examples of this phenomenon are the pneumonias that occur in patients with the cutaneous viral infections measles and varicella.

As many as 10% of influenza virus infections are associated with preexistent lower respiratory tract disease.[7] Other respiratory viruses, such as adenovirus, may also infrequently produce pneumonia in normal adults.[8,9] On very rare occasions, upper respiratory pathogens, such as rhinoviruses, may cause infection of the air spaces. The respiratory viruses function as opportunistic pathogens when they produce serious, life-threatening disease in adults. Even influenzavirus, a potent pathogen in its own right, produces pneumonia more frequently in patients with chronic cardiopulmonary disease, in elderly persons, and in women who are in the late stages of pregnancy.[1,7,10]

The predisposing factors can take a variety of forms. The patients at highest risk are those whose cellular immune system has been compromised, usually by immunosuppressive disease or chemotherapy.[11] Not unexpectedly, the most common viral infections in these patients are those produced by endogenous viruses that are periodically reactivated, especially cytomegalovirus (CMV) and herpes simplex virus.

Local host defense mechanisms are also important, as demonstrated by the predisposition to severe influenza infection in patients with chronic cardiac and pulmonary disease.[10] Herpes simplex infections often occur when the integrity of the respiratory tract has been breached by an endotracheal tube or a tracheostomy.[12] Viral pneumonia itself, usually from measles, may even serve as the predisposing factor for other viral infections.[13]

Radiologic and Pathologic Features of Viral Pneumonia

Several patterns of inflammatory reaction, which are not mutually exclusive, occur in viral infections of the lower respiratory tract.

The first of these is necrotizing bronchitis or bronchiolitis, which is produced most commonly by the influenza viruses, RSV, adenovirus, and herpes simplex virus. The inflammatory reaction to each of these agents consists primarily of mononuclear inflammatory cells, but neutrophilic leukocytes (PMNs) also participate in the inflammatory response.

On occasion, the response to a pure viral infection includes many PMNs, simulating the response to a bacterial infection.[14] The inflammatory exudate in some viral pneumonias undergoes extensive karyorrhexis and karyolysis, producing fragmented cells and

Table 12–2. Diagnostic modalities for viral respiratory disease

Virus	Culture	Antigen	Molecular	Serology	Comments
Influenza	++	+	−	+	Culture primary; antigen detection not widely practiced
Adenovirus	++	+	+	+	Culture primary
Herpes simplex	++	+	+	−	Serology not useful
Measles	+	−	−	++	Culture difficult; diagnosis clinical
RSV	++	++	−	+	Antigen detection thoroughly evaluated
Parainfluenza	++	+	−	+	Serology hard to interpret
Cytomegalovirus	++	+	+	−	Molecular probes promising; serology hard to interpret

nuclear dust that make determination of the cell types difficult. A similar phenomenon may be observed in some bacterial pneumonias, such as those produced by *Legionella* spp.[15]

A second common histologic pattern is interstitial pneumonitis with diffuse alveolar damage. Interstitial edema and lymphocytic infiltration are mixed to varying degrees with destruction and regeneration of the alveolar lining cells, intraalveolar edema and hemorrhage, and hyaline membranes. This pattern of reaction can be seen with virtually any viral infection of the lung. Unless diagnostic inclusions are present, the differential diagnosis is extensive and includes noninfectious damage to the alveolar membrane.[16]

Finally, there are focal inflammatory lesions, often centered around bronchioles or small blood vessels. These lesions may be necrotizing with an acute or chronic inflammatory response or they may resemble ischemic necrosis, perhaps because of virally induced damage to vascular endothelium. Varicella-zoster and herpes simplex viruses are the preeminent causes of this pattern, probably following hematogenous dissemination of the virus. A micronodular pattern has also been described for pulmonary infections by cytomegalovirus in immunosuppressed patients.[17]

The macroscopic and radiographic appearance of the lung is as varied as the microscopic pathology.[18] Patchy or diffuse infiltrates may be present. The chest radiograph is classically described as suggesting interstitial disease, but a pattern that indicates alveolar filling is often present.

The lungs are usually heavy and airless when visualized at surgery or at autopsy. Interstitial thickening may be evident. Hemorrhage is frequently noted. Nodular or micronodular lesions have been described pathologically. On occasion, infiltrates are segmental or even lobar, resembling bacterial pneumonia.[7,10,18]

Methods for Specific Diagnosis of Viral Infections

Infections may be diagnosed by isolation of the agent in culture, by demonstration of antigens or nucleic acid in clinical specimens, or by documenting a serological response to the virus (Table 12–2). The interested reader should consult recent textbooks of diagnostic microbiology for complete details.[19–22]

Viral Culture

Viral diagnostic facilities, which were once the province of the research laboratory, are increasingly available in clinical laboratories of academic medical centers and even in community hospitals.[23] A specimen should be submitted for culture as soon as possible, because a decrease in the number of infectious particles can be expected after storage and as the course of illness develops. The rapidity with which viruses deteriorate varies, being greatest with cytomegalovirus and respiratory syncytial virus (RSV). Although some centers prefer to inoculate cell cultures at the bedside when RSV is considered,[24] acceptable results have been achieved even with this labile virus when delays in processing did not exceed 6 h and when specimens were refrigerated during transportation.[25,26] It is quite feasible, therefore, to use a regional reference laboratory for viral cultures if facilities for culture of viruses are not available locally.[27]

In general, maintenance of the specimen at 4°C is preferable to freezing, which results in the loss of many infective particles. Once again, cytomegalovirus and RSV are particularly vulnerable to freezing and thawing. If a long delay between collection of the specimen and processing is inevitable, the specimen should be frozen quickly and maintained at −70°C. The definition of "long" is a matter of some dispute. McIntosh[28] has suggested, most reasonably, that specimens should be refrigerated unless more than 4 days will elapse before they are cultured. The worst temperature for storage of most viruses is −20°C; use of a frost-free freezer, which produces repetitive cycles of freezing and thawing, is tantamount to murder.

The major advantage of virologic diagnosis is that the procedure is relatively "broad minded," if a variety of cell cultures are infected. That is, most of the likely etiologic agents will be recovered and the prejudices of the clinician or pathologist are unlikely to misdirect the diagnostic efforts. The major disadvantage of virologic diagnosis is the length of time required for the recovery of some important pathogens, particularly cytomegalo-

Table 12–3. Viral inclusions

Virus	Intranuclear	Cytoplasmic	Comments
Influenze	−	−	Occasional reports of small cytoplasmic inclusions in exfoliated cells
Parainfluenza	−	+	Inclusions not common
Respiratory syncytial	−	+	Eosinophilic inclusions common in cell culture, less frequent in tissue
Measles	+	+	Nuclear inclusions resemble herpes; cytoplasmic inclusions may be very large
Herpes simplex, varicella-zoster	+	−	Eosinophilic; may have halo; may be multinucleate
Adenovirus	+	−	Early inclusions resemble herpes; late inclusions "smudge" cells
Cytomegalovirus	+	+	Early nuclear inclusions resemble herpes; late inclusions large and basophilic; cytoplasmic inclusions may be present

virus and respiratory syncytial virus. Innovative approaches to viral diagnosis are likely to minimize this difficulty. For example, centrifugation of the inoculum onto a monolayer of cells and subsequent detection of viral growth by immunofluorescence have resulted in recovery of most isolates of herpes simplex virus, cytomegalovirus, and respiratory syncytial virus, within 48 h.[29–31]

Direct detection of respiratory syncytial virus in clinical specimens by direct immunofluorescence or enzyme immunoassay is an acceptable substitute for viral culture.[32–34] False-positive reactions have been reported to be problems when enzyme immunoassays are used, and confirmatory blocking assays may be necessary.[35] Results may be obtained in a clinically relevant timeframe,[36] but culture techniques are still important. Other viral agents are frequently isolated from RSV-negative specimens,[37] and some authors have noted coinfections in RSV-positive patients with moderate frequency.[38]

Morphologic Diagnosis

Demonstration of viral inclusions in clinical material is the time-honored method for diagnosing viral infections rapidly (Table 12–3). All viruses produce biochemical alterations in infected cells, and morphologic abnormalities can be detected in many instances. In a few instances, the cytologic abnormalities can be visualized with the light microscope as viral inclusions. In general, the DNA-containing viruses are assembled in the nucleus and produce intranuclear inclusions, whereas the RNA-containing viruses are assembled in the cytoplasm and produce cytoplasmic inclusions.

A presumptive etiologic diagnosis can be made from the typical morphology of the inclusions. Part of the characteristic light microscopic appearance of the inclusions derives from artifacts of fixation. Strano[39] recommends fixation of material in Zenker's acetic acid or Bouin's fixative and also in formalin, if viral infection is suspected. The extent to which these fixatives are supe-

rior to formalin has not been documented, however. It is fortunate that formalin appears to be an adequate fixative, because the nature of the process is often not suspected before the tissue is fixed. Special stains for the demonstration of inclusions have been developed, but they offer no advantage over a well-done hematoxylin and eosin stain.[39]

Intranuclear inclusions must be differentiated from large nucleoli and from invaginations of cytoplasm; the differential diagnosis of cytoplasmic inclusions includes large phagolysosomes or other focal cellular abnormalities and phagocytized matter, such as red blood cells. Among the viruses that produce lower respiratory infections, herpes simplex, varicella-zoster, and adenovirus produce intranuclear inclusions; respiratory syncytial virus and parainfluenza viruses may cause cytoplasmic inclusions; both nuclear and cytoplasmic inclusions may be seen in cells infected by measles and cytomegalovirus. The inclusions may be detected in tissue sections or, in some instances, in cytologic preparations.[40,41] They are discussed under the individual infections.

Less specific cytologic alterations may also be detected in expectorated sputum or lavaged bronchial contents. Fragmented cells with enlarged, hyperchromatic nuclei and prominent nucleoli represent nonspecific responses to epithelial damage.[41] Virally induced damage to ciliated respiratory epithelial cells has been well documented.[42] Ciliocytophthoria, originally described by Papanicolaou, is a pattern of cellular degeneration in which free ciliated tufts without nuclei, nuclear degeneration, and acidophilic cytoplasmic inclusions may be found.[43] The phenomenon has been associated with viral respiratory tract infection, but may also be observed in other pulmonary diseases.[43]

The electron microscope has also been used for diagnostic purposes, although less frequently for diseases of the respiratory tract than for those of other organs such as the gastrointestinal tract. Viral particles may be demonstrated directly in clinical material or after amplification in cell culture by negative-staining electron microscopy.[44] Virions may also be demonstrated in thin sections.[45] The diagnosis may be definitive, as in the case of adenovirus. In other instances the morphology of the agents, such as those of the herpesvirus group, is identical, and electron microscopy may be of less differential value than light microscopy.

The advantages of morphologic diagnosis are that the detection of viruses is not limited by narrow specificity of reagents and that cellular or tissue damage can be documented at the time the virus is identified. However, it is often very difficult to associate viruses that produce latent infections, particularly cytomegalovirus, with clinical disease. Demonstration of cytopathology, and especially histopathology, may be a much better indicator that the agent is clinically important than the recovery of the virus in cell culture or the demonstration of viral nucleic acid in cells that appear normal structurally.

The disadvantages of morphologic diagnosis are the limited number of viruses that produce specific morphologic changes in infected cells; even in those that do, the limited number of inclusions compared to the large number of infected cells. For example, the sensitivity of detection of cytomegalic inclusions in lungs from which CMV is isolated may be as low as 38%.[46] Electron microscopy is infrequently used as a routine diagnostic tool because of the restricted availability of the equipment and the expense of examining ultrathin sections. Sampling errors are magnified when tissue is examined at the ultrastructural level. Fortunately, infectious agents are sturdy. Although the tissue may not be well preserved, the viruses are usually well preserved even after formalin fixation and paraffin embedding. Pinkerton and Carroll[47] have demonstrated that portions of a paraffin block may be successfully reembedded for electron microscopy after inclusions are identified with the light microscope.

Immunologic and Molecular Diagnosis

Immunologic and molecular diagnostic techniques can be applied to antigens and nucleic acids in solution or in tissue sections (in situ). Immunofluorescence and immunoenzymatic techniques have been used in the diagnosis of viral infections for several decades, but have received a boost in recent years from a supply of reagents that has steadily improved in quality. Monoclonal antibodies are now available for most of the viruses that infect the respiratory tract. In some instances the monoclonal antibodies represent a major improvement over their polyclonal forebears.[48] It is essential that the efficacy of the monoclonal reagent be demonstrated in clinical studies, because the restricted

antigenic site to which the monoclonal antibodies react may not be uniformly present on infecting strains.[49] The practical application of monoclonal technology to the diagnosis of viral respiratory infections is greatly increased by the efficacy of a monoclonal antibody pool against multiple viral agents.[50]

An immunoassay may be performed on imprint smears from tissue, on centrifuged fluid, or on tissue sections. If the specimen contains large amounts of mucus, which produces nonspecific fluorescence, washing of the exudate has been recommended to facilitate evaluation of the fluorescent smear,[51] but this may not be necessary to detect most infections.[52] In recent years, experience has been most extensive with RSV infections; the availability of ribavirin as effective antiviral chemotherapy has greatly stimulated the interest in rapid diagnostic tests.[36,53,54] If effective therapy becomes available for other agents, the impetus for expedited diagnosis will be increased. Although herpes simplex infections have been treated successfully with acyclovir in some instances, there are as yet no reports of therapy of herpes simplex virus infections of the lower respiratory tract.[55] The efficacy of therapy for cytomegalovirus infections has not yet been unequivocally demonstrated.

In recent years nucleic acid hybridization has been increasingly used for diagnosis of viral infections in the research laboratory.[56] Probes have been developed for a variety of viruses, including cytomegalovirus, herpes simplex, and adenovirus.[57–59] To date, most investigators have concentrated on the detection of nucleic acid in body fluids after fixation to a solid phase such as nitrocellulose.[60] Sandwich assays, in which the specimen remains in solution, are useful for testing complex biological specimens but may have reduced sensitivity.[61] Jansen and colleagues[62] approached the problem innovatively, combining molecular and immunologic methods; by absorbing the clinical specimen to a monoclonal antibody-coated surface before hybridization, they eliminated much of the nonspecific activity in highly contaminated specimens such as stool.

In situ hybridization, using tissue sections as the substrate, has been applied less frequently to the diagnosis of respiratory infections. The feasibility of the technique was demonstrated by Myerson and co-workers,[63] who detected cytomegalovirus DNA in 13 of 14 lung biopsies from which the virus was cultured; hybridization was not demonstrated in sections that contained varicella-zoster virus, herpes simplex virus, or adenovirus. One drawback of the first-generation hybridization procedures was the need to label the probe with a radiotracer, usually ^{32}P. Replacement of the radiolabel with an enzymatic colorimetric assay has been accomplished and will make the procedure more generally applicable if adequate sensitivity can be obtained. Unger and colleagues[64] have described a simplified colorimetric in situ hybridization test for CMV, which can be performed on formalin-fixed, paraffin-embedded sections; an avidin-alkaline phosphatase label can be visualized within 8 h of cutting the histologic section.

If tissue has been refrigerated or snap-frozen, there is greater flexibility in the selection of immunologic and molecular studies. In many instances enzyme immunoassays and in situ hybridization can be performed on fixed, embedded tissue. Immunofluorescence for some viral antigens can be accomplished only after the tissue section has been treated with a proteolytic enzyme such as trypsin.[65,66] Enzymatic digestion of tissue sections has been demonstrated to facilitate in situ hybridization also.[64]

These immunologic and molecular techniques facilitate the provision of more rapid etiologic diagnoses. In most instances they require such intensive or prolonged effort that it is difficult to offer them as "stat" procedures unless a therapeutic decision for a critically ill patient hangs in the balance. Even if not performed on an emergency basis, however, these tests offer greatly expedited diagnostic capability for infectious agents that are difficult to isolate, such as varicella-zoster virus, or grow slowly in isolation systems, such as respiratory syncytial virus and cytomegalovirus. There is little doubt that the nucleic acid probes will be useful diagnostically, just as immunodiagnostic procedures have been in selected situations. Adequate sensitivity and specificity must be combined with a procedure that can be performed on a routine basis before they will receive wide acceptance. The selection of the optimal nucleic acid sequence is essential for both adequate sensitivity and specificity. Although monoclonal antibodies are immunologically specific and nucleic acid probes are genetically specific, freedom from false-positive results cannot be assumed when complex clinical specimens are tested.

Approach to the Specimen in the Pathology Laboratory

If the clinician suspects an infectious etiology, many of the diagnostic procedures will have been initiated in parallel with submission of the tissue to the pathology laboratory. If an infectious process has not been suspected clinically, unfixed tissue is not likely to be reserved unless macroscopic lesions suggest an inflammatory process or a frozen section suggests an infectious cause. Increasingly, small biopsies, bronchial brushings, or bronchial washings are submitted to the laboratory, and often there is not enough residual material to refrigerate an aliquot. It is good practice, however, to preserve tissue for special studies routinely when the

patient has been subjected to the risk and trauma of a lung biopsy. Tissue fixed for electron microscopy, frozen for immunofluorescence, or refrigerated for culture is probably not often needed, but is invaluable on those few occasions.

Individual Viral Pathogens

Influenza Virus

Influenza has been and continues to be one of the great scourges of man. Influenza viruses and RSV alone produce epidemic disease annually. Irregularly, but with all-too-great frequency, widespread epidemics of influenza occur, occasionally producing a pandemic that involves virtually the whole world. Epidemics attributed to the influenza viruses have occurred throughout recorded history. In the past century, major epidemics occurred in 1890, 1900, 1918, 1957, and 1968. The great pandemic of influenza in 1918–1919 is estimated to have killed 20–40 million people and accounted for 80% of the deaths in the U.S. Army during World War I.

The influenza viruses are classified as orthomyxoviruses.[67] They contain RNA, measure 80–120 nm, have a pleomorphic shape with long filamentous forms, and acquire a lipid envelope after maturing ("budding") through the plasma membrane of an infected cell. Three antigenic types are defined by the ribonucleoprotein core of the virus. Type A is the primary pathogen of this group and is responsible for pandemic disease. Influenzavirus B is also an important pathogen and produces epidemic disease. Influenzavirus C is associated serologically with a human infection that appears to be mild and usually goes unrecognized.

Influenzaviruses A and B are additionally classified by the antigenic composition of virally specified surface projections.[68,69] Both viruses contain hemagglutinin and neuraminidase, which are important for attachment of the virus to cells and subsequent penetration of the cells. The hemagglutinin, in particular, is useful for detection of the virus in cell cultures and as a stimulus for a serologic response in infected patients. Minor changes in antigenic composition of the influenza viruses happen regularly (antigenic drift), and major changes (antigenic shift) occur periodically. Strains are described as follows: antigenic group/geographic source/host of origin if other than man/isolate number/ year, followed by the antigenic designation of the hemagglutinin and neuraminidase [e.g., Influenza-virus A/Singapore/1/57 (H2N2) or A/swine/Iowa/31 (Hsw-1N1)].

Influenzavirus was first isolated from swine in 1920 and from man in 1933. Analysis of subsequent isolates and retrospective evaluation of sera from earlier epidemics has suggested that major shifts in antigenic structure are associated with pandemic disease and that strains may recirculate. Until the 1970s, a single strain or a closely related group of strains circulated at any one time. Since 1977, however, strains with antigenic composition H3N2 and H1N1 have produced human disease concurrently.

Occasional cases of influenza infection may occur at any time of the year, but most are seen in the winter and spring months. In the northern hemisphere, most epidemics occur from January through April; from a global perspective, influenza occurs during every month of the year. There is no evidence for persistent or latent infection by influenza viruses. Although transmission of a virus from an animal to man may occur, it is presumed that the primary means for maintenance of the infection is by person-to-person transmission. As with other respiratory agents, transmission is facilitated by the crowding that occurs during the winter months. Young children are frequently responsible for dissemination of the infection to their families. It is probable that coughing and sneezing are the means of transmission of these viruses, but direct spread by contact cannot be excluded.

Experimental infection may be produced after inoculation of a variety of species, most frequently ferrets or mice. Ferrets, the species in which the initial human isolate was made, are the most susceptible host; in that species infection is usually limited to the upper respiratory tract, but the pathology of viral pneumonia appears similar to human disease.[70] Viral isolates must often be adapted to mice before damage to the tracheobronchial tree and lung results. Raut and colleagues[71] suggested that the ability of isolates to multiply in alveolar cells may confer virulence. They analyzed sections of lung that had been reacted with antiinfluenza antiserum in an indirect immunofluorescence test and suggested that alveolar macrophages were the site of viral replication. In contrast, Rodgers and Mims[72] were unable to detect any differences in the replication of virulent and avirulent isolates of influenzavirus A in macrophages. They examined macrophages that had been washed from the lungs of normal mice by bronchoalveolar lavage and infected in vitro as well as lavaged macrophages from the lungs of mice that had been previously infected in vivo. Influenzavirus A produced a cytolytic infection in alveolar macrophages, but the infection was not productive of infectious viral particles.

Influenza varies from asymptomatic infection to fatal pneumonia. The classic influenza syndrome includes the abrupt onset of headache, chills, and dry cough, followed by high fever, myalgias, malaise, and anorexia. Physical findings are usually minimal, but the patient appears toxic.[68] Fry[7] described the syndrome as follows:

The onset was dramatically sudden, the patients often being able to recall the time almost to the minute. The initial symptoms were shivering, a sensation of being chilled, headache, backache, pains in the arms and legs. Later, in a few hours, there developed symptoms referable to irritation of the respiratory tract, with nasal obstruction, rawness of the throat and chest and an irritating cough predominating. The patients felt extremely ill, with marked depression and feelings of impending doom.

The symptomatology of influenzavirus B infection is indistinguishable from that of influenzavirus A.

The symptoms in children are similar, but fever tends to be higher, febrile convulsions may occur, and gastrointestinal symptoms are more common.

Primary influenza pneumonia was first recognized during the pandemic of "Asian" influenza in 1957–1958.[10,73,74] A spectrum of pathologic lesions was recognized in that epidemic. Hers and colleagues[74] in the Netherlands described the bacteriology and pathology of 148 virologically confirmed cases of fatal Asian influenza. Pure viral lesions were present in approximately 25% of patients. Tracheobronchitis was present in all cases and was the only lesion in 4% of individuals; viral pneumonia without bacterial superinfection was demonstrated in 20%.

Primary viral pneumonia occurs predominantly in elderly individuals, in those with chronic cardiopulmonary disease, and in infants, but as many as 25% of individuals may have no recognized underlying disease.[10,75] In the typical case there is a rapid progression from the sudden onset of the influenza syndrome to a severe pneumonia with tachypnea and hypotension. Infiltrates are often found in multiple lobes by chest radiographs. Cyanosis and frothy pulmonary edema are poor prognostic signs.

Viral infection of the respiratory epithelium impairs the function of the mucociliary escalator. Impaired clearance of radiolabeled particles could be demonstrated in patients for as long as 1 month after an acute influenzavirus A infection.[76] The mechanism of the impaired clearance was presumed to be destruction of ciliated epithelial cells. Indeed, investigators have found ultrastructural evidence of ciliary damage during viral upper respiratory infection, even in epithelial cells that were not destroyed.[42]

In addition, functional impairment of phagocytes has been demonstrated in man and in experimental animals. Abramson and associates[77] found decreased middle ear pressure, decreased chemotaxis of neutrophils, and decreased chemiluminescence of stimulated leukocytes in chinchillas that had been infected with influenzavirus A. Although the phagocytic capability of alveolar macrophages is not altered after infection with influenzavirus A in vitro, an immunologically mediated defect in phagocytosis has been observed in vivo.[78] Larson and Blades[79] demonstrated that both chemotaxis and the ability to phagocytize staphylococci were impaired in infected human neutrophils.

Oropharyngeal bacteria are the main particulates of concern in a patient with influenza infection. Bacterial infection, most commonly by *Haemophilus influenzae,* was well recognized during the 1919 pandemic, although the underlying viral agent had not been documented at the time. During the 1957 pandemic *Staphylococcus aureus* was the most frequently isolated secondary pathogen in most locations, followed by *Streptococcus pneumoniae,* and, much less frequently, *Haemophilus influenzae* or *Streptococcus pyogenes.*[10,74]

Bacterial superinfection has also been demonstrated in animal models of influenzavirus infection. An increased frequency of pneumococcal otitis media occurred in chinchillas that had been experimentally infected with influenzavirus A if tympanostomy tubes were not placed in the ear.[77]

Bacterial superinfection was observed in the remaining three-quarters of the Dutch cases, bacterial tracheobronchitis in addition to a viral lesion in 5%, bacterial tracheobronchitis and pneumonia in the presence of viral tracheobronchitis in 40%, and mixed bacterial and viral pneumonia in 31%. Hers et al.[74] noted that the mixed pneumonia category might have been underrepresented, because viral lesions could have been obscured by necrotizing bacterial superinfection. Once the pathologic lesions associated with pure viral pneumonia and mixed infection were defined by bacterial and viral cultures, the presence of pathologically pure viral pneumonia during the 1918 pandemic could be recognized.

It may be very difficult to differentiate clinically the pure viral pneumonia from a mixed bacterial and viral infection unless cavitary lesions are demonstrated on chest radiographs or Gram stains of expectorated sputum suggest bacterial infection. When a bacterial superinfection complicates a resolving viral infection, there is a period of clinical improvement followed by the abrupt reappearance of fever, chills, pleuritic chest pain, and a cough productive of bloody or purulent sputum.[73,75] The mortality appears to be less than when the bacterial and viral infections are concurrent. It may be difficult to isolate the influenzavirus in this situation.

Pathologic Anatomy

In many descriptions of influenza pneumonia it is difficult to separate the viral component of the pathology from damage inflicted by secondary bacterial invaders.[80–82] Most of our knowledge about the pathology of virologically documented influenza pneumonia comes from the Asian and Hong Kong influenzavirus A epidemics of the 1950s and 1960s. There is very little information about the pathology of influenzavirus B disease, which is associated with morbidity but only rarely with mortality. Hers and Mulder[83] described a case of fatal influenzavirus B infection in which pneumonia was absent. There was a widespread degenerative change in the tracheal and bronchial epithelium without an inflammatory response, but mitotic activity was observed. These findings are compatible with more extensive data from influenzavirus A infections, but difficult to interpret in autopsy material.

Several authors have commented on the similarity of histopathology among cases from epidemics as far back as the great 1918 pandemic.[74,82] Feldman and colleagues[82] were able to compare directly the microscopic abnormalities that they observed in 1968 with those that Winternitz et al.[84] had observed at the same hospital in 1918. It appears therefore that changes in antigenic structure of the virus have not affected the interactions of virion and man in a major way.

Influenzavirus tracheobronchitis was studied by Walsh[85] and colleagues, who performed tracheal and bronchial biopsies on six young adults who had acute uncomplicated influenzavirus A disease without secondary bacterial infection. The damage to the mucosal surface was more prominent in the bronchus than in the trachea. Histologic changes ranged from cytologic abnormalities to extensive necrosis and ulceration of the epithelium. Columnar cells were vacuolated, nuclei were hyperchromatic, and cilia were absent. Desquamation of the epithelium extended to a basal cuboidal layer of cells or even to the basement membrane. Most specimens that were taken more than 24 h after onset of symptoms also demonstrated some degree of metaplasia.

The histopathology of bronchiolitis and alveolitis produced by influenzavirus A has been documented by open lung biopsy[86–88] and at autopsy.[10,80–82,89] If the cases in which bacterial superinfection occurred are eliminated, a consistent but diverse pattern of damage is evident.

The morphologic damage to the pulmonary parenchyma may be minimal even when the virus has been isolated from the lung. Hers and colleagues mentioned 13 cases between 1941 and 1953 in which the patient died in the acute stage of the infection and influenzavirus type A was isolated from the lung, but specific histologic changes were not present. They hypothesized that most of the virus had been aspirated into the distal air spaces ante mortem. Engblom and colleagues,[90] however, described a patient with an influenza syndrome followed by influenzavirus A myocarditis (proved by isolation of the virus from the myocardium) who had clear lung fields by chest radiograph and congestion of the organs at autopsy. We have observed a similar case in which the lungs showed only congestion despite isolation of influenzavirus A in pure culture from the lung. Extensive myocarditis was unsuspected clinically. It appears, therefore, that replication of the virus and serious systemic disease can occur in the absence of extensive pulmonary histopathology.

Hers and colleagues[74] described seven features of pure influenzavirus A pneumonia: (1) cytopathology of the respiratory epithelium down to the alveolar ducts; (2) cytologic damage to the alveolar lining cells; (3) capillary thrombosis and focal necrosis with leukocytic exudate; (4) capillary aneurysms and hemorrhage; (5) after 3–4 days, the appearance of a plasmatic exudate that lines the alveolar ducts and includes hyaline membranes; (6) regeneration of the epithelium of the respiratory bronchioles and alveolar ducts into a pseudostratified metaplastic epithelium after 5–7 days; and (7) regeneration of the alveolar epithelium into a continuous monolayer covering the alveolar wall. The lesions were always focal and sometimes clearly lobular in distribution.

Most recent descriptions of the pathology of influenza pneumonia have concentrated on the bronchiolitis, the interstitial pneumonia, and the reparative process. There are no viral inclusions to help distinguish this viral disease from others. In patients who died early in the course of the disease, necrosis of the ciliated and goblet cells of the epithelium was prominent.[82] Damaged epithelial cells were enmeshed in a luminal fibrin mass.[89] Even 2 weeks after onset of symptoms, patchy membranous bronchitis and bronchiolitis could be seen. The bronchiolitis is often described as necrotizing and may be observed as early as the second day of illness.[82] An acute inflammatory response in the bronchial and bronchiolar epithelium may be seen in the absence of bacterial infection and has been documented in a lung biopsy from which influenzavirus A was recovered in pure culture.[86]

The interstitium of affected areas is congested and edematous and contains a mixed cellular infiltrate. Edema fluid, fibrin, blood, and inflammatory cells fill the air spaces to a varying degree (Figs. 12–1 and 12–2). The contribution of neutrophils to the cellular response varies from scanty to extensive.[82,86,89,91] A dense, purulent inflammatory response is characteristic of bacterial superinfection. There may be areas in a pure influenza pneumonia, however, in which neutrophils are prominent. There may also be extensive fragmentation of cells, leaving a dusting of nuclear debris and making determination of the cell types more difficult (Fig. 12–1).

Hyaline membranes, which stain with periodic acid–Schiff reagent, are a prominent part of the alveolar

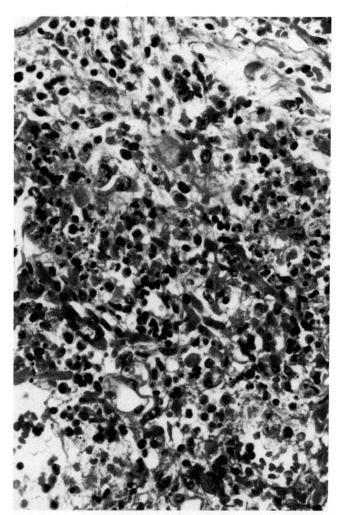

Fig. 12–1. Influenzavirus A pneumonia. Boundaries between interstitium and air space are obscured by intense inflammatory infiltrate of mononuclear cells and polymorphonuclear neutrophils. Karyolysis and karyorrhexis produce cellular debris and nuclear fragments. Influenzavirus A isolated from lung in pure culture. H and E, ×300.

reaction to influenzavirus A. They are apposed directly to the damaged alveolar walls or to the epithelium of the alveolar ducts and terminal bronchioles (Fig. 12–2). The hyaline membranes have been seen as early as the second day and as late as the third week of illness.[82] As a nonspecific response to alveolar damage, they have been noted to be more prominent when other potentially damaging influences, such as oxygen therapy, have been present.

In patients who died or were biopsied after the first week of illness, reparative changes have been prominent. Metaplastic regeneration of the epithelium has been frequent and sometimes coexistent with residual acute damage. On occasion the proliferation has produced masses of epithelium that are sometimes de-

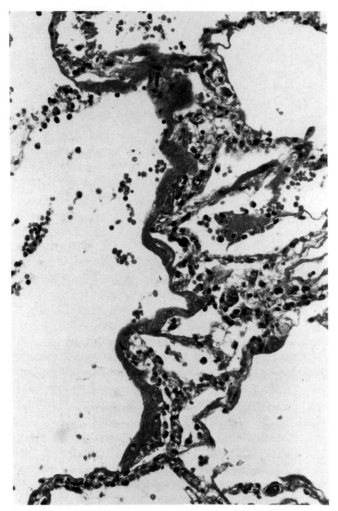

Fig. 12–2. Influenzavirus A pneumonia. Dense laminated hyaline membrane lines respiratory membrane of distal air space. Interstitium is edematous and contains scant mononuclear cell infiltrate. Red blood cells, fibrin, and few mononuclear leukocytes present in air space. Influenzavirus A isolated from lung in pure culture. H and E, ×150.

scribed as "tumorlets."[89] Interstitial fibrosis has been observed in conjunction with residual inflammation,[87] and may become prominent as the lesion heals. Restrictive pulmonary function defects have been demonstrated in uncomplicated influenza,[92] and resolution of the abnormalities may take many weeks.[93] Similarly, interstitial fibrosis and inflammation, obliterative bronchiolitis, and metaplasia may persist for weeks or months after an acute influenzavirus A infection.[94] Influenzavirus A was isolated from the lung of one child 8 weeks after the acute infection, at a time when interstitial inflammation and mild fibrosis were present.[94] The extent to which influenza infection contributes to focal or diffuse pulmonary fibrosis is unknown.

The diagnosis of influenza infection can be made by isolation of the virus, by demonstration of antigen in respiratory specimens, or by documenting a seroconversion. Isolation of influenzavirus A is made with equal facility in monkey kidney cell cultures and in embryonated eggs; influenzavirus B is more efficiently recovered in cell culture. Traditionally, washings or swabs from the nose or throat have been the specimens of choice. With improvements in virologic techniques, sputum may also provide an acceptable specimen. Antigen has been demonstrated in nasal specimens and sputum by immunofluorescence, and monoclonal antibodies have been developed, but the sensitivity of antigen detection is less than that of culture.[95,96] A common type-specific antibody to nucleoprotein antigen may be detected by complement fixation, providing a useful serologic screening tool. Strain-specific antibodies must be detected by hemagglutination inhibition.

Extrapulmonary symptoms are prominent during influenza, but inflammatory lesions outside of the respiratory tract are uncommon and identification of virus in extrapulmonary sites is even more rare. The best documented extrapulmonary inflammatory lesion is acute myocarditis, from which influenzavirus A has been isolated.[90]

Adenovirus

Adenoviruses were first recognized when spontaneous degeneration occurred in cell cultures that had been derived from tonsils and adenoidal tissue.[97] These viruses produce a variety of diseases in man and may persist for many months in a normal human host after an acute infection. Forty-one types of adenovirus have been identified. Ocular infections (including epidemic keratoconjunctivitis), acute hemorrhagic cystitis, and acute gastrointestinal disease in young children have been associated with adenoviruses. Rarely, meningoencephalitis and intussusception have been ascribed to these agents.

The most common adenovirus respiratory infections, comprising some 5% of acute respiratory disease in young children, are an exudative pharyngitis and a flu-like syndrome;[98] these diseases may be accompanied by ocular disease (pharyngoconjunctival fever). Epidemic respiratory disease has been concentrated in populations of military recruits during the winter months. Person-to-person spread by the respiratory route is presumed. Epidemics of adenovirus infection in military camps have been distinguished from influenza epidemics by limitation of disease to new recruits, other personnel presumably having become immune.[97] Similar epidemics have not occurred in civilian populations, such as college students. Nosocomial transmission of adenovirus infection has been demonstrated, however.[9]

Severe, even fatal pneumonia has occurred in recruits,[99–101] in children,* in immunosuppressed civilians,[104,105] and rarely in apparently normal adults.[8,9,106] A variety of adenovirus types has been associated with pneumonia, including types, 1,2,3,4,5,6,7,7-A, 11,21,31,35, and strains that were intermediate between two serotypes in antigenic composition. There do not appear to be any histopathologic changes that are type specific. Infection in immunosuppressed patients is similar to that in normal hosts, but is more severe and more frequently disseminated.[97,107]

Two patterns of damage have been described consistently in adenoviral infections of the lower respiratory tract: destructive infection of the bronchi or bronchioles and interstitial pneumonitis.

A necrotizing inflammation affects the bronchial and bronchiolar mucosa, which is partially or completely sloughed into an obstructive intraluminal coagulum of fibrin, necrotic tissue, and inflammatory cells. The necrosis may extend completely through the epithelium, but the muscularis is usually preserved (Fig. 12–3). Specific mention is made in multiple reports of necrotizing inflammation involving the submucosal glands of the bronchi. With time, reparative proliferative changes become evident in the surviving mucosa.

An alveolitis, which may appear necrotizing, often accompanies the bronchiolitis. Edema and cellular infiltration of the interstitium are accompanied by an alveolar exudate of fibrin, edema fluid, and cells (Fig. 12–3). Hyaline membranes are prominent in some cases. Focal necrosis of the alveolar walls has been described.

Pyknotic nuclear debris provides a necrotizing appearance to the air spaces, even in the absence of abundant inflammatory cells. Neutrophils may be virtually absent from the lesion (Fig. 12–4)[9,102] or may be a prominent part of the inflammatory response (Fig. 12–3).[3,108]

These histologic changes are not specific for adenovirus infection. A presumptive etiologic diagnosis is provided by the distinctive intranuclear inclusions that are produced by this virus (Fig. 12–5). Two types of inclusions have been described.[39,109] The first, which is eosinophilic and surrounded by a clear halo, resembles the inclusions of the herpesviruses. In its earliest form, there are multiple, small eosinophilic masses intermixed with basophilic chromatin and a prominent nucleolus. the intermixture of chromatin, eosinophilic inclusion, and clear halo may give the nucleus a honey-

* References: 2,3,47,102,103.

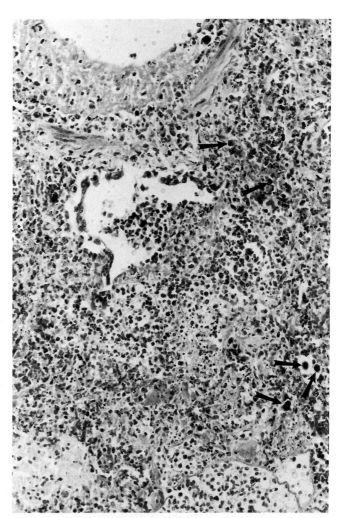

Fig. 12–3. Adenovirus pneumonia. Intensely inflammatory alveolitis in which mononuclear cells, polymorphonuclear neutrophils, and red blood cells are enmeshed in coagulum of fibrin. Extensive fragmented nuclear debris; dense adenovirus inclusions (smudge cells) can be noted even at this magnification (*arrows* indicate some obvious examples). Terminal bronchiole in left center is inflamed. At top, wall of larger, distal bronchiole is necrotic but muscularis remains intact. H and E, ×150.

comb appearance. These structures are Feulgen negative.

The second type of inclusion is often more numerous in tissue sections. This inclusion is basophilic or amphophilic and Feulgen positive. It may be surrounded by a small halo, but often fills the entire nucleus and obscures the nuclear envelope. Cells with such inclusions are often referred to as "smudge" cells. They are quite distinctive and characteristic of adenovirus infection, but must be differentiated from enlarged, hyperchromatic nuclei in regenerating epithelium. It has been suggested from study of experimentally infected hu-

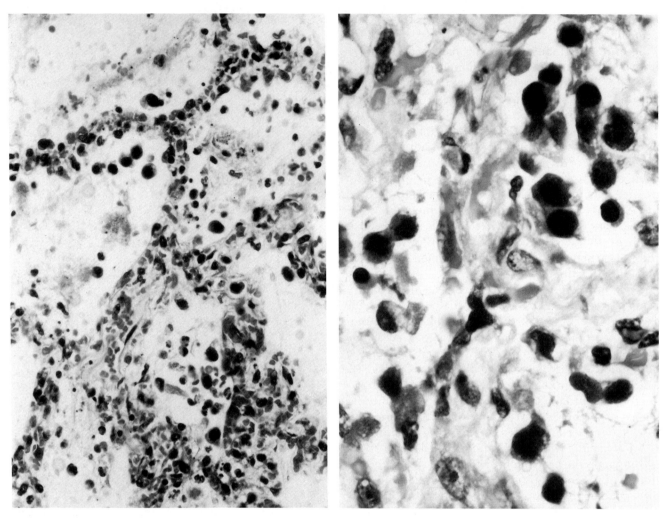

Fig. 12–4. Adenovirus, type 7 pneumonia with alveolar damage. Interstitium has increased numbers of cells; alveoli contain red blood cells, proteinaceous material, and scattered cells. Many epithelial cells appear dense because they contain mature adenovirus inclusions in nuclei. Although histopathological damage is present, this lesion is relatively noninflammatory in comparison to that pictured in Fig. 12–3. H and E, ×300.

Fig. 12–5. Adenovirus pneumonia. Virtually all cells contain mature adenovirus inclusions. Nuclei are densely basophilic, making it difficult to "see into" them. In some cases boundary between nucleus and cytoplasm is obscured. These "smudge" cells must be distinguished from nonspecifically damaged or reactive epithelial cells. H and E, ×750.

man tracheal epithelium[109] and human tissue[39] that the smudge cells are the mature form of inclusion, whereas the eosinophilic inclusion represents an earlier form. Other investigators have noted that the two types of inclusions may be physically separate in tissue sections and have suggested that they are developmentally disparate.[3]

Ultrastructurally, adenovirus inclusions consist of masses of virions packed in a paracrystalline array within the nucleus (Fig. 12–6). Adenovirus proteins are manufactured in the cytoplasm, where antigen may be demonstrated by immunofluorescence, but inclusions are not seen there. Fibrillar nuclear inclusions have

been seen in both adenovirus and influenza[91] infections in vivo, but do not have their counterpart in infected tissue culture cells.

Although adenovirus accounts for only 5% of bronchiolitis in the United States,[110] the acute inflammatory damage to the air spaces is impressive. Becroft[111] has described an equally impressive incidence of chronic complications after an epidemic of type 21 adenovirus infection. A distinctive feature of the epidemic was the protracted course of the infection, which waxed and waned over a period of several weeks; in some instances complete recovery never occurred. Similarly, Wohl and Chernick[110] noted the protracted course of adenovirus

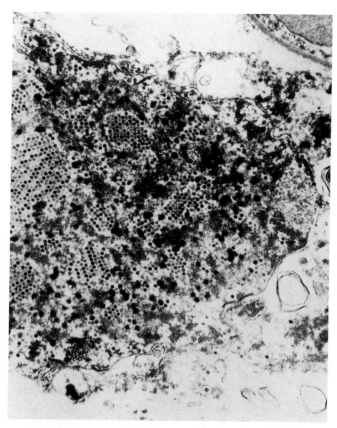

Fig. 12–6. Adenovirus pneumonia. Nucleus has been largely replaced by adenovirus virions packed in paracrystalline array. Portions of residual nuclear chromatin are pushed against nuclear membrane. Formalin-fixed lung tissue. ×12,500.

infections and development of chronic pulmonary disease in as many as 60% of infants.

Bronchiectasis, bronchiolitis obliterans, and the unilateral hyperlucent lung syndrome have been reported as serious chronic sequelae to well-documented cases of adenoviral bronchiolitis or pneumonia. The rarity of cartilage in the walls of obliterated or stenotic bronchioles suggested to Becroft[111] that the primary lesion was in the terminal bronchioles rather than the small bronchi. The mucosa and submucosa were replaced by vascular connective tissue, the nature of the structures being clarified by the residual muscularis. Distal to the obstructive lesions, the alveolar ducts were dilated.

It has been suggested that certain populations, such as those studied by Becroft,[111] are highly susceptible to severe adenovirus infection.[112] Bronchiolitis obliterans has been documented after measles, whooping cough, influenza in infants, and ingestion of foreign bodies or toxic chemicals[100] (see Chapter 5).

The diagnosis of adenovirus infections can be made by isolation of the virus from respiratory specimens, by demonstration of antigen in respiratory secretions, or by demonstration of a serological response to a common viral antigen. Inclusions have been demonstrated only infrequently in exfoliated respiratory cells.[40] Ciliocytophthoria has been described in exfoliated respiratory cells from patients with adenovirus infections.[43]

Herpes Simplex

Herpes simplex virus is the virus most commonly isolated in most hospital laboratories.[113] Two serological types have been defined, and either type of virus can produce any clinical syndrome. Gingivostomatitis, pharyngitis, esophagitis, encephalitis, and respiratory infections in adults are caused primarily by type 1 virus. Type 2 virus is the primary cause of genital infections, and may produce meningitis and disseminated neonatal infection, including pulmonary lesions. Antibody to type 1 develops during the first decade of life, whereas antibody to type 2 herpes simplex begins to appear in the teenage years.

Herpes simplex viruses occur only in man, and both types are spread by contaminated secretions. Once they have produced a primary infection, they may become latent in ganglia, from which site reactivation can occur repetitively. Asymptomatic shedding of virus is well documented in both the oral cavity[114] and in the genital tract, so that an active lesion is not required for transmission of an infection.

Herout and colleagues[115] first suggested that herpetic tracheobronchitis and pneumonia might be more common than suspected. It is unclear whether the respiratory disease is of recent occurrence or whether the diagnosis was missed previously. Nash[14] found that 9 of 10 cases of respiratory infection by herpes simplex had been missed clinically and pathologically.

Most herpetic infections of the lower respiratory tract occur in individuals whose defense mechanisms are compromised in some manner. The defects may be systemic or local. Newborn infants,[116] patients with burns,[117,118] and those with immunosuppressive diseases or treatments[119] are at increased risk of developing herpetic respiratory infection. Patients with tracheostomies or endotracheal tubes also have a greater risk of infection, although intubation is not a prerequisite for the infections.[12] The source of virus is usually the maternal vagina in neonates and the oropharynx in older children and adults. Mucocutaneous herpesvirus infection preceded respiratory disease in 17 of 20 individuals from whom herpes simplex virus was isolated at autopsy.[119]

The distribution of the pathologic lesions, prominence of tracheobronchial pathology, and association of infection with conditions that favor contamination of the lower tract all suggest that aspiration of oral secretions is the most common pathogenic mechanism.[119] Ramsey and colleagues[119] noted that diffuse interstitial pneumonia was frequently associated with disseminated infection, whereas focal pneumonia was more commonly associated with lesions in the trachea and bronchi. Focal lesions, often of a miliary nature, may also occur after disseminated infection and viremia, such as occurs in disseminated herpes simplex infections. The miliary lesions cannot be differentiated from disseminated varicella-zoster infection on morphologic grounds alone.

Several patterns of pulmonary damage occur. Ulcerative tracheobronchitis, which may also be accompanied by necrotizing pneumonia, is the most common manifestation of infection.[119] The surface of the ulcerated area is covered with a fibrinopurulent exudate containing necrotic cells, nuclear debris, fibrin, and inflammatory cells (Fig. 12–7). The infection may extend into the submucosal mucous glands. Polymorphonuclear neutrophils are a prominent part of the inflammatory response.[14] Necrosis of large portions of the epithelium may lead to sloughing of the mucosa and formation of a thick pseudomembrane, which may obstruct the airway.[12]

The accompanying pneumonitis is usually patchy, reflecting the focal endobronchial source of the infection. A necrotizing pneumonia results in a microscopic appearance that resembles the tracheal ulcers. The air spaces are filled with a coagulum of fibrin, necrotic cells, prominent fragmented nuclear debris, and inflammatory cells. The necrotizing appearance, prominence of neutrophils in the exudate, and bronchial distribution of the lesions may lead the unsuspecting pathologist to classify the lesion as bacterial in origin (Fig. 12–8). Nash[14] found 10 cases of herpetic lower respiratory infection in 1,000 consecutive autopsies at the Massachusetts General Hospital. Only 1 of the 10 cases had been diagnosed originally as a viral infection, presumably because the pathologist did not scrutinize the tissue for the characteristic inclusions.

Diffuse interstitial pneumonitis, which may also be necrotizing and hemorrhagic,[120] and miliary lesions without obvious relationship to the bronchial tree appear to be less common manifestations of herpetic lower respiratory infection (Fig. 12–9). Tuxen and colleagues,[121] however, demonstrated morphologic and virologic evidence of herpes simplex infection in the lungs of 14 patients (30%) with adult respiratory distress syndrome (ARDS).[121] The herpetic infection was associated with an increased need for prolonged respiratory support and an increased frequency of late mortality. The nature of the relationship between the herpes infection and the ARDS was not clear.

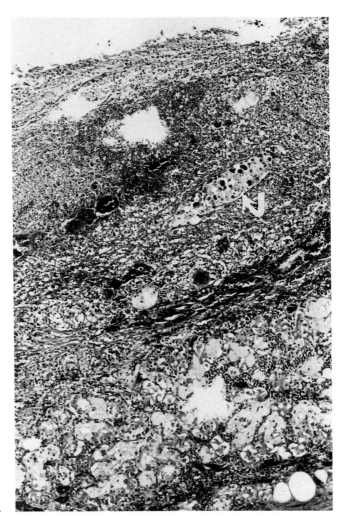

Fig. 12–7. Herpes simplex bronchitis. Mucosa and submucosa of this major bronchus are necrotic. Epithelium is replaced with coagulum of necrotic tissue, fibrin, red blood cells, mononuclear cells, and polymorphonuclear neutrophils (top). Dense, inclusion-bearing cells are visible even at this magnification (*white arrows*). Inflammation has extended from lumen through submucosal mucous glands to muscularis. H and E, ×150.

A presumptive etiologic diagnosis of herpes simplex infection may be rendered if the characteristic intranuclear inclusions are demonstrated[29] (Fig. 12–10). The inclusions of both types of herpes simplex virus and varicella-zoster virus, also a member of the herpesviridae, are identical. Initially, the nucleus enlarges and rarefies, the nucleolus is dispersed, and multiple masses of light-staining, amphophilic material are outlined by strands of basophilic chromatin. The classical Cowdry type A inclusion forms by coalescence and condensation of the smaller masses. The type A inclusion is a central, eosinophilic nuclear mass, which is surrounded by a halo and peripherally marginated, beaded chromatin.

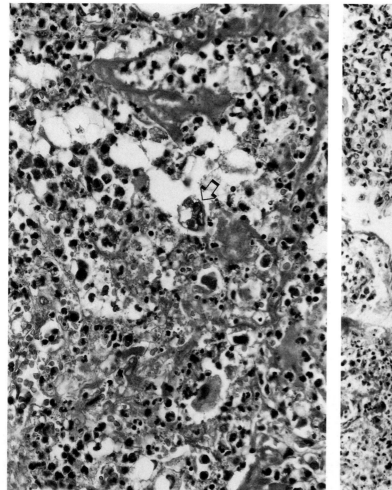

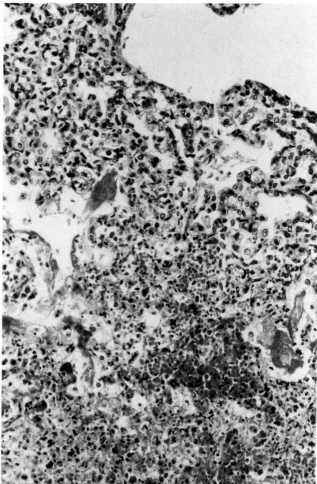

Fig. 12–8. Herpes simplex pneumonia. Alveolar structure is obliterated by necrotizing inflammation, which includes many polymorphonuclear neutrophils, fragmented nuclear debris, and fibrin. Such viral inflammatory lesions have been erroneously attributed to bacterial pathogens because of necrotizing character of inflammation. Multinucleated giant cell contains intranuclear inclusions that are surrounded by clear halo (*arrow*). Herpes simplex virus isolated from lung in pure culture. H and E, ×300.

Fig. 12–9. Neonatal herpes simplex pneumonia. Edge of miliary lesion. Lung tissue is necrotic (below) with exudate of fragmented cells, hemorrhage, and proteinaceous material. Note dilated distal airway, possibly alveolar duct (top right). Interstitium is cellular but tissue is viable. Herpes simplex isolated in pure culture. H and E, ×150.

As the inclusion becomes senescent, the central mass decreases in size, the halo widens, and the beaded character of the peripheral chromatin is lost. Ultrastructurally, the inclusion consists of viral deoxyribonucleoprotein and nucleocapsids. The naked nucleocapsids acquire a glycolipid envelope from the host cell as they pass from the nucleus to the cytoplasm (Fig. 12–11).

Multinucleation is a characteristic cellular reaction to both herpes simplex and varicella-zoster infection. Multinucleated giant cells with characteristic intranuclear inclusions are virtually diagnostic of infection by

one of these viruses. It should be remembered that parainfluenza, respiratory syncytial, and measles viruses can also produce multinucleated giant cells. Although multinucleated cells are not characteristic of cytomegalovirus (CMV) infection, their presence has been reported.[40] It has been suggested that the classical giant cells are less frequent in herpetic respiratory infection than in genital infection[122] but they are, nevertheless, commonly present both in expectorated sputum and in histologic sections.[12,40,123] The inclusions may be difficult to locate, particularly when there is a large amount of necrotic material present; they are best

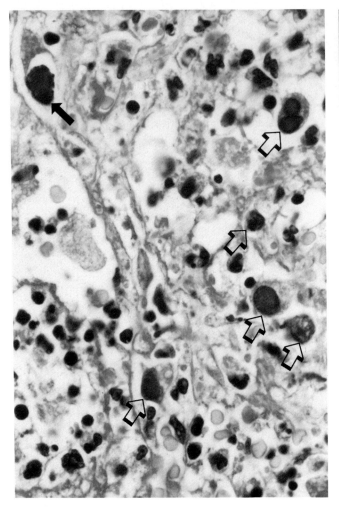

Fig. 12–10. Herpes simplex pneumonia. Multiple cells in inflammatory exudate contain intranuclear inclusions. Inclusions are eosinophilic, homogeneous, and fill virtually entire nucleus. *Open arrows* indicate several more easily identified inclusions in several phases of formation; one shows up better in color (*solid arrow*). Nuclear chromatin has been pushed to edge of nuclear membrane and is beaded in some cells. Herpes simplex virus isolated from lung in pure culture. H and E, ×750.

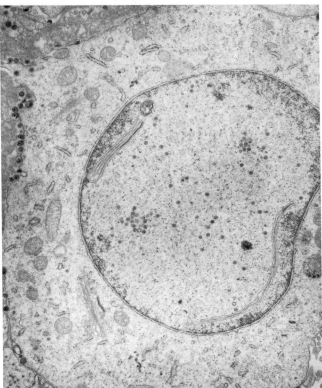

Fig. 12–11. Herpes simplex virus-infected MRC-5 fibroblast. Nucleus of tissue culture cell has been replaced by viral nucleoprotein. Scattered naked virions are evident in nucleus and nuclear chromatin has been pushed to nuclear membrane. Fully enveloped virions that have passed through nuclear membrane are evident in extracellular space at upper left of photomicrograph. ×12,000.

sought in intact cells at the periphery of ulcers or necrotic foci.

The diagnosis of herpes simplex infections is best made by a combination of viral culture or antigen detection and morphologic methods. Recovery of the virus from respiratory secretions is not of itself sufficient for a diagnosis of herpetic disease, because 1%–5% of the population excretes virus in the oropharynx.[12,114] On the other hand, demonstration of characteristic infected cells provides only presumptive identification of the etiologic agent. Serology is of little use in the diagnosis of herpes infections.

Measles Virus

Measles is a highly contagious disease that can spread only from acutely infected individuals to susceptible contacts, probably by means of respiratory secretions. The frequency of measles has decreased dramatically since the introduction of vaccines in the 1960s. Outbreaks continue to occur in populations that are inadequately immunized.[124] The diagnosis is usually so obvious clinically that specimens are not submitted to the laboratory for confirmation, but atypical cases occur, particularly in patients who received the initial killed vaccine.[125]

The most serious complications of acute measles infection are progressive infection, including pneumonia, and central nervous system disease, including postinfectious encephalitis and subacute sclerosing panencephalitis.[126] The progressive measles syndrome, in which pulmonary infection figures prominently, occurs in individuals who are immunologically compromised by underlying disease or therapy.[127] The development of the characteristic skin rash in measles coincides with the appearance of the earliest immune response; in these immunodeficient patients the rash is absent or atypical.[128] Isolation of the virus from normal individuals is virtually impossible within 48 h after development of the rash[127] whereas the virus persists in those with pneumonia. Measles pneumonia has been described, however, in apparently normal individuals who developed a rash.[129]

Measles may also be complicated by bacterial pneumonia[13] or by other viral infections.[129] *Haemophilus influenzae* was considered the cause of viral influenza in 1918 because of its frequent occurrence as a secondary invader. Similarly, a small gram-negative bacillus, possibly also *Haemophilus*, was suggested as a possible etiologic agent for measles because it was found in the lungs of patients who died shortly after the onset of the rash and had giant cell pneumonia.[130] In South Africa adenovirus and herpes simplex virus were common secondary pathogens in fatal cases of measles.[129] Goodpasture and associates[131] described a diverse group of viral pneumonias in infants. It is probable that the lesions observed in the cases of measles were caused by herpes simplex virus or by adenovirus. Cytoplasmic inclusions and giant cells were not described by these accomplished investigators; the illustrations depict structure that are compatible with or strongly suggest viral superinfection.

Macroscopically, the infiltrates of measles pneumonia are diffuse, patchy, or even nodular.[128] The nodular lesions have a distribution that is primarily peribronchial and peribronchiolar.[130] A hemorrhagic component may be present.[132] Microscopically, the small airways and alveoli are primarily affected. There is an interstitial pneumonia in which mononuclear cell infiltration predominates (Fig. 12–12). The air spaces contain fibrin and inflammatory cells; hyaline membranes may be present. The bronchioles show epithelial hyperplasia and extensive squamous metaplasia occurs, even with the formation of nodular epithelial masses. Macroscopic and microscopic pulmonary thromboemboli have been described.[133]

The most distinctive abnormality in measles pneumonia is the multinucleated giant cell, which contains eosinophilic intranuclear and intracytoplasmic inclusions (Fig. 12–13). Ultrastructurally, the inclusions consist of fibrillar viral ribonucleoprotein.[133] The giant cells are often numerous. They may be flattened against the respiratory membrane or heaped up in masses. The intranuclear inclusions are eosinophilic and resemble those of herpesviruses.[39] The cytoplasmic inclusions are brightly eosinophilic and may form very large masses[134] (Fig. 12–13).

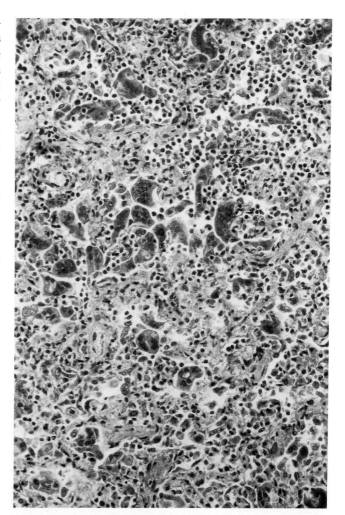

Fig. 12–12. Measles pneumonia. Architecture of air spaces has been obliterated by mixed inflammatory infiltrate, proliferation of alveolar epithelial cells, and formation of multinucleated epithelial cells. Intranuclear inclusions are easily seen in syncytial giant cells, even at low magnification; cytoplasmic inclusions also evident. H and E, ×150.

In 1910 Hecht described giant cell pneumonia in children. The similarities between Hecht's pneumonia and the lesion seen in both measles and distemper infections was recognized in 1945,[135] but the virologic association of giant cell pneumonia and measles virus was first made by Enders and colleagues.[136]

There are many other causes of giant cells in pulmonary lesions—infectious and noninfectious, viral and nonviral. The virologic differential diagnosis of interstitial pneumonia with giant cells includes respiratory syncytial virus and parainfluenza virus. A diagnosis of measles pneumonia can be made confidently if the characteristic intranuclear and intracytoplasmic inclusions are present, if there is a clinical history of measles, if the virus is isolated or identified immunologically, if a

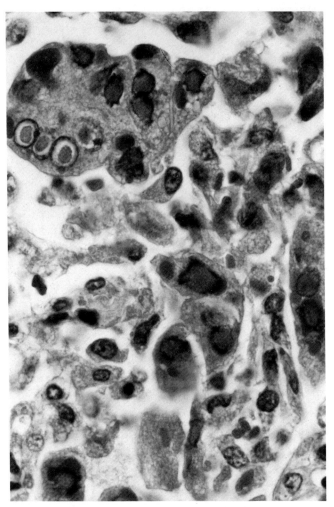

Fig. 12–13. Measles pneumonia. Many cells in air spaces, both uninucleate and multinucleate, contain inclusions. Intranuclear inclusions resemble those of herpes simplex virus; they are homogeneous and fill nucleus, pushing chromatin to periphery of nuclear membrane. Artefactual halo separates several intranuclear inclusions in multinucleated giant cells from residual chromatin. Cytoplasmic inclusions are brightly eosinophilic and vary in size. H and E, ×750.

serological response to the virus is documented, or if there are systemic abnormalities, such as lymphoid hyperplasia with Warthin–Finkeldey giant cells.

In the early 1960s, a formaldehyde-inactivated measles vaccine was introduced. Subsequently, it was recognized that children who received the vaccine developed an atypical measles syndrome in which the rash was accentuated peripherally and segmental pneumonia was prominent. This vaccine failed to induce immunity to a viral surface glycoprotein (F protein) that is essential to prevent spread of the infection.[126] Very little is known about the pathology of the atypical reaction. Annunziato and colleagues[137] described 17 patients, of

whom 15 had dense lobar or segmental pulmonary consolidation. Hilar or mediastinal lymphadenopathy and pleural effusions were seen in a minority of cases. Some infiltrates persisted and resolved into large nodular masses.[138] The differential diagnosis of nodular pulmonary infiltrates is extensive, but the lesions are sufficiently distinctive that the diagnosis of atypical measles syndrome can be suggested.[139]

Respiratory Syncytial Virus

Infection with respiratory syncytial virus occurs repeatedly throughout life including infancy to old age. Epidemics, which occur regularly in most communities, are separated by alternating long (13–16 months) and short (7–12 months) intervals.[110] Virtually all seronegative infants exposed to their first epidemic become infected. In a study of intrafamily transmission of viral infection, the secondary attack rate for RSV infection within families was 27% for all children and 45% for infants.[140] This virus is an important cause of nosocomial infection on pediatric hospital wards,[141–143] and has been reported as the cause of nosocomial pneumonia in adults.

Immunity to RSV is short lived and incomplete, although recurrent infections tend to be milder. The clinical syndrome varies from upper respiratory infection to croup, bronchitis, bronchiolitis, and interstitial pneumonia. The initial infection usually occurs in infants between 6 weeks and 6 months of age, 25%–40% of whom suffer lower respiratory tract infection (see also Chapter 8). Infection in infancy is associated with greater severity of illness; the severe involvement of bronchioles accounts for wheezing and air-trapping. Among children from whom RSV was isolated, 38% had bronchiolitis and 25%, pneumonia. Although RSV is the cause of 75% of cases of bronchiolitis, adenoviruses, rhinoviruses, parainfluenza virus (particularly type 3), mumps virus, influenza viruses, and *Mycoplasma pneumoniae* may also cause this syndrome. Immunocompromised children may develop a prolonged, sometimes fatal course of RSV pneumonia.

RSV is usually transmitted to the upper respiratory mucosa by the fingers. After an incubation period of 4–5 days, patients develop rhinorrhea and anorexia. Viral replication occurs in the nasopharynx, and during the next 1–3 days virus spreads along the airways to the lower respiratory tract. Then cough, tachypnea, low-grade fever, rales, and rhonchi occur. Signs of bronchiolar obstruction and air-trapping, including expiratory wheezes, intercostal and substernal retractions, atelectasis, and hyperresonance may also develop.[144–146] Severe illness is further characterized by dyspnea and cyanosis. The pathophysiology of bronchiolitis includes reduced pulmonary compliance, increased pulmonary resistance and end expiratory volume, and hypoxemia that is caused by decreased ventilation in the presence of normal perfusion.

Newborn infants and adults infected with RSV usually have upper respiratory infections; elderly patients often have prolonged bronchitis with tachypnea, wheezing, cough, and fever.[147] Hospitalization with RSV infection is most likely to occur during the first year of life. The mortality rate is 1% in normal children and as much as 37% in those with underlying diseases, particularly congenital heart disease and bronchopulmonary dysplasia. RSV was the most common virus isolated in a series of sudden infant deaths.[4] In developing countries, pediatric lower respiratory infections cause 4.5 million deaths annually, approximately 30% of all childhood deaths. RSV, parainfluenzaviruses, and other respiratory agents are the most frequent etiology; however, mortality occurs more often in bacterial pneumonias.[148] Fatal RSV pneumonia has also been reported rarely in adults.[142]

RSV infection is diagnosed best by viral culture or by demonstration of RSV antigen in respiratory secretions. Among infants and young children with lower respiratory tract infections, RSV is the most frequent viral isolate. Viral culture and immunologic identification of RSV antigens in washings from the nasopharynx are similar in sensitivity and specificity. Several immunologic approaches have been used, including immunofluorescence and immunoenzyme tests of aspirated epithelial cells and enzyme or radioimmunoassays on the nasopharyngeal washings.[31–34] Immunoperoxidase staining reveals RSV antigen in bronchial, bronchiolar, and alveolar epithelial cells and alveolar syncytial giant cells.[149] Recently circulating RSV antigen was also demonstrated in mononuclear cells in the peripheral circulation.[150] Serologic diagnosis may be achieved by demonstration of a fourfold or greater rise in titer of antibodies by complement fixation, neutralization, and enzyme immunoassay.

The cytoplasm of respiratory epithelial cells is the site of RSV replication. Final assembly of viral matrix proteins, nucleocapsids, and surface glycoproteins occurs at the cell membrane, which is converted into the viral envelope by the process of budding. Immunofluorescence with monoclonal antibodies to nucleocapsid proteins demonstrates cytoplasmic antigen that varies from small particles to larger inclusions.[49] These structures correspond to the cytoplasmic inclusions that are seen when infected cells are stained with H and E or by the Giemsa method (Fig. 12–14). The 1–20 μm eosinophilic inclusions in epithelial cells often have a clear halo and are located in a paranuclear cytoplasmic location (Fig. 12–15).[144,146,149]

RSV-infected cells may have a single nucleus, but are

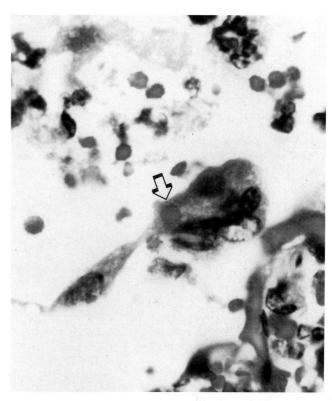

Fig. 12–14. Respiratory syncytial virus pneumonia. Air space contains proteinaceous material, red blood cells, and scant inflammatory cells. Multinucleated (syncytial) epithelial giant cell contains single, discrete cytoplasmic inclusion (*arrow*). H and E, ×750.

commonly multinucleated. The virus has a fusion protein that plays a role in the entry of virus into the host cell and the coalescence of adjacent cells to form multinucleate syncytial giant cells (Fig. 12–14). This phenomenon, which is remarkable in cell cultures infected with RSV, suggested the name of the virus. Both multinucleate syncytial and uninuclear cells show effects of cell injury, including necrosis. The syncytial giant cells are observed in vivo, and RSV infection must be included in the differential diagnosis of giant cell pneumonia, especially in the immunocompromised host. Bronchiolitis may be produced by RSV without formation of giant cells, in which case immunologic or virologic studies must be performed to elucidate the etiology of the infection.[151]

Lungs from patients with RSV bronchiolitis are overexpanded and do not collapse when the thorax is opened.[152] Chest radiographs may show a depressed diaphragm, patchy areas of atelectasis, and air-trapping, which is manifested by hyperlucency.[144] Microscopic examination reveals nipple-like projections of epithelial cells into the lumens of the airways, necrosis of the ciliated epithelium of bronchioles and bronchi,

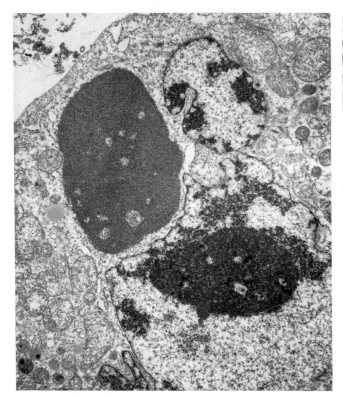

Fig. 12–15. Respiratory syncytial virus-infected HEp-2 cell. This human cell line was derived from laryngeal carcinoma and is preferred means for cultivating RSV. Large cytoplasmic inclusion is composed of fibrillar ribonucleoprotein, but difference in density between viral RNA and nucleolar RNA is evident. Remnants of cytoplasm within inclusion correspond to vacuoles in light microscopic sections. ×9,500.

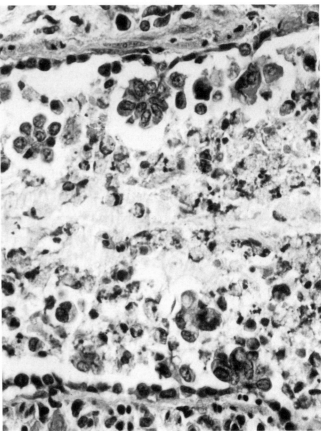

Fig. 12–16. Respiratory syncytial virus bronchiolitis. Epithelium of small bronchiole is extensively damaged, leaving intact basal layer. Several distinctive papillary projections of epithelium are present. Lumen filled with mononuclear cells, desquamated epithelial cells, and debris. H and E, ×450.

and inflammatory infiltration of the epithelium and submucosa (Fig. 12–16). The inflammation consists predominantly of lymphocytes and macrophages, which extend into adjacent alveolar septa. Necrotic cellular debris, fibrin, and mucus accumulate in the bronchiolar lumina. In the air spaces themselves there is hyperplasia of the alveolar lining cells, alveolar edema, and on occasion hyaline membranes.[144,146,151–154] Other bronchial and bronchiolar changes include a cuboidal-to-flat epithelium that represents early regeneration and a multilayered epithelium that is characteristic of regenerative hyperplasia.

Interstitial pneumonia is characterized by an infiltrate of mononuclear cells in alveoli and alveolar septa, alveolar edema, and hyaline membranes. Bronchiolar injury may also be present. RSV antigen and infectious virus are more abundant in the lungs of patients with interstitial pneumonia than with bronchiolitis.[154,155]

The pathogenesis of the bronchiolar lesions and of cellular injury by RSV in unclear. RSV does not shut off

host cell protein synthesis as do most cytopathic viruses. Yet, RSV-infected cells undergo fusion and suffer direct cytopathic injury in vitro and in vivo (see Fig. 12–14). Bronchiolitis results in part from the proclivity of the virus to infect small, easily obstructed bronchioles during the first year of life, in part from direct viral injury to respiratory epithelium, and partially because mucus accumulates in the absence of ciliary action.[156]

RSV bronchiolitis is associated with RSV-specific IgE that is bound to nasal epithelial cells, histamine, and fewer suppressor T lymphocytes.[157–159] These findings suggest that a component of the bronchiolar obstruction may be immunopathologic; IgE and histamine-mediated bronchospasm could result from a failure of the suppressor subset of T lymphocytes to limit IgE production. RSV-specific serum IgG_4 is detected at higher levels in bronchiolitis than in upper respiratory infection or pneumonia without wheezing and has been suggested as associated with hypersensitivity phenomena.[160] Leukotrienes may also play a role in the inflammatory events of RSV bronchiolitis.[161] An additional, age-dependent pathophysiologic factor is the presence of poor collateral ventilation in infant lungs, which favors atelectasis.

Acute complications of RSV infection include otitis media and bacterial superinfection, particularly by *Haemophilus influenzae*. Long-term sequelae in survivors apparently occur frequently as chronic disease of the airways. (See Bronchiectasis, Chapter 5.) Therapeutic approaches include ribavirin aerosol and intravenous neutralizing anti-RSV immunoglobulins, which may exert moderate ameliorating effects on viral replication and spread and the subsequent pathologic process.[162,163]

Parainfluenza Virus

Human parainfluenza viruses comprise the antigenically distinct types, 1, 2, 3, 4A, and 4B.[164] All types cause infections of the respiratory system; the attack rates and the frequency with which the lower respiratory tract is affected vary among the five serotypes. Parainfluenza viruses cause 8% of acute respiratory disease in hospitalized children.[165]

The clinical manifestations include upper respiratory infection, laryngotracheobronchitis (croup), bronchitis, bronchiolitis, and interstitial pneumonia. Parainfluenzavirus 3 accounts for the greatest portion of pneumonia, bronchiolitis, and bronchitis. Parainfluenzaviruses 1 and 2 are the major etiologic agents of croup. Signs and symptoms correlate with the anatomic location of the viral infection; they may include low-grade fever, rhinorrhea, hoarseness, cough, pharyngitis, stridor, rhonchi, wheezing, rales, and retractions.[166,167]

Transmission by person-to-person contact or large droplets requires only a small inoculum of this virus, which survives very poorly on environmental surfaces. After an incubation period of 2–6 days, infection of nasopharyngeal epithelium may be followed by spread to the pharynx, larynx, trachea, bronchi, bronchioles, and alveoli. Clinical, epidemiologic, and pathogenetic similarities with RSV infection are remarkable, except for the maximal occurrence of parainfluenzavirus bronchiolitis in 6- to 12-month-old children instead of at 1–3 months of age for RSV infection.[168]

Immunity to parainfluenza viruses is incomplete. Reinfections with both heterotypic and homotypic strains are frequent.[166] Definitive diagnosis of parainfluenzavirus infections requires cultivation of the virus or specific detection of viral antigens, for example, by demonstration of viral antigen in nasopharyngeal secretions, using immunofluorescence.[165,168,169] Serologic diagnosis is achieved by demonstration of a fourfold or greater rise in serum antibodies in hemagglutination inhibition, complement fixation, or neutralization tests. Heterotypic antibody responses occur often, however, and confound type-specific serologic diagnosis.

The morphology of virus-infected cells in vitro depends on the type of virus. Types 2 and 3 may cause cell fusion, multinucleated syncytial giant cells, and cell death. Some parainfluenzavirus strains cause no perceptible cytopathic effect; these strains are detected by demonstration that guinea pig erythrocytes adsorb to infected cells (hemadsorption). Neuraminic acid-containing receptors in the red blood cell membrane bind to the viral attachment protein that is inserted into the cell membrane of the infected cell. Fusion to multinucleated giant cells is mediated by the concerted effects of the viral F protein and the hemagglutinin-neuraminidase protein in the cell membrane and causes cell-to-cell spread of virus. Virus-infected cells contain cytoplasmic aggregates of viral nucleocapsids that may occur as inclusion bodies.

Human infection with parainfluenzavirus rarely results in the patient's death. The respiratory epithelium, particularly ciliated cells, is the target of the virus.[153,165,170] Viral antigen, which can be demonstrated by immunofluorescence in infected nasopharyngeal, tracheal, and bronchial epithelial cells, varies from cytoplasmic particles and poorly formed aggregates to large spherical or oval inclusions.[165,171]

Immunologically competent patients may manifest acute laryngotracheobronchitis without pulmonary parenchymal lesions (Fig. 12–17) or as bronchitis with epithelial hyperplasia, moderate hyperplasia of alveolar lining cells, and interstitial pneumonia.[153,165] Patients with T-lymphocyte deficiency who die after prolonged, progressive parainfluenzavirus infection have a different constellation of lesions. There is interstitial pneumonia, an exudative alveolar exudate, alveolar cell hyperplasia and hypertrophy, and interstitial fibrosis. The alveoli are lined by multinucleated giant cells, which may have cytoplasmic inclusions (Fig. 12–18).[142,172–174] This lesion can be differentiated from RSV infection only by immunologic or virologic identification of the etiologic agent.

Parainfluenza viruses do not shut off host cell protein synthesis[175] and are variably cytopathic. As in RSV bronchiolitis, the airways are hyperactive, and immunopathologic mechanisms appear to be important.[168,176] Virus-specific IgE appears in respiratory secretions earlier and in greater quantity in those patients who have parainfluenzavirus croup and bronchiolitis than in their counterparts who have infection of the upper airways. The amount of histamine in secretions is also greater in croup than in upper respiratory infection. There is a correlation between the severity of illness and

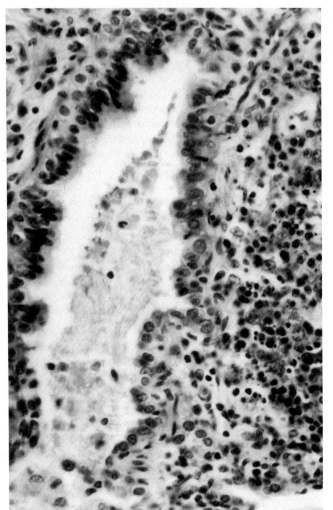

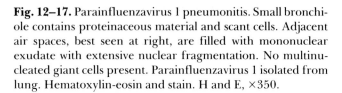

Fig. 12–17. Parainfluenzavirus 1 pneumonitis. Small bronchiole contains proteinaceous material and scant cells. Adjacent air spaces, best seen at right, are filled with mononuclear exudate with extensive nuclear fragmentation. No multinucleated giant cells present. Parainfluenzavirus 1 isolated from lung. Hematoxylin-eosin and stain. H and E, ×350.

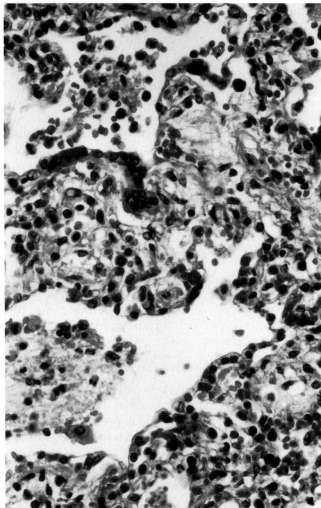

Fig. 12–18. Parainfluenzavirus 3 pneumonitis. Interstitium is edematous and heavily infiltrated by mononuclear cells. Alveoli contain fibrin, red cells, and mononuclear inflammatory cells. Several large multinucleated (syncytial) giant cells line alveolar membrane. Parainfluenzavirus 3 isolated from lung. H and E, ×300.

the maximum quantity of virus-specific IgE and histamine in nasopharyngeal secretions. It is possible that the persistent abnormalities after parainfluenzavirus-associated croup and bronchiolitis result from congenitally hyperreactive airways rather than from viral damage to the airways.

Varicella-Zoster Virus

Varicella pneumonia is a rare complication of a common disease. The annual incidence of chickenpox in the United States is 1,500 cases per 100,000 people. A history of the illness can be obtained from 70%–80% of young adults; 60%–90% of adults who do not remem-

ber the infection have antibodies to varicella-zoster virus.

In contrast, varicella pneumonia is a disease of adults and immunocompromised or newborn children. Pneumonia was diagnosed by chest radiograph in 18 (16%) of 110 previously healthy young men with chickenpox in one study and in 14% of adults in another series.[177-179] Patients who are over 19 years of age account for 90% of cases of varicella pneumonia. The severity of varicella in adults, including the frequent occurrence of pneumonia, may result from the large inoculum received from infected children. Children who have malignancies, primary or acquired immunodeficiency, or have been treated with corticosteroids or cytotoxic drugs have severe, widespread dissemination of the infection because cell-mediated immune mechanisms fail to restrict viral replication.

Although gestational chickenpox occurs in only 1 to 7 pregnancies per 10,000 pregnancies, the disease is often severe in infants who are infected in utero after their mothers develop chickenpox 5 days or less before delivery.[180,181] These babies acquire the viral infection, but do not have passively transferred antibodies from their mothers. The rash, which develops on the fifth to tenth day of life, is followed by cutaneous purpura and pneumonia. The mortality is 30%. When the vesicular rash appears in the mothers more than 5 days before delivery and antibodies to varicella-zoster virus (VZV) are presumably transferred to the infants, the rash develops in the infants before the fourth day of life and there are very few deaths.

Pregnancy itself is also a predisposing factor for varicella pneumonia,[182] and the mortality rate is 42%. A large proportion of immunocompromised patients also succumb to this infection. Even among immunocompetent patients with varicella pneumonia, however, the fatality rate is 10%.

After a mean incubation period of 14 days, a vesicular rash and mucosal lesions appear. Symptoms of pneumonia—cough, dyspnea, tachypnea, hemoptysis, and pleuritic chest pain—often begin abruptly 1–6 days later. The severity of pneumonia is usually out of proportion to the physical signs. Rhonchi and rales are detected in only 50%–60% of patients. Chest radiographs reveal a bilateral, nodular infiltrate that is often peribronchial and is more dense near the hilum. Cyanosis may occur, and death results from respiratory insufficiency.

It is unlikely that lung biopsy would be performed for varicella pneumonia because the diagnosis can usually be established on the epidemiologic basis of exposure to VZV and on the clinical appearance of the enanthem and the vesicular exanthem, which may appear in successive crops. When Tzanck preparations (scrapings of cells obtained from the base of a vesicle) are stained with H and E or by Giemsa or Papanicolau methods, multinucleated giant cells are diagnostic of either VZV or HSV infection. The nuclei appear glassy, and inclusions may be visible, especially when H and E or PAP stain have been used. The Tzanck smear from skin lesions of chickenpox and shingles is more sensitive than culture, whereas the reverse is true for herpes simplex vesicles.[183,184]

Virologic and microbiologic diagnostic methods have also been developed. A definitive diagnosis may be established by viral culture of vesicle fluid collected during the first 3 days of illness. Electron microscopy may demonstrate virions compatible with VZV and HSV, and antigen detection methods including gel diffusion, countercurrent immunoelectrophoresis, and direct immunofluorescence have been developed. Varicella-zoster virus is difficult to culture. Detection of viral antigen is a more sensitive diagnostic method than inoculation of cell cultures.[185]

A variety of serologic tests are available for documentation of VZV infection.[186] They are useful for determining the susceptibility of individuals who do not have a history of chickenpox in childhood. For the acute infection, they are all retrospective.

Cells that have been infected with VZV in vitro become refractile, then round, swell, and separate from one another before detaching from the surface of the flask. Multinucleate giant cells form. Eosinophilic intranuclear inclusions surrounded by a clear zone are observed if samples are exposed to a fixative that precipitates protein.[39] Ultrastructural examination of the nucleus reveals nucleocapsids with a dense central DNA core; the envelope is formed by budding through the nuclear membrane. Cytoplasmic virions are present in large membrane-bound vacuoles.

Cytopathology is similar in vivo. Cells swell and develop "balloon degeneration" necrosis with intranuclear inclusions. Giant cells with up to 30 nuclei often contain inclusion bodies.

The portal of entry of VZV is probably the upper respiratory tract, oropharynx, or conjunctiva, where initial replication precedes primary viremia. A second phase of viral replication then follows, possibly in the mononuclear phagocytic system, before a second viremia and clinical symptoms develop. Direct viral injury of capillary endothelium leads to thrombosis (Fig. 12–19), hemorrhage, and the spread of viral infection to cells in the adjacent tissue.

The pulmonary lesions of varicella pneumonia are multiple foci of hemorrhage and/or necrosis. They may be peribronchial, but more often appear as miliary parenchymal foci, suggesting hematogenous dissemination of virus (see Fig. 12–19). Interstitial pneumonia, including alveolar septal edema, mononuclear cell infiltration, and hyaline membranes may be present, especially adjacent to the necrotic foci. Bronchiolar exudates and even bronchial or pleural vesicles have been described. In the lungs, virally infected cells with intranuclear inclusions may be found in capillary endothelium, interstitial connective tissue, tracheobronchial mucosal epithelium, and alveolar epithelium. The intranuclear inclusions of varicella-zoster virus should be sought in viable cells at the edges of necrotic lesions. They are considerably more difficult to find than are the inclusions of herpes simplex infection. A case of neonatal VZV infection has been described as yet another form of giant cell pneumonia.[187]

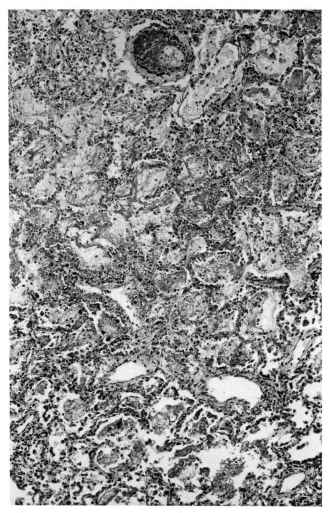

Fig. 12–19. Varicella-zoster pneumonitis. Edge of miliary, necrotic focus. At top, pulmonary arteriole contains fibrin thrombus; air spaces are necrotic. In center, alveoli contain red blood cells, abundant fibrin, and scattered inflammatory cells. At bottom, inflammation becomes less intense at edge of lesion, although no alveolus in this photomicrograph is normal. H and E, ×150.

Complications and sequelae of varicella pneumonia include secondary bacterial pneumonia, pulmonary fibrosis, diffusion abnormalities, and diffuse nodular pulmonary calcifications.[188] Treatment with acyclovir appears to ameliorate the disease.[189]

Because VZV is narrowly species specific and because simian varicella-like viruses produce infections quite different from human chickenpox, experimental elucidation of VZV pathogenesis has been difficult.

Cytomegalovirus

Human cytomegalovirus (CMV), probably the virus with the most spectacular cytopathology in the human lung, provides some of the thorniest of virologic prob-

lems in the immunocompromised host. The prevalence of infection by CMV is very high. It is difficult to establish CMV as the cause of pneumonia in the individual living patient because many CMV infections are asymptomatic. Isolation of the virus or even demonstration of viral inclusions in pulmonary cells does not establish unequivocally that CMV is responsible for clinical symptoms, because these same observations may also be made in asymptomatic infections.

Cytomegalovirus infection can be serious and even fatal. Unfortunately, there is as yet no effective antiviral chemotherapy. The severity of CMV infection depends upon the maturity and integrity of defense mechanisms, including the immune system of the host. There is increased risk of severe disease in congenitally and neonatally infected infants and in patients of all ages who are immunocompromised or are undergoing a primary infection. CMV may be transmitted transplacentally, by cervical secretions intrapartum, by aerosol droplets, by transfusion of blood or transplantation of kidney, bone marrow, liver, lung, or heart, and by contact with semen, cervical secretions, and breast milk.[190] Moreover, endogenous virus may be the source of recurrent infection, because CMV causes latent infections that may become reactivated. Reinfection with a second strain of CMV has also been observed.[191]

Congenital CMV infection occurs in 1% of infants, of whom only 5% are symptomatic.[192] Severe disease is usually characterized by jaundice, hepatosplenomegaly, thrombocytopenia, purpura, growth retardation, and less frequently by microcephaly, periventricular cerebral calcifications, chorioretinitis, optic atrophy, psychomotor retardation, and sensorineural hearing loss. Congenital CMV infection is more often severe when it is associated with primary maternal infection.[181]

Fewer than 1% of patients who are congenitally infected with CMV have pneumonia, which is incidental to widespread dissemination of virus.[193] Neonatal CMV infection is acquired from maternal cervical secretions, blood transfusion, or breast milk; although neonatal infection is usually asymptomatic, protracted pneumonia may develop.[194,195] The clinical signs—paroxysmal cough, tachypnea, intercostal retractions, rales, and bilateral pulmonary infiltrates with air-trapping—are indistinguishable from pneumonia caused by *Chlamydia trachomatis* or *Pneumocystis carinii*.[196] In fact, mixed infections of CMV and these agents occur often and are more severe than infections caused by CMV alone. Neonatal CMV pneumonia usually resolves, but virus may replicate to high titer (10^5–10^7 plaque-forming units/g) and fatal disease may result.[197,198]

CMV infection is virtually universal early in life in developing countries. In the United States 50%–90% of adults have antibodies to this virus. Infection in older children and adults is usually asymptomatic, but it is associated with an infectious mononucleosis syndrome without heterophil antibodies, particularly in patients older than 30 years of age who have received moderate-to-massive amounts of transfused blood.[199,200] Fresh donor blood may contain CMV in leukocytes. The virus may be reactivated by allogeneic interaction with histoincompatible recipient cells. Pneumonia has been observed in 6% of patients with the CMV infectious mononucleosis syndrome.

Immunocompromised patients are at greater risk for CMV pneumonia, particularly those who have the acquired immunodeficiency syndrome (AIDS) or who have received transplanted allogeneic organs or bone marrow. Nearly one-third of renal transplant patients who are treated with prednisone, cytotoxic drugs, and/or antithymocyte serum develop fever 1–3 months after transplantation. An average of 15 days later respiratory symptoms develop in 42% of these patients; these are nonproductive cough, tachypnea, dyspnea, and hypoxemia. Radiographic infiltrates usually begin as bilateral, peripheral, and basilar shadows, then spread centrally and superiorly.[201–204]

Fatalities supervene in 20% of renal transplant patients who have CMV infection, usually in those with diffuse pulmonary infiltrates and superinfection by bacteria, fungi, or P. carinii. Cell-mediated immunity, particularly cytotoxic T lymphocytes and natural killer cells, is an important host defense against CMV.[204] CMV-infected patients who are treated with high-dosage, intravenous methylprednisolone often have reduced cytotoxic T-cell activity, prolonged viremia, and a fatal outcome despite the presence of antibody to CMV before transplantation. Risk factors for overt disease in transplant patients include male sex, diabetes mellitus, transplanted kidney from parent, cadaver, nonsibling, or non-HLA identical sibling, and a donor seropositive for CMV antibodies.

The major complication of allogeneic bone marrow transplantation is pneumonia, which develops in 41% of patients.[205] The most frequently identified etiologic agent is CMV, which causes pneumonia in 16% of bone marrow recipients; the mortality rate in this population is 91%. Graft-versus-host disease, an important complication of bone marrow transplantation, is associated with an increased incidence of CMV pneumonia.

Patients with human immunodeficiency virus (HIV) infection who have AIDS are among the most immunosuppressed of patients. Almost all of these individuals develop CMV disease, often including pneumonia, at some time during their course.[206]

Lung biopsies in which CMV might be found come from immunocompromised patients with progressive pneumonia in whom the diagnosis has not been established by microbiologic and cytologic examination of respiratory specimens or by serology and in whom there has been no response to empiric therapy directed against P. carinii and common bacterial pathogens.

Virologic and immunologic methods may establish a diagnosis of CMV infection; however, they are less effective in establishing the diagnosis of CMV pneumonia. CMV infection is diagnosed by isolation of virus from urine and, less frequently, from saliva, vaginal and cervical secretions, blood, milk, semen, tears, stool, respiratory secretions, and tissue. As has been mentioned above, however, viral excretion occurs in many asymptomatic subjects so that association of an isolated virus with a pathophysiologic process may be problematic. Isolation of CMV from blood leukocytes is less sensitive than from urine, but it indicates that there is active CMV disease.[207]

There are numerous pitfalls in the interpretation of CMV serologic data. The presence of antibodies to CMV indicates only past and possibly latent infection. Transplacental transfer of IgG assures that the majority of infants have antibodies to CMV at birth even if they are not infected. Immunosuppressed patients may not mount a detectable antibody response to CMV, even in fatal cases. Transfusion with seropositive blood can lead to the appearance of passive antibodies.

A variety of serologic assays have been developed. The complement fixation test, which is not useful in the 10% of sera that are anticomplementary, is relatively insensitive. The sensitive indirect fluorescent antibody assay and even more sensitive anticomplement immunofluorescence technique are cumbersome and require a fluorescence microscope. Passive hemagglutination, enzyme immunoassay, latex agglutination, and automated fluorescence (FIAX), which are sensitive, are suitable for screening purposes. Immune adherence hemagglutination has also been used.[192,208–210]

The appearance of Fc receptors for IgG in infected cells that are employed as CMV antigens can cause problems in the indirect immunofluorescence test unless isolated nuclei are used. Assay of IgM by the indirect fluorescent antibody test is only 50% sensitive and yields false-positive results when rheumatoid factor is present. Griffiths and colleagues[211] developed a radioimmunoassay that was able to distinguish accurately primary from secondary infections in pregnant women; false-positives were found in 19 of 104 (18%) of the women when the sera were tested by indirect immunofluorescence. However, radioimmunoassay is not well suited to routine laboratory use. Enzyme immunoassays for antibody to IgM have performed in a manner similar to radioimmunoassay.[212] However, even the demonstration of IgM is not absolute assurance that the infection is primary.[213]

The diagnosis of CMV pneumonia is usually made on clinical grounds, as when there is prolonged unexplained fever followed by radiographic pulmonary infiltrates in the proper clinical setting. If there is a fourfold or greater increase in antibody titer or if CMV is isolated from secretions, the likelihood of an active infection is increased.

When a lung biopsy is obtained, viral cultures are more sensitive than histologic examination of tissue.[46,214–216] Likewise, cytologic diagnosis of CMV infection on bronchoalveolar lavage specimens is less sensitive than viral cultures. However, because viral cultures may be positive for CMV in the absence of pneumonia, cytopathologic diagnosis is, in fact, more specific. Two newer methods are immunofluorescent detection of CMV antigens and detection of CMV DNA by in situ hybridization, both of which appear comparable in sensitivity to viral culture.[57,215,217–225] When utilized effectively, the timeliness of immunofluorescence (1.5–4 h) and DNA hybridization (1–2 days) will offer advantages over viral cultures. The virologists have also made progress in the diagnosis of this infection, however. Most isolates of CMV can be detected in less than 48 h when the inoculum is centrifuged onto a monolayer of susceptible fibroblasts, which are incubated for 16 h before testing by immunofluorescence for the presence of CMV antigen in the monolayer.[29]

CMV-infected cells were described first in 1904 by Jesionek and Kiolemenoglou[226] as large protozoan-like cells. In 1921 Goodpasture and Talbot[227] reported a 2-month-old child with the same large cells, which they recognized as altered host cells. They described enlarged cells (10- to 30-µm diameter) that had large nuclei, large oval intranuclear inclusion bodies, and basophilic cytoplasmic inclusions. They suggested that these cells were spread hematogenously, and proposed the term cytomegalia for the cellular enlargement.

In 1932 Farber and Wolbach[228] described cytomegalic intranuclear and cytoplasmic inclusions in the submaxillary salivary glands of 12% of 183 infants. They pointed out the similarity of the inclusions to those found in diseases caused by filterable viruses. Cole and Kuttner[229] had already demonstrated that the cytomegalic lesions found in guinea pig salivary glands were caused by a filterable virus. Smith first successfully propagated a cytomegalovirus by serially transmitting murine CMV in mouse fibroblasts. Shortly thereafter, human CMV was isolated concurrently and independently in three laboratories.[230–232]

CMV replicates in the nucleus, where assembly into typical herpesvirus nucleocapsids occurs, corresponding to the Feulgen-stained polymerized DNA in the intranuclear inclusion.[228] The viral envelope is acquired by budding through the nuclear envelope (Fig. 12–20). Noninfectious enveloped particles contain the capsid assembly protein without viral DNA.[233] In Giemsa-stained touch preparations of lung biopsies, the cytomegalic cells measure up to 40 µm in diameter. Cellular enlargement may be related to virus-induced depolymerization of microtubules, secondary to the influx of calcium ions and breakdown of intermediate filaments.[234]

Viral inclusions are present both in the nucleus and in the cytoplasm. Intranuclear inclusions measure up to 20 µm in diameter and cytoplasmic inclusions are 1–3 µm in size.[206] In sections that have been stained with hematoxylin and eosin, the early forms of the intranuclear inclusions resemble those of herpes simplex and varicella-zoster viruses. The mature inclusions are densely stained and vary from eosinophilic to deeply basophilic (Fig. 12–20). The inclusions are usually surrounded by an artefactual halo in formalin-fixed tissue. The marginated chromatin is uniformly compressed but not beaded. A prominent, single rounded clump of peripheral chromatin is often seen protruding into the otherwise clear halo zone. This probably represents a remnant nucleolus and is characteristic of CMV.[39] Cytoplasmic inclusions appear after the intranuclear inclusions are well developed; they are not found in all cells that have intranuclear inclusions. Ganciclovir, an inhibitor of CMV DNA synthesis, has been described to alter the appearance of the CMV intranuclear inclusions which become globular and eosinophilic because of the loss of viral DNA.[235]

The cytoplasmic inclusions, which are rounded, granular, and slightly basophilic, are stained by the periodic acid–Schiff and Gomori methenamine silver procedures, but the intranuclear inclusions are not.[236] Whereas the Feulgen-positive intranuclear inclusions contain viral nucleoprotein and assembled capsids, the cytoplasmic inclusions appear to be of varied nature.[237] Some are composed of cellular elements, such as accumulations of endoplasmic reticulum, vesicles, dense bodies, mitochondria, and lysosomes; some are composed almost entirely of virions;[236] and others are a mixture of virions and cellular elements.

Hybridization with three cloned, biotinylated DNA segments that represented 56% of the CMV genomic DNA demonstrated that CMV-infected cells were not necessarily cytomegalic, nor did they always contain inclusions.[220] In fact, morphologically normal cells including fibroblasts were also virally infected. By immunofluorescence, CMV antigens are present in cells of the alveolar lining and lumen and in the endothelium. Both intranuclear and cytoplasmic inclusions contain viral antigens.[220,238]

Three different histopathological patterns have been described in the lungs of patients with CMV.[17,211,220,239] Cytomegalic cells may be found in the alveolar epithelium with minimal evidence of inflammation and injury (Fig. 12–21). Alternatively, there

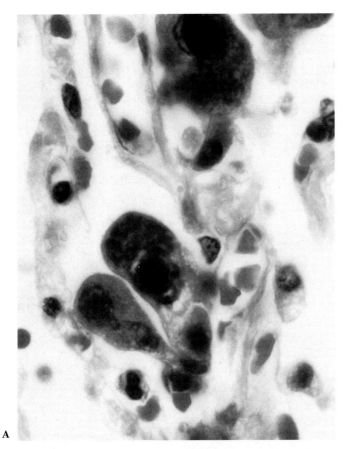

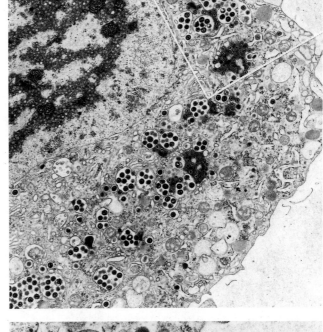

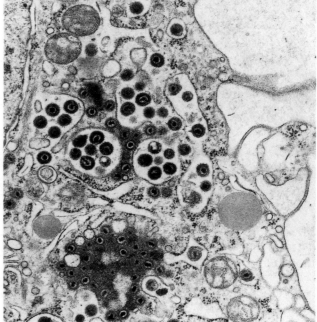

Fig. 12–20 A–C. Cytomegalovirus pneumonitis. **A.** High power: three inclusion-bearing cells are typically enlarged, containing basophilic intranuclear inclusions separated from nuclear membrane by clear space. **B,C.** Irregular, aggregated cytoplasmic inclusions are most discrete in center. Such characteristic cells are pathognomonic of cytomegalovirus infection. Cytomegalovirus isolated from lung on culture. H and E, ×750. **B.** Cytomegalovirus is seen replicating in nucleus (naked virions) and receiving coat (nucleocapsid) in cytoplasm. TEM, ×6,300. **C.** Higher power of marked area from **B.** TEM, 16,000. (**B** and **C** provided courtesy of D. Bockus, F. Remington, and S. Friedman, Mason Clinic, Electron Microscopy Laboratory, Seattle, Washington.)

may be miliary, multifocal lesions that contain cytomegalic inclusion cells. In these focal lesions the pulmonary architecture is obliterated by an exudative inflammatory response in the interstitium and in the air spaces. There may be central necrosis, hemorrhage, and an accumulation of fibrin, mononuclear cells, and neutrophils (Fig. 12–22). The third pattern is a diffuse interstitial pneumonia with lymphocytes, macrophages, and plasma cells. An exudative reaction is characterized by edema in the interstitium, serofibrinous exudates in

the alveolar spaces, and alveolar cell hyperplasia (Fig. 12–23). Hyaline membranes may be present, but are not frequent or widespread. Cytomegalic cells are scattered diffusely through the parenchyma of the lung. The miliary pattern is believed to represent hematogenous spread of virus infection to the lungs, after which slow centrifugal spread of this highly cell-associated virus produces focal lesions, just as occurs in cell monolayers.

CMV is a relatively nonvirulent virus, and infection

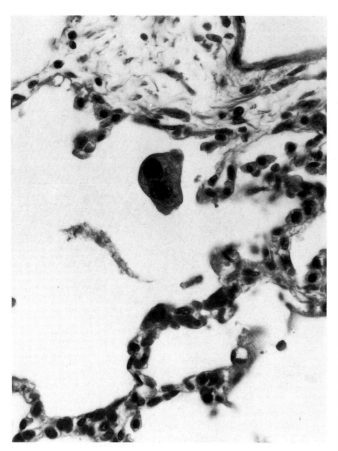

Fig. 12–21. Cytomegalovirus infection. Single inclusion-bearing cell present in air space is binucleate, an unusual finding in cytomegalovirus infection. Intranuclear inclusions present in both nuclei but cytoplasmic inclusions are absent. Minimal evidence of host reactivity: a wisp of proteinaceous material in airspace and slight increase in prominence of respiratory epithelial cells. Cytomegalovirus isolated from lung. H and E, ×300.

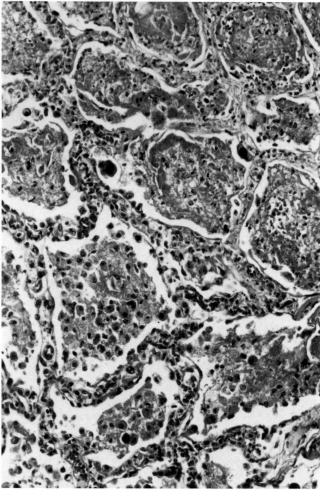

Fig. 12–22. Cytomegalovirus pneumonitis. Edge of nodular lesion depicted. Necrotic center of nodule, surrounded by damaged air spaces, is at top where alveoli are filled with coagulum of fibrin, inflammatory cells, and nuclear debris. Interstitium is edematous and contains sparse mononuclear exudate. Two large cells have dense intranuclear inclusions. Toward edge of nodule of inflammation (bottom), air spaces contain less dense collections of fibrin and mononuclear cells. Cytomegalovirus isolated from lung. H and E, ×150.

depends on defective defenses of the immunocompromised or immature host.[240–242] In vitro the virus has a relatively slow replicative cycle that produces slowly progressive lytic foci. Defective interfering particles are formed, and latent infection is established readily. In addition to direct virus-induced cytopathic effect, CMV-infected cells may be lysed by cytotoxic T lymphocytes and natural killer cells. Other possible immunopathologic mediators of tissue damage are circulating immune complexes, which are detectable in 45% of neonatal and congenital CMV cases. In some instances, deposits of IgG without CMV antigens have been observed in glomerular basement membrane.[243] Animal models of CMV must be interpreted cautiously, because cytomegaloviruses, including human CMV, have a narrow host range. In fact, human CMV shares less than 5% of its DNA with murine CMV and simian CMV.

Thus, human CMV is no more closely related to these agents than to the two serotypes of herpes simplex virus.

Primary CMV pneumonia may be fatal in its own right. In addition, this infection may be complicated by fatal bacterial, fungal, and protozoal infection. There is a close association of infection by CMV and the protozoan parasite *Pneumocystis carinii*. CMV pneumonia may resolve completely or may organize, leaving multifocal pulmonary scars.[244] Treatment with ganciclovir, foscarnet, and intravenous human immunoglobulin ameliorates the course of illness in some patients whose

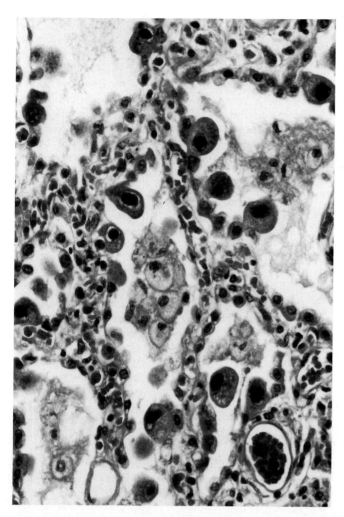

Fig. 12–23. Cytomegalovirus pneumonitis. Interstitium is edematous and contains sparse mononuclear cells. Alveolar epithelium is hyperplastic and air spaces contain macrophages and fibrin. Multiple enlarged cells contain both intranuclear and cytoplastic inclusions. Cytomegalovirus isolated from lung. H and E, ×300.

immunosuppression is transient. Severely immunocompromised patients often relapse and die despite a temporary antiviral effect.[245]

Other Viruses

Many other viruses replicate and cause disease in the upper respiratory tract. On rare occasions they may also infect the lower respiratory system, particularly in infants and children. The details of the pathologic changes are scant; for the most part the brief descriptions suggest nonspecific pulmonary damage or interstitial pneumonitis without any unique features. When the viruses produce latent infections, such as Epstein–Barr virus, or when they are frequently isolated from respiratory secretions in the absence of disease, as are enteroviruses, it may be difficult even to document the association with absolute certainty. Such viruses include rhinovirus,[246] an important etiologic agent of the common cold, Epstein–Barr virus,[247] a major cause of infectious mononucleosis, and enteroviruses,[248] which produce systemic disease, especially of the cardiac and central nervous systems.

References

1. Anderson LJ, Patriarca PA, Hierholzer JC, Noble GR. Viral respiratory illnesses. Med Clin North Am 1983; 67:1009–1030.

2. Brown RS, Nogrady MB, Spence L, Wiglesworth FW. An outbreak of adenovirus type 7 infection in children in Montreal. Can Med Assoc J 1973;108:434–439.

3. Becroft DMO. Histopathology of fatal adenovirus infection of the respiratory tract in young children. J Clin Pathol 1967;20:561–569.

4. Ferris JAJ, Aherne WA, Locke WS, McQuillin J, Gardner PS. Sudden and unexpected deaths in infants: Histology and virology. Br Med J 1973;2:439–442.

5. Hall WJ, Hall CB, Speers DM. Respiratory syncytial virus infection in adults. Clinical, virologic, and serial pulmonary function studies. Ann Intern Med 1978; 88:203–205.

6. Spelman DW, Stanley PA. Respiratory syncytial virus pneumonitis in adults. Med J Aust 1983;1:430–431.

7. Fry J. Influenza, 1959: The story of an epidemic. Br Med J 1959;2:135–138.

8. Case records of the Massachusetts General Hospital. Weekly clinicopathological exercises. Case 6–1979. N Engl J Med 1979;300:301–309.

9. Clinicopathologic Conference on adult respiratory distress syndrome. Am J Med 1971;50:521–529.

10. Martin CM, Kunin CM, Gottlieb LS, Barnes MW, Liu C, Finland M. Asian influenza A in Boston, 1957–1958. Arch Intern Med 1959;103:515–542.

11. Williams DM, Krick JA, Remington JS. State of the art: Pulmonary infection in the compromised host. Part II. Am Rev Respir Dis 1976;114:593–627.

12. Graham BS, Snell JD, Jr. Herpes simplex virus infection of the adult lower respiratory tract. Medicine (Baltimore) 1983;62:384–393.

13. Beckford AP, Kaschula ROC, Stephen C. Factors associated with fatal cases of measles. A retrospective autopsy study. S Afr Med J 1985;68:858–863.

14. Nash G. Necrotizing tracheobronchitis and bronchopneumonia consistent with herpetic infection. Hum Pathol 1972;3:283–291.

15. Winn WC Jr, Myerowitz RL. The pathology of the *Legionella* pneumonias. A review of 74 cases and the literature. Hum Pathol 1981;12:401–422.

16. Katzenstein AL, Askin FB. Surgical pathology of nonneoplastic lung disease. Philadelphia: WB Saunders, 1982.

17. Beschorner WE, Hutchins GM, Burns WH, Saral R, Tutschka PJ, Santos GW. Cytomegalovirus pneumonia in bone marrow transplant recipients: Miliary and diffuse patterns. Am Rev Respir Dis 1980;122:107–114.

18. Conte P, Heitzman ER, Markarian B. Viral pneumonia. Roentgen pathological correlations. Radiology 1970; 95:267–272.

19. Balows A, Hausler WJ Jr, Herrmann KL, Isenberg HD, Shadomy HJ, eds. Manual of clinical microbiology, 5th Ed. Washington, DC: American Society for Microbiology, 1991.

20. Lennette EH, Schmidt NJ, eds. Diagnostic procedures for viral, rickettsial and chlamydial infections. 5th ed. Washington, DC. American Public Health Association, 1979.

21. Hsiung GD. Diagnostic virology illustrated by light and electron microscopy. 3d Ed. New Haven: Yale University Press, 1982.

22. Fields BN, Knipe DM, Chanock RM, Hirsch MS, Melnick JL, Monath TP, Roizman B, eds. Virology. 2nd Ed. New York: Raven, 1990.

23. Smith TF. Diagnostic virology in the community hospital. Extent and options. Postgrad Med 1984;75:215–223.

24. Hall CB, Douglas RG, Jr. Clinically useful method for the isolation of respiratory syncytial virus. J Infect Dis 1975;131:1–5.

25. Bromberg K, Daidone B, Clarke L, Sierra MF. Comparison of immediate and delayed inoculation of HEp-2 cells for isolation of respiratory syncytial virus. J Clin Microbiol 1984;20:123–124.

26. Treuhaft MW, Soukup JM, Sullivan BJ. Practical recommendations for the detection of pediatric respiratory syncytial virus infections. J Clin Microbiol 1985;22:270–273.

27. Ray CG, Minnich LL. Regional diagnostic virology services. Are satellite laboratories necessary? JAMA 1982;247:1309–1310.

28. McIntosh K. Diagnostic virology. In: Fields BN, Knipe DM, Chenock RM, Hirsch MS, Melnick JL, Monath TP, Roizman B, eds. Virology. 2nd Ed. New York: Raven, 1990:414.

29. Gleaves CA, Smith TF, Shuster EA, Pearson GR. Comparison of standard tube and shell vial cell culture techniques for the detection of cytomegalovirus in clinical specimens. J Clin Microbiol 1985;21:217–221.

30. Gleaves CA, Wilson DJ, Wold AD, Smith TF. Detection and serotyping of herpes simplex virus in MRC-5 cells by use of centrifugation and monoclonal antibodies 16 h postinoculation. J Clin Microbiol 1985;21:29–32.

31. Smith MC, Creutz C, Huang YT. Detection of respiratory syncytial virus in nasopharyngeal secretions by shell vial technique. J Clin Microbiol 1991;29:463–465.

32. Pothier P, Nicolas JC, de Saint Maur GP, Ghim S, Kazmierczak A, Bricout F. Monoclonal antibodies against respiratory syncytial virus and their use for rapid detection of virus in nasopharyngeal secretions. J Clin Microbiol 1985;21:286–287.

33. Lauer BA, Masters HA, Wren CG, Levin MJ. Rapid detection of respiratory syncytial virus in nasopharyngeal secretions by enzyme-linked immunosorbent assay. J Clin Microbiol 1985;22:782–785.

34. Grandien M, Pettersson CA, Gardner PS, Linde A, Stanton A. Rapid viral diagnosis of acute respiratory infections: comparison of enzyme-linked immunosorbent assay and the immunofluorescence technique for detection of viral antigens in nasopharyngeal secretions. J Clin Microbiol 1985;22:757–760.

35. Ahluwalia GS, Hammond GW. Comparison of cell culture and three enzyme-linked immunosorbent assays for the rapid diagnosis of respiratory syncytial virus from nasopharyngeal aspirate and tracheal secretion specimens. Diagn Microbiol Infect Dis 1988;9:187–192.

36. Smith DW, Frankel LR, Mathers LH, Tang ATS, Ariagno RL, Prober CG. A controlled trial of aerosolized ribavirin in infants receiving mechanical ventilation for severe respiratory syncytial virus infection. N Engl J Med 1991;325:24–29.

37. Blanding JG, Hoshiko MG, Stutman HR. Routine viral culture for pediatric respiratory specimens submitted for direct immunofluorescence testing. J Clin Microbiol 1989;27:1438–1440.

38. Tristram DA, Miller RW, McMillan JA, Weiner LB. Simultaneous infection with respiratory syncytial virus and other respiratory pathogens. Am J Dis Child 1988; 142:834–836.

39. Strano AJ. Light microscopy of selected viral diseases (morphology of viral inclusion bodies). Pathol Annu 1976;11:53–75.

40. Naib ZM, Stewart JA, Dowdle WR, Casey HL, Marine WM, Nahmias AJ. Cytological features of viral respiratory tract infections. Acta Cytol (Baltimore) 1968; 12:162–171.

41. Johnston WW, Frable WJ. The cytopathology of the respiratory tract. A review. Am J Pathol 1976;84:372–424.

42. Carson JL, Collier AM, Hu SS. Acquired ciliary defects in nasal epithelium of children with acute viral upper respiratory infections. N Engl J Med 1985;312:463–468.

43. Pierce CH, Knox AW. Ciliocytophthoria in sputum from patients with adenovirus infections. Proc Soc Exp Biol Med 1960;104:492–495.

44. Almeida JD. Uses and abuses of diagnostic electron microscopy. Curr Top Microbiol Immunol 1983;104: 147–158.

45. Wang NS. Applications of electron microscopy to diagnostic pulmonary pathology. Hum Pathol 1983;14:888–900.

46. Gleaves CA, Smith TF, Wold AD, Wilson WR. Detection of viral and chlamydial antigens in open-lung biopsy specimens. Am J Clin Pathol 1985;83:371–374.

47. Pinkerton H, Carroll S. Fatal adenovirus pneumonia in infants. Correlation of histologic and electron microscopic observations. Am J Pathol 1971;65:543–548.

48. Yolken RH. Use of monoclonal antibodies for viral diagnosis. Curr Top Microbiol Immunol 1983;104:177–195.

49. Kao CL, McIntosh K, Fernie B, Talis A, Pierik L,

Anderson L. Monoclonal antibodies for the rapid diagnosis of respiratory syncytial virus infection by immunofluorescence. Diagn Microbiol Infect Dis 1984;2:199–206.

50. Stout C, Murphy MD, Lawrence S, Julian S. Evaluation of a monoclonal antibody pool for rapid diagnosis of respiratory viral infections. J Clin Microbiol 1989; 27:448–452.

51. Kim HW, Wyatt RG, Fernie BF, et al. Respiratory syncytial virus detection by immunofluorescence in nasal secretions with monoclonal antibodies against selected surface and internal proteins. J Clin Microbiol 1983;18:1399–1404.

52. Anestad G, Breivik N, Thoresen T. Rapid diagnosis of respiratory syncytial virus and influenza A virus infections by immunofluorescence: Experience with a simplified procedure for the preparation of cell smears from nasopharyngeal secretions. Acta Pathol Microbiol Immunol Scand [B] 1983;91:267–271.

53. Taber LH, Knight V, Gilbert BE, et al. Ribavirin aerosol treatment of bronchiolitis associated with respiratory syncytial virus in infants. Pediatrics 1983;72:613–618.

54. Hall CB, McBride JT, Walsh EE, et al. Aerosolized ribavirin treatment of infants with respiratory syncytial viral infection. A randomized double-blind study. N Engl J Med 1983;308:1443–1447.

55. Hirsch MS, Schooley RT. Treatment of herpesvirus infections. N Engl J Med 1983;309:963–970,1034–1039.

56. Edberg SC. Principles of nucleic acid hybridization and comparison with monoclonal antibody technology for the diagnosis of infectious diseases. Yale J Biol Med 1985;58:425–442.

57. Spector SA, Rua JA, Spector DH, McMillan R. Detection of human cytomegalovirus in clinical specimens by DNA-DNA hybridization. J Infect Dis 1984;150:121–126.

58. Virtanen M, Palva A, Laaksonen M, Halonen P, Soderlund H, Ranki M. Novel test for rapid viral diagnosis: detection of adenovirus in nasopharyngeal mucus aspirates by means of nucleic-acid sandwich hybridization. Lancet 1983;i:381–383.

59. Redfield DC, Richman DD, Albanil S, Oxman MN, Wahl GM. Detection of herpes simplex virus in clinical specimens by DNA hybridization. Diagn Microbiol Infect Dis 1983;1:117–128.

60. Chou S, Merigan TC. Rapid detection and quantitation of human cytomegalovirus in urine through DNA hybridization. N Engl J Med 1983;308:921–925.

61. Palva A, Ranki M. Microbial diagnosis by nucleic acid sandwich hybridization. Clin Lab Med 1985;5:475–490.

62. Jansen RW, Newbold JE, Lemon SM. Combined immunoaffinity cDNA-RNA hybridization assay for detection of hepatitis A virus in clinical specimens. J Clin Microbiol 1985;22:984–989.

63. Myerson D, Hackman RC, Meyers JD. Diagnosis of cytomegaloviral pneumonia by in situ hybridization. J Infect Dis 1984;150:272–277.

64. Unger ER, Budgeon LR, Myerson D, Brigati DJ. Viral diagnosis by in situ hybridization. Description of a rapid simplified colorimetric method. Am J Surg Pathol 1986;10:1–8.

65. Hondo R, Kurata T, Sato S, Oda A, Aoyama Y. Enzymatic treatment of formalin-fixed and paraffin-embedded specimens for detection of antigens of herpes simplex, varicella-zoster and human cytomegaloviruses. Jpn J Exp Med 1982;52:17–25.

66. Chandler FW, Gorelkin L. Immunofluorescence staining of adenovirus in fixed tissues pretreated with trypsin. J Clin Microbiol 1983;17:371–373.

67. Murphy FA, Kingsbury DW. Virus taxonomy. In: Fields BN, Knipe DM, Chanock RM, Hirsch MS, Melnick JL, Monath TP, Roizman B, Eds. Virology. 2nd Ed. New York: Raven, 1990:9–35.

68. Murphy BR, Webster RG. Orthomyxoviruses. In: Fields BN, Knipe DM, Chanock RM, Hirsch MS, Melnick JL, Monath TP, Roizman B, Eds. Virology. 2nd Ed. New York: Raven, 1990:1091–1152.

69. Dowdle WR, Coleman MT, Gregg MB. Natural history of influenza type A in the United States, 1957–1972. Prog Med Virol 1974;17:91–135.

70. Shope RE. The infection of ferrets with swine influenza virus. J Exp Med 1934;60:49–61.

71. Raut S, Hurd J, Cureton RJ, Blandford G, Heath RB. The pathogenesis of infections of the mouse caused by virulent and avirulent variants of an influenza virus. J Med Microbiol 1975;8:127–136.

72. Rodgers B, Mims CA. Interaction of influenza virus with mouse macrophages. Infect Immun 1981;31:751–757.

73. Louria DB, Blumenfeld HL, Ellis JT, Kilbourne ED, Rogers DE. Studies on influenza in the pandemic of 1957–1958. II. Pulmonary complications of influenza. J Clin Invest 1959;38:213–265.

74. Hers JF, Masurel N, Mulder J. Bacteriology and histopathology of the respiratory tract and lungs in fatal Asian influenza. Lancet 1958;ii:1141–1143.

75. Hall CB, Douglas RG, Jr. Nosocomial influenza infection as a cause of intercurrent fevers in infants. Pediatrics 1975;55:673–677.

76. Camner P, Jarstrand C, Philipson K. Tracheobronchial clearance in patients with influenza. Am Rev Respir Dis 1973;108:131–135.

77. Abramson JS, Giebink GS, Quie PG. Influenza A virus-induced polymorphonuclear leukocyte dysfunction in the pathogenesis of experimental pneumococcal otitis media. Infect Immun 1982;36:289–296.

78. Jakab GJ. Immune impairment of alveolar macrophage phagocytosis during influenza virus pneumonia. Am Rev Respir Dis 1982;126:778–782.

79. Larson HE, Blades R. Impairment of human polymorphonuclear leukocyte function by influenza virus. Lancet 1976;i:283.

80. Soto PJ, Jr, Broun GO, Wyatt JP. Asian influenzal pneumonitis. A structural and virologic analysis. Am J Med 1959;27:18–25.

81. Oseasohn R, Adelson L, Kaji M. Clinicopathologic study of thirty-three fatal cases of Asian influenza. N Engl J Med 1959;260:509–518.

82. Feldman PS, Cohan MA, Hierholzer WJ, Jr. Fatal Hong Kong influenza: A clinical, microbiological and pathological analysis of nine cases. Yale J Biol Med 1972;45:49–63.

83. Hers JFP, Mulder J. Changes in the respiratory mucosa resulting from infection with influenza virus B. J Pathol Bacteriol 1957;73:565–568.

84. Winternitz MC, Watson IM, McNamara FP. The pathology of influenza. New Haven: Yale University Press 1920.

85. Walsh JJ, Dietlein LF, Low FN, Burch GE, Mogabgab WJ. Bronchotracheal response in human influenza: Type A, Asian strain, as studied by light and electron microscopic examination of bronchoscopic biopsies. Arch Intern Med 1961;108:376–388.

86. Noble RL, Lillington GA, Kempson RL. Fatal diffuse influenzal pneumonia: Premortem diagnosis by lung biopsy. Chest 1973;63:644–646.

87. Pinsker KL, Schneyer B, Becker N, Kamholz SL. Usual interstitial pneumonia following Texas A2 influenza infection. Chest 1981;80:123–126.

88. Joshi VV, Escobar MR, Stewart L, Bates RD. Fatal influenza A_2 viral pneumonia in a newborn infant. Am J Dis Child 1973;126:839–840.

89. Finckh ES, Bader L. Pulmonary damage from Hong Kong influenza. Aust NZ J Med 1974;4:16–22.

90. Engblom E, Ekfors TO, Meurman OH, Toivanen A, Nikoskelainen J. Fatal influenza A myocarditis with isolation of virus from the myocardium. Acta Med Scand 1983;213:75–78.

91. Tamura H, Aronson BE. Intranuclear fibrillary inclusions in influenza pneumonia. Arch Pathol Lab Med 1978;102:252–257.

92. Johanson WG, Jr, Pierce AK, Sanford JP. Pulmonary function in uncomplicated influenza. Am Rev Respir Dis 1969;100:141–146.

93. Picken JJ, Niewoehner DE, Chester EH. Prolonged effects of viral infections of the upper respiratory tract upon small airways. Am J Med 1972;52:738–746.

94. Laraya-Cuasay LR, DeForest A, Huff D, Lischner H, Huang NN. Chronic pulmonary complications of early influenza virus infection in children. Am Rev Respir Dis 1977;116:617–625.

95. Shalit I, McKee PA, Beauchamp H, Waner JL. Comparison of polyclonal antiserum versus monoclonal antibodies for the rapid diagnosis of influenza A virus infections by immunofluorescence in clinical specimens. J Clin Microbiol 1985;22:877–879.

96. McQuillin J, Madeley CR, Kendal AP. Monoclonal antibodies for the rapid diganosis of influenza A and B virus infections by immunofluorescence. Lancet 1985;ii:911–914.

97. Horwitz MS. Adenoviral diseases. In: Fields BN, Knipe DM, Chanock RM, Hisch MS, Melnick JL, Monath TP, Roizman B, eds. Virology. 2nd Ed. New York: Raven, 1990:1723–1740.

98. Ruuskanen O, Meurman O, Sarkkinen H. Adenoviral diseases in children: A study of 105 hospital cases. Pediatrics 1985;76:79–83.

99. Dudding BA, Wagner SC, Zeller JA, Gmelich JT, French GR, Top FH, Jr. Fatal pneumonia associated with adenovirus type 7 in three military trainees. N Engl J Med 1972;286:1289–1292.

100. Levin S, Dietrich J, Guillory J. Fatal nonbacterial pneumonia associated with adenovirus type 4. Occurrence in an adult. JAMA 1967;201:975–977.

101. Loker EF, Jr, Hodges GR, Kelly DJ. Fatal adenovirus pneumonia in a young adult associated with ADV-7 vaccine administered 15 days earlier. Chest 1974;66:197–199.

102. Schonland M, Strong ML, Wesley A. Fatal adenovirus pneumonia: Clinical and pathological features. S Afr Med J 1976;50:1748–1751.

103. Chany C, Lepine P, Lelong M, Le-Tan-Vinh, Satge P, Virat J. Severe and fatal pneumonia in infants and young children associated with adenovirus infections. Am J Hyg 1958;67:367–378.

104. Zahradnik JM, Spencer MJ, Porter DD. Adenovirus infection in the immunocompromised patient. Am J Med 1980;68:725–732.

105. Wasserman R, August CS, Plotkin SA. Viral infections in pediatric bone marrow transplant patients. Pediatr Infect Dis J 1988;7:109–115.

106. Field PR, Patwardhan J, McKenzie JA, Murphy AM. Fatal adenovirus type 7 pneumonia in an adult. Med J Aust 1978;2:445–447.

107. Shields AF, Hackman RC, Fife KH, Corey L, Meyers JD. Adenovirus infections in patients undergoing bone-marrow transplantation. N Engl J Med 1985;312:529–533.

108. Myerowitz RL, Stalder H, Oxman MN, et al. Fatal disseminated adenovirus infection in a renal transplant recipient. Am J Med 1975;59:591–598.

109. Craighead JE. Cytopathology of adenoviruses types 7 and 12 in human respiratory epithelium. Lab Invest 1970;22:553–557.

110. Wohl MEB, Chernick V. State of the art: Bronchiolitis. Am Rev Respir Dis 1978;118:759–781.

111. Becroft DM. Bronchiolitis obliterans, bronchiectasis, and other sequelae of adenovirus type 21 infection in young children. J Clin Pathol 1971;24:72–82.

112. Lang WR, Howden CW, Laws J, Burton JF. Bronchopneumonia with serious sequelae in children with evidence of adenovirus type 21 infection. Br Med J 1969;1:73–79.

113. Whitley RJ. Herpes simplex viruses. In: Fields BN, Knipe DM, Chanock RM, Hirsch MS, Melnick JL, Monath TP, Roizman B, eds. Virology. 2nd Ed. New York: Raven, 1990: 1843–1887.

114. Lindgren KM, Douglas RG, Jr, Couch RB. Significance of *Herpesvirus hominis* in respiratory secretions of man. N Engl J Med 1968;278:517–523.

115. Herout V, Vortel V, Vondrackova A. Herpes simplex involvement of the lower respiratory tract. Am J Clin Pathol 1966;46:411–419.

116. Francis DP, Herrmann KL, MacMahon JR, Chivigny KH, Sanderlin KC. Nosocomial and maternally acquired herpesvirus hominis infections. A report of four fatal

cases in neonates. Am J Dis Child 1975;129:889–893.

117. Foley FD, Greenawald KA, Nash G, Pruitt BA, Jr. Herpesvirus infection in burned patients. N Engl J Med 1970;282:652–656.

118. Nash G, Foley FD. Herpetic infection of the middle and lower respiratory tract. Am J Clin Pathol 1970;54:857–863.

119. Ramsey PG, Fife KH, Hackman RC, Meyers JD, Corey L. Herpes simplex virus pneumonia: Clinical, virologic, and pathologic features in 20 patients. Ann Intern Med 1982;97:813–820.

120. Douglas RG, Jr, Anderson S, Weg JG, et al. Herpes simplex virus pneumonia. Occurrence in an allotransplanted lung. JAMA 1969;210:902–904.

121. Tuxen DV, Cade JF, McDonald MI, Buchanan MRC, Clark RJ, Pain MCF. Herpes simplex virus from the lower respiratory tract in adult respiratory distress syndrome. Am Rev Respir Dis 1982;126:416–419.

122. Jordan SW, McLaren LC, Crosby JH. Herpetic tracheobronchitis. Cytologic and virologic detection. Arch Intern Med 1975;135:784–788.

123. Cooney W, Dzuira B, Harper R, Nash G. The cytology of sputum from thermally injured patients. Acta Cytol (Baltimore) 1972;16:433–437.

124. Markowitz LE, Preblud SR, Orenstein WA, et al. Patterns of transmission in measles outbreaks in the United States, 1985–1986. N Engl J Med 1989;320,2:75–81.

125. Fulginiti VA, Eller JJ, Downie AW, Kempe CH. Altered reactivity to measles virus. JAMA 1967;202:1075–1080.

126. Norrby E, Oxman MN: Measles virus. In: Fields BN, Knipe DM, Chanock RM, Hirsch MS, Melnick JL, Monath TP, Roizman B, eds. Virology. 2nd Ed. New York: Raven, 1990:1013–1044.

127. Mitus A, Enders JF, Craig JM, Holloway A. Persistence of measles virus and depression of antibody formation in patients with giant-cell pneumonia after measles. N Engl J Med 1959;261:882–889.

128. Haram K, Jacobsen K. Measles and its relationship to giant cell pneumonia (Hecht pneumonia). Acta Pathol Microbiol Immunol Scand [A] 1973;81:761–769.

129. Kipps A, Kaschula ROC. Virus pneumonia following measles: A virological and histological study of autopsy material. S Afr Med J 1976;50:1083–1088.

130. Denton J. The pathology of fatal measles. Am J Med Sci 1925;169:531–543.

131. Goodpasture EW, Auerbach SH, Swanson HS, Cotter EF. Virus pneumonia of infants secondary to epidemic infections. Am J Dis Child 1939;57:997–1011.

132. Sobonya RE, Hiller FC, Pingleton W, Watanabe I. Fatal measles (rubeola) pneumonia in adults. Arch Pathol Lab Med 1978;102:366–371.

133. Archibald RWR, Weller RO, Meadow SR. Measles pneumonia and the nature of the inclusion-bearing giant cells: A light- and electron-microscope study. J Pathol 1971;103:27–34.

134. Hecht V. Die Riesenzellen-Pneumonie im Kindesalter. Beitr Pathol Anat 1910;48:263–310.

135. Pinkerton H, Smiley WL, Anderson WAD. Giant cell pneumonia with inclusions. A lesion common to Hecht's disease, distemper, and measles. Am J Pathol 1945;21:1–15.

136. Enders JF, McCarthy K, Mitus A, Cheatham WJ. Isolation of measles virus at autopsy in cases of giant-cell pneumonia without rash. N Engl J Med 1959;261:875–881.

137. Annunziato D, Kaplan MH, Hall WW, et al. Atypical measles syndrome: Pathologic and serologic findings. Pediatrics 1982;70:203–209.

138. Laptook A, Wind E, Nussbaum M, Shenker IR. Pulmonary lesions in atypical measles. Pediatrics 1978;62:42–46.

139. Henderson JAM, Hammond DI. Delayed diagnosis in atypical measles syndrome. Can Med Assoc J 1985;133:211–213.

140. Hall CB, Geiman JM, Biggar R, Kotok DI, Hogan PM, Douglas RG, Jr. Respiratory syncytial virus infections within families. N Engl J Med 1976;294:414–419.

141. Hall CB, Douglas G, Jr., Geiman JM, Messner MK. Nosocomial respiratory syncytial virus infections. N Engl J Med 1975;293:1343–1346.

142. Englund JA, Sullivan CJ, Jordan MC, Dehner LP, Vercellotti GM, Balfour HH, Jr. Respiratory syncytial virus infection in immunocompromised adults. Ann Intern Med 1988;109:203–208.

143. Guidry GG, Black-Payne CA, Payne DK, Jamison RM, George RB, Bocchini JA, Jr. Respiratory syncytial virus infection among intubated adults in a university medical intensive care unit. Chest 1991;100:1377–1384.

144. Adams JM, Green RG, Evans CA, Beach N. Primary virus pneumonitis. A comparative study of two epidemics. J Pediatr 1942;20:405–420.

145. Hubble D, Osborn GR. Acute bronchiolitis in children. Br Med J 1941;1:107–110.

146. Adams JM, Imagawa DT, Zike K. Epidemic bronchiolitis and pneumonitis related to respiratory syncytial virus. JAMA 1961;176:1037–1039.

147. Morales F, Calder MA, Inglis JM, Murdoch PS, Williamson J. A study of respiratory infections in the elderly to assess the role of respiratory syncytial virus. J Infect 1983;7:236–247.

148. Berman S. Epidemiology of acute respiratory infections in children of developing countries. Rev Infect Dis 1991;13(Suppl. 6):S454–S462.

149. Neilson KA, Yunis EJ. Demonstration of respiratory syncytial virus in an autopsy series. Pediatr Pathol 1990;10:491–502.

150. Domurat F, Roberts NJ, Jr, Walsh EE, Dagan R. Respiratory syncytial virus infection of human mononuclear leukocytes in vitro and in vivo. J Infect Dis 1985;152:895–902.

151. Aherne W, Bird T, Court SDM, Gardner PS, McQuillin J. Pathological changes in virus infections of the lower respiratory tract in children. J Clin Pathol 1970;23:7–18.

152. Holzel A, Parker L, Patterson WH, et al. Virus isolations from throats of children admitted to hospital with respiratory and other diseases, Manchester 1962–4. Br Med J 1965;1:614–619.

153. Zinserling A. Peculiarities of lesions in viral and myco-

plasma infections of the respiratory tract. Virchows Arch [A] 1972;356:259–273.

154. Gardner PS, McQuillin J, Court SDM. Speculation on pathogenesis in death from respiratory syncytial virus infection. Br Med J 1970;1:327–330.

155. Hall CB, Douglas RG, Jr, Geiman JM. Respiratory syncytial virus infections in infants: quantitation and duration of shedding. J Pediatr 1976;89:11–15.

156. McLean KH. The pathology of acute bronchiolitis—a study of its evolution. Aust Ann Med 1956;5:254–267.

157. Welliver RC, Ogra PL. Use of immunofluorescence in the study of the pathogenesis of respiratory syncytial virus infection. Ann NY Acad Sci 1983;420:369–375.

158. Welliver RC, Kaul TN, Ogra PL. The appearance of cell-bound IgE in respiratory-tract epithelium after respiratory-syncytial-virus infection. N Engl J Med 1980; 303:1198–1201.

159. Welliver RC, Kaul TN, Sun M, Ogra PL. Defective regulation of immune responses in respiratory syncytial virus infection. J Immunol 1984;133:1925–1930.

160. Bui RHD, Molinaro GA, Kettering JD, Heiner DC, Imagawa DT, St. Geme, JW, Jr. Virus-specific IgE and IgG$_4$ antibodies in serum of children infected with respiratory syncytial virus. J Pediatr 1987;110:87–90.

161. Ananaba GA, Anderson LJ. Antibody enhancement of respiratory syncytial virus stimulation of leukotriene production by a macrophagelike cell line. J Virol 1991;65:5052–5060.

162. Rodriguez WJ, Kim HW, Brandt CD, et al. Aerosolized ribavirin in the treatment of patients with respiratory syncytial virus disease. Pediatr Infect Dis J 1987;6:159–163.

163. Hemming VG, Rodriguez W, Kim HW, et al. Intravenous immunoglobulin treatment of respiratory syncytial virus infections in infants and young children. Antimicrob Agents Chemother 1987;31:1882–1886.

164. Chanock RM, McIntosh K. Parainfluenza viruses. In: Fields BN, Knipe DM, Chanock RM, Hirsch MS, Melnick JL, Monath TP, Roizman B, eds. Virology. 2nd Ed. New York: Raven, 1990:963–988.

165. Gardner PS, McQuillin J, McGuckin R, Ditchburn RK. Observations on clinical and immunofluorescent diagnosis of parainfluenza virus infections. Br Med J 1971;2:7–12.

166. Chanock RM, Parrott RH, Johnson KM, Kapikian AZ. Bell JA. Myxoviruses: parainfluenza. Am Rev Respir Dis 1963;88:152–166.

167. Parrott RH, Vargosko A, Luckey A, Kim HW, Cumming C, Chanock R. Clinical features of infection with hemadsorption viruses. N Engl J Med 1959;260:731–738.

168. Welliver RC, Wong DT, Sun M, McCarthy N. Parainfluenza virus bronchiolitis: Epidemiology and pathogenesis. Am J Dis Child 1986;140:34–40.

169. Waner JL, Whitehurst NJ, Downs T, Graves DG. Production of monoclonal antibodies against parainfluenza 3 virus and their use in diagnosis by immunofluorescence. J Clin Microbiol 1985;22:535–538.

170. Delage G, Brochu P, Pelletier M, Jasmin G, Lapointe N. Giant-cell pneumonia caused by parainfluenza virus. J Pediatr 1979;94:426–429.

171. Minnich L, Ray CG. Comparison of direct immunofluorescent staining of clinical specimens for respiratory virus antigens with conventional isolation techniques. J Clin Microbiol 1980;12:391–394.

172. Little BW, Tihen WS, Dickerman JD, Craighead JE. Giant cell pneumonia associated with parainfluenza virus type 3 infection. Hum Pathol 1981;12:478–481.

173. Jarvis WR, Middleton PJ, Gelfand EW. Parainfluenza pneumonia in severe combined immunodeficiency disease. J Pediatr 1979;94:423–425.

174. Frank JA, Warren RW, Tucker JA, Zeller J, Wilfert CM. Disseminated parainfluenza infection in a child with severe combined immunodeficiency. Am J Dis Child 1983;137:1172–1174.

175. Cowley JA, Barry RD. Characterization of human parainfluenza viruses. The structural proteins of parainfluenza virus 2 and their synthesis in infected cells. J Gen Virol 1983;64:2117–2125.

176. Welliver RC, Wong DT, Middleton E, Sun M, McCarthy N, Ogra PL. Role of parainfluenza virus-specific IgE in pathogenesis of croup and wheezing subsequent to infection. J Pediatr 1982;101:889–896.

177. Weber DM, Pellecchia JA. Varicella pneumonia: Study of prevalence in adult men. JAMA 1965;192:572–573.

178. Gelb LD. Varicella-zoster virus. In: Fields BN, Knipe DM, Chanock RM, Hirsch MS, Melnick JL, Monath TP, Roizman B, eds. Virology. 2nd Ed. New York: Raven, 1990:2011–2054.

179. Triebwasser JH, Harris RE, Bryant RE, Rhoades ER. Varicella pneumonia in adults. Medicine (Baltimore) 1967;46:409–423.

180. Nisenbaum C, Wallis K, Herczeg E. Varicella pneumonia in children. Helv Paediatr Acta 1969;24:212–218.

181. LaRussa P. Perinatal herpesvirus infections. Pediatr Ann 1984;13:659–670.

182. Paryani SG, Arvin AM. Intra-uterine infection with varicella-zoster virus after maternal varicella. N Engl J Med 1986;314:1542–1546.

183. Motyl MR, Bottone EJ, Janda JM. Diagnosis of herpesvirus infections: correlation of Tzanck preparation with viral isolation. Diagn Microbiol Infect Dis 1984;2:157–160.

184. Solomon AR, Rasmussen JE, Weiss JS. A comparison of the Tzanch smear and viral isolation in varicella and herpes zoster. Arch Dermatol 1986;122:282–285.

185. Drew WL, Mintz L. Rapid diagnosis of varicella-zoster virus infection by direct immunofluorescence. Am J Clin Pathol 1980;73:699–701.

186. Herrmann KL. Viral serology. In: Lennette EH, Balows A, Hausler WJ, Jr., Shadomy HJ, eds. Manual of clinical microbiology. 4th ed. Washington, DC: American Society for Microbiology, 1985;921–923.

187. Saito F, Yutani C, Imakita M, Ishibashi-Ueda H, Kanzaki T, Chiba Y. Giant cell pneumonia caused by varicella zoster virus in a neonate. Arch Pathol Lab Med 1989;113:201–203.

188. Jones EL, Cameron AH. Pulmonary calcification in viral pneumonia. J Clin Pathol 1969;22:361–366.

189. Jura E, Chadwick EG, Josephs SH, et al. Varicella-zoster virus infections in children infected with human immunodeficiency virus. Pediatr Infect Dis J 1989;8:586–590.

190. Craighead JE. Cytomegalovirus pulmonary disease. Pathobiol Annu 1975;5:197–220.

191. Chou S. Acquisition of donor strains of cytomegalovirus by renal-transplant recipients. N Engl J Med 1986;314:1418–1423.

192. Reynolds DW, Stagno S, Alford CA. Laboratory diagnosis of cytomegalovirus infections. In: Lennette EH, Schmidt NJ, eds. Diagnostic procedures for viral rickettsial and chlamydial infections. 5th Ed. Washington, DC: American Public Health Association 1979:399–439.

193. Stagno S, Pass RF, Dworsky ME, Britt WJ, Alford CA. Congenital and perinatal cytomegalovirus infections: clinical characteristics and pathogenic factors. Birth Defects 1984;20:65–85.

194. Stern H. Isolation of cytomegalovirus and clinical manifestations of infection at different ages. Br Med J 1968;1:665–669.

195. Ballard RA, Drew L, Hufnagle KG, Riedel PA. Acquired cytomegalovirus infection in preterm infants. Am J Dis Child 1979;133:482–485.

196. Stagno S, Brasfield DM, Brown MB, et al. Infant pneumonitis associated with cytomegalovirus, *Chlamydia*, *Pneumocystis*, and *Ureaplasma:* A prospective study. Pediatrics 1981;68:322–329.

197. Medearis DN. Observations concerning human cytomegalovirus infection and disease. Bull Johns Hopkins Hosp 1964;114:181–211.

198. Yeager AS, Grumet FC, Hafleigh EB, Arvin AM, Bradley JS, Prober CG. Prevention of transfusion-acquired cytomegalovirus infections in newborn infants. J Pediatr 1981;98:281–287.

199. Cohen JI, Corey GR. Cytomegalovirus infection in the normal host. Medicine (Baltimore) 1985;64:100–114.

200. Kirchner H. Immunobiology of infection with human cytomegalovirus. Adv Cancer Res 1983;40:31–105.

201. Peterson PK, Balfour HH, Marker SC, Fryd DS, Howard RJ, Simmons RL. Cytomegalovirus disease in renal allograft recipients: A prospective study of the clinical features, risk factors and impact on renal transplantation. Medicine (Baltimore) 1980;59:283–300.

202. Fiala M, Payne JE, Berne TV, et al. Epidemiology of cytomegalovirus infection after transplantation and immunosuppression. J Infect Dis 1975;132:421–433.

203. Rubin RH, Cosimi AB, Tolkoff-Rubin NE, Russell PS, Hirsch MS. Infectious disease syndromes attributable to cytomegalovirus and their significance among renal transplant recipients. Transplantation 1977;24:458–464.

204. Rook AH, Quinnan GV, Frederick WJR, et al. Importance of cytotoxic lymphocytes during cytomegalovirus infection in renal transplant recipients. Am J Med 1984;76:385–392.

205. Meyers JD, Flournoy N, Thomas ED. Nonbacterial pneumonia after allogeneic marrow transplantation: A review of ten years experience. Rev Infect Dis 1982;4:1119–1132.

206. Blumenfeld W, Wagar E, Hadley WK. Use of the transbronchial biopsy for diagnosis of opportunistic pulmonary infections in acquired immunodeficiency syndrome (AIDS). Am J Clin Pathol 1984;81:1–5.

207. Lamberson HV, Jr. Cytomegalovirus (CMV): The agent, its pathogenesis, and its epidemiology. Prog Clin Biol Res 1985;182:149–173.

208. Griffiths PD. Diagnostic techniques for cytomegalovirus infection. Clin Haematol 1984;13:631–644.

209. Moore DG, Davis BG, Oefinger PE, Carlson JR. Reactivity of serologic tests for the detection of antibody specific to cytomegalovirus. Am J Clin Pathol 1985;83:622–625.

210. McHugh TM, Casavant CH, Wilber JC, Stites DP. Comparison of six methods for the detection of antibody to cytomegalovirus. J Clin Microbiol 1985;22:1014–1019.

211. Griffiths PD, Stagno S, Pass RF, Smith RJ, Alford CA Jr. Infection with cytomegalovirus during pregnancy: specific IgM antibodies as a marker of recent primary infection. J Infect Dis 1982;145:647–653.

212. Demmler GJ, Six HR, Hurst SM, Yow MD. Enzymelinked immunosorbent assay for the detection of IgM-class antibodies to cytomegalovirus. J Infect Dis 1986;153:1152–1155.

213. Drew WL. Controversies in viral diagnosis. Rev Infect Dis 1986;8:814–824.

214. Smith TF, Holley KE, Keys TF, Macasaet FF. Cytomegalovirus studies of autopsy tissue. Am J Clin Pathol 1975;63:854–858.

215. Hackman RC, Myerson D, Meyers JD, et al. Rapid diagnosis of cytomegaloviral pneumonia by tissue immunofluorescence with a murine monoclonal antibody. J Infect Dis 1985;151:325–329.

216. Abdallah PS, Mark JB, Merigan TC. Diagnosis of cytomegalovirus pneumonia in compromised hosts. Am J Med 1976;61:326–332.

217. Woods GL, Thompson AB, Rennard SL, Linder J. Detection of cytomegalovirus in bronchoalveolar lavage specimens. Spin amplification and staining with a monoclonal antibody to the early nuclear antigen for diagnosis of cytomegalovirus pneumonia. Chest 1990;98:568–575.

218. Weiss RL, Snow GW, Schumann GB, Hammond ME. Diagnosis of cytomegalovirus pneumonitis on bronchoalveolar lavage fluid: Comparison of cytology, immunofluorescence, and in situ hybridization with viral isolation. Diagn Cytopathol 1991;7:243–247.

219. Cordonnier C, Escudier E, Nicolas J-C, et al. Evaluation of three assays on alveolar lavage fluid in the diagnosis of cytomegalovirus pneumonitis after bone marrow transplantation. J Infect Dis 1987;155:495–500.

220. Myerson D, Hackman RC, Nelson JA, Ward DC, McDougall JK. Widespread presence of histologically occult cytomegalovirus. Hum Pathol 1984;15:430–439.

221. Schrier RD, Nelson JA, Oldstone MBA. Detection of human cytomegalovirus in peripheral blood lymphocytes in a natural infection. Science 1985;230:1048–1051.

222. Hilborne LH, Nieberg RK, Cheng L, Lewin KJ. Direct in situ hybridization for rapid detection of cytomegalovirus

in bronchoalveolar lavage. Am J Clin Pathol 1987; 87:766–769.

223. Paradis IL, Grgurich WF, Dummer JS, Dekker A, Dauber JH. Rapid detection of cytomegalovirus pneumonia from lung lavage cells. Am Rev Respir Dis 1988;138:697–702.

224. Churchill MA, Zaia JA, Forman SJ, Sheibani K, Azumi N, Blume KG. Quantitation of human cytomegalovirus DNA in lungs from bone marrow transplant recipients with interstitial pneumonia. J Infect Dis 1987;155:501–509.

225. Gleaves CA, Meyers JD. Rapid detection of cytomegalovirus in bronchoalveolar lavage specimens from marrow transplant patients: Evaluation of a direct fluorescein-conjugated monoclonal antibody reagent. J Virol Methods 1989;26:345–350.

226. Jesionek KA, Kiolemenoglou B. Über einen Befund von protozoën artigen Gebilden in den Oragnen eines hereditär-luetischen. Fötus Munch Med Wochenschr 1904;43:1905–1907.

227. Goodpasture EW, Talbot FB. Concerning the nature of "protozoan-like" cells in certain lesions of infancy. Am J Dis Child 1921;21:415–425.

228. Farber S, Wolbach SB. Intranuclear and cytoplasmic inclusions ("protozoan-like bodies") in the salivary glands and other organs of infants. Am J Pathol 1932; 8:123–135.

229. Cole R, Kuttner AG. A filterable virus present in the submaxillary blands of guinea pigs. J Exp Med 1926; 44:855–873.

230. Smith MG. Propagation in tissue cultures of a cytopathogenic virus from human salivary gland virus (SGV) disease. Proc Soc Exp Biol Med 1956;92:424–430.

231. Rowe WP, Hartley JW, Waterman S, Turner HC, Huebner RJ. Cytopathogenic agent resembling human salivary gland virus recovered from tissue cultures of human adenoids. Proc Soc Exp Biol Med 1956;92:418–424.

232. Weller TH, Macauley LC, Craig JM, Wirth P. Isolation of intranuclear inclusion producing agents from infants with illnesses resembling cytomegalic inclusion disease. Proc Soc Exp Biol Med 1957;94:4–12.

233. Irmiere A, Gibson W. Isolation of human cytomegalovirus intranuclear capsids, characterization of their protein constituents, and demonstration that the B-capsid assembly protein is also abundant in non-infectious enveloped particles. J Virol 1985;56:277–283.

234. Plotkin SA, Michelson S, Alford CA, et al. The pathogenesis and prevention of human cytomegalovirus infection. Pediatr Infect Dis 1984;3:67–74.

235. Hruban Z, Kuzo R, Heimann P, Weisenberg E, Hruban RH. Globular changes in cytomegaloviral inclusions after ganciclovir treatment. Arch Virol 1989;108:287–293.

236. Gorelkin L, Chandler FW, Ewing EP, Jr. Staining qualities of cytomegalovirus inclusions in the lungs of patients with the acquired immunodeficiency syndrome: A potential source of diagnostic misinterpretation. Hum Pathol 1986;17:926–929.

237. Kanich RE, Craighead JE. Human cytomegalovirus infection of cultured fibroblasts. I. Cytopathologic effects induced by an adapted and a wild strain. Lab Invest 1972;27:263–272.

238. Iwasaki T, Satodate R, Masuda T, Kurata T, Hondo R. An immunofluorescent study of generalized infection of human cytomegalovirus in a patient with systemic lupus erythematosus. Acta Pathol Jpn 1984;34:869–874.

239. Craighead JE. Pulmonary cytomegalovirus infection in the adult. Am J Pathol 1971;63:487–504.

240. Hirsch MS, Felsenstein D. Cytomegalovirus-induced immunosuppression. Ann NY Acad Sci 1984;437:8–15.

241. Gehrz RC, Rutzick SR. Cytomegalovirus (CMV)-specific lysis of CMV-infected target cells can be mediated by both NK-like and virus-specific cytotoxic T lymphocytes. Clin Exp Immunol 1985;61:80–89.

242. Borysiewicz LK, Rodgers B, Morris S, Graham S, Sissons JGP. Lysis of human cytomegalovirus infected fibroblasts by natural killer cells: demonstration of an interferon-independent component requiring expression of early viral proteins and characterization of effector cells. J Immunol 1985;134:2695–2701.

243. Ho M. Pathology of cytomegalovirus infection. In: Greenough WB III, Merigan TC, eds. Cytomegalovirus: Biology and infection. Current topics in infectious disease. New York: Plenum, 1982:119–129.

244. Ravic C, Smith GW, Ahern MJ, McLoud T, Putman C, Milchgrub S. Cytomegaloviral infection presenting as a solitary pulmonary nodule. Chest 1977;71:220–222.

245. Faulds D, Heel RE. Ganciclovir. A review of its antiviral activity, pharmacokinetic properties and therapeutic efficacy in cytomegalovirus infections. Drugs 1990;39:597–638.

246. Craighead JE, Meier M, Cooley MH. Pulmonary infection due to rhinovirus type 13. N Engl J Med 1969; 281:1403–1404.

247. Mundy GR. Infectious mononucleosis with pulmonary parenchymal involvement. Br Med J 1972;1:219–220.

248. Grist NR, Bell EJ, Assaad F. Enteroviruses in human disease. Prog Med Virol 1978;24:114–157.

CHAPTER 13

Mycoplasmal, Chlamydial, and Rickettsial Pneumonias

DAVID H. WALKER

Mycoplasmas and the various obligate and facultative intracellular bacteria that cause significant clinical pulmonary injury are quite diverse from the point of view of microbiologic genetics and phenotypes. Molecular analysis of the DNA similarity has revealed that *Rickettsia* species of the typhus and spotted fever groups and *Ehrlichia* species are relatively closely related and that *Coxiella burnetii* and *Legionella pneumophila* are genetically related to one another.[1] However, *Rickettsia* and *Coxiella* species are only distantly related to one another and are even more distant from the genetically diverse *Chlamydia* and *Mycoplasma*.

The striking differences in the structure of the cell walls of these pneumonia agents, their target cells, and their relationships with host cells confirm the heterogeneity of these unusual bacteria (Table 13–1). Because pneumonia caused by mycoplasma, chlamydiae, coxiella, rickettsiae, ehrlichiae, various facultative intracellular bacteria (e.g., legionellae), and many viruses differ from the typical pneumonia caused by *Streptococcus pneumoniae*, these agents are often said to cause atypical pneumonia. Clinically, some of these agents (e.g., rickettsiae, *C. burnetii*, *L. pneumophila*) are usually associated with pneumonia having a nonproductive cough. However, others of these agents (e.g., *M. pneumoniae*) usually cause pneumonia with a productive cough. Thus, the clinical signs and symptoms of so-called atypical pneumonia do not constitute a distinct syndrome. The consistent feature of these agents is that, like viruses and because of their fastidious growth requirements or obligate intracellular parasitism, they are not cultivated in most hospital clinical microbiology laboratories. Thus, establishing an etiologic diagnosis in a timely manner is often difficult.

The pathologic lesions, in fact, overlap with one another and to some extent with pneumonias caused by viruses and other bacteria. The target cells and pathogenic mechanisms of mycoplasma, chlamydiae, coxiella, rickettsiae, and ehrlichiae lead to the observed histopathology and frequently explain the differences in the lesions.

Mycoplasmal Pneumonias

Mycoplasmas are extracellular bacteria that lack the structural cell wall components of gram-positive or gram-negative organisms. *Mycoplasma pneumoniae* are motile and slender, measuring 0.1 by 2 μm. They adhere to sialic acid moieties in the cell membrane of respiratory epithelium by a differentiated structure containing a specific attachment protein (Fig. 13–1).[2] *Mycoplasma pneumoniae* is perhaps the most frequent cause of pneumonia in humans. Although representing only 9% of community-acquired pneumonia isolates in preschoolers, *M. pneumoniae* constitutes 51% of isolates in 5- to 9-year-olds, 74% in 9- to 15-year-olds,[3] and 3.3%–18% in adults.[4–6] Among university students, *M. pneumoniae* causes 11% of clinically diagnosed pneumonias and 22% of radiographically confirmed pneumonias. Smoldering outbreaks begin in the fall, occurring usually in 4-year cycles.

Clinically, mycoplasmal pneumonia has a incidence of productive cough, headache, rales, and diarrhea similar to community-acquired pneumococcal pneumonia and *Legionella* pneumonia and differs in having more frequent occurrence of upper respiratory symptoms, normal leukocyte counts, and younger age.[7] After an incubation period of 2–3 weeks, the patient notes the gradual onset of malaise, headache, fever, cough, and

Table 13–1. Representative microorganisms of five different genera that cause atypical pneumonia and the microbial characteristics and host relationships which determine the lesions

	Structure	*Target cell*	*Host cell interaction*
Mycoplasma pneumoniae	Plasma membrane, but no cell wall	Respiratory epithelium	Extracellular agent attaches to luminal cell membrane and injures the cell by peroxide secretion
Chlamydia trachomatis	Cell wall contains lipopolysaccharide but no peptidoglycan; infectious form, the elementary body, has cell wall structural strength from disulfide bonds	Respiratory epithelium	Obligate intracellular agent resides in phagosome, inhibits phagolysosomal fusion, and requires host cell ATP source
Coxiella burnetti	Cell wall contains lipopolysaccharide and peptidoglycan	Alveolar macrophages	Obligate intracellular agent resides in phagolysosome
Rickettsia rickettsii	Cell wall contains lipopolysaccharide and peptidoglycan	Endothelium	Obligate intracellular agent resides free in cytosol
Ehrlichia chaffeensis	Cell wall appears to contain peptidoglycan but no lipopolysaccharide	Leukocytes	Obligate intracellular agent resides in phagosome and inhibits phagolysosomal fusion

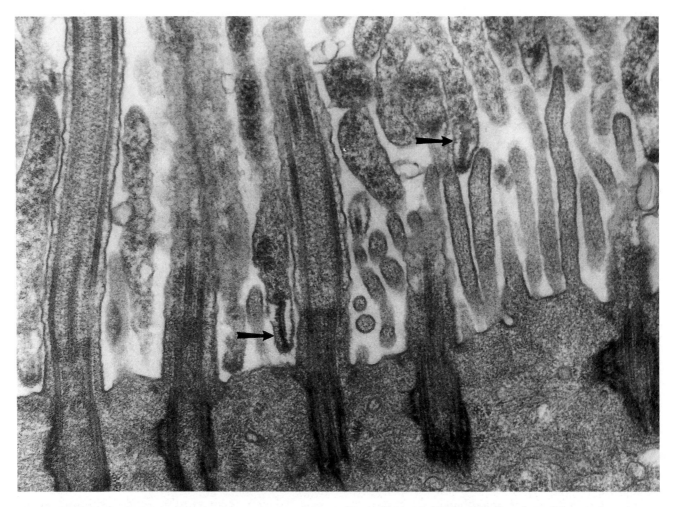

Fig. 13–1. Electron photomicrograph of *Mycoplasma pneumoniae* attached by specialized tip (*arrows*) to surface of ciliated tracheal epithelial cell in organ culture. *Arrows* point out plasma membrane; there is no outer envelope of the cell wall.

(From Clyde W.A. Kendig's disorders of the respiratory tract in children, 5th Ed. Philadelphia: Saunders, 1990, with permission.)

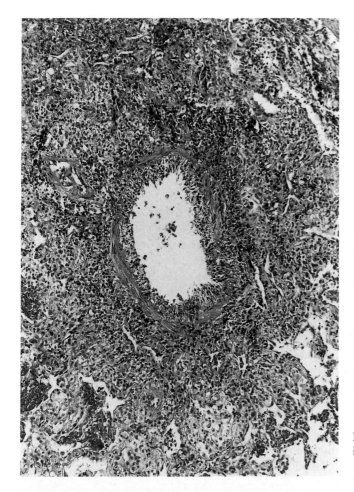

Fig. 13–2. Bronchial and peribronchial inflammation associated with *Mycoplasma pneumoniae* infection. Inflammatory infiltrate consists of lymphocytes and plasma cells.

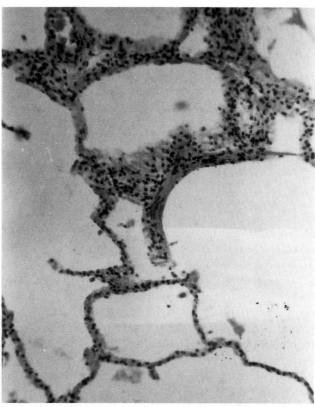

Fig. 13–3. Interstitial pneumonia with many lymphocytes infiltrated into alveolar septa of human lung with mycoplasmal pneumonia. (From Clyde W.A. Kendig's disorders of the respiratory tract in children. 5th Ed. Philadelphia: WB Saunders. 1990, with permission.)

sore throat.[8,9] *Mycoplasma pneumoniae* causes tracheobronchitis 30 times more often than pneumonia. Chest radiographs reveal bronchopneumonia usually involving one lower lobe, peribronchial thickening, subsegmental atelectasis, and streaky interstitial densities.[2]

The mycoplasmas secrete peroxide, which injures the cell membrane of the host respiratory epithelial cell to which they are attached.[9] Ciliary activity ceases, and the junctions with the adjacent cells are disrupted. The pathologic lesions in the few etiologically documented autopsies of this rarely fatal disease resemble those in the hamster model, notably peribronchial, peribronchiolar, and interstitial infiltration by macrophages, lymphocytes, and plasma cells with bronchial and bronchiolar lumina containing polymorphonuclear leukocytes, mucus, fibrin, and desquamated epithelial cells (Figs. 13–2 and 13–3).[10] Airways obstruction accounts for the frequent occurrence of segmental or subsegmental atelectasis.

Diagnosis has often rested on the demonstration of cold hemagglutinins resulting from antibodies to antigens shared by *M. pneumoniae* and the I antigen of human erythrocytes. Cold hemagglutinins are detected in only half of cases of mycoplasmal pneumonia and have also been observed in adenoviral pneumonia, measles, and infectious mononucleosis. Highly specific serologic assays that utilize mycoplasma antigens include the complement fixation test (sensitivity, 68%) and IgM-immunofluorescent antibody assay (sensitivity, 74%).[5] Because recovery of *M. pneumoniae* by culture requires 1–3 weeks, more timely methods for the detection of mycoplasma antigens or genes have been developed. An enzyme immunoassay test for *M. pneumoniae* antigen has been reported to have a sensitivity of 63%.[4] A DNA probe for detection of ribosomal RNA of *M. pneumoniae* in respiratory secretions has been shown to be highly sensitive, specific, and rapid.

Another mycoplasma, *Ureaplasma urealyticum*, has

been implicated in perinatal pneumonia. This organism was recovered from the lung in 7% of cases of perinatal pneumonia associated with chorioamnionitis and from 16%–21% of infants less than 3 months of age hospitalized with pneumonia.[11–13] The clinical syndrome and histopathology have not been distinguished from other perinatal pneumonias, and indeed mixed infections often occur.

Chlamydial Pneumonias

All three species, *Chlamydia trachomatis*, *C. pneumoniae*, and *C. psittaci*, can cause pneumonia. *Chlamydia trachomatis* is an important etiologic agent of pneumonia in infants; *C. pneumoniae* rivals *M. pneumoniae* for the major role in the incidence of atypical pneumonia; and *C. psittaci* is the etiology of a classic zoonotic pneumonia. Chlamydiae are obligate intracellular bacteria that are completely dependent on their host cells for ATP and have a distinctive developmental cycle. The compact, metabolically inactive elementary body is the infectious form that attaches to host respiratory epithelial cells, induces phagocytosis, inhibits lysosomal fusion with the phagosome, and, once within the phagosome, changes into the reticulate body. The noninfectious reticulate body is 10–100 times larger, is metabolically active, and serves the function of replication. Many of the reticulate bodies change into elementary bodies before the host cell lyses, releasing chlamydiae to initiate infection of other cells.[14]

Chlamydia trachomatis Pneumonia

Among infants 1–3 months of age who are hospitalized with pneumonia, *Chlamydia trachomatis* is the cause in 25%–36%.[12,13] Infants acquire the infection during birth through the infected endocervix of their mothers. Approximately 5% of pregnant women carry endocervical *C. trachomatis*, and 70% of their infants seroconvert; 18%–50% develop chlamydial inclusion conjunctivitis, and 17%–22% develop chlamydial pneumonia.[2,15,16] *C. trachomatis* rarely causes pneumonia in adults, even in laboratory workers or acquired immunodeficiency syndrome (AIDS) patients.[17,18]

The characteristic clinical manifestations of *C. trachomatis* pneumonia of infants include onset about 6 weeks of age of staccato cough, tachypnea, rales, roentgenographic hyperexpansion, and diffuse interstitial and patchy alveolar infiltrates, hypoxemia, and mild peripheral eosinophilia.[19] Patients are typically afebrile. Only 50% have conjunctivitis at the time of presentation with pneumonia.[16,20] In low-birth-weight neonates, *C. trachomatis* can cause severe pneumonia with onset shortly after birth.[21,22] Infantile *C. trachomatis* pneumonia is rarely fatal, and often occurs as a coinfection with other maternal genital tract agents, particularly cytomegalovirus. Thus, the histopathology of pure infantile chlamydial pneumonia is not clearly defined. A mixed picture of interstitial and alveolar pneumonia and bronchiolitis includes interstitial lymphocytes, plasma cells, eosinophils, polymorphonuclear leukocytes, germinal centers, and alveolar mononuclear cells and eosinophils.[21,23–25] Chlamydiae have been observed in human bronchiolar, bronchial, and tracheal epithelial cells.[24] Experimental infection of mice has demonstrated *C. trachomatis* reticulate bodies predominantly in type I alveolar lining cells, an early polymorphonuclear leukocytic response in alveoli and alveolar ducts, and later peribronchiolar and alveolar infiltration by lymphocytes, plasma cells, and macrophages.[26]

Chlamydia trachomatis is cultivated from respiratory secretions in cell lines such as McCoy cells, and chlamydial antigens can be demonstrated sensitively and specifically in respiratory specimens by direct immunofluorescence and enzyme immunoassay.[27–29] Molecular methods, including amplification of *C. trachomatis* DNA by polymerase chain reaction and in situ hybridization,[30] have been demonstrated to be feasible diagnostic approaches. Useful serologic assays are the complement fixation test for genus-specific antigens, enzyme-linked immunosorbent assays (ELISA), and microimmunofluorescence, including IgM-IFA (immunofluorescent antibody assay).[16]

Chlamydia pneumoniae Pneumonia

Chlamydia pneumoniae is the cause of 6%–12% of pneumonias in adults, ranking as approximately the fourth most frequent cause.[16] The infection is uncommon in the first 5 years of life and is clinically more severe in older patients. Among university students, 9% of clinically diagnosed pneumonias and 20% of radiographically confirmed pneumonias are caused by *C. pneumoniae*. Because half of adults have specific antibodies to *C. pneumoniae*, it appears to be a nearly universal infection with frequent occurrence of reinfection. Humans are the only known reservoir. Infections are nonseasonal and spread slowly even under closely confined conditions.

Clinically, 90% of *C. pneumoniae* infections are mild or asymptomatic.[16] The infection is similar to that of *M. pneumoniae*, although fever occurs less often and sore throat more often. The onset is more gradual with pharyngitis proceeding to cough and pneumonia over a period of days to a week.[31,32] The spectrum of illness includes pneumonia, bronchitis, laryngitis, pharyngitis, and sinusitis.[33] Among adults with community-acquired pneumonia caused by *C. pneumoniae*, 61% had cough; 44%, productive cough; 61%, rales; and 56%, fever.[6]

Partly because *C. pneumoniae* was discovered only recently and seldom causes fatal disease, the pathologic lesions have yet to be defined. Similarly few diagnostic tools are generally available. These chlamydiae are cultivated most effectively in HeLa-229 cells. The chlamydial complement fixation test detects antibodies to the genus-common antigen and does not distinguish among the chlamydial species. In reinfections, complement fixation serology is negative. Microimmunofluorescence serology detects species-specific antibodies. It has been reported that a fourfold rise in titer to 16 or greater, a single IgM-IFA titer of 16 or greater, or a single IgG-IFA titer of 512 or greater is diagnostic.[33]

Chlamydia psittaci Pneumonia

Chlamydia psittaci is a zoonotic agent with avian and mammalian reservoirs. The infection is transmitted to humans from pet birds and in turkey and duck processing plants. After an incubation period of 6–15 days, an influenza-like illness occurs. In Great Britain, *C. psittaci* acquired from pet birds seems to be a more frequent cause of pneumonia than *C. pneumoniae*.[34] The pulmonary histopathology of psittacosis is characterized by variation in alveolar infiltrates, polymorphonuclear leukocytes, erythrocytes, and fibrin early, and in macrophages, lymphocytes, and plasma cells later. Alveolar septa are patchily infiltrated by macrophages and lymphocytes.[35] The pathogenetic events are suggested by studies in animal models. Newborn guinea pigs inoculated intranasally with a *C. psittaci* strain indigenous to that species develop chlamydial infection of bronchial epithelial cells, bronchiolar luminal exudates of polymorphonuclear leukocytes, and interstitial and alveolar mononuclear cell infiltrates.[36]

Like other chlamydial pneumonias, the diagnosis of psittacosis is difficult to establish. Epidemiologic clues and complement fixation serology are the diagnostic mainstays. DNA probes and polymerase chain reaction technology are capable of distinguishing among the three chlamydial species.[37–39]

Q Fever Pneumonia

Coxiella burnetii has been shown by analysis of plasmid DNA, chromosomal DNA, and lipopolysaccharide to consist of six different groups of organisms. Strains of *C. burnetii* from two of these groups have been associated with acute pneumonia, while strains from some of the other groups have been associated with chronic endocarditis.[40]

Humans usually become infected by inhalation of aerosols of birth products of parturient sheep, cattle, goats, cats, and rabbits.[41,42] Infection is frequently asymptomatic. In a Swiss outbreak, only 4.4% of patients were ill enough to be hospitalized with pneumonia. Illness begins after a dose-dependent incubation period of 9–21 days with detectable bloodstream infection occurring late in the incubation period. Pneumonia varies geographically as a clinical manifestation of acute Q fever from 4%–7% in Australia to 80% of acute Q fever patients with a chest radiograph in Nova Scotia. Acute Q fever has an abrupt onset of fever, chills, fatigue, and headache. Cough that is typically nonproductive occurs in a variable proportion (4%–90%) of cases, reflecting the regional prevalence of pulmonary involvement. Chest radiographs of Q fever pneumonia demonstrate multiple, 5- to 10-cm rounded opacities, usually in the lower lobes, increased reticular markings, and atelectasis.[43] Q fever occurs occasionally as an opportunistic pneumonia in immunocompromised hosts.[44]

The major target cell of *C. burnetii* in the lung is the alveolar macrophage (Fig. 13–4).[45,46] Organisms are engulfed by macrophages and reside in the phagolysosome where they multiply and are activated metabolically by the acid milieu and multiply. *Coxiella* pneumonia is characterized by focal consolidation, microscopic bronchioloalveolitis, and interstitial and alveolar infiltration by macrophages, lymphocytes, and polymorphonuclear leukocytes (Fig. 13–5).[47,48]

Microbiology laboratories rarely attempt to isolate *C. burnetii* because of its high potential to cause laboratory-acquired infection. Nevertheless, a shell vial centrifugation-enhanced cell culture method for recovery of *C. burnetii* has been applied successfully to clinical samples of blood. The diagnosis of acute Q fever usually relies on the demonstration of antibodies to the antigens of the laboratory-derived form of the organism with truncated lipopolysaccharides (LPS) and exposed cell wall protein, referred to as *C. burnetii* phase II. The order of decreasing sensitivity of Q fever serologic assays is enzyme immunoassay, immunofluorescent antibody test, and complement fixation test.[49,50]

Pulmonary Lesions in Vasculotropic Rickettsial Diseases

Respiratory symptoms and life-threatening pneumonitis occur in rickettsial diseases as a consequence of rickettsial infection of vascular endothelium in the lung in Rocky Mountain spotted fever, boutonneuse fever,

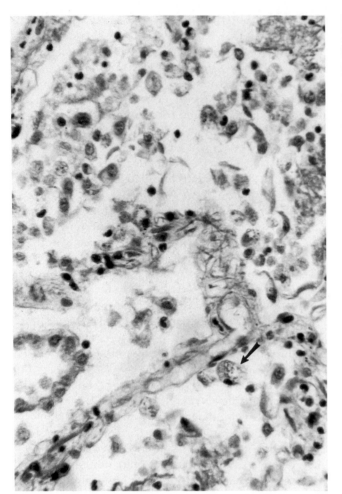

Fig. 13–4. Q Fever pneumonia with numerous alveolar macrophages containing *Coxiella burnetii* demonstrated by immunoperoxidase within large cytoplasmic vacuoles (*arrow*). (Tissue courtesy of TJ Marrie; immunoperoxidase stain prepared by JS Dumler.)

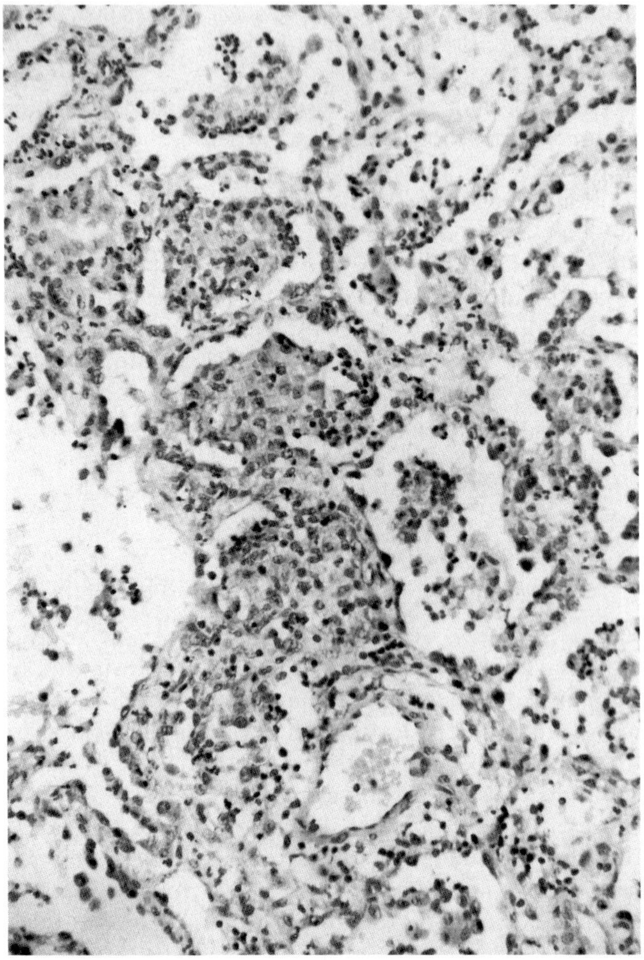

Fig. 13–5. Biopsy of lung from a patient with Q fever pneumonia contains alveoli and alveolar septa with macrophages, lymphocytes, and polymorphonuclear leukocytes. (Slide courtesy of TJ Marrie.)

epidemic typhus, murine typhus, and presumably other spotted fevers and scrub typhus.

In Rocky Mountain spotted fever, *Rickettsia rickettsii* is introduced into the skin by tick bite; rickettsiae spread via the bloodstream and establish intracellular endothelial infection throughout the body, including the lungs (Fig. 13–6). Cough, usually nonproductive and possibly related to rickettsial vascular injury in the bronchial walls, is present on hospital admission in 33%.[51] Rales, radiographic infiltrates, and abnormal gas exchange are observed frequently in hospitalized patients. Severe respiratory distress is a manifestation of noncardiogenic pulmonary edema caused by rickettsial infection of the pulmonary microcirculation and consequent increased vascular permeability. It is not unusual for patients with severe Rocky Mountain spotted fever to require ventilatory support and for respiratory failure

to be a critical life-threatening factor.[52] Histopathologic lesions include interstitial pneumonia and edema, alveolar edema, fibrin, macrophages, hemorrhages, interlobular septal edema (Fig. 13–7) and lymphohistiocytic vasculitis (Fig. 13–8).[53]

Boutonneuse fever, caused by the tick-transmitted spotted fever rickettsia *R. conorii*, is associated with cough in 10% and dyspnea in 21%.[54] Rickettsial infection of pulmonary alveolar capillaries has been demonstrated, and lesions have included perivascular lymphohistiocytic infiltrates in the lung, interstitial pneumonia, and pulmonary edema.[55,56] Other spotted fever rickettsioses are likely to have rickettsial pulmonary involvement in the most severe cases.

Typhus group rickettsioses often have respiratory signs and symptoms. Murine typhus, inoculated as infected flea feces, manifests cough in 35% of patients

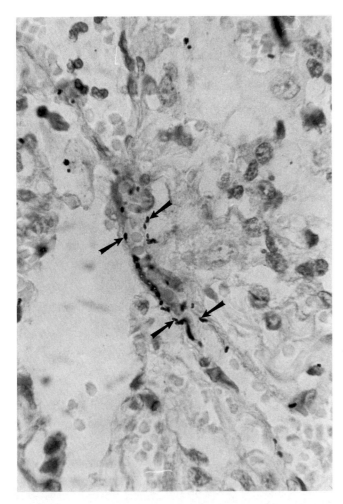

Fig. 13–6. *Rickettsia rickettsii* (at and between *arrows*) is demonstrated by immunoperoxidase in endothelial cells of blood vessel of alveolar septum. Pathophysiologic effect, interstitial and alveolar edema, the host defenses, and perivascular lymphohistiocytic infiltration constitute picture of interstitial pneumonia. (Slide courtesy of JS Dumler.)

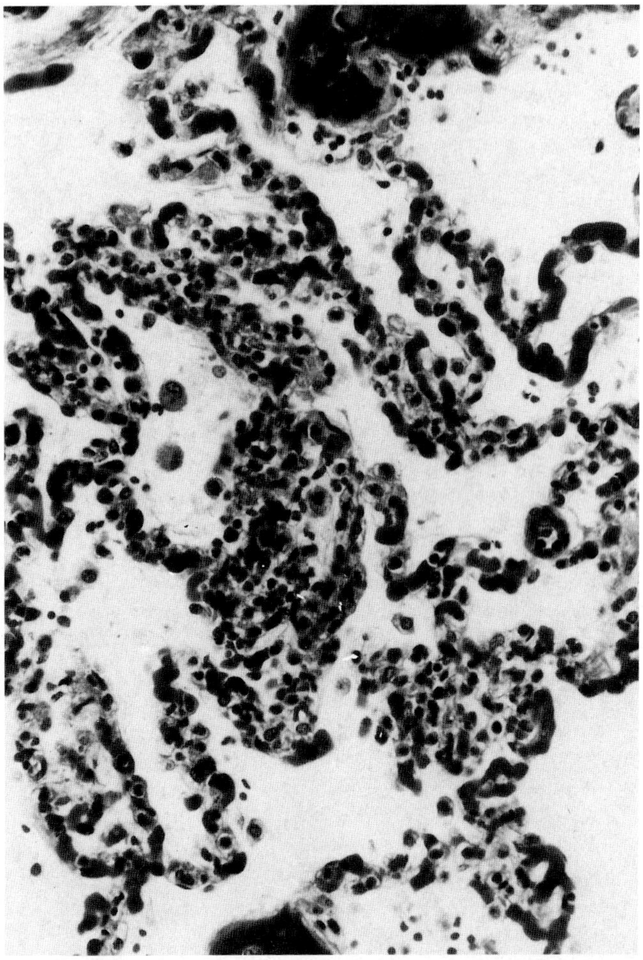

Fig. 13–7. Patchy interstitial pneumonia associated with Rocky Mountain spotted fever.

and roentgenographic pneumonitis or pulmonary edema in 14%.[57] The clinical diagnosis is so difficult that among patients with an eventually established diagnosis of murine typhus, rickettsiosis and lower respiratory tract infection represented the initial diagnosis in equal numbers of patients. Rales result from rickettsia-induced vascular leakage rather than from cardiac failure. Interstitial pneumonia is the essential histopathologic lesion and has been seen in association with diffuse alveolar damage.[58] In the preantibiotic era, patients with epidemic typhus frequently died in a coma with nosomial bronchopneumonia superimposed on *R. prowazekii*-associated interstitial pneumonia (Fig. 13–9).

Scrub typhus also has a clinically important interstitial pneumonia.[59] Macroscopic diffuse congestion, hemorrhages, and pulmonary edema reflect alveolar septal

infiltration by macrophages and lymphocytes, hyaline membranes, edema, and hemorrhage in alveolar spaces. Immunohistology or other methods for demonstration of *R. tsutsugamushi* have been lacking. Thus, these rickettsiae have not been localized in the lungs of patients with scrub typhus.

Pulmonary Involvement in Human Ehrlichiosis

A recently described, tick-transmitted infection with the novel agent *Ehrlichia chaffeensis* frequently has respiratory manifestations. Infection of mainly macrophages and lymphocytes by these obligate intracellular bacteria

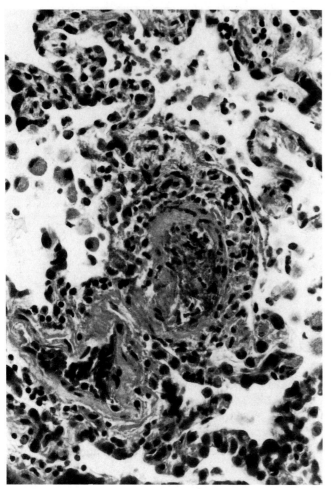

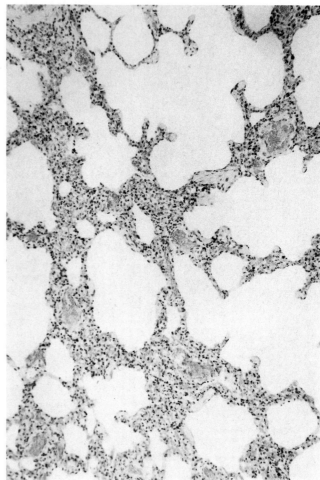

Fig. 13–8. Acute vascular injury with nonocclusive thrombus and perivascular infiltration of predominantly macrophages and lymphocytes in lung of patient with fatal Rocky Mountain spotted fever.

Fig. 13–9. Interstitial pneumonia in fatal case of epidemic typhus that occurred during World War II.

ranges from asymptomatic to fatal. Cough occurs in 39% of patients, and pulmonary infiltrates are seen in 44% of patients with chest radiographs.[60] Although *E. chaffeensis* has been demonstrated in human lung tissue by immunohistology, the pulmonary pathology is at present poorly defined.[61] Interstitial and alveolar macrophage infiltration has been observed, but not as a consistent finding. These leukocytotropic intracellular bacteria are likely to reveal future interesting insights into pulmonary pathogenic mechanisms.

References

1. Weisburg WG, Dobson ME, Samuel JE, et al. Phylogenetic diversity of the rickettsiae. J Bacteriol 1989;171:4202–4206.
2. Leigh MW, Clyde WA, Jr. Chlamydial and mycoplasmal pneumonias. Semin Respir Infect 1987; 2:152–158.
3. Murphy TF, Henderson FW, Clyde WA, Jr., Collier AM, Denny FW. Pneumonia: An eleven-year study in a pediatric practice. Am J Epidemiol 1981;113:12–21.
4. Lim I, Shaw DR, Stanley DP, Lumb R, McLennan G. A prospective hospital study of the aetiology of community-acquired pneumonia. Med J Aust 1989;151:87–91.
5. Research Committee of the British Thoracic Society, Public Health Laboratory Service. Community-acquired pneumonia in adults in British hospitals in 1982–1983: A survey of aetiology, mortality, prognostic factors and outcome. Q J Med 1987;239:195–220.
6. Marrie TJ, Grayston JT, Wang SP, Kuo CC. Pneumonia associated with the TWAR strain of Chlamydia. Ann Intern Med 1987;106:507–511.
7. Woodhead MA, Macfarlane JT. Comparative clinical and laboratory features of legionella with pneumococcal and mycoplasma pneumonias. Br J Dis Chest 1987;81:133–139.
8. Denny FW, Clyde WA, Jr., Glezen WP. *Mycoplasma pneu-*

moniae disease: Clinical spectrum, pathophysiology, epidemiology, and control. J Infect Dis 1971;123:74–92.

9. Clyde WA, Jr. Infections of the respiratory tract due to *Mycoplasma pneumoniae*. In: Chernick V, Kendig EL, Jr., eds. Kendig's disorders of the respiratory tract in children. 5th Ed. Philadelphia: WB Saunders, 1990:403–412.

10. Maisel JC, Babbitt LH, John TJ. Fatal *Mycoplasma pneumoniae* infection with isolation of organisms from lung. JAMA 1967;202:287–290.

11. Madan E, Meyer MP, Amortequi A. Chorioamnionitis: A study of organisms isolated in perinatal autopsies. Ann Clin Lab Sci 1988;18:39–45.

12. Stagno S, Brasfield DM, Brown MB, et al. Infant pneumonitis associated with cytomegalovirus, *Chlamydia*, *Pneumocystis*, and *Ureaplasma*: A prospective study. Pediatrics 1981;68:322–329.

13. Brasfield DM, Stagno S, Whitley RJ, Cloud G, Cassell G, Tiller RE. Infant pneumonitis associated with cytomegalovirus, *Chlamydia*, *Pneumocystis*, and *Ureaplasma:* Follow-up. Pediatrics 1987;79:76–83.

14. Moulder JW. Interaction of chlamydiae and host cells in vitro. Microbiol Rev 1991;55:143–190.

15. Schachter J, Grossman M, Sweet RL, Holt J, Jordan C, Bishop E. Prospective study of perinatal transmission of *Chlamydia trachomatis*. JAMA 1986;255:3374–3377.

16. Grayston JT, Thom DH. The chlamydial pneumonias. Curr Clin Top Infect Dis 1991;11:1–18.

17. Moncada JV, Schachter J, Wofsy C. Prevalence of *Chlamydia trachomatis* lung infection in patients with acquired immune deficiency syndrome. J Clin Microbiol 1986; 23:986.

18. Paran H, Heimer D, Sarov I. Serological, clinical and radiologial findings in adults with bronchopulmonary infections caused by *Chlamydia trachomatis*. Isr J Med Sci 1986;22:823–827.

19. Beem MO, Saxon EM. Respiratory-tract colonization and a distinctive pneumonia syndrome in infants infected with *Chlamydia trachomatis*. N Engl J Med 1977;296:306–310.

20. Limudomporn S, Prapphal N, Nanthapisud P, Chomdez S. Afebrile pneumonia associated with chlamydial infection in infants less than 6 months of age: Initial results of a three year prospective study. Southeast Asian J Trop Med Public Health 1989;20:285–290.

21. Griffin M, Pushpanathan C, Andrews W. *Chlamydia trachomatis* pneumonitis: A case study and literature review. Pediatr Pathol 1990;10:843–852.

22. Attenburrow AA, Barker CM. Chlamydial pneumonia in the low birthweight neonate. Arch Dis Child 1985;60: 1169–1172.

23. Frommel GT, Bruhn FW, Schwartzman JD. Isolation of *Chlamydia trachomatis* from infant lung tissue. N Engl J Med 1977;296:1150–1152.

24. Harrison HR, Alexander ER, Chiang WT, et al. Experimental nasopharyngitis and pneumonia caused by *Chlamydia trachomatis* in infant baboons: Histopathologic comparison with a case in a human infant. J Infect Dis 1979;139:141–146.

25. Arth C, Von Schmidt B, Grossman M, Schachter J. Chlamydial pneumonitis. J Pediatr 1978;93:447–449.

26. Coalson JJ, Winter VT, Bass LB, Schachter J, Grubbs BG, Williams DM. *Chlamydia trachomatis* pneumonia in the immune, athymic and normal BALB mouse. Br J Exp Pathol 1987;68:399–411.

27. Paisley JW, Lauer BA, Melinkovich P, Gitterman BA, Feiten DJ, Berman S. Rapid diagnosis of *Chlamydia trachomatis* pneumonia in infants by direct immunofluorescence microscopy of nasopharyngeal secretions. J Pediatr 1986;109:653–655.

28. Hammerschlag MR, Roblin PM, Cummings C, Williams TH, Worku M, Howard LV. Comparison of enzyme immunoassay and culture for diagnosis of chlamydial conjunctivitis and respiratory infection in infants. J Clin Microbiol 1987;25:2306–2308.

29. Hammerschlag MR, Roblin PM, Gelling M, Worku M. Comparison of two enzyme immunoassays to culture for the diagnosis of chlamydial conjunctivits and respiratory infections in infants. J Clin Microbiol 1990;28:1725–1727.

30. Ohyama M, Tanaka Y, Sasaki Y, Goto A. Detection of *C. trachomatis* by *in situ* DNA hybridization: Report of two cases with neonatal pneumonia. Acta Paediatr Jpn 1990;32:319–322.

31. Grayston JT, Kuo CC, Wang SP, Altman J. A new *Chlamydia psittaci* strain, TWAR, isolated in acute respiratory tract infections. N Engl J Med 1986;315:161–168.

32. Thom DH, Grayston JT, Wang SP, Kuo CC, Altman J. *Chlamydia pneumoniae* strain TWAR, *Mycoplasma pneumoniae*, and viral infections in acute respiratory disease in a university student health clinic population. Am J Epidemiol 1990;132:248–256.

33. Grayston JT, Wang SP, Kuo CC, Campbell LA. Current knowledge on *Chlamydia pneumoniae*, strain TWAR, an important cause of pneumonia and other acute respiratory diseases. Eur J Clin Microbiol 1989;8:191–202.

34. Wreghitt TG, Barker CE, Treharne JD, Phipps JM, Robinson V, Buttery RB. A study of human respiratory tract chlamydial infections in Cambridgeshire 1986–88. Epidemiol Infect 1990;104:479–488.

35. Lillie RD. I. The pathology of psittacosis in man. NIH Bull 1933;161:1–45.

36. Rank RG, Hough A, Jr., Jacobs RF, Cohen C, Barron AL. Chlamydial pneumonitis induced in newborn guinea pigs. Infect Immun 1985;48:153–158.

37. Rasmussen S, Timms P. Detection of *Chlamydia psittaci* using DNA probes and the polymerase chain reaction. FEMS Microbiol Lett 1991;77:169–173.

38. Watson MW, Lambden PR, Clarke IN. Genetic diversity and identification of human infection by amplification of the chlamydial 60-kilodalton cysteine-rich outer membrane protein gene. J Clin Microbiol 1991;29:1188–1193.

39. Holland SM, Gaydos CA, Quinn TC. Detection and differentiation of *Chlamydia trachomatis*, *Chlamydia psittaci*, and *Chlamydia pneumoniae* by DNA amplification. J Infect Dis 1990;162:984–987.

40. Hackstadt T. The role of lipopolysaccharides in the virulence of *Coxiella burnetii*. Ann NY Acad Sci 1990;590: 27–32.

41. Sawyer LA, Fishbein DB, McDade JE. Q fever: Current concepts. Rev Infect Dis 1987;9:935–946.

42. Pinsky RL, Fishbein DB, Greene CR, Gensheimer KF. An outbreak of cat-associated Q fever in the United States. J Infect Dis 1991;164:202–204.

43. Marrie TJ. Acute Q fever. In: Marrie TJ, ed. Q Fever. Boca Raton: CRC Press, 1990:125–160.

44. Raoult D. Host factors in the severity of Q fever. Ann NY Acad Sci 1990;590:33–38.

45. Peirce TH, Yucht SC, Gorin AB, Jordan GW, Tesluk H, Lillington GA. Q fever pneumonitis. Diagnosis by transbronchoscopic lung biopsy. West J Med 1979;130:453–455.

46. Walker DH. Pathology of Q fever. In: Walker DH, ed. Biology of rickettsial diseases, Vol II. Boca Raton: CRC Press, 1988:17–27.

47. Janigan DT, Marrie TJ. Pathology of Q fever pneumonia. In: Marrie TJ, ed. Q Fever. Boca Raton: CRC Press, 1990:161–170.

48. Janigan DT, Marrie TJ. An inflammatory pseudotumor of the lung in Q fever pneumonia. N Engl J Med 1983;308:86–88.

49. Walker DH, Peacock MG. Laboratory diagnosis of rickettsial diseases. In: Walker DH, ed. Biology of rickettsial diseases, Vol. II. Boca Raton: CRC Press, 1988:135–155.

50. Peter O, Dupuis G, Peacock MG, Burgdorfer W. Comparison of enzyme-linked immunosorbent assay and complement fixation and indirect fluorescent-antibody tests for detection of Coxiella burnetii antibody. J Clin Microbiol 1987;25:1063–1067.

51. Donohue JF. Lower respiratory tract involvement in Rocky Mountain spotted fever. Arch Intern Med 1980;140:223–227.

52. Kaplowitz LG, Fischer JJ, Sparling PF. Rocky Mountain spotted fever: A clinical dilemma. Curr Clin Top Infect Dis 1981;2:89–108.

53. Walker DH, Crawford CG, Cain BG. Rickettsial infection of the pulmonary microcirculation: The basis for interstitial pneumonitis in Rocky Mountain spotted fever. Hum Pathol 1980;11:263–272.

54. Raoult D, Walker DH. Rickettsia rickettsii and other spotted fever group rickettsiae (Rocky Mountain spotted fever and other spotted fevers). In: Mandell GL, Douglas RG, Jr., Bennett JE, eds. Principles and practice of infectious diseases, 3d Ed. New York: Churchill Livingston, 1990:1465–1471.

55. Walker DH, Gear JHS. Correlation of the distribution of Rickettsia conorii, microscopic lesions, and clinical features in South African tick bite fever. Am J Trop Med Hyg 1985;34:361–371.

56. Walker DH, Herrero-Herrero JI, Ruiz-Beltran R, Bullon-Sopelana A, Ramos-Hidalgo A. The pathology of fatal Mediterranean spotted fever. Am J Clin Pathol 1987;87:669–672.

57. Dumler JS, Taylor JP, Walker DH. Clinical and laboratory features of murine typhus in south Texas, 1980 through 1987. JAMA 1991;266:1365–1370.

58. Walker DH, Parks FM, Betz TG, Taylor JP, Muehlberger JW. Histopathology and immunohistologic demonstration of the distribution of Rickettsia typhi in fatal murine typhus. Am J Clin Pathol 1989;91:720–724.

59. Walker DH. Pathology and pathogenesis of the vasculotropic rickettsioses. In: Walker DH, ed. Biology of rickettsial diseases, Vol. I. Boca Raton: CRC Press, 1988:115–138.

60. Eng TR, Harkess JR, Fishbein DB, et al. Epidemiologic, clinical, and laboratory findings of human ehrlichiosis in the United States, 1988. JAMA 1990;264:2251–2258.

61. Dumler JS, Brouqui P, Aronson J, Taylor JP, Walker DH. Identification of ehrlichia in human tissue. N Engl J Med 1991;325:1109–1110.

CHAPTER 14

Pneumocystis Infection

Richard E. Sobonya

Pneumocystis is a microorganism that causes infection, primarily pneumonia, in immunosuppressed humans and other mammals. Both Chagas in 1909 and Carini in 1910 saw the pneumocystis organism in the lungs of experimental animals infected with trypanosomes. However, both regarded the cysts of *Pneumocystis* as part of the trypanosome's life cycle. Shortly afterward the Delanöes reviewed this material and also noted the same cyst-like organism in the lungs of Parisian sewer rats. They recognized the organism as a separate species, and proposed the name *Pneumocystis carinii* for this organism, describing it in the generic name (Greek: pneumōn, lung: kystis, "cyst") and honoring Carini in the specific designation. At this time *Pneumocystis* was not recognized as a cause of human disease, although Chagas probably had seen a case of pneumocystis pneumonia in man. Dutz has recounted the discovery of pneumocystis in detail.[1]

Is pneumocystis a fungus or a protozoan? This taxonomic controversy has extended across decades,[2,3] and the most recent evidence suggests it is a fungus. Its ribosomal RNA sequences show it to be a fungus,[4] but it lacks the protein elongation factor EF-3, which is unique to fungi.[5] The DNA content of pneumocystis nuclei is also in the range seen in protozoa.[6] Much of the difficulty in classifying *Pneumocystis* definitively stems from the inability to grow the organism continuously in culture and thus study its entire life cycle.[7] Such knowledge of pneumocystis biology would facilitate better prevention and chemotherapy of the infections it causes.

Pneumocystis, when it infects the rat, is called *Pneumocystis carinii*. Although the organism that infects man is morphologically identical to that found in the rat, some studies have indicated serologic and genetic[8] differences. It also appears that *Pneumocystis* infecting different species of mammals is fairly species specific[9] and therefore it may be imprecise to regard the human pneumocystis organism as the same species that infects the rat. Frenkel[9] has proposed naming the species *jiroveci* to honor one of the early investigators of this organism. It is easiest to refer to the organism simply as pneumocystis, a designation embracing both human infection, usually reported as *Pneumocystis carinii,* and infection in other animals.

Infection in Man

In Europe, the aftermath of World War I brought a new form of infantile pulmonary infection. Named plasma cell interstitial pneumonia because of its characteristic histologic appearance, this disease produced chronic respiratory infection, often terminating in death, in premature or severely malnourished young infants. After World War II, pneumocystis infection in orphanages became epidemic. In the decade between 1942 and 1951, investigators repeatedly noted an association between this pneumonia and the presence of pneumocystis, eventually concluding that pneumocystis was the causative organism.[10] In 1956 the first case of pneumocystis pneumonia in the United States was reported.[11] Gajdusek[12] has extensively reviewed this form of pneumoncystis infection. The clinical picture in infants is subacute, with initial symptoms of poor feeding, tachypnea, and decreased activity, progressing to dyspnea and cyanosis within 1-2 weeks of onset of the illness. Fever is not a prominent part of the illness. Approximately one-quarter of the affected infants die, and recovery in the others is prolonged.

Virtually all other patients who develop pneumocystis pneumonia can be regarded as having compromised immune status from any of several causes.[13] The disease in these patients, while producing similar symptoms to those in infants, may progress much more rapidly, depending on the immune competence of the host. Fever, cough, and dyspnea are the most common symptoms. Chest radiographs typically show alveolar infiltrates, but other patterns of disease may be seen.[14] Person-to-person transmission of pneumocystis presumably can occur following close contact, but this route of infection has not been proven.[14] Pneumocystis pneumonia is quite rare[15] in the healthy individual, and patients in apparent good health who develop pneumocystis pneumonia should be investigated for underlying disease. The spectrum of immunocompromised patients at particular risk of developing pneumocystis infection includes children with congenital immune deficiencies; patients with acquired immunosuppression, including acquired immune deficiency syndrome (AIDS); patients being treated for malignant neoplasms; and patients on immunosuppressive therapy following organ transplantation. Corticosteroid therapy itself is sufficient to allow the development of pneumocystis pneumonia, but usually cytotoxic drugs also have been administered.[16,17]

Typical forms of congenital immune deficiency associated with pneumocystis infection include agammaglobulinemia and hypogammaglobulinemia, severe combined immunodeficiency, and similar immune deficiencies.[18,19] Patients with either humoral (B-cell) or cell-mediated (T-cell) immune deficiencies are at risk for developing pneumocystis pneumonia. In acquired forms of immunodeficiency, cellular immunity usually is most severely affected, and decreased humoral immunity secondary to impaired T-cell function is often present as well.

Patients being treated for cancer, particularly lymphoma or leukemia, are prone to develop pneumocystis infection.[20] Pneumocystis infection is particularly frequent in children with acute lymphocytic leukemia or lymphosarcoma.[21,22] In one large autopsy study of children dying with malignant neoplasms,[22] 32 of 362 (9%) with lymphoreticular system neoplasia had pneumocystis at autopsy, while only 2 of 134 (1%) of those with soft-tissue, osseous, or neural tumors were infected with pneumocystis. The association of pneumocystis pneumonia with malignant neoplasms in adults shows a similar pattern: The incidence of pneumocystis pneumonia is much higher in adults with hematologic or lymphatic neoplasms, although cases associated with solid tumors have been reported.[23]

Pneumocystis infection may complicate renal transplantation.[24] The incidence of pneumocystis pneumonia in patients with transplanted kidneys is low, being 1.5% in one study.[25] However, pneumocystis pneumonia was found in 17% (9 of 54) patients dying after renal transplantation.[26] Infection with pneumocystis has been seen after orthotopic liver[27] and cardiac transplantation.[28,29] Pneumocystis pneumonia can be prevented in patients who have undergone bone marrow transplantation by prophylactic antibiotic therapy.[30] The immunosuppressive therapy given to forestall rejection is believed to suppress the host's T-lymphocyte response, allowing pneumocystis to proliferate.

The recognition of pneumocystis pneumonia in apparently healthy young men brought the acquired immunodeficiency syndrome (AIDS) to medical attention[31] and led to a sustained, striking increase in cases of pneumocystis infection. Thus, the AIDS epidemic became also a pneumocystis epidemic. In 280 patients with fatal AIDS,[32–39] 53% developed pneumocystis pneumonia that was diagnosed pre mortem. Such patients often initially respond to therapy during life, only to experience recrudescence of the disease after apparent cure or have residual pneumocystis infection at autopsy. Other cases of pneumocystis pneumonia are discovered at autopsy. The incidence of pulmonary pneumocystis infection at autopsy in patients with AIDS is variable, and reflects the extensiveness of treatment for this organism during life. In the same series of patients dying of AIDS mentioned previously,[32–39] 35% had either recurrent, progressive, or newly discovered pneumocystis at autopsy.

Subclinical infection with pneumocystis clearly exists.[40] Pneumocystis infection may persist in patients with AIDS despite apparent adequate therapy with trimethoprim-sulfamethoxozole or pentamadine, the drugs that are effective in most cases.[41,42] The organism similarly may persist in other immunosuppressed patients. Serologic testing in children has demonstrated the presence of antibodies to pneumocystis in approximately two-thirds of children by the age of 4 years.[43] Thus it is likely that most persons are exposed to pneumocystis early in life and acquire some immunity but no clinical disease. However, serologic studies of pneumocystis in humans presently are of only limited diagnostic use.[44] In one study,[45] elevations in antibody titer were not diagnostically helpful in detecting acute pneumocystis infection. Use of counterimmunoelectrophoresis to detect circulating antigen also does not yet appear to be of general clinical use.[46]

Because of inability to culture the organism and difficulties in identifying small numbers of pneumocystis in tissue using histologic means, it is difficult to document the presence of pneumocystis in the lungs of normal persons. However, pneumocystis is consistently found in the lungs of healthy rats and produces no disease until the rat's immune system is impaired.[46–48] At least some humans appear to be asymptomatic carriers of pneumocystis, and they may develop pneumocystis pneumonia if immunosuppressed or may pass the organism to a susceptible person.

Pathology

The gross appearance of pneumocystis pneumonia is not diagnostic, and may resemble bacterial pneumonia or diffuse alveolar damage. The alveolar parenchyma shows areas of a pale-grey to pale-tan, firm infiltrate that obliterates air spaces. The infiltrate may be patchy or progress to lobar or whole lung involvement (Fig. 14–1). A typical bronchopneumonic pattern is not common. Milder degrees of pneumocystis infection may produce no gross changes in tissues. When pneumocystis is associated with the histologic pattern of diffuse alveolar damage, the lung may be more pinkish-grey to focally hemorrhagic, and the process will be quite diffuse.

The histologic alterations in the lungs induced by pneumocystis are quite variable.[49,50] In extremely immunosuppressed hosts or in early infection, alterations may be minimal with only slightly increased numbers of alveolar macrophages, perhaps a few shreds of fibrin and cellular debris, and some slightly increased interstitial cellularity and capillary congestion (Fig. 14–2). Despite the lack of a significant inflammatory response as seen with most other infections, one cannot rule out pneumocystis infection without appropriate histologic stains. The more typical appearance of pneumocystis pneumonia in an immunosuppressed patient shows a foamy alveolar exudate consisting of clusters of rounded, clear spaces within eosinophilic material (Fig. 14–3). Tiny basophilic dots may be seen in the clear spaces. This vacuolated material may fill alveoli extensively. The frothy or foamy alveolar exudate is quite suggestive of pneumocystis infection, but this appearance may be mimicked by a reticular distribution of alveolar fibrin, by collections of foamy macrophages, and sometimes by other cellular debris. The blue staining dots mentioned above give pneumocysts a basophilic hue in contrast to the more monotonous eosinophilia of fibrin or hyaline membranes. Ultrastructural studies have shown that this vacuolated material is clusters of mature cysts, which do not stain well with hematoxylin and eosin, surrounded by cyst filopodia and debris, which are eosinophilic. Alveolar septa are surfaced by hyperplastic alveolar type II lining cells, and the alveolar interstitium contains a sparse-to-moderate infiltrate of histiocytes, plasma cells, and lymphocytes. Increased numbers of macrophages, many of which have a finely vacuolated, voluminous cytoplasm, may be seen in alveolar spaces. Certain histologic features associated with many other opportunistic coinfections, such as necrosis with cavitation, hemorrhage, angiitis, and airways inflammation, are less common in pneumocystis pneumonia, but occasionally occur.[51]

The entity originally described as plasma cell interstitial pneumonia[10] and now known to be caused by pneumocystis is rarely seen at present. That form of interstitial pneumonia showed a more cellular interstitial plasma cell and lymphocyte infiltrate with the typical alveolar foamy exudate containing the pneumocystis organisms.

Diffuse alveolar damage is the pathologic term for the pattern of pulmonary injury that consists of the hyaline membranes, variable interstitial inflammation, increased numbers of alveolar macrophages, and type II pneumocyte hyperplasia. While the causes of this form of acute lung injury are legion, in some cases this histologic pattern has been associated with the presence of pneumocystis.[52] Pneumocystis may be responsible for the diffuse alveolar damage in such cases, such as is shown in Fig. 14–4.

Granulomatous responses to pneumocystis have been described,[49,51,53–56] on occasion in cases in which the organism disseminates outside the lung. Granulomatous pneumocystis pneumonia is shown in Fig. 14–5. Pneumocystis has even been described as the cause of a solitary nodule in the lung consisting of a granulomatous reaction at the periphery and central fibrosis with foci of necrosis containing the pneumocystis organisms.[55] This solitary granuloma was also surrounded by small sarcoid-like satellite granulomas. While granulomatous inflammation is an atypical form of pneumocystis infection, one should still consider pneumocystis as a possible cause of pulmonary granulomas. Also, dystrophic calcification has been described in presumed longstanding cases of pneumocystis (Fig. 14–6).[57]

Typical pneumocystis infection is not associated with interstitial fibrosis in the lung. Interstitial fibrosis has been described in patients after pneumocystis infection, however, and is believed to be caused by either the injurious effects of the organism or possibly injury resulting from pentamidine therapy[51,58] (See Fig. 14–6). Treated pneumocystis infection may show variable degrees of alveolitis, and organisms may be difficult to find.

Ultrastructure

A life cycle for pneumocystis has been constructed using electron microscopic observations[59–62] as well as phase-contrast microscopy.[63] Figure 14–7 shows sev-

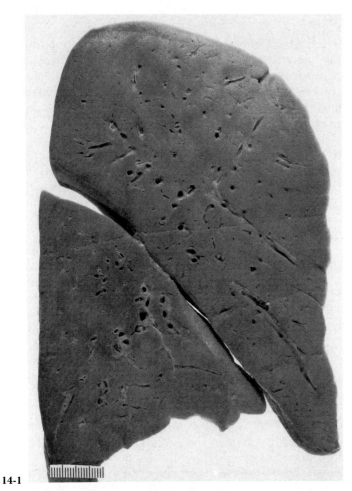

eral stages in the life cycle of pneumocystis, including a maturing trophozoite, a cyst with merozoites, and collapsed cysts. The simplest form of the organism is the trophozoite, also called the sporozoite. A trophozoite typically is amoeboid in configuration and bounded by a cell membrane called a pellicle that is 200–300Å thick; it is approximately 1–5 μm in greatest dimension. The surface of the trophozoite shows tubular extensions or filopodia. Figures 14–8 and 14–9 show trophozoites in an alveolar space, attached to type I pneumocytes. Filopodia, largely cut in transverse section, are seen in Fig. 14–9. A trophozoite contains the nucleus, nucleolus, a few mitochondria, endoplasmic reticulum, and glycogen. This organism is thought to develop into a precyst, which measures approximately 5 μm in diameter and is more ovoid in configuration. The precyst develops a thicker, trilayered wall, similar to that seen in cysts. Several masses of nucleoplasm are present. Cysts

◁ ─────────────────────────────

Fig. 14–1. Gross section of lung shows diffuse alveolar infiltrates in lung caused by pneumocystis. Scale in millimeters.

Fig. 14–2. Interstitial pneumonitis caused by pneumocystis in immunosuppressed patient. Note sparse alveolar septal inflammation and lack of exudate in alveoli. H and E, ×212.

Fig. 14–3. Interstitial pneumonitis caused by pneumocystis in child with lymphoblastic leukemia. Alveolar septal inflammation is obvious, and alveoli contain extensive frothy exudate. H and E, ×212.

14-1

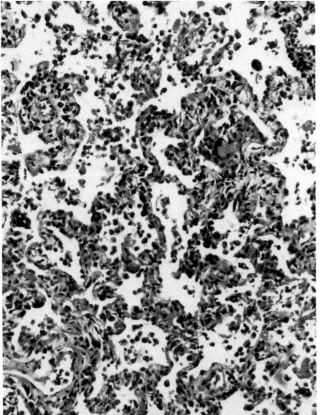

14-2

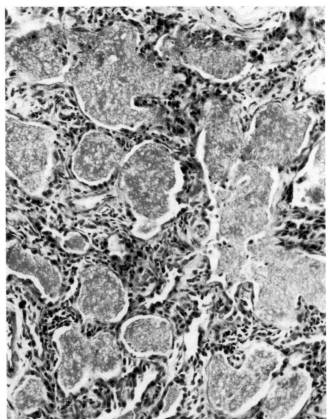

14-3

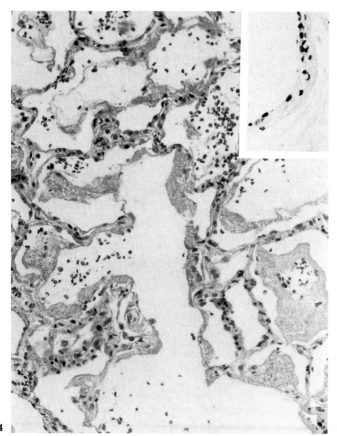

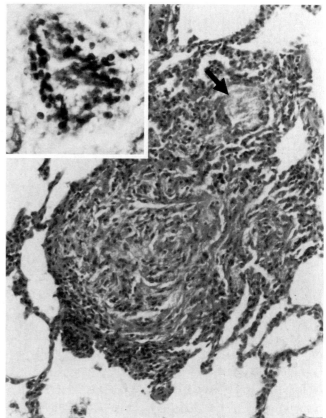

Fig. 14—4. Diffuse alveolar damage with hyaline membranes. H and E, ×212. Inset shows pneumocystis organisms in hyaline membrane. GMS, ×530.

Fig. 14—5. Loosely formed granuloma caused by pneumocystis; the bit of exudate at *arrow* contained pneumocystis organisms as shown in methenamine silver-stained inset (×600). H and E, ×212.

Fig. 14—6. Fibrosing interstitial pneumonitis within irregular dark mass of dystrophic calcification centrally. H and E, ×212.

——————————————————————————▷

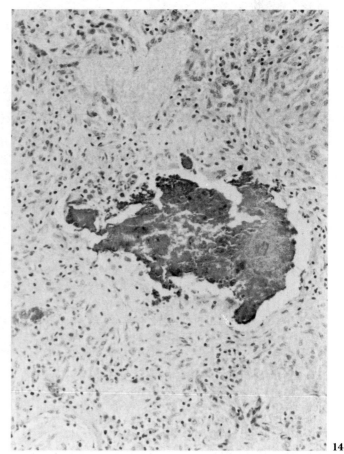

are approximately the same size but their trilayered wall shows one or two focal thickenings (Figs. 14–7 and 14–10). Several nuclear masses become defined, and additional structures referred to as intracystic bodies or merozoites eventually develop. Caution is needed in using the term introcystic body as it has been used for both merozoites with the cysts and for the focal cyst wall paired thickenings. Here it is used solely to describe merozoites. Up to eight intracystic bodies ranging from 1 to 2 μm in diameter may be found. These bodies develop a cell membrane that is sometimes continuous with the endoplasmic reticulum; they also have a nuclear mass and cytoplasmic organelles, as seen in trophozoites. The intracystic bodies develop into extracystic trophozoites following rupture of the cyst. In addition

479

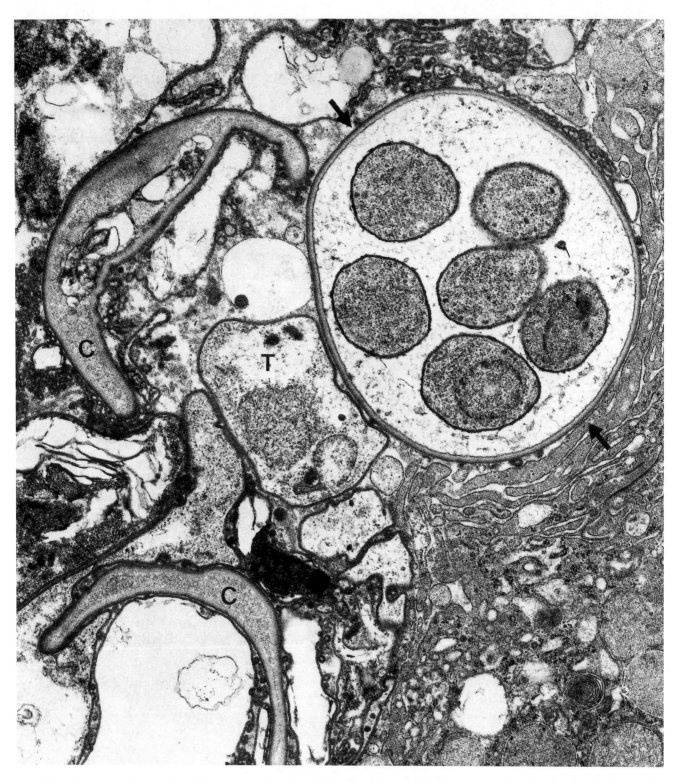

Fig. 14–7. Electron micrograph of alveolar exudate in AIDS patient with pneumocystis pneumonia. Cyst containing six merozoites is seen between *arrows*. Next to it is maturing trophozoite (T) without filopodia. Two collapsed cysts (C) are also present. Note upper cyst has discrete area of capsular thickening corresponding to darkly staining bodies seen with Gomori's methenamine silver (GMS) stain (see also Fig. 14–10). Uranyl acetate, lead citrate. ×6,400.

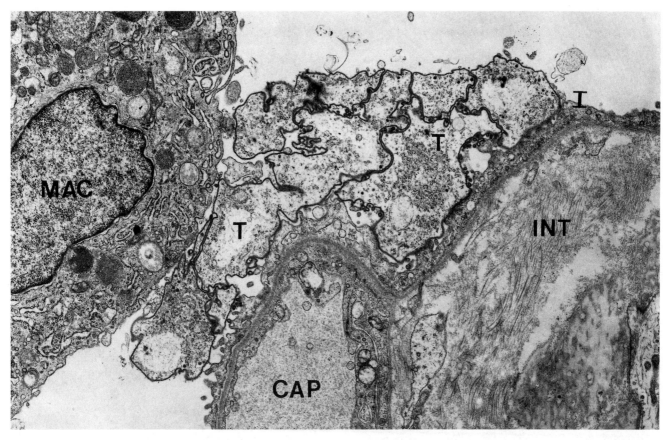

Fig. 14–8. Electron micrograph of several trophozoites (T) attached to type I pneumocyte epithelium of the alveolar wall (I). Abbrevations: macrophage, MAC; alveolar interstitium, INT; alveolar capillary, CAP. Uranyl acetate, lead citrate, ×4,100.

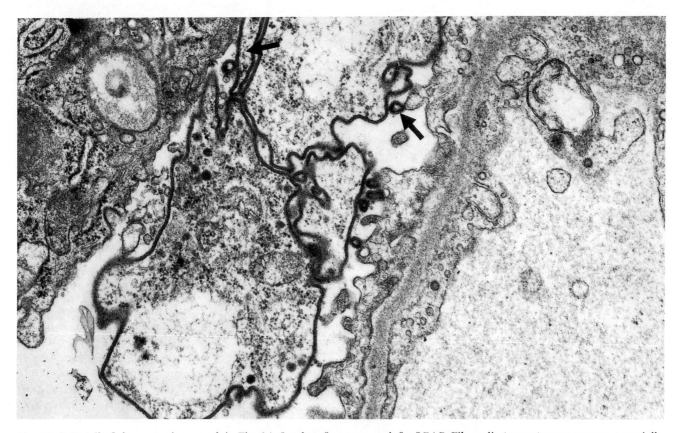

Fig. 14–9. Detail of electron micrograph in Fig. 14–8, taken from area to left of CAP. Filopodia (*arrows*) are apparent, especially in conjunction with type I pneumocyte epithelium. Uranyl acetate, lead citrate ×10,500.

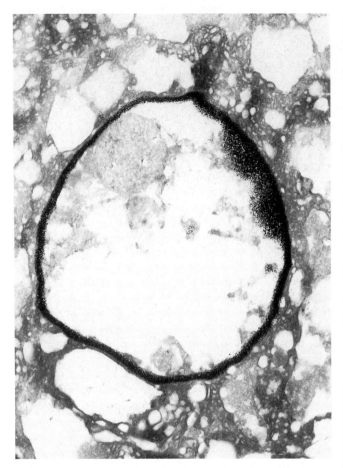

Fig. 14–10. Ultrastructure of pneumocystis cyst shows focal capsular thickenings, which appear as paired darkly staining foci with routine methenamine silver stains. Periodic acid–methenamine silver; uranyl acetate, lead citrate, ×20,500. (Courtesy of John C. Watts, M.D. Reprinted by permission of Raven Press from Watts JC, Chandler FW. Am J Surg Pathol 1985;9:744-751.

to the life cycle just described, it is likely that a trophozoite reproduces by binary fission several times before developing into a precyst.

Light Microscopy

Identification of pneumocystis in tissue is based on demonstration of the organism by histochemical stains. Routine hemotoxylin and eosin (H and E) stains do not demonstrate the organism. The bubbly or frothy intraalveolar exudate associated with the organism is virtually diagnostic of pneumocystis infection if typical and abundant. However, often this foamy material is scant or not characteristic.[64] The recommended histochemical stain for the diagnosis of pneumocystis infection is Grocott's modification[65] of Gomori's methe-

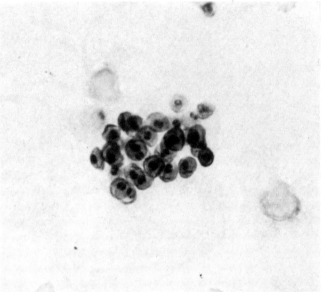

Fig. 14–11. Cluster of pneumocystis cysts in cytocentrifuge preparation of bronchoalveolar lavage fluid; note paired, comma-shaped cyst wall thickenings. GMS, ×1,355.

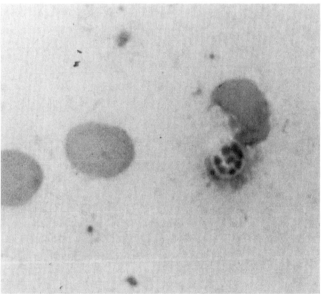

Fig. 14–12. Imprint shows eight intracystic bodies of pneumocystis in clear space, which is the nonstaining cyst; red blood cells in field indicate size. Giemsa, ×1,500.

namine silver[64,66,67] (GMS), which shows the organisms as illustrated in Fig. 14–11. This stain demonstrates the cyst wall but does not stain trophozoites or merozoites. Many cysts will show a dark-staining single structure or more commonly a pair of comma-like structures. These have also been called dark bodies, parenthesis- or apostrophe-like bodies, or darkly stained foci.[67] These struc-

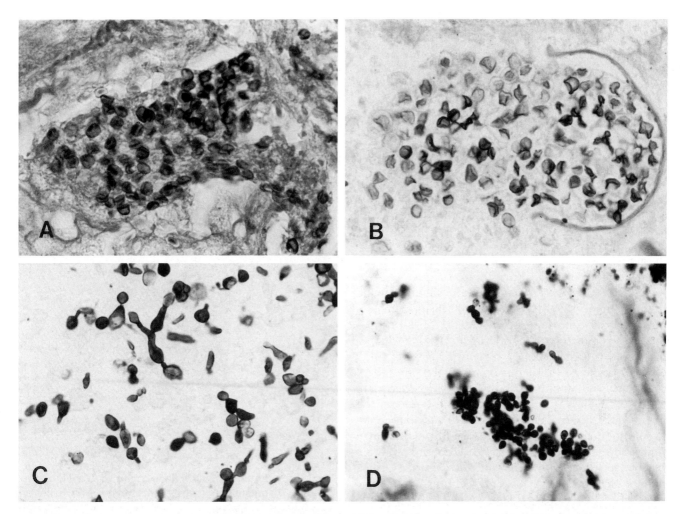

Fig. 14–13 A–D. Comparison of pneumocystis cysts and similar organisms in tissue. **A.** Pneumocystis. **B.** Ruptured spherule of *Coccidioides immitis* with endospores. **C.** Budding yeasts of *Candida* species. **D.** Yeasts of *Histoplasma capsulatum*. Some yeast forms vary in size, and some *Histoplasma capsulatum* may be as much as twice as large as pictured. **A-D,** GMS, ×846.

tures have been shown to represent foci of thickening in the cyst wall,[67] as illustrated in Fig. 14–11, and this appearance is diagnostic of the pneumocystis organism. Trophozoites, the free nonencysted form of the organism, are not stained. Giemsa or Diff-Quik stains demonstrate trophozoites and intracystic bodies but do not stain the cyst wall unless modified.[68] This clear space (the nonstaining cyst) with the eight intracystic bodies, a feature seen especially well on imprints, also is diagnostic of pneumocystis (Fig. 14–12). Routine Gomori's methenamine silver (GMS) stains require several hours to perform, but rapid GMS stains have been developed,[69–71] and GMS stains for pneumocystis now can be done within 1 h. Various modifications of the Giemsa stain can be used, such as that recommended by Dutz.[1] Periodic acid-Schiff stains (PAS) also stain the cyst walls of pneumocystis a magenta color, and intracystic bodies stain blue. However, this stain does not show the structure of the organism as well as GMS, and slides stained

by PAS are harder to screen. Toluidine blue 0 also stains the cysts well, and is recommended by some.[66] Comparison of the efficacy of these various stains[72] has not demonstrated that any one has a clear advantage over others, although the GMS stain also defines fungi well.

Organisms Confused with Pneumocystis

Pneumocystis seen in GMS-stained tissues or imprints may be confused with several small, yeast-like structures. In Fig. 14–13, pneumocystis is compared with several fungi. The cysts of pneumocystis are 3.5–5.0 μm in diameter and have a uniformly moderately thick wall. Intact cysts appear round to oval, but after they have discharged their intracystic bodies they appear collapsed and irregular or cup shaped. When using GMS stains to diagnose pneumocystis, it is extremely important to recognize the darkly stained capular focus or foci (intracystic bodies) in some of the cysts. Fungi of the genera *Candida* and *Torulopsis* may resemble pneumocystis in both size and shape.[23,73] If the organism buds, it can then be identified as a yeast. However, often the organisms are few and budding is not seen. The presence of darkly stained foci eliminates these fungi from consideration. Young et al.[73] have emphasized the ability of such fungi to mimic pneumocystis and coined the phrase "methenamine masquerade."

In areas where coccidioidomycosis is endemic, the endospores of *Coccidioides immitis* may imitate pneumocystis closely, especially in smears or in the debris of transbronchial biopsies. They are approximately the same size and do not bud, but the endospores do not contain darkly stained foci. One should look for the larger spherules with or without endospores to confirm the impression of coccidioidomycosis, but such spherules may not be seen. Other fungi, such as the yeast forms of *Histoplasma capsulatum*, are slightly smaller than pneumocystis. Differentiation of histoplasma and pneumocystis can be a problem. Again the budding of the yeast is a differential criterion.[49] Histoplasma also may show a darkly stained focus with silver stains.[67] Cryptosporidia are also approximately the same size as pneumocystis, but pulmonary infection with this organism is quite rare.[74] Cryptosporidium is acid fast and again lacks internal structure. In overstained GMS preparations, red blood cells and the nuclei of neutrophils and macrophages may also stain positively. Staining artifacts should be apparent from careful examination of the section. A positive pneumocystis control should be when staining tissues with GMS for pneumocystis.[64] Familiarity with pneumocystis morphology greatly facilitates identification of the organism, and regular scanning of the positive controls produces such familiarity.

Occurrence of Other Infections

Frequently, pneumocystis is not the only pulmonary pathogen identified in biopsies. Cytomegalovirus is the most common opportunistic pathogen associated with pneumocystis infection. An electron microscopic study has shown cytomegalovirus within pneumocystis organisms, suggesting that pneumocystis itself may serve as a reservoir or intermediate host for cytomegalovirus.[75] Pneumocystis infection has been associated with a wide variety of bacterial fungal, viral, and mycobacterial infections, particularly in patients with AIDS.[32–39] The type of opportunistic infections occurring with pneumocystis may depend on local factors. In the desert regions of Southwestern United States and Mexico, coccidioidomycosis occurs commonly with pneumocystis in patients with AIDS,[76] but this association is uncommon in other geographic areas. Pneumocystis in-

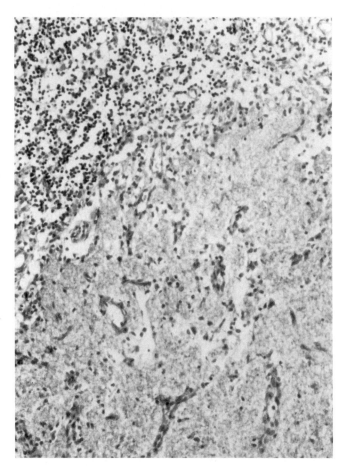

Fig. 14–14. Pulmonary lymph node largely replaced by foamy infiltrate of pneumocystis organisms. There is virtually no inflammatory response at junction of infiltrate with lymph node tissue. H and E, ×212.

fection also is associated commonly with Kaposi's sarcoma in AIDS.

Extrapulmonary Infection

Systemic dissemination of pneumocystis is uncommon,[53,57] but is being recognized with increasing frequency.[78–81] A common site for extrapulmonary pneumocystis is the pulmonary lymph nodes. Here the organism may be associated with a necrotizing, abscess-like, or granulomatous inflammatory reaction, and sometimes it appears without reaction. The typical foamy material may be seen (Fig. 14–14). Disseminated pneumocystis typically involves vertebral bone marrow, spleen, and liver, although other organs may also be involved. The histology is that of a poorly formed granulomatous response associated with areas of necrosis, or deposits of foamy material. Such dissemination usually takes place along with significant pulmonary involvement and the diagnosis therefore is facilitated by identifying the respiratory pneumocystis infection and suspecting dissemination. The organisms in extrapulmonary sites resemble those seen in the lung. Pneumocystis pneumonia can extend to involve the pleura, producing pleuritis and pneumothorax.[82–84] The organisms may then be recovered in pleural fluid.[84] However, most cases of pneumocystis pneumonia do not have pleural involvement.

Making the Diagnosis

The diagnosis of pneumocystis infection rests entirely on morphologic demonstration of the organism. Thus, to diagnose pneumocystis infection in a patient with pulmonary infiltrates, a representative sample of the alveolar exudate must be obtained in a way that causes the least harm to the patient. Pneumocystis occurring in immunosuppressed patients without AIDS is associated with a much smaller burden of pneumocystis organisms than occur in AIDS patients,[85] and studies in these patients indicated sputum examination for pneumocystis was not useful. However, examination of sputum from AIDS patients with pneumonia using histochemical stains or monoclonal antibodies identifies the organism in 15%–95% of cases; most series report success of about 70%.[86–91]

Use of hypertonic saline to induce sputum in patients without spontaneous production, experience in using the identification methods, and severity of disease can influence the success of the procedure.

Virtually all cases of pneumocystis infection can be diagnosed by bronchoscopy with a combination of bronchial washing or bronchoalveolar lavage (BAL), bronchial brushing, and transbronchial biopsy.[107–113] The concentrated sample from BAL is a particularly good source of pneumocystis organisms, and with rapid silver staining can lead to a diagnosis within an hour. This technique washes organisms out of alveoli, and they can be seen readily on GMS-stained smears of the concentrated sediment. Cytocentrifuge preparations are recommended for silver staining of bronchoalveolar lavages (see Fig. 14–11). Similarly, bronchial washings and brushings frequently demonstrate the organism.

Rapid cytologic diagnosis of pneumocystis has been improved with the recognition that the foamy alveolar casts seen in Papanicolaou- (Pap-) stained sputum or bronchoalveolar lavage fluid are diagnostic for the organism.[92–97] These casts (Fig. 14–15) are the same as the alveolar material seen histologically, consisting of masses of cysts surrounded by trophozooites and debris. The foamy casts are typically eosinophilic, and the

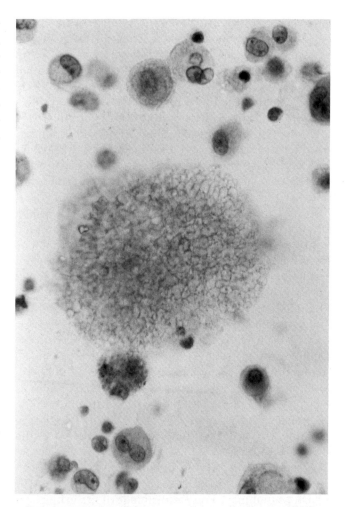

Fig. 14–15. Foamy alveolar cast of pneumocystis from bronchoalveolar lavage. Some clear spaces have central dot. Macrophages indicate size. Papanicolaou stain ×580.

clear spaces, which are nonstaining cysts, may contain basophilic dots. Mucin, especially admixed with red blood cell ghosts, may mimic this configuration, as may oral debris in a sputum sample. Of course, lack of foamy casts does not exclude pneumocystis. A histochemical stain such as GMS is recommended for confirmation and is useful for evaluation of fungal disease as well. Occasionally the GMS stain will fail to demonstrate organisms that are convincingly seen on Pap stains.[96] Thus the Papanicolaou stain is a reliable rapid stain for pneumocystis (as well as viral inclusions, malignant cells, and some fungi) and is well suited for diagnostic use outside usual laboratory hours.[96]

Monoclonal antibodies to pneumocystis cysts are commercially available and demonstrate the organism well[98–104] in either sputum or bronchoalveolar lavage fluid. Most antibodies are fluorescein labeled, but some use the immunoperoxidase technique. However, we

have seen cases with small organism burdens that were
negative by monclonal antibody studies, but a few organisms were seen with Pap or GMS stains, as well as the
converse. Such problems occur especially with small
organism burdens. The use of monoclonal antibody
techniques in addition to Pap- and GMS-stained slides
appears to maximize the identification of pneumocystis.
Pneumocystis itself is autofluorescent when stained
by the Pap method and examined with ultraviolet
light.[105–106] This method may be useful in confirming
the presence of pneumocystis in Pap-stained slides but
does not replace GMS staining.

Recently, amplification of *Pneumocystis carinii*-specific
DNA by the polymerase chain reaction (PCR) technique
has been applied to bronchoalveolar lavage specimens
to aid in the diagnosis of pneumocystis. In one study the
results of GMS staining were confirmed and a small
number of GMS-negative cases clinically thought to be
pneumocystis were positive with PCR.[114] Another study
failed to show a major advantage over morphologic
techniques.[115] Low levels of pneumocystis may be de-
tectible by PCR at a time when the patient has no clinical
pneumonia. No pneumocystis is detected by PCR following treatment of pneumocystis pneumonia, suggesting that reinfection in such patients is exogenous. The
circumstances for optimal use of PCR in diagnosing
pneumocystis infection should become evident over the
next several years.

A representative transbronchial biopsy not only can
show the organism but may show other infections or
reactions to injury. The disadvantage of tissue biopsy is
the time needed for adequate histologic processing of
the tissue. Transbronchial lung biopsies should be sampled at several levels, because the diagnostic lesion may
be quite focal (see Chapter 1). A satisfactory technique is
to examine a ribbon of sections that are stained by H
and E at multiple levels spaced throughout the biopsy.
Several slides of unstained sections adjacent to each
level are retained for additional stains.

In all possible cases of pneumocystis, the GMS stain is
performed with the initial H and E stains. Imprints
from transbronchial biopsies are not necessary because
other material such as brushings, washings, or BALs are
being studied. Making imprints from such a small
biopsy is likely to crush the biopsy and make it impossible to interpret. The coordinated analysis of the samples of pulmonary tissues and secretions obtained by
bronchoscopy allows the rapid and accurate identification of pneumocystis in nearly all cases. In unusual
forms of pneumocystis infection, such as nodular infiltrates, or in relatively indolent infection with a low
number of organisms, open lung biopsy may be needed
for definitive diagnosis.

References

1. Dutz W. Pneumocystis carinii pneumonia. Pathol Annu 1970;5:309–341.
2. Hughs WT. Pneumocystis carinii: Taxing taxonomy. Eur J Epidemiol 1989;5:265–269.
3. Walzer PD. Immunopathogenesis of Pneumocystis carinii infection. J Lab Clin Med 1991;118(3);206–216.
4. Edman JC, Kovacs JC, Masur H, Santi DV, Elwood HJ, Sogin ML. Ribosomal RNA sequence shows *Pneumocystis carinii* to be a member of the fungi. Nature (London) 1988;334(6182):519–522.
5. Jackson HC, Colthurst D, Hancock V, Marriott MS, Tuite MF. No detection of characteristic fungal protein elongation factor EF-3 in *Pneumocystis carinii*. J Infect Dis 1991;132(3):675–677.
6. Gradus MS, Gilmore M, Lerner M. An isolation method of DNA from *Pneumocystis carinii:* A quantitative comparison to known parasitic protozoan DNA. Comp Biochem Physiol 1988;89(1):75–77.
7. Smith JW, Bartlett MS. In vitro cultivation of pneumocystis. In: Young LS, ed. Pneumocystis carinii pneumonia. New York: Marcel Dekker, 1984:107–137.
8. Sinclair K, Wakefield AE, Banerji S, Hopkin JM. *Pneumocystis carinii* organisms derived from rat and human hosts are genetically distinct. Mol Biochem Parasitol 1991;45(1)183–184.
9. Frenkel JK. *Pneumocystis jiroveci* n. sp. from man: Morphology, physiology, and immunology in relation to pathology. Natl Cancer Inst Monogr 1976;43:13–27.
10. Gajdusek DC. Pneumocystis carinii: Etiologic agent of interstitial plasma cell pneumonia and premature and young infants. Pediatrics 1957;19:543–565.
11. Dauzier G, Willis T, Barnett RN. Pneumocystis carinii in an infant. Am J Clin Pathol 1956;26:787–793.
12. Gajdusek DC. Pneumocystis carinii as the cause of human disease: Historical perspective and magnitude of the problem. Introductory remarks. Natl Cancer Inst Monogr 1976;43:1–10.
13. Young LS. Clinical aspects of pneumocystosis in man: epidemiology, clinical manifestations, diagnostic approaches, and sequelae. In: Young LS, ed. Pneumocystis carinii pneumonia. New York: Marcel Dekker, 1984: 139–174.
14. Hughes WT. Pneumocystis pneumonia: A plague of the immunosuppressed. Johns Hopkins Med J 1978; 184–192.
15. Jacobs JL, Libby DM, Winters RA, Gelmont DM, Fried ED, Hartman BJ, Laurence J. A cluster of Pneumocystis carinii pneumonia in adults without predisposing illnesses. N Engl J Med 1991;324:246–250.
16. Burke BA, Good RA. Pneumocystis carinii infection. Medicine (Baltimore) 1973;52:23–51.
17. Robbins JB. Pneumocystis carinii pneumonitis: A review. Pediatr Res 1967;1:131–158.
18. Walzer PD, Schultz MG. Western KA, Robbins JB. Pneumocystis carinii pneumonia and primary immune deficiency diseases. Natl Cancer Inst Monogr 1976;

43:65–72.

19. Richmond DD, Zamvil, Remington JS. Recurrent pneumocystis carinii pneumonia in a child with hypogammaglobulinemia. Am J Dis Child 1973;125:102–103.

20. Hamlin WB. *Pneumocystis carinii.* JAMA 1968;204:171–172.

21. Johnson HD, Johnson WW. Pneumocystis carinii pneumonia with children with cancer: Diagnosis and treatment. JAMA 1970;214:1067–1078.

22. Price RA, Hughes WT. Histopathology of pneumocystis carinii infestation and infection in malignant disease in childhood. Hum Pathol 1974;5:737–752.

23. Rosen P, Armstrong D, Ramos C. *Pneumocystis carinii* pneumonia. Am J Med 1972;53:428–436.

24. Rifkind D, Faris TD, Hill RB. *Pneumocystis carinii* pneumonia. Studies on the diagnosis and treatment. Ann Intern Med 1966;65:943–956.

25. Murphy JF, McDonald FD, Dawson M, Reite A, Turcotte J, Fekety R, Jr. Factors affecting the frequency of infection in renal transplant recipients. Arch Intern Med 1976;136:670–677.

26. Washer GF, Schröter GPJ, Starzl TE, Weil R. Causes of death after kidney transplantation. JAMA 1983;250:49–54.

27. Fulginiti VA, Scribner R, Groth CG, et al. Infections in recipients of liver homografts. N Engl J Med 1968;279:619–626.

28. Copeland JG, Mammana RB, Fuller JK, Campbell DW, McAleer MJ, Sailer JA. Heart transplantation: Four year's experience with conventional immunosuppression. JAMA 1984;251:1563–1566.

29. Pomerance A, Stovin PGI. Heart transplant pathology: The British experience. J Clin Pathol 1985;38:146–159.

30. Winston DJ, Gale RP, Meyer DV, Young LS. Infectious complications of human bone marrow transplantation. Medicine (Baltimore) 1979;58:1–31.

31. Masur H, Michelis MA, Greene JB, et al. An outbreak of community-acquired pneumocystis carinii pneumonia: Initial manifestation of cellular immune dysfunction. N Engl J Med 1981;305:1431–1438.

32. Reichert CM, O'Leary TJ, Levens DL, Simrell CR, Macher AM. Autopsy pathology in the acquired immune deficiency syndrome. Am J Pathol 1983;112:357–382.

33. Guarda LA, Luna MA, Smith JL, Jr., Mansell PW, Gyorkey F, Roca AN. Acquired immune deficiency syndrome: postmortem findings. Am J Clin Pathol 1984;81:549–557.

34. Hui AN, Koss MM, Meyer PR. Necropsy findings in acquired immunodeficiency syndrome; a comparison of premortem diagnosis with postmortem findings. Hum Pathol 1984;15:670–676.

35. Nash G, Fligiel S. Pathologic features of the lung in acquired immune deficiency syndrome (AIDS): An autopsy study of seventeen homosexual males. Am J Clin Pathol 1984;81:6–12.

36. Niedt GW, Schinella RA. Acquired immunodeficiency syndrome. Clinicopathologic study of 56 autopsies. Arch Pathol Lab Med 1985;109:727–734.

37. Moskowitz L, Hensley GT, Chan JC, Adams K. Immediate causes of death in acquired immunodeficiency syndrome. Arch Pathol Lab Med 1985;109:735–738.

38. Wallace JM, Hannah JB. Pulmonary disease at autopsy in patients with the acquired immunodeficiency syndrome. West J Med 1988;149:167–171.

39. McKenzie R, Travis WD, Dolan SA, et al. The causes of death in patients with human immunodeficiency virus infection: A clinical and pathologic study with emphasis on the role of pulmonary diseases. Medicine (Baltimore) 1991;70:326–343.

40. Woodward SC, Sheldon WH. Subclinical pneumocystis carinii pneumonitis in adults. Bull Johns Hopkins Hosp 1981;109:148–159.

41. Shelhamer JH, Ognibene FP, Macher AM, et al. Persistence of pneumocystis carinii in lung tissue of acquired immunodeficiency syndrome patients treated for pneumocystis pneumonia. Am Rev Respir Dis 1984;130:1161–1165.

42. DeLorenzo LJ, Maguire GP, Wormser GP, Davidian MM, Stone DJ. Persistence of pneumocystis carinii pneumonia in the acquired immune deficiency syndrome. Chest 1985;88:79–88.

43. Pifer LL, Hughes WT, Stagno S, Woods D. Pneumocystis carinii infection: Evidence for high prevalence in normal and immunosuppressed children. Pediatrics 1978;61:35–41.

44. Jameson B. Serology of pneumocystis carinii. In: Young LS, ed. Pneumocystis carinii pneumonia. New York: Marcel Dekker, 1984;97–106.

45. Meyers JD, Pifer LL, Sale GE, Thomas ED. The value of pneumocystis carinii antibody and antigen detection for diagnosis of pneumocystis carinii pneumonia after marrow transplantation. Ann Rev Respir Dis 1979;120:1283–1287.

46. Walzer PD, Young LS. Clinical relevance of animal models of pneumocystis carinii pneumonia. Diagn Microbiol Infect Dis 1984;2:11–16.

47. Frenkel JK, Good JT, Schultz JA. Latent pneumocystis infection of rats, relapse, and chemotherapy. Lab Invest 1966;15:1559–1577.

48. Lanken PN, Minda M, Pietra GG, Fishman AP. Alveolar response to experimental pneumocystis carinii pneumonia in the rat. Am J Pathol 1980;99:561–588.

49. Weber WR, Askin FB, Dehner LP. Lung biopsy in pneumocystis carinii pneumonia: a histopathologic study of typical and atypical features. Am J Clin Pathol 1977;67:11–19.

50. Hamperl H. Variants of pneumocystis pneumonia. J Pathol Bacteriol 1957;74:353–356.

51. Travis WD, Pittaluga S, Lipschik GY. Atypical pathologic manifestations of Pneumocystis carinii pneumonia in the acquired immune deficiency syndrome. Am J Surg Pathol 1990;14(7):615–625.

52. Askin FB, Katzenstein A-LA. Pneumocystis infection masquerading as diffuse alveolar damage. Chest 1981;79:420–422.

53. LeGolvan DP, Heidelberger KP. Disseminated, granulomatous pneumocystis carinii pneumonia. Arch Pathol Lab Med 1973;95:344–348.

54. Crucikshank B. Pulmonary granulomatous pneumocystosis following renal transplantation. Am J Clin Pathol 1975;63:384–390.

55. Hartz JW, Geisinger KR, Scharyj M, Muss HB. Granulomatous pneumocystosis presenting as a solitary pulmonary nodule. Arch Pathol Lab Med 1985;102:466–469.

56. Bleiweiss IJ, Jagirdar JS, Klein JK, et al. Granulomatous Pneumocystis carinii pneumonia in three patients with the acquired immune deficiency syndrome. Chest 1988; 94:580–583.

57. Lee MM, Schinella RA. Pulmonary calcification caused by Pneumoncystis carinii pneumonia. Am J Surg Pathol 1991;15(4):376–380.

58. Whitcomb ME, Schwarz MI, Charles MA, Larson PH. Interstitial fibrosis after pneumocystis carinii pneumonia. Ann Intern Med 1970;73:761–765.

59. Huang S-N, Marshall KG. Pneumocystis carinii infection: a cytologic, histologic and electron microscopic study of the organism. Am Rev Respir Dis 1970;102:623–635.

60. Campbell WG Jr. Ultrastructure of pneumocystis in human lung: life cycle in human pneumocystosis. Arch Pathol Lab Med 1972;93:312–324.

61. Hasleton PS, Curry A, Rankin EM. Pneumocystis carinii pneumonia: a light microscopic and ultrastructural study. J Clin Pathol 1981;34:1138–1146.

62. Haque A, Plattner SB, Cook RT, Hart MN. Pneumocystis carinii. Am J Clin Pathol 1987;87:504–510.

63. Cushion MT, Ruffolo JJ, Walzer PD. Analysis of the developmental stages of Pneumocystis carinii, in vitro. Lab Invest 1988;58:324–331.

64. Katzenstein A-LA, Askin FB. Surgical pathology of nonneoplastic lung disease. In: Bennington JL, ed. Major problems in pathology. Vol. 13, 2d Ed. Philadelphia: WB Saunders, 1990:361.

65. Grocott RG. A stain for fungi in tissue sections and smears. Am J Clin Pathol 1955;25:975–979.

66. Cameron RB, Watts JC, Kasten BL. Pneumocystis carinii pneumonia: an approach to rapid laboratory diagnosis. Am J Clin Pathol 1979;72:90–93.

67. Watts JC, Chandler FW. Pneumocystis carinii pneumonitis: the nature and diagnostic significance of the methenamine silver-positive "intracystic bodies." Am J Surg Pathol 1985;9:744–751.

68. Walker J, Conner G, Ho J, Hunt C, Pickering L. Giemsa staining for cysts and trophozoites of Pneumocystis carinii. J Clin Pathol 1989;42:432–434.

69. Churukian CJ, Schenk EA. Rapid Grocott's methenamine-silver nitrate method for fungi and pneumocystis carinii. Am J Clin Pathol 1977;68:427–428.

70. Mahen CT, Sale GE. Rapid methenamine-silver stain for pneumocystis and fungi. Arch Pathol Lab Med 1978; 102:351–352.

71. Churukian CJ, Schenk EA. Dilute ammoniacal silver as a substitute for methenamine silver to demonstrate pneumocystis carinii and fungi. Lab Med 1986;17:87–90.

72. Blumenfeld W, Griffiss JM. Pneumocystis carinii in sputum. Arch Pathol Lab Med 1988;112:814–820.

73. Young RC, Bennett JE, Chu EW. Organisms mimicking pneumocystis carinii. Lancet 1976;ii:1082–1083.

74. Ma P, Villanueva TG, Kaufman D, Gillooley JF. Respiratory cryptosporidiosis in the acquired immune deficiency syndrome. JAMA 1984;252:1298–1301.

75. Wang N-S, Huang S-N, Thurlbeck WM. Combined pneumocystis carinii and cytomegalovirus infection. Arch Pathol Lab Med 1970;90:529–535.

76. Graham AR, Sobonya RE, Bronnimann DA, Galgiani JN. Quantiatative pathology of coccidioidomycosis in acquired immunodeficiency syndrome. Hum Pathol 1988;19:800–806.

77. Awen CF, Baltzan MA. Systemic dissemination of pneumocystis carinii pneumonia. Can Med Assoc J 1971; 104:809–812.

78. Cote RJ, Rosenblum M, Telzak EE, May M, Unger PD, Cartun RW. Disseminated Pneumocystis carinii infection causing extrapulmonary organ failure: clinical, pathologic, and immunohistochemical analysis. Mod Pathol 1990;3:25–30.

79. Raviglione MC. Extrapulmonary pneumocystis: The first 50 cases. Rev Infect Dis 1990;12(6):1127–1138.

80. Coker RJ, Clark D, Claydon EL, et al. Disseminated Pneumocystis carinii infection in AIDS. J Clin Pathol 1991;44(10):820–823.

81. DeRoux SJ, Adsay NV, Ioachim HL. Disseminated Pneumocystis without pulmonary involvement during prophylactic aerosolized pentamidine therapy in a patient with the acquired immunodeficiency syndrome. Arch Pathol Lab Med 1991;115:1137–1140.

82. Beers MF, Sohn M, Swartz M. Recurrent pneumothorax in AIDS patients with Pneumocystis pneumonia. Chest 1990;98:266–270.

83. McClellan MD, Miller SB, Parsons PE, Cohn DL. Pneumothorax with Pneumocystis carinii pneumonia in AIDS. Chest 1991;100:1224–1228.

84. Mariuz P, Raviglione MC, Gould IA, Mullen MP. Pleural Pneumocystis carinii infection. Chest 1991;99:774–776.

85. Limper AH, Offord KP, Smith TF, Martin WJ. Pneumocystis carinii pneumonia: Differences in lung parasite number and inflammation in patients with and without AIDS. Am Rev Respir Dis 1989;140:1204–1209.

86. Pitchenik AE, Ganjei P, Torres A, Evans DA, Rubin E, Baier H. Sputum examination for the diagnosis of pneumocystis carinii pneumonia in the acquired immunodeficiency syndrome. Am Rev Respir Dis 1986;133:226–229.

87. Bigby TD, Margolskee D, Curtis JL, et al. The usefulness of induced sputum in the diagnosis of Pneumocystis carinii pneumonia in patients with the acquired immunodeficiency syndrome. Am Rev Respir Dis 1986;133:515–518.

88. del Rio C, Guarner J, Honig EG, Slade BA. Sputum examination in the diagnosis of Pneumocystis carinii pneumonia in the acquired immunodeficiency syndrome. Arch Pathol Lab Med 1988;112:1229–1232.

89. Zaman MK, Wooten OJ, Suprahmanya B, Ankobiah W, Finch PJP, Kamholz SL. Rapid noninvasive diagnosis of Pneumocystis carinii from induced liquefied sputum. Ann Intern Med 1988;109:7–10.

90. Leigh TR, Parsons P, Hume C, Husain OAN, Gazzard B, Collins JV. Sputum induction for diagnosis of Pneumocystis carinii pneumonia. Lancet 1989;ii:205–206.

91. O'Brien RF, Quinn JL, Miyahara BT, Lepoff RB, Cohn DL. Diagnosis of Pneumocystis carinii pneumonia by induced sputum in a city with moderate incidence of AIDS. Chest 1989;95:136–138.

92. Greaves TS, Strigle SM. The recognition of pneumocystis carinii in routine papanicoalaou-stained smears. Acta Cytol 1985;29:714–720.

93. Young JA, Stone JW, McGonigle RJS, Adu D, Michael J. Diagnosing Pneumocystis carinii pneumonia by cytological examination of bronchoalveolar lavage fluid: Report of 15 cases. J Clin Pathol 1986;39:945–949.

94. Dugan JM, Avitabile AM, Rossman MD, Ernst CS, Atkinson BF. Diagnosis of Pneumocystis carinii pneumonia by cytologic evaluation of Papanicolaou-stained bronchial specimens. Diagn Cytopathol 1988;4:106–111.

95. Stanley MW, Henry MJ, Iber C. Foamy alveolar casts: Diagnostic specificity for Pneumocystis carinii pneumonia in bronchoalveolar lavage fluid cytology. Diagn Cytopathol 1988;4:112–115.

96. Naryshkin S, Daniels J, Freno E, Cunningham L. Cytology of treated and minimal Pneumocystis carinii pneumonia and a pitfall of the Grocott methenamine silver stain. Diagn Cytopathol 1991;7:41–47.

97. Sobonya RE, Barbee RA, Wiens J, Trego D. Detection of fungi and other pathogens in immunocompromised patients by bronchoalveolar lavage in an area endemic for coccidioidomycosis. Chest 1990;97:1349–1355.

98. Kovacs JA, Ng VL, Masur H, et al. Diagnosis of pneumocystis carinii pneumonia: Improved detection of sputum with use of monoclonal antibodies. N Engl J Med 1988;318:589–593.

99. Blumenfeld W, Kovacs JA. Use of a monoclonal antibody to detect Pneumocystis carinii in induced sputum and bronchoalveolar lavage fluid by immunoperoxidase staining. Arch Pathol Lab Med 1988;112:1233–1236.

100. Elvin KM, Björkman, Linder E, Heurlin N, Hjerpe A. Pneumocystis carinii pneumonia: Detection of parasites in sputum and bronchoalveolar lavage fluid by monoclonal antibodies. Br Med J 1988;297:381–384.

101. Baughman RP, Strohofer SS, Clinton BA, Nickol AD, Frame PT. The use of an indirect fluorescent antibody test for detecting Pneumocystis carinii. Arch Pathol Lab Med 1989;113:1062–1065.

102. Midgley J, Parsons PA, Shanson DC, Husain OAN, Francis N. Monoclonal immunofluorescence compared with silver stain for investigating Pneumocystis carinii pneumonia. J Clin Pathol 1991;44:75–76.

103. Minielly JA, McDuffie, Holley KE. Immunofluorescent identification of pneumocystis carinii. Arch Pathol Lab Med 1970;90:561–566.

104. Blumefeld W, McCook O, Griffiss JM. Detection of antibodies to Pneumocystis carinii in bronchoalveolar lavage fluid by immunoreactivity to Pneumocystis carinii within alveoli, granulomas, and disseminated sites. Mod Pathol 1992;5:107–113.

105. Ghali VS, Garcia RL, Skolom J. Fluorescence of pneumocystis carinii in papanicolaou smears. Hum Pathol 1984;15:907–909.

106. Wehle K, Blanke M, Koenig G, Pfitzer P. The cytological diagnosis of Pneumocystis carinii by fluroescence microscopy of Papanicolaou-stained bronchoalveolar lavage specimens. Cytopathology 1991;2(3):113–120.

107. Stover DE, Zamen MB, Hajdu SI, Lange M, Gold J, Armstrong D. Bronchoalveolar lavage in the diagnosis of diffuse pulmonary infiltrates in the immunosuppressed host. Ann Intern Med 1984;101:1–7.

108. Blumenfeld W, Wagar E, Hadley WK. Use of the transbronchial biopsy for the diagnosis of opportunistic pulmonary infections in the acquired immunodeficiency syndrome (AIDS). Am J Clin Pathol 1984;81:1–5.

109. Stover DE, White DA, Romano PA, Gellene RA. Diagnosis of pulmonary disease in the acquired immune deficiency syndrome (AIDS): role of bronchoscopy and bronchoalveolar lavage. Am Rev Respir Dis 1984;130:659–662.

110. Swinburn CR, Pozniak AL, Sutherland S, Banks RA, Teall AJ, Johnson NMCI. Early experience and difficulties with bronchoalveolar lavage and transbronchial biopsy in the diagnosis of AIDS-associated pneumonia in Britain. Thorax 1985;40:166–170.

111. Hartman B, Koss M, Hui A, Baumann W, Athos L, Boylen T. Pneumocystis carinii pneumonia in the acquired immunodeficiency syndrome (AIDS): diagnosis with bronchial brushings, biopsy, and bronchoalveolar lavage. Chest 1985;87:603–607.

112. Rorat E, Garcia RL, Skolom J. Diagnosis of pneumocystis carinii pneumonia by cytologic examination of bronchial washings. JAMA 1985;254:1950–1951.

113. Pisani RJ, Wright AJ. Clinical utility of bronchoalveolar lavage in immunocompromised hosts. Mayo Clin Proc 1992;67:221–227.

114. Wakefield AE, Pixley FJ, Banerji S, et al. Detection of Pneumocystis carinii with DNA amplification. Lancet 1990;336:451–453.

115. Blumenfeld W, McCook O, Holodniy M, Katzenstein DA. Correlation of morphologic diagnosis of Pneumocystis carinii with the presence of pneumocystis DNA amplified by the polymerase chain reaction. Mod Pathol 1992;5:103–106.

CHAPTER 15

Parasitic Infections

J. KEVIN BAIRD, RONALD C. NEAFIE, and AILEEN M. MARTY

All 42 parasites described in this chapter have been found in the lungs and associated tissues of humans. Only 2 of these parasites, however, infect human lungs by preference. The remainder are either lost in the wrong tissue or host, in transit to another organ, or disseminated (Table 15–1). Almost half of these parasites do not ordinarily infect people; the vast majority must be identified from the two-dimensional view of histologic examination. Thus, parasites in the lung present a difficult diagnostic problem for the pathologist. A specific diagnosis, when at all possible, requires demonstration of unique morphologic features of the parasite evident in tissue sections.

In this chapter we attempt to present a comprehensive listing of parasites that have appeared in human lungs. We have undertaken the task of providing the differential diagnosis for a pathologist faced with identifying a parasite in the lungs. The text and illustrations are intended to guide the pathologist to an accurate, even if nonspecific, diagnosis. We have reviewed many cases in consultation with pathologists in which inappropriate diagnosis could have been avoided by following some simple guidelines.

1. Determine if the structure in question is actually a parasite; exclude other foreign bodies and be skeptical of "parasites" in bizarre locations.
2. Decide on a kingdom: Protozoan or Metazoan. Then decide upon a phylum, e.g., Platyhelminthes, Nematoda, Arthropoda, or other?
3. Measure the maximum diameter and or length. Try to appreciate the overall dimensions. When the diagnosis is decided, check to see that the known dimensions are in agreement.
4. Based on likely taxonomic position, size, travel history, and general agreement with known specimens or illustrations, decide on a likely diagnosis.
5. Offer the specimen to colleagues for their opinion without revealing one's own diagnosis. If in conflict, understand why.
6. Remember, a specific diagnosis is often not possible on the basis of the material available.

This chapter focuses on parasites that may appear in human lungs and the lesions they provoke. The length of description given each parasite tends to reflect the available literature on each species and, to some extent, the organism's relative importance. The order of discussion reflects taxonomic affinities and not medical importance. A reader wishing more information on parasitic infections, especially on their extrapulmonary characteristics, is directed toward several general references, including: Pathology of Tropical and Extraordinary Diseases (Binford C, and Connor D, eds. Armed Forces Institute of Pathology, Washington, DC, 1976) and Clinical Parasitology, 9th Ed. (Beaver PC, Jung RC, and Cupp EW. Lea & Febiger, Philadelphia, 1984). A more recent text, Diagnostic Pathology of Parasitic Infections with Clinical Correlations (Gutierrez Y. Lea & Febiger, Philadelphia, 1990), is also helpful.

Protozoa

Toxoplasma gondii, and *Entamoeba histolytica* are the protozoans that the pathologist is most likely to encounter in the lung. *Pneumocystis carinii*, once viewed as a protozoan, is now thought to be more like a fungus; this organism is described separately in Chapter 11. *Entamoeba histolytica*, although a well-documented pulmo-

Table 15–1. Parasites found in human lung

Protozoa
    Plasmodium falciparum
    Toxoplasma gondii
    Trichomonas tenax
    Trypanosoma cruzi
    Entamoeba histolytica
    Cryptosporidium sp.
    Leishmania donovani
    Acanthamoeba sp.
Metazoa
    Dirofilaria immitis
    Wuchereria bancrofti
    Brugia malayi
    Onchocerca volvulus
    Capillaria aerophila
    Strongyloides stercoralis
    Mammomonogamus laryngeus
    Ascaris lumbricoides
    Ascaris suum
    Toxocara canis
    Mansonella perstans
    Angiostrongylus cantonensis
    Halicephalobus (Micronema) deletrix
    Metastrongylus elongatus
    Enterobius vermicularis
    Lagochilascaris minor
    Baylisascaris procyonis
    Anisakids
    Gnathostoma spinigerum
    Paragonimus spp.
    Alaria sp.
    Schistosoma spp.
    Fasciola hepatica
    Clinostomum complanatum
    Spirometra spp.
    Taenia solium
    Echinococcus granulosus
    Echinococcus multilocularis
    Echinococcus vogeli
    Mites
    Fly larvae
    Armillifer spp.
    Linguatula serrata
    Limnatis nilotica

nary pathogen in endemic regions, only infrequently invades the lungs of persons outside the endemic regions. *Toxoplasma gondii* is seen in the lungs only when the patient's infection is disseminated, which can occur in newborn infants or in adults with severe immunodeficiencies.

Other protozoans may cause severe pulmonary complications. Malaria kills about 2 million people each year, mostly children. It is one of the world's most serious public health problems. Malarial lung is relatively common among patients with malaria. Because of the extraordinary prevalence of malaria and because it is a disseminated infection, this disease and all its complications command attention.

Chronic Chagas' disease, especially in the presence of megaesophagus, may cause pulmonary disease and death. The parasite, *Trypanosoma cruzi*, may be overlooked and thus the cause of death may not be recognized. The impact of this disease on the public health, although recognized as serious, may be underestimated.

Other protozoan parasites in the lung are rare to the point of being curiosities or even unique. However, *Trichomonas tenax* may be a pulmonary infection of importance that is usually overlooked.

Malarial Lung

Pulmonary edema can occur in infection with *Plasmodium falciparum* (malignant tertian malaria). Characteristically this so-called malarial lung starts abruptly and progresses rapidly to death. Approximately 7% of nonimmune patients with falciparum malaria develop acute pulmonary insufficiency[1] that develops without cardiac decompensation or fluid overload. Further, the usual regimen of treatment for cardiogenic pulmonary edema is futile.

The pathophysiology of malarial respiratory distress is not known. Two hypotheses are cited: (1) increased capillary permeability and (2) disseminated intravascular coagulation. Malarial parasites are not directly involved; patients continue to deteriorate after chemotherapeutic clearance of parasites from peripheral blood. Delay of chemotherapy seems to contribute to development of pulmonary complications. Patients do not seem otherwise predisposed, because many victims of malarial lung, including U.S. soldiers in Vietnam, have been generally healthy before infection.[2,3]

A distinctly mild, nonfatal form of malarial lung has also been described.[4] Persons with this type have pleural effusions, interstitial edema, and lobar consolidations that resolve with antimalarial chemotherapy.

Disease

Patients with malarial lung develop shortness of breath and circumoral cyanosis 2–3 days after onset of malarial chills and fever. Respiratory rate, blood pressure, central venous pressure, radiograph, and clinical chest examination are normal at this early stage.

Within 24–48 h, however, this picture changes dramatically. The respiratory rate increases to between 40 and 70, and cyanosis spreads to the face and limbs. There may be spasmodic cough and hiccough. Hematocrit falls precipitously to between 25% and 30%. Blood pressure and central venous pressure remain normal. Patients often produce foamy, blood-tinged sputum. Chest radiography shows patchy infiltrations in lower lobes, and upper lobes have interstitial markings suggestive of pulmonary edema. Scattered rhonchi and rales may be heard at the bases of the lungs.

Administration of meperidine, digitalis, and rotating tourniquets are not helpful.[2,3,5] Patients usually die 3–8 days after onset of malaria and usually within 24 h of diagnosis of malarial lung.

Biology

Plasmodium falciparum reproduces asexually in man and sexually (by sporogony) in the mosquito. Sporozoites in mosquito salivary glands enter human blood vessels when the mosquito takes a blood meal and penetrate liver parenchymal cells minutes later. By binary fission, each sporozoite produces about 40,000 daughter cells, called merozoites. The merozoites of *P. falciparum* formed in the liver enter the bloodstream and attach on red cell surfaces and enter the cell within 1 min. The young trophozoite feeds on hemoglobin and later undergoes binary fission to produce 8–26 merozoites. The red cell containing merozoites is a schizont. Merozoites rupture the cell and enter the circulation in 36- to 48-h intervals, producing the spiking fever and chills of malignant tertian malaria. Successive generations of merozoites infect increasing numbers of red cells until the nonimmune host dies.[6]

Some merozoites within the red cell differentiate to male and female gametocytes. The mosquito ingests gametocytes at a blood meal, and sexual recombination in the gut of the mosquito follows. Within the mosquito, sporogony produces several thousand infective sporozoites per gametocyte pair, and the sporozoites migrate to the salivary glands.

Pathology

Autopsy reveals congested and edematous heavy lungs averaging 2,000 g in combined weight. There are focal hemorrhages throughout the lungs. Pink foamy fluid often fills the trachea. Pleural effusion of 100–600 ml of light-brown-to-red fluid occurs. The pericardium contains a similar fluid, and the heart may be congested or normal.

Microscopically, severe pulmonary edema, capillary congestion, hyaline membranes, and thickened alveolar septa are seen. Alveoli are edematous, and macrophages carrying malarial pigment (hemozoin) are present in the alveoli. Alveolar septa are thickened and occasionally contain trophozoites of *Plasmodium falciparum* within red cells (Fig. 15–1) and foreign body giant cells.[7] Hyaline membranes occur in about one-half of reported cases. Disseminated intravascular coagulation is seen in some patients.

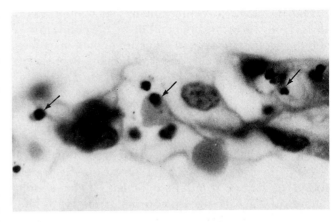

Fig. 15–1. Many trophozoites of *Plasmodium falciparum* appear in this alveolar capillary (*arrows*) in red blood cells. They are characterized by a dark spherical grain of pigment. The parasite is seen as thin rim of cytoplasm around pigment. Pigment grain, surrounding parasite, and red blood cells are all seen at this magnification. AFIP 86–6440. H and E, ×1,715.

Cardiogenic causes of malarial lung have been excluded. Increased capillary permeability or disseminated intravascular coagulation might be the underlying mechanism. If so, the relationship between malarial lung and the parasites is not understood.

Diagnosis and Treatment

Acute pulmonary insufficiency in patients with severe malaria is diagnosed from typical signs of progressive respiratory distress and pulmonary edema. Early diagnosis cannot be made from radiographs because changes do not appear until about 24 h before death.

Successful treatment includes intermittent positive pressure ventilation, dexamethasone, low molecular weight dextran, digoxin, and heparin.[8] In extreme cases pheresis and blood transfusions may save the patient. Prompt diagnosis and treatment of falciparum malaria might curtail development of malarial lung. Many patients who developed pulmonary complications were ill for at least 2–3 days before antimalarial chemotherapy was begun.

Toxoplasmosis

Toxoplasma gondii Nicolle and Manceaux 1909 is the ubiquitous coccidian that causes toxoplasmosis.[9] Disseminated infection may particularly kill patients with hematologic malignancy or acquired immunodeficiency syndrome (AIDS) or patients receiving immunosuppressive therapy.[10–13] In patients with the disseminated form of the disease, pulmonary involvement is common, occurring in more than 70% of cases.

The prevalence of infection in the United States varies from 3% to 20%, depending on the ethnic group and the geographic region. Rates are highest in eastern and central areas and in American Indians. People with healthy immune systems keep the parasite under control and remain free of symptoms. Some people, who are otherwise asymptomatic, have lymphadenopathy, a condition known as Piringer–Kuchinka lymphadenopathy. The posterior cervical nodes are most commonly involved. Other nodes may be affected, and the lymphadenopathy can be generalized. Organisms are rarely found in tissues from these patients. The lymphadenopathy may be persistent or recurrent for as long as a year. Lymphadenopathy does not usually occur in disseminated disease.

Disease

Infection of lung tissue indicates dissemination of the parasite with risk of death from bronchopneumonia or meningoencephalitis. *Toxoplasma* tachyzoites are seeded by the bloodstream and via lymphatics, and for this reason the pneumonia tends to be confluent, progressive, and fatal. Pulmonary toxoplasmosis causes dyspnea and tachypnea with or without fever. Radiographs may reveal diffuse alveolar and interstitial infiltrates. Focal pneumonia occasionally may occur; rarely, it can be cavitary.

Tachyzoites actively invade host cells by means of an anterior organelle and release of proteolytic enzymes. Within the cytoplasm, the invading organism is surrounded by a vacuole within which it multiplies. In macrophages, tachyzoites live within phagosomes and inhibit fusion with lysosomes, thereby avoiding destruction. However, cytokine-activated macrophages overcome this parasite defense and kill the intracellular parasites. The cell bursts, releasing 8–32 tachyzoites and sometimes causing focal necrosis. Some intracellular tachyzoites do not thus ripen; instead, they may transform into bradyzoites and become tolerated by the host cell. These cells eventually ripen to become true cysts (as opposed to the pseudocyst, a cell packed with tachyzoites and nearly ready to burst). True cysts persist for an indefinite period. Tachyzoites can probably multiply in any nucleated cell but lesions are most frequently seen in the brain, heart, liver, intestine, lungs, and lymph nodes.

Biology

Toxoplasma gondii is a sporozoan (Apicomplexa; Sporozoa). It is related to *Cryptosporidium*, *Sarcocystis*, and *Plasmodium*. The sporozoa alternate sexual generations; asexual multiplication (schizogony) occurs in one generation and sexual recombination with sporogony in the next.

Sporogony in *T. gondii* occurs in the intestinal epithelium of the definitive hosts, cats. Oocysts containing a sporoblast pass in feces. The oocyst (10×12 μm) is not infective when shed, and 3–4 days must pass until sporulation. There are two sporocysts in each oocyst, and each sporocyst produces four sporozoites, the infective form. Under ideal conditions in soil (moist, cool, and shady), the infective oocyst remains viable in soil for about 1 year.

Humans, who are one of many suitable intermediate hosts, acquire infection by consuming soil contaminated with oocysts from cat excrement. Eating tissue cysts in undercooked pork, mutton, and beef, and slaughtering diseased animals are high risk factors. Transmission may occur in utero, or by transplant of an infected organ.[14] Sporozoites emerge from ingested oocysts and transform into tachyzoites as they enter the gut mucosa. When the infection is acquired from undercooked meat, bradyzoites from tissue cysts become tachyzoites, penetrate the intestinal mucosa, and spread via blood and lymphatics. In intermediate hosts, *T. gondii* multiplies asexually; sexual recombination occurs only in cats. Infected cells of the intermediate host become "pseudocysts" filled with tachyzoites in the acute stages and "tissue cysts" filled with bradyzoites in the chronic stage. The tachyzoite is the proliferative form; it is crescentic and subtly pyriform. In smear preparations it is 4–8 μm but in tissue sections about one-half this size.

Pathology

At autopsy, the lungs are heavily congested, with combined weight about 2,000 g. There are petechial hemorrhages and areas of consolidation and possibly cavitation. Coagulation necrosis and an alveolar fibrinous exudate occur throughout the lungs.[15] Many alveoli are collapsed and contain cells packed with tachyzoites. Pseudocysts are abundant in areas of necrosis (Fig. 15–2). Numerous chronic inflammatory cells occupy the interstitium. Differentiating true cysts from pseudocysts may support the diagnoses of acute or chronic toxoplasmosis. Periodic acid–Schiff (PAS) and silver reagents stain true cysts; the cyst wall is argyrophilic and bradyzoites are strongly PAS positive. In contrast, pseudocyst walls and tachyzoites stain weakly with those reagents.

Diagnosis and Treatment

Diagnosis of pulmonary toxoplasmosis is established by demonstrating characteristic intracellular organisms in lung tissue. The organisms stain well with hematoxylin

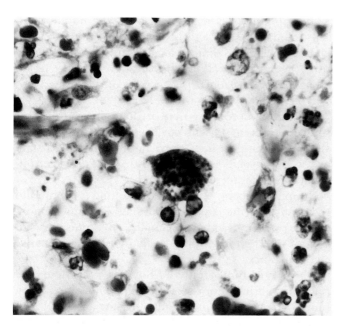

Fig. 15–2. Pseudocyst containing tachyzoites of *Toxoplasma gondii* in lung. AFIP 85–10950. H and E, ×750.

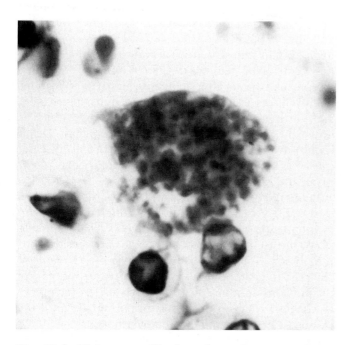

Fig. 15–3. Higher magnification of pseudocyst containing tachyzoites of *Toxoplasma gondii* in lung. AFIP 85–10950. H and E, ×2,250.

and eosin. Because of their small size, the oil immersion objective is usually required (Fig. 15–3).

For the serologic diagnosis, it is important to distinguish preexisting or passively transferred antibody from antibody associated with acute infection. A single test does not distinguish chronic from acute infec-

tion.[16,17] Serial tests demonstrating a rising antibody titer against tachyzoites support the diagnosis of acute toxoplasmosis.

The standard serologic test for acute toxoplasmosis is the Sabin–Feldman dye test. Living tachyzoites from peritoneal exudates of laboratory mice are incubated with serum from the patient. IgG or IgM directed against tachyzoites prevents staining of organellar structures by methylene blue (pH 10.8). IgM tends to be associated with acute infection, and it is not transferred in utero. Thus, it is often useful to conduct serologic tests that distinguish IgG and IgM, that is, the indirect fluorescence assay or enzyme-linked immunosorbent assay (ELISA).

Chemotherapy with pyrimethamine and sulfonamides probably kills proliferating tachyzoites but not quiescent cysts. Thus, immunocompromised patients may suffer a new wave of proliferating tachyzoites at any time following chemotherapy.

Trichomoniasis

Pulmonary trichomoniasis is infection of the respiratory tract with the flagellate protozoan *Trichomonas tenax* (O.F. Muller, 1773) Dobell 1939. Most infections in humans involve the buccal cavity. Reports of pulmonary involvement are relatively rare. First reported in 1867, only 37 infections were reported in the next 113 years. In 1980, however, a study in the then Soviet Union found 37 infections among 370 patients with chronic pulmonary disease.[18] This suggests that pulmonary trichomoniasis is an unnoticed or infrequently reported infection.

Disease

Pulmonary trichomoniasis has not been described in patients without prior chronic pulmonary disease. Tuberculosis, lobar pneumonia, putrid bronchitis, bronchiectasis, and bronchogenic carcinoma have all preceded pulmonary trichomoniasis.

Infection of the buccal cavity by *Trichomonas tenax* is associated with poor oral hygiene. Trophozoites have been cultured from the teeth, the gums, and particularly from tartar. The oral infection is transmitted by mouth-to-mouth contact or by fomites. Oral and pulmonary trichomoniasis are not usually concurrent; only one-third of cases studied had simultaneous infections.[19]

Identification of specific symptoms associated with pulmonary trichomoniasis is difficult because infection follows chronic disease. *T. tenax* has been associated with fever, empyema, and pleural effusions,[20–22] but the organism may not directly cause disease. Some investigators view *T. tenax* in the lungs as an opportunist feeding on necrotic tissue produced by chronic disease. Isolation of the organism from cavitary lesions of tuberculosis is typical of reported infections. However, at least one patient had pleural effusion specifically attributed to *T. tenax*.[23] A thorough examination of the patient for underlying chronic disease was negative, and her symptoms resolved after therapy with metronidazole.

Biology

Trichomonas tenax is a cosmopolitan parasite. Incidence of oral infections has no geographic bounds. Pulmonary infection has been reported from Europe, Asia, and North and South America.[19]

Three species of trichomonas are found in humans: *T. tenax*, *T. vaginalis*, and *T. hominis*. They can be distinguished by size, internal morphology, and characteristics of the flagellae. Only the trophozoite stage has been described in all three species. All have flagellae that originate from an anterior point. One flagellum composes the outer margin of an undulating membrane. The prominent axostyle usually protrudes through the posterior end of the trophozoite.[24,25]

Trichomonas tenax is smaller than the more familiar trichomonad, *T. vaginalis*. *T. tenax* is 5–12 μm long, averaging 6–7 μm; *T. vaginalis* is 7–23 μm long, averaging 13 μm. Also, the undulating membrane of *T. vaginalis* is relatively shorter and its cytoplasm has many more and larger siderophil granules.

Trichomonas tenax is distinguished from the common intestinal trichomonad *T. hominis* by several characteristics. *T. tenax* lacks the prominent cytostomal cleft. *T. hominis* has 3–5 but usually 4 flagellae, whereas *T. tenax* consistently has 5 flagellae, 4 free and 1 anchored to an undulating membrane. The anchored flagellum of *T. tenax* does not reach the posterior end of the body and lacks an extension beyond the undulating membrane.

Pathology

Pathologic changes caused by *T. tenax* have not been documented. The organism is usually isolated from necrotic tissue. In histologic sections, trophozoites are in both necrotic and viable tissue. A cause-and-effect relationship between the microorganism and necrosis has not been established.

Diagnosis and Treatment

Diagnosis requires identification of *T. tenax* trophozoites in sputum, bronchial washings, or pathologic specimens. The trophozoites are readily demonstrated in wet preparations as pyriform flagellated microorganisms exhibiting characteristic wobbling motility. Contamination of the clinical specimen with trophozoites from the oral cavity should be considered and excluded by obtaining a second specimen, taking care to avoid oral contamination.

Papanicolaou staining may be the stain of choice for routine screening for *T. tenax*. Cytology technicians are alert to the appearance of trichomonads in this stain because *T. vaginalis* is often diagnosed on Papanicolaou-stained vaginal smears. The organism appears as a grey body approximately 6 × 4 μm containing fine blue and red granules. The Papanicolaou stain does not demonstrate flagellae or other organelles. A Giemsa stain is superior in demonstrating the diagnostic morphologic characteristics.

The large study from the Soviet Union described pulmonary trichomoniasis without trophozoites in sputum in 16 of 37 patients, using a serologic test.[18]

Chagas' Disease

Chagas' disease is infection with the kinetoplastid flagellate *Trypanosoma cruzi* Chagas 1909. The disease is endemic to both South and Central America. *T. cruzi* invariably invades the myocardium, but other organs may be involved. Patients develop symptoms of chronic disease many years after acute infection. Complications of chronic disease include megaesophagus, megacolon, and cardiomegaly. Death in acute disease, which is unusual, is often caused by meningoencephalitis. Death is, however, the usual outcome of chronic disease; caused by pneumonia, tuberculosis, ventricular aneurysm, and cardiac arrest.

Pulmonary involvement with Chagas' disease occurs as two distinct clinical entities: (1) congenital infection of lung tissue with *T. cruzi* amastigotes (the nonflagellated, intracellular stage); and (2) a wide spectrum of pulmonary complications arising as a direct result of chagasic megaesophagus. Both forms progress to death. Consideration of pulmonary lesions secondary to chagasic megaesophagus is important because the primary cause of death is often overlooked.[26]

Disease

Infection of lung tissue with *T. cruzi* amastigotes is acquired congenitally. Pneumonitis in acute or chronic vector-transmitted disease is not known. All 15 patients with documented pulmonary Chagas' disease occurred in Brazil and Argentina. Diagnosis of infection was at autopsy of either stillborn infants or infants not surviving the first few days of life. An exception was one child who survived 41 days with pulmonary Chagas' disease.[27] These babies are born with meningoencephalitis, myocarditis, myositis, and inflammation of the gastrointestinal tract.[28]

Pneumonitis in congenital Chagas' disease is attributed to *T. cruzi* amastigotes in lung tissue. The organisms are in histiocytes in both the alveolar wall and alveolar lumen. Amastigotes are also present in the amniotic epithelium of the extraplacental membranes and umbilical cord. These sites may be infected by trypanomastigotes in the amniotic fluid. Presumably, trypanomastigotes originate in the lungs of the fetus. This process has been reported in nonhuman primates.[29]

Development of megaesophagus in chronic Chagas' disease is attributed to infection of neuroglia of the esophagus by *T. cruzi* amastigotes. Neighboring nerve cells are destroyed, and the esophagus is eventually denervated. Peristaltic motion of the organ is lost, and dilatation develops. Patients with megaesophagus cannot swallow properly. Food putrifies in the esophagus and may be aspirated. Patients with megaesophagus may develop aspiration pneumonia, tuberculosis, pulmonary abscess, bronchiectasis, asthma, and pulmonary fibrosis. Achalasia independent of Chagas' disease is rare in endemic areas.[26]

Some strains of *T. cruzi* appear to have greater affinity for the neuroglia. In essence, persons in one geographic area may develop megaesophagus while persons in another endemic area tend to develop cardiopathy.

Biology

Chagas' disease is typically transmitted by bloodsucking reduviid bugs, also called kissing or assassin bugs. These bugs are triatomid hemipterans (true bugs). The bug ingests circulating trypanosomes while feeding on human or animal blood. The trypanosome trypomastigote transforms first into an epimastigote, and then to a metacyclic trypanosome in the gut of the bug. The metacyclic trypanosome is infective to man. After an infected bug feeds, it defecates on the skin near the wound site. Metacyclic trypanosomes infect man when they are rubbed either into the wound left by the bug bite or to a mucuos membrane. Other modes of transmission include blood transfusion, breastfeeding, eating food tainted with fresh vector feces, and congenital.

Metacyclic trypanosomes in blood identify and infect susceptible host cells. Receptor–ligand endocytosis probably mediates entry into most cells. For example, fibronectin receptors of monocytes and macrophages enhance entry of parasites. The receptor ligands that may allow for penetration of other cells, for example, cardiac muscle cells and nerve cells, remain unknown. Phagocytosed trypanosomes escape the phagosome

and reside free in the cytoplasm where they avoid destruction by lysosomes. In heart and nerve cells, they transform into amastigotes and multiply by binary fission in the cavity of a cyst-like structure. Infection of other cells requires amastigote transformation to infective trypomastigotes. This usually occurs just 1 day before the infected cell ruptures. Parasites that do not differentiate are unable to leave the site and are killed by inflammatory cells.

Intracellular *T. cruzi* amastigotes are nearly round, 2–4 μm in diameter. In a Romanowsky stain, the nucleus is deep red and the rod-shaped kinetoplast is black. The kinetoplast is a tightly bound bundle of prokaryotic deoxyribonucleic acid associated with the flagellum, and its function is unknown. Both organelles are violet in hematoxylin and eosin (H and E) stains.

Pathology

Trypanosoma cruzi amastigotes cause marked interstitial abnormalities in lung tissue. The lungs appear nodular. Alveoli in areas of infiltration are obliterated. Thickened septa contain abundant histiocytes and few neutrophils. Endothelial swelling and edema of septa are present. *T. cruzi* amastigotes occur in hypertrophic macrophages in alveoli or in the alveolar walls. A single huge macrophage may contain hundreds of amastigotes. Infected macrophages in the walls of alveoli occasionally protrude into the alveoli. The nucleus of the infected macrophage may be large and hyperchromatic.

In extraplacental membranes, amastigotes are present in both cells of the amniotic epithelium and Hofbauer's cells. Necrosis of amniotic epithelium is associated with underlying infection of Hofbauer's cells.[27]

Diagnosis and Treatment

Diagnosis of acute or congenital Chagas' disease is made by identifying *T. cruzi* trypomastigotes in peripheral blood. If organisms cannot be demonstrated in a suspicious case, cultivation on special media, inoculation of susceptible laboratory animals, or xenodiagnosis (allowing laboratory-reared reduviid bugs to feed on the patient) may be helpful. In acute infection, ELISA demonstrates IgM, as does the indirect fluorescent antibody test. Complement fixation and indirect hemagglutination have been used to determine a history of exposure to *T. cruzi*. Antigen for these assays come from parasites cultivated in vitro.

Pulmonary involvement is diagnosed at autopsy with demonstration of amastigotes in tissue. *Trypanosoma cruzi* amastigotes in macrophages in the lung superficially resemble *Toxoplasma gondii* tachyzoites. Demonstration of unequivocal kinetoplasts in the microorganisms excludes toxoplasmosis and histoplasmosis. A kinetoplast does not exclude *Leishmania donovani*, the cause of visceral leishmaniasis (kala azar). The amastigotes of *L. donovani* and *Trypanosoma cruzi* are easily confused by microscopists. Some workers consider the amastigotes morphologically indistinguishable in tissue sections. However, we consider size of the amastigotes an important, albeit slight, difference; *Trypanosoma cruzi* are commonly 3–4 μm in diameter, whereas *L. donovani* amastigotes rarely exceed 3 μm in diameter. *L. donovani* does not cause neonatal disease,[28] and other species of kinetoplastid flagellates do not form amastigotes in the lungs of human beings. Therefore, demonstration of intracellular pulmonary parasites with a kinetoplast proves neonatal Chagas' disease.

Residence in an endemic area is a major diagnostic indicator, and in this setting defects in cardiac conduction, cardiomegaly, apical ventricular aneurysm, or dysphagia or constipation suggest chronic Chagas' disease. Syphilis, hypothyroidism, arteriosclerotic heart disease, primary cardiopathy, and carcinoma of the esophagus or colon may all be included in the differential diagnosis.[30]

Standard chemotherapy is indicated only for acute or congenital Chagas' disease. Two drugs are available, benznidazole (Rochagan) and nifurtimox (Lampit); they clear parasitemia and alleviate illness. However, these drugs have high toxicity and rarely eradicate the infection. Nifurtimox is available in the United States from the Centers for Disease Control in Atlanta, Georgia; benznidazole is not currently available in the United States. Treatment of congenital Chagas' disease has not been evaluated. Megaesophagus and megacolon can be relieved by surgery and sometimes by anticholinergic drugs. Symptomatic heart disease may require medication, pacemakers, or heart transplant. Corticosteroids aggravate infection.

Pulmonary Amebiasis

Pulmonary amebiasis is a complication of gastrointestinal infection with *Entamoeba histolytica* Schaudinn 1903. Unlike other amebae found in the human intestine, this ameba sometimes invades tissue and occasionally kills its host. Trophozoites of *E. histolytica* penetrate, colonize, and ulcerate intestinal epithelium and may enter the venous circulation. The liver is the most common site of secondary amebic abscess, but abscesses may arise in any organ. Pulmonary amebiasis develops either by hematogenous seeding of the lungs with viable trophozoites or by penetration of an amebic liver abscess through the liver capsule, peritoneum, diaphragm, and

pleura. Large lesions of lung and liver connect by a narrow isthmus through the hemidiaphragm, giving the complex an hourglass configuration. The lower lobe of the right lung is most commonly involved. Amebic abscesses from hematogenous spread to the lungs are relatively rare. Development of pulmonary involvement worsens the prognosis.[31]

Amebiasis is a serious public health problem in tropical and subtropical communities where inadequate sanitation and poor personal hygiene prevail. Prevalence in excess of 40% is not unusual.[32] Amebiasis is ubiquitous, however, and routinely reported even from nations with high standards of sanitation.[33]

Disease

Amebic abscess in the lower lobe of the right lung is typically contiguous with abscess in the liver. An abscess in other portions of lung develop from hematogenous spread. Abscesses in either lung may extend into the pleura. Abscesses in the left lung occasionally extend into the pericardium and cause amebic pericarditis.

Two distinct clinical manifestations occur when a hepatic amebic abscess extends into the lung. The lung is consolidated; an abscess forms, and a hepatic fistula persists. Leakage into the pleura may cause pleurisy, effusion, or empyema. The prognosis of either complication is worse than uncomplicated liver abscess, and in the case of pulmonary amebiasis, the prognosis worsens when the pleura is involved. Specifically, empyema kills one of five patients.[34] It is abrupt and difficult to treat. Vascularized serosa is exposed to necrotic debris, and septic shock rapidly develops. In Natal, South Africa, 30% of patients with thoracic amebiasis had pleural involvement; the remainder suffered less serious lesions of the lung.[31]

Communication of the hepatocontiguous abscess with a bronchus is a better prognostic sign. The patient may cough up an alarming quantity of amebic pus (as much as 4 liters) but immediately begins to feel better and usually progresses to recovery.[35]

Biology

Humans acquire amebiasis by ingesting cysts of *E. histolytica* in food or water contaminated with feces. Fecal–oral contact by any means, including fomites, poor hygiene, and sexual behavior, may lead to infection. The cyst in the small bowel is a quadrinucleate organism that yields four trophozoites. Some trophozoites penetrate the lamina propria and muscularis mucosae and cause extensive necrosis. Characteristically, as seen in tissue sections, the ulcer in the colon is "flask shaped." The mechanism of invasion and tissue lysis is incompletely understood.

The stimulus that cues trophozoites in the lumen to encyst is unknown. The trophozoite expels undigested food and spherulates, forming the "precyst." It then exudes a tough coat for protection. The cyst ripens with two meiotic divisions to produce four nuclei and is then passed in feces. Some trophozoites in colonic ulcers penetrate small veins and enter the portal circulation. From here most settle in the liver, but may seed virtually any other site. Trophozoites in tissue continue dividing asexually until they die in necrotic tissue. They do not encyst in tissue.

Moderate heat and dryness kill *E. histolytica* cysts. Cysts in moist cool soil are infective for about 2 weeks, but in water at 4°C they remain viable for several months. Flies and cockroaches carry *E. histolytica* cysts and may contaminate human food and drink.

Pathology

Amebic abscesses may be small, only a few micrometers, or large, up to 10 cm. Fluid drained from amebic abscesses is yellow brown and not malodorous. In the liver, it often has the color and consistency of anchovy sauce. The core of an amebic abscess is composed of necrotic debris containing occasional inflammatory cells and trophozoites. Trophozoites and inflammatory cells are concentrated at the margin of viable tissue around the abscess. The surrounding viable tissue is edematous and contains a mixed inflammatory cell infiltrate of neutrophils, lymphocytes, histiocytes, and plasma cells, and sometimes eosinophils.[36]

Diagnosis and Treatment

Identification of *E. histolytica* trophozoites in sputum, in aspirates of liver, or in pleural exudates confirms a diagnosis. Cysts or trophozoites in the feces of a patient suspected of having pulmonary amebiasis are presumptive evidence.

Microscopically, trophozoites of *E. histolytica* may resemble mammalian macrophages to the uninitiated, but they can usually be distinguished (Fig. 15–4) by their thicker cell membranes and the tiny central karyosome within their nucleus. Iron and hematoxylin stain, which is often recommended for demonstrating amebic trophozoites, highlights organelles, making differentiation from mammalian cells easier. Trophozoites are usually intensely periodic acid–Schiff (PAS) positive because their cytoplasm is rich with glycogen, and the stain helps locate discrete or single amebic trophozoites.[36] The PAS stain may, however, obscure details of the cytoplasm and nucleus. Therefore, after the areas where trophozoites are concentrated have been located one may revert to the H and E stain for positive

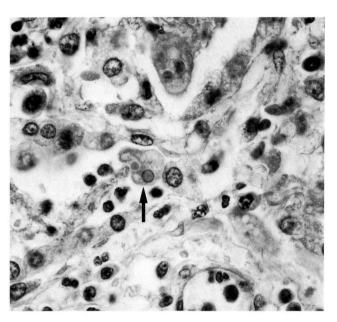

Fig. 15–4. Trophozoite of *Entamoeba histolytica* in lung (*arrow*). AFIP 79–15357. H and E, ×630.

identification. When the specimen is well fixed, H and E staining is adequate and in fact has distinct advantages. The trophozoites are usually round and have a thin but sharply limiting external membrane. The cytoplasm is amphophilic and may contain vacuoles or erythrocytes. The nucleus is small, spherical, and delicately stained. Chromatin within the nucleus is imperceptible except where the nuclear membrane is purpendicular to the slide surface. An unstained "halo" surrounds the nucleus. The karyosome is located at the precise center of the nucleus (Fig. 15–5). The karyosome of a commensal species of ameba in man, *Entameba coli*, is more eccentric within the nucleus. About 30 delicate fibrils radiate out from the karyosome to the edge of the nucleus, but these are not routinely seen. The sum of these features allows the pathologist to identify trophozoites of *E. histolytica* in tissue sections. A red blood cell in the cytoplasm of the trophozoite excludes other amebae (see Figs. 15–4 and 15–5). The diameter of *E. histolytica* varies from 10 to 60 μm, but in tissue sections most are 15–25 μm. Trophozoites from abscesses are larger than those from stool specimens.

The clinical features vary depending on the pathogenicity of the strain of *E. histolytica*, the site and intensity of the infection, and host factors. Liver abscess may arise in the presence or absence of intestinal symptoms. Only 20% of those with liver abscess will have *E. histolytica* in their stools. The clinical features often suggest a diagnosis of amebic liver abscess, but clinicians unfamiliar with hepatic amebic abscess may consider the signs and symptoms nonspecific. Most patients are febrile

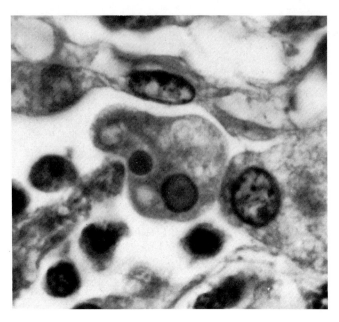

Fig. 15–5. Trophozoite has small nucleus with finely dispersed chromatin that is concentrated at nuclear membrane. Central karyosome is distinct. Cytoplasm is amphophilic, vacuolated, and contains erythrocyte. Trophozoite has sharply defined outer membrane and ameboid shape. Contrast these features with surrounding host cells. AFIP 79–15357. H and E, ×1,890.

with acute pain in the upper-right quadrant. The liver is palpable and tender, and there is localized intercostal tenderness. Pleuropulmonary amebiasis typically causes pain, cough, hemoptysis, and dyspnea. The pain is usually pleuritic and typically involves the right-lower chest.

Several reliable seroimmunologic tests are available for detection of antigens of *E. histolytica*. Cellulose acetate diffusion and agar gel diffusion methods are widely used[37]; ELISA and radioimmunoassay procedures are also available.[38,39]

Radiographs sometimes reveal empyema causing filling defects in the right chest.[34] Elevation of the right hemidiaphragm is seen with both pleural and lung involvement. Radionuclide scans of the liver may reveal a mass contiguous with the lower lobe of the right lung. The scan may appear normal from the anterior aspect.[40] Diagnosis of pleuropulmonary amebiasis is not difficult if the clinician considers amebiasis. Deaths are usually a consequence of a missed or delayed diagnosis.

Treatment requires both aspiration of the liver abscess and chemotherapy. Some investigators recommend closed thoracostomy, open thoracostomy, or decortication in conjunction with aspiration and chemotherapy.[34] Others argue that surgery is rarely neces-sary.[31] Repeated aspiration of the abscess or pleural space often is necessary.

Several chemotherapeutic regimens have been described, consisting principally of emetine, chloroquine, iodoquinol, paromomycin (Humatin), dehydroemetine, diloxanide (Furamide) or metronidazole (Flagel), and Tinidazole (Fasigyn). Metronidazole is probably the next best therapeutic agent; it has few side effects, is easy to administer, and cures concomitant amebic dysentery.[30,41] The regimen depends on the severity and site of the disease.

Miscellaneous Protozoa

Cryptosporidium species are intracellular coccidian parasites of the gastrointestinal tract of vertebrates. Water supplies contaminated with sewage of animal or human origin and contaminated uncooked vegetables are the usual source of infection. In immunosuppressed patients this infection is prolonged and involves the intestinal, respiratory, and biliary tracts. Infections with *Cryptosporidium* involving the respiratory tract have been reported in (1) the alveoli of a patient with AIDS; (2) the tracheal mucosa and glands of an immunosuppressed 12-year-old boy; (3) the bronchioles of an immunosuppressed infant;[42–44] and (4) in sputum during screening for *Mycobacterium*.[45]

Leishmania donovani causes visceral leishmaniasis (kala-azar) in Asia, Africa, and South America. The parasites multiply as amastigotes in phagocytic cells of the reticuloendothelial system, especially in spleen, lymph nodes, bone marrow, and Kupffer's cells of the liver. *L. donovani* amastigotes are usually present, in greater or lesser numbers in histiocytes of the pulmonary interstitium. They are differentiated from *Toxoplasma* and *Histoplasma* by the presence of a kinetoplast.

Acanthamoeba species are common amebae in freshwater and soil throughout the world. Human acanthamebiasis is rare but almost always fatal; approximately 60 people have died from a granulomatous amebic encephalitis caused by *Acanthamoeba* species. Trophozoites in the upper respiratory tract are probably more common than the fatal amebic encephalitis, but fewer of these have been described.[46,47] It is possible that infection of the respiratory tract precedes the fatal disease; a man who died of granulomatous amebic encephalitis had *Acanthamoeba castellanii* in his lungs.[48] Trophozoites isolated from this patient caused confluent necrotizing pneumonitis in mice.[47] Trophozoites and cysts of *Acanthamoeba* are found in the tissues of man. The trophozoites are similar in size to those of *E. histolytica*, but can be distinguished by the presence of a very large, centrally placed karyosome.

Nematoda

The nematodes, or roundworms, are an enormously successful group. *Ascaris lumbricoides*, for example, infects one-fourth of the world's human population. At any moment, there are about 20,000 tons of this worm in mankind, and this mass lays 2 thousand trillion eggs each day! Many other roundworms, such as hookworms and filariae, also infect millions of people.

In spite of this success, nematodes are only rarely detected in the lung. This may seem paradoxical at first because the larvae of many roundworm species migrate through the lungs as part of their normal life cycle. Hookworms, *Strongyloides stercoralis*, and *Ascaris lumbricoides* are examples. Their migration, maturation, and subsequent dwelling in the intestine usually causes little damage or inflammation, which is a major reason for their success. Thus, roundworms do not usually cause pulmonary lesions. Most of the lesions described here are caused by nematodes in an unusual location or in an aberrant host, such as man. In these situations the parasites tend to cause damage and provoke an intense inflammatory reaction.

Dirofilariasis

Pulmonary dirofilariasis is infection of humans with *Dirofilaria immitis* Leidy 1856, the dog heartworm. *D. immitis* infects dogs in temperate and tropical areas of the Western Hemisphere and Asia, where it is well known to veterinarians, but does not routinely occur in Europe or Africa. Prevalence of infection of dogs parallels the prevalence in man. In the United States, most infections of both humans and dogs occur in the coastal areas of southeastern states from Texas to Virginia and along the east coast from Maryland to Massachusetts. The geographic distribution of canine dirofilariasis is not as well documented in the rest of the world.

The canine population in the United States has risen rapidly during the past 15 years, and the prevalence of canine dirofilariasis has also increased. These factors have probably contributed to the increasing number of reported human infections in the United States.[49]

Disease

Humans acquire pulmonary dirofilariasis when they are bitten by mosquitoes that feed on both man and dogs. The blood of infected dogs contains microfilariae, the embryonic offspring of adult worms residing in the heart. Microfilariae ingested by a mosquito molt twice to become third-stage larvae, the infective stage. After inoculation into human skin by the mosquito they mi-

grate through subcutaneous tissue, where they molt, then enter the bloodstream and reach the heart. In man the worms die before reaching maturity, probably while clinging to the chamber of the right ventricle, and are then swept into the system of pulmonary arteries where they impact and provoke thrombosis, infarction, inflammation, and finally a granulomatous reaction surrounded by a wall of fibrous tissue. These lesions are characteristically small (2–3 cm), subpleural, spherical, and well circumscribed. Seventy percent of the patients are asymptomatic.[50] Those with symptoms have cough, chest pain, hemoptysis, fever, chills, malaise, and sometimes eosinophilia.

The disease is detected and diagnosed most often in male adults; it has not yet been seen in children. More than one-half of all infections were in men 40–60 years old,[49] who are probably the people most frequently exposed to infected mosquitos. Dog ownership is not a risk factor.

Biology

Dirofilaria immitis naturally infects a wide variety of mammals including dog, wolf, coyote, fox, bear, seals, otter, nutria, muskrat, beaver, and the domestic cat; the dog, however, is by far the most important reservoir and the definitive host. The infection is transmitted by the mosquitoes *Aedes aegypti*, *Aedes vexans*, *Aedes vigilax*, *Aedes notoscriptus*, and *Culex pipiens*.[51,52] In humans, the period of time between inoculation with infective larvae and infarction in the lung is not known, but 5–6 months are required for development to mature filariae in dogs.

Rarely, *D. immitis* has been identified in subcutaneous abscesses, in the abdominal cavity, and in the eyes.[53–55] In these locations, worms degenerate in an early stage of migration before reaching the right ventricle or pulmonary artery.

Pathology

The pulmonary lesion caused by *D. immitis* has been described radiographically as a "coin lesion" 2–3 cm in diameter, usually at the periphery, fixed to the pleura (Figs. 15–6 and 15–7). The core of the lesion consists of an area of coagulation necrosis with a ghost outline of previously viable parenchyma. Multiple histologic sections reveal the intact or degenerating worm lodged in remnants of a pulmonary arteriole (Fig. 15–8). Only immature *D. immitis* have been found in human lungs. The central area of coagulation necrosis is surrounded by a wall of fibrous tissue containing epithelioid cells, Langerhans giant cells, lymphocytes, and plasma cells.

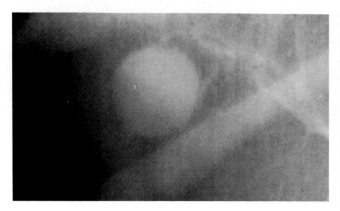

Fig. 15–6. Radiograph shows 2.5 × 2.0 cm "coin lesion" in right-lower lung. AFIP 72–10156.

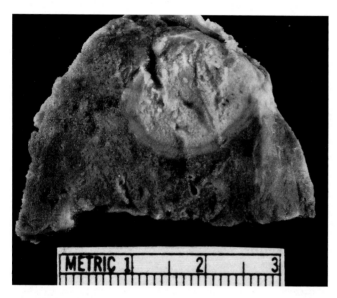

Fig. 15–7. Characteristic spherical lesion of pulmonary dirofilariasis is subpleural, sharply circumscribed, and has fibrous wall and necrotic center. AFIP 68–633. Scale in centimeters.

Even without identification of the worm, the central core of coagulation necrosis and surrounding granulomatous component in the inflammatory reaction should alert the pathologist to the possibility of pulmonary dirofilariasis. Other causes of infarction coagulation necrosis do not typically have a rim of granulomatous tissue. Antigens leaking from the worm into the tissue presumably cause the granulomatous reaction.

Diagnosis and Treatment

Pulmonary dirofilariasis is diagnosed after radiologic detection of the lesion and excision, usually done to exclude carcinoma. The histopathologic appearance of

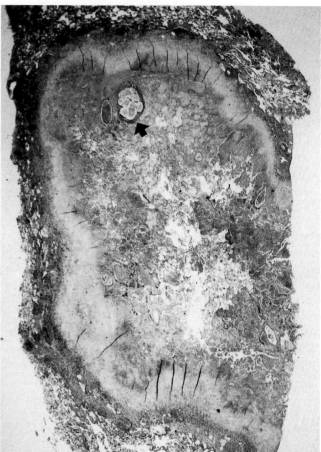

Fig. 15–8. Pulmonary dirofilariasis. Section of subpleural nodule, which is circumscribed, walled off, and contains immature *Dirofilaria immitis* in vessel (*arrow*) surrounded by necrotic tissue. Characteristically, necrotic tissue retains "ghost" outline of previously viable tissue, suggesting ischemic factor. AFIP 71–11564. Movat, ×4.5.

D. immitis permits definitive diagnosis (Fig. 15–9). Adult *D. immitis* in the dog measures 0.7–1.3 mm wide, whereas the worms found in human lungs are immature and much smaller, measuring only 100–359 μm in diameter. They have a thick cuticle (5–25 μm) with the three distinct layers characteristic of the genus *Dirofilaria*. The thick multilayered cuticle projects inwardly at the lateral chords, forming two prominent, opposing, internal longitudinal ridges.[56,57] The somatic musculature is typically prominent but the lateral chords are usually poorly preserved. Transverse sections reveal two large reproductive tubes and a much smaller intestine in female worms, and a single reproductive tube and intestine in the males. Species of *Dirofilaria* in the lung should not be confused with the many larval nematodes that also occur in the lung, because *Dirofilaria* is much larger and contains reproductive organs.

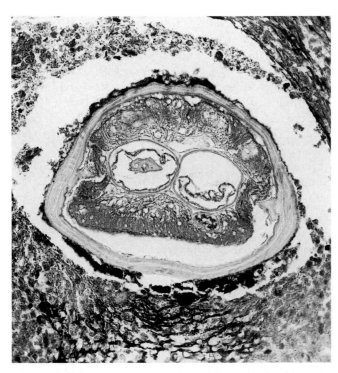

Fig. 15–9. Transverse section of immature female *Dirofilaria immitis* with pulmonary vessel. AFIP 71–1045. Movat, ×275.

Other nematodes with developed reproductive organs that are rarely found in lung (*Enterobius vermicularis*, *Wuchereria bancrofti*, and *Brugia malayi*) are much less common and are morphologically distinct from *D. immitis*.

In the absence of parasite structures, the diagnosis cannot be certain. The worm may have degenerated completely or the lesion may be a tuberculoma, histoplasmoma, or possibly a lesion of coccidioidomycosis, polyarteritis nodosa, Wegener's granulomatosis, or thromboembolism with infarction.[50] Serology, bronchoscopy, bronchial washings, or needle aspirates are not usually diagnostic. However, as pointed out previously the combination of coagulation necrosis and granulomatous reaction is characteristic and tends to exclude other possibilities. Detailed gross and histopathologic study of the lesion, and documenting the presence of the worm, are required for diagnosis; this may necessitate submitting the entire lesion for histologic study. Although immunofluorescence antibodies have been developed for tissue sections, their use is not particularly helpful.

Filariasis

Three species of filarial worms naturally infect man and may be found in the lungs: *Wuchereria bancrofti* (Cobbold 1877) Seurat 1921, *Brugia malayi* (Brug 1927)

Buckley 1958, and *Onchocerca volvulus* Railliet and Henry 1910. These worms cause bancroftian filariasis, brugian filariasis, and onchocerciasis, respectively. *Dirofilaria immitis* has been described separately because it is not a natural parasite of man.

Wuchereria bancrofti, *B. malayi*, and *O. volvulus* do not usually cause lesions in the lungs. Bancroftian and brugian filariases typically cause lymphadenopathy, lymphangitis, and, in a small percentage of chronically infected patients, elephantiasis.[58] Onchocerciasis causes a variety of changes in skin and lymph nodes,[59] and ocular involvement is a major cause of blindness worldwide.[60]

Adult worms and embryos (microfilariae) of *W. bancrofti* and *B. malayi* have been described in the lung. Adult worms cause pulmonary infarcts,[61–66] and microfilariae cause the distinct syndrome of tropical pulmonary eosinophilia.[67–70]

Most adult *O. volvulus* live in the subcutaneous tissue in what eventually becomes a walled-off nodule. Microfilariae, however, escape from the adult female, migrate through the fibrous wall, and by preference locate in the dermis, eyes, and lymph nodes. When patients are treated with diethylcarbamazine (DEC), microfilariae are mobilized and invade deep organs, including lung.[71,72]

Aberrant filarial nematodes in lung (*W. bancrofti*, *B. malayi*, and microfilariae of *O. volvulus*) are described in the next section. Tropical pulmonary eosinophilia (microfilariae of either *W. bancrofti* or *B. malayi*) is discussed separately.

Aberrant Pulmonary Filaria

Adult *Wuchereria bancrofti* or *Brugia malayi* have been reported in the lungs of six patients.[61–66] In each patient the worms caused an embolus in a small pulmonary artery, resulting in infarction. All patients had chest pain and hemoptysis. Those who had visited endemic areas developed symptoms 2–3 years after returning to a nonendemic area. Radiographs revealed patchy or well-circumscribed pulmonary lesions. The possibility of carcinoma prompted surgical excision of the nodules.

Microfilariae of *O. volvulus* appear to migrate to the lung and other deep organs after treatment with diethylcarbamazine (DEC).[71,72] Fuglsang and Anderson[72] correlated respiratory distress in a patient who had been treated with DEC with the presence of microfilariae of *O. volvulus* in sputum. Meyers et al.[71] described a patient who died of pulmonary edema after treatment with DEC whose lungs and other organs contained many microfilariae of *O. volvulus* in microabscesses (Fig. 15–10).

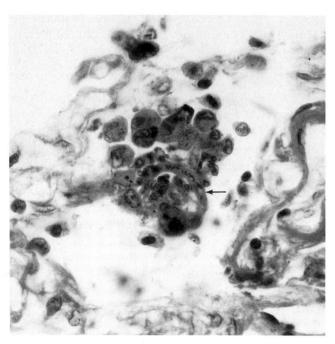

Fig. 15–10. Microfilaria of *Onchocerca volvulus* (*arrow*) in micro-abscess in lung. AFIP 86–6458. H and E, ×630.

Onchocerca volvulus is transmitted by blackflies of the genus *Simulium*, which is endemic to areas in tropical Africa, North Yemen, and Central and South America. Microfilariae of *O. volvulus* migrate within the dermis, and some are ingested when blackflies feed on humans. Treatment with DEC causes the microfilariae to leave the dermis and migrate up through the epidermis. They also migrate into the lymphatics and bloodstream, whereby they reach the deep organs such as lung, kidney, and liver. Some appear later in urine, but an immediate, vigorous, cell-mediated immune response kills many microfilariae in situ. Histopathologically, microfilariae are surrounded by eosinophilic abscesses. The clinical extreme of this massive die-off of microfilariae is itching, pain, swelling, urticaria, and sometimes systemic symptoms, collectively known as the Mazzotti reaction.

Microfilariae of *O. volvulus* are distinguished by their distinctive anterior and posterior ends. The long cephalic space is 7–13 μm, and the caudal space is 9–15 μm with a finely pointed tail.[75] Other microfilariae usually have a shorter cephalic space and a different distribution of nuclei in the tail.

Biology

Humans acquire both bancroftian and brugian filariases from the bite of infected mosquitoes. Infective larvae develop in mosquitoes after feeding on a person with microfilaremia. Both worms cause diseases that are exclusively tropical. *Brugia malayi* is found in Southeast and East Asia, and *W. bancrofti* occurs in Asia, Africa, and Central and South America.

B. malayi and *W. bancrofti* are lymphatic-dwelling worms, but aberrant infections of lung in man and infections of animals indicate a tendency for cardiopulmonary location. *Brugia buckleyi* normally inhabits the heart and pulmonary arteries of the Ceylon hare.[73] When *B. malayi* is in jirds (*Meriones unguiculatus*), the worms tend to be in pulmonary arteries.[74] *W. bancrofti* may also inhabit pulmonary arteries of experimentally infected monkeys.[74] Pulmonary arteries are aberrant sites for human lymphatic worms. Female worms identified in the lungs have been infertile, indicating this is an unnatural or inhospitable site.

Worms appear tightly coiled in pulmonary arteries. A single cross section of the artery usually contains several sections of worm. In histopathologic sections, adult *W. bancrofti* and *B. malayi* can be distinguished by their diameters, other morphologic features being virtually indistinguishable. It is difficult to assign a range of diameters for infertile female worms, but in the few patients reported *B. malayi* was about 100 μm and *W. bancrofti* was greater than 140 μm.

Pathology

In pulmonary arteries, these adult filarial worms cause thrombosis, occlusion, and a surrounding granulomatous reaction (Fig. 15–11). Nodules range in diameter from 2 to 8 cm. The center of the nodule is characterized by coagulation necrosis. Sections of the worm may extend beyond the thrombus and appear in sections of artery surrounded by normal tissue. The wall of the infarcted area is composed of dense fibrin and chronic inflammatory cells. Beyond this is a perivascular granulomatous reaction composed of eosinophils, histiocytes, epithelioid cells, and foreign body giant cells.

Diagnosis and Treatment

Filarial worms in pulmonary infarcts are diagnosed by demonstration of the parasite in histologic section.[56,75] Radiologic changes are not specific. Suspicion of carcinoma prompts surgical excision of the lesion. Specific treatment with DEC is probably unnecessary in the absence of microfilaremia. The possibility of adult filarial worms in lymphatic vessels usually prompts chemotherapy with DEC.

Tropical Pulmonary Eosinophilia

Tropical pulmonary eosinophilia (TPE) is caused by filariae, probably both *Wuchereria bancrofti* and *Brugia malayi*.[69] Adult worms have not been demonstrated in

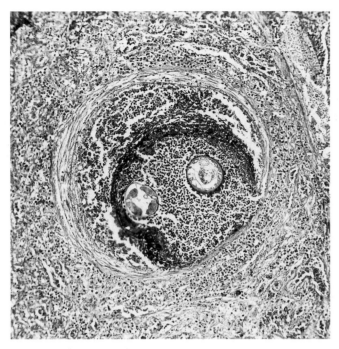

Fig. 15–11. Adult male *Wuchereria bancrofti* surrounded by thrombus obstructing pulmonary vessel. AFIP 70–9604. H and E, ×90.

patients with tropical pulmonary eosinophilia, but brugian and bancroftian filariases overlap the geographic distribution of this disease, and volunteers inoculated with *B. malayi* developed the syndrome.[76]

Tropical eosinophilia encompasses TPE and Meyers–Kouwenaar syndrome. Meyers–Kouwenaar syndrome has the same cause as TPE, but microfilariae are in lymph nodes or spleen.[69] Tropical eosinophilia is also known as Weingarten's syndrome, occult or cryptic filariasis, or filarial hypereosinophilia. TPE is also called tropical lung or eosinophilic lung (see also Chapter 16). TPE is confused with other diseases in the tropics that provoke eosinophilia, such as Loeffler's syndrome, idiopathic hypereosinophilia, chronic eosinophilic pneumonia, drug reactions, allergic aspergillosis, and some other helminthic infections.

Patients with TPE do not feel well. They have episodes of coughing, usually at night, wheezing, dyspnea, and pain or tightness in the chest. There may be low-grade fever and weight loss. Extreme eosinophilia ($>3,000/mm^3$) persists for weeks. No microfilariae can be detected in the peripheral circulation, but high titers of filarial antibodies are typical. Levels of immunoglobulin E are at least 1,000 units/ml.[70] Symptoms persist for months or they may disappear and recur years later. Pleural effusions are rare.[77]

Biology

The absence of microfilariae in the blood of patients with TPE and the presence of high levels of filarial antibody are clues to the cause of the syndrome because microfilaremic patients do not have either TPE or high levels of filarial antibody. Patients with TPE appear hypersensitive to microfilarial antigens, and it is possible that microfilariae are killed in the bloodstream and become trapped in pulmonary vessels. Adult filariae are not affected by this immune response and continue to produce microfilariae that accumulate in the lungs. This interpretation is the best rationale for the long-term symptoms associated with TPE.

Pathology

Histopathologic demonstration of microfilariae in the lungs of patients with TPE is rare. When present, they are surrounded by eosinophils. Eosinophilic abscesses eventually develop into granulomas with foreign-body giant cells and palisading epithelioid cells. Lesions are close to pulmonary venules and distant from bronchi.

Symptoms associated with TPE result from restrictive rather than obstructive defects.[70] Fewer than 30% of patients have asthma-like obstructive defects. Apparently, immediate hypersensitivity plays only a partial role in TPE.

Diagnosis and Treatment

Diagnosis of TPE in patients with typical pulmonary symptoms is made by the presence of (1) persistent hypereosinophilia; (2) high titers of filarial antibody; (3) absence of microfilariae in peripheral blood; (4) elevated IgE; (5) a history of travel to an endemic area; and (6) rapid relief of symptoms when treated with DEC.[69,70] The dosage of oral DEC is 5 mg/ml per day for 10 days.[70] Relapse resolves with another course of treatment with DEC.

Capillariasis

Capillariasis is the infection of man with one of three species of *Capillaria*: *Capillaria philippinensis*, *C. hepatica*, and *C. aerophila* Creplin 1939. Each of these worms causes a distinct form of capillariasis: intestinal, hepatic, and pulmonary, respectively.

None of the species of *Capillaria* is a natural parasite of man. *C. aerophila* is common in cats, dogs, and foxes and occurs in North and South America, Asia, Europe, and Australia. Ten infections of humans, from the Soviet Union, Iran, Morocco,[78–83] and Taiwan,[84] are known.

Disease

Patients infected with *C. aerophila* sometimes have severe dyspnea, polypnea, cough, expectoration, and fever. Eosinophilia is mild (9%–12%). Radiographs show a reticulogranular pattern and perihilar infiltrates. In humans, worms invade the mucosal epithelium of bronchioles, where they lay eggs.

Biology

Humans acquire pulmonary capillariasis by ingesting eggs of *C. aerophilia* containing infective larvae. Eggs are shed in the feces and sputa of dogs and cats, and the disease is transmitted through the soil. Eggs require 6 weeks in warm moist soil to become infective. An intermediate host may be involved, but this has not been demonstrated.

Pathology

Worms in bronchioles may provoke heavy infiltrates of eosinophils. The acute eosinophilic reaction destroys bronchioles that contain worms, and the eosinophils spill over into adjacent bronchioles and destroy them also. It should be noted that these observations are from only one patient[83]; pathologic specimens have not been collected from other patients who were successfully treated without surgery.

Diagnosis and Treatment

Diagnosis is made by identifying the characteristic eggs of *C. aerophila* in sputum. They are 65×35 μm, barrel shaped, unsegmented, and have distinctive bipolar plugs. *C. aerophila* eggs may also be found in feces, but eggs in sputum are diagnostic of *C. aerophila* because the eggs of *C. philippinensis* and *C. hepatica* are found only in feces. Thiabendazole appears to be the drug of choice. It has been used successfully to treat two patients (500 mg/day for 10 days).[82,83]

Strongyloidiasis

Strongyloidiasis is infection of man with *Strongyloides stercoralis* (Bavay 1876) Stiles and Hassall 1902, the threadworm. The infection is ubiquitous. Adult female worms usually embed in the mucosal epithelium of the upper jejunum where they lay eggs. It is speculated that the parasitic female *S. stercoralis* is parthenogenic, thus not requiring the male for reproduction. It has the uncommon ability to autoinfect its host. Although *S. stercoralis* causes most cases of strongyloidiasis, *S. fulleborni* of primates infects human beings in Africa and Papua New Guinea. The reservoir host of *S. fulleborni* on New Guinea is not known; nonhuman primates do not occur that far east of the Wallace Line (between the islands of Bali and Lombok in the Lesser Sunda Archipelago).

Migration of larvae through the lungs is obligatory in the parasitic life cycle of *S. stercoralis*, which also has a free-living cycle. Severity of pulmonary symptoms correlates with worm burden. Most infections cause epigastric or cramping abdominal pain with mild and chronic diarrhea, but have no pulmonary symptoms.

Heavy infection is common in patients with compromised immunity, including those with Hodgkin's disease, lymphocytic leukemia, cachexia, kwashiorkor, lepromatous leprosy, burns, radiation sickness, or syphilis.[85] Massive infection develops as a result of autoinfection; noninfective larvae are liberated in the gut of the host, transform into infective larvae, and penetrate the wall of the intestine. This process will overwhelm hosts unable to curtail it.

Disease

Strongyloidiasis is classified into three types: cutaneous, pulmonary, and intestinal, reflecting the course of migration of larvae through the body. Filariform larvae penetrate skin, seek blood vessels, and cause a transient and mild dermatitis.[85] Larvae migrate to the pulmonary capillaries where they immediately penetrate alveoli, causing petechial hemorrhages and infiltrates of polymorphonuclear leukocytes and monocytes.[86] Sensitized patients may experience discomfort, but usually there are no symptoms. At this stage there may be larvae in the sputum. Larvae in the lungs molt once and migrate to the trachea where they are coughed up and swallowed. Larvae reaching the gastrointestinal tract mature into adult worms and usually embed in the mucosal epithelium of the duodenum where they cause diarrhea, nausea, and vomiting.

Rhabditiform larvae emerge from eggs while still in the gut of the host. Some transform into infective larvae and penetrate the wall of the intestine. This represents autoinfection and it probably occurs in most patients with strongyloidiasis. This accounts for long-standing infections in the absence of reinfection. The reproductive activity of the worms is regulated in some manner so that the host is not in danger from an enormous worm burden. In patients with compromised immunity, however, the host–parasite regulatory mechanism is lost and autoinfection leads to life-threatening hyperinfection. In the gut of hyperinfected patients, thousands of worms produce larvae that migrate through most deep organs, particularly in the lungs. Pulmonary symptoms, correlated with the number of migrating larvae, consist of dyspnea, cough, hemoptysis, cyanosis, and respiratory distress. Eosinophilia may be present. The prognosis is poor in patients who do not have eosinophilia.

Patients with hyperinfection die of severe diarrhea, peritonitis, septicemia, or respiratory failure.[87] Some patients may have adult worms in bronchial epithelium.[86,88] These patients may have chronic bronchitis, asthma-like symptoms, or impending respiratory failure.[89,90] Dogs with adult *Strongyloides* in the lungs develop acute respiratory distress and die of pneumonitis.[88]

Biology

Adult *S. stercoralis* in warm moist soil produce rhabditiform larvae, which transform into infective larvae or mature into free-living adult worms. The conditions that regulate these alternatives are not known. Parasitic female worms are 1.5–2.5 mm long and 30–40 μm wide; rhabditiform larvae are 380 × 20 μm and filariform larvae are 600 × 16 μm. The filariform larva has a characteristic notched tail and lacks a buccal cavity.

Strongyloides stercoralis is more common in tropical and subtropical environments. Tropical soils that have an abundance of moisture and human feces favor development of *S. stercoralis*. Prevalence figures vary widely, but rural villages with poor sanitation are ideal for transmission of strongyloidiasis.

Pathology

Larvae penetrating alveoli cause petechial hemorrhages that occasionally become severe (Fig. 15–12).[88] Both cavities and abscesses of lung have been associated with filariform larvae.[91,92] When adult *S. stercoralis* invade lung they embed in bronchial epithelium, preferring higher levels where the epithelium is palisaded.[88] Adult worms in lung or rhabditiform larvae in sputum (Fig. 15–13) indicate hyperinfection. The presence of viable adult worms in lung is called pulmonary strongyloidiasis.

Diagnosis and Treatment

Diagnosis is made by identification of larvae in sputum or feces.[89–93] Fortuitous demonstration of migrating larvae in either ascitic or cerebrospinal fluid also pro-

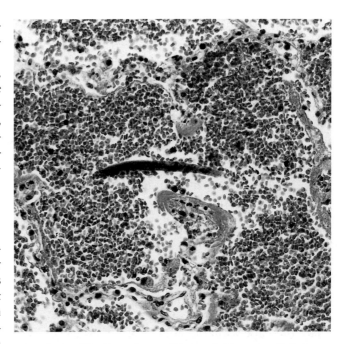

Fig. 15–12. Filariform larva of *Strongyloides stercoralis* in hemorrhagic area of lung. AFIP 75–9907. H and E, ×275.

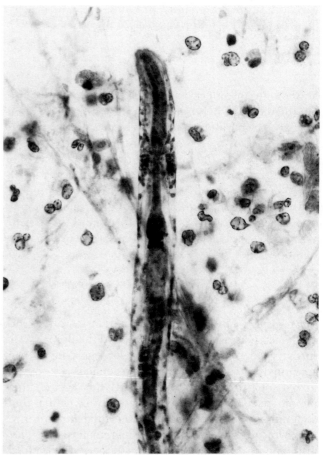

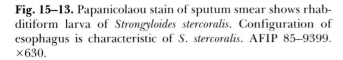

Fig. 15–13. Papanicolaou stain of sputum smear shows rhabditiform larva of *Strongyloides stercoralis*. Configuration of esophagus is characteristic of *S. stercoralis*. AFIP 85–9399. ×630.

vides the diagnosis. In hyperinfection, filariform larvae may appear in virtually any organ and must be differentiated from other parasites of man such as *Ascaris*, *Necator*, and *Ancylostoma*, as well as those causing visceral larva migrans (for example, *Toxocara* and *Baylisascaris*).[86,94] Rhabditiform larvae or eggs in sputum indicate pulmonary strongyloidiasis. These should be confirmed as *S. stercoralis*, because free-living rhabditiform larvae of other species (e.g., *Rhabditis*) occasionally contaminate laboratory specimens. The usual treatment is 25 mg thiabendazole per kilogram of body weight twice daily for 3 days. Hyperinfection requires hospitalization and prolonged courses of treatment with thiabendazole.[95]

Mammomonogamiasis

Mammomonogamiasis is the infection of humans with *Mammomonogamus laryngeus* (Railliet 1899) Ryjikov 1948, the gapeworm of cattle. More than 100 human infections have been reported, mostly in visitors to Caribbean islands: Martinique, Dominica, Puerto Rico, St. Lucia, and Trinidad. Infections have also been reported from Guyana, Brazil, and the Philippines. Most patients acquired the infection in Martinique.[96] A survey of stool specimens from 3,700 residents revealed 22 persons with eggs of *M. laryngeus*.[97]

Disease

Mammomonogamiasis is probably acquired from cattle, but the mechanism is not known. Ingestion of an intermediate or paratenic host infected with third-stage larvae of *M. laryngeus* seems most probable. Worms in humans attach to the mucosa of the throat, trachea, or bronchi, provoking the most violent symptoms in the latter site. Almost all patients have chronic cough of 1–10 months in duration.[98] The cough, frequently most intense at night, is disruptive and frightens the patient. Worms are occasionally coughed up. There may be hemoptysis.

Biology

Mammomonogamus laryngeus is common in cattle from endemic areas.[99] The worms attach to the lining of the throat where they copulate and lay eggs. Eggs from sputum or feces hatch in soil. Emergent larvae probably infect an arthropod or annelid. If this occurs, then people probably acquire the disease by eating food contaminated with the infected intermediate host.

Worms are in permanent male–female pairs. They are joined in copula, forming a characteristic Y shape

(Fig. 15–14). The male worm is much smaller than the female, 3 mm × 400 μm versus 10 mm × 650 μm. Both worms are bright red. Eggs of *M. laryngeus* are similar to those of hookworms, but are slightly larger and contain a morula (a vermiform embryo) when laid, whereas hookworm eggs contain a four- to eight-cell embryo.

Pathology

Adult worms provoke intense inflammation at the site of attachment. Pairs of worms may be encysted, but usually they are free and squirming about. There is almost always one pair of worms, but two or three pairs have been reported.[96]

Diagnosis and Treatment

Diagnosis is made by identifying eggs in sputum, although pairs of adult worms are occasionally seen in sputum. Diagnosis with fiberoptic bronchoscopy may

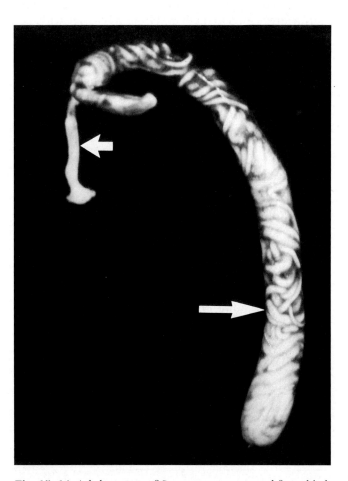

Fig. 15–14. Adult worms of *Syngamus* sp. removed from bird. Male worm (*short arrow*) is smaller than female worm (*long arrow*) to which it is permanently attached. AFIP 82–13669. ×9.

be helpful when eggs are not found in sputa of infected patients.[100] Treatment is with thiabendazole (100 mg/day for 3 days) or by bronchoscopic ablation of the attachment site of the worms.[96,100] Relief of symptoms is immediate.

Ascariasis

Ascariasis is infection of humans with *Ascaris lumbricoides* Linnaeus 1758. Prevalence in endemic areas routinely exceeds 50%. The worm is ubiquitous, but is especially common in tropical and subtropical environments with abundant moisture and human excreta in soil.

Ascariasis is ordinarily innocuous, and most people are unaware of infection. Ascariasis is an important public health problem, however, because many of the complications are life threatening.[101] Approximately 2 of every 1,000 infected persons develop intestinal obstruction, the most common complication.

The most common pulmonary complication of ascariasis is pneumonitis caused by migrating larvae, which provoke an allergic reaction that causes transient asthma. Larvae may cause bronchopneumonia (Fig. 15–15), but they are often killed and surrounded by granulomas. Rare pulmonary complications of ascariasis typify the bizarre complications caused by adult ascarids wandering through the body. An adult worm in the trachea caused death by choking[102]; an adult

worm in a pulmonary artery caused a fatal embolism[103]; a liver abscess surrounding an adult ascarid penetrated the diaphragm and caused pleural empyema[104]; and an ascarid has even been found thrashing about in lung parenchyma at thoracotomy.[105]

Disease

Pulmonary symptoms caused by migrating *A. lumbricoides* larvae are mild or absent in most patients. However, allergic or hyperinfected patients might have severe disease.

Ascaris pneumonitis is characterized by asthmatic type dyspnea with chronic cough, wheezing, low-grade fever, and a transient eosinophilia. Eosinophils and Charcot–Leyden crystals are abundant in sputum. Larvae may be in sputum, but usually they are absent. Symptoms resolve in 2–3 weeks as the larvae leave the lungs. These signs and symptoms are collectively known as acute eosinophilic pneumonia or Loeffler's syndrome (see Chapter 16). It is rare in hyperendemic areas where transmission occurs all year round.[106] In temperate areas where there is seasonal transmission, Loeffler's syndrome is relatively common among patients with ascariasis. Larvae of other worms (*Toxocara*, *Ancylostoma*, and *Necator*) also cause Loeffler's syndrome.

Infection with *Ascaris suum*, the ascarid of pigs, occurs when persons are exposed to soil containing feces from infected pigs. The infection provokes more severe symptoms than occur in patients with *A. lumbricoides*.[107] In Takata's classical experiments,[108] volunteers who swallowed eggs of *A. suum* had cough, fever, and headache, whereas those who swallowed comparable numbers of *A. lumbricoides* did not become ill.

Biology

Humans acquire ascariasis by ingesting eggs of *A. lumbricoides* containing infective larvae. Eggs in fresh feces are not infective; several weeks in soil are required before the eggs become infective. Moist shady soil 20°–30°C is ideal. Developing larvae are destroyed by sunlight, desiccation, and extreme temperature. Infective eggs in cold environments may remain viable for several years, but in tropical heat they live only a few hours. Wind, rain, and animals (e.g., dung beetles) cause eggs in soil to concentrate in certain areas and strata,[109] creating a patchy distribution of eggs in soil. Massive infection might thus be acquired from swallowing small, even inapparent, quantities of soil. Geophagia predisposes to infection, but inadvertent ingestion of soil or food contaminated with soil probably causes most infections.

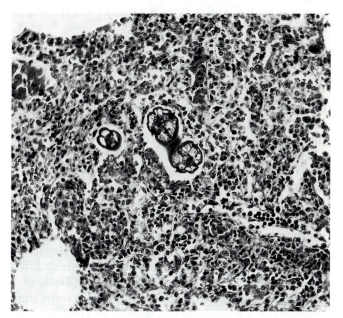

Fig. 15–15. Lung with focus of bronchopneumonia contains three transverse sections of larva of *Ascaris lumbricoides*. AFIP 68–5176. H and E, ×185.

Gnathostoma spinigerum causes gnathostomiasis in persons in Thailand, China, Malaysia, Japan, India, Java, Vietnam, the Philippines, Israel, and Mexico. Infection is acquired by drinking water contaminated with *Cyclops* containing infective larvae of *G. spinigerum*. Larvae penetrate the wall of the gut and migrate through the viscera or skin, thus causing larval migrans. Worms in the lungs or respiratory tract are rare.[140–142] Daengsvang[140] recorded 6 infections of the respiratory tract among 643 patients in Thailand with gnathostomiasis.

Trematoda

Trematodes belong to the phylum Platyhelminthes, the flatworms. Within the class Trematoda we find what is probably the most important helminthic infection of man, schistosomiasis. Of the parasitic diseases, it is second only to malaria as a cause of morbidity and mortality. As an agent of pulmonary disease, however, schistosomiasis is minor. Eggs deposited in the lungs provoke a granulomatous reaction that is generally harmless; only extraordinary infections lead to life-threatening schistosomal cor pulmonale. Most heavily infected patients die of other causes before cor pulmonale develops.

The several species of *Paragonimus* that cause paragonimiasis, especially *P. westermani*, are the only true human pulmonary parasites. They are the only parasites of which the adult worms preferentially reside in human lungs.

Alariasis is a medical curiosity in that only three people have been shown to have been infected. The disease is described in some detail because one patient who died had spectacular pulmonary lesions.

Paragonimiasis

Paragonimiasis is infection by a lung fluke of the genus *Paragonimus*. The most common lung fluke infecting man is *P. westermani* (Kerbert 1878) Braun 1899, the oriental lung fluke. These are the only helminthic parasites of man that, as adult worms, naturally infect the lungs. Worms in ectopic sites have been described in the brain, liver, gut, skeletal muscle, testes, and lymph nodes.

Paragonimiasis causes chronic lung disease and occurs in Asia, Africa, and South America. About 48 species and subspecies have been described; 9 species are believed to cause disease in humans.

In Asia paragonimiasis is caused primarily by *P. westermani*, but also by four other species. (1) *Paragonimus skrjabini* Chen, 1959 (syn. *P. szechuanensis* Chung &

Tsao 1962); (2) *P. mizayakii* Kamo, Nishida, Hatsyshika & Tomimura 1961; (3) *P. heterotremus* Chen & Hsia 1964; and (4) *P. heitungensis* Chung, Hsu, Ho, et al. 1977, or *P. philippinensis* Ito, Yokogawa, Araki, and Kobayashi 1978. Japan, Taiwan, and Korea are endemic areas. The disease is less frequent but also endemic in China, Vietnam, Laos, Cambodia, Thailand, India, Malaysia, Indonesia, Papua New Guinea, Samoa, and the Solomon Islands.

In the Western Hemisphere the species are *P. mexicanus* Miryazaki & Ishii 1968 (syn. *P. ecuadoriensis* Voelker & Arzube 1979) and *P. kellicotti* Ward 1908. Human infections have been reported in Peru, Colombia, Ecuador, Venezuela, and Costa Rica and Mexico. *P. kellicotti* is a common parasite of mink in North America.

In Africa, *P. africanus* Voelker & Vogel 1965 and *P. uterobilateralis* Voelker & Vogel 1965 infect humans, primarily in the west central portion of the continent.

Disease

Paragonimiasis causes either pulmonary disease or lesions at ectopic sites. Ectopic paragonimiasis is not a complication of pulmonary disease but a manifestation of the larvae of *Paragonimus* that lodge by chance in other tissues. Some ectopic infections are more life threatening than pulmonary paragonimiasis. The prognosis in pulmonary paragonimiasis is good, but the outcome of cerebral paragonimiasis is often fatal, even with aggressive treatment.

Humans acquire paragonimiasis by eating raw infected crabs or crayfish. Larvae penetrate the wall of the gut, then the diaphragm, and finally settle in the pleura or parenchyma of the lung (Fig. 15–23). The worms provoke leukocytic infiltrates and later fibrous encapsulation; cavities may form.[143,144] Egg laying commences in about 70 days. Cysts contain worms, eggs, and necrotic debris. When cysts perforate a bronchiole or bronchus, the contents spill out. Eggs are coughed up or become lodged in parenchyma and provoke fibrosis (Fig. 15–24).

The clinical onset is insidious. Patients usually present with hemoptysis and cough; they may have severe chest pain and night sweats. Radiography of the chest reveals transient diffuse pulmonary infiltrates and ring shadows resembling annular opacities.[145–147] Pleural effusion, which is common, was present in 48% of patients in one study.[145]

The diagnostic triad of cough, hemoptysis, and eggs in sputa or feces seen in pulmonary paragonimiasis does not occur in pleural paragonimiasis (Fig. 15–25).[148] In many patients, pleural effusion is the only clinical sign. Radiography shows normal lungs unless the infection is extraordinarily heavy.

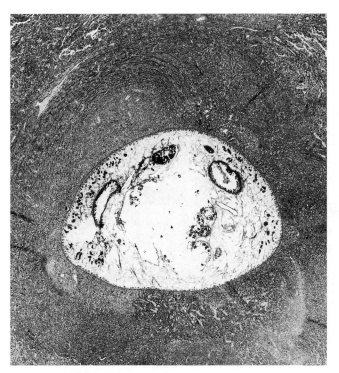

Fig. 15–23. Adult *Paragonimus westermani* in pulmonary lesion. AFIP 85–10940. H and E, ×15.

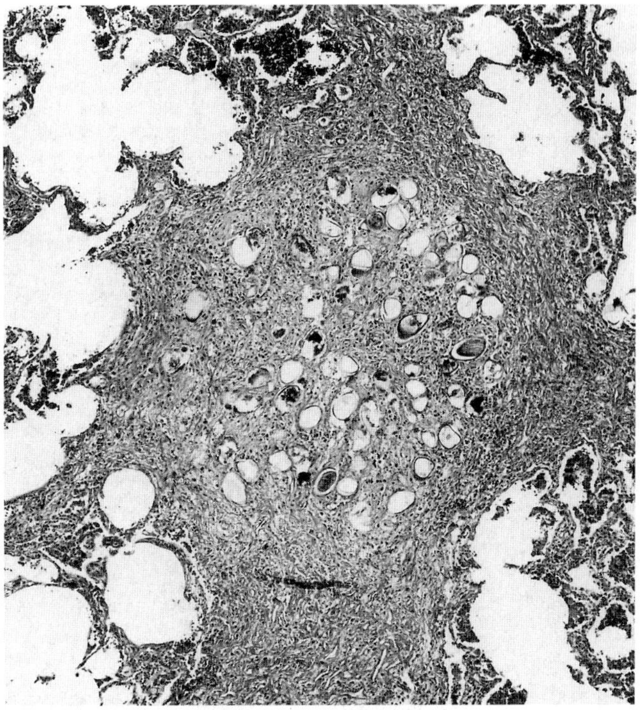

Fig. 15–24. Eggs of *Paragonimus westermani* in fibrous scar tissue of lung. AFIP 85–10941. H and E, ×60.

Biology

Eggs of *Paragonimus* are coughed up from the lungs, swallowed, and passed with feces. In water, miracidia emerge 2 weeks later and infect a molluscan intermediate host. A sporocyst and redia generation develop in the mollusc during the next several weeks. Infective cercariae emerge and penetrate the gills of a crustacean. The larvae migrate to soft tissue and encyst, and metacercariae develop in 6–8 weeks. The cyst is 0.4 mm. When a person swallows it, a pinkish metacercaria (0.7 × 0.27 mm) emerges and penetrates the wall of the stomach. The larva migrates to the diaphragm, bores through it, and settles in the lungs. Adult worms may persist in humans for 20 years.

The adult worm is plump and ovoid (Fig. 15–26), 7–12 mm long and 4–6 mm wide. Tooth-like spines cover the exterior of the worm, which is covered by a tegument (Fig. 15–27). The excretory bladder extends from the pharynx to the posterior aspect of the worm. The two deeply lobed testes are in the posterior third of the body. The ovary is lobed, posterior to the ventral sucker, and left or right of the midline, and the uterus is opposite the ovary. Vitellaria are well developed and extend the length of the worm in the lateral fields.

Eggs of *Paragonimus westermani* are ovoid, yellowish brown, operculated, and 75–110 μm long by 45–60 μm wide. The operculum is characteristically flattened

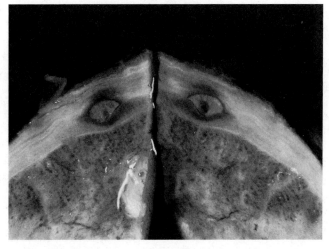

Fig. 15–25. Bisected adult *Paragonimus westermani* in pleura that is greatly thickened by fibrous tissue. AFIP 70–7295. ×3.3.

(Figs. 15–28 and 15–29). Suzuki[149] has described the differential morphology of the eggs in most *Paragonimus* species.

Pathology

Adult worms that migrate into the parenchyma of the lung usually lodge near larger bronchioles or bronchi.

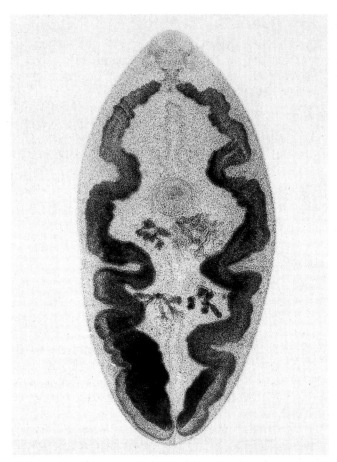

Fig. 15–26. Adult *Paragonimus westermani*. Ventral view of stained gross specimen. AFIP 76–5953. ×11.

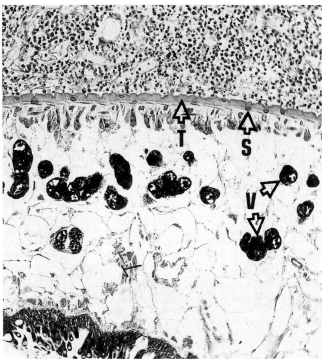

Fig. 15–27. Body wall of *Paragonimus westermani*. Symbols: T, tegument; S, spine; V, vitellaria. AFIP 74–11162. H and E, ×145.

An exudate of eosinophils and neutrophils surrounds groups of worms or, rarely, a single worm. A thin fibrous wall develops and may become several millimeters thick. Cysts are generally 1.5 cm in diameter. The center of the cyst may become necrotic, and when the cyst ruptures into a bronchiole or bronchus, this material spills out and may cause bronchopneumonia.[150]

Diagnosis and Treatment

Pulmonary paragonimiasis is frequently misdiagnosed as tuberculosis, as was done in 47% of patients in one study.[147] Eggs in sputa or feces provide the definitive diagnosis. In pleural paragonimiasis, the pleura must be aspirated to obtain eggs.

Pulmonary paragonimiasis is rarely fatal, even without treatment. Bithional is a wide-spectrum, antitrematodal drug that concentrates in lung tissue. It has a cure rate of 80%–100% and was once regarded as the drug of choice for pulmonary paragonimiasis at dosages of 30 to 50 mg/kg every other day for 2–4 weeks. Bithional is ineffective in pleural paragonimiasis. Praziquantel

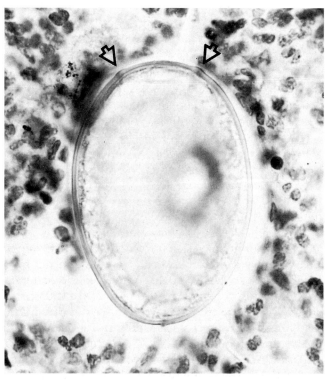

Fig. 15–28. Egg of *Paragonimus uterobilateralis* in sputum. Operculum (*arrows*) is characteristic of most trematode eggs. AFIP 83–10695. ×630.

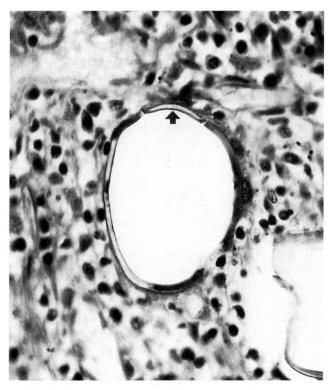

Fig. 15–29. Egg of *Paragonimus westermani* in section of lung shows operculum (*arrow*). AFIP 73–6856. H and E, ×675.

has been 100% effective against pulmonary paragonimiasis, and has cured patients who failed to respond to treatment with bithional.[151] Praziqantel is now the drug of choice. Treatment with praziquantel has caused patients to cough up living worms,[152] but otherwise there are no side effects; 25 mg/kg three times per day at 4-h intervals, after meals, for 3 days is 100% curative. Praziquantel has not been evaluated in pleural paragonimiasis. A single dose of niclofolan is curative,[153] but causes muscle pain, sweats, and lassitude.

Alariasis

Alariasis is human infection with mesocercaria larvae of species of *Alaria*. The *Alaria* species that infect humans occur in North America, where they are common parasites of canids. The intermediate hosts are usually frogs or snakes. This is the only known disease of man caused by trematode mesocercariae. The disease is rare, and only three infections are known.[154–156] We describe alariasis here because of the extraordinary pulmonary lesions reported in one patient. Also, the large number of immigrants from Southeast Asia may be predisposed to alariasis because some traditional foods consist of raw or pickled amphibians or reptiles.[157]

Disease

Of the three infections of man with *Alaria*, one was systemic, one involved the skin, and the other the eye; the systemic infection was fatal.[154] The patient was believed to have eaten frog legs heavily infected with mesocercariae of *Alaria americana*. The illness began with dyspnea, cough, hemoptysis, and tightness in the chest. Open lung biopsy revealed parasites and diffuse interstitial hemorrhage. Asphyxiation from pulmonary hemorrhage killed the patient 9 days after onset. An anticoagulant isolated from the blood of this patient was presumed to have originated from the several thousand larvae found at autopsy.

Biology

Eggs of *Alaria americana* pass in feces and hatch in freshwater, releasing ciliated miracidiae that infect snails.[158] Cercariae develop in the snail, emerge, and penetrate the skin of amphibians or reptiles. Mesocercariae develop and concentrate in the muscles of the hind legs of frogs. When the frog is eaten, mesocercariae emerge and penetrate the wall of the gut. They migrate to the diaphragm and penetrate the lung where metacercariae develop. Later they migrate to the gut to mature. In the area where the patient with fatal alariasis frequently hiked, bullfrogs contained as many as 3,500 mesocercariae each. Pathologic findings in this patient were consistent with the migratory route of mesocercariae in a canid host. Mesocercariae found in the lungs were 300–800 μm long, depending on contraction of the larva. The position of the four penetration glands, the number of rings of spines on the ventral sucker, and the pattern of spines on the dorsal surface allowed specific identification.[159]

Pathology

At autopsy, most of the deep organs were hemorrhagic. Living larvae were present in lungs, heart, liver, kidney, pancreas, spleen, lymph nodes, brain, spinal cord, and adipose tissue. Tracks of inflammatory tissue characteristic of the tracks of migrating parasites were present in the gut and diaphragm. Microscopically, there was interstitial hemorrhage and many parasites in lung tissue. Tissue surrounding the parasites was not inflamed.

Diagnosis and Treatment

Diagnosis was made by identifying larvae in an open lung biopsy specimen. Bithional, a wide-spectrum anti-trematodal drug that concentrates in lung, was administered by gastric tube with bicarbonate. It is not clear whether the drug was given too late to effect a cure or simply had no effect.

Schistosomiasis

Schistosomiasis is a tropical disease caused by blood flukes of the genus *Schistosoma*. Five species are known to infect humans: *Schistosoma mansoni* Sambon 1907, *S. haematobium* (Bilharz 1852) Weinland 1858, *S. japonicum* Katsurada 1904, and, less commonly, *S. intercalatum* or *S. mekongi*. Pulmonary lesions can occur when the metamorphosed cercariae, the schistosomula, migrate via the hemolymphatic system, through the heart to the lungs. Schistosome eggs in lung are a routine incidental finding in endemic areas,[160] but disease caused by eggs in lung tissue is relatively rare. Eggs of *S. mansoni* and more rarely of *S. japonicum* and *S. haematobium* are deposited in lung tissue from the venous circulation.

Larval pneumonitis, occurring shortly after heavy schistosome infection, and a Loeffler-like pneumonitis, are probably manifestations of allergic reactions to worm antigens. Cor pulmonale, an infrequent component of human schistosomiasis, manifests as a result of prolonged deposition of large numbers of schistosome eggs. Large numbers of eggs provoke focal perivascular granulomas and fibrosis, which cause arteritis, obstruction of vessels, and eventually cor pulmonale.[161]

Disease

Humans acquire schistosomiasis by swimming or wading through water containing infective cercariae. Cercariae penetrate the skin, enter vessels, and mature to become adult worms living together in copula in veins. The adult worms per se cause no disease, but over the years they release large numbers of eggs that lodge in tissue and provoke pathologic complications. Eggs may be shunted from mesenteric veins to the lungs through portosystemic collateral veins.

Larval pneumonitis occurs weeks to days after heavy cercarial exposure. The patient presents with a low-grade fever, a mild cough, and eosinophilia. Scattered wheezing and basilar crepitations are audible on auscultation, and chest radiographs demonstrate basilar mottling. Spontaneous resolution is common. Embolic worms may cause a similar, more localized disease or produce mass lesions in the lung.

A Loeffler-like syndrome is seen in patients during chemotherapy of heavy infections. It is believed to result from an allergic response to the sudden release of antigens from dying worms. The clinical and laboratory findings are similar to those of larval pneumonitis,

except that spontaneous resolution is usually more rapid and eosinophilia is less prominent.

Katayama fever may occur following infection of a nonimmune individual with *Schistosoma*. It is characterized by fever, chills, cough, abdominal pain, diarrhea, nausea, vomiting, headache, urticaria, hepatosplenomegaly, and lymphadenopathy. It can be life threatening. There is prominent eosinophilia and marked elevation of IgE and IgG. The clinical syndrome resembles serum sickness and usually occurs 4–6 weeks after heavy infection.

In chronic schistosomiasis, long-standing egg granuloma formation causes the majority of symptoms. When eggs lodge in arterioles, they provoke granulomatous endarteritis; pulmonary hypertension develops, and cor pulmonale follows. Schistosomal cor pulmonale, although uncommon, occurs in all schistosome-endemic areas of the world, but is most often reported in *S. mansoni* infections from Egypt and Brazil. It is mainly associated with patients with hepatosplenic schistosomiasis with portal hypertension, which allows shunting of eggs to the lungs. These patients present with easy fatigability, palpitations, dyspnea, cough, and occasional hemoptysis and right ventricular hypertrophy. The prognosis is poor.[162,163]

Biology

Schistosomiasis is transmitted from one person to another through a molluscan intermediate host. Schistosome eggs in feces or urine that are deposited in the environment release miracidiae into freshwater. Miracidiae penetrate the soft tissue of a mollusc and emerge several weeks later as infective cercariae. Fork-tailed cercariae swim until they contact skin, which they immediately penetrate, dropping off their characteristic tail. Cercariae are armed for penetration with both mechanical and chemical devices. Within 24 h of contact with skin, they reach and penetrate capillaries in the dermis. They then travel through the venous circulation through the heart and to the lungs, where they squeeze through pulmonary capillaries; and then pass back through the heart and by chance to the liver where they mature to egg-laying adults. Worm pairs eventually migrate to mesenteric veins where they remain. Extrusion of eggs into intestine, liver, or spleen, which begins 1–2 months after exposure, may cause diarrhea and fever.

Pathology

Larval pneumonitis and the Loeffler-like pneumonitis are histologically undocumented but may show an eosinophil-dominated acute inflammatory response.

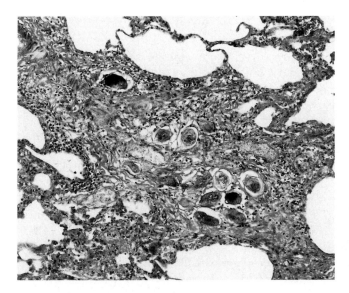

Fig. 15–30. Fibrotic lesion of lung contains eggs of *Schistosoma japonicum*. AFIP 85–10944. H and E, ×120.

In endemic areas, hypertrophy of the right ventricle (0.8–1.3 cm in thickness) suggests schistosomal cor pulmonale. Gross appearance of the lungs is normal. Microscopically, *Schistosoma* eggs cause a dumbbell-shaped granulomatous endarteritis. Eggs are surrounded by epithelioid cells and a collar of concentric collagen (Fig. 15–30). Aneurysmal dilation of the pulmonary artery may occur.[164] The lesions are angiomatoid or plexiform[165,166] (see Chapter 29). Endothelial thickening and arteriolar hypertrophy are present. Adult schistosomes are occasionally found within the lumen of pulmonary vessels (Fig. 15–31).

Diagnosis and Treatment

Egg identification is the usual method of establishing the diagnosis. The largest eggs, 140–240 by 50–85 μm, are those of *Schistosoma intercalatum*. The eggs of *S. mansoni* and *S. haematobium* are 110–175 by 40–70 μm; the eggs of *S. japonicum* are smaller, about 100 μm in greatest diameter, and those of *S. mekongi* are smaller still, about 60–70 μm in greatest diameter. The eggs of *S. mansoni* have a prominent lateral spine: the spine of *S. haematobium* is small and terminal, that of *S. intercalatum* is large and terminal, and *S. japonicum* and *S. mekongi* eggs have no significant spine. Pathologic resemblance to paragonimiasis is superficial. *Paragonimus* eggs are smaller than most schistosome eggs (100 μm), lack spines, and are operculated and birefringent. In tissue sections, however, the absence of spines or opercula may not be helpful because these features are not readily seen (Fig. 15–32). Fortuitous demonstration of these features, however, is diagnostic.

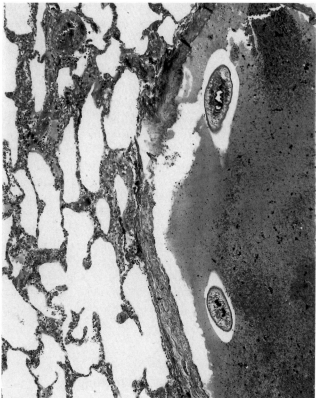

Fig. 15–31. Mature female schistosome in pulmonary artery. AFIP 91–10394. H and E, ×75.

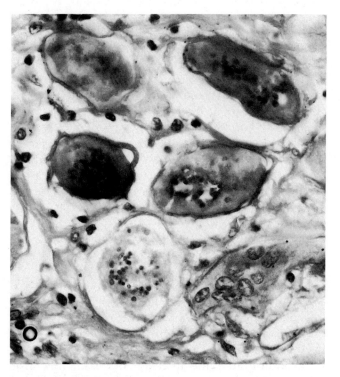

Fig. 15–32. Eggs of *Schistosoma japonicum* in pulmonary granuloma. AFIP 86–6457. H and E, ×630.

Serologic tests are available but of little practical use in endemic areas. These tests often become positive long after infection, or they become negative long after cure. Nonetheless, serology may useful for determining a history of exposure to schistosomiasis among travelers to endemic areas.

Praziquantel is the drug of choice. Amoscanate is useful and less expensive. Other drugs include furapromidum, dipterex, and niridazole. Larval pneumonitis usually resolves spontaneously. A marked Loeffler-like syndrome is an indication to temporarily discontinue chemotherapy. Treatment for Katayama fever has not been established, but antiinflammatory therapy with salicylates or corticosteroids has been used.

Schistosomal cor pulmonale is diagnosed at autopsy. Hypertrophy of the right ventricle associated with arteritis and vascular obstruction caused by schistosome eggs indicate cor pulmonale. There is no effective treatment for schistosomal cor pulmonale. Antischistosomal therapy is usually given, however, to prevent progression of disease.

Miscellaneous Trematodes

Opisthorchis viverrini is a liver fluke. It is found only in northeastern Thailand, where it infects about 25% of the population. Prijyanonda and Tandhanand[167] described a 37-year-old farmer from Thailand who died after a cyst in the liver containing parasites penetrated the diaphragm and pleura and invaded the right lung. The lower lobe of this lung contained part of a cyst with *O. viverrini* adults. Eggs of the parasites were embedded in parenchyma of the lung. The patient coughed up bile-stained sputum containing the operculated eggs of *O. viverrini* before he died. Eggs of *O. viverrini* are very small, 22–32 μm by 11–22 μm.

Fasciola hepatica is the liver fluke of sheep, but infection of humans occurs wherever sheep are raised. In man, the worm inhabits bile ducts in the liver. Migrating larvae occasionally infect ectopic sites, most commonly subcutaneous tissue. The lungs or pharynx are occasionally involved, where worms cause lung abscesses or the "halzoun" (suffocation) syndrome, respectively.[168,169] This may cause difficulty in breathing and, rarely, true suffocation.

Clinostomum complanatum is a fluke occurring in the esophagus and pharynx of herons and gulls. Three infections of man are known,[170–172] two in Japan and one in Israel. Each patient had laryngitis caused by *C. complanatum* attached to the pharynx. These patients probably acquired the infection by eating raw fish infected with metacercariae of *C. complanatum*.

Cestoda

There are three major cestode infections that cause pulmonary lesions; echinococcosis, cysticercosis, and sparganosis. Echinococcosis is the most important disease caused by cestodes, the tapeworm group, and is probably the most dreaded helminthic disease of man. It is easily acquired in endemic areas and is often fatal. Cysts in the lungs are common. We carefully distinguish the three types of echinococcosis, as these are clinically, epidemiologically, and biologically distinct.

Sparganosis and cysticercosis rarely involve the lung, and when they do, the patient's health is not seriously effected. Cysticercosis, however, occasionally causes life-threatening lesions elsewhere, particularly in the brain. Correct diagnosis of a harmless pulmonary lesion caused by cysticercosis could save the patient's life.

Sparganosis

Sparganosis is human infection with a pseudophyllidean cestode plerocercoid larva called a sparganum. The infection is aberrant because spargana in humans are *Spirometra* species, which naturally infect dogs, cats, and other carnivorous mammals.

In humans, almost all spargana cause subcutaneous nodules. Occasionally they infect other tissues including the lungs. A rare proliferative form of sparganosis can involve both skin and deep organs. Only 10 infections with proliferating spargana are known.[173] The larva causing this infection is referred to as *Sparganum proliferum* (Ijima 1905) Stiles 1908, but the adult worm has not yet been identified.

Pulmonary involvement with spargana has been reported in four patients, three with proliferative larvae and one with normal spargana. Patients with pulmonary sparganosis are not usually infected at other sites (three of four patients). Only one patient with parasites in the lung had dissemination parasitosis. Pulmonary sparganosis has been reported from Malaysia, Taiwan, Paraguay, and Pennsylvania (United States). This wide distribution reflects that of sparganosis in definitive hosts.

Disease

Humans acquire sparganosis from snakes, frogs, fish, or copepods. Eating these animals raw or drinking water contaminated with infected copepods causes sparganosis. In areas of Asia, split frogs are used as poultices; plerocercoid larvae emerge from the carcass and penetrate mucosal surfaces of humans. Eating raw pork may also cause sparganosis because pigs are infected with spargana.

A patient with pulmonary sparganosis caused by a nonproliferative sparganum had two worms in a pulmonary artery.[174] The worms probably migrated into venous circulation, passed through the heart, and created an embolus in the involved artery. A patient with a disseminated and proliferative infection died with Hodgkin's disease.[175] The parasite was thought to be a proliferating sparganum. The patient had severe bilateral pneumonia. Parasites were free in parenchyma of the lung and in giant cells. Almost every organ was invaded by this rare and peculiar parasite.

Two patients had parasites in the pleural spaces.[173,176] One had malaise and fever associated with a mediastinal mass that displaced the heart to the right. There was atelectasis of the lower lobe of the left lung. Right anterolateral thoracotomy revealed a nodular mass with extensions to the aorta, superior vena cava, bronchocephalic trunk and innominate vein. The projections adhered to these structures and could not be removed; the patient died after surgery. The other patient with pleural parasites had patchy lesions of the lungs for several years. The lesions increased in number, and eventually involved both lung fields. The parasites, removed at surgery, occupied only the pleural spaces.

Biology

Spirometra mansonoides probably causes most sparganosis in North America. Adult *S. mansonoides* live in the intestinal tract of many carnivorous mammals, including dogs and cats. Eggs passed in feces release a coracidium in freshwater that infects *Cyclops*, a ubiquitous zooplanktonic crustacean. An infective procercoid develops in the crustacean. When a snake, frog, fish, or person swallows the *Cyclops*, the procercoid larva emerges and penetrates the wall of the intestine. Larvae migrate through various tissues and organs and develop into spargana (plerocercoid larvae). If a definitive host eats infected tissue, spargana mature to an adult tapeworm in the gut. In an aberrant host like man, spargana do not mature; they migrate aimlessly through subcutaneous tissue and other organs.

Species of spargana infecting lung are not known. Unequivocal identification requires a mature worm. Thus, an intact sparganum from man is fed to a dog or cat and later the adult worm is collected and identified.[177] This, however, has not been done with spargana causing pulmonary disease. It is likely that most spargana in man are aberrant forms of the usual parasites, *S. mansonoides* in North America and *S. mansoni* in Asia.

Beaver and Rolon[173] classified proliferating spargana into three categories: (1) *Sparganum proliferum*; (2) undifferentiated cysticercus; and (3) undifferentiated sparganum or tetrathyridium (the cyclophyllidean plerocercoid larva). None of the pulmonary infections was caused by *S. proliferum*; two infections were caused by an undifferentiated sparganum, and one was caused by an undifferentiated cysticercus. The remaining infection was a nonproliferative plerocercoid larvae from Asia. The morphologic distinctions between these groups, which are subtle, are described in detail elsewhere.[173]

In general, spargana are vermiform, about 0.5×10 cm (Fig. 15–33), but the cestode larva from the lungs of the man from Pennsylvania was both a branching and cyst-like structure of indeterminate length whose width varied between 25 μm and 1 mm. Spargana are recognized as cestode larvae by their tegument, calcareous corpuscles, and the lack of both digestive and reproductive tracts. Spargana have no scolices, but the anterior end has a pronounced invagination called a bothrium.[177]

Pathology

Incision through an abscess or cyst often reveals a sluggishly motile, white sparganum. Proliferative sparganosis produces 2- to 3-cm nodular masses containing many cysts. Intact spargana provoke chronic inflamma-

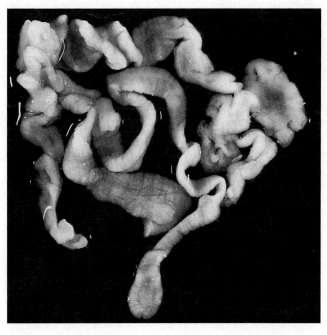

Fig. 15–33. Sparganum removed at surgery from subcutaneous nodule. AFIP 70–7392. ×2.

tion, and degenerating and necrotic worms become surrounded by dense fibrous tissue. Plasma cells, histiocytes, lymphocytes, and neutrophils are prominent, and eosinophils may be present.

Diagnosis and Treatment

The diagnosis is made by identifying the sparganum in the biopsy specimen.[178] Treatment of pulmonary sparganosis has not been evaluated. Treatment of proliferative sparganosis is difficult, and an attempt with mebendazole at 40 mg/kg per day for 4 months followed by praziquantel at 40 mg/kg per day for 2 weeks was unsuccessful in one patient with proliferative disease.[179]

Cysticercosis

Cysticercosis is human infection by the cysticercus larval stage (bladder worm) of *Taenia solium* Linnaeus 1758. People acquire the adult tapeworm, taeniasis, by consuming undercooked pork containing cysiticerci. Cysticercosis is acquired by consuming soil or food contaminated with eggs of *T. solium* from human excrement. *T. solium* is ubiquitous and can cause a serious public health problem wherever infected undercooked pork is customarily eaten.

Cysticerci may develop in virtually any tissue or organ. Intramuscular or subcutaneous sites are most common. Lesions involving the brain may be fatal. Only rarely are the lungs involved. Cysticerci in the lungs, as elsewhere, do not usually cause symptoms.

Disease

Human beings acquire cysticercosis by ingesting eggs of *T. solium* from the feces of persons with taeniasis. The eggs hatch and release oncospheres, which penetrate the wall of the gut and enter the bloodstream. The oncospheres lodge in tissue, become encysted, and differentiate into cysticerci. Cysticerci remain viable for an indefinite period of time and provoke no inflammation. As the cysticercus grows, it may compress local structures and cause symptoms. The cysticercus eventually dies and provokes a granulomatous reaction, which becomes scarred and calcified. This nodule is painless.

Biology

Man is an aberrant intermediate host and sole definitive host for *T. solium*. Only cannibalism would confer a survival advantage in human beings serving as intermediate host. The usual intermediate hosts include swine, sheep, dogs, cats, and primates.

The cysticercus is a spherical, milky-white cyst about 1 cm in diameter (Fig. 15–34). The cyst contains fluid and an invaginated scolex with four large suckers and an armed rostellum. The rostellum contains a double row of 22–32 birefringent hooklets. The cyst wall away from the scolex is 100–200 μm thick and raised into projections 10–25 μm in diameter. The tegument is 5 μm thick, and the outer surface is covered with microvilli. Smooth muscle fibers and tegumental cells subtend the tegument. Smooth muscle extends into parenchyma. The tegument is thickened in the area of the scolex (10–20 μm).[180]

Pathology

Demonstration of cysticerci in lung is usually by incidental finding. Calcified cysticerci may be seen on a radiograph. Viable cysticerci cause little reaction, but dead cysticerci first provoke neutrophils, histiocytes, and eosinophils, and eventually epithelioid cells, foreign-body giant cells, and fibrosis, sometimes with calcification.[177]

Diagnosis and Treatment

Diagnosis is usually made from identifying the morphologic features of the excised parasite. Computerized axial tomography scans reveal typical lesions.[181] Serol-

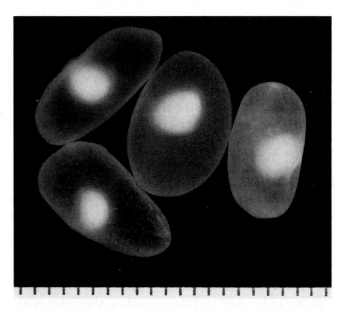

Fig. 15–34. Four cysticerci of *Taenia solium* removed from subcutaneous tissue. Each cyst has single invaginated scolex. AFIP 69–9754. ×3.5.

ogy is helpful but does not rule out hydatid disease,[182] which is usually in the differential. A history of intestinal taeniasis in the patient or a household member is a significant risk factor. Autoinfection is possible, and self-infection as the result of poor personal hygiene is common.

Echinococcosis

Echinococcosis is infection with larval tapeworms of the genus *Echinococcus*. Three are known to cause human infection: *Echinococcus granulosus* (Batsch 1786) Rudolf 1805, *E. multilocularis* (Leukart 1863) Vogel 1955, and *E. vogeli* Rausch and Berstein 1972. These larvae form cystic structures in intermediate hosts known as hydatid cysts. Echinococcosis is commonly called hydatid disease, and occasionally, hydatidosis.

Species of *Echinococcus* belong to the family Taeniidae. Adult worms live attached to the wall of the small intestine of carnivorous canids (wolf, dingo, dog, jackal, hyena). The intermediate hosts are usually grazing ungulates (sheep, goats, deer, elk, bison, moose, antelope). Echinococcosis is endemic in Australia, New Zealand, northern Europe, South Africa, the Middle East, Alaska, and Northwestern Canada, but echinococcosis is also reported from areas of the continental United States including Utah, Minnesota, the Dakotas, Iowa, Nebraska, Montana, Wyoming, and California.

Echinococcosis caused by *E. granulosus* is called cystic hydatid disease. The parasite produces unilocular slow-growing cysts in the tissues, particularly the liver and lungs. Symptoms result from the cyst mass or from a hypersensitivity reaction secondary to release of the cyst contents. There are two strains: (1) the ubiquitous parasite found in its intermediate host, the domestic sheep, and its definitive host, dogs, and (2) the strictly holoarctic worm occurring in its intermediate host, the moose, and its definitive host, the wolf. Clinical differences in human disease caused by the two strains of *E. granulosus* worms have been described. Prevalence of *E. granulosus* varies widely; the disease is often limited to restricted geographic foci. There were 77 infections reported from Great Britain between 1966 and 1972. A similar number of infections were reported from New Zealand within a 2-year period. In the United States autochthonous transmission has occurred in Alaska, Utah, Arizona, New Mexico, Minnesota, the Dakotas, California, and the lower Mississippi Valley.

Echinococcus multilocularis causes alveolar hydatid disease. The larval mass proliferates indefinitely by budding of the germinative membrane, producing an alveolar-like pattern of microvesicles. These cysts usually localize in the liver, have poorly defined borders, and infiltrate in a manner reminiscent of a neoplasm. It is endemic to Alaska, Canada, Northern Europe, Siberia, and Japan. There is a focus of infection in southern Germany and Switzerland. Relatively recent reports of infections from Minnesota and Montana (United States) suggest expanding distribution of alveolar hydatid disease.[183,184] Isolated infections have been reported from Italy, Australia, New Zealand, Argentina, and Uruguay. In Alaska, 33 infections were found in Eskimos between 1946 and 1976.[185] The parasite is common in wildlife from Montana, North Dakota, and Minnesota.

Echinococcus vogeli causes polycystic hydatid disease. This infection causes disease with clinical characteristics intermediate between those of cystic and alveolar hydatid disease. It occurs in rural areas of Colombia, Ecuador, Venezuela, Panama, and Costa Rica. The worm in humans has been mistakenly classified as *E. oligarthus* (Diesing 1863, Luke 1910). The life cycle involves wild dogs and paca.[186,187] Only 15 infections of man have been confirmed.[187]

Disease

In humans, cystic hydatid disease (*E. granulosus*) is life threatening when the cyst grows in or compresses a vital organ. The liver is the most common site of infection in adult patients (60%–70%). Cysts in the lung are common in adults (20%–25%); however, in children the lung is the most common site of infection (50%).[188] In one study, lung involvement was more frequent in boys (73%) than in girls (50%) ($p < .001$).[189] Symptoms may not appear for 5–10 years when the cyst lodges in a "roomy" site such as the lung. The cyst must become large enough to cause mechanical difficulties. Most cysts are 10 cm or less, but some may be 20 cm in diameter.

The prognosis in pulmonary cystic hydatid disease is generally good, but severe complications may develop. Several years pass before symptoms such as cough, dyspnea, and chest pain appear. If the cyst ruptures into a bronchus, much of the contents are coughed up, but suppuration may persist for several months. Cysts that rupture into the pleural space cause pneumothorax and empyema, and new cysts seed the pleura.

The most serious complications of cystic hydatid disease is pulmonary hydatid embolism, the rupture of a cyst growing in the right side of the heart. Cyst contents and pieces of the cyst wall cause pulmonary emboli (see Chapter 29). Death by anaphylactic shock, massive embolism, or valvular thrombosis may follow.[190] If the patient survives, new pulmonary cysts are the rule.

Alveolar hydatid disease, echinococcosis caused by infection by *E. multilocularis*, is perhaps the most dreadful helminthic infection of human beings.[191] Most untreated patients die (70%).[185] Surgical treatment is difficult or impossible, and chemotherapy is not often curative. Treatment extends life about 10 years (5-year survival of untreated compared to 15-year survival among those treated). Pulmonary and liver involvement with alveolar hydatid disease progresses slowly. The disease is often acquired early in life; and patients may harbor an organism for 30–40 years before dying from their disease. When the parasites lodge in the brain they can kill the host more quickly, often in less than 1 year after diagnosis.

Pulmonary disease is a complication of liver involvement. Cysts in the lung are not usually life threatening; rather, it is the underlying cyst in the liver that kills the patient. Also, cysts in the liver resist treatment whereas pulmonary cysts respond well to standard antiparasitic drugs.[192,193] Another contrast is that cysts in the liver are not usually resectable (75%), while those in the lung are easily removed.[185]

Relatively few patients infected with *E. multilocularis* have pulmonary involvement, 8 of 96 (8%) in one group. The two mechanisms for pulmonary involvement are hematogenous seeding from another cyst and penetration of the parasite through the diaphragm into the lower lobe of the right lung. These occur with about equal frequency.

Echinococcosis due to *E. vogeli*, polycystic hydatid disease, has involved the lungs or pleura in 3 of 15 known infections. Cysts in the liver are most common; these were the only lesions in 7 patients and the primary lesion in 3 others. It has been proposed, but not yet proven, that cysts in the liver may metastasize to the lung.

One patient with cysts in the parenchyma of the lungs and in the pleural spaces repeatedly spit up pus and had fever and chills. He produced 100–200 ml of expectorate daily, and had fertile polycystic hydatid cysts on the surface of both left and right lobes of the liver, the pericardium, superior vena cava, right auricle, lower and middle lobes of right lung, pleura, and diaphragm. This patient recovered after surgery. Two other patients presented with abscesses in the lungs caused by *E. vogeli*. Follow-up was incomplete, and thus the mortality caused by polycystic hydatid disease is unknown.

Biology

Humans acquire cystic hydatid disease by consuming eggs from the feces of a definitive host, such as dogs. Dogs are infected when fed internal organs of slaughtered domestic livestock, often sheep, infected with larval *E. granulosus*. Protoscolices from the cyst develop into adult worms, which attach to the wall of the small bowel of the canid. The dog may be infected with thousands of worms without apparent effect. Eggs passed in dog feces are ingested by human beings and by grazing livestock.

People acquire alveolar hydatid disease when they ingest eggs of *E. multilocularis* from the feces of foxes, the most common definitive host. Dogs and cats may also be suitable definitive hosts. A similar adaptation has occurred with *E. granulosus*; success of the parasite in dogs and sheep permitted transplantation of the parasite from the arctic wolf and moose. *E. multilocularis* has been documented in farmyard cats and rodents.[184] The chronic course of alveolar hydatid disease could mask an appreciable number of human infections that may have already occurred with increased domestication of *E. multilocularis*.[185]

Domestic dogs are only rarely infected with *E. vogeli*, the cause of polycystic hydatid disease. Nonetheless, people who get polycystic hydatid disease typically acquire their disease from domestic dogs. The cycle is maintained in the wild in bush dogs (*Speothosvenaticus* sp.) and pacas (*Cuniculus paca*). Domestic hunting dogs become infected by eating the viscera of infected game animals.[186]

Eggs of all three *Echinococcus* species that infect human beings are soilborne, originating from the feces of carnivorous definitive hosts. The eggs hatch in the small intestine, releasing invasive oncospheres that penetrate the wall of the bowel and enter the venous circulation. They lodge in virtually any tissue or organ, but most often (70%–90%) in the liver.

Development of a viable *E. granulosus* cyst (>1 cm in diameter) requires 5 months. The cyst is spherical and may eventually reach a diameter of 20 cm. The wall of the cyst is composed of a thick laminated inert layer on the outside and a thin living membrane, the germinal layer, that lines the interior (Fig. 15–35). Clusters of cells bud from the germinal layer, float freely in the interior, and eventually become brood capsules. Each brood capsule produces several infective protoscolices (Fig. 15–36). A developed cyst contains one to several daughter cysts.[194]

The alveolar hydatid cyst of *E. multilocularis* is a sterile mass of proliferative parasitic tissue. The structure is amorphous. The cut surface consists of irregular spaces, collapsed membranes, and no fluid. Man is apparently a poor host for *E. multilocularis*. The structure growing in a person will become fertile if it is experimentally fed to a more suitable intermediate host.

The polycystic hydatid cyst of *E. vogeli* is also proliferative. It proliferates by exogenous and endogenous budding. The aggregate of cysts may be 10 mm to several centimeters, and grossly resembles an irregular

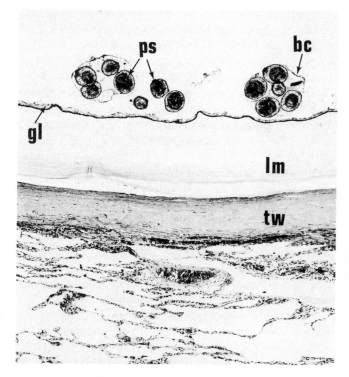

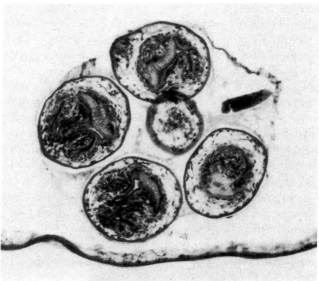

Fig. 15–36. Section of brood capsule of *Echinococcus granulosus* containing infective protoscolices. AFIP 86–6456. Movat, ×250.

Fig. 15–35. Hydatid cyst in lung, surrounded by fibrous tissue wall (tw). Germinal layer (gl) lines the laminated membrane (lm) and produces brood capsules (bc) containing protoscolices (ps). AFIP 86–6455. Movat, ×60.

cluster of grapes. The cysts are translucent, and brood capsules with infective scolices are visible through the surface. The laminated membrane of the cyst wall varies from 8 to 65 μm in thickness.

Pathology

Cysts of *E. granulosus* and *E. vogeli* are typically surrounded by a thick (3 mm) wall of the host fibrous tissue. Cysts of *E. multilocularis* are surrounded by necrotic debris and occasionally cavitate. Cysts that rupture into bronchi cause chronic suppuration and abscess. Fragments of the cyst wall that lodge in lung cause necrotizing granulomas. Cysts eventually calcify. Decay of cysts may be accompanied by bacterial infection with suppuration. Collapsed cysts of *E. granulosus* may resemble the cyst of *E. multilocularis*; the wall may be branching, sterile, and surrounded with necrotic debris.

Diagnosis and Treatment

Patients with cystic or alveolar hydatid disease of lungs may not become ill for many years after initial infection. Pulmonary cysts may be detected on routine radio-

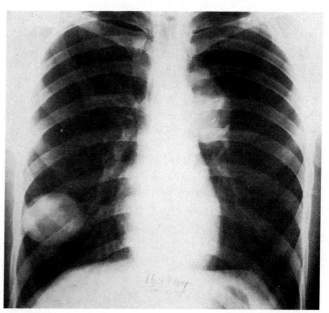

Fig. 15–37. Radiograph of chest shows hydatid cyst of *Echinococcus granulosus*. AFIP 78–8667–3.

graphs of the chest (Fig. 15–37), but they are usually detected after they rupture and produce symptoms. Coughed-up debris contains protoscolices, hooklets, or pieces of cyst wall, any or all of which may confirm the diagnosis. Polycystic hydatid disease progresses more rapidly than cystic or alveolar hydatid disease. Advanced pulmonary hydatid disease in a young patient should raise the suspicion of *E. vogeli.*

Hydatid cysts are frequently mistaken for tuberculosis or carcinoma by clinicians, although an accurate preoperative diagnosis may be made from the radiologic appearance. Cystic hydatid disease presents sharply circumscribed orbs, and the presence of daughter cysts within the larger sphere is diagnostic. Alveolar hydatid disease exhibits two distinct radiographic presentations that correspond to the mechanism of lung involvement: (1) multiple small (1–3 mm) dense foci of irregular shape located bilaterally at the periphery of the lungs; and (2) variable changes to the lower-right lobe caused by penetration of the right hemidiaphragm from the liver.[195] Computerized axial tomography scan and sonography are also helpful in locating and diagnosing alveolar hydatid disease. Radiologic studies with polycystic hydatid disease are incomplete.

Biopsy specimens taken of the cyst wall readily distinguish an echinococcus cyst from tuberculosis, carcinoma, and amebiasis. The GMS stain simplifies recognition of echinococcosis.[196] Sputum cytology can also reveal *Echinococcus.*[197] Aspiration is not recommended, because patients with echinococcosis are in danger of anaphylactic shock and metastatic proliferation when the cyst is penetrated, even with a fine needle.

Serology supports the presumptive radiologic diagnosis. All patients described by Wilson and Rausch[185] had positive indirect hemagglutination (>1:128). Schantz et al.[198] obtained similar results and determined that patients who were successfully treated became antibody negative (<1:128) within a year after beginning treatment.

Histopathologic demonstration of parasitic structures confirms the diagnosis. The pathologist often makes the diagnosis because the clinician overlooks the possibility of echinococcosis. Geographic location and history of travel may help in diagnosis. A patient with hydatid disease who has not visited an endemic area of alveolar or polycystic hydatid disease is probably infected with *E. granulosus.*

Arthropoda

The medical importance of arthropods as vectors of infectious diseases is understood by most people. However, arthropods in the capacity of an etiologic infectious agent is generally viewed as a medical curiosity. In some areas of the world arthropods routinely infect the living tissues of human beings. Pentastomiasis in Africa and Asia and myiases of the tropics are examples.

Few people have heard of pentastomes, yet in some regions of Africa and Asia virtually everyone is infected.

Pathologists are far more likely to encounter pentastomes in the lungs than any other arthropods that might occur there, namely, mites and maggots. The lungs frequently contain encapsulated nymphs, but these do not cause symptoms. Juvenile pentastomes acquired by eating raw tissues of animals attach to the throat or more deeply in the respiratory tract and cause violent symptoms. This is common in North Africa and the Middle East, where people eat raw lymph nodes from sheep.

Pulmonary acariasis, or mites in the lungs, may be a common cause of asthma worldwide but no other pulmonary lesions appear to be caused by mites. The mites probably die quickly after being inhaled and then provoke an allergic reaction. Despite some speculation, there is no evidence that they survive and cause tissue damage.

Myiasis is a rare cause of pulmonary lesions. Flies or their larvae become trapped in the lungs and die. This may happen more frequently than the four published reports indicate, and the healed or resolving lesions may be mistaken for the more commonly occurring pulmonary granulomas because the degenerated fly larvae may be difficult or impossible to identify.

Acariasis

Pulmonary acariasis is caused by inhalation of mites (Acarida). Mites act as allergens and may eventually sensitize those persons exposed. Asthma and rhinitis develop. Inhaled mites probably do not survive to infect lung tissue, although some may feed on inflammatory cells and necrotic debris. The traditional medical significance of mites is in transmission of scrub typhus or rickettsial pox. They also cause chigger sores, sarcoptic mange, and some other dermatoses.

Disease

Inhaled mites are allergens.[199] In some patients, dust inhaled with mites might be the principal allergen. Ingram et al.[200] demonstrated that storage mites themselves reduced expiratory volume. Mites are occasionally seen in tissue sections of lung,[201] but when present are an incidental finding in bronchi. Species of mites commonly involved in allergic sensitization include *Tyrophagus longior, Dermatophagoides farinae, Dermatophagoides pteronyssinus, Glycyphagus domesticus,* and *Lepidoglyphus destructor.*[199–202]

Biology

Mites in the home feed on desquamated keratin from human skin, blood, sweat, food crumbs, and fungi.

They prevail in unkempt beds, carpets, and furniture. A clean house is inhospitable to mites. Mites are barely visible to the naked eye, as they are usually less than a millimeter long. They have six or eight legs and an unarmed hypostome. In other aspects, they superficially resemble ticks.

Pathology

Kijima[203] described an eosinophilia caused by mites in the lungs. Soysa and Jayawardena[204] thought mites might cause tropical pulmonary eosinophilia, but today filarial nematodes are thought to cause tropical pulmonary eosinophilia. No other specific changes have been described.

Diagnosis and Treatment

Asthmatic or rhinitis patients with mites in sputum and a history of exposure to dust contaminated with mites may suffer type 1 hypersensitivity to mite allergens. Ingram et al.[200] established this diagnosis using cultivated mites from sites of exposure; killed and purified mite fractions were inhaled by patients and changes in expiratory volume recorded. Volumes diminished by more than 15% were considered positive.

Prevention of exposure is more practical than treatment. Mites in house dust can be eliminated with good housekeeping, particularly with thorough vacuuming. Protective breathing masks should be worn in workplaces such as hay barns, grain bins, and in other areas that are heavily contaminated with dustborne mites.

Myiasis

Myiasis is human infection with larval dipterans. A variety of flies cause myiasis by a number of strategies. Some flies deposit eggs in food that develop as the food passes through the human gut. More elaborately, a fly might capture a female mosquito and attach eggs to her underside. When the mosquito takes a blood meal, the larvae drop into the wound left by the bite of the mosquito.[205] Myiasis may involve the eyes, skin, brain, gastrointestinal tract, urogenital tract, ears, nasopharynx, or lungs. The larvae destroy surrounding tissue and provoke a vigorous host reaction. Pulmonary myiasis in man is rare. Four infections have been reported,[206–208] and many more undiagnosed infections probably occur.

Disease

A coin lesion removed from a patient's lung contained a fly larva, probably a larva that impacted in a pulmonary vessel and created a thrombus. More commonly, diffuse bilateral nodules develop that are caused by swallowing or inhaling larvae or flies. Neither of these lesions has caused significant morbidity. All infections were discovered during routine chest radiography and diagnosed in histologic section. There may be eosinophilia and a history of productive cough.

Biology

Many fly larvae migrate through the viscera (including lung) of vertebrate hosts as their course of normal development. These eventually migrate to subcutaneous tissue, creating "warbles," and eventually drop to the ground and pupate. Larvae causing pulmonary myiasis in humans do not appear to be normal pulmonary transients; rather, they appear to have been trapped after accidental deposition in lung. One patient inhaled a fly while jogging.[206]

Pathology

Encapsulated and infarcted necrotizing granulomas surround calcified larvae in parenchyma of the lung. Adjacent tissue is only slightly infiltrated with chronic inflammatory cells. One patient, who inhaled a fly, yielded 30 live larvae in a bloody aspirate from intrathoracic suction after surgery. If the fly were gravid, this would explain the many larvae.

Diagnosis and Treatment

Diagnosis is made by identifying larval dipterans in histologic section of an excised pulmonary nodule. The larvae usually exhibit the characteristic morphologic features of tracheal rings of the spiracular system (Fig. 15–38), striated muscle and sclerotized cuticular spines of unique shape and distribution. Ahmed and Miller[207] described in detail their identification of a degenerated fly larva in histologic sections of a pulmonary coin lesion.

Pentastomiasis

Pentastomiasis is infection of man with larvae, nymphs, or adult pentastomes. Pentastomes are unusual arthropods, and their taxonomic position is unsettled. Two genera of pentastomes, *Armillifer* and *Linguatula*, commonly cause disease in humans.

Pentastomiasis may be visceral or nasopharyngeal. These two forms are clinically, biologically, pathologically, and epidemiologically distinct entities. In general, *Armillifer* causes visceral disease and *Linguatula* causes nasopharyngeal disease, but exceptions are common.

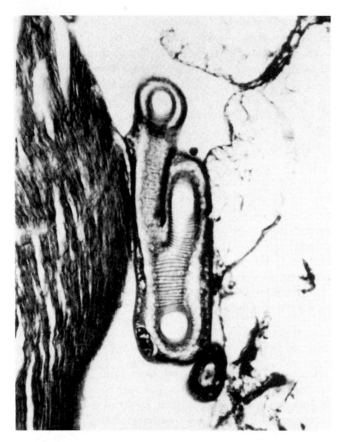

Fig. 15–38. Tracheal rings characteristic of spiracular system of larval dipterans. AFIP 72–1874. ×440.

Pentastomiasis is common in endemic areas. Prevalence of 10% is usual, and 45% has been reported.[209] *Armillifer armillatus* is probably the most common pentastome infecting man, primarily in Africa.[210] *Armillifer moniliformis* (formerly *Porocephalus moniliformis*) is common in Asia.[211] *Linguatula serrata* is widely distributed in Africa, Europe, the Middle East, and the Western Hemisphere.[212–216]

Disease

Visceral pentastomiasis rarely causes discomfort, but nasopharyngeal disease creates violent symptoms and considerable pain. The differences in these diseases caused by pentastomes reflects differing reproductive strategies at work.

People acquire visceral pentastomiasis by drinking water containing eggs of *Armillifer* species. Snakes, the definitive host, shed infective eggs at water holes. Man subsequently ingests the eggs. Eggs hatch in the human intestine releasing larvae that migrate through the viscera. The larvae eventually become encapsulated, and later transform into nymphs. Man tolerates these parasites well and there are no specific symptoms. Liver and

lungs are most frequently infected. Four types of lesions are known: (1) encapsulated nymphs, (2) encapsulated calcifying nymphs, (3) granuloma surrounding parts of degenerated nymphs, and (4) unencapsulated nymphs.

Cagnard et al.,[216] reported a fatal infection in a 5-year-old girl who apparently ate a gravid *Armillifer armillatus*. She was infected with hundreds of larval parasites, the lungs and the brain being most heavily infected.

People acquire nasopharyngeal pentastomiasis by eating organs of animals infected with encapsulated nymphs, that is, animals with visceral pentastomiasis. Nymphs emerge from digested tissue and migrate to the nasopharynx, where they firmly attach using anterior hooks. Severe symptoms follow, including pain and tightness in the throat, coughing, sneezing, dysphagia, hoarseness, lacrimation, coryza, aural pruritus and pain, dyspnea, headache, facial edema, hemoptysis, and vomiting. This is the "halzoun" syndrome. The parasites do not survive this violent reaction and are eventually coughed up or swallowed and digested, which explains the relief of symptoms within a week of onset.[217] Halzoun syndrome is well known in the Middle East and in the Sudan where people eat raw lymph nodes from sheep and goats.[218]

Biology

Pentastomes occupy a controversial taxonomic position. Some consider them annelids, and others believe they belong to a distinct phylum (Pentastomida).[219] Some think the pentastomes are arthropods. Beaver et al.[211] cited evidence for their placement in Arthropoda, Class Crustacea, Order Branchiura; we have adopted this opinion.

Pentastomes are pseudosegmented and moniliform or linguiliform. The adults are also called "tongue worms." Hooklike anterior appendages secure the "worm" in the respiratory tract of its definitive carnivorous host. The anterior end is a distinct cephalothorax, and the posterior end (the bulk of the organism) is the abdomen. The abdomen of *Armillifer* is prominently annulated (Fig. 15–39). Adult pentastomes are 1–10 cm long, and females are larger than males. Circulatory and respiratory systems are absent.

Almost all pentastomes infect reptiles, but *Linguatula serrata* parasitizes carnivorous mammals, including domestic dogs. While *Linguatula* usually causes nasopharyngeal disease, eggs are occasionally swallowed by man and cause visceral disease.[220]

Pathology

Encapsulated pentastomid nymphs are benign and do not as a rule cause necrosis.[218] When there is damage, it

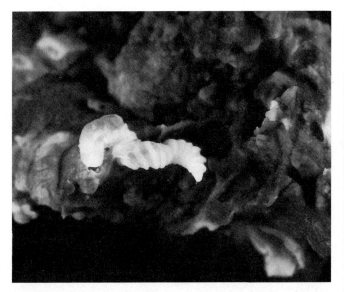

Fig. 15–39. Nonencysted larva of *Armillifer armillatus* attached to lung. AFIP 75–14497.

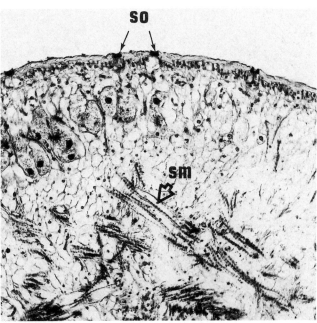

Fig. 15–41. Body wall of *Armillifer armillatus* shows characteristic sclerotized openings (so) and striated muscle (sm). AFIP 74–11161. Movat, ×210.

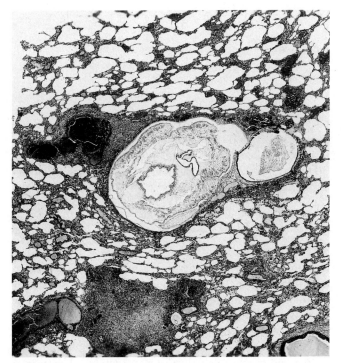

Fig. 15–40. Encysted larva of *Armillifer armillatus* in lung. AFIP 72–17643. Movat, ×12.

Diagnosis and Treatment

Diagnosis of visceral pentastomiasis is made by identifying the organisms in tissue section (Figs. 15–40 and 15–41). There is also a characteristic radiologic appearance or "C shape," and a correct size and location, which usually suffices for diagnosis in an endemic area.[222]

In tissue section, pentastomids may be confused with cysticerci, sparganga, flukes, or other arthropods. Of special help in the diagnosis are the sclerotized openings of the outer portion of the cuticle (Fig. 15–41), which no other parasite of man possesses. They are apparent with routine stains, but clearly evident with Russell's Movat pentachrome stain.[210,223] Striated muscle in the body cavity of pentastomes distinguishes them from helminths.

Treatment of visceral pentastomiasis in the absence of complications is not necessary. Generally, pentastomes in pulmonary nodules are removed for diagnosis where expert care is available.

Leeches

is usually mechanical. Larvae migrating through viscera may cause damage, as has been demonstrated in experimental pentastomiasis.[221] Sensitized people mount a vigorous immunologic reaction to migrating larvae and provoke abscesses in the affected organs.[210]

Hirundiasis is infection of humans with leeches. External hirundiasis occurs when any one of many species of leeches attaches to the skin of a person and sucks blood. In contrast, internal hirundiasis is almost always caused by *Limnatus nilotica*, which lives in freshwater through-

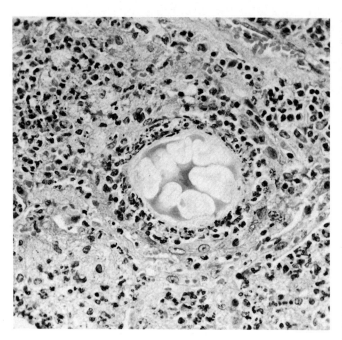

Fig. 15–42. Lentil grain in center of pulmonary granuloma. AFIP 69–9531. H and E, ×350.

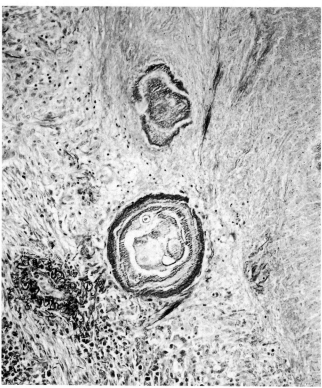

Fig. 15–43. Liesegang phenomenon in section of lung. AFIP 86–6778. ×160.

out the world. It is swallowed when man drinks from infested water. The leech attaches to the nasopharynx, pharynx, epiglottis, esophagus, larynx, trachea, or bronchi. One-third of all infections involve the pharynx or trachea.[224] Such patients present with hemoptysis, dyspnea, or loss of speech. Leeches are a common cause of halzoun syndrome (see Pentastomiasis).

False Parasites in Sections of Lung Tissue

Parasitologists and pathologists with specialized training can identify some parasites in tissue sections. A specific diagnosis, when at all possible, depends on demonstration of certain microanatomic features. These features tend to differ among groups and species of parasites. People who are unfamiliar with the microanatomy of parasites often mistake unusual structures in tissue sections for parasites.[225] For example, lentil grains and Liesegang bodies in sections of lung tissue are often mistaken for helminthic parasites.

Lentil Pneumonia

Lentil pneumonia is a multifocal inflammatory process in the lung caused by aspiration of starch grains from legumes. In tissue sections, these grains resemble eggs of helminths. The resemblance is striking to the unini-

tiated, but starch grains have a distinctive appearance (Fig. 15–42) and usually occur in microabscesses in parenchyma of lung. The walls and starch compartments are usually vividly stained with periodic acid–Schiff stain (see Chapter 5).

Liesegang Phenomenon

The structure in Fig. 15–43 resembles a section of nematode, but it is an intrinsic concretion of unknown origin; this structure is formed by a mechanism called the Liesegang phenomenon. Liesegang, a German biochemist, described this process in 1911. It is usually found in areas of necrosis. The Liesegang structures are often mistaken for exotic lesions caused by helminths or their eggs. Such a reaction in a necrotizing lesion in a kidney was misdiagnosed as a giant kidney worm, *Dioctyphyma renale*.[226] Turr and others have studied the Liesegang phenomenon in detail.[227]

References

1. Appelbaum IL, Shrager J. Pneumonitis associated with malaria. Arch Intern Med 1944;74:155–162.

2. Brooks MH, Keil FW, Sheehy TW, Barry KG. Acute pulmonary edema as a complication of acute falciparum malaria. N Engl J Med 1968;279:732–737.

3. Deaton JG. Fatal pulmonary edema as a complication of acute falciparum malaria. Am J Trop Med Hyg 1970; 19:196–201

4. Cayea PD, Rubin E, Teixidor HS. Atypical pulmonary malaria. AJR 1981;137:51–55

5. Punyagupta S, Srichaikul F, Nitiyanat P, Petchclai B. Acute pulmonary insufficiency in falciparum malaria: Summary of 12 cases with evidence of disseminated intravascular coagulation. Am J Trop Med Hyg 1974; 23:551–559.

6. Bruce-Chwatt LJ. Essential malariology. London: Heinemann, 1980:10–35.

7. Duarte MIS, Corbett CEP, Boulos M, Neto VA. Ultra-structure of the lung in falciparum malaria. Am J Trop Med Hyg 1985;34:31–35.

8. Marks S, Holland S, Getland M. Malarial lung: Report of a case from Africa successfully treated with intermittent positive pressure ventilation. Am J Trop Med Hyg 1977;26:179–180.

9. Nicolle MMC, Manceaux L. Sur un protozoaire nouveau du gondi (Toxoplasma n. sp.) Arch Inst Pasteur Tunis 1909;2:97.

10. Cheever AW, Valsamis MP, Rabson AS. Necrotizing toxoplasmic encephalitis and herpetic pneumonia complicating treated Hodgkin's disease. N Engl J Med 1965;272:26–28.

11. Cohen SN. Toxoplasmosis in patients receiving immunosuppressive therapy. JAMA 1970;211:657–660.

12. Anthony CW. Disseminated toxoplasmosis in a liver transplant patient. J Am Med Wom Assoc 1972;27:601–603.

13. Frenkel JK, Nelson BM, Arias-Stella J. Immunosuppression and toxoplasmic encephalitis: Clinical and experimental aspects. Hum Pathol 1975;6:97–111.

14. Britt RH, Enzmann DR, Remington JS. Intracranial infection in cardiac transplant recipients. Ann Neurol 1981;9:107.

15. Yermakov V, Rashid RK, Vuletin JC, Pertschuk LP, Isaksson H. Disseminated toxoplasmosis. Case report and review of the literature. Arch Pathol Lab Med 1982;106:524–528.

16. Beaver PC, Jung RS, Cupp EW. Clinical parasitology. 9th Ed. Philadelphia: Lea & Febiger, 1984:170.

17. Grandsen WR, Brown PM. Pneumocystis pneumonia and disseminated toxoplasmosis in a male homosexual. Br Med J 1983;286:1614.

18. Teras YK, Ryigas EM, Kazakova II, et al. Otdel protozoologii inst. eksperimental'noi biologii AN Estonskii SSR, Tallin, USSR. Terpapevticheskii Arkhiv 1980;52:123–125.

19. Walton BC, Bachrach T. Occurrence of trichomonads in the respiratory tract. Report of 3 cases. J Parsitol 1963; 49:35–38.

20. Rebhun J. Pulmonary trichomoniasis associated with a fever of unknown origin. Calif Med 1962;100:443–444.

21. Walzer PD, Rutherford I, East R. Empyema with Tricho-monas species. Annu Rev Respir Dis 1978;118:415–418.

22. Memick F. Trichomonads in pleural effusion. JAMA 1968;204:1145–1146.

23. Osbourne PT, Giltman LI, Uthman EO. Trichomonads in the respiratory tract: A case report and literature review. Acta Cytol 1984;28:136–138.

24. Beaver PC, Jung RC, Cupp EW. Clinical parasitology. 9th Ed. Philadelphia: Lea & Febiger, 1984:47–48.

25. Glaubach N, Guller EJ. Pneumonia apparently due to Trichomonas buccalis. JAMA 1942;120:280–281.

26. Camara EJN, Lima JAC, Olivera GB, Machado AS. Pulmonary findings in patients with Chagasic mega-esophagus. Chest 1983;83:87–91.

27. Bittencourt AL, Rodrigues de Freitas LA, Galvo de Arujo MO, Jacomo D. Pneumonitis in congenital Chagas' disease. A study of ten cases. Am J Trop Med Hyg 1981;30:38–42.

28. Bittencourt AL. Congenital Chagas' disease. A review. Am J Dis Child 1976;130:97–103.

29. Eberhard ML, D'Alessandro A. Congenital Trypanosoma cruzi in a laboratory-born squirrel monkey, Saimiri sciureus. Am J Trop Med Hyg 1983;31:931–933.

30. Edgecomb JH, Johnson CM. American trypanosomiasis. In: Binford CH, Connor DH, eds. Pathology of tropical and extraordinary diseases. Washington, DC: Armed Forces Institute of Pathology, 1976:244–251.

31. Adams EB, MacLeod IN. Invasive amebiasis. II. Amebic liver abscess and its complications. Medicine (Baltimore) 1977;56:325–334.

32. Beaver PC, Jung RC, Cupp EW. Clinical parasitology. 9th Ed. Philadelphia: Lea & Febiger, 1984:105.

33. Juniper K, Jr. Amebiasis in the United States. Bull NY Acad Sci 1971;47:448–461.

34. Ibarra-Perez C, Seiman-Lama M. Diagnosis and treatment of amebic empyema. Report of 88 cases. Am J Surg 1977;134:283–287.

35. MacLeod IN, Wilmot AJ, Powell SJ. Amebic pericarditis. Q J Med 1966;25:293–311.

36. Connor DH, Neafie RC, Meyers WM. Amebiasis. In: Binford CH, Connor DH, eds. Pathology of tropical and extraordinary diseases. Washington, DC: Armed Forces Institute of Pathology, 1976:308–316.

37. Kagan IG, Norman L. Serodiagnosis of parasitic diseases. In: Rose NR, Friedman H, eds. Manual of clinical immunology. Washington, DC: American Society for Microbiology, 1976:382–409.

38. Grundy MS. Preliminary observations using a multilayer ELISA method for the detection of Entameba histolytica trophozoite antigens in stool samples. Trans R Soc Trop Med Hyg 1982;76:396–400.

39. Pillai S, Mohimen A. A solid phase sandwich radioimmunoassay for Entameba histolytica proteins and the detection of circulating antigens in amebiasis. Gastroenterology 1982;83:1210–1216.

40. Swett HA, Greenspan RH. Thoracic manifestations of liver disease. Radiol Clin North Am 1980;18:269–279.

41. Cameron EW. The treatment of pleuropulmonary amebiasis with metronidazole. Chest 1978;73:647–650.

42. Brady EM, Margolis ML, Korzeniowski OM. Pulmonary

cryptosporidiosis in acquired immunodeficiency syndrome. JAMA 1984;252:89–90.

43. Immunodeficiency and cryptosporidiosis (Clinicopathologic Conference). Br Med J 1980;281:1123–1127.

44. Kocochis SA, Ciball ML, Davis TE, Hinton JT, Seip M, Banwell JF. Intestinal and pulmonary cryptosporidiosis in an infant with severe combined immune deficiency. J Pediatr Gastroenterol Nutr 1984;3:149–157.

45. Miller RA, Wasserheit JN, Kirihaara J, Coyle MB: Detection of Cryptosporidium oocysts in sputum during screening for Mycobacterium. J Clin Microbiol 1984;20:1192.

46. Visvesvara GS, Ballamuth W. Comparative studies on related free-living and pathogenic amebae with special reference to Acanthameba. J Protozool 1975;21:239–250.

47. Martinez AM, Markowitz SM, Duma RJ. Experimental pneumonitis and encephalitis caused by Acanthameba in mice: Pathogenesis and ultrastructural features. J Infect Dis 1975;131:692–699.

48. Visvesvara GS, Mira SS, Brandt FH, Moss DM, Mathews HM, Martinez AJ. Isolation of two strains of Acanthameba castellanii from human tissues and their pathogenicity and isoenzyme profiles. J Clin Microbiol 1983;18:1405–1417.

49. Ciferri F. Human pulmonary dirofilariasis in the United States: A critical review. Am J Trop Med Hyg 1982;31:302–308.

50. Dayal Y, Neafie RC. Human pulmonary dirofilariasis. A case report and review of the literature. Am Rev Respir Dis 1975;112:437–445.

51. Otto GF. Geographical distribution, vectors and life cycle of Dirofilaria immitis. J Am Vet Med Assoc 1969;15:370–373.

52. Yen C. Studies on Dirofilaria immitis with special reference to the susceptibility of some Minnesota species of mosquitoes to the infection. J Parasitol 1938;24:189–205.

53. Yoshimura H, Kondo K, Ohnishi Y, Kitagawa M, Kamimura K. Human dirofilariasis in Japan. Case report and review of the literature. Int J Zoonoses 1980;7:107–114.

54. Billups J, Schenken JR, Beaver PC. Subcutaneous dirofilariasis in Nebraska. Arch Pathol Lab Med 1980;104:11–13.

55. Moorehouse DE. Dirofilaria immitis: A cause of intraocular infection. Infection 1978;6:192–193.

56. Neafie RC, Connor DH, Meyers WM. Dirofilariasis. In: Binford CH, Connor DH, eds. Pathology of tropical and extraordinary diseases. Washington, DC: Armed Forces Institute of Pathology, 1976:391–396.

57. Gutierrez Y. Diagnostic features of zoonotic filariae in tissue sections. Hum Pathol 1984;15:514–525.

58. Beaver PC, Jung RC, Cupp EW. Clinical parasitology. 9th Ed. Philadelphia: Lea & Febiger, 1984:351–357.

59. Connor DH, Williams PH, Helwig EB, Winslow DJ. Dermal changes in onchocerciasis. Arch Pathol Lab Med 1969;87:193–200.

60. World Health Organization. Epidemiology of onchocerciasis. Report of a W.H.O. expert committee. Tech Rep Ser No 597, 1976.

61. Faust EC, Agosin M, Garcia-Laverde A, Sayad WY, Johnson VM, Murray NA. Unusual findings of filarial infections of man. Am J Trop Med Hyg 1952;1:239–249.

62. Spencer H. Pathology of the lung. Oxford: Pergamon, 1985:405–408.

63. Wilkey IS. Filariasis: A report of several cases. Papua New Guinea Med J 1971;14:136–138.

64. Beaver PC, Fallon M, Smith GH. Pulmonary nodule caused by a living Brugia malayi-like filaria in an artery. Am J Trop Med Hyg 1971;23:869–876.

65. Beaver PC, Cran IR. Wuchereria-like filaria in an artery associated with pulmonary infarction. Am J Trop Med Hyg 1974;23:869–876.

66. Case records of the Massachusetts General Hospital, Case 26-1974. N Engl J Med 1974;291:35–42.

67. Webb JKG, Job CK, Gault EW. Tropical eosinophilia: Demonstration of microfilaria in the lung, liver and lymph nodes. Lancet 1960;i:835–842.

68. Danaraj TJ, Pacheco G, Shanmugaratnam K, Beaver PC. The etiology and pathology of eosinophilic lung. Am J Trop Med Hyg 1966;15:183–189.

69. Beaver PC. Filariasis without microfilaremia. Am J Trop Med Hyg 1970;19:181–189.

70. Neva FA, Ottesen EA. Tropical eosinophilia. N Engl J Med 1978;298:1129–1131.

71. Meyers WM, Neafie RC, Connor DH. Onchocerciasis: Invasion of deep organs by Onchocerca volvulus. Autopsy findings. Am J Trop Med Hyg 1977;26:650–657.

72. Fuglsang H, Anderson J. Effect of diethylcarbamazine and suramin on Onchocerca volvulus microfilariae in urine. Lancet 1973;ii:321–322.

73. Dissanaike AS, Paramananthan DC. On Brugia buckleyi sp. n. from the heart and blood vessels of the Ceylon hare. J Helminthol 1961;35:209–220.

74. Vincent AL, Frommes SP, Ash LR. Brugia malayi, Brugia pahangi and Brugia patei: pulmonary pathology in jirds. Exp Parasitol 1976;40:330–354.

75. Connor DH, Neafie RC. Onchocerciasis. In: Binford CH, Connor DH, eds. Pathology of tropical and extraordinary diseases. Washington DC: Armed Forces Institute of Pathology, 1976:360–381.

76. Edeson JFB, Wilson T, Wharton RH, Laing ABG. Experimental transmission of Brugia malayi and Brugia pahangi to man. Trans R Soc Trop Med Hyg 1960;54:229–234.

77. Boornazian JS, Fagan MJ. Tropical pulmonary eosinophilia associated with pleural effusions. Am J Trop Med Hyg 1985;34:473–475.

78. Skrjabin KI, Shikhovalova NP, Orlov IV, eds. Essentials of nematology. VI. Trichocephalidae and Capillariidae of animals and man and diseases caused by them. Moscow: Academy of Sciences, USSR:420–425. (English translation; Israel Program for Scientific Translation, Jerusalem, 1970:416–419.)

79. Ananina NO. [Thominix infection of the lungs.] Sovetskaya Meditsina 1958;22:136–137. Helminthol Abstr 1961;30:288.

80. Volkov VE, Pak EM. [A case of Thominix aerophilus

complicated by asthmatic bronchitis.] Voenno- Med Zh 1973;5:84.

81. Skipina LV. A case of human thominixosis. Med Parazitol (Mosk) 1976;45:607.

82. Coudert J, Despeignes J, Battesti R. A propos d'un cas de capillariaose poumonaire. Bull Soc Pathol Exot 1972; 65:841–848.

83. Aftandelians R, Raafat F, Taffazoli M, Beaver PC. Pulmonary capillariasis in a child in Iran. Am J Trop Med Hyg 1977;26:64–71.

84. Lui JC, Whalen GE, Cross JH. *Capillaria* ova in human sputum. J Formosan Med Assoc 1970;69:80–82.

85. Meyers WM, Neafie RC, Connor DH. Strongyloidiasis. In: Binford CH, Connor DH, eds. Pathology of tropical and extraordinary diseases. Washington DC: Armed Forces Institute of Pathology, 1976:428–432.

86. Faust EC. Experimental studies on human and primate species of *Strongyloides*. IV. The pathology of *Strongyloides* infection. Arch Pathol Lab Med 1935;19:769–806.

87. Venizelos PC, Lopata M, Bardawil WA, Sharp JT. Respiratory failure due to *Strongyloides stercoralis* in a patient with renal transplant. Chest 1980;78:104–106.

88. Faust EC. The development of *Strongyloides* in the experimental host. Am J Hyg 1933;18:114–132.

89. Humphreys K, Hieger R. *Stronglyoides stercoralis* in routine Papanicolaou-stained sputum smears. Acta Cytol 1979;23:471–476.

90. Pettersson T, Stenstrom R, Kyronseppa H. Disseminated lung opacities and cavitation associated with *Strongyloides stercoralis* and *Schistosoma mansoni* infection. Am J Trop Med Hyg 1974;23:158–162.

91. Ford T, Reiss-Levy I, Clark E, Dyson AJ, Schonell W. Pulmonary strongyloidasis and lung abscess. Chest 1981;79:239–240.

92. Harris RA, Musher DM, Fainstein V, Young EJ, Clarridge J. Disseminated strongyloidiasis. Diagnosis made by sputum examination. JAMA 1980;244:65–66.

93. Rassiga AL, Lowry JL, Forman WB. Diffuse pulmonary infection due to *Strongyloides stercoralis*. JAMA 1974; 230:426–427.

94. Nichols RL. The etiology of visceral larva migrans. Comparative larval morphology of *Ascaris lumbricoides*, *Necator americanus*, *Strongyloides stercoralis* and *Ancylostoma caninum*. J Parasitol 1955;41:363–400.

95. Shumaker JD, Band JD, Lensmeyer GL, Craig WA. Thiabendazole treatment of severe strongyloidiasis in a hemodialized patient. Ann Intern Med 1978;89:644–645.

96. Mornex JF, Magdeleine J. Bronchial syngamosis as a cause of chronic cough. Lancet 1981;ii:1166.

97. Villon A, Foulon G, Ancelle R, Nguyen NQ, Martin-Bouyer G. [Prevalence of intestinal parasites in Martinique.] Bull Soc Pathol Exot 1983;76:406–416.

98. Mornex JF, Magdeleine J. Parasitic pulmonary disease: Human bronchial syngamosis. Am Rev Respir Dis 1983;127:525–526 (Letter).

99. Cordero L, Podesta M, Avalos E. [*Mammomonogamus* in Costa Rica.] Cienc Vet 1982;2(3):13–15.

100. Timmons RF, Bowers RE, Price DL. Infection of the respiratory tract with *Mammomonogamus laryngeus*: A new case in Largo, Florida, and a summary of previously reported cases. Am Rev Respir Dis 1983;128:566–560.

101. Pawlowski ZS. Ascariasis: Host pathogen biology. Rev Infect Dis 1982;4:806–814.

102. Mittal VK, Dhaliwal R, Yadav R, Saharian S. Fatal respiratory obstruction due to a roundworm. Med J Aust 1976;2:210–212.

103. Daya H, Allie A, McCarthy R. Disseminated ascariasis. A case report. S Afr Med J 1982;2:820–822.

104. Beaver PC, Jung RC, Cupp EW. Clinical parasitology. 9th Ed. Philadelphia: Lea & Febiger, 1984:316.

105. Zamora OA. Localization of *Ascaris lumbricoides* in the thoracic cavity. Report of a case. Rev Cubana Med Trop 1976;28:72–75.

106. Spillman RK. Pulmonary ascariasis in tropical communities. Am J Trop Med Hyg 1975;24:791–800.

107. Phills JA, Harrold AJ, Whiteman GV, Perelmutter L. Pulmonary infiltrates, asthma, and eosinophilia due to *Ascaris suum* infestation in man. N Engl J Med 1972; 286:965–970.

108. Takata I. Experimental infection of man with *Ascaris* of man and the pig. Kitasato Arch Exp Med 1951;23: 49–59.

109. Beaver PC. Biology of soil-transmitted helminths: the massive infection. Health Lab Sci 1975;12:116–125.

110. Baird JK, Mistrey M, Pimsler M, Connor DH. Fatal human ascariasis following secondary massive infection. Am J Trop Med Hyg 1986;35:314–318.

111. Neafie RC, Connor DH. Ascariasis. In: Binford CH, Connor DH, eds. Pathology of tropical and extraordinary diseases. Washington DC: Armed Forces Institute of Pathology, 1976:460–467.

112. Schantz PM, Weis PE, Pollard ZF, White MC. Risk factors for ocular larva migrans: A case control study. Am J Public Health 1980;70:1269–1272.

113. Beshear JR, Hendley JO. Severe pulmonary involvement in visceral larva migrans. Am J Dis Child 1973;125:599–600.

114. Snyder CH. Visceral larva migrans: Ten years experience. Pediatrics 1961;28:85–91.

115. Beaver PC, Jung RC, Cupp EW. Clinical parasitology. 9th Ed. Philadelphia: Lea & Febiger, 1984:326.

116. Nichols RL. The etiology of visceral larva migrans. I. Diagnostic morphology of infective stage *Toxocara* larvae. J Parasitol 1956;42:349–361.

117. Pollard ZF. Ocular *Toxocara* in siblings in two families. Diagnosis confirmed by ELISA test. Arch Ophthalmol 1979;97:2319–2320.

118. Gass JD, Gilbert WR, Guerry RK, Sclefo R. Diffuse unilateral subacute neuroretinitis. Ophthalmology 1978;85:521–545.

119. Aur RJA, Pratt CB, Johnson WW. Thiabendazole in visceral larvae migrans. Am J Dis Child 1971;121:226–229.

120. Meyers WM, Connor DH, Neafie RC. Dipetalonemiasis. In: Binford CH, Connor DH, eds. Pathology of tropical and extraordinary diseases. Washington DC: Armed Forces Institute of Pathology, 1976:382–389.

121. Kahn JB. Pleural effusion associated with *Dipetalonema perstans*. J Infect Dis 1983;147:166.

122. Goldwater LJ, Steinberg I, Most H, Connery J. Hemoptysis in trichiniasis. N Engl J Med 1935;213:849–851.

123. Frothingham C. A contribution to the knowledge of the lesions caused by *Trichinella spiralis* in man. J Med Res 1906;10:483–490.

124. Askanazy M. Zur lehre von der trichinosis. Virchows Archiv 1895;141:42.

125. Yii CY, Chen CY, Fresh JW, Chen T, Cross JH. Human angiostrongyliasis involving the lungs. Chin J Microbiol 1968;1:148–159.

126. Sonakal D. Pathological findings in four cases of human angiostrongyliasis. Southeast Asian J Trop Med Public Health 1978;9:220–227.

127. Beaver PC, Jung RC, Cupp EW. Clinical parasitology. 9th Ed. Philadelphia: Lea & Febiger, 1984:291.

128. Spalding MG, Greiner EC, Green SL. *Halicephalobus (Micronema) deletrix* infection in two half-sibling foals. JAVMA 1991;196:1127–1129.

129. Hoogstraten J, Young WG. Meningo-encephalitis due to a saprophagous nematode, *Micronema deletrix*. Can J Neurol Sci 1975;2:121–126.

130. Shadduck IA, Ubelacker J, Telford VQ. *Micronema deletrix* miningoencephalitis in an adult man. Am J Clin Pathol 1979;72:640–643.

131. Gardiner CH, Koh DS, Cardella TA. *Micronema* in man: Third fatal infection. Am J Trop Med Hyg 1981; 30:586–589.

132. Connor DH, Gibson DW, Zeifer A. Diagnostic features of three unusual infections: Micronemiasis, phaeomycotic cysts, and protothecosis. In: Majno C, Cotran RS, eds. Current topics in inflammation and infection. Baltimore: Williams & Wilkins, 1982:205–239.

133. Brandt M. Parasitare Lungefibrose durch *Oxyuris vermicularis*. Tuberkulosearzt 1949;3:685–688.

134. Beaver PC, Kriz JJ, Lau TJ. Pulmonary nodule caused by *Enterobius vermicularis*. Am J Trop Med Hyg 1973; 22:711–712.

135. Smith JL, Brown DD, Little MD. Life cycle and development of *Lagochilascaris sprenti* from opossums in Louisiana. J Parasitol 1983;69:736–745.

136. Botero D, Little MD. Two cases of human *Lagochilascaris* infection in Colombia. Am J Trop Med Hyg 1984; 2:345–352.

137. Huff DS, Neafie RC, Binder MJ, DeLeon GA, Brown LW, Kazakos KR. The first fatal *Baylisascaris* infection in humans: An infant with eosinophilic meningoencephalitis. Pediatr Pathol 1984;2:345–352.

138. Fox AS, Kazakos KR, Gould NS, Heydemann PT, Thomas C, Boyer KM. Fatal eosinophilic meningoencephalitis and visceral larva migrans caused by the raccoon ascarid *Baylisascaris procyonis*. N Engl J Med 1985; 312:1619–1623.

139. Kobayashi A, Tsuji M, Wilbur DL. Probable pulmonary anisakiasis accompanying pleural effusions. Am J Trop Med Hyg 1985;34:310–313.

140. Daengsvang S. A monograph on the genus *Gnathostoma* and gnathostomiasis in Thailand. Tokyo: Southeast

141. Fontan R, Beauchamp F, Beaver PC. Sur quelques helminthiasis humaines nouvelles au Laos. I. Nematodes. II. Platyhelminthes. Bull Soc Pathol Exot 1975;68:557–573.

142. Nagler A, Pollack S, Hassoun G. Human pleuropulmonary gnathostomiasis: A case report form Israel. Isr J Med Sci 1983;19:834–837.

143. Wall MA, McGhee G. Paragonimiasis. Atypical appearances in two adolescent Asian refugees. Am J Dis Child 1982;136:828–830.

144. Collins MS, Phelan A, Kim TC, Pearson RD. *Paragonimus westermani*: A cause of cavitary lung disease in an Indochinese refugee. South Med J 1980;74:1418–1420.

145. Johnson RJ, Johnson JR. Paragonimiasis in Indochinese refugees. Roentgenographic findings with clinical correlation. Am Rev Respir Dis 1983;128:534–538.

146. Vanijanonta S, Bunnay D, Harinasuta T. Radiologic findings in pulmonary paragonimiasis heterotremus. Southeast Asian J Trop Med Public Health 1984; 15:122–128.

147. Bae SK, Park YK, Rhu NS. Clinical study of pulmonary paragonimiasis. Tuberc Respir Dis 1980;27:145–150.

148. Minh V, Engle P, Greenwood JR, Prendergast TJ, Salness K, St. Clair R. Pleural paragonimiasis in a Southeast Asian refugee. Am Rev Respir Dis 1981;124:186–188.

149. Suzuki N. Color atlas of human helminth eggs. Tokyo: Southeast Asian Medical Information Center; Publ No. 2, 1975:20–21.

150. Meyers WM, Neafie RC. Paragonimiasis. In: Binford CH, Connor DH, eds. Pathology of tropical and extraordinary diseases. Washington, DC: Armed Forces Institute of Pathology, 1976:517–523.

151. Johnson RJ, Dunning SB, Minshew BH, Jong EC. Successful treatment of paragonimiasis following bithional failure. Am J Trop Med Hyg 1983;32:1309–1311.

152. Vanijanonta S, Radomyos P, Bunnag D, Harinasuta T. Pulmonary paragonimiasis with expectoration of worms: A case report. Southeast Asian J Trop Med Public Health 1981;12:104–106.

153. Kum PN, Nchinda TC. Pulmonary paragonimiasis in Cameroon. Trans R Soc Trop Med Hyg 1982;76:768–772.

154. Freeman RS, Stuart PF, Cullen JB, et al. Fatal infection with mesocercariae of the trematode *Alaria americana*. Am J Trop Med Hyg 1976;25:803–807.

155. Beaver PC, Little MD, Tucker CF, Reed RJ. Mesocercaria in the skin of man in Louisiana. Am J Trop Med Hyg 1976;26:422–426.

156. Shea M, Maberley Al, Walters J, Freeman RS, Fallis AM. Intraretinal larval nematode. Trans Am Acad Ophthalmol Otolaryngol 1973;77:784–791.

157. Shoop WL, Corkum KC. Epidemiology of *Alaria marcianae* mesocercaria in Louisiana. J Parasitol 1981; 67:928–931.

158. Shoop WL, Corkum KC. Migration of *Alaria marcianae* in domestic cats. J Parasitol 1983;69:912–917.

159. Johnson AD. *Alaria mustelae*: Description of mesocercar-

iae and key to related species. Trans Am Microsc Soc 1970;89:250–253.

160. Hill JR, Turk EP. Pulmonary schistosomiasis. Aviat Space Environ Med 1980;51:1069–1070.

161. McCully RM, Barron CN, Cheever AW. Schistosomiasis. In: Binford CH, Connor DH, eds. Pathology of tropical and extraordinary diseases. Washington, DC: Armed Forces Institute of Pathology, 1976:402–508.

162. Sadigursky M, Andrade ZA. Pulmonary changes in schistosomal cor pulmonale. Am J Trop Med Hyg 1982; 31:779–784.

163. Deloramas P, Abroise-Thomas P. Pulmonary symptoms in schistosomiasis. Arq Bras Cardiol 1980;37:107–110.

164. Miziara HL, Filomeno AP, Yunes MAF. Dissecting aneurysm of the pulmonary artery attributed to pulmonary schistosomiasis. Serv Pneumophtisiol 1981; 40:281–284.

165. Jiashun Z, Fuyuan F, Schuzhu Y. Chronic cor pulmonale due to *Schistosoma japonicum* infection. Chin Med J 1981;94:529–534.

166. Jawahiry KL, Karpas CM. Pulmonary schistosomiasis: A detailed clinicopathologic study. Am Rev Respir Dis 1963;88:517–527.

167. Prijyanonda B, Tandhanand S. Opisthorchiasis with pulmonary involvement. Ann Intern Med 1961;54:795–798.

168. Meyers W, Neafie RC. Fascioliasis. In: Binford CH, Connor DH, eds. Pathology of tropical and extraordinary diseases. Washington, DC: Armed Forces Institute of Pathology, 1976:526.

169. Watson JH, Kermin RA. Observations on the various forms of parasitic pharyngitis known as "halzoun" in the Middle East. J Trop Med Hyg 1956;59:147–154.

170. Yamashita J. *Clinostomum complanatum*, a trematode parasite new to man. Annot Zool Jpn 1983;17:563–566.

171. Witenberg G. What is the cause of the parasitic laryngitis in the Near East. Acta Med Orient 1944;3:191–192.

172. Kamo H, Ogino K, Hatsushika R. A unique infection of man with *Clinostomum* sp., a small trematode causing acute laryngitis. Yonago Acta Med 1962;6:37–40.

173. Beaver PC, Rolon FA. Proliferating larval cestode in a man in Paraguay. A case report and review. Am J Trop Med Hyg 1981;30:625–637.

174. Bonne C. A few remarks on two rare parasitic diseases in the Malayan Archipelago. A. Chromomycosis. B. Sparganosis. Trans Eighth Congr Far Eastern Assoc Trop Med 1932;2:184–188.

175. Connor DH, Sparks AK, Strano AJ, Neafie RC, Juvelier B. Disseminated parasitois in an immunocompromised patient. Possibly a mutated sparganum. Arch Pathol Lab Med 1976;100:65–68.

176. Lin TP, Su IJ, Lu SC, Yang SP. Pulmonary proliferative sparganosis. A case report. J Formosan Med Assoc 1978;77:467–472.

177. Beaver PC, Jung RC, Cupp EW. Clinical parasitology. 9th Ed. Philadelphia: Lea & Febiger, 1984:499–502.

178. Sparks AK, Neafie RC, Connor DH. Sparganosis. In: Binford CH, Connor DH, eds. Pathology of tropical and extraordinary diseases. Washington, DC: Armed Forces

Institute of Pathology, 1976:534–538.

179. Torres JR, Noya OO, Noya BA, Mouliniere R, Martinez E. Treatment of proliferative sparganosis with mebendazole and praziquantel. Trans R Soc Trop Med Hyg 1981;75:846–847.

180. Sparks AK, Neafie RC, Connor DH. Cysticercosis. In: Binford CH, Connor DH, eds. Pathology of tropical and extraordinary diseases. Washington, DC: Armed Forces Institute of Pathology, 1976:539–543.

181. Priestly SE, Wiles PG. Cysticercosis-induced epilepsy diagnosed by computerized tomography. J Soc Occup Med 1979;29:149–150.

182. Schantz PM, Schantz D, Wilson M. Serologic cross-reactions with sera from patients with echinococcosis and cysticercosis. Am J Trop Med Hyg 1980;29:609–612.

183. Gamble WG, Segal M, Schantz PM, Rausch RL. Alveolar hydatid disease in Minnesota. First human case acquired in the contiguous United States. JAMA 1979;241:904–907.

184. Leiby PD, Kritsky DC. *Echinococcus multilocularis*: A possible domestic life cycle in central North America and its public health implications. J Parasitol 1972;58:1213–1215.

185. Wilson JF, Rausch RL. Alveolar hydatid disease. A review of clinical features of 33 indigenous cases of *Echinococcus multilocularis* infection in Alaskan Eskimos. Am J Trop Med Hyg 1980;29:1340–1355.

186. Rausch RL, Bernstein JJ. *Echinococcus vogeli* sp. n. from the bush dog, *Speothos venaticus*. Z Tropenmed Parasitol 1972;23:25–34.

187. D'Alessandro A, Rausch RL, Cuello C, Aristizabal N. *Echinococcus vogeli* in man, with a review of polycystic hydatid disease in Colombia and neighboring countries. Am J Trop Med Hyg 1979;28:303–317.

188. Pineyro JR. Hydatid disease of the lung. Prog Pediatr Surg 1982;15:113–118.

189. Matsaniotis N, Karpathios T, Koutoyzis J. Hydatid disease in Greek children. Am J Trop Med Hyg 1983; 32:1075–1078.

190. Talmoudi T, Joven JC, Malmejac C. [Pulmonary hydatid embolism. Study of two personal cases and review of the literature]. Ann Chir 1980;34:245–250.

191. Beaver PC, Jung RC, Cupp EW. Clinical parasitology. 9th Ed. Philadelphia: Lea & Febiger, 1984:536.

192. Van den Brink WTJ, Van Knapen F, Van der Elst AMC. Treatment of echinococcosis with mebendazole in a woman with multiple cyst. Ned Tijdschr Geneeskd 1983;127:423–428.

193. Kern P. Human echinococcosis: Follow-up of 23 patients treated with mebendazole. Infection 1983;11:17–24.

194. Beaver PC, Jung RC, Cupp EW. Clinical parasitology. 9th Ed. Philadelphia: Lea & Febiger, 1984:527–538.

195. Treugut H, Schulze K, Hubuer KH, Andrasch R. Pulmonary involvement by *Echinococcus alveolaris*. Diagn Radiol 1980;137:37–41.

196. Marty AM, Hess SJ. Tegumental laminations in echinococci using Gomori's methenamine silver stain. Lab Med 1991;22:419–420.

197. Allen AR, Fullmer CD. Primary diagnosis of pulmonary echinococcosis by the cytologic technique. Acta Cytol 1972;16:212–216.

198. Schantz PM, Wilson JF, Wahlquist SP. Serologic tests for diagnosis and post-treatment evaluation of patients with alveolar hydatid disease. Am J Trop Med Hyg 1983; 32:1381–1386.

199. Voorhorst R, Spidksma FTM, Varekamp H, Leupen MJ, Lyklema AW. The house dust mite and the allergens it produces. J Allergy 1967;39:325–329.

200. Ingram CG, Symington IS, Jeffrey IG, Cuthbert OD. Bronchial provocation studies in farmers allergic to storage mites. Lancet 1979;ii:1330–1332.

201. Yamaguchi T. A colour atlas of clinical parasitology. London: Wolfe, 1981;22–23.

202. Cuthbert OK, Brostoff J, Wraith DG, Brighton WD. "Barn Allergy." Asthma and rhinitis due to storage mites. Clin Allergy 1979;229–236.

203. Kijima S. A case of pulmonary acariasis—histopathological findings in resected lungs. Brit Med J 1963;2: 451–452.

204. Soysa E, Jayawardena MD. Pulmonary acariasis; a possible cause of asthma. Br Med J 1945;1:1–6.

205. Ward RA, Myiasis. In: Binford CH, Connor DH, eds. Pathology of tropical and extraordinary diseases. Washington, DC: Armed Forces Institute of Pathology, 1976:626–630.

206. Komori K, Hara K, Smith KGV, Oda T, Daramine D. A case of lung myiasis caused by larvae of *Megaselia spiracularis* (Diptera: Phoridae). Trans R Soc Trop Med Hyg 1978;72:467–470.

207. Ahmed M, Miller A. Pulmonary coin lesion containing a horse bot, *Gasterophilus*. Report of a case of myiasis. Am J Clin Pathol 1969;52:414–419.

208. Betancourt VML. A case of pulmonary myiasis. Medico (Mex) 1966;15:45–47.

209. Prathap K, Lau KS, Bolton JM. Pentastomiasis: A common finding at autopsy among Malaysian aborigines. Am J Trop Med Hyg 1969;18:20–27.

210. Meyers WM, Neafie RC, Connor DH. Diseases caused by pentastomes. In: Binford CH, Connor DH, eds. Pathology of tropical and extraordinary diseases. Washington, DC: Armed Forces Institute of Pathology, 1976:546–550.

211. Beaver PC, Jung RC, Cupp EW. Clinical parasitology. 9th Ed. Philadelphia: Lea & Febiger, 1984:573.

212. Schacher JF, Saab S, Germanos R, Boustang N. The aetiology of halzoun in Lebanon: Recovery of *Linguatula serrata* nymphs from two patients. Trans R Soc Trop Med Hyg 1969;63:854–859.

213. Symmers WC, Valteris K. Two cases of human infection by larvae of *Linguatula serrata*. J Clin Pathol 1950;3:212–219.

214. Hunter WS, Higgins RP. An unusual case of human porocephaliasis. J Parsitol 1960;46:68.

215. Ali-Khan Z, Bower EJ. Pentastomiasis in western Canada: A case report. Am J Trop Med Hyg 1972;21:58–61.

216. Cagnard V, Nicolas-Randegger J, Dago Arribi A, et al. [Generalized and lethal pentastomiasis due to *Armillifer armillatus*.] Bull Soc Pathol Exot 1979;72:345–352.

217. Khalil GM, Schacher JF. *Linguatula serrata* in relation to halzoun and the marrara syndrome. Am J Trop Med Hyg 1965;14:736–746.

218. Self JT, Hopps HC, Williams AO. Pentastomiasis in Africans. Trop Geogr Med 1975;27:1–13.

219. Barnes RD. Invertebrate zoology. 3d Ed. Philadelphia, Saunders: 1974:690–691.

220. Gardiner CH, Dyke JW, Shirley SF. Hepatic granuloma due to a nymph of *Linguatula serrata* in a woman from Michigan: A case report and review of the literature. Am J Trop Med Hyg 1984;33:187–189.

221. Self JT, Hopps HC, Williams AO. Porocephaliasis in man and experimental mice. Exp Parasitol 1972; 32:117–126.

222. Azinge NO, Ogidi-Gdefbafe EG, Osunde JA, Oduah D. *Armillifer armillatus* in Bendel State (Midwest) Nigeria. Phase I. J Trop Med Hyg 1978;81:76–79.

223. Russell HK. A modification of Movat's pentachrome stain. Arch Pathol Lab Med 1972;94:187–191.

224. Beaver PC, Jung RC, Cupp EW. Clinical parasitology. 9th Ed. Philadelphia: Lea & Febiger, 1984:551.

225. Baird JK. False parasites in tissue sections. Parasitol Today 1987;3:273–276.

226. Sunn TS, Turnbull A, Lieberman PH, Sternberg SS. Giant kidney worm mimicking retioperitoneal neoplasm. Am J Surg Pathol 1986;10:508–512.

227. Turr SM, Nelson AM, Gibson DW, et al. Liesegang Rings in Tissue. How to distinguish Liesegang rings from the giant kidney worm, *Dioctophyma renale*. Am J Surg Pathol 1978;11:598–605.

CHAPTER 16

Eosinophilic Infiltrates

DAVID H. DAIL

Eosinophilic infiltrates in the lung that are discussed in this chapter include asthma, eosinophilic pneumonia, allergic bronchopulmonary aspergillosis, mucoid impaction, and bronchocentric granulomatosis. Hypereosinophilic syndrome is also mentioned. These are often manifestations of immunologically mediated reactions confined to the lungs. These entities may frequently overlap with each other because of their often-shared, common eosinophilic cell response and symptoms of asthma, and, in some cases, their common etiologies.

The Eosinophil

Several good general reviews of the eosinophilic leukocyte are available,[1–4] and several reviews have concentrated on eosinophilic infiltrates in the lung.[5–8] The eosinophilic leukocyte has a bilobed nucleus and is named for moderate-sized eosinophilic, somewhat refractile, granules in its cytoplasm. It is bone marrow derived and is beckoned locally by eosinophilic chemotactic factors such as the preformed mast cell-derived eosinophilic chemotactic factor of anaphylaxis (ECF-A) and a component of slow-reacting substance of anaphylaxis (SRS-A), leukotriene B4. Its granules contain an electron-dense central core that is alkaline at pH 10 and so has been named "major basic protein." Its high alkalinity is thought to be helpful in killing parasites. The surrounding less dense granule matrix contains cationic protein, which is harmful to parasites, peroxidase, and eosinophil-derived neurotoxin as well as other factors. Many of its enzymes modulate the mast cell enzymes of histamine, eosinophilic, neutrophilic, and monocytic chemotactic factors of anaphylaxis, hep-

arin, and chymotrypsin but it is becoming clear that the eosinophil is also a potent primary inflammatory cell on its own.[9] Even today, this cell continues to retain many of its secrets.

Asthma

Asthma is acute, usually reversible, spasmodic, diffuse airway narrowing, with persistent airway hyperreactivity. Asthma affects 3%–8% of the population[10] and causes about 2,000–3,000 deaths per year, or about 1%–2% of those with severe asthma.[11] The name is derived from the ancient Greek work for panting. As nicely reviewed by Siegel,[12] Aretaeus of Cappadocia in the second century B.C. first accurately described an asthma attack and wrote that if symptoms increase, they sometimes produce suffocation. In a twelfth-century review, the Spaniard Moses Maimoides stated death from asthma can occur "should the rules of management go unheeded and one's desires and habits be followed indiscriminately," words that ring true to this day.

Asthma is usually associated with airway inflammation and heightened sensitivity to a variety of irritants and allergens in quantity or quality that would not usually affect nonasthmatics.[13–15] Other entities can cause wheezing and shortness of breath but do not usually produce persistent airway hypersensitivity to a variety of agents or conditions. Asthma has historically been classified as "extrinsic" when an exogenous cause can be documented and "intrinsic" when no such cause(s) can be found. This division has fallen into disuse in practice. McFadden[16] classified the types of stimuli that evoke episodes of asthma as (1) infections,

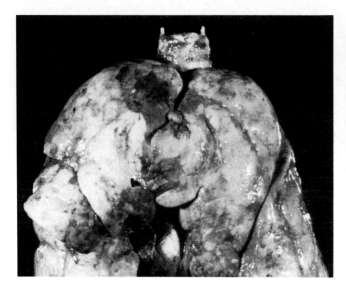

Fig. 16–1. Lungs from child who died of status asthmaticus, anterior view. Left lung is more evenly distended and is shown as a reference of more normal tissue. Right lung shows alternating areas of pale overdistension and dark atelectasis.

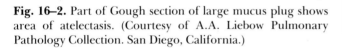

Fig. 16–2. Part of Gough section of large mucus plug shows area of atelectasis. (Courtesy of A.A. Liebow Pulmonary Pathology Collection. San Diego, California.)

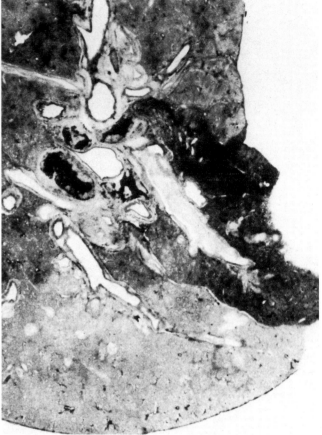

(2) exercise, (3) antigens, (4) occupational stimuli, (5) environmental causes, (6) pharmacologic stimuli, and (7) emotional stress These divisions, along with idiopathic, serve as the basis for the current classification of asthma. Cough or exertional dyspnea may at times be the only symptom of asthma.[17,18] Blood, tissue, and sputum eosinophilia are frequently present but vary in degree. Several excellent reviews of possible mechanisms of chemical and physical mediators are available.*

Pathology

Biopsies are not usually done in living asthmatic patients, so the pathology findings tend to be extrapolations of autopsy findings in cases of death from status asthmaticus.[28–37] These changes are confirmed by studying lungs of asthmatic patients dying of assorted other causes[28,33,38] and, during life, by biopsies[39–42] and cytologies,[43] including bronchoalveolar lavage.[2] Huber and Koessler in 1922[28] are credited with the first major analysis of the pathology of asthma followed by Houston et al.[29] in 1953. Much of the recent re-

*References 9,14,16,19–27.

view work has been done by Dunnill,[33–37] among others.[15,44,45]

Grossly, lungs show alternating areas of hyperexpansion and collapse (Fig. 16–1). These changes have also been seen on whole-mount lung sections.[46] Hyperexpansion, but not emphysema, is present in the distended areas. The lungs do not collapse after removal at autopsy. These gross findings are well explained by varying degrees of obstruction of the breathing tubes. If obstruction is complete, atelectasis is caused by absorption of distal air (Fig. 16–2), and if partial, air enters distal parenchyma through expanded airways in inspiration but cannot exit through the narrowed airways of expiration. Such partial obstruction leads to overexpansion by air entrapment by an almost ball-valve effect.

Soft, gelatinous, or rubbery grey mucus plugs are often seen in the cut surface of the lungs grossly, most frequently in medium to small bronchi (Fig. 16–3). These changes are usually more severe in patients dying in status asthmaticus than in asthma patients who die of other causes,[47] but, as noted, the same types of changes are seen in both. Intact or partial bronchial casts are sometimes expectorated or removed at bronchoscopy.

Microscopically, the spirally arranged bronchial smooth muscle is greatly thickened.[28,34] When mea-

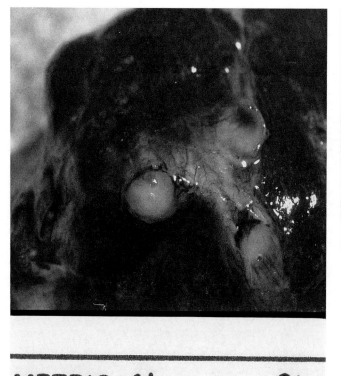

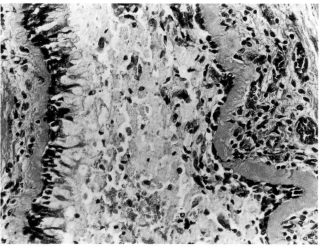

Fig. 16–4. Two sides of same bronchiolar wall in asthma. Note thick hyalinized basal lamina. On left side, intact mucosa shows increased number of goblet cells. This mucosa is degenerating on right side, and cells are sloughing as "Creola bodies." Submucosal inflammation and thickening of basal lamina are more marked in this area. H and E, ×400.

Fig. 16–3. Mucus plugs. Cut surface of teenager's lung who died from asthma. (Courtesy of Dr. Kris Sperry, Fulton County Medical Examiner's Office, Atlanta, Georgia.)

sured, it is 2.6 fold thicker in patients dying in status asthmaticus than in normal people.[34] This muscle increase is not seen in chronic bronchitis, and helps to distinguish these two diseases. The mechanisms of the muscle increase and hyperreactivity are incompletely understood and some, or perhaps most, work through neural pathways.[23,48,49]

The bronchial submucosa shows edema, vessel dilatation, and mixed inflammatory infiltrates. These inflammatory cells include eosinophils, plasma cells, lymphocytes, and some polymorphonuclear leukocytes. At times eosinophils are only minimally present or absent, and plasma cells and lymphocytes predominate. The basal lamina of the mucosa is hyalinized, pink, and thickened up to 2.5 times normal.[50,51] It appears thickest in areas of epithelial damage and submucosal inflammation (Fig. 16–4). This thickening is primarily caused by increased collagen deposition.[52] Transudation of proteins may play a role.[33] The volume of submucosal glands is also increased, but not usually to the extent that it is in chronic bronchitis.* Immunofluorescence studies have varied; some showed staining of

*References: 15,28,34,35,53–57.

immunoglobulin,[50,51] but others either failed to confirm this or indicated such staining may be nonspecific.[52]

Submucosal glands contain an increased number of mucous cells.[34] Increased numbers of goblet cells are also present in the bronchial mucosal lining, and are accompanied by a decrease in ciliated cells (Figs. 16–4 and 16–5). Normally, goblet cells in the bronchial lining are present to about the limit of cartilage in the small bronchi, which is down to about 1–2 mm in diameter, and are typically absent more peripherally (see Chapter 2). In asthmatic patients these goblet cells are seen in abundance in the more peripheral bronchioles (Fig. 16–5).

Increased mucus from both lining goblet cells and submucosal glands, and chemical changes in the mucus with a greater acid glycoprotein and DNA fiber binding[58,59] and progressive fibrin formation,[33,58] along with an altered glycoprotein:proteoglycan ratio,[45] contribute to the thick gelatinous luminal contents. Albumin[36] and other proteins leak from injured walls.[60] Such protein and mucus admixtures are demonstrated by various stains, and increasing laminations of the mucus and protein are an indication of older secretions in the bronchi. These have been studied by sections of mucus plugs or casts.[61,62] The eosinophils in asthmatic mucus are usually well preserved, presumably because they have arrived in the mucus fairly recently, in contrast to those in mucoid impaction (discussed later). They are in strands and admixed with mucus as whorls or eddies[62] (Figs. 16–4 and 16–6). Steroid therapy may

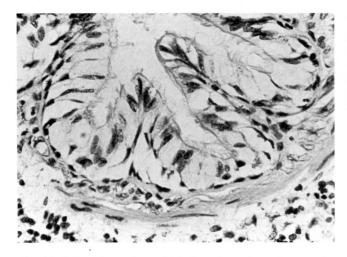

Fig. 16–5. Peripheral bronchiole in asthma shows increase in goblet cells where normally there would be none. H and E, ×500.

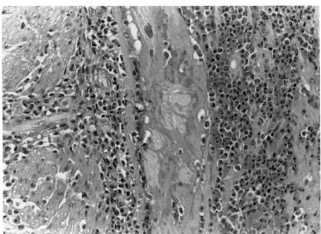

Fig. 16–6. Asthmatic mucus plug. Note thick mucus in middle and streaming of mostly intact eosinophils in lumen to right; inflamed bronchial wall with thickened smooth muscle to left. H and E, ×400. (Refer also to Figs. 16–4 and 16–7).

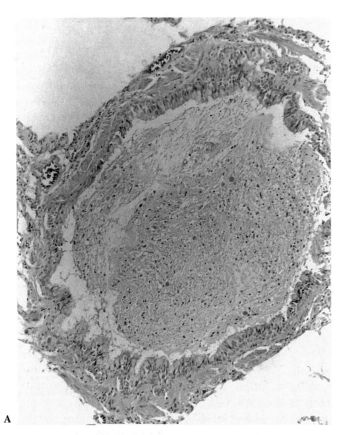

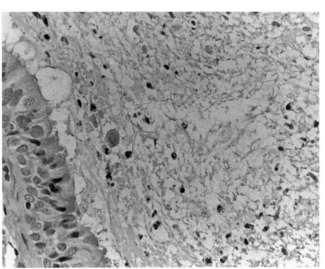

Fig. 16–7 A,B. Bronchus filled with hypocellular dense granular mucin and debris in middle-aged asthmatic woman treated with frequent steroids. **A.** Note decrease in cell content with persistence of mucus stasis. **B.** Note also return toward normal of mucus cell metaplasia as compared to Fig. 16–5.

decrease the cellular content but will not always affect mucinous plug formation (Fig. 16–7). Cilia are affected by proteinaceous fluids and some of the breakdown products of eosinophils, specifically major basic protein. Along with the tenacious material already in the lumens, these cells mobilize the luminal contents with difficulty.

Outpouchings of bronchial mucosa, probably representing dilatation of bronchial gland mouths,[33] appear to enlarge by the physical forces of increased interluminal pressure and increased muscle contraction, along with stasis of mucous passing through these areas.[63,64] (Fig. 16–8). The first description of this is attributed to Monckeberg in 1909 when he described a crypt-like

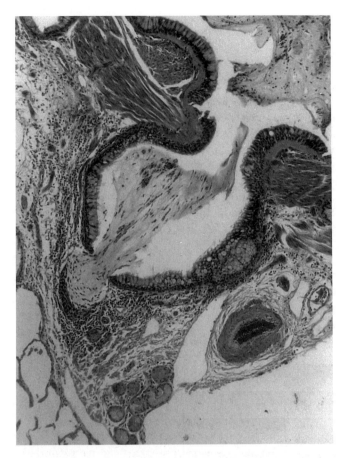

Fig. 16–8. Bronchial diverticulum. This probably represents dilatation of bronchial gland neck, with inflammatory ulceration (diverticulitis) distally. H and E, ×400. (Courtesy of Dr. L.J. Holloway, Wellington School of Medicine, New Zealand.)

protrusion of epithelium[65]; other authors have called them bronchial sacculations,[66] dilations of gland openings,[67] bronchial gland duct ectasia,[64] bronchioldiverticular[33] diverticula or diverticulosis of the epithelium,[29] or when inflamed, bronchial diverticulitis.[63]

A nice comparative study was done by Cluroe et al.[64] after encountering a 26-year-old woman who died of asthma, interstitial emphysema, and bilateral pneumothoraces. Histologically, these were traced to inflamed diverticulum,[63] and this case led to a comparative study of the 72 cases of death from asthma, with 72 cases of matched control patients.[64] Cluroe et al. histologically diagnosed asthma at autopsy when four of the following five criteria were present: mucous plugging, basement membrane thickening, epithelial shedding, submucosal eosinophil leukocyte infiltration, or smooth muscle hypertrophy. These authors described goblet cell hyperplasia but did not use that as one of their criteria. Using their criteria, the authors found histologic evidence of asthma in 53 of 72 (74%) of the asthma

deaths and 5 of 72 (7%) of the control group. In the asthma deaths, diverticulae were found in 39 of the 72 cases (54%), of which 36 of 39 (92%) were in the histologically positive asthma group. Bronchial gland neck diverticula were found in 7 of the control group, including all 5 in this group in whom there was histologic evidence of asthma changes, but in whom death was not attributed to asthma. Interstitial emphysema resulted when these diverticula ruptured; diverticula were found in 10 of the cases of fatal asthma, all of which had positive histologic asthma and gland ectasia. In none of the control group was interstitial emphysema identified.

Some interesting components are found in asthmatics' bronchioles and in their sputa. More distal bronchioles appear to produce Curshmann spirals, originally described in 1883,[68] which are small linear whorled strands twisted in a common direction with a central highly refractile densely coiled or braided coil (Fig. 16–9). The ever-tightening coil that these produce implies mucus is secreted from gland necks or flows in distal bronchioles in a common circumferential-vortical direction; otherwise, uncoiling would occur. Of note is that Curshmann spirals have been identified in cervical vaginal smears[69] and in pleural and peritoneal fluids.[70,71] On the serosal surfaces, at least, their origin is thought to be a rolling-up of a mucin-rich surface layer. In asthma, inflammatory cells may be seen admixed with mucinous and proteinaceous fluid in the lumen of the bronchi. As eosinophils degranulate, small bipyramidal hexagonal eosinophilic crystals, called Charcot–Leyden crystals, may be produced (Fig. 16–10). These are composed of pure lysophospholipase,[72] which is associated with eosinophilic membranes,[73,74] probably from eosinophilic granules. Charcot–Leyden crystals are moderately common in extracellular mucin in allergic sinusitis,[75] and have been described in pleural fluid[76–78] and in circulating blood.[79] Ayres[80] has produced these crystals using selected detergent action on eosinophils. Naylor[81] noted these crystals are not usually present in fresh and relatively warm pleural fluid, but do develop with standing and cooling. These develop only when there are eosinophils present. Their formation does not appear to have any significance in relationship to primary production of disease.

Fragments of ciliated respiratory lining undergo degeneration and detachment from the basement membrane (see Fig. 16–4). These have been called *Creola bodies* after the patient in whom they were originally described.[82] These may be seen in histologic sections, sputum specimens, or plugs and casts. The farther they travel up the bronchial tree the more difficult becomes their definite identification because of cellular degeneration. Loss of clumps of ciliated cells further hampers

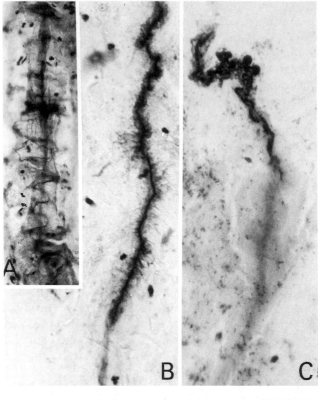

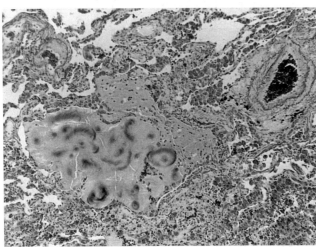

Fig. 16–9 A–D. Twisting of Curshmann spirals in asthma is seen in different views. **A.** A spiraling strand before tight coil forms (beyond this field). Papanicolaou, ×400. **B.** Long twisted core shows filaments of protruding mucus strands. Papanicolaou, ×400. **C.** More tightly coiled spiral with broad tail of spiraling mucus. Papanicolaou, ×400. **D.** Distal respiratory bronchiole-alveolar sac is distended with mucus, some of which is in whorls, suggesting possible cross sections of early Curschmann spirals. Movat's Pentachrome stain ×200.

the ciliary action in the bronchial tree. Perhaps as evidence of injury or regeneration, atypical metaplastic cells are also seen.[83] It has been proposed that the extreme transudation of proteinaceous fluid[33] or severe muscular spasm[29] may have caused this effect.

Gleich and associates[8,26,84–86] have studied the toxic effects of major basic protein on the lung. In their studies, Frigas and associates[85,86] purified major basic protein from asthmatic patients, applied this to viable explants of guinea pig and human trachea, and showed that this substance could clearly account for all of the changes in Creola body formation. These experiments showed the cells began to degenerate before detachment. Major basic protein can also primarily damage alveolar cells.[8] Considering these reactions, one might expect a high incidence of pulmonary infiltrates in asthmatics and other forms of pulmonary eosinophilia, but Ford found only 20 patients with pulmonary infiltrates with eosinophilia in a group of 5,702 consecutive asthmatic patients, for a rate of 0.35%.[87]

Status Asthmaticus

This term refers to severe asthma that is recalcitrant to the usually therapies and is characterized by extreme dyspnea, cyanosis, and exhaustion. Episodes last from a short period to a week or longer. Deaths still occur in this condition in adults and children (see introduction). As noted, most of the pathology of asthma has been described in such asthma deaths, and such patients often have extensive mucous plugging. Some of the deaths are thought to be from observable preterminal bronchoconstriction without mucous plugs,[45,88,89] and a few deaths may be caused by heart failure secondary to exogenous drugs or endogenous epinephrine, or hypoxia, or a combination of these events.[90–92]

Asthma deaths have been increasing generally two- to threefold in the past 25 years. The death rate before that was remarkably stable for the preceding 100 years.[93,94] Beginning in the 1960s in England and Wales[93,95] and also New Zealand,[96,97] a sudden increase in asthma deaths was noted. For some time it was suspected that this correlated with the release of high-dose isoproterenol preparations,[98–101] and indeed the death rate decreased to some extent in these countries after this surge.[95,97,102] However, again in the 1980s in these countries and the United States,[103] Canada,[104,105] Norway, Sweden, South Africa,[106] France,[107] and Germany,[107] another rise began that seems to be progressive and continues upward.

As noted, asthma has been described for some time. As nicely described by several authors[10,106–108] deaths from asthma were thought insignificant by many teachers even up to the early twentieth century. Such teachers as Laennec, Oliver Wendell Holmes, and William Osler downplayed the threat from this disease.[10] The large autopsy series of 21 cases described by Huber and Koessler[28] in 1922 helped dispel this notion.[106]

As reviewed by Benatar,[106] several possibilities for this rise in death rate were considered besides overdosage of drugs. In fact, 60–80% of the deaths occurred outside the hospital,[107] and rescuing techniques consist of more intense therapies once in the hospital; it is unusual to have deaths occurring under medical care. Cases of under diagnosis and under treatment were therefore considered. Teenagers, in particular with their high emotional turmoil, have conflicting concepts of infallibility, self-image, and fear of being dependent on medicines or considered sickly. Some incriminate the better criteria for diagnosing asthma,[95,109] or the more common usage of death from asthma on death certificates as related to the apparent rise. Others believe perhaps an increase in environmental pollutants has been responsible. Indeed, such chemicals known to affect asthma as metabisulfite and isocyanates have been recently increased in usage and in the atmosphere.[110] However, the double rise in the incidence of asthma in such relatively pollution-free countries as New Zealand tends to cast doubt on this, as does the fact that most known allergens for asthmatics are organic and derived from nature, while it is natural habitats that are diminishing locally and worldwide.[110] Passive tobacco smoke may be an additional environmental factor, especially for infants and children, and fortunately these factors are being given more attention today. Socioeconomically, there is a greater increase in poor people and children, and access to medical care may be a factor. Psychological factors have been carefully analyzed, including events on the day of death.[111]

None of these factors quite explains the increase in asthma deaths. I believe Whitelaw[110] has perceived the most pertinent conclusions for this rise. He stated that the patients today are better trained to use an armamentarium of drugs, many of which are very helpful and indeed are so helpful as to defer appropriate medical care and cause overdependence on home medication. Unfortunately, sometimes this leads to a high incidence of death outside hospitals. Whitelaw has pointed out that patients with such good treatment and prophylaxis often return to their harmful habitats or exposures, such as to their pet animals or workplace environments, which they might otherwise have avoided had control not been so effective. These control mechanisms work best on the acute wheezing phase but less on the delayed exudative phase, and this delay gives some patients a false sense of security.[112] A large review of such deaths by the British Thoracic Association[113] suggested preventable factors were present in many cases and that death was unavoidable in only 10 of 90 (11%) of cases.

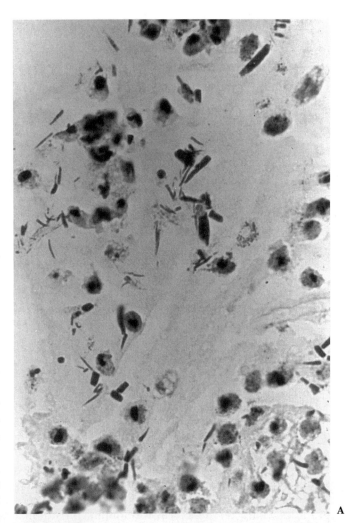

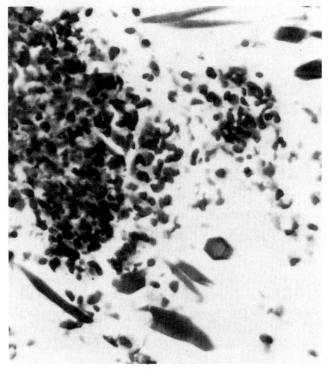

Fig. 16–10 A,B. Charcot-Leyden crystals. A. Lower power with many crystals and background eosinophils. H and E, ×400. B. Note cross-sectional hexagonal and longitudinal bipyramidal shapes. Many crystals do not form in perfect shapes. Brown and Brenn, ×1,000. (Courtesy of A.A. Liebow Pulmonary Pathology Collection, San Diego, California.)

Eosinophilic Pneumonia

Classification and History

Eosinophilic infiltrates in lung parenchyma have been subdivided into different categories. Crofton and associates[5] in 1952 used the term "pulmonary eosinophilia" to cover pulmonary infiltrations with blood eosinophilia. This excellent review, based on 16 new cases and a review of 450 cases from the literature before 1952, was the most comprehensive review in English to that date. These authors subdivided eosinophilic pulmonary diseases into (1) simple pulmonary eosinophilia, or Löffler's syndrome; (2) prolonged pulmonary eosinophilia; (3) tropical eosinophilia; (4) pulmonary eosinophilia with asthma; and (5) pulmonary eosinophilia with polyarteritis nodosa. In the same year, Reeder and Goodrich[114] used the term "pulmonary infiltration with eosinophilia" (PIE syndrome). The term "eosinophilic pneumonia" was used by Christoforidis and Molar in 1960[115] and further expanded by Liebow and Carrington[116] in 1969 to better define these pulmonary processes, as some eosinophilic infiltrates in the lung were unaccompanied by a blood eosinophilia, a necessary component of the earlier definitions.

Eosinophilic pneumonias are currently best referred to as "acute" or "chronic," with different implications for therapy. Acute eosinophilic pneumonia has also been called simple eosinophilic pneumonia,[117] and some add tropical eosinophilic pneumonia as a further subdivision[118] because of its unique filarial and geographical character. The term eosinophilic pneumonia without other qualifiers usually implies the more chronic form.

Acute Eosinophilic Pneumonia

In 1932 Löffler,[119] in Zurich, Switzerland, described 4 cases with minimal or no symptoms, transient radiographic infiltrates, and spontaneous resolution in 6–12 days without therapy. Two of 4 had elevated blood eosinophil counts of 9% and 22%; the other 2 had counts of 3.5% and 5%, respectively. As reviewed by Crofton,[5] Löffler collected 51 cases from this clinic by 1936 and 100 cases by 1944. The term Löeffler's syndrome is often used synonomously with acute eosinophilic pneumonia, but more recently another acute but more severe form has been described (see following discussion).

As symptoms in the typical Löffler's type are mild and cure is spontaneous, biopsies are not usually performed. Today it is necessary to have documented blood eosinophilia to suggest this diagnosis, although sputum or bronchoalveolar lavage eosinophilia is also

suggestive. Crofton and associates[5] further defined this syndrome as blood eosinophilia of 6% or higher, with *spontaneous cure* occurring within 1 month. Of interest, two of the original four cases described by Löffler and many of the currently described cases do not meet these criteria. Blood eosinophilia reaches its peak 3–4 days after the peak of the radiographic infiltrates.[5]

Ascaris lumbriocoides infection is a well-documented cause of this syndrome (see Chapter 15). Its prevalence in Switzerland apparently accounts for the large number of cases seen in Löffler's clinic. Von Meyenberg[120] in 1942 described autopsy findings in four young men killed accidentally who had pulmonary eosinophilia, but no or minimal symptoms in life. These presumably represented Löffler's syndrome. Noninvasive ascaris was present in the intestines of two of these men.

Ascaris was present in 23 of the 100 cases published by Löffler and Maier in 1944, according to Crofton.[5] Löffler produced this syndrome experimentally by giving ascaris larvae to guinea pigs. He was able to follow larval migration through the bowel wall, into the bloodstream, and into liver and lungs. Larvae then reached the bronchial lumens, were expectorated, swallowed, and returned to the gastrointestinal tract. Other experiments in humans confirmed this, as reviewed by Crofton.[5] The mild transient self-limited infiltrates of Löffler's syndrome associated with ascaris best fit such larval passage through lung tissue. Documenting such passage may be difficult even when adult worms are present in the bowels. Finding third-stage larvae in sputum or gastric samples helps to confirm this pulmonary passage.[121]

In 1949, Sprent[122] sensitized mice to various ascaris extracts and produced pulmonary eosinophilic infiltrates, which suggested an important role for hypersensitivity. An unfortunate prank played on four young men occurred during a university holiday in Canada. They ingested *Ascaris suum* eggs, and all became ill with diffuse pulmonary infiltrates and bloody eosinophilia 10–14 days later. The two with the highest IgE- and IgM-precipitating antibodies, worst infiltrates, and most marked eosinophilia had the least number of immature worms in their stools, which suggested an active host response or previous exposure.[123]

Spontaneous cases of ascaris infection are most frequently diagnosed in Switzerland, Germany, France, Scandinavia, the southern part of North America, South Africa, and China.[5] Crofton et al.[5] reviewed other reports of possible parasites, bacteria, and assorted inhaled antigens that may also be important. A current list of agents causing eosinophilic pneumonia is given in Table 16–1.

In developed countries today, drugs may be the most prevalent antigen suspected of causing the acute syn-

Table 16–1. Partial list of identifiable causes of eosinophilic pneumonia

Drugs		Parasites	Other infections	Other
Antibiotics	**Antihyperglycemic**	**Nematodes**	**Bacteria**	**Metal salts**
Penicillin	Chlopropamide	**(roundworms)**	Brucella	Nickel
Ampicillin	Tolbutamide	Ascaris	Staphyloccocus	Beryllium
Sulfa		Strongyloides	Pneumococcus	Zinc
Nitrofurantoin	**Antihypertensive**	Ancyclostoma	Proteus	
Streptomycin	Hydralazine	Necator	Escherchia coli	**Fumes**
Tetracycline	Mecamylamine	Toxocara	Corynebacterium	Probably nickel and
Minocycline		Trichinella	?Tuberculosis	chromium
Isoniazid	**CNS-effective**			
Aminosalicyclic	Chlorpromazine	**Filarial nematodes**	**Fungi**	**Other allergens**
acid	Desipramine	Wuchereria	Aspergillus	Pollen
Para-amino-salicylic	Imipramine	Brugia	Coccidioidomyces	Beeswax
acid	Methlphenidate	Dirofilaria	Candida	Desaturated cooking oils
	Carbamazepine		Sporotrix	Snake bite
Antineoplastic	Mephenesin	**Trematodes (flatworms**		Scorpion bite
Azathiaprine	L-tryptophan	**or flukes)**	**Viruses**	Poison ivy desensitization
Methotrexate		Schistosoma	?In children	Fire smoke
Bleomycin	**Other drugs**	Fasciola		
Procarbazine	Adrenalin		**Pneumocystis**	
	Amiodarone	**Cestodes (tapeworms)**		
Antiinflammatory	Chlofibrate	Echinococcus		
Aspirin	Dantrolene	Taenia		
Beclomethasone	Glafemine			
Naproxin	Satazopyrin			
Gold salts	Zomepirac			
Chromoglycate				

drome. Consequently, if eosinophilic pneumonia is presently considered, all drugs are temporarily discontinued to see if they may be such a cause. Because spontaneous cure is, by strict definition, an inherent part of this syndrome, cases of fleeting pulmonary infiltration in which the probable cause is removed, or effective therapy is given, no longer technically qualify as the acute form or Löffler's syndrome.

A more severe form of acute eosinophilic pneumonia is currently being described,[124–130] including some in immunosuppressed cases[124] and including AIDS[124,127] and in children.[130] This syndrome usually occurs in nonasthmatic patients without atopic history or other predisposing causes, and occurs mostly in adult men with rapid onset of symptoms, usually of less than 1 week. These symptoms are flu like and consist of cough, dyspnea, pleuritic pain and myalgia with severe hypoxia being clinically documented.[126] BAL eosinophilia in one series[126] was 28–50% and infiltrates were often patchy and bilateral, with[124,128] or without pleural effusions. The BAL fluids sometimes were eosinophilic when the transbronchial biopsies did not show eosinophilic cell infiltrates.[131,132] In one case, coccidioides was cultured from BAL fluid,[127] but only a few other associations were noted, including dusty environment,[125,126] and possible mold exposure,[125] but only rarely were medicines incriminated, such as birth control pills in one case.[126] Certainly other drugs[133] or radio-

graphic contrast material[134] can cause this (see Table 16–1). Most cases were dust- and drug exposure free.

Response is excellent to short-term steroid therapy and is usually without relapse. Acute respiratory failure has also been described in chronic eosinophilic pneumonia.[131,135,136] McEvoy[137] and others[131] have described a more subacute form, usually in asthmatics, with symptoms occurring from 4 weeks to 8 months, and these cases are sometimes included with acute but at other times chronic eosinophilic pneumonia. Some would argue that there should not be a separate entity of acute eosinophilic pneumonia other than that type described by Löffler,[138] but others state it has enough unique features, including rapid onset and severity in an apparently infectious-free setting, that it deserves some separate designation.

To complete historical review of the work of Crofton et al.,[5] in their second category, prolonged pulmonary eosinophilia, Crofton et al. included 17 cases that lasted longer than 1 month. Compared to the acute form, there was equal sex distribution, quite a variation in severity of symptoms, generally higher eosinophil count in blood, more pronounced infiltrates in the upper lobes, and greater bilaterality. Complete recovery occurred after 2–6 months. A personal or family history of allergy was present in 7 of 17 (41%). An additional 78 cases were summarized by these authors in their category of "pulmonary eosinophilia with

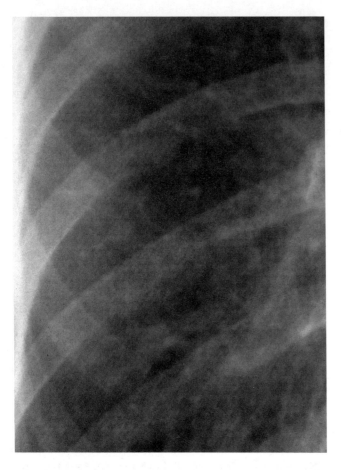

Fig. 16–11. Tropical eosinophilia. Closeup of chest radiograph highlights delicate fine nodular infiltrate in 22-year-old merchant seaman who recently returned from the Orient with high peripheral eosinophilia and positive antifilarial antibody test.

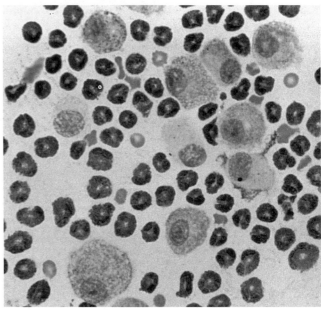

Fig. 16–12. Tropical eosinophilia. Same patient as Fig. 16–11, with abundant eosinophils. Note eosinophilic granules in alveolar macrophages.

asthma." This subdivision is no longer valid, because many of these diseases have an associated asthma that does not distinguish them from those same diseases without asthma.

Another category given by Crofton[5] covers pulmonary infiltrates and blood eosinophilia occurring with polyarteritis nodosa. Currently very few cases of classical polyarteritis nodosa have pulmonary involvement, let alone eosinophilia. Many of these cases and most of those so reported by Rose and Spencer[139] may indeed represent aspects of hypereosinophilic syndromes (see following and Chapter 30).

Crofton's other category of tropical eosinophilia requires a brief discussion. This was named by Weingarten[140] in 1943 from his studies in India, and should be considered a special variant of eosinophilic pneumonia in which tropical parasites, particularly filaria, play a role. These patients show a radiographic appearance of disseminated, 1- to 5-mm, finely nodular infiltrates in

the lung, increasing near the hilar regions and in the bases of the lungs (Fig. 16–11). Most cases occur from Pakistan to Southeast Asia; BAL specimens may be outstanding (Fig. 16–12).

Microfilariae were suspected in the original series by Weingarten[140] but could not be confirmed until a later date. Serial sections have documented filaria in the granulomatous areas.[141,142] Filaria are infrequent in the blood.[141] *Wuchereria bancrofti* and *Brugia malayi* are the species most often causing this syndrome[143,144] (see Chapter 15). Donahue,[145] on the basis of his extensive experience in the West Indies, included a positive filarial complement fixation test, a good clinical response to diethylcarbamazine, recent residence in the tropics, and pulmonary infiltrates with blood eosinophilia to fulfill his criteria of this disease. Although eosinophils and their breakdown products, such as major basic protein, may directly injure lung parenchyma, pulmonary toxicity in tropical eosinophilia may further be complicated by breakdown products of filaria and high antifilarial antibodies, the latter appear to localize to lung tissue.[146] Additional reviews are available.[147–149] Other parasites may play a role in tropical eosinophilia.[4] Multiple parasitic bowel infections often occur in the tropics and even in refugees in unlikely climates such as the northwest United States.[150] As in other eosinophilic lung disease, bronchoalveolar lavage specimens are also helpful[151] in diagnosis and following course treatment response.

Chronic Eosinophilic Pneumonia

Although Crofton et al.[5] used the term prolonged pulmonary eosinophilia, the term chronic eosinophilic pneumonia was first used by Carrington et al.[152] in 1969 to describe nine patients, all women, usually middle-aged housewives, who had a chronic and ultimately life-threatening illness with high fever, night sweats, weight loss averaging 10 kg, moderate cough, and severe dyspnea. Asthma occurred for the first time in six of these nine concurrent with or only several months before pulmonary infiltrates. Blood eosinophilia was present in four of these six, often as much as 50% or more at some time. The other three had no evidence of asthma or blood eosinophilia. No family history of similar illnesses was obtained. Four patients did have histories of allergic rhinitis. These severe constitutional symptoms with concurrent pulmonary infiltrates, frequently in the upper lobes, suggested tuberculosis. Despite negative skin tests and cultures, several patients were treated for tuberculosis. The patient in Case 1 of this series was so treated twice, much to her detriment, as her symptoms were greatly aggravated by such therapies both times this occurred. Steroid therapy led to dramatic responses in all these patients. By 4 days of steroid therapy, all symptoms were gone and the chest radiographs had begun to show clearing, which was complete by 5 weeks.

These preliminary findings have been reviewed more recently and more extensively by Jederlinc et al.[153] These authors contributed 19 new cases and surveyed published cases of chronic eosinophilic pneumonia and found twice as many women as men involved, the peak incidence was 30–39 years, with 82% being older than 30 years of age. Preexisting atopia, usually asthma, was present in one half and cough (90%), fever (87%), dyspnea (57%), and weight loss (57%) were the most frequent symptoms. Some 63% had elevated white counts and 88% had elevated eosinophil counts, with a mean value of 26%. Elevated ESR was noted in 94%. A clinical diagnosis was made in only 33%, a figure obtained mostly before BAL evaluation.

Prolonged steroid therapy is frequently required in chronic eosinophilic pneumonia. Some patients in Carrington's series required 1–3 years, and even more, of steroid therapy before being able to stop medication without recurrence.[152] A long-term follow-up study in 8 cases, 3 in men, screened from 150 cases with pulmonary infiltration and blood eosinophilia by Pearson and Rosenow,[154] showed 5 were able to discontinue steroid therapy only after an average of 4 years. One required no therapy but the other 2 were still continuing therapy for 5.5 and 8 years, respectively. Five of these had allergic reactions to penicillin and/or tetracycline, which

may have indicated a tendency toward allergic tissue reactions. Two had bilateral nasal polyps. Some 76% of Jederlinc's survey[153] required prolonged steroid therapy with 58% of these having recurrences after steroids were discontinued and an additional 21% having relapses during tapering of steroids.

The chest radiograph in patients with chronic eosinophilia pneumonia has a typical appearance, as originally suggested by Hennell and Sussman[155] in 1945. Usually the infiltrates are ground glass in density, peripheral, usually apical to axillary but occasionally lower lobe in location, and often bilateral (Fig. 16–13). Thin-walled cysts are occasionally seen. Pleural effusion is rare. Although present in less than half the cases in the literature,[153] this peripheral ground-glass radiographic appearance has a high correlative value with typical biopsy or clinical syndrome of eosinophilic pneumonia. As an additive procedure, CAT scans have been recommended (Fig. 16–13C)[152a] and may show this distribution even when routine radiographs are not so involved.[156,157] Gaensler and Carrington[158] referred to this radiographic appearance as the photographic negative of the perihilar or bat-wing appearance of acute pulmonary edema (Fig. 29-1) or alveolar proteinosis (Fig. 22–48). Crofton et al.[5] referred to this as "clouds of smoke rising after an explosion in the region of the hilum and drifting up against the chest wall peripherally" (Fig. 16–13A). Rapid radiographic clearing with steroid administration is typical (Fig. 16–13B). In Gaensler and Carrington's series,[158] clearing began in 3 days and in two-thirds of patients was complete by 10 days of therapy. This typical peripheral distribution has remained unexplained, but is perhaps related to the mast cell distribution in the lung.[143,159] The rapid clearing is attributed to the high inflammatory cell component and low destructive and organizing components, as is noted below. Barter et al.[160] have described five patients with histological evidence of bronchiolitis obliterans organizing pneumonia (BOOP; see Chapters 4 and 5) with similar peripheral densities. Two of these five patients may represent resolving chronic eosinophilic pneumonia. Incidentally, a BOOP pattern was identified histologically in 26% of Jederlinc's review.[153] Sarcoidosis may also be present with similar peripheral infiltrates.[161] At times eosinophilic pneumonia is confirmed by biopsy or BAL when chest radiographs are normal.[162,163]

The combination of blood eosinophilia present in 67%–75%, sputum eosinophilia in slightly less than 50%, BAL eosinophilia in a high percentage,[164–169] typical radiographic findings when present, CT scans, and rapid response to steroid therapy of the clinical and then the radiographic findings helps to establish this diagnosis clinically. Consequently, biopsies are no

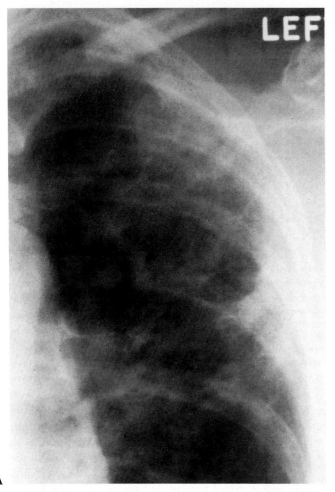

A

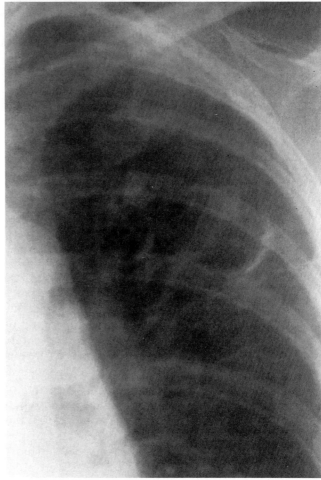

B

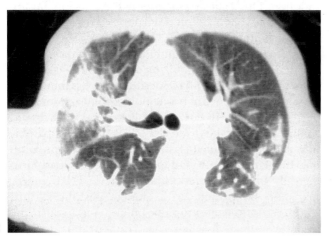

C

Fig. 16–13 A–C. Eosinophilic pneumonia (**A** and **B** plain films). **A.** Radiograph of 53-year-old housewife admitted with asthma and peripheral eosinophilia. Transbronchial biopsy confirmed charges of eosinophilic pneumonia. Note peripheral ground-glass densities. **B.** Patient after 3 days of steroid therapy. Infiltrate is significantly reduced. Radiograph 7 days later was clear. **C.** CT scan shows patchy, bilateral pneumonitis that is predominantly peripheral. (**C.** Reprinted with permission of W.B. Saunders from Radiol Clin North Am 1991; 29:1065–1084.[152a])

longer routinely done for diagnosis and are usually obtained only in atypical cases.[153]

Identified etiologies are best divided into four groups as outlined in Table 16–1. Additional etiologies are sure to continue to be added to this list.

Pathology of Acute and Chronic Eosinophilic Pneumonia

The pathology of eosinophilic pneumonia has been well defined. The original description dates to von Meyenberg in 1942.[120] A more recent case of Löffler's syn-

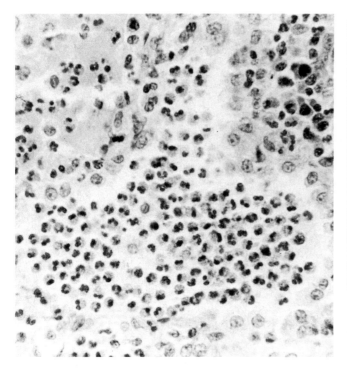

Fig. 16–14. Eosinophilic pneumonia with bilobed eosinophils and protein-rich fluid in alveoli. Note clump of interstitial plasma cells (upper right). Reactive alveolar type II cells are present lining central alveolus. H and E, ×400.

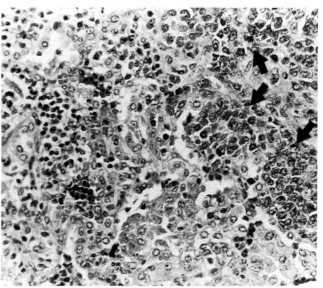

Fig. 16–15. Eosinophilic leukocytes, which are often difficult to appreciate in black and white, are present in left-middle edge. Plump macrophages rich in ingested fine eosinophilic granules are present in right-upper half (*arrows*). H and E, ×500.

drome has been studied by Bedrossian et al.[170] using electron microscopy. The pathology of the more chronic form is best summarized by Liebow and Carrington,[117] Carrington et al.,[152] and more recently Jederlinc et al.[153]

In gross appearance the involved lung tissue is airless, rubbery, and red-brown. Microscopically, the ground-glass radiographic appearance and gross appearances are attributed to flooding of air spaces by abundant eosinophils and macrophages. In half the cases there is an accompanying eosinophilic proteinaceous exudate (Fig. 16–14). Alveolar type II cells are focally hyperplastic. The interstitium is slightly to moderately broadened by an increased number of mixed inflammatory cells rich in eosinophils. Focal collections of small and medium plasma cells and lymphocytes are commonly located in the interstitum. Rarely germinal centers are present. Mild vasculitis may be observed in small veins, but is never prevalent. This may be incidental to the large number of inflammatory cells migrating across the vessel walls, yet at times small foci of vasculitis are observed apart from the most active areas.

Abundant plump phagocytic mononuclear cells in the alveoli are often more eosinophilic than usual. High-power observation of these cells shows their cytoplasm to be filled with fine eosinophilic granules com-

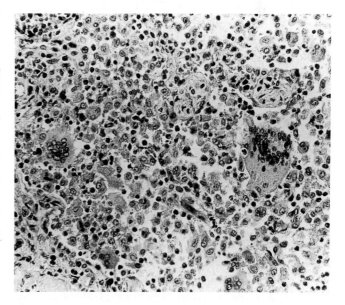

Fig. 16–16. Multinucleate giant cells are sometimes seen, usually among abundant macrophages. H and E, ×400.

ing from the nearby eosinophilic leukocytes (Figs. 16–12 and 16–15). This phagocytic action has been observed by electron microscopy by Kanner and Hammar.[171] Frequently small multinuclear cells derived from the macrophages are admixed with the mononuclear variety (Fig. 16–16). These may have an eosinophilic cytoplasm similar to that of mononuclear phago-

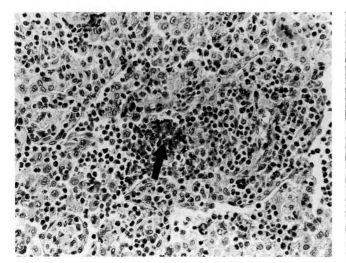

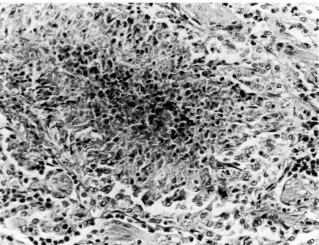

Fig. 16–17. Beginning focal degeneration of eosinophils has been called an eosinophilic abscess (*arrow*). H and E, ×400.

Fig. 16–18. Focal intraalveolar necrosis with rim of plump histiocytes represent an almost necrotizing granuloma appearance. H and E, ×400. (Courtesy of A.A. Liebow Pulmonary Pathology Collection, San Diego.)

cytes. At times, small crystals can be seen in the cytoplasms of these multinucleated cells, and these probably are precursors of Charcot–Leyden crystals.[116,152,171] However, the larger Charcot-Leyden crystals are not seen in alveoli as commonly as they are in the inspissated mucus in bronchial lumina in asthma, mucoid impaction, bronchocentric granulomatosis, or allergic bronchopulmonary aspergillosis.

Clumps of eosinophilic cells in alveoli are occasionally seen undergoing necrosis (Fig. 16–17). In the center of these areas of necrosis is degenerating basophilic debris, possibly from karyorrhectic nuclei. These have been termed eosinophilic abscesses by Liebow and Carrington.[116] About half these areas of necrosis are surrounded by a rim of plump to perpendicularly oriented and elongated epithelioid histiocytes that represent a granulomatous response (Fig. 16–18). Occasionally, small sarcoid-like granulomas are present that are not associated with areas of necrosis.

Despite the often-dense alveolar exudate, the background lung architecture is usually preserved; transeptal necrosis is uncommon. This intact architecture may be hard to recognize because of the packing of alveoli with inflammatory cells and the cellular expansion of the interstitium. Focal organization is seen microscopically in about 50% of cases, but is not very extensive. Similar small organizing fibroblastic polyps of inflammatory exudate, or bronchiolitis obliterans, are present in nearby bronchioles in some patients. The separate term "eosinophilic bronchitis" is used for eosinophilic leukocyte infiltrates in bronchial walls. The pleura·may be infiltrated by eosinophils, lymphocytes,

and plasma cells, but it is unusual to have pleural effusion or fibrinous pleuritis. Eosinophilic bronchitis is often, but not always, associated with eosinophilic pneumonia.

In summarizing the world's literature in which detailed histological description was available up to 1988, Jederlinic et al.[153] found bronchiolitis obliterans in 26%, organizing pneumonia without bronchiolitis in an additional 8%, eosinophilic microabsesses in 16%, focal intraalveolar necrosis in 18%, sarcoid-like granulomas in 13%, and Charcot–Leyden crystals in 7%.

As treatment is with steroids, it is important not to miss an infection (again see Table 16–1). Several such more recent examples with catastrophic consequences have been coccidiodomycosis[129,172] and atypical mycobacteria.[173]

The differential diagnosis of eosinophilic pneumonia includes tuberculosis, desquamative interstitial pneumonia, and pulmonary histiocytosis X (eosinophilic granuloma). The clinical setting of upper-lobe densities, fever, night sweats, and weight loss may suggest tuberculosis to the clinician. Rarely does tuberculosis present with blood or sputum eosinophilia. Histologically, necrotizing bronchial and granulomatous tuberculosis inflammatory patterns with little tissue eosinophilia help distinguish this disease. The occasional sacroid granuloma in eosinophilic pneumonia should not cause confusion.

Desquamative interstitial pneumonia may be confusing because some cases of eosinophilic pneumonia have mostly macrophages and only rare eosinophils. As at least some cases of desquamative interstitial pneumonia are caused by a hypersensitivity mechanism (see Chapter 22), this overlap in histologic appearance is understandable. In some cases it may be impossible to put a label on a histologic pattern, and it is best to describe this overlap of patterns in the pathology report. As both diseases are treated with steroids, usually with complete resolution, such a descriptive diagnosis should not change the therapy or course.

Pulmonary histiocytosis X (PHX or eosinophilic granuloma) is typically composed of varying numbers of histiocytes of the Langerhans type, with delicately convoluted nuclei, violaceous finely vacuolated cytoplasm, and a variable number of eosinophils (see Chapter 17). The number of eosinophils is usually not as great in pulmonary histiocytosis X as in eosinophilic pneumonia, but overlap does occur. Other macrophages with finely dispersed grey-tan to coarsely granular yellow, lightly iron-stained lipochrome inclusions are frequent in pulmonary histiocytosis X and not in eosinophilic pneumonia. Maturing pulmonary histiocytosis X lesions form small discrete interstitial stellate nodules in contrast to the more diffuse infiltrates of eosinophilic pneumonia. Some confusion may occur with the more acute diffuse forms of pulmonary histiocytosis X (again, see Chapter 17). Confusion may also occur with the small eosinophilic abscess or granuloma appearance of tropical eosinophilia. Langerhans cell identification can usually be suggested on hemotoxylin and eosin-stained (H and E) sections, but is easily confirmed with S100 antigen by immunoperoxidase techniques or by finding the characteristic granules by electron microscopy.

Pulmonary eosinophilia has recently been described in L-tryptophan induced eosinophilic myalgia syndrome.[174–176] The pathology here is more of an eosinophilic small vessel vasculitis and a lymphocytic interstitial pneumonia picture than eosinophilic pneumonia, although a mild degree of the latter disease has been reported.[175,176]

Hypereosinophilic Syndrome

Although cases of eosinophilic leukemia had been described earlier, Hardy and Anderson[177] in 1968 proposed the term hypereosinophilic syndrome for cases of idiopathic eosinophilia with blood and bone marrow eosinophilia with tissue infiltrates by relatively mature eosinophils accompanied by multisystem organ dysfunction. Although almost any organ can be involved; most commonly the cardiac, pulmonary, or nervous systems and skin lead the list.[178] Synonyms are eosinophilic leukemia,[179] idiopathic eosinophilia, Loeffler's fibroplastic endocarditis,[180,181] disseminated eosinophilic collagen vascular disease,[182] or eosinophilic collagenoses. In the lung the most common presentation is

with allergic granuloma and angiitis syndrome as described by Churg and Strauss[183] (see Chapter 30).

The largest series of such cases is from the U.S. National Institutes of Health. Criteria used for inclusion in this study of 26 cases reported in 1978 by Parillo et al.[184] included a persistent total eosinophil count of greater than 1500 cells/mm^3, lack of evidence of other known causes of eosinophilia, and evidence of organ specific involvement. After bone marrow and peripheral blood involvement, heart, skin, then lung and liver followed in frequency, with less involvement of gastrointestinal tract, lymph nodes, and kidney.[184] Of interest, 22 of 26 (85%) in this study were men. This study was expanded to 50 patients by Fauci et al.,[185] and the interested reader is referred to these studies and to the discussion of Churg-Strauss syndrome in Chapter 30. Of note, major basic protein studies are showing the toxic effects of this compound on human tissue, as discussed, and this may be the major mediator of tissue damage in this syndrome, as in eosinophilic syndromes with identifiable causes.[84,186] Some intriguing work on identifying major basic protein associated with a multisystem fibrosis, including that in the lung, is available.[187] Charcot–Leyden crystals have been identified in the circulatory system of one patient with hypereosinophilia syndrome.[79]

Allergic Bronchopulmonary Aspergillosis, Mucoid Impaction, and Bronchocentric Granulomatosis

The discussion of mucoid impaction (MI) and bronchocentric granulomatosis (BCG) that follows interrelates these entities with allergic bronchopulmonary aspergillosis (ABPA), as aspergillus is the most common antigen identified in each. When aspergillus is identified in mucoid impaction and bronchocentric granulomatosis, these entities may be considered aspects of allergic bronchopulmonary aspergillosis. Especially in Great Britain, where there is a high incidence of *Aspergillus,* mucoid impaction and bronchocentric granulomatosis are often thought to be solely components of allergic bronchopulmonary aspergillosis. In other countries, however, many cases of mucoid impaction and bronchocentric granulomatosis do not have proven aspergillus hypersensitivity and so are discussed as individual diseases or at least as common tissue reactions. Even in Great Britain, not all cases have proven aspergillus association (see following). Asthma is frequent in all these entities, and in representative series in the United States it occurs in some 80% of cases of mucoid impaction[188] and 43% of cases of bronchocen-

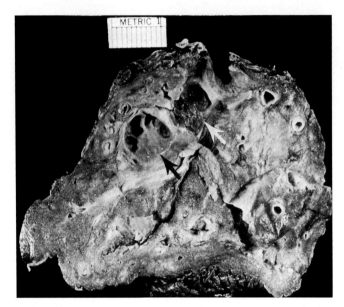

Fig. 16–19. Two areas of mucoid impaction (*arrows*). In one (*black arrow*), the plug is removed leaving a bronchiectatio-cystic-appearing cavity. (Courtesy of A.A. Liebow Pulmonary Pathology Collection, San Diego, California.)

tric granulomatosis.[189] Blood and tissue eosinophilia are present in slightly over one-half of the cases in each of these diseases in the United States. In Great Britain in cases with pulmonary eosinophilia (defined as transient radiographic lung shadows and raised blood eosino-philia), asthma is present in 97% associated with and 81% unassociated with ABPA.[190]

Mucoid Impaction

This entity was defined by Shaw[191] in 1951 in 10 cases from Texas. An expanded series of 87 cases was pub-lished in 1967 by Urschel et al..[188] The following statis-tics are based on these descriptions.

Second- to fourth-order bronchi are greatly dis-tended by tenacious, inspissated, grey to green-yellow or rusty brown mucus (Fig. 16–19). These impacted masses are round, oval or elongated, and rubbery, and vary in size up to 2.5 cm in diameter and 6 cm in length (Fig. 16–20). They are generally larger in mucoid im-paction that is non-ABPA than in those with ABPA, but there is some overlap. Others have described these as putty like or ropey and focally brown (Fig. 16–21). Fragments of these masses are coughed up by 29% of patients. They may be removed by bronchoscopy. The distended and scarred bronchus or bronchi often re-main as cystic or saccular bronchiectasis (see Fig. 16–19). Such areas of bronchiectasis are multiple in 22% of cases, and favor the upper lobe in about two-thirds of solitary cases. Because of this upper-lobe preference

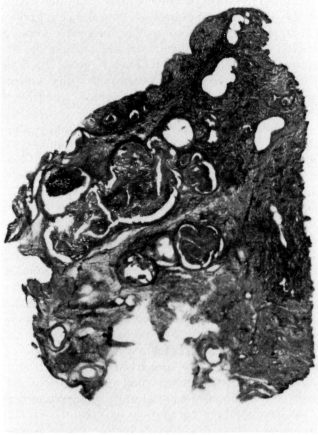

Fig. 16–20. Gough section of mucoid impaction showing cross section of "ropey" or tubular large proximal masses of mucus. Periodic acid–Schiff.

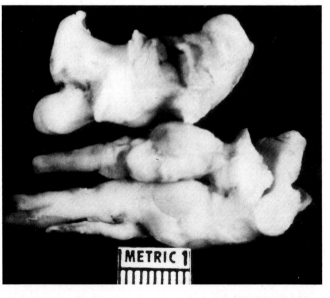

Fig. 16–21. Expectorated plugs from mucoid impaction. Scale marks are millimeters. (Courtesy of A.A. Liebow Pulmo-nary Pathology Collection, San Diego, California. Reprinted with permission of Am Rev Respir Dis 1975;111:497–537.)

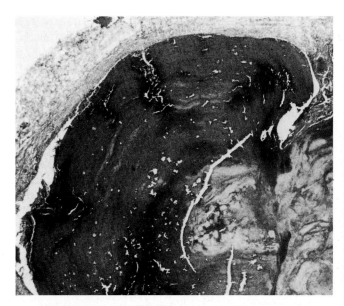

Fig. 16–22. Whorled impacted mucus in distended bronchus. Periodic acid-Schiff, ×25. (Courtesy of A.A. Liebow Pulmonary Pathology Collection, San Diego, California.)

and the focal cysts, tuberculosis was considered a likely diagnosis in the earlier cases. Cancer was also considered because of this mass effect, and their proximity to hilar nodes may suggest these nodes are involved with metastases.

Microscopically, the casts contain laminated material that stains brightly with mucin stains, especially periodic acid–Schiff (Fig. 16–22). A variable number of degenerating inflammatory cells and other entrapped debris are seen. Jelihovsky[62] detailed an arrangement of clumps of degenerating, somewhat basophilic-appearing eosinophils, inter-weaving with mucous lamellae, giving a "fir-tree" appearance as these areas are narrow centrally and more broad based peripherally. The bronchial wall is thin, as are the submucosal gland mass and surrounding cartilage. Lining cells may be ulcerated, stretched thin, or show focal basal cell hyperplasia or squamous or transitional metaplasia. Eosinophils are present in the bronchial walls in more than 50% of cases, and distal eosinophilic infiltrates in lung parenchyma may be seen in one-third of cases. Peripheral obstructive changes are common, and distal abscesses are seen in one-third of cases.

Physical removal of the masses, with possible addition of some mucolytic agents, is recommended therapy. Steroids are not effective in treating this disease. Postobstructive damage may cause permanent scarring requiring surgical excision.

Many of these cases reported in the United States in the foregoing series did not have proven etiologies. In 1952 in Great Britain, 1 year after Shaw's original

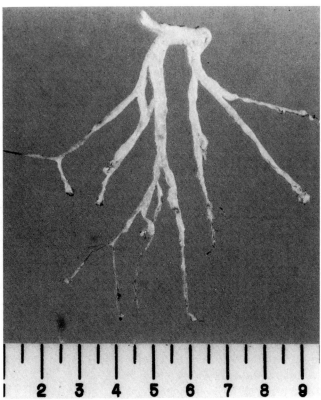

Fig. 16–23. Mucoid cast ("plastic bronchitis") extracted at bronchoscopy. Scant *Aspergillus* was identified in the case. Scale is in centimeters.

description,[191] Hinson et al.[192] described eight patients with assorted lung involvement with aspergillus fungus in which one had invasive infection as an infarct, and three had mycetomas; one had minor and three had major elements of mucoid impaction. Aspergillus was identified as small isolated fragments of hyphae in the inspissated mucoprotein substance.

Fibrinous or Plastic Bronchitis

As noted, patients dying of status asthmaticus often have thick tenacious plugs on the cut surface of their lungs at autopsy (see Figs. 16–2 and 16–3). These plugs represent casts of the bronchial system that may extend from the second- to the seventh-order bronchi[166] and as such may be expectorated and display an elaborate cast like pattern (Fig. 16–23). These plugs, or casts are smaller in diameter and softer than the larger ones of typical mucoid impaction, the casts of which are generally shorter but bigger and firmer. Occasionally these casts display dilated proximal areas representing bronchiectatic dilatations.[193] These may be seen in asthma, distal to or associated with mucoid impaction or bronchocentric granulomatosis,[194] cystic fibrosis, bronchiectasis, acute or chronic bronchitis, and possibly tuberculosis, at least in the past. As summarized by Sulavik,[193] this condition has been given the colorful names of fibrinous bronchitis,[195,196] plastic bronchitis,[194,197–200] croupous bronchitis or bronchitis croup,[201] pseudomembranous bronchitis,[195] and, in the 1920s, bronchial polyps.[197] Bettmann, in a thorough review in 1902 of the earlier literature,[195] credited Galen (A.D. 131–200) with the first description of these. The role of allergy is important in many cases but not all.[172,200] Many are part of the asthma, bronchocentric granulomatosis, mucoid impaction, and allergic bronchopulmonary fungosis portion of this chapter. Such casts or plugs do not occur in eosinophilic pneumonia alone. Eosinophils, their breakdown products of eosinophilic granular masses, Charcot–Leyden crystals, and major basic protein are evident in many associated with asthma. Fungus particles should always be searched for and cultures considered, along with possibly suggesting aspergillus serum studies. Many of the cases described as fibrinous or plastic bronchitis before 1970 probably represent a part of the allergic bronchopulmonary aspergillosis syndrome when better evaluated today.

Bronchocentric Granulomatosis

Bronchocentric granulomatosis was originally defined by Liebow[202] in 1973, and this description was expanded by Katzenstein et al.[189] in 1975. Another large series came from the United States Armed Forces Institute of Pathology by Koss et al.[203] Earlier descriptions of this type of bronchial granulomatous reaction in an allergic setting have been noted.[204,205] Other series by Saldana[206] and Lee et al.[207] are available in abstract form only (See also Chapter 30.)

This disease is confined to the lungs, specifically the bronchi, and is named for granulatomous and necrotizing replacement of bronchial mucous membrane lining. The surrounding lung parenchyma is rarely normal, as it usually has chronic inflammation and/or obstructive changes, although it does not usually exhibit granulomatous inflammation. This latter point is important in the differential diagnosis. This pattern is best considered as a tissue reaction, and is classified as a disease when all other entities in the differential diagnosis have been excluded. These entities include aspiration, chronic obstruction, invasive fungal and acid-fast infections, and, rarely, parasitic diseases, Wegener's granulomatosis, and necrotizing rheumatoid or ankylosing spondylitis lung diseases. Extrabronchial tissue reactions associated with these other diseases often help eliminate them from the differential diagnosis.

Histoplasma, blastomyces, and mycobacteria, including both *Mycobacterium tuberculosis* and *Mycobacterium avium-intracellulare*, have been shown as giving this appearance.[208] Other fungi associated with this reaction pattern[209–213] have been summarized in Table 30–9 and include *Aspergillus oryzae, Aspergillus ochaceus, Curvularia, Bipolaris, Geotrichum, Stemphylium, Penicillium,* and Candida species along with *Dreschleriosis. Helminosporium* has been added by some,[211,212] but doubt has been cast on the accuracy of fungal identification in these reports by others.[213] Because of the assorted fungal pathogens so far described, Tazelaar et al.[214] have referred to this disease pattern as bronchocentric mycosis and others as bronchocentric fungoses. In a study of solitary necrotizing granulomata of lung by Ulbright and Katzenstein,[215] granulomatous destruction of bronchioles was found in 27% of such infections caused by acid-fast bacilli and 8% from *Histoplasma capsulatum.* When those with parenchymal granulomata were eliminated, this incidence was much less. Noninvasive or minimally invasive, nonallergic aspergillus can also have this appearance.[216,217] One case of echinoccocal cysts in the lung was noted to have a similar reaction.[218] It is suspected that amoeba may give a similar appearance in its transbronchial spread.

After eliminating other possible causes, the diagnosis appears strongest in the background of asthma and eosinophilic infiltrates and, where present, mucoid impaction. Both large series mentioned above[189,203] divided patients into two groups; the first have eosinophilic infiltrates and often asthma, and the second group is much more varied and does not have these findings (see Table 16–2 and Table 30–10). One must search carefully for more typical invasive organisms.[208] When this disease does occur in a typical setting, it represents a hypersensitivity reaction to fragments of noninvasive aspergillus and so is part of the spectrum of allergic bronchopulmonary aspergillosis.

As in other hypersensitivity reactions, removal of the antigen is preferred, but as this is difficult or impossible in this entity, steroid administration is the treatment of choice. Several cases are known to this author and others[208] in which mycobacteria and invasive fungi made their presence known only after steroid therapy. Several anecdotal cases are also known in which invasive aspergillosis has developed in just this setting. Steroid therapy must be used with great caution and only after all the above criteria have been fulfilled and other diseases, particularly the infectious ones, have been eliminated to the best of one's ability.

Grossly, many sites of cheesy replacement of bronchi and larger bronchioles are present (Fig. 16–24). Microscopically, the multiple granulomas seen on a section may represent continuous replacement of adjacent bronchioles involved in continuity but cut in cross sec-

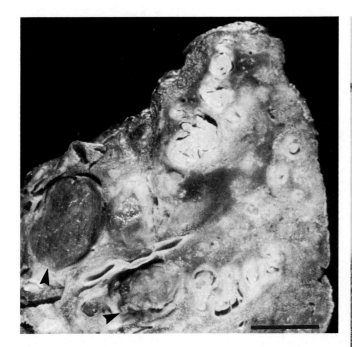

Fig. 16–24. Lung with two areas of proximal mucoid impaction (arrows) and "cheesy" replacement of more distal conducting airways, typical of gross appearance of bronchocentric granulomatosis. Bar = 1 cm. (Original contributors: TH Roberts and JD Mullins, Texas. Courtesy of A.A. Liebow Pulmonary Pathology Collection, San Diego, California. Reprinted with permission of Am Rev Respir Dis 1975;111:497–537.)

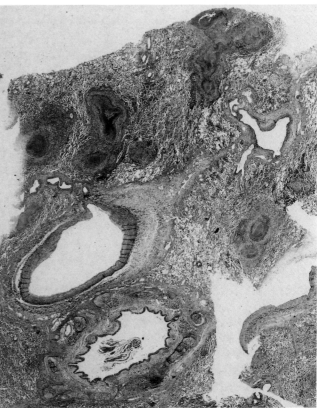

Fig. 16–25. Lung section at low power shows multifocal areas of necrosis (top and right), which correlate with gross appearance in Fig. 16–24. This case is also represented in Figs. 16–28 and 16–33. H and E, ×20. (Case used courtesy of J.C. Roberts, Jr., Torrance, California.)

tion (Figs. 16–25 and 16–26). The bronchial lumens are often filled with debris, and the bronchial walls are replaced by granulomatous inflammation or varying degrees of more mundane types of inflammation (Fig. 16–27). The granulomatous and/or necrotic replacement of bronchi appears as multiple random granulomas until one notes that these granulomas are in the location one would expect bronchi, specifically next to pulmonary arteries (Figs. 16–26 and 16–27). Elastic stains help define the internal and external elastica of the pulmonary arteries, and often remnants of the single elastic membrane of the bronchial walls are still identified around the areas of inflammation (Figs. 16–28 and 16–29). The adjacent pulmonary artery may have focal vascular involvement, but only on the side of the involved bronchus or bronchiole (Figs. 16–28 and 16–29). This is incidental to the bronchocentric destruction. Once the bronchocentric nature of this necrotizing process is identified, the differential diagnosis becomes more limited than the entire spectrum of granulomatous inflammation and includes the items already mentioned in this section.

The bronchial wall may show a sharp transition to granulomatous replacement (Fig. 16–30). In those cases with tissue eosinophilia, not only Charcot–Leyden crys-

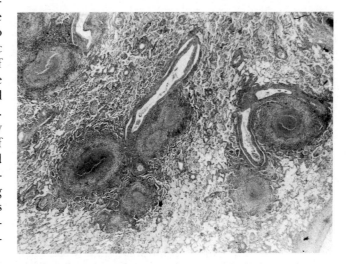

Fig. 16–26. Multiple necrotic areas appear random, but note that there are no intact bronchioles next to three segments of pulmonary arteries shown in this field. H and E, ×100.

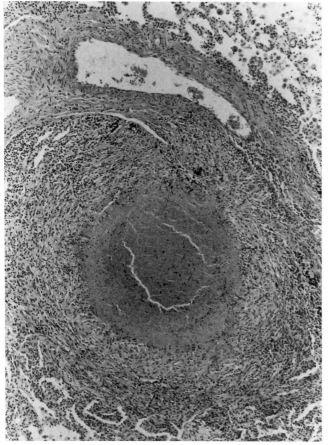

Fig. 16–27. Higher power view of involved area on right of Fig. 16–26 shows bronchiole whose lumen is filled with debris; inner wall is necrotic, followed outwardly by rim of plump histiocytes. Adjacent pulmonary artery at top is focally involved. H and E, ×400.

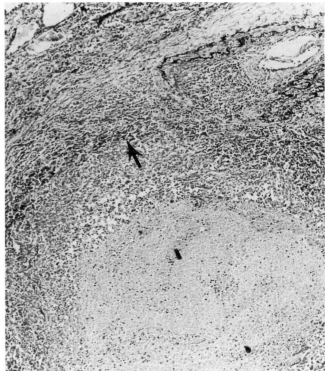

Fig. 16–28. High-power view of elastic stain. Areas of injury in pulmonary artery (note internal and external elastica) at top is toward injured bronchiole. Small amounts of remaining bronchial elastic tissue is at *arrow point*. Elastic van Gieson, ×400. (Courtesy of A.A. Liebow Pulmonary Pathology Collection, San Diego, and J.C. Roberts, Jr., Torrance, California.)

tals but also clumps of densely aggregated eosinophilic granules may be seen, which may elicit a foreign-body response (Fig. 16–31). In Katzenstein's series,[189] such aggregates were seen in 10 cases, of which 4 had a foreign-body response to them (Fig. 16–32). In those bronchi without evidence of increased eosinophils, plasma cells are dominant, and they occurred in 9 cases of 13 (69%) reported in this same series. More proximal bronchi show a dense lymphocyte and mild plasma cell infiltrate (Fig. 16–33). More distal bronchioles show chronic bronchiolitis, exudative bronchiolitis[219] (Fig. 16–34), and bronchiolitis obliterans.

When hyphae are found, they usually consist of small noninvasive fragments suggesting aspergillus (Fig. 16–35). Such patients are younger and have a higher incidence of asthma and eosinophilia than those without hyphae. (Table 16–2).[189] As noted, cases of Wegener's granulomatosis may cause bronchial injury.[220–222] Such cases may possibly account for the few cases of

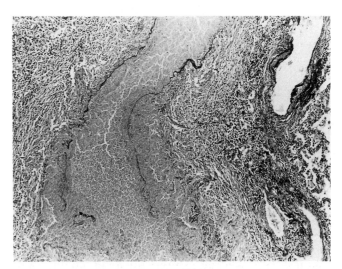

Fig. 16–29. Remaining elastica of bronchus is well outlined and is involved (in lower left field) on both of its sides by necrosis. Pulmonary artery is at right. Elastic van Gieson, ×100.

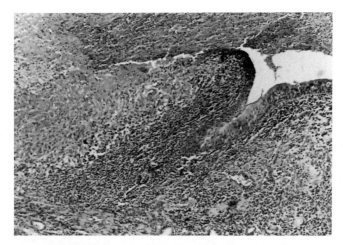

Fig. 16–30. Bronchial wall shows abrupt transition to granulomatous replacement. H and E, ×100.

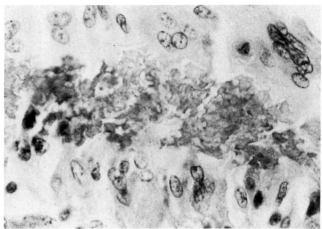

Fig. 16–32. High-power view of aggregated, almost crystalized eosinophilic granular debris with foreign body reaction. H and E, ×1,000.

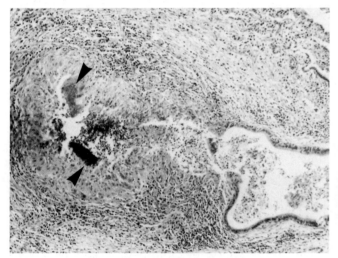

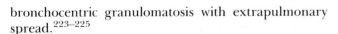

Fig. 16–31. Another bronchiole with transition to granulomatous replacement and foreign body response to eosinophilic debris (*arrows*). H and E, ×100. (Courtesy of A.A. Liebow Pulmonary Pathology Collection, San Diego, California.)

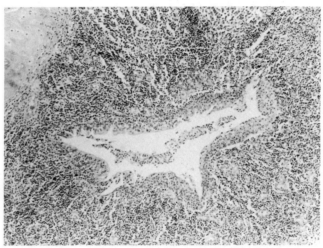

Fig. 16–33. Proximal bronchi may show intense chronic inflammation but are usually not involved with granulomatous change. H and E, ×200. (Case used courtesy of J.R. Roberts, Jr., Torrance, California.)

bronchocentric granulomatosis with extrapulmonary spread.[223–225]

Allergic Bronchopulmonary Aspergillosis

Aspergillus is notorious for its varied hypersensitivity reactions in the lung. In this chapter alone, these include all the entities discussed. As a contaminant of barley, aspergillus has caused malt worker's lung, a form of extrinsic allergic alveolitis (see Chapters 11 and 18). Invasive aspergillus and aspergilloma are discussed elsewhere (see Chapter 11). Aspergillus mold is especially prevalent in Great Britain, with higher spore counts in winter relating to increased incidence of disease in this season.[226] The spore counts in one study in the United States in Michigan showed lower counts than in Great Britain.[227] However, allergic bronchopulmonary aspergillosis (ABPA), once thought rare in the United States,[228] appears to be increasing there, perhaps because it is better recognized.[229,230]

This was first described in Great Britain in 1952 in 3 cases by Hinson et al.,[192] and the best-studied series have come from Great Britain. Henderson[231] described 32 cases in 1968, one-fourth of which had mucoid impaction. Scadding[232,233] contributed 62 cases in 1971. Also in 1971, McCarthy and Pepys[234] published a

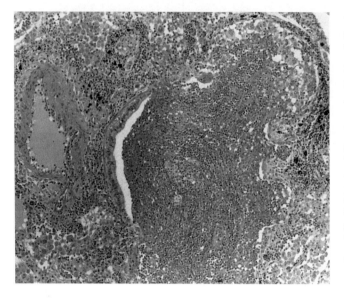

Fig. 16–34. Exudative bronchiolitis. As may be seen distal to BCG, bronchioles are distended with exudate composed of mucin, fibrin, PMNs, and eosinophils. H and E, ×100.

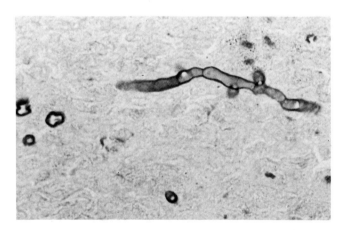

Fig. 16–35. Fragment of hyphae, which when found are in luminal contents. Septate and acute angle branching (not well shown) are typical of aspergillus. Grocott's methenamine silver (GMS), ×1,000.

Table 16–2. Bronchocentric granulomatosis[a]

	Asthmatics	Nonasthmatics
Number	10	13
Sex	7 M, 3 F	6 M, 7 F
Age	22 years (9–48)	50 years (32–76)
Asthma history	All	None
Eosinophilia	9 (6–46%)	2 (8 + 9%)
Hyphae	9	0

Modified from Katzenstein A-LA, et al. *Am Rev Respir Dis* 1975;111: 497–537, with permission.

very well studied group of 111 patients derived from a series of 143 cases of eosinophilic pulmonary infiltrates. The patients from this large series had transient pulmonary shadows, eosinophilia of blood and sputum, and immediate and delayed skin tests, and 92% had proven *Aspergillus fumigatus* precipitants in their serum samples. Ninety-six percent had asthma and 56% coughed up plugs, which often contained aspergillus hyphae, and 58% had aspergillus cultured from their sputum. The severity of asthma was unrelated to the quantity of plugs produced. Usually blood eosinophil count was greater than 1,000/mm^3. The younger patients in the series had asthma before age 10, had a higher degree of associated atopias, and on average 24 years had elapsed before allergic bronchopulmonary aspergillosis was documented after the asthma had begun, compared to 8.3 years for the age group 11–30 and 3.5 years for those older than 31. All patients had negative tests for stool ova and parasites.[234,235]

The chest radiographs from the same series were carefully described separately, and frequently showed fleeting areas of homogeneous consolidation.[236] Bronchial damage was described as delicate "tram lines," or thicker parallel lines, or tubular shadows, which were a response to infiltration, edema, and fibrosis of the walls of the breathing tubes. There were ring forms when cavities were present, and "toothpaste" and "gloved-finger" pattern when one or more bronchi were filled with material, often radiating from the hilum. Seventy-nine percent had evidence of bronchiectasis. Central or proximal saccular bronchiectasis, especially in the upper lobes, is an almost pathognomonic sign of allergic bronchopulmonary aspergillosis. More specifically, as originally described by Scadding,[237] and later confirmed by Simon,[238] the distal bronchi still retain their communications to the major area of dilatation, suggesting a local hypersensitivity that is in contrast to postinflammatory causes for bronchiectasis in which such distal connections are often destroyed. (see Bronchiectasis, Chapter 5.) These changes are all more prevalent in the upper lobes. Long-term follow-up by Safirstein et al.[239] in 50 patients showed permanent progressive damage was frequent. Fixed bronchial wall damage may account for return of fleeting parenchymal infiltrates to the same areas. The development of peripheral bronchiectasis in a patient with mucoid impaction strongly suggests bronchocentric granulomatosis may be present (Fig. 16–24). Also, blebs, bullae, and spontaneous pneumothorax may occur.[240] The findings in ABPA have been contrasted with non-ABPA eosinophile pneumonia by McCarthy and Pepys[241] and Chapman et al.[190] Occasionally, APBA is diagnosed in patients with normal chest radiographs.[242]

In the United States, Greenberger, Patterson and

co-authors[243–250] have refined criteria for diagnosing
ABPA as patients with asthma, transient pulmonary
infiltrates, blood and sputum eosinophilia, elevated
IgE, immediate skin response, with precipitating serum
antibodies and elevated IgG and IgE antibodies to
Aspergillus fumigatus antigens, along with central bronchiectasis. With the caution that most are nonspecific,
the greater the number of these findings, the more
indicative of ABPA. When all are present, this is diagnostic. These authors suggested five stages of ABPA[247]:
Stage I, Acute, when many of the findings are present,
emphasizing pulmonary infiltrates and elevated IgE,
and noting bronchiectasis may already be present in this
phase. Steroid therapy brings about significant improvement by 6 weeks.[243,251] Stage II, Remission, with
no chest infiltrates for at least 6 months. Stage III,
Exacerbation, at times with significant chest infiltrates
yet no symptoms. Stage IV, Corticosteroid-dependent
asthma.[252] Stage V, Fibrotic, with irreversible obstructive and restrictive abnormalities with fibrosis on chest
roentgenogram.[254] Not all patients have all stages or
show progression but as many as four of the five stages
may be seen in a given patient.[250] Of interest, no patient
has progressed from Stage IV to V[243] perhaps because
of intensive continuous steroid therapy required for
Stage IV. The long term role of methotrexate or other
immunosuppressives has not yet been fully evaluated in
these patients. Stage V patients usually present in this
stage.[253]

The pathology of ABPA has received some attention
in several series.[219,254] In the series by Bosken et al.,[219]
18 patients were evaluated and all showed either BCG
or MI or both, and specifically 7 had BCG, 8 had both,
and 3 MI alone. In this series then 15 of 18 (83%) had
BCG. Focal eosinophilic pneumonia was present in 13
(72%), but this was often the focal change with only one
case being more than focal. Chronic inflammation,
often with a mixture of eosinophils, was present in
bronchioles in 15 (83%) being severe in 10 (56%). In the
BCG group, 13 of 15 (87%) had a distal with a charac-
teristic-appearing exudative bronchiolitis that consisted
of bronchiolar lumens filled with necrotic neutrophils
and eosinophils in a basophilic mucinous exudate (Fig.
16–34). Noninvasive fungi were identified in 14 cases
(78%). More distal bronchiolitis obliterans and organizing pneumonia was noted in 8 (44% of total). Of
interest, despite the clinical prevalence of asthma in
ABPA only 3 (17%) had documented histologic changes
characteristic of this disease. The other series by Imbeau et al.[254] showed other secondary peripheral
changes of chronic interstitial pneumonia in half, lipoid
pneumonia in 21% and desquamative interstitial pneumonia in 14%. Bacterial pneumonia was noted in 29%
and abscess formation in 14% (and the frequency of

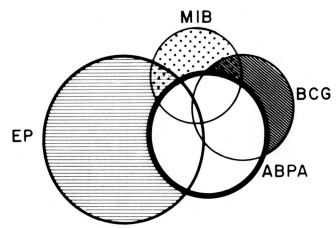

Fig. 16–36. Venn diagram of overlap and individuality of
each of eosinophilic lung diseases discussed. Abbreviations:
EP, eosinophilic pneumonia; MIB, mucoid impaction of bronchi; BCG, bronchocentric granulomatosis; ABPA, allergic
bronchopulmonary aspergillosis. (Reprinted with permission
of Am Rev Respir Dis 1975;111:497–537.)

infection has been noted by others).[233] ABPA will also
occur in the background of the cystic fibrosis, with an
incidence of 0.6%–11%.[255–259]

Overlap Syndromes

Entities of each group of eosinophilic lung diseases
discussed above may occur alone, but as already seen
may also frequently be present in combination (Fig.
16–36). For example, in Crofton's review, eosinophilic
pneumonia was 4.6 times more frequently associated
with asthma than occurred alone. Two-thirds of Carrington's original series[152] of patients with chronic
eosinophilic pneumonia had asthma of recent or concurrent onset. Preexistent asthma occurred in 80%–
96% of cases of allergic bronchopulmonary aspergillosis in Great Britain, while 80% of asthmatics in Great
Britain have precipitants to aspergillus.[233,235] Asthma
was present in 80% of those with mucoid imaction[188]
and 43% of those with bronchocentric granulomatosis[189] in the United States. Mucoid impaction occurred
in 17% of those with bronchocentric granulomatosis,[189]
and so on. ABPA (mycosis) accounts for some of the
reasons for overlap, but not all.

References

1. Beeson PB, Bass DA. The eosinophil. Vol. 14. Major
   problems in internal medicine series. Philadelphia: WB
   Saunders, 1977.
2. Nutman TB, Cohen SG, Ottesen EA. Eosinophila and
   eosinophil-related disorders. In: Middleton E, Jr., Reed

CE, Ellis EF, Adkinson NF, Yunginger JW, eds. Allergy, principles and practice. 3d ed. St. Louis: Mosby, 1988:861–890.

3. Mahmoud AAF, Austen KF. The eosinophil in health and disease. New York: Grune & Stratton, 1980.

4. Weller PF. Eosinophilia. J Allergy Clin Immunol 1984; 73:1–10.

5. Crofton JW, Livingstone JL, Oswald NC, Roberts ATM. Pulmonary eosinophilia. Thorax 1952;7:1–35.

6. Ottesen EA. Eosinophilia and the lung. In: Kirkpatrick CH, Reynolds HY, eds. Immunologic and infectious reactions in the lung. New York: Dekker, 1976:289–332.

7. Schatz M, Wasserman S, Patterson R. Eosinophils and immunologic lung disease. Med Clin North Am 1981; 65:1055–1071.

8. Ayars GH, Altman LC, Gleich G, Loegering D, Baker CB. Eosinophil and eosinophil granule-mediated pneumocytic injury. J Allergy Clin Immunol 1985;76:595–604.

9. Busse WW, Reed CE, Asthma: definition and pathogenesis. In: Middleton E, Jr., Reed CE, Ellis EF, Adkinson NF, Yunginger JW, eds. Allergy, principles and practice. 3d Ed. St. Louis: Mosby, 1988:969–998.

10. Boushey HA, Nichols J. Asthma mortality. West J Med 1987;147:314–320.

11. Strunk RC, Mrazek DA, Fuhrmann GSW, LeBresq JF. Deaths from asthma in childhood—Can they be predicted. JAMA 1985;254:1193–1196.

12. Siegel SC. History of asthma deaths from antiquity. J Allergy Clin Immunol 1987;80:458–462.

13. Nadel JA. Inflammation and asthma. J Allergy Clin Immunol 1984;73:651–653.

14. Barnes PJ. Our changing understanding of asthma. Respir Med 1989;83(suppl):17–23.

15. Thurlbeck WM, Hogg JC. Pathology of asthma. In: Middleton E, Jr., Reed CE, Ellis EF, Adkinson NF, Yunginger JW, eds. Allergy, principles and practice. 3d Ed. St. Louis: Mosby 1988;1008–1017.

16. McFadden ER, Jr. Pathogenesis of asthma. J Allergy Clin Immunol 1984;73:413–424.

17. McFadden ER, Jr. Extertional dyspnea and cough as preludes to acute attacks of bronchial asthma. N Engl J Med 1975;292:555–559.

18. Corrao WM, Braman SS, Irwin SS. Chronic cough as the sole presenting manifestation of bronchial asthma. N Engl J Med 1979;300:633–637.

19. Ishizaka T. Analysis of triggering events in mast cells for immunoglobulin E-mediated histamine release. J Allergy Clin Immunol 1981;67:90–92.

20. Ende N, Grizzanti JN, Orsi VO, Safirstein BH, Reichman L, Baturay-Smith N. Antilung antibodies in asthma. Am J Clin Pathol 1982;78:758–761.

21. Casparay FA, Feimann EL, Field EJ. Lymphocyte sensitization in asthma with special reference to the nature and identity of intrinsic form. Br Med J 1973;1:15–16.

22. Austin KF, Orange RP. Bronchial asthma; the possible role of the chemical mediators of immediate hypersensitivity in the pathogenesis of subacute chronic disease. Am Rev Respir Dis 1975;112:423–436.

23. Middleton E, Jr., Atkins FM, Fanning M. Georgitis JW. Cellular mechanisms in the pathogenesis and pathophysiology of asthma. Med Clin North Am 1981;65: 1013–1031.

24. Lee TH. The eosinophil: its role in allergic respiratory disease. Respir Med 1989;83:453–455.

25. Barnes PJ. New concepts in the pathogenesis of bronchial hyperresponsiveness and asthma. J Allergy Clin Immunol 1989;83:1013–1026.

26. Dor PJ, Ackerman SJ, Gleich GJ. Charcot–Leyden crystal protein and eosinophil granule major basic protein in sputum of patients with respiratory diseases. Am Rev Respir Dis 1984;130:1072–1077.

27. De Monchy JGR, Kauffman HF, Venge P, et al. Bronchoalveolar eosinophilia during allergen-induced late asthmatic reactions. Am Rev Respir Dis 1985;131:373–376.

28. Huber HL, Koessler KK. The pathology of asthma. Arch Intern Med 1922;30:689–760.

29. Houston JC, de Nevasquez S, Trounce JR. A clinical and pathological study of fatal cases of status asthmaticus. Thorax 1953;8:207–213.

30. Cardwell BS, Pearson RSB. Death in asthmatics. Thorax 1959;14:341–352.

31. Messer JW, Peters GA. Causes of death and pathologic findings in 304 cases of bronchial asthma. Dis Chest 1960;38:616–624.

32. Reid L. Pathological changes in asthma. In: Clark TJK, Godfrey S, eds. Asthma. London: Chapman and Hall, 1977;79–95.

33. Dunnill MS. The pathology of asthma with special reference to changes in the bronchial mucosa. J Clin Pathol 1960;13:27–33.

34. Dunnill MS, Massarella GR, Anderson JA. A comparison of the quantitative anatomy of the bronchi in normal subjects, in status asthmaticus, in chronic bronchitis and in emphysema. Thorax 1969;24:176–179.

35. Dunnill MS. The morphology of the airways in bronchial asthma. In: Stein M, ed. New directions in asthma. Park Ridge, Illinois: American College of Chest Physicians, 1975:213–221.

36. Dunnill MS. Pathology of asthma. In: Middleton E, Jr., Reed CE, Ellis EF, eds. Allergy: Principles and practice. St Louis: Mosby, 1978:678–686.

37. Dunnill MS. Pulmonary pathology. Edinburgh: Churchill-Livingtone, 1987:61–79.

38. Sobonya RE. Concise clinical study. Quantitative structural alterations in long-standing allergic asthma. Am Rev Respir Dis 1984;130:289–292.

39. Glynn AA, Michaels L. Bronchial biopsy in chronic bronchitis and asthma. Thorax 1960;23:142–153.

40. Salvato G. Some histologic changes in chronic bronchitis and asthma. Thorax 1968;23:168–172.

41. Callerame ML, Condemi JJ, Ishizaka K, Johannsson SGO, Vaughn JH. Immunoglobulins in bronchial tissue from patients with asthma, with special reference to immunoglobulin E. J Allergy 1971;47:187–197.

42. Laitinen LA, Heino M, Laitenen A, Haahtela T. Damage to the airway epithelium and bronchial reactivity in

patients with asthma. Am Rev Respir Dis 1985;131:599–606.

43. Sanerkin NG, Evans DMD. The sputum in bronchial asthma: pathopneumonic patterns. J Pathol 1965;89:535–541.

44. Kleinerman J, Adelson L. A study of asthma deaths in a coroner's population. J Allergy Clin Immunol 1987;80(3 Pt. 2):406–408.

45. Reid LM. The presence or absence of bronchial mucus in fatal asthma. J Allergy Clin Immunol 1987;80(3 Pt. 2):415–416.

46. Gough J. Correlation of radiological and pathological changes in some diseases of the lung. Lancet 1955;i:161–162.

47. Bohrod M. Pathologic manifestations of allergic and related mechanisms in diseases of the lungs. Int Arch Allergy Appl Immunol 1958;13:39–60.

48. Richardson JB. Airways smooth muscle. J Allergy Clin Immunol 1987;80(3 Pt. 2):409–411.

49. Hogg JC. Varieties of airway narrowing in severe and fatal asthma. J Allergy Clin Immunol 1987;80(3 Pt. 2):417–419.

50. Callerame ML, Condemi JJ, Bohrod MG, Vaughan JH. Immunologic reactions of bronchial tissue in asthma. N Engl J Med 1971;284:459–464.

51. Callerame ML, Condemi JJ, Ishizaka K, Johansson SGO, Vaughan JH. Immunoglobulins in bronchial tissues from patients with asthma, with special reference to immunoglobulin E. J Allergy 1971;47:187–197.

52. McCarter JH Vazquez JJ. The bronchial basement membrane in asthma. Arch Pathol Lab Med 1966;82:328–335.

53. Earle BV. Fatal bronchial asthma: Series of 15 cases with review of literature. Thorax 1953;8:195–206.

54. Reid L. Measurement of the bronchial mucous gland layer: A diagnostic yardstick in chronic bronchitis. Thorax 1960;15:132–141.

55. Leopold JG. A contrast of bronchitis and asthma. In: Symposium on the nature of asthma, King Edward VII Hospital, Midhurst, 1964:30–38.

56. Takizawa T, Thurlbeck WM. A comparative study of four methods of assessing the morphologic changes in chronic bronchitis. Am Rev Respir Dis 1971;103:774–783.

57. Takizawa T, Thurlbeck WM. Muscle and mucous gland size in the major bronchi of patients with chronic bronchitis, asthma and asthmatic bronchitis. Am Rev Respir Dis 1971;104:331–336.

58. Barton Ad, Lourenco RV. Bronchial secretions and mucociliary clearance. Arch Intern Med 1973;131:140–144.

59. Burgi H. Fibre systems in sputum. Bull Physiopathol Respir 1973;9:191–196.

60. Hulbert WC, Walker DC, Jackson A, Hogg JC. Airway permeability to horseradish peroxidase in guinea pigs. The repair phase after injury by cigarette smoke. Am Rev Respir Dis 1981;123:320–326.

61. Sanerkin NG, Evan DMD. The sputum in bronchial asthma: pathognomic patterns. J Pathol Bacteriol 1965;89:535–541.

62. Jelihovsky T. The structure of bronchial plugs in mucoid impaction, bronchocentric granulomatosis and asthma. Histopathology 1983;7:153–167.

63. Cluroe A, Beasley R, Holloway L. Bronchial diverticulitis: Complications of bronchial asthma. J Clin Pathol 1988;41:921–922.

64. Cluroe A, Holloway L, Thompson K, Purdie G, Beasley R. Bronchial gland duct ectasia in fatal bronchial asthma: Association with interstitial emphysema. J Clin Pathol 1989;42:1026–1031.

65. Mönckeberg JG. Zur Pathologischen Anatomie des Bronchialasthmas. Verh Dtsch Ges Pathol 1909;14:173–180.

66. Macdonald IG. The local and constitutional pathology and bronchial asthma. Ann Intern Med 1933;6:253–277.

67. Lamson RW, Butt EM. Fatal "asthma." A clinical and pathologic consideration of 187 cases. JAMA 1937;108:1843–1850.

68. Curschmann H. Über Bronchiolitis exsudativa und ihr verhältnis zum. Asthma nervosum. Dtsch Arch Klin Med (Leipzig) 1883;32:1–34.

69. Novak PM, Kumar NB, Naylor B. Curschmann's spirals in cervicovaginal smears. Prevalence, morphology, significance and origin. Acta Cytol 1984;28:5–8.

70. Wahl RW. Curschmann's spirals in pleural and peritoneal fluids. Report of 12 cases. Acta Cytol 1986;30:147–151.

71. Naylor B. Curschmann's spirals in pleural and peritoneal fluids. Acta Cytol 1990;34:474–478.

72. Weller PF, Goetzl EJ, Austen KF. Identification of human eosinophil lysophospholipase as the constituent of Charcot–Leyden crystals. Proc Natl Acad Sci USA 1980;77:7440–7443.

73. Weller PF, Bach D, Austen KF. Human eosinophil lysophospholipase: The sole protein component of Charcot–Leyden crystals. J Immunol 1982;128:1346–1349.

74. Ackerman SJ. Weil GJ, Gleich GJ. Formation of Charcot–Leyden crystals by human eosinophils. J Exp Med 1982;155:1597–1609.

75. Katzenstein ALA, Sale SR, Greenberger PA. Pathologic findings in allergic aspergillus sinusitis. Am J Surg Pathol 1983;7:439–443.

76. Krishnan S, Statsinger AL, Kleinman M, Bertoni MA, Sharma P. Eosinophilic pleural effusion with Charcot–Leyden crystals. Acta Cytol 1983;27:529–532.

77. Naylor B, Novak PM. Charcot–Leyden crystals in pleural fluids. Acta Cytol 1985;29:781–784.

78. Pfitzer P, Eosinophilic pleural effusion with Charcot–Leyden crystals. Acta Cytol 1985;29:906–908.

79. Dincsoy HP, Burton TJ, van der Bel-Kahn JM. Circulating Charcot–Leyden crystals in the hypereosinophilic syndrome. Am J Clin Pathol 1981;75:236–242.

80. Ayres WW. Production of Charcot–Leyden crystals from eosinophils with aerosol MA. Blood 1949;4:595–602.

81. Naylor B. Pleural, peritoneal and pericardial fluids. In:

Bibbo M, ed. Comprehensive cytopathology. Philadelphia: WB Saunders, 1991;541–614.

82. Naylor B. The shedding of the mucosa of the bronchial tree in asthma. Thorax 1962;17:69–72.

83. Cohen RC. Prentice AID. Metaplastic cells in sputum of patients with pulmonary eosinophilia. Tubercle 1959; 40:44–46.

84. Gleich GJ, Frigas E, Loegering DA, Wassom DL, Steinmuller D. Cytotoxic properties of the eosinophil major basic protein. J Immunol 1979;123:2925–2927.

85. Frigas E, Loegering DA, Gleich GJ. Cytotoxic effects of the guinea pig eosinophil major basic protein on tracheal epithelium. Lab Invest 1980;42:35–43.

86. Frigas E, Gleich GJ. The eosinophil and the pathophysiology of asthma. J Allergy Clin Immunol 1986;77:527–537.

87. Ford RM. Transient pulmonary eosinophilia and asthma: review of 20 cases occurring in 5,702 asthma sufferers. Am Rev Respir Dis 1966;93:797–803.

88. Wood DW, Lecks HI. Deaths due to childhood asthma. Are they preventable? Clin Pediatr 1976;15:677–687.

89. Hertzel MR, Clark TJH. Branthwaite MA. Asthma: Analysis of sudden deaths and ventilatory arrests in hospital. Br Med J 1977;1:808–811.

90. Drislane F, Samuels M, Kozakewich H, Schoen F, Strunk R. Myocardial contraction band lesions in patients with fatal asthma: Possible neurocardiological mechanisms. Am Rev Respir Dis 1987;135:498–501.

91. Schoen FJ. Cardiac pathology in asthma. J Allergy Clin Immunol 1987;80:419–423.

92. Robin ED, Lewiston N. Unexpected, unexplained sudden death in young asthmatic subjects. Chest 1989; 96:790–793.

93. Speizer FE, Doll R. A century of asthma deaths in young people. Br Med J 1968;3:245–246.

94. Speizer FE, Doll R, Heaf P. Observations on recent increase in mortality from asthma. Br Med J 1968; 1:335–339.

95. Burney PGJ. Asthma mortality: England and Wales. J Allergy Clin Immunol 1987;80:379–388.

96. Sears MR, Rea HH, Rothwell RPG, et al. Asthma mortality: Comparison between New Zealand and England. Br Med J 1986;293:1342–1345.

97. Sears MR, Beaglehole R. Asthma morbidity and mortality: New Zealand. J Allergy Clin Immunol 1987;80:383–388.

98. Gandevia B. Pressurized sympathomimetic aerosols and their lack of relationship to asthma mortality in Australia. Med J Aust 1973;1:273–277.

99. Inman WHW, Adelstein AM. Rise and fall of asthma mortality in England and Wales in relation to sales of pressurized aerosols. Lancet 1969;2:279–284.

100. Stolley PD, Schinnar R. Association between asthma mortality and isoproterenol aerosols: A review. Prev Med 1978;7:519–538.

101. Campbell AH. Mortality from asthma and bronchodilator aerosols. Med J Aust 1976;1:386–391.

102. Jackson RT, Beaglehole R, Rea HH, Sutherland DC. Mortality from asthma: A new epidemic in New Zealand. Br Med J 1982;285:771–774.

103. Sly RM. Increases in deaths from asthma. Ann Allergy 1984;53:20–25.

104. Bates DV, Baker-Anderson MA. Asthma mortality and morbidity in Canada. J Allergy Clin Immunol 1987; 80:395–397.

105. Mao Y, Semenciw R, Morrison H, MacWilliam L, Davies J, Wigle D. Increased rates of illness and death from asthma in Canada. Can Med Assoc J 1987;137:620–624.

106. Benatar SR. Fatal asthma. N Engl J Med 1986;314:423–428.

107. Bousquet J, Hatton F, Godard P, Micheal FB. Asthma mortality in France. J Allergy Clin Immunol 1987; 80:389–394.

108. Robin ED. Risk-benefit analysis in chest medicine: Death from bronchial asthma. Chest 1988;93:614–618.

109. Buist AS. Is asthma mortality increasing? Chest 1988; 93:449–450.

110. Whitelaw WA. Asthma deaths. Chest 1991;99:1507–1510.

111. Strunk RC. Death caused by asthma: minimizing the risks. J Respir Dis 1989;10:21–36.

112. O'Byrne PM, Dolovich J, Hargreave FE. Late asthmatic responses. Am Rev Respir Dis 1987;136:740–751.

113. Research Committee of the British Thoracic Association. Death from asthma in two regions of England. Br Med J 1982;285:1251–1255.

114. Reeder WH, Goodrich BE. Pulmonary infiltration with eosinophilia (PIE syndrome). Ann Intern Med 1952; 36:1217–1240.

115. Christoforidis AJ, Molnar W. Eosinophilic pneumonia: Report of two cases with pulmonary biopsy. JAMA 1960;173:157–161.

116. Liebow AA, Carrington CB. The eosinophilic pneumonias. Medicine (Baltimore) 1969;48:251–285.

117. Katzenstein ALA, Askin FB. Surgical pathology of non-neoplastic lung disease. 2nd Ed. Philadelphia: WB Saunders, 1990;168:213.

118. Morrissey WL, Gaensler EA, Carrington CB, Turner HG. Chronic eosinophilic pneumonia. Respiration 1975;32:453–468.

119. Löffler W. Zur differential-diagnose der lungeninfiltrier-ungen, II. Uber fluchtige succedan-infiltrate (mit eosinophile). Beitr Klin Tuberk 1932;79:368–382.

120. von Meyenburg H. Das eosinophile lungeninfiltrat. Pathologische anatomie und pathogenese. Schweiz Med Wochenschr 1942;30:809–811.

121. Gelpi AP, Mustafa M. Ascaris pneumonia. Am J Med 1968;44:377–389.

122. Sprent JFA. On the toxic and allergic manifestations produced by the tissue and fluids of *Ascaris;* effects on different tissues. J Infect Dis 1949;84:221–229.

123. Phills JA, Harrold AJ, Whiteman GV, Perelmutter L. Pulmonary infiltrates, asthma, and eosinophilia due to *Ascaris suum* infestation in man. N Engl J Med 1972; 286:965–1000.

124. Davis WB, Wilson HE, Wall RL. Eosinophilic alveolitis in acute respiratory failure: A clinical marker for a non-infectious etiology. Chest 1986;90:7–10.

125. Badesch DB, King TE, Jr., Schwarz MI. Acute eosinophilic pneumonia: A hypersensitivity phenomenon? Am Rev Respir Dis 1989;139:249–252.

126. Allen JN, Pacht ER, Gadek JE, Davis WB. Acute eosinophilic pneumonia as a reversible cause of noninfectious respiratory failure. N Engl J Med 1989;321:569–574.

127. Llibre JP, Tor J, Milla F. Acute eosinophilic pneumonia (Letter). N Engl J Med 1990;322:634–635.

128. Greenburg M, Schiffman RL, Geha DG. Acute eosinophilic pneumonia (Letter). N Engl J Med 1990;322:635.

129. Whitlock WL, Dietrick RA, Tenholder MF. Acute eosinophilic pneumonia (Letter). N Engl J Med 1990;322:635.

130. Buchheit J, Eid N, Rodgers G Jr, Feger T, Yakoub O. Acute eosinophilic pneumonia with respiratory failure: A new syndrome? Am Rev Respir Dis 1992;145:716–718.

131. Whitlock WL, Tenholder MF. Eosinophilic alveolitis? (letter). Chest 1987;91:472.

132. Davis WB. Eosinophilic alveolitis? (Reply to letter). Chest 1987;91:472–473.

133. Poe RH, Condemi JJ, Weinstein SS, Schuster RJ. Adult respiratory distress syndrome related to ampicillin sensitivity. Chest 1980;77:449–451.

134. Jennings CA, Deveikers J, Azumi N, Yeager H, Jr. Eosinophilic pneumonia associated with reaction to radiographic contrast medium. South Med J 1991;84:92–95.

135. Libby DM, Murphy TF, Edwards A, Gray G, King TK. Chronic eosinophilic pneumonia: an unusual cause of acute respiratory failure. Am Rev Respir Dis 1980;122:497–500.

136. Ivanick MJ, Donohue JF, Chronic eosinophilic pneumonia: A cause of adult respiratory distress syndrome. South Med J 1986;79:686–90.

137. McEvoy JDS, Donald KJ, Edwards RL. Immunoglobulin levels and electron microscopy in eosinophilic pneumonia. Am J Med 1978;64:529–536.

138. Anonymous. Acute eosinophilic pneumonia (editorial). Lancet 1990;335:947.

139. Rose GA, Spencer H. Polyarteritis nodosa. Q J Med 1957;26:43–81.

140. Weingarten RJ. Tropical eosinophilia. Lancet 1943;i:103–105.

141. Webb JKG, Job CK, Gault EW. Tropical eosinophilia, demonstration of microfilariae in lung, liver and lymphnodes. Lancet 1960;i:835–842.

142. Danaraj TJ, Pacheco G, Shanmugaratnam K, Beaver PC. The etiology and pathology of eosinophilic lung (tropical eosinophilia). Am J Trop Med Hyg 1966;15:183–189.

143. Beaver PC. Filariasis without microfilaremia. Am J Trop Med Hyg 1970;19:181–189.

144. Neva FA, Ottesen EA. Tropical (filarial) eosinophilia. N Engl J Med 1978;298:1129–1131.

145. Donahue DL. Tropical eosinophilia, an etiologic inquiry. N Engl J Med 1963;269:1357–1364.

146. Nutman TB, Vijayan VK, Pinkston P, et al. Tropical pulmonary eosinophilia: analysis of antifilarial antibody

localized to the lung. J Infect Dis 1989;160:1042–1050.

147. Udwadia FE. Tropical eosinophilia: A correlation of clinical, histopathologic and lung function studies. Dis Chest 1967;52:531–538.

148. Joshi UV, Udwadia FE, Gadgil RK. Etiology of tropical eosinophilia: A study of lung biopsies and review of published reports. Am J Trop Med Hyg 1969;18:231–240.

149. Udwadia FE. Tropical eosinophilia. In: Pulmonary eosinophilia: Progress in respiration research. Basal: Karger, 1975;7:35–155.

150. Parish RA. Intestinal parasites in Southeast Asian refugee children. West J Med 1985;143:47–49.

151. Pinkson P, Vijayan VK, Nutman TB, et al. Acute tropical pulmonary eosinophilia: Characterization of the lower respiratory tract inflammation and its response to therapy. J Clin Invest 1987;80:216–225.

152. Carrington CB, Addington WW, Goff AM, et al. Chronic eosinophilic pneumonia. N Engl J Med 1969;280:787–798.

152a. Hommeyer SH, Goodwin JD, Takasugi JE. Computed tomography of air-space disease. Radiol Clin North Am 1991;29:1065–1084.

153. Jederlinic PJ, Sicilian L, Gaensler EA. Chronic eosinophilic pneumonia. A report of 19 cases and a review of the literature. Medicine (Baltimore) 1988;67:154–162.

154. Pearson DJ, Rosenow EC. Chronic eosinophilic pneumonia (Carrington's), a follow-up study. Mayo Clin Proc 1978;55:73–78.

155. Hennell H, Sussman ML. The roentgen features of eosinophilic infiltrations in the lungs. Radiology 1945;44:328–334.

156. Onitsuka H, Onitsuka S, Yokomizo Y, Matsuura K. Computer tomography of chronic eosinophilic pneumonia. J Comput Assist Tomogr 1983;7:1092–1094.

157. Mayo JR, Müller NL, Road J, Sisler J, Lilligton G. Chronic eosinophilic pneumonia: CT findings in six cases. AJR 1989;153:727–730.

158. Gaensler EA, Carrington CB. Peripheral opacities in chronic eosinophilic pneumonia: The photographic negative of pulmonary edema. AJR 1977;128:1–13.

159. Selye H. The mast cells. Washington DC: Butterworths, 1965.

160. Bartter T, Irwin RS, Nash G, Balikian JP, Hollingsworth HH. Idiopathic bronchiolitis obliterans organizing pneumonia with peripheral infiltrates on chest roentgenogram. Arch Intern Med 1989;149:273–279.

161. Glazer HS, Levitt RG, Shackelford GD. Peripheral pulmonary infiltrates in sarcoidosis. Chest 1984;86:741–744.

162. Epler GR, McLoud TC, Gaensler EA, Mikus P, Carrington CB. Normal chest roentgenograms in chronic diffuse infiltrative lung disease. N Engl J Med 1978;298:934–939.

163. Dajaegher P, Derveaux L, Dubois P, Demedts M. Eosinophilic pneumonia without radiographic pulmonary infiltrates. Chest 1983;84:637–638.

164. Davis WB, Fells GA, Sun X-H, Gadek JE, Venet A, Crystal RG. Eosinophil-mediated injury to lung paren-

chymal cells and interstitial matrix: A possible role for eosinophils in chronic inflammatory disorders of the lower respiratory tract. J Clin Invest 1984;74:269–278.

165. Lieske TR, Sunderrajan EV, Passamonte PM. Broncho-alveolar lavage and technetium-99m glucoheptonate imaging in chronic eosinophilic pneumonia. Chest 1984;85:282–284.

166. Dejaegher P, Demedts M. Bronchoalveolar lavage in eosinophilic pneumonia before and during corticosteroid therapy. Am Rev Respir Dis 1984;129:631–2.

167. Prin L, Capron P, Gosset B, et al. Eosinophilic lung disease: Immunological studies of blood and alveolar eosinophils. Clin Exp Immunol 1986;63:249–257.

168. Greif J, Struhar D, Kivity S, Topilsky M. Bronchoalveolar lavage: A useful tool in the diagnosis of eosinophilic pneumonia. Isr J Med Sci 1986;22:479–480.

169. Ogushi F, Ozaki T, Kawano T, Yasuoka S. PGE_2 and $PGF_{2\alpha}$ content in bronchoalveolar lavage fluid obtained from patients with eosinophilic pneumonia. Chest 1987;91:204–206.

170. Bedrossian CWM, Greenberg SD, Williams LJ, Jr. Ultrastructure of the lung in Loeffler's pneumonia. Am J Med 1975;58:438–443.

171. Kanner RE, Hammar SP. Chronic eosinophilic pneumonia; ultrastructural evidence of marked immunoglobulin production plus macrophage ingestion of eosinophils and eosinophilic lysosomes leading to intracytoplasmic Charcot–Leyden crystals. Chest 1977;71:95–98.

172. Lombard CM, Tazalaar HD, Krasne DL. Pulmonary eosinophilia and coccidioidal infections. Chest 1987;91:734–736.

173. Wright JL, Pare PD, Hammond M, Donefan RE. Eosinophilic pneumonia and atypical mycobacterial infection. Am Rev Respir Dis 1983;127:497–499.

174. Travis WD, Kalafer ME, Robin HS, Luibel FJ. Hypersensitivity pneumonitis and pulmonary vasculitis with eosinophilia in a patient taking an L-tryptophan preparation. Ann Intern Med 1990;112:301–303.

175. Tazelaar HD, Myers JL, Drage CW, King TE, Jr., Aguayo S, Colby TV. Pulmonary disease associated with L-tryptophan-induced eosinophilia-myalgia syndrome. Chest 1990;97:1032–1036.

176. Strumpf IJ, Drucker RD, Anders KH, Cohen S, Fajolu O. Acute eosinophilic pulmonary disease associated with the ingestion of L-tryptophan-containing products. Chest 1991;99:8–13.

177. Hardy WR, Anderson RE. The hypereosinophilic syndrome. Ann Intern Med 1968;68:1220–1229.

178. Chusid MJ, Dale DC, West BC, Wolff SM. The hypereosinophilic syndrome: Analysis of fourteen cases with review of the literature. Medicine (Baltimore) 1975;54:1–27.

179. Benvenisti DS, Ultmann JE. Eosinophilic leukemia. Report of five cases and review of literature. Ann Intern Med 1969;71:731–745.

180. Roberts WC, Liegler DG, Carbone PP. Endomyocardial disease and eosinophilia. A clinical and pathologic spectrum. Am J Med 1969;46:28–42.

181. Brink AJ, Weber HW. Fibroplastic parietal endocarditis with eosinophilia. Loffler's endocarditis. Am J Med 1963;34:52–70.

182. Odeberg B. Eosinophilic leukemia and disseminated eosinophilic collagen disease—a disease entity. Acta Med Scand 1965;177:129–144.

183. Churg J, Strauss L. Allergic granulomatosis, allergic angiitis and periarteritis nodosa. Am J Pathol 1951;27:277–301.

184. Parrillo JE, Fauci AS, Wolff SM. Therapy of the hypereosinophilic syndrome. Ann Intern Med 1978;89:167–172.

185. Fauci AS, Harley JB, Roberts WC, Ferrans VJ, Gralnick HR, Bjornson BH. The idiopathic hypereosinophilic syndrome: Clinical, pathophysiologic, and therapeutic considerations. Ann Intern Med 1982;97:78–92.

186. Grantham JG, Meadows JA, III, Gleich GJ. Chronic eosinophilic pneumonia: Evidence of eosinophil degranulation and release of major basic protein. Am J Med 1986;80:89–94.

187. Noguchi H, Kephardt GM, Colby TV, Gleich GJ. Tissue eosinophilia and eosinophil degranulation in syndromes associated with fibrosis. Am J Pathol 1992;140:521–528.

188. Urschel HC, Jr., Paulson DL, Shaw RR. Mucoid impaction of the bronchi. Ann Thorac Surg 1966;2:1–16.

189. Katzenstein AL, Liebow AA, Friedman PJ. Bronchocentric granulomatosis, mucoid impaction, and hypersensitivity reaction to fungi. Am Rev Respir Dis 1975;111:497–537.

190. Chapman BJ, Capewell S, Gibson R, Greening AP, Crompton GK. Pulmonary eosinophilia with and without allergic bronchopulmonary aspergillosis. Thorax 1989;44:919–924.

191. Shaw RR. Mucoid impaction of the bronchi. J Thorac Surg 1951;22:149–163.

192. Hinson KFW, Moon JH, Plummer NS, Bronchopulmonary aspergillosis; a review and a report of eight new cases. Thorax 1952;7:317–333.

193. Sulavik SB. Bronchocentric granulomatosis and allergic bronchopulmonary aspergillosis. Clin Chest Med 1988;9:609–621.

194. Sanerkin NG, Seal RME, Leopold JG. Plastic bronchitis, mucoid impaction of the bronchi and allergic bronchopulmonary aspergillosis, and their relationship to bronchial asthma. Ann Allergy 1966;24:586–594.

195. Bettman M. Report of a case of fibrinous bronchitis with a review of the literature. Am J Med Sci 1902;123:304–329.

196. Walker IC. Two cases of fibrinous bronchitis, with a review of the literature. Am J Med Sci 1920;159:825–833.

197. Leggat PO. Plastic bronchitis. Dis Chest 1954;26:464–473.

198. Johnson RS, Sita-Lumsden EG. Plastic bronchitis. Thorax 1960;15:325–332.

199. Morgan AD, Bogomeletz W. Mucoid impaction of the bronchi in relation to asthma and plastic bronchitis. Thorax 1968;23:356–369.

200. Jett JR, Tazelaar HD, Keim LW, Ingrassia TS, III. Plastic bronchitis: An old disease revisited Mayo Clin

Proc 1991;66:305–311.

201. Streets TH: A case of croupous bronchitis: Recovery under treatment. Am J Med Sci 1980;79:148–151.

202. Liebow AA. Pulmonary angiitis and granulomatosis. Am Rev Respir Dis 1973;108:1–18.

203. Koss MN, Robinson RG, Hochholzer L. Bronchocentric granulomatosis. Hum Pathol 1981;12:632–638.

204. Chan-Yeung M, Chase WH, Trapp W, Grzybowski S. Allergic bronchopulmonary aspergillosis: Clinical and pathologic study of three cases. Chest 1971;59:33–39.

205. Warnock ML, Fennessy MB, Rippon J. Chronic eosinophilic pneumonia, a manifestation of allergic aspergillosis. Am J Clin Pathol 1974;62:73–80.

206. Saldana MJ. Bronchocentric granulomatosis: Clinicopathologic observations in 17 patients. Lab Invest 1979;40:281–282.

207. Lee JH, Joihovsky T, Yan K. Bronchocentric granulomatosis: Review of 14 patients. Thorax 1982;37:779.

208. Myers JL, Katzenstein A-LA. Granulomatous infection mimicking bronchocentric granulomatosis. Am J Surg Pathol 1986;10:317–322.

209. McAleer R, Kroenert DB, Elder JL, et al. Allergic bronchopulmonary disease caused by *Curvularia lunata* and *Drechslera hawaiiensis*. Thorax 1981;36:338–344.

210. Matthiesson AM. Allergic bronchopulmonary disease caused by fungi other than *Aspergillus*. Thorax 1981; 36:719.

211. Dolan CT, Weed LA, Dines DE. Bronchopulmonary helminthosporiosis. Am J Clin Pathol 1970;53:235–242.

212. Hendrick DJ, Ellithorpe DB, Lyon F, et al. Allergic bronchopulmonary helminthosporiosis. Am Rev Respir Dis 1982;126:935–938.

213. Travis WD, Kwon-Chung KJ, Kleiner DE, et al. Unusual aspects of allergic bronchopulmonary fungal disease: Report of two cases due to *Curvularia* organisms associated with allergic fungal sinusitis. Hum Pathol 1991;22:1240–1248.

214. Tazelaar HD, Baird AM, Mill M, Grimes MM, Schulman LL, Smith CR. Bronchocentric mycosis ocurring in transplant recipients. Chest 1989;96:92–95.

215. Ulbright T, Katzenstein A-LA. Solitary necrotizing granulomas of the lung. Am J Surg Pathol 1980;4:13–27.

216. Tron V, Churg A. Chronic necrotizing pulmonary aspergillosis mimicking bronchocentric granulomatosis. Pathol Res Pract 1986;181:621–624.

217. Nagata N, Sueishi K, Tanaka K, Iwata Y. Pulmonary aspergillosis with bronchocentric granulomas. Am J Surg Pathol 1990;14:485–488.

218. DenHertog RW, Wagenaar Sj Sc, Westermann CJJ. Bronchocentric granulomatosis and pulmonary ecchinococcosis. Am Rev Respir Dis 1982;125:344–347.

219. Boskeen CH, Myers JL, Greenberger PA, Katzenstein ALA. Pathologic features of allergic bronchopulmonary aspergillosis. Am J Surg Pathol 1988;12:216–222.

220. Travis WD, Hoffman GS, Leavitt RY, Pass HI, Fauci AS. Surgical pathology of the lung in Wegener's granulomatosis. Review of 87 open lung biopsies from 67 patients. Am J Surg Pathol 1991;15:315–333.

221. Yousem SA. Bronchocentric injury in Wegener's granulomatosis: a report of five cases. Hum Pathol 1991; 22:535–540.

222. Travis WD, Colby TV, Koss MN. Pulmonary Wegener's granulomatosis with prominent bronchocentric involvement (in manuscript).

223. Wiedemann HP, Bensinger RE, Hudson LD. Bronchocentric granulomatosis with eye involvement. Am Rev Respir Dis 1982;126:347–350.

224. Hellems SO, Kanner RE, Renzetti AD, Jr. Bronchocentric granulomatosis associated with rheumatoid arthritis. Chest 1983;83:831–832.

225. Katzenstein ALA, Askin FB. Surgical pathology of nonneoplastic lung diseases. 2d Ed. Philadelphia: WB Saunders 1990;252–289.

226. Malo JL, Hawkins R, Pepys J. Studies in chronic allergic bronchopulmonary aspergillosis: 1, Clinical and physiological findings. Thorax 1977;32:254–261.

227. Solomon WR. Burge HP. *Aspergillus fumigatus* levels in and out of doors in urban air. J Allergy Clin Immunol 1975;55:90–91.

228. Slavin RG, Stanczyk DJ. Lonigro AJ. Broun GO. Allergic bronchopulmonary aspergillosis—a North American rarity: Clinical and immunologic characteristics. Am J Med 1969;47:306–313.

229. Hoehne JH, Reed CE, Dickie HA. Allergic bronchopulmonary aspergillosis is not rare. Chest 1973;63:177–181.

230. Rosenberg M, Patterson R, Mintzer R, Cooper BJ. Roberts M, Harris KE. Clinical and immunologic criteria for the diagnosis of allergic bronchopulmonary aspergillosis. Ann Intern Med 1977;86:405–414.

231. Henderson AH. Allergic aspergillosis; review of 32 cases. Thorax 1968;12:501–512.

232. Scadding JG. Eosinophilic infiltrations of the lungs in asthmatics. Proc R Soc Med 1971;64:381–392.

233. McCarthy DS, Pepys J. Allergic broncho-pulmonary aspergillosis, clinical immunology: (1) Clinical features. Clin Allergy 1971;1:261–286.

234. McCarthy DS, Pepys J. Allergic bronchopulmonary aspergillosis, clinical immunology: (2) Skin, nasal and bronchial tests. Clin Allergy 1971;1:415–432.

235. McCarthy DS. Bronchiectasis in allergic bronchopulmonary aspergillosis. Proc R Soc Med 1968;61:503–506.

236. McCarthy DS, Simon G, Hargreave FE. The radiological appearances in allergic bronchopulmonary aspergillosis. Clin Radiol 1970;21:366–375.

237. Scadding JG. The bronchi in allergic aspergillosis. Scand J Respir Dis 1965;48:372–377.

238. Simon G. Type 1 immunologic reactions in the lung. Semin Roentgenol 1975;12:21–29.

239. Safirstein BH, D'Souza MF, Simon G, Tai EHC, Pepys J. Five-year follow-up of allergic bronchopulmonary aspergillosis. Am Rev Respir Dis 1973;108:450–459.

240. Ricketti AJ, Greenberger PA, Glassroth J. Spontaneous pneumothorax in allergic bronchopulmonary aspergillosis. Arch Intern Med 1984;144:151–152.

241. McCarthy DS, Pepys J. Cryptogenic pulmonary eosinophilias. Clin Allergy 1973;3:339–351.

242. Rosenberg M, Mintzer R, Aarouson DW, Patterson R. Allergic bronchopulmonary aspergillosis in three patients with normal chest x-ray. Chest 1977;72:597–600.

243. Greenberger PA. Allergic bronchopulmonary aspergillosis. In: Middleton E, Jr., Reed CE, Ellis EF, Adkinson NF, Yuninger JW, eds. Allergy, principles and practice. 3d Ed. St Louis: Mosby, 1988;1219–1236.

244. Patterson R, Greenberger PA, Halwig JM, Liotta JL, Roberts M. Allergic bronchopulmonary aspergillosis: Natural history and classification of early disease by serologic and roentgenographic studies. Arch Intern Med 1986;146:916–918.

245. Patterson R, Roberts M. IgE and IgG antibodies against *Aspergillus fumigatus* in sera of patients with bronchopulmonary allergic aspergillosis. Int Arch Allergy 1974; 46:150–160.

246. Rosenberg M, Patterson R, Mintzer R, Cooper BJ, Roberts M, Harris KG. Clinical and immunologic criteria for the diagnosis of allergic bronchopulmonary aspergillosis. Ann Intern Med 1977;86:405–417.

247. Patterson R, Greenberger PA, Radin RC, Roberts M. Allergic bronchopulmonary aspergillosis: Staging as an aid to management. Ann Intern Med 1982;96:286–291.

248. Ricketti A, Greenberge P, Mintzer R, et al. Allergic bronchopulmonary aspergillosis. Chest 1984;86:773–778.

249. Greenberger PA, Patterson R. Diagnosis and management of bronchopulmonary aspergillosis. Ann Allergy 1986;56:444–448.

250. Greenberger PA. Allergic bronchopulmonary aspergillosis and fungoses. Clin Chest Med 1988;9:599–608.

251. Ricketti AJ, Greenberger PA, Patterson R. Serum IgE as an important aid in management of allergic bronchopulmonary aspergillosis. J Allergic Clin Immunol 1984; 74:68–71.

252. Patterson R, Greenberger PA, Lee TM, et al. Prolonged evaluation of patients with corticosteroid-dependent asthma stage of allergic bronchopulmonary aspergillosis. J Allergy Clin Immunol 1987;80:663–668.

253. Lee TM, Greenberger PA, Patterson R, Roberts M, Liotta JL. Stage V (fibrotic) allergic bronchopulmonary aspergillosis. A review of 17 cases followed from diagnosis. Arch Intern Med 1987;147:319–323.

254. Imbeau SA, Nichols D, Flaherty D, et al. Allergic bronchopulmonary aspergillosis. J Allergy Clin Immunol 1978;62:243–255.

255. Wood RE, Boat TF, Doershuk. State of the art-cystic fibrosis. Am Rev Respir Dis 1976;113:833–878.

256. Nelson LA, Callerame ML, Schwartz RH. Aspergillosis and atopy in cystic fibrosis. Am Rev Respir Dis 1979; 120:863–873.

257. Zeaske R, Bruns WT, Fink JN, et al. Immune response to aspergillus in cystic fibrosis. J Allergy Clin Immunol 1988;82:73–77.

258. Simmonds EJ, Littlewood JM, Evans EGV. Cystic fibrosis and allergic bronchopulmonary aspergillosis. Arch Dis Child 1990;65:507–511.

259. Simmonds EJ, Littlewood JM, Evans EGV. Allergic bronchopulmonary aspergillosis. Lancet 1990;335: 1229.

CHAPTER 17

Pulmonary Histiocytosis X (Pulmonary Langerhans' Cell Granulomatosis)

Samuel P. Hammar

A conceptual understanding of pulmonary histiocytosis X, also known as pulmonary eosinophilic granuloma and pulmonary Langerhans' cell granulomatosis, is based on a knowledge of the Langerhans' cell. The Langerhans' cell was named after Paul Langerhans, a 24-year-old German medical student who identified it as a dendritic cell of the epidermis of uncertain origin and function.[1] He thought these cells represented nerve cells. In 1961, Birbeck et al.[2] discovered by electron microscopy that Langerhans' cells contained unique rod- and racquet-shaped granules that are now referred to as Langerhans' cell granules or Birbeck granules. In 1965, Basset and Turiaf[3] found that histiocytosis X cells contained the same type of unusual cytoplasmic granule that was found in Langerhans' cells, and called them histiocytosis X bodies or X bodies. Langerhans' cells and histiocytosis X cells are bone marrow derived[4,5] and have features similar but not identical to those of monocytes and macrophages[6–13]; these are shown in Table 17–1. More recent studies have shown that Langerhans' cells belong to a specific subset of macrophages, termed dendritic cells or antigen-presenting cells.[14,15] In 1986, Murphy and coworkers[16] demonstrated, in skin biopsies from patients who had undergone bone marrow transplantation, that phagocytic dermal macrophages transform into Langerhans' cells. Langerhans' cells are stated to reach normal levels 4 to 12 months after transplantation.[17]

In this author's opinion there are no significant morphologic or functional differences between Langerhans' cells and histiocytosis X cells.[18] The idea that Langerhans' cells are activated histiocytosis X cells may be correct, although Langerhans' cells in their normal locations throughout the body become activated in a variety of situations.[18] In our experience,[19] Langerhans' cells are infrequently identified in the "normal resting" lung when studied by immunohistochemistry and electron microscopy although they are frequently seen in most nonneoplastic pulmonary inflammatory conditions.

In 1941, Farber[20] proposed that Letterer-Siwe disease, Hand-Schuller Christian disease, and eosinophilic granuloma of bone represented varieties of the same basic disease process, and in 1953 Lichtenstein[21] combined these diseases under a single name, histiocytosis X. Three forms of the disease were described: (1) histiocytosis X localized to bone (essentially identical to eosinophilic granuloma of bone); (2) disseminated chronic histiocytosis X (analogous to Hand-Schuller-Christian disease); (3) disseminated acute and subacute histiocytosis X (analogous to Letterer-Siwe disease). The designation of the diseases as histiocytosis X has not been universally accepted,[22] although the ultrastructural findings showing that the "histiocytes" in these conditions are the same and essentially identical to Langerhans' cells add support to the concept. For an excellent discussion concerning the history, evolution, and controversies concerning histiocytosis X the reader is referred to the article by Vogel and Vogel.[23]

Pulmonary involvement by "lipogranulomatous" inflammation was recognized in the 1920s,[24] but it was not until 1949 that Parkinson[25] suggested that eosinophilic granuloma could solely involve the lung. He described a 56-year-old boot-repairer who was admitted to a hospital in September 1948 because of dyspnea on exertion that had become progressively worse since 1942. The patient's chest radiograph showed diffuse miliary mottling in both lung fields. Although the patient had evidence of bone involvement and diabetes insipidus, Parkinson suggested the disease could occur in an

Table 17–1. Comparison of macrophages, Langerhans' cells, and histocytosis X cells

Characteristic	Macrophates	Langerhans' cells	Histiocytosis X cells
Enzyme histochemistry			
Adenosine triphosphatase	–	+	+
Naphthyl acetate esterase	+	+	+
Naphthyl acetate esterase with NaF	–	±	±
Chloroacetate esterase	–	–	–
Acid phosphatase	+	±	±
Tartrate-resistant acid phosphatase	–	–	–
Peroxidase	–	–	–
Alkaline phosphatase	–	±	±
Frozen tissue sections			
OKT-6 (Leu 6)	–	+	+
OKT-4 (Leu 3)	±	±	+
HLA-A, B, C	+	+	+
HLA-Dr	+	+	+
Fc receptor for IgG	+	+	+
Paraffin-embedded tissue sections			
S-100 protein	–	+	+
Lysozome	+	–	–
Alpha-1-antitrypsin	+	–	–

"incomplete form" with pituitary, bone, and pulmonary disease occurring singly or in any combination.

Also in 1949, Oswald and Parkinson[26] reported on 16 patients with honeycomb lung; of these, 5 with no extrapulmonary disease, who were reviewed by Cunningham and Parkinson in 1950,[27] were thought to have a stage of eosinophilic granuloma. In July 1951, Farinacci et al.[28] reported on 2 men aged 24 and 32 with diffuse infiltrates in both lungs whose open lung biopsies showed the histologic changes of eosinophilic granuloma. Neither man had evidence of disease elsewhere, thus indicating the disease could occur as primary pulmonary disease. Mazitello[29] is credited with considering pulmonary involvement by histiocytosis X to be a nosologic entity and coined the term "primary pulmonary eosinophilic granuloma." Since then numerous reports of primary pulmonary histiocytosis X have appeared. Basset and colleagues[30] reported on 78 patients, and Friedman et al.[31] on 100 patients; we recently submitted a detailed clinicopatho-logic analysis of 31 patients.[32] In addition, Colby and Lombard[33] published an excellent review article summarizing most of the cases published to 1983 and added information on 54 cases of their own.

Etiology and Pathogenesis

The etiology of primary pulmonary histiocytosis X is unknown. The majority of patients who develop the disease are active cigarette smokers. In the study by Friedman and colleagues,[31] smoking histories were available in 69 of 100 patients studied. Of 69 patients, 67 (97%) were cigarette smokers, 12 having previously stopped. Among patients reported by Basset et al.,[30] 31 of 53 (58%) were cigarette smokers. In our study,[32] 28 of 31 (90%) were cigarette smokers.

Villar et al.[34] reported on seven patients with pulmonary eosinophilic granuloma and suggested the disease represented a form of hypersensitivity pneumonitis. Of these seven, two male patients were exposed to cement; one woman to fumes from lime kilns; one man to cotton; another woman with precipitating antibodies against bird-dropping antigens had been exposed to parakeets. In the biopsies from three patients, particulate material was identified in histiocytes in addition to the classic findings. The authors referred to the report by Girard and Bouzakoura[35] of a patient with pulmonary histiocytosis X who had a hypersensitivity to sawdust and horse serum. In addition, Auld[36] and Thompson and Langer[37] have suggested that an inhaled substance may be of etiologic importance in pulmonary histiocytosis X. Unfortunately, cigarette-smoking histories are not given for these patients.

King and colleagues[38] reported finding serum immune complexes and deposits of IgG and C3 in alveoli and vessel walls in five of six patients with pulmonary eosinophilic granuloma. The elevated serum immune complexes correlated with cellularity of the biopsy and the presence of IgG and C3 deposits. This observation is similar to that reported in cases of idiopathic interstitial pulmonary fibrosis.[39] Concerning this finding, a study published in 1979[39] failed to show that immune complexes correlated with histologic changes in cases of idiopathic interstitial fibrosis.[40]

A case of Letterer–Siwe disease with pulmonary involvement has been reported in a term stillborn male whose mother received polio vaccine in the third month of pregnancy and "Asiatic flu" vaccine in the sixth month of pregnancy.[41] Similarly, a case of histiocytosis X involvement of lymph nodes has been reported in a 9-month-old infant with congenital rubella.[42] Both these cases raise the possibility of a viral etiology of histiocytosis X.

More recently, van der Loo et al.[43] reported finding C-type virus-like particles in Langerhans' cells, indeterminate cells of the skin (possible Langerhans' cell precursors), and interdigitating reticulum cells in lymph nodes (possible Langerhans' cell precursors) in seven patients with mycosis fungoides and two patients with Sezary's syndrome. In the seven patients with mycosis fungoides, virus-containing Langerhans' cells were found in seven skin biopsies and four lymph node biopsies. The C-type particles were not found in Langerhans' cells of control biopsies of skin and lymph node. These findings relate more to the possible etiology of mycosis fungoides and Sezary's syndrome than histiocytosis X, but suggest that Langerhans' cells are capable of virus uptake.

With respect to immunologic findings in histiocytosis X, Osband et al.[44] found that 12 of 17 patients studied were considered immunologically abnormal as demonstrated by the presence of circulating lymphocytes spontaneously cytotoxic to cultured human fibroblasts or autologous red blood cells. They also found a decreased number of histamine receptors on many patients' T lymphocytes, suggesting a suppressor T-cell deficiency. Ten of 17 patients treated with injections of extracts of calf thymus showed a reversibility of these abnormal immunologic parameters. Unfortunately there was no control group, and as is discussed later, a significant number of patients show no progression of their disease or have a spontaneous remission.

Of these potential etiologies, cigarette smoke is by far the leading candidate. Cigarette-smoking individuals exhibit a variety of immunologic changes that are not found in nonsmoking persons. For example, Miller et al.[45] reported that heavy cigarette smokers (56–120 pack years and more than two packs of cigarettes per day) have an increased total number of T lymphocytes and a decreased helper-inducer/suppressor-cytotoxic T-lymphocyte ratio (T4:T8 ratio). They suggested that the observed decreased serum immunoglobulin levels in heavy cigarette smokers[46,47] were potentially caused by a decrease in helper-inducer lymphocytes, which facilitate B-lymphocyte proliferation. They also cited evidence that heavy cigarette smoking was associated with the humoral mediators of stress such as catecholamines and corticosteroids,[48] and that an increase in T-suppressor lymphocytes was seen in acute stress caused by burns and surgical trauma.[49,50] Hoogsteden et al.[51] studied the expression of CD11/CD18 cell-surface adhesion glycoprotein on alveolar macrophages in smokers and nonsmokers. As referenced by these authors, alveolar macrophages take up tobacco smoke products, which causes them to become activated and release chemotactic factors[52]; they hypothesize that these could cause an increased influx of peripheral blood monocytes into the lung. Activated alveolar macrophages produce interleukin-1,[53,54] which has been demonstrated[55] to increase the expression of CD54 intercellular adhesion molecule 1 on endothelial cells, which in turn may enhance the influx of macrophages into the lung. The findings by Hoogsteden et al.[51] that alveolar macrophages in the bronchoalveolar lavage fluid of cigarette smokers had a decreased CD11/CD18 cell-surface adhesion glycoprotein compared to nonsmokers might make it easier for these cells to reach the alveoli.

Barbers et al.[56] studied the proliferative activity of bronchoalveolar lavage macrophages obtained from tobacco and marijuana smokers. They cited published reports that alveolar macrophages are derived in part from a local proliferation of resident alveolar macrophages,[57–65] and that alveolar macrophages from tobacco or marijuana smokers showed sluggish chemotactic activity.[66,67] They suggested that published literature supported the notion that the four- to fivefold increased number of alveolar macrophages in cigarette smokers was caused by a local alveolar proliferation of these cells.[68] The replication of bronchoalveolar lavage macrophages obtained from tobacco smokers (n = 10), marijuana smokers (n = 13), and combined tobacco/marijuana smokers (n = 6) was compared to nonsmokers (n = 12) by measuring the incorporation of [^{3}H]thymidine into the DNA of dividing cells, usually counting 2000 cells on autoradiographically prepared cytocentrifuge cell preparations. Barbers et al. found an 18- to 10-fold increase in proliferative activity of tobacco- and marijuana smoker-derived macrophages compared to nonsmokers. They concluded that their study provided evidence that monocytic phagocytes with characteristics of alveolar macrophages were capable of cell division and could account for the increased macrophage population found in bronchoalveolar lavage fluid in tobacco or marijuana smokers. The exact stimulus for local alveolar macrophages proliferation remains unknown, but the findings suggest that tobacco and marijuana smoke contain substances that increase proliferative activity.

Cigarette smoking is also reported to be associated with hyperplasia of lung neuroendocrine cells, resulting in a significant increase in levels of bombesin-like peptides in the lower respiratory tract of some individuals.[69] Aguayo et al.[70] therefore postulated that bombesin-like peptides could contribute to pulmonary inflammation and fibrosis in cigarette smokers because bombesin is a chemoattractant for monocytes and a mitogen for 3T3 fibroblasts. Because pulmonary histiocytosis X occurred almost exclusively in cigarette smokers, they quantitated neuroendocrine cells with bombesin-like immunoreactivity in open lung biopsies from six patients with pulmonary histiocytosis X, and compared the results to six cigarette smokers with another type of pulmonary disease and eight patients with idiopathic pulmonary fibrosis. The six patients with pulmonary histiocytosis X exhibited a 10-fold increase in neuroendocrine cells with bombesin-like immunoreactivity, compared to smokers and patients with idiopathic pulmonary fibrosis. Somewhat surprisingly, however, the investigators found no significant difference in bronchoalveolar lavage fluid levels of bombesin-like peptides in the three conditions. The authors proposed a putative pathogenetic mechanism in which stimulation of neuroendocrine cells by cigarette smoke in certain susceptible individuals leads to an exaggerated hyperplasia of neuroendocrine cells with bombesin-like peptide immunoreactivity, increased recruitment of monocyte differentiation into dendritic Langerhans' cells, and the production of fibrosis, a common component of pulmonary histiocytosis X, from stimulation of fibroblasts by bombesin-like peptides.

Barth et al.[71] described a case of a 43-year-old cigarette-smoking man diagnosed by open lung biopsy to have pulmonary histiocytosis X; his bronchoalveolar lavage fluid contained 93% macrophages, of which 8% were CD1/OKT6 positive, suggesting they were Langerhans' cells. Northern blot analysis of RNA from bronchoalveolar lavage cells showed an exaggerated expression of macrophage colony-stimulating factor (M-CSF) gene, and of the c-*fms* gene that encodes for the corresponding receptor for macrophage colony-stimulating factor, as well as an increased level of c-sis RNA, which encodes for the beta chain of platelet-derived growth factor. With resolution of the disease as a result of corticosteroid treatment, the number of CD1/OKT6 antigen-positive Langerhans' cells decreased to 3%, and macrophage colony-stimulating factor, c-fms and c-sis gene expression were reduced to near-normal levels. The authors concluded that macrophage colony-stimulating factor and platelet-derived growth factor have a role in the initiation or maintenance of the pathologic reactions of pulmonary histiocytosis X.

A putative pathogenetic mechanism for the development of pulmonary histiocytosis X is shown in Fig. 17–1.

Incidence and Clinical Features

The exact incidence of primary pulmonary histiocytosis X is unknown. Knudson et al.[72] reported an incidence of 2.6% of 381 patients with miliary lung disease.

Gaensler and Carrington[73] identified 17 cases (3.4%) of pulmonary histiocytosis X in 502 patients who had an open lung biopsy for chronic diffuse infiltrative lung disease.

The clinical signs and symptoms of patients with pulmonary histiocytosis X are variable. The majority of the patients are between 10 and 40 years old with the sex distribution being approximately equal. In our series of 31 patients, the youngest was 15 years and the oldest 75 years old. In the study by Friedman et al.[31] of 100 patients, 23 patients were asymptomatic and were discovered because of an abnormal routine chest radiograph. In our study of 31 patients, only 2 were without symptoms.[32] The most common presenting symptoms are cough, dyspnea, chest pain, fever hemoptysis, and weight loss. Many patients will describe a flu-like illness with significant weight loss and fever suggesting an infectious process or malignancy. Spontaneous pneumothorax has been reported as the presenting finding in pulmonary histiocytosis X, but in this author's experience pneumothorax is uncommon. Some patients may have multiorgan involvement by histiocytosis X with predominantly pulmonary symptoms.

Two patients with pulmonary histiocytosis X presented with pleural effusion,[73] and Mason and Tedeschi[74] described a 17-year-old girl with pulmonary eosinophilic granuloma who had hilar and paratracheal lymphadenopathy simulating pulmonary sarcoidosis. Brambilla et al.[75] described a case of pulmonary histiocytosis X in a 33-year-old male arc welder with histologically proven mediastinal lymph node involvement. Pomeranz and Proto[76] reported seven cases of pulmonary histiocytosis X who they thought had unusual or confusing clinical and/or pathologic features. Their case six concerned a 13-year-old boy with an intratracheal mass, bilateral hilar adenopathy, and an enlarging neck mass in the region of the thyroid. He presented with shortness of breath and stridor. The patient in case seven was an 11-year-old girl who had an isolated lingular consolidation. Fichtenbaum et al.[77] reported a 58-year-old asymptomatic man with a 42-pack-year history of cigarette smoking whose preoperative chest radiograph showed a 1-cm right-middle-lobe nodule that histologically, immunohistochemically, and ultrastructurally was documented to represent eosinophilic granuloma. In our series of 31 patients,[32] 1 patient had an isolated nodule representing eosinophilic granuloma.

Sajjad and Luna[78] reported the development of primary pulmonary histiocytosis X in two patients with Hodgkin's disease who had been treated with combined radiation and chemotherapy. One of 31 patients reported by us developed the disease while being treated with chemotherapy for a disseminated non-Hodgkin's lymphocytic lymphoma.[32] In addition, a case of systemic mastocytosis and coexistent pulmonary eosino-

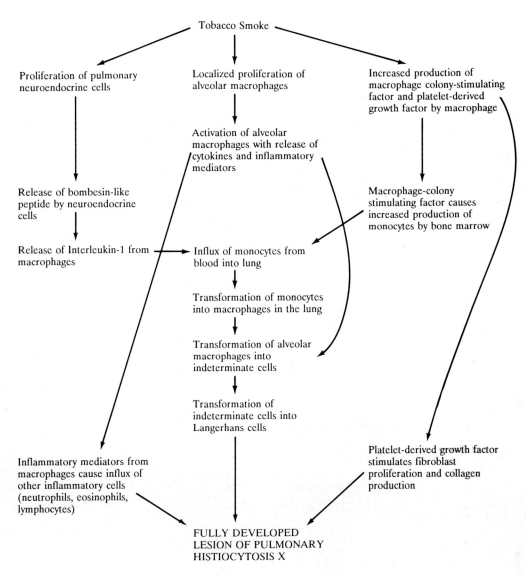

Fig. 17–1. Putative pathogenetic mechanism of pulmonary histiocytosis X

philic granuloma developed in a 22-year-old woman who had not been previously treated.[79]

More recently, Shanley et al.[80] reported a case of pulmonary histiocytosis X in an 18-year-old woman with Hodgkin's disease who was treated with eight courses of mechloretamine, Oncovin, procarbazine, prednisone, Adriamycin, bleomycin, vinblastine, and decarbazine. Coli et al.[81] also reported a case of pulmonary histiocytosis X in a 42-year-old male cigarette smoker who had been treated with cyclophosphamide, vincristine, procarbazine, and prednisone for mixed cellular Hodgkin's disease.

Physical examination findings are nonspecific and consist of diminished breath sounds, rales, wheezes, and rhonchi. In the majority of patients, routine laboratory tests such as complete blood counts or serum chemistry profiles are normal. Some patients will show a mild leukocytosis, usually less than 15,000/mm^3 or a mild anemia with a hemoglobin of 10–12 g/dl. Many who are symptomatic will have an elevated erythrocyte sedimentation rate.[37] Eosinophilia is rare.

Pulmonary function tests in patients with pulmonary histiocytosis X are usually abnormal, but the degree of abnormality varies considerably and in a few patients they may be normal. In our analysis of 31 patients,[32] all had an abnormal diffusing capacity ranging between 36% and 78% of predicted. In most patients, vital capacity and forced expiratory volume were close to normal.

The chest radiograph is abnormal in most patients and varies considerably. To some degree, the abnormality depends on the chronicity of the disease when the radiograph is taken. Various patterns described include a nodular, reticulonodular, interstitial, alveolar,

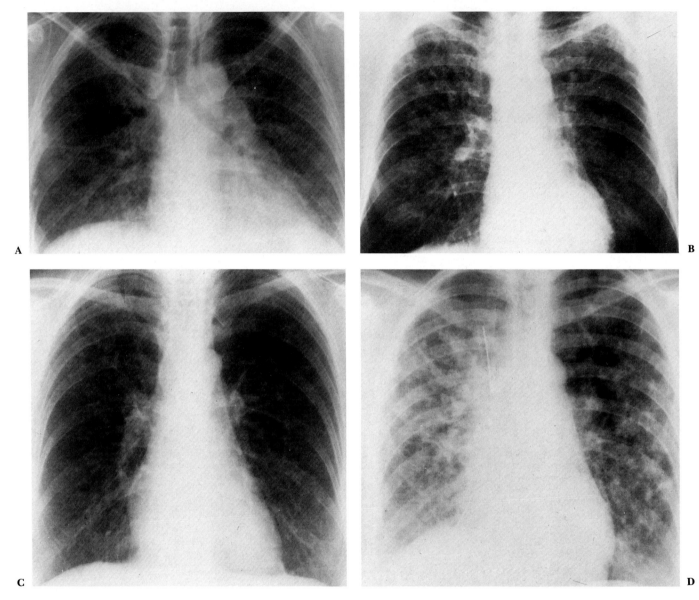

Fig. 17–2 A–D. Chest radiographs from four patients with pulmonary histiocytosis X. **A.** Diffuse reticulonodular infiltrate. **B.** Bilateral infiltrate with sparing of costophrenic angles. **C.** Bilateral micronodular infiltrate. **D.** Bilateral macronodular infiltrate, which can be mistaken for metastatic cancer.

and cystic type of change. Lacronique and colleagues[82] analyzed the radiographic changes in a semiquantitative manner by dividing the lungs horizontally and vertically and then classifying the changes according to a modification of the International Labor Organization scheme for pneumoconiosis. They used the following morphologic parameters in classifying the radiographic changes: (1) reticulation; (2) micronodules to 2 mm in diameter; (3) micronodules 2–5 mm in diameter; (4) micronodules 5–10 mm in diameter; (5) macronodules greater than 10 mm in diameter; (6) cysts to 10 mm in diameter; and (7) cysts or cavities more than 10 mm in diameter. They found that, for each type of lesion,

there was no statistical difference in the distribution of the various radiographic abnormalities between the two lungs and between central and peripheral regions of the lungs. They also found that reticulation, micronodules between 2 and 5 mm, and cysts to 10 mm in diameter were the most frequently observed abnormality and that these changes were most common in the mid- and lower lung fields, frequently sparing the costophrenic angles. From a practical point of view, the chest radiographic pattern seen in patients with pulmonary histiocytosis X varies considerably (Fig. 17–2). When the nodules approach 10 mm in diameter, a diagnosis of metastatic cancer is frequently included in the differen-

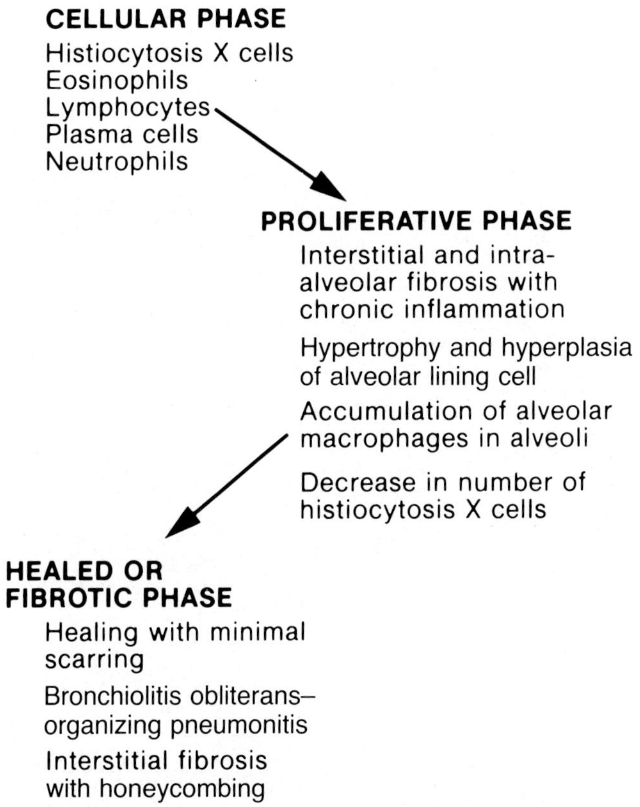

CELLULAR PHASE
Histiocytosis X cells
Eosinophils
Lymphocytes
Plasma cells
Neutrophils

PROLIFERATIVE PHASE
Interstitial and intra-
alveolar fibrosis with
chronic inflammation

Hypertrophy and hyperplasia
of alveolar lining cell

Accumulation of alveolar
macrophages in alveoli

Decrease in number of
histiocytosis X cells

**HEALED OR
FIBROTIC PHASE**
Healing with minimal
scarring

Bronchiolitis obliterans–
organizing pneumonitis

Interstitial fibrosis
with honeycombing

Fig. 17–3. Schematic diagram shows possible evolution of pulmonary histiocytosis X from cellular phase to either healing or diffuse interstitial fibrosis with honeycombing.

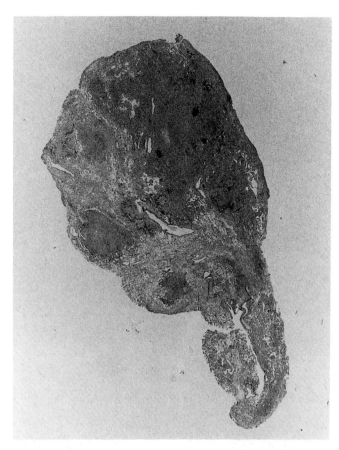

Fig. 17–4. Low-magnification view of open lung biopsy from patient with pulmonary histiocytosis X shows nodular regions of consolidation. ×3.

tial diagnosis. We evaluated standard chest radiographs, computed tomographic (CT) scans, and the results of pulmonary function tests in 17 patients with biopsy-proven pulmonary histiocytosis X and concluded that CT showed the morphology and distribution of lung abnormalities, CT findings also correlated better with diffusing capacity than plain radiographic abnormalities better than did radiography.[83] Taylor et al.[84] reported a case of pulmonary histiocytosis X in a 27-year-old, cigarette-smoking woman studied by high-resolution computed tomography that showed "cavitating" pulmonary nodules.

Pathologic Features

To understand the pathologic changes in pulmonary histiocytosis X, it is important to remember two facts: (1) As shown schematically in Figure 17–3, pulmonary histiocytosis X is a disease that may undergo a morphologic evolution; that is, it may progress from a cellular infiltrate composed of numerous histiocytosis X cells and various types of inflammatory cells to a relatively

acellular phase characterized by fibrosis and honeycombing with morphologic features identical to those seen in idiopathic pulmonary fibrosis; and (2) frequently a great deal of distortion of the usual pulmonary architecture occurs in cases of pulmonary histiocytosis X, obscuring the features that allow a definitive diagnosis. Fibrosis, a mixed inflammatory cell infiltrate, obliteration of blood vessels, and accumulation of intraalveolar macrophages may obscure aggregates of histiocytosis X cells that are the key to the histologic diagnosis.

The macroscopic features of pulmonary histiocytosis X are variable. Most frequently the peripheral lung tissue shows ovoid to irregularly shaped, well-demarcated grayish-white nodules that are separated from one another by relatively normal or slightly distorted lung tissue. These nodules are usually less than 1 cm in maximum dimension (Fig. 17–4), although occasionally they may be as large as 2 cm in diameter and be confused with metastatic tumor. The nodules of histiocytosis X cells and other inflammatory cells occasionally become cystic, but in this author's experience they do

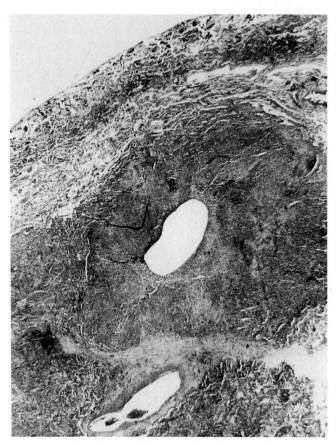

Fig. 17–5. Nodule of histiocytosis X cells and inflammatory cells shows central cystic region. ×75.

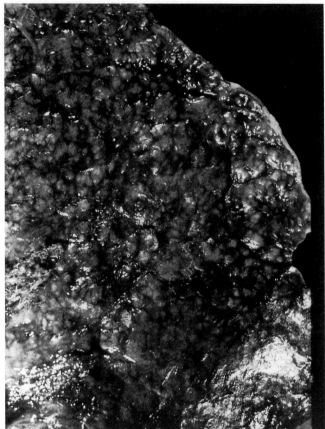

Fig. 17–7. Scarred nodular pleural surface of honeycombed lung secondary to end-stage pulmonary histiocytosis X.

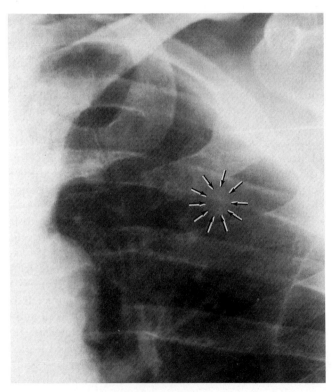

not show necrosis in the cystic areas (Fig. 17–5); the mechanism of this cystic change is uncertain. We have diagnosed one histologically proven case of pulmonary histiocytosis X presenting as an isolated pulmonary nodule (Fig. 17–6). If the disease becomes chronic there may be a progression to end-stage pulmonary fibrosis, in which the pleural surface becomes scarred and nodular (Fig. 17–7) and the parenchyma shows fibrosis and honeycombing (Fig. 17–8) just like that seen in end-stage idiopathic pulmonary fibrosis (see Chapter 20). As in any cause of pulmonary fibrosis, cor pulmonale may occur with right-ventricular hypertrophy (Fig. 17–9).

The key to the histologic diagnosis is to find aggregates of histiocytosis X cells (Figs. 17–10 through 17–12). These cells are medium to large and have pale convoluted nuclei with small-to-medium-sized nucleoli in hematoxylin and eosin-stained sections. The cytoplasm is pale pink and the cytoplasmic borders are

◁————————————————————

Fig. 17–6. Chest radiograph of 65-year-old man isolated left-upper-lobe nodule (*arrows*) that showed the histologic changes of pulmonary histiocytosis X.

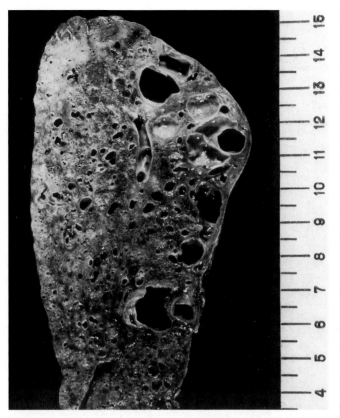

Fig. 17–8. Cut surface of lung seen in Fig. 17–7 shows diffuse interstitial fibrosis with honeycombing.

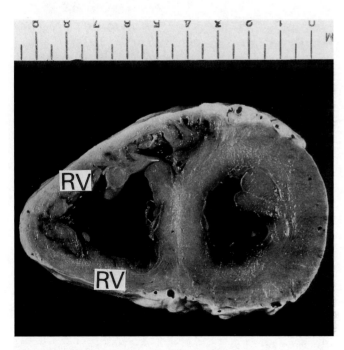

Fig. 17–9. Cross section of heart from patient whose lung is shown in Figs. 17–7 and 17–8. Note right-ventricular hypertrophy (RV).

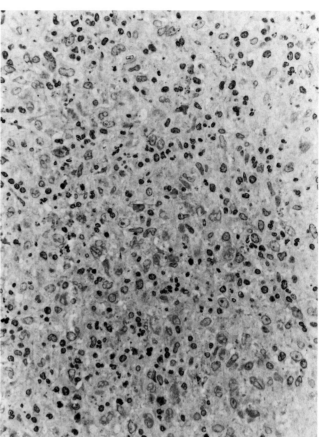

Fig. 17–10. Low-power magnification of "characteristic" nodule composed of histiocytosis X cells and various inflammatory cells. ×330.

poorly defined. In most cases the histiocytosis X cells are associated with various types of inflammatory cells, most notably eosinophils but also lymphocytes, plasma cells, and polymorphonuclear leukocytes (Figs. 17–13 and 17–14). The number of these inflammatory cells is highly variable; in some cases the histiocytosis X cells will be masked by eosinophils, which will sometimes be so numerous as to even form an eosinophilic microabscess. In other cases eosinophils and other inflammatory cells may be rare or absent.

The size, shape, and distribution of the infiltrate of histiocytosis X cells is variable from one case to the next and even within the same case. The infiltrate is frequently located around small bronchi and bronchioles, such as seen in respiratory bronchiolitis but may be interstitial away from small airways (Fig. 17–15). Histiocytosis X cells admixed with other inflammatory cells frequently infiltrate the walls of small blood vessels (Fig. 17–16) and also are found within the lumens of bronchioles and small bronchi (Fig. 17–17).

Immunohistochemical and ultrastructural identification of histiocytosis X cells has contributed to the diag-

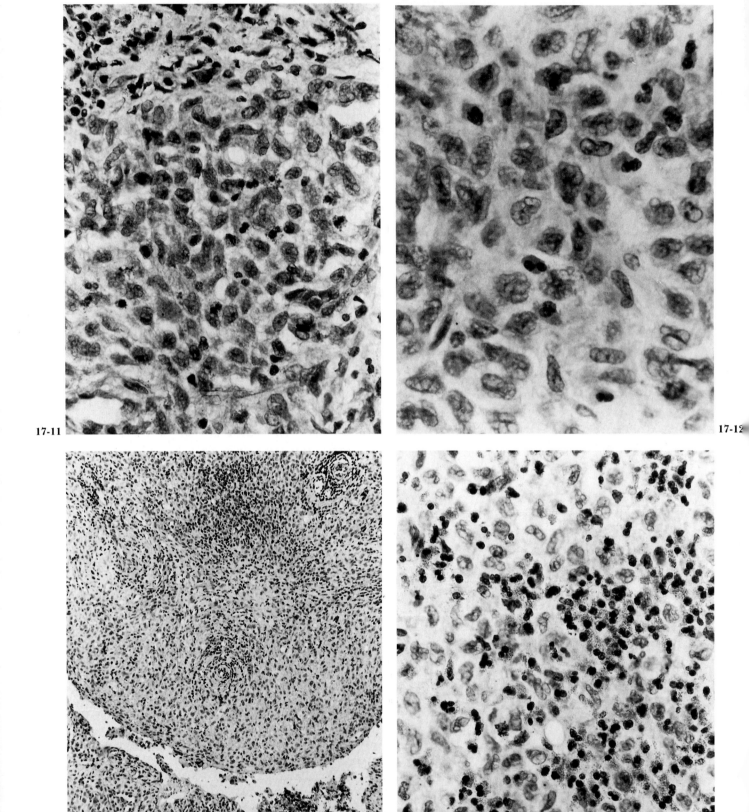

17-11

17-12

17-13

17-1

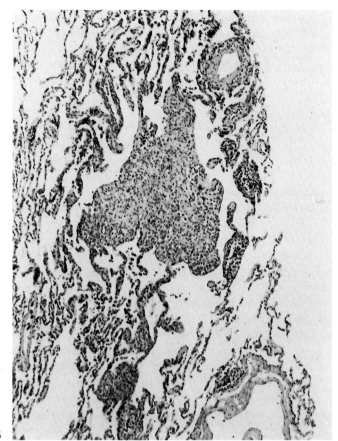

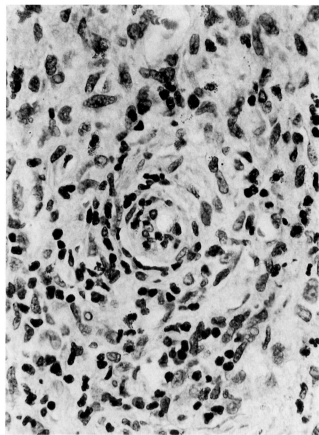

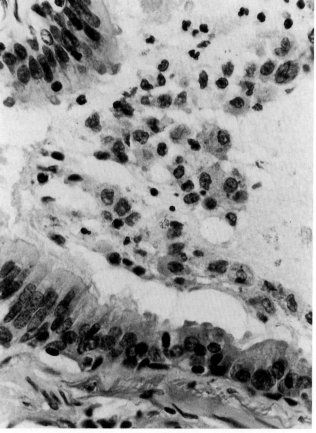

Fig. 17–15. Small interstitial nodule of histiocytosis X cells admixed with other inflammatory cells. ×75.

Fig. 17–16. Small pulmonary blood vessel is infiltrated by histiocytosis X cells and inflammatory cells. ×330.

Fig. 17–17. Bronchial lumen contains numerous histiocytosis X cells associated with a few other inflammatory cells. ×550.

◁ ————————————————

Fig. 17–11. Greater magnification of nodule composed mostly of histiocytosis X cells admixed with a few inflammatory cells. ×550.

Fig. 17–12. Histiocytosis X cells have highly convoluted nuclei with poorly defined cytoplasmic borders. A few eosinophils are admixed with histiocytosis X cells. ×775.

Fig. 17–13. Nodule is composed of histiocytosis X cells admixed with numerous inflammatory cells, most of which are lymphocytes and eosinophils. ×75.

Fig. 17–14. Histiocytosis X cells admixed with numerous eosinophils. Note granular cytoplasm of eosinophils. ×330.

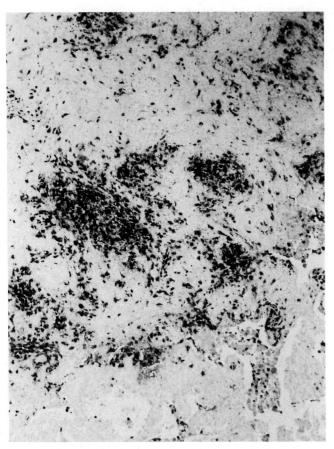

Fig. 17–18. Representative region of pulmonary histiocytosis X immunostained for S-100 protein. Black-staining S-100 protein-containing cells are easily distinguished from non-staining inflammatory cells and fibrovascular tissue. ×75.

nosis of this disease. Histiocytosis X cells contain S-100 protein, which can be easily identified in formalin-fixed paraffin-embedded tissue. Using an avidin–biotin complex immunoperoxidase technique, the number and distribution of histiocytosis X cells are easily recognized (Fig. 17–18). As discussed later, S-100 protein-containing Langerhans' cells are frequently present in other pulmonary diseases such as idiopathic pulmonary fibrosis, but do not occur in large aggregates as seen in histiocytosis X. By electron microscopy, aggregates of histiocytosis X cells are easily recognized by their highly convoluted nuclei composed of euchromatin with a prominent nuclear fibrous lamina (Fig. 17–19). In most cases they are admixed with eosinophils and other inflammatory cells (Fig. 17–20). The cytoplasm of histiocytosis X cells contains unique rod- and racquet-shaped granules (Fig. 17–21) that are identical to those seen in Langerhans' cells located in various tissues and organs of the body. These granules are present throughout the cytoplasm of the cells, but frequently may be seen budding off the Golgi membranes or in

continuity with the cell membrane. The exact function of the granules remains a mystery. The ameboid nature of the histiocytosis X cells is easily recognized ultrastructurally. These cells "infiltrate" into the alveolar epithelium, wedging themselves between alveolar lining cells and the alveolar basal lamina (Fig. 17–22), and are often present within alveolar spaces.

Variable degrees of fibrosis and distortion of the usual pulmonary architecture are usually associated with the histiocytosis X cells and other inflammatory cells. These changes can cause difficulty in making a pathologic diagnosis of pulmonary histiocytosis X. Haphazard fibrosis is seen to some degree in association with the histiocytosis X cells and other inflammatory cells (Fig. 17–23) in most cases, and as a rule seems to increase with a concomitant decrease in histiocytosis X cells. This may be part of the usual evolution of this disease, and can lead to regions of lung tissue having the appearance of organizing pneumonitis–bronchiolitis obliterans (Fig. 17–24).

The lung tissue adjacent to cellular regions of histiocytosis X is frequently abnormal. The tissue often shows some degree of interstitial fibrosis, indistinguishable from idiopathic pulmonary fibrosis, and may show a pattern identical to that described in desquamative interstitial pneumonitis[85] (Fig. 17–25). Alveolar lining cell hypertrophy and hyperplasia is frequently seen (Fig. 17–26), and may produce an adenomatous pattern (Fig. 17–27). This may lead to a false-positive cytology (Fig. 17–28). The abnormal lung parenchyma at the edges of or adjacent to regions of cellular histiocytosis X may contain Langerhans–histiocytosis X cells as demonstrated by S-100 protein staining (Fig. 17–29), but these cells are not in aggregates.

In the majority of cases of pulmonary histiocytosis X, varying numbers of smoker's macrophages are observed. These are frequently associated with the histiocytosis X cells and other inflammatory cells, and resemble alveolar macrophages except that they have tannish-brown cytoplasm in hematoxylin and eosin-stained sections (Fig. 17–30). Ultrastructurally the lysosomes of smoker's macrophages contain small needle-shaped crystals (Fig. 17–31), which represent aluminum silicate, a contaminant that is not removed from the tobacco leaves during processing. The presence of these cells in significant numbers reflects the fact that most people who develop pulmonary histiocytosis X are cigarette smokers.

Morphogenesis of Pulmonary Histiocytosis X

The morphogenesis of pulmonary histiocytosis X is poorly understood. In any given case one can find

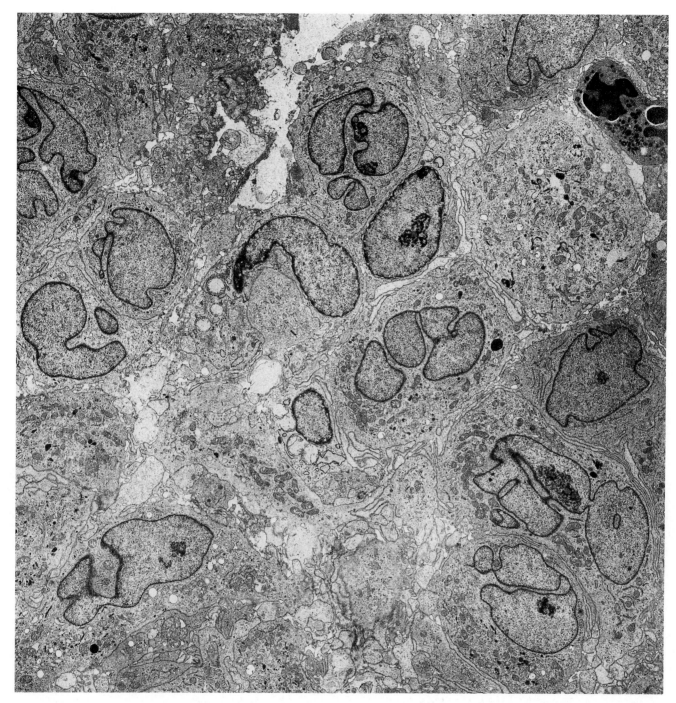

Fig. 17–19. Electron micrograph shows aggregates of histiocytosis X cells. Note convoluted nuclei and prominent nuclear fibrous lamina. ×6,400.

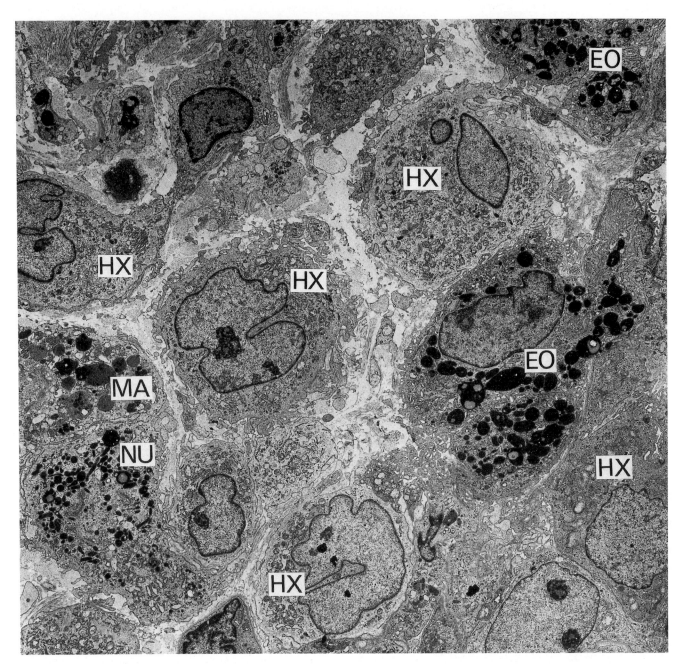

Fig. 17–20. Histiocytosis X cells (HX) are admixed with other inflammatory cells: eosinophil (EO), neutrophil (NU), and macrophage (MA). ×6,400.

Fig. 17–21. Greatly magnified histiocytosis X cell shows rod- and racquet-shaped cytoplasmic Langerhans' cell granules. ×69,000.

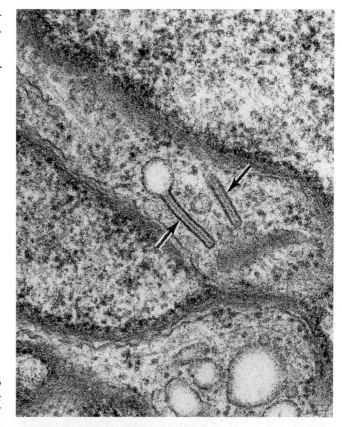

Fig. 17–22. Histiocytosis X cell (HX) is pushing between two alveolar type II cells. Note lamellar bodies in cytoplasm of type II cells (*arrows*). ×16,000.

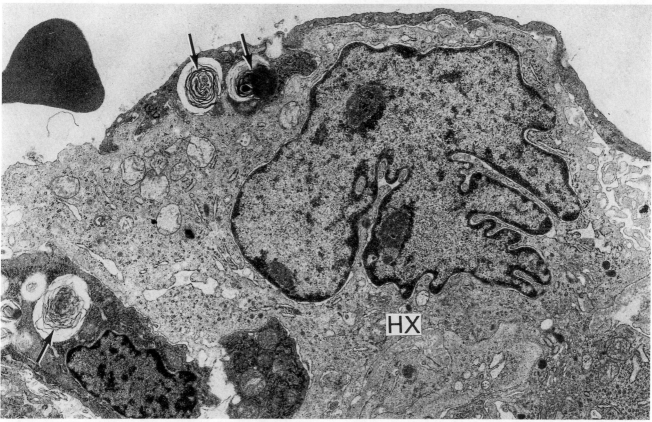

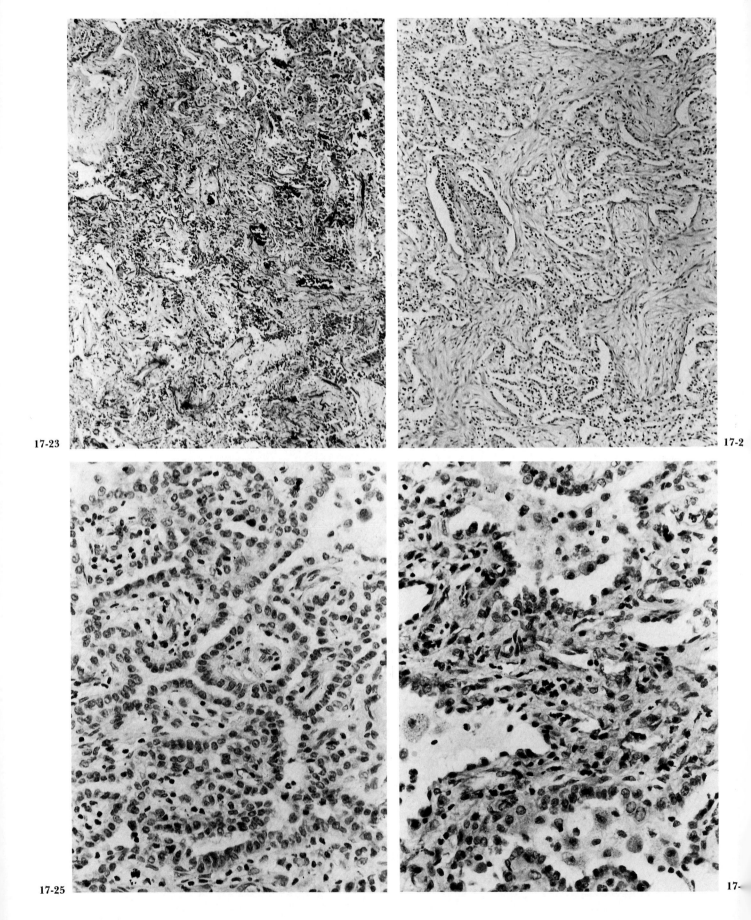

17-23

17-2

17-25

17-

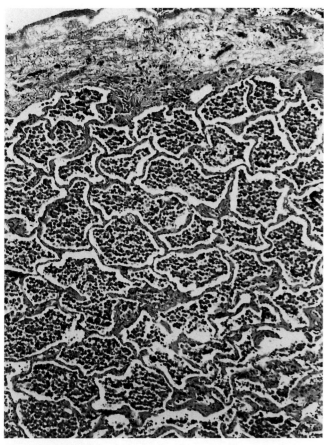

17-27

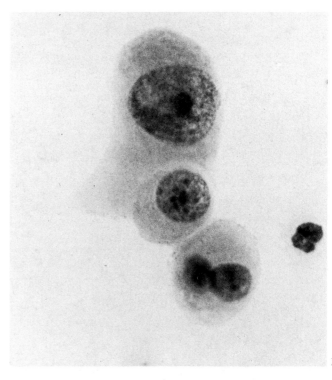

17-28

Fig. 17–27. Relative uniform hypertrophy and hyperplasia of alveolar lining cells produced this adenomatous pattern. ×330.

Fig. 17–28. Group of highly atypical alveolar cells identified in sputum from patient with pulmonary histiocytosis X. ×775.

Fig. 17–29. Region of desquamative interstitial pneumonitis adjacent to area of cellular histiocytosis X shows numerous dendritic cells immunostaining (black) for S-100 protein. ×75.

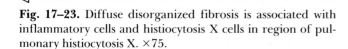

Fig. 17–23. Diffuse disorganized fibrosis is associated with inflammatory cells and histiocytosis X cells in region of pulmonary histiocytosis X. ×75.

Fig. 17–24. Region of lung tissue from case of pulmonary histiocytosis X shows organizing pneumonitis-bronchiolitis obliterans characterized by filling of alveoli and bronchioles with proliferating connective tissue. ×75.

Fig. 17–25. Area of lung tissue adjacent to region of cellular histiocytosis X shows pattern of desquamative interstitial pneumonitis characterized by accumulation of alveolar macrophages in alveolar spaces. ×75.

Fig. 17–26. Region of pulmonary histiocytosis X. Prominent alveolar lining cell hypertrophy and hyperplasia are associated with interstitial inflammation and fibrosis. ×330.

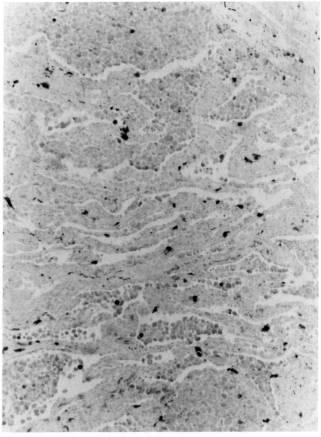

17-29

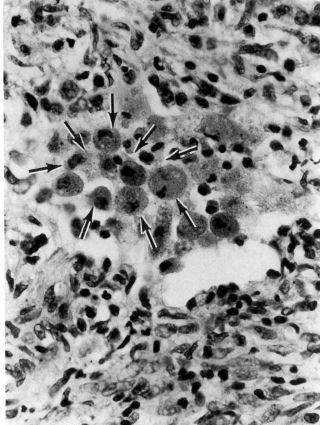

17-30

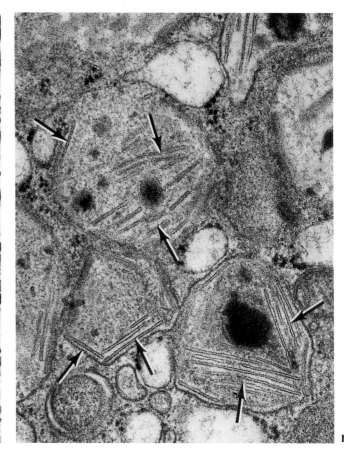

17-3

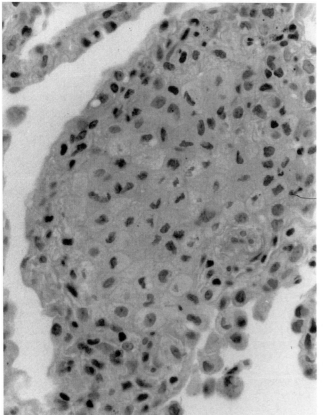

17-32

lesions composed predominantly of Langerhans' cells, others composed of a mixture of Langerhans' cells, eosinophils, neutrophils, lymphocytes, and plasma cells, and others showing these cellular elements with varying degrees of fibrosis and distortion of the usual architecture.

In this author's opinion, the initial lesions is a respiratory bronchiolitis-type change with proliferation of Langerhans' cells and transformation into indeterminate cells and Langerhans' cells (Fig. 17–32). This can be documented by immunohistochemistry using S-100 protein identification of Langerhans cells or by electron microscopy. In this location (bronchiole), the Langerhans' cells are smaller and have a slightly more convo-

Fig. 17–30. Collection of smoker's macrophages (*arrows*) admixed with histiocytosis X cells and other inflammatory cells. H and E, ×330.

Fig. 17–31. Smoker's macrophages show numerous cytoplasmic lysosomes, which contain needle-like aluminum silicate crystals (*arrows*) ×43,000.

Fig. 17–32. Lumen of respiratory bronchiole showing accumulation of histiocytes, some of which have an appearance consistent with Langerhans cells. ×300.

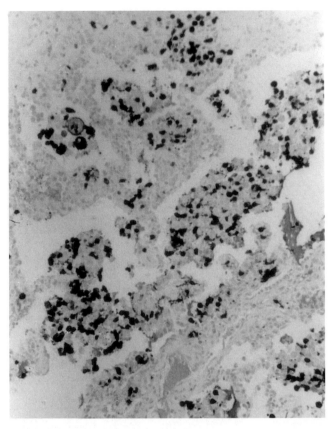

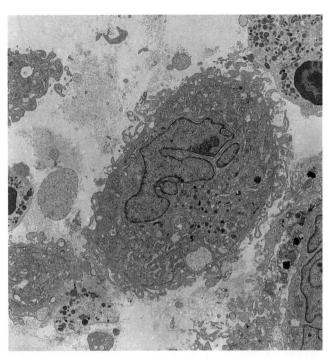

Fig. 17–34. This electron micrograph shows what we believe represents an indeterminate cells. The cell has a convoluted nucleus and a few primary lysosomes but lacks cytoplasmic Langerhans' cell granules. ×6,300.

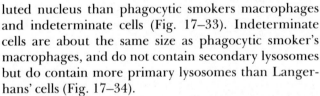

Fig. 17–33. When the section is stained for S100 protein the positive staining Langerhans' cells are easily identified. **A** × 300. ×125.

luted nucleus than phagocytic smokers macrophages and indeterminate cells (Fig. 17–33). Indeterminate cells are about the same size as phagocytic smoker's macrophages, and do not contain secondary lysosomes but do contain more primary lysosomes than Langerhans' cells (Fig. 17–34).

With the increase in the number of Langerhans' cells there appears to be a migration of these cells from within the bronchioles and alveoli into the interstitium, followed by compression and collapse of the alveoli and bronchioles (Fig. 17–35). As the lesions enlarge, the usual pulmonary architecture becomes more distorted. When the nodules of pulmonary histiocytosis X are greater than 1 cm in diameter, it becomes difficult to sort out underlying pulmonary architecture and to determine the evolution of the lesion. As described by Fukada et al.,[86] one can often see "bare" basal lamina and altered elastic tissue in the "late stage" of pulmonary histiocytosis X, as well as interstitial and intraalveolar fibrosis (Fig. 17–36). This author remains uncertain if the mechanism postulated by Fukada et al.,[86] that in the early stage of pulmonary histiocytosis X the epithelial cells are damaged and detached from base-

ment membranes, is correct. A proposed morphogenetic scheme of pulmonary histiocytosis X is shown in Fig. 17–37.

Differential Pathologic Diagnosis

Pulmonary histiocytosis X may be misdiagnosed pathologically (Table 17–2) and not included in the clinical differential diagnosis (Table 17–3). This is probably due to the relative low incidence of this disease and its variable histologic appearance, which may in part represent morphologic evolution of the disease.

By themselves, reactive endothelial cells and lipoblasts may have an appearance resembling Langerhans–histiocytosis X cells. The resemblance is primarily nuclear, and neither endothelial cells nor lipoblasts will have cytoplasmic Langerhans' cell granules. Reactive type II pneumocytes will also occasionally develop a nuclear profile resembling Langerhans–histiocytosis X cells, but will also lack Langerhans' cell granules. Most alveolar macrophages and smoker's macrophages have convoluted nuclei and can resemble Langerhans' cells.

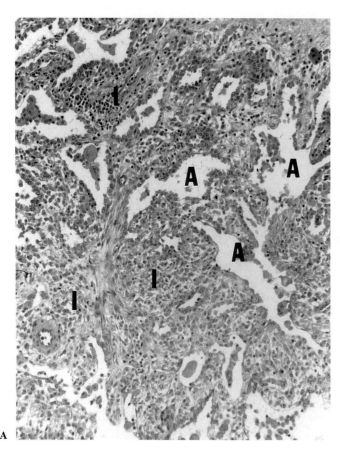

17-35A

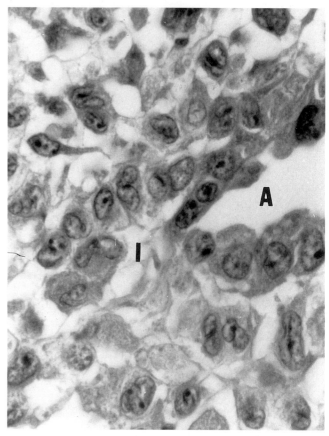

17-35

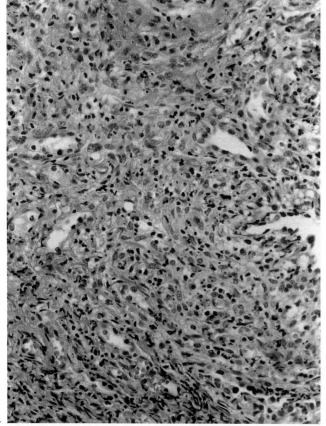

17-36A

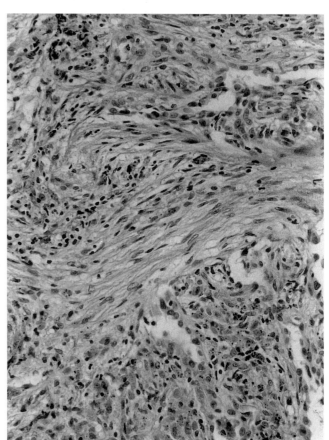

17-3

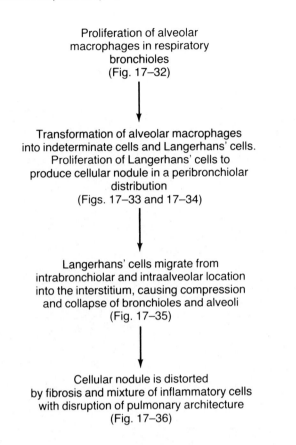

Proliferation of alveolar
macrophages in respiratory
bronchioles
(Fig. 17–32)

Transformation of alveolar macrophages
into indeterminate cells and Langerhans' cells.
Proliferation of Langerhans' cells to
produce cellular nodule in a peribronchiolar
distribution
(Figs. 17–33 and 17–34)

Langerhans' cells migrate from
intrabronchiolar and intraalveolar location
into the interstitium, causing compression
and collapse of bronchioles and alveoli
(Fig. 17–35)

Cellular nodule is distorted
by fibrosis and mixture of inflammatory cells
with disruption of pulmonary architecture
(Fig. 17–36)

Fig. 17–37. Putative morphogenesis of pulmonary histiocytosis X.

Table 17–2. Initial pathologic diagnosis in 31 cases of pulmonary histiocytosis X[a]

Diagnosis	Number of cases
Pulmonary histiocytosis X	16
Interstitial fibrosis-pneumonitis	7
Nonspecific inflammation	2
Chronic pneumonitis	1
Malignant histiocytic tumor	1
Malignant tumor-?intravascular, bronchiolar, and alveolar cell tumor	1
Lung cancer-bronchoalveolar cell carcinoma	1
Histoplasmosis	1
No pathologic diagnosis	1

[a] Reprinted with permission.[32]

Fig. 17–35 A,B. As the lesion of primary pulmonary histiocytosis X progresses, the Langerhans' cells seem to migrate from the alveoli into the interstitium (A, alveoli; I, interstitium). **A** × 125, **B** × 550.

Fig. 17–36 A. As pulmonary histiocytosis X progresses interstitial fibrous tissue often develops in association with the histiocytes and other inflammatory cells. ×125. **B.** Areas of organizing pneumonia can also develop as shown in the intraluminal fibrous tissue in this photograph. ×125.

Table 17–3. Clinical differential diagnoses in 31 cases of primary pulmonary histiocytosis X[a]

Diagnosis	Number of cases
Idiopathic interstitial fibrosis	10
Interstitial lung disease	8
Tuberculosis	7
Hypersensitivity pneumonitis	5
Sarcoidosis	4
Lung cancer	4
Pulmonary histiocytosis X	4
Drug-induced pulmonary disease	3
Wegener's granulomatosis	3
Desquamative interstitial pneumonitis	3
Collagen vascular-associated lung disease	2
Pulmonary vasculitis	2
Bronchopneumonia	1
Coccidiomycosis	1
Crytococcosis	1
Histoplasmosis	1
Fungal infection	1
Influenza pneumonia	1
Mycoplasma pneumonia	1
Psittacosis	1
Lymphangietic tumor	1
Metastatic tumor	1
Hodgkin's disease	1
Recurrent lymphoma	1
Goodpasture's syndrome	1
Pulmonary hemosiderosis	1
Pulmonary alveolar proteinosis	1
Emphysema-α-1-antitrypsin deficiency	1
Shaver's disease	1
Chronic bronchitis	1

[a] Reprinted with permission.[32]

Langerhans' cells are generally nonphagocytic and are usually smaller than smoker's macrophages. As previously discussed in the sections on pathogenesis and morphogenesis, Langerhans' cells are probably derived from alveolar macrophages that proliferate in response to cigarette smoke and it is therefore not surprising of the morphologic similarity between alveolar macrophages and Langerhans' cells.

Reactive eosinophilic pleuritis was described by Askin and colleagues[87] in 1977 as a condition to be distinguished from pulmonary eosinophilic granuloma. It is considered to be a nonspecific reaction to pleural injury and is composed of mononuclear histiocytes with convoluted nuclei resembling Langerhans'–histiocytosis X cells and other inflammatory cells including numerous eosinophils and reactive mesothelial cells (Fig. 17–38 and 17–39). The mononuclear histiocytes may have convoluted nuclei, but lack cytoplasmic Langerhans' cell granules and do not show immunostaining for S-100 protein. We have seen one case of pulmonary histiocytosis X associated with reactive eosinophilic pleuritis in which there was no clinically documented pneumothorax.[32]

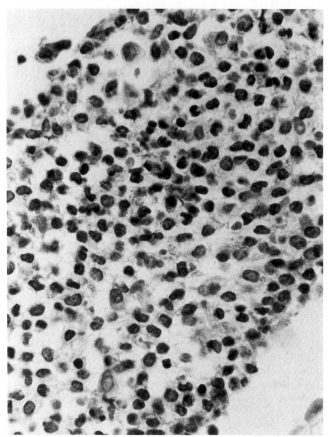

Fig. 17–38. Region of reactive eosinophilic pleuritis is composed of histiocytes with convoluted nuclei resembling histiocytosis X cells plus eosinophils and reactive mesothelial cells. ×330.

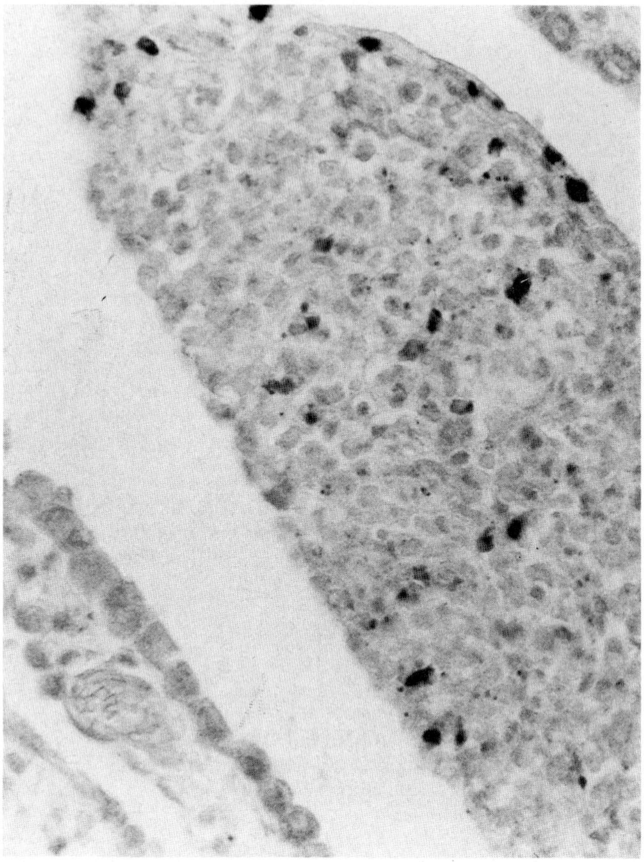

Fig. 17–39. Region of reactive eosinophilic pleuritis immunostained for S-100 protein. Histiocytes show no immunostaining. The few cells that appear positive (black) are eosinophils exhibiting endogenous peroxidase activity that was not blocked with hydrogen peroxide treatment. ×330.

In this author's experience, pulmonary histiocytosis X is most frequently misdiagnosed as interstitial pulmonary fibrosis (usual interstitial pneumonitis—idiopathic fibrosing alveolitis) (Table 17–2). This is not surprising since fibrosis is a prominent component of pulmonary histiocytosis X, and in some instances it is possible that some cases of pulmonary fibrosis represent histiocytosis X in evolution or "end-stage" histiocytosis X. Interstitial eosinophils may be observed in cases of pulmonary fibrosis, and as discussed in Chapter 20, Langerhans' cells are present in the majority of cases as shown by S-100 protein immunostaining and electron microscopy.[88] We have also observed several cases of organizing pneumonitis-bronchiolitis obliterans which, when examined by S-100 protein immunostaining or electron microscopy, contained numerous Langerhans' cells (Fig. 17–40); these cases may also represent a stage of pulmonary histiocytosis X.

In our study of 31 cases, primary pulmonary histiocytosis X was also misdiagnosed as bronchioloalveolar cell carcinoma, desquamative interstitial pneumonitis, and several other conditions[32] (Table 17–2). In the same study we identified two cases of lung cancer (one adenocarcinoma and one squamous carcinoma) coexistent with pulmonary histiocytosis X. Interestingly, the majority of pulmonary adenocarcinomas have Langerhans' cells associated with the tumor cells,[89] and we have previously postulated that some cases of bronchioloalveolar cell carcinoma of the lung may arise in regions of scarring secondary to preexisting pulmonary histiocytosis X.[90] However, Lombard et al.[91] reported 4 patients who developed pulmonary histiocytosis X and lung cancer (2 cases of large cell undifferentiated carcinoma, 1 case of adenocarcinoma, and 1 case of squamous carcinoma). They were unable to show a relationship between the fibrosis of pulmonary histiocytosis X and lung cancer and believed the cancers were more likely caused by cigarette smoking. Sadoun et al.[92] reported 5 cases of lung cancer in 93 patients with pulmonary histiocytosis X and also concluded that cig-

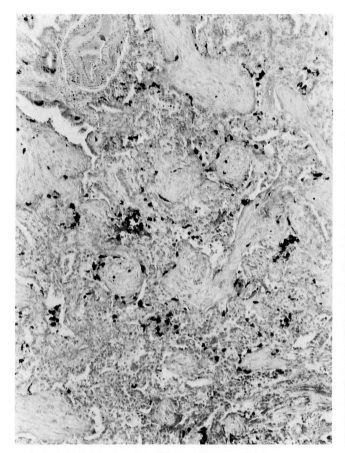

Fig. 17–40. Region of organizing pneumonitis–bronchiolitis obliterans immunostained for S-100 protein. Numerous positive-staining (black) Langerhans' cells suggest an evolving stage of histiocytosis X. ×75.

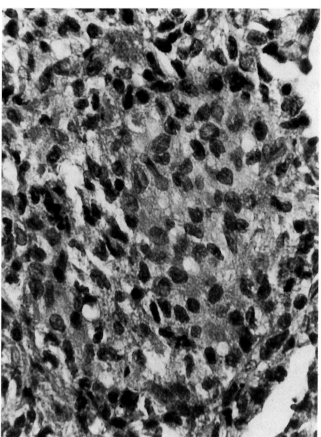

Fig. 17–41. Region of transbronchial biopsy shows collections of histiocytic-appearing cells with convoluted nuclei, suggesting diagnostic possibility of histiocytosis X. ×550.

arette smoking played the dominant role in the pathogenesis of the cancers. Tomasheski et al.[93] found a high prevalence of pulmonary and extrapulmonary neoplasms in patients with pulmonary eosinophilic granuloma. Ten of 21 patients had neoplasms, which included 3 lung carcinomas, 2 breast carcinomas, 1 transitional cell carcinoma of bladder, 1 nodular sclerosing Hodgkin's disease, 1 well-differentiated lymphocytic lymphoma, 1 metastatic large cell undifferentiated carcinoma, 1 peripheral carcinoid tumor of lung, and 1 ganglioneuroma of the mediastinum. They suggested their study showed a significantly nonrandom association between neoplasms and pulmonary histiocytosis X.

Hodgkin's disease, specifically the mixed cellular subtype, and other hematopoietic neoplasms such as malignant histiocytosis have some features that raise the possibility of pulmonary histiocytosis X. These conditions can usually be ruled out by immunostaining for S-100 protein, because neither will have significant numbers of S-100-positive Langerhans'-histiocytosis X cells.

Approach to the Diagnosis

The diagnosis of pulmonary histiocytosis X can be suspected clinically in a cigarette-smoking person 15–45 years old, with an illness characterized by cough, fever, and chest pain, whose chest radiograph shows a bilateral nodular or reticulonodular infiltrate. Most laboratory tests are normal or only mildly abnormal, and a positive diagnosis usually requires an open lung biopsy. We reported that a morphologic diagnosis of pulmonary histiocytosis X can be made in some cases from a transbronchial biopsy if the diagnosis is considered and if tissue is available for ultrastructural examination.[32] Figure 17–41 shows a portion of a transbronchial biopsy specimen from a 15-year-old boy with a bilateral reticulonodular infiltrate on chest radiograph that contains aggregates of histiocytic-appearing cells, thus raising the possibility of pulmonary histiocytosis X. When examined by electron microscopy, these cells have the typical ultrastructural appearance of histiocytosis X cells (Fig. 17–42), containing pathognomonic

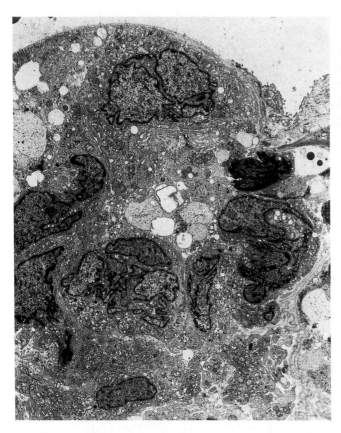

Fig. 17–42. When examined by electron microscopy, tissue shown in Figure 14–54 is composed of collections of cells with highly convoluted nuclei strongly suggestive of histiocytosis X cells. ×4,100.

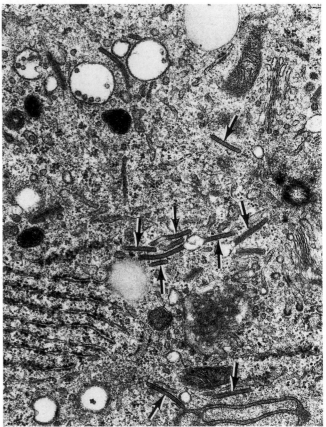

Fig. 17–43. Cytoplasm of cells shown in Fig. 14–55 contains numerous Langerhans' cell granules (*arrows*). ×26,500.

cytoplasmic Langerhans' cell granules (Fig. 17–43). In our series of 31 cases,[32] the diagnosis was made in five patients from transbronchial biopsy specimens, specifically with the aid of electron microscopy. It is for cases such as these that we routinely obtain transbronchial biopsy tissue specimens for ultrastructural examination. Contrary to our findings, Wall and colleagues[94] compared pathologic diagnoses from transbronchial biopsy specimens versus open lung biopsy specimens and found that histiocytosis X was one of the most common diseases not diagnosed by transbronchial biopsies. They did not use electron microscopy in their study.

One might logically question whether the demonstration of S-100 protein-positive cells in the transbronchial biopsy specimen would aid in the diagnosis of pulmonary histiocytosis X. Chondrocytes, fat cells and serous cells forming glands in the bronchial mucosa also show immunostaining for S-100 protein, but the main problem in using this technique as an aid to diagnosis is that small tissue specimens such as those obtained via transbronchial biopsy usually show too high levels of background staining and edge effect to be interpretable. In

the five cases of pulmonary histiocytosis X diagnosed by transbronchial biopsy cited previously,[32] we performed immunostains for S-100 protein but were unable to interpret them because of artifactual staining.

Langerhan's cells–histiocytosis X cells have been extensively evaluated immunohistochemically.[95–105] The reported immunohistochemical phenotype of Langerhans' cells/histiocytosis X cells is shown in Table 17–4. No antigen by itself, or groups of antigens, are absolutely specific for Langerhans' cells–histiocytosis X cells. Only the ultrastructural identification of Langerhans' cell granules is specific for the identification of these cells. This author strongly agrees with the comments of Baumal et al.[106] that S-100 protein is a useful but nonspecific marker in diagnostic pathology. It must be used intelligently, and in the context of other clinical and laboratory features of a given case. I also agree with the report of Cagle et al.,[99] specifically that the number of S-100 protein-positive histiocytes in a lesion can be over- or underrepresented by technical problems, and that S-100 protein-negative histiocytes are not Langerhans' cells–histiocytosis X cells. In this author's opinion, the reports indicating that in a certain percentage of

Table 17–4. Reported immunohistochemical phenotype of Langerhans' cells–histiocytosis X cells

Positive	Negative
S-100 protein	Leu-M1
CD-1$_a$ (OKT6)	LN-1
HLA-DR antigen	Leukocyte-common antigen
Peanut agglutinin^a	Epithelial membrane antigen^b
Vimentin	Pan-T cell antigen^c
LN2	CD2
LN3	CD3
LeuM1 after neuramidase	CD5
treatment^d	Pan-B cell antigen^c
Antimacrophage antibodies	CD19
KPT^e	CD22
Anti-Mac^e	
Alpha-1-antichymotrypsin^e	
Lysozome^e	
CD11$_c$^{d}	
CD$_w$32^d	
CD68^d	
Neuron-specific enolase^f	

^{a} Two of 12 cases of histiocytosis X positive.[97]
^{b} EMA reported negative in 15 cases.[98]
^{c} Sixteen cases evaluated, 5 of which had frozen sections available. Pan-T cell antigens, pan-B-cell antigens, and most macrophage antigens detected only in frozen section material.[104]
^{d} Leu-M1-positive only after pretreatment of tissue with neuramidase, which removed sialic acid.[100]
^{e} Seventeen cases evaluated, all positive for KP1 and anti-Mac in 3%–35% of cells; 11/17 cases positive for lysozyme and alpha-1-chymotrypsin in 1%–23% of cells.[101]
^{f} Eight cases evaluated, all cutaneous histiocytosis X. All cases positive for neuron-specific enolase with 70–90% of cells showing positive staining.[105]

histiocytosis X cases the Langerhan's cells–histiocytosis X cells are S-100 protein negative, or do not contain Langerhans' cell granules by ultrastructural examination, indicate either technical problems in demonstrating S-100 protein, inexperience with or sampling problems in ultrastructural identification, or incorrect diagnosis. We have found[32] that Langerhans' cell granules are fairly easy to identify in tissue retrieved from paraffin blocks and processed for ultrastructural examination.

The diagnosis of pulmonary histiocytosis X from open lung biopsy specimens may also be difficult. The diagnosis rests on the identification of aggregates of histiocytosis X cells admixed with other inflammatory cells frequently in association with varying degrees of interstitial fibrosis, inflammation, and cystic change. Immunostaining for S-100 protein can accentuate the aggregates of histiocytosis X cells, and documentation by electron microscopy can be done.

As indicated previously, pulmonary histiocytosis X is a disease that may undergo morphologic evolution, characteristically progressing from a cellular phase to a more fibrotic stage with some cases progressing to end-stage interstitial fibrosis with honeycombing. Webber and colleagues[107] studied the usefulness of S-100 protein immunostaining in the diagnosis of eosinophilic granuloma of lung. In their immunohistochemical study they assumed, on the basis of nuclear configuration and size, that the cells showing S-100 protein immunostaining were Langerhans'–histiocytosis X cells. They found Langerhans' cells in most types of nonneoplastic lung disease examined, and indicated that in cases of active or resolving pulmonary histiocytosis X there were greater than 75 Langerhans'–histiocytosis X cells per 10 high-power fields, whereas in other conditions, including end-stage fibrosis secondary to histiocytosis X, there were less than 35 Langerhans' cells per 10 high-power fields.

Soler and colleagues[108] also demonstrated the diagnostic usefulness of identifying histiocytosis X cells via an immunohistochemical demonstration of S-100 protein and OKT-6 antigen. They performed double-labeling techniques and immunoelectron microscopy to show that the same cell displayed OKT-6 antigen on the cell membrane and S-100 protein in the cytoplasm and, by electron microscopy, had Langerhans' cell granules in cytoplasm. All nine cases of pulmonary histiocytosis X showed this reactivity while control specimens of other types of interstitial lung disease did not.

These investigators subsequently examined the cells in bronchoalveolar lavage specimens for OKT-6 antingen via immunofluorescence and immunoelectron microscopy.[109] They studied lavage fluid from 131 patients including 18 with pulmonary histiocytosis X, 43 with pulmonary sarcoidosis, 67 with miscellaneous pulmonary conditions, and 3 normal controls. In the 18 patients with pulmonary histiocytosis X, 5.29 ± 1.14% of cells labeled for OKT-6, and in 13 patients these were confirmed by immunoelectron microscopy to contain Langerhans' cell granules. In 43 patients with sarcoidosis, 3 control patients, and 61 of 67 patients with miscellaneous pulmonary conditions, less than 1% of the total cells labeled for OKT-6. In the 6 remaining patients, 1.3%–2.8% of cells labeled, and by immunoelectron microscopy these had general features of Langerhans cells' but lacked Langerhans' cell granules. Their data suggest that the identification of Langerhans' cells in bronchoalveolar lavage fluid may be diagnostically helpful in identifying those patients with pulmonary histiocytosis X. Avserwald et al.[110] evaluated the percentage of Langerhans' cells in bronchoalveolar lavage fluid from 6 patients with histologically proven pulmonary histiocytosis X, 88 patients with sarcoidosis, and 97 patients with miscellaneous pulmonary conditions. All patients with pulmonary histiocytosis X had more than 5% CD-1-positive cells, whereas patients with other pulmonary conditions showed no more than 3.6% CD-

1-positive cells. They found that the dividing line of 5% CD-1-positive cells was not influenced by patients' smoking habits and that the identification of CD-1-positive cells in bronchoalveolar fluid was useful in diagnosing pulmonary histiocytosis X. Similarly, we have identified histiocytosis X cells ultrastructurally in the sputum from a patient with known pulmonary histiocytosis X.[111]

Clinicopathologic Correlations

Little is known about the natural history of pulmonary histiocytosis X. In general the disease may pursue the following possible courses: (1) spontaneous resolution with complete disappearance of pulmonary infiltrates; (2) resolution of clinical signs and symptoms but persistence of an abnormal chest radiograph; (3) persistence of clinical disease and persisting but nonprogressive abnormal chest radiograph; (4) persistence of clinical signs and symptoms with progression of pulmonary disease to end-stage interstitial fibrosis and honeycombing; and (5) a rapidly progressive fatal pulmonary disease.

The correlation of the pathologic features of pulmonary histiocytosis X with the clinical courses of the disease listed here are not well understood. Basset et al.[30] found a poor prognosis in the young, the elderly, and those with multisystem disease, especially when there was skin involvement. Four children with acute disseminated histiocytosis X who died after a short illness are similar to 2 adult patients we described,[32] 1 whose disease involved bones and the other whose disease was confined to the lungs. Basset et al. also found that a history of repeated pneumothoraces was associated with a worse prognosis as was prolonged fever and weight loss. LaCronique and colleagues[82] found in a chest radiographic study of 50 patients with histiocytosis X that those 24 patients who remained stable or improved showed sparing of their costophrenic angles. Of the 13 patients in their series who deteriorated, 4 had costophrenic angle involvement at the onset of their disease. Unlike investigators of previously reported studies, these authors found no correlation between prognosis and a history of pneumothoraces.

Friedman et al.[31] found no definite clinical pathologic correlations, with the exception that desquamative interstitial pneumonitis like cellularity, was associated with a slightly better prognosis. Colby and Lombard[33] found that more than 85% of their 54 patients and the 100 patients with pulmonary histiocytosis X reported by Friedman et al. had a good prognosis. No histologic factor was identified that was of prognostic significance.

In our study of 31 patients with primary pulmonary histiocytosis X,[32] most improved spontaneously or with therapy, although 2 died of acute disease and 2 progressed from active cellular disease to end-stage honeycombing over a period of 6 years. The patients who had fever and weight loss usually required treatment. Several patients improved clinically with or without therapy but showed no improvement of their abnormal chest radiograph.

Powers et al.[112] recently reported a patient who was diagnosed as having pulmonary eosinophilic granuloma in 1956 and who died 25 years later of end-stage pulmonary fibrosis with honeycombing. The case is of interest because the patient had stable pulmonary function tests and lacked pulmonary symptoms over the first 14 years of his disease but still progressed to end-stage fibrosis.

A question that remains unanswered is whether histiocytosis X may in some instances be a malignant disease. Ben-Ezra et al.[113] reviewed morphologic and clinical data on 31 patients with histiocytosis X (no patients had primary pulmonary histiocytosis X) and divided the patients into four groups, based on the morphologic appearance of the Langerhans' cells and clinical course of the patients. They concluded that an entity of malignant histiocytosis X existed, characterized by morphologically malignant-appearing Langerhans' cells and an aggressive clinical course. They also concluded that the morphology of Langerhans' cells was an imperfect predictor of the clinical severity of histiocytosis X. Another study[114] evaluating the relationship between the histopathology of histiocytosis X and disease outcome failed to demonstrate a correlation.

A case of cutaneous histiocytosis X was reported in which a well-defined aneuploid subpopulation of cells was identified, although clinically the patient's disease regressed during a 6-month follow-up period and there was no evidence of systemic involvement.[115] Rabkin et al.[116] performed flow cytometry on formalin-fixed, paraffin-embedded tissue from 36 patients with histiocytosis X (none with primary pulmonary histiocytosis X) and found no cases to be identified with an aneuploid stem cell population. They concluded that flow cytometric DNA content analysis was not useful in predicting the clinical stage and outcome in histiocytosis X. However, Ornvold et al.[117] evaluated the DNA content in 26 formalin-fixed, paraffin-embedded histologic specimens from 18 children with histiocytosis X by flow cytometry, and found a significant aneuploid subpopulation of cells in 2 cases with a DNA index of 1.5. Both patients had disseminated disease but without organ dysfunction. They were treated with prednisone and were without signs of disease activity 1 and 10 years, respectively, after diagnosis. The author concluded that further investigation was necessary to determine if DNA aneuploidy had any value in predicting the course and outcome of histiocytosis X in children.

Treatment

Prednisone is usually initially given in those patients thought to require therapy. If it is ineffective in controlling the signs and symptoms, methotrexate is often given. There is no evidence that combination chemotherapy is more effective than a single agent in treating the disease.[118] As correctly pointed out by Friedman et al.[31] only a prospective randomized trial could provide useful information concerning the need and efficacy of various drugs used in treating pulmonary histiocytosis X.

A more interesting approach to the treatment of pulmonary histiocytosis X is found in the report by Von Essen et al.[119] They described a 35-year-old woman with an 18-pack-year history of cigarette smoking who presented with left-sided pleuritic chest pain and a chronic, nonproductive cough; her chest radiograph showed a bilateral reticulonodular interstitial infiltrate. Her infiltrate persisted and an open lung biopsy performed 8 months after presentation showed the changes of pulmonary histiocytosis X. Smoking cessation was suggested and the patient followed this recommendation. A repeat chest radiograph 2 years after biopsy showed complete resolution of her interstitial infiltrate. The authors suggested that smoking cessation was related to resolution of her infiltrate and should be recommended for all patients with pulmonary histiocytosis X. This author agrees with this conclusion because we[32] have observed several patients whose disease resolved after they stopped smoking. This observation would further implicate cigarette smoke in the pathogenesis of pulmonary histiocytosis X.

References

1. Langerhans P. Uber die Nerven der menschlichen Haut. Virchows Arch [Pathol Anat] 1868;44:325–337.
2. Birbeck MS, Breathnach AD, Everall JD. An electron microscope study of basal melanocytes and high-level clear cells (Langerhans cells) in vitiligo. J Invest Dermatol 1961;37:51–64.
3. Basset F, Turiaf J. Identification par la microscopie electronique de particles de nature probablement virale dans les lesions granulomateuses d'une histiocytose X pulmonaire. CR Seances Acad Sci (Paris) 1965;261:3701–3703.
4. Katz SI, Tamaki K, Sachs DH. Epidermal Langerhans cells are derived from cells originating in bone marrow. Nature (London) 1979;282:324–326.

5. Wood GS, Morhenn VB, Butcher EC, Kosek J. Langerhans cells react with panleukocyte monoclonal antibody. Ultrastructural documentation using a live cell suspension immunoperoxidase technique. J Invest Dermatol 1984;82:322–325.
6. Stingl G, Wolff-Schreiner EC, Pichler WJ, Gschnait F, Knapp W. Epidermal Langerhans cells bear Fc and C3 receptors. Nature (London) 1977;268:245–246.
7. Rowden G, Lewis MC, Sullivan AK. Ia antigen expression on human Langerhans cells. Nature (London) 1977;268:247–248.
8. Murphy GF, Bhan AK, Sato S, Harrist JJ, Mihm MC. Characterization of Langerhans cells by the use of monoclonal antibodies. Lab Invest 1981;45:465–468.
9. Favara BE, McCarthy RC, Mierau GW. Histiocytosis X. Hum Pathol 1983;14:663–676.
10. Beckstead JH, Wood GS, Turner RR. Histiocytosis X cells and Langerhans cells: enzyme histochemical and immunologic similarities. Hum Pathol 1984;15:826–833.
11. Takahashi K, Isobe T, Ohtsuki Y, Sonobe H, Takeda I, Akagi T. Immunohistochemical localization and distribution of S-100 protein in human lymphoreticular system. Am J Pathol 1984;116:497–503.
12. Wood GS, Turner RR, Shiurba RA, Eng L, Warnke RA. Human dendritic cells and macrophages: in situ immunophenotypic definition of subsets that exhibit specific morphologic and microenvironmental characteristics. Am J Pathol 1985;119:73–82.
13. Franklin WA, Mason DY, Pulford K, et al. Immunohistologic analysis of human mononuclear phagocytes and dendritic cells by using monoclonal antibodies. Lab Invest 1986;54:322–335.
14. Rochester CL, Goodell EM, Stoltenborg JK, Bowers WE. Dendritic cells from rat lung are potent accessory cells. Am Rev Respir Dis 1988;138:121–128.
15. Toews GB. Pulmonary dendritic cells: Sentinels of lung-associated lymphoid tissues. Am J Respir Cell Mol Biol 1991;4:204–205.
16. Murphy GF, Messadi D, Fonferko I, Hancock WW. Phenotypic transformation of macrophages to Langerhans cells in the skin. Am J Pathol 1986;123:401–406.
17. Komp DM. Langerhans cell histiocytosis. N Engl J Med 1987;316:747–748.
18. Hammar S. Langerhans cells. Path Ann 1988 (Part 2); 23:293–328.
19. Hammar S, Bockus D, Remington F, Bartha M. The widespread distribution of Langerhans' cells in pathologic conditions: An ultrastructural and immunohistochemical study. Hum Pathol 1986;17:894–905.
20. Farber S. The nature of "solitary or eosinophilic granuloma" of bone. Am J Pathol 1941;17:625.
21. Lichtenstein L. Histiocytosis X. Integration of eosinophilic granuloma of bone. "Letterer-Siwe disease" and "Schuller-Christian disease" as related manifestations of a single nosologic entity. Arch Pathol Lab Med 1953;56:84–102.
22. Lieberman P, Jones C, Dargeon H, Begg CF. A reappraisal of eosinophilic granuloma of bone, Hand-

Schuller-Christian syndrome and Letterer-Siwe syndrome. Medicine (Baltimore) 1969;48:375–400.

23. Vogel JM, Vogel P. Idiopathic histiocytosis: a discussion of eosinophilic granuloma, the Hand-Schuller-Christian syndrome and the Letterer-Siwe syndrome. Semin Hematol 1972;9:349–369.

24. Lewis JG. Eosinophilic granuloma and its variants with special reference to lung involvement. A report of 12 patients. Q J Med 1964;33:337–359.

25. Parkinson T. Eosinophilic xanthomatous granuloma with honeycomb lungs. Br Med J 1949;1:1029–1030.

26. Oswald N, Parkinson T. Honeycomb lungs. Q J Med 1949;18:1–20.

27. Cunningham GJ, Parkinson T. Diffuse cystic lungs of granulomatous origin. A histological study of six cases. Thorax 1950;5:43–58.

28. Farinacci CJ, Jeffrey HC, Lackey RW. Eosinophilic granuloma of the lung. Report of two cases. US Armed Forces Med J 1951;2:1085–1093.

29. Mazitello WF. Eosinophilic granuloma of the lung. N Engl J Med 1954;250:804–809.

30. Basset F, Corrin B, Spencer H, et al. Pulmonary histiocytosis X. Am Rev Respir Dis 1978;118:811–820.

31. Friedman PJ, Liebow AA, Sokoloff J. Eosinophilic granuloma of lung: clinical aspects of primary pulmonary histiocytosis in the adult. Medicine (Baltimore) 1981;60:385–396.

32. Hammar SP, Hallman KO, Winterbauer RH, et al. Primary pulmonary histiocytosis X: A clinicopathologic analysis of 31 patients.

33. Colby TV, Lombard C. Histiocytosis X in the lung. Hum Pathol 1983;14:847–856.

34. Villar TG, Avila R, Marques RA. Eosinophilic granuloma of the lung and the extrinsic pulmonary granulomatoses. Ann NY Acad Sci 1976;278:612–617.

35. Girard P, Bouzakoura C. Eosinophilic granuloma of the lung with sawdust and horse serum hypersensitivity. Clin Allergy 1974;4:71–78.

36. Auld D. Pathology of eosinophilic granuloma of lung. Arch Pathol Lab Med 1957;63:113–131.

37. Thompson JR, Langer S. Eosinophilic granuloma of the lungs. Dis Chest 1964;46:553–561.

38. King TE, Schwarz MI, Dreisin RE, Pratt DS, Theofilopoulos AN. Circulating immune complexes in pulmonary eosinophilic granuloma. Ann Intern Med 1979;91:397–399.

39. Dreisen RB, Schwarz MI, Theofilopoulous AN, Stanford RE. Circulating immune complexes in the idiopathic interstitial pneumonias. N Engl J Med 1978;298:353–357.

40. Haslam PM. Circulating immune complexes in patients with cryptogenic fibrosing alveolitis. Clin Exp Immunol 1979;37:381–390.

41. Ahnquist G, Holyoke JB. Congenital Letterer-Siwe disease (reticuloendotheliosis) in a term stillborn infant. J Pediatr 1960;57:897–904.

42. Claman HN, Suvatte V, Githens JH, Hathaway WE. Histiocytic reaction in dysgammaglobulinemia and congenital rubella. Pediatrics 1970;46:89–96.

43. van der Loo FM, van Muijen GNP, van Vloten WA, Beens W, Scheffer F, Meijer CJLM. C-type virus-like particles specifically localized in Langerhans cells and related cells of skin and lymph nodes of patients with mycosis fungoides and Sezary syndrome. Virchows Arch [Cell Pathol] 1979;31:193–203.

44. Osband ME, Lipton JM, Lavin P, et al. Histiocytosis X: demonstration of abnormal immunity, T-cell histamine H2-receptor deficiency and successful treatment with thymic extract. N Engl J Med 1981;304:146–153.

45. Miller LG, Goldstein G, Murphy M, Ginns LC. Reversible alterations in immunoregulatory T cells in smoking: Analysis by monoclonal antibodies and flow cytometry. Chest 1982;82:526–529.

46. Gerard JW, Heiner PC, Mink J, Meyers A, Dosman JA. Immunoglobulin levels in smokers and non-smokers. Ann Allergy 1980;44:261–262.

47. Ferson M, Edwards A, Lind A, Milton GW, Hersey P. Low natural killer-cell activity and immunoglobulin levels associated with smoking in human subjects. Int J Cancer 1979;23:603–609.

48. Cryer PE, Haymond MW, Santiago JV, Shah SD. Norepinephrine and epinephrine release and adrenergic mediation of smoking-associated hemodynamic and metabolic events. N Engl J Med 1976;295:573–577.

49. Miller CL, Baker CC. Changes in lymphocyte activity after injury. J Clin Invest 1977;63:202–210.

50. Wang BS, Heacock EH, Wu AV, Mannick JA. Generation of suppressor cells in mice after surgical trauma. J Clin Invest 1980;66:200–209.

51. Hoogsteden HC, van Hal PThW, Wijkhuijs JM, Hop W, Verkaik APK, Hilvering C. Expression of the CD11/CD18 cell surface adhesion glycoprotein family on alveolar macrophages in smokers and nonsmokers. Chest 1991;100:1567–1571.

52. Senior RM, Kuhn C, III. The pathogenesis of emphysema. In: Fishman AP, ed. Pulmonary diseases and disorders. 2d Ed. New York: McGraw-Hill, 1988;2:1209–1219.

53. Kasama T, Kobayashi K, Fukushima T, et al. Production of interleukin 1-like factor from human peripheral blood monocytes and polymorphonuclear leukocytes by superoxide anion: The role of interleukin 1 and reactive oxygen species in inflamed sites. Clin Immunol Immunopathol 1989;53:439–448.

54. Renoux M, Lemarié E, Renoux G. Interleukin-1 secretion by lipopolysaccharide-stimulated alveolar macrophages. Respiration 1989;55:158–168.

55. Rothlein R, Czajkowski M, O'Neill MM, Marlin SD, Mainolfi E, Merluzzi VJ. Induction of intercellular adhesion molecule 1 on primary and continuous cell lines by pro-inflammatory cytokines: Regulation by pharmacologic agents and neutralizing antibodies. J Immunol 1988;141:1665–1669.

56. Barbers RG, Evans MJ, Gong H, Jr., Tashkin DP. Enhanced alveolar monocytic phagocyte (macrophage) proliferation in tobacco and marijuana smokers. Am Rev Respir Dis 1991;143:1092–1095.

57. Coggle JE, Tarling JD. The proliferation kinetics of

pulmonary alveolar macrophages. J Leukocyte Biol 1984;35:317–327.

58. Bitterman PB, Saltzman LE, Adelberg S, Ferrans VJ, Crystal RG. Alveolar macrophage replication. One mechanism for the expansion of the mononuclear phagocyte population in the chronically inflamed lung. J Clin Invest 1984;74:460–469.

59. Evans MJ, Sherman MP, Campbell LA, Shami SG. Proliferation of pulmonary alveolar macrophages during postnatal development of rabbit lungs. Am Rev Respir Dis 1987;136:384–387.

60. Evans MJ, Shami SG, Martinez LA. Enhanced proliferation of pulmonary macrophages after carbon instillation in mice depleted of blood monocytes by strontium-89. Lab Invest 1986;54:154–159.

61. Blusse Van OudAlblas A, VanFurth R. Origin, kinetics and characteristics of pulmonary macrophages in the normal steady state. J Exp Med 1979;149:1504–1518.

62. Shellito J, Esparza C, Armstrong C. Maintenance of the normal rat alveolar macrophage cell population. The roles of monocyte influx and alveolar macrophage proliferation in situ. Am Rev Respir Dis 1987;135:78–82.

63. Golde DW, Byers LA, Finley TN. Proliferative capacity of human alveolar macrophages. Nature (London) 1974;247:373–375.

64. Sawyer RT. The significance of local resident pulmonary alveolar macrophages in monocytopenic mice. J Leukocyte Biol 1986;39:77–87.

65. Sherman MP, Evans MJ, Campbell LA. Prevention of pulmonary alveolar macrophage proliferation in newborn rabbits by hyperoxia. J Pediatr 1988;112:782–786.

66. Barbers RG, Oishi J, Gong H, Jr., Tashkin DP, Wallace JM, Baker SS. Chemotaxis of peripheral blood and lung leukocytes obtained from tobacco and marijuana smokers. J Psychoact Drugs 1988;20:15–20.

67. Tashkin DP, Coulson AH, Clark VA, et al. Respiratory symptoms and lung function in habitual heavy smokers of marijuana alone, smokers of marijuana and tobacco, smokers of tobacco alone, and nonsmokers. Am Rev Respir Dis 1988;138:74–80.

68. Hunninghake GW, Crystal RG. Cigarette smoking and lung destruction. Am Rev Respir Dis 1983;128:873–878.

69. Aguayo SM, Kane MA, King TE, Jr., Schwarz MI, Graver L, Miller YE. Increased levels of bombesin-like peptides in the lower respiratory tract of asymptomatic cigarette smokers. J Clin Invest 1989;84:1105–1113.

70. Aguayo SM, King TE, Jr., Waldron JA, Sherritt KM, Kane MA, Miller YE. Increased pulmonary neuroendocrine cells with bombesin-like immunoreactivity in adult patients with eosinophilic granuloma. J Clin Invest 1990;86:838–844.

71. Barth J, Kreipe H, Radzun HJ, et al. Increased expression of growth factor genes for macrophages and fibroblasts in bronchoalveolar lavage cells of a patient with pulmonary histiocytosis X. Thorax 1991;46:835–838.

72. Knudson RJ, Badger TL, Gaensler EA. Eosinophilic granuloma of lung. Med Thorac 1966;23:248–262.

73. Guardia J, Pedreira J, Esteban R, Vargas V, Allende E. Early pleural effusion in histiocytosis X. Arch Intern Med 1979;139:934–936.

74. Masson RG, Tedeschi LG. Pulmonary eosinophilic granuloma with hilar adenopathy simulating sarcoidosis. Chest 1978;73:682–683.

75. Brambilla E, Fontaine E, Pison CM, Coulomb M, Paramelle B, Brambilla C. Pulmonary histiocytosis X with mediastinal lymph node involvement. Am Rev Respir Dis 1990;142:1216–1218.

76. Pomeranz SJ, Proto AV. Histiocytosis X. Unusual-confusing features of eosinophilic granuloma. Chest 1986;89:88–92.

77. Fichtenbaum CJ, Kleinman GM, Haddad RG. Eosinophilic granuloma of the lung presenting as a solitary pulmonary nodule. Thorax 1990;45:905–906.

78. Sajjad SM, Luna MA. Primary pulmonary histiocytosis X in two patients with Hodgkin's disease. Thorax 1982;37:110–113.

79. Wyre HW, Henrichs WD. Systemic mastocytosis and pulmonary eosinophilic granuloma. JAMA 1978;239:856–857.

80. Shanley DJ, Lerud KS, Luetkehans TJ. Development of pulmonary histiocytosis X after chemotherapy for Hodgkin disease. AJR 1990;155:741–742.

81. Coli A, Bigotti G, Ferrone S. Histiocytosis X arising in Hodgkin's disease: Immunophenotypic characterization with a panel of monoclonal antibodies. Virchows Arch A Pathol Anat 1991;418:369–373.

82. LaCronique J, Roth C, Battesti JP, Basset F, Chretien J. Chest radiological features of pulmonary histiocytosis X. A report based on 50 adult cases. Thorax 1982;37:104–109.

83. Moor ADA, Godwin JD, Müller NL, et al. Pulmonary histiocytosis X: Comparison of radiographic findings. Radiology 1989;172:249–254.

84. Taylor DB, Joske D, Anderson J, Barry-Walsh C. Cavitating pulmonary nodules in histiocytosis X: High resolution CT demonstration. Aust Radiol 1990;34:253–255.

85. Bedrossian CWM, Kuhn C III, Luna MA, Conklin RH, Byrd RB, Kaplan PD. Desquamative interstitial pneumonia-like reaction accompanying pulmonary lesions. Chest 1977;72:166–169.

86. Fukuda Y, Basset F, Soler P, Ferrans V, Masugi Y, Crystal RG. Intraluminal fibrosis and elastic fiber degradation lead to lung remodeling in pulmonary Langerhans cell granulomatosis (histiocytosis X). Am J Pathol 1990;137:415–424.

87. Askin FB, McCann BG, Kuhn C III. Reactive eosinophilic pleuritis. A lesion to be distinguished from pulmonary eosinophilic granuloma. Arch Pathol Lab Med 1977;101:187–191.

88. Hammar SP, Winterbauer RH, Bockus D, Remington F, Friedman S. Idiopathic fibrosing alveolitis: a review with emphasis on ultrastructural and immunohistochemical features. Ultrastruct Pathol 1985;9:345–372.

89. Hammar SP, Bolen JW, Bockus D, Remington F, Friedman S. Ultrastructural and immunohistochemical features of common lung tumors. An overview. Ultrastruct

Pathol 1985;9:283–318.

90. Hammar SP, Bockus D, Remington F, et al. Langerhans cells and serum precipitating antibodies against fungal antigen in bronchiolo-alveolar cell carcinomas: possible association with eosinophilic granuloma. Ultrastruct Pathol 1980;1:19–37.

91. Lombard CM, Medeiros J, Colby TV. Pulmonary histiocytosis X and carcinoma. Arch Pathol Lab Med 1987;111:339–341.

92. Sadoun D, Vaylet F, Valeyre D, et al. Bronchogenic carcinoma in patients with pulmonary histiocytosis X. Chest 1992;101:1610–1613.

93. Tomasheski JF, Khiyami A, Kleinerman J. Neoplasms associated with pulmonary eosinophilic granuloma. Arch Pathol Lab Med 1991;115:499–506.

94. Wall CP, Gaensler EA, Carrington CB, Hayes JA. Comparison of transbronchial and open biopsies in chronic infiltrative lung disease. Am Rev Respir Dis 1981;123:280–290.

95. Flint A, Lloyd RV, Colby TV, Wilson BW. Pulmonary histiocytosis X: Immunoperoxidase staining for HLA-DR antigen and S100 protein. Arch Pathol Lab Med 1986;110:930–933.

96. Ree HJ, Kadin ME. Peanut agglutinin: A useful marker for histiocytosis X and interdigitating reticulum cells. Cancer (Philadelphia) 1986;57:282–287.

97. Rabkin MS, Kjeldsberg CR. Epithelial membrane antigen staining patterns of histiocytic lesions. Arch Pathol Lab Med 1987;111:337–338.

98. Azumi N, Sheibani K, Swartz WG, Stroup RM, Rappaport H. Antigenic phenotype of Langerhans cell histiocytosis: An immunohistochemical study demonstrating the value of LN-2, LN-3, and vimentin. Hum Pathol 1988;19:1376–1382.

99. Cagle PT, Mattioli CA, Truong LD, Greenberg SD. Immunohistochemical diagnosis of pulmonary eosinophilic granuloma on lung biopsy. Chest 1988;94:1133–1137.

100. Santamaria M, Llamas L, Ree HJ, et al. Expression of silylated Leu-MI antigen in histiocytosis X. Am J Clin Pathol 1988;89:211–216.

101. Ruco LP, Pulford KAF, Mason DY, et al. Expression of macrophage-associated antigens in tissues involved by Langerhans' cell histiocytosis (histiocytosis X) Am J Clin Pathol 1989;92:273–279.

102. Rabkin MS, Kjeldsberg CR, Wittwer CT, Marty J. A comparison study of two methods of peanut agglutinin staining with S100 immunostaining in 29 cases of histiocytosis X (Langerhans' cell histiocytosis) Arch Pathol Lab Med 1990;114:511–515.

103. Fe Y, Huang S, Dong H. Histiocytosis X: S-100 protein, peanut agglutinin, and transmission electron microscopic study. Am J Clin Pathol 1990;94:627–631.

104. Ornvold K, Ralfkiaer E, Carstensen H. Immunohistochemical study of the abnormal cells in Langerhans cell histiocytosis (histiocytosis X). Virchows Arch A Pathol Anat Histopathol 1990;416:403–410.

105. Kanitakis J, Fantini F, Pincelli C, Hermier C, Schmitt D, Thivolet J. Neuron-specific enolase is a marker of cutaneous Langerhans' cell histiocytosis ("X"): A comparative study with S100 protein. Anticancer Res 1991;11:635–640.

106. Baumal R, Kahn HJ, Marks A. Role of antibody to S100 protein in diagnostic pathology. Lab Invest 1988;59:152–153 (letter).

107. Webber D, Tron V, Askin F, Churg A. S-100 staining in the diagnosis of eosinophilic granuloma of lung. Am J Clin Pathol 1985;84:447–453.

108. Soler P, Chollet S, Jacque C, Fukuda Y, Ferrans VJ, Basset F. Immunocytochemical characterization of pulmonary histiocytosis X cells in lung biopsies. Am J Pathol 1985;118:439–451.

109. Chollet S, Soler P, Dournovo P, Richard MS, Ferrans VJ, Basset F. Diagnosis of pulmonary histiocytosis X by immunodetection of Langerhans cells in bronchoalveolar lavage fluid. Am J Pathol 1984;115:225–232.

110. Averswald V, Barth J, Magnussen H. Value of CD-1-positive cells in bronchoalveolar lavage fluid for the diagnosis of pulmonary histiocytosis X. Lung 1991;169:305–309.

111. Hammar SP, Winterbauer RH, Bockus D. Diagnosis of eosinophilic granuloma by ultrastructural examination of sputum. Arch Pathol Lab Med 1978;102:606.

112. Powers MA, Askin FB, Cresson DH. Pulmonary eosinophilic granuloma. A 25-year follow-up. Am Rev Respir Dis 1984;129:503–507.

113. Ben-Ezra J, Bailey A, Azumi N, et al. Malignant histiocytosis X: A distinct clinicopathologic entity. Cancer (Philadelphia) 1991;68:1050–1060.

114. Risdall RJ, Dehner LP, Duray P, Kobrinsky N, Robison L, Nesbit ME, Jr. Histiocytosis X (Langerhans' cell histiocytosis): Prognostic role of histopathology. Arch Pathol Lab Med 1983;107:59–63.

115. Goldberg N, Bauer K, Rosen ST, et al. Histiocytosis X flow cytometric DNA-content and immunohistochemical and ultrastructural analysis. Arch Dermatol 1986;122:446–450.

116. Rabkin MS, Wittwer CT, Kjeldsberg CR, Piepkorn MW. Flow-cytometric DNA content of histiocytosis X (Langerhans' cell histiocytosis). Am J Pathol 1988;131:283–289.

117. Ornvold K, Carstensen H, Larsen JK, Christensen J, Ralfkiaer E. Flow cytometric DNA analysis of lesions from 18 children with Langerhans cell histiocytosis (histiocytosis X). Am J Pathol 1990;136:1301–1307.

118. Huhn D, Konig G, Weig J, Schneller W. Therapy in pulmonary histiocytosis X. Haematol Bluttransfus 1981;27:231–237.

119. Von Essen S, West W, Sitorius M, Rennard SI. Complete resolution of roentgenographic changes in a patient with pulmonary histiocytosis X. Chest 1990;98:765–767.

CHAPTER 18

Extrinsic Allergic Alveolitis

SAMUEL P. HAMMAR

The lung is the site of a variety of complex inflammatory reactions. In many instances the inflammation is a normal reaction against various infectious agents, such as bacteria and viruses, or is a response to necrotic tissue, such as infarcted lung parenchyma or degenerating tumor. In extrinsic allergic alveolitis, the inflammatory reaction characteristic of this condition is thought to represent a hypersensitivity process mediated by immunoglobulins, lymphokines, and immune effector cells. Although the four immunologic responses described by Gell and Coombs[1] (Fig. 18–1) are often used in characterizing various inflammatory reactions in the lungs, the immunopathogenesis of extrinsic allergic alveolitis remains poorly understood. Extrinsic allergic alveolitis, also referred to as hypersensitivity pneumonitis or microgranulomatous hypersensitivity reaction, is a predominantly chronic inflammatory disease of the peripheral gas-exchanging portion of the lung resulting from sensitization and subsequent exposure to a variety of organic dusts. The condition was first described in 1932 in farmers exposed to moldy hay.[2] Initially it was considered a mycotic process.[3,4] Pepys and colleagues[5,6] elucidated some of the initial immunologic mechanisms though to be operative in the disease. Williams[7,8] demonstrated that the disease could be produced in sensitized farmers by the inhalation of extracts of moldy hay. Farmer's lung disease was found to result from a hypersensitivity reaction against a species of thermophilic actinomyces, *Thermoactinomyces vulgarus*, that proliferated as the hay became overheated in the process of becoming moldy.[9,10] Numerous organic antigens have now been recognized as causing hypersensitivity reactions in the lung, and these are usually named after the occupation in which the patient was exposed to the organic antigen. The term extrinsic allergic alveolitis was coined by Pepys[11] to refer to the entire group of similar reactions to organic dusts.

Etiology and Prevalence

A wide variety of organic antigens derived from various microorganisms including bacteria, fungi, protozoa, and various plant or animal proteins are known causes of extrinsic allergic alveolitis (Table 18–1). Persons who develop hypersensitivity pneumonitis are usually exposed to these antigens via their occupation or avocation or in their home. In addition, several drugs such as methotrexate, procarbazine, gold sodium thiomalate, and trimethoprim can cause a hypersensitivity pulmonary reaction similar to that cased by organic dusts;[12–15] these are described in Chapter 23. New forms of hypersensitivity pneumonitis continue to be reported. Summer pneumonitis, a type of extrinsic allergic alveolitis described in Japan, is caused by *Trichosporon cutaneum*.[16] A case of mollusk shell hypersensitivity pneumonits from inhalation of dust produced during the manufacture of nacre buttons from sea-snail shells was recently described.[17] Gamboa et al.[18] reported extrinsic allergic alveolitis in a 24-year-old male plasterer caused by esparto (*Stipa tenacissima*), a grass used in the manufacture of ropes, baskets, and plaster.

In recent years, one of the most common causes of extrinsic allergic alveolitis has been contamination of air-conditioning systems, forced-air heating systems, and humidification systems by various microorganisms, most commonly thermophilic actinomycetes.[19–24] People have been exposed at work in offices or when at home from these systems.

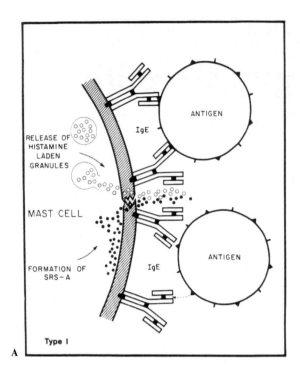

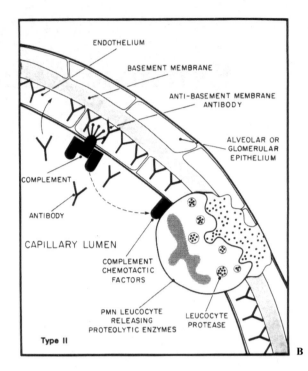

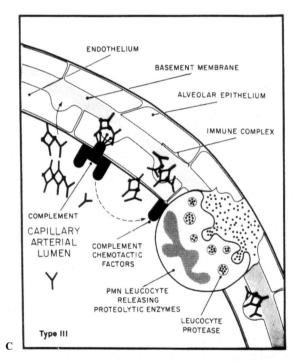

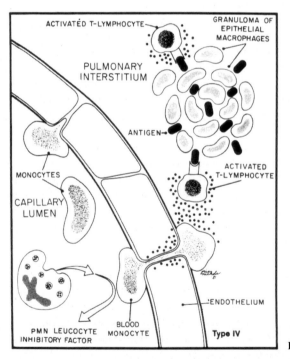

Fig. 18–1 A–D. Schematic diagram of the four basic immunologic reactions that are the basis of some lung diseases. Gell and Coombs' classification of immunopathogenic mechanisms. **A.** Type 1. Degranulation of mast cell is triggered by antigen bridging of cell-bound IgE followed by release of histamine, SRS-A, and other chemical mediators. **B.** Type II. Specific cytotoxic antibody-mediated injury. Union of antigen and antibody is followed by local activation of complement, attraction of polymorphonuclear leukocytes and release of lysosomal proteases that cause cellular destruction. **C.** Type III. Immune complexes formed in circulation become entrapped in microvasculature. Complement is activated at site of deposition, initiating a sequence of events similar to **B** above. **D.** Type IV. Cell-mediated hypersensitivity results in formation and maintenance of a granulomatous reaction through production of lymphokines by sensitized lymphocytes. The activated T lymphocyte at the top of this figure is maintaining a granuloma by secretion of macrophage inhibition factor and macrophage activation factor; one on middle right is attracting monocytes by secretion of chemotactic factor. (From Winterbauer RH, Hammar SD. Diffuse hypersensitivity disorders of the lung in Fishman AD. Update: Pulmonary diseases and disorders. New York: McGraw-Hill 1980:205–229, with permission.)

Table 18–1. Etiology of extrinsic allergic alveolitis

Disease	Antigen	Source of antigen
Farmer's lung	*Micropolyspora faeni*	Moldy hay, grain, silage
Ventilation pneumonitis	*Thermoactinomyces candidus*	Contaminated forced-air systems
Bagassosis	*Thermoactinomyces vulgaris*	Moldy sugarcane (bagasse)
Mushroom worker's lung	*Thermactinomyces sacchari*	Moldy mushroom compost
Suberosis	*Thermoactinomyces viridis*	Cork dust mold
Fungi		
Malt worker's lung	*Aspergillus fumigatus* *Aspergillus clavus*	Moldy barley
Sequoiosis	Graphium, Pullularia	Moldy wood dust
Maple bark disease	*Crypostroma corticale*	Moldy maple bark
Cheese washer's lung	*Aspergillus clavatus*	Moldy cheese
Woodworker's lung	Alternaria	Oak, cedar, and mahogany dust; pine and spruce pulp
Cheese worker's lung	*Penicillum casei*	Cheese mold
Paprika slicer's lung	*Mucor stolonifer*	Moldy paprika pods
Summer pneumonitis	*Trichosporon cutaneum*	"Contaminated old houses"
Animal protein		
Bird fancier's, breeder's, or handler's lung	Avian droppings, feathers, serum, etc.	Parakeets, budgerigars, pigeons, chickens, turkeys
Pituitary snuff taker's lung	Pituitary snuff	Bovine and porcine pituitary proteins
Fish meal worker's lung	Fish meal	Fish meal dust
Furrier's lung	Animal fur dust	Animal pelts
Bat lung	Bat serum protein	Bat droppings
Insect proteins		
Miller's lung	*Sitophilus granarius* (wheat weevil)	Dust-contaminated grain
Lycoperdonosis	Puffball spores	Lycoperdon puffballs
Unknown		
Sauna taker's lung		Contaminated sauna water
Coptic lung		Cloth wrappings of mummies
Grain measurer's lung		Cereal grain
Coffee worker's lung		Coffee bean dust
Thatched roof lung		Dead grasses and leaves
Tea grower's lung		Tea plants
Tobacco grower's lung		Tobacco plants

The prevalence or incidence of hypersensitivity pneumonitis is difficult to determine, and probably varies depending on climatic conditions, concentration of offending antigen, diagnostic accuracy, and host factors that are poorly characterized. The incidence of farmer's lung disease caused by thermophilic actinomycetes ranges between 2.3% and 8.6%; those farmers living in regions of high rainfall appear to be more susceptible to the disease.[25,26] Gruchow et al.[27] evaluated 1400 Wisconsin dairy farmers and found a prevalence of farmer's lung in 42 of 100,000. The prevalence of extrinsic allergic alveolitis in office buildings and industrial settings varies widely, but attack rates as high as 70% have been reported.[28]

Clinical Features

The disease may present in two clinical forms.[29] In the acute or subacute form in which exposure to the organic antigen is usually intermittent, signs and symptoms begin 4–6 h after inhalation of the antigen and consist of fever, malaise, chills, dyspnea, and a dry cough. The symptoms usually subside 18–24 h after exposure ceases and may recur with repeated exposure to the offending antigen. This disease is frequently mistaken clinically as an influenza syndrome.

In the chronic form of the disease in which antigen exposure is usually continuous but perhaps less intense, patients frequently complain of chronic fatigue, dyspnea on exertion, anorexia, and occasionally weight loss. The chronic disease is often progressive and may result in progressive respiratory failure. Physical examination in both forms of the disease is usually nonspecific, and rales are heard in most patients. The chest radiograph may show no change or a variety of abnormalities, depending to some degree on whether the disease is acute, subacute, or chronic[30–32]; these include a diffuse ground-glass infiltrate, diffuse finely nodular densities that are more prominent in the lower lobes,

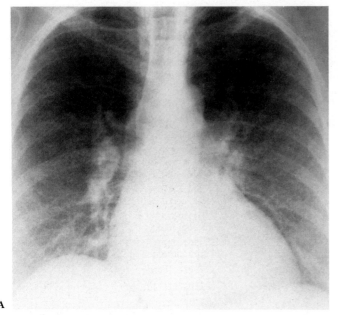

A

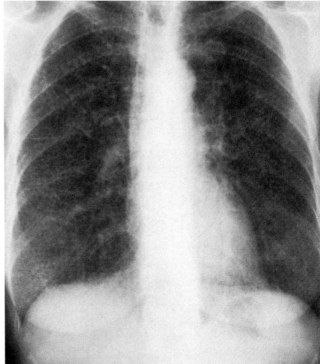

B

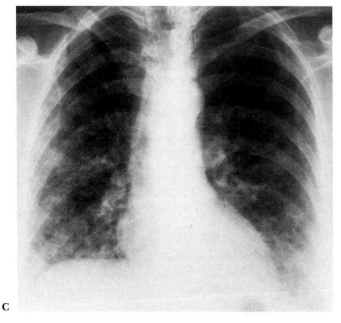

C

Fig. 18–2 A–C. Representative chest radiographs from patients with extrinsic allergic alveolitis. **A.** Mild diffuse alveolar infiltrate. **B.** Diffuse finely nodular infiltrate. **C.** Irregular coarsely nodular infiltrate.

diffuse coarse nodular densities, and diffuse interstitial infiltrates characteristic of pulmonary fibrosis (Fig. 18–2). Silver et al.[33] evaluated 13 chest radiographs and computed tomographic (CT) scans from 11 patients with hypersensitivity pneumonitis. In 7 patients who had open lung biopsies, they correlated the CT scan findings with histologic findings. Two patients with acute hypersensitivity pneumonitis showed CT scan features of air space opacification that correlated with histologic findings of noncaseating granulomas and filling of alveoli with macrophages. Nine patients with subacute hypersensitivity pneumonitis showed small rounded opacities and patchy air space opacification by

CT scan and histologic findings characteristically seen in extrinsic allergic alveolitis (see following). In those patients whose CT scans showed irregular linear opacities, there was histologic evidence of fibrosis. The authors concluded that CT scans were superior to standard chest radiographs in assessing the type and extent of abnormalities, and that high-resolution CT scans were better than conventional CT scans in showing the various changes.

Pulmonary function test abnormalities are variable depending on whether the disease is acute or chronic. In the acute form there is a decrease in forced vital capacity, a decrease in 1-s forced expiratory volume, and hypoxemia accentuated by exercise. In the chronic form there may be a moderate-to-severe restrictive impairment with a marked decrease in diffusing capacity. Other laboratory tests may be abnormal depending on the phase of the disease. In many patients laboratory tests are entirely normal. In those with acute disease, there is frequently a polymorphonuclear leukocytosis up to 25,000/mm³ with a left shift,[34] and occasionally an eosinophilia as great as 10%. An increased level of immunoglobulins, with the exception of IgE, is usually present and rheumatoid factor may be found in moderately high titers.[34]

If the offending antigen is known and relatively pure antigenic preparations are available, skin testing can be performed. In hypersensitive individuals whose skin test is positive, the antigen will produce an immediate wheal and flare followed in 4–8 h by erythema and subcutaneous swelling that resemble an Arthus reaction. A positive tuberculin-type reaction has not been described. Sera from patients with extrinsic allergic alveolitis characteristically contain an IgG-precipitating antibody against the causative antigen. This antigen can be demonstrated by an immunologic technique such as an Ouchterlony immunodiffusion (Fig. 18–3). Cell-mediated reactions to the inciting antigen can also be detected by lymphokine production and blast transformation of peripheral blood and alveolar lavage fluid lymphocytes from patients with hypersensitivity pneumonitis.[35,36]

Immunopathogenesis

Extrinsic allergic alveolitis is thought to result from a combination of a type III immune complex and a type IV cell-mediated immunologic reaction, although the exact mechanism by which these immunologic reactions produce the observed clinical and pathologic features of this disease is not clear. High titers of precipitating antibodies are present against the causative antigen, and a positive skin test 4–8 h after injection of the antigen suggests that immune complexes are formed and mediate the disease.[37] However, the 4- to 8-h delay before the onset of the skin reaction would also be consistent with a cell-mediated reaction.[38] Granulomas seen in lung biopsy specimens suggest that cell-mediated immune reactions are operative.

The antibodies present in the serum of patients with extrinsic allergic alveolitis, such as pigeon breeders' disease, are primarily of the IgG class[39] and are capable of fixing complement.[40] Smaller concentrations of IgM- and IgA-precipitating antibodies are also present. The exact significance of immune complexes in producing the disease is questionable, because asymptom-

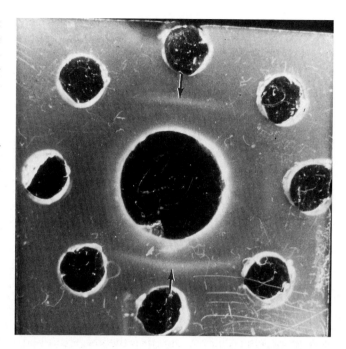

Fig. 18–3. Dense lines (*arrows*) in this Ouchterlony immunodiffusion test indicate precipitating antibodies against *Thermoactinomyces vulgarus* and *Aspergillus* antigens. Patient's serum in central well is surrounded by wells containing various antigens. Precipitin line indicates that the serum contains antibody against a given antigen.

atic persons exposed to the same antigen will exhibit similar high titers of antibodies,[39,41] and in the active disease complement levels are not depressed. In Finish farmers with farmer's lung disease, Ojanen[42] reported that the concentration of IgG, IgA, and IgE antibodies was higher in patients with the disease than their spouses and that patients had several IgG clases whereas spouses had either IgG or IgA antibodies. Their study suggested that in Finland, the serologic diagnosis of farmer's lung should include IgG antibodies against *Thermoactinomyces vulgaris* and IgA antibodies against *Aspergillus fumigatus*.

Likewise, immune complex-mediated vasculitis is usually not seen[34,43] in lung tissue sections from patients with hypersensitivity pneumonitis, although it may occasionally be found in acute disease.[44,45] Bronchoalveolar lavage fluid from pigeon breeders with extrinsic allergic alveolitis contains increased concentrations of IgG[46,47] and to a lesser extent IgM and IgA[47] but these are also found in asymptomatic pigeon breeders.[48] Antibodies to the offending antigen are present in the lavage fluid from symptomatic[49] and asymptomatic persons.

Richerson[50,51] has provided two timely reviews concerning the involvement of immune complexes in lung diseases. He stressed that in experimental studies in rabbits and guinea pigs it was found that development of alveolitis was dependent on cell-mediated immunity and not humoral mechanisms. Richerson concluded that the presence of precipitating antibodies in hypersensitivity pneumonitis represented only markers of exposure to antigen and played no definite role in the pathogenesis of extrinsic allergic alveolitis.

However, two reports published in 1985 supported the hypothesis that immune complexes are important in the pathogenesis of extrinsic allergic alveolitis. Fournier and coworkers[52] studied differential cell counts in bronchoalveolar lavage fluid in 10 patients with hypersensitivity pneumonitis and 5 control persons exposed to experimentally controlled antigen inhalation. They found that the patients with extrinsic allergic alveolitis developed an increased percentage of neutrophils in their bronchoalveolar lavage fluid, raising the possibility of immune complex formation with generation of substances such as C5a that are chemotactic for neutrophils. McSharry et al.[53] found that cigarette-smoking pigeon breeders had a significantly lower antibody response to inhaled bird antigens than those who were nonsmokers and an overall lower incidence of hypersensitivity pneumonitis. This finding suggested that antibody production and possibly immune complex formation were important in the pathogenesis of extrinsic allergic alveolitis.

Other studies have evaluated the effect of cigarette smoking and other factors on the development of hypersensitivity pneumonitis. Cormier et al.[54] studied the effect of cigarette smoking in guinea pigs with experimentally induced hypersensitivity pneumonitis. Their experimenta study showed that extrinsic allergic alveolitis resulted in an initial neutrophilic alveolitis that was significantly decreased compared to the cigarette-smoking group of animals. Kusaka and colleagues evaluated factors that caused changes in *Micropolyspora faeni* antibody titer among 92 dairy farmers in Hokkaido, Japan. The prevalence of *M. faeni* antibody was significantly higher in nonsmokers than smokers, and there was no significant change in the prevalences of *M. faeni* antibody during a 5-year period of observation. The nonsmoking farmers who remained seronegative throughout the 5-year period were older and had worked longer on the farm than the farmers who seroconverted, suggesting that in addition to cigarette smoking, age and exposure time to the antigen were also factors in the development of extrinsic allergic alveolitis. The study by Soda et al.[56] of Clq and C3 in bronchoalveolar lavage fluid from patients with summer-type hypersensitivity pneumonitis provided further support for the importance of an immune complex pathogenesis. In a study of 9 patients, they found high concentrations of Clq and C3 in the bronchoalveolar

lavage fluid whereas control patients had undetectable levels of Clq and C3. They also found that Clq, IgG, and IgA concentration in bronchoalveolar lavage fluid correlated with clinical symptoms and diffusing capacity whereas bronchoalveolar lymphocytosis did not.

Information implicating a cell-mediated type IV immunologic mechanism in extrinsic allergic alveolitis is also confusing. Several studies have shown that lymphocytes from pigeon breeders with extrinsic allergic alveolitis produced migration inhibition factor when exposed to various pigeon antigens[35,36,57] and that T lymphocytes undergo blastogenesis when exposed to antigen.[35] Bronchoalveolar lavage fluid from patients with chronic hypersensitivity pneumonitis show a marked increase in T lymphocytes,[48,49] most of which are supressor/cytotoxic lymphocytes.[48,58] Similar findings are seen in asymptomatic dairy farmers with precipitating antibodies to *Micropolyspora faeni* and surprisingly may even be present in normal farmers without precipitating antibodies.[59,60]

Keller and colleagues[61] have provided additional information concerning immunoregulation in hypersensitivity pneumonitis. They performed studies on bronchoalveolar lavage lymphocytes from four pigeon breeders with extrinsic allergic alveolitis and six equally exposed but asymptomatic pigeon breeders. They found similar numbers of T-lymphocyte subsets and helper/inducer to supressor/cytotoxic lymphocyte ratios in the symptomatic and asymptomatic group. Bronchoalveolar lavage lymphocytes from symptomatic pigeon breeders showed a significant increase in blastogenic activity to phytohemagglutinin and pigeon serum compared to asymptomatic exposed persons. When T-cell-enriched preparations of bronchoalveolar lavage lymphocytes were cultured with autologous peripheral blood lymphocytes depleted of suppressor T cells in the presence of phytohemagglutinin or pigeon serum, there was a significant increase in blastogenic activity of lymphocytes in the pigeon breeders with hypersensitivity pneumonitis as compared to the asymptomatic similarly exposed group. These findings suggested a decrease in suppressor T-cell activity in the pigeon breeders with hypersensitivity pneumonitis.

Denis and coworkers[62–64] have also added to our knowledge of the pathogenesis of hypersensitivity pneumonitis by inducing the disease in mice with *Micropolyspora faeni*. They observed a high spontaneous release of interleukin-1, interleukin-6, and tumor necrosis factor alpha in bronchoalveolar lavage fluid and an enhanced capacity for cytokine releasee by macrophages upon stimulation with *M. faeni*. Their findings suggested that hypersensitivity pneumonitis was closely linked to cytokine release in the lungs and that abrogation of the disease was correlated with a decrease in lung cytokine response. Blocking the release of tumor necrosis factor alpha with an antibody against the substance was associated with a significant decease in cellular recruitment in the lungs and a decrease in lung fibrosis. These experimental findings may be the basis for a new form of therapy for extrinsic allergic alveolitis.

Genetic factors may also be important in hypersensitivity pneumonitis. Several initial studies suggested an association between certain HLA antigens and extrinsic allergic alveolitis in pigeon breeders and farmers,[65,66] but other studies failed to confirm this association.[67,68] Observations by Benacerraf and Katz[69] that immune response genes are linked to the HLA locus may be important in this regard and explain why only 5%–15% of persons exposed to the etiologic agents of extrinsic allergic alveolitis develop the disease. Along the same lines, Allen et al.[70] found that only certain strains of inbred mice developed pulmonary granulomatous inflammation in response to intravenous Calmette–Guerin bacillus and that response was multigenic and related to immunoglobulin heavy gene complex and not the HLA complex. Ando et al.[71] recently reported an increase frequency of HLA-Dw3 antigen in 66 patients with Japanese summer-type hypersensitivity pneumonitis induced by *Trichosporon cutaneum* compared to 472 normal healthy subjects, once again suggesting a genetic factor in the development of extrinsic allergic alveolitis.

Because many of the same immunologic findings have been observed in persons with extrinsic allergic alveolitis and similarly exposed but asymptomatic persons, other factors explaining the pathogenesis of the disease have been investigated. In animals such as rabbits, treatment with soluble thermophilic actinomycete antigen will result in humoral and cellular responses but will not cause pulmonary inflammation. However, if particulate antigen is given intratracheally an extensive chronic inflammatory infiltrate will develop in alveolar septa.[72,73] In general, to produce a hypersensitivity pneumonitis-like lesion in animals requires particulate antigen and an adjuvant.

Finally, mechanisms other than immunologic may be involved in the development of extrinsic allergic alveolitis. Larson and colleagues[74] compared the concentration of hyaluronic acid and N-terminal peptide in bronchoalveolar lavage fluid from 12 farmers with no symptoms and 12 farmers admitted to the hospital with acute farmer's lung disease. They found elevated concentrations of hyaluronic acid and N-terminal peptide in the 12 symptomatic farmers and normal levels in the asymptomatic farmers. They postulated that hyaluronic acid, because it can immobilize water, was important in the development of pulmonary function impairment observed in acute farmer's lung disease. Pesci et al.[75] evaluated the number of mast cells in bronchoalveolar lavage fluid of 15 patients with farmer's lung disease and correlated this finding with the number of mast cells in transbronchial biopsy tissue specimens. Mast cell counts in bronchoalveolar lavage fluid correlated with the number of mast cells in tissue sections, and there was no correlation with other bronchoalveolar lavage fluid cells and tissue mast cells. They hypothesized that factors such as immune complexes attracted the mast cells to migrate into the alveoli. The exact significance of mast cells in farmer's lung disease remains uncertain.

Organic dusts may contain a variety of proteolytic enzymes and nonproteolytic agents capable of activating the complement and kallikrein system.[76] Also, other agents such as endotoxin and mycotoxins may cause tissue damage.[77,78] Thus it is possible that hypersensitivity pneumonitis is caused by a combination of immunologic and nonimmunologic mechanisms acting in concert.

Pathologic Features

The pathologic changes in extrinsic allergic alveolitis are essentially identical, irrespective of the causative antigen, and depend on the intensity of the antigenic exposure, and when in the course of the disease a biopsy is obtained. The first pathologic descriptions of hypersensitivity pneumonitis were of farmer's lung disease in 1958.[79–81] These reports described similar findings, consisting of chronic interstitial inflammation with occasional nonnecrotizing granulomas. Cases were also described in which acute inflammation and vasculitis were observed.[82,83]

The gross pathologic changes of extrinsic allergic alveolitis are variable depending on the stage of the disease during which the biopsy is obtained. In the acute stages, hours to days after the onset of symptoms, the lung tissue may be relatively normal or will be reddish-gray and consolidated. There may be an accentuation of the alveolar architecture. In patients with chronic disease, the lung tissue may be firm and rubbery, secondary to fibrosis, and be identical to that seen in idiopathic pulmonary fibrosis (see Chapter 20).

Histologically, open lung biopsies typically show an interstitial infiltrate of lymphocytes and plasma cells. This infiltrate can be diffuse and relatively uniform (Fig. 18–4) or patchy and of variable intensity (Fig. 18–5). The interstitial infiltrate is present around small bronchi and bronchioles, but is most uniform in alveolar septa (Fig. 18–6). The inflammatory infiltrate is frequently associated with a slight degree of interstitial fibrosis (Fig. 18–7). The intensity of the interstitial

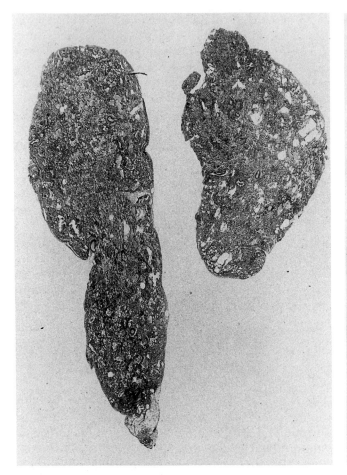

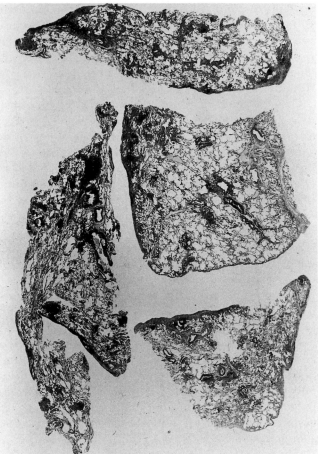

Fig. 18–4. Low-magnification view of open lung biopsy specimen from patient with hypersensitivity pneumonitis. Note relatively uniform diffuse involvement of tissue. ×4.

Fig. 18–5. Low-magnification view of open lung biopsy specimen from patient with hypersensitivity pneumonitis. Infiltrate is patchy, and frequently most intense around small bronchi and bronchioles. ×4.

infiltrate of lymphocytes and plasma cells varies considerably, and may be accompanied by an accumulation of alveolar macrophages in adjacent alveolar spaces (Fig. 18–8). The exact nature of the interstitial infiltrate is best observed by electron microscopic examination of the tissue in which lymphocytes, plasma cells, and other inflammatory cells can be clearly identified (Fig. 18–9). Hypertrophied and hyperplastic alveolar lining cells, a nonspecific reaction to injury, accompany the interstitial inflammation and can be accentuated by immunohistochemical stains for cytokeratin (Fig. 18–10).

Small, nonnecrotizing granulomata are seen in the majority of cases. They may be peribronchial or peribronchiolar but are most frequent in the alveolar parenchyma. They are located interstitially and within alveoli, and are composed of epithelioid histiocytes and Langhans' giant cells (Figs. 18–11 and 18–12). In addition, Langhans' giant cells are frequently present in association with lymphocytes and plasma cells in the interstitium (Figs. 18–13 and 18–14). Also, indistinct aggre-

gates of epithelioid histiocytes are commonly found in alveolar spaces (Fig. 18–15). In some cases, birefringent material is present within the cytoplasm of giant cells; giant cells may also contain phagocytosed organic antigen.

A variety of other pathologic changes occur in hypersensitivity pneumonitis. In some cases a pattern resembling desquamative interstitial pneumonitis is seen (Fig. 18–16). Bronchiolitis obliterans–organizing pneumonitis is also observed in some cases (Fig. 18–17). Significant interstitial fibrosis is not seen in acute cases, but is a frequent finding in those patients whose biopsy is obtained months to years after the onset of symptoms and who have had persistent exposure to the causative antigen. The histologic changes in these patients may be identical to those seen in idiopathic pulmonary fibrosis (Fig. 18–18). A pathologic finding of uncertain significance in many cases of extrinsic allergic alveolitis is the presence of Langerhans' cells.[84] These dendritic cells may be identified via electron microscopy or immuno-

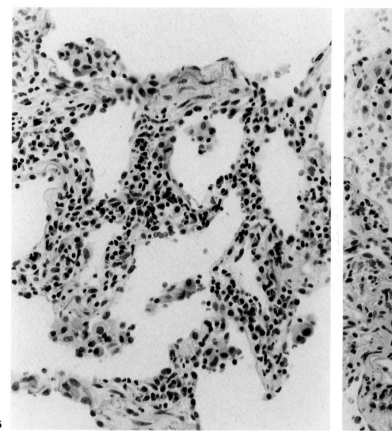

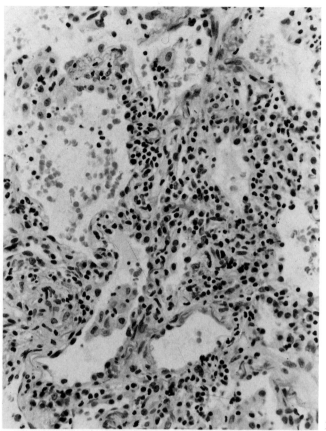

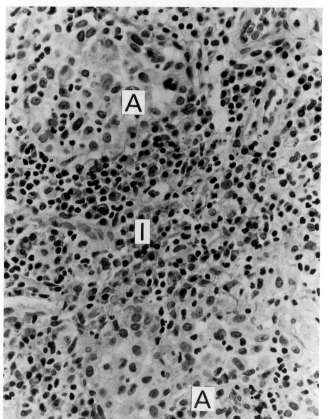

Fig. 18–6. Representative peripheral lung tissue shows diffuse moderately intense chronic inflammatory cell infiltrate characteristic of hypersensitivity pneumonitis. ×330.

Fig. 18–7. Chronic inflammatory infiltrate is frequently associated with mild interstitial fibrosis. ×330.

Fig. 18–8. In this region of extrinsic allergic alveolitis, accumulation of alveolar macrophages in alveoli (A) is adjacent to chronic interstitial inflammation (I). ×330.

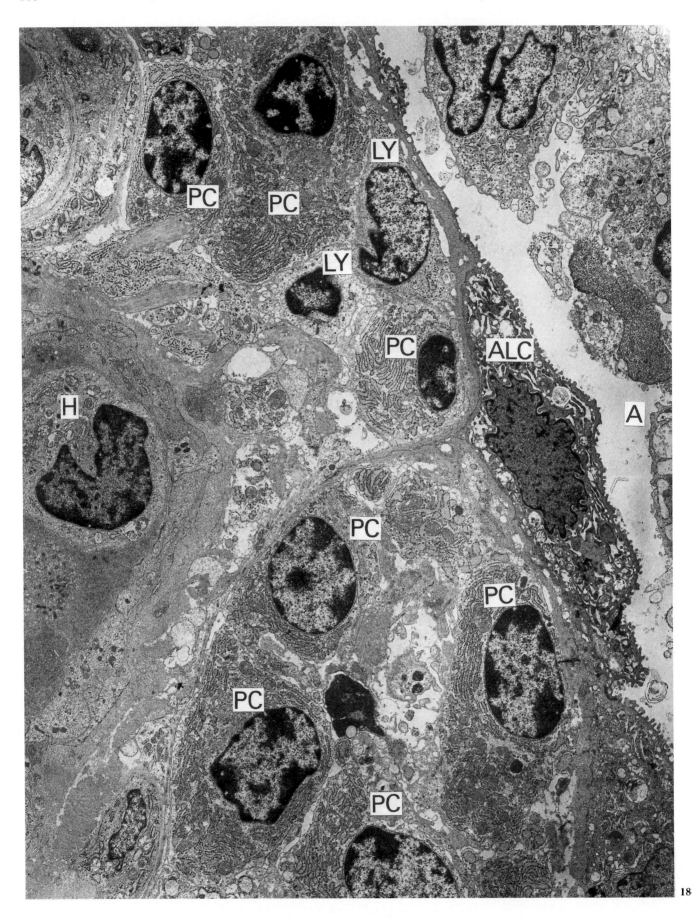

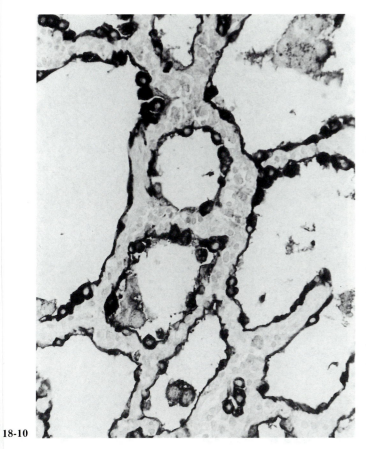

18-10

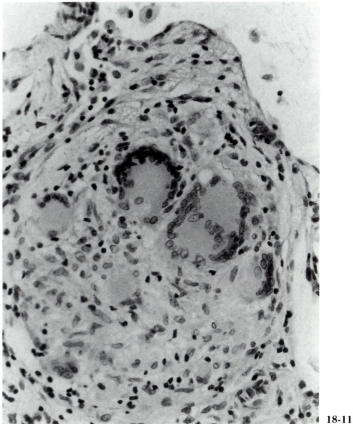

18-11

Fig. 18–10. Region of lung tissue has been immunostained for cytokeratin using immunoperoxidase technique, which accentuates hypertrophied and hyperplastic alveolar lining cells and shows lack of staining of interstitial inflammatory cells. ×330.

Figs. 18–11 and 18–12. Interstitially located small nonnecrotizing granulomata, a frequent finding in most cases of extrinsic allergic alveolitis, are composed of mononuclear histiocytes and Langhan's type giant cells with lymphocytes and plasma cells at their periphery. ×330.

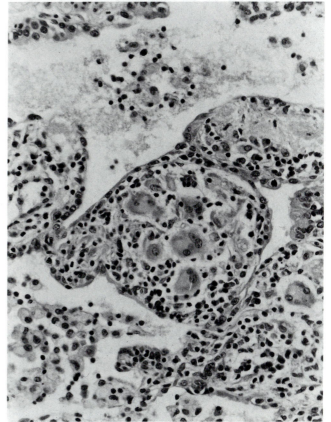

18-12

◁─────────────────────────────

Fig. 18–9. Electron micrograph shows more clearly the interstitial infiltrate of plasma cells (PC), lymphocytes (LY), and histiocytes (H). Type 1 alveolar lining cells (ALC); part of alveolus (A). ×6,400.

Table 18–2. Summary of morphologic features in pulmonary biopsies of 60 farmer's lung patients[a]

Morphologic criteria	Present	Percent	Degree of involvement[b]			
			±	1+	2+	3+
Interstitial infiltrate	60	100	0	14	19	27
Unresolved pneumonia	39	65	—	—	—	—
Pleural fibrosis	29	48	—	—	—	—
Fibrosis, interstitial	39	65	10	24	5	—
Bronchiolitis obliterans	30	50	3	—	—	—
Foam cells	39	65	6	24	6	3
Edema	31	52	—	—	—	—
Granulomas	42	70	—	—	—	—
With giant cells[c]	30	50	—	—	—	—
Without giant cells	35	58	—	—	—	—
Solitary giant cells	32	53	—	—	—	—
Foreign bodies	36	60	—	—	—	—
Birefringent[c]	28	47	—	—	—	—
Nonbirefringent	24	40	—	—	—	—

[a] Reyes et al.[43] (With permission of publisher.)

[b] Degree of involvement rated on an arbitrary but documented scale for each criterion.

[c] The discrepancy in the total numbers occurs because granulomas with and without giant cells may be found in some cases. This discrepancy also applies with the foreign bodies.

alveolitis the lymphocytic infiltrate is typically suppressor/cytotoxic lymphocytes (CD-8 cells).

Lymphocytic interstitial pneumonitis (LIP) is characterized by an interstitial infiltrate of lymphocytes and plasma cells and histologically can be very similar to hypersensitivity pneumonitis.[85] It usually does not show the small granulomata seen in extrinsic allergic alveolitis. The etiology of lymphocytic interstitial pneumonitis is unknown in most cases, but has been reported to be associated with chronic graft-versus-host disease,[86] collagen vascular diseases,[87] and recently with the acquired immune deficiency syndrome.[88–91] In lymphocytic interstitial pneumonitis associated with chronic graft-versus-host disease, the infiltrating lymphocytes are also mostly suppressor/cytotoxic lymphocytes (CD-8 cells).[86]

Idiopathic pulmonary fibrosis and interstitial fibrosis associated with collagen vascular diseases may be difficult if not impossible to differentiate from chronic extrinsic allergic alveolitis. The clinical history and a positive precipitating antibody test are helpful in differentiating these conditions. Lymphoma and lymphomatoid granulomatosis are histologically different enough from extrinsic allergic alveolitis that they usually do not cause confusion. Wegener's granulomatosis may present acutely but it is characterized by nodular infiltrates showing necrotizing granulomatous inflammation with granulomatous vasculitis. Infectious disease such as that caused by viruses, mycoplasma, mycobacteria, and some fungi may also cause an interstitial lym-

phocyte plasma cell infiltrate occasionally with granulomata, and should be considered in the differential diagnosis. Special stains for microorganisms are helpful in some instances in excluding these entities. Some drugs such as methotrexate[12] and procarbazine[13] produce a hypersensitivity lung disease with features similar to that of extrinsic allergic alveolitis. In such cases the clinical history provides the clue to making the correct diagnosis.

Rom and Travis[92] recently described a lymphocyte-macrophage alveolitis in 28 men occupationally exposed to asbestos. Open lung biopsies done in two patients showed a lymphocyte plasma cell interstitial inflammatory cell infiltrate with small nonnecrotizing granulomas, a pattern essentially identical to extrinsic allergic alveolitis. Hammar and Hallman[93] described an identical pattern in an open lung biopsy in a 63-year-old shipyard machinist who was found to have 1.38×10^6 amosite fibers and 5.52×10^6 chrysotile fibers per gram of dry lung tissue. These reports suggested that asbestos may also be capable of causing hypersensitivity like pneumonitis.

Diagnosis of Extrinsic Allergic Alveolitis

The diagnosis of extrinsic allergic alveolitis is usually made from the clinical history and the presence of a serum-precipitating antibody against the suspected antigen. The precipitating antibody can be identified using an Ouchterlony immunodiffusion technique (see Fig. 18–3). The demonstration of the antibody serves only to indicate exposure and immunologic reaction to the potential causative organic antigen and does not indicate disease. Skin testing and bronchial inhalation challenge have been performed but in general these are not standardized. A report published in 1985 suggested that using a hay extract antigen for skin testing is an effective test in diagnosing farmer's lung disease and is also helpful in separating patients with disease from asymptomatic but exposed patients.[94] Cellular analysis of bronchoalveolar lavage fluid characteristically shows a "lymphocytic alveolitis" (Fig. 18–19) with an increased number of suppressor/cytotoxic lymphocytes[95] (Fig. 18–20).

Open lung biopsy specimens from affected patients will usually show characteristic features of chronic interstitial inflammation and granulomata, strongly suggesting the diagnosis. In patients with chronic disease the pathologic changes may be nearly identical to those seen in idiopathic fibrosis, and in these cases a careful clinical history is helpful.

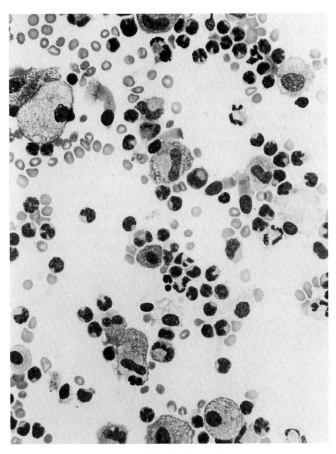

Fig. 18–19. Bronchoalveolar lavage fluid from patient with extrinsic allergic alveolitis has increased number of lymphocytes. ×330.

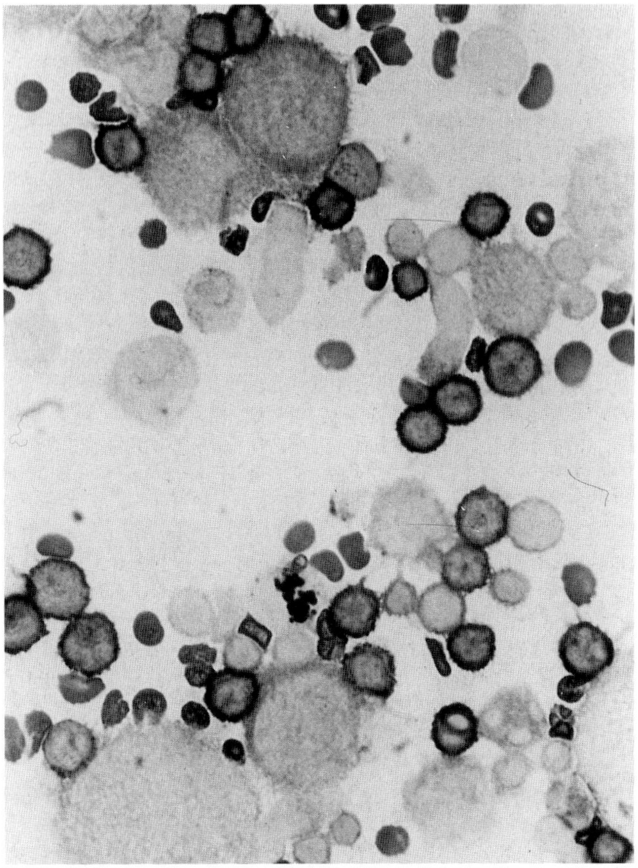

Fig. 18–20. Cytocentrifuge preparation of bronchoalveolar lavage fluid from patient with hypersensitivity pneumonitis immunostained for CD-8 antigen (marker for suppressor/cytotoxic lymphocytes). Most lymphocytes in preparation stained black for this antigen. ×550.

Clinical Pathologic Correlations

The predominant therapy for extrinsic allergic alveolitis is avoidance of the offending antigen. Various masks and filters may be helpful as well as better ventilation. Corticosteroids are frequently given therapeutically and also to prevent episodic disease.

The prognosis for patients with extrinsic allergic alveolitis depends on the amount and reversibility of damage to the lung. Chronic interstitial inflammation and granulomatous changes are reversible. If the disease is chronic and significant fibrosis has occurred, therapy of any kind may be ineffective. Anttinen and colleagues[96] evaluated two serum markers of collagen biosynthesis, galactosylhydroxylysl glucosyltransferse (S-GGT) activity and serum procollagen type III (S-PRO-III-NP), as possible indicators of irreversible pulmonary impairment in 40 patients with farmer's lung. They found that all patients with radiographic evidence of lung fibrosis after 1 year of evaluation had signifi-

cantly elevated S-GGT values at the onset of disease whereas S-PRO-III-NP was usually normal. Also, in patients with significantly elevated S-GGT values, normalization of lung function occurred more slowly or failed to equal improvement noted at the 1-year follow-up in patients with lower levels of S-GGT.

Braun et al.[97] evaluated 141 patients with farmer's lung disease and found that those patients with five or more symptomatic recurrences had significantly smaller values for vital capacity, total lung capacity, and carbon monoxide diffusing capacity than did those patients with less than five recurrences. They found no significant relationship between lung function and continued farming or length of disease. They did note that decreased carbon monoxide diffusing capacity was associated with persistently positive serum precipitins.

References

1. Gell RRA, Coombs PGH. Classification of allergic reactions responsible for clinical hypersensitivity disease. In:

Gell PGH, Coombs RRA, eds. Clinical aspects of immunology. 2d Ed. Oxford, Blackwell, 1968:575–596.

2. Campbell JM. Acute symptoms following work with hay. Br Med J 1932;2:1143–1144.

3. Fawcitt R. Fungoid conditions of the lung. Br J Radiol 1936;9:172–195; 354–378.

4. Tornell E. Thresher's lung. Acta Med Scand 1946; 125:191–219.

5. Pepys J, Riddell RW, Citron KM, Clayton YM. Precipitins against extracts of hay and moulds in the serum of patients with farmer's lung, aspergillosis, asthma and sarcoidosis. Thorax 1962;17:366–374.

6. Pepys J, Longbotton JL, Jenkins PA. Vegetable dust pneumoconiosis. Am Rev Respir Dis 1964;89:842–858.

7. Williams JV. Inhalation tests with hay and fungi in patients with farmer's lung. Acta Allergol 1961;16:77–78.

8. Williams JV. Inhalation and skin tests with extracts of hay and fungi in farmer's lung. Thorax 1963;18:182–196.

9. Corbaz R, Gregory PH, Lacey ME. Thermophilic and mesophilic actinomycetes in mouldy hay. J Gen Microbiol 1963;32:449–454.

10. Gregory PH, Fetenstein GN, Lacey ME, Skinner FA, Pepys J, Jenkins PA. Farmers lung disease: The development of antigens in moulding hays. J Gen Microbiol 1964;36:429–439.

11. Pepys J. Hypersensitivity to inhaled organic antigens. J Coll Physicians 1967;2:42–28.

12. Sostman HD, Matthay RD, Putman CE. Cytotoxic drug-induced lung disease. Am J Med 1977;62:608–615.

13. Farney RJ, Morris AH, Armstrong JD, Hammar S. Diffuse pulmonary disease after therapy with nitrogen mustard, vincristine, procarabazine and prednisone. Am Rev Respir Dis 1977;115:135–145.

14. Winterbauer RH, Wilske KR, Wheelis RF. Diffuse pulmonary injury associated with gold treatment. N Engl J Med 1976;294:919–921.

15. Higgins T, Niklasson PM. Hypersensitivity pneumonitis induced by trimethoprim. Br Med J 1990;300:1344.

16. Soda K, Ando M, Shimazu K, Sakata T, Yoshida K, Araki S. Different classes of antibody activities to *Trichosporon cutaneum* antigen in summer-type hypersensitivity pneumonitis by enzyme-linked immunosorbent assay. Am Rev Respir Dis 1986;133:83–87.

17. Orriols R, Manresa J, Aliaga J, Codina R, Rodrigo M, Morell F. Mollusk shell hypersensitivity pneumonitis. Ann Intern Med 1990;113:80–81.

18. Gamboa PM, de las Marinas MD, Antepara I, Jauregui I, Sunz MML. Extrinsic allergic alveolitis caused by esparto (*Stipa tenacissima*). Allergol Immunopathol 1990;18:331–334.

19. Banaszak EF, Theide WH, Fink JN. Hypersensitivity pneumonia due to contamination of an air conditioner. N Engl J Med 1970;283:271–276.

20. Fink JN, Banaszak EF, Thiede WH, Barboiak JJ. Interstitial pneumonitis due to hypersensitivity to an organism contaminating a heating system. Ann Intern Med 1971; 74:80–83.

21. Pickering CAC, Moore WKS, Lacey J, Holford-Stevens VC, Pepys J. Investigation of a respiratory disease associated with an air conditioning system. Clin Allergy 1976; 6:109–118.

22. Kumar P, Leech S. Hypersensitivity pneumonia due to contamination of a car air conditioner. N Engl J Med 1981;305:1531–1532.

23. Friend JAR, Gaddie J, Palmer KNV, Pickering CAC, Pepys J. Extrinsic allergic alveolitis and contaminated cooling-water in a factory machine. Lancet 1977;i:297–300.

24. Woodward ED, Friedlander B, Lesher RJ, Font W, Kinsey R, Hearne FT. Outbreak of hypersensitivity pneumonitis in an industrial setting. JAMA 1988;259:1965–1969.

25. Grant INB, Blyt W, Wardrop VE, Gordon RM, Pearson JCG, Mair A. Prevalence of farmer's lung in Scotland: a pilot survey. Br Med J 1972;1:530–534.

26. Madsen D, Klock LE, Wenzel FJ, Robbins JL, Schmidt CD. The prevalence of farmer's lung in an agricultural population. Am Rev Respir Dis 1976;113:171–174.

27. Gruchow HW, Hoffman RG, Marx JJ, Emanuel DA, Rimm AA. Precipitating antibodies to farmer's lung antigens in a Wisconsin farming population. Am Rev Respir Dis 1981;124:411–415.

28. Kreiss K, Hodgson MJ. Buildings associated epidemics. In: Walsh PJ, Dudney CS, Copenhaver ED, eds. Indoor air quality. Boca Raton, Florida: CRC Press, 1984:87–108.

29. Salvaggio JE, Karr RM, Hypersensitivity pneumonitis. Chest 1979;75(Suppl):270–274.

30. Hapke EJ, Seal RME. Thomas GO. Farmer's lung: A clinical, radiographic and serological correlation of acute and chronic stages. Thorax 1968;23:451–468.

31. Hargreave FE, Hinson KF, Reid L, Simon G, McCartney DS. The radiological appearances of allergic alveolitis due to bird sensitivity (bird fancier's lung). Clin Radiol 1972; 23:1–10.

32. Mokare S, Ikonen M, Haahtela T. Radiologic findings in farmer's lung: prognosis and correlation to lung function. Chest 1985;87:460–466.

33. Silver SF, Muller NL, Miller RR, Lefroe MS. Hypersensitivity pneumonitis: evaluation with CT. Radiology 1989; 173:441–445.

34. Fink JN. Hypersensitivity pneumonitis. J Allergy Clin Immunol 1984;74:1–9.

35. Hansen PJ, Penny R. Pigeon breeders disease. Study of the cell-mediated response to pigeon antigens by the lymphocyte culture technique. Int Arch Allergy Appl Immunol 1974;47:498–504.

36. Fink JN, Moore VL, Barboriak JJ. Cell-mediated hypersensitivity in pigeon breeders. Int Arch Allergy Appl Immunol 1975;49:831–836.

37. Pepys J. Hypersensitivity diseases of the lungs due to fungi and organic dusts. Monogr Allergy 1969;4:1–145.

38. Uhr JW. Delayed hypersensitivity. Physiol Rev 1966; 46:359–419.

39. Fink JN, Tebo T, Baraboriak JJ. Characterization of human precipitating antibody to inhaled antigens. J Immunol 1969;103:244–251.

40. Fink JN, Barboriak JJ, Sosman AJ. Immunologic studies of pigeon breeder's disease. J Allergy 1967;39:214–221.

41. Moore VL, Fink JN. Immunologic studies in hypersensitivity pneumonitis: Quantitative precipitins and complement-fixing antibodies in symptomatic and asymptomatic pigeon breeders. J Lab Clin Med 1975;85:540–545.

42. Ojanen T. Class specific antibodies in serodiagnosis of farmer's lung. Br J Ind Med 1992;49:332–336.

43. Reyes CN, Wenzel FJ, Lawton BR, Emanuel DA. The pulmonary pathology of farmer's lung disease. Chest 1982;81:142–146.

44. Barrowcliff DF, Arbuster PG. Farmer's lung: A study of an early acute fatal case. Thorax 1968;23:490–500.

45. Ghose T, Bandrigan P, Milleen R, Dill J. Immunopathological studies in patients with farmer's lung. Clin Allergy 1974;4:119–129.

46. Calvanico NJ, Ambegaonkar SP, Schlueter DP, Fink JN. Immunoglobulin levels in bronchoalveolar lavage fluid from pigeon breeders. J Lab Clin Med 1980;96:129–140.

47. Patterson R, Wang JLF, Fink JN, Calvanico JN, Roberts ME. IgA and IgG antibody activities of serum and bronchoalveolar lavage fluids from symptomatic and asymptomatic pigeon breeders. Am Rev Respir Dis 1979; 120:1113–1118.

48. Reynolds NY, Fulmer JD, Kazmierowski JA, Roberts WC, Frank MM, Crystal RG. Analysis of cellular and protein content of bronchoalveolar lavage fluid from patients with idiopathic pulmonary fibrosis and chronic hypersensitivity pneumonitis. J Clin Invest 1977;59:165–175.

49. Daniele RP, Elias JA, Epstein PE, Rossman MD. Bronchoalveolar lavage: Role in the pathogenesis, diagnosis and management of interstitial lung disease. Ann Intern Med 1985;102:93–108.

50. Richerson HB. Hypersensitivity pneumonitis: Pathology and pathogenesis. Clin Rev Allergy 1983;1:469–486.

51. Richerson HB. Immune complexes and the lung: A skeptical review. Surv Synth Pathol Res 1984;3:281–291.

52. Fournier E, Tonnel AB, Gosset Ph, Wallaer B. Ameisen JC, Voisin C. Early neutrophil alveolitis after antigen inhalation in hypersensitivity pneumonitis. Chest 1985; 88:563–566.

53. McSharry C, Banham SW, Boyd G. Effect of cigarette smoking on the antibody response to inhaled antigens and the prevalence of extrinsic allergic alveolitis among pigeon breeders. Clin Allergy 1985;15:487–494.

54. Cormier Y, Gagnon L, Berube-Genest F, Fournier M. Sequential bronchoalveolar lavage in experimental extrinsic allergic alveolitis: The influence of cigarette smoking. Am Rev Respir Dis 1988;137:1104–1109.

55. Kusaka H, Homma Y, Ogasawara H, et al. Five-year follow-up of *Microspolyspora faeni* antibody in smoking and nonsmoking farmers. Am Rev Respir Dis 1989;140:695–699.

56. Soda K, Ando M, Saka T, Sugimoto M, Nakashima H, Araki S. C1q and C3 in bronchoalveolar lavage fluid from patients with summer-type hypersensitivity pneumonitis. Chest 1988;93:76–80.

57. Caldwell JR, Pearce CE, Spencer C, Leder T, Waldman RH. Immunologic mechanisms in hypersensitivity pneumonitis. J Allergy Clin Immunol 1973;52:225–230.

58. Costabel U, Bross KJ, Marxen J, Matthys H. T lymphocytosis in bronchoalveolar lavage fluid of hypersensitivity pneumonitis: changes in profile of T-cell subsets during course of disease. Chest 1984;85:514–518.

59. Cormier Y, Belanger J, Beaudoin J, Laviolette M, Beaudoin R, Hebert J. Abnormal bronchoalveolar lavage in asymptomatic dairy farmers. Study of lymphocytes. Am Rev Respir Dis 1984;130:1046–1049.

60. Cormier Y, Belanger J, Laviolette M. Persistent bronchoalveolar lymphocytosis in asymptomatic farmers. Am Rev Respir Dis 1986;133:843–847.

61. Keller RH, Swartz S, Schlueter DP, Bar-Sela S, Fink JN. Immunoregulation in hypersensitivity pneumonitis: Phenotypic and functional studies of bronchoalveolar lavage lymphocytes. Am Rev Respir Dis 1984;130:766–771.

62. Denis M, Cormier Y, Fournier M, Tardif J, Laviolette M. Tumor necrosis factor plays an essential role in determining hypersensitivity pneumonitis in a mouse model. Am J Respir Cell Mol Biol 1991;5:477–483.

63. Denis M, Cormier Y, Laviolette M. Murine hypersensitivity pneumonitis: A study of cellular infiltrates and cytokine production and its modulation by cyclosporin A. Am J Respir Cell Mol Biol 1992;6:68–74.

64. Denis M, Cormier Y, Laviolette M, Ghadirian F. T cells in hypersensitivity pneumonitis: Effects of in vivo depletion of T cells in a mouse model. Am J Respir Cell Mol Biol 1992;5:183–189.

65. Allen DH, Basten A, Woolcock AJ. HLA and bird breeder's hypersensitivity pneumonitis. Monogr Allergy 1977; 11:45–54.

66. Flaherty DK, Iha T, Chmelik F, et al. HLA-8 and farmer's lung disease. Lancet 1975;ii:507.

67. Rittner C, Sennekamp J, Vogel F. HLA-B8 in pigeon fancier's lung. Lancet 1975;ii:1303.

68. Rodey GF, Rink J, Koethe S, et al. A study of HLA-A, B, C and DR specificities in pigeon breeder's disease. Am Rev Respir Dis 1979;119:755–759.

69. Benacerraf B, Katz DH. The nature and function of histocompatibility-linked immune response genes. In: Benacerraf B, ed. Immunogenetics and immunodeficiency. Baltimore: University Park Press, 1975:117–178.

70. Allen EM, Moore VL, Stevens JO. Strain variation in BCG-induced chronic pulmonary inflammation in mice. I. Basic model and possible genetic control by non-H-2 genes. J Immunol 1977;119:343–347.

71. Ando M, Hirayama K, Soda K, Okubo R, Araki S, Sasazuki T. HLA-DQw3 in Japanese summer-type hypersensitivity pneumonitis induced by *Trichosporon cutaneum*. Am Rev Respir Dis 1989;140:948–950.

72. Salvaggio JE, Phanuphak P, Stanford R, Bice D, Claman H. Experimental production of granulomatous pneumonitis. J Allergy Clin Immunol 1975;56:364–380.

73. Harris JD, Bice D, Salvaggio J. Cellular and humoral bronchopulmonary immune responses of rabbits immunized with thermophilic actinomycete antigen. Am Rev Respir Dis 1976;114:29–43.

74. Larson K, Eklund A, Malmberg P, Bjermer L, Lundgren R, Belin L. Hyaluronic acid (Hyaluronan) in BAL fluid distinguishes farmers with allergic alveolitis from farmers with asymptomatic alveolitis. Chest 1992;101:109–114.

75. Pesci A, Bertorelli G, Oliver D. Mast cells in bronchoalveolar lavage fluid and transbronchial biopsy specimens of patients with farmer's lung disease. Chest 1991;100: 1197–1202.

76. Berrens L, Guikers CLH, vanDijk A. The antigens in pigeon breeders disease and their interaction with human complement. Ann NY Acad Sci 1974;221:153–162.

77. Rylander R, Haglind P, Lundholm M, Mattsby I, Stenquist I. Humidifier fever and endotoxin exposure. Clin Allergy 1978;8:511–516.

78. Edwards JH, Barboriak JJ, Fink JN. Antigens in pigeon breeders disease. Immunology 1970;19:729–734.

79. Dickie HA, Rankin J. Farmer's lung: An acute granulomatous interstitial pneumonitis occurring in agricultural workers. JAMA 1958;167:1069–1076.

80. Totten RS, Reid DHS, Davies HO, Moran TJ. Farmer's lung. Am J Med 1958;25:803–809.

81. Frank RC. Farmer's lung: A form of pneumoconiosis due to organic dusts. AJR 1958;79:189–215.

82. Seal RMF, Thomas GO, Griffiths JJ. Farmer's lung. Proc R Soc Med 1963;56:271–273.

83. Seal RMF, Hapke EJ, Thomas GO, Pathology of the acute and chronic stages of farmer's lung. Thorax 1968;23: 469–489.

84. Hammar S, Bockus D, Remington F, Friedman S. The widespread distribution of Langerhans' cells in pathologic tissues: An ultrastructural and immunohistochemical study. Hum Pathol 1986;17:894–905.

85. Liebow AA, Carrington CB. Diffuse pulmonary lymphoreticular infiltration associated with dysproteinemia. Med Clin North Am 1973;57:809–843.

86. Perreault C, Cousineau S, D'Angelo G, et al. Lymphoid interstitial pneumonia after allogeneic bone marrow transplantation: A possible manifestation of chronic graft-versus-host disease. Cancer 1985;55:1–9.

87. Strimlan CV, Rosenow EC III, Divertie MB, Harrison EG Jr. Pulmonary manifestations of Sjögren's syndrome. Chest 1976;70:354–361.

88. Grieco MH, Chinoy-Acharya P. Lymphocytic interstitial pneumonia associated with acquired immune deficiency syndrome. Am Rev Respir Dis 1985;131:952–955.

89. Solal-Celingny T, Couderc LJ, Herman D, et al. Lymphoid interstitial pneumonitis in acquired immunodeficiency syndrome-related complex. Am Rev Respir Dis 1985;131:956–960.

90. Guillon J, Autran B, Denis M, et al., Human immunodeficiency virus-related lymphocytic alveolitis. Chest 1988;94:1264–1270.

91. Travis WD, Fox CH, Devaney KO, et al. Lymphoid pneumonitis in 50 adult patients with human immunodeficiency virus: Lymphocytic interstitial pneumonitis versus nonspecific interstitial pneumonitis. Hum Pathol 1992;23:529–541.

92. Rom WN, Travis WD. Lymphocyte-macrophage alveolitis in non-smoking individuals occupationally exposed to asbestos. Chest 1992;101:779–786.

93. Hammar SP, Hallman KO. Localized, acute, or unusual pulmonary disease in persons occupationally exposed to asbestos. Chest (in press).

94. Morell F, Orriols R, Molina C. Usefulness of skin test in farmer's lung. Chest 1985;87:202–205.

95. Costabel V, Bross KJ, Marxen MA, Matthys H. T-lymphocytosis in bronchoalveolar lavage fluid of hypersensitivity pneumonitis: Changes in profile of T-cell subsets during the course of disease. Chest 1984;85:514–518.

96. Anttinen H, Terho EO, Myllyla R, Savolainen E. Two serum markers of collagen biosynthesis as possible indicators of irreversible pulmonary impairment in farmer's lung. Am Rev Respir Dis 1986;133:88–93.

97. Braun SR, doPico GA, Tsiatis A, Horvath E, Dickie HA, Rankin J. Farmer's lung disease: Long-term clinical and physiologic outcome. Am Rev Respir Dis 1979;119:185–191.

CHAPTER 19

Sarcoidosis

Y. ROSEN

Sarcoidosis is a systemic disease that involves the lungs in almost all afflicted individuals. The pathologist plays a major and essential role in the management of patients with sarcoidosis because definitive establishment of the diagnosis depends on the microscopic examination of tissue. The nature of this enigmatic disease has perplexed physicians since the first description of its histologic features by Boeck in 1905. Interest in sarcoidosis has stimulated an enormous amount of research into its etiology, pathogenesis, epidemiology, abnormalities of the immune system, and clinical aspects. These efforts have resulted in thousands of publications[1,2] and 12 international conferences on sarcoidosis and other granulomatous disorders.[3–5] Yet, despite the substantial increase in knowledge about the various aspects of sarcoidosis gained during the past 100 years, its etiology remains entirely unknown. Many excellent publications present comprehensive and updated coverage of its immunological and clinical and radiographic features, epidemiology, abnormal physiology, diagnostic modalities, treatment, etc.[6–12]

Description of Sarcoidosis

Because of the current lack of knowledge about the etiology of sarcoidosis, precise definition of this disease is not possible. The following is a modification of the description of sarcoidosis adopted by the V11 International Conference on Sarcoidosis and Other Granulomatous Diseases in New York in 1975.[13]

Sarcoidosis is a multisystem granulomatous disorder of worldwide distribution whose etiology is presently unknown. Sarcoidosis may be a specific disease or it may be a syndrome. Young adults are most commonly affected and most frequently present with bilateral hilar lymphadenopathy, radiographically detectable pulmonary infiltration, skin or eye lesions. The diagnosis is established most securely when clinical and radiographic findings are supported by histologic evidence of epithelioid granulomas in more than one organ or a positive Kveim-Siltzbach skin test *and* other granulomatous diseases of known etiology are excluded. Elevation of angiotensin converting enzyme in serum and in granulomas, intrathoracic uptake of radioactive gallium and bronchoalveolar lavage fluid lymphocytosis occur in the majority of patients and are considered to be indicators of the activity of sarcoidosis rather than specific diagnostic findings. There may be hypercalciuria with or without hypercalcemia in a minority of patients. T-helper lymphocytes are present in increased numbers at sites of disease activity but not in the peripheral blood. In collaboration with cells of the mononuclear phagocytic system T-helper lymphocytes influence granuloma formation and stimulate B lymphocytes to produce antibodies resulting in raised serum immunoglobulins. There is depression of cellular immune reactions in the skin which is manifested by anergy to a variety of intradermally injected antigens. The course and prognosis of the disease correlate with the mode of onset. An acute onset, particularly with erythema nodosum and fever, usually heralds a self-limiting course with spontaneous resolution while an insidious onset may be followed by relentless progressive fibrosis. Corticosteroids relieve symptoms and suppress inflammation and granuloma formation and lead to lowering of raised serum angiotensin converting enzyme levels but their overall long-term effect on outcome is a matter of controversy.

The Etiology of Sarcoidosis

All attempts to identify the cause of sarcoidosis have been unsuccessful. Hypotheses concerning its etiology fall into two major categories: (1) Sarcoidosis is caused by one or more agents, probably of exogenous environmental origin, and is therefore a specific disease. (2) Sarcoidosis represents an abnormal host immunologic response to a variety of commonly encountered agents and is, therefore, a syndrome. This latter possibility is sometimes termed the "sarcoid diathesis." It is also possible that these may combine to play the etiologic role.

Of the numerous infectious and other agents that have been considered and investigated, none has ever conclusively been proven to be a cause of sarcoidosis. The once-popular notion that sarcoidosis is a form of tuberculosis has generally lost favor. Nevertheless, much circumstantial evidence suggests that sarcoidosis may, at least in some patients, be related to mycobacterial infection,[14-19] and this possibility cannot be easily or entirely dismissed. The extremely high incidence of lung and mediastinal lymph node involvement strongly suggests that the etiologic agent(s) are inhaled into the lungs and then disseminated to other body sites. Reports of sarcoidosis or sarcoid-like involvement of hilar and paratracheal lymph nodes in a small number of patients treated for a variety of testicular germ cell tumors[20,21] raises the possibility that tumor antigens may incite the development of sarcoidosis in some patients.

Evidence in support an underlying "sarcoid diathesis" includes the observation that sarcoidosis is more common in monozygotic twins than in heterozygotic twins,[22] the association of various manifestations of sarcoidosis with specific HLA antigens,[23,24] and reports of familial occurrence.[25]

There is some evidence to indicate that smoking may protect against development of sarcoidosis. Studies have shown a significantly lower proportion of smokers among sarcoid patients compared with nonsarcoid controls,[26-28] and evidence indicates that this relationship may be dose dependent.[28]

Immunologic Aspects of Granuloma Formation and Sarcoidosis

The Granuloma

The epithelioid granuloma is the characteristic microscopic finding in sarcoidosis (Fig. 19–1). Adams[29] defined a granuloma as "a compact (organized) collection of mature mononuclear phagocytes (macrophages or epithelioid cells) which may or may not be accompanied by accessory features such as necrosis or the infiltration of inflammatory leukocytes." He further stated that "the granuloma appears to be host's response to a high local concentration of a foreign substance which was not

destroyed by the acute inflammatory response and which is being contained and destroyed by mononuclear phagocytes in various stages of maturation or activation." James and Neville[30] have stated that "the sarcoid granuloma is the battleground between indigestible antigen and macrophages." Granuloma formation as observed under experimental conditions begins with a transient acute inflammatory reaction, which then assumes the morphologic features of nonspecific chronic inflammation. Within several days mature granulomas develop that are composed of compact aggregates of mature macrophages.[31,34-36]

The principal cellular constituents of granulomas are mononuclear phagocytes and lymphocytes. A basic understanding of the properties and functions of these two cell lines and their complex interrelationships is necessary to gain some understanding of granulomatous inflammation and the relationship of sarcoidosis to other granulomatous diseases.

Immunopathogenesis

Although very little is known about the etiology of sarcoidosis, much is now known about its immunologic aspects and immunopathogenesis. Clinical and experimental data strongly suggest that activation of the cell-mediated immune system by antigenic stimulation plays an important role both in initiating and modulating granuloma formation.[37] The formation of granulomas in sarcoidosis results from and is preceded by the presence of activated T lymphocytes and activated mononuclear phagocytes at sites of disease activity.[8,12,38-42] Mediators released by these cells appear to play a significant role in the pathogenesis of the disease and in granuloma formation.* The severity of the pulmonary disease appears to be determined by the number of T lymphocytes and macrophages in the lower respiratory tract and their state of activation.[8] Whether sarcoidosis represents an abnormal overreactivity of the immune system to antigens in general or develops only in response to a specific antigenic agent (or agents), or whether elements of both factors play a role, is not known.

Mononuclear Phagocyte System

Monocytes, tissue macrophages, inflammatory macrophages, and epithelioid cells share a common origin, morphology, and function and are regarded as belonging to the mononuclear phagocyte system.[42,45] All these cells have their origin in a bone marrow stem cell.

---

*References: 8, 38, 40, 43, 44.

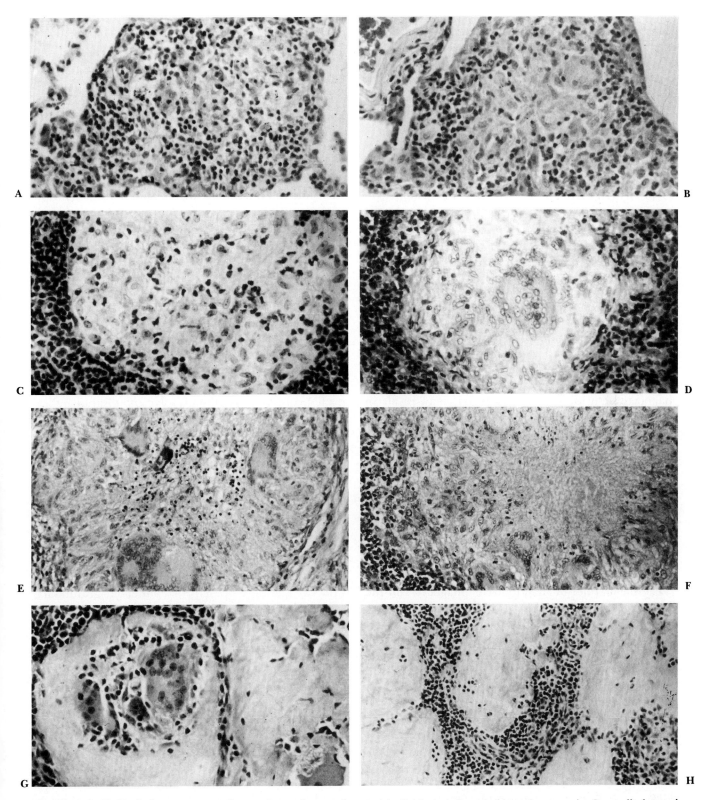

Fig. 19–1 A–H. Varied appearance of granulomas in sarcoidosis. **A.** Lung. Alveolitis with noncompact central aggregate of macrophages; early granuloma formation. **B.** Lung. Later phase of granuloma formation with alveolitis now evident predominantly at periphery. **C.** Lymph node. Epithelioid granuloma. Note sparse admixture of lymphocytes with epithelioid cells. **D.** Lymph node. Epithelioid granuloma with multinucleate foreign-body type giant cell. **E.** Lymph node. Epithelioid granuloma with early necrosis. Centrally located pyknotic, hyperchromatic nuclei (apoptotic bodies) of necrotic epithelioid cells. **F.** Lymph node. Epithelioid granuloma with well-developed central necrosis. **G.** Lymph node. Partial fibrosis (hyalinization) of granulomas. (Reprinted from Rosen et al. Pathology Annual Vol. 14. Pt. 1. Appleton-Lange, 1979, with permission.) **H.** Lymph node. Complete fibrosis (hyalinization) of granulomas.

Monocytes develop in the marrow, circulate briefly in the peripheral blood, and then migrate into the tissues. Most resident tissue macrophages arise from monocytes.[46] Mononuclear phagocytes accumulate at sites of inflammation largely as a result of varied chemotactic influences,[47,48] some of which specifically attract mononuclear phagocytes; mature mononuclear phagocytes appear to be more responsive than immature ones to chemotactic stimuli.[47]

Maturation of monoblasts to monocytes and then to mature macrophages is accompanied by distinctive morphologic and functional changes. The changes include increased cell size, decreased nuclear:cytoplasmic ratio, increased surface ruffling, and markedly increased cytoplasmic complexity as the result of development of numerous organelles.[31,49,50] These changes are accompanied by increased amounts of cytoplasmic esterase and lysozyme, pinocytosis, adherence to glass, Fc-mediated phagocytosis, number of Fc receptors,[51] and by a progressive loss of proliferative capability.[52,53] Stimulation of mononuclear phagocytes so that they are capable of killing intracellular microorganisms, parasites, and tumor cells is termed "activation."[54–57] Lymphokines appear to play a major role in mononuclear phagocyte activation,[58] and activation may result in further maturation.

Major known functions of mononuclear phagocytes include endocytosis, synthesis and secretion of a variety of proteins, and induction and regulation of the immune response.[59–61]

Mononuclear phagocytes are now recognized to have significant synthetic and secretory capability,[29,59,62] which tends to increase with maturation and with activation.[54] Angiotensin-converting enzyme (ACE), which is relevant in sarcoidosis, is one of the dozens of known secretory products of mononuclear phagocytes.

The major roles of mononuclear phagocytes in the immune response appear to be removal and catabolism of exogenous antigen, appropriate presentation of antigen to lymphocytes and secretion of soluble factors regulating lymphocytes.[29] Most antigens require interaction between macrophages and T lymphocytes to induce a lymphocyte response. The nature of this interaction has been and remains an area of intense investigation. Macrophages function to present antigen to the lymphocytes and to produce soluble mediators that act on T lymphocytes.[29] The lung macrophages in sarcoidosis are activated, and their response to antigens differs from that of alveolar macrophages in normal lungs.[8,38] Activated lung macrophages from patients with sarcoidosis appear to be capable of inducing enhanced replication and activation of T lymphocytes by means of their manner of antigen presentation and their release of a mediator, interleukin-1.[63] This has

suggested that stimulation of T-cell replication and activation is a major role of the alveolar macrophages in sarcoidosis. It is not yet known whether the response that leads to the development of disease is initiated by the lung T lymphocytes or the alveolar macrophages.

Other substances released from activated macrophages that may have a role in the pathogenesis of the lesions of sarcoidosis include cytotoxic factors, superoxide anion, type IV collagenase, gamma interferon, and tumor necrosis factor.[44]

The cells of the mononuclear phagocyte system that are found in granulomas include monocytes, macrophages, epithelioid cells, and giant cells.[36] The macrophages arise from maturation of monocytes, epithelioid cells from macrophages, and giant cells from fusion of macrophages or epithelioid cells.[31] Granulomas are considered to be either of "high-turnover" or "low-turnover" type on the basis of studies of the turnover time of their constituent cells.[64] Epithelioid granulomas are generally high-turnover granulomas. High-turnover granulomas tend to evolve into low-turnover granulomas as the inciting agent is destroyed within the macrophages.[46,64] Granulomas usually persist until the inciting agent is either destroyed or extensively degraded, and they may then resolve and disappear.[31]

Epithelioid Cells and Epithelioid Granulomas

When the inciting agent is capable of evoking extensive maturation of mononuclear phagocytes, the mature macrophages undergo transformation to epithelioid cells and epithelioid granulomas are formed[31] (see Fig. 19–1). The development of delayed hypersensitivity to the inciting agent appears to be the most important mechanism influencing the development of most epithelioid granulomas.[34,58,65] Lymphokines significantly influence the development of epithelioid granulomas because they are potent stimulants of macrophage activation in vitro. However, epithelioid granulomas may arise in the absence of delayed hypersensitivity.[31–33]

Epithelioid cells measure 25 to 40 μm in diameter and are larger than macrophages. Ultrastructural study of epithelioid cells in sarcoidosis[66] shows a centrally or eccentrically located nucleus with a prominent nucleolus; a narrow layer of heterochromatin usually is present immediately beneath the nuclear membrane. The cell periphery displays abundant, fine finger-like, cytoplasmic projections that often interdigitate with those of adjacent similar cells and are only very seldom joined by rudimentary intercellular junctions. The cytoplasmic organelles are profuse and exhibit a complex arrangement with many mitochondria, abundant rough endoplasmic reticulum and free ribosomes, and a lesser amount of smooth endoplasmic reticulum. The

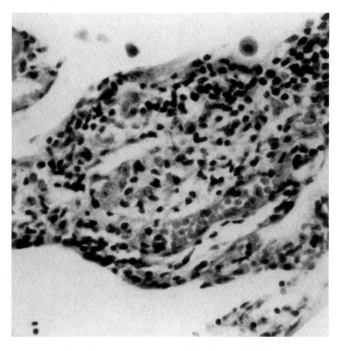

Fig. 19–2. Lung. Alveolitis in sarcoidosis.

Golgi apparatus is well developed and numerous lysosomes may be seen. The ultrastructural features of epithelioid cellls and their high content of lysosomal enzymes indicate that they have the capacity for extensive protein synthesis.[31] Compared to macrophages, epithelioid cells have increased secretory and bactericidal capability and reduced phagocytic capability.[29]

Giant Cells

Giant cells generally arise from fusion of mononuclear phagocytes[29,67–69] and are initially of foreign-body type with randomly dispersed nuclei (see Figs. 19–1D,G). They then undergo reorganization and transformation to Langhans'-type giant cells with peripherally arranged nuclei[69] (see Fig. 19–1E). Giant cells are short lived, have little phagocytic capability,[67] and may contain cytoplasmic inclusions such as asteroid bodies, Schaumann bodies, and slit-like crystals.

Lymphocytes

The marked increase in lymphocyte numbers in the lungs in sarcoidosis primarily involves T cells, largely of the helper subtype.[8,38,40,42] This T-helper lymphocytosis in the lungs occurs very early in sarcoidosis, preceding granuloma formation, and makes the main cellular contribution to the alveolitis of sarcoidosis (Figs. 19–1A and 19–2) (see later section on Alveolitis). Analysis of lymphocyte subtypes in the lungs in sarcoidosis shows a T-helper/T-suppressor ratio of 10 : 1 compared to 1.8 : 1 in the normal lung.[40,42,70] In contrast to lymphocytes in normal lung, the lung T cells in sarcoidosis are activated and release mediators (lymphokines), which appear to have a significant role in granuloma formation.[38] These include monocyte chemotactic factor,[71] migration inhibition factor, macrophage-activating factor,[72,73] leukocyte inhibitory factor,[39,74] and interleukin-2.[75]

Lymphocytes are often numerous and are well visualized by light microscopy in the peripheral cellular mantle of the sarcoid granuloma. Although lymphocytes are seldom conspicuous in the central portion of the granuloma, they can be visualized readily by electron microscopy.

Mechanism of Granuloma Formation

Granulomatous diseases, which are triggered by antigen recognition, appear to share a common pathway for granuloma formation. Activation of the two major components of the cellular immune system, lymphocytes and mononuclear phagocytes, by antigenic stimulation initiates and modulates granuloma formation via production of mediators, that is, the lymphokines and soluble macrophage factors that regulate lymphocytes. Lymphokines secreted by activated T cells have a major role in recruitment of mononuclear phagocytes. Activation of macrophages increases endocytosis and destruction of the granuloma-inciting material. Epithelioid cells and epithelioid granulomas develop under conditions that promote extreme maturation of mononuclear phagocytes. Delayed hypersensitivity plays a major role in the development of epithelioid granulomas. Cell turnover in epithelioid granulomas is initially high and tends to diminish as the inciting agent(s) are destroyed and degraded.

Function of Granulomas

Adams[29,31] has stated that "Granulomas ultimately serve to protect the host from high local concentrations of foreign or "non-self" materials of both endogenous and exogenous origin . . . by degradation, detoxification and containment of unwanted material."

Localization of the Cellular Immune Respose and Its Significance

The cellular immune response in sarcoidosis appears to be localized to sites of disease activity because the character of the inflammatory reaction in the lungs is not reflected by parallel chages in the blood. In active sarcoidosis, the inflammation in the lungs and extrapulmonary sites of involvement is characterized by large numbers of T lymphocytes whereas the number of T lymphocytes in the peripheral blood is reduced.[38,39,42] The markedly elevated number of activated T lymphocytes at sites of disease activity is probably largely responsible for the nonspecific polyclonal stimulation of the humoral immune system, resulting in hypergammaglobulinemia and production of antibodies against a variety of antigens.[76]

There is evidence that lung B lymphocytes rather than blood B lymphocytes are the source of increased immunoglobulins in sarcoidosis.[77] The apparent compartmentalization of the cellular immune response provides an explanation for various seemingly paradoxical characteristic findings, which in the past have been incorrectly interpreted as evidence of depression of the cellular immune reponse in sarcoidosis. These findings include complete or partial anergy to a variety of skin tests, impairment of the proliferative response of circulating mononuclear cells to antigens and mitogens, and lymphocytopenia. The helper/suppressor ratio of T lymphocytes in peripheral blood in sarcoidosis is only 0.8 : 1,[40] and the blood T lymphocytes are not activated.[43] Anergy is thought to be related to the reduced peripheral T-lymphocyte helper/suppressor ratio with increased suppressor effect.[8,40] It has also been suggested that reduced numbers of cutaneous Langerhans' cells in sarcoidosis may contribute to anergy.[78]

The Sarcoid Granuloma

The characteristic microscopic finding in sarcoidosis is the epithelioid granuloma (see Fig. 19–1), with or without minimal necrosis or intracytoplasmic inclusions (Fig. 19–3). From a diagnostic standpoint, granulomas of this type are considered nonspecific lesions and are a characteristic finding in many other conditions, including infections, neoplasms, chemical- and drug-induced diseases, a leukocyte oxidase defect, Crohn's disease, beryllium disease, and hypersensitivity pneumonitis.[79,80] Investigators have long sought but failed to identify some morphologic feature of granulomas that could be considered to be specific and diagnostic of sarcoidosis. At one time or another Schaumann bodies, asteroid bodies, an intact fine reticulum in granulomas, absence of necrosis, and uniform appearance of granulomas have been considered diagnostically important and subsequently shown to be nonspecific findings. Electron microscopic examination of granulomas does not generally contribute to diagnosis.

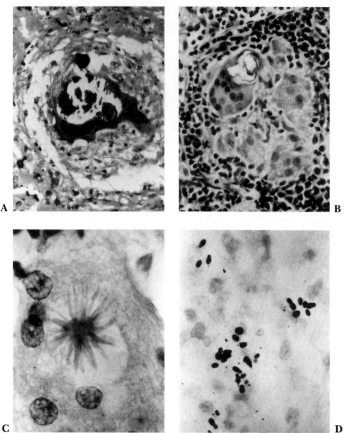

Fig. 19–3 A–D. Inclusions in sarcoidosis. **A.** Schaumann (conchoidal) body. **B.** Schaumann body containing a large amount of birefringent crystalline material within a giant cell (polarized light). **C.** Asteroid body in giant cell (oil immersion). **D.** Hamazaki–Wesenberg bodies with yeastlike pseudobudding appearance. Methenamine silver stain (oil immersion). (**C** and **D** reprinted from Rosen et al. Pathology Annual, Vol. 14, Pt. 1. Appleton-Lange, 1979, with permission.)

Localization of T Lymphocyte Subsets

Studies with immunohistochemical techniques using monoclonal antibodies against T lymphocytes and T lymphocyte subsets[81–84] and B lymphocytes[85] in frozen tissues containing epithelioid granulomas of diverse etiology have shown relatively large numbers of lymphocytes admixed with epithelioid cells in the central portion of the granulomas as well as in the peripheral mantle. Most studies have shown that in the epithelioid granulomas of sarcoidosis, tuberculoid leprosy, and tuberculosis, cells of the suppressor/cytotoxic subtype are seen almost exclusively in the outer peripheral mantle whereas cells of the helper/inducer subtype are seen throughout the granuloma and in the inner area of the peripheral mantle, representing almost all the lymphocytes that are admixed with epithelioid cells in the central portion.[81-84]

Although the significance of this striking arrangement of T-lymphocyte subsets in epithelioid granulomas is not known, it seems likely that the intimate contact of helper T cells with mononuclear phagocytes results in epithelioid maturation and effective antigen presentation, and that the presence of suppressor T cells at the periphery may reflect their possible role in localizing and modulating the granulomatous reaction.[82-84] By contrast, in inflammatory reactions where macrophages are the predominating cell type and epithelioid cells and granulomas are not formed (lepromatous leprosy, rhinoscleroma), the suppressor and helper T lymphocytes are diffusely distributed and admixed throughout the lesion; there is no peripheral lymphocyte mantle.[82] Usually very few bacteria are found in the epithelioid granulomas of tuberculoid leprosy and tuberculosis compared to the very large number of bacteria usually seen in the lesions of lepromatous leprosy and rhinoscleroma, which seems to indicate that the specific locations of T-cell subpopulations and their ratios may reflect the effectiveness of the granulomatous inflammatory response in eliminating the inciting agent.[82,83]

Necrosis in Sarcoid Granulomas

Although the granulomas in sarcoidosis are generally regarded as being nonnecrotizing, necrosis is actually a frequent finding. Ricker and Clark,[86] who reported necrosis in 35% of cases of sarcoidosis in 1949, drew attention to this finding. Subsequent reports by other investigators confirmed this observation and indicated that necrosis can be seen in granuloma-containing tissues from patients with sarcoidosis in 6%–39% of cases.[87] The necrosis that has been observed in the granulomas of sarcoidosis has been variously described as fibrinoid, granular, eosinophilic granular, and coagulative, and its resemblance to "caseous" necrosis has been noted. Necrosis seen in sarcoidosis usually differs only quantitatively from that seen in tuberculosis and other granulomatous diseases in which it is more extensive and is regarded as a characteristic feature. The necrosis in sarcoidosis is usually minute, spotty, and inconspicuous, involving the central portions of only a small proportion of the granulomas (see Figs. 19–1E,F). Ovoid cells with condensed, hyperchromatic, and fragmented nuclei and acidophilic cytoplasm (apoptotic bodies) are often seen in the central portion of granulomas in sarcoidosis and other diseases[88] (see Fig. 19–1E). These represent individual and isolated necrotic epith-

lioid cells that may occur in either the presence or absence of focal necrosis. Necrosis in tuberculosis and other infectious diseases may appear identical to that seen in sarcoidosis. Rare cases of sarcoidosis may exhibit larger and even confluent areas of necrosis. Carlens et al.[89] noted an association of fever, erythema nodosum, and arthralgia with necrosis in mediastinal lymph nodes of patients with sarcoidosis. Zettergren[15] found necrosis to be more prevalent in biopsy material obtained from patients with recent onset of sarcoidosis.

Necrosis in granulomas occurs when the granuloma-inciting agent is highly toxic to the macrophages or when a vigorous delayed hypersensitivity response is evoked,[34] and is probably related to secretion of hydrolytic and proteolytic enzymes and activated oxygen intermediates by macrophages.[90] Ischemic (coagulative) necrosis in granulomatous lesions secondary to granulomatous angiitis probably also occurs, but this is not well documented.

The term "caseous necrosis" and related terms often used in diagnoses and discussions of granulomatous lesions exhibiting necrosis have proven to be a source of substantial confusion for both pathologists and clinicians. Concerning the definition of "caseation," Medlar[91] stated:

The term caseation is applied to the gross characteristics of the necrotic material commonly seen in tuberculous infection. This necrotic tissue can easily be removed from the surrounding living tissue, leaving a cavity. It has no texture and varies in consistence from thick pus to a crumbly material not unlike cottage cheese.

This description stresses that the term caseation describes only the gross appearance of necrotic tissue as well as the common association of this gross appearance with tuberculosis. Microscopic examination of tissue that grossly appears "caseous" shows partial autolysis of the necrotic cells, which fuse with intercellular materials to become a formless and coagulated inspissated mass.[92] The "caseous" appearance results from incomplete digestion of necrotic tissue, probably because of local inhibition of proteolytic enzymes.[92] Many physicians erroneously consider the mention of "caseation" or "caseating" in a pathology report to be tantamount to a diagnosis of tuberculosis, but "caseation" appears in numerous other diseases including fungal infections, pulmonary angiitis and granulomatosis, malignant neoplasms, parasitic infections, aspiration of cod liver oil, syphilis, tularemia, and typhoid fever.[92] On the other hand, suppuration, liquefactive necrosis, and coagulative necrosis may occur in tuberculosis in addition to the more usual caseous necrosis.

It is evident that "caseation" is difficult to define and

that its description is imprecise and based on highly subjective criteria. Moreover, it does not describe a microscopic appearance and has no particular diagnostic relevance. The terms "caseation," "caseating," "noncaseating," and "caseous" are gross descriptive terms only. As they serve no relevant purpose as diagnostic terms or modifiers in human pathology and may even be diagnostically misleading, these terms should be avoided in pathology reports. It is appropriate to describe granulomas as being either "necrotizing" or "nonnecrotizing" or as "exhibiting minimal necrosis."

Intracytoplasmic Inclusions in Sarcoid Granulomas

Schaumann (Conchoidal) Bodies

Schaumann bodies, also called "conchoidal bodies," are very large (25–200 μm), concentrically lamellated bodies seen predominantly within giant cells in the granulomas of sarcoidosis in hypersensitivity pneumonitis and other granulomatous diseases (see Figs. 19–3A,B). They are formed within the cytoplasm of epithelioid cells and giant cells and are composed of a mucopolysaccharide matrix impregnated with calcium salts and some iron.[93] As the bodies enlarge, cell rupture may result in their extrusion into the extracellular space. A crystalline component that is colorless, intensely birefringent, and spiculated may be seen frequently, either alone or in combination with the conchoidal body[94] (see Fig. 19–3B). As many as 70% of conchoidal bodies have crystals associated with them. The crystals range from 1 to 20 μm and are usually found in clumps within the cytoplasm of giant cells. They stain positively for iron and calcium salts.

It is possible that these crystals act as a nidus for the formation of the conchoidal body. Jones Williams[94] reported finding crystalline and conchoidal bodies in 88% of cases of sarcoidosis, 62% of chronic beryllium disease, and 6% of tuberculosis. Conchoidal bodies alone may be seen in approximately 50% of cases of sarcoidosis.[87] Crystalline bodies occurring without conchoidal bodies have been reported in 41% of cases of sarcoidosis, 15% of chronic beryllium disease, and 3% of tuberculosis.[94] Crystalline inclusions within granulomas have been reported in approximately two-thirds of biopsy specimens containing nonnecrotizing granulomas (mostly sarcoidosis) when routine slide examination was supplemented by polarized light examination.[95] Histochemical analysis of the crystalline inclusions indicates that the majority are composed of calcium oxlate.[95,96]

Asteroid Bodies

Asteroid bodies are stellate inclusions that are found only in the cytoplasm of multinucleated giant cells in sarcoidosis and a variety of other granulomatous diseases including tuberculosis, leprosy, histoplasmosis, schistosomiasis, lipoidal granulomas, and foreign-body granulomas.[86] These structures vary from 5 μm to 30 μm in size and contain as many as 30 or more rays radiating from a central core (see Fig. 19–3C). Asteroid bodies may be seen in granuloma-containing tissues in 2%–9% of patients with sarcoidosis.[86,87]

Ultrastructural examination of asteroid bodies shows that they are composed of microfilaments, microtubules, mature centrioles, paracentrioles, and an intervening amorphous matrix.[97] There is no evidence that they contain collagen. It has been postulated that asteroid body formation is related to the process of cell fusion and internal organization involved in the formation of giant cells from epithelioid cells.[97] Cain and Kraus[97] stated that "the forces required for this end are provided by the microfilaments and microtubules which evolve under the regulation of the centrioles with hypertrophy of the system which later on "solidifies" in a star shaped configuration." Asteroid bodies may thus be viewed as composed of cell organelles that are, in all likelihood, functionally obsolescent.

Hamazaki–Wesenberg Bodies

Spindle-shaped bodies, generally called Hamazaki–Wesenberg bodies (see Fig. 19–3D), are frequently seen in the granulomatous lymph nodes from patients with sarcoidosis and in nongranulomatous lymph nodes from patients with sarcoidosis and a variety of other disorders.[98–106] These structures are variously named yellow bodies,[102] yellow-brown bodies,[103] curious bodies,[100] spiral bodies,[106] and spindle bodies.[99] They are oval or spindle shaped, pleomorphic, and range from 0.5 to 0.8 μm in size. They appear yellow-brown in sections stained with hematoxylin and eosin (H and E). Histochemically the yellow-brown pigment has the characteristics of lipofuscin.

The bodies are seen both intracellularly and extracellularly, predominantly at or near the peripheral sinus of the lymph node, and almost invariably outside the granulomas. They have been reported in 11% to 68% of sarcoid lymph nodes,[103,107] in 11.5% to 15% of nongranulomatous lymph nodes that were either normal or involved with various diseases,[102,107] and in 16% of open lung biopsy specimens from patients with sarcoidosis.[107] By light microscopy these structures often exhibit an appearance that is similar to yeast-like budding, and they stain well with methenamine silver stains (see Fig. 19–3D); for these reasons, they can easily be mistaken for fungi (budding yeasts). Recognition of their pleomorphism and acid-fastness with the Ziehl–Neelsen stain and the fact that they elicit no host response readily facilitate their distinction from fungi. Positive staining reactions are also obtained with the following stains: Fontana–Masson, Oil Red O, Sudan Black B, and periodic acid–Schiff (PAS), with and without diastase.[108] Ultrastructural examination shows that the Hamazaki-Wesenberg bodies are giant, intracellular and extracellular lysosomes and residual bodies.[103–105,107,109] The appearance of budding is caused by conglomeration.

Slit-Like Crystals

Elongated needle-shaped birefringent crystals having physical and chemical properties of cholesterol derivatives may be seen in giant cells in as many as 17% of cases of sarcoidosis and in other granulomatous diseases.[87] Schaumann bodies have, on rare occasion, been observed forming around these crystals.[93]

Centrospheres

Poorly defined clusters of vacuoles of uncertain origin found within the cytoplasm of giant cells.[110] These structures many sometimes resemble fungi when stained with H and E.

Lung Involvement in Sarcoidosis

Prevalence and Radiographic Aspects

A worldwide review of several thousand patients with sarcoidosis[111] showed radiographic evidence of intrathoracic involvement in 87% of cases: lungs (41%) and hilar lymph nodes (80%) being the sites most frequently involved. Open lung biopsy studies have shown that the lungs are involved in nearly 100% of patients with intrathoracic sarcoidosis even when the lungs appear normal by radiography.[112–114] Clinical staging of intrathoracic sarcoidosis is based on radiographic findings: stage 0, normal chest radiograph; stage 1, mediastinal lymphadenopathy only; stage 2, mediastinal lymphadenopathy and lung infiltrates; stage 3, lung infiltrates only. The presence of cystic lesions in sarcoidosis patients with chronic fibrotic lung disease is sometimes designated as stage 4.

The radiographic patterns do not necessarily represent sequential progression of the disease. Throughout this chapter the term intrathoracic sarcoidosis is used to designate only involvement of the lungs, airways, or mediastinal lymph nodes; involvement of the heart or other intrathoracic structures is not considered.

Clinical Aspects

Data combined from sarcoidosis treatment centers throughout the world show the following stages at presentation: stage 0, 8%; stage 1, 51%; stage 2, 29%; stage 3, 12%.[111] Approximately 50% of patients with intrathoracic sarcoidosis are asymptomatic, and their disease is usually first detected by chest radiography performed as part of a routine physical examination or chest disease screening program.[11] Uveitis and erythema nodosum are among the most commmon causes of presenting symptoms.

Patients with stage 1 disease are almost all asymptomatic and without evidence of extrathoracic lesions. The hilar lymphadenopathy is bilateral in 96% of these patients.[115] The combination of bilateral hilar lymphadenopathy and erythema nodosum in the same patient is known as Löfgren's syndrome.[116] Some patients with Löfgren's syndrome may also have uveitis, parotitis, and fever. The prognosis is excellent for these patients, and the lesions undergo spontaneous resolution in almost all cases. Although malignant neoplasms of various types may also present with bilateral hilar lymphadenopathy, this finding is most characteristic of sarcoidosis. Winterbauer and Moore[117] reported bilateral hilar lymphadenopathy as a presenting finding in 9.4% of patients with lymphoma and in 0.8% and 0.2% of patients with bronchogenic carcinoma and extrathoracic malignancies, respectively, compared with 74% of patients with sarcoidosis.

Symptomatology and Pulmonary Function

Dyspnea is the most frequent symptom produced by lung involvement. Cough is an infrequent feature, and pleuritic chest pain, wheezing, pleural effusions, and clubbing of the fingers are rare.[118] Hemoptysis, reported in 4%–6% of patients with sarcoidosis,[119,120] most frequently occurs in association with advanced fibrous and cystic changes in the lungs. When hemoptysis of major or massive degree occurs, the underlying cause is almost invariably a mycetoma (aspergilloma)[120] Measurements of lung function in patients with sarcoidosis are of no diagnostic value, but they do serve to assess the degree of disability and to monitor the course of the disease and the patients' response to therapy. The degree of measurable abnormality of lung function depends on the severity and location of granulomatous inflammation, alveolitis. and fibrosis. It is well known that in sarcoidosis it is difficult to correlate clinical status, radiographic findings, results of pulmonary function studies, and results of pathologic examination. The reduction in diffusing capacity appears to correlate best with the severity of lung disease as determined by pathologic examination.[121,122]

Extrathoracic Involvement

Extrathoracic lesions occur with significant frequency among patients with intrathoracic sarcoidosis; they are seen mostly in those with chronic disease and only infrequently in patients with stage 1 disease. Approximately 70% of patients exhibit clinical evidence of extrathoracic lesions at some time in the course of their disease.[123] The distribution of extrathoracic involvement in patients with intrathoracic sarcoidosis, as observed in clinical studies, is as follows: peripheral lymph nodes, 59%; eye, 30%; liver, 28%; skin, 26%; spleen, 23%; salivary glands, 7%; bone, 10%–15%; heart, 5%; and kidneys, 5%.[124,125] By contrast an autopsy series of 30 cases of sarcoidosis showed the following distribution of extrathoracic involvement: peripheral lymph nodes, 77%; liver, 47%; spleen, 33%; heart, 13%; and kidneys, 13%.[126]

Distribution and Gross and Microscopic Appearance of Lesions

Granulomas are seen thoughout both lungs and have a tendency to occur preferentially in the upper two-thirds. The opportunity to study the gross appearance of pulmonary sarcoidosis is rare except at autopsy in patients with very advanced disease. Consequently, there is little information available on gross appearances in relatively early pulmonary sarcoidosis. The granulomas may be small, discrete, and of uniform size, or they may be confluent and form nodular masses. Confluent granulomas may be seen in as many as 27% of open lung biopsies from patients with sarcoidosis.[127] Poorly defined granulomas are often seen within alveoli. In addition to granulomas, nongranulomatous interstitial pneumonitis (alveolitis) (see Figs. 19–1A and 19–2) is often seen in early disease and has been identified in approximately two-thirds of open lung biopsy specimens[41] (see section on **Alveolitis**).

Although the granulomas may occur anywhere in the lung parenchyma and its airways, blood vessels, and pleural coverings (Fig. 19–4), as many as 75% of granulomas may be localized in alveolar walls and connective tissue around fixed structures, that is, blood vessels, bronchioles, pleura, and fibrous septae.[128] Because

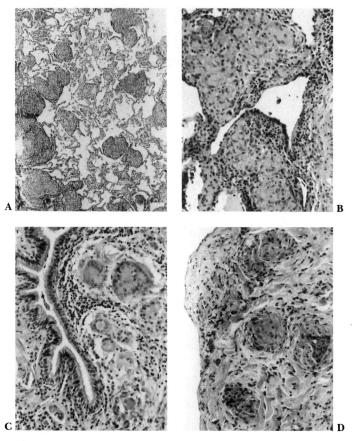

Fig. 19–4 A–D. Lung involvement in sarcoidosis. **A** and **B.** Epithelioid granulomas within alveolar walls at low (**A**) and high (**B**) magnification. **C.** Granulomatous involvement of bronchiole. **D.** Granulomatous involvement of visceral pleura.

these are the areas of the lung that contain lymphatic channels, the distribution of granulomas in the lungs in sarcoidosis is often referred to as "perilymphatic." The distribution of granulomas in the lungs in sarcoidosis is similar to the distribution of inhaled minute particles, for example, silica, and suggests that the etiologic agent(s) of sarcoidosis are minute particles inhaled from the atmosphere and that the lungs are the "portal of entry" for the disease-inciting agent(s). The high density of granulomas in hilar lymph nodes compared to lung parenchyma in early stages of sarcoidosis is consistent with minute particle inhalation, and suggests that such particles are promptly and easily transported from the lungs to lymph nodes. Evidence suggesting that the conjunctiva may be a primary site of involvement in sarcoidosis[129] further supports the concept of airborne transmission.

Granulomatous involvement of peribronchial and mediastinal lymph nodes is almost always identifiable on microscopic examination (see Figs. 19–1C–H). The extent of enlargement of these lymph nodes varies

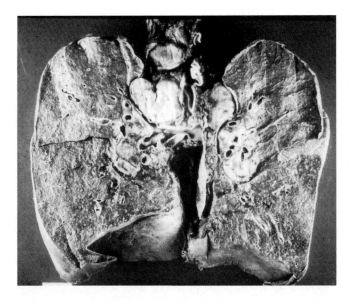

Fig. 19–5. Lung (post mortem) in sarcoidosis exhibiting massive bilateral hilar lymphadenopathy.

inversely with the duration of disease and the radiographic stage. Many patients with early disease exhibit marked enlargement of intrathoracic lymph nodes (Fig. 19–5), whereas patients with long-standing sarcoidosis tend not to exhibit intrathoracic lymphadenopathy.

Alveolitis

On the basis of studies of open lung biopsy specimens,[41,121,128] inflammatory and immune effector cells obtained by bronchoalveolar lavage,[38,130,131] and experimental granuloma formation in laboratory animals,[34,132,133] it is generally accepted that alveolitis (nongranulomatous interstitial pneumonitis) is the earliest pulmonary lesion in sarcoidosis and precedes granuloma formation. The alveolitis of sarcoidosis is characterized by an interstitial cellular infiltrate in which lymphocytes constitute approximately 90% of the cells (see Figs. 19–1A,B and 19–2). It is frequently and readily observed in open lung biopsy specimens[41,121,128] but is not often recognized in small transbronchial biopsy specimens. In a study of 128 open lung biopsy specimens from patients with sarcoidosis by Rosen et al.,[41] alveolitis was found to be either the predominating or a prominent microscopic finding, together with granulomas, in 62% of specimens and was absent in 38%. Alveolitis is considered to be critical in influencing the evolution and ultimate outcome of interstitial lung diseases.

Bronchoalveolar lavage has been a major factor in facilitating studies of the alveolitis of sarcoidosis.[130] With the lavage technique, inflammatory and immune

effector cells from the lower respiratory tract can be readily obtained and studied. Comparison of the effector cell population recovered by lavage and that isolated from tissue obtained during open lung biopsy in the same subjects has shown that lavage accurately indicates the types and state of activation of the effector cells present in the lower respiratory tract.[7,8,134–136] In the normal lung, alveolar macrophages constitute more than 90% of the effector cells[137–139] and lymphocytes almost all the remaining 10%.[138] The distribution of lymphocyte subtypes in normal lung is approximately similar to that in blood, and most lymphocytes in the normal lung are not activated.[38,42,138] Interstitial lung disorders are characterized by a marked change in the the normal proportion of effector cells, and certain patterns of inflammation are characteristically associated with certain diseases.[7] Bronchoalveolar lavage studies in patients with active untreated sarcoidosis show a fourfold increase beyond normal in the total number of inflammatory and immune effector cells and a significant shift in their relative proportions. In sarcoidosis, lymphocytes constitute 36% of the effector cells compared to 10% or less in the normal lung, and macrophages are 55% of the effector cells compared to the normal value of 90%. Although the proportion of macrophages is reduced compared to normal, their actual numbers are increased.

Neutrophils and eosinophils together constitute 5% or less of the cells in the alveolitis of sarcoidosis.[8] Eosinophils are present in larger numbers than neutrophils and what role, if any, either of these cells play in the pathogenesis of sarcoidosis is unknown.

The alveolitis tends to diminish in intensity and resolve as the disease resolves, progresses, or becomes chronic.[41,140] On the basis of studies of cells obtained by bronchoalveolar lavage, there is some evidence that in sarcoidosis the intensity[140] and duration[141] of the alveolitis, and the magnitude of the helper/suppressor ratio of T lymphocytes in the lung,[142] are inversely related to a good prognosis. There have been a small number of reports of an alveolitis-like inflammatory infiltrate preceding granuloma formation in extrapulmonary sites in sarcoidosis.[39,42,143] Teilum's statement[144] that "it seems clear that granuloma formation is preceded by a diffuse mononuclear cell infiltration in all sites where granulomas are found . . ." is probably correct and reflects the immunopathogenesis of sarcoidosis and·other granulomatous diseases.

Granulomatous Pulmonary Angiitis

Granulomatous involvement of pulmonary blood vessels in sarcoidosis (Fig. 19–6) is a frequent finding in open lung biopsy[121,145,146] and autopsy material. Gran-

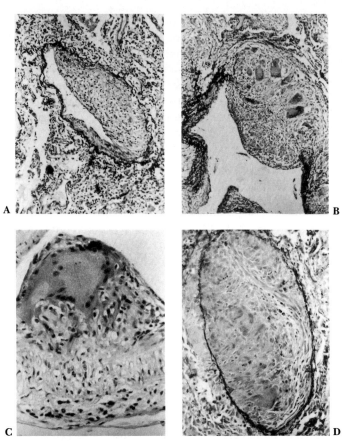

Fig. 19–6 A–D. Granulomatous pulmonary angiitis in sarcoidosis. **A.** Pulmonary vein with marked narrowing of lumen. (Reprinted from Rosen et al. Pathology annual, Vol. 14, Pt. 1. Appleton-Century-Crofts, with permission.) **B.** Pulmonary vein. Transmural granulomatous phlebitis with focal elastica destruction and pronounced giant cell reaction. **C.** Pulmonary artery. Granuloma limited to intima (transbronchial biopsy specimen). **D.** Pulmonary vein with complete obliteration of lumen.

ulomatous angiitis is, in the author's experience, an unusual finding in transbronchial biopsy specimens. However, a large study reported from Japan[147] showed granulomatous angiitis in transbronchial biopsy specimens in 53% of cases in which extravascular granulomas were present. Examples of extrapulmonary granulomatous angiitis in sarcoidosis have also been documented.[146] The most extensive study of this lesion[146] showed that granulomatous angiitis was present in 69% of 128 open lung biopsy specimens from patients with sarcoidosis in all clinical stages. Most of the vascular lesions were detectable with routine H and E staining, but some were seen only with the aid of elastica stains.

Venous granulomas, much more common than arterial granulomas, were seen in 92% and 39% of positive biopsies, respectively. Of the positive biopsy specimens,

31% showed both arterial and venous granulomas, 61% had venous granulomas only, and 8% had arterial granulomas only. Granulomas involving lymphatic vessels may be seen but are rare.

The likelihood of finding granulomatous angiitis varies in direct proportion to the number of granulomas present in the lung tissue. In many instances the vascular granulomas appear to be the result of extension of perivascular parenchymal granulomas into the vessel walls, but in the majority the granulomas clearly appear to have an intravascular origin. Occasionally the location of granulomas appears limited to the intima of the blood vessel (see Fig. 19–6C).

Granulomatous angiitis may cause marked destructive changes in the vessel walls (see Fig. 19–6B) as well as stenosis (see Fig. 19–6A) or complete obliteration (see Fig. 19–6D) of the lumen. Thrombosis or aneurysm formation is not encountered despite severe destructive vascular changes. Parenchymal necrosis (infarction) is rare even in the presence of extensive granulomatous angiitis. A small number of case reports[147–151] indicate that pulmonary hypertension is a definite, although probably rare, complication of granulomatous pulmonary angiitis in sarcoidosis. A condition simulating pulmonary veno-occlusive disease has been reported as a result of selective and severe venous involvement.[149–151] Rare instances of granulomatous angiitis of large proximal pulmonary blood vessels in patients with sarcoidosis have been reported.[152] The true incidence of large proximal pulmonary blood vessel granulomas in sarcoidosis is not known.

In addition to being a feature of sarcoidosis, granulomatous pulmonary angiitis is encountered in tuberculosis, Wegener's granulomatosis, necrotizing sarcoid granulomatosis (see later description), schistosomiasis, foreign-body embolization associated with intravenous substance abuse and cardiac catherization, and in association with mineralization and fragmentation of blood vessel elastica seen in patients with extensive pulmonary hemorrhage and pulmonary veno-occlusive disease. In areas where sarcoidosis is prevalent it is probably the most common cause of granulomatous pulmonary angiitis. Although granulomatous pulmonary angiitis has been regarded as extremely rare in beryllium disease,[121,153] one report has described its presence in four of six open lung biopsy specimens from patients with chronic beryllium disease.[154] Granulomatous pulmonary angiitis is not, however, a known feature of hypersensitivity pneumonitis.

Other Vascular Lesions

Systemic[155] and pulmonary[156,157] nongranulomatous microangiopathies of undertermined pathogenesis and significance have been reported to occur with high frequency in patients with sarcoidosis.

Bronchial and Bronchiolar Involvement

Granulomatous lesions in the airways, a frequent finding in sarcoidosis (see Fig. 19–4C), are detectable by bronchial wall biopsy in 15%–55% of patients with sarcoidosis.[158] Bronchial or bronchiolar granulomas may be seen in as many as 57% of open lung biopsy specimens in sarcoidosis.[87] Bronchoscopy reveals normal-appearing mucosa in approximately half of patients with sarcoidosis. The most frequent abnormality visualized by bronchoscopy is thickened, edematous, and hyperemic mucosa. The likelihood of detecting granulomas in abnormal-appearing bronchial mucosa is about twice as great as in normal-appearing mucosa. Siltzbach and Cahn[159] found granulomas in 44% of bronchial biopsy specimens taken from normal-appearing areas and in 82% of specimens taken from abnormal-appearing areas. Pulmonary function studies have shown that airways obstruction is common in all stages of sarcoidosis[160] and may be detected in as many as 75% of patients having radiographic evidence of pulmonary fibrosis.[161] The incidence of airways obstruction is variable and appears to be influenced by racial and genetic factors.[160]

Symptoms referable to bronchial involvement are unusual and are most likely to occur when bronchostenosis is present. Bronchostenosis is an unusual complication of granulomatous airway involvement in sarcoidosis that is detectable by bronchoscopy in as many as 8% of patients with intrathoracic sarcoidosis.[162,163] The stenotic lesions are usually multiple and may be seen in lobar, segmental, or subsegmental bronchi. Although bronchostenosis is almost invariably seen in patients having radiographic evidence of pulmonary fibrosis, it has also been reported in the absence of radiographic pulmonary infiltrates.[164] Symptoms referable to bronchostenosis include expiratory wheezing, dyspnea, and cough; occasionally patients with this lesion are asymptomatic. Atelectasis may be visible on chest radiography. Bronchostenosis in sarcoidosis may be caused by a locally severe granulomatous process or fibrosis or, very rarely, by external bronchial compression by enlarged hilar lymph nodes.

Pleural Involvement

Although visceral pleural granulomas may be seen in as many as 35% of open lung biopsies from patients with sarcoidosis (see Fig. 19–4D), clinical/radiographic manifestations of granulomatous pleuritis are far less frequent. Early reports indicated clinical/radiographic manifestations of pleural involvement in only approximately 1% of sarcoidosis patients.[126,165] A large study of pleural involvement reported in 1974 indicated a 10.1% incidence of radiographically detectable pleural reactions in 227 patients with pulmonary sarcoidosis.[166] Pleural effusion and pleural thickening are the usual radiographic manifestations of pleural involvement, with pleural effusion being the more frequent.[166,167] A large proportion of those cases reported in the literature as examples of pleural involvement in sarcoidosis lack histologic confirmation of pleural granulomas. Sarcoidosis patients who develop pleural effusion should be investigated with pleural biopsy to document the presence of pleural granulomas and to investigate the distinct possibility of other causes of pleural reactions such as neoplasm, tuberculosis, or fungal infection.

Pulmonary Fibrosis

Fibrosis occurs when the severity and duration of alveolar wall injury prevent reconstitution of normal structure. The factors that influence the development of fibrosis are not well understood. One factor may be destruction of the epithelial basement membrane, because repopulation of alveolar epithelium following lung injury appears to depend on the presence of an intact basement membrane.[168] Fibrosis is characterized by the presence of increased numbers of fibroblasts and collagen, predominantly of type 1.[169,170] Mononuclear phagocytes probably play an important role in fibrosis by modulating the local accumulation and replication of fibroblasts through release of mediators such as fibronectin[7,171,172] and alveolar macrophage-derived growth factor.[173]

"End-Stage" Changes: Other Complications

The end stage of pulmonary sarcoidosis is characterized by severe fibrosis (Figs. 19–7 and 19–8) of lung parenchyma, and often of pleura (Fig. 19–7), with bronchiolectasis (Fig. 19–8) and destruction of lung parenchyma producing large nonfunctional air-filled spaces that result in "honeycombing" (Fig. 19–8). These changes tend to be most severe in the upper portions of the lungs and subpleurally. Pulmonary vascular changes attributable to pulmonary hypertension may be present. Granulomas may be difficult to find within lung tissue at this stage, and the hilar lymph nodes may be extensively scarred. Bronchiectasis or bronchostenosis may occur secondary to granulomatous airway involvement and superimposed infection. Atelectasis has been reported in less than 1% cases of chronic sarcoidosis and has been attributed to bronchostenosis.[125] Bron-

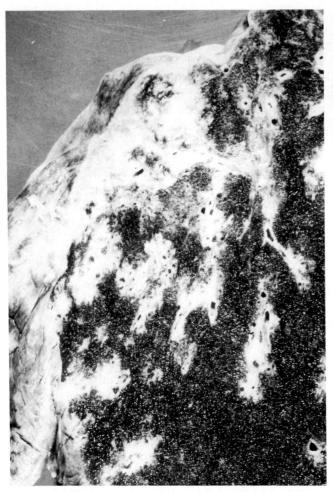

Fig. 19–7. Lung in sarcoidosis exhibiting extensive focal parenchymal fibrosis and marked pleural fibrosis.

chiectasis may be of the cylindrical or saccular types. Emphysema is also seen in end-stage sarcoidosis and may, in some instances, be caused by bronchostenosis resulting from fibrosis of bronchial wall granulomas.[110] Spontaneous pneumothorax is an unusual complication that is probably related to rupture of an emphysematous bulla. The cystic lung changes seen radiographically in some patients with advanced pulmonary sarcoidosis are undoubtedly produced by emphysematous bullae or large foci of saccular bronchiectasis. True cavitation, which is rare in sarcoidosis, may be the result of ischemic necrosis.[174] Some reported cases of cavitation in sarcoidosis likely represent preexisting cysts, foci of saccular bronchiectasis, emphysematous bullae, or infection. One should be skeptical that sarcoidosis is the cause of a true cavitary lung lesion.

Aspergillomas occur with moderate frequency in sarcoidosis patients with marked cystic parenchymal disease, and often produce hemoptysis, which may be life threatening in some patients.[175] Major or massive hemoptysis in patients with chronic sarcoidosis almost

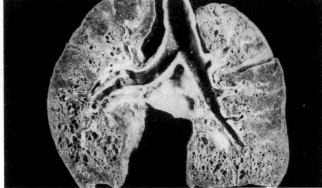

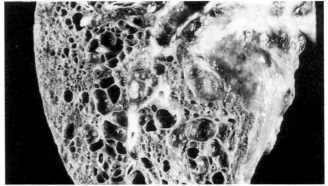

Fig. 19–8. "End-stage" lung in sarcoidosis (post mortem) exhibits extensive diffuse fibrosis and "honeycombing."

always reflects the presence of an aspergilloma. However, aspergilloma was also reported in 42% of sarcoidosis patients with only minor hemoptysis.[120] Superimposed infection may produce a variety of alterations in the lungs that are unrelated to the underlying granulomatous disease. Systemic amyloidosis is an extremely rare occurrence in sarcoidosis.[176–178]

Although it has been stated that sarcoidosis may predispose to the development of certain malignant neoplasms, particularly lung cancer and malignant lymphomas, there is currently no definite statistical support for such an association.[179]

Course and Prognosis

The overall prognosis for recovery and survival in sarcoidosis is excellent, and the chest radiographic abnormalities completely resolve in 54% of all patients.[111]

The prognosis varies inversely with the stage of the disease. A retrospective study of 818 patients with intrathoracic sarcoidosis[180] showed complete resolution of chest radiographic abnormalities within 2 years of presentation in 61% of patients presenting in stage 1, 39% in stage 2, and 38% in stage 3. There was no evidence that corticosteroid therapy in some patients influenced the ultimate chest radiographic changes. Of stage 1 patients, 14% developed stage 2 disease before resolution of the radiograph abnormality and 7% developed pulmonary infiltrates that persisted beyond 2 years despite resolution of the hilar adenopathy, that is, they developed stage 3 disease. Of the patients with stage 2 disease, 2.4% developed stage 3 disease that subsequently resolved, and an additional 5.3% developed stage 3 disease that persisted beyond 2 years.

Approximately 65% of patients with sarcoidosis recover completely or have minimal residual disease.[125] It is assumed that complete or near complete resolution and disappearance of granulomas occur in these patients. Some degree of permanent disability remains in 20%–25% of patients,[125] mainly as a result of pulmonary fibrosis. Chronic involvement of the eyes, skin, kidneys, heart, central nervous system, and musculoskeletal system contributes to permanent disability in many patients.

Factors that tend to be associated with a good prognosis include an abrupt onset of disease, erythema nodosum, female gender, age under 30, and stage 1 disease at presentation. A poor prognosis is associated with insidious onset, lupus pernio, involvement of the upper respiratory tract, bone cysts, nephrocalcinosis and cor pulmonale.[115]

Mortality in Sarcoidosis

The overall mortality of patients with sarcoidosis has generally been estimated to be between 3.8% and 10%.[125,174,180,181] A worldwide study of sarcoidosis[111] reported an overall mortality of approximately 4%; 55% of the deaths were attributed to sarcoidosis and 45% to other unrelated diseases. Deaths in Western countries are usually the result of pulmonary fibrosis with respiratory failure, cardiac failure secondary to cor pulmonale, or a combination of these. In Japan, autopsy data[182] showed cardiac involvement as the leading cause of death. A small number of patients die as a result of renal failure and uremia associated with nephrocalcinosis. Evidence of chronic cor pulmonale is found at autopsy in 28%–36% of sarcoid patients dying with advanced pulmonary fibrosis.[174,183,184] Autopsy studies in the United States[185] and Japan[182] show that the diagnosis of sarcoidosis is not made pre mortem in approximately two-thirds of patients diagnosed as having sarcoidosis at autopsy.

Biopsy in the Diagnosis of Sarcoidosis

The demonstration of granulomas in tissue to provide proof of granulomatous disease is essential for the definitive establishment of the diagnosis of sarcoidosis.

Kent et al.[186] emphasized that clinical criteria for the diagnosis of sarcoidosis, even when supported by demonstration of granulomas in peripheral lymph node biopsy, may be very unreliable. They studied 30 patients with typical clinical and radiographic features of sarcoidosis who had peripheral lymph node biopsy, mostly of scalene lymph nodes, that demonstrated nonnecrotizing granulomas. As a result of further diagnostic studies, 27 of 30 patients were found to have a disease other than sarcoidosis: 19 had tuberculosis; 3, nontuberculous mycobacterial infection; 2, metastatic carcinoma; and 1 each had histoplasmosis, beryllium disease, and hemosiderosis.

On the other hand, the reliability of clinical criteria for the diagnosis of stage 1 sarcoidosis was stressed by Winterbauer et al.[117] In their study of 100 patients with bilateral hilar lymphadenopathy, they found that all 30 asymptomatic patients had sarcoidosis and that 50 of 52 patients with completely negative physical examinations had sarcoidosis. On the basis of their findings they concluded that "bilateral hilar lymphadenopathy in asymptomatic patients with negative physical examinations or in association with erythema nodosum or uveitis should be considered a priori evidence of sarcoidosis, and biopsy confirmation of the diagnosis is not necessary."

Although the main purpose of biopsy in patients suspected to have sarcoidosis is to demonstrate the presence of granulomas and to stain and examine these lesions for the presence of microorganisms, there are other important reasons: (1) to provide lesional tissue to culture for microorganisms, and (2) to provide lesional tissue for additional diagnostic and investigative procedures including electron microscopy, immunohistochemical studies, enzyme determinations, and chemical analysis.

Small transbronchial biopsy specimens are adequate for demonstration of granulomas and even for culture of microorganisms, but larger specimens are needed for more extensive morphologic and biochemical studies. The amount of information that can be obtained from the biopsy specimen is directly related to its size.

Choice of Biopsy Site

The choice of a biopsy site should be dictated by both the likelihood of obtaining a diagnosis and the morbidity and mortality associated with the biopsy procedure. Because sarcoidosis is a systemic disease, diagnostically useful biopsy specimens may be obtained from diverse body sites. The lungs and hilar lymph nodes are the sites most frequently involved,[111] and therefore most biopsy efforts are directed toward either or both of these tissues. Granulomas are demonstrable in nearly 100% of open lung biopsy specimens from patients with intrathoracic sarcoidosis even when the lungs appear normal radiographically.[112,113] In approximately two-thirds of patients with stage 1 sarcoidosis, the lungs appear completely normal to the surgeon at the time of open lung biopsy.[113] The diagnostic accuracy of mediastinal lymph node biopsy is almost as high as that of open lung biopsy.[145] Cytologic examination of sputum in patients with sarcoidosis may show evidence of a granulomatous disease,[187] but information derived from sputum cytology is usually of very limited diagnostic value in granulomatous disorders.

It is desirable to demonstrate the presence of granulomas in more than one organ system to establish that one is dealing with a "multisystem" disease rather than a "local sarcoid reaction." This is often not practical, however, and is probably not done in most patients.

Biopsy Procedures

Open Lung Biopsy

Because its diagnostic yield is nearly 100% and because sufficient tissue is generally obtained for culture and other special studies, the open lung biopsy is, theoretically, the biopsy procedure of choice for the diagnosis of sarcoidosis. However, open lung biopsy is a major surgical procedure that requires general anesthesia and relatively long hospitalization and may be associated with significant morbidity. Because of the success and popularity of transbronchial lung biopsy via the flexible fiberoptic bronchoscope, open lung biopsy has virtually disappeared as a modality for diagnosis of sarcoidosis and is used only in those cases where diagnosis by other means is not possible. Much of our present knowledge about the morphologic aspects of pulmonary sarcoidosis has been derived from study of open lung biopsy material. Unfortunately, the smaller transbronchial biopsy specimens now available are generally unsuitable for any purposes relative to sarcoidosis beyond identification of granulomas and staining to attempt identification of microorganisms.

Mediastinal Lymph Node Biopsy

Mediastinal lymph node biopsy performed via the mediastinoscope has a diagnostic yield almost as high as open lung biopsy and entails a much lower degree of risk to the patient. However, general anesthesia and several days of hospitalization are usually required, and usually less tissue is obtained than from open lung biopsy.

Percutaneous Lung Biopsy Procedures

Percutaneous lung biopsy procedures performed with a cutting needle or trephine drill provide very small specimens. Because these procedures are associated with a high incidence of complications including pneumothorax, hemorrhage, and air embolism, as well as some mortality, they are considered dangerous and are rarely utilized.

Fine-Needle Aspiration Biopsy Procedures

Transthoracic[188] or transbronchial[189] fine-needle aspiration biopsy may be used as to aid in diagnosis when the patient presents with nodular lesions. Fine-needle aspiration biopsy has also been reported to be useful in the diagnosis of sarcoidosis in cervical lymph nodes, salivary glands,[190] and spleen.[191] Great caution must be observed in interpretation of findings in these minute aspiration specimens when they suggest granulomatous diseases. When fine-needle aspiration biopsy of a nodular lung lesion shows evidence of granulomas, the possibility of infection or neoplasm-associated granulomatous reaction cannot be excluded, and the lesion should be further evaluated by other methods.

Transbronchial Lung Biopsy

Transbronchial lung biopsy performed via the flexible fiberoptic bronchoscope is currently considered as the biopsy procedure of choice in patients suspected of having intrathoracic sarcoidosis. This procedure is very safe and relatively easy to perform, and may, in some cases, be done as an outpatient procedure. Transbronchial lung biopsy is complicated by pneumothorax in 5.5% of patients and hemorrhage in 1%–4% of patients who are not immunodeficient or uremic.[192] Hemorrhage occurs in 25% of immunodeficient patients and in 45% of uremic patients.[192] The overall incidence of "major" complications is 2%, and the mortality associated with this procedure is 0.2%.[192] Transbronchial lung biopsy is especially well suited to the workup of patients suspected to have sarcoidosis because the highest diagnostic yield with this procedure is obtained in those diseases in which specific diagnostic structures are likely to be found (granulomas, microorganisms, tumor cells, etc.).

The yield of granulomas in patients suspected to have sarcoidosis, on the basis of combined data from four series,[193–197] is 78% in all stages combined, 69% in stage 1, 82% in stage 2, and 86% in stage 3. It is evident that although the diagnostic yield of granulomas with transbronchial biopsy is high, it is less than that of open lung or mediastinoscopic lymph node biopsy. Its main disadvantage is the small size of the biopsy specimens, usually about 2 mm. The average greatest dimension of open lung biopsy specimens reported in one series was 21 mm.[112] The problem of sampling error from small specimen size can be overcome, to some extent, by obtaining multiple specimens. Gilman and Wang[198] demonstrated that in sarcoidosis the chance of obtaining a positive biopsy result increased from 46% with a single biopsy specimen to 90% with 4 specimens. It has been shown that the diagnostic accuracy of transbronchial lung biopsy in sarcoidosis approaches 100% when 10 biopsy specimens are obtained in stage 1 disease[199] and 5 to 6 specimens in stages 2 and 3.[198,199] However, it is usually not possible or practical to obtain this many specimens.

In addition to specimen size, the likelihood of obtaining a positive transbronchial biopsy result in sarcoidosis depends on whether alveoli are present in the biopsy specimen. In one study, granulomas were found in 58% of alveoli-containing specimens and in only 18% of specimens not containing alveoli.[198]

Granulomas identified in transbronchial lung biopsy specimens are often few in number, and little if any lesional tissue may be available for stains and cultures for microorganisms and other studies. The presence of only a few nonnecrotizing granulomas in a small biopsy specimen provides no assurance that necrotizing granulomas, more characteristic of tuberculosis or fungal infection, are not present nearby. Fechner et al.[200] have reviewed the problems encountered by pathologists in examination of transbronchial lung biopsy specimens.

Examination and Evaluation of Biopsy Specimens

The main purposes of microscopic examination of biopsy specimens in patients suspected to have sarcoidosis are

1. to determine whether granulomas are present
2. to exclude, insofar as limitations of available techniques permit, an infectious or other diagnosable etiology, and
3. to determine whether some other diagnosable condition is present that may explain the patient's clinical problem if granulomatous lesions are not found.

A minimum of three microscopic sections should be cut from different levels of the tissue block and stained with H and E or other routinely used tissue stain. If no granulomas or other diagnostic lesions are found, additional sections should be prepared and examined. The routine use of an elastic tissue stain is recommended to facilitate identification of vascular lesions and distorted or obliterated bronchioles.

If epithelioid granulomas of inapparent etiology are identified on routinely stained sections, demonstration of a possible infectious etiologic agent must be attempted. All biopsy specimens obtained from patients who may have an infectious disease should be stained for microorganisms and cultured if sufficient tissue is available. If the biopsy specimen is received in the laboratory unfixed, direct smears or imprints can be prepared and stained for microorganisms. Routine stains for microorganisms include the methenamine silver and the periodic acid–Schiff (PAS) stains for fungi, the Ziehl–Neelsen or Auramine-O stains for acid-fast bacilli, and the Gram stain. Giemsa and spirochete stains should be performed if indicated. Specimens for culture should be handled with sterile technique and sent to the microbiology laboratory in sterile containers *by the physician who obtained the specimen(s) from the patient.* This will minimize the possibilities of contamination, undue delay, and inadvertent fixation that may occur if the specimen is first sent to the surgical pathology laboratory. Cultures for mycobacteria, fungi, and aerobic and anaerobic bacteria should be routinely requested. If there is sufficient tissue, some should be frozen (or placed in holding media) in the event that viral culture is indicated.

The microscopic examination of tissue sections and smears for acid-fast bacilli is tedious and time consuming, but it is the most rapid way to establish a presumptive diagnosis of mycobacterial infection. Because mycobacteria range up to 10 μm in length, most can be seen at $400\times$ magnification. It is not necessary to use the oil immersion objective, which tends to slow down the examination substantially. If the Ziehl–Neelsen stain is used, removal of the blue filter from the microscope's illumination system increases the contrast between the pink-staining, acid-fast bacilli and the background and facilitates their identification. Many reports have indicated that Auramine-O staining and examination with the fluorescence microscopy has a substantially higher yield of positive results than the Ziehl–Neelsen stain.[201–203] Immunohistochemical[204] and nucleic acid probe methods[205] show great promise for improving the detection and identification of mycobacteria. The failure to identify acid-fast bacilli in tissue sections or smears does not constitute strong evidence against mycobacterial infection, because the yield of positive stains in proven infections with *Mycobacterium tuberculosis* is very low. A positive stain for acid-fast bacilli does not distinguish between or permit definitive identification of *M. tuberculosis*, atypical mycobacteria, and saprophytic mycobacteria; this can only be accomplished by culture.

Saprophytic mycobacteria from tap water, stored distilled water, and other sources in the laboratory may contaminate tissue sections and result in "false-positive" stains for acid-fast bacilli.[206] Because of the many opportunities for laboratory contamination by acid-fast bacilli, it is strongly recommended that a negative control always be examined in addition to the standard positive control and that areas of the unknown slide

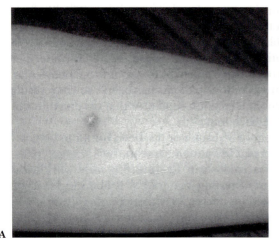

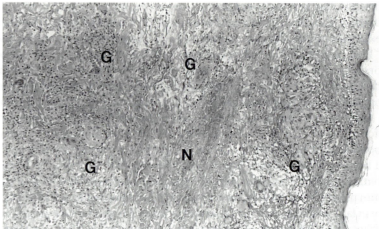

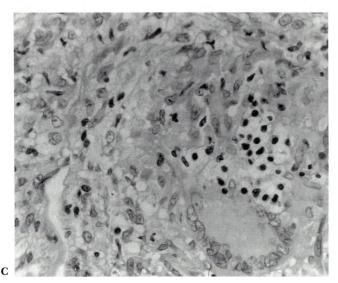

Fig. 19–9 A–C. Kveim test. **A.** Very reactive site of injection on forearm 6 weeks after injection. **B.** Abundant granulomas (G) surrounding a focally necrotic center (N) in the most active Kveim reactions. H and E × 60. **C.** High-power view shows epithelioid histiocytes, a giant cell, and lymphocytes. H and E × 250.

cially available. For these reasons as well as the relative ease of performance and high diagnostic yield of transbronchial lung biopsy, routine testing with satisfactory validated Kveim–Siltzbach test suspensions has decreased and is limited to relatively few centers throughout the world where it is utilized primarily as an investigative tool. It seems clear that a simpler laboratory test for the diagnosis of sarcoidosis that could be readily available to all physicians is needed.

Angiotensin-Converting Enzyme

Angiotensin-converting enzyme (ACE), a glycoprotein component of the renin-angiotensin system, catalyzes the cleavage of carboxyterminal dipeptides from a vareity of peptides including the decapeptide angiotensin I, which is converted to the octapeptide angiotensin II, a potent pressor, aldosterone regulator, and dipsogen. ACE is localized predominantly at the luminal surface of endothelial cells. Development of clinically applicable spectrophotometric[221] and sensitive, rapid, and rel-

atively simple fluorometric assays[222] for serum angiotensin-converting enzyme (SACE) has aided clinical studies.

Serum ACE (SACE) levels are found to be elevated in 50%–60% of all patients with sarcoidosis and in as many as 85% of patients with active sarcoidosis.[223] SACE levels have been reported to be elevated in 27% of sarcoidosis patients in stage 0, 56% in stage 1, 72% in stage 2, and 56% in stage 3 (223). In sarcoidosis, SACE activity correlates well with the total body granuloma load as assesed by ^{67}Ga scans.[224] SACE levels in sarcoidosis tend to decrease with increasing duration of disease[225] and usually following corticosteroid therapy.[221,225]

Studies seeking to determine the source of elevated SACE in sarcoidosis have revealed markedly elevated ACE levels in virtually all granulomatous lymph nodes in sarcoidosis.[226] The lymph node ACE levels do not correlate well with SACE levels.[226] Indeed, ACE and its cleavage product angiotensin II can be identified by immunohistochemical techniques in the cytoplasm of epithelioid cells of granulomas in more than 90% of granuloma-containing tissues from patients with sarcoidosis.[227,228] These studies failed to demonstrate ACE in tissue containing nonsarcoid granulomas or in tissue without granulomas. Ultrastructural study of sarcoid granulomas reacted with an immunoperoxidase-labeled anti-ACE antibody showed localization of ACE along the plasma membrane of the epithelioid cells.[229]

Although it appears likely that ACE is manufactured by cells of the mononuclear phagocytic system in the sarcoid granulomas, the reason for this and the mechanism of induction of ACE biosynthesis are unknown. Experimental studies suggest that human peripheral monocytes in culture, and presumably the epithelioid cells and macrophages of the sarcoid granuloma, are stimulated to increase their synthesis of ACE by T-cell lymphokine.[230]

It appears that elevation of SACE and tissue ACE is not an inherent feature of all diseases characterized by epithelioid granulomas or increased mononuclear phagocytes. Although it is elevated in some conditions associated with increased mononuclear phagocytes (sarcoidosis, Gaucher's disease, leprosy), SACE is generally not elevated in patients with tuberculosis, beryllium disease, and Crohn's disease. The mechanism of induction of ACE biosynthesis in the epithelioid cells in sarcoidosis is not known.

SACE has also been found to be significantly elevated in a small percentage of patients with conditions that may be confused with sarcoidosis on both clinical and morphologic grounds. These include tuberculosis, histoplasmosis, primary biliary cirrhosis, leprosy, beryllium disease, silicosis, asbestosis, Hodgkin's disease, farmer's lung, and chronic granulomatous disease.[223,231] Significant elevation of SACE has also been observed in Gaucher's disease and in some cases of Paget's disease of bone.[87]

Measurement of serum ACE levels initially appeared to have the potential for becoming a specific, easily performed, and reliable diagnostic test for sarcoidosis. Further experience has now shown that elevation of SACE is a nonspecific finding that may nevertheless be extremely helpful in diagnosis when considered with other findings. SACE appears to be a marker of disease activity in sarcoidosis, and as such its greatest value lies in monitoring the progress of the disease and its response to corticosteroid therapy and in following treated patients for evidence of relapse.

Bronchoalveolar Lavage

Bronchoalveolar lavage, introduced in the early 1970s,[137] is an investigative tool that has facilitated the acquisition of data pertaining to the alveolitis of sarcoidosis and other interstitial lung diseases. The analysis of cells obtained by bronchoalveolar lavage does not promise to assume a significant role in diagnosis of sarcoidosis, but there is some evidence that this procedure may provide information relating to disease activity, prognosis and response to therapy.[130,232]

Gallium Scanning

Gallium-67 citrate, given intravenously, localizes in areas of acute or chronic inflammation for reasons that are unknown, and may be demonstrated in various body sites with a scanning technique.[7] The normal lung accumulates little ^{67}Ga whereas patients with active alveolitis exhibit a diffuse or patchy accumulation of the isotope in the lung parenchyma.[7] Evaluation of the lung scan is based on the extent of parenchymal involvement and the intensity of uptake.[233] Examination of cells obtained by bronchoalveolar lavage after ^{67}Ga administration shows most of the isotope to be associated with mononuclear phagocytes.[234] In vitro studies have shown that uptake of ^{67}Ga by macrophages is enhanced when they are activated.[234]

A multinational study of the usefulness of ^{67}Ga scanning in sarcoidosis[235] concluded: (1) in 16% of untreated patients, this appeared to be the only noninvasive method capable of detecting clinical activity; (2) gallium scanning may be useful in identifying sites for lung biopsy and in selecting lung segments for bronchoalveolar lavage; and (3) gallium scan is more sensitive than chest radiography in detecting improvement and predicting relapses.

Differential Diagnosis of Sarcoidosis

From a diagnostic standpoint, epithelioid granulomas with or without minimal necrosis or cytoplasmic inclusions are considered to be nonspecific lesions that are a characteristic finding in many other conditions besides sarcoidosis.[236]

The major categories of disease that the pathologist must consider in the differential diagnosis of sarcoidosis are (1) infectious granulomas, (2) hypersensitivity pneumonitis (extrinsic allergic alveolitis), (3) chronic beryllium disease, and (4) necrotizing sarcoid granulomatosis.

Infectious Granulomas

A study of a large number of granulomatous lesions seen in routine surgical pathology practice[203] showed that infectious granulomas and sarcoidosis represented approximately 30% each of all granulomas encountered. Mycobacterial, fungal, and parasitic infection accounted for 64%, 30%, and 6%, respectively, of the infectious granulomas. The importance of using all available techniques to exclude an infectious etiology cannot be overemphasized because these two major categories of granulomas very often cannot be separated on morphologic grounds alone.   -

Hypersensitivity Pneumonitis and Chronic Beryllium Disease

The pulmonary lesions in these two conditions may closely resemble each other, and the lesions of sarcoidosis and tend to differ from sarcoidosis in a quantitative rather than a qualitative manner.[121] Compared to sarcoidosis, alveolitis and nongranulomatous inflammation of bronchioles are generally more prominent features; granulomas and granulomatous angiitis are less prominent. Although hilar lymph nodes are not usually enlarged on radiography, they may contain granulomas. The key to the diagnosis of hypersensitivity pneumonitis is a history of exposure to aerosolized organic antigen, observation of clinical improvement when the patient is removed from the source of exposure, and, if possible, appropriate serologic tests. An occupational history of exposure is important for suspecting and establishing the diagnosis of chronic beryllium disease. The diagnosis is confirmed by the demonstration of beryllium in tissue or body fluids or of sensitization of patient lymphocytes to beryllium.

Necrotizing Sarcoid Granulomatosis

Necrotizing sarcoid granulomatosis (NSG), first described in 1973 by Liebow,[237] is a pulmonary disease of unknown etiology and uncertain relationship to sarcoidosis that is characterized by confluent masses of granulomas in lung tissue, necrosis within the granulomatous masses, and destructive vasculitis that is predominantly of granulomatous type. The 11 patients that Liebow initially described were young and middle-aged adults who had varying clinical and radiographic manifestations. Most of the patients were symptomatic, with complaints attributable to lung involvement and constitutional symptoms suggestive of an infectious disease. One was a metalworker who was exposed to mercury fumes and probably to beryllium as well. With the exception of 1 patient who may have had transient hilar lymphadenopathy, none exhibited any of the characteristic clinical features of sarcoidosis. The lung lesions were most often multiple, and bilateral and granulomas were said to involve bronchi and bronchioles frequently as well as the pleura in some cases. Granulomas were seen in some mediastinal lymph nodes even though they were not enlarged. With regard to the nature of NSG, Liebow stated that "the problem is whether the disease represents necrotizing angiitis with sarcoid reaction, or sarcoidosis with necrosis of the granulomas and of the vessels." This question still remains unanswered. He chose the term "necrotizing sarcoid granulomatosis" as a tentative one encompassing both possibilities.

Subsequent to Liebow's initial report of 11 cases of NSG in 1973, approximately 75 additional cases have been published in three relatively large series[238-240] and a few case reports.[241-250] The topic of NSG and its differential diagnosis have also been discussed in review articles about the pathology of granulomatous diseases and pulmonary angiitis and granulomatosis.[251-253] On the basis of the information provided by the cases of NSG thus far reported, the following generalizations appear to be justified:

1. The lung lesions are usually mutiple and bilateral and present a nodular radiographic appearance with or without evidence of pleural effusion.
2. The majority of patients are symptomatic and may experience cough, dyspnea, pleuritic chest pain, fever, hemoptysis, night sweats, weight loss, and malaise. Those having solitary pulmonary lesions tend to be asymptomatic.
3. Patients with NSG tend not to have other clinical features of sarcoidosis. With the exception of one series[239] in which hilar lymphadenopathy was found in 50% of the cases, this finding has been reported in only 7%–9% of the cases.[237,238,240] Only four patients with NSG have been reported to have uveitis.[239,240,254] Granulomatous skin lesions have not been reported in association with NSG.
4. Necrosis tends to occur in areas of confluent granulomas and to be quite variable in extent. In some cases it may be massive or extensive (infarct-like) and in others it may be limited to single or multiple small punctate foci. The published descriptions give the impression that massive or extensive necrosis is seen in only a minority of the cases. The necrosis generally appears bland, but suppuration is possible.[244] Radiographic evidence of cavitation, presumably the result of necrosis, is occasionally seen.[238,240]
5. Vasculitis involves both veins and arteries, is predominantly granulomatous, and very closely resembles the vasculitis that is so frequently seen in the lungs in sarcoidosis. Destruction of vascular elastic tissue is frequently seen, but thrombosis or aneurysm formation has not been reported.
6. Extrapulmonary lesions are extremely rare.[245,255]
7. The prognosis is extremely favorable. Many of the patients have shown improvement following corticosteroid therapy, but spontaneous resolution following biopsy and apparent cures following surgical

excision of solitary lesions are well documented. There have been recurrences in a small number of patients.

Kveim tests performed in five patients were negative in four.[245,256] Serum angiotensin-converting enzyme has been measured in only five patients with NSG, and in all the level was found to be normal.[239,244,247] Angiotensin II was not found in granulomas in fresh lung tissue in three cases of NSG when sought by immuno-histochemical means.[254] Fresh-frozen lung tissue from one case of NSG studied for the presence of ACE with immunohistochemistry was negative.[244]

It seems quite unlikely that NSG is an infectious disease that is caused by a well-known microorganism, because stains for microorganisms and culture of fresh tissues performed in a large number of cases of NSG have been negative. However, it appears quite certain that mycobacterial and fungal infections can produce lesions identical to NSG. Of the cases in one series,[239] 20% that fulfilled the morphologic criteria for NSG had to be excluded from publication because cultures of specimens from biopsy yielded mycobacteria or fungi. One group[240] has presented evidence indicating the possibility that hypersensitivity to *Aspergillus* antigens may have been etiologically related to NSG in one patient.

Is it possible that NSG may be part of the spectrum of sarcoidosis? The morphology of the disease is certainly bears close resemblance to sarcoidosis except for the extensive necrosis that is seen in some cases. Small scattered foci of necrosis in sarcoidosis are a frequent finding, and occasionally apparently bona fide cases of sarcoidosis may show larger and even somewhat confluent areas of necrosis (see previous section on **Necrosis**). The other morphologic features seen in NSG are also frequently seen in sarcoidosis.[127] Confluent granulomas were seen in 27% of 128 open lung biopsies from patients with sarcoidosis; necrosis was seen in 20% of those specimens with confluent granulomas; vasculitis was seen in 86% of specimens with confluent granulomas; and vasculitis and necrosis occurring together were seen in 17% of specimens with confluent granulomas. Confluent granulomas, vasculitis, and necrosis, the morphologic findings of NSG, were seen in 6 of 128 (4.7%) open lung biopsy specimens from patients with sarcoidosis

The characteristic nodularity of the lung lesions is certainly not typical of sarcoidosis. However 1.5%–4% of sarcoid patients reported in large series present with nodular lesions on chest radiograph, and many of these individuals do not have hilar lymphadenopathy.[257–261] The entity of "nodular sarcoidosis" has not been well studied either clinically or morphologically. Informa-tion gathered from a limited number of patients indicates that somewhat less than half of patients with nodular sarcoidosis have hilar lymphadenopathy; a minority have uveitis and arthralgias, Kveim tests performed on a very small number have been positive, and biopsy studies show confluent granulomas that occasionally exhibit necrosis.[258,262] Cavitation has also been reported in nodular sarcoidosis.[263–267]

On the basis of what is presently known about NSG and sarcoidosis, a reasonable conclusion is that NSG is part of the spectrum of sarcoidosis and may be identical to the lesion that has been termed "nodular sarcoidosis." In this respect, it may be significant that approximately 5% of open lung biopsy specimens from patients with sarcoidosis show morphologic features of NSG.[127] This closely approximates the proportion of sarcoidosis patients who initially present with nodular lesions on chest radiography. The extremely favorable prognosis of patients with NSG also suggests that this lesion is more akin to sarcoidosis than to one of the varieties of pulmonary angiitis and granulomatosis.

There is, however, no proof for this conclusion, and it certainly begs the question of whether the lesion that is now called "nodular sarcoidosis" is itself part of the spectrum of sarcoidosis. Evidence suggesting that NSG may be an entity apart from sarcoidosis includes the generally low incidence of hilar adenopathy and other clinical features of sarcoidosis, the typical bilateral multinodular radiographic appearance, the rarity of extrathoracic involvement, the failure to demonstrate elevation of SACE or presence of ACE or one of its reaction products in granulomas, and negative Kveim tests in the very small number of patients in whom these studies have been done.

The true nature of necrotizing sarcoid granulomatosis and nodular sarcoidosis, and their possible relationship to each other and to sarcoidosis, still remain to be determined.

References

1. Mandel W, Thomas JH, Carman CT, McGovern JP. Bibliography on sarcoidosis 1878–1963. Washington, D.C.: U.S. Public Health Service Publication No. 1213, 1964.
2. Ito Y. Bibliography on sarcoidosis. Tokyo: World Education, 1981.
3. Chrétien J, Marsac J, Saltiel JC, eds. Sarcoidosis and other granulomatous disorders. Ninth international conference on sarcoidosis and other granulomatous disorders. Paris: Pergamon Press, 1983.
4. Johns CJ, ed. Tenth international conference on sarcoidosis and other granulomatous disorders. Ann NY Acad Sci 1986;465.
5. Grassi C, Rizzato G, Pozzi E, eds. Sarcoidosis and other

granulomatous disorders. Proceedings of the XI world congress on sarcoidosis and other granulomatous disorders. Amsterdam: Excerpta Medica, 1988.

6. James DG, Jones Williams W. Sarcoidosis and other granulomatous disorders. Philadelphia: WB Saunders, 1985.

7. Crystal RG, Bitterman PB, Rennard SI, Hance AJ, Keogh BA. Interstitial lung diseases of unknown cause, Part 1. N Engl J Med 1984;310:154–166.

8. Crystal RG, Bitterman PB, Rennard SI, Hance AJ, Keogh BA. Interstitial lung diseases of unknown cause, Part 2. N Engl J Med 1984;310:235–244.

9. Fanburg BL, ed. Sarcoidosis and other granulomatous diseases of the lung. New York: Marcel Dekker, 1983.

10. Berkmen YM. Radiologic aspects of intrathoracic sarcoidosis. Semin Roentgenol 1985;20:356–375.

11. Sharma OP. Sarcoidosis. DM 1990;36:474–535.

12. Thomas PD, Hunninghake GW. Current concepts of the pathogenesis of sarcoidosis. Am Rev Respir Dis 1987; 135:747–760.

13. James DG, Turiaf J, Hosoda Y, et al. Description of sarcoidosis: Report of the committee on classification and definition. In: Siltzbach LE, ed. Seventh international conference on sarcoidosis and other granulomatous disorders. Ann NY Acad Sci 1976;278:742.

14. Scadding JG. Further observations on sarcoidosis associated with *M. tuberculosis* infection. In: Levinsky L, Macholda F, eds. Proceedings of the fifth international conference on sarcoidosis and other granulomatous disorders. Prague: Universita Karlova, 1971:89–92.

15. Zettergren L. Lymphogranulomatosis benigna. Acta Soc Med Ups (suppl 5) 1954;5:1–180.

16. Vănek J, Schwarz J. Demonstration of acid-fast rods in sarcoidosis. Am Rev Respir Dis 1970;101:395–400.

17. Mankiewicz E, van Walbeek M. Mycobacteriophages: Their role in tuberculosis and sarcoidosis. Arch Environ Health 1962;5:122–128.

18. Chapman, JS, Speight M. Further studies of mycobacterial antibodies in the sera of sarcoidosis patients. Acta Med Scand (Suppl) 1964;425:61–66.

19. Siltzbach LE. Sarcoidosis and mycobacteria. Am Rev Respir Dis 1968;97:1–8.

20. Kok TC, Haasjes JG, Splinter TAW, ten Kate FJ. Sarcoid-like lymphadenopathy mimicking metastatic testicular cancer. Cancer 1991; 68:1845–1847.

21. Toner GC, Bosl GL. Sarcoidosis, "sarcoid-like lymphadenopathy," and testicular germ cell tumors. Am J Med 1990;89:651–56.

22. Familial associations in sarcoidosis: A report to the Research Committee of the British Thoracic and Tuberculosis Association. Tubercle 1973;54:87–98.

23. Brewerton DA, Cockburn C, James DCO, James DG, Neville E. HLA antigens in sarcoidosis. Clin Exp Immunol 1977;27:227–229.

24. James DG, Jones Williams W. Sarcoidosis and other granulomatous disorders. Philadelphia: WB Saunders, 1985:220.

25. Sharma OP, Neville E, Walker AN, James DG. Familial sarcoidosis: A possible genetic influence. In: Siltzbach

LE, ed. Seventh international conference on sarcoidosis and other granulomatous disorders. Ann NY Acad Sci 1976;278:386–400.

26. Harf RA, Ethevenaux C, Gleize J, Perrin-Fayolle M, Guerin JC, Ollagnier C. Reduced prevalence of smokers in sarcoidosis: Results of a case control study. In: Johns CJ, ed. Tenth international conference on sarcoidosis and other granulomatous disorders. Ann NY Acad Sci 1986;465:625–631.

27. Valeyre D, Soler P, Clerici C, et al. Smoking and pulmonary sarcoidosis: Effect of cigarette smoke on prevalence, clinical manifestations, alveolitis and evolution of the disease. Thorax 1988;43:516–524.

28. Bresnitz EA, Israel H, Stolley PD, Soper K. Possible risk factors for sarcoidosis: A case control study. In: Johns CJ, ed. Tenth international conference on sarcoidosis and other granulomatous disorders. Ann NY Acad Sci 1986;465:632–642.

29. Adams DO. The biology of the granuloma. In: Ioachim HL, ed. Pathology of granulomas. New York: Raven Press, 1983:1–20.

30. James DG, Neville E. Pathobiology of sarcoidosis. Pathobiol Annu 1977;7:31–61.

31. Adams DO. The granulomatous inflammatory response. Am J Pathol 1976;84:163–192.

32. Tanaka A, Emori K, Nagao S, et al. Epithelioid granuloma formation requiring no T-cell function. Am J Pathol 1982;106:165–170.

33. Jagadha V, Andavolu RH, Huang CT. Granulomatous inflammation in the acquired immune deficiency syndrome. Am J Clin Pathol 1985;84:598–602.

34. Boros DL. Granulomatous inflammation. Prog Allergy 1978;24:184–267.

35. Epstein WL. Granuloma formation in man. Pathobiol Annu 1977;7:1–30.

36. Spector WG. The macrophage: Its origins and role in pathology. Pathobiol Annu 1974;4:33–64.

37. Spector WG. Granulomatous hypersensitivity. Prog Allergy 1967;11:36–88.

38. Crystal RG, Roberts WC, Hunninghake GW, Gadek JE, Fulmer JD, Line BR. Pulmonary sarcoidosis: A disease characterized and perpertuated by activated lung T lymphocytes. Ann Intern Med 1981;94:73–94.

39. Hunninghake GW, Fulmer JD, Young RC, Gadek JE, Crystal RG. Localization of the immune response in sarcoidosis. Am Rev Respir Dis 1979;120:49–57.

40. Hunninghake GW, Crystal RG. Pulmonary sarcoidosis: A disorder mediated by excess helper T-lymphocyte activity at sites of disease activity. N Engl J Med 1981;305:429–434.

41. Rosen Y, Athanassiades TJ, Moon S, Lyons HA. Nongranulomatous interstitial pneumonitis in sarcoidosis: relationship to the development of epithelioid granulomas. Chest 1978;74:122–125.

42. Semenzato G, Pezzutto G, Chilossi M, Ossi E, Angi MR, Cipriani A. Immunohistological study in sarcoidosis: evaluation at different sites of disease activity. Clin Immunol Immunopathol 1984;30:29–40.

43. Hunninghake GW, Crystal RG. Mechanisms of hyper-

gammaglobulinemia in pulmonary sarcoidosis: Site of increased antibody production and role of T lymphocytes. J Clin Invest 1981;67:86–92.

44. Semenzato G. The sarcoid granuloma formation—immunology. In: Grassi C, Rizzato G, Pozzi E, eds. Sarcoidosis and other granulomatous disorders. Proceedings of the XI world congress on sarcoidosis and other granulomatous disorders. Amsterdam: Excerpta Medica, 1988:73–87.

45. van Furth R, Cohn ZA, Hirsch JG, Humphrey JH, Spector WG, Langevoort HL. The mononuclear phagocyte system: A new classification of macrophages, monocytes and their precursor cells. Bull WHO 1972;46:845–852.

46. Spector WG. Chronic inflammation. In: Zweifach BW, Grant L, McCluskey RT, eds. The inflammatory process, Vol.3, 2d Ed. New York: Academic Press, 1974:277–290.

47. Wilkinson PC. Chemotaxis and inflammation. Edinburgh: Churchill Livingston, 1974.

48. Ward PA, Becker EL. Biology of leukotaxis. Rev Physiol Biochem Pharmacol 1977;77:125–148.

49. van Furth R, Fedorko ME. Ultrastructure of mouse mononuclear phagocytes in bone marrow: colonies grown in vitro. Lab Invest 1976;34:440–450.

50. Nichols BA, Bainton DF. Ultrastructure and cytochemistry of mononuclear phagocytes. In: van Furth R, ed. Mononuclear phagocytes in immunity, infection and pathology. Oxford: Blackwell, 1975:17–56.

51. van Furth R. Mononuclear phagocytes in inflammation. In: Vane JR, Ferreira SH, eds. Handbook of experimental pharmacology, Vol. 50, Part 1. Berlin: Springer Verlag, 1978:68–108.

52. Stewart CC, Lin HS. Macrophage growth factor and its relationship to colony stimulating factor. J Reticuloendothel Soc 1978;23:269–285.

53. van der Zeijst BAM, Stewart CC, Schlesinger S. Proliferative capacity of mouse peritoneal macrophages in vitro. J Exp Med 1978;147:1253–1266.

54. Cohn ZA. The activation of mononuclear phagocytes: Fact, fancy and future. J Immunol 1978;121:813–816.

55. Nelson DS. Macrophages and cell-mediated immunity. In: Gadebusch HH, ed. Phagocytes and cellular immunity. Cleveland: CRC Press, 1979:57–100.

56. Keller R. Mononuclear phagocytes and antitumor resistance: A discussion. In: James K, McBride A, Stuart A, eds. Symposium on the macrophage and cancer. Edinburgh: University of Edinburgh, 1979:31–49.

57. North RJ. The concept of the activated macrophage. J Immunol 1978;121:806–809.

58. Meltzer MS, Ruco LP, Boraschi B, Nacy CA. Macrophage activation for tumoricidal toxicity: analysis of intermediary reactions. J Reticuloendothel Soc 1979;26:403–416.

59. Lasser A. The mononuclear phagocytic system. Hum Pathol 1983;14:108–126.

60. Pierce CW. Macrophages: Modulators of immunity. Am J Pathol 1980;98:10–28.

61. Unanue ER. The regulatory role of macrophages in antigen stimulation, Part 2: symbiotic relationships between lymphocytes and macrophages. Adv Immunol 1981;31:1–136.

62. Unanue ER. Secretory function of mononuclear phagocytes. Am J Pathol 1976;83:396–417.

63. Hunninghake GW. Release of interleukin-1 by alveolar macrophages of patients with active pulmonary sarcoidosis. Am Rev Respir Dis 1984;129:569–572.

64. Spector WG, Mariano M. Macrophage behaviour in experimental granulomas. In: van Furth R, ed. Mononuclear phagocytes in infection, immunity and pathology. Oxford; Blackwell, 1975:927–942.

65. Hirsch BC, Johnson WC. Concepts of granulomatous inflammation. Int J Dermatol 1984;23:90–100.

66. Soler P, Basset F, Bernaudin JF, Chrétien J. Morphology and distribution of the cells of a sarcoid granuloma: Ultrastructural study of serial sections. In: Siltzbach LE, ed. Seventh international conference on sarcoidosis and other granulomatous disorders. Ann NY Acad Sci 1976;278:147–160.

67. Chambers TJ. Multinucleate giant cells. J Pathol 1978;126:125–148.

68. Papadimitriou JM, Sforsina D, Papaelias L. Kinetics of multinucleate giant cell formation and their modification by various agents in foreign body reactions. Am J Pathol 1973;73:349–364.

69. Black MM, Epstein WL. Formation of multinucleate giant cells in organized epithelioid cell granulomas. Am J Pathol 1974;74:263–274.

70. Ginns LC, Goldenheim PD, Burton RC et al. T-lymphocyte subsets in peripheral blood and lung lavage in idiopathic pulmonary fibrosis and sarcoidosis: Analysis by monoclonal antibodies and flow cytometry. Clin Immunol Immunopathol 1982;25:11–20.

71. Ward PA, Remold HG, David JR. Leukotactic factor produced by sensitized lymphocytes. Science 1969; 163:1079–1081.

72. Oppenheim JJ. Lymphokines. In: Oppenheim JJ, Rosenstreich M, Potter M, eds. Cellular functions in immunity and inflammation. New York: Elsevier/North Holland, 1981:259–282.

73. David JR, Rocklin RE. Lymphocyte mediators "the lymphokines". In: Samter M, ed. Immunological diseases, Vol. 1. Boston: Little, Brown, 1978:307–324.

74. Rocklin RE. Products of activated lymphocytes: Leukocyte inhibitory factor (LIF) distinct from migration inhibition factor (MIF). J Immunol 1974;112:1461–1466.

75. Hunninghake GW, Bedell GN, Zavala DC, Monnick M, Brady M. Role of interleukin-2 release by lung T cells in active pulmonary sarcoidosis. Am Rev Respir Dis 1983;128:634–638.

76. Byrne EB, Evans AS, Fouts DW, Israel HL. Serological hyperreactivity to Epstein-Barr virus and other viral antigens in sarcoidosis. In: Iwai K, Hosoda Y, eds. Proceedings of the sixth international conference on sarcoidosis. Baltimore: University Park Press, 1974: 218–225.

77. Lawrence EC, Martin RR, Blease RM, et al. Increased bronchoalveolar IgG secreting cells in interstitial lung

diseases. N Engl J Med 1980;302:1186–1188.

78. Berman B, Fox JL, Teirstein AS. Quantitation of cutaneous Langerhans cells of sarcoidosis patients. In: Johns CJ, ed. Tenth international conference on sarcoidosis and other granulomatous disorders. Ann NY Acad Sci 1986;465:250–259.

79. James DG. Granulomatous disorders which mimic sarcoidosis. In: Iwai K, Hosoda Y, eds. Proceedings of the sixth international conference on sarcoidosis. Baltimore: University Park Press, 1974:132–135.

80. James DG. Sarcoidosis. DM 1970:February (special issue).

81. Semenzato G, Pezzutto A, Chisoli M, Pizzola G. Redistribution of lymphocytes in the lymph nodes of patients with sarcoidosis. N Engl J Med 1982;306:48–49.

82. Modlin RL, Hofman FM, Meyer PR, Sharma OP, Taylor CR, Rea TH. In situ demonstration of T lymphocyte subsets in granulomatous inflammation: Leprosy, rhinoscleroma and sarcoidosis. Clin Exp Immunol 1983; 51:430–438.

83. Modlin RL, Hofman FM, Sharma OP, Gottlieb B, Taylor CR, Rea TH. Demonstration in situ of subsets of T-lymphocytes in sarcoidosis. Am J Dermatopathol 1984; 6:423–427.

84. van Maarsseven A, Mullink H, Alons C, Stam J. Distribution of T-lymphocyte subsets in different portions of sarcoid granulomas: Immunohistologic analysis with monoclonal antibodies. Hum Pathol 1986;17:493–500.

85. Van Den Oord JJ, DeWolf-Peeters C, Facchetti F, Desmet VJ. Cellular composition of hypersensitivity type granulomas. Hum Pathol 1984;15:559–565.

86. Ricker W, Clark M. Sarcoidosis: a clinico-pathologic review of 300 cases, including 22 autopsies. Am J Clin Pathol 1949;19:725–749.

87. Rosen Y, Vuletin JC, Pertschuk LP, Silverstein E. Sarcoidosis from the pathologist's vantage point. Pathol Annu 1979; 14(part 1):405–439.

88. Cree IA, Nurbhai S, Milne G, Swanson Beck J. Cell death in granulomata: The role of apoptosis. J Clin Pathol 1987;40:1314–1319.

89. Carlens E, Hanngren A, Ivemark B. The concomitance of feverish onset of sarcoidosis and necrosis formation in the lymph nodes. In: Iwai K, Hosoda Y, eds. Proceedings of the sixth international conference on sarcoidosis. Baltimore: University Park Press, 1974:409–412.

90. Dannenberg AM, Jr., Sugimoto M. Liquefaction of caseous foci in tuberculosis. Am Rev Respir Dis 1976;113:257–259.

91. Medlar EM. A study of the process of caseation in tuberculosis. Am J Pathol 1926;2:275–290.

92. Rich AR. The pathogenesis of tuberculosis, 2d Ed. Springfield: Thomas, 1951:734–742.

93. Zak F. Contribution to the origin, development and experimental production of laminated calcino-siderotic Schaumann bodies. Acta Med Scand (suppl) 1964;425:21–24.

94. Jones Williams W. The nature and origin of Schaumann bodies. J Pathol Bacteriol 1960;79:193–201.

95. Visscher D, Churg A, Katzenstein AA. Significance of crystalline inclusions in lung granulomas. Mod Pathol 1988;1:415–419.

96. Reid JD, Andersen ME. Calcium oxalate in sarcoid granulomas. Am J Clin Pathol 1988;90:545–558.

97. Cain H, Kraus B. The ultrastructure and morphogenesis of asteroid bodies in sarcoidosis and other granulomatous disorders. In: Williams JW, Davies BH eds. Eighth international conference on sarcoidosis and other granulomatous diseases. Cardiff:Alpha Omega, 1980:30–37.

98. Jones Williams W, Williams D. "Residual bodies" in sarcoid and sarcoid-like granulomas. J Clin Pathol 1967;20:574–577.

99. Hamazaki T. Über ein Neues, säuerfeste Substanz führendes Spindelkörperchen der Menschlichen Lymphdrüsen. Virchows Arch (Pathol Anat) 1938;301:490–522.

100. Carter CJ, Gross MA. The selective staining of curious bodies in the lymph nodes as a means for the diagnosis of sarcoid. Stain Technol 1969;44:1–4.

101. Baro C, Butt CG. Hamazaki-Wesenberg bodies in sarcoidosis. Lab Med Bull Pathol 1970;102:281.

102. Boyd JF, Valentine JC. Unidentified yellow bodies in human lymph nodes. J Pathol 1970;102:58–60.

103. Doyle WF, Brahman HD, Burgess JH. The nature of the yellow-brown bodies in peritoneal lymph nodes. Histochemical and electron microscopic evaluation of these bodies in a case of suspected sarcoidosis. Arch Pathol 1973;96:320–326.

104. Sieracki JC, Fisher ER. The ceroid nature of so-called "Hamazaki-Wesenberg" bodies. Am J Clin Pathol 1973;59:248–253.

105. Boutet M. Étude ultrastructurale et histochimique des corps d'Hamazaki-Wesenberg dans la sarcoidose ganglionaire. Ann Anat Pathol 1975;20:201–212.

106. Wesenberg W. On acid-fast Hamazaki spindle bodies in sarcoidosis of lymph nodes and on double refractile cell inclusions in sarcoidosis of the lungs. Arch Klin Exp Dermatol 1966;227:101–107.

107. Vuletin JC, Rosen Y. Nature of pseudo-fungal budding structures (Hamazaki-Wesenberg bodies) and asteroid bodies in sarcoidosis (abstract). Am J Clin Pathol 1977;68:99.

108. Senba M, Kawai K. Nature of yellow-brown bodies. Histochemical and ultrastructural studies on the brown pigment. Zentralbl Allg Pathol Anat 1989; 135:351–355.

109. Hall M, Eusebi V. Yellow-brown spindle bodies in mesenteric lymph nodes: A possible relationship with melanosis coli. Histopathology 1978;2:47–52.

110. Spencer H. Pathology of the lung. 4th Ed. Oxford: Pergamon Press, 1985:828–829.

111. James DG, Neville E, Siltzbach LE, et al. A worldwide review of saroicdosis. In: Siltzbach LE, ed. Seventh international conference on sarcoidosis and other granulomatous disorders. Ann NY Acad Sci 1976;278:321–334.

112. Rosen Y, Amorosa JK, Moon S, Cohen J, Lyons HA. Occurrence of lung granulomas in patients with stage 1

sarcoidosis. AJR 1977;129:1083–1085.

113. Eule H. Findings by lung biopsy in patients with Löfgren's syndrome. In: Levinsky L, Macholda F, eds. Proceedings of the fifth international conference on sarcoidosis and other granulomatous disorders. Prague: Universita Karlova, 1971;469–471.

114. Freiman DG. The pathology of sarcoidosis. Semin Roentgenol 1985;20:327–339.

115. James DG, Jones Williams W. Sarcoidosis and other granulomatous disorders. Philadelphia: WB Saunders, 1985:46–53.

116. Löfgren S. Erythema nodosum: studies on aetiology and pathogenesis in 185 adult cases. Acta Med Scand 1946(suppl 174);124:1–197.

117. Winterbauer RH, Moore KD. A clinical interpretation of bilateral hilar adenopathy. Ann Intern Med 1973; 78:65–71.

118. James DG, Jones Williams W. Sarcoidosis and other granulomatous disorders. Philadelphia: WB Saunders, 1985:49.

119. Chang JC, Driver AG, Townsend CA, Kataria YP. Hemoptysis in sarcoidosis. Sarcoidosis 1987;4:49–54.

120. Johns CJ, Schonfeld SA, Scott PP. The course and management of 53 patients with hemoptysis in sarcoidosis. In: Grassi C, Rizzato G, Pozzi E, eds. Sarcoidosis and other granulomatous disorders. Proceedings of the XI world congress on sarcoidosis and other granulomatous disorders. Amsterdam: Excerpta Medica, 1988:417–420.

121. Carrington CB, Gaensler EA, Mikus JP, Schachter AW, Burke GW, Goff AM. Structure and function in sarcoidosis. In: Siltzbach LE, ed. Seventh international conference on sarcoidosis and other granulomatous disorders. Ann NY Acad Sci 1976;278:265–283.

122. Huang CT, Heurich AE, Rosen Y, Moon S, Lyons HA. Pulmonary sarcoidosis. Roentgenographic, functional and pathologic considerations. Respiration 1979;37: 337–345.

123. Smellie H, Hoyle G. The natural history of pulmonary sarcoidosis. Q J Med 1960;29:539–558.

124. Daniel TM. Sarcoidosis. In: Baum GL, Wolinsky E, eds. Textbook of pulmonary diseases. 3rd Ed. Boston: Little Brown, 1983:685–701.

125. Fraser RG, Pare JAP. Diagnosis of disease of the chest. 2d Ed. Philadelphia: WB Saunders, 1979:1675–1689.

126. Longcope WT, Freiman DG. A study of sarcoidosis. Medicine (Baltimore) 1952;31:1–132.

127. Rosen Y, Moon S. Unpublished data.

128. Lacronique J, Bernaudin JF, Soler P, et al. Alveolitis and granulomas: Sequential course in pulmonary sarcoidosis. In: Chrétien J, Marsac J, Saltiel JC, eds. Sarcoidosis and other granulomatous disorders. Ninth international conference on sarcoidosis and other granulomatous disorders. Paris: Pergamon, 1983:36–42.

129. Angi MR, Ossi E, Secchi AG, et al. The conjunctiva as a primary site of involvement in sarcoidosis. In: International Committee on Sarcoidosis, 10th international conference on sarcoidosis and other granulomatous disorders (abstracts). Baltimore, 1984:77.

130. Daniele RP, Elias JA, Epstein PE, Rossman MD. Bronchoalveolar lavage: Role in the pathogenesis, diagnosis and management of interstitial lung disease. Ann Intern Med 1985;102:93–108.

131. Campbell DA, Poulter LW, Du Bois RM. Immunocompetent cells in bronchoalveolar lavage reflect the cell populations in transbronchial biopsies in pulmonary sarcoidosis. Am Rev Respir Dis 1985;132:1300–1306.

132. Unanue ER, Benacerraf B. Immunologic events in experimental hypersensitivity granulomas. Am J Pathol 1973;71:349–364.

133. Spector WG, Heesom N. The production of granulomata by antigen–antibody complexes. J Pathol 1969;98: 31–39.

134. Hunninghake GW, Kawanami O, Ferrans VJ, Young RC, Roberts WC, Crystal RG. Characterization of the inflammatory and immune effector cells in the lung parenchyma of patients with interstitial lung disease. Am Rev Respir Dis 1981;123:407–412.

135. Halsam PL, Turton CWG, Heard B, Lukoszek A, Collins JV. Bronchoalveolar lavage in pulmonary fibrosis: Comparison of cells obtained with lung biopsy and clinical features. Thorax 1980;35:9–18.

136. Paradis IL, Rogers RM, Rabin BS, Dauber JH. Lymphocyte phenotypes in bronchoalveolar lavage and lung tissue in sarcoidosis. In: Johns CJ, ed. Tenth international conference on sarcoidosis and other granulomatous disorders. Ann NY Acad Sci 1986;465:148–156.

137. Reynolds HY, Newball HH. Analysis of proteins and respiratory cells obtained from human lungs by bronchial lavage. J Lab Clin Med 1974;84:559–573.

138. Hunninghake GW, Gadek JE, Kawanami O, Ferrans VJ, Crystal RG. Inflammatory and immune processes in the human lung in health and disease: Evaluation by bronchoalveolar lavage. Am J Pathol 1979;97:149–206.

139. Crapo JD, Barry BE, Gehr P, Bachofen M, Weibel ER. Cell number and cell characteristics of the normal human lung. Am Rev Respir Dis 1982;126:332–337.

140. Keogh BA, Hunninghake GW, Line BR, Crystal RG. The alveolitis of pulmonary sarcoidosis: Evaluation of natural history and alveolitis dependent changes in lung function. Am Rev Respir Dis 1983;128:256–265.

141. Israel-Biet D, Venet A, Chrétien J. Persistent high alveolar lymphocytosis as a predictive criterion of chronic pulmonary sarcoidosis. In: Johns CJ, ed. Tenth international conference on sarcoidosis and other granulomatous disorders. Ann NY Acad Sci 1986;465:395–406.

142. Costabel U, Bross KJ, Guzman J, Nilles A, Rühle KH, Matthys, H. Predictive value of bronchoalveolar T cell subsets for the course of pulmonary sarcoidosis. In: Johns CJ, ed. Tenth international conference on sarcoidosis and other granulomatous disorders. Ann NY Acad Sci 1986;465:418–426.

143. Takahashi M. Histopathology of sarcoidosis and its immunological bases. Acta Pathol Jpn 1970;20:171–182.

144. Teilum G. Morphogenesis and development of sarcoid lesions. Similarities to the group of collagenosis. Acta Med Scand (Suppl) 1964;425:14–18.

145. Addrizzo JR, Minkowitz S, Lyons HA. Triple biopsy in

the diagnosis of sarcoidosis. In: Levinsky L, Macholda F, eds. Proceedings of the fifth international conference on sarcoidosis and other granulomatous disorders. Prague: Universita Karlova, 1971:476–479.

146. Rosen Y, Moon S, Huang CT, Gourin A, Lyons HA. Granulomatous pulmonary angiitis in sarcoidosis. Arch Pathol Lab Med 1977;101:170–174.

147. Levine BW, Saldana M, Hutter AM. Pulmonary hypertension in sarcoidosis. Am Rev Respir Dis 1971;103: 413–417.

148. Smith LJ, Lawrence JB, Katzenstein AA. Vascular sarcoidosis: a rare cause of pulmonary hypertension. Am J Med Sci 1983;285:38–44.

149. Crissman JD, Koss M, Carson RP. Pulmonary veno-occlusive disease secondary to granulomatous venulitis. Am J Surg Pathol 1980;4:93–99.

150. Hoffstein V, Ranganathan N, Mullen JBM. Sarcoidosis simulating pulmonary veno-occlusive disease. Am Rev Respir Dis 1986;134:809–811.

151. Portier F, Lerebours-Pigeonniere G, Thiberville L, et al. Sarcoïdose simulant une maladie veino-occlusive pulmonaire. Rev Mal Resp 1991;8:101–102.

152. Turiaf J, Battesti P, Marland P, Basset F, Amouroux F. Sarcoidosis involving large pulmonary arteries. In: Williams JW, Davies BH, eds. Eighth international conference on sarcoidosis and other granulomatous diseases. Cardiff:Alpha Omega, 1980:3–8.

153. Freiman DG, Hardy HL. Beryllium disease. Hum Pathol 1970;1:25–44.

154. Kitaichi M, Izumi T. Comparative pulmonary pathology of sarcoidosis, chronic beryllium disease and hypersensitivity pneumonitis based on open lung biopsy specimens. In: International Committee On Sarcoidosis, 10th international conference on sarcoidosis and other granulomatous disorders (abstracts). Baltimore, 1984;65.

155. Mikami R, Sekiguchi M, Ryuzin Y, et al. Changes in peripheral vasculature of various organs of patients with sarcoidosis—possible role of microangiopathy. Heart Vessels 1986;2:129–139.

156. Mochizuki I, Kobayashi T, Wada R, et al. Vascular lesions in the biopsied bronchus of patients with sarcoidosis: Changes of the endothelial cells in aggregation of eosinophils. Sarcoidosis 1990;7:35–41.

157. Takemura T, Matsui Y, Oritsu M, et al. Pulmonary vascular involvement in sarcoidosis: Granulomatous angiitis and microangiopathy in transbronchial lung biopsies. Virchows Archiv [A] 1991;418:361–368.

158. Littler LPW. Bronchoscopy in sarcoidois. In: Levinsky L, Macholda F, eds. Proceedings of the fifth international conference on sarcoidosis and other granulomatous disorders. Prague: Universita Karlova, 1971:463–465.

159. Siltzbach LE, Cahn LR. Random biopsy of bronchial and palatal mucosa in the diagnosis of sarcoidosis. In: Lofrgren S, ed. Proceedings of the third international conference on sarcoidosis. Acta Med Scand 1964(suppl); 425:230–233.

160. Sharma OP, Izumi T. The importance of airway obstruction in sarcoidosis. Sarcoidosis 1988;5:119–120.

161. Miller A, Teirstein AS, Jackler I, Siltzbach LE. Evidence of airway involvement in late pulmonary sarcoidosis using flow-volume curves and nitrogen washout. In: Iwai K, Hosoda Y, eds. Proceedings of the sixth international conference on sarcoidosis. Baltimore: University Park, 1974:421–424.

162. Olsson T, Björnstad-Petersen H, Stjernberg NL. Bronchostenosis due to sarcoidosis. Chest 1979;75:663–666.

163. Miller A, Brown LK, Teirstein AS. Fixed upper airway obstruction (UAO) caused by bilateral bronchial stenosis in sarcoidosis. In: International Committee On Sarcoidosis. Tenth international conference on sarcoidosis and other granulomatous disorders. Abstracts. Baltimore, 1984:86.

164. Hadfield JW, Page RL, Flower CDR, Stark JE. Localized airways narrowing in sarcoidosis. Thorax 1982;37:443–447.

165. Chusid E., Siltzbach LE. Sarcoidosis of the pleura. Ann Intern Med 1974;81:190–194.

166. Wilen SB, Rabinowitz JG, Ulreich S, Lyons HA. Pleural involvement in sarcoidosis. Am J Med 1974;57:200–209.

167. Beekman JF, Zimmet SM, Chun BK, Miranda AA, Katz S. Spectrum of pleural involvement in sarcoidosis. Arch Intern Med 1976;136:323–330.

168. Vracko R. Significance of basal lamina for regeneration of injured lung. Virchows Arch (Pathol Anat) 1972;355: 264–274.

169. Madri JA, Furthmayr H. Collagen polymorphism in the lung: An immunochemical study of pulmonary fibrosis. Hum Pathol 1980;11:353–366.

170. Editorial. Collagen in idiopathic pulmonary fibrosis. Lancet 1979;ii2:1277–1278.

171. Rennard SI, Hunninghake GW, Bitterman PB, Crystal RG. Production of fibronectin by the human alveolar macrophage: Mechanism for the recruitment of fibroblasts to the site of tissue injury in interstitial lung diseases. Proc Natl Acad Sci USA 1981;78:7147–7151.

172. Ruoslahti E, Enegvall E, Hayman EG. Fibronectin: current concepts of its structure and functions. Collagen Rel Res 1981;1:95–128.

173. Bitterman PB, Rennard SI, Hunninghake GW. Human alveolar macrophage growth factor for fibroblasts: regulation and partial characterization. J Clin Invest 1982;70:806–822.

174. Mayock RL, Bertrand P, Morisson CE, Scott JH. Manifestations of sarcoidosis. Am J Med 1963;35:67–89.

175. Israel HL, Ostrow A. Sarcoidosis and aspergilloma. Am J Med 1969;47:243–250.

176. Fresko D, Lazarus SS. Reactive systemic amyloidosis complicating long-standing sarcoidosis. NY State J Med 1982;82:232–234.

177. Swanton RH, Peters DK, Burn JI. Sarcoidosis and amyloidosis. Proc R Soc Med 1971;64:1002–1003.

178. Sharma OP, Koss M, Buck F. Sarcoidosis and amyloidosis: is the association causal or coincidental? Sarcoidosis 1987: 4:139–141.

179. Rømer FK. Sarcoidosis and cancer: A prospective study. In: Grassi C, Rizzato G, Pozzi E, eds. Sarcoidosis and other granulomatous disorders. Proceedings of the XI

world congress on sarcoidosis and other granulomatous disorders. Amsterdam: Excerpta Medica, 1988:327–328.

180. Neville E, Walker AN, James DG. Prognostic factors predicting the outcome of sarcoidosis; an analysis of 818 patients. Q J Med 1983;52:525–533.

181. Huang CT, Heurich AE, Sutton AL, Rosen Y, Lyons HA. Mortality in sarcoidosis. In: Williams JW, Davies BH, eds. Eighth international conference on sarcoidosis and other granulomatous diseases. Cardiff: Alpha Omega, 1980:522–526.

182. Iwai K, Taschibana T, Hosoda Y, Matsui Y. Sarcoidosis autopsies in Japan. Sarcoidosis 1988;5:60–65.

183. Sones M, Israel HL. Course and prognosis of sarcoidosis. Am J Med 1960;29:84–93.

184. Battesti JP, Georges R, Basset F, Saumon G. Chronic cor pulmonale in sarcoidosis. Thorax 1978;33:76–84.

185. Sharma OP, Klatt E. Factors which adversely affect the course of sarcoidosis: An analysis of 111 autopsied cases of sarcoidosis. In: Grassi C, Rizzato G, Pozzi E, eds. Sarcoidosis and other granulomatous disorders. Proceedings of the XI world congress on sarcoidosis and other granulomatous disorders. Amsterdam: Excerpta Medica, 1988:421–422.

186. Kent DC, Houk VN, Elliot RC, Sokolowisi JW, Baker JH, Sorensen K. The definitive evaluation of sarcoidosis. Am Rev Respir Dis 1970;101:721–727.

187. Aisner SC, Gupta PK, Frost JH. Sputum cytology in pulmonary sarcoidosis. Acta Cytol 1977;21:394–398.

188. Vernon SE. Nodular pulmonary sarcoidosis: diagnosis with fine needle aspiration biopsy. Acta Cytol 1985;29:473–476.

189. Shure D, Fedullo PF. Transbronchial needle aspiration of peripheral masses. Am Rev Respir Dis 1983;128:1090–1092.

190. Frable MA, Frable WJ. Fine needle aspiration biopsy in the diagnosis of sarcoid of the head and neck. Acta Cytol 1984;28:175–177.

191. Selroos O. Fine needle aspiration biopsy of the spleen in diagnosis of sarcoidosis. In: Siltzbach LE, ed. Seventh international conference on sarcoidosis and other granulomatous disorders. Ann NY Acad Sci 1976;278:517–521.

192. Fulkerson WJ. Current concepts: Fiberoptic bronchoscopy. N Engl J Med 1984;311:511–515.

193. Teirstein AS, Chuang M, Miller A, Siltzbach LE. Flexible-bronchoscope biopsy of lung and bronchial wall in intrathoracic sarcoidosis. In: Siltzbach LE, ed. Seventh international conference on sarcoidosis and other granulomatous disorders. Ann NY Acad Sci 1976;278:522–527.

194. Koerner SK, Sakowitz AJ, Appelman RI, Becker NH, Schoenbaum SW. Transbronchial lung biopsy for the diagnosis of sarcoidosis. N Engl J Med 1975;293:268–270.

195. Koontz CH, Joyner LR, Nelson RA. Transbronchial lung biopsy via the fiberoptic bronchoscope in sarcoidosis. Ann Intern Med 1976;85:64–66.

196. Khan MA, Corona F, Masson RG. Transbronchial biopsy for sarcoidosis. N Engl J Med 1976;295:225.

197. Poletti V, Patelli M, Spiga L, Ferracini R, Manetto V. Transbronchial lung biopsy in pulmonary sarcoidosis; Is it an evaluable method in detection of disease activity? Chest 1986;89:361–365.

198. Gilman MJ, Wang KP. Transbronchial lung biopsy in sarcoidosis. An approach to determine the optimal number of biopsies. Am Rev Respir Dis 1980;122:721–724.

199. Roethe RA, Fuller PB, Byrd RB, Hafermann DR. Transbronical lung biopsy in sarcoidosis. Chest 1980;77:400–402.

200. Fechner RE, Greenberg SD, Wilson RK, Stevens PM. Evaluation of transbronchial biopsy of the lung. Am J Clin Pathol 1977;68:17–20.

201. Koch ML, Coté RA. Comparison of fluorescense microscopy with Ziehl–Neelsen stain for demonstration of acid fast bacilli. Am Rev Respir Dis 1965;91:283–294.

202. Wellman KF, Teng KP. Demonstration of acid fast bacilli in tissue sections by fluorescense. Can Med Assoc J 1962;87:837–841.

203. Woodard BH, Rosenberg SI, Farnham R, Adams DO. Incidence and nature of primary granulomatous inflammation in surgically removed material. Am J Surg Pathol 1982;6:119–129.

204. Wiley EL, Mulhollan TJ, Beck B, Tyndall JA, Freeman RG. Polyclonal antibodies raised against *Bacillus Calmette-Guerin*, *Mycobacterium duvalii* and *Mycobacterium paratuberculosis* used to detect mycobacteria in tissue with the use of immunohistochemical techniques. Am J Clin Pathol 1990;94:307–312.

205. Eisenach KD, Crawford JT, Bates JH. Repetitive DNA sequences as probes for *Mycobacterium tuberculosis*. J Clin Microbiol 1988;26:2240–2245.

206. Lin CS, Ruiz A. Contamination by saprophytic acid-fast bacilli in the histology laboratory. Lab Med 1977;8:11–13.

207. Ulbright TM, Katzenstein AA. Solitary necrotizing granulomas of the lung. Am J Surg Pathol 1980;4:13–28.

208. Grange JM. Tuberculosis. In: Wilson G, Miles A, Parker MT, eds. Topley and Wilson's principles of bacteriology, virology and immunity, Vol 3. Baltimore: Williams & Wilkins, 1983:42–43.

209. Boyd WA. A textbook of pathology. 3d Ed. Philadelphia: Lea & Feibiger, 1938.

210. Gottlieb JA, Fanburg BL, Pauker SG. A decision analytic view of the diagnosis of sarcoidosis. In: Fanburg BL, ed. Sarcoidosis and other granulomatous diseases of the lung. New York: Marcel Dekker, 1983:349–380.

211. Williams RH, Nickerson DA. Skin reactions in sarcoid. Proc Soc Exp Biol Med 1935;33:403–405.

212. Siltzbach LE. The Kveim test in sarcoidosis. Am J Med 1961;30:495–501.

213. Chase MW. The preparation and standardization of Kveim antigen. Am Rev Respir Dis 1961;84(Part 2):86–88.

214. Chapman J. The Kveim test. Arch Pathol Lab Med 1977;101:515–517.

215. Kataria YP. Cutaneous granulomata in response to in-

jection with autoclaved bronchoalveolar lavage cell preparation in sarcoidosis patients. In: Grassi C, Rizzato G, Pozzi E, eds. Sarcoidosis and other granulomatous disorders. Proceedings of the XI world congress on sarcoidosis and other granulomatous disorders. Amsterdam: Excerpta Medica, 1988:139–142.

216. Siltzbach LE. Qualities and behavior of satisfactory Kveim suspensions. In: Siltzbach LE, ed. Seventh international conference on sarcoidosis and other granulomatous disorders. Ann NY Acad Sci 1976;278:665–669.

217. Teirstein AS, Brown LK. The Kveim Siltzbach test in 1987. In: Grassi C, Rizzato G, Pozzi E, eds. Sarcoidosis and other granulomatous disorders. Proceedings of the XI world congress on sarcoidosis and other granulomatous disorders. Amsterdam: Excerpta Medica, 1988:7–18.

218. Mishra BB, Poulter LW, Sherlock S, James DG. The Kveim . Siltzbach granuloma: A model for sarcoid granuloma formation. In: Johns CJ, ed. Tenth international conference on sarcoidosis and other granulomatous disorders. Ann NY Acad Sci 1986;465:164–175.

219. Kataria YP, Park HK. Dynamics and mechanism of the sarcoidal granuloma: Detecting T cell subsets, non T cells and immunoglobulins in biopsies at varying intervals of Kveim–Siltzbach test sites. In: Johns CJ, ed. Tenth international conference on sarcoidosis and other granulomatous disorders. Ann NY Acad Sci 1986;465:221–232.

220. Cohn ZA, Fedorko ME, Hirsch JG, Turiaf J, Chabot J. In: Turiaf J, Chabot J, James DG, Zatouroff MA, eds. La Sarkoidose. Report of the 4th international conference on sarcoidosis. Paris: Masson et Cie, 1967:141–149.

221. Lieberman L. Elevation of serum angiotensin converting enzyme (ACE) in sarcoidosis. Am J Med 1975;59:365–372.

222. Friedland J, Silverstein E. Sensitive fluorometric assay for serum angiotensin-converting enzyme with the natural substrate angiotensin 1. Am J Clin Pathol 1977;68:225–228.

223. Studdy PR, James DG. The specificity and sensitivity of serum angiotensin converting enzyme in sarcoidosis and other diseases. Experience in twelve centres in six different countries. In: Chrétien J, Marsac J, Saltiel JC, eds. Sarcoidosis and other granulomatous disorders. Ninth international conference on sarcoidosis and other granulomatous disorders. Paris: Pergamon Press, 1983:332–344.

224. Muthuswamy PP, Lopez-Majano V, Ranginwala M, Trainor WD. Serum angiotensin-converting enzyme (SACE) activity as an indicator of total body granuloma load and prognosis in sarcoidosis. Sarcoidosis 1987;4:142–148.

225. Silverstein E, Friedland J, Lyons HA. Serum angiotensin converting enzyme in sarcoidosis: Clinical significance. Isr J Med Sci 1977;13:1001–1006.

226. Silverstein E, Friedland J, Lyons HA, Gourin A. Markedly elevated angiotensin converting enzyme in lymph nodes containing nonnecrotizing granulomas in sarcoidosis. Proc Natl Acad Sci USA 1976;73:2137–2141.

227. Pertschuk LP, Silverstein E, Friedland J. Detection of angiotensin-converting enzyme in sarcoid granulomas. Am J Clin Pathol 1981;75:350–354.

228. Pertschuk LP, Stanek AE, Silverstein E, Friedland J. Immunocytochemical detection of angiotensin-converting enzyme in sarcoidosis granulomas. In: DeLellis RA, ed. Monographs in diagnostic pathology. Vol. 7. Advances in immunohistochemistry New York: Masson, 1984:311–323.

229. Stanek AE, Silverstein E, Friedland J. Angiotensin converting enzyme is localized in the plasma membrane of the epithelioid cell of the sarcoidosis granuloma. Clin Res 1982;30:438A.

230. Silverstein E, Friedland J. Pathogenesis of sarcoidosis; T lymphocyte modulation of induction of angiotensin converting enzyme in human monocytes in culture. Evidence of mediation by lymphokine. In: International committee on sarcoidosis. 10th international conference on sarcoidosis and other granulomatous disorders (abstracts). Baltimore, 1984:96.

231. Ryder KW, Stephen JJ, Saleem KO, Meredith HT. Serum angiotensin converting enzyme activity in patients with histoplasmosis. JAMA 1983;249:1888–1889.

232. Check IJ, Gowitt GT, Staton GW. Bronchoalveolar lavage cell differential in the diagnosis of sarcoid interstitial lung disease: Likelihood ratios based on computerized data base. Am J Clin Pathol 1985;84:744–747.

233. Line BR, Fulmer JD, Reynolds HY, et al. Gallium-67 citrate scanning in the staging of idiopathnic pulmonary fibrosis; correlation with physiologic and morphologic features and bronchoalveolar lavage. Am Rev Respir Dis 1978;118:355–365.

234. Hunninghake GW, Line BR, Szapiel SV, Crystal RG. Activation of inflammatory cells increases the localization of gallium-67 at sites of disease. Clin Res 1981;29:171A.

235. Rizzato G, Blasi A. A European survey on the usefulness of gallium-67 lung scans in assessing sarcoidosis: Experience in 14 research centers in seven different countries. In: Johns CJ, ed. Tenth international conference on sarcoidosis and other granulomatous disorders. Ann NY Acad Sci 1986;465:463–478.

236. Hirsh BC, Johnson WC. Pathology of granulomatous diseases. Epithelioid granulomas, Part 1. Int J Dermatol 1984;23:237–246.

237. Liebow AA. The J Burns Amberson Lecture. Pulmonary angiitis and granulomatosis. Am Rev Respir Dis 1973;108:1–118.

238. Saldana MJ. Necrotizing sarcoid granulomatosis: Clinico-pathologic observations in 24 patients. Lab Invest 1978;38:364 (abstract).

239. Churg A, Carrington CB, Gupta R. Necrotizing sarcoid granulomatosis. Chest 1979;76:406–413.

240. Koss MN, Hochholzer L, Feigin DS, Garancis JC, Ward PA. Necrotizing sarcoid-like granulomatosis: Clinical, pathologic and immunopathologic findings. Hum Pathol 1980;2(Suppl):510–519.

241. Stephen JG, Baimbridge MV, Corrin B, Wilkinson SP, Day D, Whimster WF. Necrotizing "sarcoidal" angiitis

and granulomatosis of the lung. Thorax 1976;31:356–360.

242. Menon MPS, Beohar PC, Jain SK, Narayanan SK. Necrotizing sarcoid angiitis and granulomatosis of the lung. Indian J Chest Dis Allied Sci 1980;22:123–127.

243. Fisher MR, Christ ML, Bernstein JR. Necrotizing sarcoid-like granulomatosis: radiologic-pathologic correlation. J Canad Assoc Radiol 1984;35:313–315.

244. Rolfes DB, Weiss MA, Sanders MA. Necrotizing sarcoid granulomatosis with suppurative features. Am J Clin Pathol 1984;82:602–607.

245. Gibbs AR, Jones William W. Necrotising sarcoidal granulmatosis. In: International Committee on Sarcoidosis. Tenth international conference on sarcoidosis and other granulomatous disorders. Abstracts. Baltimore, 1984:1–2.

246. Rühl GH, Schlanstein A, Hartung W. Nekrotisierende sarkoidale Granulomatose der Lunge. Prax Klin Pneumol 1985;39:284–287.

247. Weiss M, Gokel JM. Die nekrotisierende sarkoide Granulomatose der Lunge. Pathologe 1990;11:178–182.

248. Sugama Y, Matsuoka R, Kitamura S. A case of necrotizing sarcoid granulomatosis diagnosed by open lung biopsy. Jpn J Thorac Dis 1989: 27:75–80.

249. Armbruster C, Vetter N. Zur Differentialdiagnose der nekrotisierenden sarkoidalen Angiitis: Nekrotisierende sarkoidale Angiitis und Kollagenerkrankung-ein Fallbericht. Pneumologie 1991;45:63–66.

250. Gordon CI. Necrotizing sarcoid granulomatosis: Report of a case. J Am Osteopath Assoc 1986;584–588.

251. Katzenstein AA. The histologic spectrum and differential diagnosis of necrotizing granulomatous inflammation in the lung. In: Fenoglio CM, Wolff M, eds. Progress in surgical pathology. Vol. 2. New York: Masson, 1980:42–70.

252. Cole SR, Johnson KJ, Ward PA. Pathology of sarcoidosis, granulomatous vasculitis and other idiopathic granulomatous diseases of the lung. In: Fanburg BL, ed. Sarcoidosis and other granulomatous diseases of the lung. New York: Marcel Dekker, 1983:149–202.

253. Churg A. Pulmonary angiitis and granulomatosis revisited. Hum Pathol 1983;14:868–883.

254. Cole SR. Personal communication.

255. Singh N, Cole SR, Krause PJ, Conway M, Garcia L. Necrotizing sarcoid granulomatosis with extrapulmonary involvement. Am Rev Respir Dis 1981;124:189–191.

256. Dail DH. Personal communication.

257. Kirks DR, McCormick VD, Greenspan RH. Pulmonary sarcoidosis. Roentgenologic analysis of 150 patients. AJR 1973;117:777–786

258. Sharma OP, Hewlett R, Gordonson J. Nodular sarcoidosis: an unusual radiographic appearance. Chest 1973;64:189–192.

259. Sharma OP. Sarcoidosis: unusual pulmonary manifestations. Postgrad Med 1977;61:67–73.

260. Rømer FK. Sarcoidosis with large nodular lesions simulating pulmonary metastases: an analysis of 126 cases of intrathoracic sarcoidosis. Scand J Respir Dis 1977;58:11–16.

261. Rose RM, Lee RGL, Costello P. Solitary nodular sarcoidosis. Clin Radiol 1985;36:589–592.

262. Onal E, Lopata M, Lourenco RV. Nodular pulmonary sarcoidosis. Chest 1977;72:296–300.

263. Tellis CJ, Putman JS. Cavitation in large multinodular pulmonary disease. A rare manifestation of sarcoidosis. Chest 1977;71:792–793.

264. Ohsaki Y, Abe S, Yahara O, Murao M. Bilateral hilar lymphadenopathy and cystic lung lesion. Chest 1977;71:81–82.

265. Cavallo A, Perin B, Perini L, Natale F. Rara complicanza della sarcoidosi: Cavitazione polmonare. Radiol Med 1987;73:589–590.

266. Tada H, Yasumizu R, Yuasa S, Sato M, Mizuno Y. Annular lesion of the lung in sarcoidosis. Thorax 1989;44:756–757.

267. Dorcier F, Grenier N, Dubroca J, Lacoste D, Beylot J, Grelet PH. Sarcoïdose thoracique avec «cavitation» pulmonaire. Radiologie 1987;68:451–454.

CHAPTER 20

Idiopathic Interstitial Fibrosis

SAMUEL P. HAMMAR

Fibrosis is a nonspecific reaction to injury typically occurring in association with or after a significant inflammatory process. In the case of a myocardial infarct, for example, the region of ischemic necrosis is eventually replaced by a dense fibrous scar. In skin, regions of surgical incision or traumatic laceration undergo fibrosis as part of the normal healing process. Similarly, the lung is an organ in which fibrotic reactions occur. In some instances, such as pulmonary infarcts, fibrosis may be part of a normal healing process, and the mechanism of fibrosis is relatively well understood. In other conditions, such as asbestosis, the etiology is apparent but the mechanism of fibrosis is poorly understood. In myocardial infarcts and wound healing, fibrosis serves a useful purpose. When it occurs in the interstitium of peripheral lung tissue, it has a deleterious effect, interfering with normal physiologic functions such as blood flow and gas diffusion.

Interstitial lung disease refers to a condition in which the predominant tissue abnormality is in the alveolar septa, in contrast to intrabronchial and intraalveolar locations. More than 100 known causes of interstitial lung disease are recognized, and most are associated with some degree of interstitial fibrosis.[1–3] In approximately two-thirds of cases, the cause is unknown and the morphogenesis is poorly understood.[4] This unknown group of interstitial lung diseases has a prevalence in the United States of 5–10 cases/100,000 population and results in 10,000 admissions to hospitals each year.[4] Some cases of interstitial lung disease are acute,[5,6,7] and may be caused by viral or mycoplasma infections,[8] but most have an insidious onset over months to years, have no obvious cause, and result in diffuse interstitial pulmonary fibrosis. The features of idiopathic pulmonary fibrosis are discussed in this chapter.

History and Nosology

The recognition of diffuse interstitial pulmonary fibrosis as a distinct entity can be traced to the publications of Louis Hamman and Arnold Rich.[9,10] Between 1931 and 1935, they encountered four patients aged 21, 37, 47, and 68 years who developed a rapidly progressive pulmonary illness and died between 20 days and 3 months after admission to hospital. At autopsy, the lungs were described as being firm and consolidated, and showed the following similar microscopic changes: (1) inflammatory infiltrates, which were mostly interstitial and contained few polymorphonuclear leukocytes; (2) alveolar lining cell hypertrophy and hyperplasia; (3) necrosis of alveolar and bronchiolar epithelium; (4) formation of hyaline membranes that lined alveoli; (5) marked edema and fibrin deposits in alveolar walls; (6) extensive diffuse and progressive interstitial proliferation of fibrous tissue throughout all lobes of both lungs, associated with focal organization of intraalveolar exudate; (7) the presence of eosinophils in the interstitial tissue in three of four cases; and (8) the absence of stainable bacteria in the tissue. The changes they described are similar to those described in acute alveolar damage[5] and those seen in the lungs of patients dying from adult respiratory distress syndrome.[11] The acuteness of the clinical syndrome, and most of the pathologic changes such as hyaline membranes and necrosis of epithelium, are not characteristically seen in most cases of idiopathic pulmonary fibrosis. Olson et al.[12] reported on 29 cases of acute interstitial pneumonitis which they considered synonymous with Hamman-Rich Syndrome and reviewed three of the original cases reported by Hamman and Rich.[9,10] As correctly pointed out by Olson and colleagues,[12] the pathologic changes observed by Hamman and Rich were those of acute diffuse alveolar damage (see Chapter 4) and not what is currently referred to as idiopathic pulmonary fibrosis or a variety of other names to be discussed (see following). Nevertheless, when the topic of pulmonary fibrosis is discussed, the term Hamman–Rich syndrome is inevitably mentioned.

In the 1960s, Liebow and Carrington[13] began a study of interstitial lung disease that resulted in the histologic typing of these diseases into five distinct groups: (1) usual interstitial pneumonitis (UIP); (2) usual interstitial pneumonitis with bronchiolitis obliterans (BIP); (3) desquamative interstitial pneumonitis (DIP); (4) lymphocytic interstitial pneumonitis (LIP); and (5) giant cell interstitial pneumonitis (GIP). Usual interstitial pneumonitis was described as a lesion with histologic features that extended from acute diffuse alveolar damage with hyaline membrane formation to interstitial fibrosis and predominantly chronic inflammation. Usual interstitial pneumonitis with bronchiolitis obliterans was characterized as having features of usual interstitial pneumonitis with superimposed damage to bronchioles and organizing exudate in the lumens of bronchioles. Desquamative interstitial pneumonitis was initially described in 1965[14] as a relatively uniform lesion characterized by accumulation of large mononuclear cells in alveolar spaces, prominent lymphoid follicles and lack of necrosis, exudation and hyaline membrane formation, and minimal interstitial fibrosis. Lymphocytic interstitial pneumonitis was characterized histologically as showing an interstitial infiltrate of mature lymphocytes and plasma cells without germinal center formation, lymph node involvement, or nodular parenchymal masses of lymphocytes.[15] Giant cell interstitial pneumonitis was described as a rare lesion characterized by the accumulation of bizarre giant cells in alveolar spaces.

The term idiopathic fibrosing alveolitis was suggested by Scadding[16] on the advice of Alfred Fishman[17] to refer to the gamut of histopathologic changes ranging from the acute disease described by Hamman and Rich to more frequently observed diffuse interstitial pulmonary fibrosis with inflammation. A similar name, chronic diffuse idiopathic fibrosing alveolitis, was offered by Gough.[18] Scadding and Hinson[19] suggested that the histologic patterns of desquamative interstitial pneumonitis and usual interstitial pneumonitis represented the early and late stages of a single disorder and that there was not a sharp clinical or pathologic distinction between these forms of "interstitial pneumonia." They also proposed the terms "mural fibrosing alveolitis" to be equivalent to usual interstitial pneumonitis and "desquamative fibrosing alveolitis" to be equal to

Table 20–1. Terms used for chronic fibrosis

Idiopathic interstitial pulmonary fibrosis
Idiopathic fibrosing alveolitis
Usual interstitial pneumonitis
Diffuse interstitial pulmonary fibrosis
Diffuse alveolar fibrosis of the lungs
Idiopathic pulmonary fibrosis
Idiopathic fibrosing alveolitis (mural type)
Chronic Hamman–Rich syndrome
Hamman–Rich syndrome
Cryptogenic fibrosing alveolitis

desquamative interstitial pneumonitis. Even though usual interstitial pneumonitis (UIP) as described by Liebow and Carrington and cryptogenic fibrosing alveolitis as described by Scadding included an acute phase process presumably analagous to that described by Hamman and Rich,[9,10] these two terms are currently understood by pathologists to refer to diffuse interstitial fibrosis and not to acute diffuse alveolar damage or acute interstitial pneumonitis.

In the few years following the publication by Hamman and Rich in 1944, several reports described a chronic form of "interstitial" lung disease.[20–24] It soon became apparent that this chronic form was more frequent than acute disease, and several review articles describing its clinical, pathologic, and physiologic features were published in the late 1950s and early 1960s.[25–27] Livingstone et al.[27] presented clinical, radiologic, and pathologic information on 45 patients and thoroughly reviewed the relevant literature to 1964. Scadding[28] subsequently reviewed some of the controversies concerning pulmonary fibrosis, including a discussion of problems inherent in using the term "interstitial." Despite Scadding's valid reasons for not using this descriptive but perhaps imprecise designation, it is ingrained in the medical literature and (in the United States) is used more than any other term to describe this disease). Even Scadding, in an article published in 1960,[29] used interstitial in referring to pulmonary fibrosis. Various names are currently used to describe a chronic disease of unknown cause whose predominant pathologic features are alveolar septal fibrosis and chronic inflammation; these are listed in Table 20–1.

Etiology

The designation *idiopathic* indicates an unknown cause. In approximately 10%–20% of cases, interstitial fibrosis is associated with a systemic disease, most notably a collagen vascular disease such as rheumatoid arthritis, polymyositis-dermatomyositis, systemic lupus erythematosus, Sjögren's syndrome, scleroderma, or mixed connective tissue disease. Most of the pertinent references concerning pulmonary involvement in the collagen vascular diseases until 1979 are listed in the review by Hunninghake and Fauci[30] (see Chapter 21). Additional reports of pulmonary disease in these conditions have appeared since 1979.[31–51] Pulmonary fibrosis has also been reported in association with various liver disorders.[52–55]

Several reports have described interstitial pulmonary fibrosis in families, thus suggesting the importance of genetic factors.[56–61] This author has seen two such examples of familial pulmonary fibrosis, one involving three brothers and the other two sisters, which suggest that familial occurrence may be more common than reported. Also, the possible association of pulmonary fibrosis with specific HLA types would suggest a genetic predisposition of the disease,[62–67] although the validity of this association remains uncertain.[68]

Cigarette smoking is a potentially significant factor that is infrequently mentioned in discussions concerning pulmonary fibrosis. In 1963, Auerbach[68,69] suggested that cigarette smoking can cause interstitial fibrosis, resulting in an abnormal chest radiograph. The potential fibrogenic effect of cigarette smoking was recently commented on by Weiss[70] in the context of its association with asbestos in causing pulmonary fibrosis. It is of interest that Carrington et al.,[71] in their comparison of usual interstitial pneumonitis and desquamative interstitial pneumonitis, stated that 90% of patients diagnosed as having desquamative interstitial pneumonitis and 71% with usual interstitial pneumonitis had a cigarette smoking history of greater than 10 pack-years.

Other clinical studies have reported a relatively high frequency of cigarette smoking in persons who develop pulmonary fibrosis.[72–77] De Cremoux et al.[78] evaluated the effect of cigarette smoking on idiopathic interstitial fibrosis. They found several different features in noncigarette smokers that were not seen in the cigarette-smoking group of persons who developed idiopathic interstitial fibrosis. These included an aggressive onset, a higher lymphocyte count in bronchoalveolar lavage fluid, and a better response to prednisolone therapy. However, noncigarette smokers with interstitial fibrosis did not exhibit a survival advantage.

Viral pneumonitis typically produces acute changes, but may rapidly lead to a chronic condition with pathologic changes indistinguishable from idiopathic pulmonary fibrosis.[79–81] Verganon et al.[82] recently identified antibodies with titers greater than 1:160 to various Epstein–Barr virus antigens in bronchoalveolar lavage fluid from 10 of 13 patients with cryptogenic fibrosing alveolitis. In contrast, none of 12 patients with other types of interstitial lung disease (6 with extrinsic allergic alveolitis, 3 with drug-induced disease, 2 with collagen vascular disease, 1 with asbestosis) had IgG antibodies against Epstein–Barr virus antigens in lavage fluid. These findings suggested that Epstein–Barr virus may play a role in causing idiopathic fibrosing alveolitis.

Roggli[83] evaluated the mineral fiber content of lung parenchyma in 24 cases of diffuse pulmonary fibrosis of unknown cause via scanning electron microscopy, and compared his findings with those of 36 autopsy cases of histologically confirmed asbestosis and 20 autopsy cases of patients with normal lungs. He concluded that most patients with advanced pulmonary fibrosis, whose tissue samples did not meet the histologic criteria for asbestosis (see Chapter 28) did not have asbestos-induced fibrosis, even though there may have been a history of exposure to asbestos. However, in Roggli's case 23, the asbestos fiber concentration in a patient thought to have idiopathic pulmonary fibrosis was within the range for mild asbestosis, which may have been obscured by superimposed radiation-associated fibrosis. Roggli's case 24 concerned an 85-year-old man who developed fatal pulmonary fibrosis 20 years after retirement from his occupation as a brake grinder. Although the uncoated fiber content was relatively low, the patient had asbestos body counts by light microscopy and scanning electron microscopy, which made it difficult to exclude the diagnosis of asbestosis. Thus, it seems possible that some cases diagnosed as idiopathic pulmonary fibrosis may, in fact, represent examples of asbestosis. Unless one has a very accurate history or identifies asbestos bodies in histologic sections of lung tissue, most of these cases will continue to be classified as "idiopathic."

Pathogenesis and Morphogenesis of Pulmonary Fibrosis

The pathogenesis of idiopathic pulmonary fibrosis is poorly understood, although much basic information exists concerning such cells as neutrophils, pulmonary alveolar macrophages, lymphocytes, and pulmonary epthelial cells, cell products such as fibrnectin and lymphokines/cytokines, and collagen production, all of which are thought to be important in the development of pulmonary fibrosis. The normal number, the turnover rates, and the alveolar surface area covered by normal lung cells are listed in Table 20–2.[84–87] (Also see Chapter 2.)

In pulmonary fibrosis, the number and character of these cells are markedly altered. Pulmonary alveolar macrophages are bone marrow derived, but a population of immature cells exists in the interstitium of the

Table 20–2. Normal lung cells

Cell type	Total alveolar cells (%)	Alveolar surface area covered (%)	Average turnover rate (days)
Type I pneumocyte	8–10	90	7–35
Type II pneumocyte	12–16	10	7–35
Endothelial cell	30–40	NA[a]	77
Interstitial cell	30–36	NA	?
Macrophages	2–10	NA	21(?)

[a] NA, not applicable.

lung that may give rise to a normal number of alveolar macrophages in the absence of bone marrow precursors.[88] The interaction between alveolar macrophages, neutrophils, and lymphocytes appears important in the pathogenesis and morphogenesis of pulmonary fibrosis. Alveolar macrophages produce a chemotactic factor that induces migration of polymorphonuclear leukocytes into the lung and another factor that stimulates bone marrow production of granulocytes and monocytes.[89–91] The observed increase in neutrophils in lavage fluid from patients with idiopathic fibrosis may be caused by these factors. In addition, alveolar macrophages produce fibronectin, a 440-kilodalton glycoprotein that recruits fibroblasts to regions of inflammation and causes the attachment of fibroblasts to collagenous matrix.[92,93] Fibronectin is increased in bronchoalveolar lavage fluid from patients with pulmonary fibrosis.

Pulmonary alveolar macrophages are the source of many cytokines, which are also known as peptide growth factors or biologic response modifiers. They are important in normal tissue growth, and also seem to be important in a variety of disease states such as idiopathic pulmonary fibrosis, sarcoidosis, and hypersensitivity pneumonitis. These cytokines are thought to be mediators of cellular communication and behavior, and their function includes stimulation of mitoses, angiogenesis, cytoskeleton differentiation, and immunomodulation and the production of extracellular matrix.[94] They are listed with some of their functions in Table 20–3, and many of their complex interactions are shown in Fig. 20–1. Vignaud et al.[95] evaluated alveolar macrophages obtained by bronchoalveolar lavage from normal individuals and individuals with idiopathic pulmonary fibrosis. They found that platelet-derived growth factor was present in normal and fibrotic lungs and was specifically associated with macrophages. They also found that macrophages and alveolar epithelial cells expressed the platelet-derived growth factor beta-chain gene, in idiopathic pulmonary fibrosis, and that the accumulation of platelet-derived growth factor in the lung preceded the fibrotic process. They concluded that platelet-derived growth factor may play a role in normal lung mesenchymal cell turnover and in the pathogenesis of lung fibrosis. This subject has also been reviewed by Marinelli,[96] who also provided information on the platelet-derived growth factor in the development of pulmonary fibrosis. Tumor necrosis factor has also been reported to be important in the development of bleomycin-induced pulmonary fibrosis in rats.[97,98]

Interleukin-8 was evaluated in bronchoalveolar lavage fluid by Lynch et al.[99] They found that bronchoalveolar lavage cells from patients with idiopathic pulmonary fibrosis expressed messenger RNA for interleukin-8, and the amount of interleukin-8 messenger RNA was correlated with the percent of neutrophils in the bronchoalveolar lavage fluid. Isolated cells from healthy subjects did not express messenger RNA for interleukin-8, and only low levels of interleukin-8 messenger-RNA were found in cells from patients with pulmonary sarcoidosis. These authors concluded that the expression of interleukin-8 may be a feature of idiopathic pulmonary fibrosis and support a role for

Table 20–3. Selected cytokine effects on target cells[a]

Cytokine	Target cells		Other effects
	Promitogenic for	Antimitogenic for	
PDGF	Mesenchymal cells		
bFGF	Mesenchymal cells, endothelial cells	Cancer cells	Pituitary, ovarian function
TGF-β	Fibroblasts, osteoblasts	Fibroblasts, epithelial cells, osteoblasts, T and B lymphocytes	adrenal steroidogenesis, immunoglobulin synthesis
EGF/TGF-α	Lymphocytes, fibroblasts, keratinocytes	Cancer cells	
IL-1	T-lymphocytes, fibroblasts, keratinocytes	Cancer cells	Bone resorption fever
IL-6	Fibroblasts, epithelial cells		Ig synthesis cell-surface antigen, acute-phase reactants
TNF-α	Fibroblasts, epithelial cells	Cancer cells	collagenase, lipoprotein lipase, cachexia
IGF-I	Mesenchymal cells and many other cell types		

[a] Modified from Kelley J. Cytokines of the lung. Am Rev Respir Dis 1990;141:765–788.

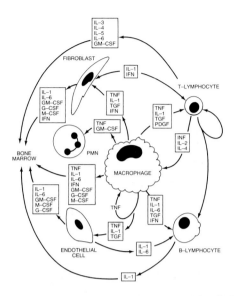

Fig. 20–1. Schematic shows multiple potential cellular interactions involving cytokines as elucidated through in vitro studies. Not all pathways shown have been documented in the lung. Some cytokine interactions are constitutive; others are observed only after induction. From Kelley J. Cytokines of the lung. Am Rev Respir Dis 1990;141:765–788.

interleukin-8 in the development of neutrophilic alveolitis thought to occur in idiopathic pulmonary fibrosis.

Alveolar macrophages from patients with interstitial fibrosis also release an 18,000-dalton molecular weight growth factor, termed alveolar macrophage growth factor, or basic fibroblast growth factor, that causes proliferation of fetal fibroblasts in cell culture.[100] This factor is not produced by alveolar macrophages from normal persons; it is distinct from other growth factors such as insulin-like growth factor, appears to exert its effect by stimulating target cells to synthesize DNA, and acts in concert with fibronectin. The synthesis and release of this factor is stimulated by activated T lymphocytes and immune complexes. Immune complexes have been demonstrated by direct immunofluorescence in the lung tissue from some patients with pulmonary fibrosis.[101] Most of the factors produced by alveolar macrophages are done so by "activated macrophages." The demonstration of DR or Ia antigen on the cell surface of alveolar macrophages indicates they are activated and thus potentially capable of producing these various substances.[102]

Several factors produced by lymphocytes are also thought to be important in the pathogenesis of pulmonary fibrosis. Immune complexes identified in lung tissue and lavage fluid are believed to be derived from immunoglobulin-producing resident B lymphocytes, which are increased in absolute numbers in patients with pulmonary fibrosis.[103] T lymphocytes are also increased in absolute numbers in lung tissue from

patients with fibrosing alveolitis, although their exact function in this condition is uncertain.[104] They do not spontaneously release lymphokines and the ratio of helper/inducer to suppressor/cytotoxic T cells is normal.[104] Several studies have shown they may be important in causing fibrosis. In bleomycin-induced pulmonary fibrosis, athymic nude mice deficient in T cells show less cellular infiltration, less fibroblast proliferation, and less collagen deposition than euthymic mice with normal T lymphocytes.[105] Activated human peripheral blood lymphocytes produce a factor that stimulates proliferation of dermal fibroblasts and synthesis of collagen and noncollagenous proteins.[106]

Polymorphonuclear leukocytes and their products may also play a role in interstitial pulmonary fibrosis. Polymorphonuclear leukocytes and neutrophil collagenase are increased in bronchoalveolar lavage fluid from patients with fibrosing alveolitis.[107–109] Neutrophils contain a variety of proteolytic enzymes in their lysosomes, such as elastase and collagenase, which are capable of producing tissue injury. However, in a recent experimental study, beige mice, which have a selective inability to degranulate their neutrophils and consequently do not release hydrolytic enzymes, showed no amelioration of the fibrogenic response to bleomycin.[110] Neutrophils and alveolar macrophages also produce toxic oxygen metabolites such as hydrogen peroxide, which may be more important than proteolytic enzymes in causing tissue injury and subsequent fibrosis in mice.[111,112]

Other factors may also be important in the development of idiopathic pulmonary fibrosis. Nettleblatt and Halgren[113] evaluated hyaluronic acid in bronchoalveolar lavage fluid in the development of bleomycin-induced alveolitis in rats. They found increased concentrations of hyaluronic acid in bronchoalveolar lavage fluid 3 days after bleomycin administration, with peak values being present at 5 days in a range about 75 fold higher than those seen in control animals. They found that the increased concentration of hyaluronic acid in bronchoalveolar lavage fluid could not be explained by plasma leakage, and that it progressively decreased after day 5 and returned to normal values within 3 weeks after bleomycin treatment. They suggested that hyaluronic acid was involved in the influx of polys into the bronchoalveolar lavage fluid, and that it may be important in the early inflammatory phase of bleomycin-induced pulmonary fibrosis. Montano et al.[114] evaluated lung collagenase inhibitors and spontaneous latent collagenase activity in patients with idiopathic pulmonary fibrosis and hypersensitivity pneumonitis. They studied tissue samples from 5 patients with idiopathic pulmonary fibrosis and 6 patients with chronic hypersensitivity pneumonitis, and found that in both diseases the inhibitor levels were higher in patients with idiopathic pulmonary fibrosis and hypersensitivity pneumonitis than in control subjects. They also found low amounts of collagenase in patients with idiopathic pulmonary fibrosis, and also excessive enzyme inhibitors, which may have resulted in decreased collagen catabolism. Noguchi et al.[115] studied tissue eosinophilia and eosinophil degranulation in 34 patients with inflammatory fibrosis, 12 with idiopathic retroperitoneal fibrosis, 7 with sclerosing mediastinitis, 4 with sclerosing cholangitis, and 11 with pulmonary fibrosis. Eosinophil infiltration or extracellular major basic protein deposition was observed in 8 of the 11 cases of pulmonary fibrosis. In contrast, eosinophil infiltration and major basic protein deposition were not observed in 16 patients with noninflammatory fibrous proliferations. These results suggested that eosinophil infiltration and release of major basic protein commonly occurred in inflammatory fibrosis and were important in the pathogenesis of fibrosis. The authors discussed the previous work in this area, showing that eosinophil extracts stimulate fibroblast proliferation, and supported the concept that eosinophils possess a fibroblast-stimulating factor. Also of interest along these same lines is the report that dog mastocytoma cells in culture secrete a growth factor for fibroblasts that may contribute to pathologic fibrosis.[116]

Another area of uncertainty in idiopathic pulmonary fibrosis is the question of whether there is a definite increase in collagen concentration in the lung or only a variation in the types of collagen. Currently, six polymorphic types of collagen are recognized. In normal lung, types I and III collagen are predominantly in alveolar septa whereas type II collagen is associated with the trachea and bronchi. In normal lung, the ratio of type I to type III collagen in alveolar septa is 2:1, and collagen constitutes about 15% of the dry weight of lung parenchyma. Although the results of one study suggested there was no increase in collagen content in fibrotic lung,[117] another study showed an absolute increase in collagen content and an increase in the ratio of type I to III collagen in cases of idiopathic pulmonary fibrosis.[118] In the latter study, collagen accounted for 25% of the dry weight of lung parenchyma. The discrepancy in these two studies may have resulted from the larger tissue sample used in the latter study. Raghu and colleagues[119] studied lung tissue from patients with pulmonary fibrosis with fluorescein-labeled polyclonal antibodies against human collagens types I, III, IV, and laminin. They found that type III collagen was initially dominent in fibrotic alveolar septa and was replaced by type I collagen as the disease progressed.

A theoretic immunopathogenic mechanism for the development of pulmonary fibrosis, which is proposed by the author, is shown in Fig. 20–2.

The exact mechanism by which fibrosis forms in the peripheral lung tissue is poorly understood. In 1985, Corrin and colleagues[120] studied lung tissue ultrastructurally from 17 patients with cryptogenic fibrosing alveolitis and 8 patients with asbestosis, and found evidence of endothelial cell injury characterized by swelling and reduplicated basal lamina and necrosis of alveolar type I cells with loss of these cells and exposure of the underlying basal lamina. They postulated that the loss of epithelial cells was important in the development of fibrosis, perhaps by loss of epithelial inhibitors of connective tissue proliferation. It is interesting that the ultrastructural changes were the same in the cryptogenic cases of fibrosis and asbestosis.

Basset and co-workers in 1986[121] published a histologic-ultrastructural study regarding the mechanism of fibrosis occurring in a variety of interstitial lung diseases, including those observed in 92 patients with idiopathic pulmonary fibrosis. They showed intraluminal organization of exudate with fibrosis to be a common finding in several different diseases. Fibroblasts and myofibroblasts migrated through defects in the alveolar wall, leading to "intraluminal buds" that could progress to obliteration of the alveolus and fusion of adjacent alveolar structures. Basset et al. found intraluminal buds in 13 of 92 patients and mural incorporation in 69 of 92 patients with idiopathic pulmonary fibrosis. The mechanism of fibrosis in idiopathic pulmonary fibrosis may in part result from coalescence of collapsed alveolar septa and incorporation of organizing intraalveolar exudate into the interstitium.[5]

Kuhn and colleagues[122–124] have also studied the morphogenesis of idiopathic pulmonary fibrosis and have suggested that fibrosis in chronic idiopathic pulmonary fibrosis results mainly from organization of exudate within air spaces, just as it does in acute lung injury. The morphogenesis and pathogenesis have been recently reviewed, with a discussion of uncertain areas, by MacDonald.[125] His schematic concept of this change is shown in Fig. 20–3. Hyde et al.[126] and Ward[127] have reviewed the literature stating that alveolar septal epithelial and endothelial cell injury are critical factors in the development of pulmonary fibrosis. Kuhn has described the formation of fibroblastic foci in usual interstitial pneumonitis (idiopathic pulmonary fibrosis), which are similar to Masson bodies in bronchiolitis obliterans–organizing pneumonitis. They are composed of parallel-arranged, fibroblastic-appearing cells (Fig. 20–4) that have immunohistochemical and ultrastructural features of myofibroblasts. They are usually enmeshed in a matrix of fibronectin-containing fibrils that linked cells and collagen bundles. These cells are contractile and are thought to play a role in the remodeling of the lung. That this mechanism of fibrosis

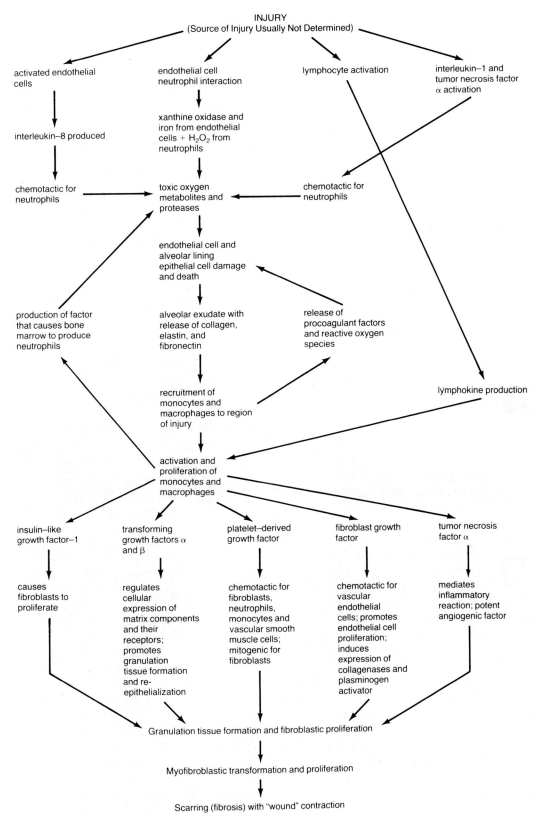

Fig. 20–2. Diagram of possible relationships between immunopathogenic factors thought to be important in development of pulmonary fibrosis.

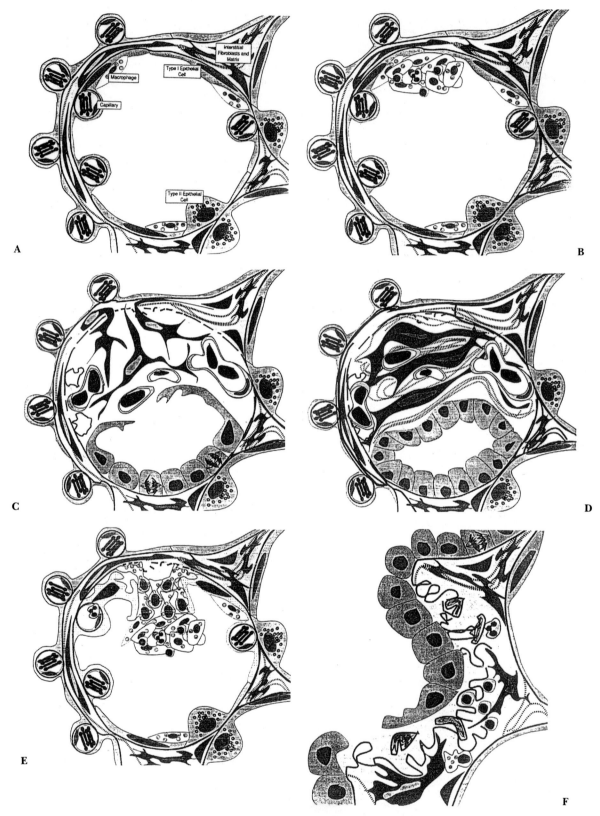

Fig. 20–3 A–F. A. Normal alveolus and its structures. **B.** Formation of an intraalveolar inflammatory exudate, the earliest histologically detectable lesion in idiopathic pulmonary fibrosis. **C.** Alveolar ulceration after formation of an exudate. **D.** Alveolar organization phase in idiopathic pulmonary fibrosis. **E.** Fibrosis, the end stage of unresolved alveolar injury. **F.** Alveolar collapse, a component in the pathogenesis of restrictive lung disease. From McDonald JA. Idiopathic pulmonary fibrosis: A paradigm for lung injury and repair. Chest 1991;99(suppl):87S–93S.

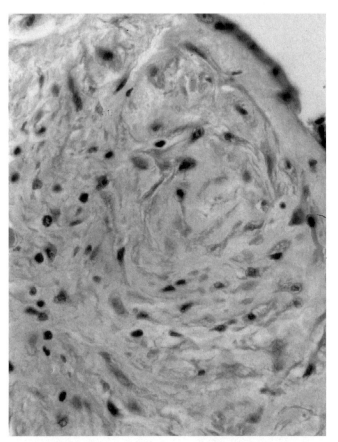

Fig. 20–4. Focal area of proliferation of fibroblastic-appearing cells underlying an epithelial lining of a distorted alveolus. These cells show expression of actin, and by electron microscopy have features of myofibroblasts. They are thought to represent areas of organization of exudate. ×550.

occurs in idiopathic fibrosis seems somewhat paradoxical because it is the same mechanism of organization that takes place in acute interstitial pneumonitis.

Clinical Features

Idiopathic pulmonary fibrosis usually occurs in middle-aged men and women. The insidious onset of dyspnea, the most common symptom, is usually progressive to a point at which patients may become unable to perform the activities of daily living. Clubbing of the digits and inspiratory rales are common signs. Extrapulmonary symptoms such as fatigue, weight loss, and arthralgias occur in 25%–40% of patients, especially in those whose pulmonary fibrosis is associated with a collagen vascular syndrome.

Abnormalities appearing in laboratory tests may include a low-titer positive antinuclear antibody, abnormal liver function tests, and an elevated erythrocyte sedimentation rate. When associated with a collagen

vascular disease, laboratory test abnormalities are more frequent and depend on which specific syndrome is involved, such as systemic lupus erythematosus, dermatomyositis, or mixed connective tissue disease.

Pulmonary function tests typically show a restrictive defect that is characterized by a decrease in total lung capacity, forced vital capacity, residual volume, diffusion capacity of carbon monoxide, and arterial oxygen concentration. The reduction in diffusion capacity and decreased arterial oxygen saturation is thought to be caused by a decrease in pulmonary capillary volume and by ventilation-perfusion abnormalities. With exercise, the arterial oxygen saturation decreases sharply.

Chest radiographs usually show diffuse bilateral infiltrates that appear most severe at the bases of the lungs with sparing of the apices, and are often referred to as interstitial, alveolar, or reticulonodular. There is always some variability in radiographs from patient to patient (Fig. 20–5), and we have shown that the apparent increased involvement in the lower lobes results from only the greater lung volume in the lower lobes and not from more severe disease in this region.[128] Conventional and high-resolution CT scans of the lungs can[129–131] more clearly show the abnormalities that are seen macroscopically by the pathologist (Figs. 20–6 and 20–7).

Pathologic Features

The gross pathologic changes of the lungs from patients with idiopathic pulmonary fibrosis vary, depending on which stage of the disease the lung is biopsied. In the early stages there may be few discernible macroscopic changes. The lungs from a person dying from pulmonary fibrosis show reproducible abnormalities. The lungs are two to three times their usual weight and are stiff. The pleural surface is diffusely nodular, much like the surface of a cirrhotic liver (Fig. 20–8). When sectioned, the most peripheral 2–3 cm of lung tissue is strikingly abnormal, with the more proximal or central parenchyma appearing normal or only mildly abnormal (Fig. 20–9). The peripheral parenchyma shows obliteration of the delicate alveolar lung architecture, with replacement by dense grayish-white to yellow-tan fibrous tissue. The nodular pleural surface is due to irregular scarring of the underlying parenchyma. The irregular scarring with obstruction of bronchi and bronchioles and destruction of parenchyma leads to cystically dilated spaces in the scarred parenchyma, referred to as honeycombing.

As shown in Figs. 20–8 and 20–9, the changes are just as severe in the upper as in the lower lobes, but the greater volume of lung tissue in the lower lobes accounts for the apparent localization of the disease to the

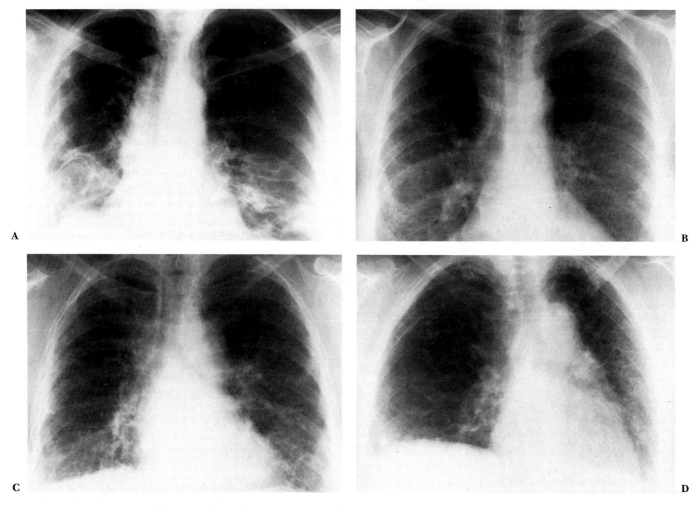

Fig. 20–5 A–D. Chest radiographs from four patients with idiopathic pulmonary fibrosis. Note variability and that infiltrate appears most prominent in lower lobes.

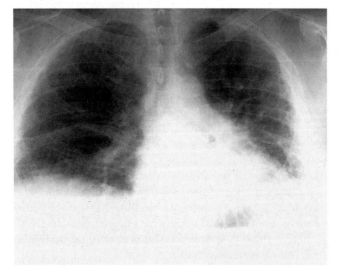

Fig. 20–6. Radiograph of idiopathic pulmonary fibrosis shows markedly reduced lung volumes and coarse fibrosis concentrated peripherally and at lung bases. (Courtesy of Dr. D. Godwin, Dept. of Radiology, University Hospital, Seattle, Washington.)

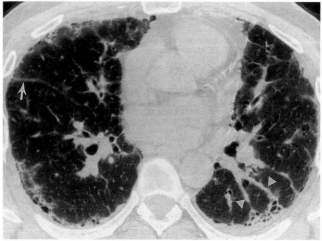

Fig. 20–7. High-resolution CT scan of idiopathic pulmonary fibrosis shows patchy, peripheral, subpleural honeycombing. Note thickening of major fissure (*arrow*), and thickening and nodularity of vessel interfaces in left lung base (*arrowheads*). (Courtesy of Dr. D. Godwin, Dept. of Radiology, University Hospital, Seattle, Washington.)

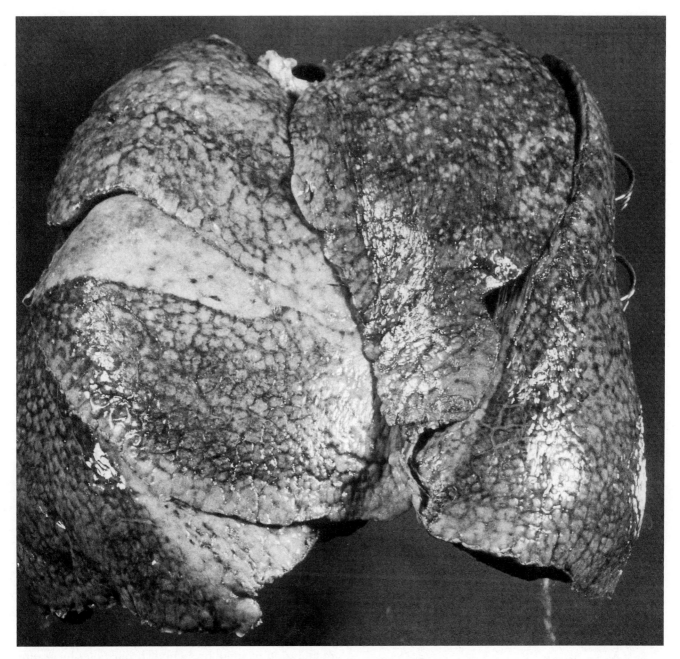

Fig. 20–8. Right and left lung from person dying of idiopathic interstitial pulmonary fibrosis. Note nodular pleural surface, which is similar to surface of cirrhotic liver.

lower lobes in chest radiographs. That the disease is most severe in the peripheral parenchyma means that any open lung biopsy is, to some degree, nonrepresentative. In a diffuse disease such as pulmonary fibrosis, our surgeons are specifically requested to not biopsy the region that shows the greatest gross abnormality. Although Newman et al.[132] found that the lingula may show mild fibrosis and other abnormalities in patients without diffuse lung disease, in our experience this alteration is usually mild. In this author's experience,

the lingula is as abnormal as other peripheral lung tissue in patients with idiopathic pulmonary fibrosis, an observation supported by the report of Wetstein showing that lingular biopsies are representative in several types of lung disease including idiopathic interstitial fibrosis.[133]

The most conspicuous histologic feature of idiopathic pulmonary fibrosis is its variability. In every open lung biopsy or autopsy lung section, there is a wide spectrum of changes. The pleura is frequently thickened, and

658 S.P. HAMMAR

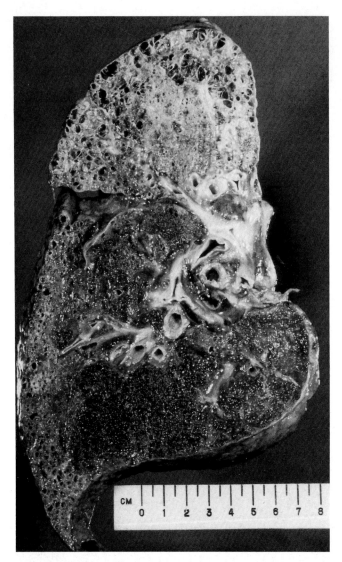

Fig. 20–9. Cut surface of right lung shown in Fig. 20–8. Note fibrosis and honeycombing in peripheral 2–3 cm and that more central parenchyma, especially in lower lobe, is relatively normal. Scale in centimeters.

shows an increase in vascularity with hypertrophy and hyperplasia of mesothelial lining cells (Fig. 20–10). The peripheral lung tissue shows a haphazard pattern of fibrosis, inflammation, occasional smooth muscle proliferation, elastic tissue fragmentation and/or synthesis, alveolar and bronchiolar lining cell hypertrophy, and hyperplasia and honeycoming (Figs. 20–11 through 20–16).

In this author's opinion, the suggestion that the disease necessarily progresses from an "active cellular phase" to an end stage relatively "acellular fibrotic phase" is not borne out by the histologic changes. In our study of open lung biopsies from 37 lobes in 20 patients, we found significant variation in histologic changes.

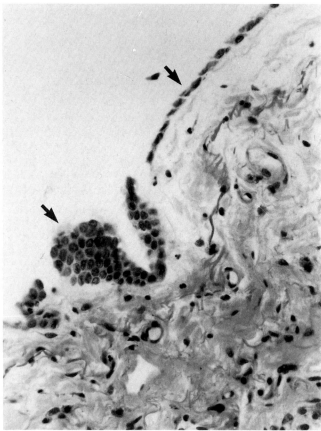

Fig. 20–10. Visceral pleura is slightly thickened. Note reactive hypertrophy and hyperplasia of surface mesothelial cells (*arrows*). ×330.

Individual regions of the same biopsy frequently show more than one of the patterns of interstitial pneumonitis as described by Liebow and Carrington[11] (Fig. 20–17). In each open biopsy we give a semiquantitative estimation of the average severity of fibrosis on an arbitrary 0 to 4+ scale (Fig. 20–18). Intimal fibrosis and medial hypertrophy of small pulmonary arteries are seen in most cases (Fig. 20–19). Likewise, occasional obliteration of small bronchi or bronchioles by granulation or fibrous tissue, bronchiolitis obliterans (Fig. 20–20), is a common finding. This author prefers the Movat pentachrome stain to delineate the histologic changes; with this stain, elastic tissue stains black, young

Fig. 20–11 and Fig. 20–12. Representative sections of open lung biopsy shows distortion of usual pulmonary architecture and variability of the abnormality. Fig. 20–11, ×4; Fig. 20–12, ×8.

Fig. 20–13 and Fig. 20–14. At slightly greater magnifications, disorganization of peripheral lung tissue is evident. Moderate interstitial fibrosis is associated with chronic inflammatory cell infiltrate. ×75.

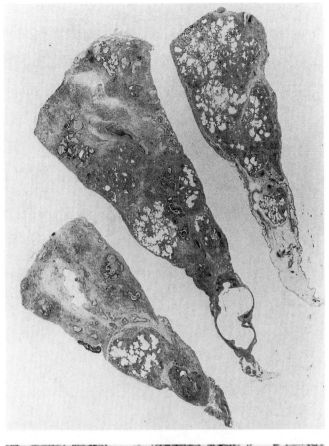

20-11

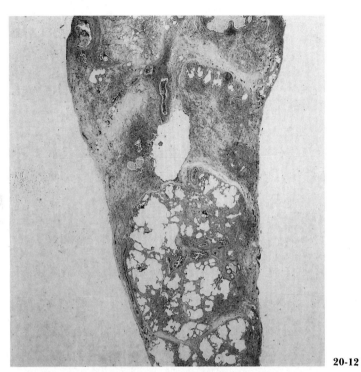

20-12

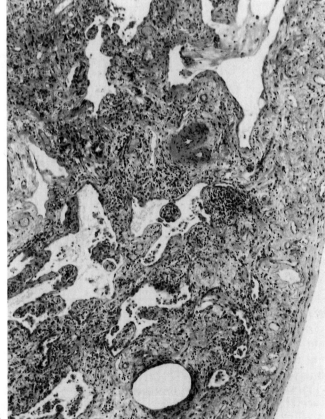

20-13

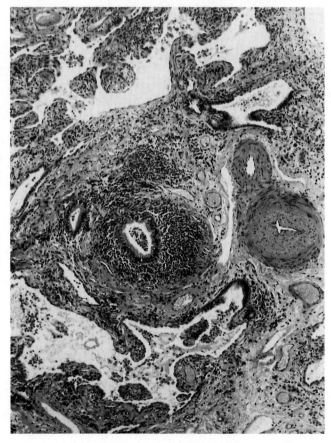

20-14

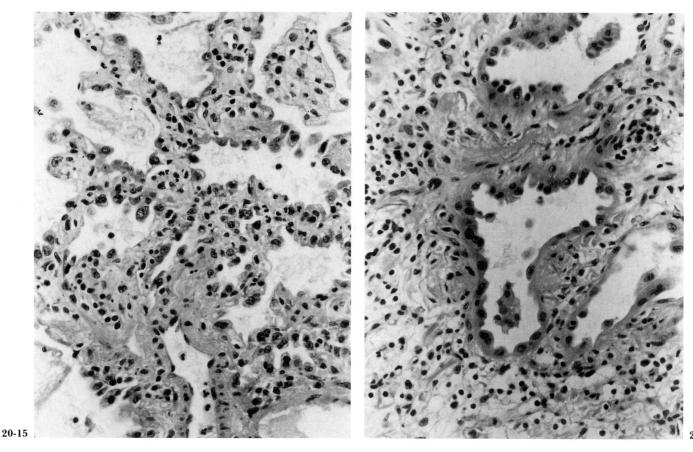

Fig. 20–15 and 20–16. Interstitial fibrosis and chronic inflammation are obvious at this magnification. Note alveolar lining cell hypertrophy and hyperplasia. ×330.

connective tissue green, collagen yellow, and smooth muscle red. The most dramatic histologic feature using this stain is the marked fragmentation and/or increase in elastic tissue (Fig. 20–21). In some cases, smooth muscle proliferation is a prominent feature (Fig. 20–22).

Immunohistochemistry and electron microscopy are effective tools in further characterizing the pathologic changes in idiopathic fibrosis. Using monoclonal antibodies directed against low or high molecular weight cytokeratin, epithelial membrane antigen, or human milk fat globule protein, the hypertrophied and hyperplastic alveolar and bronchiolar lining cells are accentuated (Fig. 20–23). Ultrastructurally, the marked disorganization of the lung tissue is better seen (Figs. 20–24 and 20–25). Atypia of alveolar lining cells is prominent (Fig. 20–26), with most of these atypical cells representing alveolar type II cells (Fig. 20–27). As they become reactive, the number of lamellar bodies usually decreases. Some will show intranuclear tubular inclusions, which can also be seen by light microscopy (Figs. 20–28 and 20–29). Occasionally these cells will engulf other

cells such as erythrocytes and polymorphonuclear leukocytes, and some will show accumulation of "alcoholic hyaline," which represents aggregates of intermediate cytokeratin filaments (Fig. 20–30). A neoplastic proliferation of these reactive cells probably accounts for the increased incidence of peripheral lung adenocarcinoma in patients with idiopathic fibrosis.[134–137]

Immunohistochemical identification of the intermediate filaments vimentin and desmin, panleukocyte antigen, and muscle-specific actin is helpful in identifying alveolar macrophages, interstitial mesenchymal cells, inflammatory cells, and smooth muscle cells. Demonstration of these cells via immunohistochemistry is usually not necessary for diagnosis but is useful in identifying various cell types (Figs. 20–31 and 20–32). An experimental study of bleomycin-induced pulmonary fibrosis in rats showed that the interstitial cells exhibited immunostaining for vimentin and not desmin, suggesting that these cells are of fibroblast and not smooth muscle origin.[138]

Other cells that can be identified in the interstitium of

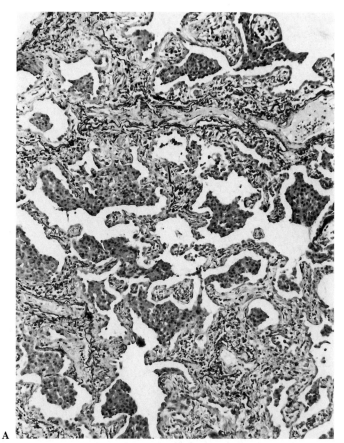
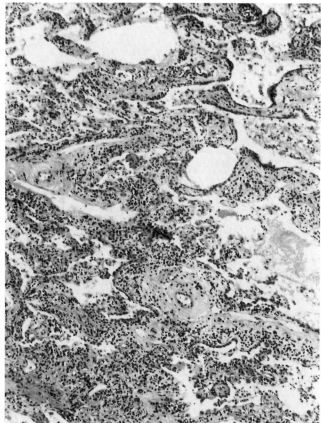

Fig. 20–17 A,B. Open lung biopsy shows significant variability in histologic appearance. **A.** Note "desquamative" pattern with accumulation of intraalveolar macrophages. **B.** Note more lymphocytic interstitial pneumonitis pattern characterized by intense interstitial infiltrate of lymphocytes and plasma cells. ×75.

fibrotic lungs ultrastructurally or immunohistochemically but are not observed in hemotoxylin and eosin-stained light microscopic sections are mast cells (Fig. 20–33) and Langerhans' cells. Mast cell hyperplasia has recently been noted in cases of bleomycin-induced pulmonary fibrosis, although its exact role in the development of fibrosis is uncertain.[139] Langerhans' cells are unique dendritic histiocytes of bone marrow origin that occur normally in the skin and other organs[140] and are present in most cases of idiopathic pulmonary fibrosis.[141–144] They can be identified ultrastructurally because of their pathognomonic cytoplasmic Langerhans' cell granules or immunohistochemically by the presence of S-100 protein (Figs. 20–34 and 20–35). Unlike pulmonary histiocytosis X in which Langerhans' cells (histiocytosis X cells) usually occur in nodular aggregates,[145–147] (see Chapter 17) these cells are typically associated with reactive alveolar lining cells or are in association with interstitial lymphocytes. Langerhans' cells function by presenting antigens to T lymphocytes, and in the skin are important in sensitization to and perhaps eradication of contact antigens. Their exact function in idiopathic pulmonary fibrosis is unknown but presumably is immunologic.

As previously stated, as many as 20% of cases of pulmonary fibrosis may be associated with a collagen vascular disease. We have recently found that those cases associated with a collagen vascular syndrome or with a viral infection showed marked alveolar septal capillary endothelial cell swelling with intracellular tubuloreticular structures and cylindrical confronting cisternae (Figs. 20–36 and 20–37).[148,149] As reviewed, these changes are caused by inferferon,[148–149] and we have postulated that the primary mechanism of injury in collagen vascular disease and viral-associated pulmonary fibrosis is endothelial cell damage.[144]

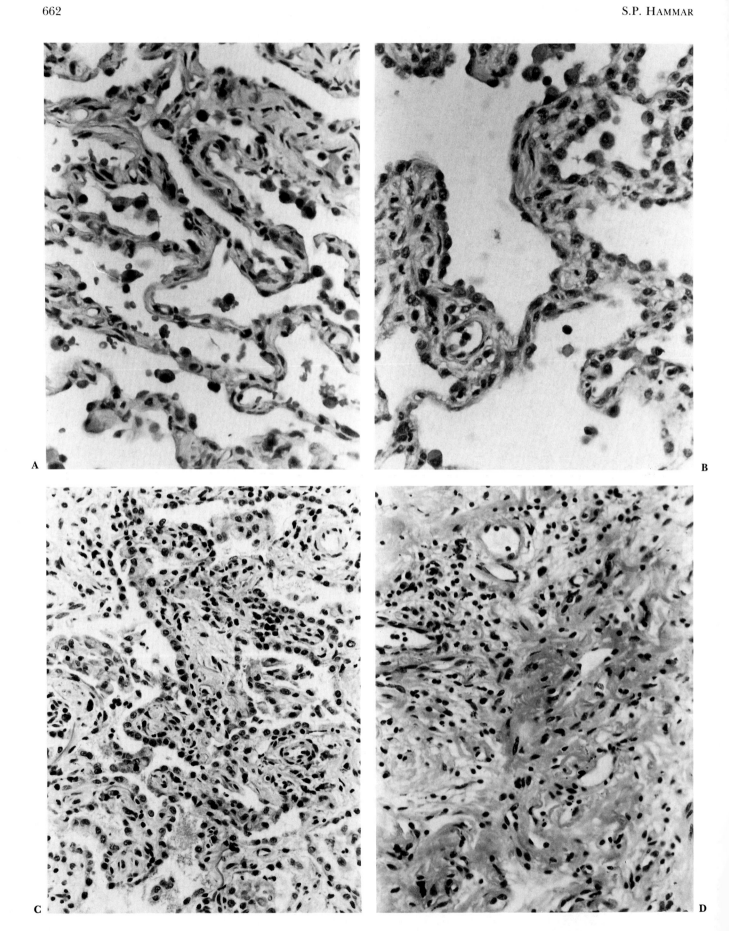

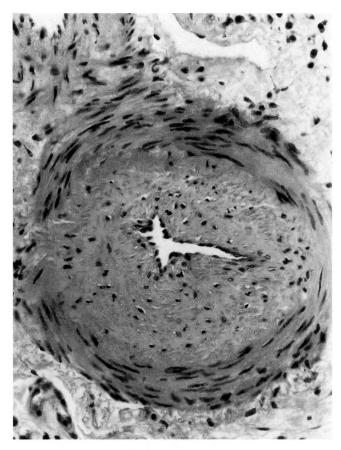

Fig. 20–19. In most cases of pulmonary fibrosis, small pulmonary arteries and veins show some degree of muscular hypertrophy and intimal fibrosis. ×550.

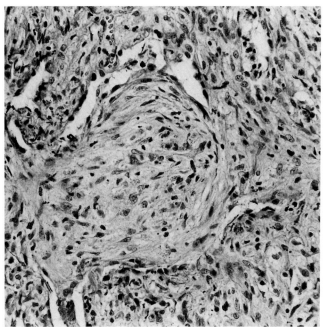

Fig. 20–20. Focal bronchiolitis obliterans characterized by granulation tissue or fibrous tissue in lumen of bronchiole, is a common finding in cases of idiopathic pulmonary fibrosis. ×330.

Fig. 20–21. Peripheral lung tissue stained for elastic tissue (*black*) shows apparent increase and/or fragmentation of the elastic fibers, which could be secondary to collapse of parenchyma. ×330.

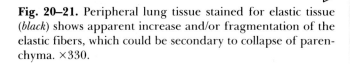

Fig. 20–18 A–D. In each open biopsy showing histologic changes of interstitial pulmonary fibrosis, we assess average degree of fibrosis on an arbitrary scale of 0 to 4+; 0, normal tissue with no interstitial fibrosis; 1+, interstitial fibrosis (**A**) is characterized by slight widening of alveolar septa with relatively normal alveoli; 2+, interstitial fibrosis (**B**) is characterized by slight-to-moderate fibrous thickening of alveolar septa; 3+, fibrosis (**C**) shows moderate to marked septal thickening with a moderate distortion of the usual architecture including obliteration of alveoli; 4+, fibrosis (**D**) is characterized by complete obliteration of alveoli by dense fibrous tissue. In each grade of fibrosis there usually is some degree of chronic inflammation and alveolar lining cell hypertrophy and hyperplasia. ×330.

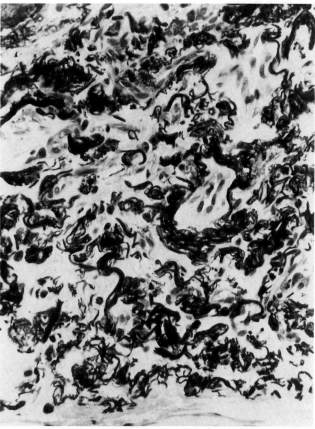

20-21

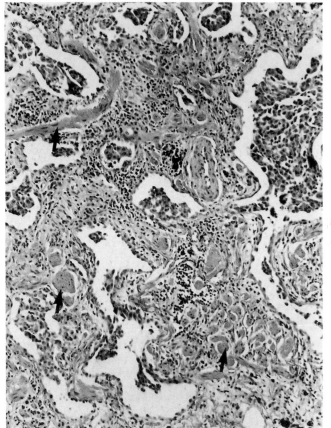

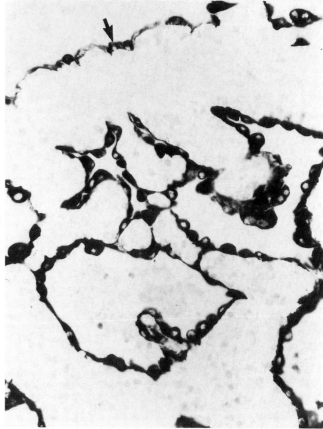

20-22

20-2

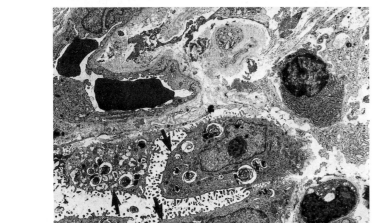

20-24

Fig. 20–22. Regions of smooth muscle proliferation (*arrows*) not obviously associated with vessels or bronchi are seen in some cases of pulmonary fibrosis. ×75.

Fig. 20–23. Peripheral fibrotic lung tissue immunostained for low molecular weight cytokeratin vividly shows hypertrophied and hyperplastic alveolar lining cells and accentuates thickened interstitium. Pleural mesothelial cells (*arrow*) are also seen. ×550.

Fig. 20–24. Low-power electron micrograph shows marked disorganization of peripheral lung tissue characteristic of idiopathic pulmonary fibrosis. In this region is seen a mixed interstitial inflammatory cell infiltrate with hypertrophy and hyperplasia of alveolar lining cells, most of which are alveolar type II cells (*arrows*). Interstitial collagen (COL) and elastic tissue (ET) are increased in interstitium. ×6,500.

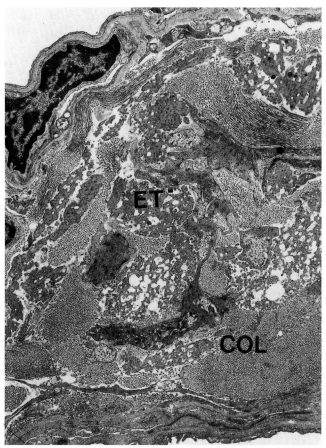

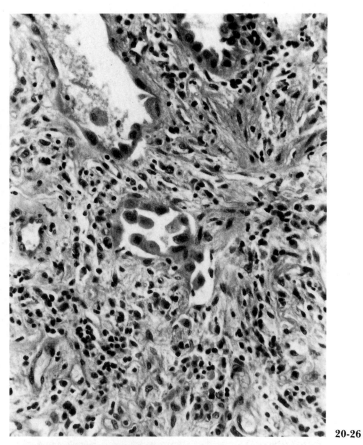

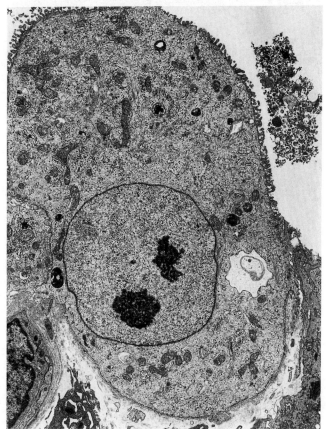

Fig. 20–25. Lung tissue shows dense interstitial collagen (COL) and elastic tissue (ET) formation with little inflammation and no alveolar lining cell changes. ×6,500.

Fig. 20–26. Atypical alveolar lining cells, obvious in this peripheral lung tissue, can result in a false-positive sputum cytology. ×330.

Fig. 20–27. Reactive alveolar lining cell with large nucleus and prominent nucleoli probably represents a type II pneumocyte although it lacks well-formed lamellar bodies in its cytoplasm. ×10,500.

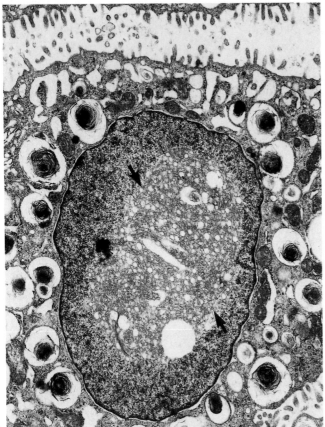

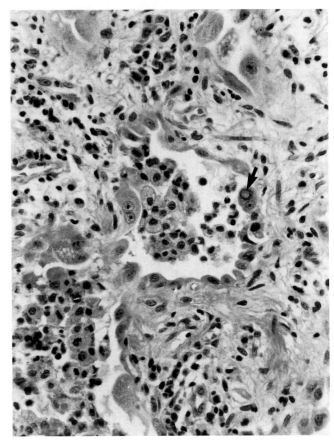

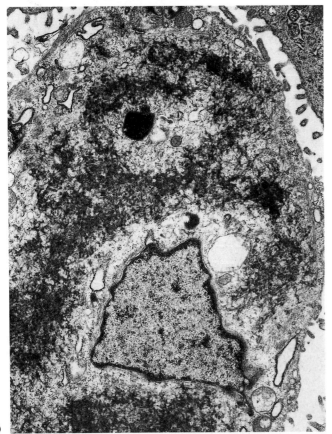

Fig. 20–28. Reactive alveolar type II cell contains intranuclear tubular inclusion (*arrows*). Thought to be derived from the inner nuclear membrane, these are frequently seen in bronchiolo-alveolar cell carcinomas but are not specific for malignancy. ×10,500.

Fig. 20–29. Intranuclear inclusion seen in Fig. 20–28 can be recognized by light microscopy as a ground glass-like inclusion (*arrow*) that may stain with periodic acid–Schiff reagent. ×330.

Fig. 20–30. Reactive alveolar lining cell contains aggregates of electron-dense intermediate filaments that represent cytokeratin. In H and E-stained sections, these have the appearance of "alcoholic hyaline" as seen in liver cells. ×16,500.

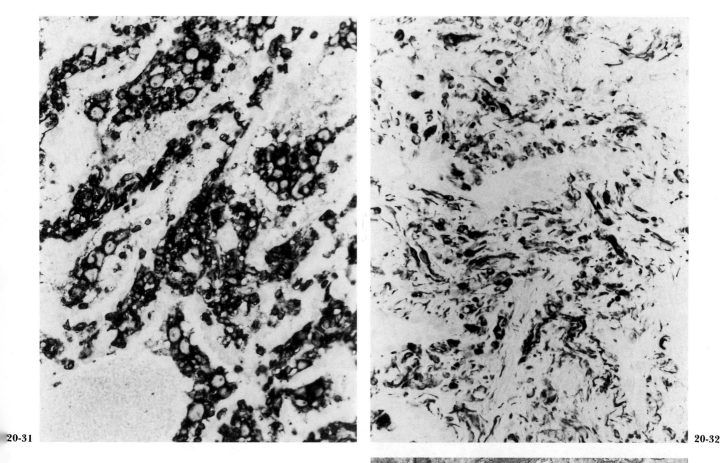

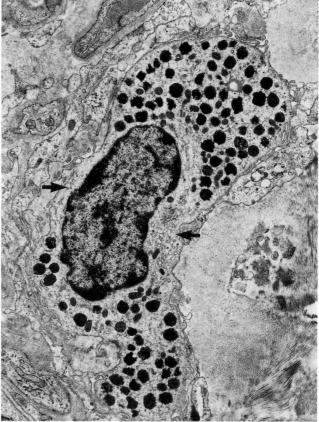

Fig. 20–31. Lung tissue immunostained for pan leukocyte antigen shows numerous, predominantly interstitial, "positive" (*black*) staining cells, mostly lymphocytes and macrophages. ×330.

Fig. 20–32. Lung tissue immunostained for the intermediate filament vimentin shows numerous "positive" (*black*) cells, a combination of fibroblasts, endothelial cells, and inflammatory cells. ×330.

Fig. 20–33. Mast cell (*arrows*) seen by electron microscopy is frequent in most cases of pulmonary fibrosis but is usually not visible in H and E stained sections. ×6,500.

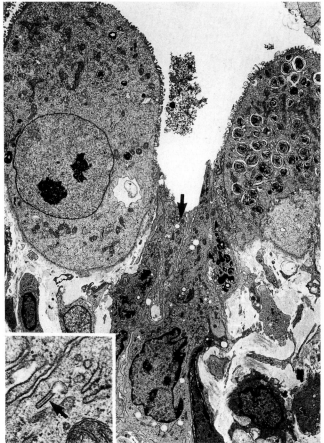

20-34

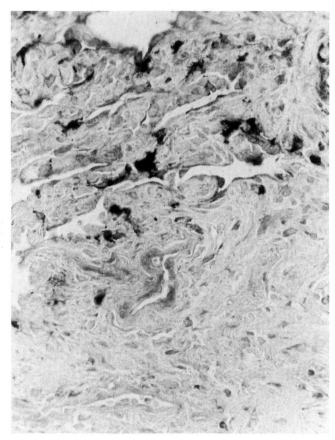

20-35

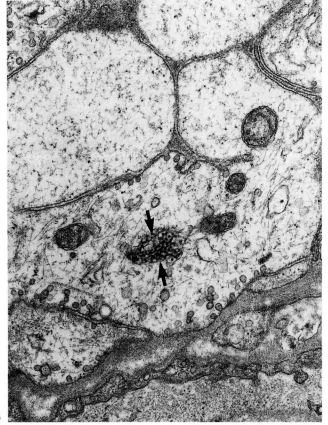

20-36

Fig. 20–34. Langerhans' cell (*arrow*) wedges between reactive alveolar type II cells in this example of pulmonary fibrosis. ×6,500. Inset: Typical Langerhans' cell granule (*arrow*) present in cytoplasm of Langerhans' cell at higher magnification. ×26,500.

Fig. 20–35. Fibrotic lung tissue immunostained for S-100 protein shows several "positive" (*black*) cells with dendritic processes that represent Langerhans' cells as shown in Fig. 20–34. ×330.

Fig. 20–36. Tubuloreticular structure (*arrows*) in cytoplasm of swollen endothelial cell from patient with interstitial fibrosis associated with mixed connective tissue disease. ×16,500.

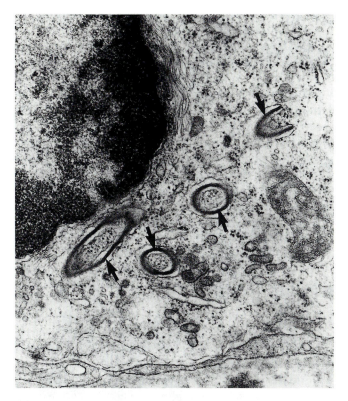

Fig. 20–37. Cylindrical confronting cisternae (*arrows*), also known as test tube and ring-shaped structures, are present in cytoplasm of endothelial cell from patient with interstitial pulmonary fibrosis associated with systemic lupus erythematosus. Cylindrical confronting cisternae and tubuloreticular structures are formed in response to elevated levels of interferon in these conditions. × 16,500.

Differential Diagnosis

In most instances, the diagnosis of idiopathic pulmonary fibrosis is straightforward. The clinical history of insidious dyspnea of unknown cause, a diffuse bilateral interstitial infiltrate on chest radiograph, and the typical pathologic changes described in this chapter all add up to the diagnosis.

The problem for clinician and pathologist is to exclude other known causes of fibrosis. Chronic hypersensitivity pneumonitis can progress to chronic fibrosis indistinguishable from idiopathic fibrosis; a careful clinical history is most important. The end stages of pulmonary histiocytosis X can macroscopically and microscopically be identical to idiopathic fibrosis. In pulmonary histiocytosis X, the disease usually occurs in a younger age group and is frequently biopsied in the acute stage of the disease. In the end stages it may be difficult, if not impossible, to identify aggregates of histiocytosis X cells. Viral pneumonia can progress rapidly or insidiously to pulmonary fibrosis. Again, the

history is critical and serologic or viral culture studies may help elucidate this etiology. Also, ultrastructural examination will characteristically show endothelial cell swelling and intracytoplasmic tubuloreticular structures. Another potential cause, or association, of pulmonary fibrosis is the acquired immune deficiency syndrome (AIDS). A case of pulmonary fibrosis without superimposed opportunistic infection has been reported,[150] as has lymphocytic interstitial pneumonitis.[151,152] The same ultrastructural features seen in collagen vascular disease and viral-associated fibrosis, namely endothelial cell swelling, tubuloreticular structures and cylindrical confronting cisternae, may also be seen in the lung tissue from patients with AIDS. In AIDS, this is also probably caused by interferon, which is elevated in the serum of patients with this syndrome.[153]

In chronic, postobstructive pneumonitis, histologic changes identical to those seen in idiopathic pulmonary fibrosis may be present. There may also be, however, a significant number of foamy macrophages. Such a change is usually unilateral and the cause of the obstruction, such as a neoplasm, is usually obvious. Bronchiolitis obliterans organizing pneumonia, an entity that may have several etiologies or be idiopathic, may be confused with idiopathic fibrosis.[154,155] Unlike patients with pulmonary fibrosis, there is complete recovery in 65% of subjects. Histologically there is more intraalveolar and intrabronchiolar organizing fibrous tissue than is seen in cases of idiopathic fibrosis.

A description of the patterns of pulmonary fibrosis seen in various disease conditions was published in 1986 and is helpful to the pathologist because it contrasts the patterns of fibrosis seen in many diseases and tells which patterns are specific and which are not.[156]

In acute alveolar damage or acute interstitial pneumonitis, the problem is usually ruling out known causes of these conditions rather than considering a different diagnosis.

Approach to the Diagnosis

The handling of an open lung biopsy specimen is critical to making an accurate diagnosis (see Chapter 1). At our institution open lung biopsy specimens are received in sterile containers from the operating rooms. With today's surgical techniques, the cut edge or edges of the specimen are usually closed with metal staples. Often, there is enough tissue in association with the staples that can be used for routine bacteriologic and viral cultures. Most biopsy specimens that show the changes of interstitial fibrosis will be sufficiently stiff so that no inflation-type procedure will be necessary to maintain the overall architecture.

symptoms at the onset of the disease. In our study[128] of 20 patients with diffuse interstitial pneumonitis treated with prednisone and/or azathioprine, we found that the degree of interstitial fibrosis was the single most important factor in separating those who responded to therapy versus those who did not. In the study of Carrington et al.[71] of the natural history and treated course of 40 patients with "desquamative interstitial pneumonitis" and 53 patients with "usual interstitial pneumonitis," approximately 22% with desquamative interstitial pneumonitis and none with usual interstitial pneumonitis showed spontaneous improvement without therapy. With prednisone therapy, 61.5% of desquamative interstitial pneumonitis patients and 11.5% with usual interstitial pneumonitis improved clinically. The mean survival in patients with desquamative interstitial pneumonitis was 12.2 years, and in usual interstitial pneumonitis patients it was 5.6 years. Their findings are similar to ours in that the patients with desquamative interstitial pneumonitis, according to their definition, lacked significant interstitial fibrosis.

In the study by Gelb and colleagues,[168] only 2 of 16 patients with "cellular disease" and none of 4 with a "pure fibrotic reaction" showed a response to corticosteroids. In the study by Rudd and co-workers[173] of 120 patients with cryptogenic fibrosing alveolitis, of whom 91 were treated, lymphocyte counts were significantly higher in bronchoalveolar lavage fluid in responders versus nonresponders, while neutrophils and eosinophils were highest in those who did not respond to therapy. Haslam et al.[174] found a similar negative therapeutic correlation with the number of neutrophils and eosinophils in lavage fluid. If our hypothesis is correct that polys are seen in distorted bronchi possibly obstructed secondary to fibrosis, this may also be a manifestation of the degree of fibrosis.

Winterbauer[175] has provided an excellent current review of the treatment of idiopathic fibrosis. The response to treatment of idiopathic pulmonary fibrosis is inconsistent. As pointed out by Winterbauer, patients with disease of less than 1 year duration; those whose bronchoalveolar lavage fluid shows greater than 5% lymphocytes, less than 10% neutrophils, and 5% eosinophils; and those whose open biopsy specimen demonstrates more inflammation and less fibrosis have the greatest potential for improvement with therapy. A separate study conducted by Winterbauer suggested that azathioprine was useful in treating idiopathic pulmonary fibrosis and statistically prolonged survival time without increasing side effects. Cyclosphamide was also found to be effective, especially in the group of patients with collagen vascular disease-associated pulmonary fibrosis.

Several studies have addressed the clinical significance of serum immune complexes in patients with idiopathic fibrosis. In 1978, Dreisin and colleagues[101] found a correlation between the degree of inflammation in lung tissue and the the presence of circulating immune complexes. Those with elevated levels of circulating immune complexes and significant pulmonary inflammation showed a better response to corticosteroid therapy than those who lacked these features. In 1979, Haslam et al.[174] found no correlation between histologic changes in lung tissue and the presence or absence of immune complexes. Gelb et al.[168] also studied the association between serum immune complexes, histologic changes in lung tissue, and response to corticosteroid therapy in 20 patients with pulmonary fibrosis. They found elevated levels of immune complexes in 12 of 14 patients whose lung tissue showed significant inflammation. In all 12 patients, the elevated titers of immune complexes returned to normal within 2 months after beginning steroid therapy regardless of response to therapy. Only 2 of 16 patients whose lung biopsy showed significant inflammation and none of those with "pure fibrosis" improved with therapy. The authors concluded that immune complexes were associated with increased inflammation in the biopsy specimens but did not predict response to therapy.

More recently, Martinet et al.[176] performed a study to determine the clinical significance of circulating immune complexes in 16 patients with cryptogenic fibrosing alveolitis and 24 patients with collagen vascular-associated interstitial lung disease. Clq binding, a measure of immune complexes in serum, was elevated in 62.5% of patients with collagen vascular disease and 31.3% of patients with idiopathic pulmonary fibrosis. Those patients with serum immune complexes tended to be younger and have a shorter duration of symptoms and less evidence of radiographic disease, but had similar mean values for total lung capacity, forced vital capacity, and forced expiratory volume than those without immune complexes in their serum. There was no correlation between responsiveness to corticosteroid therapy or length of survival with the presence of serum immune complexes.

We have found that patients with interstitial fibrosis associated with collagen vascular syndromes, whose lung tissue and peripheral blood lymphocytes contain tubuloreticular structures, will frequently not respond to prednisone therapy but may show dramatic improvement with cyclophosphamide therapy.[177] When these patients clinically improve, the tubuloreticular structures seen in their lymphocytes disappear. The role of cyclophosphamide in treating idiopathic pulmonary fibrosis is still being evaluated.

In summary, idiopathic pulmonary fibrosis is a chronic progressive pulmonary syndrome usually occurring in middle-aged men and women. It is known by a variety of names, such as usual interstitial pneumonitis or fibrosing alveolitis, and may be associated with a collagen vascular disease or be a consequence of viral pneumonitis. Histologically, the lung shows a highly variable pattern of change including fibrosis, inflammation, alveolar lining cell hypertrophy, and thickening of small pulmonary vessels. The disease is usually progressive, leading to respiratory insufficiency and death, although patients whose disease is associated with a collagen vascular disease may show a dramatic therapeutic response to cyclophosphamide.

References

1. Fulmer JD, Crystal RG. Interstitial lung disease. Curr Pulmonol 1797;1:1–65.
2. Keogh BA, Crystal RG. Chronic interstitial lung disease. Curr Pulmonol 1981;3:237–340.
3. Crystal RG, Gadek JE, Ferrans VJ, Fulmer JD, Line BR, Hunninghake GW. Interstitial lung disease: Current concepts of pathogenesis, staging and therapy. Am J Med 1981;70:542–568.
4. Crystal RG, Bitterman PB, Rennard SI, Hance AJ, Keogh BA. Interstitial lung diseases of unknown cause. Disorders characterized by chronic inflammation of the lower respiratory tract. N Engl J Med 1984;310:154–166, 235–244.
5. Katzenstein AA. Pathogenesis of "fibrosis" in interstitial pneumonia. An electron microscopic study. Hum Pathol 1985;16:1015–1024.
6. Katzenstein AA, Myers JL, Mazur MT. Acute interstitial pneumonia. A clinicopathologic, ultrastructural and cell kinetic study. Am J Surg Pathol 1986;10:256–267.
7. Pratt DS, Schwarz MI, May JJ, Dreisin RB. Rapidly fatal pulmonary fibrosis: The accelerated variant of interstitial pneumonitis. Thorax 1979;34:587–593.
8. Spencer H. Pneumonias due to rickettsiae, chlamydia, viruses and mycoplasma. In: Pathology of the lung. 4th Ed. Oxford: Pergamon, 1985:222–259.
9. Hamman L, Rich AR. Fulminating diffuse interstitial fibrosis of the lungs. Trans Am Clin Climatol Assoc 1935;51:154–163.
10. Hamman L, Rich AR. Acute diffuse interstitial fibrosis of the lungs. Bull Johns Hopkins Hosp 1944;74:177–212.
11. Hasleton PS. Adult respiratory distress syndrome—a review. Histopathology 1983;7:307–332.
12. Olson J, Colby TV, Elliot CG. Hamman–Rich syndrome revisited. Mayo Clin Proc 1990;65:1538–1548.
13. Liebow AA, Carrington CB. The interstitial pneumonias. In: Simon M, Potchen EJ, Lemay M, eds. Frontiers of pulmonary radiology. New York: Grune & Stratton, 1969:102–141.
14. Liebow AA, Steer A, Billingsley JG. Desquamative interstitial pneumonia. Am J Med 1965;39:369–404.
15. Carrington CB, Liebow AA. Lymphocytic interstitial pneumonia. Am J Pathol 1966;48:36a.
16. Scadding JG. Fibrosing alveolitis. Br Med J 1964;2:686.
17. Fishman AP. UIP, DIP and all that. N Engl J Med 1978;298:843–845.
18. Gough J. Fibrosing alveolitis. Br Med J 1964;2:818.
19. Scadding JG, Hinson KFW. Diffuse fibrosing alveolitis (diffuse interstitial fibrosis of the lungs). Correlation of histology at biopsy with prognosis. Thorax 1967;22:291–304.
20. Potter BP, Gerber IE. Acute diffuse interstitial fibrosis of the lungs: report of a case. Arch Intern Med 1948;82:113–124.
21. Stursa M. Interstitial pneumonia with chronic course. Cas Lek Ces 1949;88:464–466.
22. Beams AJ, Harmos O. Diffuse progressive interstitial fibrosis of lungs. Am J Med 1949;7:425–430.
23. Ferrari M, Cavbarrére NL, Botinelli MD, Mendilaharsu C, Giudice D. Neumofibrosis intersticial evolutiva: Una neuva entidad? Hoja Tisiol 1949;9:207–221.
24. Golden A, Tullis IF, Jr. Diffuse interstitial fibrosis of lungs. Mil Surg 1949;105:130–137.
25. Rubin EH, Lubliner R. The Hamman-Rich syndrome: review of the literature and analysis of 15 cases. Medicine (Baltimore) 1957;36:397–463.
26. Kourilsky R, Decroix G, Verley B, Voisin G, Matossy Y. Primary diffuse interstitial pulmonary fibrosis (Hamman-Rich syndrome). J Fr Med Chir Thorac 1959;13:637–674.
27. Livingstone JL, Lewis JG, Reid L, Jefferson KE. Diffuse interstitial pulmonary fibrosis: A clinical, radiological and pathological study based on 45 patients. Q J Med 1964;33:71–103.
28. Scadding JC. Diffuse pulmonary alveolar fibrosis. Thorax 1974;29:271–281.
29. Scadding JC. Chronic diffuse interstitial fibrosis of the lung. Br Med J 1960;1:443–448.
30. Hunninghake GW, Fauci AS. Pulmonary involvement in the collagen vascular diseases. Am Rev Respir Dis 1979;119:471–503.
31. Epler GR, Snider GL, Gaensler EA, Cathcart ES, Fitzgerald MX, Carrington CB. Bronchiolitis and bronchitis in connective tissue disease: A possible relationship to the use of penicillamine. JAMA 1979;242:528–532.
32. Cordier JF, Falconnet M, Moulin J, Brune J, Touraine R. Brochiolite severe et polyarthrite rheumatoide: Role tres probable de la d-penicillamine dans deux observations. Lyons Med 1980;224:113–114.
33. Athreya BH, Doughty RA, Bookspan M, Schumacher HR, Sewell EA, Chatten J. Pulmonary manifestations of juvenile rheumatoid arthritis. Clin Chest Med 1980;1:361–374.
34. Herzog CA, Miller RA, Hoidal JR. Bronchiolitis and rheumatoid arthritis. Am Rev Respir Dis 1981;124:636–639.
35. Salmeron G, Greenberg SD, Lidsky MD. Polymyositis and diffuse interstitial lung disease: A review of the pulmonary histopathologic findings. Arch Intern Med 1981;141:1005–1110.
36. Turton CW, Williams G, Green M. Cryptogenic obliter-

ative bronchiolitis in adults. Thorax 1981;36:805–810.

37. Murphy KC, Atkins CJ, Offer RC, Hogg JC, Stein HB. Obliterative bronchiolitis in two rheumatoid arthritis patients treated with penicillamine. Arthritis Rheum 1981;24:557–560.

38. Wiener-Kronish JP, Solinger AM, Warnock ML, Churg A, Ordonez N, Golden JA. Severe pulmonary involvement in mixed connective tissue disease. Am Rev Respir Dis 1981;124:499–503.

39. Lahdensuo A, Mattila J, Vilppula A. Bronchiolitis in rheumatoid arthritis. Chest 1984;85:705–708.

40. Lyon MG, Bewtra C, Kenik JG, Hurley JA. Tubuloreticular inclusions in systemic lupus pneumonitis: Report of a case and review of the literature. Arch Pathol Lab Med 1984;108:599–600.

41. Kallenberg CGM, Jansen HM, Elema JD. The TH. Steroid-responsive interstitial pulmonary disease in systemic sclerosis. Monitoring by bronchoalveolar lavage. Chest 1984;86:489–492.

42. Constantopoulos SH, Papadimitriou CS, Moutsopoulous HM. Respiratory manifestations in primary Sjogren's syndrome: a clinical, functional and histologic study. Chest 1985;88:226–229.

43. Konig G, Luderschmidt C, Hammer C, Adelmann-Grill BG, Braun-Falco O, Fruhmann G. Lung involvement in scleroderma. Chest 1984;85:318–324.

44. Yousem SA, Colby TV, Carrington CB. Lung biopsy in rheumatoid arthritis. Am Rev Respir Dis 1985;131:770–777.

45. Rossi GA, Bitterman PB, Rennard SI, Ferrans VJ, Crystal RG. Evidence for chronic inflammation as a component of the interstitial lung disease associated with progressive systemic sclerosis. Am Rev Respir Dis 1985;131:612–617.

46. Askin FB. Pulmonary disorders in the collagen vascular diseases. Hum Pathol 1990;21:465–466.

47. Helmers R, Galvin J, Hunninghake GW. Pulmonary manifestations associated with rheumatoid arthritis. Chest 1991;100:235–238.

48. Tazelaar HD, Viggiano RW, Pickersgill J, Colby TV. Interstitial lung disease in polymyositis and dermatomyositis: Clinical features and prognosis is correlated with hisologic findings. Am Rev Respir Dis 1990;141:727–733.

49. Yousem SA. The pulmonary pathologic manifestations of the CRST syndrome. Hum Pathol 1990;21:467–474.

50. Weinrib L, Sharma OP, Quismorio FP, Jr. A long term study of interstitial lung disease in systemic lupus erythematosus. Semin Arthritis Rheum 1990;20:48–56.

51. Cervera R, Ramirez G, Fernandez-Sola J, D'Crox D, et al. Antibodies to endothelial cells in dermatomyositis: Association with interstitial lung disease. Br Med J 1991;302:880–881.

52. Capron JP, Marti R, Rey JL, et al. Fibrosing alveolitis and hepatitis B surface antigen-associated chronic active hepatitis in a patient with immunoglobulin A deficiency. Am J Med 1979;66:874–878.

53. Turner-Warwick M. Fibrosing alveolitis and chronic liver disease. QJ Med 1968;37:133–149.

54. Lynne-Davies P, Sproule BJ. Pulmonary fibrosis and hepatitis. Can Med Assoc J 1967;96:1110–1112.

55. Jonard P, Geubel A, Wallon J, Rahier J, Dive C, Meunier H. Primary sclerosing cholangitis and idiopathic pulmonary fibrosis: A case report. Acta Clin Belg 1989;44:24–30.

56. Hughes EW. Familial interstitial pulmonary fibrosis. Thorax 1964;19:515–525.

57. Bonanni PP, Frymoyer JW, Jacox RF. A family study of idiopathic pulmonary fibrosis. Am J Med 1965;39:411–421.

58. Adelman AG, Chertokow G, Hayton RC. Familial fibrocystic pulmonary dysplasia: A detailed family study. Can Med Assoc J 1966;95:603–610.

59. Swaye P, VanOrdstrand HS, McCormack LJ, Wolpaw SE. Familial Hamman-Rich syndrome: report of eight cases. Dis Chest 1969;55:7–12.

60. Solliday NH, Williams JA, Gaensler EA, Coutu RE, Carrington CB. Familial chronic interstitial pneumonia. Am Rev Respir Dis 1973;108:193–204.

61. Davies BH, Tuddenham EGD. Familial pulmonary fibrosis associated with oculocutaneous albinism and platelet function defect: A new syndrome. Q J Med 1976;45:219–232.

62. Crystal RG, Fulmer JD, Roberts WC, Moss ML. Line BR, Reynolds HV. Idiopathic pulmonary fibrosis: Clinical, histologic, radiologic, physiologic, scintigraphic, cytologic, and biochemical aspects. Ann Intern Med 1976;85:769–788.

63. Evans CC, Evans JM. HL-A in farmer's lung. Lancet 1975;ii:975–976.

64. Turton CWG, Morris LM, Lawler SD, Turner-Warwick M. HLA in cryptogenic fibrosing alveolitis. Lancet 1978;i:507–508.

65. Varpela E, Tiilikaine A, Varpela N, Tukiainen P. High prevalences of HLA-B15 and HLA-DW6 in patients with cryptogenic fibrosing alveolitis. Tissue Antigens 1979;14:68–71.

66. Strimlan CV, Taswell HF, DeRemee RA, Kueppers F. HL-A antigens and fibrosing alveolitis. Am Rev Respir Dis 1977;116:1120–1121.

67. Briggs DC, Vaughan RW, Welsh KI, Myers A, du Bois RM, Black CM. Immunogenetic prediction of pulmonary fibrosis in systemic sclerosis. Lancet 1991;338:661–662.

68. Auerbach O, Stout AP, Hammond EC, Garfinkel L. Smoking habits and age in relation to pulmonary changes: Rupture of alveolar septums, fibrosis and thickening of walls of small arteries and arterioles. N Engl J Med 1963;269:1045–1054.

69. Auerbach O, Garfinkel L. Hammond EC. Relation of smoking and age to findings in the lung parenchyma: A microscopic study. Chest 1974;65:29–35.

70. Weiss W. Cigarette smoke, asbestos and small irregular opacities. Am Rev Respir Dis 1984;130:293–301.

71. Carrington CB, Gaensler EA, Coutu RE, Fitzgerald MX, Gupta RG. Natural history and treated course of usual and desquamative interstitial pneumonia. N Engl J Med 1978;298:802–809.

72. Turner Warwick M, Burrows B, Johnson A. Cryptogenic fibrosing alveolitis: Clinical features and their influence on survival. Thorax 1980;35:171–180.

73. Turner Warwick M, Burrows B, Johnson A. Cryptogenic fibrosing alveolitis and their influence on survival. Thorax 1980;35:593–599.

74. Rudd RM, Haslam PL, Turner Warwick M. Cryptogenic fibrosing alveolitis: Relationships of pulmonary physiology and bronchoalveolar lavage to treatment and prognosis. Am Rev Respir Dis 1981;124:1–8.

75. Stack BHR, Choo-Kang YFJ, Heard BE. The prognosis of cryptogenic fibrosing alveolitis. Thorax 1980;35:535–542.

76. Turner Warwick M, Lebowitz M, Burrows B, Johnson A. Cryptogenic fibrosing alveolitis and lung cancer. Thorax 1980;35:496–499.

77. Haslam PL, Turton CWG, Lukoszek A, et al. Bronchoalveolar lavage fluid cell counts in cryptogenic fibrosing alveolitis and their relation to therapy. Thorax 1980;35:328–329.

78. de Cremoux H, Bernaudin J, Laurent P, Brochard P, Bignon J. Interactions between cigarette smoking and the natural history of idiopathic pulmonary fibrosis. Chest 1990;98:71–76.

79. Winterbauer RH, Ludwig WR, Hammar SP. Clinical course, management and long term sequelae of respiratory failure due to influenza viral pneumonia. Johns Hopkins Med J 1977;141:148–155.

80. Pinsker KL, Schneyer B, Becker N, Kamholz SL. Usual interstitial pneumonia following Texas A2 influenza infection. Chest 1981;80:123–126.

81. Martin WJ II, McDougall JC. Cytomegalovirus infection with idiopathic pulmonary fibrosis: Diagnosis suggested by bronchoalveolar lavage. Chest 1983;84:500–502.

82. Verganon JM, De The G, Weynants M, Vincent JF, Mornex JF, Brone J. Cryptogenic fibrosing alveolitis and Epstein-Barr virus: An association?. Lancet 1984;ii:768–771.

83. Roggli VL. Scanning electron microscopic analysis of mineral fiber content of lung tissue in the evaluation of diffuse pulmonary fibrosis. Scanning Microsc 1991;5:71–83.

84. Gail DB, Lenfant CJM. Cells of the lung: Biology and clinical implications. Am Rev Respir Dis 1983;127:366–387.

85. Crapo JD, Barry BE, Gehr P, Bachofen M, Weibel ER. Cell number and cell characteristics of the normal human lung. Am Rev Respir Dis 1982;125:740–745.

86. Crapo JD, Young SL, Fram EK, Pinkerton KE, Barry BE, Crapo RD. Morphometric characteristics of cells in the alveolar region of mammalian lungs. Am Rev Respir Dis 1983;128:S42–S46.

87. Bowden DH. Cell turnover in the lung. Am Rev Respir Dis 1983;128:S46–S48.

88. Golde DW, Finley TN, Cline MJ. The pulmonary macrophage in acute leukemia. N Engl J Med 1974;290:875–878.

89. Kazmierowski JA, Gallin JI, Reynolds HY. Mechanism for the inflammatory response in primate lungs: Demonstration and partial characterization of an alveolar macrophage-derived chemotactic factor with preferential activity for polymorphonuclear leukocytes. J Clin Invest 1977;59:273–281.

90. Hunninghake GW, Gallin JI, Fauci AS. Immunologic reactivity of the lung: The in vivo and in vitro generation of a neutrophil chemotactic factor by alveolar macrophages. Am Rev Respir Dis 1978;117:15–23.

91. Golde DW, Finley TN, Cline MJ. Production of colony stimulating factor by human macrophages. Lancet 1972;ii:1397–1399.

92. Postlethwaite AE, Keski-Oja J, Balian G, Kung AH. Induction of fibroblast chemotaxis by fibronectin: Localization of the chemotactic region to a 140,000 molecular weight non-gelatin binding region. J Exp Med 1981;153:494–499.

93. Klebe RJ. Isolation of a collagen dependent cell attachment factor. Nature 1974;250:248–251.

94. Kelley J. Cytokines of the lung. Am Rev Respir Dis 1990;141:765–788.

95. Vignaud J, Allam M, Martinet N, Pech M, Plenat F, Martine Y. Presence of platelet-derived growth factor in normal and fibrotic lung is specifically associated with interstial macrophages, while both interstitial macrophages and alveolar epithelial cells express the c-sis protooncogene. Am J Respir Cell Mol Biol 1991;5:531–538.

96. Marinelli WA, Polunovsky VA, Harmon KR, Bitterman PB. Role of platelet-derived growth factor in pulmonary fibrosis. Am J Respir Cell Mol Biol 1991;5:503–504.

97. Everson MP, Chandler DB. Changes in distribution, morphology and tumor necrosis factor alpha secretion of alveolar macrophage subpopulations during the development of bleomycin-induced pulmonary fibrosis. Am J Pathol 1992;140:503–512.

98. Warren JS, Yabroff KR, Remick DG, et al. Tumor necrosis factor participates in the pathogenesis of acute immune complex alveolitis in the rat. J Clin Invest 1989;84:1873–1882.

99. Lynch JP, III, Standiford TJ, Rolfe MW, Kunkel SL, Strieter RM. Neutrophilic alveolitis in idiopathic pulmonary fibrosis. Am Rev Respir Dis 1992;145:1433–1439.

100. Bitterman PB, Adelberg S, Crystal RG. Mechanisms of pulmonary fibrosis: spontaneous release of alveolar macrophage derived growth factor in the interstitial lung disorders. J Clin Invest 1983;72:1801–1813.

101. Dreisen RB, Schwarz MI, Theofilopoulous AN, Stanford RE. Circulating immune complexes in the idiopathic interstitial pneumonias. N Engl J Med 1978;298:353–357.

102. Razma AG, Lynch JP, Wilson BS, Ward PA, Kunke SL. Expression of Ia-like (DR) antigen on human alveolar macrophages isolated by bronchoalveolar lavage. Am Rev Respir Dis 1984;129:419–424.

103. Hunninghake GW, Kawanami O, Ferrans VJ, et al. Characterization of the inflammatory and immune effector cells in the lung parenchyma of patients with interstitial lung disease. Am Rev Respir Dis 1981;123:407–412.

104. Hunninghake GW, Gudek JE, Young RC, Jr, Kawanami

O, Ferrans VJ, Crystal RG. Maintenance of granuloma formation in pulmonary sarcoidosis by T-lymphocytes within the lung. N Engl J Med 1980;302:594–598.

105. Schrier DJ, Phan SH, McGarry BM. The effects of nude (nu/nu) mutation on bleomycin-induced pulmonary fibrosis. A biochemical evaluation. Am Rev Respir Dis 1983;127:614–617.

106. Wahl SM, Wahl LM, McCarthy JB. Lymphocyte mediated activation of fibroblasts proliferation and collagen production. J Immunol 1978;121:942–946.

107. Reynolds HY, Fulmen JD, Kazmierowski JA, Roberts WC, Frank MM, Crystal RG. Analysis of cellular and protein content of bronchoalveolar lavage fluid from patients with idiopathic pulmonary fibrosis and chronic hypersensitivity pneumonitis. J Clin Invest 1977;59:165–175.

108. Weinberger SE, Kelman JA, Elson NA, et al. Bronchoalveolar lavage in interstitial lung disease. Ann Intern Med 1978;89:459–466.

109. Gadeck JE, Kelman JA, Fells G, et al. Collagenase in the lower respiratory tract of patients with idiopathic pulmonary fibrosis. N Engl J Med 1979;301:737–742.

110. Phan SH, Schrier D, McGarry B, Duque RE. Effect of the beige mutation on bleomycin induced pulmonary fibrosis in mice. Am Rev Respir Dis 1983;127:456–459.

111. Snider GL. Interstitial pulmonary fibrosis—which cell is the culprit? Am Rev Respir Dis 1983;127:540–544.

112. Strausz J, Müller-Quernheim J, Steppling H, Ferlinz R. Oxygen radical production by alveolar inflammatory cells in idiopathic pulmonary fibrosis. Am Rev Respir Dis 1990;141:124–128.

113. Nettelbladt O, Hällgren R. Hyaluronan (hyaluronic acid) in bronchoalveolar lavage fluid during the development of bleomycin-induced alveolitis in the rat. Am Rev Respir Dis 1989;140:1028–1032.

114. Montano M, Ramos C, Gonzalez G, Vadillo F, Pardo A, Selman M. Lung collagenase inhibitors and spontaneous and latent collagenase activity in idiopathic pulmonary fibrosis and hypersensitivity pneumonitis. Chest 1989;96:1115–1119.

115. Noguchi H, Kephart GM, Colby TV, Gleich GJ. Tissue eosinophilia and eosinophil degranulation in syndromes associated with fibrosis. Am J Pathol 1992;140:521–528.

116. Pennington DW, Ruoss SJ, Gold WM. Dog mastocytoma cells secrete a growth factor for fibroblasts. Am J Respir Cell Mol Biol 1992;6:625–632.

117. Fullmer JD, Biekowski RS, Cowan MJ, et al. Collagen concentration and rates of synthesis in idiopathic pulmonary fibrosis. Am Rev Respir Dis 1980;122:289–301.

118. Madri JA, Furthmayr H. Collagen polymorphism in the lung: An immunochemical study of pulmonary fibrosis. Hum Pathol 1980;11:353–366.

119. Raghu G, Striker LJ, Hudson LD, Striker GE. Extracellular matrix in normal and fibrotic human lungs. Am Rev Respir Dis 1985;131:281–289.

120. Corrin B, Dewar A, Rodriguez-Roisin R, Turner-Warwick M. Fine structural changes in cryptogenic fibrosing alveolitis and asbestos. J Pathol 1985;147:107–119.

121. Basset F, Ferrans VJ, Soler P, Takemura T, Fukuda Y, Crystal RG. Intraluminal fibrosis in interstitial lung disorders. Am J Pathol 1986;122:443–461.

122. Kuhn C, III, Boldt J, King TE, Jr., Crouch E, Vartio T, McDonald JA. An immunohistochemical study of architectural remodeling and connective tissue synthesis in pulmonary fibrosis. Am Rev Respir Dis 1989;140:1693–1703.

123. Kuhn C. Patterns of lung repair: A morphologist's view. Chest 1991;99:11S–14S.

124. Kuhns C, McDonald JA. The roles of myofibroblasts in idiopathic pulmonary fibrosis: Ultrastructural and immunohistochemical features of sites of active extracellular matrix synthesis. Am J Pathol 1991;138:1257–1265.

125. MacDonald JA. Idiopathic pulmonary fibrosis: A paradigm for lung injury and repair. Chest 1991;99(Suppl.) 87S–93S.

126. Hyde DM, Nakasima JM, Harris JA, Giri SN. Epithelial injury is a critical factor in the development of pulmonary fibrosis following multiple episodes of inflammation. Chest 1991;99:28S.

127. Ward PA. Overview of the process of cellular injury in interstitial lung disease. Chest 1991;100:230–232.

128. Osborne DR. The Lung: Segmental anatomy and nonneoplastic diseases. In: Godwin JD, ed. Computed tomography of the chest. Philadelphia: JB Lippincott Co, 1984;160–186.

129. Müller NL, Miller RR. Computed tomography of chronic diffuse infiltratitive lung disease. Am Rev Respir Dis 1990;142:1206–1215.

130. Swensen SJ, Aughenbaugh GL, Brown LR. High resolution computed tomography of the lung. Mayo Clin Proc 1989;64:1284–1294.

131. Gamsu G. High-resolution computed tomography of diffuse lung disease. Invest Radiol 1989;24:805–812.

132. Newman SL, Michael RP, Wang NS. Lingular lung biopsy: Is it representative? Am Rev Respir Dis 1985;132:1084–1086.

133. Wetstein L. Sensitivity and specificity of lingular segmental biopsies of the lung. Chest 1986;90:383–386.

134. Meyer EC, Liebow AA. Relationship of interstitial pneumonia, honeycombing and atypical epithelial proliferation to cancer of the lung. Cancer (Phila) 1965;18:322–351.

135. Haddad R, Maasaro D. Idiopathic diffuse interstitial pulmonary fibrosis (fibrosing alveolitis), atypical epithelial proliferation and lung cancer. Am J Med 1968;44:211–219.

136. Fraire AE, Greenberg SD. Carcinoma and diffuse interstitial fibrosis of lung. Cancer 1973;31:1078–1086.

137. Turner-Warwick M, Lebowitz M, Burrows B, Johnson A. Cryptogenic fibrosing alveolitis and lung cancer. Thorax 1980;35:496–499.

138. Woodcock-Mitchell J, Adler KB, Low RB. Immunohistochemical identification of cell types in normal and in bleomycin-induced fibrotic rat lung: Cellular origins of interstitial cells. Am Rev Respir Dis 1984;130:910–916.

139. Goto T, Befus D, Low R, Bienstock J. Mast cell hetero-

geneity and hyperplasia in bleomycin-induced pulmonary fibrosis of rats. Am Rev Respir Dis 1984;130:797–802.

140. Rowden G. The Langerhans cell. CRC Crit Rev Immunol 1981;3:95–180.

141. Basset F, Soler P, Wyllie L, Mazin F, Turiaf J. Langerhans cells and the lung interstitium. Ann NY Acad Sci 1976;278:599–611.

142. Kawanami O, Basset F, Ferrans VJ, Soler P, Crystal RG. Pulmonary Langerhans cells in patients with fibrotic lung disease. Lab Invest 1981;44:227–233.

143. Hammar S, Bockus D, Remington F, Bartha M. The widespread distribution of Langerhans cells in pathologic tissues: An ultrastructural and immunohistochemical study. Hum Pathol 1986;17:894–905.

144. Hammar SP, Winterbauer RH, Bockus D, Remington F, Friedman S. Idiopathic fibrosing alveolitis: A review with emphasis on ultrastructural and immunohistochemical features. Ultrastruct Pathol 1985;9:345–372.

145. Colby TV, Lombard C. Histocytosis X in the lung. Hum Pathol 1983;14:847–856.

146. Basset F, Corrin B, Spencer H, et al. Pulmonary histiocytosis X. Am Rev Respir Dis 1978;118:811–820.

147. Hammar S, Winterbauer RH, Gilmore T, Hallman KO, Bush W, Dail DH. Pulmonary histiocytosis X: A clinicopathologic study of 3 cases. (manuscript submitted to Ultra Pathol)

148. Hammar SP, Winterbauer RH, Bockus D, Remington F, Sale GE, Myers JD. Endothelial cell damage and tubuloreticular structures in interstitial lung disease associated with collagen vascular diseases and viral pneumonia. Am Rev Respir Dis 1983;127:77–84.

149. Bockus D, Remington F, Luu J, Friedman S, Bean M, Hammar SP. Induction of cylindrical confronting cisternae (AIDS inclusions) in Daudi lymphoblastoid cells by recombinant alpha interferon. Hum Pathol 1988;19:78–82.

150. Ramaswamy G, Jagadha V, Tchertkoff V. Diffuse alveolar damage and interstitial fibrosis in acquired immunodeficiency syndrome patient without concurrent pulmonary infection. Arch Pathol Lab Med 1985;109:408–412.

151. Grieco MH, Chinoy-Acharya P. Lymphocytic interstitial pneumonia associated with the acquired immune deficiency syndrome. Am Rev Respir Dis 1985;131:952–955.

152. Solal-Celingny T, Couderc LJ, Herman D, et al. Lymphoid interstitial pneumonitis in acquired immunodeficiency syndrome-related complex. Am Rev Respir Dis 1985;131:956–960.

153. DeStefano E, Friedman RM, Friedman-Klein AE, et al. Acid labile human leukocyte interferon in homosexual men with Kaposi's sarcoma and lymphadenopathy. J Infect Dis 1982;146:451–455.

154. Epler GR, Colby TV, McLoud TC, Carrington CB, Gaensler EA. Bronchiolitis obliterans organizing pneumonia. N Engl J Med 1985;312:152–158.

155. Katzenstein AA, Myers JL, Prophet WD, Corley LS, Shin MS. Bronchiolitis obliterans and usual interstitial pneumonia: A comparative clinocpathologic study. Am J Surg Pathol 1986;10:373–381.

156. Colby T, Churg AC. Patterns of pulmonary fibrosis. In: Sommers SC, Rosen PP, Fechner RE, eds, Pathology annual. Norwalk: Appleton-Century-Crofts, 1986, Part 2:277–310

157. DeHoratius RJ, Abruzzo JL, Williams RC. Immunofluorescent and immunologic studies of rheumatoid lung. Arch Intern Med 1972;129:441–446.

158. Clinicopathologic conference. N Engl J Med 1975;293:136–144.

159. Wiener-Kronish JP, Solinger AM, Warnock ML, Churg A, Ordonez N, Golden JA. Severe pulmonary involvement in mixed connective tissue disease. Am Rev Respir Dis 1981;124:499–503.

160. Hogan PG, Donald KJ, McEvoy JDS. Immunofluorescence studies of lung biopsy tissue. Am Rev Respir Dis 1978;118:537–545.

161. Levin DC, Wicks AB, Ellis JH. Transbronchial lung biopsy via the fiberoptic bronchoscope. Am Rev Respir Dis 1974;110:4–12.

162. Smith CW, Murray GF, Wilcox BR, Starek PJK, Delany DJ. The role of transbronchial lung biopsy in diffuse pulmonary disease. Ann Thorac Surg 1977;24:54–58.

163. Jenkins R, Myerowtiz RL, Kavic T, Slasky S. Diagnostic yield of transbronchoscopic biopsies. Am J Clin Pathol 1979;72:926–930.

164. Wall CP, Gaensler EA, Carrington CB, Hayes JA. Comparison of transbronchial and open biopsies in chronic infiltrative lung disease. Am Rev Respir Dis 1981;123:280–290.

165. Reynolds HY, Newball HH. Analysis of proteins and respiratory cells obtained from human lungs by bronchial lavage. J Lab Clin Med 1974;84:559–573.

166. Dohn MN, Baughman RP. Effect of changing instilled volume for bronchoalveolar lavage in patients with interstitial lung disease. Am Rev Respir Dis 1985;132:390–392.

167. Cantin A, Begin R, Rola-Pleszczynski M, Boyleau R. Heterogeneity of bronchoalveolar lavage cellularity in stage III pulmonary sarcoidosis. Chest 1983;83:485–486.

168. Gelb AF, Dreisen RB, Epstein JD, et al. Immune complexes, gallium lung scans and bronchoalveolar lavage in idiopathic interstitial pneumonitis-fibrosis: A structure–function clinical study. Chest 1983;84:148–153.

169. Davis GS, Brody AR, Craighead JE. Analysis of airspace and interstitial mononuclear cell populations in human diffuse interstitial lung disease. Am Rev Respir Dis 1978;118:7–16.

170. Hunninghake GW, Kawanami O, Ferrans VJ, Young RC, Jr, Roberts WC. Crystal RG. Characterization of inflammatory and immune effector cells in the lung parenchyma of patients with interstitial lung disease. Am Rev Respir Dis 1981;123:407–412.

171. Haslam PL, Turton C, Heard B, et al. Bronchoalveolar lavage in pulmonary fibrosis: Comparison of cells ob-

tained with lung biopsy and clinical features. Thorax 1980;35:9–18.

172. Stack BH, Choo-Kang YF, Heard BE. The prognosis of cryptogenic fibrosing alveolitis. Thorax 1972;27:435–542.

173. Rudd RM, Haslam PL, Turner-Warwick M. Cryptogenic fibrosing alveolitis: Relationships of pulmonary physiology and bronchoalveolar lavage to response to treatment and prognosis. Am Rev Respir Dis 1981;124:1–8.

174. Haslam PL. Circulating immune complexes in patients with cryptogenic fibrosing alveolitis. Clin Exp Immunol 1979;37:381–390.

175. Winterbauer RH. The treatment of idiopathic pulmonary fibrosis. Chest 1991;100:233–235.

176. Martinet Y, Haslam PL, Turner-Warwick M. Clinical significance of circulating immune complexes in "lone" cryptogenic fibrosis alveolitis and those with associated connective tissue disorders. Clin Allergy 1984;14:491–497.

177. Winterbauer RH, Hammar SP. Tubuloreticular structures: An electron microscopic marker of cyclophosphamide responsive fibrosing alveolitis. Am Rev Respir Dis 1982;125:91A.

CHAPTER 21
Rheumatic Connective Tissue Diseases

J.T. LIE

The terms rheumatic *connective tissue diseases* and *collagen-vascular diseases* are synonymous, both referring to a large heterogeneous group of immunologically mediated inflammatory disorders (Table 21–1). In this chapter, emphasis is directed to a discussion of pulmonary involvement in nine selected rheumatic connective tissue disorders: rheumatic fever, rheumatoid arthritis (RA), systemic lupus erythematosus (SLE), dermatomyositis-polymyositis (DPM), mixed connective tissue disease (MCT), Sjögren syndrome, ankylosing spondylitis (AS), and relapsing polychondritis (RP) (Table 21–2).

The Concept of Rheumatic Connective Tissue Diseases

The idea that the characteristic organ and tissue alterations in rheumatic fever and rheumatoid arthritis reflect a systemic involvement of the entire connective tissues of the human body was first conceived by the German pathologist Fritz Klinge in the 1930s.[1,2] In 1942, the American pathologists Paul Klemperer, Abou Pollack, and George Baehr[3] proposed that both systemic lupus erythematosus and scleroderma were characterized microscopically by "a fundamental alteration of the collagenous tissue" and could be viewed as "systemic diseases of the connective tissues." They expressed this concept by the phrase *diffuse connective disease*.[3] Klemperer[4] later emphasized that this phrase was a metaphor in which collagen stood for connective tissue in its entirety.

The term *diffuse vascular disease* was used by Banks[5] in 1941 to include scleroderma, dermatomyositis, disseminated lupus erythematosus, and polyarteritis nodosa on the basis that "all of which represent a widespread vascular involvement, differing usually in the extent of the pathologic change, the size of the vessels involved, and the organs chiefly affected." The hybrid name *collagen-vascular disease* was introduced by another pathologist, A.R. Rich,[6] in 1946 to unify the two views (*collagen* and *vascular* diseases) of the pathology of periarteritis nodosa, rheumatic fever, disseminated lupus erythematosus, and rheumatoid arthritis. Neither the pathologic anatomy nor the clinical features of collagen-vascular diseases define a perfectly discrete and distinctive group of disorders. The proliferation of the number of entities for inclusion to the group (see Table 21–1) justifies Klemperer's warning, in 1950, that *collagen-vascular disease* "may become a catch-all term for maladies with puzzling clinical and anatomical features."[4]

Pulmonary Involvement in Rheumatic Diseases

Although musculoskeletal manifestations are the most noted clinical features of rheumative connective tissue diseases, pulmonary involvement is not uncommon and has been the subject of several excellent reviews in the past decade.[7–12] Involvement of the lungs is known to occur in virtually every variety of rheumatic connective tissue diseases, and their histopathologic features frequently overlap (see Table 21–2). The frequency and type of pulmonary involvement in each rheumatic disorder vary according to whether clinical, roentgenographic, or histologic criteria are used to document the lung disease. Interstitial pneumonitis, diffuse or multifocal and often accompanied by fibrosis, is the most common pulmonary parenchymal manifestation of connective tissue disorders and the one most frequently fatal. This type of pulmonary involvement accounts for an estimated 1,600 deaths per year, or about 25% of all deaths from interstitial lung disease.[13] Pulmonary involvement in rheumatic diseases is rare in the neonates but occurs almost as commonly in children as in adults.[14,15]

The diagnosis of pulmonary disease in rheumatic disorders is fraught with several intrinsic problems. First, the pathogenesis of lung disease in rheumatic disorders remains incompletely understood, and the histologic features are diverse and often overlap in different disorders. Second, the possibility exists that the pulmonary abnormalities and the rheumatic disorder may be entirely coincidental. Third, pulmonary complications of the general drug hypersensitivity and specific antirheumatic drug therapy are diverse and may be histologically indistinguishable from pulmonary disease arising *de novo* in the underlying rheumatic disorder.[16,17] Fourth, the sampling problem in biopsy diagnosis cannot always be avoided, especially with small transbronchial biopsies, even when multiple step sections are used.[18,19] In open biopsies, a tissue sample no smaller than 2–3 cm in any dimension is usually recommended. The surgeon should select lung tissue that is abnormal, but not the most abnormal, because nonspecific endstage fibrosis or honeycombing might be the only finding from such a biopsy[11,20] (see Chapter 1).

In recent years, bronchoalveolar lavage (BAL) has become a useful adjunctive diagnostic tool in the evaluation of lung disease in rheumatic connective tissue disorders,[21–28] as has the gallium scanning technique.[29–32] BAL has proved to be of great value in the diagnosis of infections in immunocompromised hosts,[21,32] and in influencing clinical management of

Table 21–1. Expanding family of connective tissue diseases

Original Members
  Rheumatic fever
  Rheumatoid arthritis
  Systemic lupus erythematosus
  Scleroderma (progressive systemic sclerosis)
  Dermatomyositis-polymyositis
  Polyarteritis nodosa
  Gouty and other crystal arthritis
  Ankylosing spondylitis
Additional Members
  Serum sickness
  Anaphylactoid (Schönlein-Henoch) purpura
  Pulmonary infiltration with eosinophilia (Löffler syndrome)
  Disseminated eosinophilic collagen disease/eosinophilic fasciitis
  Chronic relapsing nonsuppurative panniculitis
    (Weber-Christian syndrome)
  Sjögren syndrome
  Cogan syndrome
  Behçet syndrome
  Mixed connective tissue disease
  Relapsing polychondritis
  Essential mixed cryoglobulinemia
  Familial Mediterranean fever
  Amyloidosis
  Sarcoidosis
  Primary pulmonary hypertension
  Idiopathic retroperitoneal/mediastinal fibrosis

Table 21–2. Comparative pathologic spectrum of pulmonary involvement in rheumatic connective tissue diseases[a]

Type of disease	RA[b]	SLE	PSS	DPM	MCT	SS	AS	RP
Pleural inflammation	++	+++	+	0	+	+	+	0
Lung parenchymal disease								
Acute interstitial pneumonitis	0	++	0	++	++	0	0	0
Chronic pneumonitis/fibrosing alveolitis	++	+	++	++	++	++	0	0
Upper-lobe fibrosis	+	0	0	0	0	0	+++	0
Lymphocytic interstitial pneumonitis	++	++	+	+	+	+++	0	0
Diffuse alveolar hemorrhage/capillaritis	+	++	+	+++	+	0	0	+
Necrobiotic nodules	++	0	0	0	0	0	0	0
Amyloidosis	+	+	0	0	0	+	0	0
BOOP	++	+	+	++	+	+	0	0
Blood vessel disease								
Vasculitis	++	++	0	+	+	+	0	0
Proliferative intimal sclerosis	+	+	+++	+	++	0	0	0
Pulmonary hypertension	+	++	++	+	+	0	0	0
Laryngeal/tracheal abnormalities	++	+	+	0	0	+	0	+++
Respiratory muscle abnormalities	0	0	0	++	+	0	0	0
Esophageal muscle dysfunction	0	0	+++	+	++	0	0	0

[a] Modified from Wiedemann and Matthay[10] and Colby,[11] with permission.

[b] Abbreviations: AS, ankylosing spondylitis; BOOP, bronchiolitis obliterans organizing pneumonia; DPM, dermatopolymyositis; MCT, mixed connective tissue disease; PSS, progressive systemic sclerosis; RA, rheumatoid arthritis; RP, relapsing polychondritis; SLE, systemic lupus erythematosus; SS, Sjögren syndrome; 0, nonexistent or rare; +, unusual or only occasionally; ++, intermediate frequency and may be clinically important; +++, frequent and clinically significant.

patients with a variety of interstitial lung diseases.[26–28] The detection of abnormally increased numbers of neutrophils, eosinophils, or lymphocytes and macrophages in BAL, and the finding of immune complexes, immunoglobulins, complements, lymphokines, and various macrophage secretory factors have been shown to be associated with active lung involvement that is theoretically more amenable to aggressive corticosteroid or immunosuppressive therapy.*

Rheumatic Fever

Not much is known about pulmonary involvement in rheumatic fever, and little has been written on this association in the past 25 years. "Rheumatic pneumonias" have been the subject of sporadic reports between 1888 and 1966[33–35] describing both lobar and multilobar consolidation of the lungs.[33] In 1926 Von Glahn and Pappenheimer[34] found pulmonary arteritis in 20% of patients with rheumatic fever with concentric thickening of blood vessels and vascularization of the intima. In 1966 Massumi and Legier[35] described three cases of pneumonitis in rheumatic fever, two with histologic confirmation. In all three patients, the hospital course was progressively downhill with death ensuing in weeks to months. The clinical picture corresponded with active rheumatic carditis, complicated by the adult respiratory distress syndrome (ARDS). At autopsy, the lungs were heavy and showed an organizing pneumonia with interstitial edema and focal vasculitis. Chronic lung disease as a sequela of rheumatic fever appears to be an even more questionable nosologic entity, and probably cannot be distinguished from secondary pulmonary changes seen in chronic severe congestive heart failure of rheumatic mitral valve disease.[36,37]

Rheumatoid Arthritis

Rheumatoid arthritis (RA) is a systemic disease with prominent symmetric, deforming, and nonsuppurative arthritis of the small peripheral joints. A. B. Garrod[38] coined the term *rheumatoid arthritis* in 1858 to separate it from gout, and pulmonary involvement in RA was first described by Ellman and Ball[39] 90 years later, in 1948. By the late 1960s, five major manifestations of rheumatoid lung disease were recognized,[40–42] including (1) pleuritis with or without effusion; (2) necrobiotic (rheumatoid) nodules; (3) rheumatoid pneumoconiosis, or Caplan syndrome; (4) diffuse interstitial pneumonitis

---

*References: 22–24, 26, 28, 30, 32.

and fibrosis including fibrosing alveolitis; and (5) pulmonary vasculitis. The more recent addition of lymphocytic interstitial pneumonitis and bronchiolitis obliterans organizing pneumonia,[43–48] further broadens the clinicopathologic spectrum of rheumatoid lung disease, which is probably among the best known and most extensively studied pulmonary manifestations of rheumatic connective tissue diseases.[7–12,39–50]

Despite the predilection of rheumatoid arthritis in women, pleuropulmonary involvement occurs more commonly in men.[7,50] Although pulmonary involvement may be asymptomatic, as many as 40% of patients with rheumatoid arthritis tested have restrictive pulmonary function test abnormalities and nearly that many have some clinical evidence of pleural involvements.[49–55] On the other hand, only about 9% of patients with biopsy-proven interstitial lung disease have normal chest roentgenograms,[56] and perhaps no more than 5% of adults with rheumatoid arthritis have clinically significant parenchymal pulmonary disease[41,53,57–59]; however, perhaps half of the autopsied patients appeared to have evidence of active or old pleuropulmonary involvement.[7,60] Thus, the incidence and prevalence of pleuropulmonary disease in rheumatoid arthritis varies greatly, depending on whether the method of assessment is by the clinical presentation, abnormal pulmonary function tests, abnormal chest roentgenographs, or abnormal lung histology.[7,47]

Pleuritis with or Without Effusion

Initially described in 1943 by Baggenstoss and Rosenberg[61] in an autopsy series, pleuritis is the most common but least specific pulmonary manifestation of rheumatoid arthritis and is found in 20%–40% of patients examined at autopsy.[61–63] The incidence of pleural effusion during the life of patients with rheumatoid arthritis is probably only 3%–5%[62,63] and, in one series of 309, clinical radiographic evidence of pleural inflammation (pleural thickening and scarring) was identified in 24% of men and 16% of women.[64]

Pleural effusions are usually associated with manifestations of active rheumatoid disease, including peripheral arthritis, subcutaneous necrobiotic nodules, and high titers of rheumatoid factor.[7] The pleural fluid in rheumatoid arthritis is usually an exudate with low pH, low glucose, and high concentrations of protein and lactate dehydrogenase.[45,63,65–68] In most rheumatoid effusions, RA cells can be identified. These cells have cytoplasmic inclusions representing phagocytized IgM rheumatoid factor in immune complex form. The presence of RA cells in pleural fluid is not specific for rheumatoid arthritis, however, and may also be found in pleural effusions associated with other collagen-

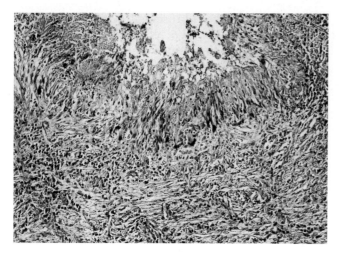

Fig. 21–1. Pulmonary necrobiotic nodule in rheumatoid arthritis, opened out to surface of visceral pleura (*top*) in pleural biopsy. Note orientation of palisading histiocytes and multinucleated giant cells. H and E, ×160.

vascular diseases, tuberculosis, and malignancy, and in idiopathic or primary pleural effusions.[67]

Open pleural biopsies usually show only nonspecific inflammatory and fibrotic changes, but occasionally a granulomatous lesion that has been described as an opened-out necrobiotic (rheumatoid) nodule (Fig. 21–1) with palisading epithelioid cells is found on the visceral pleura as well as the pericardium.[7,68–70] A needle biopsy of the pleura is seldom diagnostic, and is helpful only insofar as it may exclude tuberculous or malignant diseases that have biochemical constituents in pleural effusions similar to those of rheumatoid arthritis.[66–68]

Necrobiotic (Rheumatoid) Nodules

Subcutaneous necrobiotic nodules were first described to occur in rheumatic fever in 1812[71] and almost a century later in rheumatoid arthritis.[72] The reported prevalence of subcutaneous rheumatoid nodules varies greatly, from 13.5% to 53%,[73,74] probably because cases of ankylosing spondylitis or osteoarthritis among the rheumatoid patients, series of atypical rheumatoid arthritis and perhaps geographic variations have been included.[75]

Pulmonary necrobiotic nodules, single or multiple, are the most characteristic and least common type of lung lesions associated with rheumatoid arthritis.[41,42,64,76] Walker and Wright[41] reported only 3 cases in a series of 516 patients with rheumatoid arthritis; and in a radiographic series of 309 rheumatoid arthritis patients, Jurik et al.[64] found only 1 person with pulmonary nodules. Pulmonary rheumatoid nodules usually

are found in men with advanced seropositive rheumatoid arthritis who frequently also have subcutaneous nodules, but the pulmonary nodules can also appear before the onset of arthritis[42,76–78] and in patients without rheumatoid arthritis.[47,79,80] When solitary, these nodules may be confused with malignant tumors radiographically[81]; when they occur in endobronchial locations, they must be distinguished from carcinoma by biopsy.[82]

The pathologic features of the pulmonary nodules are identical to those of necrobiotic nodules in the skin and viscera.[47,63,83–85] Typically, three histologic zones can be identified: surrounding a central zone of acellular fibrinoid necrosis is a zone of palisading epithelioid cells, which in turn are surrounded by a collar of lymphocytes, plasma cells, and fibroblasts.[63,83–85] Stages in the development and maturation of the rheumatoid nodules may be identified and delineated (Fig. 21–2). The nodules may cavitate, occasionally leading to hemoptysis or hemothorax, clinically and radiographically mimicking pulmonary tuberculosis.[86,87] Secondary infection of cavitating nodules may further confuse the diagnosis of rheumatoid lung disease.[88–90]

Rheumatoid Pneumoconiosis (Caplan Syndrome)

Rheumatoid pneumoconiosis, or Caplan syndrome, was originally described in 1953 as a characteristic chest radiographic appearance in coalworkers with rheumatoid arthritis.[91] Currently, the concept of Caplan syndrome has been broadened to include rheumatoid arthritis patients whose lungs have been exposed to inhaled silica.[92–94] Clinical and radiological investigations in a group of coal miners showed that there was an increased prevalence of rheumatoid arthritis in miners with small nodules defined as nodular simple pneumoconiosis and also in miners having a mixture of nodular and irregular opacities that are normally included in the category of progressive massive fibrosis.[92] In addition, independent immunologic studies revealed that miners with these chest radiographic appearances or the classic radiographic changes of Caplan syndrome who had no history, symptoms, or signs of rheumatoid arthritis had a high proportion of positive rheumatoid factor tests.[92,93] It has been suggested that inhaled silica is a weak stimulus for the formation of rheumatoid factor. The mechanism by which silica leads to pulmonary fibrosis is unknown.[63,94]

Histologically, the nodules described by Caplan in pneumoconiosis are similar to simple rheumatoid pulmonary nodules, with the occasional addition of black coal dust in stranded lines in the central necrotic area[95,96] (See Chapter 27).

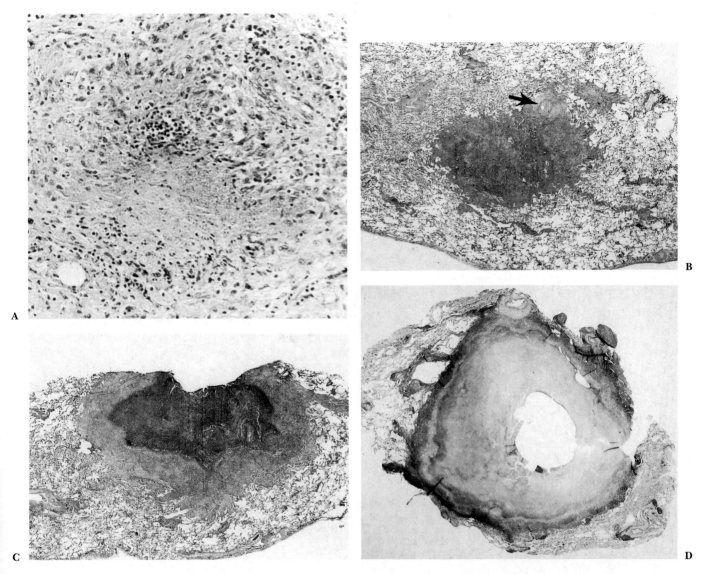

Fig. 21–2 A–D. A. Early pulmonary rheumatoid nodule with palisading histiocytes surrounding central zone of necrobiosis. H and E, ×160. B–D. Stages in rheumatoid nodule formation. **B.** Earlier focus shows inflammatory and fibrous nodule with almost obliterated blood vessel at edge (*arrow*). **C.** Midstage of development with central zone of necrosis. **D.** Well-developed sclerotic nodule with spherical contour and central cavitation. H and E, ×6.

Diffuse Interstitial Pneumonitis and Fibrosis

Diffuse interstitial lung disease associated with rheumatoid arthritis was first described by Ellman and Ball in 1948.[39] The reported prevalence of interstitial lung disease ranges from 16% in clinical surveys of unselected series of rheumatoid arthritis patients[51] to 60% of open lung biopsies done on unselected volunteers with rheumatoid arthritis.[45] It is obvious that the true incidence of interstitial lung disease in rheumatoid arthritis is unknown and varies according to the method of assessment. In radiographic studies, the reported incidence of parenchymal rheumatoid lung disease varies from 1.5% to 4.5%[64,97] although as many as 40% of patients tested may exhibit abnormal pulmonary function tests.[52–54] Such variations suggest that the chest roentgenogram is relatively insensitive in detecting the early stage of interstitial lung disease and pulmonary fibrosis.[56,98]

Interstitial lung disease in rheumatoid arthritis tends to be gradual and steadily progressive. The histologic features of rheumatoid interstitial lung disease are indistinguishable from those of the idiopathic type of interstitial pneumonia,* spanning the spectrum of des-

*References: 42, 45, 47, 97, 99.

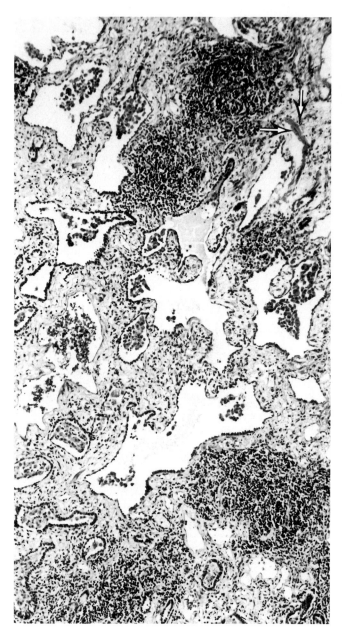

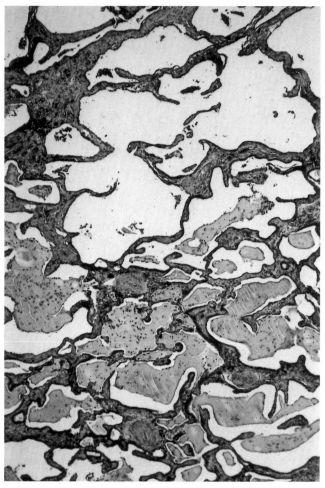

Fig. 21–4. Honeycombing in end-stage diffuse interstitial fibrosis of rheumatoid lung disease. H and E, ×40.

Fig. 21–3. Diffuse pulmonary interstitial fibrosis in rheumatoid arthritis: Normally delicate alveoli have been altered by broadened septal fibrosis lined by cuboidal cells resembling terminal bronchioles with lymphocytic infiltrate and smooth muscle fibers at top right (*arrows*). H and E, ×100.

quamative interstitial pneumonia to usual interstitial pneumonia to septal fibrosis resulting in patchy destruction of the alveoli and honeycombing (Figs. 21–3 and 21–4). Between these two extremes are the sequential changes of diffuse alveolar damage and fibrosing alveolitis, bronchiolitis obliterans organizing pneumonia, and lymphocytic interstitial pneumonitis (Fig. 21–5).[43–49,97–101] Biopsy specimens often showed a mixed

histologic pattern, and the prognosis of rheumatoid interstitial lung disease is correlated with the severity and extent of irreversible fibrosis and honeycombing.[47] Open biopsy is the preferred and definitive procedure for the diagnosis of rheumatoid interstitial lung disease,[47,48] and the biopsy may be complemented or supplemented by fiberoptic bronchoscopy and serial bronchoalveolar lavages.[26–28,32,102]

Pulmonary Vasculitis and Pulmonary Hypertension

Vasculitis is a recognized systemic manifestation of seropositive rheumatoid arthritis and plays an important role in the morbidity and mortality of the disease.[103–105] Pulmonary vasculitis (Fig. 21–6) occurs infrequently but it may be the principal manifestation of pulmonary involvement in rheumatoid arthri-

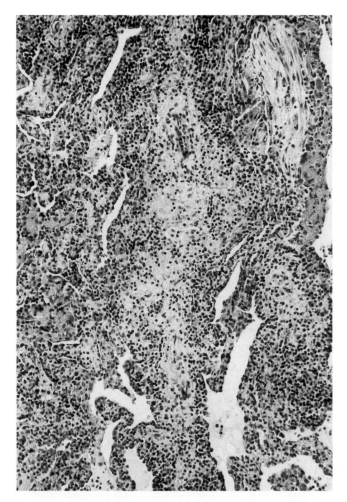

Fig. 21–5. Bronchiolitis obliterans organizing pneumonia and lymphocytic interstitial pneumonitis with early septal fibrosis in rheumatoid lung disease. H and E, ×160.

tis.[41,99,105,106] It is important to distinguish these patients from those with systemic polyarteritis nodosa. Increased levels of serum IgM have been reported in rheumatoid arthritis and 7S IgM levels have been associated with rheumatoid vasculitis,[99,107,108] suggesting that specific types of immune complexes may be responsible for the development of rheumatoid vasculitis by deposition in vessel walls. Rarely, pulmonary vasculitis occurs in the absence of significant parenchymal disease in the lungs.[109,110] Pulmonary vasculitis-related pulmonary hypertension without parenchymal disease or systemic vasculitis is uncommon but has been reported.[109–114] Immunofluorescence studies in these patients did not show deposition of immunoglobulins or complement.[109] Plexiform vascular lesions of primary pulmonary hypertension have been demonstrated in one case.[114]

Juvenile Rheumatoid Arthritis

In contrast to the classic rheumatoid arthritis in adults, there have been relatively few descriptions of pulmonary involvement in juvenile rheumatoid arthritis,* and only a handful of those cases had histologic documentation.[118] That abnormal pulmonary function tests can be detected in more than 50% of patients with juvenile rheumatoid arthritis indicates lung disease may be more prevalent than the small number of cases reported would suggest. The documented histologic changes appeared to run the whole gamut of pulmonary lesions seen in adult rheumatoid arthritis, including pleuritis, pleural adhesions, lymphoid hyperplasia, and follicular bronchitis (Fig. 21–7), interstitial lung disease with or without fibrosis, pulmonary hemosiderosis, pulmonary vasculitis, and pulmonary hypertension.[115–118]

Systemic Lupus Erythematosus

Kaposi, in 1872,[119] mentioned intercurrent pneumonia in his original account of the visceral lesions of disseminated lupus erythematosus. This was followed by Osler's description, at the turn of the century, of persistent lower-lobe infiltrates and hemoptysis in a 24-year-old woman with systemic lupus erythematosus (SLE).[120] Specific pulmonary lesions in SLE were first described by Rakov and Taylor in 1942[121]; since then, pulmonary manifestations of SLE have been the topic of many reports and reviews.[7–13,122–146]

Pleuropulmonary involvement is generally believed to be more common in SLE than any of the other rheumatic connective tissue diseases, occurring in 50%–70% of patients.[7–10,134,143] The reported incidence, however, ranges from as low as 9%[147] to as high as 98%,[128] and the number of patients with histologically documented significant pulmonary parenchymal lesions is probably closer to 20%.[10,130,140–150]

In SLE, there are no pathognomonic pleuropulmonary findings, but there is virtually an inexhaustibly long list of lung disorders of variable reported frequencies (Table 21-3). Hematoxylin bodies are diagnostic of SLE but they have been found in the lungs of only 1 of 120 patients in one study.[140] Generally, infections are the most frequent cause of pulmonary infiltrates in SLE patients[8–10,140,144]; acute interstitial pneumonitis resembling idiopathic usual interstitial pneumonia is uncommon and accounts for only 1%–6% of cases.[13] Interstitial pulmonary fibrosis is common in other con-

---

*References: 41, 50, 58, 98, 115–118.

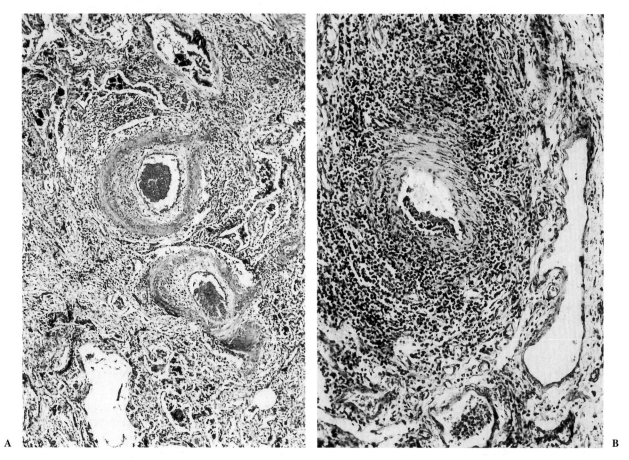

Fig. 21–6 A, B. Pulmonary vasculitis of medium-sized and small arteries in open lung biopsy that also shows changes of usual interstitial pneumonia. H and E, ×64, ×160, respectively.

nective tissue diseases, such as rheumatoid arthritis, systemic sclerosis, and dermato-polymyositis, but is much less prevalent in SLE and is clinically insignificant.[130,140,143] When diffuse pulmonary fibrosis is present in SLE patients, one should question whether an overlap syndrome or other connective tissue disease might be the correct diagnosis. Pulmonary vascular disease, on the other hand, is quite common in SLE.* Pulmonary capillaritis with diffuse alveolar hemorrhage (Fig. 21–8), pulmonary vasculitis (Fig. 21–9), and pulmonary hypertension (Fig. 21–10) are major causes of morbidity and mortality in SLE patients.

Immune complexes are thought to play an important role in the pathogenesis of pulmonary vascular disease in SLE patients.[141,157] Immune deposits are demonstrated mainly in the alveolar interstitium and vessel walls.[13,141] Most studies have shown granular deposits of IgG, IgM, IgA, and C3.[134,141,144] IgE has also been

found in the lungs of SLE patients with acute bronchiolitis.[150,158] Ultrastructurally, cytoplasmic tubuloreticular inclusions (Fig. 21–11) have been detected in pulmonary endothelial cells of SLE patients.[159,160] Although such inclusions are morphologically similar to the nucleoprotein strands of myxoviruses, they are considered to be products of nonspecific cellular injury and are specifically induced by acid-labile alpha interferon.

Among the less common pulmonary manifestations in SLE patients are bronchiolitis obliterans (Fig. 21–12) and lymphocytic interstitial pneumonitis (Fig. 21–13); both are of unknown etiology but are probably immune-mediated diseases.[131,136,150,158] Another interesting and controversial pulmonary manifestation of SLE is the "shrinking lung syndrome,"[13,148,161–166] which refers to SLE patients who have dyspnea associated with a restrictive ventilatory defect but have small, clear lungs on chest radiographs. There are no diagnostic histologic abnormalities in the lungs, and the cause of this shrinking lung syndrome is unknown. Initially, the syndrome was attributed to diffuse microatelectasis of

*References: 123, 128, 131, 134, 135, 137, 140, 141, 151–156.

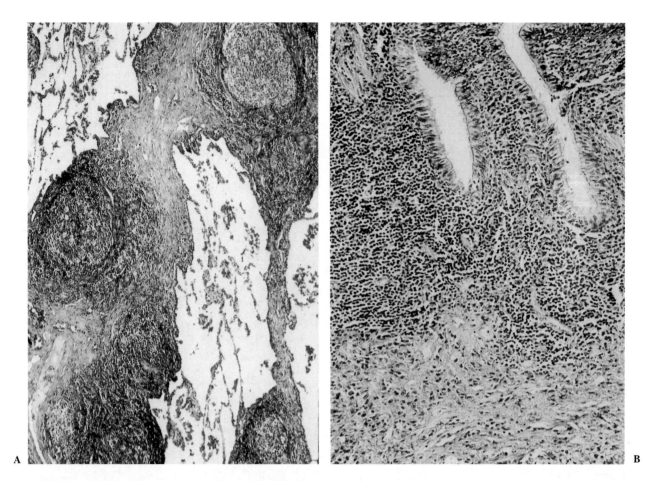

Fig. 21–7 A,B. Open lung biopsy in juvenile rheumatoid arthritis. **A.** Septal lymphocytic interstitial pneumonitis with prominent lymphoid follicles and germinal centers. H and E, ×64. **B.** Follicular bronchiolitis indistinguishable from that occurring in Sjögren syndrome with lung involvement. H and E, ×160.

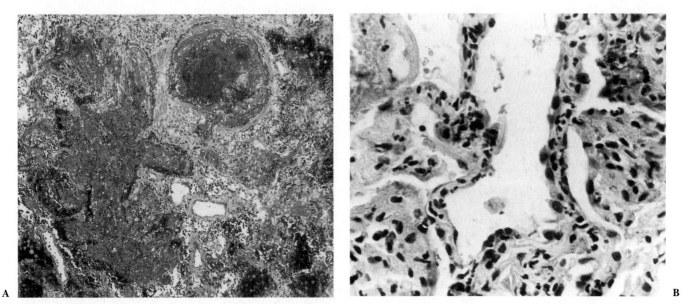

Fig. 21–8 A,B. Lupus lung. **A.** Diffuse alveolar hemorrhage. H and E, ×64. **B.** Alveolar capillaritis associated with pulmonary hemorrhage in systemic lupus erythematosus. H and E, ×600.

Table 21–3. Pleuropulmonary manifestations of systemic lupus erythematosus in a combined series of 266 autopsy patients[a]

Type of involvement	Percent of patients affected[b]
Pleural thickening	54
Bronchopneumonia	52
Pulmonary edema	51
Pulmonary congestion	47
Pulmonary atelectasis	41
Alveolar hemorrhage/capillaritis	40
Chronic interstitial infiltrates	36
Pleural effusion	35
Pleuritis	31
Acute bronchitis	28
Distal airway alterations	22
Interstitial pulmonary fibrosis	21
Pulmonary vasculitis and pulmonary hypertension	18
Bronchiolitis obliterans organizing pneumonia	17
Lung abscesses	17
Pulmonary tuberculosis	17
Opportunistic infection	7
Diffuse alveolar damage	7
Pulmonary infarction	6
Pulmonary empyema	4
Lobar pneumonia	2

[a] Adapted from Miller et al.[143] with data from references 122, 123, 126, 128, 133, and 140.

[b] Calculation was based on those autopsy series in which data were given; not all autopsy series described every type of pleuropulmonary involvement listed in this table.

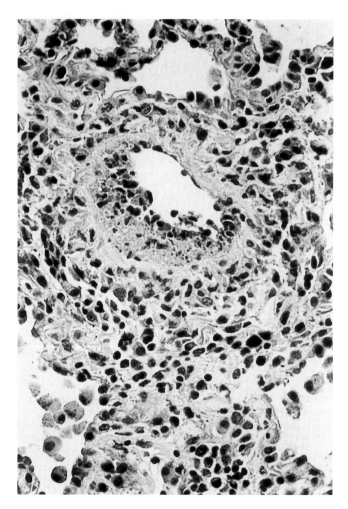

Fig. 21–9. Small-vessel pulmonary angiitis in systemic lupus erythematosus may be associated with pulmonary hypertension. H and E, ×400.

the lung[161] or to pleural adhesions that prevented diaphragmatic descent.[162] This seems unlikely because conditions such as asbestosis-related pleural fibrosis and therapeutic pleuridesis do not have significant effects on diaphragm function. Although neuropathy and myopathy can occur in SLE, the diaphragmatic dysfunction appears to be unrelated to these disorders and may improve or remain stable over time without specific treatment.[164,166]

Systemic Sclerosis (Scleroderma) and the CREST Syndrome Variant

Hippocrates (*History of Epidemics*, Book 5, Case 9) purportedly first described a patient with scleroderma who also had cor pulmonale.[167] Clinical evidence of pulmonary disease in scleroderma and the CREST (calcinosis–Raynaud's phenomenon–esophageal dysmotility–sclerodactyly–telangiectasia) syndrome is common, and abnormal autopsy findings in the lungs are almost universal.[7,13,168–185] Although the majority of patients

with scleroderma will develop pulmonary symptoms during the course of their disease, pulmonary symptoms are rarely (less than 1% or 2%) the initial manifestation of scleroderma.[181,182]

Systemic sclerosis patients with pulmonary involvement had significantly poorer survival prospects than did patients with gastrointestinal involvement but without renal, cardiac, or pulmonary disease. The results of a multicenter cooperative follow-up study of 264 patients showed that patients with pulmonary systemic sclerosis (without renal or cardiac disease) survived a median of 28 ± 17 months, but 60 of 104 (58%) died before the last follow-up (average, 5.2 years).[186] One of the earliest descriptions of systemic sclerosis, in 1870,[187] emphasized respiratory symptoms as a prominent feature of the advanced disease and considered this the result of restrictive skin thickening of the chest wall. Contemporary studies showing normal compliance of

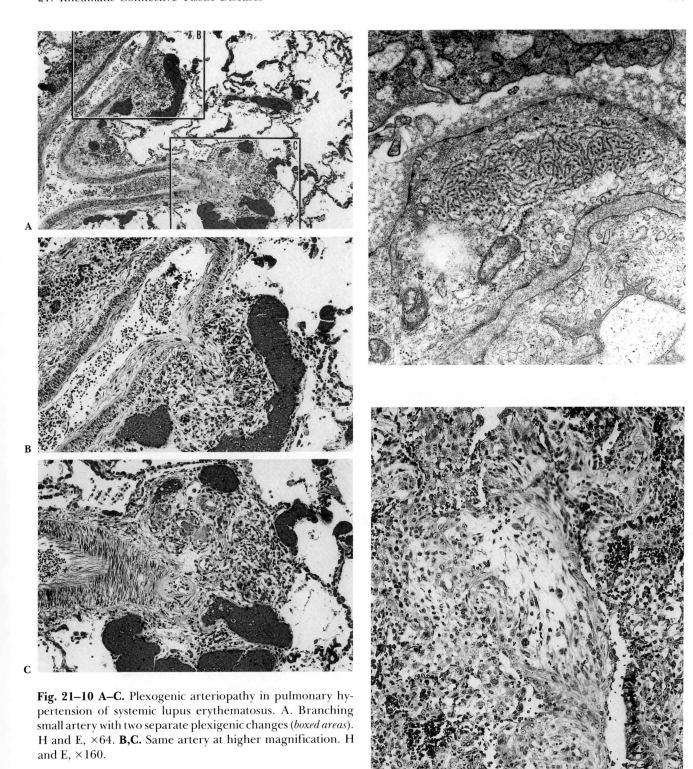

Fig. 21–10 A–C. Plexogenic arteriopathy in pulmonary hypertension of systemic lupus erythematosus. A. Branching small artery with two separate plexigenic changes (*boxed areas*). H and E, ×64. **B,C.** Same artery at higher magnification. H and E, ×160.

Fig. 21–11. Tubuloreticular structure in alveolar endothelial cells of lupus lung. H and E, ×16,000.

Fig. 21–12. Bronchiolitis obliterans in systemic lupus erythematosus. H and E, ×160.

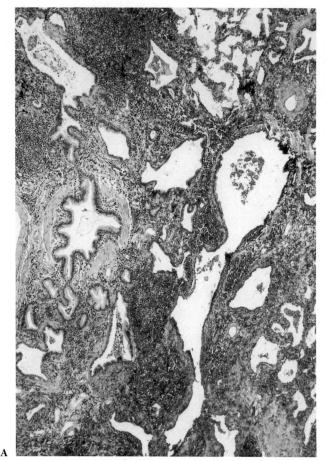

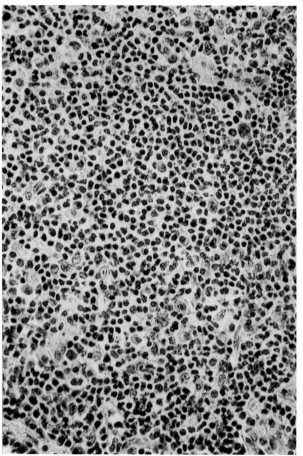

Fig. 21–13 A,B. A. Lymphocytic interstitial pneumonitis. H and E, ×64. **B.** Higher power view of benign lymphoid cells in pseudolymphoma; both are indistinguishable from those oc- curring in Sjögren syndrome with lung involvement. H and E, ×400.

the chest wall in scleroderma make this supposition an unlikely cause of symptomatic lung disease. The major complications of systemic sclerosis are interstitial pul- monary fibrosis and pulmonary hypertension.[171–185]

Interstitial Pulmonary Fibrosis

According to a study of 73 patients with systemic sclero- sis and its various subgroups, chest roentgenographic evidence of interstitial fibrosis was present at the time of diagnosis of the connective tissue disease in 18% of patients with the classic systemic sclerosis, in none of the patients with the CREST syndrome variant, and in 75% of patients with the scleroderma-overlap syndrome.[188] However, interstitial lung disease in the scleroderma- overlap group was usually basilar and mild on the initial chest film; while the classic scleroderma group had a less frequent radiographic evidence of lung disease, it was usually more diffuse and severe.

Histologic evaluation of lung disease in systemic scle-

rosis has mainly been derived from autopsy se- ries,[168,171,172,177] which emphasize the end-stage fibro- sis with bronchiectasis and subpleural honeycombing (Fig. 21–14). In general, interstitial fibrosis in systemic sclerosis is indistinguishable from that of the idiopathic usual interstitial pneumonia, but the interstitial fibrosis in scleroderma appears to be more indolent and more slowly progressive than usual interstitial pneumonia. Rapidly progressive type of interstitial pneumonitis (Fig. 21–15), on the other hand, has also been report- ed,[189] as has diffuse pulmonary hemorrhage.[176] Pleural fibrosis is a common finding in scleroderma lungs.[172] Bronchoalveolar carcinoma arising in the fibrotic lung of scleroderma patients has been described,[190] and lung cancers of other cell types and the association of extra- pulmonary malignancy are also known.[191,192] In one study, the relative risk of lung cancer in patients with scleroderma was 16.5[193]; in another, it was 4.4, without a clear relationship to smoking.[194] Reports of rapid onset of systemic sclerosis associated with either breast

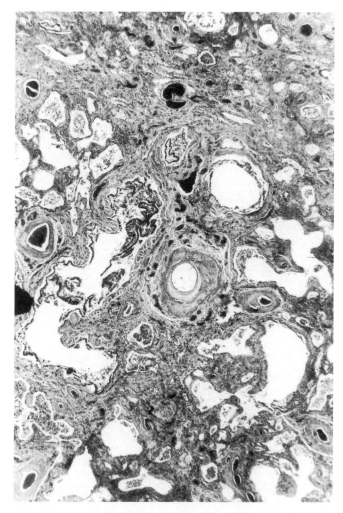

Fig. 21–14. Diffuse interstitial fibrosis with early honeycombing in scleroderma lung. Pulmonary vasculitis involving small to medium-sized artery is seen in center of figure; other arterial branches show occlusive intimal fibrosis. H and E, ×40.

or lung cancer suggest that systemic sclerosis may be a paraneoplastic syndrome in some patients.[195,196] Rarer pulmonary complications of systemic sclerosis include spontaneous pneumothorax,[197] hemoptysis from endobronchial telangiectasia,[198] and alveolar hypoventilation from respiratory muscle weakness.[199,200]

Pulmonary Hypertension

Pulmonary hypertension occurs in 10%–33% of patients with systemic sclerosis and in 40%–65% of patients with the CREST syndrome variant, depending on the criteria of diagnosis selected.* In CREST patients,

*References: 175, 179, 182, 201, 202.

pulmonary hypertension is frequently not associated with interstitial fibrosis.[181] The vascular changes of the scleroderm and CREST lungs are similar, consisting of some medial hypertrophy and, most typically, concentric intimal proliferation (Fig. 21–16).[169,171,177] Fibrinoid necrosis and plexiform lesions of primary pulmonary hypertension are usually not seen in scleroderma and CREST,[177] but there are occasional exceptions.[184] Interstitial fibrosis and pulmonary vascular disease are often present in the same lung, but they do not appear to be causally related except in the rare instances of pulmonary hypertension secondary to widespread and severe interstitial fibrosis.[177]

The cause of pulmonary hypertension in systemic sclerosis and the CREST syndrome variant is unknown, but endothelial injury has been implicated as the initial lesion.[203,204] Some investigators have suggested that the pulmonary hypertension that occurs in systemic sclerosis might be similar to Raynaud's phenomenon of the lung, an increase in cold vasoreactivity.[205–207] Others, however, were unable to demonstrate consistently neither the heightened cold vasoreactivity nor a sustained beneficial response to vasodilators in patients with systemic sclerosis.[208–210]

Dermatomyositis—Polymyositis

Dermatomyositis and polymyositis (DPM) are considered subgroups of the same inflammatory myopathy of unknown etiology that affect principally the limb girdles, neck, and pharynx, associated with a characteristic skin rash in about 40% of patients.[211] DPM is a relatively uncommon disease with an incidence of 5–5.5 cases per million in the United States.[212,213] It occurs twice as frequently in women as men in all age groups, with two ages of peak onset in the first decade of life and in the fifth and sixth decades.[212]

The first description of pulmonary involvement in DPM, by Mills and Matthews[214] in 1956, was that of a 52-year-old woman with diffuse interstitial pneumonitis, confirmed at autopsy.[214] Radiographic evidence of interstitial lung disease in DPM varies widely according to different investigators: Frazier and Miller[215] identified 10 (5%) of a series of 213 DPM patients; Salmeron et al.[216] found 10 (9.5%) in 105 patients; but Bohan et al.[217] did not find any cases in 153 patients. Higher prevalence figures were reported in other series with smaller numbers of patients. Songcharoen et al.[218] found 7 of 15 patients (47%) patients had roentgenographic evidence of interstitial lung disease in DPM; Dickey and Myers[219] described 12 of 42 (28.6%) patients with possible interstitial lung disease radiographically or by lung function testing, but considered only 4

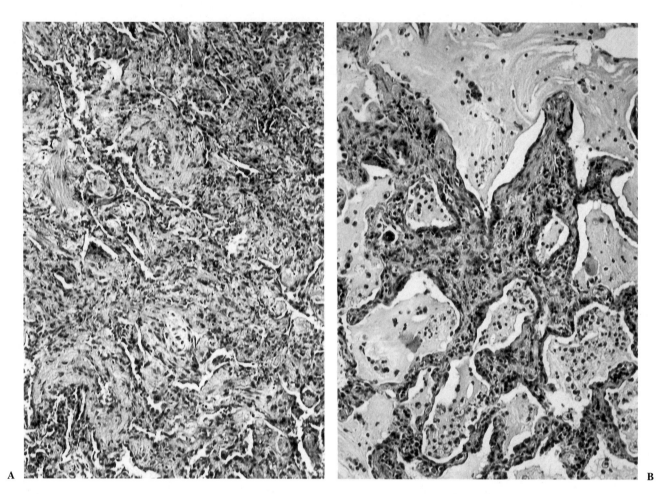

Fig. 21–15 A,B. Scleroderma lung. **A.** Rapidly progressive type of usual interstitial pneumonitis. H and E, ×64. **B.** Septal fibrosis and honeycombing. H and E, ×160.

(9.5%) had probable interstitial lung disease; and Takizawa et al.[220] reported a remarkably high prevalence of 9 in 14 (64%) Japanese patients; the diagnosis of interstitial lung disease was confirmed histologically in 8 of 9 patients.

Three types of pulmonary involvement in DPM were described initially:[221,222] (1) a primary form of usual interstitial pneumonitis (UIP); (2) ventilatory insufficiency caused by respiratory muscle weakness; and (3) aspiration pneumonia. Subsequent studies showed that diffuse alveolar damage (DAD) and fibrosing alveolitis (Fig. 21–17) also occurred frequently in patients with DPM,[223–225] as did bronchiolitis obliterans organizing pneumonia (BOOP).[226] Pulmonary vasculitis (Fig. 21–18) and pulmonary hypertension are recognized only rarely in patients with DPM.[225–228] Clinically significant respiratory muscle weakness is also uncommon.[229]

The prognosis for DPM patients with evidence of lung disease is poor. The case fatality rate for patients with histologically proven interstitial fibrosis and myo-

sitis was 62% over a 2-year period.[230] UIP is the most common type of pulmonary involvement in DPM and has been found in 41% of autopsy patients.[225] Clinically, the interstitial lung disease may precede the evidence of myositis, or the characteristic lung disease may precede the evidence of myositis or the characteristic skin rash of DPM in at least one-third of patients reported in the literature.[222–226] Patients with BOOP had a more favorable prognosis than did those with UIP, and patients with DAD or pulmonary vascular disease had a uniformly poor prognosis.[225–228]

Mixed Connective Tissue Disease

Almost all shades of connective tissue disease "overlap" occur; some claim that as many as 25% of patients with connective tissue disease may fall into one or other overlap group.[231] The term mixed connective tissue disease (MCT) was coined by Sharp et al.[232] in 1972, to

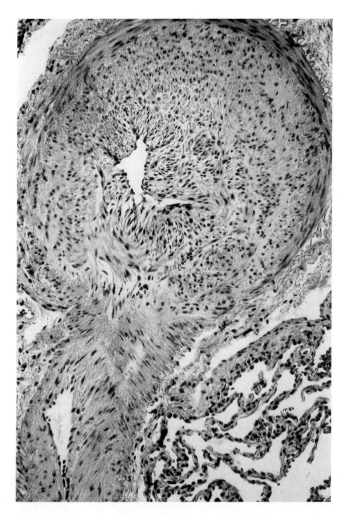

Fig. 21–16. Artery with marked intimal proliferative occlusive disease of scleroderma lung associated with severe pulmonary hypertension. H and E, ×160.

describe patients whose clinical manifestations represent an "overlap syndrome" of systemic lupus erythematosus, progressive sclerosis, and dermatopolymyositis, and the syndrome was strongly associated with the presence of antibodies to nuclear ribonuclear protein. In some patients, the clinical overlap may also include rheumatoid arthritis and Sjögren syndrome.[233]

The original description of MCT[232] made no reference to the pulmonary manifestations of the disease, but subsequent studies[234–237] have documented the frequent occurrence of lung involvement in MCT. A detailed prospective study of 34 patients with MCT by Sullivan et al.[234] diagnosed respiratory disease in 85%, whereas Prakash et al.,[236] in a retrospective analysis of 81 MCT patients, found pleuropulmonary manifestations in 25%.

The types of lung disease in MCT include pleuritis with effusion; interstitial pneumonitis, often involving the lower lung fields; and pulmonary hypertension similar to that of systemic lupus erythematosus and systemic sclerosis.[236–240] Respiratory muscle dysfunction does not appear to be a factor in MCT.[235] Unlike systemic lupus erythematosus, immune complexes have not been demonstrated in the pulmonary vascular disease of MCT patients.[238] The prognosis of pulmonary disease in MCT is variable; some cases are steroid responsive while others are steroid resistant and require treatment with cytotoxic agents.[238–240] Death from pulmonary vasculitis and plexogenic pulmonary hypertension (Fig. 21–19), although rare, has been well documented.[239,240]

Sjögren Syndrome

Sjögren syndrome is a chronic autoimmune inflammatory disease that affects mainly exocrine glands. Sjögren syndrome can occur alone (*primary Sjögren syndrome*), or in association with other autoimmune diseases, such as rheumatoid arthritis, systemic lupus erythematosus, and systemic sclerosis (*secondary Sjögren syndrome*).[241–243] A number of visceral organs, including the lungs, may be affected in primary or secondary Sjögren syndrome.[241] Pulmonary manifestations of Sjögren syndrome include small and large airway disease, pleuritis, interstitial pneumonia, alveolitis, lymphocytic interstitial pneumonitis, and lymphoma.[244–252] Occasionally, Sjögren lung disease may be associated with systemic, pulmonary, or cerebral vasculitis.[253,254]

The patients with Sjögren syndrome and lung disease were characterized by a number of immunologic serologic markers irrespective of the presence or type of associated connective tissue disorder. The commonest found were speckled antinuclear antibody, antibodies to the acidic nuclear antigen B, increased serum DNA binding, raised levels of circulating immunoglobulins, high titers of rheumatoid factor, and circulating soluble immune complexes.[244,245] Pulmonary function tests showed a restrictive ventilatory impairment or low diffusion capacity, or both, in almost all patients studied.[244–248]

A review of 343 patients with classic Sjögren syndrome seen at the Mayo Clinic revealed pulmonary involvement in 31 patients (9%); the types of involvement were diverse (Table 21–4).[244] Others have reported up to 15% of pulmonary involvement in Sjögren syndrome.[7] Diffuse interstitial lung disease, including lymphocytic interstitial pneumonitis (Fig. 21–20) was most common, followed by small and large airway obstruction, and desiccation of upper respiratory tract. It has been suggested that the lymphocytic interstitial pneumonitis is the consequence of Sjögren syndrome

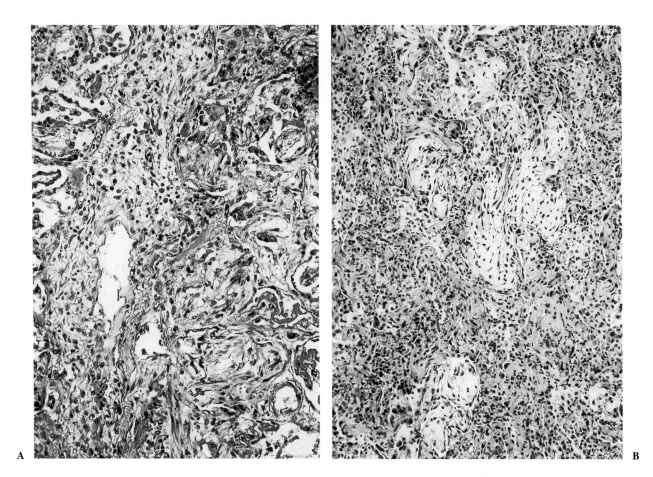

Fig. 21–17 A,B. Pulmonary manifestations of dermatopolymyositis. **A.** Diffuse alveolar damage progressing to fibrosing alveolitis. H and E, ×160. **B.** Bronchiolitis obliterans organizing pneumonia. H and E, ×160.

and that diffuse interstitial fibrosis is the result of associated connective disease,[7] but this has not been supported by either recent biopsy or bronchoalveolar lavage studies.[246–251] In a series of 50 patients with Sjögren syndrome and associated low- to high-grade non-Hodgkin's lymphoma seen at the Mayo Clinic, 10 (20%) had pulmonary involvement, and high-grade lymphomas were associated with increased mortality; 4 of the 10 patients died 8–48 months after the diagnosis of lymphoma.[252] As in pulmonary lymphomas in general, angioinvasion or "pulmonary vasculitis" (Fig. 21–21) is not uncommon in pulmonary lymphoma associated with Sjögren syndrome but it has no direct bearing on the prognosis.[252]

Ankylosing Spondylitis

Ankylosing spondylitis, like psoriatic arthritis and Reiter's disease, is an autoimmune disorder of the axial skeleton associated with the HLA phenotype HLA-B27,[255] which is found in 90% of ankylosing spondylitis patients.[255] Other hereditary or environmental factors are also important, because ankylosing spondylitis will develop in only 2% of HLA-B27-positive person and in 20% of HLA-B27-positive relatives of ankylosing spondylitis patients.[256]

The first description of lung disease in ankylosing spondylitis is often attributed to Hamilton,[257] but Dunham and Kautz[258] probably deserve this credit. Other descriptions of this association soon followed.[259–266] Pleuropulmonary manifestations of ankylosing spondylitis are uncommon. In a review of 2,080 patients with ankylosing spondylitis seen at the Mayo Clinic, Rosenow et al.[262] found only 28 patients (1.3%) with lung disease. The intrathoracic manifestations of ankylosing spondylitis are principally of two types: upper-lobe fibrobullous disease[259–266] and chest wall restriction.[267–270] Less frequently, organizing pneumonia, lymphocytic interstitial pneumonitis, and septal fibrosis have been observed,[265] as have fungal and mycobacterial infections.[262] Pulmonary manifestations usually appear late

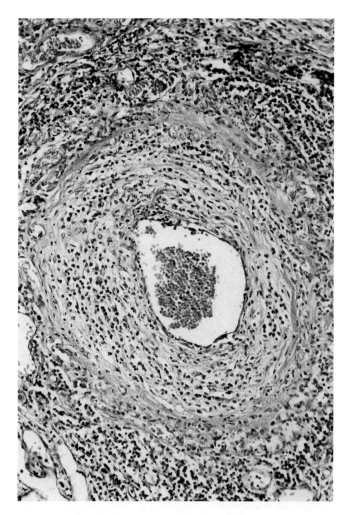

Fig. 21–18. Pulmonary vasculitis in dermatopolymyositis with lung involvement that occurs infrequently (5 in 65 autopsy cases[225]). H and E, ×160.

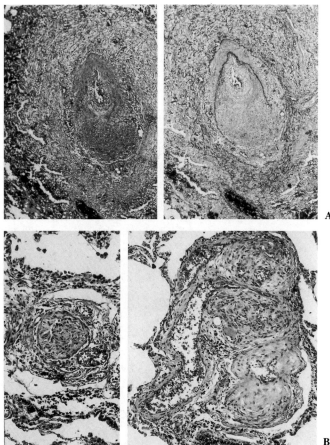

Fig. 21–19 A,B. A. Pulmonary vasculitis. H and E, ×64. **B.** Plexogenic pulmonary hypertension in fatal case of mixed connective tissue disease with lung involvement. H and E, ×160. Histologic features are indistinguishable from those of primary pulmonary hypertension.

in the disease when the inflammatory arthropathy has become quiescent.[266] The morphologic features of lung disease in ankylosing spondylitis are nonspecific. Upper-lobe bullae and honeycombing are the characteristic gross findings, and histologically interstitial fibrosis with epithelial metaplasia, chronic inflammatory infiltrate, mucus retention, and bronchiectasis are found.[259–272]

Relapsing Polychondritis

Relapsing polychondritis is an autoimmune disease often associated with other connective tissue disorders. The disease is characterized by episodic inflammation and destruction of cartilaginous structures such as ears,

Table 21–4. Pleuropulmonary manifestations of Sjögren syndrome[a]

Upper respiratory tract
    Atrophic rhinitis
    Xerostomia
Lower respiratory tract
    Pleuritis with and without effusions
    Tracheobronchitis
    Recurrent infectious (bronchitis, bronchiectasis and pneumonia)
    Pulmonary discoid atelectasis
    Diffuse interstitial fibrosis
    Lymphocytic interstitial pneumonitis
    Pseudolymphoma or lymphoma
    Pulmonary vasculitis
    Amyloidosis
Diaphragmatic/respiratory myopathy

[a] Modified from Strimlan et al.,[244] with permission.

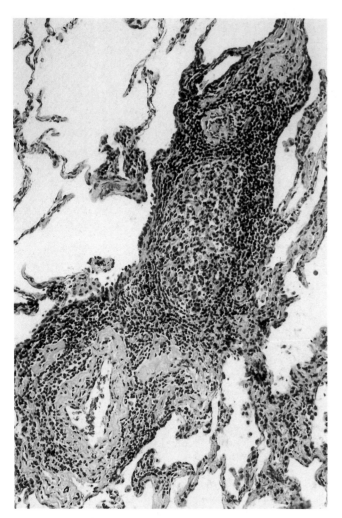

Fig. 21–20. Lymphocytic interstitial pneumonitis with prominent lymphoid follicle and germinal center in Sjögren syndrome lung disease. H and E, ×160.

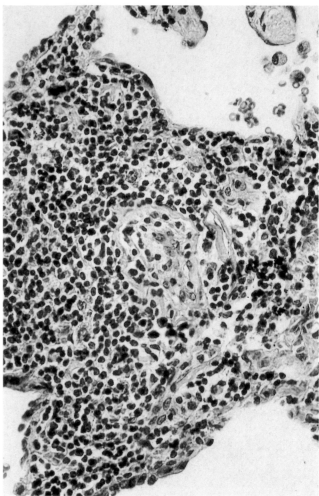

Fig. 21–21. Low-grade pulmonary lymphoma in Sjögren syndrome with characteristic angioinvasion of small blood vessels; distinguish from true vasculitis, which also occurs in Sjögren syndrome. H and E, ×400.

nose, larynx, trachea, and joints. Other tissue with high contents of glycosaminoglycans such as the heart, blood vessels, inner ear, cornea, and sclera also can be affected.[273–280] Although the term *relapsing polychondritis* was first introduced in 1960,[273] clinical cases of a similar type have been described as "polychondropathia" by Jaksch-Wartenhorst[281] in 1923 and as "chondromalacie" by Atherr[282] and von Meyerburg[283] in 1936. (See also Chapter 22).

Relapsing polychondritis is not quite as uncommon as it was once considered; at least 565 cases have been reported in the literature up to 1991.[280] In a study of 112 patients seen at one institution,[279] by using covariate analysis early manifestations of relapsing polychondritis were identified that predicted mortality. The 5- and 10-year probabilities of survival after diagnosis

were 74% and 55%, respectively. The most frequent causes of death were infection, systemic vasculitis, and malignancy. Although respiratory tract complications may occur at some point in about half of the patients with relapsing polychondritis,[277–288] only 10% of the deaths could be attributed to airway involvement.[279] The larynx, trachea, and bronchi may all be affected by fixed or dynamic obstruction with increased risk of pulmonary infection. Fixed obstruction is caused by inflammatory edema, fibrosis, or stricture formation. Dynamic obstruction is associated with the loss of cartilaginous support and large airway collapse and may vary with the respiratory cycle.[8] (See Fig. 22–21.)

Airway obstruction can be a serious complication of relapsing polychondritis and requires early recognition and aggressive treatment with immunosuppressive agents,[277,280,289-292] including oral corticosteroids and pulse methylprednosolone,[292] azothioprine or 6-mercaptopurine,[277] cyclophosphamide,[280] penicillamine,[291] and cyclosporin A.[277,289] Because humoral autoimmunity appears to be important in the pathogenesis of the disease, plasmapheresis may have a role in the management of these patients.[290] The lung parenchyma is seldom involved in relapsing polychondritis unless there is an associated connective tissue.

Summary and Conclusion

The rheumatic connective tissue diseases include a large and diverse group of systemic disorders that can affect the lung almost as frequently as the joints and muscles. Pleuropulmonary manifestations are often an important cause of morbidity and mortality in almost all rheumatic connective tissue diseases. For diagnostic purposes, histologic evidence is usually needed to document pulmonary involvement of the rheumatic diseases. For each of the major connective tissue disorders, certain characteristic pulmonary pathologic changes tend to predominate over others. In rheumatoid arthritis, it is interstitial fibrosis; in systemic lupus erythematosus, it is capillaritis and pulmonary vasculitis; in systemic sclerosis and the CREST variant, it is proliferative vascular disease and pulmonary hypertension; in Sjögren syndrome, it is lymphocytic interstitial pneumonitis and lymphoma; in dermato-polymyositis, it is diffuse alveolar damage and bronchiolitis obliterans; in mixed connective tissue disease, it is acute interstitial pneumonitis; in ankylosing spondylitis, it is upper lobe fibrosis; and in relapsing polychondritis, it is large and small airway obstruction. Although different connective tissue diseases may represent distinct clinical entities, considerable overlap in the histopathologic features of pulmonary manifestations exists among them, and apparently similar morphologic changes may respond in different manners to the same treatment regimen. Close and frequent communication between the clinician, radiologist, and pathologist is the key to success in the management of rheumatic disease patients with pulmonary involvement.

References

1. Klinge F. Der Rheumatismus. Pathologisch-anatomische und experimentell-pathologische Tatsachen und ihre Auswertung für das änztliche Rheumaproblem. Ergeb Allg Pathol 1933;27:1–351.
2. Klinge F. Zur pathologischen Anatomie des Rheumatismus. Verh Dtsch Orthop Ges 1934;28:44–50.
3. Klemperer P, Pollack AD, Baehr G. Diffuse collagen disease: Acute disseminated lupus erythematosus and diffuse scleroderma. JAMA 1942;119:331–332.
4. Klemperer P. The concept of collagen diseases. Am J Pathol 1950;26:505–519.
5. Banks BM. Is there a common denominator in scleroderma, dermatomyositis, disseminated lupus erythematosus, the Libman-Sack syndrome and polyarteritis nodosa? N Engl J Med 1941;225:433–444.
6. Rich AR. Hypersensitivity in disease, with special reference to periarteritis nodosa, rheumatic fever, disseminated lupus erythematosus and rheumatoid arthritis. Harvey Lect 1947;42:106–147.
7. Hunninghake GW, Fauci AS. Pulmonary involvement in the collagen vascular diseases. Am Rev Respir Dis 1979;119:471–503.
8. Boulware DW, Weissman DN, Doll NJ. Pulmonary manifestations of the rheumatic diseases. Clin Rev Allergy 1985;3:249–267.
9. Harmon KR, Leatherman JW. Respiratory manifestations of connective tissue disease. Semin Respir Infect 1988;3:258–273.
10. Wiedemann HP, Matthay RA. Pulmonary manifestations of collagen vascular disease. Clin Chest Med 1989;10:677–722.
11. Colby TV. Lung pathology. In: Cannon GW, Zimmerman GA, eds. The lung in rheumatic diseases. New York: Marcel Dekker, 1990:145–178.
12. Wise RA. Pulmonary complications in collagen-vascular disease. In: Lynch JP III, DeRemee RA, eds. Immunologically mediated pulmonary diseases. Philadelphia: JB Lippincott, 1991:40–88.
13. Eisenberg H. The interstitial lung diseases associated with the collagen-vascular disorders. Clin Chest Med 1982;3:565–578.
14. Coleman WP, III, Coleman WP, Derbes VJ, Jolly HW, Jr., Nesbitt LT, Jr. Collagen disease in children: A review of 71 cases. JAMA 1977;237:1095–1100.
15. Goldsmith DP. Neonatal rheumatic disorders: views of the pediatrician. Rheum Dis Clin North Am 1989;15:287–305.
16. Cannon GW. Pulmonary complications of antirheumatic drug therapy. Semin Arthritis Rheum 1990;19:353–364.
17. Walker Smith GJ. The histopathology of pulmonary reactions to drugs. Clin Chest Med 1990;11:95–117.
18. Wall CP, Gaensler EA, Carrington CB, Hayes JA. Comparison of transbronchial and open biopsies in chronic infiltrative lung disease. Am Rev Respir Dis 1981;123:280–285.
19. Nagata N, Hirano H, Takayama K, Miyagawa Y, Shigematsu N. Step section preparation of transbronchial lung biopsy. Chest 1991;100:959–962.
20. Gaensler EA, Carrington CB. Open biopsy for chronic diffuse infiltrative lung disease: clinical, roentgenographic and physiological correlation in 502 patients. Ann Thorac Surg 1980;30:411–426.
21. Meduri GU, Stover DE, Greeno RA, Nash T, Zaman MB. Bilateral bronchoalveolar lavage in the diagnosis of

opportunistic pulmonary infections. Chest 1991; 100:1272–1276.

22. Jansen HM, Schutte AJ, van der Giessen M, The TH. Immunoglobulin classes in local immune complexes recovered by bronchoalveolar lavage in collagen vascular diseases. Lung 1984;162:287–296.

23. Rossi GA, Bitterman PB, Rennard SI, Ferrans VJ, Crystal RG. Evidence for chronic inflammation as a component of the interstitial lung disease associated with progressive systemic sclerosis. Am Rev Respir Dis 1985;131:612–617.

24. Garcia JGN, Wolven RG, Garcia PL, Keogh BA. Assessment of interlobar variation of bronchoalveolar lavage cellular differentials in interstitial lung diseases. Am Rev Respir Dis 1986;133:444–449.

25. Chamberlain DW, Braude AC, Rebuck AS. A critical evaluation of bronchoalveolar lavage: criteria for identifying unsatisfactory specimens. Acta Cytol 1987; 31:599–605.

26. Stoller JK, Rankin JA, Reynolds HY. The impact of bronchoalveolar lavage cell analysis on clinicians' diagnostic reasoning about interstitial lung disease. Chest 1987;92:839–943.

27. Turner-Warwick M, Haslam P. The value of serial bronchoalveolar lavages in assessing the clinical progress of patients with cryptogenic fibrosing alveolitis. Am Rev Respir Dis 1987;135:26–34.

28. Reynolds HY. Bronchoalveolar lavage. Am Rev Respir Dis 1987;135:250–263.

29. Siemsen JK, Grebe SF, Waxman AD. The use of gallium-67 in pulmonary disorders. Semin Nucl Med 1978;8:235–249.

30. Line BR, Fulmer JD, Reynolds HY, et al. Gallium-67 citrate scanning in the staging of idiopathic pulmonary fibrosis: correlation with physiologic and morphologic features and bronchoalveolar lavage. Am Rev Respir Dis 1978;118:355–365.

31. Greene NB, Solinger AJ, Baughman RP. Patients with collagen-vascular disease and dyspnea: The value of gallium scanning and bronchoalveolar lavage in predicting response to steroid therapy and clinical outcome. Chest 1987;91:698–703.

32. Elstad MR. Lung biopsy, bronchoalveolar lavage, and gallium scanning. In: Cannon GW, Zimmerman GA, eds. The lung in rheumatic diseases. New York: Marcel Dekker, 1990:117–143.

33. Ellman P, Cudkowicz L. Pulmonary manifestations in the diffuse collagen diseases. Thorax 1954;9:46–57.

34. Von Glahn WC, Pappenheimer AM. Specific lesions of peripheral blood vessels in rheumatism. Am J Pathol 1926;2:235–250.

35. Massumi RA, Legier JF. Rheumatic pneumonitis. Circulation 1966;33:417–425.

36. Gouley BA. The evolution of the parenchymal lung lesions in rheumatic fever and their relationship to mitral stenosis and passive congestion. Am J Med Sci 1938;196:1–10.

37. Muirhead EE, Haley AE. Rheumatic pneumonitis: A case of widespread chronic (proliferative) type with acute (exudative) foci. Arch Intern Med 1947;80:328–342.

38. Garrod AB. The great practical importance of separating rheumatoid arthritis from gout. Lancet 1982; ii:1033–1037.

39. Ellman P, Ball RE. "Rheumatoid disease" with joint and pulmonary manifestations. Lancet 1948;ii:816–820.

40. Petty TL, Wilkins M. The five manifestations of rheumatoid lung. Dis Chest 1966;49:75–82.

41. Walker WC, Wright V. Pulmonary lesions and rheumatoid arthritis. Medicine (Baltimore) 1968;47:501–502.

42. Scadding JG. The lungs in rheumatoid arthritis. Proc R Soc Med 1969;62:227–238.

43. Strimlan CV, Rosenow EC, III, Weiland LH, Brown LR. Lymphocytic interstitial pneumonitis: Review of 13 cases. Ann Intern Med 1978;88:616–621.

44. Epler GR, Suider GL, Gaensler EA, Cathcart ES, Fitzgerald MX, Carrington CB. Bronchiolitis and bronchitis in connective tissue disease. JAMA 1979;242:528–532.

45. Cervantes-Perez P, Toro-Perez AH, Rodriguez-Jurado P. Pulmonary involvement in rheumatoid arthritis. JAMA 1980;243:1715–1719.

46. Herzog CA, Miller RR, Hoidal JR. Bronchiolitis and rheumatoid arthritis. Am Rev Respir Dis 1981;124:636–639.

47. Yousem SA, Colby TR, Carrington CB. Lung biopsy in rheumatoid arthritis. 1985;131:770–777.

48. Hakala M, Pääkko P, Huhti E, Tarkka M, Sutinen S. Open lung biopsy of patients with rheumatoid arthritis. Clin Rheumatol 1990;9:452–460.

49. Turner-Warwick M, Evans RC. Pulmonary manifestations of rheumatoid disease. Clin Rheum Dis 1977; 3:549–564.

50. MacFarlane JD, Dieppe PA, Rigden BG, Clark TJ. Pulmonary pleural lesions in rheumatoid disease. Br J Dis Chest 1978;72:288–300.

51. Popper MS, Bogdonoff ML, Hughes RI. Interstitial rheumatoid lung disease. Chest 1972;62:243–249.

52. Frank ST, Weg JG, Harkelroad LE, Fitch RF. Pulmonary dysfunction in rheumatoid disease. Chest 1973;63:27–34.

53. Laitinen O, Nissila M, Salorinne Y, Aalto P. Pulmonary involvement in patients with rheumatoid arthritis. Scand J Respir Dis 1975;56:297–304.

54. Geddes DM, Webley M, Emerson PA. Airway obstruction in rheumatoid arthritis. Ann Rheum Dis 1979; 38:222–225.

55. Hill EA, Davies S, Geary M. Frequency dependence of dynamic compliance in patients with rheumatoid arthritis. Thorax 1979;34:755–761.

56. Epler GR, McLoud TC, Gaensler EA, Mikus JP, Carrington CB. Normal chest roentgenograms in chronic diffuse infiltrative lung disease. N Engl J Med 1978;298:934–939.

57. Patterson CD, Harville WE, Pierce JA. Rheumatoid lung disease. Ann Intern Med 1965;62:685–697.

58. Martel W, Abell MR, Mikkelsen WM, Whitehouse WM. Pulmonary and pleural lesions in rheumatoid disease. Radiology 1968;90:641–653.

59. Walker WC, Wright V. Diffuse interstitial pulmonary fibrosis and rheumatoid arthritis. Ann Rheum Dis 1969;28:252–259.

60. Cruickshank B. Interstitial pneumonia and its consequences in rheumatoid disease. Br J Dis Chest 1959;53:226–236.

61. Baggenstoss AH, Rosenberg EF. Visceral lesions associated with chronic infectious (rheumatoid) arthritis. Arch Pathol 1943;35:503–516.

62. Walker WC, Wright V. Rheumatoid pleuritis. Ann Rheum Dis 1967;26:467–474.

63. Shiel WC, Jr., Prete PE. Pleuropulmonary manifestations of rheumatoid arthritis. Semin Arthritis Rheum 1984;13:235–243.

64. Jurik AG, Davidsen D, Graudal H. Prevalence of pulmonary involvement in rheumatoid arthritis and its relationship to some characteristics of the patients: A radiological and clinical study. Scand J Rheumatol 1982;11:217–224.

65. Sahn SA, Kaplan RL, Maulitz RM, Good JT. Rheumatoid pleurisy, observations on the development of low pleural fluid pH and glucose level. Arch Intern Med 1980;140:1237–1238.

66. Patterson T, Klockars M, Hellstrom PE. Chemical and immunological features of pleural effusion: comparison between rheumatoid arthritis and other diseases. Thorax 1982;37:354–361.

67. Faurschou P. Decreased glucose in RA cell-positive pleural effusion, correlation of pleural glucose, lactic dehydrogenase and protein concentration to the presence of RA cells. Eur J Respir Dis 1984;65:272–277.

68. Faurschou P, Francis D, Faarup P. Thoracoscopic, histological and clinical findings in nine cases of rheumatoid pleural effusion. Thorax 1985;40:371–375.

69. Champion GD, Robertson MR, Robinson RG. Rheumatoid pleurisy and pericarditis. Ann Rheum Dis 1968; 27:521–530.

70. Aru A, Engel U, Francis D. Characteristic and specific histological findings in rheumatoid pleurisy. Acta Pathol Microbiol Immunol Scand Sect A (Suppl) 1986;94:57–62.

71. Wells WC. On rheumatism of the heart. Trans Soc Improv Med Chirug Knowl 1812;3:373–424.

72. Osler W, McCrae T, eds. Modern medicine: Its theory and practice. New York: Lea & Febiger 1909:501–509, 534–536.

73. Duthie JJR, Brown PE, Truelove LH, et al. Course and prognosis in rheumatoid arthritis: A further report. Ann Rheum Dis 1964;23:193–204.

74. Gordon DA, Stein JL, Broder I. The extra-articular features of rheumatoid arthritis: A systematic analysis of 127 cases. Am J Med 1973;54:445–452.

75. Benedek TG. Subcutaneous nodules and the differentiation of rheumatoid arthritis from rheumatic fever. Semin Arthritis Rheum 1984;13:305–321.

76. Eraut D, Evans J, Caplan M. Pulmonary necrobiotic nodules without rheumatoid arthritis. Br J Dis Chest 1978;72:301–306.

77. Hull S, Mathews JA. Pulmonary necrobiotic nodules as a presenting feature of rheumatoid arthritis. Ann Rheum Dis 1982;41:21–24.

78. Nusslein HG, Rodl W, Giedel J, Missmahl M, Kalden JR. Multiple peripheral pulmonary nodules preceding rheumatoid arthritis. Rheumatol Int 1987;7:89–91.

79. Baumer HM, Van Belle CJ. Pulmonary nodules in rheumatoid arthritis. Respiration 1972;29:556–563.

80. Kaye B, Kaye R, Bobrove A. Rheumatoid nodules: Review of the spectrum of associated conditions and proposal of a new classification, with a report of four seronegative cases. Am J Med 1984;76:279–292.

81. Burrows FG. Pulmonary nodules in rheumatoid disease: A report of two cases. Br J Radiol 1967;40:256–261.

82. Johnson TS, White P, Weiss ST, et al. Endobronchial necrobiotic nodule antedating rheumatoid arthritis. Chest 1982;82:199–200.

83. Ellman P, Cudkowicz L, Elwood JS. Widespread serous membrane involvements by rheumatoid nodules. J Clin Pathol 1954;7:239–244.

84. Walters MN, Ojeda VJ. Pleuropulmonary necrobiotic rheumatoid nodules: A review and clinicopathologic study of six patients. Med J Aust 1986;144:648–651.

85. Ziff M. The rheumatoid nodule. Arthritis Rheum 1990;33:761–767.

86. Crisp AJ, Armstrong RD, Graham R, Dussek JE. Rheumatoid lung, pneumothorax and eosinophilia. Ann Rheum Dis 1982;41:137–140.

87. Yue CC, Park CH, Kushner I. Apical fibrocavitary lesions of the lung in rheumatoid arthritis: Report of two cases and review of the literature. Am J Med 1986;81:741–746.

88. McConnochie K, O'Sullivan M, Khalil JF, Pritchard MH, Gibbs AR. Aspergillus colonization of pulmonary rheumatoid nodule. Respir Med 1989;83:157–160.

89. Pillemer SR, Webb D, Yocum DE. Legionnaire's disease in a patient with rheumatoid arthritis treated with cyclosporin. J Rheumatol 1989;16:117–120.

90. Watkin SW, Bucknall RC, Nisar M, Agnew RA. Atypical mycobacterial infection of the lung in rheumatoid arthritis. Ann Rheum Dis 1989;48:336–338.

91. Caplan A. Certain radiological appearances in the chest of coal miners suffering from rheumatoid arthritis. Thorax 1953;8:29–37.

92. Caplan A, Payne RB, Withey JL. A broader concept of Caplan's syndrome related to rheumatoid factors. Thorax 1962;17:205–212.

93. Benedik TG. Rheumatoid pneumoconiosis. Am J Med 1973;55:515–524.

94. Crystal RG, Rennard S. Pulmonary connective tissue and environmental lung disease. Chest 1981;80(1):33S–38S.

95. Sluis-Cremer GK. Respiratory manifestation of rheumatoid arthritis. S Afr Med J 1970;44:843–846.

96. Wagner JC. Pulmonary fibrosis and mineral dusts. Ann Rheum Dis 1977;36(Suppl):42–46.

97. Roschmann RA, Rothenberg RJ. Pulmonary fibrosis in rheumatoid arthritis: A review of clinical features and therapy. Semin Arthritis Rheum 1987;16:174–185.

98. Wagener JS, Taussig LM, DeBenedetti C, et al. Pulmo-

CHAPTER 22

Metabolic and Other Diseases

DAVID H. DAIL

The entities discussed in this chapter are diverse. Many come under the heading of metabolic diseases, which may be congenital or acquired. Others are, or act through, an immunologic basis. A few have a single identifiable cause. Some represent a common tissue response to multiple identified causes, while others appear to have no known cause.

For the sake of discussion, these entities are organized roughly into anatomic compartments, starting with those of the tracheobronchial system, continuing into the pulmonary interstitium, and ending with diseases involving intraavelolar bodies and macrophages. Some cross over these anatomic designations, as in the case of amyloid, which presents as tracheobronchial, or parenchymal, (nodular, or diffuse interstitial) disease. Some, such as Goodpasture's disease or primary hemosiderosis, obviously affect one compartment, but are most noted for secondary involvement of another area, as with alveolar hemorrhage in these two examples. Some are solely lung diseases and others are pulmonary components of systemic diseases. Some readers may think different components of this chapter belong elsewhere in this book; however, for various reasons these are presented or reviewed here while referring to discussions elsewhere as appropriate.

Tracheobronchial Abnormalities

The entities covered in this part of the chapter consist of relapsing polychondritis or chondromalacia, tracheobronchopathia osteochondroplastica, tracheomegaly, tracheal stenosis, lipoid proteinosis, and various pigments in bronchial mucosa. Mucoviscidosis is covered in Chapters 5 and 7. Amyloid will serve as a transition from this compartment to the next group, those principally involving the interstitium.

Relapsing Polychondritis

This is a rare disease affecting cartilage but also other tissues with a high glycosaminoglycan content, specifically, sclera, cornea, aorta, and noncartilaginous ear parts.[1] It was first described by Jaksch-Wartenhorst[2] in 1923 under the name "polychondropathia." In 1960, Pearson and associates[3] suggested the name used in this section. A nice review of 23 personal cases with literature review of 136 other cases was published by Mc-Adam et al.,[4] and many of the following comments are based on this review. In addition to the histologic confirmation of chondritis from some site, these authors proposed criteria of which at least three are usually present. These include: (1) recurrent chondritis of both auricles; (2) nonerosive seronegative inflammatory polyarthritis; (3) nasal chondritis; (4) ocular inflammation; (5) chondritis of the respiratory tract; and (6) cochlear and/or vestibular damage. Tissue for histologic confirmation of chondritis is most often obtained from biopsies of the ear, nose, or respiratory tract.

This disease is episodic, but generally progressive, with each episode leading to more severe damage. The first episode is usually the most severe individual episode. This disease entity affects both sexes equally and involves all ages, but is most prevalent in the 20- to 70-year-old period, with many cases in the 40- to 60-year-old range and an average age in the early forties. About half the cases begin with chondritis of the auricles followed by migratory arthritis. Nasal, ocular, and respiratory chondritis each account for about an equal number of presentations following these. The best-

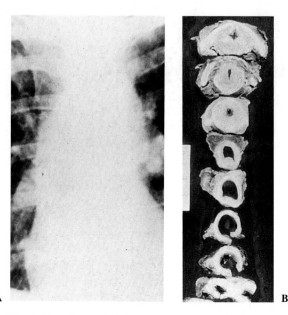

Fig. 22–1. Chondromalacia. **A.** Radiograph shows absence of tracheal air shadow. **B.** Cross-sectioned trachea shows narrowing caused by collapse. (Courtesy AA Liebow Pulmonary Pathology Collection, San Diego, California.)

described onset is in the external ear, where the disease starts suddenly with marked redness, swelling, and tenderness. The patient is hesitant to lie on, or to have other pressure against, the involved area. The inflammation usually subsides in 5–10 days with or without therapy. Approximately 30% of cases have an associated "autoimmune" disease that often precedes the chondritis itself.

Most often, early respiratory symptoms center on the larynx, with hoarseness being most marked. Some present with stridor, asthma-like dyspnea, and cough resulting from flaccidity of the larynx, trachea, and bronchi. Eventually some 56% of patients have laryngeal and/or tracheal chondritis that most often results in tracheal stenosis (Fig. 22–1). usually diffuse but also focal.

Histologically the first apparent effect is a loss of acid mucopolysaccharides in the matrix of the cartilage, with loss of its normal basophilia and replacement by a degree of eosinophilia. Perichondrial inflammation with lymphocytes and plasma cells follows, with eventual replacement of cartilage by fibrous tissue (Figs. 22–2 and 22–3). The border between the cartilage and connective tissue becomes indistinct. Chondrocytes become vacuolated and pyknotic with eventual loss of cell and lacunar outline. Dystrophic ossification may occur (Fig. 22–4), but does not provide support in the same manner as does native cartilage. Linck et al.[5] noted that the cartilage near the areas of damage has a normal

appearance, with normal basophilia, glycogen content, and elastic fiber configuration. There are, however, a few empty lacunae in these surrounding areas. Electron microscopy on ear cartilage shows progressive signs of cell death of both chondrocytes and perichondral cells.[5]

Strictly speaking, the term "tracheomalacia" covers any cause of softening of the trachea; this spectrum is covered in Chapter 7 (see **tracheomalacia** and **tracheobronchomegaly**). Iatrogenic causes have particular importance, especially in the immature neonate (see **tracheomalacia,** Chapter 8). In the setting of generalized polychondritis in the adult, respiratory tract involvement in the trachea may be focal, but is more often diffuse. In this disease the trachea becomes soft (tracheomalacia) because of dissolution of cartilage; therefore the tracheal diameter shrinks, and at times may approach collapse with resulting disappearance of tracheal air shadow on chest radiographs, wheezing-type symptoms, and current pneumonias. Fifty-nine percent of persons with relapsing polychondritis die a respiratory death.[4] Those cases initially presenting with respiratory tract involvement have a worse prognosis, needing tracheostomy more often (11 of 14, or 79%) and dying more frequently, than those presenting with extrapulmonary chondritis who later develop respiratory chondritis necessitating tracheostomy (15 of 58, or 28%).[4]

As Neild and associates[6] have pointed out, the lack of a family history, peak incidence in middle age, and patchy involvement suggest an acquired disease rather than a congenital disease. Immunologic studies do not show consistent circulating anticartilage antibodies. Valenzuela and associates[7] have shown granular deposits of immunoglobulin and C3 component of complement at the chondrofibrous junction, suggesting a possible specific test for this disease.

Subglottic involvement of the trachea is seen in 15% of cases of Wegener's granulomatosis cases with head and neck involvement (see Chapter 30, Table 30–2). This disease may also involve bronchial cartilage[8] and is distinguished from chondromalacia in that more widespread involvement of vasculitis and necrotizing granulomatosis, lack of auricular chondritis, and presence of antineutrophilic cytoplasmic antibodies (ANCA) are found in Wegener's granulomatosis. Other etiologies such as radiation therapy should be distinguished by history and localization of radiation fields. Likewise, lung transplantation damage to cartilage[9] should be in a narrow segment corresponding to the surgical anastamosis. Bronchocentric granulomatosis (BCG) injures cartilage but does so more in relationship to mucosal disease. BCG also does not typically involve the trachea (see Chapters 16 and 30).

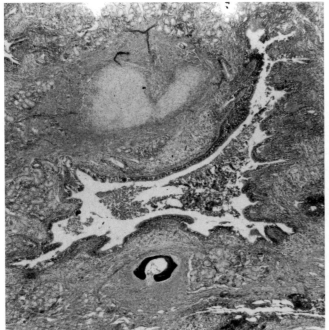

22-2

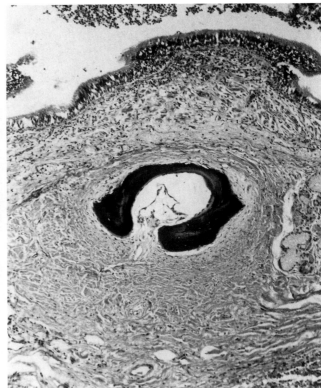

22-4

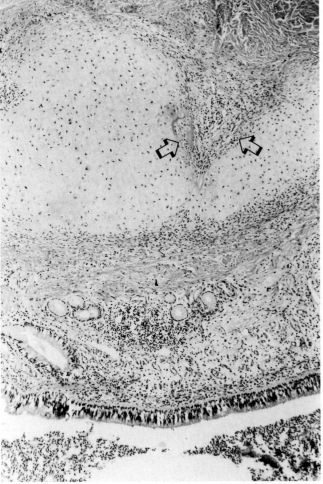

22-3

Fig. 22–2. Chondromalacia. Bronchus shows loss of support, with collapse. Note paucity of cartilage for bronchus of this size. H and E, ×25.

Fig. 22–3. Chondromalacia. Higher power view of upper part of bronchus shown in Fig. 22–2. Cartilage is being replaced by inflammatory, vascular, and fibrous tissue. One wedge (*arrows*) is deeply erosive, but similar reaction is present around much of remaining cartilage. H and E, ×250.

Fig. 22–4. Chondromalacia. Higher power view of Fig. 22–2, opposite that shown in Fig. 22–3, shows dystrophic calcification and mature collagen totally replacing once-present cartilage. H and E, ×250.

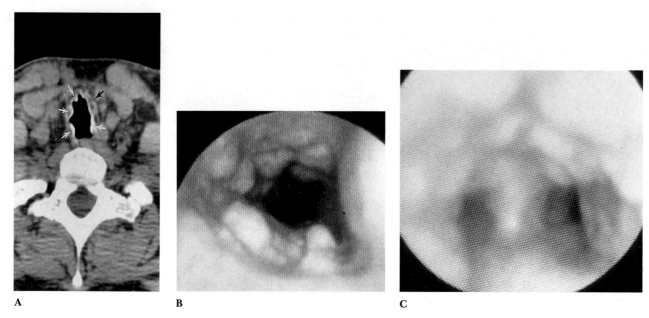

A   **B**   **C**

Fig. 22–5 A–C. Tracheobronchopathia osteochondroplastica. **A.** CT scan shows calcified nodules protruding into tracheal air space (*white arrows*). *Black arrow* indicates area of more generalized thickening. **B,C.** Bronchoscopy picture of same case shows impressive excrescences in (**B**) trachea and (**C**) carina. (**B,C.** Contributed by Dr. Ken Casey, Virginia Mason Clinic, Seattle, Washington.)

Tracheobronchopathia Osteochondroplastica

The histology of this disease was originally described by Wilks in 1857,[10] although several other authors were mentioning it in their clinical findings in the preceding several years.[11] It was originally named tracheopathia osteoplastica in 1910[12] but its name has been modified as just mentioned because it also involves the bronchi and proliferation of not only bone but cartilage. It is distinguished from senile osseous metaplasia of cartilaginous rings by its degree of proliferation and extent beyond the original tracheal cartilaginous rings.

Obtaining the true incidence of this disease is difficult. In the past, as reviewed by Nienhuis et al.[11] and Prakash et al.,[13] more than 90% were incidental findings at autopsy. Dalgaard[14] reported 90 cases up to 1947, and by 1974 the largest recent series of 26 cases was added to the 219 cases in the literature for a total of 245 cases.[15] The incidence in bronchoscopies varies between none in 25,000[16] to 5 in 3,500.[17] In another series of 1,500 bronchoscopies,[18] 25 cases had bronchoscopy for refractory cough, and 7 of those had identifiable diseases in which tracheobronchopathia osteoplastica was identified in 2, an incidence of 29%. Prakash et al.[13] estimated a good working average is 1 case per 2,000 bronchoscopies. As reviewed by Nienhuis et al.,[11] the bronchoscopic appearance has been given various descriptions including rock garden, stalactite cave, cobblestoned appearance, or veritable mountainscape (Fig. 22–5). More cases are likely to be discovered with more frequent bronchoscopies and with better imaging techniques. Tomography shows a typical scalloped or beaded appearance and CT scans accentuate the calcification, which is often inapparent by routine chest radiograph (Fig. 22–5). In one series[11] some 35% were suggested by laryngoscopy alone. It is a disease that is typically been strongly male predominant, but several series have reported more women.[13,19] It usually involves patients over the age of 50, but the youngest was reported as age 12.[20] This is a very slowly progressive disease, as we do not know its starting point. The older age spectrum may reflect the time of death rather than the time of onset.[13]

Symptoms include dry throat, dry cough, changes in voice, moderate dyspnea, hemoptysis, wheezing, and sometimes recurrent obstructive effects. Right-middle-lobe collapse has been attributed to this disease.[21]

The osseous, often cartilaginous overgrowths appear to begin in or adjacent to cartilaginous rings.[22] The disease is most striking in the area of preexistent tracheal cartilage, and often spares the trachealis muscle posteriorly,[11] although exceptions with total encasement do occur.[15] The epithelium overlying these nodules is usually intact, metaplastic, and sometimes dysplastic or ulcerated. Microscopically benign bony and cartilaginous growths replace the submucosa of the bronchus and crowd out bronchial glands. Bone marrow may be present in some of the bony portions.

Biopsing such hard nodules may be difficult. Laser bronchoscopy helps clear obstruction when necessary. The disease appears to progress quite slowly. Radiation has been used occasionally, but without dramatic response.

Some believe this is an end stage of tracheobronchial amyloid,[23–25] and indeed some cases do appear to have this relationship (see following section). Other cases must have other etiologies because some 200 cases were described by 1972 while only about 30 cases of all forms of respiratory tracheobronchial amyloid had been described by that time.[23] Only 2 of 14 cases of Hui's series[26] of tracheobronchial amyloid have osseus metaplasia. Other theories of genesis, reviewed by Martin[15] and Neinhuis et al.,[11] include benign neoplasias (enchondroses and exostoses) and genetic anomalies, degenerative or metabolic processes, inflammatory, chemical, or mechanical irritation, and metaplasia of elastic tissue. As these conditions are only rarely associated with calcifications outside the chest, they probably represent background incidence alone.[13]

Tracheobronchomegaly

This entity can be congenital, or at least evident in early life, when it is called Mounier–Kuhn syndrome (see Chapter 7). It has occurred in several cases of Ehler–Danlos syndrome,[27] suggesting it may be related to poor elastic support, or perhaps to loss of other support such as in chondromalacia. It occurs in adults, mostly in men in their thirties and forties, and can be acquired later in life secondary to a number of inflammatory conditions affecting the trachea, such as chronic bronchitis secondary to tobacco abuse, cystic fibrosis, trauma, emphysema, or pulmonary fibrosis.

A good review and an intriguing study of various pulmonary fibrotic reactions associated with this entity was reported by Woodring et al.[27] They evaluated tracheal diameters on plain films in a series of 34 cases of fibrotic lung reactions, and enlargement of the trachea was present in 10 (29%). The associated lung diseases were idiopathic pulmonary fibrosis in 4, sarcoid in 4, and chronic progressive histoplasmosis in 2. In 7 of these cases the tracheomegaly progressed with time, and a similar progression was seen even in 9 of 24 (38%) of those without tracheomegaly by strict measurements. These changes were usually associated with moderate-to-severe restrictive pulmonary defects, and it was proposed that shrinkage of the lung tissue retracts all adjacent spaces including trachea in a manner similar to bronchectasis within the lung (see Chapter 5).

The dilatation from whatever cause may extend into the bronchial tree, and therefore the name tracheobronchomegaly is given. In the lungs it may give the appearance of bronchectiasis, and in either bronchi or lungs drainage and infection are complications which may in themselves may induce secondary bronchectiasis.[27]

Tracheal Stenosis

This condition may occur in either an extended or focal segment of the trachea. With extended disease, it is more often related to generalized disease such as chondromalacia or secondary to pulmonary diseases described previously. Intubation is a common iatrogenic cause for focal disease, as is malignancy. Endophytic malignancy is often difficult to diagnose and is not very common in the trachea (see Chapter 33), but extrinsic compression in the mediastinum or lung by tumor, infections, fibrosis, vascular anomalies, or other space-occupying lesions may compress the trachea. Primary diseases causing this are discussed in other sections; when biopsies are obtained of nonspecific inflammation of fibrosis, correlation with the clinical setting and radiographic findings is advisable.

Lipoid Proteinosis

Care must be taken not to confuse this entity with pulmonary alveolar (phospholipo)proteinosis. Lipoid proteinosis presents mainly with skin, upper respiratory tract, and oral cavity involvement, and has also been called "hyalinosis (or lipidosis) cutis et mucosae" or Urbach–Wiethe syndrome. It was originally described in 1929 by the authors for whom the syndrome is named.[28] Visceral involvement has been summarized by Caplan.[29] Often internal viscera have only mild perivascular or perineural deposits, and almost any site may be involved, including the lung. Occasionally the trachea and bronchi may be extensively involved in a manner similar to the larynx and oropharynx. Submucosal deposits may also occur in the esophagus, especially toward its upper end. There may be intraocular involvement, and peculiar hippocampal calcification may be accompanied by epilepsy.

The disease follows an autosomal-recessive inheritance pattern, and the deposited substance is a lipoglycoprotein that has not been further characterized. Lipid and PAS stains outline these deposits. Lipid stains on frozen section material are more sensitive than PAS stains on permanent sections for detecting such small deposits.

The disease frequently presents in infancy, typically as a child with a weak cry, or in childhood as persistent hoarseness followed by progressive skin involvement. Usually the disease is noted by age 20 years if it is to become clinically significant. The patient seen by the

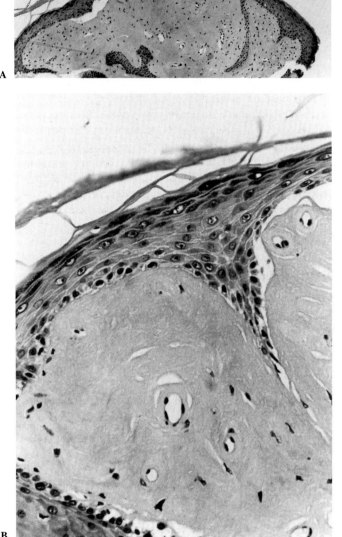

Fig. 22–6 A,B. Lipoid proteinosis. Biopsy of carina shows **(A)** surface squamous metaplasia replacing respiratory mucosa and dense submucosal infiltrate of hyalinized substance, which in **(B)** also infiltrates vessel walls. **A,** H and E, ×100; **B,** H and E, ×400.

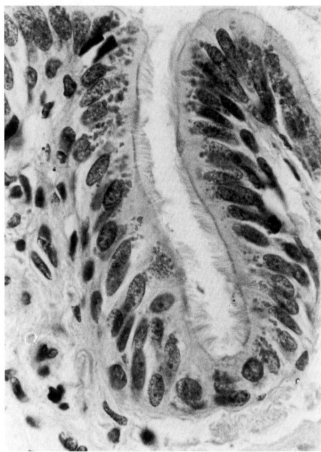

Fig. 22–7. Lipochrome. Bronchial wall shows many small to medium-sized golden-yellow supranuclear inclusions, which stain as lipochrome. Note cilia on surface of many of involved cells. Goblet cells are not clearly seen. H and E, ×100.

author (Fig. 22–6) had an emergency tracheostomy at age 17 for unknown circumstances; a permanent tracheostomy was placed at age 58, and the biopsy of his carina as illustrated was taken at age 70. Repeat bronchoscopy at age 72 (in 1986) showed persistent grey-pink nodules throughout the trachea, involving the midlateral and posterior extent and extending from the tracheostomy site ot the carina. These were as seen 2 year previously and persisted without significant

change. Previous examination of his oropharynx had shown multiple "cobblestone"-type lesions, and his skin was involved with plaques. Biopsy of the skin showed changes quite similar to those illustrated in the carina. In 1985, a 1.2-cm, poorly differentiated carcinoma with mixed glandular and neuroendocrine features was found in his left-upper lobe, and the patient died of disseminated lung cancer in 1988 at age 74.

Pigment in Bronchial Mucosa

Incidental lipochrome is occasionally observed in bronchial mucosal cells (Fig. 22–7), and occurs without other associations. It is usually composed of variously sized, tan-to-golden, round-to-oval inclusions between the nuclei and borders of ciliated respiratory lining cells. It stains as does lipofuscin elsewhere. Some distinguish subtle differences in the terms "lipofuscin," "lipochrome," and "ceroid,"[30] while others consider them part of a spectrum of PAS-positive, acid-fast, lipid degradation products usually located in lysosomes. (Also see Hamazaki–Wesenberg bodies in sarcoid granulomata, Chapter 19, and Hermansky–Pudlak syndrome at the end of this chapter.)

Melanin might theoretically be found in normal bronchial mucosa, but none has been described.[31] It has been described next to bronchial melanomas, where it has been termed "the melanoma flare".[32,33] It may occur in pulmonary carcinoid tumors (see Chapter 32) and possibly in perivertebral melanotic schwannomas arising in the posterior mediastinum.[34]

Amyloid

Various classifications for both systemic and pulmonary amyloid have been proposed. The most generally accepted one for systemic amyloid, by Reiman in 1935,[35] consists of primary, secondary, multiple myeloma-associated, and senile types.

Primary amyloid is that which occurs without known cause or association. This term should not be used for localized involvement of one organ by amyloid. Primary amyloid is type AL (see following), derived from immunoglobulin light chain, and therefore is usually (some authors say always[36]) associated with monoclonal plasma cell proliferations. In those not so associated, Isobe and Osserman[37] suspected that most such cases may be associated with unrecognized plasma cell dyscrasias, although unproven by current techniques.

The lungs were involved in primary systemic amyloidosis, in different series, in 36%,[38] 44%,[39] 88%,[40] 91%,[41] and 92%.[42] In one series, Celli and associates[42] showed prominent alveolar septal deposits in 11 of 12 cases of primary systemic amyloid, of which 4 had accompanying pulmonary symptoms; in 1 of these, the pulmonary involvement was severe enough to have been the cause of death. The degree of lung involvement in primary amyloidosis is always worse than in the secondary amyloidosis.

A well-studied series of 153 primary systemic amyloidosis cases by Gertz and Kyle[36] contained an unusually low incidence of pulmonary involvement (1.5%). This series excluded overt myeloma cases and cases with only carpal tunnel syndrome from consideration. The lungs were involved in secondary systemic amyloidosis in 1%,[40] 10%,[43] 20%,[44] 50%,[41] 71%,[42] and 73%.[45] The associated diseases in secondary cases now are most often rheumatoid arthritis, chronic osteomyelitis, and malignancies. Now that more patients with mucovisidosis are living to adulthood, cases of secondary amyloid in this group are being described.[46] In the past, chronic tuberculosis and other chronic suppurative diseases such as bronchiectasis were more prevalent than today, and accounted for more cases of secondary amyloid.

With better antibiotic therapy, the overall incidence of secondary systemic amyloid in these cases is decreasing.[40] In parts of the world, secondary amyloid is common in leprosy patients.[47] When amyloid is found, its possible relationship with multiple myeloma should always be considered.

Senile amyloid is mild, occurs most frequently as an incidental finding in patients over the age of 80, and is estimated to occur in approximately 10% of those over 80 years of age and 50% of those over 90 years of age. Lung involvement parallels heart involvement and is usually without serious symptoms.[48]

Involvement of the lung in the various forms of systemic amyloid is usually in the diffuse interstitial form as detailed in following sections. Occasionally, nodular amyloid is associated with systemic involvement.[49,50] Several good reviews of lung involvement in systemic disease are available.[40–42,51] Before more thoroughly discussing the forms of pulmonary involvement, a brief review of the basics of amyloid is offered.

Basics of Amyloid

Amyloid was so named because it stained with iodine, a common carbohydrate reagent in earlier times.[36] The base word *amyl* derives from the Greek *amylon*, meaning starch. Amyloid is a waxy pink material that until recently was quite resistant to investigation. It can be induced experimentally, especially with casein injections. It stains best with Congo red and has a characteristic *apple-green* birefringence with polarization.[52] Collagen, with which it is most often confused, is not as deeply orangophilic on Congo red stain and polarizes straw-yellow. Amyloid presents a somewhat unusual light to medium blue-gray color with Mallory's trichrome stain in contrast to the more definite deep blue color of collagen. Using high-quality light microscopy and polarization, connective tissue and blood vessels occasionally will show a nonspecific apple-green birefringence.[53] These same areas do not show the waxy orangophilic deposits on nonpolarized examination. Thioflavin-T or -F fluorescence is less specific but more sensitive for such deposits.[53] Amyloid also stains metachromatically with crystal or methyl violet. A good review of the basics of amyloid is that by Glenner[54]; an early history was presented by Gertz and Kyle.[36]

These staining reactions are apparently dependent on the beta pleated-sheet arrangement of the individual fibrils.[41] This is an unusual molecular arrangement in mammals, although some human prealbumin shows this configuration.[54] Electron microscopy shows a tangled or felt-like mass of very long tubular nonbranching hollow fibrils 7.5–10 nm (75–100 Å) in diameter, perhaps some 800 nm (8000 Å) long.[54,55] About 10% of the components consist of a pentagonal substance (P component) that is a glycoprotein and accounts for any periodic acid–Shiff (PAS) staining. Amyloid fibrils have now been subclassified as those of immunoglobulin origin, usually representing the variable N-terminal end of light chains (AL), the type commonly found in primary amyloidosis, those of unique protein-determined origin, called protein A (AA), senile type (AS or SSA), caused by transthyretin (see following), and that associated with endocrine tumors, especially medullary carcinoma (AE). Familial amyloidosis is designated AF and is related to a variant of transthyretin in the prealbumin area. Isolated atrial amyloid (IAA) is derived from atrial natriuretic polypeptide. Cerebral vascular amyloid, called cerebral amyloid angiopathy (CAA), is caused by a B or A4 subunit protein and carpal tunnel syndrome by a B_2 microglobulin deposition. Type II diabetes mellitus amyloid (IAPP) is the result of an islet polypeptide deposition. Other subtypes with appropriate letter designations are being described.

Most cases of AA types have been found in typical secondary amyloid conditions, along with the few cases of familial Mediterranean fever. Potassium permanganate and, to a lesser degree, trypsin, have been used as pretreatments before Congo red staining to help separate AA, the predominant secondary type, from that occurring in primary, multiple myeloma-associated or senile types.[54,56] Elimination of staining by predigestion is typical of protein A. Page et al.[57] were the first to type pulmonary nodular amyloid as AL. Others have now confirmed this finding.[56,58] All forms of pulmonary amyloid as listed here are most commonly found to be AL type.[36,59,60] Hui et al.[26] detailed such analysis on 23 of their 48 cases. Three of 5 tracheobronchial and 9 of 18 nodular amyloid cases were resistant to digestion, suggesting these were composed of amyloid of immunoglobulin origin (AL). Five showed total digestion, suggesting protein A derivation. Hui et al.[26] also noted that 18 of 26 patients typed with light chains were clearly polyclonal, while only 2 suggested some lambda light chain predominance. This is unlike the monoclonality often found in primary systemic amyloidosis.

The classification for amyloid used here (Table 22–1) is based on that of Rubinow.[51]

Amyloid localized to the pulmonary system is rare. Some articles published on amyloid emphasize pulmonary disease, but on careful reading one notes that other organs are frequently involved or sampling of other organs is insufficient to exclude such involvement.

One hundred fifty-seven cases of lower respiratory tract amyloid, including 31 (20%) with secondary pulmonary deposits, were summarized in 1983 by Thompson and Citron[61] in Great Britain. The largest single

Table 22–1. Classification of pulmonary amyloid

I. Tracheobronchial
   A. Isolated, localized or nodular
   B. Multifocal or diffuse
II. Parenchymal
   A. Nodular
      1. Solitary
      2. Multiple
   B. Interstitial, septal, or vascular

series from one institution is based on 48 referral cases seen at the U.S. Armed Forces Institute of Pathology (AFIP), Washington, D.C., published in 1986 by Hui et al.[26] Another large single institution series of 21 cases is from France, by Cordier et al.[59] and another more recent literature review is that by Chen.[62] Depending on the series, either tracheobronchial[51] or nodular[26] is more common or of about equal frequency,[61] while all authors agree the diffuse form limited to the lungs is least common as a primary presentation in the lung.

Lesser[63] in 1877 is credited with the first description of amyloid localized to the lung. A good historical review was provided by Prowse.[64] Eliminating the proven secondary cases, the 1983 literature review by Thompson and Citron[61] contained 126 cases presenting predominantly in the pulmonary system. Sixty-seven were tracheobronchial (10 of which were of the isolated or nodular tracheobronchial form), 55 were discrete pulmonary nodules, and 10 were diffuse interstitial forms. The other 31 with focal amyloid deposits in a more typical secondary setting included 11 with associated neoplasia; of these, 5 had an admixture of small cell or carcinoid tumor with amyloid in the tumors themselves. The same review noted 8 cases of hilar and mediastinal node involvement with amyloid, but only 2 cases of isolated or mediastinal or cervical node without lung involvement are included.[61] The series by Hui et al.[26] included 14 cases of tracheobronchial amyloid (4 localized and 10 multifocal or diffuse), 28 cases of nodular (10 solitary, 10 multiple and bilateral, 4 multiple and unilateral, 4 undetermined), and 6 of diffuse interstitial forms. The reader is referred to both these series for more details.

In the differential of amyloid is systemic light chain disease.[65–72] This has been described as both pulmonary reticulonodular,[65,70] and delicate interstitial thickening[66,67] is usually PAS positive and refractile blue on Giemsa but negative by polarization with all the amyloid stains, and is composed of dark, dense, granular deposits by electron microscopy. Other cases with systemic light chain disease have had interstitial pulmonary amyloid.[71,72] Some cases of nodular paramyloid discussed are yet to be better classified (see next).

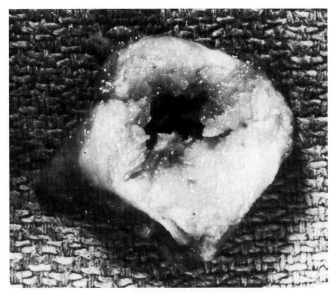

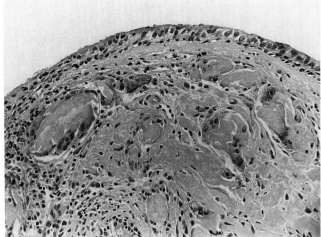

Fig. 22–8. Tracheobronchial amyloid. Cross section of left-mainstream bronchus is extensively infiltrated by amyloid. (Courtesy A.A. Liebow Pulmonary Pathology Collection, San Diego, California. Original source, Lawrence and Memorial Hospitals, New Haven, Connecticut.)

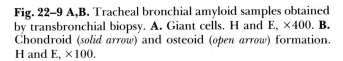

Fig. 22–9 A,B. Tracheal bronchial amyloid samples obtained by transbronchial biopsy. **A.** Giant cells. H and E, ×400. **B.** Chondroid (*solid arrow*) and osteoid (*open arrow*) formation. H and E, ×100.

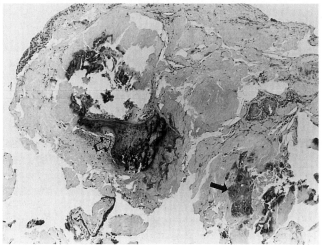

Tracheobronchial Amyloid

Amyloid limited to the tracheobronchial system was first described by Balser in 1883.[73] Tracheobronchial involvement in a patient has been documented as lasting for as long as 30 years.[74] The average age of involvement is about 53 years, with a range of about 16 to 76 years.[51] The youngest patient, a 16-year-old boy, had recurrent endobronchial polypoid amyloid deposits.[75] Only 3 cases of lower respiratory tract amyloid in the AFIP series of 48 cases occurred in people less than 40 years of age, and these were all of the tracheobronchial type.[26]

Obstruction and constriction (partial obstruction) are frequent occurrences. Focal tracheobronchial disease is obviously easier to resect and cure or control than the diffuse tracheobronchial form, but it is unfortunately not as common. Cough, stridor, dyspnea, and hemoptysis are frequent presenting complaints.[61] Bleeding may be massive or cause death, as may stridor.[51,61] Bleeding may be spontaneous or secondary to biopsy.

One person with posttransbronchial biopsy hemorrhage also died during the procedure of air embolism.[76] Another had hemorrhage believed caused by medial dissection of involved pulmonary arteries.[77] Recurrent pneumonia and bronchiectasis may be present and are explained by the airway narrowing. Polypoid masses are usually solitary, with rare exceptions, and occur in the major bronchi.

Microscopically, amyloid deposits occur in the submucosa (Fig. 22–8). Multinucleated cells are frequently seen (Fig. 22–9A). Calcifications, chondrification, and ossification occur with some regularity in this form (Figs. 22–9 and 22–10). As previously discussed, the entity of tracheobronchopathia osteochondroplastica, as originally described by Wilks in 1857,[10] is thought to possibly be an end stage of trancheobronchial amyloid.[23,24,78–81] As already noted, more than 200 cases of tracheobronchopathia osteochondroplastica, generally without any associated amyloid, were described by 1972 compared with only about 30 cases of all other forms of respiratory tract amyloid by that time.[23] Only 2 of 14

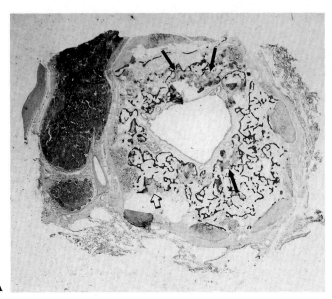

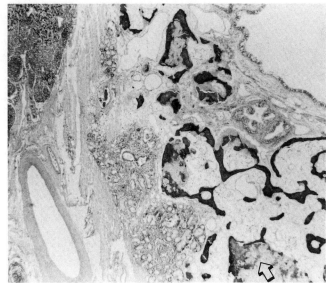

Fig. 22–10 A,B. Tracheobronchial amyloid with extensive ossification. **A.** Remnant amyloid is present (*arrows*), but extensive ossification approaches appearance of tracheobron-

chopathia osteoplastica. H and E. ×4. **B.** Higher power view with amyloid and ossification is shown (compare *open arrow* here and area of *open arrow* on Fig. 22–10A). H and E. ×15.

cases (14%) in Hui's series[26] of tracheobronchial amyloid has osseous metaplasia. Some cases of tracheobronchopathia osteochondroplastica must occur by alternate routes such as by metaplasia, as a reaction to injury or degeneration. (See earlier discussion.)

Nodular Amyloid

Nodular amyloid in the lung presents as tumor-like masses and has been called "amyloidomas." Several good series are available.[49,82–84] Lesser's description in 1877 still retains the record for the largest such tumor mass, being 15 cm in maximum dimension.[63] The nodules vary in size from millimeters to this 15 cm, but most are 0.4–5 cm,[82] averaging 3 cm,[26] and are about equally divided between solitary and multiple forms,[26,28] with occasional exceptions such as the series by Saab et al.[85] in which multiple nodules outnumbered solitary nodules by 27 to 10 (2.7:1). They are more frequent in the lower lobes and are 2.5 times more frequent in the right lung, with the right-lower lobe being the site most frequently involved.[26] When bilateral, they are usually asymmetrical.[84] More than 40 individual amyloid nodules have been described in a single person,[86] and a rare case described bilateral nodular confluence.[49,87] One case also showed adjacent thoracic structure involvement (vertebral body cortex, epicardial fat, and hilar nodes).[49] Patients with nodular pulmonary amyloid are usually older, averaging mid- to late sixties,[26,83] but the youngest is a 16-year-old.[88] Most patients are asymptomatic, and the nodules are found incidentally. This form of pulmonary amyloid has a good prognosis.

These nodules are typically described as waxy, lardaceous, or rock hard (Fig. 22–11); the term lardaceous here refers to the texture of cold lard, not to a greasy appearance. They are semitranslucent gray with varying degrees of focal yellow opacities; the latter usually correlate with calcium deposits. Grossly, they stain with iodine (Fig. 22–11B). Irregular densities of more or less confluent amyloid deposits are seen (Fig. 22–12). As noted also in tracheobronchial amyloid metaplastic bone, calcification and sometimes cartilage may occur in these nodules (Fig. 22–13), and were found in 28% in one series[26] and almost all in another.[89] Calcification may be reflected as a "cloud-like" calcification on radiography; it appears stippled on tomograms and is seen in some 50% of chest radiographs.[90] Such nodules may show cavitation.[59,91] At times these nodules coexist with other lung diseases, such as multiple bullae in Sjögren's syndrome,[92] Sjögren's associated lymphoid interstitial pneumonia[93] or pulmonary lymphoma.[94] They often have sharp gross borders, but microscopic amyloid deposits are frequently found in the immediately adjacent lung parenchyma[26,87] (Fig. 22–12). Multinucleated foreign-body-type giant cells are frequently seen and often appear to be ingesting amyloid (Fig. 22–14). Plasma cells are moderate in number and sometimes are present in clusters. The background lung architecture in the nodules is generally lost, but exceptions occur.[89] Some extend directly into pleura (Fig. 22–15). Hilar nodal amyloid may be present with or without lung parenchymal involvement,[95–104] and is bilateral in 89% of all cases.[95] An occasional nodule appears peculiar by light microscopy but is typical amyloid by ultrastructure (Fig. 22–16).

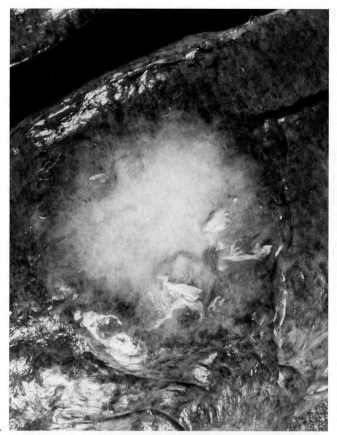

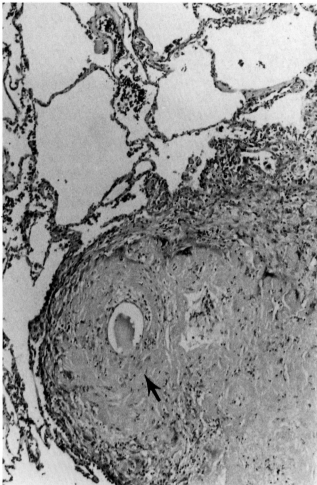

Fig. 22–12. Nodular amyloid. Edge of nodule shows involved vessel (*arrow*) within mass of amyloid, but no significant vessel or interstitial involvement is seen in adjacent lung. H and E, ×100. (Contrast with Fig. 22–17).

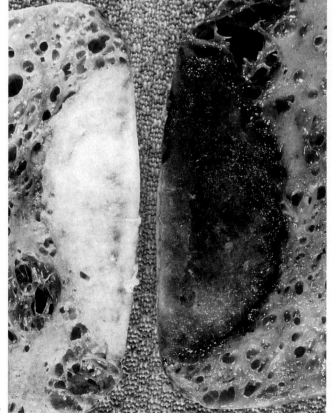

◁

Fig. 22–11 A,B. Amyloid nodule in lung. **A.** Surface view. **B.** Sectioned nodule, one half stained with iodine. (Courtesy of Robert E. Tank, M.D., Providence Hospital, Seattle, Washington.)

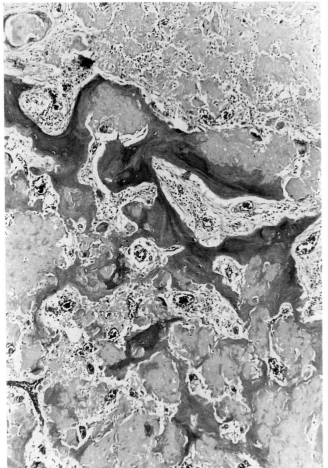

22-13

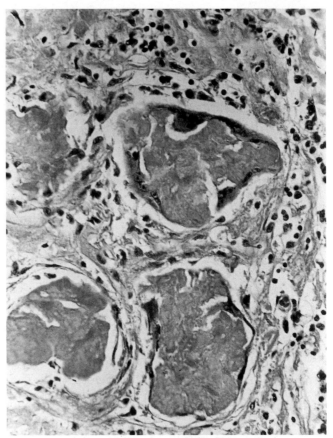

22-1

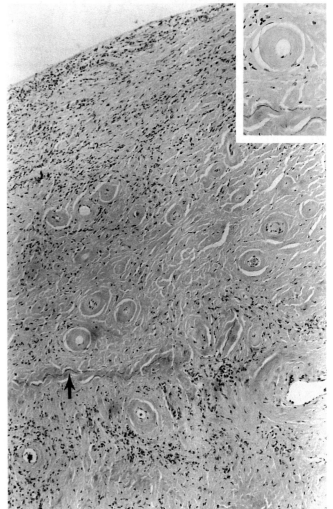

22-

Fig. 22–13. Nodular amyloid. Dystrophic calcification is occurring within nodule of amyloid. H and E, ×100.

Fig. 22–14. Multinucleate giant cells surrounding amyloid fragments. H and E, ×200.

Fig. 22–15. Pleural spread of amyloid. Low-power view with pleural elastica highlighted with *arrow*. H and E, ×100. **Inset.** Area at higher power shows vessels also involved. H and E, ×400.

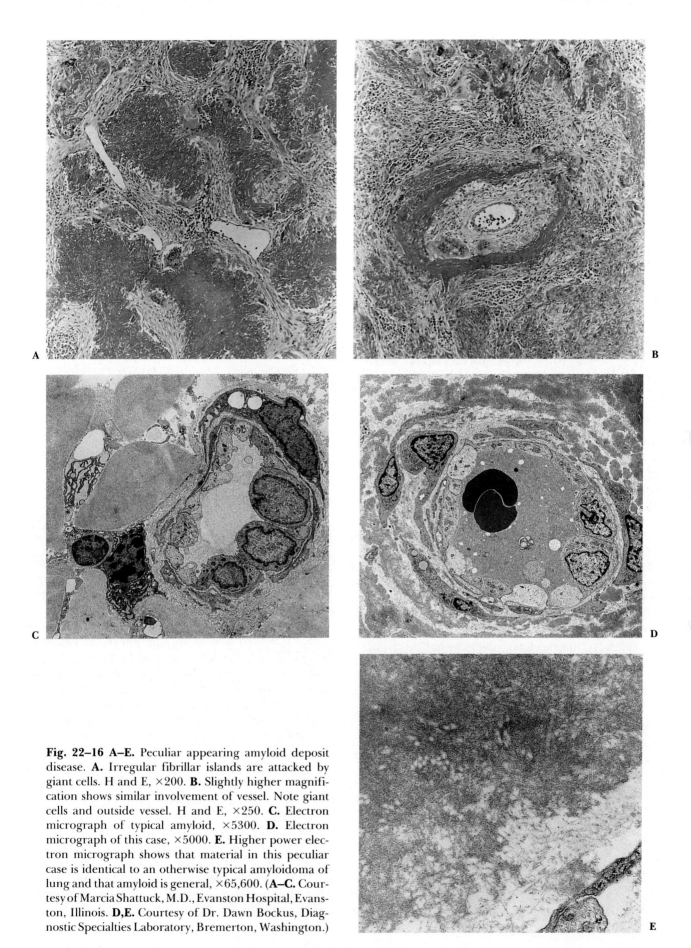

Fig. 22–16 A–E. Peculiar appearing amyloid deposit disease. **A.** Irregular fibrillar islands are attacked by giant cells. H and E, ×200. **B.** Slightly higher magnification shows similar involvement of vessel. Note giant cells and outside vessel. H and E, ×250. **C.** Electron micrograph of typical amyloid, ×5300. **D.** Electron micrograph of this case, ×5000. **E.** Higher power electron micrograph shows that material in this peculiar case is identical to an otherwise typical amyloidoma of lung and that amyloid is general, ×65,600. (**A–C.** Courtesy of Marcia Shattuck, M.D., Evanston Hospital, Evanston, Illinois. **D,E.** Courtesy of Dr. Dawn Bockus, Diagnostic Specialties Laboratory, Bremerton, Washington.)

Diffuse Parenchymal Amyloid (Interstitial, Septal, or Vascular)

Diffuse interstitial amyloid is widespread and bilateral, and in its isolated form is the least common but most serious of the types presenting in the lower respiratory tract. One series[59] of pulmonary amyloid had a disproportionately high percentage (71%) of interstitial amyloid. The average age for those involved is in the mid-fifties, close to the age range for tracheobronchial form but some 10 years younger than the nodular form. Symptoms are frequent, and death usually occurs within 2 years of diagnosis,[26] although exceptions occur.[77,105] Pulmonary arterial hypertension can occur, presumably because of these vascular deposits.[106] In cases that come to autopsy or otherwise have extensive evaluation, systemic involvement of amyloid is frequent, but some cases do appear to be limited to the lungs.[26,61] This form is sometimes divided into interstitial and vascular subtypes,[40] but often both compartments are involved. Rarely is the pleura predominately involved in this form.[107–112]

Gross and subgross (hand lens and dissecting microscope) appearance of diffuse pulmonary amyloid has been likened to a remarkably "uniform rubber sponge-like appearance."[113] In this form, the vessel walls and interstitial compartments are often both involved[113–115] (Fig. 22–17). Giant cells and plasma cells are rarely observed and are far less outstanding than in tracheobronchial and nodular forms. Osseous metaplasia does not usually occur in the interstitial form.

Interstitial amyloid may present as fine interstitial involvement, reticulonodular, and at times nodular patterns on radiography. The "nodular" appearance in this form is distinguished from the true nodular form by the usually smaller sized nodules and by the bilaterally extensive internodular parenchymal involvement in the diffuse form.

In the differential diagnosis of interstitial amyloid is fibrosis, which is often more cellular, confluent, and irregular. Electrocautery effect must also be considered (Fig. 22–18); this is more often focal-zonal, along the edge of tissue. Systemic light chain disease as already discussed early in this section, should also be excluded. Congo red stains can easily be done if assistance in separating these entities is needed.

Interstitial Diseases

The next group consists of diseases of interstitial vascular and lining cell subcompartments, and covers myxedema, vascular diseases of Goodpasture's disease and idiopathic pulmonary hemosiderosis, iron encrustation of elastic tissue, assorted calcifications and ossifications,

and ends with cytoplasmic hyaline of alveolar lining cells.

Myxedema

In a 1963 study by Naeye[116] of the lungs from 14 autopsy cases of patients with severe hypothyroidism receiving insufficient or no replacement thyroid therapy, 4 had characteristic amorphous pale-pink material about pulmonary capillaries and small veins on H and E stain (Fig. 22–19). Unlike more typical fibrous tissue in this location, this material rarely compressed these vessels or caused changes of pulmonary hypertension. A change similar to this was seen in the glomerular capillaries in this study. Histochemical studies showed this mucoprotein to be PAS- and acid mucosubstance positive.

These deposits may cause the arterial oxygen desaturation that sometimes occurs in myxedema subjects. No such lesions were identified in cases of hypothyroidism with adequate replacement therapy. Myxedematous deposits in the skin may disappear after only several weeks of adequate therapy,[117] but this could not be evaluated in the lungs on Naeye's[116] autopsy study. When other etiologies are excluded, there may be pleural effusions solely caused by myxedema,[118] perhaps related to vascular malfunction.[119]

Goodpasture's Syndrome

Goodpasture's syndrome is a condition characterized by the association of pulmonary hemorrhage and rapidly progressive (crescentic) glomerulonephritis. Stanton and Tange[120] reported a series of patients who died from pulmonary hemorrhage and nephritis, and named this syndrome in recognition of Goodpasture, who published the first report of pulmonary hemorrhage and renal disease in 1919.[121] Of interest, Goodpasture's original cases were associated with systemic vasculitis during the major flu epidemic in 1918, and today this syndrome is limited to those with antibasement membrane antibodies (ABMA), and only rarely is there associated systemic vasculitis. Of all the cases with ABMA, 60%–80% have both pulmonary and renal disease, 20%–40% have glomerulonephritis, and fewer than 10% have pulmonary disease only.[122]

The best, more recent clinical reviews are those by Leatherman et al.[123] and Young.[124] More than 75% of these cases occurred in the age range 16–30 years. Tobacco use was correlated with 37 of 47 cases (78.7%) of ABMA with pulmonary hemorrhage and only 2 of 10 (20%) with renal disease alone.[125] Men outnumber women by two- to ninefold, and this variance is thought to be related to how many men smokers are in each

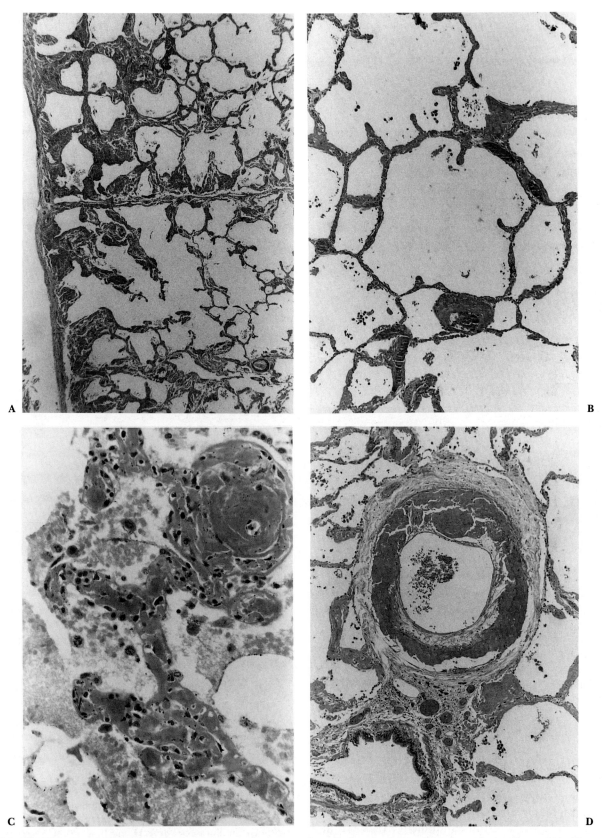

Fig. 22–17 A–D. Interstitial amyloid. **A.** Low power shows more interstitial amyloid toward pleura in this case. **B.** Even at higher power, the least involved areas in this case show interstitial amyloid. H and E, ×400. **C.** Another view of more heavily involved interstitium and small vessel(s). H and E, ×600. **D.** Same case shows dense vascular involvement. H and E, ×200.

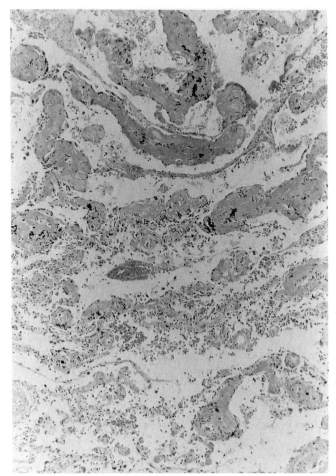

Fig. 22–18. Electrocautery artifact in the differential of interstitial amyloid is worse along top half; more normal interstitium appears below left. H and E, ×200. Compare least involved area with Fig. 22–17B.

series.[124] Pulmonary manifestations usually precede evidence of renal disease, and hemoptysis is stated to occur as the initial symptom in 80%–90% of patients accompanied by chest infiltrates in 80%, often with dyspnea on exertion, weakness, and fatigue.[126,127] Most patients have iron deficiency anemia with hemoglobin of less than 12 g/dl, elevated white blood cell counts (greater than 10,000 per mm³) cubic, and proteinuria with red cell and white cell casts. At presentation, some 55% are azotemic, 75% have proteinuria, and 83% have microscopic hematuria.[127] Although rapidly progressive glomerulonephritis is the usual renal disease, only 20% of those cases have ABMA,[128] and as reviewed by Young,[124] the antibasement membrane antibodies recognize an epitope of α3 (IV) chain of type IV collagen, the latter a major component of basement membrane. Some heterogeneity of this component exists and may account for the renal, pulmonary, and choroid plexus capillary networks being favored for this disease while other type IV collagen basement membranes are

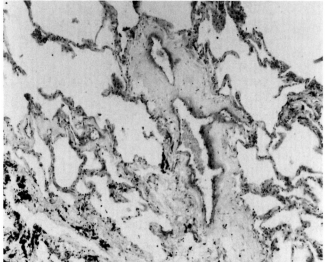

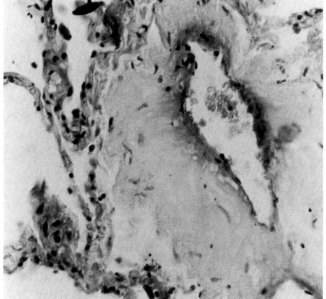

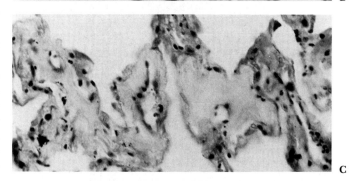

Fig. 22–19 A–C. Myxedema. **A.** Low-power view shows pale hyaline substance around vein in center and around smaller vessels in midleft area. H and E, ×100. **B.** Vein in **A.** H and E. ×200. **C.** Smaller vessel in **A.** H and E. ×200. (Courtesy of AA Liebow Pulmonary Pathology Collection, San Diego, California. Original source, Richard L. Naeye, M.D., Hershey Medical Center, Hershey, Pennsylvania.)

spared. Reese and coworkers[129] found a marked increase in HLA-DR2 haplotype in patients with Goodpasture's syndrome as compared to controls plus a slight increase in HLA-B7 haplotype.

Experimental evidence with ABMA has shown production of consistent renal disease, but there is difficulty in reproducing pulmonary deposits and pulmonary disease unless the lungs are injured by 100% oxygen,[130,131] tracheal installation of gasoline,[132] or other components that increase permeability of unfenestrated alveolar endothelium, such as a combination of interleuken 2 and α-interferon.[133] Interestingly, there is no definite relationship between ABMA titers and episodes or severity of pulmonary hemorrhage.[134–136] In pulmonary hemorrhage in humans, approximately 50%[123] follow an episode of presumed pulmonary infection.[133,135,136] Perhaps smoking is one such cofactor. T and B lymphocytes together appear to play a role in Goodpasture's disease.[124]

Grossly the lungs are heavy and hemorrhagic (Figure 22–20), at least in tissue examined in acute-phase disease. Microscopic pathology of ABMA (Fig. 22–21) has recently been reviewed by Lombard et al.[137] and Travis et al.[138] As Lombard et al.[137] discuss, other authors have described hemorrhage alone[139–144] and in combination with alveolar damage with hyaline membranes,[145–147] mononuclear infiltrates,[148–150] alveolitis,[139,151] eosinophilic infiltration,[152] and in cases associated with Wegener's granulomatosis.[153,154] ABMA has also been associated with pulmonary eosinophilic vasculitis.[155] Lombard et al.[137] made a thorough study of four cases (excluding their case five, which seems to be an outlyer) that showed mostly acute hemorrhage with intact red blood cells and alveoli with variable amounts of hemosiderin-laden macrophages always identified in the background. No case contained only acute hemorrhage; all had areas of neutrophilic capillaritis that were focal in three cases and more extensive in one.

Pulmonary leukocytic or neutrophilic capillaritis has been carefully described by Mark and Ramirez[156] as having the following: (1) fibrin thrombin in capillaries in interalveolar septa; (2) sessile fibrin clots attached to alveolar septa projecting into alveoli; (3) fibrinoid necrosis of capillary walls; (4) neutrophils and nuclear dust in fibrin in both the interstitium and the immediately adjacent alveolar blood; and (5) interstitial red blood cells and hemosiderin (see Figure 22–21). They noted that not all these findings were present in each case and warned that recognizing this entity is challenged by the delicacy of the interstitium and the fact that when the capillaries are destroyed they are hard to identify; further, blood, fibrin and PMNs easily leak out of the alveolar walls into adjacent alveoli. Certainly with some attention to detail, even on a low- or medium-power microscopic examination, a clue to this disease is

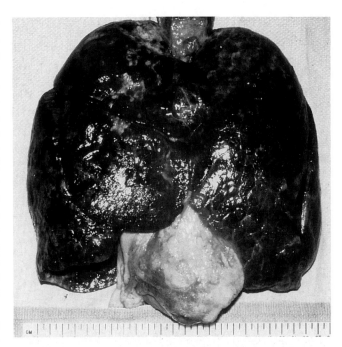

Fig. 22–20. Goodpasture's syndrome. Death in acute phase; autopsied lungs show abundant bilateral hemorrhage. Pale heart is in lower midline.

lines of PMNs, representing past alveolar septa, appearing in blood-filled alveolar spaces. Even as recently as 1986 Goodpasture's disease was thought not to be an active vasculitis component.[157] This entity is described more thoroughly in Chapter 30.

An elaborate study was done by Travis et al.[138] of 34 cases of diffuse pulmonary hemorrhage, 31 of which were confirmed by open lung biopsy and 3 by transbronchial biopsy. This series, worthy of discussing in some detail, included 4 cases of ABMA, 4 of idiopathic pulmonary hemorrhage including 2 of idiopathic pulmonary hemosiderosis and 2 additional that appeared similar but with immune complexes identified, 5 of definite and 6 of probable Wegener's granulomatosis, 3 of systemic necrotizing vasculitis, 2 of lupus, and 1 each of rheumatoid disease, seronegative juvenile rheumatoid disease, and IGA nephropathy, along with 2 of idiopathic glomerulitis and 5 of unclassified pulmonary hemorrhage. Therefore, 41% of these cases had vasculitis and 32% were difficult to subclassify. Pulmonary leukocytic capillaritis was present in 88% of these cases, was extensive in only 24% of the total, and was found in all categories listed. Hyaline membranes were focally identified in 1 case each of ABMA, idiopathic pulmonary hemorrhage, systemic necrotizing vasculitis, and IGA nephropathy, and in these cases could not otherwise be explained. Hyaline membranes have been described by others[145–47] and were present in 3 of 4 cases by Lombard et al.[137] These are generally focal but were

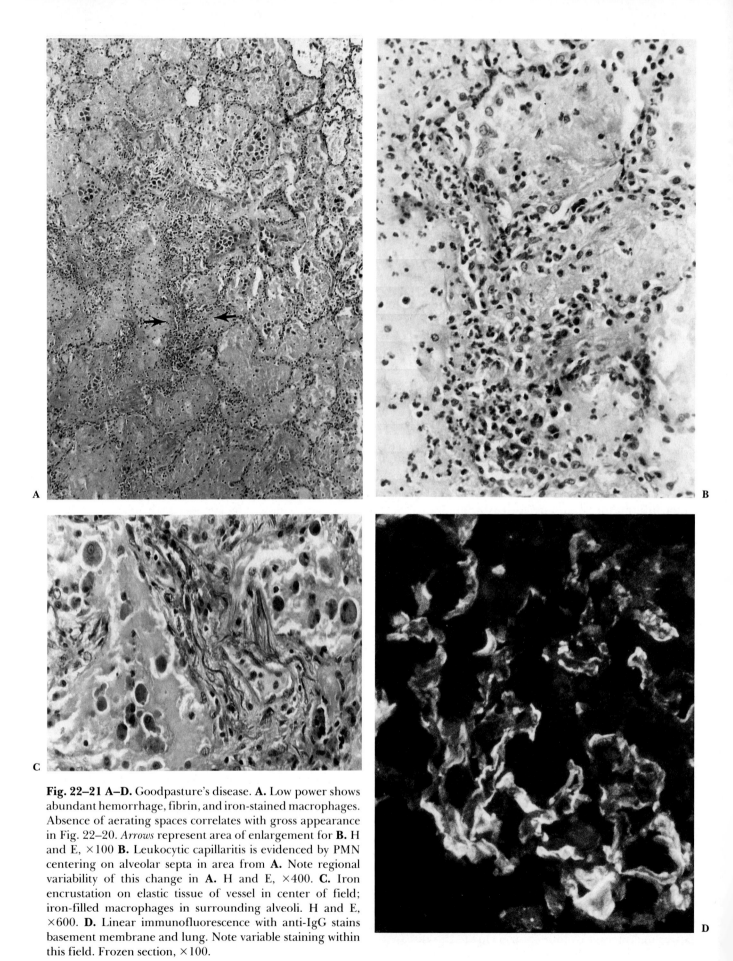

Fig. 22–21 A–D. Goodpasture's disease. **A.** Low power shows abundant hemorrhage, fibrin, and iron-stained macrophages. Absence of aerating spaces correlates with gross appearance in Fig. 22–20. *Arrows* represent area of enlargement for **B.** H and E, ×100 **B.** Leukocytic capillaritis is evidenced by PMN centering on alveolar septa in area from **A.** Note regional variability of this change in **A.** H and E, ×400. **C.** Iron encrustation on elastic tissue of vessel in center of field; iron-filled macrophages in surrounding alveoli. H and E, ×600. **D.** Linear immunofluorescence with anti-IgG stains basement membrane and lung. Note variable staining within this field. Frozen section, ×100.

724

extensive in one case. Alveolar and septal damage is often reflected in edematous, widened interstitium with reactive alveolar type II cell hyperplasia. Organizing fibroblastic polyps are sometimes present, but only rarely are sufficient to reflect the entity of bronchiolitis obliterans organizing pneumonia (BOOP). Mononuclear cell infiltrates are focal and mild in degree, and occasionally occur around small venules; more often they appear in the interstitium and around the bronchioles.

Leukocytic capillaritis is apparently transient. In two cases reported by Travis et al.[138] an active leukocytic capillaritis was documented by biopsy in an autopsy in one case 7 days after steroids and in another case 10 days after only antibiotic therapy; no vasculitis was present. I have seen a similar case in which the patient died within 2 weeks of biopsy and was surprised not to have confirmed the disease at autopsy. Leukocytic capillaritis may correlate with episodes of hemorrhage, and its tombstone may be past hemorrhage as evidenced by the hemosiderin in the background of ABMA, and certainly in cases of idiopathic pulmonary hemosiderosis, as discussed next.

Antimembrane antibodies are best confirmed by serum analysis. Indirect immunofluorescent evaluation of renal biopsies is less reliable but still helpful, and immunofluorescence of lung tissue may be positive but is likely to have a high nonspecific background.[158,159] Usually linear deposits of IgG and the C3 component of complement are present,[158] while less often IgA and rarely IgM are detected (Fig. 22–21D). Electron microscopy confirms linear deposits.[123,124,160,161]

In the past few years, diffuse alveolar hemorrhage originating from capillaries in the alveolar septa has been described as occurring in association with a variety of diseases, many of which have an associated glomerular lesion. These syndromes have frequently been referred to as "pulmonary renal syndromes",[162] and have been reviewed and classified in detail by Albelda and co-workers[163] and also by Leatherman et al.[123] The classification by Albelda et al.[163] into six groups depending on the immunologic nature (or lack thereof) and type (or lack thereof) of renal disease is appealing (Fig. 22–22 and Table 22–2). It has become obvious, for example, that immune complex disease caused by a type III immunologic reaction[164] and other diseases can masquerade as Goodpasture's syndrome and, therefore, in the purest sense, the term "Goodpasture's syndrome" should perhaps best be reserved for those cases of diffuse alveolar hemorrhage and associated crescentic nephritis in which a serum antibody is identified by immunofluorescence that causes linear deposits in a basal lamina distribution along alveolar septa and in renal glomeruli.

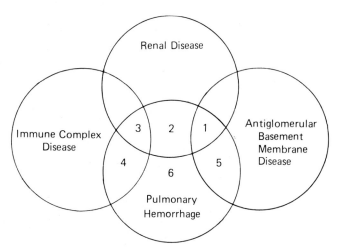

Fig. 22–22. Diagram shows interrelationship of factors in classification of diffuse pulmonary hemorrhage. *Group 1.* Pulmonary hemorrhage associated with glomerulonephritis and anti-GBM antibody. *Group 2.* Pulmonary hemorrhage associated with renal disease without demonstrable immunologic abnormalities. *Group 3.* Pulmonary hemorrhage associated with glomerulonephritis and immune complex disease. *Group 4.* Pulmonary hemorrhage and immune complex disease without renal disease. *Group 5.* Pulmonary hemorrhage associated with anti-GBM antibodies without renal disease. *Group 6.* Pulmonary hemorrhage without demonstrable immunologic associations or renal disease. (From Albelda et al.[163] with permission.)

Primary Pulmonary Hemosiderosis

These cases are considered primary or idiopathic as no cause for the accumulation of pulmonary hemosiderin is apparent. When other causes are known, the disease is best classified otherwise. Such associations as neurodynamic abnormalities or coagulopathy, or systemic disorders such as vasculitis, ABMA, or lupus, need to be excluded.[122]

Most of these cases occur in infancy and childhood;[165] the latter are discussed in Chapter 8, and the reader is referred to that chapter to complement the current discussion. The disease does occur in adults, and Waldenström[166] is credited with the first description in an adult. By 1956 Wynn-Williams and Young[167] added 1 case to 15 collected from the literature; in 1959 Boyd[168] added 3 cases to 26 reported; in 1960 Bronson[169] added 1 to 37 collected cases in the literature, and by 1963 Ognibene and Johnson[170] added 1 to 52 cases. Morgan and Turner-Warwick[171] have more recently summarized these cases. Usually the disease is not familial, and only rarely are geographic clusters of cases identified.[172]

Most adults with this disease experience their first episode in their late teens or twenties,[165] but episodes

Table 22–2. Classification of diffuse pulmonary hemorrhage[a]

Group	Characteristics	Examples
Group 1	Pulmonary hemorrhage associated with glomerulonephritis and anti-GBM antibody	"Classic" Goodpasture syndrome
Group 2	Pulmonary hemorrhage associated with renal disease without demonstrable immunologic abnormalities	
Group 2A	Probably nonimmunologic	Legionnaires' disease, uremic lung bleeding
Group 2B	Probably immunologic	Crescentic glomerulonephritis without evidence of anti-GBM antibodies or immune complexes
Group 3	Pulmonary hemorrhage associated with glomerulonephritis and immune complex disease	Lupus erythematosus, Wegener granulomatosis, cryoglobulinemia, Henoch–Schonlein purpura, mixed connective-tissue disease, and immune-complex-associated "systemic vasculitis"
Group 4	Pulmonary hemorrhage and immune complexes without associated renal disease	Lupus, Wegener granulomatosis, immune-complex-associated "systemic vasculitis"
Group 5	Pumonary hemorrhage associated with anti-GBM antibodies without renal disease	Early Goodpasture syndrome of Goodpasture "variant"
Group 6	Pulmonary hemorrhage without demonstrable immunologic associations or renal disease	
Group 6A	Idiopathic pulmonary hemosiderosis	
Group 6B	Bleeding disorders	Anticoagulant use, disseminated intravascular, coagulation, thrombocytopenia, leukemia
Group 6C	Acute lung injury	Adult respiratory distress syndrome, toxic inhalation, oxygen toxicity
Group 6D	Miscellaneous causes	Aspiration of blood, drugs, blunt trauma, mitral stenosis

[a] From Albelda et al.,[163] with permission.

have been reported in people in their fifties.[171] The disease in adults is similar to that in children, except that it is usually milder,[171] as is so often true of the adult form of diseases occurring in more fulminant form at an earlier age. In contrast to the equal sex distribution in children, men are 2.5 times as frequently involved as women.[169] Attacks may be as frequent as in childhood, but in adults may be separated by up to 20 years.[169] A chronic anemia with continued production of iron-stained macrophages in the sputum between attacks suggest that the disease may be ongoing.[123] Bleeding problems outside the lung are rare. Iron deficiency anemia develops, despite the paradoxical excess of iron in the lungs, which is apparently unavailable for hematopoiesis. Iron is increased some 5- to 2000 fold in the lungs.[173] Pulmonary infiltrates are usually patchy and described as bilateral small nodular to reticular type, especially in the perihilar and basilar portions of the lung.[170] Because they are probably related to the less severe disease in adults, infiltrates are often not as confluent in adults as they are in children.

The lungs and regional lymph nodes may be grossly dark red to orange-brown. Early cases have not been documented in adults, so most tissue sections show mild-to-moderate fibrosis. The most striking finding is abundant acute hemorrhage and hemosiderin-laden macrophages in alveoli (Fig. 22–23). The alveolar septa are broadened not only by fibrosis but by dilated capillaries and some lymphocytes and reactive alveolar type II cells. Recently, leukocytic capillaritis has rarely been identified.[138] Peribronchial and pleural lymphoid sump areas contain increased numbers of lymphocytes and plasma cells, and iron-stained macrophages. The lymphatic spaces show some dilatation, perhaps related to some obstruction caused by the cellular infiltrates. Interlobular septa are sometimes fibrotic. Tissue necrosis, granulomas, interstitial hemorrhage, vasculitis, thromboemboli, or old vascular scars are not usually seen. Only rarely is there organizing pneumonia. The bronchial arteries usually show mild-to-moderate fibrosis without dilatation in chronic cases.[173]

Electron microscopic studies have found no consistent lung defects. Focal rupture of the capillary basement membrane has been described by some[174,175] but not by others.[176,177] Multiplication and thickening of the basement membrane was described in one case.[178] The loss of alveolar type I cells, and hyperplasia of alveolar type II cells and fibrosis, appear to be reactive changes.

By definition, no antibodies to basement membranes are present. In one series reported by Morgan and Turner-Warwick,[171] eight cases were studied without antibasement membrane antibodies; three were found to have antinuclear antibodies and two had positive rheumatoid factors. It is unclear whether any patient had both of these. It has long been suspected that this disease may be immunologic. An intriguing association with celiac disease (sprue) has been reported in 10

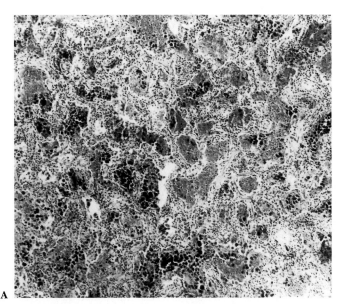

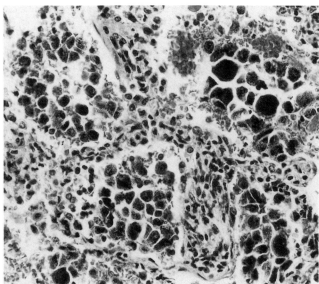

Fig. 22–23 A,B. Primary pulmonary hemosiderosis. **A.** Extensive acute and chronic intraalveolar hemorrhage obscures airspaces. H and E, ×100. **B.** Higher power shows darkly staining, heavily hemosiderin-laden intraaveolar macrophages, with focal acute hemorrhage and moderate cellular interstitial thickening. H and E, ×400.

cases,[179–186] and in 9 with follow-up, the lung disease has improved with treatment even though the gastrointestinal disease was only improved in 3.[180,183,185,186] A finding that needs more correlation in idiopathic pulmonary hemosiderosis (IPH) is the 78% with antireticulin and 95% with antigliadin antibodies in sprue.[187] In more than 50% of pediatric cases of IPH, IgG levels are elevated,[188] but this is only rarely found in adults.[171] IgA deposits have been found in glomeruli of such a young man when the glomeruli appeared normal by light microscopy.[189] Previous studies of IPH have not studied renal glomeruli with immunofluorescence.[123]

Most of the cases of primary pulmonary hemosiderosis in children and adults were described before 1964, when immunologic techniques were not as well advanced as they are currently.[163] It is expected that some (or perhaps many) of these cases may fit into one of the other six variations as proposed by Albelda et al.[163] and noted in the preceding section on Goodpasture's disease.

As well outlined in the discussion of the pediatric primary pulmonary hemosiderosis in Chapter 8, this is very much a disease of exclusion after all other known causes of pulmonary hemorrhage have been excluded. While trying to extend knowledge in this area, all such cases should have the best immunologic evaluation possible. At some point renal biopsies may be suggested[123] to further refine this diagnosis of exclusion or fit into one of the six categories mentioned. Although most patients are younger than the "young-to-middle-aged" spectrum of Goodpasture diseases, primary pulmonary hemosiderosis comes closest to that disease in many investigators' opinions. Perhaps some new marker antibodies will be discovered in this disease in the future, comparable to antineutrophilic cytoplasmic antibodies noted in Wegener's granulomatosis.

Iron Encrustation of Pulmonary Elastic Tissue

Any condition causing chronic and persistent hemorrhage in the lung can be associated with iron encrusting on elastic tissue in the lung. Most often this is seen in primary pulmonary hemosiderosis[173] and pulmonary venoocclusive disease.[190] It has been described only rarely in severe congestive heart failure, mostly notably in a child.[191] It is uncommon but does occur in Goodpasture's disease (Fig. 22–21C) or pulmonary hypertension.[191,192] I have rarely identified it focally around sclerosing hemangiomas of lung (see Chapter 33) and a large cell-giant cell carcinoma. It is similar to Gamna–Gandy body formation in the spleen, but has not been associated with old infarcts in the lung as is often the case in the spleen. It has erroneously been referred to as "endogenous pneumoconiosis."[193] At times this reaction has been mistaken for asbestos bodies, but does not have the circumferential rings or dumbbell-shaped ends or clear cores of asbestos bodies.

Iron accumulates on the elastic tissues of smaller arteries and veins, and less frequently on bronchiolar elastic tissue. It rarely encrusts on alveolar septal elastic tissue. As elastic tissue becomes more severely encrusted, it may become thicker, more brittle, and yellow

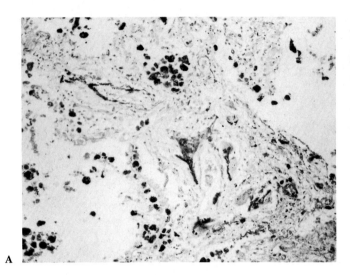
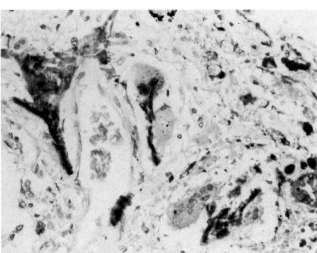

Fig. 22–24 A,B. Elastic tissue encrustation with iron. **A.** Iron accumulates on elastic tissue of vessel (left, top) and causes foreign body response (below, right). Iron-stained macro- phages are in adjacent alveoli. Prussian blue, ×100. **B.** High-power view of foreign-body effect of encrusted elastic tissue from **A.** Note foreign-body giant cells. Prussian blue, ×400.

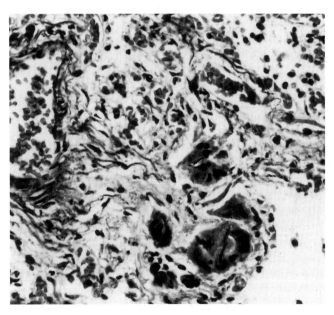

Fig. 22–25. Elastic tissue encrustation with iron on H and E stain. Iron stains are not usually necessary to see blackened elastic fibers. Individual fibers from larger vessel to left and smaller vessel above are being individually attacked by small foreign-body giant cells. H and E, ×400.

in appearance (Fig. 22–24), and may fracture with tissue sectioning. This may also be blue-black on H and E-stained sections, almost appearing to be an elastic tissue stain (Figs. 22-21c and 22–25). These coated fibers act as foreign bodies, and are attacked by small multinucleate giant cells (Figs. 22–24 and 22–25). The differential diagnosis is encrustation of elastic and con- nective tissue by DNA in oat cell carcinoma and by

calcium in interstitial calcification. Brightly staining on iron stain helps to distinguish this from the other two, as does the chronic hemorrhage in the background. Spe- cial stains for iron, DNA, and calcium are also distin- guishing. Similar to that seen in the spleen, it is expected that heavily encrusted areas in an exceptional case will cease to stain brightly with iron stains.

Dystrophic Calcification

This form of calcification occurs as a chronic reaction to various injuries such as granulomas, old infarcts and emboli, chronic pneumonias (such as adult chicken pox), pleural plaques, and slowly growing tumors. Such calcification is not associated with altered serum calcium or phosphorus levels; it is usually of little significance and is discussed further under the individual entities.

Interstitial or Metastatic Calcification

This is also called calcinosis of the lung, and generally but not always involves altered serum calcium and phosphorus metabolism. This was originally described by Virchow in 1855[194] and was nicely reviewed in 1947 by Mulligan,[195] who classified the associated conditions into those with parathyroid neoplasms and hyperplasia, chronic renal diseases, primary and secondary condi- tions of bone including myeloma and leukemia, hyper- vitaminosis D, and those of uncertain association. To this group should be added therapies that alter calcium or phorphorus metabolism.[196] Many of the recent, better studied groups have been dialysis patients.[196–200] The presence and severity of metastatic calcification

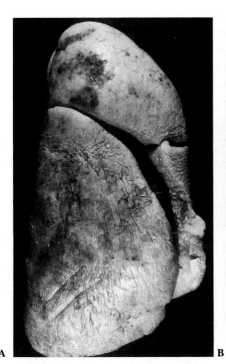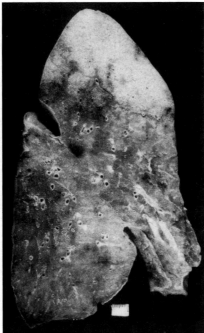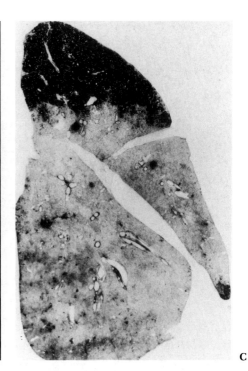

Fig. 22–26 A–C. Interstitial metastatic calcification. Interesting case of 27-year-old woman with acute lymphocytic leukemia who died with tumor-induced hypercalcemia. Upper-lobe location is discrete and extensive. **A.** Surface view shows no collapse of "stony-hard" upper lobe. **B.** Cut surface. **C.** Gough sections stained with von Kossa stain. (Courtesy of M Bonin and K Miyai, San Diego, California.)

correlates poorly with serum calcium and phosphorus levels, degree of parathyroid hyperplasia or activity, type of primary disease, or length of dialysis.[196–201]

Metastatic calcification is often bilateral and diffuse, but may be focal or nodular.[196–204] An unusual case reported by Bonin and Miyai[204] showed interstitial calcification limited to both upper lobes in a 27-year-old leukemic patient (Fig. 22–26). Other cases favoring the upper lobes have been described,[195,200,205–207] which is thought to be related to a higher ventilation perfusion ratio with higher oxygen content, lower carbon dioxide content, and therefore increased alkalinity of the upper lobes. Most other focal distributions are irregular and not as zonal as this one. Deposits of calcification may be reversible, at least in some cases.[203]

Most cases are not detected until death. The calcification is so delicate that it may not be detected by routine radiography.[198] Even if it is, it is often misinterpreted as edema[208–209] or pneumonia.[210,211] In at least one case, bilateral chylous pleural effusion and massive breast and leg enlargement suggested a generalized lymphatic abnormality.[212] Dual-energy digital radiography has been used and was successful in detecting metastatic calcifications in 40% of hemodialysis cases in one series.[200] CT scanning is also very effective[207] and may detect all types of calcification and ossification.[207] Specimen radiographs are helpful at the time of autopsy if

this is suspected (Fig. 22–27). Noting a negative or black pleural shadow may help detect some early increases in lung density,[213] but this finding could be caused by multiple types of infiltrates. (See also black pleura in pulmonary alveolar microlithiasis.) Bone-scanning isotopes sometimes are helpful, and highlight bilateral lung calcifications, even in conditions without deposits of osteoid.[214] These isotopes include technetium-99m, strontium-85, fluorine (^{18}F), and labeled phosphates.

Most patients are asymptomatic, but a few develop respiratory failure.[199] Pulmonary involvement may progress rapidly.[198] Other organs may be involved by metastatic calcification; most often the heart, stomach, and kidney are so involved. Wells,[215] in 1911, and later Hueper[216] in 1927, proposed that the lungs, stomach, and kidney represent three alkaline areas of the body that would favor calcium deposition. Death from metastatic calcification is most often cardiac.[196,210] Calcification may be deposited in and affect the conducting pathways.[197] Whether accelerated atherosclerosis is prominent in these cases is undecided.[197,217] The lungs are most frequently involved of all the organs just cited. In general, involvement of the various body sites is roughly parallel, although exceptions do occur.

In a series of 56 chronically dialyzed and 18 nondialyzed chronic uremic patients, Kuzela et al.[197] found the lungs were involved in 75% of the dialysis group,

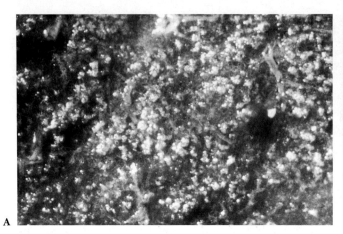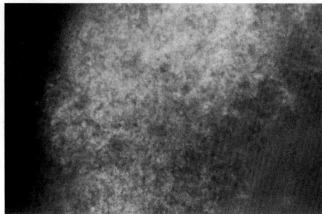

Fig. 22–27 A,B. Interstitial metastatic calcification. **A.** Gross picture of lung of 63-year-old woman who died in terminal renal failure. Focal nature of interstitial calcification in this case gives it a fine nodular grittiness. **B.** Specimen radiograph shows superimposition of areas of calcification.

including severe involvement of 48% of the total number of dialyzed patients. The lungs were involved in only 44% of the nondialyzed group, and involvement was severe in only 17% of the total of this group.

Grossly, the lungs involved with metastatic calcification may be heavy and yet retain their original architecture. The areas of involvement are usually dry; they vary from spongy to firm to brittle, do not collapse even on sectioning, and have a fine sharpness or grittiness (Figs. 22–26 and 22–27A). Their color varies from light grey to grey-yellow. Microscopically, mild-to-moderate involvement may be quite patchy, and the areas involved have alveoli fixed in a rigid open appearance, in contrast to nearby collapsed lung (Figs. 22–28 and 22–29). Calcium is deposited principally on the elastic tissue of alveolar septa, arteries, veins, bronchioles, and bronchi (Fig. 22–22). Early deposition consists of fine stippled basophilic granules, usually in mildly edematous septa.

As deposition continues, the areas of involvement become more fibrotic and calcium is more platelike (Fig. 22–29B). Alveoli may show a fibrinous edema, and the calcified deposits sometimes appear to fracture with processing. Also, a foreign-body response to some of the calcified elastic tissue may be present.[197–199] The calcified areas stain with von Kossa and Alizarin red S stains. Scanning electron microscopy gives a graphic high-power appearance.[201] Several transmission electron microscopy studies have been done.[218,219] The calcium is usually deposited as a phosphate,[199,201] but occasionally as a carbonate.[196] Calcium may be increased some 55 times over normal values.[218]

Neff and associates[196] have described metaplastic ossification in the interstitium in such cases. Their case is well illustrated, and the areas of involvement were multifocal and progressively involved over at least 3 years. These were associated with near-confluent fibrosis in adjacent alveoli. Kuzela et al.[197] mentioned metastatic ossification in 4 of 56 dialysis patients, but these cases were not illustrated. Several similar cases are available in the A.A. Liebow Pulmonary Pathology Collection (San Diego, California), and the descriptive words "ossifying pneumonia" have been used in reference to some of these cases (see following). Also, several cases of a peculiar calcification of intraalveolar amorphous-appearing material have been accumulated in the A.A. Liebow Pulmonary Pathology collection. In one such case (Fig. 22–30), the calcified lines form an interesting conchus-like pattern. In this case there is no evidence of ossification. This, and one other similar case, presented with focally dense radiographic infiltrates. This might represent dystrophic calcification in areas of confluent organizing pneumonia, but more cases need to be studied to explore this hypothesis.

Ossification

Ossification in the lung may occur in several situations. It may be an incidental metaplastic change in the tracheobronchial cartilaginous rings as a part of aging effect. It may occur in dystrophic situations in chronic necrosis and/or slowly growing tumor masses. It may occur in pulmonary alveolar microlithiasis or nodular or tracheobronchial amyloid, or tracheobronchopathia osteochondroplastica, as discussed in this chapter. It may also be associated with malignancy, as in metastatic osteosarcomas.

Another form of benign ossification occurs in the lung, most often in the parenchyma, that cannot be specifically related to necrosis or tumor masses. Given

Fig. 22–28 A–C. Interstitial calcification. **A.** Low-power view shows abundant calcification. H and E. ×30. Note it is irregular and does not involve all the alveolar septa. **B.** Note fine calcification of the elastic tissue about bronchiole and in alveolar septa. Von Kossa, ×150. **C.** Calcification may end abruptly, as seen in this transition zone to more normal lung. Von Kossa, ×400.

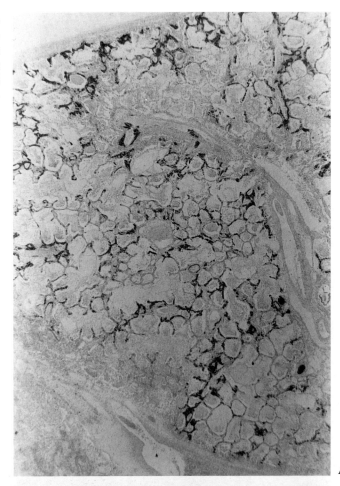

A

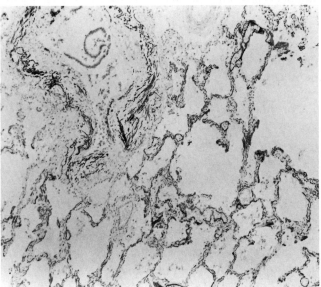

B

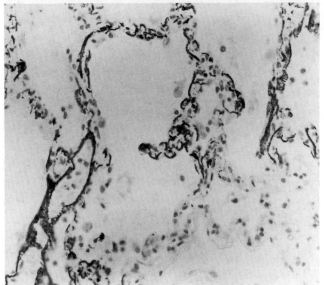

C

the designation of "ossification of the lung," this entity was first reported in 1859 by Wagner.[220] Its common association with mitral valve disease was noted in 1932 by Salinger.[221] Much of the early work was published in German, including a review of 33 cases by Janker[222] in 1936, and a nice review in English of this literature was done by Wells and Dunlap in 1943.[223]

Generally, two types of ossification are described, nodular or circumscribed and dendriform or branching types. The most common form of ossification is the

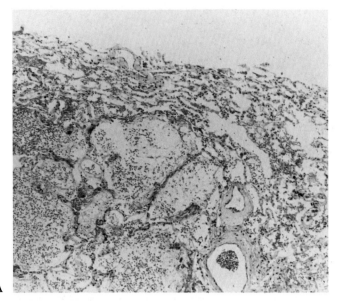

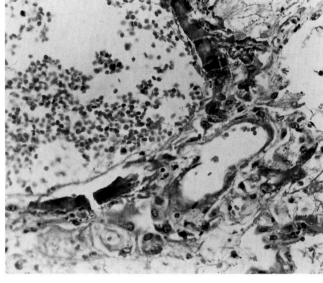

A   B

Fig. 22–29 A,B. Interstitial metastatic calcification. More severely involved case than in Fig. 22–28. **A.** Calcification in alveolar septal walls holds alveoli open. Note difference in size between those fixed open and surrounding more atelectatic uninvolved parenchyma. Also note fibrin and blood in involved areas. H and E, ×100. **B.** High-power view shows dense plate-like calcification in alveolar septal walls and less dense vascular involvement. H and E, ×400.

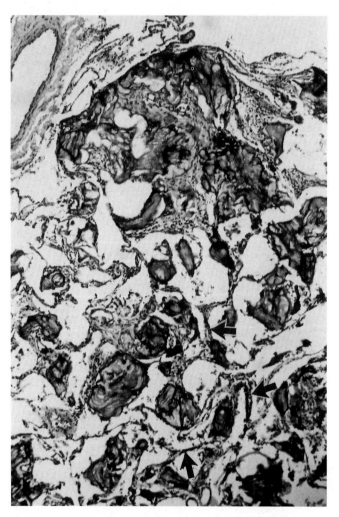

dendriform type.[223] This type is distinguished by its evolution from fibrosis and it contains marrow spaces as described next, and is sometimes confused on cross section with the nodular form, which has neither of those components. Both forms are composed of mature lamellar bone without much osteoblastic or osteoclastic activity and without evidence of pre- or coexistent cartilage. In only one case of which I am aware has cartilage been identified.[224] There is also usually no interstitial calcification in either type. Both types appear more commonly in the lower lobes and emphasize the periphery.

The dendriform form consists of linear and branching bony deposits, usually within the interstitium, often probably in alveolar septa that are greatly expanded. This form usually contains marrow elements composed of mature fat and hematopoietic cells, although rarely the marrow is involved with systemic diseases such as one case reported with leukemic involvement.[224] It is sometimes referred to as "diffuse" or "disseminated,"[223] but it is almost always localized. Besides dendriform (derived from the Greek *drys*, tree) and branching, other terms applied to this form are racemose (from Latin *racemosus*, full of clusters),[223] net-like,

◁————————————————————————

Fig. 22–30. Calcifying "pneumonia." Laminated calcium without ossification is present in intraalveolar pattern in this unusual case. Original matrix for calcium deposit is no longer identifiable. Interstitial calcification is present focally in midst of pattern (*arrows*, bottom right). H and E, ×100.

coral tree, or dichotomic.[225] Müller et al.,[225] in a study of four cases and a nice review of the literature, documented these spicules to be 2–8 mm in diameter and exhibiting regular dichotomous branching at angles of 60°–70° every 2 cm. Certainly the overall appearance (Figs. 22–31 and 22–32) suggests forms following some anatomic pathways in the lung, such as bronchopulmonary rays, veins, interlobular septa, or lymphatics, but as yet this cannot be proven.[225]

Dendriform ossification has been reported most commonly in older men, averaging age 67,[226] but I have seen two recent cases in men both in their thirties. This can produce rather spectacular lacy-appearing specimen radiographs[225,227] (Fig. 22–31) and interesting digestion specimens[224,228] (Fig. 22–32). In 1929, Daust[226] suggested this form may be a senile metaplasia of interstitial connective tissue, perhaps similar to that in the tracheobronchial cartilage. One case occurred in a patient treated for 13 years with busulfan therapy for chronic myelogenous leukemia.[227] Many other cases reported earlier did not have consistent associations other than with chronic inflammation. As reviewed by Joines and Roggli,[224] this has also been seen in cases of cystic fibrosis, histoplasmosis, and chronic abscess. These authors also described the case illustrated in Fig. 22–32A, an asbestos-exposed patient. Bone appears to rise out of peculiar nodular fibrosis.[225] (Fig. 22–32C,D) distinct from that of idiopathic pulmonary fibrosis.

The nodular circumscribed form of pulmonary ossification consists of small nodules 2–8 mm in maximum dimension. Grossly these nodules are detected as local grittiness, and are most often found in the subpleural areas of the lower lobes[229] but can be found in upper lobes. On cut surface these may simulate the appearance shown in Fig. 22–27 and even Fig. 22–31B. Specimen radiographs have been used in their study,[230–232] and occasionally these are beautifully illustrated in three dimensions[231] (Fig. 22–33).

These ossified (or ossific) bodies usually found free in alveolar space[233] (Fig. 22–32B), are composed of mature bone and usually do not contain marrow elements. When smaller, they are often round to oval, but may be irregular in shape and sometimes appear to conform to alveolar contours. When larger, they have a mulberry shape,[223,232,233] (Fig. 22–33). Elastic stains sometimes show stainable fibers in them (Fig. 22–33C), but whether this is native to lung or arises in the process of osteogenesis is unclear. I favor the former. They are usually composed of mature lamellar bone throughout, but remnant lung architecture has occasionally been demonstrated in some, as if the nodule had formed in a confluent fashion in adjacent alveoli.[234] Rarely, small ossific nodules appear to be attached to or arising in the interstitium[235] (Fig. 22–34), and whether this is a step in their evolution or a separate entity is unknown.

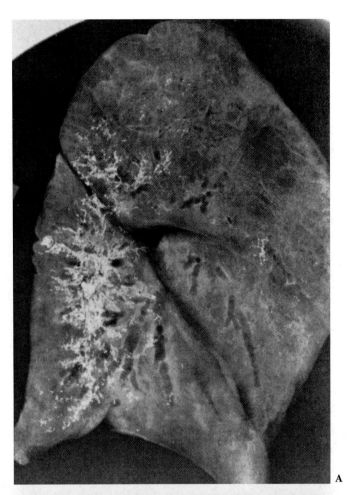

A

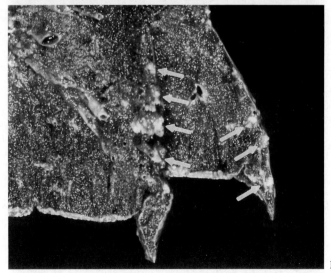

B

Fig. 22–31 A,B. Dendriform ossification. **A.** Specimen radiograph shows extensive network of branching ossification. (From Kuplic et al.,[227] with permission of the American Lung Association.) **B.** Cross-cut gross appearance of lower lobe showing subpleural ossifications (*arrows*).

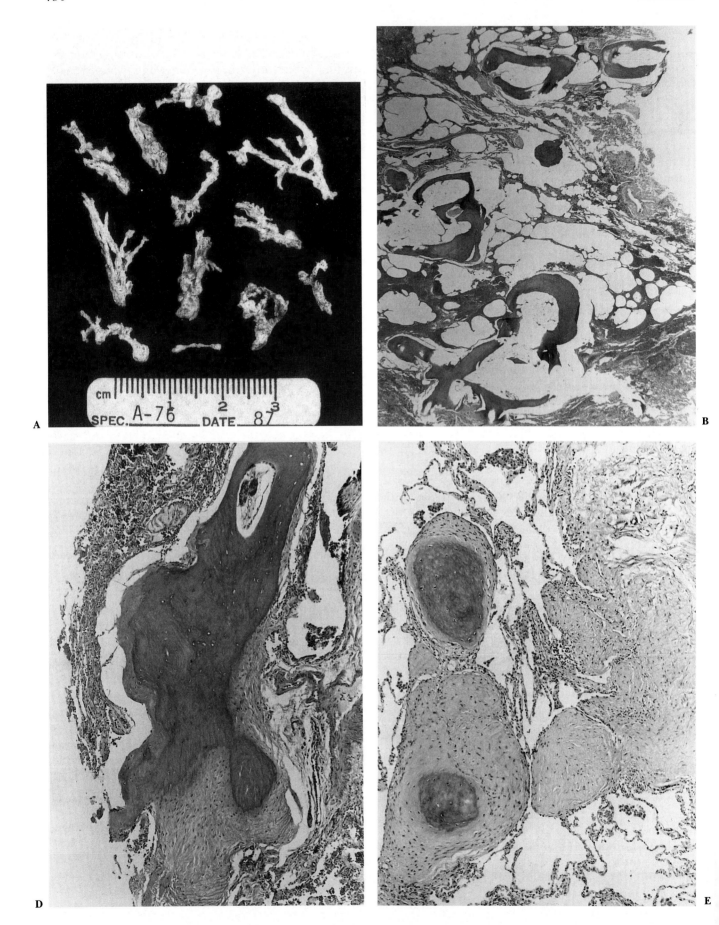

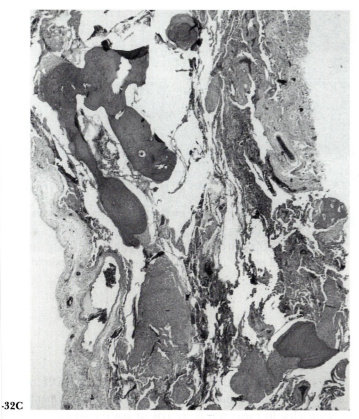

-32C

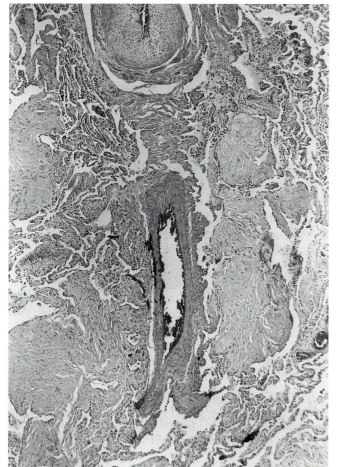

2F

Men are predominantly affected by this form of ossification as in the dendritic form, but these nodular ossified bodies occur in a younger age group, usually from 20 to 50 years. They have most frequently been described in cases of pulmonary venous hypertension, especially with mitral stenosis.[232,234] Galloway and associates[232] studied chest radiographs of 204 patients with mitral valve disease, and found 27 with definite and 9 with probable ossified nodules. This is an underestimate of the incidence; these authors also studied 8 additional patients who died with mitral valve disease but did not have radiographic evidence of ossified nodules, and all 8 had ossific nodules in their lungs at autopsy.

Other conditions in which these nodules are seen are mostly associated with pulmonary venous hypertension, and include cardiac abnormalities of mitral ring calcification, aortic valve disease, left-ventricular failure from old infarcts or other causes of myocardial fibrosis, left-atrial myxoma, core triatriatum, and constrictive pericarditis. Other extracardiac causes include assorted causes for pulmonary venous hypertension.[223,231,232] One case radiographically appeared to develop rather rapidly over a 1-month period in a patient with "shock lung."[235] At autopsy 2 years later, ossified nodules were present in the upper and lower lobes, and the background airspaces showed 44–48% obliteration by point score. Sometimes no associated abnormalities are identified.[229,236]

Nodular ossific formation in the lower lobes, most commonly in a setting of venous hypertension, suggests possible roles of both increased tissue acidity and injury. Circumstances of tissue calcification and ossification were well explored by Wells in 1911.[215] Lendrum and associates[237] suggested these nodules might form on areas of persistent intraalveolar edema. Wells and Dunlap[223] have described beginning ossification of intraalveolar exudate and organizing fibrosis. See the previous discussion of "ossifying pneumonia" with interstitial calcification and mention of similar cases by others.[225,238]

◁—————————————————————————

Fig. 22–32 A–F. Dendriform ossification. **A.** Gross fragments retrieved from sodium hypochlorite digestion of lung. (From Joines and Roggli,[224] with permission.) **B.** Microscopic detail highlights mature lamellar bone with fat-filled marrow spaces. H and E, ×60. **C.** Low-power view of metaplastic bone being produced in areas of nodular fibrosis. H and E, ×60. **D.** Precursor areas of nodular fibrosis at bottom with lamellar bone. Note marrow space at top. H and E, ×240. **E.** Early bone in nodules of fibrosis. H and E, ×240. **F.** Peculiar fibrous nodules or cords adjacent to area in **E** before bone metaplasia. H and E, ×100. (Original contributor of **C–F**: Dr. Lora Shehi, Halifax Medical Center, Daytona Beach, Florida.)

Intraalveolar Bodies and Macrophage Abnormalities

The following discussion covers many diseases related to assorted intraalveolar macrophage dysfunctions. Intraalveolar bodies of different types are included, because macrophages may play a role in their formation. Some of these macrophage abnormalities also occur in the interstitium.

Pulmonary Alveolar Microlithiasis

This is a rare disease of undermined cause. Approximately 169 cases had been published through 1987.[246,247] It is characterized by calcium phosphate microliths, sometimes called calcospherites, filling alveoli. The backbone matrix is similar to corpora amylacea in the lung and elsewhere,[248] but calcium-rich rings, the enlarged size of some of these bodies, the somewhat irregular contours at times, a lack of central nidus or inclusion, and the extent of involvement help to histologically distinguish this disease from the usually incidental corpora amylacea.

Harbitz first described this disease in 1918,[249] and Puhr[250] in 1933 coined the term "mikrolithiasis alveolaris pulmonum." Several good reviews are available.[246,247,251–254] The single largest series of 23 cases was reported by Sosman et al.[251] A complete review by Prakash and colleagues[246] in 1983 added 8 cases to their literature review of 120 published cases, and pediatric cases were reviewed in 1987.[247]

A family history is present in about half of the cases.[251] In the familial cases siblings are predominantly involved with up to four siblings being involved in one family.[251] One case involved a parent and child,[255] another two siblings and an offspring of one of them.[256] There is equal gender incidence in sporadic cases with a 2:1 female predominance in siblings. The disease has been reported in premature twins[252] and although the pictures in this report[257] are not clearly typical, it does occur in the very young. It also occurs up to age 80.[258] About 85% are diagnosed before age 50, with a mean age at diagnosis of 35.[253] Of interest, the peak incidence for diagnosis in Japan is between 4 and 9 years of age.[257] Most patients are asymptomatic (70%) when diagnosed. Cough is the most common symptom;[246,251] rarely is there clubbing.[251,259] There may be a mild restrictive defect that correlates with the degree of fibrosis. Most patients are stable, or show only very slow progression over many years. Moderate progression is rare, and rapid deterioration is exceptional.[260]

The chest radiograph shows a "sandstorm" appearance (Figs. 22–37 through 22–39), with increased granular density most striking over the mid- and lower lung

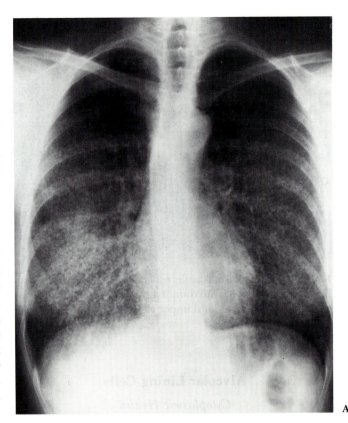

A

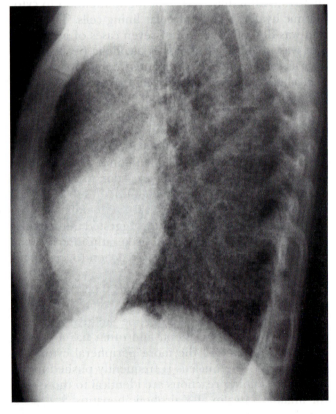

B

Fig. 22–37 A,B. Pulmonary alveolar microlithiasis. Chest radiographs in **A.** posterior to anterior and **B.** lateral views show grainy or sandy-appearing lung. No "black" pleura is seen here. (Courtesy of Reilly Kidd, M.D., The Virginia Mason Clinic, Seattle, Washington.)

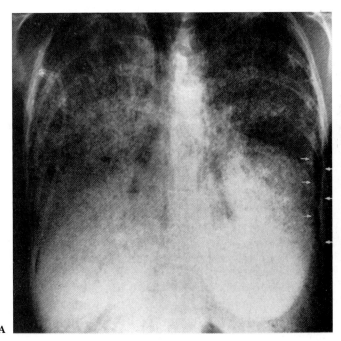

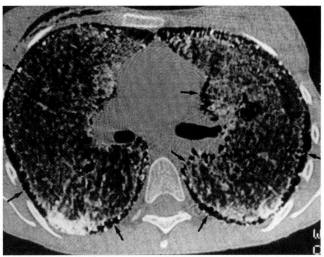

Fig. 22–38 A,B. Radiographic imaging of "black pleura." **A.** Highlighted with *white arrows* on routine chest radiograph. **B.** CT scan shows subpleural cysts (*black arrows*) accounting for black pleura. (From Korn et al.,[226] with permission.)

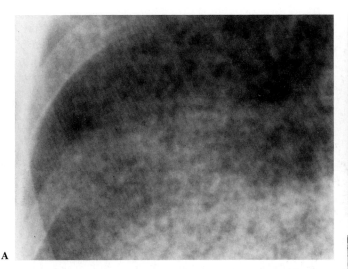

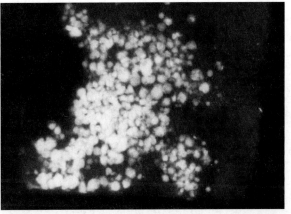

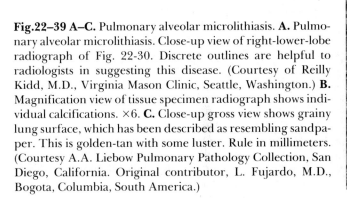

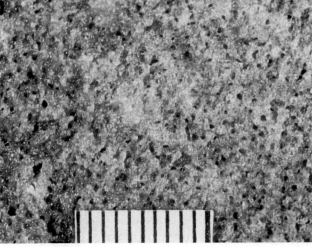

Fig.22–39 A–C. Pulmonary alveolar microlithiasis. **A.** Pulmonary alveolar microlithiasis. Close-up view of right-lower-lobe radiograph of Fig. 22-30. Discrete outlines are helpful to radiologists in suggesting this disease. (Courtesy of Reilly Kidd, M.D., Virginia Mason Clinic, Seattle, Washington.) **B.** Magnification view of tissue specimen radiograph shows individual calcifications. ×6. **C.** Close-up gross view shows grainy lung surface, which has been described as resembling sandpaper. This is golden-tan with some luster. Rule in millimeters. (Courtesy A.A. Liebow Pulmonary Pathology Collection, San Diego, California. Original contributor, L. Fujardo, M.D., Bogota, Columbia, South America.)

fields. Sometimes the entire lung is involved.[213,251] The lungs are moderately to extremely opacified by miliary densities. Computerized axial tomography (CT) nicely demonstrates widespread involvement.[247,261,262] The pleura in some cases, in contrast to the underlying lung, has been called "black pleura" radiographically,[213] but white pleura has also been described.[263–267] The latter finding was thought to be caused by calcification but in one series[265] only fibrohyaline change in pleura was noted histologically. The "black pleura" (Fig. 22–38A) has now been shown by high-resolution CT scans to result from 5- to 10-mm subpleural cysts[268] (Fig. 22–38B). These scans also show there is a gradient of distribution of these bodies, with more in the lower lobes, especially posteriorly.[268] The heart and diaphragm outlines are often obscured by the sandy parenchymal densities, but may be seen with over-penetrated films. Cor pulmonale can develop. Technetium-99 isotope bone scans indicate bilateral dense uptake.[246,261,262]

The degree of pulmonary involvement radiographically and pathologically is much worse than the patient's clinical symptoms. Approximately half the cases in the past were originally considered to result from miliary tuberculosis,[254] but the absence of significant clinical symptoms is against such a disease. Other miliary patterns, as with pneumoconiosis, lymphangiitic cancer, and, less likely, fungi, have been considered in the differential, but the particular appearance is so striking as to be diagnostic. Newer imaging techniques also help confirm the calcified nature if any question persists.[268–270]. As with pulmonary alveolar proteinosis, the discordance of the chest radiograph and the patient's symptoms may be a clue to diagnosis. Occasionally microliths are produced in the sputum and lavage specimens.[271,272]

Grossly, the lungs are heavy and cut with great difficulty, and sometimes require sawing! They are gritty, have a white-tan to yellow-grey color (Fig. 22–39), and retain their whole-organ shape when sectioned. Gough sections "look virtually like sandpaper."[273] The microliths generally vary between 0.01 and 0.5 mm in diameter, with most being about 0.2 mm.[246,273] One series measured microliths up to 2.8 mm![246] These bodies fall out of the gross tissue easily, indicating they are usually not trapped in the lung by fibrous tissue. This coincides with the microscopic appearance.

Microscopically the liths are round to elongate to slightly irregular, have distinctly amphiphilic to basophilic accentuation of their onion-like rings, and have find radial striations (Fig. 22–40). These bodies can fracture on sectioning, and often some of their substance is removed in tissue processing. On frozen section they are polarizable and sudanophilic, suggesting a lipid content.[273] They stain with periodic acid–Schiff and iron stains. They do not have black, crystalline, or other core ingredients such as are present in corpora amylacea. Several liths may occupy a single alveolus, or a large one may fill an entire alveolus (Fig. 22–41). They do not appear to fuse with each other. The lung architecture in less involved areas is normal, but fibrosis and chronic inflammation accompany increasing involvement by these bodies. Occasionally ossification is present in more severe cases[273] (Fig. 22–40B). Rarely, similar bodies are within bronchiolar walls.[258,274]

Scanning electron microscopy shows peculiar scale-like formations on the surface.[246,275] Transmission electron microscopy shows the rings and radial striations and many small matrix vesicles of undetermined origin.[246,276] Except for these small vesicles and the calcification, the backbone is similar to corpora amylacea.[246,248] Chemical analysis has shown these bodies to be composed predominantly of calcium phosphate, the major calcium salt of bone,[246,253,273,277] in a hydroxyapatite crystalline arrangement.[276] Calcium carbonate and very small amounts of magnesium and iron have also been found.

This disease is not usually associated with stone-forming tendency elsewhere, but rare exceptions have been reported.[264] These exceptions probably fall within the spectrum of findings in the general population. The serum calcium and phosphate levels are usually normal, as is vitamin D metabolism. There are histologic similarities in these bodies and psammomatous calcifications in papillary adenocarcinomas, but these similarities may only represent limited responses of the host. One author[278] suggested four cases observed in Saudi Arabia may be variants of desert lung syndrome (nonoccupational dust pneumoconiosis); specifically, that fine sand particles may act as nidi. This is unproven, and most cases in the world's literature have no such association documented. A careful dust exposure and other exposure history is, however, always warranted. The greatest association is with familial incidence, but the cause or mechanism(s) remains undetermined. No therapy has proven helpful. Bronchoalveolar lavage has been tried but without success.[272]

Corpora Amylacea

Corpora amylacea are intraalveolar spherical bodies first described by Friedreich[279] in 1856 and named because their staining characteristics are similar to those of starch (see naming of amyloid in this chapter). Lubarsch and Plenge[280] summarized many of their features in 1931, and noted their occurrences in cases of

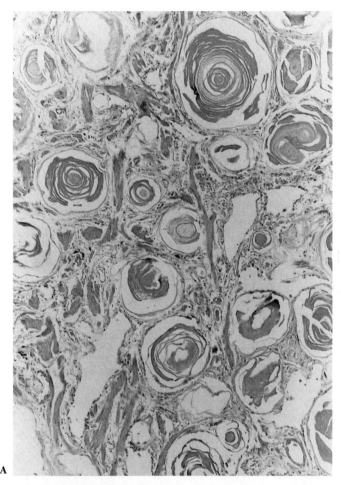

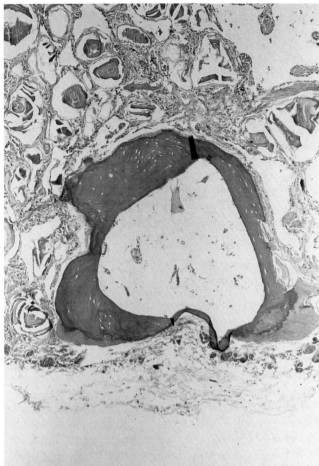

A

B

Fig. 22–40 A,B. Pulmonary alveolar microlithiasis. **A.** Multiple intraalveolar microliths show some shattering artefact with tissue processing and sectioning. **B.** Note ossification with marrow space in subpleura and absence of subpleural cysts here.

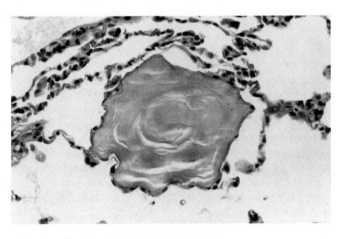

Fig. 22–41. Pulmonary alveolar microlithiasis. At times microliths assume slightly irregular contour and carry with them contour of adjacent septa. Rings in this case are not as well calcified as in Fig. 20–30. H and E, ×200.

emphysema, chronic bronchitis, congestion, infarction, atelectasis, and pneumonia.

In an unselected autopsy series of 1,070 cases, Michaels and Levene[281] found corpora amylacea in 3.8%. These were not present before age 20, occurred in limited frequency and number between ages 20 and 60, and were more frequent after 60 years of age. The authors did not find any particular lobe was favored, nor did they find any particular site within acini prone to collect these bodies. In another large review by Hollander and Hutchins,[282] 37 cases were found in 6,500 unselected autopsies, an incidence of 0.6%, and these occurred in the age range of 48 to 87 years, with an average of 70 years of age. Neither series could document any particular disease association as had been suggested by Lubarsch and Plenge in 1931.[280]

The staining characteristics were well described by Baar and Ferguson[283] and others.[281,284] These are very

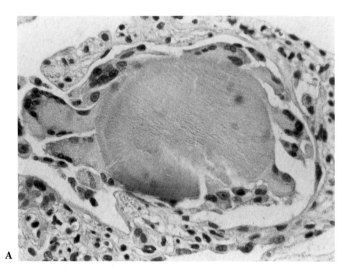 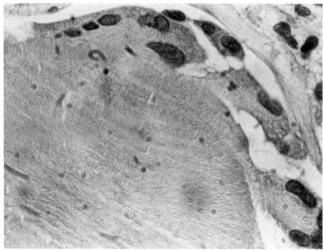

A   B

Fig. 22–42 A,B. Corpora amylacea. **A.** Matrix of corpora amylacea has radiating fibrillar lines and one delicate circumferential line. H and E, ×400. **B.** Higher magnification shows rim of multinucleate cells H and E, ×1000.

similar to such inclusions in prostate duct lumens,[283] except that in the lung they are more often about the same size, are more generally spherical, have somewhat better developed layers, and contain various inclusions when compared to prostate.

The corpora amylacea vary between 30 and 200 μm, and are usually 60–100 μm.[281] These bodies are composed of glycoprotein and are free of lipid, calcium, and iron. Little of their substance is altered by tissue processing, unlike pulmonary alveolar microlithiasis or blue bodies. They have closely applied layers of circumferentially laminated fine lines crossed occasionally by some delicate radiating lines. These bodies stain pink to slightly amphophilic on H and E, blue on Mason's trichrome, and magenta on PAS stains. Although not always present, a rim of macrophages around their perimeter occurs in some. One could argue that these cells are reacting to the presence of these bodies, but it seems more logical that they are playing a role in their formation[281] (Fig. 22–42). Corpora amylacea appear to be "free floating" in the alveoli. They have a maltese cross pattern with polarization, and stain nonspecifically with Congo red, giving an alternating yellow and green cross pattern.

Inclusions, often present in the center of these bodies (Fig. 22–43), may consist of black fragments and ring forms, or of small polarizable crystals that are organic in nature and disappear on incineration (Figs. 22–44 and 22–45). Some of the black fragments probably represent carbon fragments, but Hollander and Hutchins[282] found a certain number were rather monotonous ring forms, which they proposed correspond to the plant spores of *Lycopodium*, used in dusting and facial powders. These ring forms are 15–20 μm, and occurred in

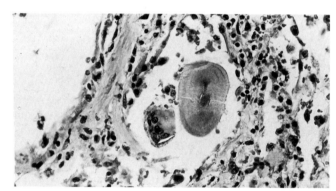

Fig. 22–43. Corpora amylacea. Crystalline material, usually needle shaped, may be in center of these bodies as shown in larger central body. Smaller multinucleate cell near this contains a larger but similar body, suggesting one possible mechanism for early corpora amylacea formation. Circumferential rings are similar to those of alveolar microliths but are not calcified. H and E, ×200.

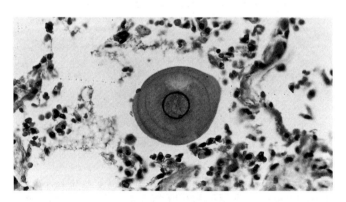

Fig. 22–44. Corpora amylacea. Darkly staining ring forms may be in center of these bodies. H and E, ×400.

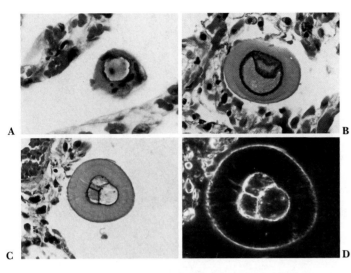

Fig. 22–45 A–D. Corpora amylacea. Other variations are shown. **A.** Early nidus is suggested. H and E, ×400. **B.** Complex ring form. H and E, ×200. **C.** Tripartite ring form. H and E, ×200. **D.** Phase microscopy of Fig. 20–45C. H and E, ×300.

one-third of their patients with corpora amylacea, although they were only present in a small number of these bodies (3%). The ring-form inclusions did not stain with periodic acid–Schiff (PAS), methenamine silver, or Alizarin red.

It seems probable that many of these concretions form around assorted small inhaled particles or other foci of irritation to the alveolus and macrophage. Central crystals may be formed in a process similar to their formation in macrophages, and may then be nonspecific. Some of these bodies may form to irritating products that have since been degraded, or possibly to certain foci of inspissated mucus or other secretions that are not apparent on inspection at a later time. The latter is the presumed route of their formation in the prostate, and would account for those cases with no inclusions.

At times there may be confusion with pulmonary alveolar microlithiasis,[283] but these two types of bodies should be easily distinguished. The nonspecific term "microlith" may apply to either of these bodies and to assorted other bodies.

Blue Bodies

This term was proposed by Dr. Averill A. Liebow in 1965, for want of a better term, to describe small roughly ovoid-to-spherical irregularly laminated structures in the cytoplasm of alveolar macrophages.[285] These were described by Michaels[286] in 1967 as probable wood dust in the lungs of 2 lumber workers, but were not present in 21 autopsies of other workers in the same industry. The largest series of 19 cases, by Dail and Liebow,[285] is available in abstract form only. One of the cases summarized by them was reported separately by Gardiner and Uff.[287] The best-evaluated series of 10 cases is by Koss et al.,[288] and 1 of their cases was separately published by Kim and associates.[289] Ninety percent of the patients involved were men, and the age range is 28 to 76, with an average of 48 years.

These blue bodies have a highly refractile polarization pattern on frozen[285] and unstained deparaffinized section appearance.[288] Tissue processing reduces the polarization, but does not always totally eradicate it[285] (Fig. 22–46). Where some substance is lost, there are as many as three or four, light to medium blue-grey rings inside clear spaces inside the cytoplasm of macrophages. These rings are weakly iron positive, strongly PAS positive, and von Kossa positive. Koss et al.[288] have proved this dissolved matrix is calcium carbonate, which is dissolved by acid solutions in many histochemical stains. These bodies have been analyzed in sputum, further confirming this component.[290] The individual inclusions are 15–40 μm in diameter, and the larger ones may form by junctions with smaller bodies. Electron microscopic studies have shown these not to be membrane bound or to have core material as might be seen in corpora amylacea. The rings consist of electron-dense granules, probably iron, with some fine radiating fibrillar material, perhaps mucopolysaccharide matrix.[287,288] Electron probe analysis has not identified exogenous minerals, as would occur in pneumoconiosis.[287]

Blue bodies are patchy in distribution, but when several are found, more are likely nearby. They are frequently associated with hemosiderin-laden macrophages and are most frequently described in a histologic background of the reaction of desquamative interstitial pneumonitis (DIP).[285] Because they are small and often not obvious, they are easily missed, but sometimes they are alarmingly obvious (Fig. 22–46). Once the pathologist is sensitized to the possibility of their presence, they may be seen with some frequency around tumor masses, and this author estimates they are found in approximately 1 of 20 lungs resected for tumor, usually in the immediate vicinity of the tumor. Of interest, they are not usually a component of primary hemosiderosis, passive congestion, Goodpasture's disease, exogenous lipid pneumonia, or the histiocytic reaction associated with pulmonary histiocytosis X.

Blue bodies appear to be a product of histiocyte metabolism, especially in chronic histiocyte stasis. They do not represent exogenous pneumoconiosis, but as noted they can sometimes be quite abundant. In the differential diagnoses are conchoidal and Schaumann bodies, but these are usually larger, up to 100 μm,

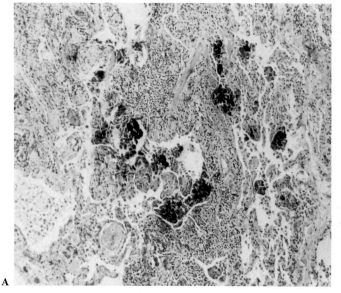

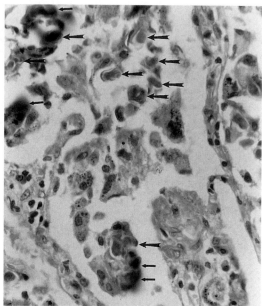

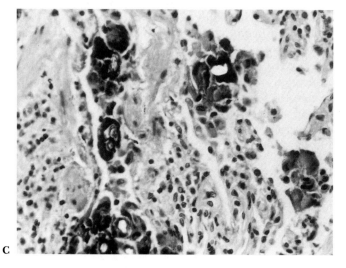

Fig. 22–46 A–C. Blue bodies. **A.** Calcified bodies are clustered in alveoli. **B.** Multiple laminated irregular blue bodies are seen (*arrows*). Note laminar whorled character in some. More are out of plane of focus (*small arrows*). H and E, ×400. **C.** Partial polarization shows some refractile material. Note irregularly laminated areas in less densely calcified zones. (H and E, ×250.

contain lipid, and are in the interstitium in giant cells.[288,291,292] Blue bodies are unlike oxalate crystals, which have a different polarizable appearance, and maintain this appearance after tissue staining. Oxalate crystals are usually larger and lack the internal blue lines of blue bodies. Pulmonary alveolar microlithiasis and corpora amylacea are much larger, and each has easily distinguished characteristics.

Other Inclusions

Other inclusions, calcified bodies, or microliths have been noted, especially in the sputum. These include inspissated mucus and calcified broken loops of Curschmann's spirals. Tao[293] described microliths of varying sorts in 26 of 100 patients with assorted chronic obstructive pulmonary diseases, 7 of which appeared to be calcified fragments of Curschmann's spirals. By con-

trast, in the same study Tao also reviewed 100 patients with other pulmonary diseases and 1 of these (with tuberculosis) had sputum microliths, but none of the third group of 100 without pulmonary problems had microliths. Other conditions producing sputum microliths of different sorts have been reviewed by Pritzker et al.[294] Polarizable inclusions may be a nonspecific part of granulomatous inflammation[295] (see Chapter 19).

Minute myelin lamellar type bodies are sometimes recognized by light microscopy in pulmonary alveolar proteinosis.[296] Larger whorled or delicately laminated spherical bodies may represent giant lamellar bodies, similar to these and are sometimes seen in other conditions. This author has seen them in cases of so-called "alveolar adenomas" and "sclerosing hemangioma of the lung" (Fig. 22–47). Sclerosing hemangiomas contain large blood-filled cysts, and such figures may be the result of chronic breakdown of cell membranes. Other

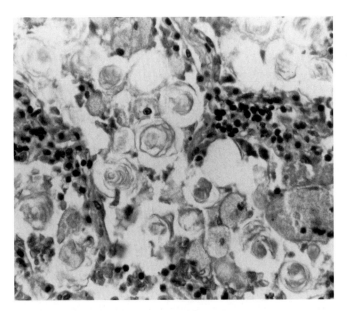

Fig. 22–47. Whorled or giant lamellar bodies may occur in areas of chronic trapped hemorrhage or other areas of chronic cell breakdown. This case represents one field in a so-called "sclerosing hemangioma" of lung. Note granular lipid-filled macrophages, which presumably have role in forming these bodies. H and E, ×400.

by-products of these would be cholesterol clefts and crystals, and these two are commonly seen in this tumor.

Other macrophage inclusions such as asteroid bodies, giant lysosomes of Hamazaki–Wesenberg, asteroid, conchoid, and Schaumann bodies are discussed in Chapter 19.

Pulmonary Alveolar (Phospholipo)Proteinosis

Rosen et al.[296] in 1958 named and published "27 cases of a remarkable disease of the lung that consists of the filling of the alveoli by a PAS-positive proteinaceous material, rich in lipid." The name alveolar proteinosis or lipoproteinosis, or perhaps most accurately phospholipoproteinosis, applies equally to this entity. It should not be confused with lipoid proteinosis of the trachea, which is discussed elsewhere in this chapter.

About half the patients in this original series had some exposure to dusts, including wood dust, or fumes, as did a similar proportion of the 139 cases reviewed by Davidson and MacLeod[297] in 1969. In humans, fine silica,[298–302] aluminum,[303] and kaolin[304] dust exposures have caused this reaction. In experimental animals, silica[305–308] (including volcano dust,[309]) aluminum,[310,311] and fiberglass dusts,[312] iprindole,[313] cholphentermine,[314–316] and 100% oxygen exposure,[317] welding fumes,[318] bentonite, talc, or kaolin[319] have induced this reaction. Many of these experimental models evolve through an endogenous lipid pneumo-

nia, which at times is almost desquamative in type. McEuen and Abraham[320] found increased dust particles using backscatter electron microscopy in 78% of their cases. These particles were predominantly less than 1 μm in diameter, so were impossible to see by light microscopy. They were found in both alveolar contents and interstitium. Specific particle analysis from this series was added later.[321] There was good correlation in some individuals; for example, silica in a sandblasting worker, cement particles in cement workers, and metal fumes in a welder. Tobacco use had been suspiciously high (27 of 29 involved individuals) in one series,[322] but the analyses of McEuen and Abraham[320,321] did not identify the spectrum of soil components as might be needed to confirm an unusually high percentage of tobacco users. Three of five infants with this disease have been shown to have an increased amount of silicates, especially talc, in their lungs. Another had many fume-sized cadmium and selenide particles, possibly from overheated red paint from some object. The fifth, who never left the hospital after birth, had a high content of silica and iron of unknown origin. In a review of 34 cases from one institution (Mayo Clinic), Prakash et al.[323] noted a history of dust or chemical exposure in only 4 (12%) but comment that is by retrospective review. Although multiple minerals were identified, there was no difference in minerals identified from lungs samples of this disease compared to other pulmonary diseases.[323]

Alveolar proteinosis occurs in other situations, many suggesting altered immunity. It has occurred with extensive bilateral involvement in patients with chemotherapy[321] with various hematologic abnormalities[324–326] and in other immunosuppressed cases such as children with congenital alymphoplasia,[327–329] hypogammaglobulinemia,[330] or juvenile dermatomyositis.[331] Rarely, newborns have the disease without proven defects.[332,333] It has also been described focally around cases of tuberculosis[334] and at times as more widespread disease during therapy for tuberculosis.[335,336] In cases of tuberculosis and proteinosis, tuberculosis usually preceded the alveolar proteinosis except in two cases.[336] In a series of 26 patients with *Pneumocytis carinii* pneumonia, BAL fluids were examined by electron microscopy and in all showed myelin figures identical to that seen in PAP, but in only 9 (34.6%) was the appearance of PCP suggested on H and E stain.[337] Whether this is a shared reaction or was considered a diagnostic possibility in any case as PAP is not clear (see following). Focal area in postobstructive endogenous lipid pneumonia sometimes suggest alveolar proteinosis by light and electron microscopy. It is proposed this change might be related to oxygen and/or carbon dioxide content locally.[338]

Clinical Setting

The original description of 27 cases and the inclusive reviews of 85 cases in 1965 by Larsen and Gordinier,[322] 139 cases in 1969 by Davidson and MacLeod,[297] along with the several larger institutional reviews by Prakash et al.[323] and Kariman et al.[339] are useful in summarizing the clinical setting. There is a male predominance that varies from 1.8:1 to 4.3:1. The age range is from newborn[327,332,333] to 79 years.[340] The peak incidence is between 20 and 50 years, but 18% of cases occur in infants and children.[341] The younger age group has a higher mortality than do adults.[329] Familial occurrence is rare, although four siblings in one family died of this entity, three by the age of 6 months.[342]

Patients usually present with insidious onset of slowly progressive dyspnea. Almost half have a premonitory, low-grade febrile illness. Some have a dry cough, sometimes with streaky hemoptysis; others have pleuritic pain and some have clubbing. Minimal physical findings, despite significant radiographic changes, may be a clue to the diagnosis. Other symptoms include fatigue, chest pain, and some weight loss. Some 18% are asymptomatic.[323] Most are treated with antibiotics, and some show initial response.

Laboratory Findings

Usually the hemoglobin is normal, but in some 15%–25%, a polycythemia with hemoglobin greater than 17 gm/dl is present, probably related to chronic hypoxia. Serum proteins may be slightly altered, usually with a decreased albumin and increased alpha^1-globulin and alpha$_2$-globulin. A few patients have elevated beta or gamma globulins. Serum lipids are normal. Cultures do not show consistent organisms but are valuable in detecting superinfections, as noted below. Skin tests for the standard infections reflect the population as a whole.

Pulmonary function tests generally show an impaired diffusion defect with moderate shunting. This is more restrictive in type without obstructive elements. There is also a mild to moderate reduction in lung volume.

Lavage fluids are cloudy white, tan, or gray. Smear preparations may disrupt the typical appearance of the material, but cytospin concentrations may show preservation of the finely to focally slightly coarse PAS-positive granularity. The grossly observed cloudiness is a clue that must be explained if no history is given or no other explanation is plausible.

Radiographs

The classical radiographic appearance consists of fine, diffuse, feathery to vaguely nodular bilateral infiltrates centering around the hilar regions, usually sparing the most peripheral lung zones and including the costophrenic angles (Fig. 22–48A). This is similar to the "butterfly" or "batwing" pattern of severe acute pulmonary edema. CT findings have been described by Godwin et al.[343] (Fig. 22–48B,C). Not only the typical fluffy appearance (Fig. 22–48B) but also an interstitial pattern is seen. (Fig. 22–48C); the latter has not been explained histologically yet, but may be interstitial edema. When it occurs, resolution proceeds irregularly from the periphery toward the hila. Preger[344] also noted alternate radiographic appearances of bibasilar densities, lobar consolidation or separate nodules. Prakash et al.[323] noted asymmetric bilateral densities in 18% and unilateral involvement in 15%. Rarely, an interstitial pattern has been described.[331] Air bronchograms may be prominent. Occasionally biopsy may yield fairly extensive disease despite a normal chest radiograph.[322] Prior chest radiographs are usually normal unless involved in a similar fashion, the latter suggesting prior episodes. There is no pleural effusion nor hilar node enlargement and only rare blebs or pneumothorax. Cavitation occurs only when there is secondary infection.

Pathology

Grossly, the involved areas contain multiple firm yellow-tan to gray-white nodules, each a few millimeters to 2 cm in maximum dimension (Fig. 22–49). Whole lung examination at autopsy shows heavy lungs, usually two to five times that expected.[322] A viscid yellow fluid, sometimes described as milky or pus-like, has been noted to exude from the cut surface.[296,297,325,336]

Microscopically the dominant feature is filling of preserved or slightly expanded alveoli with finely granular periodic acid–Schiff diastase-resistant (PASD) acellular material (Fig. 22–50). This same material may be seen in terminal and respiratory bronchioles, but is not present in the interstitium. It is alcian- and mucicarmine negative. Frozen section examination shows abundant lipid, which is best stained with Oil Red O or Sudan Black, but lipid can also be seen on water-based rapid stains such as Goodpasture's or Terry's stains. Chemical analysis of tissue reveals even more lipid than evident by stains.[296] The intraalveolar material is usually eosinophilic on permanent and frozen sections, but may appear more basophilic than expected on some frozen sections.[345] This material stains with surfactant apoprotein by immunoperoxidase techniques.[346]

Focally, cholesterol crystals are seen that are doubly refractile on frozen section but dissolve with processing and leave clefts in the granular material (Fig. 22–50). Larger, denser, more solid clumps of PASD-positive material are also sometimes noted focally among the fine granularity (Figs. 22–50 and 22–51). After fixation, the alveolar contents have a dried appearance on high-power examination. Focally degenerating cells are present, sometimes foamy, sometimes only seen as ghosts. Collections of more viable foamy macrophages are seen, especially at the periphery, and may show transitions into degenerating forms and accumulated debris (Fig. 22–52). Most evident in the periphery, alveolar type II cells may be hyperplastic. There are no small bubble-like, cyst-like spaces, or basophilic stippling as might be seen with *Pneumocystis carinii* infection, and there is no or minimal fibrosis and no associated hyaline membrane formation unless complications have occurred. Fibrin is not evident, except in a few cases with immunosuppression.[325] Calcification is extremely unusual.[347] Acute extravasation of red cells may be present, but there is no generalized congestion, either of the blood vessels or the lymphatic spaces. Nodes rarely, if ever, have similar materials in them.[348] Any increase in inflammatory cells either acute or Any increase in either acute or chronic inflammatory cells may indicate infection. If typical areas are included diagnosis can be made by transbronchial biopsies.[323,349]

Singh et al.[346,350] and Bedrossian et al.[326] suggested dividing this disease histologically into primary and secondary forms, the secondary having much less intense surfactant apoprotein or PAS staining, although these authors do show differences in staining intensity, and others[324] have trouble with that concept, as many cases of anything once thought primary (idiopathic) have their etiologies or associations better defined with time, and the same cases then become secondary. However, secondary cases may be more focal and not have the same presentation or course as the typical primary cases.

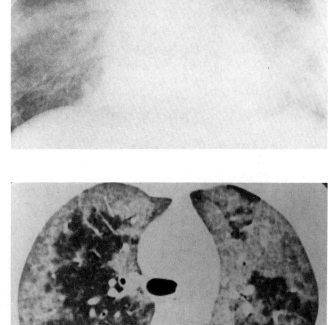

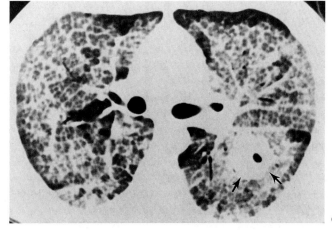

Fig. 22–48 A–C. Pulmonary alveolar proteinosis. **A.** Typical chest radiographic pattern with bilateral perihilar and basilar infiltrates. Pulmonary edema may be similar, but has vascular shunting with prominence of upper lobe vessels not seen in this disease. **B.** High-resolution CT scan shows patchy air space opacification, concentrated peripherally. Margins of patches are sharp, indicating that the opacities are bordered by interlobular septa. **C.** High-resolution CT scan shows widespread air space opacification with superimposed reticular pattern indicating thickening of interlobular septa, presumably by edema, in view of its later resolution following bronchoalveolar lavage. In addition, there is a nocardial abscess (*arrows*) in the left-lower lobe. (**B,C.** Courtesy of Dr. David Godwin, University of Washington School of Medicine, Seattle, Washington. From Radiology 1988;169:609–613, with permission.)

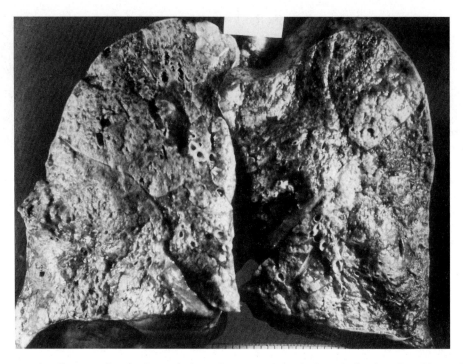

Fig. 22–49. Pulmonary alveolar proteinosis. Frontal view of both lungs shows more confluent involvement on right and more focal involvement on left. (Courtesy A.A. Liebow Pul- monary Pathology Collection, San Diego, California. Original contributor, M. Kartub, M.D., St. Lukes Hospital, Phoenix, Arizona.)

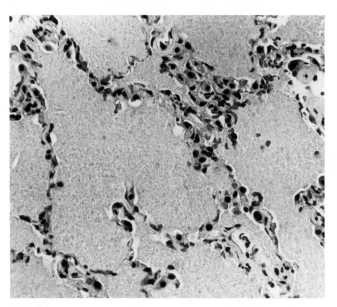

Fig. 22–50. Pulmonary alveolar proteinosis. Typical material in alveoli. Note granular "dried" appearance with some slightly larger fragments and small needle-like empty clefts. Interstitum and alveolar type II cells show only minimal changes. H and E, ×400.

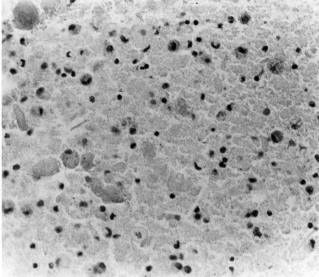

Fig. 22–51. Pulmonary alveolar proteinosis. Lavage fluid shows fine granular and larger globular fragments, possibly in macrophages. More multinucleated cells are present here than in middle of tissue reaction shown in Fig. 22–50 and may come from periphery of involved zones shown in Fig. 20–52. Cell block. H and E, ×600.

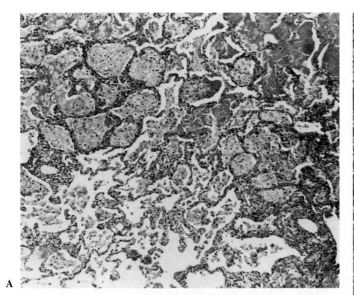

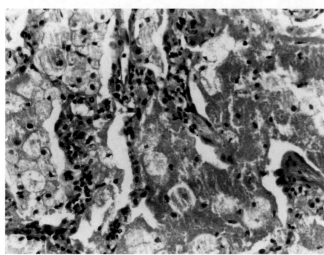

Fig. 22–52 A,B. Pulmonary alveolar proteinosis. Edge of reaction shows foamy macrophages. **A.** More typical granular material is at upper right Interstitial lymphocytes are more prevalent than toward center of reaction. H and E, ×100. **B.** High-power view of transition from intact foamy macrophages into granular debris. H and E, ×600.

Mechanisms

The original description suggested that the accumulated material in the alveoli may result from degenerating cell products; Rosen et al.[296] described small laminated bodies seen by light microscopy and illustrated their appearance. Kuhn et al.[351] confirmed that there are cell breakdown products in this material, including some structures relating to the bodies described. Larsen and Gordinier[322] in 1965 proposed that the material was surfactant. Electron microscopy has now confirmed that lamellar bodies seen by microscopy are surfactant[352,353] (Figs. 22–53 and 22–54). This has further

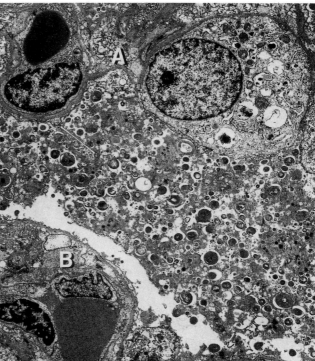

Fig. 22–53. Pulmonary alveolar proteinosis. Transmission electron micrograph shows one alveolar septum marked A, with capillary to left. Basal lamina is just below and alveolar type II cell to right of marker A. B indicates second alveolar septum; between A and B is intraalveolar space filled with material of alveolar proteinosis. ×2,500.

been substantiated by specific surfactant apoprotein stains.[346,350] The material extracted from lung specimens or lavage material is high in (di)palmityl lecithin, the major component of surfactant, but does not have its usual surface-active properties.[351,354] However, such activity can be restored by ethanol treatment.[355]

Although present in increased quantities, the various types of lipid and their percentage distribution, including the individual phospholipids, were the same when compared to normal lungs.[354,355] When alveolar proteinosis material is added to (di)palmityl lecithin, it inhibits the normal surface tension reducing action of this compound.[351,354] Surfactant extracted from uninvolved areas of a person's lung sample have shown normal surfactant activity. There is also some protein material present, reflecting mostly fibrinogen and other proteins from the serum.[355,356] However, some of these components appear in altered form when compared to their native serum counterparts.[354,356,357] Transudation accounts for most of this protein.[356,358–360]

There is dispute whether this tissue reaction is caused by increased production,[317,322,336] decreased clearance

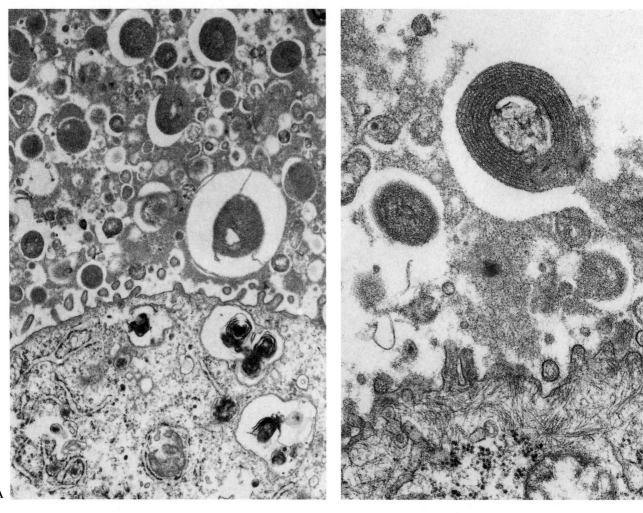

Fig. 22–54 A,B. Pulmonary alveolar proteinosis. **A.** Alveolar type II cell at bottom with lamellar surfactant bodies near surface. TEM, ×6,000. Some intraalveolar bodies are granular; others are laminar membranous, as in **B.** TEM, ×16,000.

of this surfactant material.[351,354] or a combination of these,[336,361] It is even wondered whether this reaction results from defective production of surfactant.[362] Ramirez,[354] using radiolabeled lipids, showed surfactant production in humans was not increased. Heppleston et al.[361] thought that synthesis in experimental animals was increased over the ability to remove this material. Perhaps increased activity is present in the earlier stage and not in the later.[363] A good biochemical review of this problem is that by Smith,[363] who concluded that in considering experimental production of this disease, the dosage of instigator, route of administration, and choice of animal species are critical to the experimental model as no single agent produces the disease over wide dose ranges or in all species.

Macrophages from these patients have been shown to be defective in many macrophage activities and have decreased proliferative activity.[364,365] The material

from alveolar lipoproteinosis can produce macrophage dysfunction in normal human blood monocytes[364] and mouse peritoneal macrophages.[366] The lymphocytes have also been shown experimentally to become less active.[367]

Opportunistic Infections

Infections are common and represent the major complication of alveolar proteinosis. Forty of about 260 cases (15%) reviewed in 1980[325] were found to be involved with opportunistic infections. This is in contrast to 5 of 120 cases (4%) of desquamative interstitial pneumonia to that time.[325] Fungi and *Nocardia asteroides* are most frequently identified (see Fig. 22–48B), but mycobacteria and viruses have also been seen. One review indicated the rate approaches 60% when all types of infections are considered.[322] This rate seems far too high and may reflect publication of complex cases only. The lipoproteinaceous material added to routine culture material has augmented growth of several different groups of organisms, including *Nocardia, Aspergillus,* and atypical mycobacteria.[368] Of note, infectious complications were more common in case reports before therapeutic bronchoalveolar lavage, and have become rare today.[324] Also, use of steroids with or without antibodies is more restricted. The possibility of infection or superinfection, however, should always be kept in mind and appropriate cultures and special stains done if it is suspected.

Treatment and Prognosis

Steroid therapy has not been beneficial and may aggravate or induce secondary infection, so is contraindicated. Antibiotics and steroids have been given in the past. There is some relief in a number of patients with antibiotics, but this seems to be only temporary. Specific antimicrobial therapy should be directed toward isolated organisms. Bronchopulmonary lavage is now the accepted therapy.[369,370] This usually needs to be repeated periodically over a course of years, and one patient had 21 lavage treatments.[324]

Based on prelavage series, about 30% of these patients died of their disease, 20–50% persisted with this process, and 25%–45% improved while the rest lived but did poorly. Prolonged and recurrent episodes are documented and are moderately common. Although spontaneous remissions do occur,[324,333] this reaction is commonly considered a subacute to chronic one. The review of 85 cases to 1965 documented the average age of death as 40.7 years.[323] Again, this precedes therapy with bronchopulmonary lavage. Two series address outcome with lavage[324,339] and show a favorable but not unusually good outcome. A few cases have progressive fibrosis.[296,297,371] Other cases have been shown to remain the same with repeat biopsies.[372]

Conclusions

It was suggested in the original report that the entity may be a common tissue reaction to assorted irritants. This has now been well documented. The descriptive term of pulmonary alveolar proteinosis (or alveolar phopholipoproteinosis), however, delineates a characteristic setting of extensive radiographic infiltrates and symptoms, usually of insidious onset, that are much less severe clinically than would be implied by the degree of radiographic involvement. Often there is a prolonged course needing treatment by repeated lavage.

Desquamative Interstitial Pneumonia

Historical Aspects

Desquamative interstitial pneumonia (DIP) is a term proposed by Liebow in 1962[373] to describe a condition with monotonous appearance of alveoli filled with abundant nonvacuolated macrophages, with mild interstitial thickening but no necrosis or fibrin. The original detailed series by Liebow et al.[374] in 1965 reviewed 18 cases seen between 1960 and 1964. An addendum to this article noted an additional 14 cases seen by this group in the next 6 months. Attention was also brought to this pattern in 1962 by Herbert et al.,[375] who noted an unusual pattern of abundant histiocytes rich in hemosiderin in 2 cases of a series of 12 with interstitial fibrosis. Gaensler et al.[376] presented an expanded series of 12 cases in 1966, several with long-term follow-up.

As this disease can be produced by various causes and may be a component of many other reactions, it is now rightfully considered a pattern of tissue reaction and not a distinct disease. Scadding and Hinson[377] in 1967 were the first to propose that it is a cellular phase of the more usual type of interstitial fibrosis (see following). There are some benefits to using this term as a descriptive pattern, as it has a characteristic appearance, response to therapy, and prognosis that differs from interstitial fibrosis.

In his original consultation correspondence, Liebow was not sure whether the intraalveolar cells were histiocytes or lining cells, and so referred to this entity as desquamative histiocytic interstitial pneumonitis (DHIP). This term was referred to in one case discussed by Bates and Christie in their text in 1964.[378] Liebow ultimately chose alveolar lining cells for his 1962 presentation and modified this name to desquamative interstitial pneumonia. This proved to be a less appropriate name as the cells in the alveoli have now been proven by electron microscopy to be predominantly macrophages, admixed with a few alveolar type II cells.[379–383] This has been confirmed by enzyme histochemical markers in experimental[383] and human studies.[384,385] Little has been added to the original description except for (1) identifying the cell type as macrophage, (2) noting assorted conditions causing this type of reaction, (3) broadening its "typical" radiographic description, and (4) noting its high frequency and overlap with tobacco abuse.

Clinical Setting

The following descriptions refer to the type of involvement noted in the original paper. About equal numbers of men and women are involved, most frequently in the 35- to 55-year-old group, while 10% of the cases occur

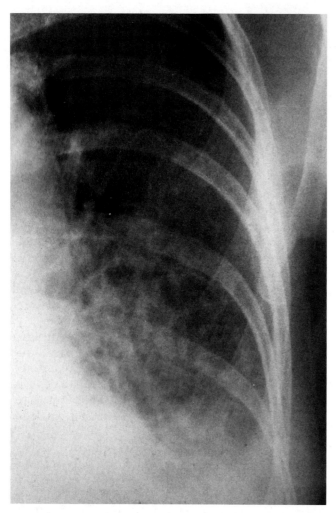

Fig. 22–55. Desquamative interstitial pneumonia. Typical chest radiographic appearance of this reaction was originally described as wedge- or pyramid-shaped infiltrate from hilum to base, as illustrated here.

Radiographs

The typical radiographic appearance as originally described consisted of bibasilar ground-glass triangular infiltrates with their bases toward the diaphragm and their apices toward the pulmonary hila (Fig. 22–55). This is still very characteristic of this reaction but is present in only one-sixth of cases.[389–392] Assorted nonpathognomonic patterns are more frequent than the "classical" appearance, and even normal chest radiograph findings are described, occurring in 26% of 47 cases in the best studied series.[391] Biopsies may still be done because of these nonspecific clinical and radiographic presentations. As this is a reaction pattern, transbronchial biopsies may not exclude other more central lesions.[393,394] However, the clinician may wish to give a trial of steroids before proceeding to open lung biopsy if the radiographic pattern is typical and the transbronchial biopsy is consistent. CT scans suggest this disease when there are patchy peripheral densities and is more accurate in follow-up than routine radiography.[395]

Pathology

Grossly the involved lungs are nodular, indurated, and airless. Involved areas vary from red-gray to pasty yellow. The histologic appearance shows consolidation of 10%–98% of the distal air spaces; in 50% of the Liebow series, more than 90% of air spaces were involved on biopsy.[374] One must remember that these statistics probably apply to some of the most involved zones preferentially selected for biopsy. The free alveolar cells are usually densely packed, while retaining cytoplasmic borders. These have been referred to as squamoid cells[374] or epithelioid histiocytes.[396] With slight artifactual retraction from tissue processing, these have been compared to "paving stones"[393] (Fig. 22–56). Sometimes this retraction artifact is not present (Fig. 22–56C).

The cytoplasm is dense, eosinophilic to slightly amphophilic, and often has a brown hue, part of which results from an increased number of phagolysosomes and some of which is from finely particulate iron, which is present in one-half of cases. Periodic acid–Schiff (PAS) stains accentuate this fine granularity in some cases. Heavy deposits of hemosiderin are not typical and should make one search for other causes especially as related to bleeding. No vacuoles or foamy appearance is present. The macrophages have a generally monotonous appearance and may have a slight admixture of eosinophils, lymphocytes, and polymorphonuclear leucocytes (PMNs). Multinucleated cells are formed from the individual macrophages. Fine polariz-

in infants and children.[385] There is no familial occurrence. Most are afebrile and present with progressive dyspnea. Other organs are usually not involved, so symptoms are pulmonary related. Cough, nonproductive in most, or chest pain may be present. Sometimes weight loss occurs. Cyanosis and clubbing occur in about one-third of cases. Physical examination is generally unremarkable except for finding fine rales in less than half of these cases. Only rarely is there pleural or pericardial fluid or pneumothorax, and there is no lymph node enlargement. Pulmonary function tests show diffusion defects, which may cause an elevated hemoglobin. There may be a mild leukocytosis with increased polymorphonuclear leukocytes, presumably stress related. DIP can present as sudden death in infants[386]; recurrences at 7 and 12 years after resolution have been documented.[387,388]

Fig. 22–56 A–C. Desquamative interstitial pneumonia. **A.** Low-power view of multiple alveoli filled with enlarged macrophages shows some retraction artifact. H and E, ×100. **B.** Desquamative interstitial pneumonia. Many somewhat enlarged macrophages with rather solid-looking cytoplasm fill alveoli. Fixation artefact has led to retraction, which has been called a "cobblestone" effect. H and E, ×400. **C.** Desquamative interstitial pneumonia. In children, macrophages may be more confluent. H and E, ×400.

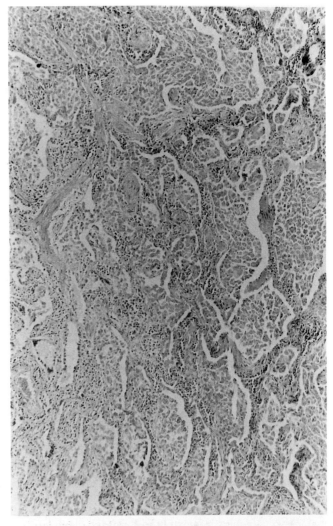

A

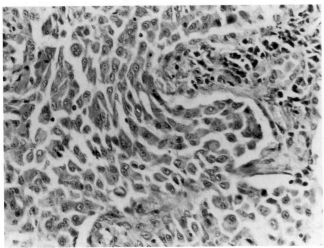

B

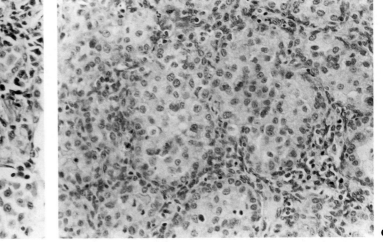

C

able needle-shaped crystals are present in a moderate number of cases. Basophilic laminated inclusions called "blue bodies" are sometimes seen in the giant cells (see **Blue Bodies** elsewhere in this chapter). The macrophage nuclei are only focally indented, or are oval, and are generally larger than the usual alveolar macrophage. Mitoses are more often identified in the free alveolar macrophages than in the alveolar type II cells. Nucleoli are sometimes prominent. Necrosis, fibrin, or hyaline membranes are not present.

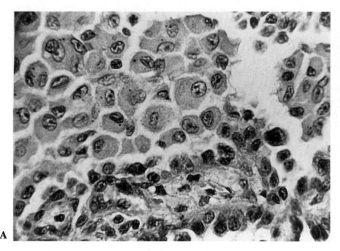

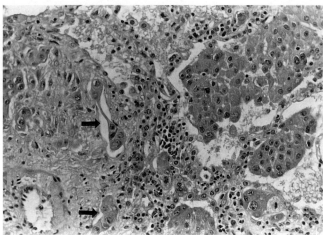

Fig. 22–57 A,B. DIP-lookalike carcinomas. In the differential of DIP-like reaction are some malignancies. **A.** Bronchioloalveolar carcinoma of true alveolar type II (nonmucinous) type. H and E, ×800. **B.** Squamous carcinoma. Individual cells to the right suggest DIP but their presence in lymphatics (*arrows*) about the vessel helps in the differential diagnosis, as does its more focal distribution when seen at lower power. H and E, ×400.

Although the term "interstitial" is used in the name of this reaction pattern, the interstitium is usually only mildly thickened by mixed inflammatory cells and young or established fibrous tissue. More significant thickening or honeycombing indicates the term interstitial fibrosis may be more appropriate, although recognizing some cases of this entity do progress to fibrosis. The alveolar type II lining cells are hyperplastic and may have intranuclear inclusions in them. When the process is focal it is remarkably peribronchiolar in location, suggesting a possible reaction to inhaled material. Also, alveolar macrophages tend to migrate to these areas. Bronchiolar walls are slightly thickened by an increased number of plasma cells, some mast cells, and small lymphoid collections. Occasionally, small lymphoid collections are noted in adjacent alveolar septa. The free cells focally extend into adjacent terminal bronchioles. Similar cells are not located in the interstititium or in nearby lymph nodes.[374] Vessels in the involved area are focally thickened but are normal in less involved areas. No thrombi are noted. In classical cases without significant fibrosis, the overall lung architecture is usually preserved, and only rarely are organizing intraalveolar or endobronchial fibroblastic polyps of inflammation present.

If the term desquamative interstitial pneumonia is used to describe a widespread tissue reaction with monotony and not much destruction, this retains its usefulness for communication. However, focal collections of intraalveolar cells are seen in many entities, including interstitial fibrosis as noted above. The latter entity has a more progressive downhill course, and therefore the components of each should be described.

Course

Of note, interstitial fibrosis is also a common tissue reaction to assorted injuries and in various diseases. Further evaluation of a large series of 40 cases of desquamative interstitial pneumonitis (DIP) and 53 cases of the more usual interstitial fibrosis (UIP) by Carrington et al.[389] showed the DIP cases had a 22% improvement without therapy compared to none of the UIP cases, 61.5% of DIP improved with steroids compared to 11.5% of UIP, and only 27% of DIP worsened compared to 69.2% of UIP cases. Death occurred in 27.5% of the DIP cases, with a mean survival of 12.2 years, compared to 66% of the UIP cases with a mean survival of 5.6 years. Cases with a predominantly desquamative interstitial pneumonia pattern were, on an average, 8 years younger in this series, and 20 years younger in Valdivia's series,[396] than those with interstitial fibrosis. Although some cases of DIP progress to UIP, most cases of UIP do not appear to progress through DIP, as best as can be determined. Therefore, it seems unwise to think of DIP as a cellular or early form of UIP as a usual event.

Therapy

Steroids are the treatment of choice. The more cellular the pattern, the better the response, while those with more fibrosis do less well. Some patients do well with no therapy.[384,389] Of interest, one patient responded to the antiviral medication, ribaflavin, after he responded poorly to steroids and immunosuppressive therapies.[397]

Differential Diagnosis

The differential diagnosis consists of excessive tobacco smoke response, nonspecific reactions, as a variation of *Pneumocystis carinii* (see Fig. 6–8) an artefact of atelectasis, eosinophilic pneumonia, eosinophilic granuloma, and, rarely, pulmonary hemosiderosis, alveolar proteinosis, or malignancy. Foamy macrophage diseases such as lipid pneumonia, either secondary to aspiration or obstruction, lipid storage diseases, or other foamy cells, as with amiodarone reactions, should be easily distinguished. Respiratory bronchiolitis (see Chapters 4, 5, 25, and 26) may be present in some cases of DIP. I have seen 3 cases where the differential diagnosis was DIP or DIP-like reaction versus respiratory bronchiolitis in patients in their thirties or forties where this distinction could not be made. This is also discussed in Chapter 4 and by Myers[398,399] and Yousem et al.[400] In comparison of 18 cases of respiratory bronchiolitis associated interstitial lung disease (RB/ILD) and 36 cases of typical DIP, Yousem et al.[400] concluded DIP tends to occur in older individuals, be more symptomatic, have ground-glass infiltrates radiographically, and have worse pulmonary function, with more progress than RB/ILB. Lesser degress of involvement are sure of occur in DIP and a careful correlation with tobacco use may be helpful in any case of DIP. Tobacco may have an underexamined and underrated association with DIP. The patient with this, or for that matter, any lung disease, is well advised to discontinue smoking and exposure(s) to any dusty or otherwise unhealthy respiratory environment. Several cases have been described with transitions between desquamative interstitial pneumonitis and alveolar proteinosis.[401,402] Overlap with eosinophilic pneumonia is also seen. As some cases of DIP have eosinophils in them, estimated to be 3%–5% in touch preparations in one series,[393] and as some cases of eosinophilic pneumonia have abundant eosinophilic nonfoamy macrophages and lesser numbers of eosinophiles, such cases may be difficult to subclassify. Both these reactions will be treated with steroids, so that distinction may not be critical. A descriptive diagnosis explaining this overlap may be necessary. Cases in which this overlap has been described tend classically to be neither of these patterns and reflect the limited responses of the lung.

Of other differential diseases, iron and hemorrhage are much more abundant in pulmonary hemosiderosis and more often these patients are teenaged males. (see **Primary Pulmonary Hemosiderosis** elsewhere in this chapter.) Eosinophilic granuloma, in the usual form, causes nodular histiocytic proliferations in the interstitium, sometimes in a stellate form, with lipochrome or dust pigment or varying numbers of eosinophils. However, the acute form may be peribronchiolar and in-volve adjacent alveoli, and be somewhat confusing. The Langerhans, cells can be identified by electron microscopy or S-100 protein in difficult cases. The typical Langerhans' cells are lightly violaceous, finely vacuolated, and have more delicate convolutions to the nuclei than in the usual case of desquamative interstitial pneumonitis (see Chapter 17). Of interest, eosinophilic granuloma also has a high association with tobacco use (see Chapters 4 and 17).

A rare case of malignancy may cause confusion, such as a true alveolar type II cell adenocarcinoma (Fig. 22–57A; see Chapter 32) or poorly differentiated adenocarcinoma or squamous carcinoma (Fig. 22–57B). These should generally not cause confusion except perhaps in transbronchial biopsies, because findings of nearby malignancy are usually obvious in larger biopsies. In troublesome cases, more tissue or other evidence of malignancy should be sought. Also with the possible exception of bronchioloalveolar carcinoma, most malignancies are more focal than DIP.

Possible Etiologies

As noted in the original article,[374] the pattern of desquamative interstitial pneumonia (DIP) is a reaction to multiple assorted insults. Gray lung virus disease in rats and mice suspected as caused by a pleuropneumonia-like organism (PPLO), and progressive ovine pneumonia are spontaneous animal diseases that have a similar appearance. Freund's adjuvant has produced such a pattern in experimental animals.[403,404] Deodhar and Bhagwat[403] compared this to desquamative interstitial pneumonitis, which in their model eventually progressed to true granulomatous inflammation. Of interest in humans, Valdivia et al.[396] compared the alveolar macrophages to loose epithelioid histiocytes. The drug iprindole has induced this lesion in rats only, a species with a high rate of spontaneous pulmonary histiocytosis.[382]

In humans this has been seen in chronic nitrofurantoin use,[405] in patients exposed to wood dust,[374] asbestos,[383,406] talc,[393,407,408] graphite and silica,[408] silicates,[408] hard metals including cobalt and tungsten carbide,[409–411] and aluminum dust.[412] In one large series of 93 cases drawn from the A.A. Liebow Pulmonary Pathology Collection (San Diego, California), 17 cases were qualitatively analyzed for dusts and fumes by Abraham and Hertzberg.[407] These authors found increased particulates in 92% of cases, the particulates being on an average 72.5 times greater when compared to background control patient levels. More than half these cases did not show increased polarizable material by light microscopy, generally indicating the very small size of most of the particles. Of interest the only statistical difference in analysis of these cases with those with alveolar proteinosis was that no cases of desquamative interstitial pneumonitis contained silicates (SiO_2) as a major particulate.

The desquamative pneumonia pattern has been described in tuberculosis.[413] and around intraparenchymal lesions of eosinophilic granuloma, lymph nodes, rheumatoid nodules, and chondromas.[392] It frequently occurs to some degree in atelectatic areas, mostly or solely because of artifactual collapse of lung around the macrophages. It certainly appears more prevalent in areas of collapse, perhaps artefactually emphasized by the lack of distended air spaces. Its possible association with tobacco smoke has been noted.

Intranuclear inclusions have been identified in many cases, primarily in lining cells, and were first thought to suggest possible virus infections.[374,376] These have been the subject of several studies[414,415] and probably represent surfactant inclusions. No viruses have been found in any of the electron micrographic studies[415-418] nor have any viruses been detected in at least eight cases cultured in one series.[393] None of the routine microbiologic cultures have proven significantly positive. Macrophages from DIP cases obtained from bronchopulmonary lavage in two cases proved to have normal antibacterial properties.[419]

Immunoglobulin and immune reactant staining in cases of DIP have shown variable results. Valdivia et al.[393] found no specific staining in four cases. In one of four cases of Hogan et al.[420] some IgG was present in the interstitium in an unidentified location. Dreisin et al.[421] found increased circulating immune complexes and third component of complement (C3) with granular IgG deposits in lung capillaries and along aveolar walls in most of their seven cases. These were also found in eight cases of "cellular interstitial fibrosis," but not in eight or more cases of advanced fibrosis. Finding IgG and C3 in humans is similar to experimental studies inducing this disease using bovine albumin complexes formed in antigen equivalents.[422,423] Bone et al.[402] documented IgG and C3 in the interstitium in their case.

Stachura et al.,[384] in a well-controlled study, found increased IgG and C3 on macrophage surfaces in the airways in four cases of DIP. Those were rich in lysozyme, an enzyme that increases with activated macrophages. The receptor sites for immunoglobulin were also increased on activated macrophages. In their best studied case, negative cultures or serologies were found for aerobic and anaerobic bacteria, *Legionella*, mycobacteria, adenovirus, herpes virus, cytomegalovirus (CMV), and coxsackie virus. This patient had circulating immune complexes and decreased serum IgG, but

normal complement C3 and C4 components, during the acute phase when there were bilateral basilar pulmonary infiltrates. Two weeks later the patient's dyspnea and infiltrates had cleared without treatment, the serum IgG had returned to normal, and the circulating immune complexes could no longer be detected. These authors suggested that immune complexes are formed to an unknown antigen, resulting from or causing stimulated macrophages which then release digestive enzymes and cause focal tissue and macrophage.

Giant Cell Interstitial Pneumonia (GIP)

This unusual disease was first described by Liebow in 1967[424] and was mentioned by him again in 1968[425] and 1975.[426] Early reports were by Reddy et al.[427] in 1970, Sokolowski et al.[428] in 1972, and Hendrycy and Dail[429] in 1978. These cases are rare, and most are now thought to result from cobalt exposure[409,430-436] and perhaps other components from hard metal (tungsten carbide) production.[435] Other aspects of hard metal pneumoconioses are discussed in Chapter 27, and hard metal exposure may cause asthma, extrinsic allergic alveolitis, interstitial fibrosis or desquamative interstitial pneumonia.[437]

This reaction has been induced experimentally with cobalt.[438] Cobalt is quite soluble in solutions, including human fluids, and successful documentation of its presence in tissue is usually difficult. Positive tissue analysis or a history of exposure to the tungsten carbide industry was noted in 13 of 16 cases studied by Abraham by 1985.[431] Affected patients usually range from the middle of the seventeenth year to age 72 years,[434,439] and many are in their twenties to forties, perhaps representing the age of industrial exposure.[432]

The tissue reaction is quite striking, principally because of the size of the giant cells. These large multinucleate cells vary up to 40–60 μm in diameter, and may contain as many as 20–30 nuclei in any one tissue plane (Fig. 22–58). These nuclei vary, may be tightly packed around the periphery of the cells, may be multifocally around the periphery of the cell, or may cluster together toward the center of the cell. There are no viral inclusions in the nuclei or the cell cytoplasm, but asteroid bodies may be present, as may be abundant dust in the cytoplasm. The giant cells have an irregular shape. Reddy and associates[427] described these as having a "splashed" appearance, with peripheral pseudopod-like projections. A striking feature is the frequent presence of cells that appear to be intact in the multinucleate cell cytoplasm, often surrounded by a retraction space. These cells are usually mononuclear and sometimes are smaller multinucleate cells, but even polymorphonu-

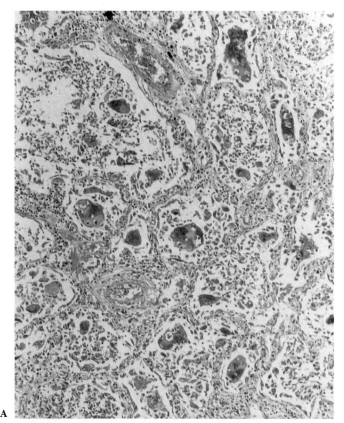

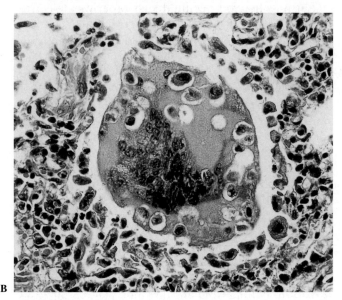

Fig. 22–58 A,B. Giant cell interstitial pneumonia. **A.** Low-power view shows very enlarged giant cells. Multiple other alveolar macrophages fill alveoli; some interstitial thickening with chronic inflammation. H and E, × 64. **B.** Giant cell interstitial pneumonia. Large multinucleate giant cells may almost fill alveoli in this reaction. Note enlarged nuclei in syncytial cluster. Many cells appearing to be migrating into or through cytoplasm. No viral inclusions are found in this disease. H and E, ×400.

clear cells have been identified. Giant cells have been observed in bronchoalveolar lavage specimens.*

At times the same cells are seen in the surrounding alveolar space and appear to be "chasing" a frayed edge of a giant cell cytoplasm. Perhaps some of these are aiding in the formation and/or growth of these multinucleate cells, but at other times the cells appear to be distinctly intact and migrating through the giant cell cytoplasm (emperiopolesis). These cells have, at times, been identified as being intact by electron microscopy.[431] At times the alveolar lining cells may become syncytial and slightly enlarged, and electron microscopy has confirmed that some of the giant cells in lung tissue sections are composed of alveolar type II cells; however, the multinucleate cells seen cytologically are composed entirely of macrophages.[431] Most of the individual intraalveolar mononuclear cells and the larger multinucleate cells in tissue sections also have characteristics of macrophages.[431] In the largest single series of 22 cases by Abraham[431] (reported in abstract form), of those eventually proven to have this disease, autopsy lungs were diagnostic in 7 of 7 (100%), and open lung biopsies in 13 of 14 (93%), but only 3 of 6 (50%) of transbronchial biopsies were positive and BALs in 2 were positive.

The main entity in the differential diagnosis is viral pneumonia, especially measles pneumonia. Other viral-induced giant cells such as in parainfluenza[443,444] or respiratory syncytial virus[445] (see Chapter 12) are usually smaller than those of GIP.[436] Measles usually follows an onset of rash, and a typical clinical syndrome, follows an acute course and often occurs in people younger than those seen with giant cell interstitial pneumonia. Histologically it is necessary to see viral inclusions to confirm measles pneumonia, unless culture or electron microscopy are used. These inclusions may not be present in the early formation of multinucleate giant cells, but when present are cytoplasmic and intranuclear and are glassy red on H and E stains. They may also be stained with Lendrum viral stain or specific DNA probes. When measles giant cells are well developed, they can be quite striking, with abundant nuclear and cytoplasmic inclusions (see Chapter 12).

Measles pneumonia also involves alveolar lining cells, which also become syncytial and show viral inclusions similar to those in the alveolus. These syncytial lining cells are usually evenly contoured about the alveolus and do not show the polypoid excrescences as seen in respiratory syncytial virus. Also, this latter virus is usually more prevalent in infants and young children; histologically it is most obvious in bronchioles and has fewer inclusions. Rarely, extreme desquamative inter-

_____

*Reference numbers: 430, 433, 434, 440–442.

stitial pneumonia-type pattern can have some multinucleate cells without viral inclusions. This type of reaction is especially seen in infants.[402] Other reactions, such as aspiration and eosinophilic pneumonias, are usually easily distinguished. There is no necrosis or granuloma formation in GIP as might be seen in tuberculosis or fungal infections.

At times aspiration may elicit giant cells, but these are usually in areas of confluent fibrosis with destruction of lung architecture and not occurring discretely as in alveoli.

Malakoplakia

This is an unusual disease of poor macrophage digestion. It was first described by von Hansemann[446] and Michaelis and Gutmann[447] in 1901–1903. It was named by von Hansemann for the soft yellow tumor-like plaques in the bladder of a man with tuberculosis. An excellent general review of this entity is by Damjanov and Katz[448] and many of the following details are drawn from this review article.

The disease is most common in the bladder, but can occur almost anywhere. It can be confused with malignant tumor masses wherever it occurs. Seventy-five percent of cases are related to *Escherichia coli*, but other gram-negative and gram-positive bacteria, fungi, and even mycobacteria have been involved.

Seven cases have been described in the lung. Multiple lower-lobe nodules that seemed to center on bronchi were present in the first case reported by Gupta et al.[449] in 1972. This case is illustrated here (see following). Two cases were reported by Colby and associates[450] in 1980 in immunosuppressed hosts. Their first case occurred as a persistent left-upper-lobe nodule 3 years after heart transplantation. Malakoplakia in this case was diagnosed on needle aspiration and confirmed at autopsy. Their second case occurred in a setting of recurrent Hodgkin's disease, was endobronchial, and obstructed the right-middle lobe. Here the diagnosis was by transbronchial biopsy. In 1984 Hodder et al.[451] reported a renal transplant patient with a cavitary 4-cm, right-lower-lobe mass, again diagnosed by transbronchial biopsy. Decreasing the patient's immunosuppressive therapy lead to complete clearing. Also in 1984, Crough and co-workers[452] used x-ray spectroscopic analysis to study this disease in an alcoholic patient with bilateral lower-lobe 0.5- to 2.5-cm nodules.

More recently, malakoplakia has been associated with *Rhodococcus equi* in the lungs in AIDS cases.[450,453,454] This is an equine organism; it is uncommon in humans, and most (90%–95%) human cases are in immunosuppressed patients and present as pneumonia, often cavitary, with empyema and favoring the upper lobes. In AIDs cases, as with other infections, this can be a very persistent organism despite appropriate therapy. It may rarely involve extrapulmonary sites.[455] Even when not described as characteristic malakoplakia, finely granular smaller macrophages filled with gram-positive coccobacillary, vividly PAS-positive organisms reminiscent of Whipple's and even *Mycobacterium avium-intracellulare* histiocytoses are seen. *Rhodococous equi* organisms are usually acid fast with Fite stain and Gormori methenamine silver (GMS) negative. (See Whipple's disease next, *Mycobacterium avium-intracellulare* in Chapter 10, and more about R. equi in Chapter 9.)

Grossly, the soft yellow plaques for which the disease is named occur predominantly in hollow organs. In other organs, including the lung, these areas vary from grey-tan and yellow. Smaller nodules are more solid, but necrosis is frequent even in these, and may lead to cavitation. Some lesions extend across pulmonary fissures.[450]

Histologically the background architecture may be obliterated, but at the edges alveolar filling may be seen (Fig. 22–59). Multiple granular-to-vacuolated "von Hansemann's histiocytes" are seen better at higher power (Fig. 22–59B,C). These consist of histiocytes with distinct cytoplasmic borders and cytoplasmic granules that vary greatly in size. These granules are PAS- and PASD positive and are lipid rich on frozen sections. Round intracytoplasmic blue-grey "target-like" or "owl-eye-like" Michaelis–Gutmann bodies are important findings in confirming this disorder (Fig. 22–59). They range from 3 to 20 μm in diameter, and may be round, oval, or slightly indented on one side. Most are intracellular but some may be extracellular. They tend to have a central or eccentric dark mass surrounded by a clear zone with peripheral accentuation. They may stain with iron and calcium stains. Analysis by Crough et al.[452] has shown some variation in the amounts of calcium, phosphorus, and iron among individual bodies examined. This variability has lead this group to suggest that carbonates may be present along with organic phase lipids and polysaccharides. About 95% of the bodies are organic.

Careful search may yield some histiocytes containing gram-staining or acid-fast organisms, but these are usually not numerous and are not seen in all cases. Electron microscopy indicates that many cells have assorted lysosomes, and some have identifiable bacteria in their cytoplasm. Along with the characteristic histiocytic infiltration, plasma cells and lymphocytes are present. Multinucleate giant cells are absent or infrequent. Granulation tissue and fibrosis are common at the edges of the areas of inflammation, but they may be mixed with histiocytes.

Underlying diseases are common and immunosup-

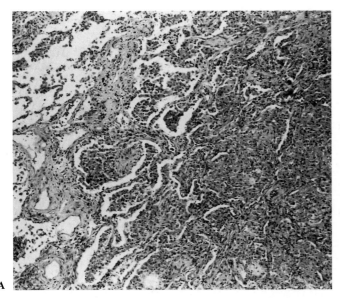

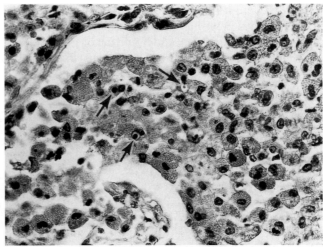

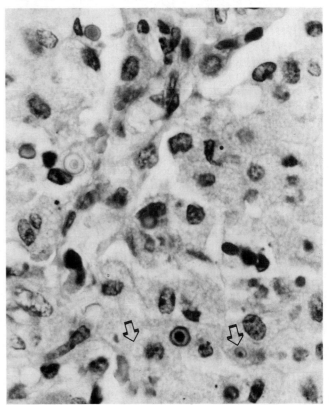

Fig. 22–59 A–C. Malakoplakia. **A.** Edge of reaction shows interstitial and alveolar filling by cells. H and E, ×250. **B.** High-power view shows granular glistening macrophages in Michaelis–Guttman bodies (*arrows*). H and E, ×400. **C.** Various types of central densities in Michaelis-Guttman bodies. Note two smaller ones at bottom (*arrows*) in addition to three or four obvious ones. (Courtesy A.A. Liebow Pulmonary Pathology Collection, San Diego, California. Original contributor, R.K. Gupta, M.D., St. Catherine General Hospital, Ontario, Canada.) H and E, ×1,000.

pression may play a role in malakoplakia, as seen even in the lung cases mentioned above. However, many cases occur without these associations.

Careful search for Michaelis–Gutmann bodies may be necessary, but once these are found, the pathologist will be rewarded with a more secure diagnosis. The diagnosis of malakoplakia should be preserved for those cases with identifiable Michaelis–Gutman bodies.[456] Clear, foamy, and granular macrophage diseases are in the differential diagnosis, and include endogenous lipid pneumonia, Whipple's disease, *Mycobacterium*

avium-intracellulare, Niemann–Pick, Gaucher's, and other storage diseases. None of these has been reported to contain Michaelis–Gutmann bodies. The distinguishing characteristics of these other diseases are discussed separately.

Whipple's Disease

This disease was described in 1907 by G.H. Whipple,[457] who noted fatty deposits in intestines and mesenteric nodes in a patient with diarrhea, abdominal pain, weight loss, and arthralgia. He called this "intestinal lipodystrophy." This has also been called "lipogranulomatosis." As the intestinal and lipid part of the name do not fully describe the variety of organs that can be involved or the true character of the process, most authors now refer to this simply as Whipple's disease. Whipple himself originally noted that the fat present was mostly extracellular and was probably secondary to chylous drainage obstruction. He also astutely noted some argyrophilic-staining bodies on Levaditi silver stain and suggested these might be bacteria.

Many theories and associations have been advanced to explain this disease. In 1949 Black-Schaffer[458] noted vivid PAS staining in the typical Whipple's disease macrophages. Sieracki[459] called these "sickleform particle-containing" (SPC) cells. Whipple's original case was stained some years later with PAS stain, confirming the presence of these particles.[460] Two separate studies in 1960, using early electron microscopy, interpreted these sickle-shaped bodies as either a protein carbohydrate complex of some type[461] or possibly a virus.[462] In 1961 two studies, by Chears and Ashworth[463] and by Yardley and Hendrix,[464] determined that these bodies were most likely bacteria. They were called "bacillary"[464] or "bacilliform"[460] bodies. In 1952 a case was reported to respond to chloramphenicol,[465] and in 1964[466] another was reported to respond to tetracycline. Early literature review of 33 cases reported between 1907 and 1948,[467] and a more comprehensive review of 114 patients in 1970[468] characterized much of the history and clinical presentation. One group of investigators thought the organism was a cell wall-deficient alpha hemolytic *Streptococcus*,[469] but the organism's classification and culture requirements are still undetermined. As noted in the preceding section on malakoplakia, *Rhodococcus equi* is vividly PAS positive, and of interest, *Corynebacterium* (the genus to which *R. equi* was originally thought to belong) are among the organisms cultured from patients with Whipple's disease.[468,470–472] One case of Whipple-like disease in an AIDs patient was thought to be due to *R. equi*.[469]

The disease occurs most frequently in the intestinal tract, especially in jejunum, but can occur in any location along this organ system. It also may occur in many other organs. One of the best-detailed studies of multiorgan involvement is by Sieracki and Fine.[473] Lymph nodes and serosa are involved with some regularity.

Concerning pulmonary involvement, cough has been noted in some 50% of patients in a review of 98 cases by Enzinger and Helwig.[474] They believed this was probably secondary to nonspecific pleuritis, which was present in 72% of those autopsies reviewed in the patients with cough. Pericarditis was present at autopsy in 73% in their series, but was rarely diagnosed during

life. Pleuripericarditis may precede gastrointestinal tract involvement by some time; in one report, this was 4 years.[475] In the three cases with lung tissue available for examination in a series of five cases by Sieracki and Fine,[473] all three contained typical PAS-positive histiocytes in the interstitium, including in alveolar septa. Rarely a few free macrophages contained these typical organisms. Grossly, these porous lymph nodes have holes up to 2 mm in diameter and are yellow to tan-orange to red, with small yellow flecks in them. These macrophages have been described in the tracheobronchial lymph nodes, and the nodes show the typical histologic changes of Whipple's disease as elsewhere.

Apperly and Copley[476] first reported granulomatous change in lungs in patients with Whipple's disease. Rodarte and associates[477] reported a case of granulomatous inflammation in the lungs, pleura, and peripheral nodes, but with no evidence of PAS-staining organisms. Three years later the patient had transient gastrointestinal tract symptoms, and shortly thereafter died of a massive gastrointestinal hemorrhage while on large doses of steroids for presumed sarcoid. At autopsy typical Whipple's cells were present in the jejunum, regional nodes, liver, spleen, lung, pleura, pericardium, and heart. These authors wondered if there might be a PAS-negative early phase of the disease. Other pulmonary findings included two cases with typical organisms in pulmonary arteries, as reported by James and Bulkley.[478] Spain and Kliot[479] reported on typical Whipple's cells in pulmonary emboli in one case.

Winberg et al.[480] carefully studied the case illustrated in Fig. 22–60 with electron microscopy. This patient had a progressively worsening cough over 2 years before he developed diarrhea for the first time. His chest radiograph showed bilateral peribronchiolar basilar infiltrates and a diffuse accentuation of an interstitial pattern. Transbronchial biopsy was not diagnostic, but

———————————————————————————→

Fig. 22–60 A–E. Whipple's disease. **A.** Reticulonodular infiltrates consist of predominantly interstitial collections of typical macrophages about bronchioles, infiltrating muscle coat (*open arrow*) at bottom edge, with extension into submucosa. *Solid arrow* is site of higher power view in B. H and E, ×100. **B.** Higher power shows granular macrophages in submucosa and outside muscularis. H and E, ×400. **C,D.** Periodic acid-Schiff stain intensely stains bacteria. **C.** Area indicated by *arrows* is lymphoid nodule. PAS, ×100. **D.** Higher power view of transition from PAS-positive macrophages to unstained lymphoid nodule from C. PAS, ×400. (Courtesy of M.E. Rose, M.D., and R.E. Horowitz, M.D. St. Joseph Medical Center, Burbank, California, and C.D. Winberg, M.D. City of Hope National Medical Center, Duarte, California.) **E.** Oil immersion of PAS stain shows how minute and delicate are the organisms. ×1000.

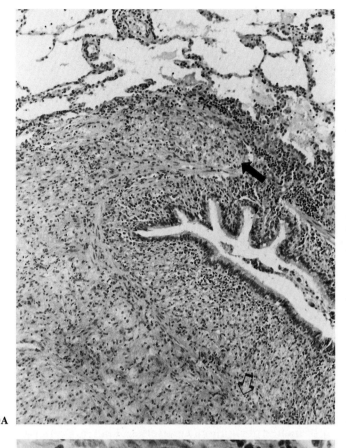

-60A

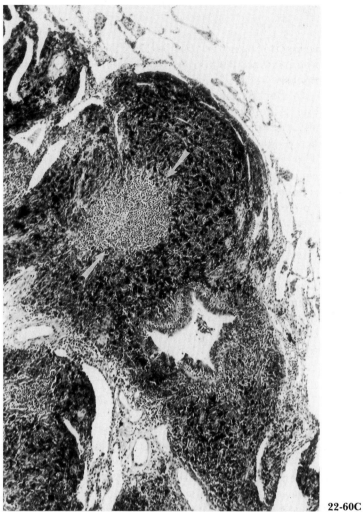

22-60C

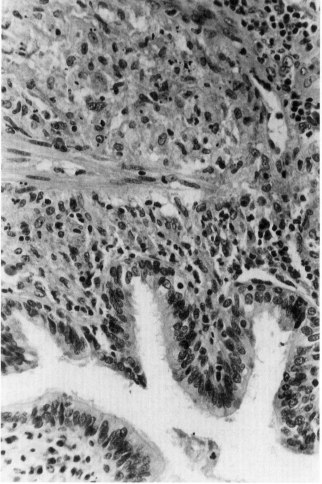

50B

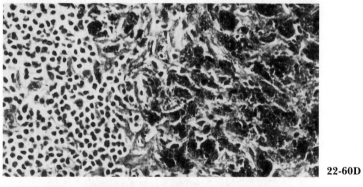

22-60D

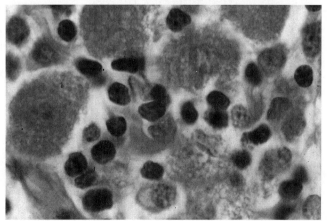

22-60E

an open lung biopsy showed the diagnostic lesions. A follow-up gastrointestinal biopsy confirmed Whipple's disease.

In this case the involved cells formed nodules in the interstitium about bronchioles and to a lesser degree, about vessels of all sizes (Fig. 22–60). Grossly, these were described as firm, white, and up to 5 mm in diameter. The typical PAS-positive enlarged histiocytic cells infiltrated both the bronchiolar smooth muscle and bronchiolar mucosa (see Fig. 22–60). Plasma cells and lymphocytes were scattered among these cells, but were limited in number. There were no giant cells, and no evidence of necrosis or vasculitis. In this case, a large number of typical PAS-positive histiocytes were also noted in the pleural connective tissue, and it was proposed by these authors that pleural biopsy might have been used to make the diagnosis. It seems likely that transbronchial biopsy may also have been positive. Electron microscopy showed $0.2 \times 1.0 \times 1.5$ μm bacilliform structures.

The histochemical staining of these organisms shows fine pale to light-blue vacuolation on H and E staining. They are brightly PAS- and PASD positive and stain with PAS component of Gridley's PAS stain or other PAS-containing stains. They are moderately to intensely GMS positive and acid-fast negative.

The differential diagnosis of Whipple's disease in the lung includes malakoplakia and, less often, *Pneumocystis Legionella*, endogenous lipid pneumonia, other xanthogranulomatous inflammation, Niemann–Pick, and Gaucher's disease. These diseases more often have alveoli filled with distended macrophages, while Whipple's disease is more interstitial. A PAS stain should help distinguish the organisms in Whipple's disease, but some of the other diseases also have PAS staining. Care must be taken in other infections such as *Mycobacterium avium-intracellulare*, as these can present as foamy to granular interstitial macrophages with PAS-positive organisms in them. These organisms are larger than those of Whipple's disease and are vividly acid-fast.

Niemann–Pick Disease

This disease results in an accumulation of sphingomyelin. Its histochemistry has been evaluated by several authors.[481–484] The radiographic appearance has been covered by Lachman et al.[484] Involved cells in the lung have been studied by electron microscopy.[485]

The gross appearance of extensively involved lungs shows a grey-brown color, and a frothy greasy material exudes from the cut surface, but the lungs themselves do not float on water.[486] The nodes may be similarly involved, and be described as "spongy" or "rubbery." Lesser degrees of involvement manifest as smaller nodules in the range of 1 to 2 mm. Histologically there are

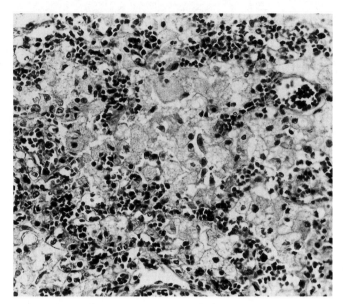

Fig. 22–61. Niemann–Pick disease. Macrophages are filled with vacuoles of various sizes. H and E, ×200.

foamy cells, usually in alveoli (Fig. 22–61), but the same cells are also located in lymphatic spaces and sometimes in branches of pulmonary arteries. They are less frequently seen in alveolar septa. They stain positively with lipid and PAS stains. The storage cells are usually 20–90 μm in diameter and often have one but may have as many as two to four nuclei scattered around within the cell cytoplasm. Cell cytoplasm may stain as cleared droplets or, because of lipofuscin, may have varying tinctures, varying from tan to yellow to green to brown. Lipid stains are more vivid when there is a greater quantity of lipofuscin. With Giemsa stain there is a blue-green tint, and many cases of "sea-blue" histiocyte syndrome may represent adult Niemann–Pick disease.[187] Cell contents may be weakly acid-phosphatase positive, in contrast to the strong reaction in Gaucher's disease, and may be Schultz reaction positive in Niemann–Pick whereas they are negative in Gaucher's cells. The lung involvement in this disease is in general not as severe as that described in Gaucher's disease. However, exceptions do occur, and a case of cor pulmonale resulting from adult Niemann–Pick has been described.[488]

Adult Niemann–Pick-Like Lipidosis

Certain acquired conditions may lead to excess lipid accumulations in systemic histiocytes and sometimes in other cells that give an appearance like Niemann–Pick disease. Some disease may be induced by excess breakdown of cell membranes, such as anemias, leukemias, or thrombocytopenias.[489,490] There may also be lipid storage problems caused by groups of drugs that have a

763

common pathway of inability of the lysosomes to totally degredate the phospholipids. Amiodarone is one such example (see Chapter 23). This was nicely evaluated in the Japanese literature as reviewed by Lüllman et al. in Germany.[491] These drugs have in common amphophilic characteristics consisting of closely associated highly hydrophilic and hydrophobic portions. These common characteristics seem to interfere with intralysosomal lipid degredation when they combine with lipid products.

Gaucher's Disease

Lungs in Gaucher's disease can be extensively involved with both interstitial and alveolar macrophage accumulation of glucocerebroside because of a deficiency in lysomal β-glucosidase. Capillary plugging from Gaucher's cells also has been described.[492] These have been classified as infantile, juvenile, and adult forms, and the adult form is characterized by lack of neurologic involvement. Cases reported as "adults" are in this category solely by this criteria, and one series of three cases demonstrated extreme pulmonary involvement in patients who died at ages 4 and 10, and another who was alive but on oxygen therapy at age 9 years.[492] In "over one-third" of the largest series of 89 autopsied cases of Gaucher's disease, significant lung involvement was noted.[493] At times there may be pulmonary hypertension,[494] and right heart failure may aggravate the cirrhosis seen in some of these cases.[493] Treatment has been attempted with bone marrow transplantation but is high risk. One study showed moderate pulmonary function improvement in two patients treated with mannose-terminated glucocerebrosidase.[495]

The storage cells vary between 20 and 100 μm, have small slightly eccentric nuclei that may be multinucleated with as many as five to eight nuclei, and have cytoplasm that stains pink on H and E stain. The cytoplasm has been described as "wrinkled tissue paper," "crumpled silk," or "striated small rod-like" in appearance (Fig. 22–62). This cytoplasm stains PAS positive, and weakly lipid- and iron positive. It is autofluorescent, and has a typical electron microscopic appearance of twisted membranous bilayers 60 Å thick. Radiographic appearance have been described by Wolson.[496] An excellent general review by Peters et al.[497] is available.

Other Storage Disorders

Fabry's Disease

Assorted other storage diseases have been described in the lung. Fabry's disease has also been called "angiokeratoma corpora diffusum universale." It is an

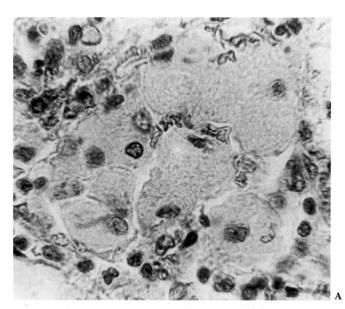

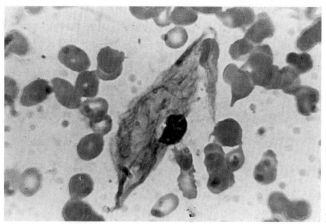

Fig. 22–62 A,B. Gaucher's disease. At low-power magnification this is very similar to Letterer–Siwe disease, but examination at higher power is distinctive. **A.** High-power view shows striated cytoplasm. H and E, 600. **B.** Intracytoplasmic detail is best seen on touch preparation with Giemsa stain. Oil. Giemsa, ×1,000.

X-linked deficiency of alpha-galactosidase A that leads to deposits of crystalline glycosphingolipid. This material polarizes with a Maltese cross-type pattern. It accumulates in endothelial cells, smooth muscle cells, and perithelious cells, and to a lesser degree in histiocytes throughout the body, and has been described as affecting the lung.[498–500] In a review in 1972 by Bartimmo et al.[498] little functional defect was noted in most of the patients reported, with some exceptions.[499,500] Tobacco smoking greatly aggravates bronchitis and emphysema in these patients. A study of lipids in the lung in this disease was conducted by Bagdade et al.[501] Death is usually more commonly from renal failure, cardiac, or cerebrovascular disease.

Hermansky–Pudlak Syndrome

In Hermansky–Pudlak syndrome,[502] or oculocutaneous albinism syndrome, lung involvement of five patients with a ceroid-like storage disorder, restrictive function defects, and open lung biopsy showed interstitial fibrosis and accumulation of ceroid-laden macrophages in two cases.[503] Two other cases in the study presented with inflammatory bowel disease with similar ceroid-like storage cells, as discussed by Schinella et al.[504] Patients ranged in age from 20 to 43 years. Cells stained PAS positive, weakly acid-fast positive, Fontana positive, and negative for iron and fluoresce orange by ultraviolet examination. In an update of these series, Schinella et al.[505] noted pulmonary fibrosis is fairly common. Lavage findings have been noted by White et al.[506]

Diabetic Xanthogranuloma in Lung

One particularly extensive study of diabetic xanthogranuloma in lung by Reineilä[507] examined multiple sections of autopsies from diabetic patients' lungs, and found perivascular collections of foamy histiocytes in 6% of diabetic patients compared with 2% of control patients. The nodular collections averaged 176 μm, and the average size of vessel surrounded was 205 μm. However, a third of vessels were in the range of 60 to 100 μm. These did not stain with PAS or iron stain and did not cause functional defects.

Glycogen Storage

Occasionally, persons with severe glycogen storage disease have glycogen-filled macrophages in the lung. Caplan[508] described one case in an 11-month-old infant with presumed von Gierke's disease.

References

1. Hughes RAC, Berry CL, Seifert M. Relapsing polychondritis. Three cases with a clinicopathological study and literature review. QJ Med 1972;41:363–380.
2. Jaksch-Wartenhorst R. Polychondropathia. Wien Arch Intern Med 1923;6:93–100.
3. Pearson CM, Kline HM, Newcomer VD. Relapsing polychondritis. N Engl J Med 1960;263:51–58.
4. McAdam LP, O'Hanlan MA, Bluestone R, Pearson CM. Relapsing polychondritis: Prospective study of 23 patients and a review of the literature. Medicine (Baltimore) 1976;55:193–215.
5. Linck G, Porte A, Mantz JM, et al. Light and electron microscopic study of ear cartilage in a case of relapsing polychondritis evolving under corticoid treatment. Virchows Arch [A] 1981;391:301–308.
6. Neild GH, Cameron JS, Lessof MH, Ogg CS, Turner DR. Relapsing polychondritis with crescentic glomerulonephritis. Br Med J 1978;1:743–745.
7. Valenzuela R, Cooperrider PA. Gogate P, Deodhar SD, Bergfeld WF. Relapsing polychondritis: Immunomicroscopic findings in cartilage of ear biopsy specimens. Hum Pathol 1980;11:19–22.
8. Yousem SA. Bronchocentric injury in Wegener's granulomatosis. Hum Pathol 1991;22:535–540.
9. Yousem SA, Dauber JA, Griffith BP. Bronchial cartilage alterations in lung transplantation. Chest 1990;98:1121–1124.
10. Wilks S. Ossific deposits on larynx, trachea and bronchi. Trans Pathol Soc (London) 1857;8:88.
11. Nienhuis DM, Prakash UBS, Edell ES. Tracheobronchopathia osteoplastica. Ann Otol Rhinol Laryngol 1990;99:689–694.
12. Aschoff-Freiburg L: Über Tracheopathia osteoplastica. Verh Dtsch Pathol Ges 1910;14:125–127.
13. Prakash UBS, McCullough AE, Edell ES, Nienhuis DM. Tracheopathia osteoplastica: Familial occurrence. Mayo Clin Proc 1989;64:1091–1096.
14. Dalgaard JB. Tracheopathia chondro-osteoplastica: A case elucidating the problems concerning development and ossification of elastic cartilage. Acta Pathol Microbiol Scand 1947;24:118–134.
15. Martin CJ. Tracheobronchopathia osteochondroplastica. Arch Otolaryngol 1974;100:290–293.
16. Elmind K. Tracheopathia chondro-osteoplastica. Nord Med 1964;72:1029–1031.
17. Jepsen O, Sorensen H. Tracheopathia osteoplastica and ozaena. Acta Otolaryngol (Stockh) 1960;51:79–83.
18. Sen RP, Walsh TE. Fiberoptic bronchoscopy for refractory cough. Chest 1991;99:33–35.
19. Carr DT, Olsen AM. Tracheopathia osteoplastica. JAMA 1954;155:1563–1565.
20. Härmä RA, Suurkari S. Tracheopathia chondro-osteoplastica: A clinical study of thirty cases. Acta Otolaryngol (Stockh) 1977;84:118–123.
21. Hodges MK, Israel E, Tracheobronchopathia osteochondroplastica presenting as right middle lobe collapse. Diagnosis by bronchoscopy and computerized tomography. Chest 1988;94:842–844.
22. Pounder DJ, Pieterse AS. Tracheopathia osteoplastica: A study of minimal lesions. J Pathol 1982;138:235–239.
23. Alroy CG, Lichtig C, Kaftori JK. Tracheobronchopathia osteoplastica: End stage of primary pulmonary amyloidosis: Chest 1972;61:465–468.
24. Sakula A. Tracheobronchopathia osteoplastica: Its relationship to primary tracheobronchial amyloidosis. Thorax 1968;23:105–110.
25. Shuttleworth JS, Self CL, Pershing HS. Tracheopathia osteoplastica. Ann Intern Med 1960;52:234–242.
26. Hui AN, Koss MN, Hochholzer L, Wehunt WD. Amyloid presenting in the lower respiratory tract. Arch Pathol Lab Med 1986;110:212–218.
27. Woodring JH, Barrett PA, Rehm SR, Nurenberg P. Acquired tracheomegaly in adults as a complication of diffuse pulmonary fibrosis. AJR 1989;152:743–747.

28. Urbach E, Wiethe C. Lipoidosis cutis et mucosae. Virchows Arch Pathol Anat 1929;273:285–319.

29. Caplan RM. Visceral involvement in lipoid proteinosis. Arch Dermatol 1967;95:149–155.

30. Moscovic EA. Sarcoidosis and mycobacterial L-forms: A critical reappraisal of pleomorphic chromogenic bodies (Hamazaki corpuscles) in lymph nodes. Pathol Annu 1978;13:69–164.

31. Carstens PHB, Kuhns JG, Ghazi C. Primary malignant melanomas of the lung and adrenal. Hum Pathol 1984;15:910–914.

32. Salm R. A primary malignant melanoma of the bronchus. J Pathol Bacteriol 1963;85:121–123.

33. Allen MS Jr, Drash EC. Primary melanoma of the lung. Cancer 1968;21:154–159.

34. Mennemeyer RP, Hammar SP, Tytus JS, Hallman KO, Raisis JE, Bockus D. Melanotic schwannoma: Clinical and ultrastructural studies of three cases with evidence of intracellular melanin synthesis. Am J Surg Pathol 1979;3:3–10.

35. Reiman HA, Koucky RF, Ecklung CM. Primary amyloidosis limited to tissue of mesodermal origin. Am J Pathol 1935;11:977–988.

36. Gertz MA, Kyle RA. Primary systemic amyloidosis: A diagnostic primer. Mayo Clin Proc 1989;64:1505–1519.

37. Isobe T, Osserman EF. Patterns of amyloidosis and their association with plasma-cell dyscrasia, monoclonal, immunoglobulins and Bence-Jones proteins. N Engl J Med 1974;290:473–477.

38. Duff GL, Murray EGD. Primary systemic amyloidosis. Am J Med Sci 1954;328:317–333.

39. Dahlin DC. Primary amyloidosis, with report of six cases. Am J Pathol 1949;25:105–123.

40. Smith RRL, Hutchins GM, Moore GW, Humphrey RL. Type and distribution of pulmonary parenchymal and vascular amyloid: Correlation with cardiac amyloidosis. Am J Med 1979;66:96–104.

41. Toriumi J. The lung in generalized amyloidosis. Acta Pathol Jpn 1972;22:141–153.

42. Celli BR, Rubinow A, Cohen AS, Brody JS. Patterns of pulmonary involvement in systemic amyloidosis. Chest 1978;74:543–547.

43. Dahlin DC. Secondary amyloidosis. Ann Intern Med 1949;31:105–119.

44. Briggs GW. Amyloidosis. Ann Intern Med 1961;44:943–957.

45. Kuhlback B, Wegelius O. Secondary amyloidosis: A study of clinical and pathological findings. Acta Med Scand 1966;180:737–745.

46. McGlennen RC, Burke BA, Dehner LP. Systemic amyloidosis complicating cystic fibrosis. Arch Pathol Lab Med 1968;110:879–884.

47. Jayalakshmi P, Looi LM, Lim KJ, Rajogopalan K. Autopsy findings in 35 cases of leprosy in Malaysia. Int J Lepr 1987;55:510–514.

48. Pitkanen P, Westermark P, Cornwell GG. Senile systemic amyloidosis. Am J Pathol 1984;117:391–399.

49. Laden SA, Cohen ML, Harley RA. Nodular pulmonary amyloidosis with extrapulmonary involvement. Hum Pathol 1984;15:594–597.

50. Monreal FA. Pulmonary amyloidosis: Ultrastructural study of early alveolar septal deposits. Hum Pathol 1984;15:388–390.

51. Rubinow A, Celli BR, Cohen AS, Rigden BG, Brody JS. Localized amyloidosis of the lower respiratory tract. Am Rev Respir Dis 1978;118:603–611.

52. Cohen AS, Amyloidosis. N Engl J Med 1967;177:522–530;574–583;628–638.

53. Klaskin G. Nonspecific green birefringence in Congo red-stained tissues. Am J Pathol 1969;56:1–12.

54. Glenner CG. Amyloid deposits and amyloidosis. The beta fibrilloses. N Engl J Med 1980;302:1283–1291, 1333–1343.

55. Kyle RA, Bayrd ED. Amyloidosis: Review of 236 cases. Medicine (Baltimore) 1975;54:271–299.

56. Wright JR, Calkins E, Humphrey RL. Potassium permanganate reaction in amyloidosis: A histological method to assist in differentiating forms of disease. Lab Invest 1977;235:274–281.

57. Page DL, Isersky C, Harada M, Glenner GG. Immunoglobulin origin of localized nodular pulmonary amyloidosis. Res Exp Med (Berl) 1972;159:75–86.

58. van Rijswijk MH, van Heusden CWGJ. The potassium permanganate method: A reliable method for differentiating amyloid AA from other forms of amyloid in routine laboratory practice. Am J Pathol 1979;79:43–54.

59. Cordier JF, Loire R, Brune J. Amyloidosis of the lower respiratory tract. Clinical and pathologic features in a series of 21 patients. Chest 1986;90:827–831.

60. Gertz MA, Greipp PR. Clinical aspects of pulmonary amyloidosis (editorial). Chest 1986;90:790–791.

61. Thompson PJ, Citron KM. Amyloid and the lower respiratory tract. Thorax 1983;38:84–87.

62. Chen KTK. Amyloidosis presenting in the respiratory tract. Pathol Annu 1989;24(Pt. 1):253–273.

63. Lesser A. Ein Fall von Enchondroma osteiodes mixtum der Lunge mit partieller Amyloidentartung. Virchows Arch Pathol Anat 1877;69:404–408.

64. Prowse CB. Amyloidosis of the lower respiratory tract. Thorax 1958;13:308–320.

65. Kijner CH, Yousem SA. Systemic light chain deposition disease presenting as multiple pulmonary nodules. A case report and review of the literature. Am J Surg Pathol 1988;12:405–413.

66. Linder J, Croker BP, Vollmer RT, Shelburne J. Systemic kappa light chain deposition: An ultrastructural and immunohistochemical study. Am J Surg Pathol 1983;7:85–93.

67. Seymour AE, Thompson AJ, Smith PS, Woodruffe AJ, Clarkson AR. Kappa light chain glomerulosclerosis in multiple myeloma. Am J Surg Pathol 1980;101:557–579.

68. Cohen JJ, Colvin RB. Case records of the Massachusetts General Hospital. N Engl J Med 1981;304:33–43.

69. Silver MM, Hearn SA, Ritchie S, et al. Renal and systemic kappa light chain deposits and their plasma cell origin identified by immuno electron microscopy. Am J Pathol 1986;122:17–27.

220. Wagner E. Zahlreiche kleine Knochen in den Lungen. Arch Physiol Heilk (Stuttg) 1859;35:411.

221. Salinger H. Die Knochenbildungen in der Lunge mit besonderer Berücksichtigung der tuberösen Form. Fortschr Geb Röntgenstr 1932;46:269–275.

222. Janker R. Dei verästelten Knockenbildungen in der Lunge. Fortschr Röntgenstr 1936;53:840–860.

223. Wells HG, Dunlap CE. Disseminated ossification of the lungs. Arch Pathol Lab Med 1943;35:420–426.

224. Joines RW, Roggli VL. Dendriform pulmonary ossification. Report of two cases with unique findings. Am J Clin Pathol 1989;91:398–402.

225. Müller KM, Kriemann J, Stichroth E. Dendriform pulmonary ossification. Pathol Res Pract 1980;168:163–172.

226. Daust W. Über verästelte Knochenspangenbidung in der Lung. Frankfurt Z Pathol 1929;37:313–327.

227. Kuplic JB, Higley CS, Niewoehner DE. Pulmonary ossification associated with long-term busulfan therapy in chronic myelogenous leukemia. Am Rev Respir Dis 1972;106:759–762.

228. Ndimbie OK, Williams CR, Lee MW. Dendriform pulmonary ossification. Arch Pathol Lab Med 1987;111:1062–1064.

229. Wilson WR, Sasaki R, Johnson CA. Disseminated nodular pulmonary ossification in patients with mitral stenosis. Circulation 1959;19:323–331.

230. Pear BL. Idiopathic disseminated pulmonary ossification. Radiology 1968;91:746–748.

231. Epstein EJ, Chapman R, Coulshed N, Galloway RW. Pulmonary ossific nodule formation in the absence of mitral valve disease: A report of four cases. Am J Heart 1963;65:816–825.

232. Galloway RW, Epstein EJ, Coulshed N. Pulmonary ossific nodules in mitral valve disease. Br Heart J 1961;23:297–307.

233. Daugavietis HE, Mautner LS. Disseminated nodular pulmonary ossification with mitral stenosis. Arch Pathol Lab Med 1957;63:7–12.

234. Elkeles A, Glynn LE. Disseminated parenchymatous ossification in the lungs in association with mitral stenosis. J Pathol Bacteriol 1946;58:517–522.

235. Popelka CG, Kleinerman J. Diffuse pulmonary ossification. Arch Intern Med 1977;137:523–525.

236. Green JD, Harle TS, Greenberg SD, Weg JG, Nevin H, Jenkins DE. Disseminated pulmonary ossification: A case report with demonstration of electron microscopic features. Am Rev Respir Dis 1970;101:293–298.

237. Lendrum AC, Scott LDW, Parks SDS. Pulmonary changes due to cardiac diseases, with special reference to hemosiderosis. Q J Med 1950;19:249–262.

238. Katzenstein A-L A, Askin FB. Surgical pathology of non-neoplastic lung disease. Philadelphia: WB Saunders, 1982;371.

239. Kuhn C, III, Kuo T-T. Cytoplasmic hyalin in asbestosis: A reaction of injured alveolar epithelium. Arch Pathol Lab Med 1973;95:190–194.

240. Phillips MJ, Mallory bodies and the liver. Lab Invest 1982;47:311–313.

241. Warnock ML, Press M, Churg A. Further observations on cytoplasmic hyaline in the lung. Hum Pathol 1980;11:59–65.

242. Personal communication. Samuel P. Hammar, M.D., Seattle, Washington, 1986.

243. Denk A, Franke WW, Eckerstrofer R, Schmid E, Kerjaschdi D. Formation and involution of Mallory bodies "alcoholic hyalin" in marine and human liver revealed by immunofluorescence microscopy with antibodies to prekeratin. Proc Natl Acad Sci USA 1979;76:4112–4116.

244. Michel RP, Limacher JJ, Kimoff RJ. Mallory bodies in scar adenocarcinoma of the lung. Hum Pathol 1982;13:81–85.

245. Dekker A, Krause JR. Hyaline globules in human neoplasms: A report of three autopsy cases. Arch Pathol Lab Med 1973;95:178–181.

246. Prakash UBS, Barham SS, Rosenow EC, III, Brown ML, Payne WS. Pulmonary alveolar microlithiasis: A review including ultrastructural and pulmonary function studies. Mayo Clin Proc 1983;58:290–300.

247. Nolle E, Kaufmann HJ. Pulmonary alveolar microlithiasis in pediatric patients. A revew of the world literature and two new observations. Pediatr Radiol 1987;17:439–442.

248. Michaels L, Levene C. Pulmonary corpora amylacea. J Pathol Bacteriol 1957;74:49–56.

249. Harbitz F. Extensive calcification of the lungs as a distinct disease. Arch Intern Med 1918;21:139–146.

250. Puhr L, Mikrolithiasis alveolaris pulmonum. Virchows Arch Pathol Anat 1933;290:156–160.

251. Sosman MC, Dodd GD, Jones WD, Pillmore GU. The familial occurrence of pulmonary alveolar microlithiasis. AJR 1957;77:947–1012.

252. Caffrey PR, Altman RS. Pulmonary alveolar microlithiasis occurring in premature twins. J Pediatr 1965;66:758–763.

253. Thurairajasingam S, Dhrmasena BD, Kasthuriratna T. Pulmonary alveolar microlithiasis. Australas Radiol 1975;19:175–180.

254. Thind GS, Bhatia JL. Pulmonary alveolar microlithiasis. Br J Dis Chest 1978;72:151–154.

255. Drinkovic I, Strohal K, Sabljica B. Mikrolithiasis alveolaris pulmonum. Fortschr Geb Röntgenstr Nuklearmed Erganzungsband 1962;97:180–185.

256. Mikhailov V. Pulmolithiasis endoalveolaris et interstitialis diffusa. Klin Med (Mosk) 1954;32:31–36.

257. Kino T, Kohara Y, Tsuji S. Pulmonary alveolar microlithiasis: A report of two young sisters. Am Rev Respir Dis 1972;105:105–110.

258. Sears MR, Chang AR, Taylor AJ. Pulmonary alveolar microlithiasis. Thorax 1971;26:704–711.

259. Puleihan FJD, Abboud RT, Balikian JP, Nucho CFN. Pulmonary alveolar microlithiasis: Lung function in five cases. Thorax 1969;24:84–90.

260. Biressi PC, Casassa PM. La microlitiasi polmonare endoalveolare. Minerva Med 1956;47:930–939.

261. Shigeno C, Fukunaga M, Morita R, Maeda H, Hino M, Torizuka K. Bone scintigraphy in pulmonary alveolar

microlithiasis: A comparative study of radioactivity and density distribution. Clin Nucl Med 1982;7:103–107.

262. Brown ML, Swee RG, Olson RJ, Bender CE. Pulmonary Uptake of ^{99m}Tc diphosphonate in alveolar microlithiasis. AJR 1978;131:703–704.

263. Balkian JP, Fuleihan FJD, Nucho CKN. Pulmonary alveolar microlithiasis: report of 5 cases with special reference to roentgen manifestations. AJR 1968;103:509–518.

264. Pant K, Shah A, Mathur RK, Chhabra SK, Jain SK. Pulmonary alveolar microlithiasis with pleural calcification and nephrolithiasis (letter). Chest 1990;98:245–246.

265. Petit MA. Pulmonary alveolar microlithiasis (letter). Chest 1991;100:290.

266. Cole WR. Pulmonary alveolar microlithiasis. J Fac Radiol 1959;10:54–56.

267. Winzelberg GG, Boller M, Sachs M, Weinberg J. CT evaluation of pulmonary alveolar microlithiasis. J Comput Assist Tomogr 1984;8:1029–1031.

268. Korn MA, Schurawitzki H, Klepetko W, Burghober OC. Pulmonary alveolar microlithiasis: Findings on high-resolution CT. AJR 1992;158:981–982.

269. Chalmers AG, Wyatt J, Robinson PS. Computed tomographic and pathological findings in pulmonary alveolar microlithiasis. Br J Radiol 1986;59:408.

270. Winzelberg GG, Boller M, Sachs M, Weinberg J. CT evaluation of pulmonary alveolar microlithiasis. J Comput Assist Tomogr 1984;8:1029–1031.

271. Tao L-C. Microliths in sputum specimens and their relationship to pulmonary alveolar microlithiasis. Am J Clin Pathol 1978;69:482–485.

272. Palombini BC, da Silva Porto N, Wallau CU. Camargo JJ. Bronchopulmonary lavage in alveolar microlithiasis. Chest 1981;80:242–243.

273. Sharp ME, Danino EA. An unusual form of pulmonary calcification: "Microlithiasis alveolaris Pulmonum." J Pathol Bacteriol 1953;389–399.

274. Kent G, Gilbert ES, Meyer HH. Pulmonary microlithiasis: Microlithiasis alveolaris pulmonum. Arch Pathol Lab Med 1955;60:536–562.

275. Kawakami M, Sato S, Takashima T. Electron microscopic studies on pulmonary alveolar microlithiasis. Tohoku J Exp Med 1978;126:343–361.

276. Bab I, Rosenmann E, Ne'eman Z, Sela J. The occurrence of extracellular matrix vesicles in pulmonary alveolar microlithiasis. Virchows Arch [A] 1981;391:357–361.

277. Greenberg MJ. Miliary shadows in the lungs due to microlithiasis alveolaris pulmonum. Thorax 1957;12:171–174.

278. Nouh MS. Is the desert lung syndrome (nonoccupational dust pneumoconiosis) a variant of pulmonary alveolar microlithiasis? Report of 4 cases and review of the literature. Respiration 1989;55:122–126.

279. Friedreich N. Kleinere mittheilungen: I. Corpora amylacea in den lungen. Virch Arch Pathol Anat 1856;9:613–618.

280. Lubarsch O, Plenge K. Die corpora amylacea. In: Hemke E, Lubarsch O, eds. Handb der spezielle pathol

Anat u Hist. Vol. 3. Part 3. Berlin: Springer-Verlag, 1931:607–654.

281. Michaels L, Levene C. Pulmonary corpora amylacea. J Pathol Bacteriol 1957;74:49–56.

282. Hollander DH, Hutchins GM. Central spherules in pulmonary corpora amylacea. Arch Pathol Lab Med 1978;100:629–630.

283. Baar HS, Ferguson FF. Microlithiasis alveolaris pulmonum: Association with diffuse interstitial pulmonary fibrosis. Arch Pathol Lab Med 1963;76:659–666.

284. Steele HD, Kinley G, Leuchtenberger C, Lieb E. Polysaccharide nature of corpora amylacea. Arch Pathol Lab Med 1952;54:94–97.

285. Dail DH, Liebow AA. Intraalveolar conchoidal bodies. Am J Pathol 1974;76:43A (abstr.).

286. Michaels L. Lung changes in woodworkers. Can Med Assoc J 1967;96:1150–1155.

287. Gardiner IT, Uff JS. "Blue bodies" in case of cryptogenic fibrosing alveolitis (desquamative type)—an ultrastructural study. Thorax 1978;33:806–813.

288. Koss MN, Johnson FB, Hochholzer L. Pulmonary blue bodies. Hum Pathol 1981;12:258–266.

289. Kim CK, Goyal PC, Payne CB, Jr. Pulmonary blue bodies. Hum Pathol 1983;14:739–740.

290. Kung ITM, Johnson FB, So S-Y, Lam W-K, Hsu C. Blue bodies in cytology specimens in a case of pulmonary talcosis. Am J Clin Pathol 1984;81:675–678.

291. Williams WJ. The nature and origin of Schaumann bodies. J Pathol Bacteriol 1960;79:193–201.

292. Williams WJ, Williams D. The properties and development of conchoidal bodies in sarcoid and sarcoid-like granulomas. J Pathol Bacteriol 1968;96:491–496.

293. Tao L-C. Microliths in sputum specimens and their relationship to pulmonary alveolar microlithiasis. Am J Clin Pathol 1978;69:482–485.

294. Pritzker KPH, Desai SD, Patterson MC, Cheng P-T. Calcite sputum with characterization by analytic scanning electron microscopy and x-ray diffraction. Am J Clin Pathol 1981;75:253–257.

295. Koss MN, Huchholzer L, Feigin DS, Gavancis JC, Ward PA. Necrotizing sarcoid-like granulomatosis: Clinical, pathologic and immunopathologic findings. Hum Pathol 1980;11:510–519.

296. Rosen SH, Castleman B, Liebow AA. Pulmonary alveolar proteinosis. N Engl J Med 1958;258:1123–1142.

297. Davidson JM, MacLeod WM. Pulmonary alveolar proteinosis. Br J Dis Chest 1969;63:13–28.

298. Gough J. Silicosis and alveolar proteinosis. Br Med J 1967;1:629.

299. Buechner HA, Ansari A. Acute silicoproteinosis: A new physiologic variant of acute silicosis in sandblasters, characterized by histologic features resembling alveolar proteinosis. Dis Chest 1969;55:274–284.

300. Hoffman EO, Lamberty J, Pizzolato P. The ultrastructure of acute silicosis. Arch Pathol Lab Med 1973;96:104–107.

301. Xipell JM, Ham KN, Price CG, Thomas DP. Acute silicolipoproteinosis. Thorax 1977;32:104–111.

302. Suratt PM, Winn WC Jr, Brody AR, Bolton WK, Giles

RD. Acute silicosis in tombstone sandblasters. Am Rev Respir Dis 1977;115:521–529.

303. Miller RR, Churg AM, Hutcheon M, Lam S. Pulmonary alveolar proteinosis and aluminum dust exposure. Am Rev Respir Dis 1984;130:312–315.

304. Abraham JL, Auchincloss JH. Pulmonary alveolar proteinosis and kaolin exposure. Am Rev Respir Dis 1985;131:A203 (abstr.).

305. Gross P, deTreville RTP. Alveolar proteinosis: Its experimental production in rodents. Arch Pathol Lab Med 1968;86:255–261.

306. Corrin B, King E. Experimental endogenous lipid pneumonia and silicosis. J Pathol 1969;97:325–330.

307. Heppleston AG, Wright NA, Stewart JA. Experimental alveolar lipoproteinosis following the inhalation of silica. J Pathol 1970;101:293–307.

308. Heppleston AG, Young AE. Alveolar lipo-proteinosis: An ultrastructural comparison of the experimental and human forms. J Pathol 1972;107:107–117.

309. Martin TR, Wehner AP, Butler J. Pulmonary toxicity of Mt. St. Helens volcanic ash. Am Rev Respir Dis 1983; 128:158–162.

310. Corrin B, King E. Pathogenesis of experimental alveolar proteinosis. Thorax 1970;25:230–236.

311. Gross P, Harley RA, Jr, de Treville RTP. Pulmonary reaction to metallic aluminum powders: An experimental study. Arch Environ Health 1973;26:227–255.

312. Lee KP, Barris CE, Griffith FD, Waritz RS. Pulmonary response to glass fiber to inhalation exposure. Lab Invest 1979;40:123–133.

313. Vijeyaratnam GS, Corrin B. Pulmonary alveolar proteinosis developing from desquamative interstitial pneumonia in long term toxicity studies of iprindole in the rat. Virchows Arch [A] 1973;358:1–10.

314. Lüllmann-Rauch R, Reil GH, Rossen E, Seiler KU. The ultrastructure of rat lung changes induced by an anorectic drug (Chlorphentermine). Virchows Arch [Zellpathol] 1972;11:167–181.

315. Heath D, Smith P, Hasleton PS. Effects of chlorphentermine on the rat lung. Thorax 1973;28:551–558.

316. Smith P, Heath D, Hasleton PS. Electron microscopy of chlorphentermine lung. Thorax 1973;28:559–566.

317. Schober R, Kosek JC, Bensch KG. Origin of the membraneous intraalveolar material in pulmonary alveolar proteinosis. Lab Invest 1974;30:388–389.

318. Likhaechev IuP, Batsura IuD. Direev VI. The role of some occupational factors in the development of pulmonary alveolar proteinosis. Arkh Patol 1975;37:63–69.

319. Vallyathan V, Reasor M, Schwegler D. Stettler L. Comparative in vitro cytotoxicity and relative pathogenicity of mineral dusts. Ann Occup Hyg (in press).

320. McEuen DD, Abraham JL. Particulate concentrations in pulmonary alveolar proteinosis. Environ Res 1978; 17:334–339.

321. Abraham JL, McEuen DD. Inorganic particulates associated with pulmonary alveolar proteinosis: SEM and x-ray microanalysis results. Appl Pathol 1986;4:138–146.

322. Larson RK, Gordinier R. Pulmonary alveolar proteino-

sis: report of six cases, review of the literature, and formulation of a new theory. Ann Intern Med 1965;62:292–312.

323. Prakash UBS, Barham SS, Carpenter HA, Dines DE, Marsh HM. Pulmonary alveolar phospholipoproteinosis: experience with 34 cases and a review. Mayo Clin Proc 1987;62:499–518.

324. Lakshiminarayan S. Schwartz MI, Standford RE. Unsuspected pulmonary alveolar proteinosis complicating acute myelogenous leukemia. Chest 1976;69:433–435.

325. Bedrossian CWM, Luna MA, Conklin RH, Miller WC. Alveolar proteinosis as a consequence of immunosuppression: A hypothesis based on clinical and pathologic observations. Hum Pathol 1980;11:527–535.

326. Doyle AP, Balcerzak SP, Wells CL, Crittenden JO. Pulmonary alveolar proteinosis with hematologic disorders. Arch Intern Med 1963;112:940–946.

327. Haworth JC, Hoogstraten J, Taylor H. Thymic alymphoplasia. Arch Dis Child 1967;42:40–54.

328. Jean R, Nezelof C, Bonnett H, et al. Protéinose alvéolaire et inclusions cytomégaliques pulmonaires au cours de l'alymphoplasie thymique. Arch Franc Pediatr 1968; 25:1009–1021.

329. Colon AR, Lawrence RD, Mills SD, O'Connell EJ. Childhood pulmonary alveolar proteinosis (PAP): report of a case and review of the literature. Am J Dis Child 1971;121:481–485.

330. Webster JR Jr, Battifora H, Furey C, Harrison RA, Shapiro B. Pulmonary alveolar proteinosis in two siblings with decreased immunoglobulin A. Am J Med 1980;69:786–789.

331. Samuels MP, Warner JO. Pulmonary alveolar lipoproteinosis complicating juvenile dermatomyositis. Thorax 1988;43:939–946.

332. Coleman M, Dehner LP, Sibley SK, Burke BA, L'Heureux PR, Thompson TR. Pulmonary alveolar proteinosis: an uncommon cause of chronic neonatal distress. Am Rev Respir Dis 1980;121:583–586.

333. Knight DP, Knight JA. Pulmonary alveolar proteinosis in the newborn. Arch Pathol Lab Med 1985;109: 529–531.

334. Steer A. Focal pulmonary alveolar proteinosis in pulmonary tuberculosis. Arch Pathol Lab Med 1969;87: 347–352.

335. Payseur CR, Konwaler BE, Hyde L. Pulmonary alveolar proteinosis. Am Rev Tuberc 1958;79:906–915.

336. Reyes JM, Putong PB. Association of pulmonary alveolar lipoproteinosis with mycobacterial infection. Am J Clin Pathol 1980;74:478–485.

337. Tran Van Nhieu J, Vojtek A-M, Bernaudin J-F, Escodier E, Fleury-Feith J. Pulmonary alveolar proteinosis associated with Pneumocystis carinii: Ultrastructural identification in bronchoalveolar lavage in AIDS and immunocompromised non-AIDS patients. Chest 1990;98: 801–805.

338. Verbeken EK, Demedts M, Vanwing J, Deneffe G, Lauweryns JM. Pulmonary phospholipid accumulation distal to an obstructed bronchus. Arch Pathol Lab Med 1989;113:886–890.

339. Kariman K, Kylstra JA, Spock A. Pulmonary alveolar proteinosis: Prospective clinical experience in 23 patients for 15 years. Lung 1984;162:223–231.

340. Sanguigno N, Campesi G. Proteinosi alveolare ad evoluzione in sclerosi polmonare di tipo clinicamente idiopatico. Riv Tuberc Mal 1961;9:463.

341. Sunderland WA, Campbell RA, Edward MJ. Pulmonary alveolar proteinosis and pulmonary cryptococcosis in an adolescent boy. J Pediatr 1972;80:450–456.

342. Teja K, Cooper PH, Squires JE, Schnatterly PT. Pulmonary alveola proteinosis in four siblings. N Engl J Med 1981;305:1390–1392.

343. Godwin JD, Müller NL, Takasugi JE. Pulmonary alveolar proteinosis: CT findings. Radiology 1988;169:609–613.

344. Preger L. Pulmonary alveolar proteinosis. Radiology 1969;92:1291–1295.

345. Corsello BF, Choi H. Basophilic staining in pulmonary alveolar proteinosis: Report of three cases. Arch Pathol Lab Med 1984;108:68–70.

346. Singh G, Katyal SL, Bedrossian CWM, Rogers RM. Pulmonary alveolar proteinosis: Staining of surfactant apoprotein in alveolar proteinosis and in conditions simulating it. Chest 1983;83:82–86.

347. William GE, Medley DR, Brown R. Pulmonary alveolar proteinosis. Lancet 1960;i:1385–1388.

348. Sieraki JL, Horn RC Jr, Kay S. Pulmonary alveolar proteinosis: Report of three cases. Ann Intern Med 1959;51:728–739.

349. Rubinstein I, Mullen JBM, Hoffstein V. Morphologic diagnosis of idiopathic pulmonary alveolar lipoproteinosis–revisited. Arch Intern Med 1988;148:813–816.

350. Singh G, Katyal S. Surfactant apoprotein in normalignant pulmonary disorders. Am J Pathol 1980;101:51–62.

351. Kuhn C III, Gyorkey F, Levine BE, Ramirez-Rivera J. Pulmonary alveolar proteinosis, a study using enzyme histochemistry, electron microscopy and surface tension measurement. Lab Invest 1966;15:492–509.

352. Basset F, Soler P, Turiaf J. Étude ultrastructurale du contenu alvéolaire dans la protéinose alvéolaire pulmonaire et dans les pseudoprotéinoses. Am Med Interne (Paris) 1973;24:279–290.

353. Costella JF, Moriarity DC, Branthwaite A, Turner-Warwick M, Corrin B. Diagnosis and management of alveolar proteinosis: the role of electron microscopy. Thorax 1975;30:121–132.

354. Ramirez J, Harlan WR, Jr. Pulmonary alveolar proteinosis, nature and origin of alveolar lipid. Am J Med 1968;45:502–512.

355. McClenahan JB, Mussenden R. Pulmonary alveolar proteinosis. Arch Intern Med 1974;133:284–287.

356. Hawkins JE, Savard EV, Ramirez-Rivera J. Pulmonary alveolar proteinosis: origin of proteins in pulmonary washings. Am J Clin Pathol 1967;48:14–17.

357. Hook GER, Bell DY, Gilmore LB, Nadeau D, Reasor MJ, Talley FA. Composition of bronchoalveolar lavage effluents from patients with pulmonary alveolar proteinosis. Lab Invest 1978;39:342–357.

358. Stansifer PP, Bourgeois C. Pulmonary alveolar proteinosis: Histochemical observations. Am J Clin Pathol 1965;44:539–545.

359. Ray RL, Salm R. A fatal case of pulmonary alveolar proteinosis. Thorax 1962;17:257–266.

360. Bell DY, Hook GER. Pulmonary alveolar proteinosis: Analysis of airway and alveolar proteins. Am Rev Respir Dis 1979;119:979–990.

361. Heppleston AG, Fletcher K, Wyatt I. Changes in the composition of the lung lipids and the "turnover" of diplmitoyl lecithin in experimental alveolar lipo-proteinosis induced by inhaled quartz. Br J Exp Pathol 1974;55:384–395.

362. Hook GER, Gilmore LB, Talley FA. Multilamellated structures from the lungs of patients with pulmonary alveolar proteinosis. Lab Invest 1984;50:711–725.

363. Smith FB, Alveolar proteinosis: atypical pulmonary response to injury. NY State J Med 1980;80:1372–1380.

364. Golde DW, Territo M, Finley TN, Cline MJ. Defective lung macrophages in pulmonary alveolar proteinosis. Ann Intern Med 1976;85:304–309.

365. Harris JO. Pulmonary alveolar proteinosis: Abnormal in vitro function of alveolar macrophages. Chest 1979;76:156–159.

366. Nugent KM, Pesanti EL. Macrophage function in pulmonary alveolar proteinosis. Am Rev Respir Dis 1983;127:780–781.

367. Ansfield MJ, Kaltreider HB, Benson BJ, Shalaby MR. Canine surface active material and pulmonary lymphocyte functon: Studies with mixed lymphocyte culture. Exp Lung Res 1980;1:3–11.

368. Ramirez-R J, Savard EV, Hawkins JE. Biological effects of pulmonary washings from cases of alveolar proteinosis. Am Rev Respir Dis 1966;94:244–246.

369. Ramirez-R J. Bronchopulmonary lavage: New techniques and observations. Dis Chest 1966;50:581–588.

370. Ramirez-R J. Alveolar proteinosis: Importance of pulmonary lavage. Am Rev Respir Dis 1971;103:666–678.

371. Claque HW, Wallace AC, Morgan WKC. Pulmonary interstitial fibrosis associated with alveolar proteinosis. Thorax 1983;38:865–866.

372. Fraimow W, Cathcart RT, Kirshner JJ, Taylor RC. Pulmonary alveolar proteinosis: A correlation of pathological and physiological findings in a patient followed up with serial biopsies of the lung. Am J Med 1960;28:458–467.

373. Liebow AA. Desquamative interstitial pneumonia. Am J Pathol 1962;41:127 (title only).

374. Liebow AA, Steer A, Billingsley JG. Desquamative interstitial pneumonia. Am J Med 1965;39:369–404.

375. Herbert FA, Nahmias BB, Gaensler EA, McMahon HE. Pathophysiology of interstitial pulmonary fibrosis. Arch Intern Med 1962;110:626–648.

376. Gaensler EA, Goff AM, Prowse CM. Desquamative interstitial pneumonia. N Engl J Med 1966;274:113–128.

377. Scadding JG, Hinson KFW. Diffuse fibrosing alveolitis (diffuse interstitial fibrosis of the lungs): Correlation of histology at biopsy with prognosis. Thorax 1967;22:291–304.

378. Bates DV, Christie RV. Respiratory function in disease. Philadelphia: WB Saunders, 1964:298–303.

379. Leroy EP. The blood-air barrier in desquamative interstitial pneumonia (D.I.P.). Virchows Arch Pathol Anat 1969;348:117–130.

380. Brewer DB, Heath D, Asquith P. Electron microscopy of desquamative interstitial pneumonia. J Pathol 1969; 97:317–323.

381. Farr GH, Harley RA, Hennigar GR. Desquamative interstitial pneumonia: An electron microscopic study. Am J Pathol 1970;60:347–354.

382. Vijeyaratnam GS, Corrin B. Pulmonary histiocytosis simulating desquamative interstitial pneumonia in rats receiving oral iprindole. Thorax 1972;108:105–113.

383. Corrin B, Price AB. Electron microscopy studies in desquamative interstitial pneumonia associated with asbestos. Thorax 1972;27:324–331.

384. Stachura I, Singh G, Whiteside TL. Mechanisms of tissue injury in desquamative interstitial pneumonia. Am J Med 1980;68:733–740.

385. Rosenow EC, O'Connell EJ, Harrison EG, Jr. Desquamative interstitial pneumonia in children. Report of two cases. Am J Dis 1970;120:344–348.

386. Golden IL, Sherwin RP. Desquamative interstitial pneumonia in an infant. Mimicry of sudden infant death syndrome. Am J Forensic Med Pathol 1989;10:344–348.

387. Hunter AM, Lamb D. Relapse of fibrosing alveolitis (desquamative interstitial pneumonia) after twelve years. Thorax 1979;34:677–679.

388. Lipworth B, Woodcock A, Addis B, Turner-Warwick M. Late relapse of desquamative interstitial pneumonia. Am Rev Respir Dis 1987;136:1253–1255.

389. Carrington CB, Gaensler EA, Coutu RE, FitzGerald MX, Gupta RG. Natural history and treated course of usual and desquamative interstitial pneumonia. N Engl J Med 1978;298:801–809.

390. Feigin DS, Friedman PJ. Chest radiography in desquamative interstitial pneumonitis: A review of 37 patients. AJR 1980;134:91–99.

391. Epler GR, McLoud TC, Gaensler EA, Mikus JP, Carrington CB. Normal chest roentgenograms in chronic diffuse infiltrative lung disease. N Engl J Med 1978;298:934–939.

392. Bedrossian CWM, Kuhn C, III, Luna MA, Conklin RH, Byrd RB, Kaplan PD. Desquamative interstitial pneumonia-like reaction accompanying pulmonary lesions. Chest 1977;72:166–169.

393. Valdivia E, Helsney G, Wu J, Leroy EP, Jaeschke W. Morphology and pathogenesis of desquamative interstitial pneumonitis. Thorax 1977;32:7–18.

394. Gaensler EA, Carrington CB, Coutu RE. Chronic interstitial pneumonias. Clin Notes Respir Dis 1972;10:3–16.

395. Vedal S, Welsh EV, Miller RR, Muller NL, Desquamative interstitial pneumonia. Computed tomographic findings before and after treatment with corticosteroids. Chest 1988;93:215–217.

396. Valdivia E, Hensley G, Wu J, LeRoy EP, Jaeschke W. Desquamative interstitial pneumonitis. Am J Pathol 1976;82:44a–45a (Abstr.)

397. Prieto J, Sangro B, Beloqui O. Ribavirin in desquamative interstitial pneumonia. Chest 1988;93:446–447.

398. Myers JL, Veal CF, Shin MS, Katzenstein ALA. Respiratory bronchiolitis causing interstitial lung disease. Am Rev Respir Dis 1987;135:880–884.

399. Myers JL. Respiratory bronchiolitis with interstitial lung disease. Semin Respir Med 1991;13:134–139.

400. Yousem SA, Colby TV, Gaensler EA. Respiratory bronchiolitis and its relationship to desquamative interstitial pneumonia. Mayo Clin Proc 1989;64:1374–1380.

401. Bhagwat AG, Wentworth P, Conen PE. Observations on the relationship of desquamative interstitial pneumonia and pulmonary alveolar proteinosis in childhood: A pathologic and experimental study. Chest 1970;58: 326–332.

402. Wigger HJ, Berdon WE, Ores CN. Fatal desquamative interstitial pneumonia in an infant: Case report with transmission and scanning electron microscopical studies. Arch Pathol Lab Med 1977;101:129–132.

403. Deodhar JD, Bhagwat AG. Desquamative interstitial pneumonia-like syndrome in rabbits. Arch Pathol Lab Med 1967;84:54–58.

404. Moore RD, Schoenberg MD. The response of histiocytes and macrophages in the lungs of rabbits injected with Freund's adjuvant. Br J Exp Pathol 1964;45:488–497.

405. Bone RC, Wolfe J, Sobonya RE, et al. Desquamative interstitial pneumonia following long-term nitrofurantoin therapy. Am J Med 1976;60:697–701.

406. Freed JA, Miller A, Gordon RE, Fischbein A, Kleinerman J, Langer AM. Desquamative interstitial pneumonia associated with chrysotile asbestos. Br J Ind Med 1991;48:332–337.

407. Abraham JL, Hertzberg MA. Inorganic particulates associated with desquamative interstitial pneumonia. Chest 1981;80:675–705.

408. FitzGerald MX, Carrington CB, Gaensler LA. Environmental lung disease. Med Clin North Am 1973;57:593–622.

409. Coates EO, Watson JHL. Diffuse interstitial lung disease in tungsten carbide workers. Ann Intern Med 1971;75:709–716.

410. Ohori MP, Sciurba FC, Owens GR, Hodgson MJ, Yousem SA. Giant cell interstitial pneumonia and hard-metal pneumoconiosis. A clinicopathologic study of four cases and review of the literature. Am J Surg Pathol 1989;13:581–587.

411. Cugall DW, Morgan WK, Perkins DG, Rubin A. The respiratory effects of cobalt. Arch Intern Med 1990;150:177–183.

412. Herbert A, Sterling G, Abraham J, Corrin B. Desquamative interstitial pneumonia in an aluminum welder. Hum Pathol 1982;13:694–699.

413. Canetti G. The tubercle bacillus in the pulmonary lesions of man. New York: Springer, 1955.

414. Patchefsky AS, Banner M, Freundlich IM. Desquamative interstitial pneumonia: Significance of intranuclear viral-like inclusion bodies. Ann Intern Med 1971; 74:322–327.

415. McNary WF, Jr., Gaensler EA. Intranuclear inclusion

bodies in desquamative interstitial pneumonia: Electron microscopic observations. Ann Intern Med 1971; 74:404–407.

416. Shortland JR, Durke CS, Crane WAJ. Electron microscopy of desquamative interstitial pneumonia. Thorax 1969;24:192–208.

417. Tubbs RR, Benjamin SP, Reich NE, McCormack LJ, VanOstrand HS. Desquamative interstitial pneumonitis: Cellular phase of fibrosing alveolitis. Chest 1977; 72:159–165.

418. Tubbs RR, Benjamin SP, Oborne DG, Barenberg S. Surface and transmission ultrastructural characteristics of desquamative interstitial pneumonitis. Hum Pathol 1978;9:693–703.

419. Fromm GB, Dunn LJ, Harris JO. Desquamative interstitial pneumonitis: Characterization of free intraalveolar cells. Chest 1980;77:552–554.

420. Hogan PG, Donald KJ, McEvoy JDS. Immunofluorescence studies of lung biopsy tissue. Am Rev Respir Dis 1978;118:537–545.

421. Dreisin RB, Schwarz MI, Theofilopoulos AN, Stanford RE. Circulating immune complexes in the idiopathic interstitial pneumonias. N Engl J Med 1978;298: 353–357.

422. Brentjens JR, O'Connell DW, Pawlowski IB, Hsu KC, Andres GA. Experimental immune complex disease of the lung: The pathogenesis of a laboratory model resembling certain human interstitial lung diseases. J Exp Med 1974;140:105–125.

423. Scherzer H, Ward P. Lung injury produced by immune complexes of varying composition. J Immunol 1978; 121:947–952.

424. Liebow AA. New concepts and entities in pulmonary disease. In: Liebow AA, ed. The lung International Academy of Pathology Monograph No 8. Baltimore: Williams & Wilkins, 1967:332–365.

425. Liebow AA, Carrington CB. The interstitial pneumonias. In: Simon M, Potchen EJ, LeMay M, eds. Frontiers of pulmonary pathology. New York: Grune and stratton, 1968:102–141.

426. Liebow AA. Definition and classification of interstitial pneumonias in human pathology. Prog Respir Dis (Basel) 1975;8:1–33.

427. Reddy PA, Gorelick DF, Christianson CS. Giant cell interstitial pneumonia (GIP). Chest 1970;58:319–325.

428. Sokolowski JW, Cordray DR, Cantow EF, Elliott RC, Seal KB. Giant cell interstitial pneumonia. Report of a case. Am Rev Respir Dis 1972;105:417–420.

429. Hendrycy P, Dail DH. Giant cell interstitial pneumonia. Lab Invest 1978;38:348 (abstr.).

430. Davison AG, Haslam PL, Corrin B, et al. Interstitial lung disease and asthma in hard metal workers: Bronchoalveolar lavage, unltrastructural and analytical findings and results of bronchial provocation tests. Thorax 1983;38:119–128.

431. Abraham JL. Exposure to hard metal. Chest 1985; 87:554 (letter).

432. Ohori NP, Sciurba FC, Owens GR, Hodgson MJ, Yousem SA. Giant-cell interstitial pneumonia and hard-metal pneumoconiosis: A clinicopathologic study of four cases and review of the literature. Am J Surg Pathol 1989;13:581–587.

433. Cugell DW, Morgan WKC, Perkins DG, Rubin A. The respiratory effect of cobalt. Arch Intern Med 1990;150:177–183.

434. Demedts M, Gheysens B, Nagels J, et al. Cobalt lung in diamond polishers. Am Rev Respir Dis 1984;130: 130–135.

435. Cullen MR. Exposure to hard metal. Chest 1985;87:554 (answer to letter).

436. Daroca PJ, Jr. George WJ. Giant cell pneumonia. South Med J 1991;84:257–263.

437. Sprince NL, Chamberlin RI, Hales CA, Weber AL, Kazemi H. Respiratory disease in tungsten carbide production workers. Chest 1984;84:549–557.

438. Schepers GWH. The biological action of particulate cobalt metal: Studies on experimental pulmonary histopathology. AMA Arch Ind Health. 1955;12:127–133.

439. Abrahams JL. Lung pathology in 22 cases of giant cell interstitial pneumonia (GIP). Chest 1987;91:312 (Abstr.).

440. Valicenti JF, McMaster KR III, Daniell CJ. Sputum cytology of giant cell interstitial pneumonia. Acta Cytol 1979;23:217–221.

441. Abraham JL, Spragg RG. Documentation of environmental exposure using open biopsy, transbronchial biopsy, and bronchopulmonary lavage in giant cell interstitial pneumonia (GIP). Am Rev Respir Dis 1979; 119:A197(Abstr.).

442. Tabatowski K. Giant cell interstitial pneumonia in a hard-metal worker: Cytologic, histologic and analytical electron microscopic investigation. Acta Cytol 1988; 32:240–246.

443. Delage G, Brochu P, Pelletier M, et al. Giant cell pneumonia caused by parainfluenza virus. J Pediatr 1979; 94:426–429.

444. Weintrub PS, Sullender WM, Lombard C, Link MP, Arvin A. Giant cell pneumonia caused by parainfluenza type 3 in a patient with acute myelomonocytic leukemia. Arch Pathol Lab Med 1987;111:569–570.

445. Delage G, Brochu P, Robillard L, Jasmin G, Jones JH, Lapointe N. Giant cell pneumonia due to respiratory syncytial virus. Arch Pathol Lab Med 1984;108:623–625.

446. von Hansemann D. Uber malakoplakie der Harnblase. Virchows Arch Pathol Anat 1903;173:302–308.

447. Michaelis L, Gutmann C. Uber einschluse in Blasentumoren. Z Klin Med 1902;47:208–215.

448. Damjanov I, Katz SM. Malakoplakia. Pathol Annu 1981;16:103–126.

449. Gupta RK, Schuster RA, Christian WD. Autopsy findings in a unique case of malakoplakia: A cytoimmunohistochemical study of Michaelis-Gutmann bodies. Arch Pathol Lab Med 1972;93:42–48.

450. Colby TW, Hunt S, Pelzmann K, Carrington CB. Malakoplakia of the lung: A report of two cases. Respiration 1980;39:295–299.

451. Hodder RV, St. George-Hyslop P, Chalvardjian A, Bear

RA, Thomas P. Pulmonary malakoplakia. Thorax 1984;39:70–71.

452. Crouch E, White V, Wright J, Churg A. Malakoplakia mimicking carcinoma metastatic to lung. Am J Surg Pathol 1984;8:151–156.

453. Scannell KA, Portoni EJ, Finkle HI, Rice M. Pulmonary malacoplakia and *Rhodococcus equi* infection in a patient with AIDS. Chest 1990;97:1000–1001.

454. Schwartz DA, Ogden PO, Blumberg HM, Honig E. Pulmonary malacoplakia in a patient with acquired immunodeficiency syndrome. Arch Pathol Lab Med 1990;114:1267–1272.

455. Fierer J, Wolf P, Seed L, Gay T, Noonan K, Haghighi P. Nonpulmonary *Rhodococcus equi* infections in patients with acquired immune deficiency syndrome. J Clin Pathol 1987;40:556–558.

456. Colby TV, Lombard C, Yousem SA, Kitaichi M. Atlas of pulmonary surgical pathology. Philadelphia: WB Saunders. 1991;162.

457. Whipple GH. A hitherto undescribed disease characterized anatomically by deposits of fat and fatty acids in the intestinal and mesenteric lymphatic tissues. Bull Johns Hopkins Hosp 1907;18:382–391.

458. Black-Schaffer B. The tinctorial demonstration of a glycoprotein in Whipple's disease. Proc Soc Exp Biol Med 1949;72:225–227.

459. Sieracki JC. Whipple's disease: Observation on systemic involvement: I. Cytologic observations. Arch Pathol Lab Med 1958;66:464–467.

460. Yardley JH, Fleming WH II. Whipple's disease: A note regarding PAS-positive granules in the original case. Bull Johns Hopkins Hosp 1961;109:76–79.

461. Haubrich WS, Watson JHL, Sierachi JC. Unique morphologic features of Whipple's disease. A study by light and electron microscopy. Gastroenterology 1960;30:459–467.

462. Cohen AS, Schimmel EM, Holt PR, Isselbacher KJ. Ultrastructural abnormalities in Whipple's disease. Proc Soc Exp Biol Med 1960;205:411–414.

463. Chears WC, Jr., Ashworth CT. Electron microscopic study of the intestinal mucosa in Whipple's disease. Demonstration of encapsulated bacilliform bodies in the lesion. Gastroenterology 1961;41:129–138.

464. Yardley JH, Hendrix TR. Combined electron and light microscopy on Whipple's disease: Demonstration of "bacillary bodies" in the intestine. Bull Johns Hopkins Hosp 1961;109:80–98.

465. Paulley JW. A case of Whipple's disease (intestinal lipodystrophy). Gastroenterology 1952;22:128–133.

466. Bacillus-like bodies in Whipple's disease; Disappearance with clinical remission after antibiotic therapy. Am J Med 1964;37:481–490.

467. Plummer K, Russi S, Harris WH, Jr., Caravati CM. Lipophagic intestinal granulomatosis (Whipple's disease): Clinical and pathologic study of thirty-four cases, with special reference to clinical diagnosis and pathogenesis. Arch Intern Med 1950;86:280–310.

468. Maizel H, Ruffin JM, Dobbins WO III. Whipple's disease: A review of 19 patients from one hospital and a review of the literature since 1950. Medicine (Baltimore) 1970;49:175–205.

469. Clavey RL, Tomkins WAF, Muckle TJ, Anderson H, Rawls WE. Isolation and characterization of an aetiologic agent in Whipple's disease. Br Med J 1975;3:568–570.

470. Caroli J, Julien C, Bonneville B. La Maladie de Whipple: revue générale et acquisitions récentes. Rev Fr Edut Clin Biol 1965;10:362–380.

471. Fleming JL, Wiesner RH, Shorter RG. Whipple's disease: Clinical, biochemical, and histopathologic features and assessment of treatment in 29 patients. Mayo Clin Proc 1988;63:539–551.

472. Wang HH, Tollerud D, Danar D, Hanff P, Gottesdiener K, Rosen S. Another Whipple-like disease in AIDS? N Eng J Med 1986;314:1577–1578.

473. Sieracki JC, Fine G. Whipple's disease—observations on systemic involvement. II. Gross and histologic observations. AMA Arch Pathol 1959;67:81–93.

474. Enzinger FM, Helwig EB. Whipple's disease. A review of the literature and report of fifteen cases. Virchows Arch Path Anat 1963;336:238–269.

475. Pastor BM, Geerken RG. Whipple's disease presenting as pleuripericarditis. Am J Med 1973;55:827–831.

476. Apperly FL, Copley EL. Whipple's disease (lipophagia granulomatosis). Gastroenterology 1943;1:461–470.

477. Rodarte JR, Garrison CO, Holley KE, Fontana RS. Whipple's disease simulating sarcoidosis: A case with unique clinical and histological features. Arch Intern Med 1972;129:479–482.

478. James TN, Bulkley BH. Whipple bacilli within the tunica media of pulmonary arteries. Chest 1984;86:454–458.

479. Spain DM, Kliot DA, PAS and Sudan positive pulmonary emboli in Whipple's disease. Gastroenterology 1962;43:202–205.

480. Winberg CD, Rose ME, Rappaport H. Whipple's disease of the lung. Am J Med 1978;65:873–880.

481. Crocker AC, Farber S. Niemann-Pick disease: a review of 18 patients. Medicine (Baltimore) 1958;37:1–95.

482. Lynn R, Terry RD. Lipid histochemistry and electron microscopy in adult Niemann-Pick disease. Am J Med 1964;37:987–994.

483. McCusker JJ, Parsons DB. Niemann-Pick disease: Report of two cases in siblings including the necropsy and histochemical findings in one. Arch Pathol Lab Med 1962;74:127–136.

484. Lachman R, Crocker A, Schulman J, Strand R. Radiological findings in Niemann-Pick disease. Radiology 1973;108:659–664.

485. Skikne MI, Prinsloo I, Webster I. Electron microscopy of lung in Niemann-Pick disease. J Pathol 1972;106:119–122.

486. Terry RD, Sperry WM, Brodoff B. Adult lipidosis resembling Niemann-Pick disease. Am J Pathol 1954;30:263–285.

487. Long RG, Lake BD, Pettit JE, Scheuer PJ, Sherlock S. Adult Niemann-Pick disease: Its relationship to the syndrome of the sea-blue histiocyte. Am J Med 1977;62:627–635.

488. Lever AML, Ryder JB. Cor pulmonale in an adult secondary to Niemann-Pick disease. Thorax 1983; 38:873–874.

489. Rywlin AM, Hernandez JA, Chastain DE, Pardo V. Ceroid histiocytosis of spleen and bone marrow in idiopathic thrombocytopenic purpura (ITP): A contribution to the understanding of the sea-blue histiocyte. Blood 1971;37:587–593.

490. Beltrami CA, Bearzi I, Fabris G. Storage cells of spleen and bone marrow in thalassemia: An ultrastructural study. Blood 1973;41:901–912.

491. Lüllmann H, Lüllmann-Rauch R, Wasserman O. Drug-induced phospholipidoses. CRC Crit Rev Toxicol 1975;4:185–218.

492. Schneider EL, Epstein CJ, Kaback MJ, Brandes D. Severe pulmonary involvement in adult Gaucher's disease: Report of three cases and review of the literature. Am J Med 1977;63:475–480.

493. Lee RE, Yousem SA. The frequency and type of lung involvement in patients with Gaucher's disease. Mod Pathol 1988;1:54A (Abstr.).

494. Smith RRL, Hutchins GM, Sack GH Jr, Ridolfi RL. Unusual cardiac, renal and pulmonary involvement in Gaucher's disease: Interstitial glucocerebrosidal accumulation, pulmonary hypertension and fatal bone marrow embolization. Am J Med 1978;65:352–360.

495. Beutler E, Kay A, Saven P, et al. Enzyme replacement therapy for Gaucher's disease. blood 1991;78:1183–1189.

496. Wolson AH. Pulmonary findings in Gaucher's disease. AJR 1975;123:712–715.

497. Peters SP, Lee RE, Glew RH. Gaucher's disease: A review. Medicine (Baltimore) 1977;56:425–442.

498. Bartimmo EE Jr, Guisan M, Moser KM. Pulmonary involvement in Fabry's disease: A reappraisal. Follow-up of a San Diego kindred and review of the literature. Am J Med 1972;53:755–764.

499. Rosenberg DM, Ferrans VJ, Fulmer JD, et al. Chronic airflow obstruction in Fabry's disease. Am J Med 1980; 68:898–905.

500. Kariman K, Singletary WV Jr, Sieber HO. Pulmonary involvement in Fabry's disease. Am J Med 1978;64: 911–912.

501. Bagdade JD, Parker F, Ways PO, Morgan TE, Lagunoff D, Eidelman S. Fabry's disease: A correlative clinical, morphologic and biochemical study. Lab Invest 1968;18:681–688.

502. Hermansky F, Pudlak A. Albinism associated with hemorrhage diathesis and unusual pigmented reticular cells in the bone marrow: Report of two cases with histochemical studies. Blood 1959;14:162–169.

503. Garay SM, Gardella JE, Fazzini EP, Goldring RM. Hermansky-Pudlak syndrome: Pulmonary manifestations of a ceroid storage disorder. Am J Med 1979;66: 737–747.

504. Schinella RA, Greco MA, Cobert BL, Denmark LW, Cox RP. Hermansky-Pudlak syndrome with granulomatous colitis. Ann Intern Med 1980;92:20–23.

505. Schinella RA, Greco MA, Garay SM, Lackner H, Wolman SR, Fazzini EP. Hermansky-Pudlak syndrome: A clinicopathologic study. Hum Pathol 1985;16:366–376.

506. White DA, Smith GJW, Cooper JAD, Jr., Glickstein M, Rankin JA. Hermanski-Pudlak syndrome and interstitial lung disease: Report of a case with lavage findings. Am Rev Respir Dis 1984;130:138–141.

507. Reinelä A. Perivascular xanthogranulomatosis in the lungs of diabetic patients. Arch Pathol Lab Med 1976;100:542–543.

508. Caplan H. A case of endocardial fibroelastosis with features of glycogen storage disease. J Pathol Bacteriol 1958;76:77–82.

CHAPTER 23

Iatrogenic Injury: Radiation and Drug Effects

RODNEY A. SCHMIDT

Virtually all therapies of modern medicine carry the potential for harm. Fortunately, the potential is usually low and the consequences are mild. Nevertheless, iatrogenic disease is common and can result in the death of patients. For example, it is estimated that the incidence of adverse drug reactions most likely lies between 10% and 20% but may range as high as 28%.[1] Drug reactions cause between 2.9% and 6.2% of all hospital admissions and as many as 0.31% of all hospital deaths.[1,2] A substantial fraction of drug reactions involve the respiratory system. Radiation therapy is also associated with adverse effects. Estimates of radiation pneumonitis range from 5% to 20% for patients given tumoricidal doses of thoracic radiation.[3–5]

Some iatrogenic disease (e.g., radiation pneumonitis) can be anticipated and can be managed effectively. Most drug reactions and most other iatrogenic injuries are relatively mild and are diagnosed and treated without any help from the pathologist. Occasionally, however, the injury is unusual, severe, or unexpected or is clinically indistinguishable from infection or neoplasm and the pathologist becomes involved. In the following pages we review the characteristic clinical and morphologic features of the more common manifestations of iatrogenic injury.

Consequences of Thoracic Irradiation

The adverse pulmonary effects of high-energy x irradiation have been known since the 1920s. Groover et al. are credited with the first descriptions in 1922, which were followed soon thereafter by reports from other authors.[6–9] In 1925, Evans and Leucutia divided the clinical consequences of radiation into acute radiation pneumonitis and chronic fibrosis.[10] Desjardins described the histologic features of radiation pneumopathy the following year.[11] The pathology has been reviewed more recently by Fajardo and Berthong[12] and Schuh and Kemmer,[13] among others. The pathophysiology of radiation lung injury has been the subject of several excellent reviews.[3,5,14–16] The sequential effects of radiation of the lung have been well documented for experimental animals and, although the data are necessarily less complete for humans, the same events seem to occur.

Adverse pulmonary effects of radiation are relatively common. Estimates of the incidence of radiation pneumonitis range from 5% to 20%[3–5] but may be higher in some settings. Although the effects are not usually fatal, patients may die of either acute pneumonitis, chronic fibrosis, or delayed reactions.[14] Pulmonary radiation injury is most commonly seen following cancericidal doses to tumors in the lung or mediastinum; however, because x rays readily penetrate through the thorax, it may also be seen following radiation of the breast, chest wall, or whole body.[17–22] Acute pneumonitis can be avoided by using low doses or fractionated schedules, but fibrosis appears unavoidable.[15,23]

Symptoms and Pathologic Abnormalities

Few clinical symptoms appear during or immediately after radiation exposure. Humans generally tolerate 200–300 cGy of x irradiation to the chest per day without clinical symptoms attributable to the lungs, but some patients may need to have their therapy interrupted after 2–3 weeks of daily radiation because of desquamation of the esophageal mucosa.[24] Bronchial secretions may become more tenacious transiently, and a nonproductive cough may develop that can persist for life. The lungs of experimental animals examined immediately after radiation therapy show minimal histologic abnormalities. Even humans who die within days of massive radiation injury show only congestion, edema, and increased numbers of intraalveolar macrophages on histologic examination.[4] Biochemically, there is evidence for transient alterations that occur immediately following pulmonary irradiation. These include loss of surfactant granules from type II pneumocytes, changes in alveolar fluid composition,[25,26] and endothelial cell dysfunction.[27–31] The alterations in surfactant production are transient, but evidence of endothelial dysfunction (angiotensin-converting enzyme activity, plasminogen activator activity, prostacyclin synthesis, and thromboxane production) may persist until the pneumonitis phase in lethally irradiated rats.[15] In humans given cancericidal doses of radiation, the functional changes that occur within the first 6–12 weeks are clinically silent.[3,15]

The clinical symptoms of acute radiation pneumonitis typically begin 6–12 weeks after the completion of radiation therapy, although the onset may be delayed 6 months or more.* In 90% of cases, symptoms begin between 1 and 7 months after radiation (Fig. 23–1). There is a tendency toward earlier onset of pneumonitis with increasing total dose of fractionated radiotherapy.[3,33] Patients develop insidious dyspnea on exertion and a cough that is nonproductive or productive of scanty sputum. Shortness of breath may progress to dyspnea at rest. A low-grade fever is common but occasional patients may exhibit a high spiking fever. If large volumes of lung have been irradiated, symptoms may progress to acute respiratory failure and death.[9] Although the chest radiograph may initially be normal, radiographic changes soon appear and in fact radiologic manifestations are more common than are clinical symptoms of radiation pneumonitis. Some radiographic abnormalities can be found in 50% of all irradiated patients.[34] Computed tomography (CT) is probably more sensitive than conventional radiographs at detecting radiographic evidence of pneumonitis.[35,36] An important radiographic finding is that the abnormalities in radiation pneumonitis are confined to the radiation field in 85% of cases.[3,37] Clinically and radiologically, acute radiation pneumonitis may be difficult to distinguish from pulmonary infection or progressive neoplasm in some patients.

Biopsies obtained during the acute pneumonitis phase typically show edema and sparse intraalveolar and interstitial chronic inflammation in a pattern of

*References: 13,14–16,24,32.

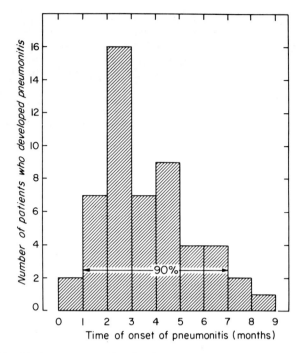

Fig. 23–1. Frequency distribution of time of onset of radiation pneumonitis in patients receiving single doses of thoracic irradiation. (Reprinted with permission of Pergamon Press, Inc., Van Dyk et al. Int J Radiat Oncol Biol Phys. 1981;7:461–467.)

acute lung injury.[3,4,12,14] Intraalveolar proteinaceous exudates are usually present, which may be organized as hyaline membranes (Fig. 23–2). Intraalveolar macrophages are numerous, and there are lesser numbers of other inflammatory cells within the exudates. Type II pneumocyte hyperplasia is typically present. Frequently, the proliferating pneumocytes are enlarged and have abundant cytoplasm. They may be multinucleated and may possess macronuclei, features that can be confused with viral cytopathic effect. The interstitium typically contains variable edema, predominantly mononuclear inflammatory cell infiltration, and fibrosis. Spindle cell proliferations composed of fibroblasts and myofibroblasts are usually present, both within the interstitium and in the intraalveolar exudates. Platelet thrombi and microemboli may be found within small blood vessels. Vascular endothelial cells are often plump, and the walls of vessels, particularly arterioles, may be thickened and hyalinized. Foam cells may be found within the intima and atypical fibroblasts may be present in the interstitium. The conducting airway epithelium may exhibit focal necrosis and squamous metaplasia.[3,4]

Radiation fibrosis develops in nearly all patients following radiation pneumonitis and in most patients who receive lung irradiation, even if they do not develop acute pneumonitis.[3,15] Radiologically, radiation fibrosis

Fig. 23–2. Radiation pneumonitis. Patient died 12 weeks after radiation therapy for lung cancer. Note hyaline membranes, loss of epithelial cells, interstitial edema, and sparse mononuclear inflammatory cell infiltrate. H and E, ×315.

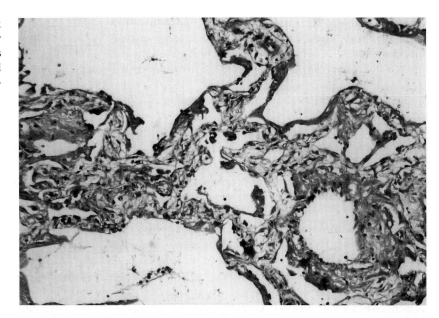

Fig. 23–3. Radiation fibrosis. Patient died 5 years after receiving radiation therapy for breast cancer. Note diffuse fibrosis filling all former air spaces, preservation of elastic tissue network, and thick-walled blood vessels. Movat pentachrome, ×80.

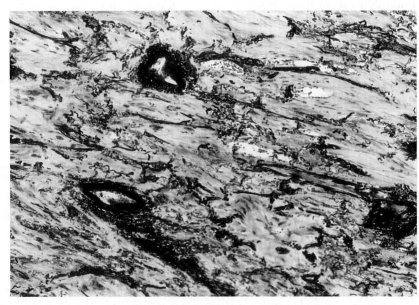

is centered on the radiated field but, in contrast to acute pneumonitis, structural alterations usually extend outside the radiation port.[4,15,16] Retraction and distortion of surrounding lung tissue are common and compensatory hyperinflation of adjacent or contralateral lung tissue may occur. The likelihood of clinical symptoms is most directly related to the volume of lung that becomes fibrotic and to the patient's pulmonary reserve.[3,15] Most often, radiation fibrosis is a radiologic finding. When symptoms are present, they include dyspnea on exertion and reduced exercise tolerance, but chronic respiratory failure may supervene in some patients.

Lungs with radiation fibrosis are grossly firm and airless in the affected region. The cut surface is depressed, and the architecture may be obliterated by dense scar tissue; fibrosis may be milder, in which case the interstitium simply appears accentuated. Histologically, fibrosis involves all compartments of the lung.[12] Alveolar spaces are collapsed and obliterated by fibrosis (Fig. 23–3). Fibrosis also involves alveolar septa and the interstitium surrounding blood vessels and bronchi. Vascular changes, including intimal sclerosis, mural hyalinization, and fibrosis, are particularly prominent and involve both arteries and veins although venous involvement tends to be milder. Secondary epithelial changes include bronchiolar metaplasia and squamous metaplasia. Cytologic atypia may be present in both epithelial and mesenchymal cells. Pleural adhesions and fibrosis are also typical of late radiation fibrosis.

Unusual consequences of radiation therapy include

reactions outside the radiation port, acute respiratory distress syndrome, pleural effusions, spontaneous pneumothorax, acute airway obstruction, hyperlucent lung, rib fractures, tracheoesophageal fistula, pericardial effusion, and pericarditits.[3,16,38–40] Bronchiectasis may develop in areas of radiation fibrosis and may lead to recurrent infections.

Occasionally, pulmonary alterations radiographically suggestive of radiation pneumonitis appear outside the radiation port and even in the contralateral lung.[35,36,41,42] The observed incidence of these abscopal effects seems to depend on the technology with which they are sought. They are rare when assessed by conventional chest x-ray examinations,[3,15] but acute pneumonitis has been reported outside the apparent radiation field in 4 of 17 cases examined by computed tomography (CT).[36] Explanations that have been advanced to explain these effects have included significant radiation exposure outside the ports, vascular damage distal to the radiation field, generalized inflammation (cellular to humeral), lymphatic obstruction, and infectious agents such as viruses.

Radiation exposure outside the presumed ports can be caused by orientation of the radiation beam or by generation of secondary energetic particles within the target tissue. When radiation is given in multiple fractions, the radiation fields may be imperfectly aligned or even deliberately angled. Further, the radiation beams diverge from a small source so that the cross-sectional area of the beam is appreciably smaller at the entrance surface than at the exit surface. Together, these factors serve to blur the margins of the radiation field and may result in significant exposure outside an idealized port. Wechsler et al.[43] found that by carefully computing the dose to the lung from all ports, including angled fields, they could explain all posttherapy radiographic infiltrates on the basis of radiation exposure in most cases. Secondary particles may be generated within the irradiated lung tissue and may in turn interact with adjacent lung tissue outside the radiation port. This may be particularly important for neutron beam therapy, which generates numerous energetic secondary particles.

Bell et al.[35] obtained evidence of subclinical vascular damage outside the radiation field. They carefully studied pulmonary perfusion following radiation therapy in 39 patients using CT and single photon emission computed tomography (SPECT) with ^{99}Tc-labeled microspheres as a marker of intravascular volume. Following therapeutic irradiation, perfusion and vessel caliber decreased in the radiation field, but similar changes were also noted in large areas of lung perfused by vessels that passed through the radiation port. The changes could be seen by both CT and SPECT but

SPECT was the more sensitive technique. It is notable that abscopal vascular changes were only observed when the hila of the lungs or the mediastinum had been irradiated. Bell et al. suggested three possibilities for their observations: (1) irradiation of the main pulmonary arteries might cause progressive downstream vascular sclerosis; (2) perivascular fibrosis might cause extrinsic compression and thereby decrease vascular perfusion; and (3) peribronchial fibrosis might cause decreased ventilation and reflexive decreased perfusion. Although none of Bell's patients were reported to have radiation pneumonitis, it is possible that the vascular changes they observed are related to abscopal radiation pneumonitis reported in other patients. Interestingly, many of the patients reported by others with pneumonitis outside the radiation field have had hilar or mediastinal irradiation.[41,42]

Others have suggested that lymphatic obstruction from mediastinal or hilar irradiation and posttherapy infections may underlie some cases of abscopal radiation pneumonitis. The evidence supporting these explanations is not strong.[3,16]

Finally, some cases of apparent abscopal radiation pneumonitis may result from inflammation, either through the release of humeral mediators from irradiated tissue or via a generalized cellular inflammatory reaction. Support for this notion derives in part from the studies of Gibson et al.,[42] who showed that bronchoalveolar lavage fluid from irradiated and contralateral lungs showed a similar absolute lymphocytosis. Bilateral increases in gallium uptake were also present. These findings were interpreted as evidence of hypersensitivity pneumonitis but they might also represent a generalized response to circulating mediators. Powerful mediators known to be released by cells in the lung in response to radiation include tumor necrosis factor alpha, interleukin-1, platelet-derived growth factor, and fibroblast growth factor.[44] Which, if any, of these are functionally important in the development of either radiation pneumonitis or fibrosis is not yet clear.

Patients have developed adult respiratory distress syndrome (ARDS) after thoracic radiation.[45,46] The clinical syndrome differs from the usual radiation pneumonitis in that it occurs earlier after radiation therapy (latency of a day to weeks instead of months), follows a rapid, fulminant course unresponsive to oxygen or steroid therapy, and is not limited to the irradiated fields. The described histopathologic features (hyaline membranes, intimal and medial proliferative changes within the vasculature, and some degree of interstitial inflammation) are not strikingly different from those of radiation pneumonitis. The relationship between ARDS and radiation pneumonitis in this setting is not clear. It is interesting to note that all reported cases have followed extensive radiation to the mediastinum or hila.[45,46]

Effects of Radiation Dose and Delivery

The likelihood of a patient developing an adverse response to radiation therapy relates to individual sensitivity to radiation, the radiation delivery schedule, the difficulty of precisely calculating the radiation dose delivered to the lung, and the tendency to deliver the highest dose of radiation for which most patients do not develop serious complications. Patients who have previously received pulmonary irradiation and those treated with certain drugs (see following) are also at increased risk. Five percent of patients will exhibit radiation pneumonitis following a single dose of 820 cGy delivered to the whole lung in a single fraction (Fig. 23–4A), and 50% and 90% will develop injury at 930 and 1100 cGy, respectively.[32] Radiation tolerance is markedly increased if the same total radiation dose is delivered in multiple smaller fractions (Fig. 23–4B). Thus, 5% and 50% of patients will not exhibit pneumonitis until 2,560 and 3,000 cGy, respectively, if the radiation is given in multiple fractions.[16] The slope of the dose-response curve is steep in both humans and animals, and small differences in dose near the tolerance threshold result in significant differences in the number of patients developing complications.[16,47] Accurate estimates of radiation delivery to the lung are difficult to make and must be corrected for pulmonary transmission. Such correction factors may be as much as 15%–20%, suggesting that failure to correct for lung transmission could result in a higher incidence of radiation toxicity.[15,32] Dose rate is also important. Radiation delivery at 5 cGy/min is less toxic than 30 cGy/min, which in turn is less damaging than 200–300 cGy/min. Taken together, these considerations may explain some cases of radiation injury that are initially considered unlikely to be caused by radiation effect.

Pathogenesis

The pathogenesis of radiation injury is the subject of numerous ongoing studies. The major questions have to do with the immediate effects of radiation on tissue (i.e., what the target molecules are and how radiation causes injury) and how the immediate effects of radiation ultimately are translated into organ dysfunction. Radiation can cause injury to macromolecules either directly or by way of the intermediate generation of free radicals. The former is important for high linear energy transfer (LET) radiation (e.g., neutrons) whereas the latter predominates for low-LET radiation (gamma rays, x rays).[48] In either case, the immediate damage to

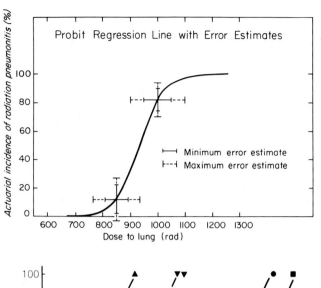

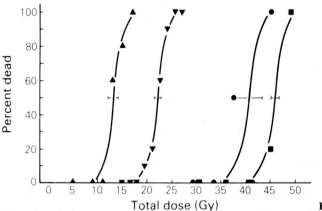

Fig. 23–4. Dose–response curves for radiation pneumonitis in humans and mice. **A.** Actuarial incidence of radiation pneumonitis in 150 patients receiving single doses of radiation. Horizontal error bars reflect uncertainties in estimating actual dose to lung (±5%–10%); vertical error bars indicate likely errors in estimation of incidence of pneumonitis (±10%–15%). Actual incidence of radiation pneumonitis is likely to be slightly less than actuarial incidence because some patients die of other causes before they experience radiation pneumonitis. (Reprinted with permission of Pergamon Press, Inc., from Van Dyk et al. Int J Radiat Oncol Biol. Phys 1981;71:461–467.) **B.** Effect of fractionation on radiation tolerance. Groups of at least 10 mice were radiated once (▲), weekly (▼), daily (●), or twice daily (■) to total doses shown. Mortality was assessed at 28 weeks. Note similar shapes of mortality curves and marked shift to right with increasing fractionation. (Reprinted from Siemann et al. Br J Cancer 1986;53(Suppl. VII):365–367, with permission.

macromolecules can be manifest as increased membrane permeability or fragmentation of molecules such as DNA or connective tissue. The theoretical possibility that long-lived matrix macromolecules such as elastin might serve as internal dosimeters has not found clinical application. If the dose of radiation is sufficiently high

(>1000 cGy in a single dose), cells may be killed immediately and directly.[14] At the typical doses used clinically, however, radiation injury does not result in cell death until the first, second, or third postirradiation mitosis.[14] Because focal damage to macromolecules such as DNA can be repaired while massive damage cannot, a single large dose of radiation is considerably more damaging than the same total dose administered in several fractions.[3]

All cells in the lung presumably suffer sublethal injury at the time of irradiation, but clinical symptoms are delayed. The delay is usually attributed to the turnover and repair kinetics of the major cell populations in the lung because the cells do not die until they attempt replication.[3,4,14–16] Replication rates are problematic to measure in humans, but in growing mice type II pneumocytes are replaced every 28–35 days. Type I cells are replaced solely through replication and differentiation of type II cells. Regenerating capillary endothelial cells appear to proliferate at the same rate as regenerating type II pneumocytes. Bronchial epithelial cells turn over every 1–3 weeks. Presumably, as cells attempt replication and die, they leave a void and fail to maintain the structure and function of the lung in their vicinity. The clinical extent and severity of pneumonitis are then dependent on the degree to which cell renewal has been abrogated by radiation.

The response of cells to radiation is very complex, and the development of clinical symptoms may not be adequately explained by simple cell kinetics. It is known for example that irradiated cells coordinately regulate many genes, including some that are related to cell growth, metabolism, and proliferation.[49,50] Cellular proto-oncogenes, such as *fos, jun,* and *egr-1,* are induced by radiation.[50] Radiated endothelial cells change their metabolism of arachadonic acid and in addition produce mitogens such as platelet-derived growth factor and basic fibroblast growth factor.[50,51] Radiation also causes monocytes and some cultured sarcoma cell lines to produce cytokines such as tumor necrosis factor alpha and interleukin-1.[50] The clinical significance of these alterations is not yet clear, but therapies directed at one or more of these alterations may some day ameliorate the deleterious effects of radiation.

Drug Interactions

Some, but not all, chemotherapeutic drugs increase the likelihood of radiation lung toxicity at standard radiation doses (Table 23–1). Actinomycin D, cyclophosphamide, bleomycin, and mitomycin C are the drugs for which this relationship has been best established,[15,16,52] but certain interferons also appear to enhance radiosensitivity. Fluorouracil, methotrexate, *cis*-platinum,

Table 23–1. Documented influence of drugs on the incidence of radiation pneumonitis[a]

Increased risk of radiation pneumonitis	No definite increased risk
Actinomycin D	5-Fluorouracil
Bleomycin[72]	Carboplatin[53]
Busulfan[73]	Cisplatinum
Cyclophosphamide	Etoposide[53]
Doxorubicin	Methotrexate
Mitomycin C (possible)[74,75]	
Interferons	
Human leukocyte interferon	
R-Human betaser	
Vincristine (lesser risk)	

[a] Revised from references 15, 16, and others as indicated. These data are for drugs used as single agents.

carboplatin, and etoposide (VP-16) do not appear to enhance radiation toxicity when given as single agents.[15,53] There have been relatively few controlled studies of the radiation-enhancing effects of chemotherapeutic agents (either individually or in combination) and it seems likely that other agents will be found to enhance radiation toxicity.

In some circumstances, therapeutic irradiation appears to cause latent damage that may be unmasked later. Examples include the increased sensitivity of previously irradiated tissue to further irradiation[3] and the "radiorecall" phenomenon elicited by bleomycin and (possibly) mitomycin C.[51,54,55] Radiorecall was described among patients with testicular cancer who were treated with high-dose bleomycin for metastases. Five of 12 patients who had received thoracic irradiation within the year before chemotherapy developed pulmonary toxicity whereas only 4 of 89 nonirradiated patients developed pneumotoxicity. Their disease might not represent a classic radiorecall phenomenon, however, because the pulmonary manifestations were not confined to the radiation ports and because disease appeared during a time period when subclinical acute radiation pneumonitis might still have been active. Cyclophosphamide, actinomycin D, busulfan, vincristine, doxorubicin, and 5-fluorouracil (drugs that potentiate radiation pneumonitis) have not been reported to elicit a radiorecall phenomenon.

Diagnosis

The diagnosis of radiation pneumonitis is indirect and is based on compatible pathologic findings, an appropriate clinical context, and an absence of confounding factors. The pathologic features described previously are characteristic but not specific for radiation pneumopathy. Radiation pneumonitis closely resembles diffuse alveolar damage, which may be caused by many agents. Many of the features of radiation fibrosis are nonspecific characteristics of pulmonary fibrosis. In surgical or autopsy tissue, the features of radiation pneumonitis (hyaline membranes and edema) may be superimposed on radiation fibrosis. This combination of features has been regarded as particularly suggestive of radiation injury.[41,56] An appropriate clinical context is one in which a sufficient dose of radiation has been delivered to the lung and the latency period is appropriate (6 weeks to 6 months after completion of therapy for acute pneumonitis and more than 6 months for radiation fibrosis). Confounding factors such as infiltrating neoplasm or infection can usually be ruled out by light microscopy, special stains, and cultures. Certain drugs may enhance or mimic the toxic effects of radiation, and it may be impossible to separate their effects from those of radiotherapy. Lung injury may be ascribed to the combined effects of drugs and radiation in those cases where the patient is known to have received a drug that increases radiosensitivity.

Two histologic features of radiation injury that are relatively distinctive are vascular "foam cells" and interstitial atypical stromal cells ("radiation fibroblasts"). Lipid-rich foam cells may be found in the intima of arterioles from any irradiated organ.[4,12] Some authors consider them to be pathognomonic of radiation injury. Unfortunately, they are not always present and they have been reported in nonirradiated vessels from nonpulmonary sites such as the gallbladder, uterus, and placenta.[12] Presumably, the "foam cells" are modified macrophages and smooth muscle cells similar to the foam cells that accumulate in fatty streaks and atheromatous plaques. They may represent a nonspecific response to endothelial injury.

Atypical stromal cells are another consequence of radiation injury that may occur in any tissue.[12] The cells have abundant, usually basophilic cytoplasm that is attributable to accumulations of rough endoplasmic reticulum. The nuclei are enlarged, hyperchromatic, and may have prominent nucleoli. Mitotic figures are rare, however. Atypical stromal cells are not specific for radiation; they are well known to occur in the bladder, vagina, and pharynx, for example. They are also not a reliable marker of radiation injury because similar cells may be found in areas of active inflammation or repair. To our knowledge, there are no features that distinguish radiation-induced atypical fibroblasts from those unrelated to radiation.

Therapy

Acute radiation pneumonitis is frequently treated with corticosteroids. Symptoms often but not always respond dramatically. If steroids are abruptly withdrawn symptoms may recur.[57,58] Cases of postradiation steroid-withdrawal pneumonitis have also been reported in patients who had not previously exhibited radiation pneumonitis.[57,59] There is no efficacious therapy for radiation fibrosis.

Secondary Neoplasms

Radiation, whether from environmental or iatrogenic sources, can induce cancers in the lung. Studies of atomic bomb survivors, uranium miners, and British radiologists have all demonstrated an increased risk of lung carcinomas.[14,60,61] As for most radiation-induced cancer, the induction period is usually more than 10 years. Diagnostic radiologic procedures carry a small theoretical risk of inducing lung cancer but no studies have actually demonstrated such an increased incidence. For example, studies of women and men who were examined fluoroscopically an average of 71 and 91 times, respectively, during lung collapse therapy for tuberculosis did not show an increased risk of lung cancer, but the women had an increased risk of developing breast cancer.[62,63] The average total dose (91 cGy) was low compared to therapeutic doses. Patients therapeutically irradiated for ankylosing spondylitis have an increased incidence of lung cancer that becomes apparent more than 9 years after irradiation.[64] Patients treated with radiotherapy for Hodgkin's disease also appear to have a 1.6- to 5-fold relative risk of developing lung cancer.[65–67] Lung cancer was the most common second tumor in this population and it usually occurred in the radiation field. In contrast to other patients, Hodgkin's disease patients did not always exhibit a long latency period before their lung cancer appeared.[66] Secondary radiation-induced lung cancers may also appear after radiation therapy for a primary lung cancer, but it is usually difficult to prove that the second tumor is caused by radiation and is not related to the first.[65]

Tumors other than carcinoma of the lung may also be induced by radiation. Breast carcinomas were mentioned, and pleural and peritoneal mesotheliomas have been reported to occur with latency periods of 7–36 years.[54,68] Other radiation-induced thoracic tumors include esophageal cancer,[69] malignant fibrous histiocytoma of trachea or pulmonary artery,[70,71] and leukemia and lymphoma.[62,67]

Drug Reactions

The number of drugs with adverse effects on the bronchopulmonary system is large and everexpanding.

More than 75 drugs, including drugs of all pharmacologic classes, are currently known to cause respiratory reactions.[76] Clinically, drug reactions may be divided into those that are predictable based on the known pharmacology of the drug and those that are unpredictable.[1,77] The latter, including toxic reactions, hypersensitivity reactions of all types, and idiosyncratic reactions, and are the primary focus here. There are many excellent recent reviews of pulmonary drug reactions with clinical[52,76,78–83] or pathologic[84–87] orientation; these are organized by drug[52,76,78–84] or by tissue reaction.[85–87]

Drug reactions can be classified in many ways but a scheme based on tissue site and pattern of reaction is perhaps the most useful to the pathologist. Unfortunately, the respiratory system is only moderately complex and is capable of only a limited number of patterns of response; necessarily, then, many different and unrelated drugs will cause the same morphologic changes in tissue. Few if any of these changes are distinctive for a particular drug or even for a class of drugs, and in fact none are even pathognomonic of drug toxicity. The diagnosis of drug reaction, therefore, requires knowledge of not only the tissue reaction but also of the clinical context. The following discussion emphasizes morphologic features that characterize different types of drug reactions. Examples of drugs commonly causing each pattern of injury are also discussed with their characteristic clinical presentations.

Bronchospasm and Cough

The adverse effects of therapeutic drugs on the airways are manifest clinically as bronchospasm and cough. The many drugs that can cause these symptoms may be grouped by mechanism of action or pharmacologic class (Table 23–2). Meeker and Wiedemann[88] have comprehensively reviewed this topic, which has also been summarized by Israel-Biet et al.[79] and Demeter et al.[80]

The association of aspirin with nasal polyps and asthma [the acetylsalicylic acid (ASA) triad] was first described in 1967[89] and has been studied extensively and reviewed since then.[79,80,88] Aspirin sensitivity has an estimated prevalence of 0.3% in the normal adult population.[90] Aspirin-sensitive bronchospasm is acquired during life, usually appears in the third or fourth decade, and may follow the development of aspirin-induced vasomotor rhinitis and nasal congestion. After aspirin is ingested, bronchospasm appears within minutes to hours and is often preceded by conjunctival irritation, rhinorrhea, and facial flushing. Interestingly, patients with bronchospasm do not usually display other symptoms of aspirin sensitivity such as urticaria and angioedema.[91]

Table 23–2. Drug-related bronchospasm[a]

Aspirin Sensitivity
  Aspirin
  NSAIDS (ibuprofen, naproxen, fenoprofen, indomethacin, flufenamic acid, phenylbutazone, etc.)
  Hydrocortisone
  Acetaminophen
  Tartrazine (FD&C #5)
β-Blockers
  Propranolol, metroprolol, atenolol, pindolol, oxypenolol, acebutolol
Cholinesterase Inhibitors (rarely)
Angiotensin-Converting Enzyme Inhibitors
  Captopril, enalapril
Neuromuscular Blocking Agents
  Tubocurarine, alcuronium, atracurium, vecuronium
Radiographic Contrast Media
Inhaled Agents
  Metered dose inhalers, nebulizers, aerosolized pentamidine
Anaphylactic, Anaphylactoid, and Asthmatic Reactions
  Iodinated radiographic contrast media
  Penicillins, cephalosporins, trimethoprim-sulfamethoxazole (172), streptomycin, bromsulphothalein, dextran, iron dextran, procaine, insulin, demeclocycline, lidocaine, nitrofurantoin, cimetidine, aminophylline, ACTH, trypsin, ketamine, alphamethyldopa, carbamazepine, dyazide, psyllium, vitamins K_1 and B_{12}
  Vaccines[111]
  Antilymphocyte globulin[111]
  L-asparaginase,[77] cyclophosphamide,[111] cytarabine,[111] bleomycin, vinca alkaloids with mitomycin[52]

[a] Compiled from references 79, 87, 88, and others as noted.

Aspirin-sensitive asthmatics are almost always sensitive to other nonsteroidal inhibitors of cyclo-oxygenase and vice versa.[88] A few also react to agents such as acetaminophen and hydrocortisone that do not inhibit cyclo-oxygenase directly but which may indirectly alter arachadonic acid metabolism.[92,93] These observations have led to the hypothesis that aspirin-induced bronchospasm results from either an imbalance in the production of, or sensitivity to, the bronchodilating and bronchoconstricting cyclo-oxygenase products (prostaglandins) or from a shunting of arachadonic acid metabolites through the lipoxygenase pathway to form bronchoconstrictive leukotrienes.[88]

Pathologic changes in the airways of aspirin-induced bronchospasm have not been described. Treatment consists of desensitization or avoidance of aspirin and nonsteroidal antiinflammatory drugs.

Beta-adrenergic drugs act as bronchodilators, and some individuals (particularly those with a family history of atopy or asthma) may develop bronchospasm after being given β-blockers. The effects seem to be less pronounced for cardioselective β-blockers, such as metoprolol and atenolol, but any of the β-blockers may induce bronchospasm, particularly in patients with greater degrees of airway hyperreactivity or when used in higher doses.[88,94-96] Normal individuals do not demonstrate decreased expiratory flows with β-blockers,[97] and bronchospasm was not reported in four cases of massive propranolol intoxication.[98] This suggests that some underlying factor (heritable or acquired) must be present for β-blockers to induce bronchospasm.

Cholinesterase inhibitors might be expected to cause bronchoconstriction but the reported incidence is remarkably low.[88] Neuromuscular blocking agents may also rarely cause bronchospasm.[99] It is proposed that the neuromuscular blockers act by releasing histamine from basophils or mast cells, but this mechanism remains to be proven.[88] The angiotensin-converting enzyme inhibitors captopril and enalapril seem to cause bronchospasm in some individuals, particularly those with underlying bronchial hyperreactivity.[88] The mechanism is unknown.

Clinically significant bronchospasm is a recognized but rare complication of intravenous radiographic contrast media administration. Patients develop a transient, subclinical decline in expiratory air flow within 4–5 min.[100-102] The incidence of measurable airflow restriction is similar in those with and without an allergic history, although the magnitude of the airflow restriction tends to be higher in those with an allergic history.[102] Agents with low osmolality cause less airflow restriction than agents with high osmolality.[101]

Bronchospasm has also been described for inhaled agents of all types, including those given via metered dose inhalers and nebulizers. The effect may be caused by inert propellants and dispersants, because similar effects were reported with a placebo inhaler containing only inert ingredients.[103] Some nebulized bronchodilator solutions contain sulfites; sulfite sensitivity may thus explain some cases of paradoxical bronchospasm after nebulized bronchodilator therapy.[104-107] Cough and bronchospasm are frequently reported side effects of aerosolized pentamidine therapy.[108] The mechanism is uncertain but may include nonspecific irritation due to inhaled particles, histamine release, or inhibition of cholinesterases by pentamidine.[96,109,110]

Probably the most common mechanisms of drug-induced bronchospasm involve allergic and pseudo-allergic reactions. The bronchial symptoms may be isolated or may occur as part of a more generalized anaphylactic reaction. Anaphylactic reactions only occur in patients who have become sensitized to the drug. Following an initial exposure, patients develop IgE antibodies that are then displayed on the surfaces of mast cells. Subsequent reexposure to the offending drug results in the massive release of inflammatory mediators and clinical symptoms. These develop within seconds to minutes of exposure and consist of bronchoconstriction, urticaria, pruritis, vascular collapse,

and shock. Anaphylactoid reactions are clinically similar but are apparently not mediated through IgE. It is thought that the offending drugs cause mast cell degranulation directly or through other nonimmunologic mechanisms.[77,111] Drug-induced asthmatic reactions are relatively uncommon but may be caused by virtually all classes of drugs.[77,79] Among cytotoxic agents, L-asparaginase is the most likely to cause anaphylactic reactions, and the combination of vinblastine with mitomycin is particularly likely to cause bronchospasm.[52,77]

The pathology of anaphylactic and anaphylactoid reactions has been reported infrequently and then only at autopsy.[111,112] The reported changes include increased bronchial secretions, submucosal edema, peribronchial vascular engorgement, and eosinophilic infiltrates in the bronchial walls. A more recent large series of fatal cases of drug-induced anaphylaxis suggested that there are six distinguishable patterns of morphologic abnormalities.[113]

Cough is a common manifestation of many types of pulmonary disease, including disturbances of the airways. Cough has been described with particular frequency following administration of angiotensin-converting enzyme inhibitors, inhaled agents of all types, and radiographic contrast media.[79,88]

Pleural Manifestations

Drug-related pleural disease usually presents as pleuritic chest pain or pleural effusions. It is most frequently seen as drug-related lupus (DRL; or lupoid reaction) or with concurrent parenchymal reactions, but may also be seen as an isolated finding (Table 23–3). Patients receiving anticoagulant therapy may develop hemorrhage effusions.

A partial list of the many drugs that can cause a lupus-like syndrome is given in Table 23–3. Symptoms are particularly common with procainamide, isoniazide, hydralazine, and diphenylhydantoin, which together may account for 90% of all cases of DRL.[82,87,114] The syndrome typically begins after several months of drug therapy and will usually disappear after the drug is withdrawn.[115] As in systemic lupus, symptoms are usually those of a polyserositis, including arthritis, pleuritis, pericarditis, and peritonitis, although some patients will present with fever and myalgia.[116] Pleuropulmonary reactions (pleuritis, pleural effusions, and parenchymal lung infiltrates) are particularly frequent and are present in more than 50% of cases.[79] In contrast to systemic lupus erythematosus (SLE), central nervous system (CNS), renal, and skin involvement are much less common in DRL.[79,116] Also, drug-related lupus does not show the marked female predominance seen

Table 23–3. Drug-related pleural disease[a]

Drug-Related Lupus (DRL)
  Most common: diphenylhydantoin, hydralazine, isoniazid,
    procainamide
  Acebutolol, atenolol, captopril, carbamazepine,[163]
    chlorpromazine, chlorthalidone*, D-penicillamine, digitalis,
    ethosuximide, gold*, griseofulvin*, guanoxan*, hydrazine,
    hydrochlorothiazide, isoguinazepan*, labetalol, levodopa,
    lithium carbonate, lovostatin,[174] mephenytoin, methimazole,
    methylthiouracil, methyldopa, metoprolol, nitrofurantoin, oral
    contraceptives, oxyphenistatin, oxyprenolol, penicillin,
    phenylbutazone, phenytoin, pindolol, practolol, primidone,
    propranolol, propylthiouracil, quinidine, reserpine*,
    streptomycin*, sulfonamides*, tetracycline*, tolazamide,
    trimethadione
Concurrent Parenchymal Disease
  Amiodarone,[163] bleomycin, bromocriptine, busulfan,
    dantrolene,[175] gold salts, ibuprofen, methotrexate,
    methysergide, mitomycin, nitrofurantoin, nitromycin,
    paraaminosalicylic acid, penicillin, procarbazine
Isolated Pleural Disease
  Bleomycin,[134,137] methotrexate,[52,79] methysergide,[120]
    nitrofurantoin[77]
Hemorrhagic Effusions Associated with Anticoagulants

[a] Compiled from references 79, 86, 87, 116, and others as noted.
Drugs considered by Solinger[116] to have an unlikely association to
lupus have either been omitted or marked with an asterisk.

Table 23–4. Patterns of parenchymal
drug reactions

Pulmonary edema
Cytotoxic injury and fibrosis
Cellular inflammation
  Lymphocytes, monocytes, and macrophages
  Eosinophils
Distinctive reaction patterns
  Alveolar macrophages (amiodarone)
  Obliterative bronchiolitis (penicillamine)
  Bronchiolitis obliterans with organizing pneumonia
  Pulmonary alveolar proteinosis
Vascular disease
  Pulmonary hypertension
  Vasculitis
  Pulmonary renal syndrome (penicillamine)

Parenchymal Drug Reactions

Parenchymal drug reactions can be logically separated into those marked purely by pulmonary edema, those with evidence of cytotoxic injury, those where cellular inflammation predominates, and those classified on the basis of unusual and distinctive patterns of reaction (Table 23–4). This scheme has the intellectual attraction of correlating with the mechanism of injury and with prognosis (reversibility). It does not necessarily correlate well with the type of drug causing the injury because: (1) the same drug may cause different patterns of injury in different patients; (2) the pattern of injury may evolve over time within a single patient; and (3) unrelated drugs may cause histologically identical injury. Nevertheless, the classification is useful for characterizing the type of injury seen in lung tissue and has the additional advantage of at least partially avoiding the myriad of overlapping diagnostic labels that have been applied to inflammatory lung diseases.

in idiopathic SLE, and blacks are apparently less likely to exhibit DRL.[117]

The diagnosis is usually established on the basis of characteristic clinical symptoms, history of exposure to an appropriate drug, and serologic tests. The patients have antinuclear antibodies and have a much higher frequency of antihistone antibodies than do patients with idiopathic SLE.[79,116,118] There have been few studies of the range of pathologic alterations in pleural DRL because the lung and pleura are rarely biopsied unless there is clinical concern for infection or neoplasm. Pleural fibrosis and effusions (clear or sometimes hemorrhagic) have been reported.[119] The few cases we have examined have shown mild chronic inflammation and fibrosis. Parenchymal alterations have included eosinophilic pneumonia and nonspecific interstitial pneumonitis.

Pleural effusions or fibrosis may accompany parenchymal drug reactions such as pulmonary edema, hypersensitivity pneumonitis, and interstitial fibrosis. A few drugs, such as the cytotoxic drugs methotrexate and bleomycin, can cause pleural symptoms in the absence of parenchymal changes. Methysergide has also been linked to retroperitoneal fibrosis, to fibrosis at other anatomic sites, and to pleural effusion and fibrosis.[79,120]

Pulmonary Edema

The literature regarding drug-induced pulmonary edema is confusing because all pulmonary inflammatory reactions are associated with edema and because the clinical appellation of noncardiogenic pulmonary edema is applied freely regardless of whether the actual tissue reaction pattern is known. Moreover, because patients with pure pulmonary edema can usually be diagnosed and managed without an open lung biopsy, pure pulmonary edema reactions tend not to be documented histologically.

Table 23–5 lists the drugs for which there is the most solid evidence that they can cause pure pulmonary edema. Salicylate-induced pulmonary edema has been studied extensively following its first description by

Table 23–5. Drugs causing isolated pulmonary edema[a]

Cytotoxic drugs
  Cytosine arabinoside, cyclophosphamide*, methotrexate
    (intrathecal)
Salicylates and related drugs
  Aspirin, ibuprofen[83]
Narcotics, antagonists, and sedatives
  Heroin, propoxyphene, methadone, naloxone, ethchlorvynol,
    chlordiazepoxide
Other drugs
  Terbutaline, ritodrine, lidocaine*, hydrochlorothiazide,
    colchicine*, fluorescein
Interleukin-2[131,132]

[a] Compiled from references 52, 82, 87, 139, and others as noted.
*Single case.

Reid et al.[80,82,83,121] It may be seen in either acute or chronic overdose but requires serum levels of greater than 30–40 mg/dl (more than twice the therapeutic range).

Not all patients with salicylate overdose necessarily develop pulmonary edema. The frequency of edema is increased in older patients, smokers, and those taking salicylates chronically.[83] Patients typically present with dyspnea and have diffuse interstitial or acinar infiltrates that are consistent with pulmonary edema on chest radiographs. Lethargy and confusion are usually present and are attributable to the toxic effects of salicylates on the CNS. The edema fluid was studied in two patients and found to be similar to plasma in terms of electrolyte composition and oncotic pressure, thus suggesting the edema fluid accumulates because of increased vascular permeability.[122] Measurements of the pulmonary capillary wedge pressure have been normal. The edema may be sufficiently profound as to require mechanical ventilation but the overall prognosis for salicylate-induced pulmonary edema is very good if the correct diagnosis is made promptly. The chest x-ray abnormalities may take 3–8 days to clear.[80]

The histopathological alterations of salicylate-induced pulmonary edema have not been described except for one early autopsy report that documented "fluid-filled lungs."[83] A similar syndrome of pulmonary edema has been ascribed to ibuprofen but not to any of the other nonsteroidal antiinflammatory agents.[83]

Pulmonary edema from opiate intoxication was first described by Osler in 1880.[82,123,124] The syndrome is perhaps most common in heroin addicts but also occurs after overdoses of propoxyphene and methadone. Edema occurs only in the setting of drug overdose and may occur with the first exposure or after chronic use. One study found that as many as 33% of patients admitted with heroin overdose had clinical evidence of pulmonary edema.[125]

Clinically, patients with edema from opiate overdose are usually obtunded and may exhibit cyanosis, hypoventilation, and pulmonary crackles.[124] Systemic hypotension is rare. Pulmonary function tests show a restrictive deficit, and chest radiographs show a pattern consistent with pulmonary edema. Treatment is generally supportive, and the chest radiographs usually improve within 5 days unless there is superimposed pneumonia.[80]

Lung tissue that has been examined has exhibited generalized edema with focal consolidation but without cellular inflammation.[123] In the case of i.v. drug abuse, talc and other particulate material may also be present in the lungs.[80,126,127]

The mechanism of opiate-induced edema seems to involve increased vascular permeability because the edema fluid has a similar composition to plasma and there is no evidence of cardiac dysfunction.[82] Proposed mechanisms include direct opiate-induced mast cell degranulation, endothelial damage from complement activation, and neurogenic pulmonary edema.[82]

The opiate antagonist naloxone was reported to cause noncardiogenic pulmonary edema in two cases, only one of which was well documented.[82,128] Ethchlorvynol[129] and chlordiazepoxide[87] have both been reported to cause pulmonary edema after drug overdose. Chlordiazepoxide-induced edema was linked to i.v. injection of an oral preparation.

The tocolytic beta-sympathomimetic drugs ritodrine and terbutaline have been reported to cause noncardiogenic pulmonary edema in small numbers of patients when used intravenously to treat premature labor.[82] Symptoms consisting of dyspnea and cough begin after 48–72 h of i.v. therapy and may be quite severe. Chest radiographs and physical examination findings are consistent with pulmonary edema. Measurements of pulmonary capillary wedge pressure have been normal, consistent with a noncardiogenic cause. Treatment consists of discontinuation of the drug. Rapid recovery is expected and mortality is low. In one case, pulmonary edema was found at autopsy.[82]

Interleukin-2 (IL-2) has been given to patients with or without in vitro lymphokine-activated killer lymphocytes as an antitumor therapy in phase II clinical trials. IL-2 causes a consistent, profound, multisystem capillary leak syndrome that occurs during IL-2 infusion and resolves after the infusion ceases. In the lung, this is manifest as pulmonary edema, pleural effusions, and occasionally bronchospasm.[130,131] Interstitial patterns of edema are most frequent (76%), but air space disease is seen in 20% of patients.[131] Increased vascular permeability is probably not due to IL-2 itself but to cytokines such as gamma interferon, interleukin-1, tumor necro-

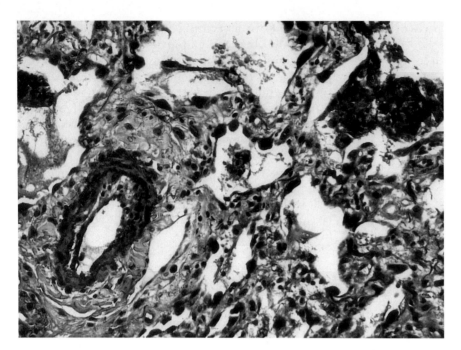

Fig. 23–5. Cytotoxic injury. Patient died 8 weeks after bone marrow transplantation where CDDP, BCNU, and VP-16 were used in conditioning regimen. Note loss of epithelial cells, hyaline membranes, interstitial edema, atypia of remaining epithelial cells, and paucity of inflammation. H and E, ×260.

sis factor, and lymphotoxin that are secreted by lymphocytes in response to IL-2.[130] The frequency of pulmonary edema seems to be decreased if IL-2 is given as continuous intravenous infusion rather than as i.v. boluses.[132]

Cytotoxic Injury and Fibrosis

Cytotoxic lung injury includes a spectrum of clinical presentations ranging from acute, rapidly progressive respiratory distress to chronic, slowly progressive interstitial lung disease with insidious onset.[52,82] The unifying feature is that it results from direct toxicity of the drug to parenchymal cells. Pathologically, the lungs of patients with acute, fulminant disease show hyaline membranes, epithelial cell necrosis, edema, and fibroblastic proliferation in a pattern closely resembling diffuse alveolar damage from other causes.[78] A distinctive feature that is often present is remarkable enlargement and atypia of the alveolar lining cells (Fig. 23–5). The cells have hyperchromatic, enlarged, and irregular nuclei, features which may raise concern about viral cytopathic effect, radiation injury, or even malignancy. Fibrosis predominates in the lungs of patients with slowly progressive disease, and the pathologic findings may be indistinguishable from usual interstitial pneumonitis. Some mononuclear inflammatory cells are always present in cytotoxic lung injury but, in contrast to hypersensitivity pneumonitis, they are sparse and do not form granulomas. Vascular endothelial cells may also be affected but endothelial changes are relatively inconspicuous by light microscopy.

Cytotoxic lung injury is usually caused by antineoplastic drugs, particularly alkylating agents, but it can also occur with other drugs (Table 23–6). In either case, it can present clinically as noncardiogenic pulmonary edema. One significant difference, however, is that noncardiogenic pulmonary edema (NCPE) from antineoplastic agents tends to have significant mortality and to leave survivors with residual lung deficits, while NCPE from other drugs has an excellent prognosis once the inciting agent is removed.[82] Symptoms of cytotoxic injury are usually insidious and slowly progressive. Dry cough, dyspnea, and fever are common complaints. The chest radiographs characteristically show fine bibasilar interstitial and alveolar infiltrates that may progress to consolidation.[78]

Bleomycin is the best-known and most extensively studied cause of cytotoxic lung injury. It is an antitumor antibiotic isolated from *Streptomyces verticillus* that causes

Table 23–6. Drugs that cause cytotoxic injury and fibrosis[a]

Antineoplastic agents
  Alkylating agents
    Busulfan, cyclophosphamide, chlorambucil, melphalan, nitrosoureas (e.g., BCNU)
  Antimetabolites
    Azathioprine, methotrexate
  Cytotoxic antibiotics
    Bleomycin, mitomycin C
Other drugs
  Amiodarone,[151,152] gold, nitrofurantoin, penicillamine*

[a] Compiled from references 52, 78, 82, and others as indicated. *, Single case.

Fig. 23–6. Nodular bleomycin fibrosis. Incidental lung nodule in 28-year-old woman who had received bleomycin for choriocarcinoma. Smooth muscle hyperplasia is prominent within fibrotic nodule. H and E, ×50.

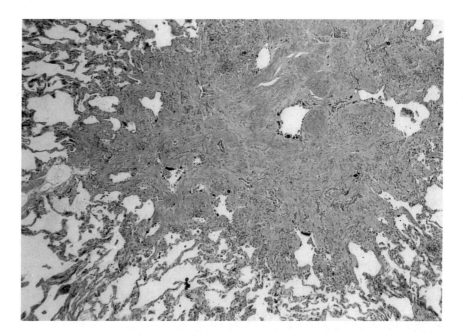

pneumonitis and fibrosis in both humans and experimental animals.[133] In animal models, it causes disease whether given intravenously, intratracheally, subcutaneously, or intraperitoneally.[52,133] Much has been learned about the action of bleomycin from animal studies, and it is presumed that its deleterious effects in humans are similar to those in the animal models.

Bleomycin is concentrated in the lung. It is inactivated by a hydrolase but the enzyme is relatively deficient in the lung compared to other tissues, which may explain the relative sensitivity of the lung to bleomycin. At least in part, bleomycin toxicity appears to be mediated through the production of reactive oxygen species such as superoxide.[52] Bleomycin produces superoxide when incubated with iron and oxygen in vitro. In animals, hypoxia protects against bleomycin toxicity, and in humans, bleomycin toxicity is potentiated by oxygen therapy.[52,134] Superoxide dismutase also protects against bleomycin toxicity in some experimental systems. Other mechanisms that may be important in initiating or propagating lung injury include production of factors that are chemotactic for neutrophils, lymphocyte-mediated interstitial fibrosis, and direct effects on fibroblast metabolism.[52]

Pathologically, a sequence of alterations occurs that is best studied in experimental animals and seems to be similar in humans.[52,134] The first evidence of injury in mice is intracellular edema and blebbing of endothelial cells. Necrosis of type I pneumocytes and loss of lamellar inclusions in type II pneumocytes then occurs. Later, macrophages and type II pneumocytes proliferate at a time when increased amounts of surfactant can be recovered from bronchoalveolar lavage fluid. Pneu-

mocyte atypia (described previously) is characteristic but not specific for bleomycin toxicity. Fibroblast proliferation and fibrosis follow the acute injury and may be the dominant feature in slowly progressive disease. Bleomycin fibrosis may be nonuniform, focal, or nodular (Fig. 23–6).[135,136]

The reported incidence of bleomycin toxicity ranges from 2% to 40% in different series but in the largest series is less than 5%.[78,134] Factors that influence toxicity include dose, concommitant oxygen or drug therapy, and radiation therapy. At total doses of less than 400–500 units, there is a constant low incidence of toxicity. At more than 400–500 units, however, the incidence rises.[78] Patients who have received bleomycin may be at increased risk for respiratory distress if high oxygen concentrations are given later.[134] Bleomycin may be synergistic with other chemotherapeutic drugs, particularly cyclophosphamide, for lung injury.[52,78] Concommitant radiation therapy is associated with enhanced lung injury, and previous thoracic radiation may also be a risk factor.[134] The role of bleomycin in a possible "radiorecall" phenomenon was discussed previously (see p. 784).

Decreased diffusion capacity appears to be an early manifestation of bleomycin toxicity and may indicate that further therapy should be withheld.[78,134] Steroids have been used to treat bleomycin toxicity. In addition to cytotoxic injury, bleomycin may cause hypersensitivity pneumonitis and an acute chest pain syndrome.[137]

Busulfan, an alkylating agent, was the first cytotoxic drug to be identified as a cause of pulmonary injury.[138] The incidence of disease appears to be less than 4%, but there is a strong dose dependence.[78,79,139] Adverse reactions are rare at total doses of less than 500 mg/m^2 unless other cytotoxic agents or radiation therapy have been given. The interval between initiation of therapy and onset of symptoms is usually greater than 4 years, which is longer than for most other chemotherapeutic agents.[139]

The histologic findings in busulfan injury resemble those of bleomycin toxicity. Interstitial fibrosis is usually present, and the alveolar pneumocytes often appear enlarged with markedly hyperchromatic and atypical nuclei.[81,139] Organizing fibrinous exudates may also be present. Unusual pathologic alterations include pulmonary ossification and pulmonary alveolar proteinosis.[140,141]

Cyclophosphamide-induced pulmonary toxicity is rare when cyclophosphamide is used as a single agent but is more common in combination chemotherapy regimens.[139] There is no clear relationship to dose or delivery schedule. The pathologic changes are similar to those induced by bleomycin.[78,142] High-dose cyclophosphamide therapy seems to sensitize the lung to radiotherapy and increase the incidence of radiation fibrosis.[78,139]

BCNU (carmustine) causes lung injury more frequently than do other nitrosoureas. There is a well-established dose dependency.[78,143,144] The risk of pulmonary injury increases slowly up to a cumulative dose of approximately 1500 mg/m^2 and thereafter rises more steeply. The incidence of lung injury is approximately 50% at 1500 mg/m^2, and most cases are apparent within 4 years after therapy. Other risk factors include preexisting lung disease, abnormal lung function, and possibly concomitant cyclophosphamide therapy.[78,79,139]

A recently recognized consequence of BCNU therapy is the late development of pulmonary fibrosis.[145,146] O'Driscoll et al.[145] studied 11 survivors among patients who were treated with BCNU as children for brain tumors. All had clinical evidence of restrictive disease and all lung biopsy material (transbronchial biopsies) showed pulmonary fibrosis when assessed 13–17 years later. Ultrastructural studies demonstrated type I cell lucency, foci of bare epithelial basement membranes, and degenerative changes in endothelial cells.[146] Late BCNU fibrosis is distinctive in its late onset, apparent universality, and predilection for the apices and subpleural regions of the lungs. There is no obvious dose dependence. In some cases, CT scans and chest radiographs are normal despite clinical and functional evidence of pulmonary fibrosis.

Methotrexate causes cytotoxic injury, acute pleuritis, pulmonary edema, and hypersensitivity pneumonitis.[81,83,139] Pleuritis and pulmonary edema have been reported only with antineoplastic therapy.[83] Cytotoxic injury appears to be less common than hypersensitivity reactions. Biopsies from patients with cytotoxic injury reveal hyaline membranes and prominent, sometimes atypical, alveolar lining cells.[81,147,148] Interstitial fibrosis may also be present and may be progressive.[149,150] The prognosis for methotrexate pneumonitis is generally good but is probably not as favorable for patients with cytotoxic injury as it is for hypersensitivity reactions (see following).

Amiodarone causes diffuse alveolar damage in approximately one-third of patients with drug reactions.[151] It is thought that these changes are caused by a direct toxic effect of the drug in most cases.[152] In contrast to other cytotoxic agents, epithelial cell atypia is not prominent.

Nitrofurantoin causes several patterns of injury including diffuse alveolar damage.[153,154] There is experimental evidence of direct injury, probably mediated through the production of oxygen radicals.[82]

Cellular Inflammation

Cellular inflammatory reactions are probably the most common drug reactions observed in biopsy material. The category is broadly defined to include reactions with patterns labeled as lymphocytic interstitial pneumonitis, chronic interstitial pneumonia (some cases), hypersensitivity pneumonitis, nonspecific interstitial pneumonitis, and eosinophilic pneumonia, among other terms.[84–86] The unifying concept is that the morphologic features suggest activation of the immune system, particularly the cellular immune system, as the dominant pathologic process. All probably represent hypersensitivity reactions, although proof that hypersensitivity mechanisms are involved is not always available.

The list of drugs that cause cellular inflammatory reactions is long and evergrowing. It is probably true that any drug can cause such a reaction in some patient. An abbreviated list of the drugs most frequently linked to hypersensitivity reactions is given in Table 23–7. Drugs less frequently implicated have been listed by Wykoff.[155]

Mononuclear Cell and Granulomatous Reactions

Morphologically, cellular inflammatory reactions fall into two broad, somewhat overlapping categories: those in which lymphocytes, monocytes, and macrophages predominate, and those containing a significant infiltrate of eosinophils. The former comprise a spectrum that is similar to that of hypersensitivity reactions to inhaled antigens (extrinsic allergic alveolitis, EAA).[85,156,157] Both extrinsic and noneosinophilic drug-induced hypersensitivity reactions are characterized by a cellular alveolitis composed of lymphocytes

Table 23–7. Drugs frequently reported to cause cellular inflammatory infiltrates[a]

Antibiotics
  Erythromycin, isoniazid, nitrofurantoin, para-aminosalicylate,
    penicillins, sulfonamides, tetracycline
Antiepileptics
  Phenytoin, carbamazepine
Antiinflammatory and analgesic drugs
  Gold, ibuprofen, naproxen, sulindac
Cytotoxic agents
  Bleomycin, methotrexate, procarbazine
Psychotropic drugs
  Imipramine, methylphenidate
Other drugs
  Chlorpropamide, cromolyn sodium, hydralazine, mecamylamine,
    mephenesin, sulfasalazine

[a] Compiled from references 82, 85, 155, 158, and 159.

and other mononuclear cells. In many cases (80% for EAA), loose nonnecrotizing granulomas are present (Fig. 23–7). In contrast to sarcoidal granulomas, they are small, poorly cohesive, and centered in alveolar septa instead of along lymphatic routes. In contrast to infectious granulomas, they do not become large or acquire central necrosis. One difference between extrinsic and drug-induced reactions is that the former usually display cellular bronchiolitis whereas the latter do not. Either may lack granulomas and have the appearance of nonspecific interstitial pneumonitis. Interstitial fibrosis may develop in either case, usually after long exposure to the offending agent.

Characteristically, hypersensitivity has a subacute onset (hours to days) of dyspnea, nonproductive cough, fever, chills, myalgias, skin rash, and headache.[158] Peripheral blood eosinophilia is present in as many as 40% of patients. Chest radiographs often show diffuse acinar infiltrates; pleural effusions may also be present. Pulmonary function tests usually show mild restriction and decreased diffusion capacity. Treatment consists of steroids and withdrawal of the offending agent. The prognosis is excellent unless fibrosis has developed.

The diagnosis of a drug reaction is based on clinical correlation with histopathological features. Clinical and laboratory tests, such as skin tests, serum antibody determinations, and lymphocyte transformation assays, may be helpful in some circumstances but are not routinely used.[79] The pathogenesis of drug-induced hypersensitivity reactions is not clearly understood but there is evidence that endothelial cells, macrophages, neutrophils, and lymphocytes may all be important under some circumstances.[82,158]

Methotrexate is the drug most widely recognized to cause hypersensitivity reactions among the antineoplastic agents. The onset of symptoms tends to be more delayed and of more insidious onset than most hyper-

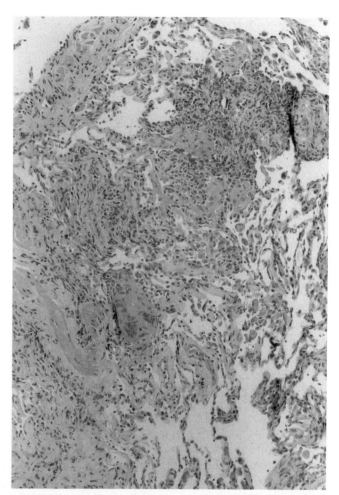

Fig. 23–7. Hypersensitivity pneumonitis caused by methotrexate. Patient was receiving 5 mg methotrexate thrice weekly for 2 years as treatment for mycosis fungoides. Transbronchial biopsy shows mononuclear cell infiltrate that involves alveolar septa. Note multinucleate giant cell. H and E, ×165.

sensitivity drug reactions.[79,83,139,148] Clinical symptoms are similar, however. Peripheral blood eosinophilia is present in half of patients. Radiographic infiltrates are usually interstitial or interstitial/alveolar in appearance. Tissue biopsies reveal a cellular infiltrate that is usually composed of mononuclear cells with occasional granulomas. Eosinophils may be present in some patients. In contrast to hypersensitivity reactions to most other drugs, some cases of methotrexate pneumonitis will resolve even if the patient continues to take the drug.

Eosinophilic Reactions

The presence of eosinophils in lung biopsy material is a relatively distinctive finding and is suggestive, but not pathognomonic, of a drug reaction.[85] Virtually all the drugs listed in Table 23–7 have been reported to cause pulmonary eosinophilia.[82,85,159] An even larger group of drugs causes peripheral blood eosinophilia in association with radiographic pulmonary infiltrates, the so-called pulmonary infiltrates with eosinophilia (PIE) syndrome.[155]

Two patterns of pulmonary eosinophilia may be seen histologically.[85,160] One is an eosinophilic pneumonia with exudative flooding of alveoli by an inflammatory infiltrate that is rich in eosinophils. The overall architecture is preserved, and eosinophils are also present in the interstitium and around airways. Patients with this pattern of involvement tend to have acute disease with fleeting and variable infiltrates on chest radiographs. Abnormalities respond quickly to drug withdrawal or corticosteroid therapy. The reaction is most often caused by antibiotics.

The other pattern is that of an interstitial pneumonitis with fewer eosinophils and with the cells in an interstitial location. Fibrosis is often present in a pattern of usual interstitial pneumonia. Clinically, this pattern is seen with more chronic disease and presumably reflects persistent low-grade injury. The prognosis and response to therapy are less salutary than with eosinophilic pneumonia. Agents such as nitrofurantoin and gold are most clearly associated with this histologic picture.

The differential diagnosis of pulmonary eosinophilia is essentially that of the "pulmonary infiltrates with eosinophilia" syndrome.[155,160] Allergic reactions to fungal airway colonization and helminthic infections are the other most common causes of PIE. Pulmonary eosinophilia may also be seen in the hypereosinophilia syndrome, angiitis and granulomatosis (Churg–Strauss syndrome, Wegener's granulomatosis, etc.), sarcoidosis, Hodgkin's disease, and unusual non-small cell carcinomas.

Eosinophils have phagocytic, antiinflammatory, and cytotoxic antihelminthic properties, but little is known about why they participate in some but not all pulmonary drug reactions. The cells have surface receptors for complement components, IgG, and IgE, and it may be that they are attracted and activated through these receptors.[160–162] Eosinophils can modulate type I (mast cell-mediated) hypersensitivity reactions, secrete mediators such as platelet-activating factor and arachidonic acid metabolites, and act as antigen-presenting cells under certain conditions.

Nitrofurantoin causes an acute hypersensitivity reaction more frequently than the cytotoxic effect discussed previously.[153,154,158] The incidence is probably less than 1% but adverse reactions are relatively common because the drug has been widely used. Patients present with dyspnea, fever, rashes, and pulmonary acinar infiltrates within 1 month of therapy. Peripheral blood eosinophilia is common. Lung biopsies show interstitial inflammation, usually with eosinophils; granulomas may be present. The prognosis is excellent if the drug is withdrawn.

Fewer patients experience chronic pneumonitis and fibrosis from nitrofurantoin. The onset tends to be later and is more insidious. Radiographs suggest pulmonary fibrosis, and indeed fibrosis is present in lung biopsy material. Eosinophils are often present. The prognosis is poorer and mortality may reach 10%.

Distinctive Parenchymal Reactions

Accumulation of Intraalveolar Macrophages

Intraalveolar macrophages accumulate in amiodarone toxicity but may also accumulate focally in rare reactions to methotrexate, mitomycin, cyclophosphamide, nitrofurantoin, and bleomycin.[85] *Amiodarone* is an oral antiarrythmic drug used as long-term therapy for patients with cardiac arrythmias.[79,163] Between 2% and 15% of patients develop pulmonary toxicity. Clinically, they develop dyspnea and dry cough and may have fevers and chills. The most characteristic finding in lung biopsy or autopsy material is a chronic mononuclear cell interstitial pneumonitis accompanied by accumulations of intraalveolar foamy macrophages[151] (Fig. 23–8). Endothelial cells and interstitial cells are also affected but are not conspicuous. The pattern may resemble desquamative interstitial pneumonitis. Ultrastructurally, the macrophages contain large numbers of membrane-bound inclusions filled with laminated stacks of phospholipid (Fig. 23–9). Characteristic cells can be recovered by bronchoalveolar lavage (BAL) and, in the right clinical context, BAL material can be diagnostic.[79,163]

Experimental and analytical work indicates that phospholipid accumulates in cells because of direct inhibition by amiodarone of phospholipid degradation in lysosomes.[152] Amiodarone has been shown to inhibit cellular phospholipases. Biochemical analysis of BAL fluid and macrophages from affected patients demonstrates an increase in all classes of phospholipids. Amiodarone is an amphiphilic molecule that is concentrated in lipid-rich tissues and may act by inserting into phospholipid membranes.

Foamy macrophages may be found in the lung tissue of patients taking amiodarone regardless of whether the patients have symptoms of amiodarone toxicity.[151] They are increased in patients with toxicity, however.[152] The effect is dose dependent in experimental animals[164] and probably in humans, although the slow elimination of the drug (45- to 60-day half-life) tends to mask differences of oral intake.[152,163] Patients taking

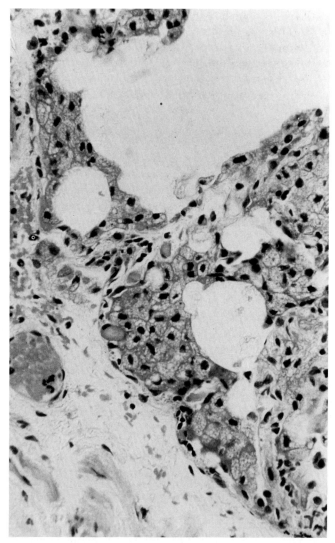

Fig. 23–8. Amiodarone pulmonary toxicity. Foamy macrophages and alveolar lining cells have accumulated in distal air spaces. Rare foamy interstitial cells are also apparent. H and E, ×400.

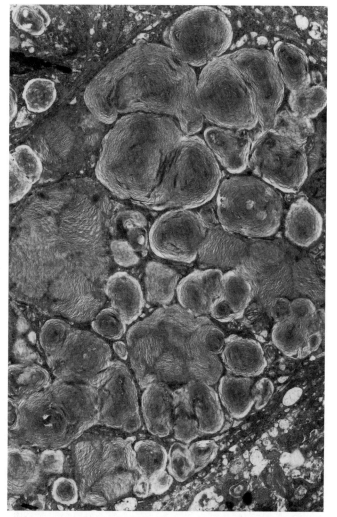

Fig. 23–9. Electron micrograph of amiodarone toxicity. Cytoplasm of macrophage contains lamellated lysosomal inclusions typical of phospholipidoses. ×10,000.

less than 400 mg/day seem to have a lower risk of toxicity.[82] Amiodarone toxicity is treated by discontinuation of the drug, and most patients recover.[82,84,163]

Other patterns of amiodarone toxicity include rare cases of cytotoxic injury, organizing pneumonia with or without bronchiolitis obliterans, and hypersensitivity reactions.[151,152,163]

Obliterative Bronchiolitis

Obliterative bronchiolitis (OB), sometimes called constrictive bronchiolitis, is an unusual process characterized by bronchial inflammation and circumferential intraluminal scarring leading to narrowing and ultimate obliteration of the airway. It has been reported to occur following penicillamine and gold salt therapy in patients with rheumatoid arthritis.[82,83] However, because OB has been reported in rheumatoid patients not treated with either drug, one must be cautious about attributing the reaction to the drug. Thirteen cases of OB have been associated with penicillamine and 2 with gold therapy.[83] The clinical symptoms and histopathological features are identical to those of OB patients without drug exposure.

Obliterative bronchiolitis is seen following lung transplantation, where it is considered to result from chronic rejection.[165] Rare bone marrow transplantation patients also develop OB[109] (Fig. 23–10). Symptoms generally begin with cough approximately 3–6 months after transplantation but progress to severe respiratory

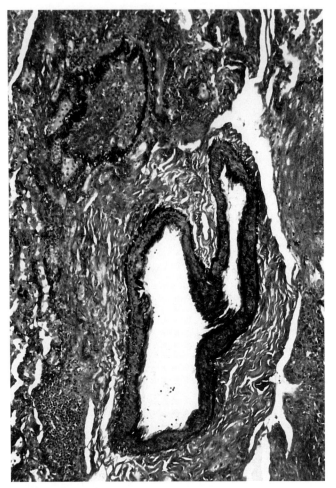

Fig. 23–10. Obliterative bronchiolitis (OB) following bone marrow transplantation. Note completely stenotic bronchiole adjacent to pulmonary artery. Verhoff van Gieson, ×125. (Case courtesy of Dr. H. Shulman.)

insufficiency and death. OB is associated with chronic graft-versus-host disease (GVHD) and is thought to represent an unusual form of GVHD.[166,167] Its recent description in two autologous bone marrow transplant patients suggests that it may have other causes as well.[168]

Bronchiolitis Obliterans with Organizing Pneumonia

Bronchiolitis obliterans with organizing pneumonia (BOOP) is now recognized to be histologically and clinically distinct from OB. It is a relatively common tissue reaction pattern characterized by luminal polypoid masses of granulation tissue that seem to emanate from respiratory bronchioles and extend into alveolar ducts and alveolar sacs (classic histologic bronchiolitis obliterans). Also present is effacement of alveolar air spaces by tufts of fibrous tissue (organizing pneumo-

nia). BOOP may be idiopathic or caused by infections, toxic gases, and other agents.[169] In addition, it is a common microscopic finding next to larger focal abnormalities such as granulomas or neoplasms. It has been reported with reactions to sulfasalazine,[82] amiodarone,[151] and numerous other drugs.[84]

Pulmonary Alveolar Proteinosis

Pulmonary alveolar proteinosis (PAP) occurs in some patients with hematologic malignancies, as well as those who are immunosuppressed or have occupational exposures to certain dusts. PAP has also been reported as a possible reaction to cytotoxic agents in rare patients with chronic myelogenous leukemia or lymphoma[86,170] but it is uncertain whether the observations reflect fortuitous coincidences or true drug reactions. PAP has also been reported in patients receiving chemotherapy for solid tumors.[85] In most of these cases it appears to be an incidental microscopic finding in patients who come to open lung biopsy or autopsy for other reasons. The radiographic appearance is different than for patients presenting with idiopathic or leukemia-associated disease. Symptoms seem to relate to their coexistent pathology rather than to PAP. Implicated drugs include cyclophosphamide, busulfan, and chlorambucil.

Vascular Disease

Drug-induced alterations of the pulmonary vasculature include pulmonary hypertension, vasculitis, and a pulmonary-renal syndrome. Pulmonary hypertension has been associated with aminorex and with alpha-adrenergic nasal sprays.[79,87] *Aminorex,* an appetite suppressant, is epidemiologically linked to a wave of cases of pulmonary hypertension, primarily in Europe. The clinical symptoms were similar to those of idiopathic pulmonary hypertension. The disease was progressive, and 10%–20% of affected patients died of their disease. The pathologic findings were indistinguishable from idiopathic plexiform pulmonary arteriopathy. The drug is no longer available for therapeutic use. Pulmonary hypertension is also a well-known complication of intravenous drug abuse.[127] In this setting, hypertension develops as a consequence of occlusive vascular damage from embolic drug and foreign material.

Pulmonary vasculitis is often listed as a potential complication of drug therapy, but the diagnosis is usually a presumptive one based on pulmonary infiltrates in a patient with a concurrent drug-related cutaneous vasculitis.[85,87] Cases of biopsy-proven pulmonary vasculitis are rare, perhaps because patients respond well to conservative management and biopsies are not obtained. The drugs most commonly linked to pulmonary vasculitis are hydralazine, phenylbutazone, propylthio-uracil, quinidine, promazines, and sulfa and hydantoin derivatives.[85] This list includes many that cause hypersensitivity reactions and drug-related lupus erythematosis.

Leukocytoclastic capillaritis occurs in drug reactions[85,171,172] but large vessel vasculitis is distinctly uncommon.[85] Patients tend to have relatively mild pulmonary symptoms and respond to drug withdrawal with or without corticosteroid therapy.

A syndrome of pulmonary hemorrhage and renal failure has been reported in 11 patients on penicillamine therapy for rheumatoid arthritis, Wilson's disease, or primary biliary cirrhosis.[79,83] Patients suffer acute onset of dyspnea, cough, hemoptysis, and hematuria. Chest radiographs reveal diffuse alveolar infiltrates. Hypoxemia often occurs and may require mechanical ventilatory support. Evidence of renal failure includes elevations in blood urea nitrogen (BUN) and creatinine along with hematuria and urinary red cell casts.

Lung biopsies disclose alveolar hemorrhage without vasculitis or significant inflammation. Renal biopsies reveal segmental necrotizing glomerulonephritis. Despite the resemblance to Goodpasture's syndrome, circulating antibasement membrane antibodies have been reported in only one case. Immunofluorescent studies for immune complex deposits have usually been negative on both lung and kidney. There are no obvious risk factors but patients tend to be on long-term therapy. Prognosis is variable; 4 of 11 patients have died but others have recovered with plasmapheresis and immunosuppressive therapy. The pathogenesis is unknown.

Complications of Drug Abuse

Abusers of drugs are theoretically susceptible to all the adverse drug reactions discussed previously. In practice, however, the usual adverse drug reactions are outnumbered by a special set of complications related to the route and method of administration of the abused substance and to the inherent toxicity of the drug. Intravenous (i.v.) drug abuse, especially of tablets intended for oral use, is associated with infectious and distinctive noninfectious complications. Drugs that are inhaled, such as cocaine and marijuana, also cause pulmonary injury.

Intravenous Drug Abuse

All i.v. drug abusers have an increased risk of infectious disease.[176,177] It is widely recognized that the risk of human immunodeficiency virus (HIV) infection is in-creased in i.v. drug users compared to nonabusers of similar socioeconomic class. The prevalence of HIV seropositivity has increased rapidly, and between 61,000 and 398,000 i.v. drug abusers in the United States were seropositive in 1989.[176] The prevalence of HIV positivity varies widely among cities and countries and between ethnic groups within single cities.[176] Factors that increase the risk of HIV infection (and which may account for the variable seropositivity rates among subsets of drug abusers) include sharing drug injection equipment, withdrawal of blood into the syringe to mix with the drug, and injections of cocaine with or without heroin.[176] Many HIV-positive drug users will develop the acquired immunodeficiency syndrome (AIDS), with all the attendant respiratory infections and complications.

The most common pulmonary infectious complication among i.v. drug abusers is community-acquired pneumonia.[176,177] The relative risk is increased 10 fold and is further increased if the patients are also HIV seropositive. The responsible organisms and their antibiotic sensitivities are similar to those of community-acquired pneumonias in general. Pulmonary tuberculosis is also more common in i.v. drug abusers, regardless of HIV infection. The pathologic spectrum of tuberculosis in HIV-negative drug abusers is similar to that of the general population, but the incidence of atypical presentations and disseminated disease is increased in drug abusers with AIDS.[177]

Septic pulmonary emboli and hematogenously acquired pneumonia are also common among i.v. drug abusers. The incidence is attributable to nonsterility of the drug and injection equipment as well as to the tendency among addicts not to sterilize the skin before injecting the drugs. The infectious organism is almost invariably *Staphylococcus aureus* or *Staphylococcus albus*.[176] The source of infection is usually in the skin at the injection site or endocarditis on the tricuspid valve.[176] Radiologically, patients may have either diffuse infiltrates or peripheral nodules; pleural effusions may also be present. Pathologically, a bacterial pneumonia is present that is often necrotizing and which may develop into a frank lung abscess. The diagnosis is certain if the embolus is identified and found to contain organisms and inflammation. In some cases, empyema, bronchopleural fistula, tension pneumothorax, or diffuse alveolar damage may develop.[176] If there is a pulmonary infarct, it may cavitate within days.[178] Mycotic aneurysms of pulmonary arteries or veins are a rare development.[176,179] Septicemia from *Candida albicans*, *Aspergillus* spp., or other organisms also occurs in i.v. drug abusers, even in the absence of thrombophlebitis or septic emboli.[176]

In addition to infection, i.v. drug abusers are at risk

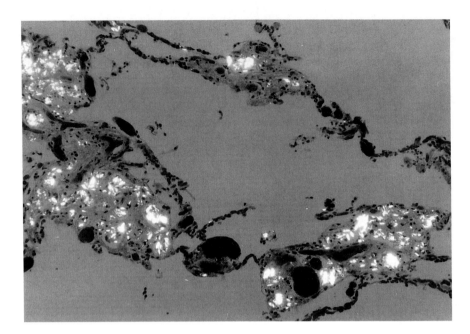

Fig. 23–11. Pulmonary talc granulomatosis from case of emphysema secondary to IV Ritalin abuse. Note brightly birefringent talc particles tend to cluster at confluence of alveolar septa. Multinucleate giant cells are relatively sparse in this case. Photographed using partially crossed polarizers. H and E, ×165. (Reprinted with permission from Schmidt et al. Am Rev Respir Dis 1991;143:649–656. With permission.)

for asthmatic reactions and wheezing immediately after drug injections.[180] Sudden death sometimes occurs and may be attributed to drug toxicity, drug overdose, reaction to the drug, or reaction to foreign material used to "cut" the drug.

Drug abusers who inject material intended for oral use are at risk for a unique set of pathology. Tablets and oral preparations commonly contain inert materials, such as talc, corn starch, microcrystalline cellulose, etc., that act to bind the tablet together and give it volume. The substances are poorly biodegradable and may elicit a foreign-body giant cell reaction. When i.v. drug abusers inject suspensions of tablets intended for oral use, this material embolizes to the lungs where it lodges because the particles are generally larger than the capillaries.

The simplest consequence is the formation of foreign-body granulomas ("talc granulomas").[127,181,182] These appear to form intravascularly and then migrate through the vessel wall so that they come to lie in both intravascular and extravascular compartments.[127] Associated vascular lesions resemble the findings in plexogenic pulmonary arteriopathy in some respects. They include angiothrombosis, "plexiform-like" lesions, arterial dilatation, and angiomatoid lesions.[127] Most tablet fillers and binders are brightly birefringent so that the foreign material can be visualized easily using crossed polarizers (Fig. 23–11). When the pulmonary burden of embolic material is large, chest radiographs may exhibit a fine reticulonodular pattern or may display millimeter-sized nodules.[177,180,182] It is not certain that "talc" granulomatosis in itself is clinically important, although

it has been associated with decrements of pulmonary diffusion capacity (D$_L$CO).[177,180,182]

In some patients, pulmonary hypertension develops as a result of vascular obstruction. Patients suffer from progressive dyspnea and may exhibit pulmonary artery enlargement on chest x-ray examinations. Inhaled talc may cause a pneumoconiosis-like disorder in some patients. A few patients with talc granulomatosis from i.v. drug use have been described who eventually developed fibrotic lesions resembling progressive massive fibrosis (PMF).[177,182,183] Fibrosis tends to occur in the mid- to upper lungs and is progressive with time. Histologically, birefringent foreign material is embedded in broad fibrous scars. The reported patients were not occupationally exposed to talc dust, and many of the recovered talc particles were larger than 5 μm in diameter, that is, larger than respirable dust particles.

Emphysema, with or without bullae, is another underrecognized manifestation of i.v. abuse of drugs intended for oral use. Obstructive lung disease is infrequent in cross-sectional studies of i.v. drug abusers, but a long-term follow-up study of i.v. methadone abusers with talc granulomatosis documented the emergence of obstructive lung disease.[184] All six patients in that report had bullae; four had PMF-like lesions and three had panacinar emphysema. Panacinar emphysema has also been noted in individual i.v. methadone abusers by others.[185,186] Sherman et al.[187] noted severe obstructive lung disease (probably emphysema) in a cohort of young IV Ritalin tablet abusers. Subsequent pathologic study of Ritalin abusers who died of their lung disease showed severe panacinar emphysema (Fig. 23–12) with

Fig. 23–12. Panacinar emphysema in an intravenous Ritalin (R) abuser. The lung slice is a transverse section taken through the lower lobe of an inflated, dried lung specimen. Scale is in cm. (Reprinted with permission from Schmidt et al, Am Rev Respir Dis 1991;143:649–656.)

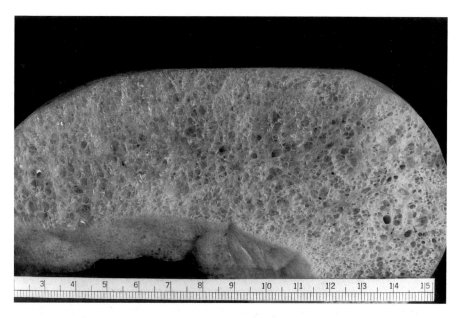

lower lobe predominance indistinguishable clinically from alpha-1-antitrypsin (AAT) deficiency.[126] Measured AAT levels were normal, however. In contrast to the reported i.v. methadone abusers,[184] the Ritalin abusers did not have significant fibrosis and had few bullae. Together these studies suggest that panacinar emphysema in i.v. drug abusers results from the filler in the tablets and not from the specific drug. The mechanism is uncertain but is probably related to localized protease–antiprotease imbalances around the innumerable granulomas.

Inhaled Drug Abuse

Two of the most commonly abused inhaled drugs are marijuana and cocaine. Marijuana has documented effects on the conducting airways.[177,188] Marijuana smokers experience an acute bronchodilation to which they become habituated. Chronic smokers develop symptoms of chronic bronchitis similar to those of cigarette smokers. Bronchial biopsies of habitual tobacco and marijuana smokers show similar changes of basal cell hyperplasia, goblet cell hyperplasia, cellular disorganization, and basement membrane thickening.[188] The changes are more frequent in marijuana smokers than in tobacco smokers despite differences in the amount of material smoked (3–4 joints compared to >20 cigarettes). This apparent difference in potencies may be because marijuana generates about twice as much tar per unit weight as does tobacco, marijuana joints are usually unfiltered whereas most cigarettes are filtered, and because marijuana smokers tend to inhale more deeply than tobacco smokers.[188] An increased risk of lung cancer has not yet been demonstrated for marijuana, possibly because marijuana smoking by a sizable segment of the population is a phenomenon sufficiently recent that the effect has not yet become obvious. Marijuana smoke is mutagenic and tumorogenic in in vitro and animal systems, however.[188]

Pathologic complications of cocaine abuse are determined by the form of the drug and the route of administration. Nasal insufflation ("snorting") of cocaine hydrochloride is associated with symptoms of chronic rhinitis and sinusitis as well as an acute chest pain syndrome.[189] Nasal septal necrosis may occur,[177,189] and there have even been reports of pulmonary granulomatosis from the talc and cellulose that contaminated the cocaine.[190] Acute chest pain occurs within hours of the dose and spontaneously remits; it is more common in those who smoke freebase ("crack") cocaine than in those who snort cocaine hydrochloride. The pathogenesis is not well understood but cardiac ischemia is probably not responsible in most patients.[189]

Pulmonary abnormalities are more common among crack smokers than other cocaine users.[189] Acute complications include pneumomediastinum and pneumothorax, pulmonary edema (apparently noncardiogenic), diffuse alveolar hemorrhage, bronchiolitis obliterans with organizing pneumonia, diffuse alveolar damage, asthma, pulmonary infiltrates with eosinophilia, and thermal burns of the conducting airways.* The true incidence of these complications is unknown because most reports have been of single patients or small groups of patients. The mechanisms of pulmo-

---

*References: 177,188,189,191–193.

nary injury remain to be determined; in a minority of cases there is evidence of immune-mediated lung injury.[193]

Crack cocaine smoking may cause chronic lung abnormalities. Although lung volumes and flows do not seem to be affected, pulmonary diffusing capacity (D_LCO) is reduced in freebase cocaine smokers.[191,192] Decreased D_LCO persists for weeks to months after the most recent drug use and is not explained by concurrent tobacco smoking or i.v. drug abuse.[192] It may result from injury to the alveolar-capillary membrane or to reduction in capillary blood volume from vascular injury. Susskind et al.[194] documented an increased clearance of radiolabeled diethylenetriamine pentaacetate (DTPA) from the lungs of habitual crack smokers, suggesting increased permeability of the alveolar-epithelial membrane.[194] Murray et al.[195] documented medial hypertrophy in small and medium pulmonary arteries in the lungs of 20% of drug abusers dying of acute cocaine intoxication.[195]

References

1. Davis DM, ed. Textbook of adverse drug reactions. 3d Ed. New York: Oxford University Press, 1985:1–38.

2. Turner WM, Milstein JB. Drug induced diseases. In: Pharmacotherapy: A pathophysiologic approach. 1st Ed. New York: Elsevier, 1989:60–67.

3. Gross NJ. Pulmonary effects of radiation therapy. Ann Intern Med 1977;86:81–92.

4. White DC. Lung. In: *An atlas of radiation histopathology.* Technical Information Center, Office of Public Affairs, U.S. Energy Research and Development Administration, 1975:106–125.

5. Gross NJ. The pathogenesis of radiation-induced lung damage. Lung 1981;159:115–125.

6. Groover TA, Christie AC, Merritt EA. Observations on the use of the copper filter in the roentgen treatment of deepseated malignancies. South Med J 1922;15:440–444.

7. Hines LE. Fibrosis of the lung following roentgen-ray treatments for tumor. JAMA 1922;79:720–722.

8. Tyler AF, Blackman JR. Effect of heavy radiation on the pleurae and lungs. J Radiol 1922;3:469–475.

9. Rubin P, Casarett GW. Clinical radiation pathology. Philadelphia: WB Saunders, 1968.

10. Evans WA, Leucutia T. Intrathoracic changes induced by heavy radiation. AJR 1925;13:206–220.

11. Desjardins AU. The reaction of the pleura and lungs to roentgen rays. AJR 1926;16:444–453.

12. Fajardo LF, Berthong M. Radiation injury in surgical pathology: Part I. Am J Surg Pathol 1978;2(2):159–199.

13. Schuh D, Kemmer C. Radiation pneumonitis. Morphology and pathogenesis. Zentralbl Allg Pathol Pathol Anat 1988;134(7):611–626.

14. Coggle JE, Lambert BE, Moores SR. Radiation effects in the lung. Environ Health Perspect 1986;70:261–291.

15. McDonald S, Rubin P, Maasilta P. Response of normal lung to irradiation: Tolerance doses/tolerance volumes in pulmonary radiation. In: Vaeth JM, Meyer JL, eds. Radiation tolerance of normal tissue. Front Radiat Ther Oncol 1989;23:255–276.

16. Rosiello RA, Merrill WW. Radiation-induced lung injury. Clin Chest Med 1990;11(1):65–71.

17. Lingos TI, Recht A, Vicini F, Abner A, Silver B, Harris JR. Radiation pneumonitis in breast cancer patients treated with conservative surgery and radiation therapy. Int J Radiat Oncol Biol Phys 1991;21(2):355–360.

18. Prince A, Jack WJ, Kerr GR, Rodger A. Acute radiation pneumonitis after postmastectomy irradiation: Effect of fraction size. Clin Oncol (R Coll Radiol) 1990;2(4):224–229.

19. Newman G, Bell J, Goddard P, Bullimore JA. Pulmonary changes in breast cancer patients treated by three different radiotherapy techniques. Clin Oncol (R Coll Radiol) 1989;1(2):91–96.

20. Weshler Z, Breuer R, Or R, et al. Interstitial pneumonitis after total body irradiation: Effect of partial lung shielding. Br J Haematol 1990;74(1):61–64.

21. Coscina WF, Arger PH, Mintz MC, Coleman BG. CT demonstration of pulmonary effects of tangential beam radiation. J Comput Assist Tomogr 1986;10(4):600–602.

22. Keane TJ, Van Dyk J, Rider WD. Idiopathic interstitial pneumonia following bone marrow transplantation: The relationship with total body irradiation. Int J Radiat Oncol Biol Phys 1981;7:1365–1370.

23. Siemann DW, Rubin P, Penney DP. Pulmonary toxicity following multifraction radiotherapy. Br J Cancer 1986;53(Suppl VII):365–367.

24. Minna JD, Pass H, Glatstein E, Ihde DC. Cancer of the lung. In: De Vita VT, Jr., Heldman S, Rosenberg SA, eds. *Cancer: Principles and practice of oncology.* 3d Ed. Philadelphia: JB Lippincott, 1989:591–705.

25. Rubin P, Shapiro DL, Finklestein JN, Penney DP. The early release of surfactant following lung irradiation of alveolar type II cells. Int J Radiat Oncol Biol Phys 1980;6:75–77.

26. Hallman M, Maasilta P, Kivisaari L, Mattson K. Changes in surfactant in bronchoalveolar lavage fluid after hemithorax irradiation in patients with mesothelioma. Am Rev Respir Dis 1990;141:998–1005.

27. Ward WF, Molteni A, Solliday SH, Jones GR. The relationship between endothelial dysfunction and collagen accumulation in irradiated rat lung. Int J Radiat Oncol Biol Phys 1985;11:1985–1990.

28. Gross NJ, Narine KR, Colletti-Squinto L. Replicative activity of lung type 2 cells following lung X-irradiation. Radiat Res 1987;111:143–150.

29. Ward WF, Solliday NH, Molteni A, Port CD. Radiation injury in rat lung. II. Angiotensin-converting enzyme activity. Radiat Res 1983;96:284–293.

30. T'sao CH, Ward WF, Port CD. Radiation injury in rat lung. III. Plasminogen activator and fibrinolytic inhibitor activities. Radiat Res 1983;96:294–300.

31. Ward WF, Molteni A, T'sao C, Solliday NH. Pulmonary

endothelial dysfunction induced by unilateral as compared to bilateral thoracic irradiation in rats. Radiat Res 1987;111:101–106.

32. Van Dyk J, Keane TJ, Kan S, Rider WD, Fryer CJH. Radiation pneumonitis following large single dose irradiation: A re-evaluation based on absolute dose to the lung. Int J Radiat Oncol Biol Phys 1981;7:461–467.

33. Stover DE. Pulmonary toxicity. In: De Vita VT, Jr., Heldman S, Rosenberg SA, eds. Cancer: Principles and practice of oncology. 3d Ed. Philadelphia: JB Lippincott, 1989:591–705.

34. Gross NJ. The pathogenesis of radiation-induced lung damage. Lung 1981;159:115–125.

35. Bell J, McGivern D, Bullimore J, Hill J, Davies ER, Goddard P. Diagnostic imaging of post-irradiation changes in the chest. Clin Radiol 1988;39(2):109–119.

36. Ikezoe J, Morimoto S, Takashima S, Takeuchi N, Arisawa J, Kozuka T. Acute radiation-induced pulmonary injury: Computed tomography evaluation. Semin Ultrasound CT MR 1990;11(5):409–416.

37. Lichtenstein H. X-ray diagnosis of radiation injuries of the lung. Dis Chest 1960;38:294–297.

38. Pezner RD, Horak DA, Sayegh HO, Lipsett JA. Spontaneous pneumothorax in patients irradiated for Hodgkin's disease and other malignant lymphomas. Int J Radiat Oncol Biol Phys 1990;18(1):193–198.

39. Cameron SJ, Grant IWB, Lutz W, et al. The early effect of irradiation on ventilatory function in bronchial carcinoma. Clin Radiol 1969;20:12–18.

40. Libshitz HI, Southard ME. Complications of radiation therapy: The thorax. Semin Roentgenol 1974;9:41–49.

41. Bennett DE, Million RR, Ackerman LV. Bilateral radiation pneumonitis, a complication of the radiotherapy of bronchogenic carcinoma. Cancer (Philadelphia) 1969; 23:1001–1018.

42. Gibson PG, Bryant DH, Morgan GW, et al. Radiation-induced lung injury: A hypersensitivity pneumonitis? Ann Intern Med 1988;109(4):288–291.

43. Wechsler RJ, Ayyangar K, Steiner RM, Yelovich R, Moylan DM. The development of distant pulmonary infiltrates following thoracic irradiation: The role of computed tomography with dosimetric reconstruction in diagnosis. Comput Med Imaging Graph 1990; 14(1):43–51.

44. Sherman ML, Datta R, Hallahan DE, Weichselbaum RR, Kufe DW. Regulation of tumor necrosis factor gene expression by ionizing radiation in human myeloid leukemia cells and peripheral blood monocytes. J Clin Invest 1991;87:1794–1797.

45. Fulkerson WJ, Mclendon RE, Prosnitz LR. Adult respiratory distress syndrome after limited thoracic radiotherapy. Cancer (Philadelphia) 1986;57:1941–1946.

46. Byhardt RW, Abrams R, Almagro U. The association of adult respiratory distress syndrome (ARDS) with thoracic irradiation (RT). Int J Radiat Oncol Biol Phys 1988;15:1441–1446.

47. Hendry JH. Response of human organs to single (or fractionated equivalent) doses of irradiation. Int J Radiat Biol 1989;56(5):671–700.

48. Hellman S. Principles of radiation therapy. In: De Vita VT, Jr., Heldman S, Rosenberg SA, eds. Cancer: Principles and practice of oncology. 3d Ed. Philadelphia: JB Lippincott, 1989:247–275.

49. Fornace AJ, Jr., Nebert DW, Hollander MC, et al. Mammalian genes coordinately regulated by growth arrest signals and DNA-damaging agents. Mol Cell Biol 1989;9(10):4196–4203.

50. Weichselbaum RR, Hallahan DE, Sukhatme V, Dritschilo A, Sherman ML, Kufe DW. Biological consequences of gene regulation after ionizing radiation exposure. J Natl Cancer Inst 1991;83(7):480–488.

51. Eldor A, Vlodavsky I, Fuks Z, Matzner Y, Rubin DB. Arachidonic metabolism and radiation toxicity in cultures of vascular endothelial cells. Prostaglandins Leukot Essent Fatty Acids 1989;36(4):251–258.

52. Cooper JAD, Jr., White DA, Matthay RA. Drug-induced pulmonary disease: Part 1:Cytotoxic drugs. Am Rev Respir Dis 1986;133:321–340.

53. Glaholm J, Repetto L, Yarnold JR, et al. Carboplatin (JM8), etoposide (VP16) and thoracic irradiation for small cell lung cancer (S.C.L.C.): An evaluation of lung toxicity. Radiother Oncol 1988;12(1):31–7.

54. Roggli VL, Kolbeck J, Sanfilippo F, Shelburne JD. Pathology of human mesothelioma: Etiologic and diagnostic considerations. Pathol Annu 1987;22(Pt. 2):91–132.

55. Samuels ML, Johnson DE, Holoye PY, Lanzotti VJ. Large-dose bleomycin therapy and pulmonary toxicity. A possible role of prior radiotherapy. JAMA 1976; 235:1117–1120.

56. Warren S, Spencer J. Radiation reaction in the lung. AJR 1940;43:682–701.

57. Pezner RD, Bertrand M, Cecchi GR, Paladugu RR, Kendregan BA. Steroid-withdrawal radiation pneumonitis in cancer patients. Chest 1984;85(6):816–817.

58. Castellino RA, Glatstein E, Turbow MM, et al. Latent radiation injury of lungs or heart activated by steroid withdrawal. Ann Intern Med 1974;80:593–599.

59. Fryer CJH, Fitzpatrick PJ, Rider WD, Poon P. Radiation pneumonitis: Experience following a large single dose of radiation. Int J Radiat Oncol Biol Phys 1978;4:931–936.

60. Smith PG, Doll R. Mortality from cancer and all causes among British radiologists. Br J Radiol 1981;54:187–194.

61. Sources and effects of ionizing radiation. United Nations Scientific Committee on the Effects of Atomic Radiation 1977 Report to the General Assembly, with annexes. United Nations, New York, 1977. [Official Records of the General Assembly, 32d Session, Suppl. No. 40 (A/32/40).]

62. Boice JD, Jr. Carcinogenesis—a synopsis of human experience with external exposure in medicine. Health Phys 1988;55(4):621–630.

63. Davis FG, Boice JD, Kelsey JL, Monson RR. Cancer mortality after multiple fluoroscopic examinations of the chest. J Natl Cancer Inst 1987;78(4):645–652.

64. Smith PG, Doll R. Mortality among patients with ankylosing spondylitis after a single treatment course with X-rays. Br Med J 1982;284:449–460.

65. Klastersky J, Leleux A. Secondary neoplasms following cancer treatment with a special emphasis on lung tumors. Neoplasma 1991;38(3):253–256.

66. Travis LB, Curtis RE, Boice JD, Hankey BF, Fraumeni JF. Second cancers following non-Hodgkin's lymphoma. Cancer (Philadelphia) 1991;67:2002–2009.

67. Van Leeuwen FE, Somers R, Tall BG, et al. Increased risk of lung cancer, non-Hodgkin's lymphoma, and leukemia following Hodgkin's disease. J Clin Oncol 1989;7(8):1046–1058.

68. Lerman Y, Learman Y, Schacter P, Herceg E, Lieberman Y, Yellin A. Radiation-associated malignant pleural mesothelioma. Thorax 1991;46:463–464.

69. Okazaki A, Matsuura M, Noda M, et al. Esophageal cancer developing 13 years after radiotherapy of lung cancer. Gann No Rinsho 1988;34(6):787–793.

70. Louis S, Cross CE, Amott TR, Cardiff R. Postirradiation malignant fibrous histiocytoma of the trachea. Am Rev Respir Dis 1987;135(3):761–762.

71. Shah IA, Kurtz SM, Simonsen RL. Radiation induced malignant fibrous hitiocytoma of the pulmonary artery. Arch Pathol Lab Med 1991;115(9):921–925.

72. Einhorn L, Krause M, Hornback N, Furnas B. Enhanced pulmonary toxicity with bleomycin and radiotherapy in oat cell cancer. Cancer (Philadelphia) 1976;37:2414–2416.

73. Soble AR, Perry H. Fatal radiation pneumonia following subclinical busulfun injury. AJR 1977;128:15–18.

74. Buzdar AU, Legha SS, Luna MA, Tashima CK, Hortobagyi GN, Glumenschein GR. Pulmonary toxicity of mitomycin. Cancer (Philadelphia) 1980;45:236–244.

75. Orwoll ES, Kiessling P, Patterson R, et al. Interstitial pneumonia from mitomycin. Ann Intern Med 1978;89:352–355.

76. Rosenow EC, III. Drug-induced bronchopulmonary pleural disease. J Allergy Clin Immunol 1987;80:780–787.

77. DeSwarte RD. Drug allergy: An overview. Clin Rev Allergy 1986;4:143–169.

78. Ginsberg SJ, Comis RL. The pulmonary toxicity of antineoplastic agents. Semin Oncol 1982;9:34–51.

79. Israel-Biet D, Labrune S, Huchon GJ. Drug-induced lung disease: 1990 review. Eur Respir J 1991;4:465–478.

80. Demeter SL, Ahmad M, Tomashefski JF. Drug-induced pulmonary disease: Part 2. Categories of drugs. Clevel Clin Q 1979;46(3):101–112.

81. Demeter SL, Ahmad M, Tomashefski JF. Drug-induced pulmonary disease: Part 3. Agents used to treat neoplasms or alter the immune system including a brief review of radiation therapy. Clevel Clin Q 1979; 46(3):113–124.

82. Cooper JAD, Jr., White DA, Matthay RA. Drug-induced pulmonary disease: Part 2. Noncytotoxic drugs. Am Rev Respir Dis 1986;133:488–505.

83. Zitnik RJ, Cooper JAD, Jr. Pulmonary disease due to antirheumatic agents. Clin Chest Med 1990;11:139–150.

84. Myers JL. Pathology of drug-induced lung disease. In: Katzenstein ALA, Askin FB, eds. Surgical pathology of non-neoplastic lung disease. 2d Ed. Philadelphia: WB Saunders, 1990;13:97–127.

85. Smith GJW. The histopathology of pulmonary reactions to drugs. Clin Chest Med 1990;11:95–117.

86. Bedrossian CWM. Pathology of drug-induced lung diseases. Semin Respir Med 1982;4(2):98–105.

87. Demeter SL, Ahmad M, Tomashefski JF. Drug-induced pulmonary disease: Part 1. Patterns of response. Clevel Clin Q 1979;46(3):89–99.

88. Meeker DP, Wiedemann HP. Drug-induced bronchospasm. Clin Chest Med 1990;11:163–175.

89. Samter M, Beers RF, Jr. Concerning the nature of intolerance to aspirin. J Allergy 1967;40:281–293.

90. Zeitz HJ. Bronchial asthma, nasal polyps, and aspirin sensitivity: Samter's syndrome. Clin Chest Med 1988;9:567–576.

91. Slepian IK, Mathews KP, McLean JA. Aspirin-sensitive asthma. Chest 1985;87:386–391.

92. Spector SL, Wangarrd CH, Farr RS. Aspirin and concomitant idiosyncrasies in adult asthmatic patients. J Allergy Clin Immunol 1979;64:500–506.

93. Szceklik A, Nizankowska E, Czerniawska-Mysik G, Sek S. Hydrocortisone and airflow impairment in aspirin-induced asthma. J Allergy Clin Immunol 1985;76:530–536.

94. Decalmer PBS, Chatterjee SS, Cruickshank JM, et al. Beta-blockers and asthma. Br Heart J 1978;40:184–189.

95. Gulekas D, Georgopoulos D, Papakosta D, et al. Influence of pindolol on asthmatic and effect of bronchodilators. Respiration 1986;50:158–166.

96. Mattson K, Poppius II. Controlled study of the bronchoconstriction effect of pindolol administered intravenously or orally to patients with unstable asthma. Eur J Clin Pharmacol 1978;14:87–92.

97. Grieco MH, Pierson RN, Jr. Mechanisms of bronchoconstriction due to beta-adrenergic blockage. J Allergy Clin Immunol 1971;48:143–152.

98. Frishman W, Jacob H, Eisenberg E, Ribner H. Clinical pharmacology of the new beta-adrenergic blocking drugs. Part 8. Self-poisoning with beta-adrenoceptor blocking agents: Recognition and management. Am Heart J 1979;98:798–811.

99. Beemer GH, Dennis WL, Platt PR, et al. Adverse reactions to atracurium and alcuronium. Br J Anaesth 1988;61:680–684.

100. Bertrand P, Rouleau P, Alison D, Chastin I. Use of peak expiratory flow rate to identify patients with increased risk of contrast medium reaction. Results of preliminary study. Invest Radiol 1988;23:S203–S205.

101. Dawson P, Pitfield J, Britton J. Contrast media and bronchospasm: A study with iopamidol. Clin Radiol 1983;34:227–230.

102. Littner MR, Ulreich S, Putman CE, et al. Bronchospasm during excretory urography. Lack of specificity for the methylglucamine cation. AJR 1981;137:477–481.

103. Yarbrough J, Mansfield LE, Ting S. Metered dose inhaler-induced bronchospasm in asthmatic patients. Ann Allergy 1985;55:25–27.

104. Koepke JW, Selner JC, Dunhill AL. Presence of sulfur

dioxide in commonly used bronchodilator solutions. J Allergy Clin Immunol 1983;72:504–508.

105. Koepke JW, Christopher KL, Chai H, Selner JC. Dose-dependent bronchospasm from sulfites in isoetharine. JAMA 1984;251:2982–2983.

106. Trautlein J, Allegra J, Field J, Gillin M. Paradoxic bronchospasm after inhalation of isoproterenol. Chest 1976;70:711–714.

107. Cocchetto DM, Sykes RS, Spector S. Paradoxical bronchospasm after use of inhalation aerosols: A review of the literature. J Asthma 1991;28:49–53.

108. Montgomery AB, Debs RJ, Luce JM, et al. Aerosolised pentamide as sole therapy for *Pneumocystis carinii* pneumonia in patients with acquired immunodeficiency syndrome. Lancet 1987;ii:480–483.

109. Alston TA. Inhibition of cholinesterases by pentamide [letter]. Lancet 1988;ii:1423.

110. Paton WD. Aerosolised pentamidine [letter]. Lancet 1987;ii:1146.

111. Ligresti DJ. Anaphylaxis. Clin Dermatol 1986;4:40–49.

112. James LP, Jr., Austin KF. Fatal systemic anaphylaxis in man. N Engl J Med 1964;270:597–603.

113. Shkutin AE, Naresheva KA, Donchenko VS. Morphology and pathogenesis of changes in the lungs during drug-induced anaphylactic shock in humans. Arkh Patol 1989;51:48–54.

114. Rosenow EC. Drug-induced pulmonary disease. Clin Notes Respir Dis 1977;16(1):3–11.

115. Ginsburg WW. Drug-induced systemic lupus erythematosus. Semin Respir Med 1980;2:51–58.

116. Solinger AM. Drug-related lupus. Clinical and etiologic considerations. Rheum Dis Clin North Am 1988;14:187–202.

117. Hess EV. Drug-related lupus: The same or different? In: Lahita RG, ed. Systemic lupus erythematosus. New York: Wiley, 1987:869–880.

118. Jain KK. Systemic lupus erythematosus (SLE)-like syndromes associated with carbamazepine therapy. Drug Safety 1991;6(5):350–360.

119. Haas C, Hugues FC, Le-Jeunne C. Drug-induced pleural pathology (excluding antineoplastic chemotherapy). Ann Med Interne 1989;140(7):589–592.

120. Hindle W, Posner E, Sweetnam MT, Tan RSH. Pleural effusion and fibrosis during treatment with methysergide. Br Med J 1970;1:605–606.

121. Reid J, Watson RD, Sproull DH. The mode of action of salicylate in acute rheumatic fever. Q J Med 1950;19:261–268.

122. Hormaechae E, Carlson RW, Rogove H, Uphold J, Henning RJ, Weil MH. Hypovolemia, pulmonary edema and protein changes in severe salicylate poisoning. Am J Med 1979;66:1046–1050.

123. Osler W. Oedema of the lung complicating morphia poisoning. Montreal Gen Hosp Rep 1880;1:291–293.

124. Steinberg AD, Karliner JS. The clinical spectrum of heroin pulmonary edema. Arch Intern Med 1968;122:122–127.

125. Smith WR, Wells ID, Glauser FL, Novey HS. Immuno-

logic abnormalities in heroin lung. Chest 1975;68:651–653.

126. Schmidt RA, Glenny RW, Godwin JD, Hampson NB, Cantino ME, Reichenbach DD. Panlobular emphysema in young intravenous Ritalin abusers. Am Rev Respir Dis 1991;143:649–656.

127. Tomashefski JF, Hirsch CS. The pulmonary vascular lesions of intravenous drug abuse. Hum Pathol 1980;11:133–145.

128. Flacke JW, Flacke WE, Williams GD. Acute pulmonary edema following naloxone reversal of high-dose morphine anesthesia. Anesthesiology 1977;47:376–378.

129. Glauser FL, Smith WR, Caldwell A, et al. Etchlorvynol (Placidyl)-induced pulmonary edema. Ann Intern Med 1976;84:46–48.

130. Margolin KA, Rayner AA, Hawkins MJ, et al. Interleukin-2 and lymphokine-activated killer cell therapy of solid tumors: Analysis of toxicity and management guidelines. J Clin Oncol 1989;7:486–498.

131. Saxon RR, Klein JS, Bar MH, et al. Pathogenesis of pulmonary edema during interleukin-2 therapy: Correlation of chest radiographic and clinical findings in 54 patients. AJR 1991;156(2):281–286.

132. Thompson JA, Shulman KL, Benyunes MC, et al. Prolonged continuous intravenous infusion interkeukin-2 and lymphokine-activated killer cell therapy for metastatic renal cell carcinoma. J Clin Oncol 1992;10:960–968.

133. Cantor JO. Bleomycin-induced pulmonary fibrosis: In: Cantor JO, ed. CRC handbook of animal models of pulmonary disease. Vol. I. Boca Raton: CRC Press, 1989:117–130.

134. Jules-Elysee K, White DA. Bleomycin-induced pulmonary toxicity. Clin Chest Med 1990;11:1–20.

135. Santrach PJ, Askin FB, Wells RJ, Azizkhan RG, Merten DF. Nodular form of bleomycin-related pulmonary injury in patients with osteogenic sarcoma. Cancer (Philadelphia) 1989;64:806–811.

136. Cohen MB, Austin JHM, Smith-Vaniz A, Lutzky J, Grimes MM. Nodular bleomycin toxicity. Am J Clin Pathol 1989;92:101–104.

137. White DA, Schwartzberg LS, Kris MG, Bosl GJ. Acute chest pain syndrome during bleomycin infusions. Cancer (Philadelphia) 1987;59:1582–1585.

138. Oliner H, Schwartz R, Rubio F, Dameshek W. Interstitial pulmonary fibrosis following busulfan therapy. Am J Med 1961;31:134–139.

139. Twohig KJ, Matthay RA. Pulmonary effects of cytotoxic agents other than bleomycin. Clin Chest Med 1990;11:31–54.

140. Kuplic JB, Higley CS, Niewoehner DE. Pulmonary ossification associated with long-term busulfan therapy in chronic myeloid leukemia. Am Rev Respir Dis 1972;106:759–762.

141. Aymard JP, Gyger M, Lavallee R, et al. A case of pulmonary alveolar proteinosis complicating chronic myelogenous leukemia. A peculiar pathologic aspect of busulfan lung? Cancer (Philadelphia) 1984;53:954–956.

142. Gould VE, Miller J. Sclerosing alveolitis induced by

cyclophosphamide. Am J Pathol 1975;81:513–520.

143. Aronin PA, Mahaley MS, Rudnick SA, et al. Prediction of BCNU pulmonary toxicity in patients with malignant gliomas. An assessment of risk factor. N Engl J Med 1980;303:183–191.

144. Smith AC. The pulmonary toxicity of nitrosoureas. Pharmacol Ther 1989;44:443–460.

145. O'Driscoll BR, Hasleton PS, Taylor PM, Poulter LW, Gattamaneni HR, Woodcock AA. Active lung fibrosis up to 17 years after chemotherapy with carmustine (BCNU) in childhood. N Engl J Med 1990;323:378–382.

146. Hasleton PS, O'Driscoll BR, Lynch P, et al. Late BCNU lung: A light and ultrastructural study on the delayed effect of BCNU on the lung parenchyma. J Pathol 1991;164:31–36.

147. Bedrossian CWM, Miller WC, Luna MA. Methotrexate-induced diffuse intersitial pulmonary fibrosis. South Med J 1979;72:313–318.

148. Sostman HD, Matthay RA, Putman CE, Walker-Smith GJ. Methotrexate-induced pneumonitis. Medicine (Baltimore) 1976;55:371–388.

149. Kaplan RL, Waite DH. Progressive interstitial lung disease from prolonged methotrexate therapy. Arch Dermatol 1978;114:1800–1802.

150. Phillips TJ, Jones DH, Baker H. Pulmonary complications following methotrexate therapy. J Am Acad Dermatol 1987;16(2 Pt. 1):373–375.

151. Myers JL, Kennedy JI, Plumb VJ. Amiodarone lung: Pathologic findings in clinically toxic patients. Hum Pathol 1987;18:349–354.

152. Martin WJ, II. Mechanisms of amiodarone pulmonary toxicity. Clin Chest Med 1990;11:131–138.

153. Holmberg L, Boman G. Pulmonary reactions to nitrofurantoin. Eur J Respir Dis 1981;62:180–189.

154. Sovijärvi ARA, Lemola M, Stenius B, Idänpään-Heikkilä J. Nitrofurantoid-induced acute, subacute and chronic pulmonary reactions. Scand J Respir Dis 1977;58:41–50.

155. Wykoff RF. Eosinophilia. South Med J 1986;79(5):608–612.

156. Kawanami O, Basset F, Barrios R, Lacronique JG, Ferrans VJ, Crystal RG. Hypersensitivity pneumonitis in man: Light and electron-microscopic studies of 18 lung biopsies. Am J Pathol 1983;110:275–289.

157. Coleman A, Colby TV. Histologic diagnosis of extrinsic allergic alveolitis. Am J Surg Pathol 1988;2:514–518.

158. Cooper JA, Jr., Matthay RA. Drug-induced pulmonary disease. Dis Mon 1987;33(2):61–120.

159. Goodwin SD, Glenny RW. Nonsteroidal antiinflammatory drug-associated pulmonary infiltratres with eosinophilia: Review of the literature and FDA adverse drug reaction reports. Arch Intern Med 1992;152:1521–1524.

160. Geddes DM. Pulmonary eosinophilia. J R Coll Physicians Lond 1986;20(2):139–145.

161. Kay AB. Biological properties of eosinophils. Clin Exp Allergy 1991;21(Suppl. 3):23–29.

162. Weller PF. The immunobiology of eosinophils. N Engl J Med 1991;324:1110–1118.

163. Kennedy JI, Jr. Clinical aspects of amiodarone pulmo-nary toxicity. Clin Chest Med 1990;11:119–129.

164. Wilson BD, Clarkson CE, Lippman ML. Amiodarone-induced pulmonary inflammation: Correlation with drug dose and lung levels of drug, metabolite and phospholipid. Am Rev Respir Dis 1981;143:1110–1114.

165. Yousem SA, Berry GJ, Chamberlain D, et al. A working formulation for the standardization of nomenclature in the diagnosis of heart and lung rejection: Lung rejection study group. J Heart Lung Transplant 1990;9:593–601.

166. Holland HK, Wingard JR, Beschorner WE, Saral R, Santos GW. Bronchiolitis obliterans in bone marrow transplantation and its relationship to chronic graft-v-host disease and low serum IgG. Blood 1988;72:621–627.

167. Epler GR. Bronchiolis obliterans and airways obstruction associated with graft-versus-host disease. Clin Chest Med 1988;9:551–556.

168. Paz HL, Crilley P, Patchefsky A, Schiffman RL, Brodsky I. Bronchiolitis obliterans after autologous bone marrow transplantation. Chest 1992;101:775–778.

169. Epler GR, Colby TV, McLoud TC, Carrington CB, Gaensler EA. Bronchiolitis obliterans organizing pneu-monia. N Engl J Med 1985;312:152–158.

170. Aymard J-P, Gyger M, Lavallee R, Legresley L-P, Desy M. A case of pulmonary alveolar proteinosis complicat-ing chronic myelogenous leukemia: A peculiar manifes-tation of busulfan lung? Cancer (Philadelphia) 1984;53:954–956.

171. Myers JL, Katzenstein AA. Wegener's granulomatosis presenting with massive pulmonary hemorrhage and capillaritis. Am J Surg Pathol 1987;11:895–898.

172. Colby TV. Diffuse pulmonary hemorrhage in Wegen-er's granulomatosis. Semin Respir Med 1989;10:136–140.

173. Johnson MP, Goodwin SD, Shands JW, Jr. Tri-methoprim-sulfamethoxazole anaphylactoid reactions in patients with AIDS: Case reports and literature re-view. Pharmacotherapy 1990;10:413–416.

174. Ahmad S. Lovastatin-induced lupus erythematosus. Arch Intern Med 1991;151(8):1667–1668.

175. Miller DH, Haas LF. Pneumonitis, pleural effusion and pericarditis following treatment with dantrolene. J Neu-rol Neurosurg Psychiatry 1984;47(5):553–554.

176. Hind CRK. Pulmonary complications of intravenous drug misuse—2: Infective and HIV related complica-tions. Thorax 1990;45:957–961.

177. Heffner JE, Harley RA, Schabel SI. Pulmonary reac-tions from illicit substance abuse. Clinics Chest Med 1990;11(1):151–162.

178. Libby LS, King TE, LaForce FM, Schwartz MI. Pulmo-nary cavitation following pulmonary infarction. Medi-cine (Baltimore) 1985;64(5):342–348.

179. Navarro C, Dickinson PCT, Kondlapoodi P, Hagstrom JWC. Mycotic aneurysms of the pulmonary arteries in intravenous drug addicts: Report of three cases and review of the literature. Am J Med 1984;76:1124–1131.

180. Hind CRK. Pulmonary complications of intravenous drug misuse—1: Epidemiology and non-infective com-plications. Thorax 1990;45:891–898.

181. Hopkins GB. Pulmonary angiothrombotic granulomatosis in drug offenders. JAMA 1972;221(8):909–911.

182. Paré JAP, Fraser RG, Hogg JC, Howlett JG, Murphy SB. Pulmonary 'mainline' granulomatosis: Talcosis of intravenous methadone abuse. Medicine (Baltimore) 1979; 58(3):229–239.

183. Crouch E, Churg A. Progressive massive fibrosis of the lung secondary to intravenous injection of talc. A pathologic and mineralogic analysis. Am J Clin Pathol 1983;80:520–526.

184. Paré JP, Cote G, Fraser RS. Long-term follow-up of drug abusers with intravenous talcosis. Am Rev Respir Dis 1989;139:233–241.

185. Groth DH, Mackay GR, Crable JV, Cochran TH. Intravenous injection of talc in a narcotics addict. Arch Pathol 1972;94:171–178.

186. Vevaina JR, Civantos F, Viamonte M, Jr., Avery WG. Emphysema associated with talcum granulomatosis in a drug addict. South Med J 1974;67:113–116.

187. Sherman CB, Hudson LD, Pierson DJ. Severe precocious emphysema in intravenous methylphenidate (Ritalin) abusers. Chest 1987;92:1085–1087.

188. Tashkin DP. Pumonary complications of smoked substance abuse. West J Med 1990;152:525–530.

189. Brody SL, Slovis CM, Wrenn KD. Cocaine-related medical problems: Consecutive series of 233 patients. Am J Med 1990;88:325–331.

190. Oubeid M, Bickel JT, Ingram EA, Scott GC. Pulmonary talc granulomatosis in a cocaine sniffer. Chest 1990; 98:237–239.

191. Ettinger NA, Albin RJ. A review of the respiratory effects of smoking cocaine. Am J Med 1989;87:664–668.

192. Tashkin DP, Khalsa M-E, Gorelick D, et al. Pulmonary status of habitual cocaine smokers. Am Rev Respir Dis 1992;145:92–100.

193. Forrester JM, Steele AW, Waldron JA, Parsons PE. Crack lung: An acute pulmonary syndrome with a spectrum of clinical and histopathologic findings. Am Rev Respir Dis 1990;142:462–467.

194. Susskind H, Weber DA, Volkow ND, Hitzemann R. Increased lung permeability following long-term use of free-base cocaine (crack). Chest 1991;100:903–909.

195. Murray RJ, Smialek JE, Golle M, Albin RJ. Pulmonary artery medial hypertrophy in cocaine users without foreign particle microembolization. Chest 1989; 96:1050–1053.

CHAPTER 24

Transplantation Pathology

DEAN W. CHAMBERLAIN

Serious consideration of lung transplantation as a treatment option for various forms of advanced pulmonary disease began with the first human lung transplant which was performed by Dr. James Hardy in 1963.[1] However, there was little subsequent clinical success in this area until cyclosporin became available in 1981. Thirty-eight lung transplants had been carried out worldwide up to 1980, with only 2 patients surviving more than 1 month; the median survival was 8.5 days.[2,3] Death usually occurred as a result of infection, complications in relation to the airway anastomosis, or rejection.

The introduction of cyclosporin made improved immunosuppression possible. As well, cyclosporin use reduced the dependence on steroids thereby minimizing adverse effects on airway anastomosis healing.[4] The first successful heart-lung transplant (HLT) was carried out in 1981 at Stanford University Medical Center. This was followed by the first successful single-lung transplant (SLT) in 1983 and double-lung transplant (DLT) in 1986, both by the Toronto Lung Transplant Group.[5-7] Through the 1980s, lung transplantation became increasingly explored as a possible treatment option for advanced disease such as pulmonary hypertension, emphysema, pulmonary fibrosis, cystic fibrosis, and bronchiectasis. For example, the Toronto Lung Transplant Group carried out 123 procedures through 1991 (Fig. 24–1). Actuarial survivals of 62%–78% and 61%–70% at 1 and 2 years post transplantation, respectively, are now expected.[8,9]

Surgical Methods of Transplantation

Considerations relevant to management in lung transplantation include recipient selection, donor selection, selection of transplant procedure and technique, and, finally, medical treatment. Transplantation is generally reserved for patients under the age of 60 years who have terminal lung disease with a predicted life expectancy of 1–2 years. Recipients should not be on steroid therapy going into the procedure, and there should be no significant extrathoracic disease or psychosocial contraindications.

The availability of acceptable donor lungs is a serious limiting factor. Lungs when made available may be unacceptable, for example, through infection, other forms of acute lung injury occurring in the terminal period, or logistical problems. As well, there is still no good method of preserving lungs once harvested. Lungs from patients who are under the age of 50 years who have not been heavy cigarette smokers and who have clear chest radiographs with a $Pa_{O_2} > 300$ mm Hg while receiving 100% oxygen with 5 cm water end-expiratory pressure may be used. The donor and recipient must be ABO blood group compatible and exhibit only minimal lung size mismatch as assessed radiologically. The selection of procedure is in part a matter of institutional bias although recipient bilateral lung infection such as that which occurs in cystic fibrosis tends to contraindicate SLT, and pulmonary hypertension associated with significant cardiac disease (primary or secondary) tends to indicate HLT.

Methods of lung preservation are undergoing intensive research, and currently there is no optimal or consensus method employed. At present, on evisceration the donor pulmonary artery is usually flushed with cold Euro-Collins solution preceded by an injection into the artery of prostaglandin E_1 to maximize pulmonary perfusion. The extracted organ is immediately immersed in Euro-Collins solution and kept cold until implantation. Cooper[10] reported success with ischaemic periods as long as 9.5 h using modifications of this method.

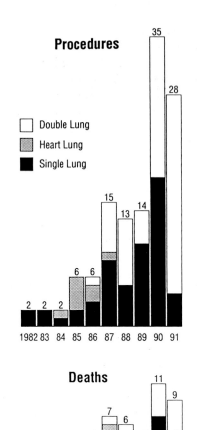

Fig. 24–1. Number and types of transplant procedures at Toronto Hospital, 1982–1991 inclusive, carried out on 110 patients with 45 deaths.

HLT is achieved through en bloc implantation with end-to-end tracheal anastomosis, circumferential right atrial anastomosis, and end-to-end aortic anastomosis.[5] SLT utilizes end-to-end bronchial and common pulmonary artery anastomosis and circumferential anastomosis of the donor left atrial cuff to recipient left atrium.[11] DLT is similar to SLT but initially employed end-to-end tracheal anastomosis.[7] Because of complications at the tracheal anastomosis with an associated 25% mortality rate, the method currently favored is that of sequential single lung transplantation known as the "bilateral lung transplant".[10,12]

The airway anastomosis is vulnerable to ischaemia in all these procedures because the bronchial systemic vessels, severed during the procedure, are never reestablished. One method commonly employed to both protect the airway anastomosis and promote revascularization is to circumferentially wrap the airway in pedicled omentum.[13] Severed lymphatics and nerves are also left interrupted.

Medical management consists of immunosuppres-

sion, initially utilizing cyclosporin, azathioprine, and antilymphocyte globulin with little or no steroid in the early posttransplant period, and antimicrobials as indicated plus pneumocystis and cytomegalovirus (CMV) prophylaxis.[10]

Lung Allograft Rejection

Immunopathology

The immunologic basis for rejection, particularly that involving lung, is complicated and needless to say not fully understood. Unlike most other solid organs, lung allografts retain a degree of immune competence for several months[14] post transplantation and therefore graft-versus-host disease may contribute to the early rejection process. As well, infections such as CMV infection, to which the lung is particularly prone, are capable of intensifying T-cell- and antibody-mediated responses. This may occur through stimulation of interferon production and result in increased donor cell major histocompatibility complex (MHC) antigen expression, effector cell Fc receptor expression and enhanced natural killer (NK) cell activity.[15] Because of this, it is often difficult to evaluate the relative contributions of infection and rejection per se in the overall resulting inflammatory process.

This account is intended only as an overview; more detailed accounts can be found elsewhere.[16–18] Discussion also is limited to the lung, although one must also consider the heart in combined heart-lung transplantation.

The ability to differentiate between self and nonself is basic to an organism's system of self-defense. This largely depends on the recognition by surveillance cells of cell-surface markers called the major (MHC) and minor (minor HA) histocompatibility antigens, which are genetically coded. MHC antigens are the more powerful in inducing a rejection response; less is known about the minor HA system. MHC antigens include class I antigens (HLA-A, HLA-B, and HLA-C), which are found in varying quantity on the surface of most nucleated cells, and class II antigens (HLA-DR, HLA-DQ, and HLA-DP), which are normally restricted to B lymphocytes, monocytes/macrophages, Langerhans cells/dendritic cells, endothelial cells, and activated T lymphocytes. MHC class II antigens may also be expressed on airway epithelial cells.[19] In addition, class II antigen expression is inducible and can be unregulated in the presence of immune interferon in almost any cell type.

At transplantation, recipient T lymphocytes infiltrate the graft and, through interaction with donor cell-surface alloantigen and the monocyte/macrophage system, interleukin-1 (IL-1), necessary for T-cell proliferation, is released. With CD4 helper cells binding to class II MHC antigens, cell activation occurs, resulting in the synthesis and release of a number of lymphokines that include interleukin-2 (IL-2) and B-cell growth factor. CD8 cytotoxic T cells bind to class I MHC antigens and also become activated. The activated T cells express newly synthesized cell-surface receptors with binding affinities for IL-2 and subsequent IL-2-mediated clonal proliferation of activated T-helper and cytotoxic cells occurs.

Through this progression, the cytotoxic cells mature and differentiate into alloantigen-specific effector cells. IL-2 amplifies the process further by stimulating release of immune interferon, which increases expression of class II MHC antigen. All this results in T-cell-mediated graft injury through direct cytotoxicity and through the release of lymphokines. Direct cytotoxicity is therefore mediated mainly by helper-dependent cells, which become the predominant cell and the major effector cell of tissue destruction in cellular rejection. As indicated, cellular rejection requires cooperation between helper T and cytotoxic T subsets, and therefore the cellular nature of each rejection process will depend, in turn, on the relative quantities of MHC class I and II antigens expressed on the target donor cell population. In addition, it is likely that a population of helper-independent cytotoxic T cells participates in the process, and that T cells not expressing CD4 or CD8 cell-surface markers reacting to alloantigen other than MHC antigens may be involved.

B-cell growth factor enables B cells to be activated by target antigen, resulting in production of antigraft antibodies. Antigen–antibody binding may result in cell injury through complement fixation and antibody-dependent cell-mediated cytotoxicity (ADCC). ADCC effector cells include polymorphonuclear leukocytes, monocytes/macrophages and lymphocytes, both T cells and natural killer (NK) cells, all of which have surface receptor for the Fc portion of IgG. These cells, therefore, can bind nonspecifically to surface-bound, antiallograft-specific IgG.

Clinical Manifestations

Clinical indications of rejection are generally divided into two types: acute rejection and bronchiolitis obliterans, the latter an expression of chronic rejection.[20] Acute rejection should be considered in patients who develop pyrexia in association with decreased exercise tolerance or decreased oxygen saturation with exercise, bilateral alveolar radiologic infiltrates, and peripheral leukocytosis. However, infection can produce a similar clinical picture and must always be a prime consideration in differential diagnosis. Biopsy support is therefore required. Further, the chest radiograph and blood gas analysis in rejection may show no abnormality.[21] The diagnostic clinical gold standard of rejection is generally considered to be a response within hours to a pulse dose of intravenous corticosteroid.

Most patients experience two or three significant episodes of acute rejection in the first 3–4 weeks following transplantation, with a peak incidence in the second week. However, acute rejection has been seen as early as 48 h post transplantation and may occur at any time.

Bronchiolitis obliterans should be considered when patients develop insidious onset of dyspnea, often with a dry cough, in association with increasing airways obstruction on pulmonary function testing. This may occur any time from 1 month post transplantation, with a peak incidence at 4–6 months.

Morphology

Before the use of cyclosporin and the resulting increase in the numbers of lung transplant procedures, little had been written concerning the pathology of rejection. In 1972 Veith and Hagstrom[22] described two patterns of rejection that they called "classic" rejection and "alveolar" rejection. Yochum Prop[23,24] later described the pathologic phases and mechanisms of rejection in a rat model. The former oversimplifies the picture of rejection that is now emerging and the latter, although informative, has limited practical application to the human context. It became clear from reports issuing from the various centers carrying out lung transplants that there was little uniformity in classification and grading schemes being used for rejection. There was also little agreement as to the methods used for monitoring rejection. In the early 1980s attention centered on endomyocardial biopsy, which had shown its usefulness in monitoring for rejection in heart transplantation. Unfortunately it quickly became clear that in combined heart-lung transplantation the lung and heart do not react synchronously and that the pathology of each must be assessed separately.[25–28] Bronchoalveolar lavage was thought to be another possibility, but evaluation of cells harvested from lavage lack specificity for rejection.[29]

Subsequently, transbronchial biopsy emerged as the most reliable method of investigating rejection. It is safe and repeatable.[30–33] For example, an overall sensitivity of 84% and specificity of 100% for rejection has been reported by the Papworth Hospital program using this method.[34] The same group later showed the predictive value of grading the degree of acute rejection.[35a,35b] However, to compare experience from one institution

Table 24–1. Classification and grading of rejection[a]

A. Acute rejection
    Grades 0 ⎤ modifiers
        1 | (a) bronchiolar involvement
        2 | (b) no bronchiolar involvement
        3 | (c) bronchial involvement
        4 ⎦   (d) bronchioles not represented
B. Active airway inflammation without scarring
    1. Lymphocytic bronchitis
    2. Lymphocytic bronchiolitis
C. Bronchiolitis obliterans
            modifiers
    1. Subtotal ⎤ (a) active
    2. Total   ⎦ (b) inactive
D. Chronic vascular rejection
E. Vasculitis

[a]Modified from Yousem SA, Berry GJ, Brunt EM et al. J Heart Transplant 1990;9:593–601,[36] with permission.

to another, a consensus classification and grading system was clearly needed: this was accomplished following discussions involving seven member institutions called the Lung Rejection Study Group (Table 24–1).[36]

The classification of rejection proposed by this group is described here. It is based simply on histology rather than immunopathogenesis. The classification reflects the experience of the member institutions in the evaluation of human lung allografts, principally through transbronchial biopsy. The classification is equally applicable to the lung of heart-lung and isolated lung procedures in that the patterns of rejection have shown no significant differences.[37]

Acute Rejection

Acute rejection describes progressive, predominantly lymphocytic, infiltration of the allograft. Initially, this is most marked in relation to small vessels, particularly venules. This perivascular infiltrate includes small round lymphocytes, larger and more active-appearing lymphocytes, plasmacytoid lymphocytes, macrophages, and occasionally small numbers of eosinophils (Fig. 24–2). These cells may be seen infiltrating the vessel wall to a varying degree, and the vessel may exhibit

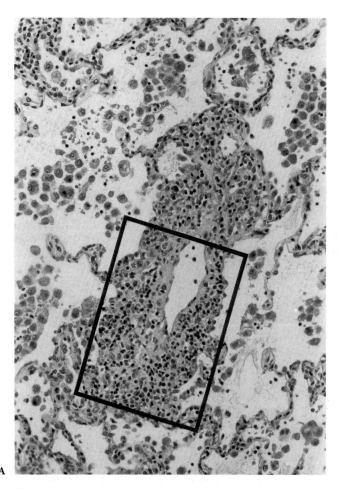

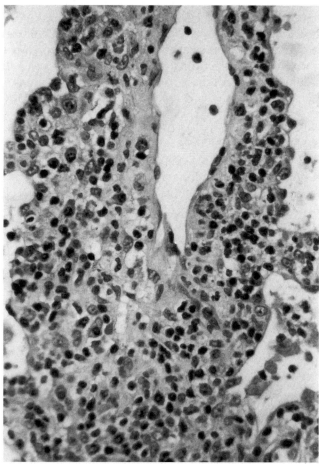

Fig. 24–2A,B. A. Perivenous mixed lymphocytic infiltrate typical of acute rejection. H and E, ×160. **B.** Enlargement of boxed area in **A**. H and E, ×400

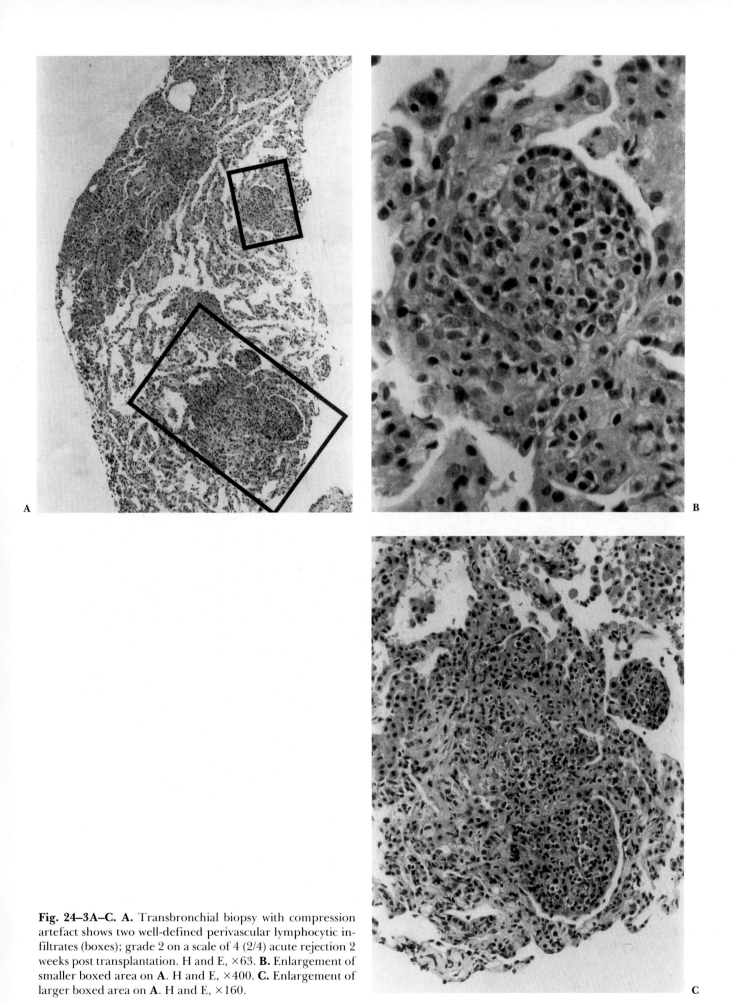

Fig. 24–3A–C. A. Transbronchial biopsy with compression artefact shows two well-defined perivascular lymphocytic infiltrates (boxes); grade 2 on a scale of 4 (2/4) acute rejection 2 weeks post transplantation. H and E, ×63. **B.** Enlargement of smaller boxed area on **A**. H and E, ×400. **C.** Enlargement of larger boxed area on **A**. H and E, ×160.

reactive intimal or endothelial changes ("endothelialitis"). A similar infiltrate may also be seen in relation to airways. In grade 1 rejection the infiltrates are infrequent, but it is believed that at least two such foci should be seen in a transbronchial biopsy before concluding that the finding reflects rejection. In grade 2 rejection, the pattern of the infiltrates is similar in that they remain more or less confined to vessels with or without airway involvement. However, they are more numerous and easier to identify on low-power microscopy (Figs. 24–3 and 24–4).

Grade 3 rejection is reflected by a change in the pattern of infiltration. Here the infiltrates extend beyond the perivascular and airway areas within the interstitium so that areas of alveolitis are produced in addition to the perivascular and airway foci (Fig. 24–5). Varying spillover of the infiltrate into air spaces also occurs. In grade 4 rejection, there is obvious lung injury at the alveolar level as reflected by any of the following: hyaline membrane formation, cellular alveolar exudates including varying numbers of polymorphonu-

clear leukocytes, parenchymal necrosis, and epithelial reactive/regenerative changes (Fig. 24–6). With immunosuppressive therapy today, this is a rare event; it likely corresponds to what Veith called "alveolar" rejection.[22]

As mentioned, the term acute rejection as described here bears no fixed relationship to timing; it may be observed at any time after transplantation. The changes are patchy in distribution as well and vary quantitatively from field to field, with a tendency for greater severity in grade in the lower lung zones.

The Lung Rejection Study Group (LRSG) recommended, when acute rejection is accompanied by airway involvement without airway wall fibrosis, that this be noted although this is not intended to imply that the changes are necessarily related in immunopathogenesis.

Unfortunately, many other conditions can produce very similar histological findings, and therefore the diagnosis depends as much on ruling out look-alikes as ruling in rejection. This is particularly so at each end of

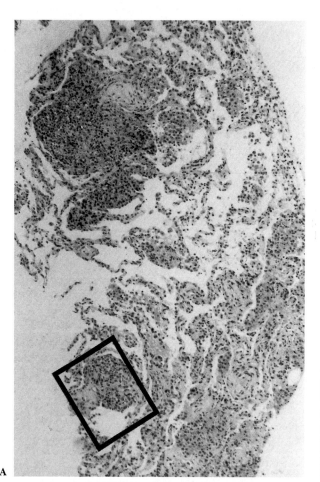

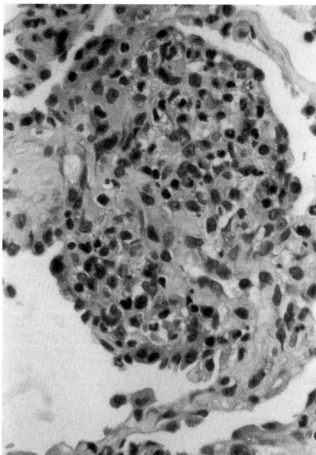

A

B

Fig. 24–4A,B. A. Transbronchial biopsy. Lymphocytic infiltrates of varying size remain confined to perivascular zone. Grade 2/4 acute rejection 5 weeks post transplantation. H and E, ×63. **B.** Enlargement of boxed area on **A**. H and E, ×400.

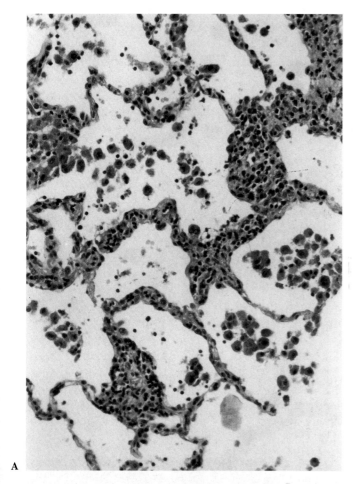

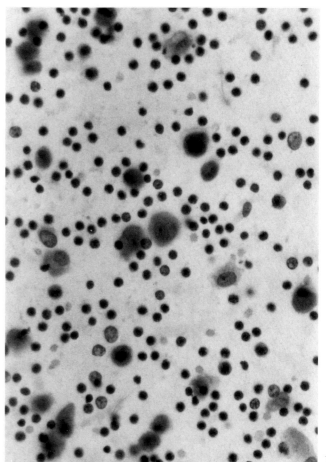

Fig. 24–5A,B. A. Grade 3/4 acute rejection with accompanying bronchoalveolar lavage. Lymphocytic infiltrates are no longer confined to perivascular zone: instead, there is extension into adjacent interstitium. H and E, ×160. **B.** BAL shows relative lymphocytosis of 68%. Millipore filter Papanicolaou, ×400.

the severity spectrum. Very rare perivascular lymphocytic infiltrates may be incidental and meaningless while, at the other extreme, severe lung injury such as diffuse alveolar damage (DAD) has a long differential diagnosis (see Chapter 4). Perivascular interstitial rejection-like lymphocytic infiltrates are relatively common in a wide variety of infections, particularly CMV infection and pneumocystis pneumonia (PCP).[38] Tazelaar[39] emphasized the importance of ruling out infection before accepting biopsy findings as rejection. However, infection and rejection may coexist, and speculation concerning relative impact on clinical disease in this instance ranges from difficult to impossible. Further, when perivascular lymphocytic infiltrates are prominent, particularly when associated with large "active-appearing" cells and vasoinfiltration, one must consider the possibility of posttransplant lymphoproliferative disease (see **Complications**).[40]

Active Airway Inflammation Without Scarring

This pattern of rejection, also called chronic inflammation of the bronchi (CIB),[41] is reflected by mixed mononuclear inflammatory cell infiltrates involving airway mucosa with lymphocytes of varying morphology being the predominant cell class (Fig. 24–7). Epithelial regenerative or metaplastic changes may be seen in association with the infiltrates, but there should be no mural or intraluminal fibrosis. The process should also be disproportionate to changes of coexistent acute rejection rather than simply appearing to be a component of acute rejection.

Again, one must recognize the relative nonspecificity of this inflammatory process. Infection, particularly viral, is a prime consideration. Hruban et al.[42] have suggested using immunoperoxidase staining for Leu-7-positive lymphocytes as a way of increasing the sensitiv-

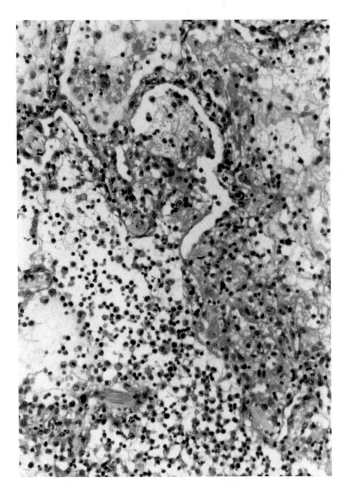

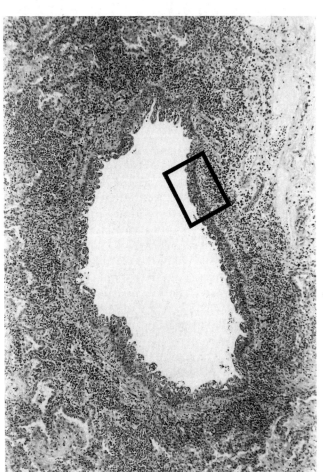

A

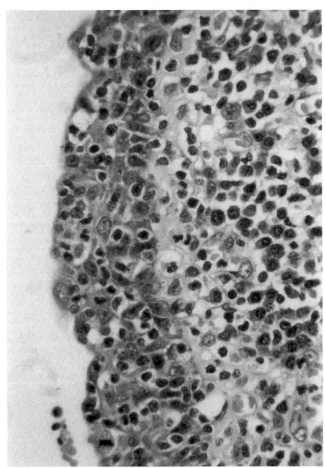

B

Fig. 24–6. Open lung biopsy shows fibrinoexudative lymphocyte-dominant pneumonia 4 weeks post transplantation. Clinical course supported diagnosis of grade 4/4 acute rejection. After appropriate antirejection therapy, patient is well at 19 months. H and E, ×160.

◁———————————————————

ity and specificity of the biopsy for rejection. Leu-7 is a cell-surface antigen present in a subpopulation of cytotoxic T cells thought to be effector cells in rejection.

Bronchiolitis Obliterans

Bronchiolitis obliterans (BO) is a term used to describe inflammatory bronchiolar disease which is associated with mural or intraluminal fibrosis. This may take the form of asymmetric or concentric mural fibrosis of varying degree or total obliteration of the airway which, even with the help of elastic stains, may be difficult to identify (Figs. 24–8 through 24–10). Airways often can be seen occluded with granulation tissue (Fig. 24–11). Some of these may exhibit epithelial-lined channels

———————————————————

Fig. 24–7A,B. A. Open lung biopsy shows lymphocytic bronchiolitis without scarring. Dense mixed lymphocytic infiltration of mucosa includes surface epithelium. Patient was 7 months post transplantation. H and E, ×63. **B.** Enlargement of boxed area in **A.** H and E, ×400. ▽

varying in size and shape reminiscent of the process of recanalization of a thrombus (Fig. 24–12). In an analysis of open lung biopsy and autopsy material of four cases of rejection-mediated BO (herein designated BO®) from the Toronto program, there did not appear to be any zonal predilection for the lesion. The percentage of membranous and respiratory bronchioles involved from patient to patient varied from 38.7% to 78.6% (mean, 58.0%). The possibility of BO should be considered on finding endogenous lipidosis in a transbronchial biopsy specimen.

Again, the nonspecificity of the lesion for rejection must be recognized. Injury as diverse as that caused by drug reactions to those of collagen vascular disease have been causally implicated in BO (see Chapter 5). In the posttransplant context, airway injury caused by inhib-

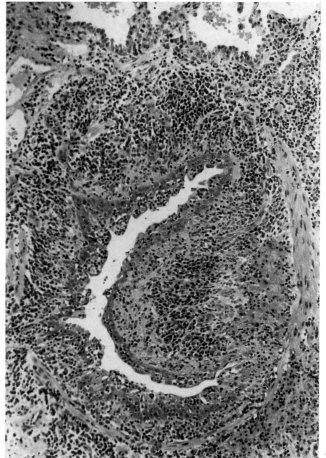

24-8

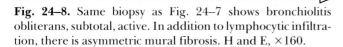

Fig. 24–8. Same biopsy as Fig. 24–7 shows bronchiolitis obliterans, subtotal, active. In addition to lymphocytic infiltration, there is asymmetric mural fibrosis. H and E, ×160.

Fig. 24–9. Same biopsy as Figs. 24–7 and 24–8 shows another pattern of bronchiolitis obliterans, subtotal, active. H and E, ×160.

Fig. 24–10. Same biopsy as Figs. 24–7 through 24–9 shows bronchiolitis obliterans, total, active. H and E, ×160.

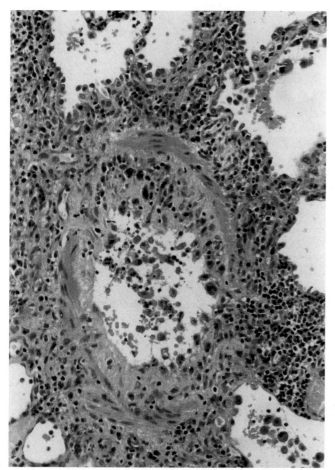

24-9

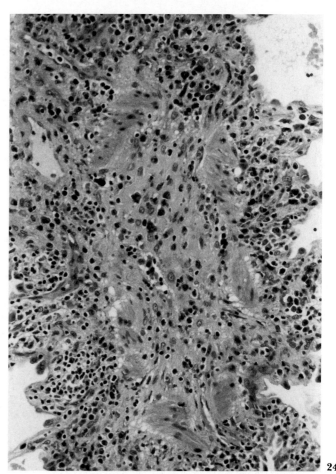

24-10

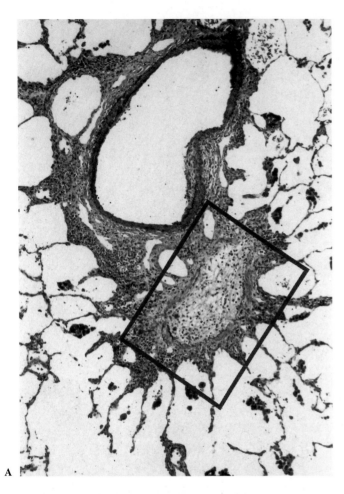

A

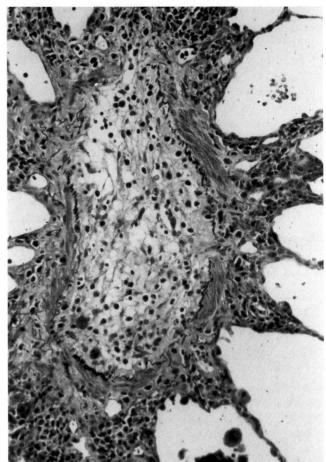

B

Fig. 24–11A,B. A. Open lung biopsy 5 months post transplantation shows bronchiolitis obliterans, total, active. Elastic trichrome, ×63. **B.** Enlargement of boxed area in **A**. Elastic trichrome, ×160. △

ited clearance relating to the severing and reanastomosis of the bronchus, aspiration, and infection must particularly be considered. Attributing BO to rejection in transbronchial biopsy samples requires clinical support.

Chronic Vascular Rejection

Chronic vascular rejection is also referred to a accelerated arteriosclerosis, graft arteriosclerosis (GAS),[43] and vascular occlusive disease (VOD).[44] It is manifested by fibrointimal thickening, which is usually more or less circumferential, involving pulmonary arteries of all sizes and veins, particularly small pulmonary veins and venules. The process tends to be patchy, like the other changes of rejection. Varying degrees of activity may be seen as reflected by accompanying mural mononuclear inflammatory cell infiltrates (Figs. 24–13 and 24–14).

◁

Fig. 24–12. Same biopsy as Fig. 24–11 shows bronchiolitis obliterans, total, inactive, with evolving "recanalization." H and E, ×160.

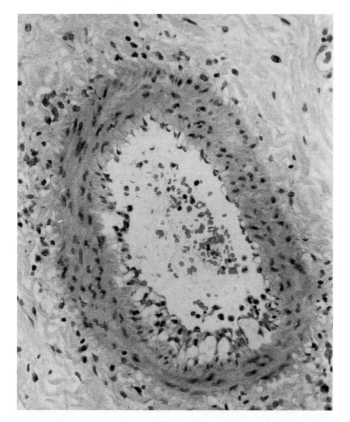

Fig. 24–13. Muscular pulmonary artery shows chronic vascular rejection. Early lesion with active lymphocytic infiltrates involves intima 9 months post transplantation. H and E, ×160.

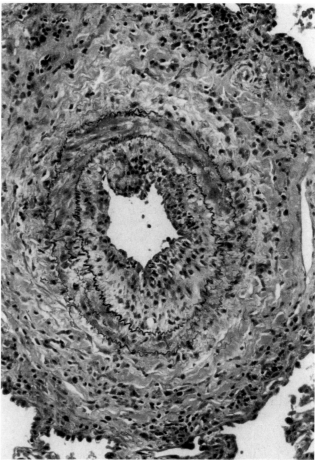

Fig. 24–14. Same biopsy as Fig. 24–13 shows more advanced arterial involvement with intimal fibrosis. Elastic trichrome, ×160.

When inactive this change is the least specific of the proposed patterns of rejection (Figs. 24–15 and 24–16). It can result from a wide variety of injuries that include regional and generalized pulmonary hypertension. In transbronchial biopsy material in particular, inactive fibrointimal thickening is best reported as simply a morphologic finding without implying that it is rejection mediated. Active vascular inflammation with intimal lymphocytic infiltrates appears to be far more specific and, in contrast, may be the most specific of the proposed patterns of rejection.

Vasculitis

Vasculitis was proposed by the Lung Rejection Study Group as a form of vascular rejection although, to that point in 1990, it had been observed by only one of the member institutions (Toronto). Subsequently, experience has shown a spectrum of vessel changes varying in activity and intensity analogous to that seen in chronic airway-directed rejection. Therefore we now consider this to be an active form of chronic vascular rejection.

Immunopathology and Morphology: A Synthesis

The immunopathogenesis of each of the recognized morphologic patterns of rejection is at present open to speculation. The manifestations described in the Lung Rejection Study Group classification suggest cell-mediated rather than humoral mechanisms. Hyperacute humoral rejection caused by the presence of preexisting circulating antibodies and acute humoral rejection, both of which result in vasculitis from either complement fixation or ADCC, have not as yet been clearly described in human lung allografts; however, hyperacute rejection is suspected as the cause of intraoperative graft failure within minutes of revascularization in one of the Toronto single lung transplants. Further, some episodes classified as rejection occurring in the early posttransplant period may actually be the result of graft-versus-host disease.[14]

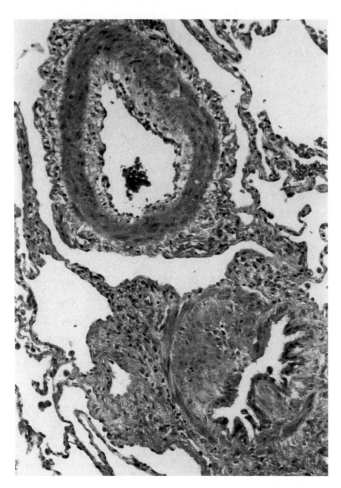

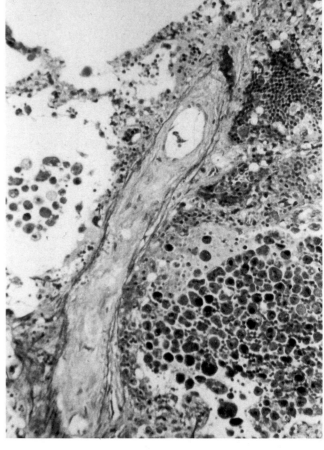

Fig. 24–15. Autopsy of case shown in Figs. 24–13 and 24–14 exhibits less active chronic vascular rejection and subtotal inactive bronchiolitis obliterans. Patient died at 15 months. H and E, ×160.

Fig. 24–16. Open lung biopsy shows inactive chronic vascular rejection involving small vein. Elastic trichrome, ×160.

Acute rejection may therefore result from more than one immunopathogenic pathway or be multicomponent immune mediated, and this is reflected by the heterogeneous nature of the cellular infiltrates that the process exhibits. To simplify, however, the most important component in acute rejection appears to be cell-mediated rejection and the presumed prime target cell population is allograft endothelium.

Active airway inflammation without scarring [lymphocytic bronchitis, or chronic inflammation of the bronchi (CIB)] and BO® appear to be related in terms of timeframe as manifestations of chronic rejection and in terms of immunopathogenesis.[41,45] This is shown by Figs. 24–7 through 24–10, which depict the same lung biopsy. BO® was first described by Burke et al.;[46] they observed this complication in 35.7% of long-term survivors in Stanford's first 19 heart-lung transplants. It now is recognized as a major cause of late morbidity and mortality with incidences of 8%, 50%, and 54% in

long-term heart-lung transplants being reported from Papworth Hospital (near Cambridge, England),[30] and from Stanford[47] and Pittsburgh[37] in the United States, respectively. BO® has been observed in 23.1% of 39 single-lung transplants (SLT) and 5.4% of 37 double-lung transplants (DLT) surviving longer than 3 months in Toronto. In contrast, Pittsburgh quotes an incidence of 62% in isolated lung transplant patients.[37] The reasons for this great variation remain to be resolved, but Keenan et al.[37] suggested that too great an emphasis is being placed on clinical deterioration in making this diagnosis, noting that 25% of the Pittsburgh group cases were asymptomatic and had no deterioration of lung function. BO® may occur at any time from 2 months after transplantation, but usually is seen at 4–12 months.

Rejection-mediated broncholitis obliterans (BO®) is generally considered to be a form of chronic rejection caused by augmented expression of MHC class II antigens on airway epithelium and mediated by T cells.[48] However, there is still controversy as to the value of evaluating MHC class II antigen expression on bronchial epithelial cells as a marker of rejection.[48,49] This upregulation of antigen expression may be induced by episodes of acute rejection and infection, particularly pneumocystis pneumonia and viral infection such as CMV.[48,50–54a] It is clear, therefore, that treating acute rejection and infections early and completely is important in minimizing the risk of BO®, and this may further explain the reported interinstitutional differences in incidence. Recently, using donor antigen-specific primed-lymphocyte-test reactivity of bronchoalveolar lavage lymphocytes, Reinsmoen et al.[54b] found that a predominant donor-specific class II-directed pattern of reactivity correlated with acute rejection episodes and that a predominant class I-directed pattern of reactivity correlated with bronchiolitis obliterans.

Lymphocytic bronchitis commonly accompanies BO®. It is likely that this simply is the morphologic expression of airway epithelium-directed, cell-mediated chronic rejection in large airways while in small airways the result is mural fibrosis with or without BO.[41,45]

Less is known about chronic vascular rejection. This effect often coexists with BO®, and recurrent severe and persistent acute rejection appears to be a predisposing factor as in the case of BO®.[44] Colvin[15] suggested that chronic vascular rejection may result from either T-cell or humoral mechanisms.

Pulmonary Complications

There is no organ more vulnerable to complications following transplantation than the lung. Opportunistic infection, rejection, particularly chronic rejection, and pathology in relation to the airway anastomosis such as stenosis and dehiscence continue to be the main problem areas. This is not surprising when one considers the events that have occurred through transplantation. The donor organ or organs have been harvested from a terminally ill patient and have been inadequately preserved during the period before reimplantation. The donor lungs are frequently the site of infection or organism colonization.

The transplant procedure, even under ideal circumstances, is associated with significant morbidity. It leaves an implanted organ with impaired clearance mechanisms as a result of permanently severed nerves (therefore inhibited cough reflex) and of severed lymphatics, in addition to interruption of mucosal continuity at the airway anastomosis. As well, permanent severing of the bronchial systemic vessels jeopardizes bronchial mucosal viability (therefore mucociliary function) and

healing of the airway anastomosis. Differences in the MHC antigens expressed by recipient immune effector cells interfere with interaction of these cells with donor parenchymal cells. This interference, plus the impaired lymphatic circulation, result in an inhibited immune response. Together, these factors produce an impressive local opportunistic state. This condition is worsened by systemic medical immunosuppression, which is necessary to minimize rejection.

Understandably, the complications that occur after transplantation are virtually limitless. While these difficulties principally involve thoracic structures, extrathoracic complications such as those resulting from cyclosporin toxicity are nevertheless very significant. This discussion is limited to the more common and relatively specific problems that affect the lung.

Infection is the most common serious complication. For example, infection was responsible for 75% of all deaths in the Pittsburgh transplant program up to early 1989.[55] Infection also potentiates other serious complications such as chronic rejection and lymphoproliferative disease.[40,56]

Bacterial Pneumonia

Although bacterial pneumonia may occur at any time, it is particularly common in the early postoperative period. If the patient is still intubated there may be considerable difficulty in distinguishing bacterial colonization from infection and this, in turn, from acute rejection and pulmonary edema. Routine antibacterial prophylaxis and specific treatment for organisms cultured from the donor airway at harvesting have reduced the risk of infection somewhat. Enterobacteriaceae and pseudomonas followed by staphylococcus aureus and hemophilus pneumoniae are the most usual organisms.

Patients with cystic fibrosis (CF) present a unique problem because the upper respiratory tract including sinuses is almost always colonized by various strains of *Pseudomonas aeruginosa* and/or *cepacia*. Of 13 CF patients who underwent DLT in the Toronto program, 12 had at least one significant complicating infection in the first postoperative month.[57] Three of these patients died perioperatively as a result of *P. aeruginosa* and/or *P. cepacia* pneumonia (Fig. 24–17).

Pneumocystis carinii

Pneumocystis carinii pneumonia (PCP) does not usually occur until several months post transplantation. Until the routine use of antibiotic prophylaxis was instituted, the incidence of infection was high, but PCP now appears to be relatively uncommon. Surveillance for

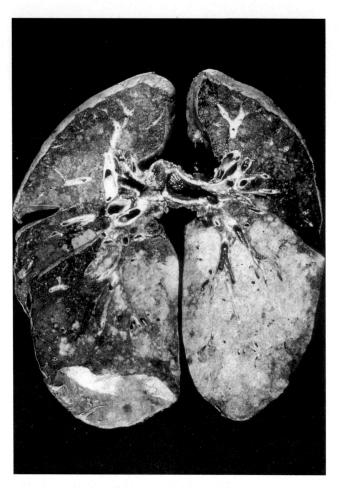

Fig. 24–17. Anterior view of double lung transplant shows widespread *Pseudomonas* pneumonia with lobar distribution in left-lower lobe. Autopsy of cystic fibrosis patient 2 weeks post transplantation.

this is largely dependent on bronchoalveolar lavage (BAL), which is rapid and has shown sensitivities ranging from 89% to 97%.[58,59]

Cytomegalovirus Pneumonia

Cytomegalovirus (CMV) pneumonia is widely recognized as a major cause of morbidity and death in lung allograft recipients.[60–62] It is the most common cause of infection in the 1- to 2-month postoperative interval. Seronegative recipients receiving donor positive organs are at greatest risk through primary infection. However, significant risk is also present with both donor positive-recipient positive and donor negative-recipient positive situations, because of either reinfection by a different strain of virus in the former or reactivation of endogenous virus in either of these situations.[63] To reduce the risk of primary infection and reinfection,

seronegative blood products and donors are used where possible, and acyclovir/ganciclovir and CMV hyperimmune globulin prophylaxis is instituted.

The diagnosis of CMV pneumonia is difficult in that it can mimic acute rejection clinically including the effect on BAL cell profile. Few would argue that the diagnostic gold standard is the finding of typical CMV-infected cells by conventional light microscopy in a tissue context of interstitial inflammation in the absence of other infectious agents (Fig. 24–18). Unfortunately, this is often not the case, and the criteria used to establish a diagnosis short of this vary from center to center, complicating discussions concerning the incidence and significance of this disease.[61] Because immunohistochemistry using monoclonal antibodies, DNA in situ hybridization, and the shell vial culture technique are now available, rapid detection of virus is possible.[64,65] However, test sensitivity and specificity tend to be inversely related so that no one test can be considered diagnostic of CMV pneumonia. The pathologist should realise that the finding of CMV inclusion-containing cells in BAL material by conventional light microscopy has high specificity, but sensitivities of only 21%[64] and 29%[65] have been reported by experienced centers.

Fungal Infection

Fungal infection of any type can occur in the setting of lung transplantation, as in any opportunistic state, but *Candida* and *Aspergillus* species are the most common. Either may colonize the upper respiratory tract, and distinguishing colonization from infection may be difficult. We have had two SLT patients with aspergillus colonization of end-stage cystic areas of the native lung in the posttransplant period. One patient later developed disseminated invasive aspergillosis (Fig. 24–19). Kahn et al.[66] reported that the finding of hyphae in BAL material of immunocompromised patients with new pulmonary infiltrates has a 75% predictive value for invasive disease.

Acute Lung Injury

Acute lung injury from causes other than acute rejection and infection is another major cause of morbidity in the first posttransplant month. Differential diagnosis is difficult, clinically and pathologically. The pathology is usually that of nonspecific diffuse alveolar damage (DAD) and the aetiologic possibilities are numerous. These include pathology originating in the terminal period of the donor, problems related to poor organ preservation, reperfusion injury after periods of ischaemia, and continuing impairment of perfusion postoperatively. These may individually or in combination

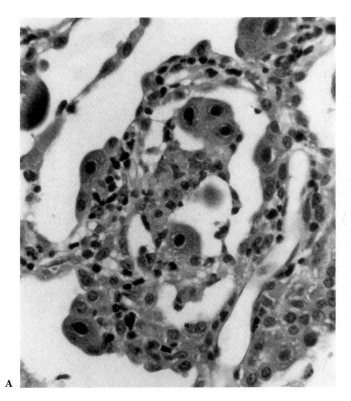

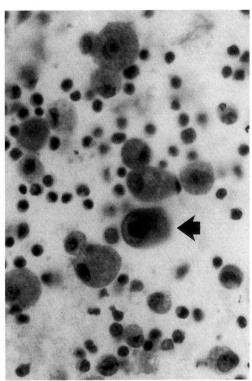

Fig. 24–18A,B. A. Transbronchial biopsy at 3 months post transplantation shows alveolitis with typical cytomegalic inclusion (epithelial) cells. H and E, ×400. **B.** Associated BAL shows relative lymphocytosis and scattered inclusion cells (*arrow*). Millipore filter Papanicolaou, ×400.

cause or contribute to lung injury. The exact cause of injury is often unknown and therapy simply supportive. However, reperfusion injury, also called postperfusion syndrome, may soon be an exception. This is thought to occur through complement activation with resultant neutrophil release of enzymes and oxygen-derived free radicals. The therapeutic roles of free radical scavenger therapy[67] and corticosteriods[68] are currently being investigated. At this point, however, the term acute lung injury should be viewed as an aetiologically nonspecific diagnosis, which nevertheless implies that infection and rejection have been ruled out.

Problems with the Airway Anastomosis

The availability of cyclosporin in 1981 meant that corticosteroid use in the early postoperative period could be diminished. Before this, inhibited healing at the airway anastomotic site caused by corticosteroids was a common cause of graft failure. As described, the systemic arterial supply to the lung is not reconnected at the time of transplantation, and, until tissue revascularization occurs, donor airway viability is entirely dependent on collateral blood flow from the pulmonary circulation. Systemic revascularization may take several weeks and during this time the anastomotic site, requiring good perfusion for healing, is at high risk. Ischaemia may lead to mucosal necrosis, which may in turn be complicated by colonization/infection at the anastomosis, distal opportunistic infection, and, with healing, stricture. Panmural ischaemic necrosis causes partial or complete dehiscence, which is frequently complicated by abscess formation or mediastinitis (Fig. 24–20).

It is now common to wrap the anastomotic site with a pedicled flap of omentum (omentopexy), a procedure introduced by Dr. J.D. Cooper in 1982.[69] This has the double advantage of promoting revascularization through development of collateral blood flow and acting as a barrier should dehiscence occur. Prolonged systemic hypotension and lung parenchymal disease such as pneumonia, both of which interfere with collateral flow from the pulmonary circulation, have been shown to be significant risk factors.[12] Lung preservation before implantation is likely another relevant factor. Reported incidences of significant airway complications are for combined heart-lung transplantation, 8.7% (discussion of Dr. R.L. Hardesty, Pittsburgh[12]) and for the bronchial anastomosis in a combined study of SLT and DLT, 14.0%.[70] Trachea-to-trachea anastomosis, which was employed originally in the Toronto

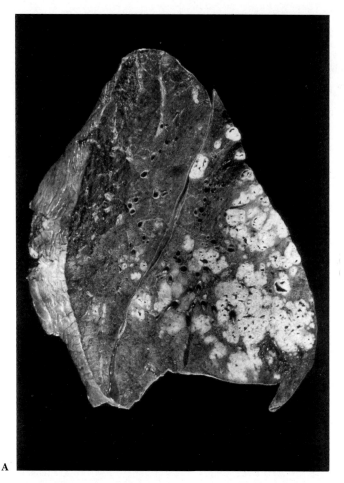

A

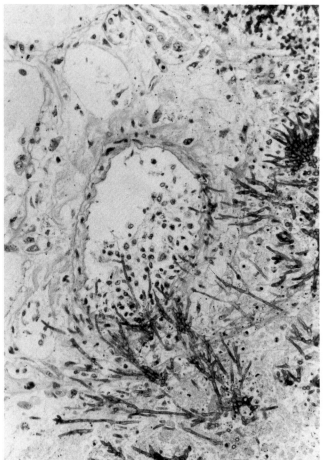

B

Fig. 24–19A,B. A. Sagittal view of allograft 4 months post single lung transplant shows widespread fungal abscesses. **B.** Microscopy shows necrosis and vasoinvasion by *Aspergillus.* Infection occurred secondary to colonization of contralateral emphysematous native lung. Haematoxylin Phloxine Saffron, ×160.   △

DLT program, has been replaced in this procedure by bilateral bronchial anastomoses because of an unacceptably high incidence of complications.[12]

Bronchiectasis

Cylindrical ectasia of proximal bronchi (also see Chapter 5) appears to be relatively common in long-term lung transplant survivors. In studying alterations in bronchial cartilage in patients surviving 45 days or more after transplantation, Yousem et al.[71] have shown that abnormalities in cartilage are common and likely result from poor perfusion of these airways. Similarly, poor perfusion may adversely affect the integrity of the entire bronchial wall, therefore predisposing to bronchiectasis. Other likely components of the pathogenesis are denervation and recurrent airway infection or

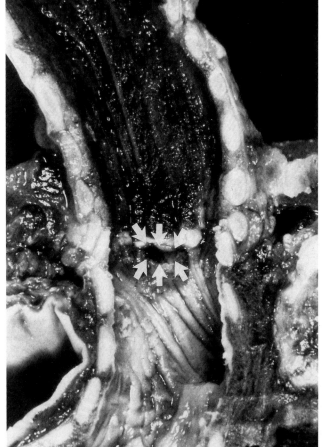

24-20

◁ ─────────────────────────────

Fig. 24–20. Anterior view shows bronchial anastomosis of double lung transplant with focal dehiscence (*arrows*). Note marked congestion of recipient bronchus.

chronic airway colonization, often by *Pseudomonas*. A vicious cycle results with bronchiectasis predisposing to infection and infection making the bronchiectasis worse.

In addition to rendering the patient at risk for opportunistic infection, this scenario may well increase the risk of chronic rejection. In an autopsy study of HLT recipients, Tazelaar and Yousem[72] found that all the patients with bronchiolitis obliterans had evidence of proximal bronchiectasis. The relationship of infection and rejection has been discussed, but it is pertinent to recognize that bronchiolitis obliterans may also occur distal to bronchiectasis as a complication of impaired clearance rather than rejection.

Lymphoproliferative Disease

Posttransplant lymphoproliferative disease (PTLD) consists of a spectrum of B-lymphocyte proliferative conditions that occur in immunosuppressed patients after transplantation.[73a] These may be more common following lung transplantation than after solid organ transplantation. For example, the Pittsburgh program reports an incidence of 7.8% (5/64) in lung transplant recipients surviving more than 30 days as compared to 3.4% (15/439) in their heart transplant program.[56] However, the incidence in Toronto lung transplant survivors of more than 30 days is 3.5% (3/86).

PLTD appears to result from B-lymphocyte proliferation in response to Epstein–Barr virus (EBV) infection, which is allowed to go unchecked by cytotoxic T-cell regulation because of selective suppression by cyclosporin.[40,56,73a,73b] The differences in reported incidence may simply reflect differences in the use of immunosuppressive therapy from organ to organ and center to center.

PTLD most frequently develops as a nodular infiltrate or infiltrates in the lung allograft, although some develop in extrapulmonary sites. This usually occurs 2–4 months postoperatively. The proliferative spectrum ranges from polymorphous hyperplasia to monomorphous neoplasia. The term polymorphous is used to describe the variation in lymphocytes that make up the infiltrate. B lymphocytes, seemingly at all stages of differentiation from small lymphocytes to plasma cells, are characteristically seen. Variable numbers of large abnormal lymphoid cells referred to as "atypical immunoblasts" also can be seen in addition to reactive polymorphonuclear leukocytes and histiocytes. This polymorphous process may be either polyclonal or monoclonal/oligoclonal. When monomorphous, PTLD is composed of uniform lymphoid cells, which appear to be predominantly at one stage of differentiation, giving a picture indistinguishable from that of typical non-Hodgkin's lymphoma (Fig. 24–21). Immunogenotypic/immunophenotypic analysis reveals monoclonality or oligoclonality.

Both processes tend to show a propensity for angiocentric, angioinvasive growth in the lung. When polymorphous, therefore, the process may be difficult to distinguish from florid acute rejection in transbronchial biopsy samples. Conventional light microscopic criteria that help one in recognizing PTLD in this context are the number of atypical immunoblasts present, necrosis, and airway invasion with destruction. Clinical and radiological information should also be sought for support in addition to genotypic study. This distinction is important because rejection requires augmentation of immunosuppressive therapy whereas PTLD, particularly when presenting early and as a polymorphous lesion, often responds to a reduction in immunosuppression. Antiviral therapy is also recommended.

Diagnostic Methods

It is clear from the foregoing that lung transplant recipients require close surveillance concerning the development of infection, rejection, and PTLD. All would agree that the most reliable test is the examination of a representative open lung biopsy. Unfortunately, this is not readily repeatable, and the cost in terms of morbidity is too great for routine use. Transbronchial lung biopsy (TBB) complemented by bronchoalveolar lavage (BAL) has emerged as the surveillance method of choice.[30–33] However, it is important to recognize that total disease representation has been compromised in employing this method. Findings, regardless of how specific, may only represent a component of a larger picture; findings lacking high specificity may not be representative. Any final conclusion therefore should take into account all the information available, both clinical and radiographic.

Before its use in monitoring lung transplants, the utility of TBB had been investigated in diffuse lung disease. For example, Gilman and Wang[74] found that four TBB specimens could achieve a 90% diagnostic yield in pulmonary sarcoidosis and therefore recommended this number of biopsies to ensure adequate representation. The Papworth Hospital group has led discussion on the number of biopsies and sampling adequacy in transplant monitoring. They have stated that a minimum of five peripheral biopsies are needed for a diagnosis of rejection and that accurate assessment of grade requires more.[35a,35b] The Lung Rejection Study Group recommended that a minimum of five transbronchial specimens containing lung parenchyma should be obtained under fluoroscopic control.[36] The

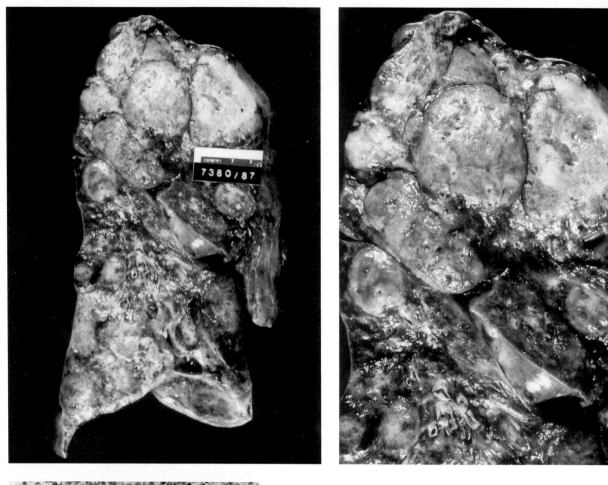

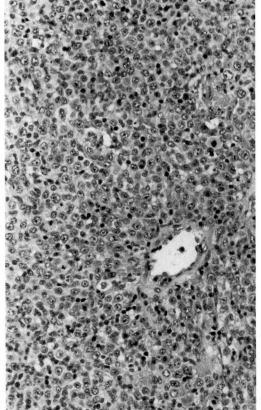

Fig. 24–21A–C. A,B. Sagittal view of native lung following pneumonectomy 4 months after single lung transplant. **C.** Microscopy shows diffuse large cell immunoblastic non-Hodgkin's lymphoma. Further study showed that malignant cells were EBV-transformed B lymphocytes. Patient died 7 months later with widespread respiratory tract and intestinal involvement. H and E, ×160.

biopsies should represent areas of maximal radiographic abnormality or, if no abnormality exists, two lobes should be sampled randomly.

Our routine is to place the biopsies immediately into 10% neutral buffered formalin and serially section these to give five sections on each of 10 slides. A preliminary report is given following examination of 2 H and E-stained slides and elastic trichrone- and silver methenamine-stained slides. The remaining slides are then stained as appropriate utilizing histochemistry or immunohistochemistry. Each TBB series is accompanied by a BAL that undergoes cytologic assessment including differential cell count by conventional light microcopy,[75,76] smears and culture for bacteria including mycobacteria, and culture for fungi and viruses. The procedures are generally carried out as a routine every 1–4 weeks in the first 3 months post transplant; thereafter, the schedule is every 3 months for the first year and every 6–12 months after the first year. Sampling also occurs when clinically indicated.

Transbronchial Biopsy

There is now a clear consensus, despite some criticism,[38,39] that transbronchial biopsy (TBB) has a high degree of sensitivity and specificity for acute rejection. Figures of 84% and 100%, respectively, as reported by the Papworth Hospital group[34] are fairly representative. However, the procedure is less valuable in the investigation of infection and chronic rejection. Before its use in lung transplantation, the diagnostic accuracy of TBB in the immunocompromised host with infection was reported to be in the 26%–36% range.[77,78] A similar sensitivity is now reported in lung transplant recipients (Fig. 24–22).[34] Without fluoroscopic guidance, diagnostic yields as low as 13% can be anticipated.[79] Chronic rejection, specifically rejection-mediated bronchiolitis obliterans (BO®), is another frequent and important complication for which TBB has low sensitivity. Although Yousem[80a] showed, in a small number of patients, that a series of four TBB specimens had a 66% sensitivity for BO®, others have suggested that open lung biopsy is a more appropriate test in this situation.[31] Open lung biopsy allows better evaluation of the morphologic nature and context of bronchiolitis obliterans. This is important in the determination of aetiology.[80b] In 591 TBB series averaging 2.8 specimens per series, we found evaluable membranous bronchioles or proximal respiratory bronchioles in only 26.8% of the series. We therefore anticipate a sensitivity of 15.5% for a series of 2.8 specimens given the percentage mentioned previously of small airways that show involvement by the process when present. Hruban et al.[45] have suggested that changes in proximal bronchial biopsies reflect distal airway disease and that this therefore may offer an alternative method of investigation. Although

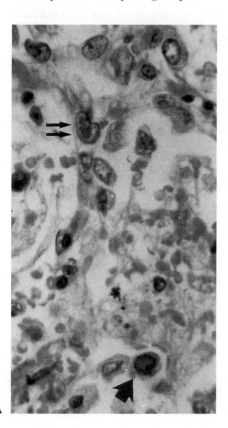

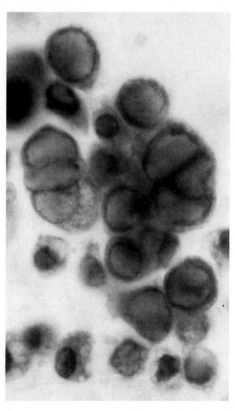

Fig. 24–22A,B. Transbronchial biopsy shows allograft herpes simplex pneumonia. **A.** Note homogenous type inclusion (*single arrow*) and intranuclear inclusion with halo (*double arrow*). H and E, ×400. **B.** Accompanying BAL shows multinucleation of cells with homogeneous inclusions. Millipore filter Papanicolaou, ×1000.

A

B

they showed that immunostaining for MHC class II antigen expression on bronchial epithelial cells does not appear to be useful,[49] staining for intraepithelial lymphocytes expressing Leu-7 antigen may add further to the specificity of the biopsy.[42]

Bronchoalveolar Lavage

Bronchoalveolar lavage complements the use of TBB in monitoring the lung allograft and therefore these tests should be done together. BAL has greater sensitivity and specificity for infection and TBB has greater sensitivity and specificity for acute rejection. It appears that conventional total and differential cell counts do not reliably distinguish rejection from other inflammatory processes in the lung. However, there is reason to hope that phenotypic and functional analysis of the cells will eventually enable this distinction to be accomplished with accuracy.[29,81,82] We nevertheless think that a relative lymphocytosis supports a diagnosis of acute rejection if infection can be ruled out. The sensitivity of BAL for infection, excluding culture, has been discussed. This ranges from 21%[64] for CMV pneumonia using conventional light microscopy to 89%[58] for pneumocystis pneumonia. These results can be further improved through the use of immunohistochemistry and DNA in situ hybridization.

Primed Lymphocyte Testing

Primed lymphocyte testing (PLT) is a test for donor-specific alloreactive T cells. It measures the proliferative response of recipient lymphocytes induced by irradiated donor lymphocytes from either the donor spleen or lymph node tissue. The Pittsburgh group[83] has shown that PLT performed on separated BAL lymphocytes and lymphocytes grown from TBB, but not peripheral blood lymphocytes, correlates well with a clinical diagnosis of acute rejection. As well, they have shown a correlation with BO®. Further, the group has suggested that donor-specific alloreactivity of BAL and TBB cells is predictive of BO® in clinically stable patients.[84] Interestingly, they report positive testing in 28% of patients with infection again implying a relationship between infection and rejection.[50] More studies using PLT by more institutions are needed to fully evaluate the practical usefulness of this method of surveillance. The specificity of this test might be enhanced by using homozygous typing cells representing the MHC class I and II antigens expressed by the recipient and donor cells to better define the PLT reactivity observed when testing BAL-derived cells from recipients.[54b]

Conclusion

The rapid developments in organ transplantation that have occurred since the advent of cyclosporin have few parallels in medical history. Lung transplantation presents a unique challenge. The viability of the lung is dependent on the maintenance of adequate ventilation and perfusion. It is particularly vulnerable to infection. Infection and rejection appear to behave synergistically. However, the problems are not prohibitive. With continuing progress, lung transplantation will doubtless become a successful and widely practiced method of treating end-stage pulmonary disease.

References

1. Hardy JD, Webb WAS, Dalton ML, Walker GR. Lung homotransplantation in man. JAMA 1963;186:1065–1074.
2. Kamholz SL. Current perspectives in clinical and experimental single lung transplantation. Chest 1988;94:390–396.
3. Nelems JMB, Rebuck AS, Cooper JD, Goldberg M, Halloran PF, Vellend H. Human lung transplantation. Chest 1980;78:569–573.
4. Griffin BP, Hardesty RL, Bahnson HT. Powerful but limited immunosuppression for cardiac transplantation with cyclosporin and low-dose steroid. J Thorac Cardiovasc Surg 1984;87:35–42.
5. Reitz BA, Wallwork JL, Hunt SA, et al. Heart-lung transplantation: Successful therapy for patients with pulmonary vascular disease. New Engl J Med 1982;306:557–564.
6. The Toronto Transplant Group. Unilateral lung transplantation for pulmonary fibrosis. N Engl J Med 1986;314:1140–1145.
7. Patterson GA, Cooper JD, Goldman B, et al. Technique of successful clinical double-lung transplantation. Ann Thorac Surg 1988;45:626–633.
8. Atkinson JB. The pathology of heart-lung transplantation. Hum Pathol 1988;19:1367–1368.
9. Hutter JA, Despins P, Higenbottam T, Stewart S, Wallwork J. Heart-lung transplantation: Better use of resources. Am J Med 1988;85:4–11.
10. Cooper JD. Current status of lung transplantation. Transplant Proc 1991;23:2107–2114.
11. Cooper JD, Pearson FG, Patterson GA, et al. Technique of successful lung transplantation in humans. J Thorac Cardiovasc Surg 1987;93:173–181.
12. Patterson GA, Todd TR, Cooper JD, Pearson FG, Winton TL, Mauer J. Airway complications after double lung transplantation. J Thorac Cardiovasc Surg 1990;99:14–21.
13. Dubois P, Choiniere L, Cooper JD. Bronchial omentopexy in canine lung allotransplantation. Ann Thorac Surg 1984;38:211–214.

14. Paradis IL, Marrari M, Zeevi A, et al. HLA phenotype of lung lavage cells following heart-lung transplantation. Heart Transplant 1985;4:422–425.

15. Colvin RB. The pathogenesis of vascular rejection. Transplant Proc 1991;23:2052–2055.

16. Bach FH, Sachs DH. current concepts: Transplantation immunology. N Engl J Med 1987;317:489–492.

17. Ettenger R, Ferstenberg LB. Basic immunology of transplantation. Perspect Pediatr Pathol. 1991;14:9–40.

18. Hall BM. Cells mediating allograft rejection. Transplantation 1991;51:1141–1151.

19. Glanville AR, Tazelaar HD, Theodore J, et al. The distribution of MHC class I and II antigens on bronchial epithelium. Am Rev Respir Dis 1989;139:330–334.

20. Lawrence EC. Diagnosis and management of lung allograft rejection. Clin Chest Med 1990;11:269–278.

21. Sleiman C, Groussard O, Mal H, et al. Clinical use of transbronchial biopsy in single-lung transplantation. Transplantation 1991;51:927–929.

22. Veith FG, Hagstrom JWC. Alveolar manifestations of rejection: An important cause of the poor results with human lung transplantation. Ann Surg 1972;175:336–348.

23. Prop J, Wildevuur CRH, Nienwenhuis P. Lung allograft rejection in the rat lung: Corresponding morphological rejection phases in various rat strain combinations. Transplantation 1985;40:132–136.

24. Prop J, Tazelaar HD, Billingham ME. Rejection of combined heart-lung transplants in rats. Am J Pathol 1987;127:97–105.

25. Scott WC, Haverich A, Billingham ME, Dawkins KD, Jamieson SW. Lethal rejection of the lung without significant cardiac rejection in primate heart-lung allotransplants. Heart Transplant 1984;4:33–39.

26. McGregor CGA, Baldwin JC, Jamieson SW, et al. Isolated pulmonary rejection after combined heart-lung transplantation. J Thorac Cardiovasc Surg 1985;90:623–630.

27. Hutter JA, Stewart S, Higenbottam T, Scott JP, Wallwork J. The characteristic histological changes associated with rejection in heart-lung transplant recipients. Transplant Proc 1989;21:435–436.

28. Starnes VA, Theodore J, Oyer PE, et al. Evaluation of heart-lung transplant recipients with prospective, serial transbronchial biopsies and pulmonary function studies. J Thorac Cardiovasc Surg 1989;98:683–690.

29. May RM, Cooper DKC, Dutoit ED, Reichart B. Cytoimmunologic monitoring after heart and heart-lung transplantation. J Heart Transplant 1990;9:133–135.

30. Hutter JA, Stewart S, Higenbottam T, Scott JP, Wallwork J. Histologic changes in heart-lung transplant recipients during rejection episodes and at routine biopsy. J Heart Transplant 1988;7:440–444.

31. Stewart S, Higenbottam TW, Hutter JA, Penketh ARL, Zebro TJ, Wallwork J. Histopathology of transbronchial biopsies in heart-lung transplantation. Transplant Proc 1988;20:764–766.

32. Higenbottam T, Stewart S, Wallwork J. Transbronchial lung biopsy to diagnose lung rejection and infection of heart-lung transplants. Transplant Proc 1988;20:767–769.

33. Starnes VA, Theodore J, Oyer PE, et al. Pulmonary infiltrates after heart-lung transplantation: Evaluation by serial transbronchial biopsies. J Thorac Cardiovasc Surg 1989;98:945–950.

34. Higenbottam T, Stewart S, Penketh A, Wallwork J. Transbronchial lung biopsy for the diagnosis of rejection in heart-lung transplant patients. Transplantation 1988;46:532–539.

35a. Clelland C, Higenbottam T, Otulana B, et al. Histologic prognostic indicators for lung allografts of heart-lung transplants. J Heart Transplant 1990;9:177–186.

35b. Scott JP, Fradet G, Smyth RL et al. Prospective study of transbronchial biopsies in the management of heart-lung and single lung transplant patients. J Heart Lung Transplant 1991;10:626–637.

36. Yousem SA, Berry GJ, Brunt EM, et al. A working formulation for the standardization of nomenclature in the diagnosis of heart and lung rejection: Lung Rejection Study Group. J Heart Transplant 1990;9:593–601.

37. Keenan RJ, Bruzzone P, Paradis IL, et al. Similarity of pulmonary rejection patterns among heart-lung and double-lung transplant recipients. Transplantation 1991;51:176–180.

38. Cagle PT, Truong LD, Holland VA, Lawrence EC, Noon GP, Greenberg SD. Lung biopsy evaluation of acute rejection versus opportunistic infection in lung transplant patients. Transplantation 1989;47:713–715.

39. Tazelaar HD. Perivascular inflammation in pulmonary infections: Implications for the diagnosis of lung rejection. J Heart Lung Transplant 1991;10:437–441.

40. Yousem SA, Randhawa P, Locker J, et al. Posttransplant lymphoproliferative disorders in heart-lung transplant recipients: Primary presentation in the allograft. Hum Pathol 1989;20:361–369.

41. Yousem SA, Paradis IL, Dauber JA. Large airway inflammation in heart-lung transplantation recipients—its significance and prognostic implications. Transplantation 1990;49:654–656.

42. Hruban RH, Beschorner WE, Baumgartner WA, et al. Diagnosis of lung allograft rejection by bronchial intraepithelial Leu-7 positive T lymphocytes. J Thorac Cardiovasc Surg 1988;96:939–946.

43. Yousem SA, Paradis IL, Dauber JH, et al. Pulmonary arteriosclerosis in long-term human heart-lung transplant recipients. Transplantation 1989;47:564–569.

44. Scott JP, Higenbottam TW, Clelland C, et al. The natural history of obliterative bronchiolitis and occlusive vascular disease of patients following heart-lung transplantation. Transplant Proc 1989;21:2592–2593.

45. Hruban RH, Beschorner WE, Hutchins GM. Lymphocytic bronchitis and lung allograft rejection. Transplantation 1990;50:723.

46. Burke CM, Theodore J, Dawkins KD, et al. Post-transplant obliterative bronchiolitis and other late lung sequelae in human heart-lung transplantation. Chest

1984;86:824–829.

47. Burke CM, Baldwin JC, Morris AJ, et al. Twenty-eight cases of heart-lung transplantation. Lancet 1986;i:517–519.

48. Burke CM, Glanville AR, Theodore J, Robin ED. Lung immunogenicity, rejection and obliterative bronchiolitis. Chest 1987;92:547–549.

49. Hruban RH, Beschorner WE, Baumgartner WA, et al. Evidence that the expression of class II MHC antigens is not diagnostic of lung allograft rejection. Transplantation 1989;48:529–530.

50. Griffith BP, Paradis IL, Zeevi A, et al. Immunologically mediated disease of the airways after pulmonary transplantation. Ann Surg 1988;208:371–378.

51. Gryzan S, Paradis IL, Zeevi A, et al. Unexpectedly high incidence of pneumocystis carinii infection after lung-heart transplantation. Am Rev Respir Dis 1988; 137:1268–1274.

52. Taylor PM, Rose ML, Yacoub MH. Expression of MHC antigen in normal human lungs and transplanted lungs with obliterative bronchiolitis. Transplantation 1989; 48:506–510.

53. Yousem SA, Dauber JA, Keenan R, Paradis IL, Zeevi A, Griffith BP. Does histologic acute rejection in lung allografts predict the development of bronchiolitis obliterans. Transplantation 1991;52:306–309.

54a. Keenan RJ, Lega ME, Dummer JS, et al. Cytomegalovirus serologic status and postoperative infection correlated with risk of developing chronic rejection after pulmonary transplantation. Transplantation 1991;51: 433–438.

54b. Reinsmoen NL, Bolman RM, Savik K, Butters K, Hertz M. Differentiation of class I and classII-directed donor-specific alloreactivity in bronchoalveolar lavage lymphocytes from lung transplant recipients. Transplantation 1992;53:181–189.

55. Dauber JH, Paradis IL, Dummer JS. Infectious complications in pulmonary allograft recipients. Clin Chest Med 1990;11:291–308.

56. Armitage JM, Kormos RL, Stuart RS. Posttransplant lymphoproliferative disease in thoracic organ transplant patients: Ten years of cyclosporin-based immunosuppression. J Heart Lung Transplant 1991;10:877–887.

57. deHoyos A, Ramirez J, Patterson A, Mauer J. Infectious complications after double lung transplantation for cystic fibrosis. Am Rev Respir Dis 1991;143:A455.

58. Ognibene FP, Shelhamer J, Gill V, et al. The diagnosis of pneumocystis carinii pneumonia in patients with the acquired immunodeficiency syndrome using subsegmental bronchoalveolar lavage. Am Rev Respir Dis 1984; 129:929–932.

59. Golden JA, Hollander H, Stulbarg MS, Gamsu G. Bronchoalveolar lavage as the exclusive diagnostic modality for pneumocystis carinii pneumonia. Chest 1986;90:18–22.

60. Wreghitt, T. Cytomegalovirus infections in heart and heart-lung transplant recipients. J Antimicrob Chemother 1989;23(suppl E):49–60.

61. Smith CB. Cytomegalovirus pneumonia. State of the Art. Chest 1989;95(suppl):182S–187S.

62. Sissons JGP, Borysiewicz LK. Human cytomegalovirus infection. Thorax 1989;44:241–246.

63. Smyth RL, Sinclair J, Scott JP et al. Infection and reactivation with cytomegalovirus strains in lung transplant recipients. Transplantation 1991;52:480–482.

64. Paradis IL, Grgurich WF, Dummer JS, Dekker A, Dauber JH. Rapid detection of cytomegalovirus pneumonia from lung lavage cells. Am Rev Respir Dis 1988;138:697–702.

65. Crawford SW, Bowden RA, Hackman RC, et al. Rapid detection of cytomegalovirus pulmonary infection by bronchoalveolar lavage and centrifugation culture. Ann Intern Med 1988;108:180–185.

66. Kahn FW, Jones JM, England DM. The role of bronchoalveolar lavage in the diagnosis of invasive pulmonary aspergillosis. Am J Clin Pathol 1986;86:518–523.

67. Paull DE, Keagy BA, Entwistle T, Wilcox BR. Effect of superoxide dismutase and catalase infusion at reflow on cardiopulmonary function after lung ischaemia in dogs breathing room air. Curr Surg 1988;45:292–294.

68. Jansen NJG, van Oeveren W, Broek LVD. Inhibition by dexamethasone of the reperfusion phenomena in cardiopulmonary bypass. J Thorac Cardiovasc Surg 1991; 102:515–525.

69. Lima O, Goldberg M, Peters WJ, Ayabe H, Townsend E, Cooper JD. Bronchial omentopexy in canine lung transplantation. J Thorac Cardiovasc Surg 1982;83:418–421.

70. Schafers, H, Haydock DA, Cooper JD. The prevalence and management of bronchial anastomotic complications in lung transplantation. J Thorac Cardiovasc Surg 1991;101:1044–1052.

71. Yousem SA, Dauber JH, Griffith BP. Bronchial cartilage alterations in lung transplantation. Chest 1990;98: 1121–1124.

72. Tazelaar HD, Yousem SA. The pathology of combined heart-lung transplantation: an autopsy study. Hum Pathol 1988;19:1403–1416.

73a. Nalesnik MA, Jaffe, R, Starzl TE, et al. The pathology of posttransplant lymphoproliferative disorders occurring in the setting of cyclosporin A—prednisone immunosuppression. Am J Pathol 1988;133:173–192.

73b. Berg LC, Copenhaver CM, Morrison VA. B-cell lymphoproliferative disorders in solid-organ transplant patients: detection of Epstein-Barr virus by in situ hybridization. Hum Pathol 1992;23:159–163.

74. Gilman MJ, Wang KP. Transbronchial lung biopsy in sarcoidosis—an approach to determine the optimal number of biopsies. Am Rev Respir Dis 1980;122:721–724.

75. Reynolds HY. Bronchoalveolar lavage. Am Rev Respir Dis 1987;135:250–263.

76. Chamberlain DW, Braude AC, Rebuck AS. A critical evaluation of bronchoalveolar lavage: Criteria for identifying unsatisfactory specimens. Acta Cytol 1987;31: 599–605.

77. Nishio JN, Lynch JP. Fiberoptic bronchoscopy in the immunocompromised host: The significance of a "nonspecific" transbronchial biopsy. Am Rev Respir Dis

1980;121:307–312.

78. Katzenstein AA, Askin FB. Interpretation and significance of pathologic findings in transbronchial lung biopsy. Am J Surg Pathol 1980;4:223–234.

79. Jenkins R, Myerowitz RL, Kavic T, Slasky S. Diagnostic yield of transbronchial biopsies. Am J Clin Pathol 1979;72:926–930.

80a. Yousem SA, Paradis IL, Dauber JH, Griffith BP. Efficacy of transbronchial lung biopsy in the diagnosis of bronchiolitis obliterans in heart-lung transplant recipients. Transplantation 1989;47:893–895.

80b. Abernathy EC, Hruban RH, Baumgartner WA, Reitz BA, Hutchins GM. The two forms of bronchiolitis obliterans in heart-lung transplant recipients. Hum Pathol 1991;22:1102–1110.

81. Gryzan S, Paradis IL, Hardesty RL, Griffith BP, Dauber JH. Bronchoalveolar lavage in heart-lung transplantation. Heart Transplant 1985;4:414–416.

82. Shennib H, Nguyen D. Bronchoalveolar lavage in lung transplantation. Ann Thorac Surg 1991;51:335–340.

83. Rabinowich H, Zeevi A, Paradis IL, et al. Proliferative responses of bronchoalveolar lavage lymphocytes from heart-lung transplant patients. Transplantation 1990;49:115–121.

84. Zeevi A, Rabinowich H, Yousem SA, et al. Presence of donor-specific alloreactivity in histologically normal lung allografts is predictive of subsequent bronchiolitis obliterans. Transplant Proc 1991;23:1128–1129.

CHAPTER 25

Tobacco

RUSSELL A. HARLEY, JR.

History of Tobacco

Nicotiana tabacum is America's most famous plant. There is little evidence to support the thesis that mandrake of the Old Testament (Genesis 30) was tobacco, but the evidence is strong that tobacco was smoked in the new world 2,000 years ago by Mayan Indians. Columbus and other early European explorers described Indians chewing tobacco, using tobacco as snuff, and smoking tobacco in pipes and large and small cigars. The name was derived from the Haitian Indian word for a forked tubular inhaler called a "tabac"[1] (Fig. 25–1). The forked end of the tabac was placed in the nostrils while the other end held the burning leaf or snuff. Central and South American Indians called tobacco "zig," and the word for smoking was "zikar." While searching for the great Chinese Khan, Luis de Torres and Jerez, members of Christopher Columbus' first expedition, found Indian men and women smoking cigars on Hispanola 500 years ago. Jerez bears the distinction of being described as the first European habituated to tobacco.[2,3]

There are more than 60 species of tobacco, but *Nicotiana tabacum* and *N. rustica* are the only two that have been widely used. *N. tabacum* originated as a hybrid in Central and South America while the stronger tasting *N. rustica* originated in North America. Friar Pane, sailing with Columbus, introduced the new weed to the Old World by importing it into Portugal. Cardinal Santa Croce brought tobacco into Italy from Portugal in the mid-1500s and Andre Threvet brought it into France at about the same time. Jean Nicot sent tobacco to the French Court as a panacea; the genus *Nicotiana* and the nicotine found in the plant were named for him. To-

bacco also became popular in England, but much more so following John Rolfe's introduction of the milder *N. tabacum*, which replaced the native North American tobacco grown by early settlers and thus established a new industry in Virginia. Tobacco was widely accepted, and its export provided a major source of funding for the American Revolution. Tobacco accounted for more than 50% of total colonial American exports.[4] However, the early use of tobacco was not without its critics, including James I of England, who described it as "a vile, stinking habit." It could have been worse: The ancients reported the smoking of cow dung for the treatment of melancholy.[5] Snuff temporarily replaced smoking in the 1700s and was called the "final reason for the human nose."[6]

Czar Michael Romanov threatened tobacco users with dire punishments including cutting off their noses, castration, and beating their feet until bloody. Persistent violators were executed.[5] Needing money, however, Czar Michael eventually established a government monopoly of tobacco sales.

Indians of Mexico and Peru cultivated various plants 5,000 to 6,000 years B.C. Tobacco seeds have been found in the remains of permanent settlements dating to approximately 3500 B.C.[7] Snuff tubes of various simple and ornamental shapes have been recovered from widely divergent areas of Central and South America and the West Indies.[8]

There have been many unusual religious, medicinal, and practical uses of tobacco over the centuries. Teotlacualli (food of God) was prepared by mixing large amounts of tobacco with the ashes of burnt poisonous animals collected by young boys, one seed of ololiuhqui, and a number of black hairy worms. Priests smeared themselves with this, became absolutely fearless, and

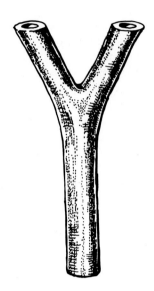

Fig. 25–1. Tabac. Forked tube used primarily for inhaling snuff.

wrought general havoc.[9] In a more helpful mood, North American Indians treated drowning by hanging the victim upside down and performing a massive tobacco smoke enema.[7] This procedure continued to be used at least until the negative experimental studies of Daniel Legare in the early nineteenth century. Among the attempted practical uses of tobacco, along with smoking it to drive away gnats and mosquitoes and applying chewed tobacco to salve wasp stings, smoking was used to overcome the odor of decaying bodies during the Great Plague of 1665.

The Nature of Tobacco Smoke: Its Deposition and Clearance

Tobacco smoke is an aerosol of gases, organic vapors, and particulates. The U.S. Surgeon General's 1979[10] report on smoking and health defines "mainstream" smoke as that which "emerges from the tobacco product while being drawn through the tobacco during puffing." It defines "sidestream" smoke as that which "rises from the burning cone of tobacco." As such, mainstream smoke may have an effect on, and be affected by, the smoker, and also contributes to the environment as the smoker's exhaled smoke. This latter component has been referred to as "exhaled mainstream smoke."[10]

"Passive," involuntary," or "secondary" smoking usually applies to exposure of a nonsmoker to tobacco smoke products. The smoker also is exposed to passive smoke from the environment.

Combustion, pyrolysis, and vaporization of paper and tobacco occur in the burning cone of a cigarette.

Combustion yields products of both complete and partial oxidation, many in unpredictable amounts. Tobacco combustion occurs at temperatures as low as 200°C but rises to more than 900°C. The most typical heating rates during a cigarette puff are between 200° and 500°C per second. The formation of large amounts of carbon monoxide (CO) depends on a rapid heating rate with 90% of CO occurring at temperatures close to 900°C. Thus, the faster the cigarette is smoked, the more CO is produced. Carbon monoxide (CO) and carbon dioxide (CO_2) account for about 60% by weight of the products in tobacco smoke.[11] One cigarette produces about 800 cm^3 gas, mostly CO and CO_2, but aldehydes, furfurals, and ammonia are also present.

Air inhaled through the burning cone and an additional 20% (by volume) of gases produced by the cone result in a stream of gas traveling the length of the cigarette. This stream is primarily nitrogen (N) with small amounts of oxygen (O_2), CO_2, and CO and even smaller amounts of organic vapor. Entrained, suspended, and moving in this stream of gas is a mass of particles that vary between 0.1 and 1.0 μm in diameter. These particles are globular droplets of water with central dark resinous cores. The watery rim contains such substances as will dissolve in water at the various temperatures encountered from cone to lung. The water is volatile at the high temperatures near the burning cone, but rapidly cools as it passes through the compressed tobacco cylinder. These smoke particles, approximately 0.2 μm in diameter, are widely separated by about the diameter of a red blood cell, 7 μm, and would thus be about 35 diameters apart were it not for the obstacles in their path and the turbulence of the airstream as they move with a forward velocity of about 40 cps (some 2 million diameters per second). The average deviation from the flow line for particles of the 0.2-cm size range is about 2 μm, or 10 diameters, which is a relatively violent motion even if moving through the clean architecture of a filter. Semivolatile substances dissolved or suspended in the aqueous rim of a smoke particle may escape through the surface of the particle or alternatively may encounter the resinous core at the center of the particle. If these semivolatile substances escape, they may be adsorbed by surrounding structures, such as tobacco, paper, filter, or epithelial surfaces, once the smoke is inhaled. If the condensate from the smoke of a cigarette were collected to form a single 25-mg droplet, the surface area of the droplet would be about 40 mm^2. However, as it is divided into 60 trillion 0.2-μm particles, the surface area increases to more than 7 million mm^2, or 7 m^2.

The particulate matter in cigarette smoke is commonly measured by one of two basic techniques. In one, smoke particles are collected and measured; in the other, the physical properties of the aerosol are studied. The results of the techniques are generally in fairly good agreement, suggesting a mean diameter of particles of approximately 0.2–0.4 μm. The single particle aerodynamic relaxation time (SPART) analyzer suggests a mass median aderodynamic diameter (MMAD) of 0.46 μm for cigarette-smoke particles.[12] Using a different technique, Hinds[13] found MMAD of 0.37 to 0.52 μm, and refined light scattering methods[14,15] show a mean diameter of 0.18 μm. Particle concentrations measure about 3×10^9 or 3×10^{10}/ml.[11,13] Particulate concentration increases by more than 50% as the smoked cigarette shortens.[16]

Deposition of inhaled particulates varies depending on a number of factors, but probably averages about 50% of particulate mass.[17] Organic compounds in smoke particles are fairly evenly distributed, indicating that it would not be feasible to remove selected organic substances by selective filtration of particles of a particular size.[15]

On entering the mouth and pharynx, the swirling stream of smoke is usually mixed with a following bolus of inhaled air and driven down the trachea and lower airways. Air flow in these beautifully constructed passages is generally laminar, and at some point in the trachea and upper airways, the particles concentrate near the center of the diluted smoke stream, following the airways as they divide. Unlike blood, which flows in a circle and can maintain a forward velocity, air flow stops as inhalation ceases and reverses itself with exhalation.

When airways divide, the combined cross-sectional diameter of the two new divisions is usually greater than that of the parent tube, and as the volume of airways enlarges, the rate of flow slows. A puff of smoke combined with the gasp that follows it may reach the volume of a liter. This liter of dilute smoke, traveling through a $2 \times 3 \times 15$ cm trachea with a volume of nearly 100 cm³, must move at 2500 cps, but the same liter moving through bronchioles having a cross-sectional area of 1000 m² hardly moves at all. A small puff of a few hundred cubic centimeters (milliliters) would remain entirely in the airways.

When mass air flow stops, the tiny smoke particles (watery globes with resinous centers) still bounce around violently because of Brownian motion and, when forward motion comes to a standstill in the to-and-fro of respiration, the particles still tend to collide with the walls of airways and air spaces. Once they hit an airway wall, they are immediately adsorbed and caught in the watery stream propelled by cilia moving back toward the mouth. When particles in the inhaled airstream are relatively heavy, and when the airstream divides at a point of bronchial branching, these heavy particles may fail to make the turn and may be carried into the wall at the point of division.

However, smoke particles are relatively light and not much affected by such inertial deposition. Many particles stay suspended when air flow stops instead of settling out by gravitational pull. This is obvious when one watches exhaled smoke, which diffuses fairly evenly through the atmosphere of a room. The smoker may think "what goes in, comes back out." However, between 30% and 90% of inhaled smoke particles may be deposited. The exact figure is difficult to ascertain,[18,19] but probably more than half the smoke particles inhaled are actually deposited in the lung. "Cloud behavior" has been postulated as one cause of unexpectedly heavy intrapulmonary deposition.[18]

From examination of quantitative models of the bronchial tree, it can be calculated that forward mass air flow during ordinary breathing essentially stops in or just beyond the respiratory bronchioles.[20,21] Oxygen and CO_2 diffuse to zones of lesser concentration, their molecules presumably passing each other in opposite directions along alveolar ducts.

Approximately 98% of smoke particles that land in bronchi are removed by ciliary activity within 24 h. Some particles may penetrate the mucosa. It has been shown that gaps appear between bronchial epithelial cells of smokers through which particles penetrate.[22] This raises the possibility that allergenic particles such as pollens could breach the smoke-damaged mucosal barriers of the respiratory tract, initiating and perpetuating allergic reactions.

Because forward mass air flow essentially stops in the respiratory bronchioles and proximal alveolar ducts, a cloud of particles remains there for a time before moving back out. The 0.2-μm particles occupy respiratory chambers that range from about 200 to 600 μm in diameter. If Brownian motion moves the particles 2 μm randomly, most particles 1–2 μm from an alveolar wall would be expected to encounter a wall and be adsorbed. In a chamber of 200 μm in diameter with one wall missing, which approximates an alveolus, if particles are 0.2 μm in diameter and separated by 7 μm, approximately 30,000 particles would be present of which about 3,000 (10%) might be close enough to a wall to encounter it in any instant. Deposition would depend to a great extent on the time course of the respiration. Particles would remain until dissolved, engulfed by a macrophage, removed to lymphatics, or transported by surface fluid movement to the ciliary escalator.

Insoluble particles may remain for years; most are engulfed by macrophages. Some macrophages move into the interstitium, lymphatics, and nodes, but many remain in alveoli. It is thus in the respiratory bronchiole at the proximal end of the cone-shaped acinus that cigarette-smoke particles have their longest contact with lung tissue. These accumulations of dust are easily seen with the naked eye as small, 1- to 3-mm black spots in the lung, predominantly in the upper parts of the lobes. A pack of cigarettes per day at 20 of mg "tar" per cigarette amounts to 400 mg or about 150 g (1/3 pound) of "tar" inhaled per year. A nonsmoking city dweller might be expected to inhale 1 g of particulate matter per year. About half the particles inhaled are deposited. Thus, the personal pollution (cigarette smoking) is more than a hundred times worse than general air pollution in terms of simple particulates. Persons regularly exposed to environmental tobacco smoke might deposit less than 1 g of particulate matter per year.[23]

Connective tissue septa extend into the lung for short distances from the pleura. The pleural origins of these septa are visible through the visceral pleura, often outlined in black by dust in lymphatics. If the lung is sectioned near and parallel to the pleura, these connective tissue septa mark the boundaries of lobules (the secondary lobules of Miller). Sizes of such lobules vary, and a varying number of acini can fit into a lobule. The black spots marking the respiratory bronchioles are seen near the midportion of the lobule, a roughly centrilobular position. Because centrilobular emphysema (CLE), also known as centriacinar emphysema or proximal acinar emphysema, affects the respiratory bronchioles as well, the black spots often serve to focus the eye on the lesions of CLE.

"Respirable" dust is dust composed of particles smaller than about 7 μm in mean aerodynamic diameter. Most respirable dust will behave much like tobacco-smoke particles, either landing on bronchi and being rapidly cleared or concentrating in respiratory bronchioles of the proximal acinus. Many dusts are "nontoxic," creating a macrophage response but causing no interstitial damage. Hematite dust from iron mining and soft coal dust are examples. These rusty or black spots mark respiratory bronchioles. No emphysema or focal emphysema may be seen within these, the latter only with great concentrations of dust. However, tobacco smoking is often associated with severe emphysema appearing out of proportion to the amount of dust present. Inhaled gases, vapors, and fumes are distributed fairly evenly throughout the lung whereas, as demonstrated, particles that remain in respiratory bronchioles are not.[24]

Cigarettes produce quite a lot of CO. As previously noted, the amount increases with the rate at which the cigarette is smoked. The highest concentrations of CO occur with inhaled cigar smoke; pulmonary concentrations amount to 0.04%. After one cigar has been smoked and inhaled, 5% of the blood could not func-

tion as an oxygen carrier. This is equivalent to the loss of 250 ml of blood.

Chemical Composition of Tobacco and Tobacco Smoke

The chemical composition of tobacco and tobacco smoke has been studied intensively and has been found to be extraordinarily complex. More than 4,000 components have been detected in tobacco smoke, and more continue to be added. The index of any major toxicology book contains far fewer entries.

The pH of smoke from U.S. commercial cigarettes averages 5.6, despite the presence of ammonia in concentrations as great as 300 μg in the smoke of one cigarette.[25,26] Sidestream smoke ammonia is more than twice that in mainstream smoke. Cigar and pipe smoke tend to be more alkaline than cigarette smoke.

From 20 to 40 μg of formaldehyde per cigarette may be present, and combustion of glycerol may also produce the tear gas acrolein, which occurs at concentrations of 100 μg per cigarette in smoke. Methyl alcohol, phenols, hydrocyanic acid, anthracenes, and pyrenes are present. Benzo[a]pyrene, 3.5×10^{-5} mg per cigarette, occurs in mainstream smoke, a higher level than in sidestream smoke. Cadmium is present in concentrations of 12.5×10^{-5} mg per cigarette in mainstream smoke but is also higher in sidestream smoke. Benzo[a]pyrene is known to be a potent carcinogen, and cadmium has been linked to emphysema in some studies, although not in all. Arsenic, lead, and radioactive plutonium from fertilizers and insecticides may appear in tobacco smoke: Arsenic concentration in tobacco smoke ranges from 3.3 to 10.5 mg/m^3 of smoke; the amounts of arsenic and lead inhaled are probably below the level of toxicity, but plutonium is potentially carcinogenic. It is estimated that 1300 rems from polonium-210 would account for cancers occurring in 2-pack-per-day smokers.[27] The estimated smoker's dose during 40 years of smoking, including indoor radon progeny (decay products), may be considerably greater than that (1600–2000 rems).[28]

Tobacco, it seems, may be a unique plant in containing precursors that produce smoke containing high concentrations of carcinogenic alkylated polynuclear aromatic hydrocarbons (PAH). These substances include complete carcinogens. 2-(p-hydroxyphenyl)-ethanol (PHPE) and m-hydroxybenzyl alcohol (MHBA) are alcoholic subfractions that are major components of the tumor promoting component of cigarette-smoke condensate. PHPE occurs in unburned tobacco, and MHBA compound is formed during combustion.[29]

Only certain fractions of the neutral portion of cigarette smoke condensate contain PAH and other tumor initiators.[30–32] Benzanthracenes, benzophenanthrenes, benzopyrenes, benzofluoranthenes, dibenzopyrenes, and alkylated fluoranthenes and chrysenes are probably the important tumor initiators in tobacco smoke. N-alkylated carbazoles seem to be important accelerators. The acidic portions of the condensate contains significant tumor-promoting activity. Alkyl-2-cyclopenten-2-ol-1-ones appear to be active promotors in the weakly acidic fraction.[33]

Nicotine

Nicotine is a colorless oily fluid with an unpleasant odor that is very soluble in water and becomes brown on exposure to air. It is one of the few natural liquid alkaloids.[34] It is elaborated by the root of the tobacco plant and constitutes of 0.5%–8% of the weight of the dried leaf, existing in the form of an organic salt. When tobacco is burned, these salts are volatilized. The faster a cigarette is smoked, the more nicotine is found in mainstream smoke, but an average figure might be 1% of smoke. About 85% of the nicotine present in smoke is absorbed in the lungs, amounting to 2.5–3.5 mg of nicotine. The symptoms produced are similar to those caused by an injection of 1 mg nicotine intravenously. Cardiovascular alterations include an increase in heart rate, blood pressure, cardiac output, stroke volume, velocity of contraction, contractile force, and myocardial oxygen consumption. Arrhythmias may develop.

Morphologic Changes: Chronic Obstructive Pulmonary Disease and Cancer

Morphologic changes include:

1. Macrophage accumulation, other inflammatory cell changes, and pigmentation
2. Airways disease and emphysema
3. Pulmonary vascular disease
4. Preneoplastic changes and cancer
5. Pleural disease.

Macrophages and Pigment Accumulation

Tobacco-smoke particles deposited in airways are cleared by ciliary action and coughing. Most particles landing in alveoli are phagocytosed by macrophages although some, especially smaller ones, penetrate epithelial membranes and are deposited in the interstitium or removed by lymphatics and occasionally blood vessels. Macrophages accumulate in great numbers and collect in the alveoli of respiratory bronchioles. Bronchoalveolar lavage produces roughly 10,000 macrophages per milliliter from nonsmokers and 40,000 per milliliter from smokers. They often contain brown or black particulate matter, and substances characteristic of the soil in which some tobaccos are grown may be found by electron microscopy (Fig. 25–2).[35] These alveoli often collapse about the macrophages and dust, entrapping them. When macrophages die, they may deliver their particulate load to ensuing generations. Clearance occurs gradually in the interstitium through Macklin's lymphatic sumps or continues on the surface over the ciliated terminal bronchioles.

Particles in the periphery of the acinus delineate subpleural lymphatic pathways and outline them in black visible to the naked eye. The geometric patterns resembling pentagons and hexagons are familiar to all students of gross pathology. Less often noticed are spots of pigment located in the centers of the geometric patterns. With mixed dust exposure, and especially with congestive heart failure, the central spots may be of a different color, such as brown rather than black. Pleural blebs and centrilobular emphysema may occur in association with such central spots. Although most dust in lymphatics goes to hilar and mediastinal lymph nodes, some goes to the parietal pleura and even beyond. Thoracic and upper abdominal periaortic nodes may be pigmented; pigmented lymph nodes are commonly found on the superior surface of the midpancreas. Black dust may be found in association with malpighian corpuscles of the spleen, adjacent to portal tracts in the liver, and in the bone marrow. Although much dust is swallowed, it is seldom found in mesenteric nodes suggesting it seldom penetrates the thick intestinal mucosal barrier in quantities sufficient to be seen.

Airways Disease

Tobacco smoke causes large and small airways disease (see Chapter 26). Morphologic changes in both sets of airways are complex and as yet incompletely described, although much has been written about them. At first it seems surprising that so few changes are noted in the trachea. However, when it is noted that all inhaled air passes through progressively smaller tubes, the question arises whether the proximity of the central laminar airstream and the slowing of flow rates does not expose progressively smaller airway walls to progressively more particulates. In any case, the tracheal mucosa is spared relative to subsequent larger bronchi. The same cannot be said of the larynx, which is subject to impaction of

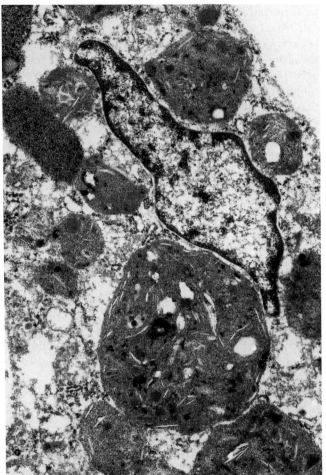

25-2

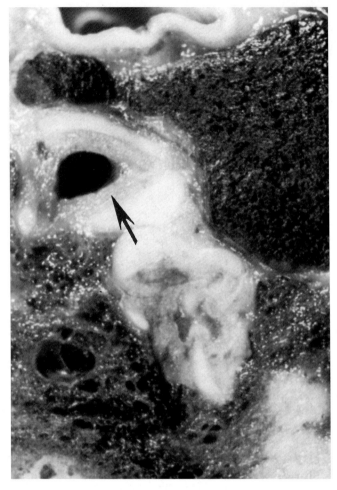

25-

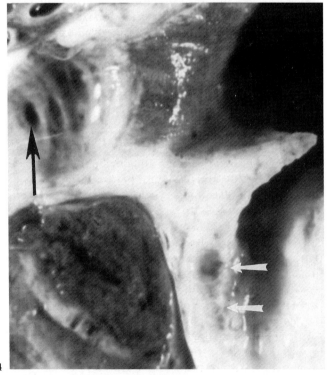

25-4

Fig. 25–2. Smoker's macrophage shows multiple phagolysosomes containing thin, clear-appearing plates of kaolinite. Transmission electron microscopy, ×16,000.

Fig. 25–3. Severe chronic bronchitis in heavy smoker. Note thickness of bronchial mucosa (*arrow*).

Fig. 25–4. Chronic bronchitis in heavy smoker. Note greatly dilated openings of ducts from bronchial mucus glands. (*Black arrow* from surface; *white arrows* in profile.)

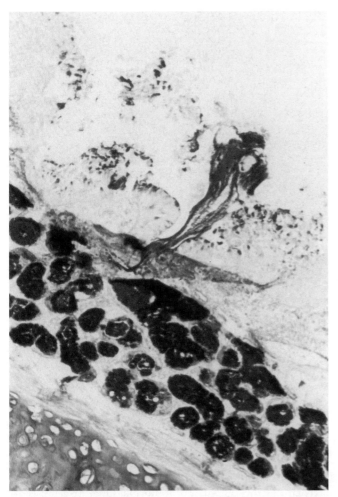

Fig. 25–5. Chronic bronchitis. Alcian blue diastase–PAS–hematoxylin stain. Note strand of tenacious mucus stuck in mouth of mucous gland.

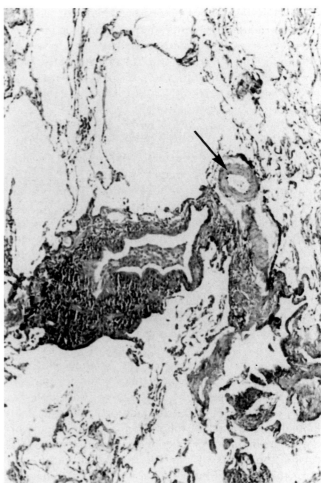

Fig. 25–6. Chronic bronchiolitis with lymphoid hyperplasia and adjacent centrilobular emphysema. Wall of muscular pulmonary artery appears thickened (*arrow*).

tobacco-smoke particles and other pollutants (see Chapter 33). Hyperplasia of the bronchial mucous apparatus is a major change found in large bronchi (Figs. 25–3 and 25–4). Goblet cell hyperplasia may be pronounced. However, more than 90% of the mass of mucous cells in the airways are in the bronchial mucous glands, not on the bronchial surface. These glands become distinctly hypertrophied and also hyperplastic in cigarette smokers. Not only is the gland mass enlarged, accounting for increased secretions, but a relative loss of serous cells and a relative increase of mucous cells account for the increased viscosity of secretions (Fig. 25–5).

Chronic inflammatory cell infiltration may be seen, but the pathologist must be wary of using the term "chronic bronchitis" to describe this because the term carries a connotation of a clinically defined entity: "Chronic bronchitis" has been described as productive cough for at least 3 months of the year for at least 2 years in a row.[36] (see Chapter 26). An increase in bronchial

mucous gland volume and mucous metaplasia in these glands correlates well with increased sputum production, but does not define the precise clinical entity, and inflammatory cell infiltrates may be altogether absent. Tobacco smoke also causes submucosal edema, with epithelial cell damage and increased particle penetration through the bronchial mucosa.

Small airways disease (SAD) is a term used by clinicians to describe obstruction to airflow denoted by such functional events as early closing times, reduced midexpiratory flow rate (FEF-25–75), and frequency dependence of dynamic compliance. The pathologic counterparts explaining these changes include mucosal edema, mucous metaplasia, mucous plugging, peribronchiolar fibrosis, and complete obliteration and disappearance of small airways, as well as "respiratory bronchiolitis" with accumulations of macrophages in respiratory bronchioles (Fig. 25–6). To effect a general change in pulmonary function tests, such changes must be widespread and therefore cannot be evaluated with certainty in biopsy material. Quantitative morphologic methods are necessary.[37] The small airways have been known to pulmonary physiologists as the "silent area" of the lung. To pathologists, they are the inscrutable area, easy to see but hard to assess.

Emphysema

Emphysema involves destruction of alveolar walls without fibrosis. The anatomic classification, reviewed in Chapter 26, is based on the secondary lobule or the acinus, for example, centrilobular emphysema (CLE) or centriacinar or proximal acinar emphysema. CLE is the form commonly seen in cigarette smokers. It occurs most often in the upper parts of the lung, including the superior segment of the lower lobe, which probably reflects the effects of gravity in the upright human on pulmonary air and blood distribution and on alveolar clearance. CLE is characterized by grossly visible foci of destruction (holes), usually several millimeters in diameter and usually associated with a focus of black pigmentation. The foci may enlarge and become confluent (Fig. 25–7). The black pigmented spots seen in the smoker's lung mark the respiratory bronchioles in which masses of dust-laden macrophages occur. Panlobular (panacinar, peripheral acinar) emphysema often occurs in the lower lobes of smokers and may be less conspicuous than CLE but is functionally important nevertheless. Mild emphysema is seen occasionally in nonsmokers, but severe emphysema very rarely occurs in nonsmokers. In an analysis of several pathologic studies, only 3 of 227 patients with severe emphysema were nonsmokers (19, p. 244). When severe emphysema does appear in nonsmokers, it is often a result of homozygous alpha-1-antitrypsin deficiency, which occurs in less than 1% of the general population. Smoking may unduly accelerate the development of emphysema in such deficient subjects. In two brothers in their early thirties who had equally severe alpha-1-antitrypsin deficiency, the man who had smoked for 10 years had advanced chronic obstructive pulmonary disease (COPD) whereas the other, 2 years older, had no disability. In 1861, Waters[38] concluded that a metabolic fault caused emphysema, but it was not until the discoveries of Laurell and Ericksson[39] and of Gross et al.[40] a century later that the proteolytic basis of emphysema was unmasked. Laurell and Ericksson[39] noted the absence of alpha-1-antitrypsin in certain patients with emphysema, and Gross et al.,[40] after finding that papain injected intratracheally into rodents caused emphysema, suggested that an endogenous enzyme might do the same to humans. An explosion of research then demonstrated that proteolysis was a basic mechanism

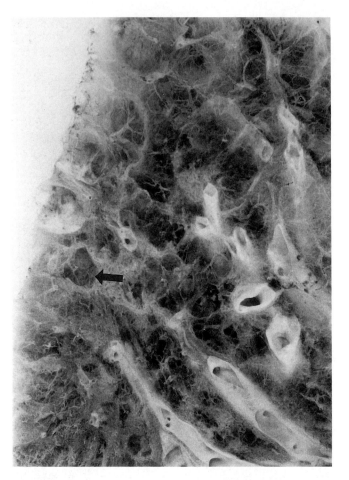

Fig. 25–7. Confluent centrilobular emphysema with focal alveolar destruction adjacent to normal lung. *Arrow* rests on normal tissue and points to focus of destruction. (Formalin-inflated lung photographed under water.)

and that neutrophils, and to a lesser extent macrophages, contained elastase-like proteases.[41–45] The lung, with its catch-trap vascular architecture, is one of the graveyards of the circulating neutrophil. Septic and other inflammatory conditions can concentrate the presence of neutrophils in the lung, and smoking may cause a chronic elevation in neutrophils.[46]

Pulmonary Vascular Disease

Emphysema destroys alveolar capillaries and disrupts tissues that support larger vessels. These changes may contribute to pulmonary hypertension. Both emphysema and chronic airways disease may cause hypoxia, and hypoxia causes constriction of pulmonary arteries. This also contributes to pulmonary hypertension.

Sleep apnea syndrome occurs most commonly in overweight smokers. Smoking irritates the soft tissues of the pharynx, which causes obstruction to air flow and snoring during sleep. Associated hypoxia is well documented and can cause pulmonary vasoconstriction during sleep. Some degree of pulmonary hypertension is thus a feature of several smoking-related diseases, and it is not surprising that muscular thickening and intimal hyperplasia should be seen in smokers. It is a bit surprising, however, that vascular changes can be found in smokers whose airways and alveolar disease is not severe.[47]

Preneoplastic Changes and Cancer

Slow progression from minor atypia to in situ carcinoma to invasive carcinoma is best known in the uterine cervix. Similar changes occur in the tobacco-smoke-exposed bronchus. In the cervix, the squamocolumnar junction is the usual site of these changes. In larger bronchi, the ridges at points of branching and the borders of bronchial mucous gland duct ostia are commonly sites of preneoplastic changes, but these may occur anywhere. Bronchial epithelium is often injured by infectious agents as well as other noxious agents such as those in tobacco smoke. Increased numbers of dividing cells in the regenerating epithelium probably accelerate the risk of neoplastic transformation. Smokers' lung cancers are usually in the upper lobes or upper segments of the lower lobes and are usually associated with emphysema. They may be of any major histologic type: squamous, adenocarcinoma, small cell, or large cell.

Peripheral lung adenocarcinomas show a less definite relationship to tobacco smoking. As noted, smoke particulates and gaseous elements do penetrate to the alveoli, suggesting the potential for tobacco-smoke-related peripheral tumors. It is possible that carcinogens are more concentrated on the mucosa of large bronchi, or perhaps the more rapidly dividing mucosal cells are more susceptible to the effects of the carcinogens.

Pleural Disease

Pigmentation of the pleura is commonplace among smokers, but seems relatively harmless. Blebs and bullae occur among smokers, mostly in association with emphysema. These sometimes rupture causing pneumothorax. Mesotheliomas and other primary pleural tumors are not associated with smoking.

Experimental Pathology

Many experiments have exposed a variety of animals to cigarette smoke in an effort to reproduce such diseases in man. These studies have met with remarkably little success, probably in large part because of the chronicity of smoking necessary to cause cancer and COPD in humans. Emphysema has been reproduced in smoking dogs although the gross patterns are not the same as in the upright human.[48,49] Hamsters exposed to low-dose cigarette smoke or to low-dose elastase do not develop emphysema, but exposure to both agents together does cause measurable change.[50]

Murine K-*ras* oncogenes are activated by carcinogens found in tobacco smoke; G:T transversions are the changes most frequently detected in benzo[a]pyrene-induced tumors. G:T transversion are also the *ras* gene mutations most frequently detected in human adenocarcinomas or large cell carcinomas. It has been suggested that bulky or aromatic hydrophobic DNA adducts resulting from exposure to mutagens in tobacco smoke are responsible for *ras* gene activation in many adenocarcinomas and large cell carcinomas of the lung. These bulky DNA adducts can be found in large numbers in smokers' lungs, and are detectable as long as several years after cessation of smoking.[51]

Epidemiology

As of 1984, approximately 30% of adult Americans and 15% of American adolescents were smokers.[52] Both prospective and retrospective studies have shown, to the satisfaction of most of the scientific community, a clear causal relationship between cigarette smoking and bronchogenic cancer and between cigarette smoking and COPD. The prospective studies of more than 17 million person-years of examination, including more than 330,000 deaths, show an increased mortality among cigarette smokers ranging from 2- to 14-fold the expected rate.[53–56]

The carcinogenic effects of tobacco were first recognized some 200 years ago.[57,58] A number of studies have shown a clear-cut dose response between lung cancer mortality and number of cigarettes smoked per day, with heavy smokers having 25 times as many lung cancers as nonsmokers. The use of filters results in a small but detectable difference.[59] The latency period between beginning smoking and the beginning of a rise in lung cancer rates is about 20 years.[60] A study of smoking and nonsmoking twins showed that those who smoked developed lung cancer about five times as often as those who did not.[61] Fifteen percent of lung cancers occur in nonsmokers. It has been suggested that passive smoking may account for 20 to 100% of these; the role of passive smoking in carcinogenesis is still confusing but is becoming more clear cut (see section on *Environmental Tobacco Smoke*).

Bronchogenic carcinoma is far and away the most

common deadly cancer of American men and recently surpassed breast cancer as a cause of death in women. The most frightening aspect has been the rate at which it is increasing. In men, this seems to be leveling off; however, in women the death rate continues to accelerate at an alarming rate. As the national decline in smoking takes effect, we expect to see a decline in the rate of male deaths during the next decade and in the rate of female deaths perhaps by the year 2010.

Mortality ratios from emphysema and bronchitis in prospective studies have shown an increase of 10- to 15 fold excess mortality among smokers as compared with nonsmokers.[62] Unlike cancer, COPD frequently causes significant disease without causing death, and is present in even greater numbers among smokers when compared with nonsmokers. Studies by Thurlbeck et al.[63] and by Pratt et al.[64] are among those showing dramatically increased severity of emphysema with heavy smoking.

Environmental Tobacco Smoke

Environmental tobacco smoke (ETS) or secondhand smoke is derived from two sources, sidestream smoke and exhaled smoke. The former, from burning cigarettes, cigars, or pipes, is the major ingredient of ETS. Sidestream smoke from one cigarette yields approximately 20 mg of particulate matter, 50 mg of carbon monoxide, 2 mg of nicotine, 2 mg of oxides of nitrogen, and a considerable number of volatile hydrocarbons. Many polycylic aromatic hydrocarbons (PAHs) are present in sidestream smoke, including more than 1 mg of fluoranthene per cigarette. Carcinogenic nitrosamines are present in much higher concentrations in sidestream smoke than in mainstream. The alpha emitter polonium 210, as well as other radioisotopes, is present in tobacco.

The major importance of ETS, however, may be in providing respirable particles to which charged radon progeny can be attached. Sidestream tobacco smoke approximately doubles the equilibrium concentrations of radon decay products in an enclosed room, whatever the initial concentration may be. Thus, ETS increases the risk of carcinoma posed by *atmospheric* radon progeny.[65] In an overview of the chemical composition and genotoxic components of ETS, Lofroth[66] summarized measurements in smoking sections of restaurants as compared with control sites. Elements of tobacco smoke, including carcinogens, were elevated in smoking areas as might be expected. But do these compounds pose a health risk in these still relatively small concentrations? Hirayama[67] found that nonsmoking wives of heavy smokers were 2.4 fold more likely to develop lung cancer than were nonsmoking wives of nonsmokers.

Other epidemiologic studies have generally supported a carcinogenic effect of ETS, and the National Research Council in 1986 estimated that the adjusted risk of lung cancer in nonsmokers from passive smoke exposure was about 25%.[68] Claxton et al.[69] assembled a nine-page table summarizing mainstream, sidestream, and indoor air concentrations of compounds found in tobacco smoke and have studied the mutagenicity of particulate, semivolatile, and volatile fractions of tobacco smoke; they found no mutagenicity associated with the volatile fraction. They estimated that 40% of mutagenicity from cigarette smoke was found in sidestream particulates, 30% in mainstream particulates, 20% in sidestream semivolatile components, and 10% in the mainstream semivolatile fraction. It has been estimated that each cigarette smoked in a household contributes approximately 1 μg of particulate matter per cubic meter, about 40 μg/day in a 2-pack-per-day household. Peak levels, however, may be several times this high. Interestingly, particulate levels in dwellings in developing countries are much higher because indoor burning of biofuels is more prevalent.[70]

Markers of Tobacco Smoke Exposure

As summarized by Jarvis,[71] carbon monoxide, thiocyanate, nicotine, and cotinine are most commonly used as markers of exposure. The first two are easy to measure and thiocyanate has the longest half-life (1–2 weeks) of the markers, but these suffer from nonspecificity. Nicotine, which has a half-life in blood of 1–2 h, may be used for documenting acute exposure; cotinine has a half-life of 12–20 h, which may give an estimate of daily exposure. It is estimated that approximately 4 h of exposure to an atmosphere heavily contaminated with ETS are required to produce the equivalent of smoking a single cigarette. Exposure to the more usual concentrations of ETS in household or workplace would require approximately 30 h of exposure to equal that of smoking one cigarette. Conversely, carbon monoxide is absorbed so much more readily that one cigarette-equivalent can occur in less than 2 h of passive smoking. Jarvis[71] has pointed out that ETS exposure is so prevalent in today's society that most urban dwellers have detectable levels of specific tobacco smoke markers in blood, urine, and saliva amounting to an average of about 1% of the dose resulting from active cigarette smoking. Using nicotine and cotinine as markers of exposure to the more toxic particulate fraction of ETS, Jarvis suggested ballpark figures for nonsmokers of about 0.5% the levels found in smokers. In 1987, 87,261 males died of lung cancer in the United States; 42,748 lung cancer deaths occurred among females for a total of 130,009. Approximately 85%, or 110,508; probably occurred in smokers. If Jarvis' ballpark estimate is correct, this suggests about 500 lung cancer deaths may have occurred as a result of passive smoking in 1987. This is only a small percentage, approximately 3%, of the 19,500 lung cancers that occurred in nonsmokers. Conversely, Vainio and Partanen[72] estimated that ETS causes 20%–30% of the lung cancers that occur among nonsmokers.

Smokers have increased risk of developing carcinomas other than bronchogenic forms, including cancers of the mouth, esophagus, pancreas, and bladder. The total may outnumber bronchogenic carcinomas, although many of these are not so deadly. Tobacco-smoke carcinogens with target organs other than lung and bronchi include the aromatic amines known to cause bladder cancer and N-nitrosamines, which affect many organs. In the 1984 study by Hirayama,[73] women with husbands who smoked developed excessive numbers of brain and nasal carcinomas as well as lung cancers.

These figures cannot necessarily be applied to conditions in other developed countries because the concentrations of tobacco smoke in these households may be excessively high. Matsukura et al.[74] noted very high urinary cotinine excretion among exposed Japanese nonsmokers. Nasopharyngeal carcinomas are also more common in the Orient than elsewhere. The effects of ETS on a population possibly more susceptible could bias the data for neoplasms.

Doll[75] has estimated that 85% of deaths caused by cancer of the lung, COPD, and aortic aneurysm are attributable to smoking; 25% of deaths caused by ischemic heart disease and cancer of the pancreas and bladder are caused by smoking. Does ETS contribute to morbidity or mortality related to atherosclerosis or COPD? There is evidence on both sides. Because ETS can cause an increase in respiratory infections, asthma, rhinitis, and sinusitis, it seems possible that the airways components of COPD, chronic bronchitis, and small airways disease might to a limited extent be caused by ETS. This would especially be true in sensitive populations such as asthmatics. It seems unlikely that the approximately 1% dose a passive smoker might inhale as compared with the dose of an active smoker could cause noticeable emphysema, except possibly in individuals with alpha-1-antitrypsin deficiency.

The U.S. Environmental Protection Agency issued a draft report in May 1990 classifying ETS as a known human carcinogen. The National Institute of Occupational Safety and Health (NIOSH) has classified ETS as a potential occupational carcinogen. Consideration of ETS as a clear cause of harm to nonsmokers may well serve, more than any previous factor, to promote the social unacceptability of smoking. Estimates by opponents of smoking have suggested that secondhand tobacco smoke is responsible for 53,000 deaths each year in the United States, more than motor vehicle accidents or breast cancer. Most of these deaths are suggested to be caused by smoke-related heart disease.

Interaction with Other Pulmonary Conditions

Lung disease caused by tobacco smoke is often admixed with diseases of other causes. In fact, this happens so commonly that it is difficult to study lung disease not caused by tobacco smoke because of the frequency of the confounding problem of smoking. Studies of byssinosis show severe accentuation of COPD among cotton textile workers who smoke.[76] Likewise, asbestos workers' bronchogenic carcinoma occurs almost entirely in the smoking population. Hammond et al.[77] found that smokers who were not exposed to asbestos had about 10 times as many lung cancers as nonsmokers also not exposed to asbestos. Nonsmokers who were exposed to asbestos had 5 times as many lung cancers, and smoking plus asbestos exposure resulted in a more than 50 fold increase in lung cancer. This is clearly more than an additive effect, and Saracci,[78] after analyzing five such studies, concluded that smoking plus asbestos were multiplicative. One reason for this may be that asbestos particle clearance is inhibited by smoking.[79] Much of the scientific literature regarding the interaction between smoking and asbestos has been summarized by Burns.[80]

Tobacco, Allergy, and the Immune System

The tobacco plant is antigenic in man, but good evidence of the antigenicity of tobacco *smoke* is lacking. Respiratory infections are more common among children of smoking parents, and there is evidence that environmental tobacco smoke increases the risk of asthma and atopy.[81–84] This evidence and other aspects of the relationship of smoking to asthma to allergy and to the immune system have been reviewed in detail elsewhere.[85,86] Bronchoalveolar lavage fluid contains increased absolute numbers of suppressor T cells among smokers resulting in a halving of the CD4/CD8 ratio, but absolute numbers of lymphocytes in smokers are actually elevated.[87] Whether this and other such changes constitute an immunologic threat to the defense against viral infection can be debated, but it is generally agreed that smokers suffer more severely from respiratory viral infections.

Habituation and Economics

Tobacco smoking is a most powerful habit and once acquired, can only be broken with difficulty. The habit is frequently acquired at an early age. At present, fewer Americans are smoking than in recent decades, but more young women are becoming habituated. Physicians, professional medical groups, voluntary health organizations, and the Surgeon General's office (in the United States) are leading the fight against smoking, but are meeting great pressure from an entrenched multibillion dollar industry with enormous annual advertising expenditures. Tobacco smoking is increasing rapidly in the Third World.

In the United States, tobacco is heavily taxed, and until recently it could be argued that state and federal income roughly balanced smoking-associated health expenditures. With the continued frightening rise in the prevalence of lung cancer and evidence from more recent epidemiology studies showing an increase in other health risks, the cost of health care for tobacco-induced disease appears to have outstripped income derived from tobacco taxes.

More of the financial burden of smoking-related diseases is being shifted to the smoker by insurance companies that offer reduced rates to nonsmokers. Property losses from fires set by cigarettes are a significant factor costing millions of dollars per year. Smokers lose more time from work than do nonsmokers, which has been estimated to account for additional millions of dollars in lost production. These and many other data can be used to suggest that tobacco exacts an enormous economic toll on the country, perhaps in excess of 50 billion U.S. dollars.[85,88,89] No monetary value can be suggested for the suffering experienced by smokers with severe and often deadly illness or by their families. Even though tobacco helped support the American Revolution and has provided pleasure and comfort to millions, we now see more clearly the true nature of this plant, which is killing more Americans each year than were lost in all of World War II and that has been exported to the entire world.[89,90,91]

Freud was addicted to cigars and continued smoking them even after the resultant cancer and surgery had destroyed most of his face. Alcohol and drug programs are more often than not characterized by excesses of coffee and cigarettes, and psychiatry texts often give more space to glue sniffing than to tobacco addiction. Nevertheless the psychological aspects of smoking and its cessation and prevention are of utmost importance. The best cessation programs are characterized by only mediocre results, and recidivism is more common than not. Like lung cancer, smoking is difficult to treat but should be eminently preventable. Pathologists, among other physicians, have important roles to play in efforts for smoking prevention and cessation, chief among which is assisting health organizations in educational programs. The pathologist is in a unique position to provide material for purposes of demonstration. An ounce of prevention is worth a pound of cure, and while such community service efforts can be troublesome and take a bit of time, they are worthwhile.

On June 24, 1992, the U.S. Supreme Court ruled in favor of Cippolone in the case of *Cippolone v. Ligget Group, Inc.* Recognizing that nicotine is addictive and robs its victim of the right to choose, the tobacco industry may be held legally responsible for medical harms caused by smoking, a radical change from the traditional view that a smoker is responsible for his own conduct. Combined with the national mood, the potential of this decision is enormous.

References

1. Stewart GG. A history of the medicinal use of tobacco 1942–1860. Med Hist 1967;11:228–268.
2. Massie IE. Tobacco leaf—a look at history. In: Recent advances in tobacco science, Vol. 7, Tobacco leaf chemistry: Its origin, understanding, and current trends. Proceedings of 35th Tobacco Chemists Research Conference, October 1981, Winston Salem, North Carolina.
3. Ochsner A. Smoking and health. New York: Julian Messner, 1954.
4. Best J. Economic interests and the vindiction of deviance: Tobacco in seventeenth century Europe. Soc Q 1979; 20:171–182.
5. Van Lancker JL. Smoking and disease. In: Research on smoking behavior, Research monograph Ser. 17. National Institute on Drug Abuse, 1977:230–280.
6. Christen AG, Swanson BZ, Glover ED, Henderson AH. Smokeless tobacco: The folklore and social history of sniffing, sneezing, dipping, and chewing. J Am Dent Assoc 1982;105:821–829.
7. Voges E. Pleasures of tobacco—How it all began and the whole story. Tobacco encyclopedia. Tob Coun Int 1984;1:80–82.
8. Wassen S.H. Anthropological survey of the use of South American snuffs. Enthnopharmacologic Search for Psychoactive Drugs. Public Health Service Publ. 1645. Washington, DC: U.S. Government Printing Office, 1967:233–289.
9. Duran D. Historia de las indias de Nueva Espana. Libro de las ritos y ceremonias en las fiestas de las dioses y celebracion de ellas. Mexico: Editorial Porrua, 1967. Quoted by Elferink JGR. The narcotic and hallucinogenic

use of tobacco in pre-Columbian Central America. J Ethnopharmacol 1983;7:111–122.

10. Smoking and health: A report of the Surgeon General. Washington DC: U.S. Government Printing Office, 1979:11–15.

11. Baker RR. Product formation mechanisms inside a burning cigarette. Progr Energ Combust Sci 1981;7:135–153.

12. McCusker K, Hiller FC, Wilson JD, Mazunder MK, Bone R. Aerodynamic sizing of tobacco smoke particulate from commercial cigarettes. Arch Environ Health 1983; 38:215–218.

13. Hinds WC. Size characteristics of cigarette smoke. Am Ind Hyg Assoc J 1978;39:48–54.

14. Okada T, Matsunuma K. Determination of particle-size distribution and concentration of cigarette smoke by a light-scattering method. J Colloid Interface Sci 1974; 48:461–469.

15. Morie GP, Baggett MS. Observations on the distribution of certain tobacco smoke components with respect to particle size. Beitr Tobakforsch 1977;9:72–78.

16. Keith CH, Derrick JC. Measurement of the particle size distribution and concentration of cigarette smoke by the "conifuge." J Colloid Sci 1960;15:340–356.

17. Hinds W, First MW, Huber GL, Shea JW. A method for measuring respiratory deposition of cigarette smoke during smoking. Am Ind Hyg Assoc J 1983;44:113–118.

18. Phalen RF. Inhalation studies: Foundations and techniques. Boca Raton: CRC Press, 1984:7–9.

19. Chronic obstructive lung disease: A report of the surgeon general. Washington, DC: U.S. Government Printing Office, 1984:422.

20. Weibel ER. Design and structure of the human lung. In: Fishman AP, ed. Pulmonary diseases and disorders. New York: McGraw-Hill, 1980:224–271.

21. Horsefield K, Dart G, Olsen DE, Cumming G. Models of the human bronchial tree. J Appl Physiol 1971;31:207–217.

22. Simani AS, Inoue S, Hogg JC. Penetration of the respiratory epithelium of guinea pigs following exposure to cigarette smoke. Lab Invest 1974;31:75–81.

23. Hiller FC, McCusker KT, Mazumder MK, Wilson JD, Bone RC. Deposition of sidestream cigarette smoke in the human respiratory tract. Am Rev Respir Dis 1982;125:406–408.

24. West JB. Ventilation/blood flow and gas exchange. Oxford: Blackwell, 1965:28–30.

25. Elson LA, Betts TE. Sugar content of the tobacco and pH of the smoke in relation to lung cancer risks of cigarette smoking. J Natl Cancer Inst 1972;48:1885–1890.

26. Stedman RL, Lakritz L, Strange ED. Composition studies on tobacco. XXXIII. Changes in smoke composition and filtration by artificial alteration of smoke pH: Pyridine and nicotine. Beitr Tabakforsch 1969;5:13–17.

27. Radford EP, Jr., Hunt VR. Polonium-210, a volatile radioelement in cigarettes. Science 1964;143:247–249.

28. Martell EA. Radiation at bronchial bifurcations of smokers from indoor exposure to radon progeny. Proc Natl Acad Sci USA 1983;80:1285–1289.

29. Hecht SS, Carmella S, Hoffman D. Chemical studies on Tobacco Smoke. LIV. Determinations of hydroxybenzyl alcohols and hydroxyphenyl ethanols in tobacco smoke. J Anal Toxicol 1978;2:56–59.

30. Bock FG, Swain AP, Steadman RL. Composition studies on tobacco. XLIV. Tumor-promoting activity of subfractions of the weak acid fraction of cigarette smoke condensate. J Natl Cancer Inst 1971;47:429–436.

31. Schmeltz I, Hoffman D. Nitrogen-containing compounds in tobacco and tobacco smoke. Chem Rev 1977;77:295–311.

32. Hoffman D, Wynder EL. A study of tobacco carcinogenesis. XI. Tumor initiators, tumor accelerators, and tumor-promoting activity of condensate fractions. Cancer (Philadelphia) 1971;27:848–864.

33. Hecht SS, Thorne RL, Maronpot RR, Hoffman D. A study of tobacco carcinogenesis. XIII. Tumor-promoting subfractions of the weakly acidic fraction. J Natl Cancer Inst 1975;55:1329–1336.

34. Taylor P. Ganglionic stimulating and blocking agents. In: Gilman AG, Goodman LS, Gilman A. The pharmacological basis of therapeutics. New York: Macmillian, 1980:211–219.

35. Brody AR, Craighead JE. Cytoplasmic inclusions in pulmonary macrophages of cigarette smokers. Lab Invest 1975;32:125–132.

36. Fletcher CM, ed. Terminology, definitions, and classification of chronic pulmonary emphysema and related conditions. A report of the conclusions of a CIBA guest symposium. Thorax 1959;14:286–299.

37. Niewoehner DE, Kleinerman J, Rice DB. Pathologic changes in the peripheral airways of young cigarette smokers. N Engl J Med 1974;291:755–758.

38. Waters ATH. Emphysema of the lungs. London: Churchill, 1862.

39. Laurell CB, Eriksson S. The electrophoretic alpha. Globulin pattern of serum. Scand J Clin Lab Invest 1963;15:132–140.

40. Gross P, Babyak MA, Tolker E, Kaschak M. Enzymatically produced pulmonary emphysema. A preliminary report. J Occup Med 1964;6:481–484.

41. Gross P, Pfitzer EA, Tolker E, Babyak MA, Kaschak M. Experimental emphysema: Its production with papain in normal and silicotic rats. Arch Environ Health 1965;11:50–58.

42. Marco V, Mass B, Meranze DR, Weinbaum G, Kimbel P. Induction of experimental emphysema in dogs using leukocyte homogenates. Am Rev Respir Dis 1971; 104:595–598.

43. Janoff A. Elastase-like proteases of human granulocytes and alveolar macrophages. In: Mittman C, ed. Pulmonary emphysema and proteolysis. New York: Academic Press, 1972:205–224.

44. Senior RM, Tegner H, Kuhn C, Ohlsson K, Starcher BC, Pierce JA. The induction of pulmonary emphysema with human leukocyte elastase. Am Rev Respir Dis 1977; 116:469–479.

45. Janoff A. Elastases and emphysema. Current assessment of the protease-antiprotease hypothesis. Am Rev Respir Dis 1985;132:417–433.

46. Hunninghake GW, Crystal RG. Cigarette smoking and lung destruction: Accumulation of neutrophils in the lungs of cigarette smokers. Am Rev Respir Dis 1983;128:833–838.

47. Hale KA, Niewoehner DE, Cosio MG. Morphologic changes in the muscular pulmonary arteries: Relationship to cigarette smoking, airways disease, and emphysema. Am Rev Respir Dis 1980;122:273–278.

48. Auerbach O, Hammond EC, Kirman D, Garfinkel L. Emphysema produced in dogs by cigarette smoking. J Am Med Assoc 1967;199:89–94.

49. Zwicker GM, Filipy RE, Park JF, et al. Clinical and pathological effects of cigarette smoke exposure in beagle dogs. Arch Pathol Lab Med 1978;102:623–628.

50. Hoidal JR, Niewoehner DE. Cigarette smoke inhalation potentiates elastase-induced emphysema in hamsters. Am Rev Respir Dis 1983;127:478–481.

51. Reynolds SH, Anderson MW. Activation of proto-oncogenes in human and mouse lung tumors. Environ Health Perspect 1991;93:145–148.

52. Cigarette smoking and health: Official statement of the American Thoracic Society. American Lung Association, 1984.

53. Hirayama T. Smoking in relation to the death rates of 265,118 men and women in Japan. National Cancer Center, Research Institute, Epidemiology Division. Tokyo: 1967.

54. Best EWR, Josie GH, Walker CB. A Canadian study of mortality in relation to smoking habits. Can J Public Health 1961;52:99–106.

55. Doll R, Peto R. Mortality in relation to smoking: 20 years observation on male British doctors. Br Med J 1976;2(6051):1525–1536.

56. Hammond EC, Seidman H. Smoking and cancer in the United States. Prev Med 1980;9:169–173.

57. Redmond DE. Tobacco and cancer: The first clinical report, 1761. N Engl J Med 1970;282:18–23.

58. Soemmerring ST. De morbis vasorum absorbentium corporis humani. Pars pathologica, p. 109. Verrentrapp et Wener, Traiecti ad Moenum 1795. Quoted by Shimkin MB, Triolo VA. History of chemical carcinogenesis: Some prospective remarks. Prog Exp Tumor Res 1969;2:1–20.

59. Wynder EL, Stellman SD. Comparative epidemiology of tobacco related cancers. Cancer Res 1977;37:4608–4622.

60. Doll R. Etiology of lung cancer. Adv Cancer Res 1955;3:1–50.

61. Cederlof R, Frieberg L, Lundman T. The interactions of smoking, environment and heredity and their implications for disease etiology. Acta Med Scand (suppl) 1977;612:1–128.

62. Kahn HA. The Dorn study of smoking and mortality among U.S. veterans: Report on eight and one half years of observation. In: Haenszel W, ed. Epidemiological approaches to the study of cancer and other chronic diseases. National Cancer Institut Monograph No. 19. Washington, DC: U.S. Public Health Service, 1966:1–125.

63. Thurlbeck WM, Ryder RC, Sternby N. A comparative study of the severity of emphysema in necropsy populations in three different countries. Am Rev Respir Dis 1974;109:239–248.

64. Pratt PC, Vollmer RT, Miller JA. Prevalence and severity of morphologic emphysema and bronchitis in nontextile and cotton textile workers. Chest 1980;77:323–325.

65. Harley NA, Pasternack BS. A model for predicting lung cancer risks induced by environmental levels of radon daughters. Health Phys 1981;40:307–316.

66. Lofroth G. Environmental tobacco smoke: Overview of chemical composition and genotoxic components. Mutat Res 1989;222:73–80.

67. Hirayama T. Non-smoking wives of heavy smokers have a higher risk of lung cancer: a study from Japan. Br Med J 1981;282:183–185.

68. U.S. National Research Council. Environmental tobacco smoke: Measuring exposures and assessing health effects. Washington, DC: National Academy Press, 1986.

69. Claxton LD, Morin RS, Hughes TJ, Lewtas J. A genotoxic assessment of environmental tobacco smoke using bacterial bioassays. Mutat Res 1989;222:81–99.

70. Pandey MR, Boleij JSM, Smith KR, Wafula EM. Indoor air pollution in developing countries and acute respiratory infection in children. Lancet 1989;i(8635):427–429.

71. Jarvis MJ. Application of biochemical intake markers to passive smoking measurement and risk estimation. Mutal Res 1989;222:101–110.

72. Vainio H, Partanen T. Population burden of lung cancer due to environmental smoke. Mutat Res 1989;222:137–140.

73. Hirayama T. Cancer mortality in non-smoking women with smoking husbands based on a large-scale cohort study in Japan. Prev Med 1984;13:680–690.

74. Matsukura S, Taminato T, Kitano N, et al. Effects of environmental tobacco smoke on urinary cotinine excretion in non-smokers: Evidence for passive smoking. N Engl J Med 1984;311:828–832.

75. Doll R. Tobacco: An overview of health effects. In: Zaridze D, Peto R, eds. Tobacco—A major international health hazard. IARC Scientific Publications No. 74. Lyon: International Agency for Research on Cancer, 1986:11–22.

76. Merchant JA, Lumsden JC, Kilburn KH, et al. An industrial study of the biological effects of cotton dust and cigarette smoke exposure. J Occup Med 1973;15:212–221.

77. Hammond EC, Selikoff IJ, Seidman H. Asbestos exposure, cigarette smoking and death rates. Ann NY Acad Sci 1979;330:473–490.

78. Saracci R. Asbestos and lung cancer: An analysis of the epidemiological evidence on the asbestos-smoking interaction. Int J Cancer 1977;20:323–331.

79. McFadden D, Wright JL, Wiggs B, Churg A. Smoking inhibits asbestos clearance. Am Rev Respir Dis 1986;133:372–374.

80. Burns DM, ed. Asbestos, smoking and disease. The Scientific Evidence. Boston: Commercial Union Insurance Companies, 1982.

81. Norman-Taylor W, Dickinson VA. Dangers for children in smoking families. Community Med (London) 1972;128:32–33.

82. Colley JRT, Holland WW, Corkhill RT. Influence of passive smoking and parental phlegm on pneumonia and bronchitis in early childhood. Lancet 1974;ii(3886):1031–1034.

83. Cameron P, Kostin JS, Zahs JM, et al. The health of smokers' and nonsmokers' children. J Allerg Clin Immunol 1969;43:336–341.

84. Tager IB, Wass ST, Rosner B, Speizer FE. Effect of parental cigarette smoking on the pulmonary function of children. Am J Epidemiol 1979;110:15–26.

85. The health consequences of smoking: Chronic obstructive lung disease. A report of the Surgeon General. Washington, DC: U.S. Government Printing Office, 1984.

86. The health consequences of involuntary smoking. A report of the Surgeon General. DHHS Publication No. (CDC) 87-8398. Washington, DC: U.S. Government Printing Office, 1986.

87. Costabel U, Bross KJ, Reuterc, Ruhle K, Matthys H. Alterations in immunoregulatory T-cell subsets in cigarette smokers. Chest 1986;90:39–44.

88. Schultz JM. Perspectives on the economic magnitude of cigarette smoking. NY State J Med 1985;85:302–306.

89. Warner KE. The economics of smoking: Dollars and sense. NY State J Med 1983;83:1273–1274.

90. Fielding JE. Smoking: Health effects and control. N Engl N J Med 1985;313:491–498.

91. Blum A, ed. The cigarette underworld. Secaucus: Lyle-Stuart, 1985:70–71.

CHAPTER 26

Emphysema and Chronic Airways Disease

Philip C. Pratt

Pulmonary emphysema is among the most prevalent of all diseases. On the basis of examination of properly inflation-fixed lungs from consecutive autopsy series, it is present in at least one-third of the adult male population and in half or more of those men who smoke.[1–5] This high prevalence is partly the result of the gradual evolution and progression of the lesions, which on average probably take some 30 or more years from the asymptomatic onset to the final lethal episode of respiratory failure. The prolonged course also gives many individuals the opportunity to die of other diseases so that the death rate from emphysema is far lower than the prevalence rate. Therefore, the major societal impact of the disease results not so much from total prevalence or deaths, as from the many years of disability and loss of productivity experienced by the many cases who become symptomatic in their late forties and survive with impairment throughout their fifties and sixties. The disease is less common in women, but the incidence in women has increased in recent years.[5]

These principles are illustrated in Fig. 26–1 in which is presented the regression line of the correlation between age at death and morphologic extent (percentage) of emphysema in a consecutive series of 173 autopsies of men with emphysema who had been regular smokers. This study, which is reviewed later in this chapter, was made at the Durham Veteran's Administration Medical Center, Durham, North Carolina (United States). Most individuals with less than 25% of the lung destroyed by emphysema are unaware of respiratory illness, while most of those above this level are symptomatic with the clinical syndrome of "chronic obstructive pulmonary disease" (COPD). The graph shows that, on average, an emphysema extent of 25% occurred in smokers at age 56, and the progression was

linear at the rate of about 7.0% per 10 years. Following the regression line to the zero point suggests that the beginning of emphysema occurred at about the age of 18 years, which clearly coincides with the mean age at which this group of individuals became regular smokers.[6] Emphysema was also found in nonsmokers, but was much less prevalent (11% compared to about 50%) and also less severe, with the mean extent of destruction for all nonsmokers with emphysema being only 7%, in contrast to 25% in smokers with emphysema. Because of its prevalence, the possibility of emphysema should be considered in almost every clinical patient. Its contributory role in symptomatology and prognosis may often be significant even when emphysema is not the primary diagnosis.

Emphysema is defined here as a group of pulmonary diseases characterized by abnormal enlargement of the air spaces distal to terminal bronchioles with destruction of alveolar walls. This slight modification of the definition proposed by the World Health Organization[7,8] is intended to emphasize that the several forms of emphysema are not simply different morphologic versions of a single disease but need to be considered as separate diseases.

It must be noted that emphysematous lungs cannot be examined adequately unless they have been prepared by inflation fixation. Various techniques for this purpose have been described. Those which involve drying of the lung are very convenient for gross observations and specimen portability but provide poor histologic results. Liquid formalin pressure-fixation,[9] used for the specimens described in this chapter, requires that lung slices be examined and photographed while submerged in liquid, but has the advantage of producing excellent histology because the distended state

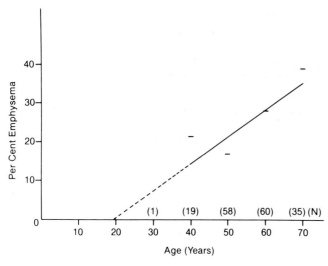

Fig. 26–1. Regression of correlation between age at death and percentage of lung involvement by centrilobular emphysema, determined by point-counting, in 173 autopsies of smokers who had the disease. Slope represents disease progression at rate of 7% per 10 years. Correlation coefficient is .27, and probability that this trend might have occurred by chance is less than .001. Equation for the regression line is: Emphysema extent = .69 × age − 13.2. Values in parentheses represent number of cases seen in each 10-year age group. Horizontal bars represent average extent of emphysema per group.

persists during dehydration, paraffin embedding, and sectioning.

No discussion of the pathology of emphysema can be considered complete without also detailing the accompanying lesions and effects on large and small airways, specifically bronchi and bronchioles. The commonly paired appellations of "emphysema and chronic bronchitis" give credit to these coexistent partners in disease yet also acknowledge that each may occur independent of the other. However, the clinical term bronchitis is unsatisfactory because it tends to obscure the important distinction between involvement of the large airways and the small airways and the separate role each plays in symptomatology and functional impairment. These roles are explained in the following section.

Chronic Airways Disease

Large and small airway disease are both present in many lungs, but either disease can occur in the absence of the other. It is therefore important to characterize them separately.

Chronic large airways disease is recognized morphologically as an increase in the proportion of goblet cells in the surface mucosa[10] and as an increase in the volume of submucosal mucous gland acini (Fig. 26–2). Surface

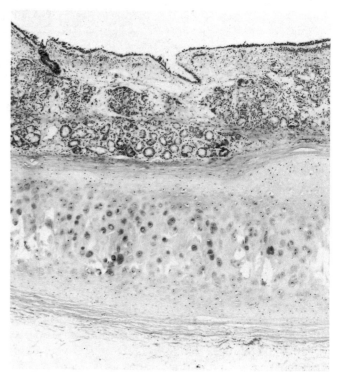

Fig. 26–2. Chronic large airways disease in main bronchus to left lung of 68-year-old smoker with history of chronic cough and sputum production. Surface epithelium has been partially lost but does have increased proportion of mucus-secreting cells. Submucosal gland layer represents at least two-thirds of distance for basement membrane to perichondrium. Note mild chronic inflammatory infiltrate in submucosa and among gland acini. H and E, ×25.

mucosal goblet cells normally average about 1 per 20 ciliated cells in the trachea and are progressively fewer in lobar and segmental bronchi. In large airways disease they can become more numerous than the ciliated cells. An increase in the surface goblet cell number usually correlates with an increase in submucosal gland mass. The ratio of the width of the submucosal gland (bronchial gland) mass to the distance between the basal lamina of the mucosa and inner perichondrium is the "Reid Index."[11] This measurement has been shown to correlate well with the volume of sputum produced daily by the patient.[11] The index is normally less than 0.4, and any higher number indicates gland enlargement.

A common but less constant finding is infiltration of the submucosal stroma and submucosal glands by a chronic inflammatory cell infiltrate, especially lymphocytes[10] (see Fig. 26–2). Focal fibrosis in the submucosa and adventitia and focal squamous metaplasia and more diffuse reserve cell hyperplasia in the mucosa may also be observed. The fact that inflammation and its

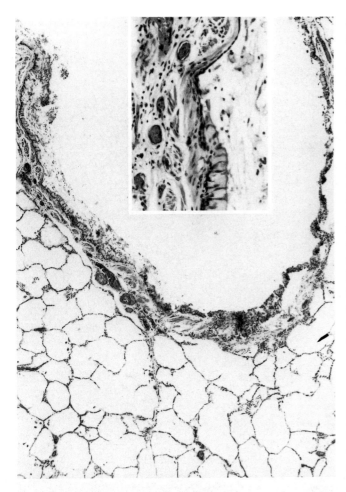

Fig. 26–3. Chronic small airways disease in cross section of 2-mm, noncartilage-containing airway of 48-year-old smoker who had reduced forced expiratory flow but only mild centrilobular emphysema. Surface epithelium contains more mucus-secreting than ciliated cells. Layer of mucus overlies epithelium. Inflammatory infiltration in wall is minimal. Lung was fixed in inflation. Note intact alveoli and alveolar ducts adjacent to bronchiole. H and E, ×25. Inset: Close-up view of epithelium and wall of bronchiole. Note goblet cell preponderance and slight chronic inflammatory cell infiltrate. H and E, ×100.

reactive effects can be absent is one of the reasons for avoidance of the term chronic bronchitis. Recalling that this has been defined as "chronic cough and sputum production for at least three consecutive months in at least two consecutive years,"[8] it is apparent that chronic large airway disease is the lesion associated with clinical chronic bronchitis.

Small airways disease is described separately because the small airways are not necessarily involved when large airways disease is present and can have lesions when large airways are normal.[12] Noncartilage-containing channels (bronchioles) 2.0–0.5 mm in diameter are considered as small airways. Normally, mucus-secreting

cells are absent from this region,[13] but they are present and may even be the predominant surface cell type in chronic small airways disease,[14,15] and mucus is often seen in the lumens (Fig. 26–3). Here, too, chronic inflammation may or may not be present. Careful quantification of the number and size distribution of small airways suggests that few if any of them are totally effaced.[12]

The symptoms and signs resulting from small airways disease differ from those of large airways disease.[16] Instead of cough and sputum production, patients with small airways disease have reduction in maximum forced expiratory flow. Because their lumens are small, any encroachment, either by inflammation in the wall or mucus in the lumen, can produce increased resistance to airflow. This is most severe during exhalation because all airway lumens are smaller in this phase of the respiratory cycle. This functional difference is another reason for separation of large and small airways disease and for the substitution of these terms for the clinically defined "chronic bronchitis."[17]

Emphysema

The remainder of this chapter is devoted to the classification, morphology, and functional effects of the various types of emphysema. The types of emphysema that are described and illustrated are listed in Table 26–1. The terms used are the same as those in other classifications, but the descriptions and criteria for recognition are somewhat different. The result is that the number of classes required to encompass all cases is smaller than in other systems. Other terms that are synonymous with those used in this chapter are listed in parentheses.

Before describing the characteristics of the various types of emphysema it is necessary to review the terms *lobule* and *acinus* (also see Anatomy, Chapter 2). The lobule, as used in the first workable classification of the emphysemas,[18] is the secondary lobule identified by W.S. Miller[19] and represents a group of air spaces surrounded by fibrous septa. The problem in using this concept and terminology for identifying the emphysemas is that, in human lungs, the fibrous septa are highly variable in their prominence, not only in different lung specimens, but even in different zones of a single lung. They are usually well seen in the apical half of the upper lobes, but become less conspicuous and are often com-

Table 26–1. Types of emphysema

Centrilobular (centriacinar, proximal acinar)
Panlobular (panacinar, generalized)
Localized (bullous, distal acinar, paraseptal)
Perifocal (paracicatricial, irregular)

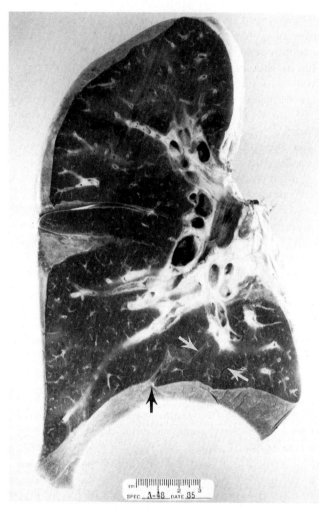

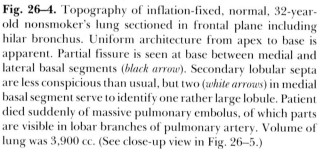

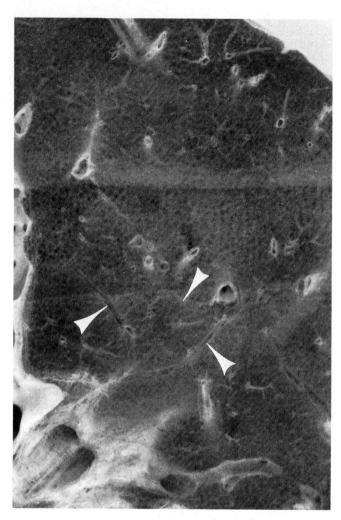

Fig. 26–4. Topography of inflation-fixed, normal, 32-year-old nonsmoker's lung sectioned in frontal plane including hilar bronchus. Uniform architecture from apex to base is apparent. Partial fissure is seen at base between medial and lateral basal segments (*black arrow*). Secondary lobular septa are less conspicuous than usual, but two (*white arrows*) in medial basal segment serve to identify one rather large lobule. Patient died suddenly of massive pulmonary embolus, of which parts are visible in lobar branches of pulmonary artery. Volume of lung was 3,900 cc. (See close-up view in Fig. 26–5.)

Fig. 26–5. Close-up view of area in normal upper lobe of Fig. 24–4. Several secondary lobular septa are seen; in lower center, one lobule is completely outlined (*arrowheads*). Here and throughout field, hundreds of orifices are cross sections of alveolar ducts. Apparent solid tissue between each of these is alveoli, which are not resolvable at this magnification. Approximately ×3.3.

pletely absent in the lower portion of the upper lobes and in the lower lobes. The resulting difficulty in ascertaining the limits of lobules was one of the reasons for proposing the term acinus as the basis for classifying the emphysemas. The acinus is defined solely in terms of airway architecture, is smaller than the secondary lobule, and is that portion of lung tissue supplied by one terminal bronchiole. Thus one acinus consists of those respiratory bronchioles, alveolar ducts, alveolar sacs, and alveolar spaces distal to each terminal bronchiole. The number of acini per secondary lobule is variable, averaging 3 to 8, and can range up to about 20. In fact,

the distinction between acini and lobules is not important for the purpose of recognizing the types of emphysema. Choosing one, the original lobular term, centrilobular, is used here.[18]

Centrilobular Emphysema

The key observation for recognition of centrilobular emphysema (CLE) is that one must demonstrate multiple grossly visible sites on the cut surface of a lung where both normal alveolar architecture (Figs. 26–4 and 26–5) and enlarged spaces with alveolar wall destruction are

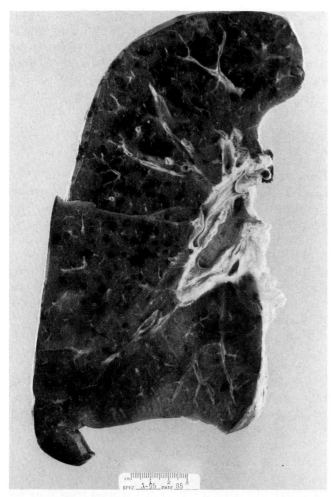

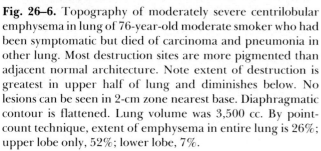

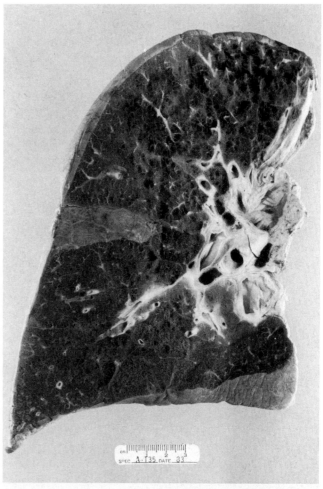

Fig. 26–6. Topography of moderately severe centrilobular emphysema in lung of 76-year-old moderate smoker who had been symptomatic but died of carcinoma and pneumonia in other lung. Most destruction sites are more pigmented than adjacent normal architecture. Note extent of destruction is greatest in upper half of lung and diminishes below. No lesions can be seen in 2-cm zone nearest base. Diaphragmatic contour is flattened. Lung volume was 3,500 cc. By point-count technique, extent of emphysema in entire lung is 26%; upper lobe only, 52%; lower lobe, 7%.

Fig. 26–7. Topography of centrilobular emphysema in lung from 74-year-old heavy smoker who died in respiratory failure from centrilobular emphysema and small airways disease. Alternating pattern of destruction and normal architecture is apparent in most areas, although some lobules in upper lobe have no remaining normal architecture. Lung volume was 3,900 cc. By point-counting, extent of disease is 44%; upper and lower lobes, respectively, are 66% and 24%. (See close-up view in Fig. 26–8.)

situated immediately adjacent to each other (Figs. 26–6 through 26–8). When this requirement is met it does not matter whether one can recognize a lobule or an acinus as such; this definition is equally applicable to the terms centriacinar or proximal acinar emphysema.[5]

Centrilobular emphysema is undoubtedly a gradually progressive disease, as noted earlier, and progression occurs both by extension of individual sites and by development of new sites of destruction. When destruction has occurred in an area of lung where lobular septa are present, it can often be recognized that such destruction has extended to involve all the alveoli within a

lobule (see Fig. 26–6). However, such a lobule should not then be considered to represent panlobular emphysema, nor should such a lung be interpreted as having both centrilobular and panlobular emphysema. Instead the observer should examine less severely involved areas of the specimen to determine the type of emphysema. If such areas show the pattern of adjacent sites of normal architecture and destruction, the entire lung should be classified as having only centrilobular emphysema. In such a lung one can confidently expect to find some areas with this characteristic pattern because it is not possible for centrilobular emphysema to progress to

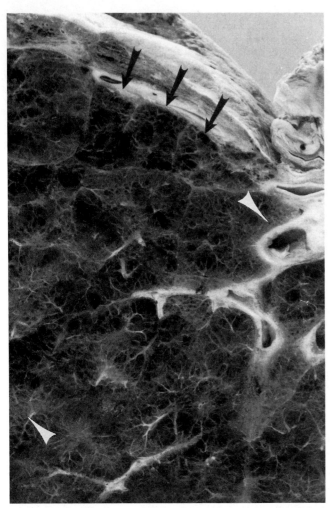

Fig. 26–8. Close-up view of centrilobular emphysema in upper lobe of Fig. 26–7. Lobular architecture is more readily seen here than in other figures. Many lobules show destruction throughout (for example, three adjacent to vein near top margin) *(black arrows)*, while others show small zones of persistent normal architecture (for example, near lower-left margin or cross-sectioned bronchi at right) *(white arrowheads)*. Approximately ×3.3.

the point of complete involvement of all lobules. Patients begin to die of respiratory failure with about 60% involvement, and the greatest extent seen in the author's series of 192 lungs with centrilobular emphysema was 90%. Centrilobular emphysema is usually less severe in lower lobes, and correct classification may only be possible by examining these areas.

Defining centrilobular emphysema in this way leads to a simplification of certain other concepts regarding emphysema. For example, some classifications include a group with diffuse paraseptal or distal acinar involvement with destruction adjacent to lobular septa or the pleura.[5] In this author's experience no lungs show only

this form of destruction, as it is always accompanied by other lesions in the centrilobular distribution. These cases are therefore logically included as examples of centrilobular emphysema. Further, because no distinctive clinical phenomena have been proposed for the cases with paraseptal lesions, there seems to be no compelling reason to place them in a separate class.

Panlobular Emphysema

Panlobular emphysema implies that the enlargement of spaces with destruction of alveolar septal tissue is evenly distributed from the center to the periphery of the lobule, or acinus. This is true at the onset of the disease and throughout its progression to the point of lethal respiratory failure. Further, in most cases the involvement is rather evenly distributed over the entire lung (Figs. 26–9 and 26–10), although often somewhat more severe in the lower lobes in contrast to the upper-lobe predominance in centrilobular emphysema. This even distribution was emphasized in the original presentation of the classification of the emphysemas in which the name generalized emphysema was proposed.[18]

A moment's thought will lead the reader to realize that centrilobular and panlobular emphysema, as defined here, are almost totally mutually exclusive. Even if the centrilobular form becomes so severe as to destroy all alveoli in some lobules, there will always be other lobules, usually in the less involved lower lobes, where both destruction and normal alveolar architecture coexist. Since the panlobular form involves the lobules uniformly from center to margin, even at its onset, and is usually more severe in lower lobes, neither disease can duplicate the other at any stage.

Conceptually it is possible that an individual might have both centrilobular emphysema and panlobular emphysema. This coexistence could only be recognized if both lesions were very mild and the accentuation of destruction in the deeper portions of lobules (mainly in upper lobes) were still apparent. The author has seen rare examples of this combination. Because both lesions are of necessity mild, all such patients have been unaware of respiratory illness and have died of nonpulmonary disease.

Localized Emphysema

The term localized emphysema is used to identify cases in which there is only one, or at most a few, sites of severe destruction of alveoli and the remaining pulmonary architecture is normal. Commonly, this lesion is found in the extreme apex of both upper lobes, but it can occur in any other location, even at the base of a lower lobe (Fig. 26–11). Small lesions of this type are

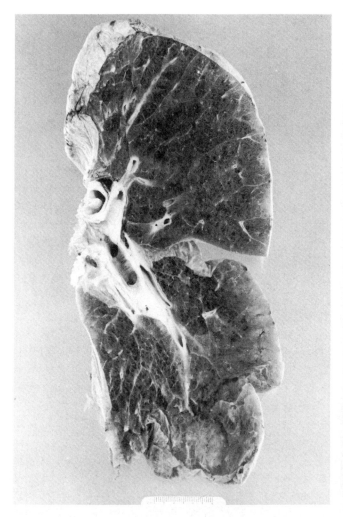

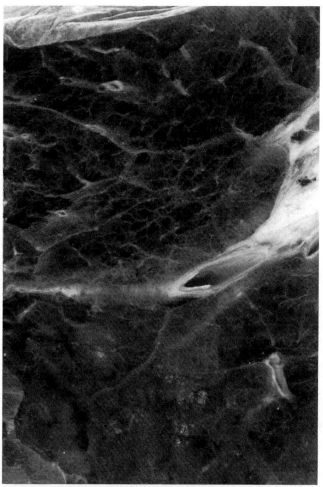

Fig. 26–9. Topography of severe panlobular emphysema in 73-year-old heavy smoker who died in respiratory failure with history of obstructive pulmonary disease. Note destruction extends evenly across all secondary lobules and is more severe in lower lobe than upper. Secondary lobular septa are prominent. Severity of this disease cannot be measured by point-counting because the count would be 100% in either upper or lower lobe. Volume of lung was 3,400 cc. (See close-up in Fig. 26–10).

Fig. 26–10. Close-up view of panlobular emphysema in lower lobe of Fig. 26–9. Note prominence of secondary lobular septa and uniform involvement extending across all lobules to septa. Approximately ×3.3.

usually inconsequential, but may lead to spontaneous pneumothorax and are the most likely cause of spontaneous pneumothorax in young adults.[5,20]

This disease also is progressive and can lead to sizable zones of destruction, often called bullae. The term bulla can be applied to any single site of destruction larger than some arbitrary diameter, often given as 2 cm. Such lesions can range upward to the size of an entire hemithorax. Because bullae can occur in cases of centrilobular and panlobular emphysema, the term "bullous emphysema" is nonspecific and should be avoided. Instead, the observer should identify the type of emphysema (centrilobular, panlobular, localized, or peri-

focal) and add "with bullae" if the latter are large enough to be significant.

In some classifications the term paraseptal or distal acinar emphysema has been used for the lesions named localized emphysema in this chapter.[5] Because those terms are also applied to diffuse lesions in those classifications, such use tends to obscure the existence of the distinctive localized process.

Perifocal Emphysema

The term perifocal emphysema, sometimes called paracicatricial emphysema, refers to the air space enlargement and septal destruction that usually occurs in the vicinity of focal lesions in the lung such as scarring granulomas or other scars from any cause such as infarcts or organized pneumonia. The destruction is not present at the time the scar is formed but gradually

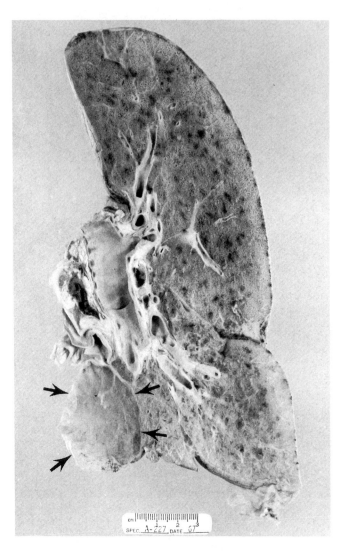

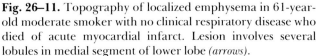

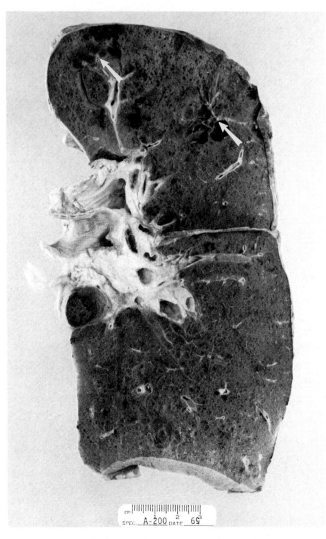

Fig. 26–11. Topography of localized emphysema in 61-year-old moderate smoker with no clinical respiratory disease who died of acute myocardial infarct. Lesion involves several lobules in medial segment of lower lobe *(arrows)*.

develops over a period of years. In most cases, there are only a few sites of fibrosis, and the resulting perifocal emphysema has little functional significance (Figs. 26–12 and 26–13). However, if the lesions are multiple, for example as after healing of an extensive tuberculous dissemination, the distortion and volume changes may interfere with function in a manner comparable to that associated with centrilobular emphysema.[21]

Other Terms

Many terms other than the four just described (and their synonyms) have been applied to the emphysemas. Most of these others have in fact probably been used to identify the disease presented here as centrilobular

Fig. 26–12. Topography of mild perifocal (paracicatricial) emphysema in 38-year-old patient with glomerulonephritis who died of renal failure. No clinical respiratory disease was present. Several sites of markedly enlarged thin-walled spaces appear to surround central dense foci *(arrows)*. A few sites of mild centrilobular emphysema are also present. (See close-up view in Fig. 26–13.)

emphysema. However, the definitions have not been clearly stated and often the specimens were inadequately prepared and illustrated. This writer recommends complete abandonment of all such terms and the use of a simple classification, such as given here, with as few separate forms of emphysema as possible. Terms to be discarded include *diffuse obstructive, vesicular, bullous, primary, hypertrophic, atrophic, generalized, senile, Laennec's, paraseptal, distal acinar,* and *irregular.*

So-called focal emphysema or coalworkers' pneumoconiosis is ostensibly an occupational disease and is presented in Chapter 27, Pneumoconioses. However, it

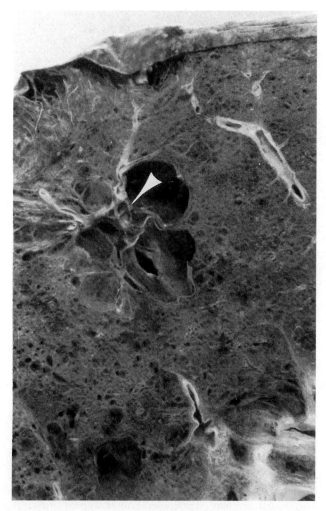

Fig. 26–13. Close-up view of perifocal (paracicatricial) emphysema in Fig. 26–12. Central site of scar formation also incorporated bronchus and pulmonary artery *(arrowhead)*. Although spaces are partially walled, fenestrations and communications into surrounding more normal tissue are seen. There is also some associated subpleural emphysema. Approximately ×3.3.

Pathology

The external *gross* appearance of a lung with moderate-to-severe centrilobular emphysema shows it to be larger than normal, even after removal from the chest. The contours are distorted with rounded protruding subpleural bullae that are often several centimeters in diameter. These bullae are commonly conceptualized as sites of "trapped air" resulting from a ball-valve-like distortion and obstruction of the supplying bronchus or bronchiole. In fact, they can almost always be shown to be in free communication with the adjacent lung tissue, which is demonstrated by applying finger pressure to the bulla and observing that air can be displaced from it into adjacent lung. After release of pressure the bulla promptly reinflates to its original size. The bullae are distended because they are more compliant, due to their reduced elastic recoil and lack of internal support, than the adjacent more normal alveoli. Because the bullae and the surrounding lung communicate, the air in both sites must be at the same pressure, and the bulla distends until the tension in its pleural surface equalizes the pressure in the bulla to that in the underlying pulmonary tissue.

The air pressure just noted is present in all excised lungs, provided the pleura is intact, and is created in the following way: When the pleural space is opened, lungs collapse because of elasticity and surface tension but always stop deflating before all air has been expelled. This occurs because small airways, probably bronchioles, close before all the air is out, and the lung then is airtight so that remaining air cannot even be squeezed out.[23] Because alveoli still contain air and their surfaces are moist, their surface tension plus the small alveolar radius create positive pressure within the lung.[24,25] The same surface tension is also present in the bulla, but because its radius is much larger than the alveoli, air is displaced into it until its wall becomes tense.

The excised collapsed lung with centrilobular emphysema is large, if its pleura is intact, because the intrapulmonary airways close and make the lung airtight at a larger lung volume than is the case for normal lungs. In both cases, the amount of retained air is closely comparable to the in vivo residual volume. (Volume and pressure relationships between normal and emphysematous lungs are discussed further in a following section.) Excised panlobular emphysema lungs also are large for the same reasons. Lungs with perifocal emphysema are less likely to be large, because the required scars tend to reduce lung size even though the emphysema, if severe, could cause some increase in size.[21]

The *subgross* morphology of emphysematous lungs is best observed by examining the cut surface of inflation-fixed tissue with a dissecting microscope. Several tech-

is worth noting that the distribution of the destructive lesions in these cases is very similar to that of centrilobular emphysema. One might be tempted to suggest that when centrilobular emphysema occurs in a coalworker, it is coalworkers' pneumoconiosis. The implication of this term is that the occupation is causally related to the disease. However, as will be discussed, centrilobular emphysema is caused predominantly by tobacco smoking. Since many coal miners also smoke and because there is no reason to suggest that any pneumoconiosis would prevent this effect of smoking, it follows that some "focal emphysema" is indeed centrilobular emphysema caused by smoking. This is supported by the fact that nonsmoking coalworkers rarely develop any type of emphysema to a disabling degree.[22]

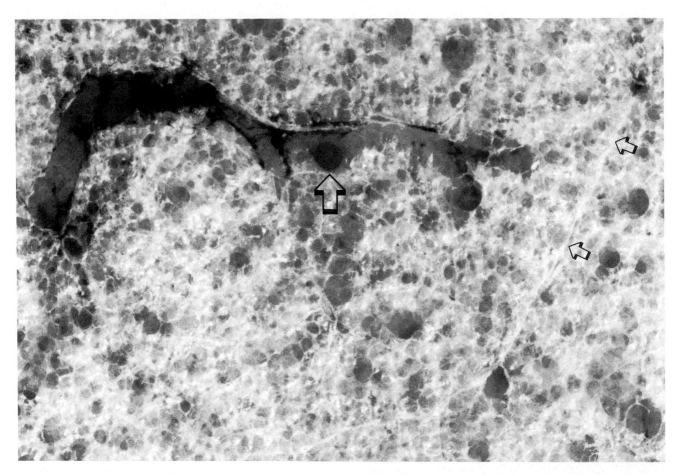

Fig. 26–14. Dissecting microscope subgross view of normal lung tissue prepared by freeze-drying after air inflation. Bronchiole lumen can be seen at left extending across upper center. Round opening in center *(large arrow)* is branch bronchiole projecting into tissue. From this point on structure is a respiratory bronchiole with alveoli on its lower surface. This branches to become alveolar duct. Other alveolar ducts are seen as cross sections; structures between ducts are alveoli. Secondary lobular septum extends diagonally at right *(small arrows)*. All alveolar septal membranes appear intact; no fenestrations are seen. Black streaks are inhaled dust, accumulated in adventitia of bronchiole and associated vessels. ×15.

niques have been described for preparation of such lung specimens.[25–30] At magnifications of 10–25×, the enlargement of air spaces and destruction of walls are readily apparent (Figs. 26–14 and 26–15). Destruction is seen by the presence of holes or *fenestrations*[31] in alveolar septa, which must be distinguished from the normal interalveolar openings known as pores of Kohn (see Chapter 2). These pores are uniformly small and are difficult to detect at the given magnifications. Therefore, if openings are easily seen and vary in size, they constitute absolute evidence for the tissue destruction required by the accepted definition of emphysema.

Fenestrations can be present in occasional specimens that appear entirely normal to the naked eye,[27–29,33] and they also can be seen in areas of grossly emphysematous lungs that appear uninvolved to the naked eye.

Thus, the fenestration can be considered one of the earliest manifestations of the disease.

When fenestrations in an individual alveolar septum are large, the septal tissue is reduced to a network of thin strands. These too can be destroyed so that two alveoli coalesce into a single larger space. Fenestrations are often present in the septa of such coalesced alveoli, and thus destruction creates progressively larger spaces until they become visible to the naked eye. Using the dissecting microscope, one often can see long thin strands of tissue extending across the lumen of such spaces (see Fig. 26–15). These strands often have the branching pattern of a vascular tree, and indeed they are the persisting vessels that originally supplied blood to the capillaries of the destroyed septa. Even the walls of grossly visible lesions have fenestrations (Figs. 26–8

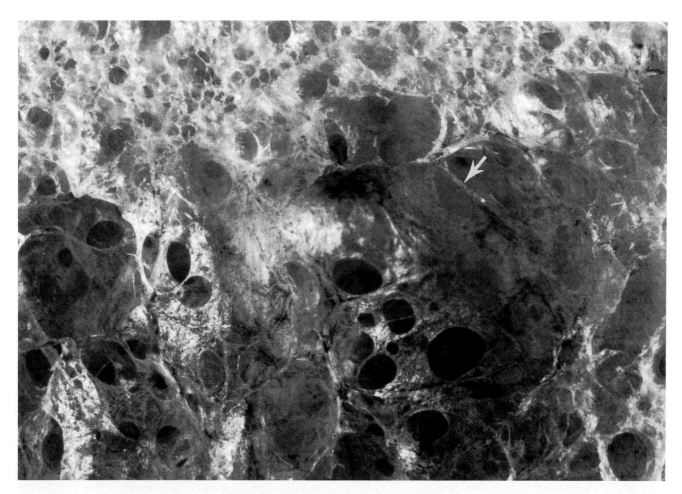

Fig. 26–15. Dissecting microscope subgross view of margin of centrilobular emphysema lesion, prepared as in Fig. 26–14. At top, adjacent more normal architecture of alveolar ducts and alveoli can be seen. Some alveoli near lesion show fenestrations. In lower portion, architecture has been completely destroyed leaving empty space, a bleb, demarcated by membranes that also show many small and large fenestrations. Residual strands of tissue extend across many of these, and sometimes branching pattern of vessels can be seen *(arrow)*. Black streaks are in adventitia of larger vessels; minute black granules are macrophages filled with phagocytized dust. ×15.

and 26–15) and can thus coalesce with adjacent alveoli or adjacent sites of emphysema.[32,33]

The presence of emphysematous destruction is also recognizable by light microscopy of histologic sections. The mere presence of spaces larger than normal is not absolutely diagnostic, because such an appearance can result from overdistension alone. The characteristic histologic evidence for emphysema is the finding of isolated or "free-lying" segments of viable alveolar septal tissue or isolated cross sections of pulmonary vessels. The architecture of normal lung tissue requires all alveolar septal tissue to connect with other septal tissue at least on one end if not both (Fig. 26–16). This is true because all normal alveoli consist of intersecting sheets of tissue and the plane of a histology section cannot produce an isolated fragment. However, the strands of tissue produced by emphysematous destruction (Figs.

26–6 through 26–8, 26–10, 26–15) will often be seen histologically as cross sections, apparently unattached at either end (Fig. 26–17). These structures are viable and often contain blood cells in the capillary or larger vessel lumen. The finding of such fragments is absolutely diagnostic of emphysema. It is impossible, however, to estimate microscopically the extent or severity of the disease from histologic sections because they represent only small samples of the entire lung. Panlobular, localized, and perifocal emphysema at the subgross and light microscopic level all manifest most of the findings described for centrilobular emphysema.

Electron microscopy has been carried out occasionally in emphysematous lungs. The scanning mode, using the freeze-substitution technique, reveals the fenestrations described as seen under the far simpler dissecting microscope. It is of course possible to use much

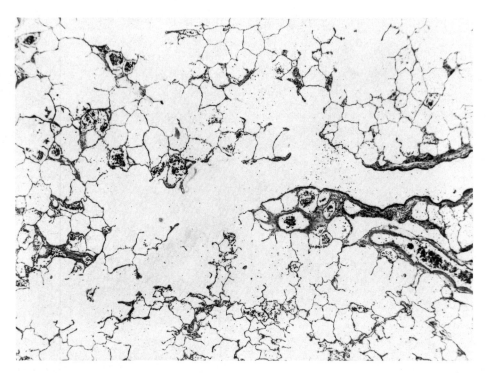

Fig. 26–16. Normal alveolar histology in 56-year-old non-smoker with lymphoma who died of massive pulmonary embolus. Respiratory bronchiole seen at right extends into branching alveolar duct surrounded by alveoli. Note that every alveolar septum is continuous and is attached to surrounding tissue. Septa along duct project into lumen and therefore are attached on only one end. This appearance is normal and does not indicate "rupture" of septa. Three-dimensional status is apparent in Fig. 26–14. Clustered cells in alveoli and in lumen of bronchiole are erythrocytes. H and E, ×18.

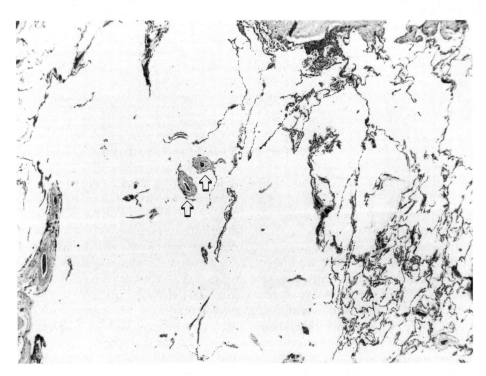

Fig. 26–17. Histopathology of centrilobular emphysema in 79-year-old smoker who had progressive respiratory impairment for years before death of respiratory failure. Intact alveolar architecture is seen at lower right. Central large space contains many isolated strands of alveolar septal tissue and several cross sections of small vessels *(arrows)* representing strands of tissue seen in Fig. 26–15. H and E, ×18.

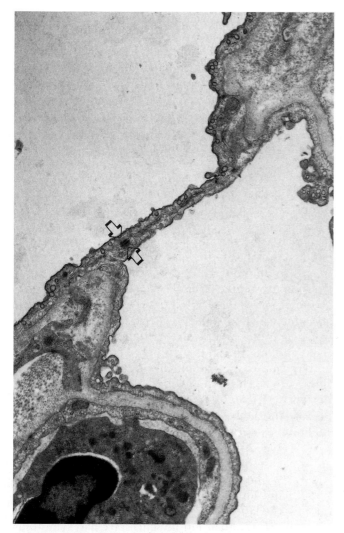

Fig. 26–18. Electron microscopic view of alveolar septum shows segment in which epithelial basement membrane and other stromal components (collagen, elastic tissue) are absent and type I cells lining two adjacent alveoli are in direct contact. They are actually connected by a desmosome (between *arrows*). At top and bottom, all normal components of alveolar septum can be seen, including capillary and leukocyte at bottom. ×15,000. (Kindly loaned by Dr. T. Takaro, Chief of Staff, Asheville V.A. Medical Center, Asheville, North Carolina.)

higher magnifications, but because only the surface can be examined, little of added significance can be seen. Transmission electron microscopy reveals abnormalities in alveolar septa that may precede the development of complete fenestrations. These lesions consist of focal loss of basement membrane and stroma in a segment of septum between capillaries.[34] This produces foci in which alveolar type 1 cell cytoplasm from the opposite sides of the septum comes into direct contact (Fig. 26–18). Such lesions are said to be more commonly seen

in emphysematous lungs than in normals. While it is impossible to observe directly the sequence from cytoplasmic contact to actual fenestration, it seems likely that it may occur at such sites. Sections of completed fenestrations regularly show that they are lined by intact alveolar type 1 cell cytoplasm, which appears continuous from one side to the other. Sometimes a cell junction is seen in the vicinity of the fenestration.

Experience at Author's Institution

It was indicated in the introduction that emphysema is an extraordinarily common disease, and this has been shown in several published studies using lungs obtained from hospital autopsy services and medical examiner cases.[1–5] In these reports, proper inflation-fixation methods were used and background information from hospital records or interviews with close relatives was obtained. However, the classification systems were not consistent and all were different from that described in this chapter. Therefore, the epidemiologic study carried out at the author's hospital will be presented in some detail to illustrate the high prevalence, especially for centrilobular emphysema, and the etiologic role of smoking.

One lung from each autopsy is submitted for inflation-fixation. This is accomplished in most cases using the established system of intrabronchial cannulation and formalin instillation at a hydrostatic pressure of 18–20 cm.[9] The fixation pressure is maintained for at least 2 days before dissection, and a specimen from each lung is preserved in liquid formalin. These procedures assure a permanent state of inflation. Each lung is cut into complete slices about 2 cm thick, extending from apex to base of the lung in the frontal plane and including the hilar bronchi, vessels, and lymph nodes.

Groups of specimens are examined at random intervals after the autopsy to separate them into "normal" and emphysema groups and to classify the emphysemas. This is purposely done without reference to clinical information or other autopsy findings. In each case with centrilobular emphysema, the extent of involvement is measured using a "point-counting" system that permits determination of the percentage of the entire lung volume involved by emphysematous destruction as visible to the naked eye.[35]

At another time, purposely avoiding knowledge about the autopsy specimen, each patient's clinical record is reviewed for information as to age, occupation, smoking and drinking experience, and the nature of the illness responsible for hospitalization and death. All these data are coded and stored in computer memory for automated analysis and statistical evaluation. The following data were collected over a 4-year period

Table 26–2. Effect of smoking on prevalence and extent of centrilobular emphysema (CLE)

Group	n	Mean age	CLE (%)[a]	Mean % of CLE[b]
All	469	55.5	42	9.7
Nonsmoker	95	57.1	18	1.7
Moderate smoker[c]	210	55.3	48	12.6
Heavy smoker[d]	76	54.4	61	16.5
Unknown[e]	88	55.8	38	5.8

[a] Prevalance of any degree of CLE.

[b] Average opf measured extent ;(%) of CLE for all cases in group, counting each case without emphysema as "0."

[c] 10–30 cigarettes per day.

[d] More than 30 cigarettes per day.

[e] Smoking history not recorded in clinical chart.

during which 873 autopsies were performed and 659 suitable lung specimens (75%) were prepared. Information was available for smoking and other factors in 565 (86%) of these cases.

The 565 cases for which complete information was available were classified into three groups: normal (209 cases, 37% of study), centrilobular emphysema (231 cases, 41%), and "other" (125 cases, 22%). The latter group included lungs with other forms of emphysema, pulmonary fibrosis, carcinoma, or other processes that prevented identification or quantification of centrilobular emphysema. Among these were 81 cases with panlobular, localized, or perifocal emphysema. Together these amounted to 14% of the entire series of 565 cases as compared to 41% with centrilobular emphysema. Many lungs with acute terminal processes such as edema, pneumonia, and infarcts without liquefaction were still classifiable as structurally normal or emphysematous and were usable in the study.

Reliability of background information in hospital records is often questioned. However, the data obtained in this study seem to indicate that the information is applicable. For example, Table 26–2 contains highly significant evidence for a dose–response connection between recorded smoking intensity and both prevalence and severity of centrilobular emphysematous lung destruction. Prevalence of centrilobular emphysema (of any degree from trace to most severe) was 18% among patients who stated that they had never smoked regularly, 48% among those who had smoked regularly but admitted to no more than 1.5 packs of cigarettes per day, and 61% for those who admitted having smoked more than 1.5 packs per day (chi-square value, 35.9; DF, 2; $p < .001$). The average amount of emphysema as determined by point counting was 1.7% for nonsmokers, 12.6% for moderate smokers, and 16.5% for heavy smokers.

One further point revealed in Table 26–2 deserves emphasis: even in the heavy smoking group, the prevalence of centrilobular emphysema only reached 61%. Thus, some 39% of heavy smokers did not have even a trace of centrilobular emphysema while some died of respiratory failure with as much as 90% of their lungs involved by emphysematous destruction. Perhaps some of the nonemphysema cases were not inhalers of smoke, but this could not account for all 39% as noninhalers are by no means this common, especially among heavy smokers. Therefore, one must conclude that some individuals simply are not susceptible to emphysema. While reasons for such "immunity" are almost completely unknown, data do show that alcohol use is one such protective factor (see following, including Table 26–4).

In the following epidemiologic tables, smoking information is used on an all-or-none basis: each patient either has or has not been a regular smoker, without regard to amount. Table 26–3 shows data for prevalence of any degree of emphysema and of emphysema involving more than 25% of the lung in nonsmokers and smokers. The smokers are also separated into those using cigarettes and those who stated they had limited their smoking to cigars or pipes. The mean extent of emphysema in the patients having emphysema is also shown for each of the groups. Numbers of cases reported in Table 26–3 are larger than in Table 26–2 because the analysis in Table 26–2 was carried out as a preliminary study while data were still being collected.

In Table 26–3, in this series of 565 consecutive autopsies the prevalence of centrilobular emphysema was 37.2% and that of emphysema involving more than 25% of the lung volume was 13.5%. The reason for quoting the latter value is that most cases with 25% or more of centrilobular emphysema have had symptoms of respiratory impairment during life.[37] This frequency of 13.5% is more striking if expressed in the terms used for the lung carcinoma death rate, which is currently about 70 per 100,000 males. Converting the prevalence of symptomatic emphysema to those terms gives the value 13,500 per 100,000 males.

The differences in centrilobular emphysema prevalence between smokers and nonsmokers are striking, and all are statistically significant with probabilities less than .0001. Note that only 1% of nonsmokers had as much as 25% involvement, and this was a single case among the 105 nonsmokers. Perhaps this individual did falsely deny having been a smoker. The data for pipe and/or cigar smokers are of special interest. The prevalence of centrilobular emphysema falls between that for cigarette smokers and for nonsmokers ($p < .05$ for both), while the average amount of involvement in the cases who have emphysema (23.0%) is very close to the average for cigarette smokers (26.6%). These data suggest that the lower prevalence in pipe/cigar smokers may result from a lower proportion of smoke inhalers in

Table 26–3. Prevalence and mean extent of centrilobular emphysema (CLE)

Group	n	Age (years)	CLE (%)[a]	CLE (%)[b]	Mean % of CLE[c]
All	565	56.5	37.2	13.5	24.9
All smokers	460	56.3	42.2	16.3	26.4
			$(p < .0001)$[d]	$(p < .0001)$	$(p < .0001)$
Nonsmokers	105	57.3	16.2	1.0	6.7
			$(p < .0001)$	$(p < .0001)$	$(p < .0001)$
Cigarette smokers	427	55.6	43.6	16.9	26.6
			$(p < .05)$[e]	$(.05 < p < /10)$[e]	$(p < .5)$
Pipe/cigar smokers	33	65.1	24.2	9.1	23.0

[a] Prevalence of lungs with trace or more of CLE.
[b] Prevalence of lungs with 25% or more of CLE.
[c] Mean extent of CLE in all cases with CLE.
[d] Probability values are located between the items compared.
[e] Probability for nonsmokers versus pipe/cigar smokers is same as this.

Table 26-4. Effect of alcohol consumption on prevalence and extent of centrilobular emphysema in smokers

Alcohol use	n	Age	Prevalence of CLE		Mean % of CLE	
			Trace or more	More than 25%	All cases	Cases with CLE
None	57	59	56.1	25.9	16.9	30.2
Slight to moderate	59	58	52.5	17.0	12.2	23.1
Heavy	57	55	35.1	10.5	8.6	24.6
Mean	173	57.3	47.9	17.8	12.6	25.9

this group. Among those who do inhale and develop emphysema, the extent of the tissue destruction is the same as for cigarette smokers.

In Table 26–4 is presented an unexpected finding that alcohol use tends to reduce both prevalence and severity of centrilobular emphysema in the entire population, especially in smokers. The population presented here consists of those shown in Table 26–3 for whom both smoking and drinking information was available. These data also reveal a dose-response relationship in that both prevalence and extent of emphysema decrease progressively among nondrinkers, slight-to-moderate drinkers, and heavy drinkers. Slight-to-moderate drinkers were those who reported "social drinking," or regular consumption of no more than two drinks (cans of beer, glasses of wine, or cocktails) daily. Individuals consuming more than these amounts were classified as heavy drinkers. Further details of this study have been published.[36]

The other forms of emphysema are not sufficiently common to permit statistically valid epidemiologic evaluation. Note, however, that every 1 of the 20 patients with panlobular emphysema was a smoker. Their mean age at death was lower than that of the centrilobular emphysema cases. At the time of this study, serum antitrypsin levels were not being measured at this hospital, but this deficiency is a well-established risk factor for panlobular emphysema (see later, **Etiology and Pathogenesis**).

Clinical Correlation

The clinical manifestations of centrilobular emphysema include the presence of a "barrel chest," an increase in residual volume, reduction in flow rates during forced exhalation, and reduction in the diffusion capacity for oxygen or carbon monoxide. The ways in which the lesions described above can produce these problems are reviewed in this section.

Studies with excised lungs in which lung volumes can be measured have shown that total lung capacity of emphysematous lungs is larger than normal, even when the patient did not have respiratory symptoms during life and died of a nonpulmonary disease.[37,38] Thus, increase in volume is an integral aspect of centrilobular emphysema, and it does not develop as a result of airflow obstruction. Volume does increase progressively as the severity of the emphysema increases.[37,39] It is this progressive increase in volume that causes the barrel chest as well as widened retrosternal space, and flattening of the diaphragm as seen in chest radiographs.[40,41]

Residual volume is also increased, especially in symptomatic cases of emphysema. This phenomenon was demonstrable in the same excised lungs as were used for total volume measurements. As was noted previously, it was found that when the excised lungs were allowed to collapse from full inflation they would not deflate to airlessness but would always retain air, and the volume

5. Thurlbeck WM. Chronic airflow obstruction in lung disease. Philadelphia: WB Saunders, 1976.

6. U.S. Department of Health and Human Services. Reducing the Health Consequences of Smoking. A report of the Surgeon General. Office on Smoking and Health. DHHS Publication Number 89-8411. 1989:299.

7. World Health Organization Report. Chronic cor pulmonale: Report of an expert committee. WHO Tech. Rep. Ser. 312, 1961:15.

8. American Thoracic Society. Chronic bronchitis, asthma and pulmonary emphysema: A statement by the committee on diagnostic standards for nontuberculous respiratory diseases. Am Rev Respir Dis 1962;85:762–768.

9. Heard BE, Esterly JR, Wootliff JS. A modified apparatus for fixing lungs to study the pathology of emphysema. Am Rev Respir Dis 1967;95:311–312.

10. Reid L. Pathology of chronic bronchitis. Proc R Soc Med 1956;49:771–773.

11. Reid L. Measurement of the bronchial mucous gland layer. A diagnostic yardstick on chronic bronchitis. Thorax 1960;15:132–141.

12. Matsuba K, Thurlbeck WM. Disease of the small airways in chronic bronchitis. Am Rev Respir Dis 1973;167:552–558.

13. Krahl V. Microstructure of the lung. Arch Environ Health 1963;6:37–42.

14. Karpick RJ, Pratt PC, Asmundsson T, Kilburn KH. Pathologic findings in respiratory failure: Goblet cell metaplasia, alveolar damage and myocardial infarction. Ann Intern Med 1970;72:189–197.

15. Fletcher CM, Pride NB. Definitions of emphysema, chronic bronchitis, asthma and airflow obstruction: 25 years on from the Ciba symposium. Thorax 1984;39:81–85.

16. Peto R, Speizer FE, Cochrane AL, et al. The relevance in adults of air-flow obstruction, but not of mucus hypersecretion, to mortality from chronic lung disease. Am Rev Respir Dis 1983;128:491–500.

17. Atsushi N, West WW, Thurlbeck WM. The National Institutes of Health intermittent positive-pressure breathing trial: Pathology studies. II. Correlation between morphologic findings, clinical findings, and evidence of expiratory air-flow obstruction. Am Rev Respir Dis 1985;132:946–953.

18. Ciba Guest Symposium Report: Terminology, definitions and classification of chronic pulmonary emphysema and related conditions. Thorax 1959;14:286–299.

19. Miller WS. The lung. 2d Ed. Springfield: Thomas, 1947.

20. Lichter L, Gwynne JF. Spontaneous pneumothorax in young subjects. A clinical and pathological study. Thorax 1971;26:409–417.

21. Tomashefski JF, Lancaster JF. Tuberculosis–A cause of emphysema. Am Rev Respir Dis 1963;87:435–437.

22. Rom WN, Kanner RE, Renzetti AD, et al. Respiratory disease in Utah coal miners. Am Rev Respir Dis 1981;123:372–377.

23. Miller JA, Pratt, PC, Capp MP. Human bronchial and bronchiolar compressibility measured by postmortem bronchography. Lab Invest 1973;29:465–477.

24. Radford EP. Static mechanical properties of mammalian lungs. In: Fenn WO, Balen H, eds. Handbook of physiology, Section 3, Respiration. Vol. 1. Washington DC: American Physiological Society, 1964:429–449.

25. Mead J, Whittenberger JL, Radford EP. Surface tension as a factor in pulmonary volume-pressure hysteresis. J Appl Physiol 1957;10:191–196.

26. Hartroft WD, Macklin CC. Intrabronchial fixation of the human lung for purposes of alveolar measurements, using 25 μ microsections made therefrom. Trans R Soc Can (Biol) 1943;37:75–80.

27. Blumenthal BJ, Boren HG. Lung structure in three dimensions after inflation and fume fixation. Am Rev Respir Dis 1959;79:165–171.

28. Pratt PC, Klugh GA. A technique for the study of ventilatory capacity, compliance, residual volume of excised lungs and for fixation, drying and serial sectioning in the inflated state. Am Rev Respir Dis 1961;83:690–696.

29. Weibel ER, Vidone RA. Fixation of the lung by formalin steam in a controlled state of air inflation. Am Rev Respir Dis 1961;84:856–862.

30. Sills B. A multidisciplinary method for study of lung structure and function. Am Rev Respir Dis 1962;86:238–243.

31. Boren HG. Alveolar fenestrae: Relationship to pathology and pathogenesis of pulmonary emphysema. Am Rev Respir Dis 1962;85:328–344.

32. Pratt, PC, Haque A, Klugh GA. Correlation of postmortem function and structure in normal and emphysematous lungs. Am Rev Respir Dis 1961;83:856–865.

33. Pratt PC, Kilburn KH. A modern concept of the emphysemas. Hum Pathol 1970;1:443–463.

34. Takaro T, Gaddy LR, Pirra S. Thin alveolar epithelial partitions across connective tissue gaps of the human lung: ultrastructural observations. Am Rev Respir Dis 1982;126:328–331.

35. Weibel ER. Morphometry of the human lung. New York: Academic Press, 1963.

36. Pratt, PC, Vollmer RT. The beneficial effect of alcohol consumption on the prevalence and extent of centrilobular emphysema: A retrospective autopsy analysis. Chest 1984;85:372–377.

37. Pratt PC, Jutabha O, Klugh GA. Quantitative relationship between structural extent of centrilobular emphysema and postmortem volume and flow characteristics of lungs. Proceedings of the seventh Aspen conference on research in emphysema. Med Thorac 1965;22:197–208.

38. Thurlbeck WM. Postmortem lung volumes. Thorax 1979;34:735–739.

39. Pratt PC, Klugh GA. Chronic expiratory airflow obstruction—cause or effect of centrilobular emphysema? Dis Chest 1967;52:342–349.

40. Sutinen S, Christoforidis AJ, Klugh GA, Pratt PC. Roentgenologic criteria for the recognition of nonsymptomatic pulmonary emphysema. Am Rev Respir Dis 1965;91:69–76.

41. Pratt PC. The role of conventional chest radiography in diagnosis and exclusion of emphysema. Am J Med 1987;82:998–1006.

42. Nagai A, Yamawaki I, Takizawa T, Thurlbeck WM. Alveolar attachments in emphysema of human lungs. Am Rev Respir Dis 1991;144:888–891.

43. Dayman H. Mechanics of air flow in health and disease. J Clin Invest 1951;30:1175–1190.

44. Pratt PC, Klugh GA. Intrapulmonary radial traction: measured. US Public Health Serv Rep 1968;1717:125–137.

45. Pratt PC. Intrapulmonary radial traction. In: Bouhuys A, ed. Airway dynamics: Physiology and pharmacology. Springfield: Thomas, 1970:109–122.

46. Hentel W, Longfield AH, Vincent TN, Filley GF, Mitchell RS. Fatal chronic bronchitis. Am Rev Respir Dis 1963; 87:216–224.

47. Pratt PC, Thong-Yai K. The relative importance of bronchiolitis and extent of centrilobular emphysema in pulmonary ventilatory interference. US Public Health Serv Rep 1967;1787:339–356.

48. Forster RE. Diffusion of gases. In: Fenn WO, Balen H, eds. Handbook of physiology, Section 3, Respiration. Vol. 1. Washington DC: American Physiological Society, 1964:839–872.

49. Thurlbeck WM. Internal surface area and other measurements in emphysema. Thorax 1967;22:483–496.

50. Jenkins DE, Greenberg SD, Boushy SF. Correlation of morphologic emphysema and pulmonary function parameters. Trans Assoc Am Physicians 1965;107:50–63.

51. Gelb AF, Gold WM, Wright RR, Breech HR, Nadel JA. Physiologic diagnosis of clinically unsuspected pulmonary emphysema. Am Rev Respir Dis 1973;107:50–63.

52. Anderson JA, Dunnill MS, Ryder RC. Dependence of the incidence of emphysema on smoking history, age and sex. Thorax 1972;27:547–551.

53. Thurlbeck WM, Ryder RC, Sternby N. A comparative study of the severity of emphysema in necropsy populations in three different countries. Am Rev Respir Dis 1974;109:239–248.

54. Laurell CB, Eriksson S. The electrophoretic alpha 1-globulin pattern of serum in alpha 1-antitrypsin deficiency. Scand J Clin Lab Invest 1963;15:132–140.

55. Gross P, Pfitzer EA, Toker E, Babyak MA, Kaschak M. Experimental emphysema. Its production with papain in normal and silicotic rats. Arch Environ Health 1965; 11:50–58.

56. Snider GL. The pathogenesis of emphysema. Twenty years of progress. Am Rev Respir Dis 1981;124:321–324.

57. Cohen AB, ed. Proteases and antiproteases in the lung. Am Rev Respir Dis 1983;127(Part 2):S2–S59 (suppl).

58. Janoff A. Elastases and emphysema: current assessment of the protease–antiproteast hypothesis. Am Rev Respir Dis 1985;132:417–433.

59. Morrow PE, Gibb FR, Giazioglu KM. A study of particulate clearance from the human lungs. Am Rev Respir Dis 1967;96:1209–1221.

60. Sachs CW, Christensen RH, Pratt PC, Lynn WS. Neutrophil elastase activity and superoxide production are diminished in neutrophils of alcoholics. Am Rev Respir Dis 1990;141:1249–1256.

CHAPTER 27

Pneumoconioses, Mineral and Vegetable

Victor L. Roggli and John D. Shelburne

The term *pneumoconiosis*, originally coined by Zenker,[1] literally means dust in the lung. Because various types of dust can be found in the lungs of virtually all adults, this term has come to mean the accumulation of abnormal amounts of dust in the lungs and the pathologic response to this dust. A great variety of dust particles have been identified which, when inhaled in sufficient amounts, are capable of producing disease in man. The sources of these particles are diverse, ranging from occupational to environmental exposures. Factors important in determining the pathologic response to a given dust exposure include the number, size, and physiochemical properties of the inhaled particles; the route and efficiency of clearance of the particles from the respiratory tract; the nature and intensity of the host's inflammatory response to the particles deposited in the lung; the duration of the exposure and interval since initial exposure; and interactions between the inhaled particles from multiple sources and other environmental pollutants, such as cigarette smoke.

Deposition and subsequent clearance of particles from the lung is extremely important in determining the pathologic response to a given particulate exposure. Particles that have the greatest probability of deposition and retention in the air-exchanging portions of the lung are in the size range of 1 to 5 μm. These particles deposit primarily by inertial impaction at bronchial, bronchiolar, or alveolar duct bifurcations.[2] Particles less than 0.5 μm in maximum dimension are deposited by diffusion and Brownian motion; particles greater than 10 μm in diameter are largely removed by impaction in the nasopharynx and gravitational settling. Deposition patterns may be quite different for nose versus mouth breathing, and are also influenced by tidal volume and respiratory rate. Clearance of deposited particles occurs via the mucociliary escalator for particles deposited on ciliated surfaces and by alveolar macrophage phagocytosis, epithelial uptake and translocation to the interstitium, or lymphatic drainage for particles deposited in the air-exchanging regions. Dissolution may also be important for particle clearance, although this process is very slow for most inhaled inorganic particulates. Nevertheless, this mechanism of removal may be important for particles trapped in the interstitium, where residence time may be prolonged. The relative importance of the various mechanisms for particle clearance depends on the anatomic site of particle deposition, particle solubility, and efficiency of the host's phagocytic system. Various factors such as cigarette smoking interfere with particle clearance from the lower respiratory tract.[3]

A wide variety of pathologic reactions to inhaled dusts have been described ranging from a minimal response (nuisance dusts) to florid and lethal scarring of the lung parenchyma. This chapter presents a survey of lung diseases related to exposure to mineral and metallic particles and to vegetable dusts, with emphasis on specific diagnostic features and differential diagnosis from pathologically similar conditions; asbestos-associated diseases (Chapter 28) and hypersensitivity pneumonitis (Chapter 18) are discussed elsewhere in this volume. At the end of the chapter is presented a summary of special diagnostic procedures useful in investigating known or suspected mineral pneumoconioses.

Silicosis

Silica is the mineralogic term for the oxide of the element *silicon*—SiO_2. Silica occurs in both crystalline and amorphous forms. Crystalline polymorphs of silica

Table 27–1. Occupations with exposure to crystalline silica[a]

Sandblasting
Quarry work
Stone masonary
Pottery and ceramic manufacture
Boiler scaling
Fire-brick manufacturing
Abrasive powder manufacture
Foundry work, molding and grinding
Mining: coal, copper, gold, graphite, lead, mica, tin

[a] Modified with permission from Spencer H, ed. The pneumoconioses and other occupational lung diseases. In: Pathology of the lung, 4th Ed., Vol. 1. Copyright 1985, Pergamon Books Ltd.

include quartz, tridymite, cristobalite, coesite, and stishovite.[4] Quartz is by far the most common of these, and is one of the most common components of the earth's crust. Diatomaceous earth is a familiar example of amorphous (noncrystalline) silica. *Silicates*, on the other hand, are higher oxidized forms of the element silicon (SiO_4) combined with various metallic cations.

When one considers the abundance of silica in the earth's crust, it is not surprising that exposure to crystalline silica occurs in many types of mining operations. An important source of exposure in the past has been sandblasting. The severe toxicity of the dust generated in this procedure has led to the development of a number of abrasive substitutes. A partial listing of some important occupational sources of silica exposure[5] is provided in Table 27–1. Silica also occurs in a biogenic form (phytoliths) in some plants[6] and has been identified in urban air samples and tobacco smoke.[7] Silica is often a component of coal dust as well (see later discussion).

The biologic activity of silica particles is complex and depends on a number of particle and host factors. Crystalline forms of silica are much more toxic than amorphous forms.[8] Particle size is important; quartz particles in the size range of 0.5–2.0 μm are the most fibrogenic. The presence of impurities within the crystal, such as iron or aluminum, reduces its toxicity. Quartz particles often contain a soluble amorphous surface layer, the Beilby layer, which reduces their biologic activity. The toxicity of quartz particles is enhanced when this layer is removed by acid washing or when freshly cleaved crystal surfaces are exposed (as in sandblasting). Tridymite, which is the most fibrogenic form of crystalline silica, lacks a Beilby layer.[4]

Current concepts of the mechanism of tissue injury by crystalline silica have focused on surface activity of the crystal. SiOH groups on the hydrated surface of the crystal are thought to form hydrogen bonds with cellular macromolecules, including phospholipids and pro-

teins. This bonding can lead to protein denaturation and damage to lipid membranes. Free radical generation from freshly fractured silica particles may also play a role in silica–induced cytotoxicity.[9] The alveolar macrophage is central in the tissue injury caused by silica. Phagocytized silica particles interact with lysosomal and/or plasmalemmal membranes of the macrophage, leading to cell injury and death. Injured or dying macrophages release a soluble protein factor that stimulates fibroblast proliferation and collagen synthesis.[10] Direct interaction between silica and fibroblasts may be important as well.[11] Immunologic factors resulting from exposure of antigenic sites of denatured proteins have been suggested to play a role in the pathogenesis of silica-related tissue injury.[4] The silicic acid theory of tissue damage by silica is untenable, because amorphous silica, which produces silicic acid most readily, is the least active biologically.[4]

Silicosis is the pulmonary disease that results from exposure to crystalline silica, often not becoming manifest until 20–40 years after the initial exposure. The disease may develop after only 10–15 years and occasionally occurs more acutely in individuals with particularly heavy exposures. The characteristic lesion is the hyalinized nodule, which ranges in size from a few millimeters to more than a centimeter in diameter. The lesions are firm, spherical, and slate gray to black in appearance, depending on what other dusts were inhaled along with the silica, and may be found anywhere in the lung, although they tend to be more numerous in the upper lobes. The nodules may coalesce to form black, irregular firm masses 2 cm or more in maximum dimension, usually in the upper lobes and often bilaterally. These coalescent lesions are referred to as conglomerate silicosis. Such masses may cavitate centrally as a result of ischemia (Fig. 27–1), although when this occurs, superimposed tuberculosis should be suspected (see later). Perifocal emphysema may be identified adjacent to fibrotic lesions. Nodules often extend to the pleura, and there may be extensive pleural adhesions.[12]

Hilar lymph nodes are virtually always involved in silicosis. Abnormalities in the hilar nodes may be found in the absence of parenchymal nodules, especially in early or mild disease. The lymph nodes are black, enlarged, and have an extremely firm consistency similar to that of vulcanized rubber. Calcifications may be present, and may result in the familiar radiographic appearance of "eggshell" calcification of hilar nodes. This radiographic finding may be diagnostic of silicosis, especially when combined with the presence of small rounded opacities in the upper lung zones. Extrathoracic lesions may also be found, especially in cases with heavy and prolonged exposures.[13] The most common sites for extrathoracic silicotic nodules are spleen, liver,

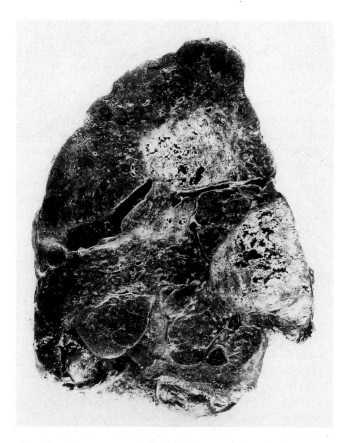

Fig. 27–1. Gross photograph of conglomerate silicosis with ischemic cavitation. This patient used abrasive powders containing silica to polish bathroom fixtures. (Courtesy Dr. S.D. Greenberg, Houston, Texas.)

bone marrow, and abdominal nodes. The silica particles producing these lesions are transported from the lung to extrathoracic sites hematogenously or through lymphatics, where they are then phagocytized by fixed tissue histiocytes in the spleen, liver, bone marrow, or lymph nodes.

Silicotic nodules are characterized histologically by concentric, acellular, whorled bundles of dense hyalinized collagen fibers (Fig. 27–2). Calcification may be present, and variable amounts of black pigment are present centrally or at the periphery.[12] The nodules often occur in perivascular or peribronchiolar locations but may occur anywhere within the lung parenchyma. The appearance within lymph nodes is identical. Silicotic nodules must be distinguished microscopically from old healed tuberculous or fungal granulomas. The differential diagnostic features are summarized in Table 27–2. Examination of sections with polarized light is of limited use in this regard, because silica particles are weakly birefringent and small particles in tissue sections may be difficult or impossible to visualize.[14]

The brightly birefringement, platy or needle-shaped particles sometimes seen in silicotic nodules are not silica but silicate particles, which are inhaled along with the silica dust. Conglomerate silicosis shows more extensive fibrosis, sometimes with ischemic cavitation. Examination of elastin stains may demonstrate obliterated vessels, which in turn are responsible for the ischemic necrosis.[12]

An unusual reaction to silica dust is alveolar lipoproteinosis. This consists of abundant granular eosinophilic material that accumulates in the alveolar spaces (Fig. 27–3), and is identical morphologically to idiopathic pulmonary alveolar proteinosis (see Chapter 22). The eosinophilic material stains positively with periodic acid–Schiff (PAS) but negatively with alcian blue. This disease occurs in some individuals within a few years of intense exposures to very fine silica particles, and many of the reported cases have been in sandblasters.[15] The lesion has also been reproduced in experimental animals exposed to high levels of silica dust.[16] The lungs become consolidated with proteinaceous material that chemically resembles surfactant but lacks surface-tension-reducing properties. It is postulated that the dust injures macrophages and alveolar epithelium, altering surfactant production or degradation or both. A similar lesion has been reported in an individual exposed to high levels of fine aluminum dust.[17] The diagnosis of alveolar proteinosis should prompt an investigation into the patient's occupational history.

Patients with simple silicosis are often asymptomatic, and may even have normal chest radiographs.[18] However, conglomerate silicosis is often associated with restrictive changes on pulmonary function tests, perifocal emphysema, and hypoxia. Pulmonary hypertension and cor pulmonale may then supervene. Patients with silicosis have impaired resistance to tubercle bacilli, with 0.5%–5.0% of cases complicated by tuberculosis. Conglomerate silicosis may be complicated by tuberculosis in 40%–60% of cases.[12] Cavitary lesions in patients with silicosis should always raise the possibility of tuberculosis. Impaired resistance to tubercle bacilli may be caused by silica-induced injury to macrophages, which then are unable to contain and kill the organisms.

A currently controversial issue is the putative association between silica dust exposure and bronchogenic carcinoma in humans.[19,20] Such an association has been suggested in a number of epidemiologic studies. However, most of these studies have not been properly controlled for confounding factors, such as cigarette-smoking among exposed workers or radon exposure in underground mining operations.[21] It is the authors' opinion that current evidence is inconclusive with regard to a causal association between silica exposure and bronchogenic carcinoma in humans.

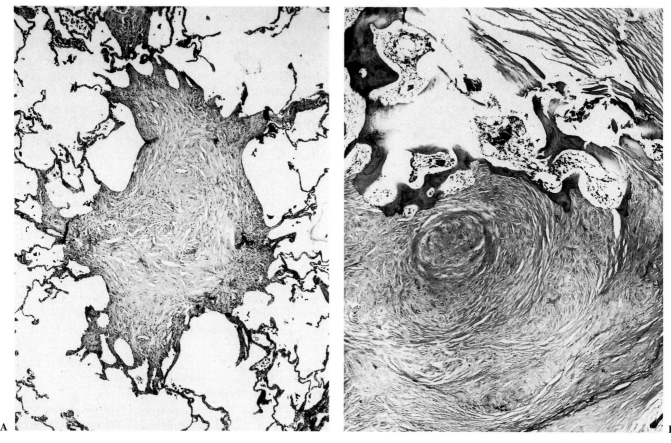

Fig. 27–2 A,B. A. Silicotic nodule in lung parenchyma. Note slight adjacent perifocal emphysema. **B.** Silicotic nodule in hilar lymph node with focal osseous metaplasia.

Table 27–2. Differentiating pathologic features for silicotic nodules, coal workers' pneumoconiotic (CWP) nodules, and healed tuberculous or fungal granulomas

	Healed granuloma	Silicotic nodule	CWP nodule
Location	Unilateral, often solitary	Bilateral, multiple	Bilateral, multiple
Pigment	Absent to slight	Slight to moderate	Marked
Caseous necrosis	Often present	Absent	Absent
Giant cells	Usually present	Rarely present	Rarely present
Silica particles[a]	Scant	Numerous	Numerous
Occupational exposure to silica	None[b]	Yes	Yes[c]

[a] Best demonstrated by electron microscopy. See section on particle analysis.

[b] Note: Tuberculosis may complicate silicosis or coalworkers' pneumoconiosis, as is suggested by the presence of caseous necrosis and more than occasional giant cells in association with otherwise typical lesions of silicosis or coalworkers' pneumoconiosis.

[c] Certain types of coal dust may contain up to 3% silica be weight, and mine dust may contain even more. See text.

Coalworkers' Pneumoconiosis

Coal dust consists mainly of amorphous, noncrystalline carbon together with varying amounts of crystalline silica (quartz), kaolin, mica, and other silicates. The quartz content of coal dust is an important determinant of the pathologic response. The content varies from one mine to another, with anthracite (hard) coal usually containing a higher percentage than bituminous (soft) coal. Quartz exposure also varies with different jobs within a mine. For instance, individuals engaged in drilling into the ceiling of a shaft or in construction of communicating shafts between adjacent coal seams are exposed to higher levels of crystalline silica than individuals working at the coal face or loading coal for transport. Although quartz is highly fibrogenic, amor-

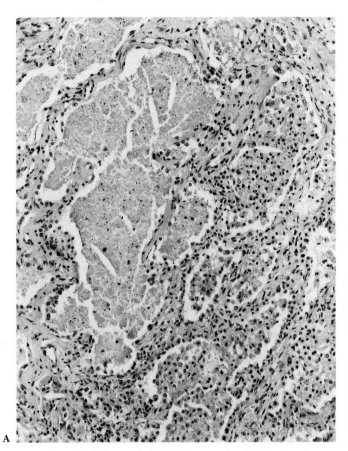

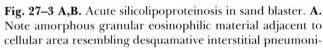

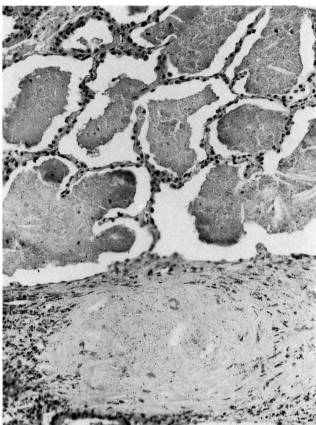

Fig. 27–3 A,B. Acute silicolipoproteinosis in sand blaster. **A.** Note amorphous granular eosinophilic material adjacent to cellular area resembling desquamative interstitial pneumoni- tis. **B.** Amorphous eosinophilic material in alveolar spaces adjacent to interstitial silicotic nodule. (Courtesy Dr. Howard Buechner, New Orleans, Louisiana.)

phous carbon per se is innocuous and is therefore classified as a nuisance dust. Intratracheal instillation of amorphous carbon in experimental animals results in a substantial influx of macrophages into alveolar spaces, but no appreciable fibrosis.[22] The cytoplasm of these macrophages becomes stuffed with clumps of carbon particles, which in the case of inhaled coal dust range up to about 3 μm in maximum dimension.[7,14]

A number of abnormalities may be found in the lungs of coalworkers, depending on the quantity and quality of inhaled dust, occupation within the mine, duration of exposure and interval since last exposure, and additional factors such as cigarette smoking. The characteristic lesion of coalworkers' pneumoconiosis is the coal dust macule. In well-prepared specimens, these nonpalpable macular lesions appear as black areas 1–4 mm in diameter (Fig. 27–4) distributed more or less evenly throughout the lung. Together with a diffuse increase in background pigmentation they impart a black appearance, giving rise to the popular term "black lung disease." Macular lesions are usually more numerous in the upper lobes, and blackening also occurs along the

secondary lobular septa and subpleurally. The presence of palpable nodular lesions indicates a change in the pathologic response, most likely related to the silica content of the inhaled dust. This process is sometimes referred to as anthracosilicosis. The spherical nodules are generally similar in appearance and distribution to those observed in silicosis, except that they are generally more darkly pigmented. The nodular lesions of coalworkers' pneumoconiosis are arbitrarily classified into micronodules, which are as large as 0.7 cm in diameter; macronodules, which range in size from 0.7 to 2 cm; and progressive massive fibrosis, which is more asymmetrical in distribution and irregular in shape, with lesions by definition at least 2 cm in one or more dimensions.[14] The latter resembles conglomerate silicosis, most often involves upper lobes, and may extend across fissures to involve adjacent lobes. Cavitation may occur, and its presence should suggest superimposed tuberculosis, although ischemic necrosis also occurs. Liquified material within these cavities has the appearance of India ink.

Histologically, the macular lesion consists of focal

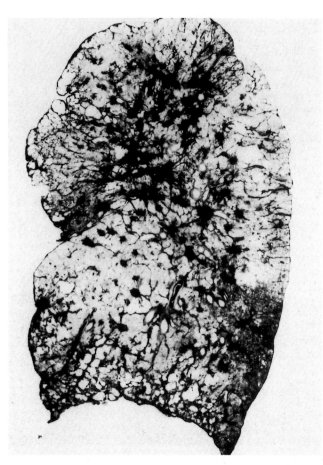

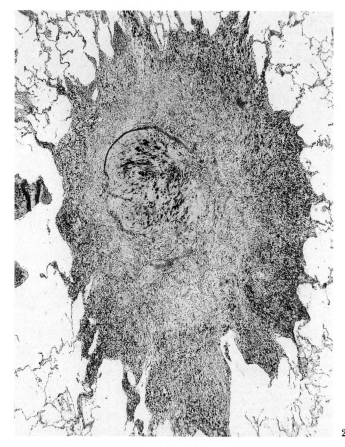

27-5

Fig. 27–4. Whole lung section prepared from 75-year-old coal miner shows macronodules, micronodules, and occasional dust macules with focal emphysema. (From Kleinerman J, Green F, Laquer W. Pathology standards for coal workers pneumoconioses. Arch Pathol Lab Med 1979;103:413, with permission. Copyright 1979, American Medical Association.)

collections of coal dust-laden macrophages at the division of respiratory bronchioles that often extend into and fill adjacent alveolar spaces as well as involving the peribronchiolar interstitium.[14] These collections of macrophages may be associated with a few reticulin fibers, but mature collagen is inconspicuous. The macrophages may form a mantle around respiratory bronchioles and the small pulmonary arteries that accompany them. Nodular lesions, both micro- and macronodules, contain a collagenous center that may be

$\longrightarrow$ $\triangleright$

Fig. 27–5 A,B. A. Micronodule in lung from coal miner. Central nodule of whorled collagen is deeply pigmented and surrounded by stellate mantle of dust-laden macrophages and collagen fibers. (Reprinted from Roggli and Shelburne. Semin Respir Med 1982;4:138–148, Fig. 4, with permission.) **B.** Silicotic nodules beneath the capsule of hilar lymph node from coalworker.

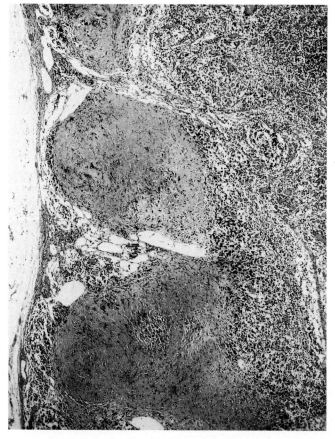

27-5

hyalinized. Pigmented macrophages may be present in the center of the nodules as well as in the stellate mantle surrounding the lesion (Fig. 27–5A). The similarity of the histologic appearance of these nodules to the silicotic nodule suggests that they are related to the silica content of the coal dust (Table 27–2). The regional lymph nodes are jet black, often enlarged (Fig. 27–4), and may contain silicotic nodules (Fig. 27–5B).

Progressive massive fibrosis contains collagen fibers characteristically arranged in a haphazard fashion and separated by large amounts of coal dust. Vascular structures are often obliterated. Variable amounts of necrosis may be associated with lipid debris and cholesterol clefts. Caseous necrosis and giant cells should suggest tuberculosis (Fig. 27–6), although the typical histologic picture of tuberculosis may be lacking even in cases in which mycobacteria are demonstrable. Examination of sections with polarized light may demonstrate fairly numerous brightly birefringent, platy silicate particles, but particles of silica are difficult to visualize with this technique.[14] Factors that are thought to be important in the evolution of simple coalworkers' pneumoconiosis into progressive massive fibrosis include silica content of the mine dust, infection with *Mycobacterium tuberculosis*, and immunologic factors. Although the relative contribution of each of these factors to progressive massive fibrosis is at present controversial,[5,14] there is evidence that the silica content in areas of massive fibrosis is greater than in adjacent nonfibrotic lung.[23]

Patients with simple coalworkers' pneumoconiosis may be asymptomatic. However, patients with progressive massive fibrosis often have restrictive and obstructive defects on pulmonary function tests, perifocal emphysema, and hypoxia, as is also the case for conglomerate silicosis. Pulmonary hypertension and cor pulmonale may then follow. Coalworkers also have an increased risk for tuberculosis, especially those patients with progressive massive fibrosis. In the past, as many as 40% of patients with progressive massive fibrosis have had superimposed tuberculosis.[14] Currently, the incidence of complicating tuberculosis is thought to be less frequent, but precise estimates are not readily found.

An unusual pathologic response known as Caplan's lesion may be seen in the lungs of some coal miners who also have rheumatoid arthritis. These appear as giant silicolic nodules up to 5 cm or more in diameter, with smooth borders and concentric internal laminations (Fig. 27–7). Microscopically, they may show histiocytic palisading at the periphery and focal areas of necrobiosis, as occur in rheumatoid nodules in other sites. At the margin of the nodules, a perivascular infiltrate of plasma cells is often demonstrable. Caplan's lesions thus appear to be a peculiar combination of silicotic nodules and rheumatoid nodules.

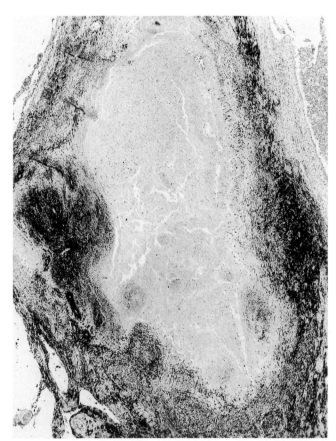

Fig. 27–6. Area of caseous necrosis surrounded by mantle of coal dust in coalworker with progressive massive fibrosis complicated by tuberculosis.

Emphysematous changes often occur in the zone immediately adjacent to the coal dust macule. Some authorities consider this a specific and integral part of simple coalworkers' pneumoconiosis, and refer to this lesion as *focal emphysema*.[24] This lesion is limited in its extent to a small zone in the proximal part of the pulmonary acinus. It closely resembles centrilobular emphysema in its gross and histologic features, differing only in its limited extent and invariable association with the dust macule. Perifocal emphysema may also occur, especially adjacent to areas of progressive massive fibrosis. A form of bronchitis known as industrial bronchitis is thought to occur in individuals working in a dusty environment, but this entity has not been well studied pathologically. Patients with simple coalworkers' pneumoconiosis may show pathologic changes of emphysema or bronchitis, and the effects of cigarette smoking and dust exposure appear to be additive in the production of obstructive changes.[25] However, those who develop symptomatic and incapacitating chronic obstructive pulmonary disease almost invariably have been cigarette-smoking miners.[26] Coalworkers are at no apparent increased risk for developing lung cancer,[27]

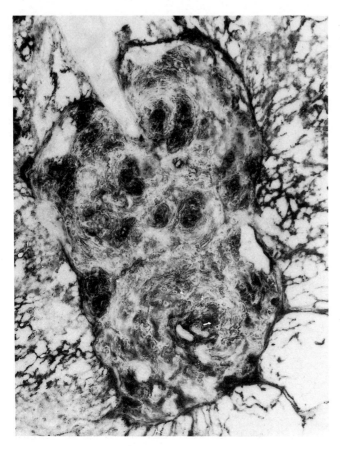

Fig. 27–7. Close-up of whole lung section prepared from coal miner with rheumatoid arthritis shows 4.5 × 3.5 cm Caplan's lesion in upper lobe. (Courtesy Dr. Val Vallyathan, Appalachian Laboratory, Morgantown, West Virginia.)

and the cancers that do occur are histologically no different from those that occur in nonminers who smoke.[28]

Coalworkers' pneumoconiosis must be distinguished histologically from anthracosis secondary to cigarette smoking and urban living, from graphite worker's lung, and from carbon electrode-maker's pneumoconiosis. Some pigmentation can be found in the lungs of virtually all adults in industrialized nations. Although pigment accumulation is related both to age and amount of cigarette smoking, there is considerable variation from individual to individual in efficiency of particle clearance.[29] Simple anthracosis resulting from smoking and urban living appears as pigment-laden macrophages located interstitially adjacent to bronchioles and pulmonary arteries, subpleurally, and within hilar nodes. It differs from coalworker's pneumoconiosis both in degree of pigmentation and absence of carbon-laden macrophages consolidating alveolar spaces.

Dust from graphite, which is mined principally in

Ceylon, Austria, South Africa, and Siberia, consists of approximately 50% crystalline carbon or graphite and 25% quartz; the remainder is various silicates. Graphite miners may show the same pathologic changes observed in silicosis and coalworkers' pneumoconiosis. One histologic difference is the presence of giant cells within alveolar spaces in the graphite workers.[5] Carbon electrode makers are exposed to a dust containing crushed coke and anthracite, and may show pathologic changes indistinguishable from simple coalworkers' pneumoconiosis and, occasionally, progressive massive fibrosis.[30] Silica particles were not identified in the lesions in two fatal cases, and tuberculosis was thought to have played a part in the development of massive fibrosis. Nevertheless, a possible role for quartz has not been excluded, because anthracite coal was used in the electrode manufacture.

Talcosis (Talc Pneumoconiosis)

Talc is a hydrated magnesium silicate that occurs in platy, granular, and fibrous forms. Its basic structure consists of two sheets of silica tetrahedra between which a magnesium hydroxide layer is sandwiched. Important contaminants that often accompany talc are quartz and noncommercial varieties of amphibole asbestos, such as tremolite, and anthophyllite. In tissue sections examined with polarized light, talc particles are seen as brightly birefringent, needle-shaped particles 0.5–10 μm in length that represent plates of talc viewed "edge on." Occasional plates viewed en face may be seen as well. Experimental animal studies have demonstrated that the amphibole contaminants of talc, tremolite and anthophyllite, are markedly fibrogenic in guinea pigs, whereas "pure talc" produces primarily a cellular macrophage response.[31] The pathogenicity of relatively pure forms of talc in man has been described only recently.[32] The purity of talc varies with its source.[33]

Exposure to talc, which is used in a number of manufacturing processes because of its lubricant properties, occurs in a variety of ways. Occupational exposure may result from mining and milling of talc. In the United States, talc is mined and milled in California, Montana, New York, North Carolina, Texas, and Vermont. Other occupations associated with exposure to talc include leather, rubber, paper and textile industries; manufacture of ceramics, cosmetics, paints, pharmaceuticals, soaps, toiletries, and refractory and roofing materials; plate casting in which molds are dusted with talc before pouring; and dusting of life rafts with talc.[33,34] A substantial amount of personal exposure may occur in individuals who use, and abuse, cosmetic talc. In addition, talc particles may embolize to the lung when tablets containing talc as a filler are crushed and injected intravenously (intravenous drug abuse).[35]

Talcosis develops primarily in individuals with prolonged and heavy exposure to talc dust. Pleural thickening and dense pleural adhesions are described in many cases. Parietal pleural plaques were first described in talc miners, and probably result from contaminating tremolite and anthophyllite asbestos. The lung may contain tiny discrete palpable nodules[34] or may show diffuse interstitial fibrosis.[33,36] In some cases, progressive massive fibrosis, which manifests as circumscribed, bilateral, irregular gray to gray-black masses with a firm, often gritty consistency, has been described.[37] These lesions involve the central portions of the upper lobes and superior portions of the lower lobes. Occasionally these areas of progressive massive fibrosis undergo central cavitation.[33]

The histologic appearance of talcosis includes three types of lesions: interstitial fibrosis, which may be focal or diffuse, poorly defined fibrotic nodules, and foreign body granulomas.[32] The degree of fibrosis appears to correlate with duration of exposure and dust content of the lung parenchyma. Milder lesions consist of dust-laden macrophages and connective tissue in the peribronchiolar and perivascular interstitium. Prolonged exposure to high concentrations of talc dust is associated with diffuse fibrosis and variable numbers of multinucleated giant cells. Birefringent particles are observed with polarized light microscopy within giant cells, within macrophages, or free within the interstitium.[32] Poorly defined fibrotic nodules are less well circumscribed than typical silicotic nodules, but may represent modification of the response to crystalline silica caused by the presence of large amounts of silicate. Nonnecrotizing foreign body granulomas may resemble those seen in sarcoidosis, but can be distinguished by the presence of birefringent platy particles (Fig. 27–8). The latter are more numerous and larger than the occasional small birefringent calcite particles observed in giant cells in sarcoidosis.[7,38] The differentiating

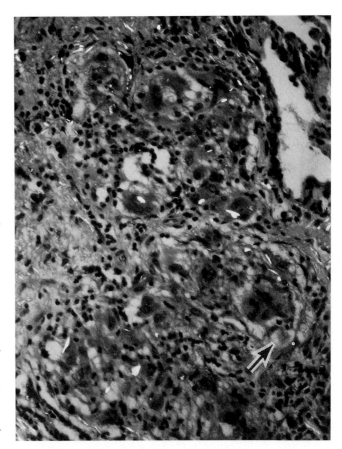

Fig. 27–8. Granulomatous inflammation with numerous giant cells and birefringent platy particles in individual with talcosis. Partially crossed polarized light. Asteroid body is present in one giant cell *(arrow).*

pathologic features of talcosis, intravenous talc injection, and sarcoidosis are shown in Table 27–3.

Patients with intravenous drug abuse have a unique histologic response to embolized talc particles. Intravascular and interstitial granulomas occur and may be associated with variable degrees of fibrosis.[35] Giant cells within the granulomas contain birefringent talc parti-

Table 27–3. Differentiating pathologic features for inhalational talcosis, intravenous talc injection, and sarcoidosis

	inhalation talcosis	*Talc injection (IV)*	*Sarcoidosis*
Distribution of granulomas	Randomly within lung parenchyma and interstitium	Intravascularly and within pulmonary interstitium	Along lymphatic pathways (peribronchiolar, perivascular, subpleural)
Size of particles[a]	0.5–10 μm	0.5–50 μm	1–5 μm
Numbers of particles[a]	Numerous	Numerous	Occasional
Types of particles[a]	Talc	Talc	Calcium carbonate (calcite)
Sources of particles	Exogenous, inhaled	Exogenous, injected	Endogenous
Giant cells	Moderate to numerous	Moderate to numerous	Moderate to numerous

[a] This table refers only to those particles that are birefringent when viewed with polarized light. Schaumann bodies, consisting of amorphous calcium phosphate particles, appear as laminated blue concretions within giant cells on H and E sections, are nonbirefringent, and may be found in giant cells in all three conditions listed. (See Chapter 19, Sarcoidosis.)

cles, many of which are too large to have been inhaled.[39] Pulmonary hypertension and cor pulmonale may be the initial presentation in these individuals. Several cases with progressive massive fibrosis from intravenous injection of talc have been described.[37,40] The average size of particles in the areas of massive fibrosis was greater than that of particles in adjacent lung or in other organs and suggested that the larger size of the talc particles was responsible for the development of progressive massive fibrosis.[37] However, a case with progressive massive fibrosis containing talc particles less than 0.5 μm in diameter and detectable only by electron microscopy has been reported in an individual exposed to aerosolized talc dust.[34] The talc in this case was contaminated with anthophyllite asbestos. Quartz was not mentioned. As is the case for silicosis and coalworkers' pneumoconiosis, the factors responsible for development of progressive massive fibrosis in talcosis are complex.

A fourfold increase in lung cancer risk for talc miners in New York State in 1944–1949 was detected in one study.[41] In a later period, lung cancer mortality returned to the expected level coincident with improved dust control at the mine. The lung cancer excess was attributed to asbestos contamination of the talc dust. Pulmonary tumors have not been produced in experimental animals exposed to pure talc.[33]

Kaolin Pneumoconiosis

Kaolinite, a hydrated aluminum silicate, is a member of the group of sheet silicates known as phyllosilicates. It is the major component of kaolin (china clay), which in the United States occurs in deposits extending from central Georgia to west central South Carolina. Deposits are also mined in Great Britain, Germany, Japan, Czechoslovakia, and Egypt. In addition to kaolinite, smaller amounts of mica and quartz may be present. Kaolin is used in the manufacture of paper products, refractory materials, and ceramics, and as a filler in paints, plastics, and rubber.[42] Occupational exposure to kaolin dust can occur in persons employed in any of these industries, but the most intense exposures occur in individuals employed in the mining and processing of kaolin.[43] Kaolinite has also been identified on tobacco leaves and in cigarette smoke as well as in alveolar macrophages obtained from the lungs of cigarette smokers.[44]

Kaolinite is cytotoxic in vitro for peritoneal and alveolar macrophages, as determined by release of the enzyme lactate dehydrogenase into the culture medium.[45] Elastase secretion is augmented in peritoneal macrophages exposed to kaolinite, but decreased in alveolar macrophages. Kaolin has been shown to stim-

ulate secretion of the toxic metabolites hydrogen peroxide and superoxide anion in a murine model of kaolin-induced inflammation.[46] Nevertheless, the firogenicity of kaolinite appears to be minimal, and fibroplasia is not observed in the lungs of experimental animals exposed to kaolinite.[47,48]

Pneumoconiosis has been reported in kaolin miners and processing plant workers.[43] The lungs show greybrown discoloration in the form of nonpalpable macules and numerous firm, grey-brown nodules. These range in size from 0.5 cm to firm rubbery masses as much as 12 cm in diameter, replacing large portions of parenchyma. Strands of grey-white connective tissue extend from these large masses into the adjacent lung. Perifocal emphysema may be present. In some nodules, the centers may be yellow with a pasty consistency because of necrosis. The hilar lymph nodes are often enlarged, secondary to accumulation of masses of dust-laden macrophages.[43] In some cases, 20–40 g of dust can be recovered from these lungs.[5]

Microscopically, the macular lesions consist of massive amounts of intracellular and extracellular deposits of fine golden-brown particulates, primarily in a peribronchiolar distribution. The appearance and distribution of the lesions is reminiscent of that seen in coalworkers' pneumoconiosis. Particle-laden macrophages distend the interstitium (Fig. 27–9) and, in cases with recent exposure, are found in large numbers within alveolar spaces. A delicate reticulin network surrounds dust-laden cells within the interstitium. The nodular masses consist largely of dust deposits traversed by occasional randomly distributed bands of collagen. Obliterative vascular lesions caused by transmural infiltration by dust-laden macrophages are commonly seen within nodules and may result in central ischemic necrosis. Whorled dense collagenous deposits have been described in some cases, but not in cases in which dust recovered from the lung showed no detectable quantities of quartz.[43] Such lesions should be attributed to contaminating quartz rather than kaolinite.

Kaolin exposure rarely produces symptomatic changes except in advanced disease.[49] Progressive massive fibrosis may occur in individuals exposed concomitantly to significant amounts of quartz as in firebrick manufacture or in individuals with superimposed tuberculosis.[43] Kaolin deposits in the southeastern United States are relatively free of quartz (<1%).

Berylliosis

Beryllium is a lightweight metal that has many industrial uses. The main source of beryllium is the mineral beryl, which is beryllium aluminum silicate. In the United

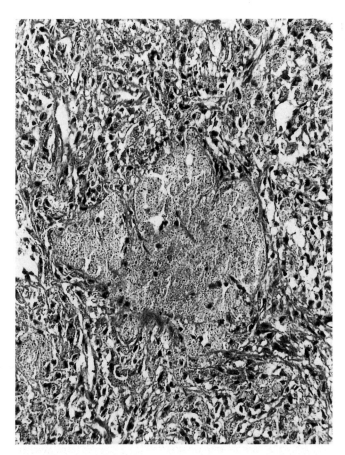

Fig. 27–9. Lung tissue from kaolin worker. Interstitial macrophages are stuffed with kaolin particles with no apparent fibrotic response. (Courtesy Dr. Val Vallyathan, Appalachian Laboratory, Morgantown, West Virginia.)

States, deposits occur in Colorado, New Mexico, and Utah. In the past, the principal industrial use of beryllium was in the manufacture of fluorescent lights. The manufacturing process resulted in exposure not only to beryllium silicate but to beryllium oxide, hydroxide, fluoride, chloride, and sulfate as well.[50] Currently, the usage of beryllium has shifted to the aerospace industries, where it is used in structural materials, guidance systems, optical devices, rocket motor parts, and heat shields. It is also used in the electronics industry in ceramic parts, in the manufacture of thermal couplings and crucibles, and in atomic reactors.[6,7] Exposure also occurs during mining and extraction of beryllium ores. The first ambient air quality standard ever established was that set in 1949 for beryllium, which preceded all others by about 25 years.[50]

Berylliosis is the term used for pulmonary disease resulting from exposure to beryllium. It occurs in both acute and chronic forms. Acute berylliosis is a form of chemical pneumonitis resulting from short-term exposure to high levels of soluble salts of beryllium (>25

$\mu g/m^3$), with symptoms beginning a few hours to several days after exposure. About 10% of individuals with acute berylliosis will go on to develop the chronic form of the disease, which may also occur in individuals with no history of acute berylliosis.[51] Patients with chronic berylliosis have an insidious onset of dyspnea, which may first become manifest 15 or more years after initial exposure. Only about 0.4%–2.0% of individuals at risk develop berylliosis implying that host susceptibility is an important factor.[5] It has been suggested that beryllium toxicity is a hypersensitivity phenomenon, although the mechanism of toxicity remains obscure despite extensive study.[6,7] This disease has largely been brought under control as a result of the establishment of air quality standards limiting exposure and discontinuance of use of beryllium in fluorescent lights. A Berylliosis Case Registry, to which new cases may be reported, has been established in the United States at the Massachusetts General Hospital, Boston, Massachusetts, for the study of this disease.[52] There is evidence that exposure to beryllium results in an increased risk of lung cancer.[53,54]

The lungs in acute berylliosis are wet, heavy, and congested. Microscopically, there is diffuse alveolar damage, with pulmonary edema, congestion, swollen epithelial cells, and scattered inflammatory cells within the interstitium and alveolar spaces. The pathologic features are entirely nonspecific and resemble any acute chemical pneumonitis. In chronic berylliosis, the lungs are small, fibrotic, and may show honeycomb changes. Bilateral hilar lymphadenopathy may be present.[55] Histologic examination shows interstitial lymphocytic infiltration and nonnecrotizing granulomatous inflammation, which may progress to diffuse interstitial fibrosis. Granulomas may be inconspicuous or absent in some cases. Giant cells often contain inclusions such as Schaumann bodies, which are basophilic, laminated calcospherites, or asteroid bodies (Fig. 27–10).[56]

In cases where lymphocytic interstitial infiltrates are prominent and granulomas are scattered and poorly formed, berylliosis may be difficult to distinguish from hypersensitivity pneumonitis (see Chapter 18). Indeed, it has been proposed that chronic berylliosis is a form of hypersensitivity pneumonitis.[6,57] In cases with abundant nonnecrotizing granulomas, berylliosis must be distinguished from sarcoidosis (see Chapter 19). The pathologic diagnosis depends on the finding of one of the previously described histologic patterns together with an appropriate exposure history or elevated tissue levels of beryllium. Beryllium has classically been identified in lung tissue by wet chemical spectrographic techniques, but more recently individual particles have been detected in situ by means of laser microprobe or

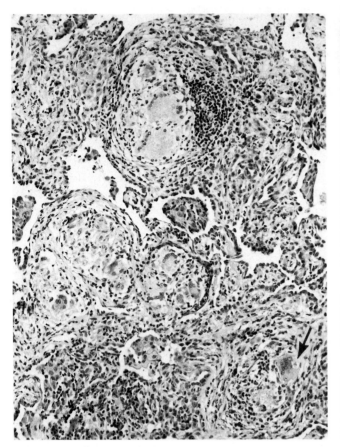

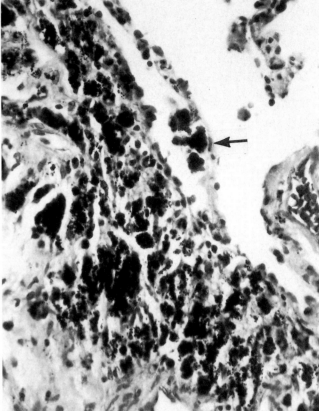

Fig. 27–10. Granulomas within pulmonary interstitium of individual with berylliosis. Note asteroid body within giant cell *(arrow)*. (Courtesy Dr. F.B. Askin, Baltimore, Maryland.)

Fig. 27–11. Numerous aggregates of iron oxides are present within pulmonary interstitium of welder. Few pseudoasbestos bodies with sheet silicate cores are present in nearby alveolus *(arrow)*.

ion microprobe mass spectrometry, and by electron energy loss spectrometry[7] (see section at the end of this chapter).

Welders' Pneumoconiosis

Welders are exposed to fumes, the composition of which varies with the type of welding that is done.[58] Fumes consist of particles in the range of 0.1-1 μm in diameter. Welding fumes consist of a variety of metal oxides, including iron, titanium, manganese, and aluminum, together with various silicates and carbonates. The nature of the reaction of the lung to welding fumes depends on the duration and intensity of exposure as well as the predominant component of the fumes. Aluminum oxides have been associated with a variety of tissue changes, whereas titanium and iron oxides appear to be relatively inert.[7]

On gross inspection, the lungs appear deeply pigmented, but in most instances there is little or no fibrosis. A metallic sheen resembling tarnished aluminum has been described in the lungs of aluminum arc welders. Chest radiographs may show prominent interstitial markings, which may be misinterpreted as interstitial fibrosis. Interstitial markings may result from the presence of extensive deposits of metal oxides within alveolar macrophages and the pulmonary interstitium, although diffuse fibrosis may occur with exposure to aluminum oxides. The identification of pleural thickening or interstitial fibrosis on gross inspection should arouse suspicion of exposure to an additional agent, such as asbestos in shipyard welders.

The predominant microscopic feature in welders' pneumoconiosis is the presence of large amounts of dust within the interstitium, with little if any accompanying fibrotic response. The dust consists of dark brown to black spherical particles, often occurring in aggregates, in a peribronchiolar or perivascular distribution (Fig. 27–11). A characteristic feature of the dust is the presence of a golden-brown outer layer with dark centers in some particles. This probably represents in situ conversion of iron oxide to iron hydroxide, commonly referred to as hemosiderin.[5] Various sheet silicates may also be found in the lungs, and may be partially coated with iron to form pseudoasbestos bodies or nonasbestos ferruginous bodies. The presence of true asbestos bodies and appreciable amounts of fibrosis indicate concomitant exposure to asbestos. Diffuse interstitial fibrosis,[59] granulomatous inflammation,[60] and desquamative interstitial pneumonitis[61] have been described in aluminum arc welders.

Some studies have suggested that welders have an increased risk for developing bronchogenic carcinoma.[58] A study from the Danish Welding Institute in Copenhagen indicated that the excess lung cancer risk for welders can be accounted for by cigarette smoking, asbestos exposure (shipyard welders), and exposure to hexavalent chromium (welders of stainless steel).[62]

Hematite Miner's Lung

Hematite, or iron sesquioxide (Fe_2O_3), is a type of iron ore that is mined in Belgium, Sweden, England, and the western end of Lake Superior in the United States.[5] The ore contains varying amounts of silica and silicates. The predominant component is iron oxide, so that miners exposed to hematite may develop a form of siderotic lung disease similar to that of welders. Although iron oxide per se is considered to be inert, the presence of crystalline silica may result in varying degrees of fibrosis, a process sometimes referred to as siderosilicosis.

The gross features of hematite miners' lung are reminiscent of those seen in coalworkers' pneumoconiosis. This should not be surprising, considering that both iron oxide and coal dust exert a modifying influence on silica. Macroscopically, hematite miners' lungs may be classified into one of three gross categories: diffuse, nodular, and massively fibrotic. In the diffuse variety, the lung has a brick-red appearance. Fibrosis is diffuse but minimal, and there may be varying degrees of perifocal or focal emphysema analogous to simple coalworkers' pneumoconiosis. The nodular form is characterized by the presence of firm reddish-black nodules up to 1 cm in diameter, predominantly in the upper lobes. These nodules are superimposed on a background of diffuse brick-red coloration. The nodules may undergo central necrosis. Pleural adhesions are frequently observed. The massive fibrotic form is similar to progressive massive fibrosis in coalworkers' pneumoconiosis. The irregular, sharply circumscribed masses of fibrotic tissue occur primarily in the upper lobes, have a brownish-red color, and may undergo central cavitation that is either tuberculous or ischemic.

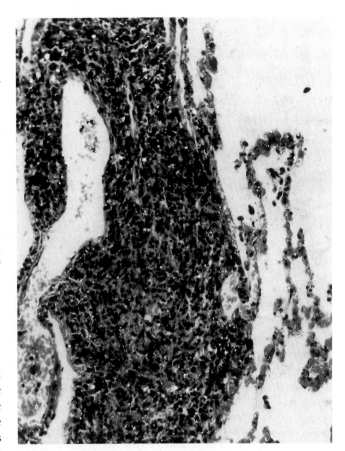

Fig. 27–12. Hematite dust (iron oxides, silicates, and silica) within pulmonary interstitium of hematite miner, viewed with partially crossed polarized light. (From Vallyathan et al.,[59] with permission.)

The hilar lymph nodes are often enlarged and fibrotic, with a mottled brick-red-to-black appearance.

Microscopic examination of pulmonary tissues in hematite miners shows large amounts of dark dust particles within the pulmonary interstitium and within alveolar spaces. Occasional birefringent dust particles (probably silicates) are observed with polarized light microscopy (Fig. 27–12). Iron oxide does not stain with the Prussian blue reaction,[63] but varying amounts of hemosiderin may be observed, especially around the periphery of silicotic nodules.[5] Interstitial fibrosis is often present, and may be diffuse or in the form of whorled silicotic nodules composed of hyalinized collagen. In cases with massive fibrosis, bands of haphazardly arranged collagen fibers are separated by accumulations of dust particles. Necrosis in these areas may be related to fibrous obliteration of blood vessels, but should alert the pathologist to the possibility of superimposed tuberculosis. The occurrence of the nodular lesions and massive fibrosis is related to the silica content of the hematite ore.[5,55]

The complications of exposure to hematite, similar to those seen with coal dust, include cor pulmonale in patients with massive fibrosis and tuberculosis. An unexpected prevalence of lung cancer has been observed in hematite miners in west Cumberland, United Kingdom, where the mines are contaminated with radon gas.[5,9] The resulting radiation exposure may offer an explanation for the occurrence of lung cancer in these miners.

Silver Polishers' Lung

In addition to welders and hematite miners, a third form of siderotic lung disease occurs in silver polishers. The final stages in the manufacture of silverware involve a polishing procedure. The abrasive material used consists of iron oxide powder, and the procedure generates a dust consisting of fine particles of iron oxide and silver. The iron particles accumulate within the pulmonary interstitium in a perivascular and subpleural distribution. The silver, however, combines with the tissues, staining elastic tissue of pulmonary vessels and alveolar septa black. A fibrotic response does not occur around the deposits of iron oxides, and the latter do not stain with Prussian blue. Although silica is not believed to be present in the dust employed in silver polishing, cases of massive fibrosis have been observed in silver polishers.[5] The mechanism of massive fibrosis in these cases is unknown, and analyses of dust recovered from the lungs of affected individuals using modern techniques have not been reported.

Silicon Carbide Pneumoconiosis

Silicon carbide (Carborundum) is a synthetic abrasive that is widely used because of its hardness, which is just slightly below that of diamond. It is used for abrasive wheels and in the manufacture of refractory materials for boilers and foundry furnaces. Silicon carbide is made by fusing high-grade sand, finely ground carbon, common salt, and wood dust in an electric furnace at 2,400°C. The fused product is then crushed and milled to remove impurities. Silicon carbide is thought to be inert in humans, and does not produce fibrosis in experimental animals.[64] Silicosis has been described in silicon carbide workers, and is attributed to the use of quartz dust in the production process.

Although radiographic studies have been reported in a number of workers exposed to pure silicon carbide, only one pathologic study has been described.[65] This was in an individual who worked on a conveyor belt loading powdered silicon carbide for 14 years. The patient's chest radiography showed bilateral reticulonodular densities and hilar prominence. Open lung biopsy showed dust-laden macrophages in a peribronchiolar and perivascular distribution as well as in alveolar spaces. Birefringent needle-shaped particles were visible with polarized light microscopy. Ferruginous bodies with an appearance similar to that described in hamsters exposed to silicon carbide whiskers[66] were also observed. Although fibrosis was said to be present,[65] the published micrographs show mostly interstitial accumulation of dust-laden phagocytes with little fibrotic response. X-ray diffraction studies of the dust recovered from the lung showed predominantly silicon carbide with minor traces of quartz and tungsten carbide. Many particles were less than 0.1 μm in diameter.

Hard-Metal Lung Disease (Tungsten Carbide Pneumoconiosis)

Tungsten carbide is a metal with properties of extreme strength, rigidity, and heat resistance[67] that are useful in the manufacture of cutting tools, drilling equipment, armaments, alloys, and ceramics. Tungsten carbide is produced in a process of powdered metallurgy in which tungsten and carbon are heated and blended in the presence of a binder, which is cobalt. Most particles generated during this process are less than 2.0 μm in diameter and therefore in the respirable range. The finished product contains 5%–25% cobalt by weight.

Workers exposed to tungsten carbide may develop an obstructive airways disease resembling asthma or an interstitial pneumonitis. The latter is referred to as tungsten carbide pneumoconiosis or hard-metal lung disease.[5] The lungs in fatal cases show a severe diffuse interstitial fibrosis. Lung biopsies at earlier stages of the disease show interstitial pneumonitis, which may represent giant cell interstitial pneumonitis (see Chapter 16) or idiopathic pulmonary fibrosis. In some cases, the microscopic appearance may resemble that of hypersensitivity pneumonitis or desquamative interstitial pneumonitis. Epithelial hyperplasia may be exuberant, with multinucleate giant cells attached to alveolar walls (Fig. 27–13). Alveolar macrophages may fuse to form giant cells, which are sometimes recovered in bronchoalveolar lavage fluid.[68] Cells recovered from lavage fluid may also be analyzed to detect the presence of tungsten carbide and cobalt. Interstitial fibrosis is the predominant feature in more advanced cases.

Cobalt, rather than tungsten carbide, is thought to be the injurious agent in hard-metal lung disease. Experimental animal studies have shown that intratracheal

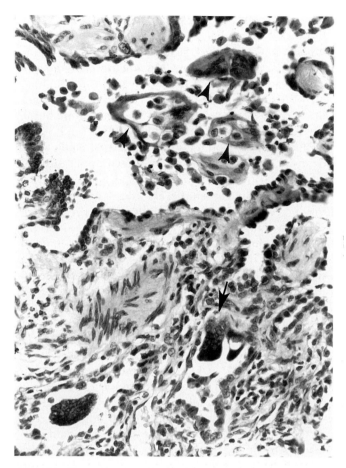

Fig. 27–13. Open lung biopsy from 25-year-old man who worked in manufacture of carbide cutting tools. Histologic features are typical for giant cell interstitial pneumonitis, including multinucleated cells within alveoli *(arrowheads)* as well as lining alveolar spaces *(arrow)*. Particles containing tungsten, tantalum, and titanium were identified within lung tissue.

instillation of tungsten carbide is innocuous, whereas a mixture of tungsten carbide and cobalt produces a chemical pneumonitis.[69] The occurrence of interstitial lung disease in tungsten carbide production workers has been associated with elevated peak air concentrations of cobalt in excess of 500 μg/m^3,[67] although some cases have occurred following exposures of less than 50 μg/m.[3] Interstitial lung disease occurred in less than 1% of individuals at risk in cross-sectional studies of current workers. The obstructed airways syndrome in tungsten carbide workers has also been correlated with colbalt exposure, and occurs in about 10% of workers at risk.[69] It has been suggested that cobalt interacts with tissue or serum proteins to form a hapten, which can then lead to immunologically induced lung injury. The resemblance of the histologic lesion to hypersensitivity pneumonitis is consistent with this proposal.

Tungsten carbide pneumoconiosis must be distin-guished histologically from hypersensitivity pneumonitis and idiopathic pulmonary fibrosis, which it may closely resemble. The distinction is based on the exposure history and the finding of tungsten carbide particles in lung tissue. The finding of giant cell interstitial pneumonitis is almost pathognomonic of hard-metal lung disease and should provoke an investigation of occupational exposure history.[71] Although Spencer[5] noted that cobalt, which is water soluble, is not usually found in the lungs in fatal cases of hard-metal lung disease, we have noted the presence of both tungsten and cobalt containing particles in lung tissue from an exposed worker. Coates and Watson[72] reported that mass spectroscopy identified the presence of tungsten carbide, cobalt, and titanium in lung tissue of tungsten carbide workers with interstitial fibrosis. The detection of cobalt in tissues of these individuals probably depends on both the sensitivity of the technique employed and the time since last exposure.

Titanium Lung

Titanium dioxide is a white powder that is used extensively in the dye industry. Grinding of titanium oxide generates particles in the size range of 0.5–1.0 μm that are therefore respirable. Exposure of experimental animals to titanium-containing dusts does not produce fibrosis, and titanium dioxide is considered to be an inert nuisance dust. Inspection of the lungs of former titanium workers shows deposits of white pigment that may have a greenish hue.[5,73] Fibrosis is not observed. Microscopic examination shows dust-laden macrophages in a perivascular and peribronchiolar distribution. The particles are birefringent when viewed with polarized light. Particles are also transported to the hilar nodes. Rutile is a form of titanium dioxide that may occur in a fibrous form in association with silica. These fibers may become coated with iron to form pseudoasbestos bodies with dark central cores[74] (see section on **Nonasbestos Mineral Fibers**). Titanium carbide is used in the hard-metal industry (see previous section), and like tungsten carbide is considered to be biologically inert.

Fuller's Earth Lung

Fuller's earth generally refers to calcium montmorillonite, a calcium aluminum silicate with adsorbent properties. It was originally used to remove grease from wool, a process known as fulling. Currently, fuller's earth is used principally as a filtering and decolorizing agent for mineral oils, as a filler for paper and cosmetic preparations, and as a binder for molding sands. Deposits of calcium montmorillonite, found in Germany, Great Britain, and the United States, are obtained by strip mining. A small amount of quartz is usually present in the dust. Exposure to fuller's earth may occur through mining, drying, crushing, or milling of this substance or during its industrial application.

The lungs of individuals with fuller's earth pneumoconiosis contain irregular black macules up to 2 cm in diameter. Massive fibrosis has been described in the upper lobes in some cases. Microscopically, numerous dust particles may be found in alveoli and in a perivascular and peribronchiolar distribution. The dust particles produce yellow birefringence when viewed with polarized light. Relatively few macrophages are found in these lesions, and reticulin and collagen fibers envelop the dust particles. The fibrotic reaction is probably attributable to the quartz content of the dust. This disease is considered to be a relatively benign pneumoconiosis, and in many respects resembles the changes related to exposure to kaolin.

Stannosis

Tin is a silver-white metal of industrial importance because of its pliability and because of its ability to readily form alloys with other metals. It is mined principally as tin dioxide ore (cassiterite), and deposits are often closely associated with quartz-containing rock. In the past, miners of tin ore often developed silicosis (see Table 27–1), but the risk has decreased greatly with the introduction of wet drilling procedures. The pneumoconiosis related to exposure to tin is called *stannosis*, and the greatest exposure occurs during bagging of processed tin ore or during the smelting procedure. Accumulation of tin within the lung results in striking interstitial opacities visible by chest radiography because of its high atomic number ($Z = 50$). As is the case in welders' siderosis, the radiographic changes are caused by the dust itself rather than by fibrosis. The lungs of workers with stannosis show gray-to-black, 2- to 5-mm macules distributed fairly evenly throughout the lungs. Secondary lobular septa may stand out in bold relief as a result of dust accumulation; massive fibrosis does not occur. As much as 3 g of tin dioxide may be recovered from individual lungs. Microscopic examination shows dust-laden macrophages in a perivascular and peribronchiolar location, subpleurally, within secondary lobular septa, and within hilar lymph nodes.[5] The dust particles are brightly birefringent. There is little if any fibrous reaction to the particles of tin, which is therefore categorized as a nuisance dust.

Barium Lung (Baritosis)

Barium sulfate, or *barytes*, is a relatively insoluble salt of barium that is mined in the United States in Mississippi, Nevada, and Georgia.[55] It is often found in combination with other minerals such as calcite, fluorite, and silica (quartz). Barium sulfate is used in the manufacture of paint, vulcanized rubber, glass, and radiographic contrast media. Exposure to barium may occur during mining or during its industrial application. In addition, barium sulfate used in upper-gastrointestinal radiographic contrast studies may be aspirated into the lungs.[5,7] Accumulation of barium within the lung results in striking opacities visible on chest radiographs because of high atomic number ($Z = 56$). On gross inspection of the lung, white patches may be observed in areas where the barium has accumulated. Microscopically, most of the particles occur in alveolar spaces with few in the interstitium. They are refractile and brightly birefringent when viewed with polarized light. A few particles may assume a fibrous shape. Many particles are phagocytized by alveolar macrophages. Little if any fibrotic response occurs, and its presence should lead to a search for a contaminating fibrogenic agent, such as quartz. When barium sulfate is aspirated into the lung, evidence of simultaneous aspiration of other materials may be found in the form of foreign-body giant cells, meat fibers, or vegetable matter[7] (Fig. 27–14). Particle size is of limited value in this regard, because barium particles used in radiographic contrast media are in the respirable size range.

Dental Technicians' Pneumoconiosis

Dental laboratory workers may be exposed to a dusty environment that may include a number of different particulates potentially injurious to the lungs. Prosthetic devices made of metal alloys are polished with high-speed abrasive wheels, which may generate dust composed of particulate silica or silicon carbide in the respirable size range. In addition, asbestos molds are used in the process of dental gold casting, and exposure to substantial levels of aerosolized asbestos fibers may occur when these molds are dismantled. Recent studies have suggested that chromium–cobalt–molybdenum alloys may be found in the lungs of some dental technicians and may be an important factor in the development of pneumoconiosis.[75] These alloys may cleave into elongated fragments that subsequently become coated with iron to produce a type of nonasbestos ferruginous body (see later section). Other investigators have suggested a pathogenic role for acrylic resins used in the

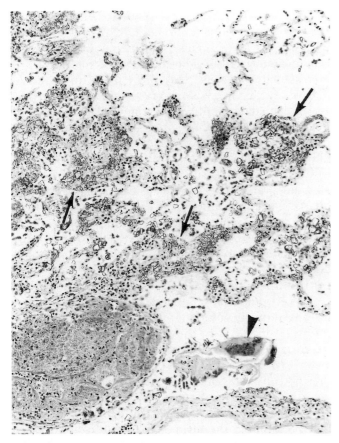

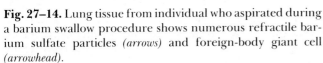

Fig. 27–14. Lung tissue from individual who aspirated during a barium swallow procedure shows numerous refractile barium sulfate particles *(arrows)* and foreign-body giant cell *(arrowhead).*

Fig. 27–15. Open lung biopsy from 76-year-old dental technician who used silica to grind dental prostheses for more than 20 years. Cellular areas (above) consisted of fibroblasts and histiocytes, acellular areas (below) consisted of dense bundles of hyalinized collagen. Numerous tiny, faintly visible particles were visible with polarizing microscopy. (Courtesy Dr. Fred Askin, Johns Hopkins, Baltimore, Maryland.)

preparation of dental prostheses,[76] or alginate impression powder in the case of an elderly dentist with pneumoconiosis.[77]

We have examined an additional example of dental technician's pneumoconiosis that occurred in a 76-year-old worker who presented with bilateral irregular upper lobe masses. He had used silica to grind dentures for more than 20 years. An open biopsy from the left upper lobe showed dense areas of acellular collagen alternating with more cellular areas composed of indistinct granulomas (Fig. 27–15). The latter contained a few small multinucleated cells and many tiny particles when viewed with polarizing microscopy. This histologic appearance is indicative of progressive massive fibrosis. Examination of tissue sections using a scanning electron microscope equipped with backscattered electron imaging and an energy-dispersive spectrometer indicated that half the particles were composed of silicon only, consistent with either silica or silicon carbide. Other particles identified included gold, tin, titanium, aluminum, and chromium–cobalt–iron. These observations confirmed the exposure to substantial numbers of particulates that presumably derived from metals and metal alloys in dental prostheses and the abrasives used to polish them.

Fly Ash Lung

Fly ash is the particulate residue of smoke produced by burning coal. It consists of spherical particles with an outer amorphous glass phase and with central mullite (an aluminum silicate) and quartz particles.[78] When combustion is incomplete, the particles have a lacy black appearance from the presence of soot. Elemental analysis may also reveal the presence of titanium, iron, calcium, and phosphate. Many particles are less than 3 μm in diameter and are therefore respirable. Fly ash is used commercially as a filler material in construction and in cement, but most of the fly ash recovered is placed in land fills. Fly ash particles have been shown to be mutagenic in the Ames bacterial assay, probably because of adsorbed polycyclic aromatic hydrocarbons,[79] and are capable of activating complement in vitro.[80]

A single case of fly ash lung has been reported.[78] The individual was a steel-mill worker and shipyard boilermaker who developed progressive interstitial fibrosis and squamous cell carcinoma of the lung. He had smoked a package of cigarettes daily for 43 years. Macroscopically, the lung parenchyma showed patchy pale-gray interstitial fibrosis with honeycomb changes subpleurally. Histologic sections showed patchy interstitial fibrosis with scattered mononuclear inflammatory cells. In areas of pigment deposition, occasional lacy black fly ash particles were identified. They were also noted in alveolar macrophages and within intraalveolar corpora amylacea. Analysis of lung tissue demonstrated the presence of 6 million fly ash particles per gram of wet lung tissue. In addition, there were 140,000 asbestos fibers per gram of wet lung, which is at the lower end of the range of values we have observed for cases of asbestosis.[81] The relative contribution of the asbestos fibers and the fly ash particles to this patient's interstitial fibrosis is unknown.

Volcanic Ash Lung

The eruption of Mount St. Helens in the state of Washington (United States) on May 18, 1980, spewed hundreds of millions of tons of volcanic ash into the atmosphere, exposing a substantial segment of the population of the northwestern United States to this dust. This event generated considerable interest in the scientific community regarding the possible health effects of volcanic ash. Volcanic ash consists of a mixture of glass and crystals in several mineral phases. Amorphous silicates constitute about 65% of the dust, and there are varying quantities of iron and aluminum oxides, lime, soda, and potash. Crystalline silica, which constitutes 1%–6% of the ash, may include the polymorphs cristobalite, tridymite, and quartz.[82,83] The respirable fraction of particles varies considerably from one volcanic eruption to another, but for the May 18, 1980, eruption of Mt. St. Helens, 85% of sedimented ash particles collected 155 miles from the volcano were in the respirable range.[83]

The cytotoxic and fibrogenic potential of volcanic ash has been examined in a number of experimental studies. In vitro studies have shown that the hemolytic activity and macrophage cytotoxicity of volcanic ash is intermediate between that of an inert dust control (barite) and highly cytotoxic crystalline silica, quartz.[83] In vivo inhalation studies at relatively low doses (10 mg/m³) have shown no appreciable physiologic or pathologic effects for Mt. St. Helens volcanic ash.[84] However, inhalation of high doses (100 mg/m³) of ash resulted in mild interstitial fibrosis, although considerably less than that produced by similar doses of quartz.[82] The conclusion of all these studies is that high doses of volcanic ash may produce lung damage in the form of fibrosis, but that the cytotoxic and fibrogenic potential of volcanic ash is considerably less than that of quartz.

Investigation of the deaths related to the Mt. St. Helens eruption showed that death could be attributed to inhalation of volcanic dust and either thermal or traumatic injury.[85] In the former instance, death resulted from asphyxiation from blockage of the major airways by dust-laden mucus. There was no evidence that persons with chronic respiratory disease experienced acute exacerbations consequent to the inhalation of the dust. Similarly, there has been no apparent long-term effect on the respiratory function of the general population in the vicinity of the eruption. In addition, longitudinal studies of loggers in areas of heavy dust fallout showed evidence of mucus hypersecretion and airway inflammation that reversed when exposure levels decreased.[86]

Lung Disease Caused by Nonasbestos Mineral Fibers

A fiber is generally defined as a mineral particle with an aspect (length-to-diameter) ratio of 3:1 or greater and roughly parallel sides. A variety of nonasbestos mineral fibers have been identified in the human lung[87–89] (Table 27–4). Some of these have been discussed in previous sections: for example, silica, talc, kaolinite, rutile (titanium dioxide), and barium sulfate. Others have been identified in human lung tissue but not implicated in disease: for example, apatite, feldspar, gypsum, illite, mullite, pyroxene, pyrophyllite, sericite, and sillimanite. The remaining nonasbestos mineral fibers listed in Table 27–4 are the subject of this section. It should be noted that most of these minerals occur in both fibrous and nonfibrous forms; a wide range of pathogenic potential is associated with these mineral fibers, and mechanisms of tissue injury are in general poorly understood.

Table 27–4. Nonasbestos mineral fibers found in human lung[a]

Apatite	Pyroxene
Attapulgite	Pyrophyllite
Barium sulfate	Rock wool
Carbon	Rutile
Ceramic fibers	Sericite
Chromium	Silica
Feldspar	Sillimanite
Fiberglass	Talc
Gypsum	Tin
Illite	Vermiculite
Kaolinite	Wollastonite
Mullite	Zeolite

[a] Modified with permission from Churg[87] and Scanning Electron Microsc 1985; II:659–680.[88]

Man-Made Mineral Fibers

This group includes fibrous glass, rock wool, and ceramic fibers, cylindrical amorphous silicates that tend to break perpendicular to their length rather than separating longitudinally in the manner of asbestos fibers. Fibrous glass is manufactured from borosilicate and low alkaline silicate glasses mixed with various amounts of silica, soda, lime, aluminum, and titanium.[90] Rock wool is made by melting and drawing out into fibrous form naturally occurring rock. Ceramic fibers are made from refractory materials used in the ceramics industry. Man-made mineral fibers have the properties of high tensile strength and resistance to heat, cold, and chemicals. Because of these properties, they have a wide range of industrial applications. Rock wool and fibrous glass wool are used in thermal insulation. Glass fibers are used to reinforce plastics, rubber, and paper, in fabrics, and in filter products. Ceramic fibers are used in materials requiring high thermal or chemical resistance. Man-made mineral fibers have a wide range of fiber diameters; depending on the particular industrial application, they vary from microfibers 0.05 μm in diameter to coarse glass fibers 254 μm in diameter.[90] Similarly, the lengths of individual fibers may range from less than a micron to many hundreds of microns.

Dimensional considerations are very important in any analysis of the biologic activity of fibers. Because of the tendency of fibers to line up with their long axes parallel to the flow of air, the aerodynamic behavior of fibers is dependent primarily on their diameter and is relatively independent of fiber length. Fibers with a diameter of 3.5 μm or less may penetrate to the lung periphery, whereas larger diameter fibers impact for the most part in the upper airways. However, fibers with lengths ranging well over 200 μm can penetrate

into respiratory bronchioles and alveolar ducts, provided they have an appropriately thin diameter. Experimental studies with fibrous glass have shown that long fibers are more fibrogenic than shorter ones.[91] In addition, long (>8 μm) and thin (<1.5 μm) glass fibers are the most carcinogenic in an animal model of pleural mesothelioma.[92] Thus, long and thin fibers are particularly dangerous because of their access to distal airways and biologic activity. Other considerations in the pathogenicity of fibrous glass include the relative brittleness of the fibers, especially in comparison to asbestos, and the solubility of the fibers in vivo. Long glass fibers tend to break up into shorter fibers, which are then transported to regional nodes. Further, fiberglass will dissolve in tissues, particularly in an alkaline environment.[93] This tendency to dissolve and break up into smaller fibers probably accounts to some extent for the lesser fibrogenicity of fiberglass as compared with asbestos fibers of comparable dimensions.[91]

Most epidemiologic studies have indicated that man-made mineral fibers do not produce chronic respiratory disease in exposed workers,[90,94,95] although an excess of nonmalignant respiratory disease in a group of fiberglass workers was reported in one study.[96] Gross et al.[97] found no significant difference in the fiber content of lungs from individuals who had worked for as long as 30 years in the fiberglass industry as compared to controls. One epidemiologic study showed a slightly increased risk of malignant mesothelioma in fiberglass workers,[98] although this finding has not been confirmed.

Zeolite

Zeolites are hydrated aluminum silicates that include approximately 40 distinct mineral species. Two of the forms of zeolite, mordenite and erionite, occur as predominantly fibrous species. Natural deposits of zeolites are found in the western United States. Because of their hydrophilic nature and selective adsorption and ion-exchange capabilities, zeolites are used in the petrochemical industry, wastewater treatment, water filtration, cement production, and in animal litter. Commercial interest in both natural and synthetic zeolites appears to be increasing.[90]

Erionite, a fibrous zeolite found naturally in volcanic tuff in Turkey, has physical characteristics that closely resemble those of amphibole asbestos.[99] These fibers may have a high aspect ratio, and most have diameters less than 0.25 μm. Experimental studies have shown that intraperitoneal injection of erionite results in the production of peritoneal mesotheliomas and fibrosis.[100] The author concluded that the carcinogenic and fibrogenic effects of fibrous erionite are similar to those of asbestos. However, many of the zeolites that are used commercially are nonfibrous or granular particles, and their pathogenic potential, although unknown, is probably nil.

Interest in the pathologic effects of zeolites can be largely attributed to the discovery of an epidemic of malignant pleural mesothelioma in two small villages in the Anatolian region of Turkey.[101] These villages, Karain and Tuskoy, have combined population of less than 3,000 and the highest rates of mesothelioma of any population yet encountered, whereas other villages only a few kilometers away had no detected mesotheliomas. Karain and Tuskoy are situated on volcanic tuffs rich in fibrous erionite, and the mineral is ubiquitous in the local environment. Surveys of the villages have shown striking prevalence of pleural calcification and plaque formation as well as diffuse interstitial fibrosis.[90] Fibrous erionite has been identified in lung tissue from villagers who died of mesothelioma.[102] Thus fibrous erionite is associated with a range of pathologic changes similar to those that occur in individuals exposed to asbestos (see Chapter 28).

Wollastonite

Wollastonite is a fibrous monocalcium silicate. Deposits of this mineral are found in Austria, Finland, Mexico, and New York. Wollastonite has insulating and fire-retarding properties, and has been used as an asbestos substitute in wallboards, insulation, and brake linings. It is also used extensively as a filler in the ceramics industry.[90] The quartz content of wollastonite mined in New York is less than 2%. Little is known concerning the pathogenicity of wallastonite fibers. In vitro studies have shown that alveolar macrophages exposed to wollastonite fibers have normal surface characteristics but a diminished phagocytic capacity. Furthermore, wollastonite fibers are capable of activating complement.[103] Wollastonite can produce pleural mesotheliomas in rats, but is less effective in this regard than are many other fibrous dusts.[92]

There are few epidemiologic studies of the health effects of wollastonite in man. Respirable fibers with diameters in the range of 0.2–0.3 μm can be found in airborne dust in areas where wollastonite is mined or processed. One study of wollastonite miners in New York showed an increased prevalence of chronic bronchitis but no evidence of obstructive or restrictive ventilatory changes.[104] However, a study of Finnish wollastonite quarry workers showed increased interstitial markings on chest radiographs in some workers, as well as pleural thickening and calcification.[105] There was also an increased prevalence of chronic bronchitis. The exposure to quartz was probably greater in the Finnish

than in the New York workers, although nodular opacities were not observed. Pathologic studies are not available, nor was the possible carcinogenicity of wollastonite and mortality of exposed workers studied in detail.

Vermiculite

Vermiculite is a hydrated aluminum-iron-magnesium-silicate that includes 19 distinct mineral species. As vermiculite is heated, the fiber expands to become curved or worm like, hence its name. Deposits of this mineral are found in South Africa, and, in the United States, in Montana, Virginia, and South Carolina. In addition to vermiculite, a number of other minerals including quartz, feldspar, apatite, corundum, chlorite, talc, and asbestos occur in these deposits. Contamination with tremolite, actinolite, or anthophyllite asbestos fibers has raised concerns regarding the potential health effects of vermiculite exposure.[106] Vermiculite may occur in a tubular form that closely resembles chrysotile.[90] Vermiculite is used as an aggregate in cement, wallboards, and plasters, as a filler in plastic, rubber, roofing, and flooring material, as a soil additive, and as a bulking agent in animal feeds. It is also used as a carrier for various industrial chemicals.[90]

Neither fibrogenic nor carcinogenic properties of vermiculite have been demonstrated in animal studies. Workers in the vermiculite industry have been shown to have benign pleural effusions that were correlated with cumulative fiber exposure, but no abnormalities were seen on pulmonary function tests. These pleural abnormalities are thought to be related to the contamination of vermiculite by asbestos fibers. Vermiculite miners have an increased risk of pleural mesothelioma and carcinoma of the lung, and analysis of lung tissue samples has revealed large numbers of high-aspect-ratio tremolite asbestos fibers.[107] The health effects of pure vermiculite are unknown.[98]

Carbon

Carbon particles occasionally occur in a fibrous form and have been described in coal workers[7] and in individuals with no known occupational exposure.[74] Ramage et al. described a unique case of an elderly woman with dyspnea and interstitial changes on chest radiography from whom numerous black fibers (some coated with iron) were recovered by bronchoalveolar lavage. Open lung biopsy showed patchy interstitial fibrosis associated with numerous black fibers (Fig. 27–16). Digestion studies of the biopsy specimen demonstrated more than 2 million black fibers per gram of lung tissue, and energy-dispersive x-ray analysis showed them to contain no elements with atomic number greater than

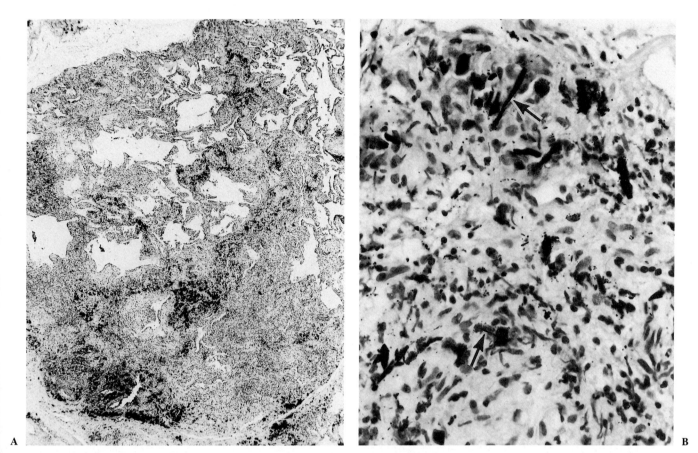

Fig. 27–16 A,B. Open lung biopsy from individual exposed to woodstove dust. **A.** Patchy interstitial fibrosis. **B.** Higher magnification shows elongated black carbon fibers, some coated with iron *(arrows)*, embedded in fibrous matrix.

or equal to 11. The black fibers included lathe-like and grid-like structures, and bizarre forms. The composition and appearance of these particles fits that described in woodstove dust.[109] Asbestos fibers were not identified. The source of the fibers was believed to be an old woodstove with a poorly sealed door in her home, a small trailer that was inadequately ventilated. The relationship of these intrapulmonary fibers to the interstitial fibrosis is unclear. However, recent studies regarding the cytotoxicity of certain carbon fiber composites indicate that some of these fibers are not inert, causing irreversible injury to alveolar macrophages and large increases in airway cells and neutrophils in rat lungs.[110]

Chromium

Chromium fibers have not been previously identified in human tissues. A case studied by one of the authors (V.L.R.) was a patient who at autopsy had large cell carcinoma of the right-upper lobe and bilateral parietal pleural plaques. Digestion studies showed more than 600,000 fibers per gram of wet lung tissue, more than 90% of which had an elemental composition of chro-

mium. The fibers were generally curved or semicircular, with irregular borders. A few particularly long chromium fibers were iron coated. The patient's occupation had been that of a metal polisher, although he had been retired for some 12 years. The relationship of this man's lung cancer and pleural plaques to the chromium fibers is unknown. A rare chrysotile fiber was encountered in the lung tissue. Chromate workers have been shown to have an increased risk for lung cancer, but there are no reports of increased lung cancer risk in metal polishers.

Nonasbestos Ferruginous Bodies

The coating of asbestos fibers with an iron-protein mucopolysaccharide matrix in the formation of asbestos bodies is well known. Not as well appreciated is the fact that a number of other types of fibrous dusts may also be coated with iron to become ferruginous bodies. The coating material is deposited by alveolar macrophages on fibers that are generally 20 μm or more in length. Experimental studies have shown that a number of fibrous dusts, including talc, fiberglass, ceramic fibers, and silicon carbide whiskers, can become coated.[66] In humans, a number of fibrous dusts may form the cores of ferruginous bodies, including diatomaceous earth, sheet silicates (broad yellow core fibers), carbon, iron oxide, chromium, rutile, silicon carbide, and chromium–cobalt–molybdenum alloys (black cores).[65,74,75,111] These structures have been referred to as pseudoasbestos bodies, and are usually distinguishable from true asbestos bodies by light microscopy. On the other hand, ferruginous bodies with zeolite[102] cores may be indistinguishable from true asbestos bodies by light microscopy.

Lung Diseases Caused by Metal Fumes

Fumes are particles less than 1 μm and as small as 0.2 μm in diameter. Such particles behave like vapors or gases, and hence penetrate readily into the air-exchanging regions of the lung. There they rapidly enter the alveolar walls and, if irritative, can lead to a chemical pneumonitis that may eventuate in diffuse interstitial fibrosis. The initial chemical pneumonitis has the microscopic features of diffuse alveolar damage.

Bauxite Lung

Bauxite lung, or Shaver's disease, results from exposure to fumes generated during the manufacture of alumina abrasives. This material, also known as corundum, is made by finely grinding bauxite, iron, and coke and fusing the mixture in an electric furnace. The resulting fumes consist of particles less than 1 μm in diameter with a composition of aluminum oxide (50%), amorphous silica (36%), ferric oxide (3%–4%), and traces of titanium oxide and other constituents.[112] Individuals exposed to these fumes may become short of breath and show radiographic changes as soon as 3 months after exposure. In fatal cases, the lungs are heavy, greyish black, and have dense fibrotic areas scattered throughout. Dense pleural adhesions and large subpleural emphysematous bullae may be present and may lead to spontaneous pneumothorax. Microscopically, there is diffuse alveolar septal fibrosis associated with aggregates of black dust particles. This may progress to diffuse fibrosis with obliteration of alveolar spaces. Analyses of lungs show the same constituents that are present in the bauxite fumes.[5] Interstitial fibrosis has also been described among aluminum smelters, aluminum arc welders and aluminum polishers.[59,113]

Cadmium Pneumonitis

Cadmium is used in the manufacture of alloys and alkaline accumulators, in electroplating, and in the control of atomic reactors. Cadmium oxide fumes can be generated in these processes, and also during welding of steel plated with cadmium as an anticorrosive.[5] Symptoms begin within 8 h of exposure, starting with throat irritation and progressing to dyspnea. Death occurs in about 16% of cases. In acutely fatal cases, the lungs are heavy and microscopically show diffuse alveolar damage. In cases with chronic cadmium pneumonitis, the lungs show emphysematous changes. Microscopically, there is edema, perivascular fibrosis, and chronic lymphocytic infiltration. These changes are nonspecific, and diagnosis requires a careful occupational history and analysis of lung tissue for cadmium.[5]

Mercury Pneumonitis

Mercury vapors are produced during the volatilization of mercury and its subsequent condensation to metallic liquid mercury. Exposure to these vapors has been reported to produce a chemical pneumonitis with gradual development of dyspnea and chills that progresses to frank pulmonary edema. Pathologic findings in fatal cases have been those of diffuse alveolar damage.[5]

Mixed Pneumoconiosis and Mixed-Dust Pneumoconiosis

Mixed pneumoconiosis is lung disease that results from exposure to two or more types of inorganic dusts and has pathologic features characteristic of each component. An example alluded to previously in this chapter is siderosilicosis in hematite miners, in which diffuse interstitial deposits of iron oxides may be seen in combination with typical silicotic nodules. Another example is asbestosilicosis, in which peribronchiolar interstitial fibrosis and asbestos bodies may be seen juxtaposed with typical silicotic nodules. This is a fairly common finding in workers in shipyards, where sandblasting, boiler-scaling, and insulating activities may be going on simultaneously in a confined space. One case of mixed pneumoconiosis was reported in which four separate dust-related processes were identified: silicosis, asbestosis, talcosis, and berylliosis.[114] It is anticipated that more instances of mixed pneumoconiosis will be identified with careful attention to pathologic features and use of sophisticated methods of analysis of lung dust burdens.

Mixed-dust pneumoconiosis has been less precisely defined.[115] In the author's opinion, this term should be reserved for patients who have been exposed to a dust mixture with multiple components (usually including silica and silicates), demonstrate a nonspecific pattern of diffuse interstitial fibrosis and alveolar and macrophage response, and whose lesions do not fit into any of the other categories described above. An example is the silicate pneumoconiosis of farm workers.[116] The fibrotic response may result in part from the silica (quartz) content with modification of the response due to the silicate component. The role of the more numerous silicate particles in the fibrotic process is unclear. Diagnosis of mixed-dust pneumoconiosis requires a careful and detailed occupational history and the finding of diffuse interstitial markings on chest radiography. If lung tissue is obtained, it should be analyzed for inorganic particulate content (see following) and the results correlated with the exposure history.

Vegetable Pneumoconioses

Several disorders have been described as a result of inhalation of organic dusts. Some of these are related to hypersensitivity to antigens in the dusts and are thus immune mediated. The pathologic features and various etiologic agents of hypersensitivity pneumonitis are discussed in Chapter 18. Other pulmonary disorders related to inhalation of organic dusts are not thought to be mediated by immune mechanisms. These include pulmonary mycotoxicosis and byssinosis, which are the subjects of the following sections.

Pulmonary Mycotoxicosis (Organic Dust Toxic Syndrome)

Mycotoxins are toxic products produced by a wide variety of fungi.[117] Some familiar examples of mycotoxins include ergot alkaloids, aflatoxin (associated with hepatocellular carcinoma), and the hepatotoxin produced by *Amanita phalloides* (poison mushrooms). Exposure to mycotoxins by inhalation may occur among some workers during the removal of silage from silos or, less commonly, of corn from corn cribs.[118] During storage of these grains, fungi and bacteria grow profusely in the upper few feet of the layers of grain, where a relatively high pH and aerobic conditions prevail. This upper layer must be removed before the silo (or corn crib) can be emptied, and it is during this process that workers may be exposed to very high levels of organic dust containing large numbers of fungal spores and hyphae.

Such exposures have been associated with a characteristic clinical syndrome known as pulmonary myco-

toxicosis[119] or organic dust toxic syndrome.[118] Within a few hours of exposure, the worker complains of fever, myalgias, chest tightness, cough, headache, malaise, or dyspnea.[118] Crackles are often heard on physical examination. The duration of illness ranges from a few hours to several days, and the disease is self-limiting.[120] Bronchoalveolar lavage fluid contains increased numbers of neutrophils within the first few days of the onset of symptoms, and shows a relative lymphocytosis 1 to 7 months post exposure. Fungal spores may also be present within the lavage fluid, and several different species may be recovered in culture.[121] A similar illness has been described among some cotton workers as "mill fever" and among storage elevator workers as "grain fever." One outbreak was described among several members of a college fraternity, related to a party held in a poorly ventilated room with several inches of moldy straw on the floor.[120]

The pathologic features of pulmonary mycotoxicosis have been described in only a small number of cases.[121] There is a nonspecific obliterative bronchiolitis with neutrophils in the terminal bronchioles, alveoli, and pulmonary interstitium (Fig. 27–17). Fibrinous intraalveolar exudates in various stages of organization may be observed, and many fungal spores may be noted as well. Interstitial pneumonitis with scattered multinucleate giant cells, as seen in farmer's lung or other types of hypersensitivity pneumonitis, is not observed in pulmonary mycotoxicosis.

Pulmonary mycotoxicosis must be distinguished from farmer's lung and silo filler's disease. In addition to the pathologic features just described, these disorders differ with respect to a number of clinical features. Pulmonary mycotoxicosis is characterized by normal chest radiographs, absence of serum precipitins, lavage fluid immunoglobulins within the normal range, and clustering of cases when several workers are exposed simultaneously. The seasonality of exposures ranges from July to October. In contrast, farmer's lung disease is characterized by reticulonodular infiltrates on chest roentgenograms, positive serum precipitins to fungal antigens, elevated lavage fluid immunoglobulins, and absence of clustering.[118,120] The seasonality of exposures for farmer's lung disease ranges from October to May. Silo filler's disease is associated with alveolar infiltrates on chest x ray and a history of exposure to brownish smoke (nitrogen oxides).[120]

The mechanism of injury in organic dust toxic syndrome is unknown, although the term pulmonary mycotoxicosis suggests that mycotoxins are involved in the pathogenetic sequence. In fact, there are no published accounts on the effects of mycotoxin inhalation in experimental animals.[117] Other suggested mechanisms

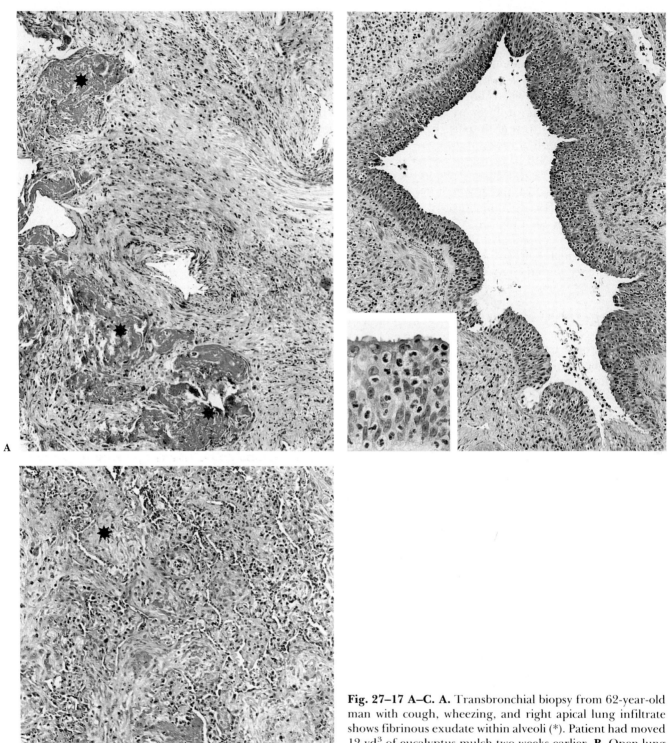

Fig. 27–17 A–C. A. Transbronchial biopsy from 62-year-old man with cough, wheezing, and right apical lung infiltrate shows fibrinous exudate within alveoli (*). Patient had moved 12 yd³ of eucalyptus mulch two weeks earlier. **B.** Open lung biopsy from same patient 2 weeks later shows acute inflammation (inset) within wall of bronchiole. Diffuse alveolar damage, fungal hyphae, and oxalate crystals were also identified in sample. Several fungal species were cultured from both biopsy specimen and eucalyptus mulch. **C.** Open lung biopsy from 68-year-old farmer, who presented with dyspnea 2 days after cleaning out dusty corncrib, shows organizing exudate consisting of edematous plugs of connective tissue within alveoli or alveolar ducts (*) and focal residual fibrin (*arrowhead*). (Courtesy Dr. Tom Colby, Mayo Clinic, Rochester, Minnesota.)

include activation of the alternative complement pathway by organic dusts or exposure to bacterial endotoxins also present within the dust.

Byssinosis

Byssinosis is a form of obstructive lung disease associated with the inhalation of cotton dust among cotton textile workers. This disorder is best characterized by a decrease in the forced expiratory volume at 1 sec (FEV_1) during the first workday after a weekend off or a vacation. The reduction in FEV_1 is less pronounced on subsequent days of the workweek. As a worker with this disorder continues in his job, the degree of reduction in the FEV_1 often increases and the effect is observed on more days of the workweek. In some workers, the effect on the FEV_1 can eventually be observed every day, and some may develop chronic respiratory failure with total disability.[122] Symptoms related to the decrease in FEV_1 include cough, chest tightness, and dyspnea. A dose–response relationship has been demonstrated for the acute phase of byssinosis, with a positive correlation between higher dust levels and increased risk of acute symptoms.[123] There is some variation in the occurrence of byssinosis in various locations within the textile mill, with the highest risk associated with the "carding" operation, which tends to be a particularly dusty area. Lesser risk is associated with the less dusty procedures of "spinning" and "weaving."[122]

Relatively few studies have examined the pathologic features of byssinosis.[124,125] The histologic features observed, which are not specific for cotton dust exposure, include mucous gland hyperplasia in the large airways (bronchi) and goblet cell metaplasia in the small airways (bronchioles).[124] These morphologic features are illustrated in the chapter on Emphysema and Chronic Bronchitis (Chapter 26). There is no evidence of an increased prevalence of emphysema among cotton mill workers as compared to nontextile workers,[124,125] although there is a strong association between the prevalence of emphysema and a history of cigarette smoking.[124] This implies that, among nonsmoking cotton textile workers, the obstructive changes are potentially reversible following cessation of exposure to cotton dusts.

An additional finding reported to be present in the lungs of some workers is the so-called byssinosis body. This structure consists of dark, irregularly shaped strands embedded in a dense collagenous matrix and measuring up to 200 μm in maximum dimension.[5] The dark core material is deeply hematoxyphilic and is partially coated by a golden-brown substance, probably hemosiderin. Histochemical and ultrastructural studies indicate that the core material is cellulose, and the byssinosis body thus probably represents cotton fibers that are deposited in the lung and incite an inflammatory response with subsequent calcification and ferruginization.

The mechanism of tissue injury in byssinosis continues to be elusive. It is known that dust derived from cotton bract, the thin brittle leaves surrounding the cotton ball, probably contains the responsible agent.[126] Aqueous extracts of cotton bracts have been shown to produce decrements in lung function 1–2 h after administration, and such extracts have chemotactic activity for neutrophils.[127] It has been suggested that endotoxin derived from bacterial contamination of cotton dust is the causative agent of byssinosis, and exposure to increasing levels of airborne endotoxin has been shown to increase the risk of pulmonary abnormalities among cotton workers.[123] However, it is unlikely that endotoxin can explain all the airway epithelial changes in byssinosis, and further research seems warranted to identify other biologically active agents in cotton dust.[123,126]

Methods of Analysis of Mineral Dust in Lung Tissue

Indications and Medicolegal Implications

Just as clinical investigation of a patient with suspected pneumoconiosis should begin with a thorough and complete occupational history, so should the pathologic examination begin with a review of the available details regarding gross morphologic features and of routinely stained histologic sections. The latter should include examination of sections with polarized light. In most instances, the combination of occupational history, gross morphologic features including chest radiographic findings, and histology will result in the correct pathologic diagnosis (Table 27–5). However, in some cases the patient may not be able to provide the required information or may even be unaware of exposure to a noxious agent. In addition, analysis of lung tissue for the presence of putative injurious agents may provide important evidence in medicolegal circumstances. Moreover, the histologic appearance in many instances is nonspecific and additional studies are required to arrive at a correct pathologic diagnosis. In this section we review analytical techniques that may be applied to the detection and quantification of inorganic particulates in lung tissue. It must be emphasized that the *quantification* of inorganic particulates in lung tissue requires knowledge of the content of the constituents of interest in the lungs of the general population, specifi-

Table 27–5. Pathologic features of selected common mineral pneumoconioses

Dust	Disease	Pathologic features	Tuberculosis[a]
Silica	Silicosis	Hyalinized nodules, solitary or conglomerate, upper lobes and lymph nodes	Yes
Coal dust	Coalworkers' pneumoconiosis	Macule, micro- and macronodules, progressive massive fibrosis, focal emphysema	Yes
Talc	Talcosis	Nonnecrotizing granulomas, diffuse interstitial fibrosis, progressive massive fibrosis (rare)	No
Kaolin	Kaolin pneumoconiosis	Macules and nodules consisting of collections of dust-laden macrophages, minimal fibrosis	No
Beryllium	Berylliosis	Nonnecrotizing granulomas, interstitial pneumonitis, diffuse interstitial fibrosis	No
Welding fumes	Welder's pneumoconiosis	Peribronchiolar and perivascular accumulation of dust particles, minimal fibrosis	No
Hematite	Hematite miners' lung	Peribronchiolar and pervascular dust deposits, diffuse and nodular fibrosis, progressive massive fibrosis	Yes

[a] Increased host susceptibility to tuberculosis.

cally, individuals with no occupational exposure to the particulate under investigation.

Tissue Preparation

Techniques have been described for analyzing elemental content of routine paraffin sections, which require a minimum of tissue preparation.[128] Paraffin sections 5-7 μm thick can be cut onto carbon supports, deparaffinized in xylene, and if desired coated with a conducting material such as carbon or gold. These sections can then be examined by analytical scanning electron microscopy as discussed subsequently. Areas of dust content can be identified on adjacent hematoxylin and eosin-stained (H and E) sections and readily compared with the scanning electron microscopy image to localize the dust. While procedures for quantitating the particulate content in paraffin sections have also been devised,[129] they are not widely used at present. In some instances, paraffin blocks are not available or the area of interest is localized to a single region of one slide. Techniques are available to transfer tissue from a glass slide to a carbon disc, allowing the investigator to study by analytical scanning electron microscopy a particular cell or particulate observed in an H and E section.[130] These methods of examining paraffin sections have the advantages of being nondestructive, of preserving the pulmonary architecture and the anatomic distribution of dusts, and of having retrospective application to materials readily available to the pathologist, especially paraffin blocks. They have the disadvantages of potential interference with particle identification or localization because of matrix effects and because of difficulty in identification and measurement of fibers.[129]

As a result of these latter disadvantages, techniques have been developed for extracting inorganic particulates from lung tissue. The particles may then be concentrated and characterized more readily. Potential problems with these techniques include loss of particles during the isolation procedure or contamination by particles not originally in the tissue. In addition, the particles themselves may be altered by the extraction process. For example, ashing lung tissue in a muffle furnace at 400°–500°C may cause fracture of fibers (resulting in a falsely elevated total fiber count and altering their length distribution), fracture of the iron coating of fibers (decreasing the ratio of coated to uncoated fibers), and altering the crystal structure of some inorganic particulates. These problems are greatly reduced by using a low-temperature plasma asher.[131] Wet chemical techniques that have been devised for recovering particulates from lung tissue include digestion with hot potassium hydroxide, hydrogen peroxide, formamide, concentrated acids, or proteolytic enzymes. A popular technique in the United States is digestion in commercial bleach, which is a 5.25% sodium hypochlorite solution.[132] This technique has little effect on most inorganic particulates found in lung tissue.[63] The extraction techniques enumerated are best applied to wet formalin-fixed lung tissue, and the particulate content can be related to the wet or dry weight of lung tissue examined. If one uses such techniques to analyze paraffin blocks, the removal of lipids during the embedding process will reduce the wet and dry weight of the sample, and this decrease in the denominator will alter the concentration of particles per gram of tissue.[81]

Transmission Electron Microscopy

This technique is more expensive and time consuming than light microscopy, but offers a number of advantages over that technique. Particles beyond the resolution of light microscopy can be readily identified by

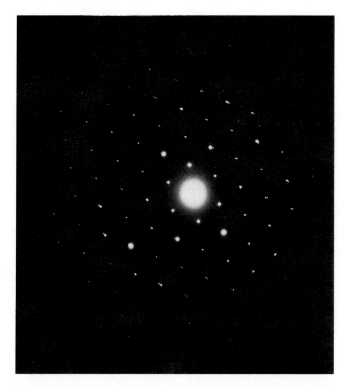

Fig. 27–18. Selected-area electron diffraction pattern obtained from kaolinite particle shows pseudohexagonal pattern.

beam produces x rays with energies characteristic of the elements of which the particle is composed. The energies of the x rays can be analyzed with a siliconlithium semiconductor detector and displayed as a spectrum showing the relative abundance of all elements with an atomic number of 11 (sodium) or greater. This process is referred to as energy-dispersive x-ray analysis.[133] Diffraction of the electron beam passing through a selected area of the specimen can provide information regarding the crystallographic structure of a particle, as is discussed later. Selected-area electron diffraction produces a pattern of dots characteristic of the particular lattice geometry of the crystal (Fig. 27–18). The combination of transmission electron microscopy, energy-dispersive x-ray analysis, and selected area electron diffraction has been used to identify various types of inorganic fibers isolated from human lungs[87] as well as a variety of nonfibrous inorganic particulates[134] (Table 27–6). Many of these particles require both chemical composition and crystallographic structural information for reliable identification. One of the limitations of transmission electron microscopy is the small volume of tissue that can be analyzed. This technique is primarily applicable to particles extracted from tissue, because ultrathin sections contain such a small volume as to be insensitive for the detection and identification of some particulates.[135]

transmission electron microscopy, and their morphologic details are more readily apparent. Chemical and crystallographic information can be obtained on particles as small as 0.1 μm in maximum dimension. Bombardment of a particle with a finely focused electron

Scanning Electron Microscopy

The technique of scanning electron microscopy also permits identification of particles beyond the resolution of the light microscope, but its resolution is somewhat

Table 27–6. Analytical techniques for identification of inorganic particulates in lung tissue

Technique	Parameter measured	Application
Energy-dispersive x-ray analysis (EDXA)	Elemental composition of inorganic particulates ($Z \geq 11$)	Identification of most inorganic particulates, including silica, silicates, etc.
Selected-area electron diffraction (SAED)	Crystallographic structure of individual particle	Supplemental information (along with EDXA) for identification of silicates and other inorganic particulates
X-ray diffraction	Crystallographic structure of extracted dust	Identification and quantification of talc, mica, kaolinite, etc. (independently or complementary to EDXA)
Electron energy-loss spectrometry (EELS)	Elemental composition of inorganic particles, especially for $Z < 11$	Identification of beryllium and occasionally other light elements
Secondary ion mass spectrometry (SIMS)	Elemental and isotopic composition of tissue, with sensitivity in ppm range	Identification of beryllium, cobalt, mercury, cadmium, and other trace elements
Laser microprobe mass analyzer (LAMMA)	Elemental and isotopic composition of tissue, with sensitivity in ppm range	Identification of beryllium, cobalt, mercury, cadmium, and other trace elements
X-ray fluorescence (XRF)	Elemental composition of inorganic particulates ($Z \geq 11$), with sensitivity greater than EDXA	Identification of cobalt, mercury, cadmium, and other trace elements

less than that of transmission electron microscopy. Several imaging modes are possible with the scanning electron microscope. Secondary electron imaging utilizes the low-energy secondary electrons scattered from the surface of the specimen to provide the familiar "three-dimensional" images of the specimen with considerable depth resolution (Fig. 27–19). Backscattered electron imaging utilizes elastically scattered, high-energy primary electrons to provide an image that contrasts high atomic number particles within a low atomic number matrix. This imaging mode is ideal for locating inorganic particulates within paraffin sections of lung.[63,129,131] In addition, x rays produced by bombardment of the specimen with the electron beam may be imaged to show the topographic distribution of a single element in a dot map or of all elements with atomic number greater than or equal to 11. This is referred to as total rate imaging with x rays.[132] Spot-mode analysis of individual particles may also be used to obtain energy-dispersive x ray spectra (Fig. 27–20) and hence a chemical profile of the particle. Scanning electron microscopy has the advantage over transmission electron microscopy in that it can be applied to a wide variety of samples, ranging from paraffin sections, as described previously, to bulk tissue samples with a volume up to 3 cm^3, to extracted particles on a membrane filter, to cell monolayers, etc. In addition, automated-image x-ray analyzers are commercially available that can be interfaced with the scanning electron microscope and are capable of automatically analyzing as many as 1,000 inorganic particulates per hour on a suitable substrate.[132] Information can thus be obtained

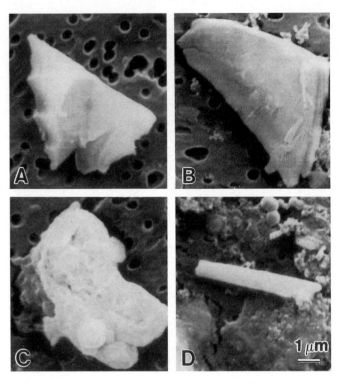

Fig. 27–19 A–D. Secondary electron images of particles commonly found in lung tissue extracts. **A.** Silica. **B.** Talc. **C.** Kaolinite. **D.** Rutile or titanium dioxide fiber. Scanning electron microscopy. Scale bar = 1.0 μm.

concerning chemical composition, physical dimensions, and concentration of particles per unit area at a rate many times greater than is attainable by manual operation.[136] Disadvantages of scanning electron microscopy

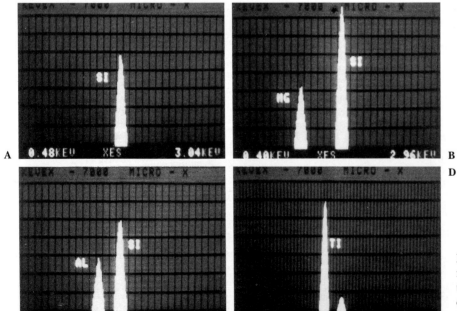

Fig. 27–20 A–D. Energy-dispersive x-ray analysis spectra obtained from particles commonly found in lung tissue extracts. **A.** Silica. **B.** Talc. **C.** Kaolinite. **D.** Rutile or titanium dioxide fiber.

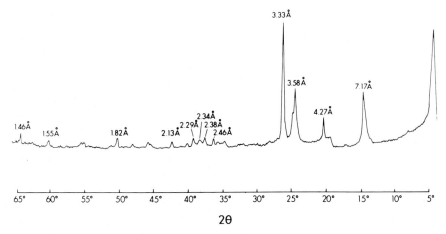

Fig. 27–21. X-ray diffraction spectrum obtained from dust isolated from lung of patient in Fig. 27–1. Note numerous peaks for alpha quartz. Peaks for several silicates are also present.

include lack of crystallographic data, as obtained by selected-area electron diffraction, and inability to detect some morphologic features of particles that may be observed with the transmission electron microscope.[63,132]

X-Ray Diffraction Techniques

Crystallographic information is often necessary for the accurate identification of some inorganic particulates. Although selected-area electron diffraction can provide structural information pertaining to an individual particle, x-ray diffraction can provide similar information for a bulk sample. Dust extracted from lung tissue is placed on an appropriate substrate in an x-ray diffractometer, and the data are recorded either as a series of peaks on a strip chart (Fig. 27–21) or as series of rings on a photographic film using a Debye–Scherer camera.[137] The lattice parameters of each crystalline substance in the extracted dust can be measured from the diffraction pattern and compared with the known values of thousands of crystalline materials as indexed by the American Society for Testing Materials.[138] The area under the peaks in the diffraction pattern is proportional to the quantity of the material that is present, and this relationship has been used to quantitatively measure inorganic materials such as quartz and chrysotile asbestos using x-ray diffraction.[139,140] We have used x-ray diffraction to measure the silica content of lung tissue, and found 10-100 mg total of quartz for both lungs combined, in both smokers and nonsmokers from the general population.[7] Patients with silicosis typically have several hundred to several thousand milligrams of quartz in both lungs.

Other Techniques

Most of the inorganic particulates discussed in this chapter can be identified by one or more of the tech-

niques described (Table 27–6). Occasionally techniques with greater sensitivity are required, such as for the detection of beryllium in lung tissue of patients with suspected berylliosis. In addition to wet chemical spectrographic techniques, some of the newer microanalytical techniques that have been employed to detect beryllium in tissue sections include electron energy loss spectrometry, secondary ion mass spectrometry, and laser microprobe mass analysis. Some toxic metals such as cadmium, mercury, and cobalt may be identified using x-ray fluorescence, secondary ion mass spectrometry, or laser microprobe mass analysis. Often overlooked is the utilization of bulk chemical techniques, particularly for trace element analysis. These techniques, which are sensitive for many elements at the part per billion level, include atomic absorption spectrometry, atomic emission spectroscopy, and neutron activation analysis. The details of these analytical techniques and their specific applications have been discussed elsewhere.[132,137]

The analytical approach used by a pathologist in the investigation of a particular case will depend somewhat on the equipment and expertise available in his institution. Not only may different analytical approaches be used from one institution to another, but most of these techniques have not been standardized for biologic samples. Hence results may differ from one institution to another even when the same technique is used. Further, normal ranges have not been established for most inorganic particulates in human lung tissue, for example, silicates, metals, and other xenobiotics with known toxic potential. Even in the case of mineral fibers for which some data are available with respect to levels in the general population, the methods of analysis of human tissues are not nearly as well standardized as the U.S. Environmental Protection Agency's methods of fiber analysis of water or air samples. One should therefore interpret mineralogic analyses of tissues with caution, and the mere identification of a given particulate in lung tissue does not necessarily imply the presence of disease or that the particulate identified is the cause of any abnormalities present. In other words, mineralogic analyses of tissues should be interpreted in the context of all clinical and pathologic data available to the investigator. Standardization of techniques and determination of normal ranges would be facilitated by establishment of regional centers, and long-term stable funding in this regard is highly desirable.

References

1. Zenker FA. Staubinhalations Krankheiten der lungen. 1866.

2. Brody AR, Roe MW. Deposition pattern of inorganic particles at the alveolar level in the lungs of rats and mice. Am Rev Respir Dis 1983;128:724–729.

3. Raabe OG. Deposition and clearance of inhaled particles In: Gee JBL, Morgan WKC, Brooks SM, eds. Occupational lung disease. New York: Raven, 1984:1–37.

4. Langer AM. Crystal faces and cleavage planes in quartz as templates in biological processes. Q Rev Biophys 1978;2:543–575.

5. Spencer H, ed. The pneumoconioses and other occupational lung diseases. In: Pathology of the lung. 4th Ed., Vol. 1. Oxford: Pergamon Press, 1985:413–510.

6. Abraham JL. Recent advances in pneumoconiosis: The pathologists' role in etiologic diagnosis. In: Thurlbeck M, ed. The lung: Structure, function, and disease. IAP Monogr. 19. Baltimore: Williams & Wilkins, 1978:96–137.

7. Roggli VL, Mastin JP, Shelburne JD, Roe M, Brody AR. Inorganic particulates in human lung: relationship to the inflammatory response. In: Lynn WS, ed. Inflammatory cells and lung disease. Boca Raton: CRC Press, 1983:29–62.

8. Pratt PC. Lung dust content and response in guinea pigs inhaling three forms of silica. Arch Environ Health 1983;38:197–204.

9. Vallyathan V, Shi X, Dalal NS, Irr W, Castranova V. Generation of free radicals from freshly fractured silica dust: Potential role in silica-induced lung injury. Am Rev Respir Dis 1988;138:1213–1219.

10. Heppleston AG: Pulmonary repair and fibrosis. In: Glynn LE, ed. Tissue repair and regeneration. Amsterdam: Elsevier/North Holland, 1981:393–456.

11. Absher M, Mortara M. Effect of silica on the proliferative behavior of human lung fibroblasts. In Vitro 1980;16:371–376.

12. Kleinerman J. The pathology of some familiar pneumoconioses. Semin Roentgenol 1967;2:244–264.

13. Slavin RE, Swedo JL, Brandes D, Gonzalez-Vitale JC, Osornio-Vargas A. Extrapulmonary silicosis: A clinical, morphologic, and ultrastructural study. Hum Pathol 1985;16:393–412.

14. Kleinerman J, Green F, Laquer W, et al. Pathology standards for coal workers pneumoconiosis. Arch Pathol Lab Med 1979;103:375–432.

15. Buechner HA, Ansari A. Acute silico-proteinosis. Dis Chest 1969;55:274–284.

16. Heppleston AG, Wright NA, Steward JA. Experimental alveolar lipoproteinosis following the inhalation of silica. J Pathol 1970;101:293–307.

17. Miller RR, Churg AM, Hutcheon M, Lam S. Pulmonary alveolar proteinosis and aluminum dust exposure. Am Rev Respir Dis 1984;130:312–315.

18. Craighead JE, Vallyathan NV. Cryptic pulmonary lesions in workers occupationally exposed to dust containing silica. JAMA 1980;244:1939–1941.

19. Craighead JE, Kleinerman J, Abraham JL, et al. Diseases associated with exposure to silica and nonfibrous silicate minerals. Arch Pathol Lab Med 1988;112:673–720.

20. Goldsmith DF, Winn DM, Shy CM, eds. Silica, silicosis, and cancer: Controversy in occupational medicine. Cancer Research Monographs. New York: Praeger, 1986.

21. Craighead JE. Do silica and asbestos cause lung cancer? Arch Pathol Lab Med 1992;116:16–20.

22. Adamson IYR, Bowden DH. Role of monocytes and interstitial cells in the generation of alveolar macrophages. II. Kinetic studies after carbon loading. Lab Invest 1980;42:518–524.

23. Pratt PC. Role of silica in progressive massive fibrosis. Arch Environ Health 1968;16:734–737.

24. Heppleston AG. The pathological anatomy of simple pneumoconiosis in coal workers. J Pathol Bacteriol 1953;66:235–246.

25. Marine WM, Gurr D, Jacobsen M. Clinically important respiratory effects of dust exposure and smoking in British coal miners. Am Rev Respir Dis 1988;137:106–112.

26. Rom WN, Kanner RE, Renzetti AD, et al. Respiratory disease in Utah coal miners. Am Rev Respir Dis 1981;123:372–377.

27. Ames RG, Amandus H, Attfield M, Green FY, Vallyathan V. Does coal mine dust present a risk for lung cancer? A case-control study of U.S. coal miners. Arch Environ Health 1983;38:331–333.

28. Vallyathan NV, Green FHY, Rodman NF, Boyd CB, Althouse R. Lung carcinoma by histologic type in coal miners. Arch Pathol Lab Med 1985;109:419–423.

29. Pratt PC, Kilburn KH. Extent of pulmonary pigmentation as an indicator of particulate environmental air pollution. Inhaled Part Vap 1971;2:661–670.

30. Watson AJ, Black J, Doig AT, Nagelschmidt G. Pneumoconiosis in carbon electrode makers. Br J Ind Med 1959;16:274–285.

31. Schepers GWH, Durkan TM. Experimental study of the effects of talc dust on animal tissue. Arch Ind Health 1955;12:317–328.

32. Vallyathan NV, Craighead JE. Pulmonary pathology in workers exposed to nonasbestiform talc. Hum Pathol 1981;12:28–35.

33. Vallyathan NV. Talc pneumoconiosis. Respir Ther 1980;10:34–39.

34. Miller A, Teirstein AS, Bader MD, Bader RA, Selikoff IJ. Talc pneumoconiosis: Significance of sublight-microscopic mineral particles. Am J Med 1971;50:395–402.

35. Tomashefski JF, Hirsch CS. The pulmonary vascular lesions of intravenous drug abuse. Hum Pathol 1980; 11:133–145.

36. Berner A, Gylseth B, Levy F. Talc dust pneumoconiosis. Acta Pathol Microbiol Scand 1981;89A:17–21.

37. Crouch E, Churg A. Progressive massive fibrosis of the lung secondary to intravenous injection of talc. A pathologic and mineralogic analysis. Am J Clin Pathol 1983; 80:520–526.

38. Williams WJ. The pathology of pulmonary sarcoidosis. Proc R Soc Med 1967;60:986–988.

39. Abraham JL, Brambilla C. Particle size for differentiation between inhalation and injection pulmonary talcosis. Environ Res 1980;21:94–96.

40. Paré JP, Cote G, Fraser RS. Long-term follow-up of drug abusers with intravenous talcosis. Am Rev Respir Dis 1989;139:233–241.

41. Kleinfeld M, Messite J, Zaki MH. Mortality experiences among talc workers: A follow-up study. J Occup Med 1974;16:345–349.

42. Sepulveda M-J, Vallyathan V, Attfield MD, Piacitelli L, Tucker JH. Pneumoconiosis and lung function in a group of kaolin workers. Am Rev Respir Dis 1983; 127:231–235.

43. Lapenas D, Gale P, Kennedy T, Rawlings W, Dietrich P. Kaolin pneumoconiosis: Radiologic, pathologic, and mineralogic findings. Am Rev Respir Dis 1984;130:282–288.

44. Brody AR, Craighead JE. Cytoplasmic inclusions in pulmonary macrophages of cigarette smokers. Lab Invest 1975;32:125–132.

45. White R, Kuhn C. Effects of phagocytosis of mineral dusts on elastase secretion by alveolar and peritoneal exudative macrophages. Arch Environ Health 1980;35: 106–109.

46. Huber W, Saifer MG. Orgotein, the drug version of bovine Cu-Zn superoxide dismutase. I. A summary account of safety and pharmacology in laboratory animals. In: Michelson AM, McCord JM, Fridovich I, eds. Superoxide and superoxide dismutases. New York: Academic Press 1977;517–536.

48. King EJ, Harrison CV. The effects of kaolin on the lungs of rats. J Pathol Bacteriol 1948;60:435–440.

48. Sabu AP, Shanker R, Zaidi SH. Pulmonary response to kaolin, mica and talc in mice. Exp Pathol 1978;16:276–282.

49. Morgan WKC, Donner A, Higgins ITT, Pearson MG, Rawlings W, Jr. The effects of kaolin on the lung. Am Rev Respir Dis 1988;138:813–820.

50. Eisenbud M. Origins of the standards for control of beryllium disease (1947–1949). Environ Res 1982;27: 79–88.

51. Katzenstein A-L A, Askin FB. Pneumoconiosis: In: Surgical pathology of non-neoplastic lung disease. Philadelphia: WB Saunders, 1982:101–102.

52. Kriebel D, Brain JD, Sprince NL, Kazemi H. The pulmonary toxicity of beryllium. Am Rev Respir Dis 1988; 137:464–473.

53. Mancuso TF. Occupational lung cancer among beryllium workers. In: Lemen R, Dement DM, eds. Dusts and disease: Occupational and environmental exposures to selected fibrous and particulate dusts. Park Forest South: Pathotox, 1979:463–471.

54. Infante PF, Wagoner JK, Sprince NL. Bronchogenic cancer and nonneoplastic respiratory disease associated with beryllium exposure. In: Lemen R, Dement JM, eds. Dusts and disease: Occupational and environmental exposures to selected fibrous and particulate dusts. Park Forest South: Pathotox, 1979:473–482.

55. Morgan WKC, Seaton A. Occupational lung diseases, 2d Ed. Philadelphia: WB Saunders, 1984:449–497.

56. Vorwald AJ. The beryllium problem: The chronic or delayed disease: Pathologic aspects. In: Vorwald AJ, ed. Pneumoconiosis: Beryllium, bauxite fumes, compensation. New York: Hoeber, 1950:190–207.

57. Newman LS, Kreiss K, King TE, Jr., Seay S, Campbell PA. Pathologic and immunologic alterations in early stages of beryllium disease: Re-examination of disease definition and natural history. Am Rev Respir Dis 1989;139:1479–1486.

58. Sferlazza SJ, Beckett WS. The respiratory health of welders. Am Rev Respir Dis 1991;143:1134–1148.

59. Vallyathan V, Bergeron WN, Robichaux PA, Craighead JE. Pulmonary fibrosis in an aluminum arc welder. Chest 1982;81:372–374.

60. Chen W-J, Monnat RJ, Chen M, Moffett NK. Aluminum induced pulmonary granulomatosis. Hum Pathol 1978;9:705–711.

61. Herbert A, Sterling G, Abraham J, Corrin B. Desquamative interstitial pneumonia in an aluminum welder. Hum Pathol 1982;13:694–699.

62. Stern RM. The assessment of risk: Application to the welding industry lung cancer. The International Institute of Welding Commission, VIII: Safety and Health Doc. IIW, VIII:2034–2083. Copenhagen: Danish Welding Institute, 1983:1–26.

63. Vallyathan NV, Green FHY, Craighead JE. Recent advances in the study of mineral pneumoconiosis. Pathol Annu 1980;15:77–104.

64. Gardner LU. Studies on the relationship of mineral dusts to tuberculosis. Am Rev Tuberc 1923;71:344–357.

65. Funahashi A, Schlueter DP, Pintar K, Siegesmund KA, Mandel GS, Mandel NS. Pneumoconiosis in workers exposed to silicon carbide. Am Rev Respir Dis 1984;129:635–640.

66. Gross P, de Treville RTP, Cralley LJ, Davis JMG. Pulmonary ferruginous bodies: Development in response to filamentous dusts and a method of isolation and concentration. Arch Pathol 1968;85:539–546.

67. Sprince NL, Chamberlin RI, Hales CA, Weber AL, Kazemi H. Respiratory disease in tungsten carbide production workers. Chest 1984;86:549-557.

68. Tabatowski K, Roggli VL, Fulkerson WJ, Langley RL, Benning T, Johnston WW. Giant cell interstitial pneumonia in a hard-metal worker: Cytologic, histologic, and analytical electron microscopic investigation. Acta Cytol 1988;32:240–246.

69. Schepers GWH. The biological action of tungsten car-

bide and cobalt: Studies on experimental pulmonary histopathology. Arch Ind Health 1955;12:140–146.

70. Sprince NL, Oliver LC, Eisen EA, Greene RE, Chamberlin RI. Cobalt exposure and lung disease in tungsten carbide production: A cross-sectional study of current workers. Am Rev Respir Dis 1988;138:1220–1226.

71. Ohori NP, Sciurba FC, Owens GR, Hodgson MJ, Yousem SA. Giant-cell interstitial pneumonia and hard metal pneumoconiosis: A clinicopathologic study of four cases and review of the literature. Am J Surg Pathol 1989;13:581–587.

72. Coates EO, Watson JHL. Diffuse interstitial lung disease in tungsten carbide workers. Ann Intern Med 1971;75:709–716.

73. Ophus EM, Rode L, Gylseth B, Nicholson DG, Saeed K. Analysis of titanium pigments in human lung tissue. Scand J Work Environ Health 1979;5:290–296.

74. Crouch E, Churg A. Ferruginous bodies and the histologic evaluation of dust exposure. Am J Surg Pathol 1984;8:109–116.

75. De Vuyst P, Vande Weyer R, De Coster A, et al. Dental technicians pneumoconiosis: A report of two cases. Am Rev Respir Dis 1986;133:316–320.

76. Barrett TE, Pietra GG, Maycock RL, Rossman MD, Minda JM, Johns LW. Acrylic resin pneumoconiosis: Report of a case in a dental student. Am Rev Respir Dis 1989;139:841–843.

77. Loewen GM, Weiner D, McMahan J. Pneumoconiosis in an elderly dentist. Chest 1988;93:1312–1313.

78. Golden EB, Warnock ML, Hulett LD, Churg AM. Fly ash lung: A new pneumoconiosis? Am Rev Respir Dis 1982;125:108–112.

79. Fisher GL, Chrisp CE, Raabe OG. Physical factors affecting the mutagenicity of fly ash from a coal-fired power plant. Science 1979;204:879–881.

80. Hill JO, Rothenberg SJ, Kanapilly GM, Hanson RL, Scott BR. Activation of immune complement by fly ash particles from coal combustion. Environ Res 1982;28:113–122.

81. Roggli Vl, Pratt PC, Brody AR. Asbestos content of lung tissue in asbestos-associated diseases: A study of 110 cases. Br J Ind Med 1986;43:18–28.

82. Martin TR, Chi EY, Covert DS, et al. Compared effects of inhaled volcanic ash and quartz in rats. Am Rev Respir Dis 1983;128:144–152.

83. Vallyathan V, Robinson V, Reasor M, Stettler L, Bernstein R. Comparative in vitro cytotoxicity of volcanic ashes from Mount St. Helens, El Chichon, and Galunggung. J Toxicol Environ Health 1984;14:641–654.

84. Raub JA, Hatch GE, Mercer RR, Grady M, Hu P-C. Inhalation studies of Mt. St. Helens volcanic ash in animals: II. Lung function, biochemistry, and histology. Environ Res 1985;37:72–83.

85. Craighead JE, Adler KB, Emerson RJ, Mossman BT, Woodworth CD. Health effects of Mount St. Helens volcanic dust. Lab Invest 1983;48:5–12.

86. Buist AS, Vollmer WM, Johnson LR, Bernstein RS, McCamant LE. A four-year prospective study of the respiratory effects of volcanic ash from Mt. St. Helens.

Am Rev Respir Dis 1986;133:526–534.

87. Churg A. Nonasbestos pulmonary mineral fibers in the general population. Environ Res 1983;31:189–200.

88. Baker D, Kupke KG, Ingram P, Roggli VL, Shelburne JD. Microprobe analysis in human pathology. In: Johari O, ed. Scanning electron microscopy, Vol. II. Chicago: SEM, 1985:659–680.

89. Roggli VL. Nonasbestos mineral fibers in human lungs. In: Russell PE, ed. Microbeam Analysis—1989. San Francisco: San Francisco Press, 1989:57–59.

90. Lockey JE. Nonasbestos fibrous minerals. Clin Chest Med 1981;2:203–218.

91. Wright GW, Kuschner M. The influence of varying lengths of glass and asbestos fibres on tissue response in guinea pigs. In: Walton WH, ed. Inhaled particles IV. Oxford: Pergamon, 1977:455–474.

92. Stanton MF, Layard M, Tegeris A, et al. Relations of particle dimensions to carcinogenicity in amphibole asbestos and other fibrous minerals. J Natl Cancer Inst 1981;67:965–975.

93. Morgan A, Holmes A, Davison W. Clearance of sized glass fibres from the rat lung and their solubility in vivo. Ann Occup Hyg 1982;25:317–331.

94. Enterline PE, Marsh GM. Environment and mortality of workers from a fibrous glass plant. In: Lemen R, Dement JM, eds. Dusts and disease: Occupational and environmental exposures to selected fibrous and particulate dusts. Park Forest South: Pathotox, 1979:221–231.

95. Wright GW. Proceedings of the second symposium on occupational exposure to fibrous glass. Washington D.C.; US Government Printing Office, 1976:126.

96. Bayliss D, Dement J, Wagoner JK, Blejer HP. Mortality patterns among fibrous glass production workers. Ann NY Acad Sci 1976;271:324–335.

97. Gross P, Tuma J, de Treville TP. Lungs of workers exposed to fiber glass: A study of their pathologic changes and their dust content. Arch Environ Health 1971;3:67–76.

98. McDonald AD, McDonald JC. Malignant mesothelioma in North America. Cancer 1980;46:1650–1656.

99. Pooley FD. Evaluation of fiber samples taken from the vicinity of two villages in Turkey. In: Lemen R, Dement JM, eds. Dusts and disease: Occupational and environmental exposures to selected fibrous and particulate dusts. Park Forest South: Pathotox, 1979:41–44.

100. Suzuki Y. Carcinogenic and fibrogenic effects of zeolites: Preliminary observations. Environ Res 1982;27:433–445.

101. Baris YI, Artvinli M, Sahin AA. Environmental mesothelioma in Turkey. Ann NY Acad Sci 1979;330:423–432.

102. Sebastien P, Gaudichet A, Bignon J, Baris YI. Zeolite bodies in human lungs from Turkey. Lab Invest 1981;44:420–425.

103. Warheit DB, Hill LH, Brody AR. In vitro effects of crocidolite asbestos and wollastonite on pulmonary macrophages and serum complement. In: Johari O, ed. Scanning electron microscopy. Vol. II. Chicago: SEM, 1984:919–926.

104. Shasby DM, Peterson M, Hodous T, Boehlecke B, Merchant J. Respiratory morbidity of workers exposed to wollastonite through mining and milling. In: Lemen R, Dement JM, eds. Dusts and disease: Occupational and environmental exposures to selected fibrous and particulate dusts. Park Forest South: Pathotox, 1979:251–256.

105. Huuskonen MS, Tossavainen A, Koskinen H, et al. Wollastonite exposure and lung fibrosis. Environ Res 1983;30:291–304.

106. Moatamed F, Lockey JE, Parry WT. Fiber contamination of vermiculites: A potential occupational and environmental health hazard. Environ Res 1986;41:207–218.

107. McDonald JC, Armstrong B, Case B, et al. Mesothelioma and asbestos fiber type: Evidence from lung tissue analyses. Cancer 1989;63:1544–1547.

108. Ramage JE, Jr., Roggli VL, Bell DY, Piantadosi CA. Interstitial lung disease and domestic wood burning. Am Rev Respir Dis 1988;137:1229–1232.

109. McCrone WC, ed. The particle atlas. Vols V and VI. 2d Ed. Ann Arbor: Ann Arbor Science, 1980:1336, 1634.

110. Martin TR, Meyer SW, Luchtel DR. An evaluation of the toxicity of carbon fiber composites for lung cells in vitro and in vivo. Environ Res 1989;49:246–261.

111. Dodson RF, O'Sullivan MF, Corn CJ, Williams MJ, Hurst GA. Ferruginous body formation on a nonasbestos mineral. Arch Pathol Lab Med 1985;109:849–852.

112. Jephcott CM. Chemical aspects of Shaver's disease. In: Vorwald AJ, ed. Pneumoconiosis: Beryllium, bauxite fumes, compensation. New York: Hoeber, 1950:489–497.

113. Abramson MJ, Wlodarczyk JH, Saunders NA, Hensley MJ. Does alumium smelting cause lung disease? Am Rev Respir Dis 1989;139:1042–1057.

114. Mark GJ, Monroe CB, Kazemi H. Mixed pneumoconiosis: Silicosis, asbestosis, talcosis, and berylliosis. Chest 1979;75:726–728.

115. Mason GR, Abraham JL, Hoffman L, Cole S, Lippman M, Wasserman K. Treatment of mixed-dust pneumoconiosis with whole lung lavage. Am Rev Respir Dis 1982;126:1102–1107.

116. Sherwin RP, Barman ML, Abraham JL. Silicate pneumoconiosis of farm workers. Lab Invest 1979;40:576–582.

117. Taylor G. Acute systemic effects of inhaled occupational agents. In: Merchant JA, ed. Occupational respiratory diseases. DMHS (NIOSH) Publ. No. 86102, Washington, DC. U.S. Government Printing Office, 1986:618.

118. May JJ, Stallones L, Darrow D, Pratt DS. Organic dust toxicity (pulmonary mycotoxicosis) associated with silo unloading. Thorax 1986;41:919–923.

119. Emanuel DA, Wenzel FJ, Lawton BR. Pulmonary mycotoxicosis. Chest 1975;67:293–297.

120. Brinton WT, Vastbinder EE, Greene JW, Marx JJ, Jr., Hutcheson RH, Schaffner W. An outbreak of organic dust toxic syndrome in a college fraternity. JAMA 1987;258:1210–1212.

121. Lecours R, Laviolette M, Cormier Y. Bronchoalveolar lavage in pulmonary mycotoxicosis (organic dust toxic syndrome). Thorax 1986;41:924–926.

122. Pratt PC. Comparative prevalence and severity of emphysema and bronchitis at autopsy in cotton mill workers vs. controls. Chest 1981;79:495–535.

123. Kennedy SM, Christiani DC, Eisen EA, et al. Cotton dust and endotoxin exposure-response relationships in cotton textile workers. Am Rev Respir Dis 1987;135:194–200.

124. Pratt PC, Vollmer RT, Miller JA. Epidemiology of pulmonary lesions in nontextile and cotton textile workers: A retrospective autopsy analysis. Arch Environ Health 1980;35:133–138.

125. Moran TJ. Emphysema and other chronic lung disease in textile workers: An 18-year autopsy study. Arch Environ Health 1983;38:267–276.

126. Cloutier MM, Rohrbach MS. Effects of endotoxin and tannin isolated from cotton bracts on the airway epithelium. Am Rev Respir Dis 1986;134:1158–1162.

127. Ainsworth SK, Neuman RE. Chemotaxins in cotton mill dust: Possible etiologic agent(s) in byssinosis. Am Rev Respir Dis 1981;124:280–284.

128. Brody AR, Vallyathan NV, Craighead JE. Distribution and elemental analysis of inorganic particulates in pulmonary tissue. In: Johari O, ed. Scanning electron microscopy, Vol. III. Chicago: IIT Research Institute, 1976:477–484.

129. Abraham JL, Burnett BR. Quantitative analysis of inorganic particulate burden *in situ* in tissue sections. In: Johari O, ed. Scanning electron microscopy, Vol. II. Chicago: SEM, 1983:681–696.

130. Pickett JP, Ingram P, Shelburne JD. Identification of inorganic particulates in a single histologic section using both light microscopy and x-ray microprobe analysis. J Histotechnol 1980;3:155–158.

131. Gylseth B, Ophus EM, Mowe G. Determination of inorganic fiber density in human lung tissue by scanning electron microscopy after low temperature ashing. Scand J Work Environ Health 1979;5:151–157.

132. Ingram P, Shelburne JD, Roggli VL, eds. Microprobe analysis in medicine. New York: Hemisphere, 1989.

133. Marshall AJ. Electron probe x-ray microanalysis. In: Hayat MA, ed. Principles and techniques of scanning electron micrscopy, Vol. 4. New York: Van Nostrand-Reinhold, 1975:103–173.

134. Berry JP, Henoc P, Galle P, Pariente R. Pulmonary mineral dust: A study of ninety patients by electron microscopy, electron microanalysis and electron microdiffraction. Am J Pathol 1976;83:427–456.

135. Shelburne JD, Wisseman CL, Broda KR, Roggli VL, Ingram P. Lung—nonneoplastic conditions. In: Trump BF, Jones RJ, eds. Diagnostic electron microscopy, Vol. 4. New York: Wiley, 1983:475–538.

136. Johnson GG, White EW, Strickler D, Hoover R. Image analysis techniques. In: Asher IM, McGrath PP, eds. Symposium on electron microscopy of microfibers: Proceedings of the first FDA Office of Science summer symposium. Washington DC: U.S. Government Printing Office, 1976:76–82.

137. Roggli VL, Ingram P, Linton RW, Gutknecht WF, Mas-

tin P, Shelburne JD. New techniques for imaging and analyzing lung tissue. Environ Health Perspect 1984;56:163–183.

138. A.S.T.M. Index: Index to the powder diffraction file. Philadelphia: American Society for Testing Materials.

139. Barrow RE. X-ray diffraction analysis of quartz in lung tissue. Tex Rep Biol Med 1974;32:441–448.

140. Lange BA, Haartz JC. Determination of microgram quantities of asbestos by x-ray diffraction: Chrysotile in thin dust layers of matrix material. Anal Chem 1979;51:520–525.

CHAPTER 28

Asbestos

SAMUEL P. HAMMAR and RONALD F. DODSON

Few substances have created as much interest, fear, and misunderstanding as asbestos. In 1971, asbestos became the first material to be regulated by the Occupational Safety and Health Administration. In 1982, lawsuits filed on behalf of workers suffering from asbestos-related pulmonary disease led one asbestos products producer to file for bankruptcy, primarily as a result of claims for asbestos injury from asbestos products his company produced. Even as of the 1990s, controversies still exist concerning the toxicity and potential health effects of asbestos.

Asbestos Mineralogy and Definitions

The word "asbestos" is defined in Websters's Medical Dictionary[1] as "a mineral (as amphibole) that readily separates into long flexible fibers suitable for use as a non-combustible, nonconducting, chemically resistant material." With such properties, it is not surprising that asbestos has been referred to as a "magic or miracle mineral." Practically speaking, asbestos is best thought of as a generic term applied to a group of silicate minerals with a fibrous crystalline structure that have among their properties a high tensile strength, a resistance to heat, a high aspect ratio (length-to-width ratio), and a resistance to many chemicals. Asbestos is sometimes simply defined as a group of fibrous hydrated silicate minerals with high aspect ratios. The several minerals constituting "asbestos" vary in fiber size, crystal structure, and chemical composition (Table 28–1). They share what mineralogists sometimes refer to as an asbestiform "habit" in that the minerals crystallize into bundles of thousands of flexible fibrils that look like

organic fibers. Terms that are sometimes used to describe asbestos or similar minerals include fiber, fibrous, asbestiform, and acicular. The term fiber is usually used in the context that it resembles an organic fiber; the term fibrous is used to describe a crystallization habit in which a mineral appears to be composed of fibers. "Asbestiform" is defined as a special fibrous habit in which the fibers have a higher tensile strength and flexibility than crystals in other parts of the same mineral; asbestiform is generally synonymous with fibrous, or sometimes is meant to mean "like asbestos"; and "acicular" refers to a crystal that has a needle-like form.

All major types of asbestos have silicon tetroxide (SiO_4) tetrahedra as the backbone of the crystal lattice, and silicate minerals are classified according to their crystal structure. Asbestos occurs as two main groups: the serpentine and the amphibole minerals. Chrysotile, the only member of the serpentine group, is a magnesium silicate in which the layers of the linked silica tetrahedra alternate with layers of magnesium oxide–hydroxide octahedra. In general, in serpentine rock, the double layers tend to produce crystals that cleave into sheets like mica. However, in the asbestos form variety of serpentine rock, the double layer rolls up onto itself, pearling as it grows, to form long hollow tubes that are characteristic of chrysotile. The commercial amphiboles, amosite and crocidolite, belong to the amphibole group, which is composed of aggregates of cations (usually calcium, sodium, iron, magnesium, or aluminum) sandwiched between strips of linked silica tetrahedra in the form of parallel chains. All the amphiboles have the same basic structure, but are substituted with different cations. Amphiboles usually grow as single crystals, often in veins of massive nonfibrous

Table 28–1. Asbestos compounds

Mineral	Major group	Chemical formula	Common name
Serpentine	Serpentine	$3MgO \cdot 2SiO_2 \cdot 2H_2O$	Chrysotile, white asbestos
Riebeckite	Amphibole	$Na_2O \cdot Fe_2O_3 \cdot 3FeO \cdot 8SiO_2 \cdot H_2O$	Crocidolite, blue asbestos
Cummingtonite (grunerite)	Amphibole	$7FeO \cdot 7MgO \cdot 8SiO_2 \cdot H_2O$	Amosite, brown asbestos
Tremolite-actinolite	Amphibole	$2CaO \cdot 4MgO \cdot 8SiO_2 \cdot H_2O$	Tremolite-actinolite asbestos
Anthophyllite	Amphibole	$7MgO \cdot 8SiO_2 \cdot H_2O$	Anthophyllite asbestos

rock. Only two amphiboles, amosite and crocidolite, have been used commercially to any significant degree.

A recent troublesome issue that has arisen is the mineralogic distinction between fibers and cleavage fragments and whether this distinction has any biologic implications. Tremolite, a type of noncommercial amphibole asbestos, often a component (contaminant) of chrysotile ore, has been in the spotlight with respect to this issue of the importance of cleavage fragments as opposed to asbestiform fibers. As recently reported,[2] the main issue is whether two fibrous particles of identical size and shape have different biologic properties if the particles are pieces of mineral that have broken off a larger sample parallel to a crystal face (cleavage fragment), as opposed to particles that originally grew in a fibrous habit (asbestiform fibers). As concluded by a task force on the health effects of tremolite,[2] "the distinction between cleavage fragments and asbestiform fibers, although theoretically clear, is in practice extremely murky." As further stated by the committee, another problem is that the distinction should not be between cleavage fragments and asbestiform fibers, but between asbestiform and nonasbestiform fibers. As of June 8, 1992, the U.S. Department of Labor, Occupational Safety and Health Administration,[3] determined that substantial evidence was lacking to conclude that nonasbestiform tremolite, anthophyllite, and actinolite presented the same type or magnitude of health effects as asbestos. They further concluded that substantial evidence did not support a finding that exposed persons would be at a significant risk if nonasbestiform tremolite, anthophyllite, or actinolite were not regulated in the workplace.

Historical Aspects of Asbestos

The historical aspects of asbestos have been reviewed by Henderson et al.[4] and by Pooley,[5] and readers are referred to these excellent reviews for a detailed discussion. According to Pooley, Pliny was the first author to use the word "asbestos" to refer to a fibrous mineral. The word is of Greek derivation, and meant "inextinguishable" or "unquenchable," a meaning somewhat opposite of its true nature of being incombustible.

Anthophyllite asbestos was identified in clay used to make 4000-year-old pottery in Finland. Asbestos was used as a cremation cloth in 445–425 B.C., and the Romans used asbestos in the wicks of lamps made between 30 B.C. and 175 A.D. Marco Polo recorded that asbestos cloths were used by Tartars in the Khanate Province of Ghinghintalas during the Yuan Dynasty. Chevalier Jean Aldini (1762–1834) used asbestos cloth to make a fire-resistant suit that he exhibited in several European cities, including London in 1829.

The commercial production of asbestos did not begin until the nineteenth century. Between 1710 and 1720, asbestos was discovered in the Ural Mountains of Russia, and a variety of asbestos products were made in a factory operated during the reign of Peter the Great. The products produced included textiles, socks, gloves, and handbags. The first commercial use of asbestos originated in Italy in approximately 1810. In 1860, chrysotile asbestos was discovered near St. Joseph, Quebec, Canada, and it is chrysotile asbestos that has been used extensively for weaving. Chrysotile deposits were subsequently discovered near Danville, Quebec, and mining started in 1878. There was a great demand for asbestos in England and the United States, which led to rapid development of the mines near Danville and Thetford Mines. Crocidolite asbestos was discovered on the Orange River of South Africa in 1815, but commercial development did not occur until about the end of the 1800s. Amosite was discovered in the Central Transvaal region of South Africa in 1907. The name "amosite" was applied to the fiber in 1918, and the name originated from the letters of "asbestos mines of South Africa." Commercial production of amosite began in 1960. Chrysotile was mined in Rhodesia beginning in 1907, and centered around Mashaba deposits. Chrysotile was also discovered in the Shabani area of Rhodesia in 1906, but was not mined until about 1950.

Manufacture of Asbestos Products

In the United States, spinning and weaving of chrysotile asbestos for the production of textiles began about 80 years ago. The early products included fireproof items such as coats, helmets, gloves, and shoes. Asbestos brake lining products were made in the United States in 1906 and had first been made in England in about 1886. Asbestos paper used as a form of heat insulation material was first manufactured in North America in 1878, using first Italian and then Canadian asbestos. About the same time, pipe and boiler coverings containing 15% asbestos were manufactured. Asbestos cement products appeared in Europe in about 1896 and were introduced in North America in about 1903. Asbestos cement pipes were first manufactured in Italy in 1913. Because of the use of asbestos in so many different products, persons working in a variety of different occupations and industries have been exposed to asbestos[6] (Tables 28–2 and 28–3).

Geographic Location of Asbestos

Chrysotile asbestos is found worldwide in any geological area in which serpentine rocks are found. It is a common mineral, and may be present in certain environments as a natural background mineral dust. Chrysotile asbestos has been mined commercially in a variety of locations, including Quebec, South Africa, Eastern United States, California, and the Ural Mountains region of the Commonwealth of Independent States. Crocidolite asbestos was mined predominantly in South Africa and Western Australia. Amosite asbestos was mined only in the Eastern Transvaal region of South Africa. Anthophyllite asbestos has been found in many locations throughout the world, but the only deposits of commercial significance were those in the United States and in Finland. Tremolite asbestos is a relatively little importance, although it has been mined in Italy, Turkey, Pakistan, and South Korea.

Ferruginous Bodies

Historical Background

The use of the term "ferruginous body" in a literal sense means an "iron-rich" entity. These golden-brown structures were first reported in lung tissue by Marchard in 1906.[7] While Marchand[7] was the first to report golden-brown bodies in the human lung, it remained for Cooke[8] to emphasize the relationship of exposure to asbestos dust with the formation of these bodies. Gloyne[9] subsequently applied a coat removal procedure and confirmed the core to be asbestos fibers. These ferruginous structures when seen in tissue sections are routinely classified as asbestos bodies. Their presence in tissue is a hallmark of past asbestos exposure.[10,11]

Asbestos is not the only inhaled particulate that stimulates the disposition of a surrounding "iron-protein"

coat. Gross et al. have shown in an animal model that an exposure to fibrous dust of several types can stimulate formation of ferruginous bodies.[12,13] In an additional study using human lung material, Gross et al.[13] observed ferruginous bodies formed on both nonfibrous and fibrous particles and therefore suggested the use of the general term ferruginous body to describe all such structures. His argument is based on the fact that when such bodies are formed on nonasbestos fibers, the appearance is often morphologically similar to those formed on asbestos cores. Further clarification about the suggested use of the terms ferruginous body and asbestos body is presented in a later portion of the chapter that discusses core composition.

Formation

Asbestos dust is composed of components that can vary appreciably both in length and width (Figs. 28–1A and 28–1B). The respirable fraction of any fibrous dust is based on aerodynamic characteristics associated with its free-falling speed, which is determined largely by its diameter rather than length.[14] Therefore, in theory both shorter fibers and those longer than 100 μm can reach the lower respiratory tract. However, the turbulence created as air traverses the various bends and branches of the respiratory system provide an efficient mechanism for entrapment of the longer fibers. Those longer fibers (≥8 μm) that do reach the respiratory bronchiole/alveolar level provide the potential stimuli for ferruginous body formation (Fig. 28–2).

Much of our understanding of the process by which a fiber becomes coated comes from experimental animal models. Once the fibers reach the lower respiratory tract, an alveolitis occurs that includes an initial response of both macrophages and neutrophils.[15,16] The short fibers are phagocytized by the defense cells[15,17] (Fig. 28–3) and are eventually "packaged" within the phagosomes of the macrophages. Short fibers are occasionally seen in type I pneumocytes (Fig. 28–4).[18] The longer fibers, however do not completely fit within the phagocyte, and as a result several macrophages may simultaneously be reacting with different portions of the same fiber. This process continues until the fiber is cleared, or if the fiber remains in the lung, this can lead to the deposition of a coating.

The experimental animal models have shown that this sequence of events is important in the formation of "mature" ferruginous bodies. Over time, the generations of macrophages that interact with these longer fibers leave an iron-protein deposit on the fibers. The iron component has been suggested to be ferritin[19] or hemosiderin[19–21], interspersed within a matrix composed of mucopolysaccharides.[16]

Table 28–2. Estimates of probability of asbestos exposure according to job title[a]

	Category		
	Likely		Possible
U.S. census code	Job title	U.S. census code	Job title
[b]012	Electrical and electronic engineer	006	Aeronautical and astronautical engineer
013	Industrial engineer	011	Civil engineer
014	Mechanical engineer	022	Sales engineer
404	Boilermaker	023	Engineer, n.e.c.[c]
[b]486	Railroad and car shop	056	Personnel and labor relations workers
[b]522	Plumbers and pipefitters	140	Teachers, college and university
[b]525	Power station operator	142	Elementary school teachers
[b]534	Roofers and slaters	[b]151	Chemical technicians
[b]601	Asbestos and insulation workers	152	Draftsmen
615	Dry wall installers and lathers	173	Technicians, n.e.c.[c]
622	Furnacemen, smelter-men, and pourers	190	Painters and sculptors
[b]751	Construction laborers, excluding carpenters' helpers	216	Managers and superintendents, building
		221	Officers, pilots, and pursers; ship
		326	Insurance adjusters, examiners and investigators
		403	Blacksmiths
		410	Brickmasons and stonemasons
		413	Cabinetmakers
		415	Carpenters
		424	Cranemen, derrickmen, hoistmen
		[b]430	Electricians
		[b]433	Electric power linemen and cablemen
		436	Excavating, grading, and road machine operators; exc. bulldozer
		441	Foremen, n.e.c.[c]
		442	Forgemen and hammermen
		446	Heat treaters, annealers, and temperers
		454	Job and die setters, metal
		[b]455	Locomotive engineer
		461	Machinists
		471	Mechanics and repairmen; aircraft
		[b]473	Automobile mechanics
		481	Heavy equipment mechanics, including diesel
		482	Household appliance and accessory installers and mechanics
		483	Loom fixers
		492	Miscellaneous mechanics and repairmen
		495	Not specified mechanics and repairmen
		502	Millwrights
		503	Molders, metal
		[b]510	Painters, construction and maintenance
		514	Pattern and model makers, excluding paper
		533	Rollers and finishers, metal
		535	Sheetmetal workers and tinsmiths
		545	Stationary engineers
		550	Structural metal craftsmen
		552	Telephone installers and repairmen
		561	Tool and die makers
		610	Checkers, examiners, and inspectors; manufacturing
		611	Clothing ironers and pressers
		621	Filers, polishers, sanders, buffers
		[b]623	Garage workers and gas station attendants
		641	Mixing operatives
		650	Drill press operatives
		651	Grinding machine operatives
		661	Sailors and deckhands
		662	Sawyers
		[d]670	Carding, lapping and combing operatives

Table 28–2. *Continued*

Category			
Likely		Possible	
U.S. census code	*Job title*	*U.S. census code*	*Job title*
		[d]672	Spinners, twisters and winders
		[d]673	Weavers
		[d]674	Textile operatives, n.e.c.
		[d]680	Welders and flame-cutters
		[d]681	Winding operatives, n.e.c.
		690	Machine operatives, miscellaneous specified
		[b]694	Miscellaneous operatives
		695	Not specified operatives
		710	Motormen; mine, factory, logging camp, etc.
		753	Freight and material handlers
		[b]760	Longshoremen and stevedores
		944	Hairdressers and cosmetologists

[a] Reprinted with permission from Teta MJ, Lewinsohn HC, Meigs MW, Vidone RA, Mowad LZ, Flannery JT. Mesothelioma in Connecticut, 1955–1977. J Occup Med 1983;25:749–756.

[b] An occupation identified in reference sources as having potential for asbestos exposure or actually described in conjunction with a case in the literature.

[c] n.e.c., not otherwise classified.

[d] Occupations in textile factories that need further investigation to determine whether asbestos textiles were involved as distinct from cotton, wool, or manmade fibers.

The length of time required from first exposure to the development of mature ferruginous bodies in lung tissue has been reported in animal models. Identifiable bodies have been found within intrapleural granulomas at 14 days post exposure in guinea pigs, at 3–4 weeks in mice,[16] and in other models at post exposure intervals of 30 days,[22] 2 months,[23] and 6 months.[20] Studies by Holt and colleagues using a guinea pig model[24] have shown that ferruginous body formation occurs in similar sequences whether the stimulus was chrysotile, anthophyllite, crocidolite, or amosite. Davis[16] did not observe ferruginous body formation in rats for the duration of a study that included 6 months post exposure. This and other studies offer an interesting observation that various reactions to the same particulates can occur in different species. The animal models also illustrated the importance of the length of a fiber in defining its potential for becoming "coated." As is discussed in the section on tissue burden, the ferruginous bodies represent varying percentages of this population of fibers.

The data from animal models, therefore, offer reasonable assumptions that can be applied to the formation of ferruginous bodies in humans. One of these is the requirement of some latency period from first exposure to the development of "mature" ferruginous bodies. During this interval, the same phagocyte–fiber interactions occur as described in animal models and continue to occur on the residual fibers. Evidence for this is found in biopsy and autopsy tissue analyses from asbestos-exposed individuals.

Composition and Relevance in Tissue

An important question is, What purpose is served by the initial and prolonged interaction of macrophages with asbestos fibers that results in the deposition of a coating on some of the longer fibers? An overview of these interactions offers perspectives on the issue. Macrophages are the primary defense cells in the airways and alveoli. Their roles for protecting the surface of the lung include the ability to isolate, detoxify, and assist in the clearance of inhaled particles. The first objective can be more readily achieved for smaller fibers in that these fit within cellular compartments. However, the attempt to isolate and clear the longer fibers can involve generations of macrophages over an extended period of time. Data from animal studies, therefore, have shown that the shorter fibers are located in intracellular compartments (phagosomes). The longer fibers, which are more likely to stimulate ferruginous body formation, are physically in contact with both intra- and extracellular regions (Figs.28–5A and 28–5B).[16] The sequence of interactions with the longer fibers can result in a layered deposition as reflected in the internal structure of the coating material (Fig. 28–6). The multiple interactions with generations of cells also offer a

Table 28–3. Estimate of probability of exposure according to industry title.[a]

Category			
Likely		*Possible*	
U.S. census code	*Industry title*	*U.S. census code*	*Industry title*
057	Nonmetallic mining and quarrying except fuel	127	Cement, concrete, gypsum, and plaster products
067	General building contractors	128	Structural clay products
068	General contractors, except building	158	Fabricated structural metal products
069	Special trade contractors	289	Beverage industries
138	Miscellaneous nonmetallic mineral and stone products	318	Miscellaneous textile mill products
139	Blast furnaces, steel works, rolling and finishing mills	328	Pulp, paper, and paperboard mills
147	Other primary iron and steel industries	337	Paperboard containers and boxes
148	Primary aluminum industries	348	Plastics, synthetics and resins, excluding fibers
149	Other primary nonferrous industries	379	Rubber products
168	Miscellaneous fabricated metal products	407	Railroads and railway express service
177	Engines and turbines	417	Trucking service
199	Household appliances	419	Water transportation
207	Radio, TV, and communication equipment	427	Air transportation
208	Electrical machinery, equipment and supplies, n.e.c.[b]	567	Alcoholic beverages—wholesale
209	Not specified electrical machinery, equipment and suppliers	609	Department and mail order establishments
227	Aircraft and parts	627	Miscellaneous general merchandise stores
228	Shipbuilding and boat building and repairing	648	Gasoline service stations
229	Railroad locomotives and equipment	649	Miscellaneous vehicle dealers
239	Scientific and controlling instruments	758	Electrical repair shops
258	Ordnance	759	Miscellaneous repair services
467	Electric light and power	857	Elementary and secondary schools
477	Water supply	858	Colleges and universities
529	Electrical goods—wholesale	867	Educational services, n.e.c.
539	Machinery equipment and suppliers—wholesale	888	Engineering and architectural services
558	Petroleum products—wholesale		
568	Paper and its products—wholesale		
569	Lumber and construction materials—wholesale		
607	Lumber and building material retailing		
639	Motor vehicle dealers		
647	Tire, battery, and accessory dealers		
668	Household appliances, TV and radio stores		
757	Automobile repair and related services		
779	Laundering, cleaning, and other garment services		
917	Federal public administration		
927	State public administration		
937	Local public administration		

[a] Reprinted with permission from Teta MJ, Meigs MW, Vidone RA, Mowad LZ, Flannery JT. Mesothelioma in Connecticut, 1955–1977. J Occup Med 1985;25:749–756.
[b] n.e.c., not otherwise classified.

reasonable explanation for the segmented appearance of mature ferruginous bodies (Fig. 28–7).

The longer fibers, because of their needle-like characteristics, can be thought of as a physical irritant. Thus, one explanation for the coating process is that it offers protective isolation from the tissue.[16,23,25] Does this imply that a mature ferruginous body is an "inert" entity? An increasing base of data suggests this is not the case and that the ferruginous coating may carry its own potential for producing harmful reactions. These data are discussed in the section on fiber and ferruginous body toxicity.

Once a ferruginous body is formed, it is physically more difficult to clear from the lung than an uncoated fiber of equal length. With exception of those occasionally cleared, such mature bodies are assumed to remain as permanent entities within the tissue. This statement is supported by findings that confirm tissue ferruginous body burdens years after the last occupational exposures.[26]

Fragmented ferruginous bodies may be observed and explained because of several causes. These include actual fragmentation of bodies as may occur within the tissue or during some isolation or preparative procedures. Fragments seen in tissue sections may in reality be complete ferruginous bodies formed on a nonfila-

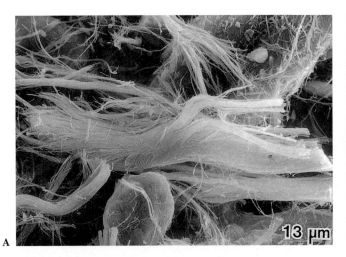

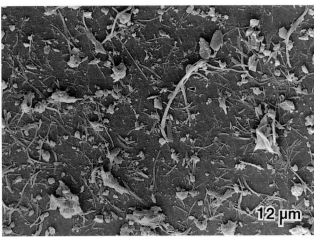

Fig. 28–1 A,B. A. Bulk material in scanning electron micrograph illustrates typical insulation sample made up of asbestos and other nonfibrous components. SEM. **B.** Another important use of asbestos has been in brake linings. Chrysotile bundles (*arrowhead*) as well as other nonfibrous dusts collected from worn brake linings. SEM.

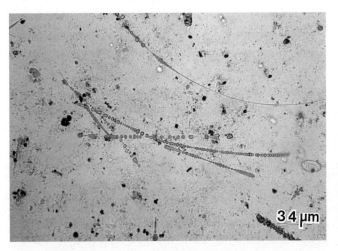

Fig. 28–2. Isolated ferruginous bodies typify various patterns of ferruginous coating.

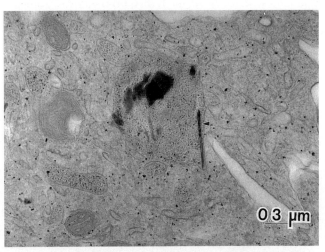

Fig. 28–3. Shorter fibers of amosite are readily phagocytized by macrophages and "packaged" within siderosomes (*arrowhead*); 18 days post exposure, guinea pig model. TEM.

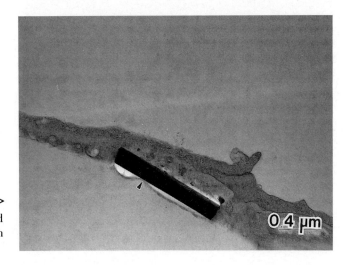

Fig. 28–4. Amosite fiber in type I pneumocyte is separated from alveolar space by thin layer of cytoplasm (*arrowhead*); 2 h post exposure, guinea pig model. TEM.

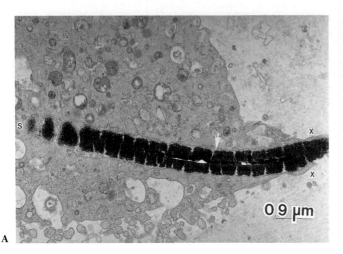

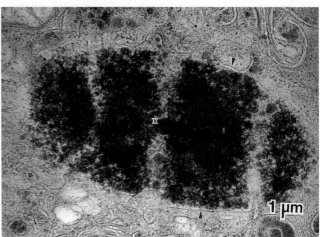

Fig. 28–5 A,B. A. Plane of section through amosite-cored ferruginous body permits identification of cellular membrane of the macrophage (*arrowhead*), which in some areas comes quite close to dense ferruginous coat; in other areas, granular material being released from macrophage forms separate interface. Ferruginous body extends into macrophage and, most likely due to average length, on other side of field (s). At opposite end, cytoplasmic extension of macrophage is at-tempting to surround this tip of ferruginous body (X). Human sputum sample collected 8 years from last exposure. TEM. **B.** Cross-sectional view of amosite-cored ferruginous body shows another perspective of cell membrane–ferruginous body relationship. Labeled components include cell membrane (*arrowhead*) and amosite core (X). Human sputum sample collected 13 years from last exposure. TEM.

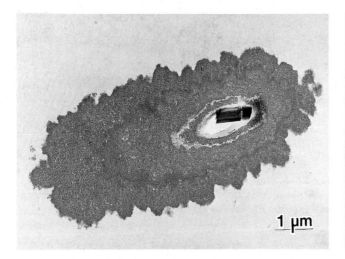

Fig. 28–6. Thin section of ferruginous body isolated from human tissue shows "ring-like" deposits that form ferruginous coat around amosite core. TEM.

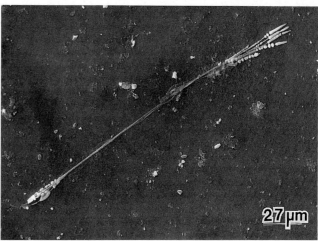

Fig. 28–7. Frayed ends of bundles have also resulted in coating process in which deposits of ferruginous material appear as "fanned-type" effect. Body isolated from human lung. SEM.

mentous dust or represent only the visible portion of the body, because it is not unusual for only a small portion of the fiber to have a ferruginous coating or be in the plane of section.

As noted earlier, Gross et al.[12] suggested the more generic term ferruginous body could be used to de-scribe fibrous and nonfibrous golden-brown coated structures as seen by light microscopy. Because nonas-bestos fibers have been shown in animals to induce ferruginous body formations that are similar to asbestos bodies,[12,27] Gross suggested the name "pseudoasbestos bodies."[12]

The Pneumoconiosis Committee of the College of American Pathologists and the National Institute for Occupational Safety and Health[10] recommended that the term "asbestos body" be interchanged with "ferruginous body" if the bodies have colorless, transparent cores by light microscopy. This position has been stated because most ferruginous bodies from human material, when analyzed by electron microscopy techniques, contain a high percentage of asbestos cores. This observation was consistent whether the cohorts in the study were from an environmental setting[28–32] or from occupational or paraoccupational settings where exposures to asbestos and various types of nonasbestos fibers could be expected.[33–36] The assumption that ferruginous bodies with straight, colorless cores are asbestos bodies is based on a large amount of data; however, the question remains whether special exposure situations may exist in which appreciable numbers of "classical ferruginous bodies" may be formed on nonasbestos fibers.

The diagnostic importance of finding or not finding ferruginous bodies in tissue sections follows several lines of argument. The Pneumoconiosis Committee of the College of American Pathologists[10] has stated that the minimal findings that permit a diagnosis of asbestosis (interstitial fibrosis induced by asbestos) are "the demonstration of discrete foci of fibrosis in the walls of respiratory bronchioles associated with the accumulation of asbestos bodies." What is overlooked by this position is the relative insensitivity of tissue section analysis for detecting ferruginous bodies, even in cases of individuals with heavy occupational exposures.[37] Thus, sampling through tissue sections offers limited insight into the total asbestos tissue burden.

Other techniques permit isolation of coated fibers and uncoated fibers from larger tissue samples and thus offer a more objective assessment of overall tissue burden.[38] This is particularly true in cases of individuals who, like certain animal species, do not effectively coat fibers even when abundant fibers are present in the tissue.[39] Techniques used for preparing larger samples and the correlation of fibers/body with exposure are discussed in a following section.

Previous studies using core analysis have shown that an appreciable percentage (usually the majority) of ferruginous bodies are formed on amphibole cores.* There are physical reasons why the longer amphiboles (Fig. 28–8A) are more likely to reach the lower airways than a similar length chrysotile structure (Fig. 28–8B). Thus, they are potentially more likely candidates for ferruginous body formation. The processes described for macrophage–fiber interactions preferentially result in the coating of a portion of the longer fiber burden (≥8 μm). However, the first prerequisite is that the fibrous dusts reach the respiratory bronchioles and

---

*References: 29,30,33,34,40.

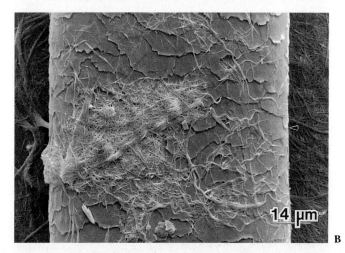

Fig. 28–8 A,B. A. Amosite fibers are of various lengths. However, even the longest fibers tend to remain straight and thus are more aerodynamically likely to be inhaled than comparable length but curved chrysotile fiber. For size comparison, preparation was made with human hair (*arrowhead*). SEM. **B.** Chrysotile fibers, in contrast to those of amosite **(A)** tend to coil or bend with increasing length. As **(A)**, human hair (*arrowhead*) shows contrast in dimension. SEM.

alveolar areas. The potential for a fiber to traverse the various levels of the respiratory tract is in large part determined by its diameter[14] and not its length. Chrysotile "fibrils" (the thinnest unit of structure) are often less than 50 nm (Fig. 28–9A) while a similar amphibole structure (Fig. 28–9C) is approximately 500 nm.[41] Logic would seem to argue that more long chrysotile fibers than long amphiboles should reach the lung and, therefore, more chrysotile-cored ferruginous bodies should be observed. Also, this reasoning is supported by the exposure potential because most of the commercial asbestos in use (based on percent used) is chrysotile or in chrysotile-containing products.[42,43] In

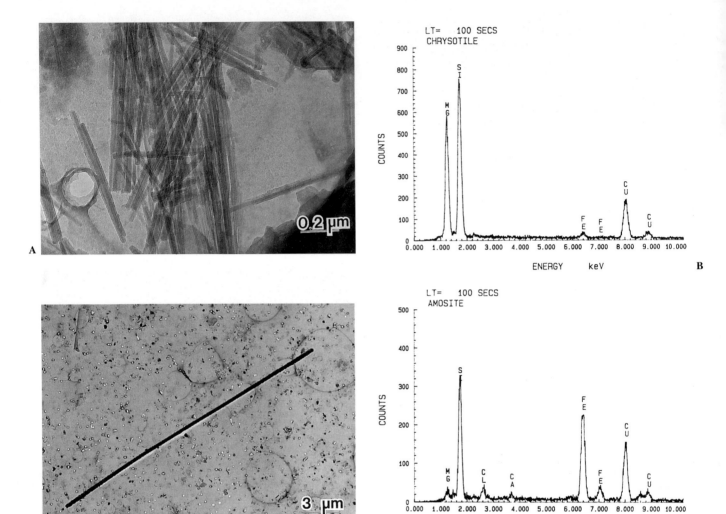

Fig. 28–9 A–D. Individual "fibrils" can be recognized within bundles of chrysotile in this replica preparation. Filter used for collection of sample was 0.2-μm Nucleopore. TEM. **B.** Typical chrysotile spectrum. **C.** Isolated amosite fiber can be compared in size to pores in background replica, 0.2-μm Nucleopore filter. TEM. **D.** Typical x-ray energy-dispersive spectrum of amosite.

actual comparison, however, a chrysotile fiber has a much larger functional diameter because of its curved or coiled morphology than amphibole fiber of equal length. Thus, the longer amphiboles are less likely to be intercepted when aligned with the air flow streams because they offer smaller collision cross sections[44] than chrysotile fibers.

The physical characteristics that favor long amphiboles over long chrysotile reaching the lung do not imply that ferruginous bodies are not formed on chrysotile cores. Such ferruginous bodies are occasionally seen in samples from the general population[28,29] and more commonly in workers when the workplace includes a higher population of long chrysotile fibers (Fig. 28–10).[36]

Thus, an appreciable percentage of ferruginous bodies is formed on chrysotile in environments where the characteristics and quantity of chrysotile overcome the inherent protective mechanisms of the respiratory system. Holden and Churg[36] reported 64% of the isolated bodies from chrysotile workers are formed on chrysotile while examples from our own facility include an individual with exposure as a clutch repairman (Dodson, unpublished data) in which 72% of the ferruginous bodies were formed on chrysotile cores (Figs. 28–11A and 28–11B). While length is an obvious predictor of which fibers have the greatest likelihood of becoming coated, width and surface irregularities (Figs. 28–12A and 28–12B) also appear to be factors in the selection process.[45]

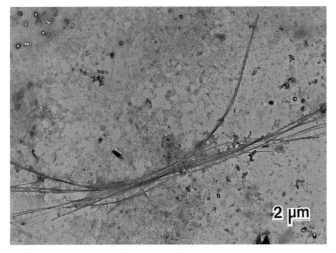

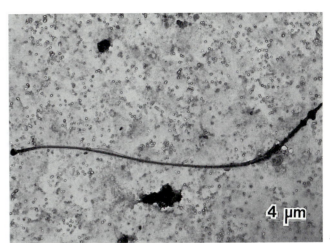

Fig. 28–10. Bundle of long chrysotile fibers found in lavage sample that contained chrysotile-cored ferruginous bodies. TEM.

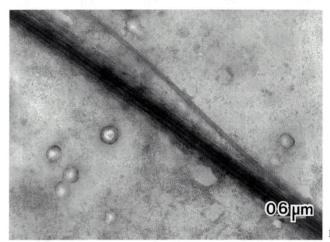

Fig. 28–11 A,B. A. Chrysotile-cored ferruginous body was isolated from the lung of individual whose work history included clutch manufacturing. TEM. **B.** High magnification of exposed central area of ferruginous body reveals typical tubular morphology of fibrils in chrysotile core. TEM.

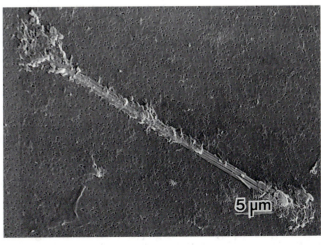

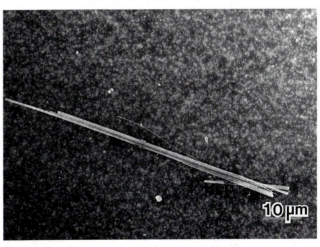

Fig. 28–12 A,B. A. As with chrysotile-cored ferruginous body, partially removed core of amphibole-cored ferruginous body reveals multifibrilar composition. SEM. **B.** Total coat removal from isolated amosite-cored ferruginous body reveals several unique features. Core is composed of multifibrillar bundles of varying lengths; surface variations as well as end irregularities present. SEM.

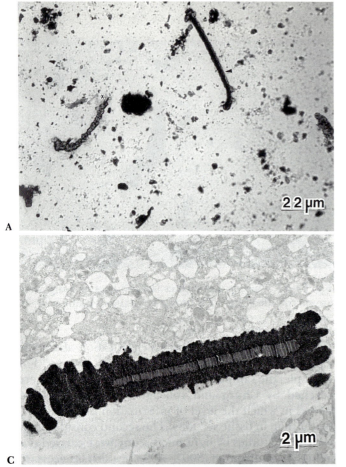

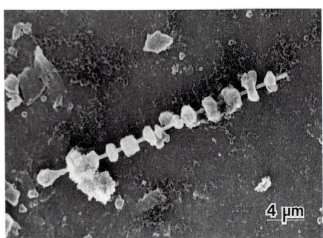

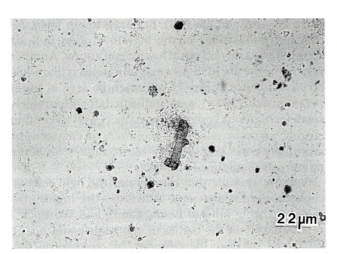

Fig. 28–14 A–C. **A.** One ferruginous body (*arrowhead*) can easily be distinguished from asbestos body by its black "rod-like" core material. Other ferruginous body appears to be typical for most of its length, but slender black filament (core material) can be seen extending from one end of body (X). **B.** Core of isolated ferruginous body was confirmed by analytical electron microscopy to be an "iron-rich" fiber. SEM. **C.** Thicker core of ferruginous body in this tissue section was determined to be of "organic" material. TEM.

Fig. 28–15. Although core material in this isolated ferruginous body is elongated, thickened yellowish material suggests composition is sheet silicate.

copy are met? The data suggest this is a reasonable position so long as the assessments are made with the awareness that the material was not obtained from an exposure setting in which a nonasbestos cohort inhaled fibers, resulting in a tissue response similar to those described in animal models by Gross.[12]

The use of the term pseudoasbestos body for classifying those without asbestos cores[12] has fallen in disfavor because of the argument that a "classical" ferruginous body seen by light microscopy is an asbestos body.[64] The external features of such elongated ferruginous bodies are, however, similar to those of asbestos bodies. The distinction between the forms is dependent on identifying characteristics of the core material. Those with broad black cores or thin black filaments, when analyzed by electron microscopy techniques, were concluded to be formed on carbon-rich cores.[40] Such black-cored ferruginous bodies have been reported in coal miners,[65] and it is proposed that occurrences in tissue from the general population have resulted from the widespread use of coal for heating purposes.[40] Black-cored ferruginous bodies have also been reported in tissue from silicon carbide workers by Masse et al.[66] and in various forms in material from foundry workers.[67] The latter have subsequently been shown to have formed cores that were either iron fibers (see Fig. 28–14B), "carbon" (see Fig. 28–14C), or fiberglass (Fig. 28–19).

Various types of sheet silicates also stimulate ferruginous body formation. It is relatively simple to distinguish these by light microscopy when the core material is wide, exposed, and bright yellow in color. However,

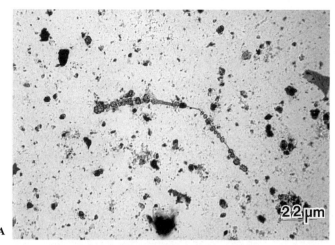

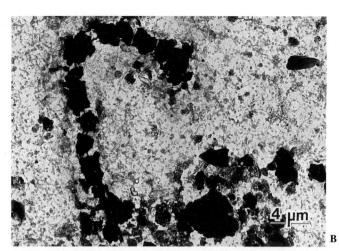

Fig. 28–16 A,B. A. Isolation of ferruginous body via digestion permits evaluation on flat plane with cleared background. At this enhanced level of resolution, identification of thin black filament (which differentiates this body from those formed on asbestos core) is possible. One can readily appreciate the complexities associated with making this same distinction at

either lower magnification or with increased confusion associated with seeing a body in tissue section. **B.** Core of ferruginous body is comparable to thin filament that forms core in **A.** Analysis of core by analytical transmission electron microscopy indicated core to be "organic." TEM.

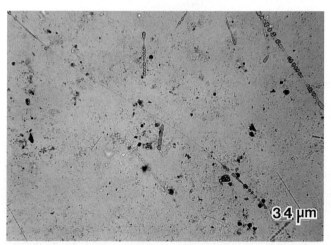

Fig. 28–17. Diversity of forms and lengths of ferruginous bodies shown in example from digested tissue from occupationally exposed individual. Some apparently uncoated fibers are in fact covered with thin ferruginous coat not readily distinguished by light microscopy.

when the cores of such bodies are thin, which also reduces the yellow intensity, the "distinction between these bodies and asbestos bodies is not always possible with the light microscope"[40] (Fig. 28–20). There are large numbers of nonasbestos fibers within our environments which, once inhaled, are potential stimuli for ferruginous body formation. Limited data exist on this subject because of the complexity of carrying out tissue burden assessment by electron microscopy. However, studies have reported the nonasbestos uncoated fiber burden is an appreciable percentage and in some cases the majority of fiber types in lung.[39,68–70] The large numbers of such fibers illustrate that nonasbestos fibers are available and may become cores of ferruginous bodies. A major characteristic of the nonasbestos fibers

in each of these reports is that the fibers are generally very short and therefore do not meet the minimum criteria (>8 μm) for being suitable cores of ferruginous bodies. This would change dramatically if a cohort was exposed in a work environment to longer forms of these fibers.

Uncoated Fibers

Instruments and Methods Used in Quantitation

Asbestos, as found in nature, consists of veins (Fig. 28–21) that are separated through processing into a more purified form. All asbestos types are composed at a more microscopic level of stacks of units not unlike logs in a woodpile (Fig. 28–22). When the material is disturbed, a tendency exists for fragmentation into thinner and shorter units. This begins at initial mining stages and continues through product fabrication and use. The thinner the fiber, the greater is its likelihood of staying suspended in air, which increases its potential for being respirable.[14]

The amphibole forms of asbestos (amosite, tremolite, actinolite, crocidolite, anthophyllite) are formed with internal repeating subunits (Fig. 28–23). The magnesium hydroxide layer is interfaced on the silicate matrix in the chrysotile fibril in such a way to create a "scroll" type of appearance when seen at the electron microscopic level (Fig. 28–24). This chrysotile structure results in an increased flexibility, which is proportional in part to the length of the fiber. Therefore, such a tendency to coil makes a chrysotile fiber have an appreciably greater functional diameter as related to respirability than an equivalent-length amphibole. This phenomena in large part explains why it is common to find greater numbers of long amphibole fibers rather than

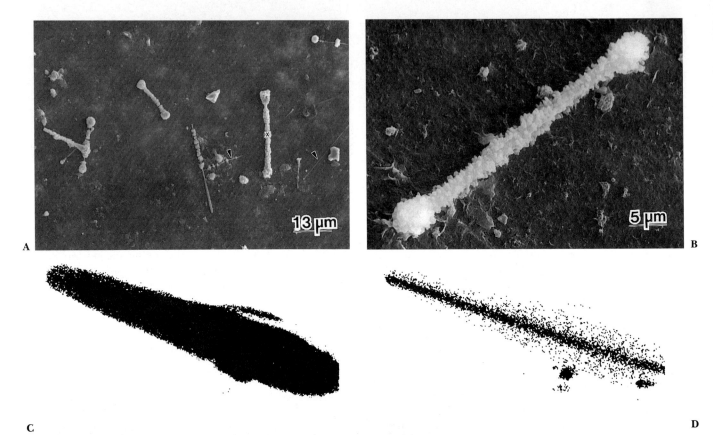

C   D

Fig. 28–18 A–D. A. Isolated ferruginous bodies (prepared from digested tissue) typify variations in surface coatings from limited coverage of core material (*arrowhead*) to those with total coating (X). SEM. **B.** Core material in isolated ferrugi- nous body is totally coated, making identification more com- plex. SEM. **C.** Iron–x-ray map of totally coated head of ferruginous body. TEM. **D.** Silica–x-ray map of head in **C** marks amosite core within coat. TEM.

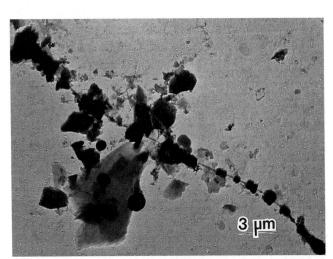

Fig. 28–19. Fiberglass-cored ferruginous body isolated from lavage material from foundry worker. TEM.

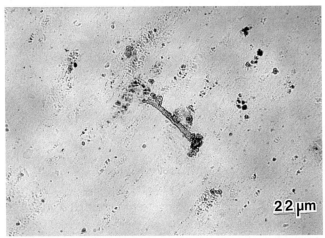

Fig. 28–20. Patient from whom this ferruginous body was isolated had been exposed to both sheet silicates and asbestos, as confirmed by core analysis through analytical transmission electron microscopy. Light microscopy distinction of those ferruginous bodies formed on sheet silicates, as in Fig. 28–15, cannot be easily applied here because core material is elon- gated and narrow.

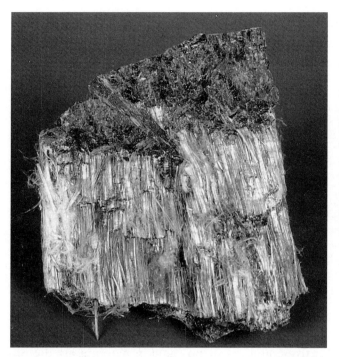

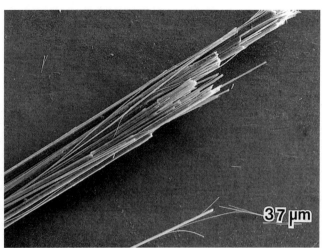

Fig. 28–22. Bundle of amphibole fibers shows inherent "stacking" configuration. SEM.

Fig. 28–21. Parallel veins of chrysotile are conspicuous in this serpentine rock.

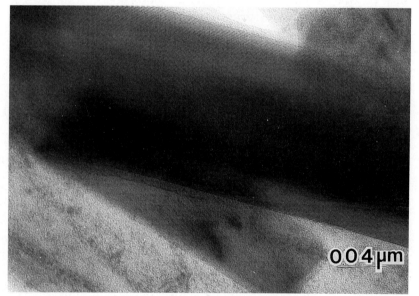

Fig. 28–23. High-resolution transmission electron microscopy of thin section through amosite asbestos fiber permits identification of repeating subunits that form internal structure of amphiboles. TEM.

chrysotile in tissue. This is in spite of the fact that chrysotile constitutes more than 90% of the asbestos used in commercial products and, therefore, logically is prevalent in most exposures.[42,43]

The diameters of the thinnest units of asbestos can be less than 50 nm for chrysotile and 500 nm for amphiboles.[41] Asbestos fibers, therefore, have very small dimensions and their detection is highly dependent on the resolution of the instrument used for making the assessment. The resolutions for instruments available

for counting fibers include 0.2 μm for the phase contrast microscope, 50Å for the scanning electron microscope, and 5Å for the transmission electron microscope.[71] While the use of light microscopy is important in determining the presence of ferruginous bodies in samples, uncoated amphiboles and chrysotile fibers are often sufficiently thin that even the long fibers are invisible by light microscopy because of their small diameter.[72–74]

It is critical when assessing any data to define clearly

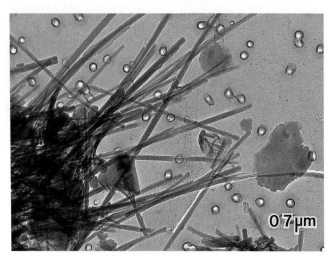

Fig. 28–24. "Scroll-type" formation of chrysotile unit structures creates fibril that appears as hollow tube. TEM.

the parameters used in obtaining that data. When evaluating information about uncoated fiber burden in tissue, fiber length and width and the counting rules must be considered because they define those fibers which are included in the count. Background quality assurance data must also be provided to give meaning to the results. The latter include critical issues necessary for assuring that fibers were not contributed from sources of contamination, that is, water, solvents, filters, or other tissue fluids.

The scanning electron microscope is a superior instrument for fiber and particulate analysis when compared to the light microscope because it offers better resolution and, when equipped with x-ray spectrometers, can provide elemental composition for separation of individual asbestos and nonasbestos fibers (an achievement not possible with the light microscope). There are, however, still appreciable numbers of fibers (particularly chrysotile fibrils) that are at or below this instrument's practical working resolution. A second difficulty is that the slow scanning speeds required to achieve this type of resolution can greatly limit the size of the area analyzed.

The transmission electron microscope offers the best available resolution and enables the user to detect the smallest particulate. As with scanning electron microscopy, elemental composition of particles can be obtained by x-ray energy dispersive spectroscopy.[75] Additionally, with proper orientation of the fiber, an electron diffraction pattern can be obtained by transmission electron microscopy. This pattern results from the interaction of the electron beam with the internal crystalline configuration of the asbestos. The result is a specific "fingerprint" for a given mineral.

Transmission electron microscopy is classified as a "state-of-the-art" instrument for analysis of air samples for asbestos under the Asbestos Hazard Emergency Response Act (Title II of the Toxic Substance Control Act 15, U.S.C. Sections 2641 through 2654). The basis of this position as applicable to tissue quantitation for uncoated fibers is that in both applications "all" fibers can be "seen" and analyzed. The guidance document also emphasized that fiber analysis should be done by rigid quality control. The use of electron microscopes for analysis must be done with the recognition summarized by Omenn et al. that "counting fibers is an exercise in probability theory."[71] It is, therefore, mandatory that the best possible tissue sampling techniques and fiber distribution be achieved in preparations. It is also important that multiple areas be analyzed on a preparation and these be scanned at different magnifications if random sampling errors are to be overcome to provide the most representative information of tissue burden.

As already discussed, tissue sections provide a very insensitive method for confirming ferruginous bodies in tissue and are of no value in determining the uncoated fiber burden because of limits of resolution and random sampling problems. Thus, several approaches have been used for isolating particulates from tissue. These include sample filtration,[76] low-temperature ashing,[77] and high-temperature ashing.[78,79] Tissue digestion with ozone,[80,81] strong bases,[31,82] and hydrogen peroxide[83–85] have also been used. Some of these procedures alter the chemical composition of asbestos while others may fragment or break fibers, bundles of fibers, or ferruginous bodies.[86–88]

Drying the tissue before digestion[82] has been suggested to cause breakage. Therefore, many investigators believe the most advantageous method incorporates a wet digestion procedure of multiple samples. One sample from each site can be dried and provide data for determining wet to dry weight ratios while an adjacent second sample from the site is used as a "wet sample" through the procedure.[86] The multiple sites for the wet sample from each lobe are pooled and digested. The resultant aliquot permits sampling with an inherent compensation for random sampling errors. The choice of collection membrane is important in meeting the desired objectives. Mixed cellulose ester filters can be cleared via acetone vapor and ferruginous bodies easily quantified by light microscopy, but a smooth-surfaced polycarbonate filter is preferred for transmission electron microscopy analysis. Selected filters from each lot should be screened for contamination and establishment of background levels.

The choice of pore sizes should be determined after assessing the amount of digest to be filtered and the information level sought in the analysis. While larger pore sizes are appropriate for collecting ferruginous bodies, it should be recognized that considerable uncoated fiber loss can occur unless 0.2-μm-pore-size filters are used.[89]

One of the more widely used digestion procedures incorporates chemical treatment of tissue with laundry bleach.* Some of these procedures work reasonably well for isolating larger structures such as ferruginous bodies but leave appreciable residue from samples with a high mucous content. This layer can cover the surface of the collection filter and obscure smaller particulates, including asbestos fibers. A modified bleach procedure of Williams et al.[92] permits even samples that are particularly mucous rich (such as sputum and lavage) to be analyzed for ferruginous bodies and uncoated fibers.

A wet procedure such as bleach digestion offers the best opportunity for minimizing fiber loss and allows sampling of multiple sites through tissue pools and aliquots. This digestion procedure is straightforward and can be used when necessary on small samples directly on the filter.

Locations in Body

The lung constitutes one of three surfaces in man exposed to the aerosolized contaminants. Unlike the skin and digestive tract, the respiratory system is a closed system that requires entering particles to exit via the same airways. This system is not without protection; its efficiency for entrapping larger particles from the incoming air stream is very good. Most particles larger than 5 μm in diameter (many asbestos fibers are less) are caught on the surface of the larger airways by impaction or sedimentation. The mucociliary escalator further contributes to the cleansing process by moving mucus-entrapped particles to the back of the throat where they can be swallowed or expelled in sputum. The system of clearance works sufficiently well that Gross et al.[93] suggested a 98%–99% removal efficiency. Many inhaled asbestos fibers, as with dust in general, are also effectively entrapped or cleared. A study by Evans et al.[94] in an animal model suggested that two-thirds of the inhaled fibers were trapped in the larger airways, thus greatly limiting the potential peripheral burden. By the end of the first month, it was further observed that clearance had eliminated three-fourths of the particles that reached the distal airways. The process as studied in other animal models indicates a highly effective clearance of short asbestos fibers and appreciably slower clearance of larger fibers.[95,96]

As discussed, the most efficient removal is of the small short fibers because this size can be phagocytized by

*References: 12,40,83,90,91.

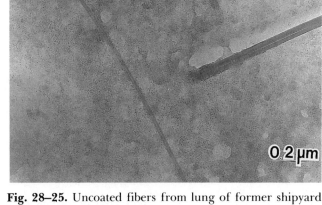

Fig. 28–25. Uncoated fibers from lung of former shipyard workers. Longer chrysotile (65 μm) was too small in diameter to have been resolved by light microscopy. TEM.

macrophages and therefore carried within their cytoplasmic compartments from the alveoli to the escalator level. Another route of clearance is by fiber penetration into the circulation of either the bloodstream or pulmonary lymphatics.[97] The lymphatic circulation provides a vehicle for relocation of inhaled soot and silica dust to extrapulmonary areas such as lymph nodes, spleen, and liver where granulomatous lesions occur.[98] Similarly, in an animal model exposed to mixed dusts, McMillan et al.[99] have shown the relocation of titanium dioxide and quartz particles from the lung parenchyma to lymph nodes.

While clearance via the respiratory airways consists of an active and rather rapid process, clearance based on flow through the lymphatics is a slow process.[100] The potential exists via this route for particulates to contribute to the pathogenesis within the tissue because the slow rate of particle movement allows time for maximum interactions to occur.[100]

While ferruginous bodies are in tissues outside the lung (see section on ferruginous bodies), little is known about the presence or numbers of the more easily relocated uncoated fibers in the extrapulmonary areas. A quantitative analysis by light and electron microscopy for coated and uncoated fibers from parenchyma (Fig. 28–25), thoracic lymph nodes (Fig. 28–26), and pleural plaques (Fig. 28–27) from former shipyard workers was reported from our laboratory. Appreciable numbers of uncoated fibers of both chrysotile and amphibole types were found in the extrapulmonary sites (see Table 28–4).[50,74]

The highest concentration of uncoated asbestos fibers occurred outside of the original site of deposition, the parenchyma. In six subjects, this occurred in the

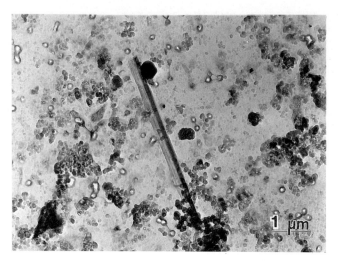

Fig. 28–26. Amosite fiber from lymph node of former shipyard worker. TEM.

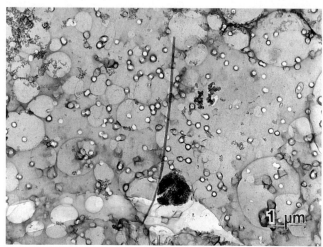

Fig. 28–27. Chrysotile fiber, as well as amphiboles, found in pleural plaques from shipyard workers. TEM.

Table 28–5. Percentage of uncoated asbestos fibers conforming to the Stanton hypothesis (length, ≥8 μm)[a]

Location	Chrysotile (%)	Amphiboles, %
Plaque	0.3	10
Lung	6	23
Node	0	3

[a] Data reprinted with permission from Dodson RF, Williams MG, Corn CJ, Brollo A, Bianchi C. A comparison of asbestos burden in lung parenchyma, lymph nodes, and plaques. Ann NY Acad Sci 1991;643:53–60.

Table 28–6. Percentage of total uncoated asbestos fibers resolvable by light microscopy (fibers >5 μm)[a]

	Resolution	
	0.2 μm	0.25 μm
Amphiboles	10%	5%
Chrysotile	0%	0%

[a] Data reprinted with permission from Dodson RF, Williams MG, Corn CJ, Brollo A, Bianchi C. A comparison of asbestos burden in lung parenchyma, lymph nodes, and plaques. Ann NY Acad Sci 1991;643:53–60.

nodes, whereas in two subjects the highest concentration was in the plaques. While most uncoated fibers in nodes and plaques were 5 μm or less in length, some fibers conforming to the more carcinogenically active fibers of the "Stanton hypothesis," long (≥8-μm) thin fibers were present in both the plaques and nodes (Table 28–5).[74] It should be noted that tissue analysis carried out by transmission electron microscopy included all fibers of 0.5 μm or more in length. This study emphasizes the limitations of the resolution limit of light microscopy and to some degree scanning electron microscopy when assessing uncoated fiber burden because all the chrysotile fibers and 95% of all amphibole fibers were less than 0.25 μm in diameter (Tables 28–6 and 28–7).[50,74] This included some fibers of appreciable length which, because of their thin diameter (see Fig. 28–25), require the resolution capability of transmission electron microscopy for identification.

A mechanism to explain the route of relocation, which includes flow to the lymph node and eventually to the parietal pleura via lymphatics, has been supported through findings in animal models by Kanazawa et al.[55] Viallat et al.[101] showed a physical shift of chrysotile

fibers following interstitial injection in rats. The retrieval of fibers in the pleural fluid in this study suggests that a mechanical penetration of the tissue barrier has occurred and may be an event that is independent of relocation within a carrier cell (phagocyte). Godwin and Jagatic[26] also concluded, in a study using human material, that fiber relocation occurs via the lymphatics and bloodstream.

The fact that asbestos fibers are sufficiently small to cross many barriers has been shown not only in the previous studies, but also in that asbestos ingested in water can pass from the body in the urine.[102,103] The fibers apparently also can pass the placental barrier. Haque et al.[104] reported chrysotile fibers in one of three tissue sites from each of five stillborns. The uncoated asbestos burden ranges from 71,000 to 357,000 fibers/g wet tissue.

Uncoated Fibers: Methods of Analysis and Sampling Schemes

As discussed previously, the literature on uncoated fiber and asbestos body burden in tissue can best be

Table 28–7. Uncoated asbestos fiber burden[a]

	Average length[b]	Average width[b]	Percentage >5 μm[c]	Percentage >10 μm[c]
Uncoated chysotile fibers				
Plaque	1.34 ± 1.50 (0.85)	0.09 ± 0.15 (0.06)	3.1	0.00
Lung	2.87 ± 1.07 (1.51)	0.07 ± 0.06 (0.05)	14.0	4.00
Node	1.27 ± 1.07 (0.94)	0.08 ± 0.06 (0.06)	0.0	0.0
Uncoated amphibole fibers				
Plaque	1.98 ± 3.13 (1.05)	0.15 ± 0.07 (0.14)	10.0	8.0
Lung	5.82 ± 6.71 (3.39)	0.19 ± 0.21 (0.14)	41.0	20.0
Node	2.22 ± 3.36 (1.55)	0.21 ± 0.12 (0.18)	6.0	2.5

[a] Data reprinted with permission from Dodson RF, Williams MG, Corn CJ, Brollo A, Bianchi C. Asbestos content of lung tissue, nodes, and pleural plaques from former shipyard workers. Am Rev Respir Dis 1990;142:843–847. Data reprinted with permission from Dodson RF, Williams MG, Corn CJ, Brollo A, Bianchi C. A comparison of asbestos burden in lung parenchyma, lymph nodes, and plaques. Ann NY Acad Sci 1991;643:53–60.
[b] All dimensions in μm; numbers in parentheses are geometric means.
[c] Length.

understood when like procedures and instruments are used to obtain the data. For example, an analysis of a tissue sample by light microscopy may provide useful data about ferruginous body content; however, uncoated fiber burden would be of little value when compared to the information gained by analysis of the same sample by scanning electron microscopy or preferably by transmission electron microscopy. Even when the best available resolution is used in the study, additional questions must be answered about the model. These include the necessity that quality assurance methods were used in the lab for sample preparation, for filter assessment, and in each step used in preparing grids for transmission electron microscopy. Digestion procedures offer advantages of evaluating larger tissue samples via sampling of multiple sites. Following sample collection, a determination must be made whether to prepare the digested sample for transmission electron microscopy evaluation by the indirect or direct method. The indirect procedure involves taking a sample of the digest and dropping the liquid on a previously coated grid. The coating film may be formvar, parlodian, or carbon. The droplet then dries and the grid is evaluated. The concern for such a technique is in the variation in the distribution of particles due to surface tension as associated with drying properties (similar to that of a droplet drying on a pane of glass) and the possibility that fibers may fragment during drying or preparation. The more gentle direct method of sample preparation was recommended for asbestos analysis at a recent workshop.[105]

In the direct method, a solution of the digest is filtered through a membrane-type filter. In theory, the pores within the polycarbonate membrane maintain a dispersed flow on the digest solution and create an equal distribution of its content. Thus, a randomized collection of material is possible as based on the suspension in the solution. Such solutions can also be collected via a similar filtration procedure on mixed cellulose ester filters. These filters can be "cleared" or made transparent by using acetone vapors, thus allowing unobstructed light microscopy assessment for ferruginous bodies. In the preparation for transmission electron microscopy analysis, the polycarbonate filters are carbon coated or the mixed cellulose ester filters are collapsed and surface etched.[106] This process entraps the surface particulates in place within the carbon replica of the surface. After the filter matrix is dissolved, sections of this replica are placed on grids for evaluation by transmission electron microscopy.

As additional quality control measures, all solutions used in the procedure should be prefiltered to eliminate possible sources of contamination. Likewise, batches of polycarbonate filter should be screened for establishment of background levels because some series contain short asbestos fibers. When counting schemes include only fibers 5 μm and longer, this becomes a rather moot point as these fibers are generally less than 5 μm. The selection of pore sizes must also be based on the size of particulates you choose to screen and the volume of the sample you plan to filter. Appreciable numbers of thin short fibers can be lost through even a 0.45-μm pore size.[89] The more efficient filtration achieved with a 0.2-μm pore size has limitations in that saturation (via trapping of more particulates) will more rapidly restrict the total volume one can filter as opposed to a filter with larger pore sizes.

As noted, the tissue sampling scheme should permit examining parenchymal tissue at multiple sites when possible. This enables the preparation of an aliquot that compensates for random sampling errors.[107] The objectives of an analysis and the availability of tissue will dictate the options for preparation. These include dividing each sample into portions used for (1) pathologic classification of the region, (2) pooled areas for fiber analysis, and (3) equivalent areas used to assess wet and dry weight as needed to quantify tissue burden per gram of ferruginous bodies and uncoated fibers. The wet-to-dry-weight ratio will vary with the extent of fibrosis and tissue reactions in an area. The weighed wet samples and fluid are used in the digestion procedure.

Concentrations of Ferruginous Bodies and Fiber Burden in Tissue

Data from some of the studies that have used particulate isolation procedures for reporting fiber/ferruginous body burden in man are shown in Table 28–8. The number of uncoated fibers and ferruginous bodies tend to stratify according to the types of past exposures and fall into the three following groups: (1) general populations, (2) blue-collar workers, and (3) occupationally exposed individuals. Less information is known about the tissue burden among members of the general population than the more heavily exposed cohorts. Churg and Warnock[83] reported uncoated asbestos fiber burden in a study of 21 urban dwellers. The majority of the uncoated burden was reported to be chrysotile (80%), and 90% of these fibers were less than 5 μm in length. The average concentration for chrysotile was determined to be 130×10^3 fibers/g wet weight while the mean total amphibole concentration was 25×10^3 fibers/g wet weight. Two-thirds of these were less than 5 μm long, and 95% of the amphiboles were noncommercial forms. This and similar studies[74,108] emphasize the importance of using transmission electron microscopy and a counting scheme that includes short and thin fibers; the alternative is to risk presenting data that represent only a fraction of the uncoated fiber burden. It should be noted that the individuals in the study of Churg and Warnock[83] were urban dwellers in large metropolitan areas where background exposures should have existed because of the reasonable expectation that asbestos-containing products were components of many buildings. Indeed, establishment of lev-

els of asbestos fibers in the general population is complicated in that all members of our society have exposure to asbestos. However, if we exclude blue-collar exposures (which is sometimes difficult due to incomplete histories), a variation in background level should be expected on the basis of differing environmental factors. For example, while the tissue levels reported by Churg and Warnock[83] are from individuals who had lived in larger older cities, such exposures may not represent environmental exposures that occur in newer urban settings or rural environments. Churg and Warnock[83] concluded that because most uncoated fibers were short (≤5 μm), the presence of longer fiber populations may suggest occupational or occupational-like exposures. In many instances the longer population of fibers is represented by ferruginous bodies. Thus, if the level of asbestos bodies per gram of wet tissue is 20 or higher,[109] past exposure to occupational or paraoccupational exposures should be suspected. Elevated total fiber burden has been reported in individuals with asbestos-induced diseases. Churg[110] when comparing a mean number of 1×10^6 fibers/g dry lung for general population levels (80% of which were chrysotile, <5 μm in length), concluded that individuals in the general population with pleural plaques had similar total fiber burden for their group, but a 50-fold increase in long thin commercial amphiboles; however individuals with asbestos-induced diseases (asbestosis and mesotheliomas) had 100 to 200×10^6 fibers/g dry lung.

In a study of chrysotile workers with mesothelioma, Churg and colleagues[111] reported elevated levels of total fiber burden when compared to "control" miners (without disease). However, they suggested that the ratio of the tremolite levels in the mesothelioma cases may suggest the importance of the amphibole burden to the pathogenesis of tumors. A report by McDonald and associates[112] further suggested the importance of exposure to amphiboles and risk of cancer. This study reviewed a series of mesotheliomas and noted that elevated tissue levels of amosite-crocidolite are often found. Warnock and Isenberg[35] argued that large burdens of asbestos do not always cause pulmonary fibrosis and thus asbestosis may be a poor marker for fiber-related lung cancer. The suggestion made is that the presence of more than 500,000 total amphibole fibers/g of dry lung signifies that interstitial fibrosis is caused by asbestos.[38]

The point that exposure to longer amphiboles carries an increased risk for cancer should not be used as an argument to exclude longer chrysotile or short and long fibers of both types from concern. In fact, a mixture of types and lengths of uncoated fibers in tissue is the rule rather than the exception.

For example, the study of tissue from eight former

Table 28–8. Asbestos bodies and fiber in various populations[a]

Reference	Population	Method[b]	FB/g wet[c]	FB/g dry[c]	ASB type[d]	F/g wet[e]	F/g dry[e]
136	Homogeneously exposed shipyard or insulation workers with at least 300,000 amosite F/g dry; no histologic asbestosis; and one normal lung	TEM					
	Twenty persons with mesothelioma, average age 65; average exposure, 17 yr						
	Site:						
	Peripheral upper lobe		—	—	Amosite	—	6.3×10^6
	Peripheral lower lobe		—	—	Amosite	—	6.7×10^6
	Central upper lobe		—	—	Amosite	—	5.2×10^6
	Central lower lobe		—	—	Amosite	—	6.5×10^6
	Ten persons with carcinoma; average age, 68; average exposure, 25 yr						
	Site:						
	Peripheral upper lobe		—	—	Amosite	—	5.5×10^6
	Peripheral lower lobe		—	—	Amosite	—	5.6×10^6
	Central upper lobe		—	—	Amosite	—	11.5×10^6
	Central lower lobe		—	—	Amosite	—	3.7×10^6
137	Ten persons from nonurban general population; 12 amosite workers (average exposure, 3.7 yr)	LM/SEM	—	17.9	Chrysotile	—	0.058×10^6
					Amphibole	—	0.204×10^6
			—	208×10^3	Chrysotile	—	1.2×10^6
					Amphibole	—	45×10^6
107a	Male accident victims from general population:	LM/TEM					
	Fifteen persons, ≤18 yr			120	Chrysotile	—	0.050×10^6
					Amphibole	—	0.006×10^6
	Thirty-three persons, 19–40 yr		—	270	Chrysotile	—	0.033×10^6
					Amphibole	—	0.014×10^6
	Nineteen persons, 41–60 yr		—	350	Chrysotile	—	0.089×10^6
					Amphibole	—	0.113×10^6
	Fourteen persons, 61+ yr		—	530	Chrysotile	—	0.062×10^6
					Amphibole	—	0.024×10^6
107b	Fourteen males with asbestosis, average age, 72 yr; average exposure, 22 yr	LM/TEM	1190×10^3		Chrysotile[f]	—	0.932×10^6
					Amphibole[f]	—	1.31×10^6
	Nineteen males without asbestos exposure, average age, 64 yr		—		Chrysotile[f]	—	0.687×10^6
					Amphibole[f]	—	0.141×10^6
68	Fourteen males with lung cancer; no occupational asbestos exposure; 11 blue-collar, 3 white-collar; average age, 63 yr	TEM	—	—	Chrysotile	—	0.4×10^6
					Amphibole	—	0.72×10^6
	Fourteen males without lung cancer; 11 blue-collar, 3 white-collar; average age, 63 yr		—	—	Chrysotile	—	0.2×10^6
					Amphibole	—	0.61×10^6
69	Nine chrysotile miners with early asbestosis; average exposure, 34 yr; average age, 66 yr	LM/TEM	—	46×10^3	Chrysotile	—	47×10^6
					Amphibole	—	106×10^6
	Nine chrysotile miners without asbestosis; average exposure, 32 yr, average age, 61 yr		—	20×10^3	Chrysotile	—	23×10^6
					Amphibole	—	58×10^6

[a] The synopsis of data shown in this table was prepared by M.G. Williams, Jr.
[b] Method: TEM, transmission electron microscopy; LM, light microscopy; SEM, scanning electron microscopy.
[c] FB/g, ferruginous bodies/g wet or dry tissue weight.
[d] ASB, asbestos type.
[e] F/g, fibers/g wet or dry tissue weight.
[f] Median.

shipyard workers from Dodson's laboratory showed the total uncoated asbestos burden (chrysotile and amphiboles) in the lung ranged from 480,000 to $192,000 \times 10^3$ uncoated fibers/g dry lung with mixed populations of various fibers (see Table 28–4).

Significance of Ferruginous Bodies in Tissue

As noted, the ferruginous body burden varies with the types of exposures and, to a lesser degree, with individual responses to that exposure. The latter include the impact of clearance and variation in coating efficiencies. Ferruginous body burden in the general population (urban dwellers), in a study of 29 persons by Churg and Warnock,[28] was reported to be fewer than 100 such bodies/g dry weight of lung. A later publication by the same investigators reported members of the general population as having 0–500 ferruginous bodies/g wet weight of lung, but with a further qualifier that most persons have between 0 and 50 ferruginous bodies/g wet weight.[30] The lower figure is more consistent with levels reported by Roggli,[109] Roggli and Benning,[51] and Breedin and Buss[113] for cohorts from North Carolina and the Dodson et al. findings from the general population in east Texas and Houston (0–20 asbestos bodies/g wet weight).[114]

The ferruginous bodies, therefore, serve as a marker for past exposure to longer fibers and, for reasons already discussed, the cores are often amphiboles.[83] The cores can be chrysotile if the exposure includes fibers that meet the criteria for ferruginous body formation.[36] The relationship of ferruginous bodies to the uncoated fiber burden varies greatly even when the only occupational exposure is to pure amphiboles.[39] Furthermore, individual variation in the efficiency for coating inhaled particulates exists in humans just as in some species of animals. Thus, ferruginous bodies may be absent or rare even when the tissue contains an appreciable number of suitable length amphiboles.[39,114]

Uncoated Fibers and Extrapulmonary Sites

Becklake[115] has summarized the relationship between pleural plaques and asbestos exposure for both occupational or nonoccupational exposure. The concept of asbestos fibers from the parenchyma of the lung eventually reaching the pleura in sufficient numbers to elicit a response could be explained by two mechanisms: the first was that the actual fibers reached this target site, and the second option was that inhaled fibers triggered a reaction in the lung that resulted in changes in the pleura without the asbestos fibers being present at the site. Hillerdal[116] offered a reasonable explanation for pleural involvement following asbestos exposure that incorporates the basic physiology of the lung and pleura and involves lymphatic drainage. His explanation is as follows:

Some of the small fibers will spread toward the visceral pleura of the lung, just like all inhaled dusts. Once in the visceral pleura, some of them will penetrate to the pleural space. The fibers will then follow the normal lymph flow from the pleural space, which is exclusively through the parietal pleura. Finally, in passing through the parietal pleura, a portion will

remain in macrophages there, causing a low-grade stimulation of the submesothelial fibroblasts. After some decades, this will result in visible pleural plaques.

If this concept is valid, then asbestos fibers should be found within the plaques. A "state-of-the-art" assessment of historical data on this subject led Churg and Green to conclude in 1987[117] that "the asbestos fiber content of plaques and pleurae appears to be quite different from that of the lung, and these sites are not useful for mineral fiber analysis." Thus, the lack of existing data confirming the presence of asbestos bodies or fibers in plaques seems to nullify the explanation offered by Hillerdal.[116] If one works within the resolution limits of light microscopy, at lower magnification by electron microscopy, or with a counting scheme, which preferentially excludes short or thin fibers, we have found the statement to be accurate.

However, when applying transmission electron microscopy, the instrument recommended[17,72,118] for identifying thin or short fibers, to count all fibers 0.5 μm or longer in plaques from former shipyard workers, an appreciable uncoated asbestos burden was observed (see Table 28–4).[50] Both uncoated amphibole and chrysotile fibers of various lengths were in the plaques.

When the uncoated fiber burden from lymph nodes was also taken into account with data from the plaques, the greatest number of uncoated fibers per gram was found in one of these extrapulmonary sites.[74] In two of the cases, this occurred in the plaques. Most fibers were short, with 0.3% of the chrysotile and 10% of the amphiboles being more than 8 μm in length, and all were thin. Because of the thin diameter of fibers in the extrapulmonary sites, none of the chrysotile and only a small percentage of the amphiboles would have been resolved by light microscopy (see Table 28–6). Appreciable fibers including some long fibers 8 μm or greater were shown to reach the parietal pleura, but little was known about the content of the "way stations" in the "Hillerdal concept" of relocation,[116] the lymph nodes. Two studies in 1990 provided the first quantitative data concerning asbestos content in lymph node. Roggli and Benning[51] reported three cases in which hilar node ferruginous body levels were 21,800, 15,500, and 3,200 asbestos bodies/g by light microscopy and lung burdens of 22,000, 481,000, and 5,470 asbestos bodies/g, respectively. A fourth lymph node sample, for which there was no companion lung sample, contained 322,000 asbestos bodies/g. Asbestos bodies were in lymph nodes in 6 of 14 control cases with the burden being higher in the nodes than the lung tissue in four of the cases.

Dodson and colleagues[50] compared the light and transmission electron microscopy data from tracheal lymph nodes of former shipyard workers in addition to the tissue and pleura burdens as discussed (see Table 28–4). Ferruginous bodies were found in the nodes of seven of the eight cases. The total number of ferruginous bodies per gram was greater in three of the subjects than in their parenchymal samples. Uncoated asbestos fibers of both the chrysotile and amphibole forms were found in the nodes. Their total concentration exceeded that of the lung in six of the eight subjects. Obviously, the ferruginous bodies represented a portion of the larger amphibole fibers (≥8 μm); however, most uncoated amphibole fibers within the nodes were 5 μm long or less. A small percentage (2.5%) of the amphiboles were longer than 10 μm.

The reports of Roggli and Benning[51] and Dodson et al.[50] showed that appreciable numbers of fibers including some longer than 8 μm reach the lymph nodes, as shown by the ferruginous body[50,51] and uncoated fiber burden.[50] A comparison of residual uncoated fiber burden of parenchyma, nodes, and plaques[50] suggests a possible difference over time of the influence of clearance on lung burden as opposed to more static areas such as lymph nodes. These studies raise the question as to whether extrapulmonary areas may offer a better monitor of past exposures because there is less impact of clearance on short fibers in these areas than on the burden in lung tissue. More studies must be carried out to test this hypothesis. However, final conclusions regarding uncoated fiber burdens in any sample are heavily dependent on the instrument and counting scheme used. The data presented must state whether short and thin fibers are analyzed to accurately assess total fiber burden.

Ferruginous Bodies and Uncoated Fibers in Body Fluids

Bronchoalveolar Lavage Sample

Bronchoalveolar lavage (BAL) offers a method for sampling the lower respiratory tract.[119–121] The procedure provides useful information for determining the diagnosis of several pulmonary diseases, possibly including those caused by dust.[122]

The most extensive work to date for assessing lavage samples for ferruginous bodies and relating the significance of their numbers to disease states is a series of studies by De Vuyst and colleagues.[123–127] Their work shows a correlation between the numbers of asbestos bodies in BAL fluid and tissue.[124] While realizing that finding an asbestos body in lavage is not proof of disease, the investigators concluded that "asbestos bodies in BAL fluid correlates with occupational risk and can disclose unknown exposure better than a questionnaire."[126] A companion study reported a correlation of

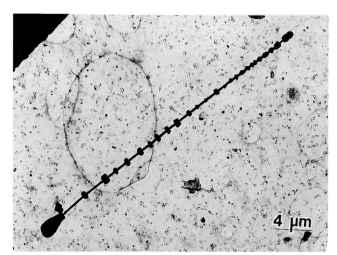

Fig. 28–28. Amosite-cored ferruginous body obtained from digested lavage sample from individual occupationally exposed to this form of asbestos. TEM.

asbestos bodies in lavage to radiologic evidence of disease.[125] Use of the lavage samples analyzed for ferruginous body content has also been the basis of a report on a "nonoccupationally exposed" individual with disease[127] and cited in a case of an individual who had inhaled asbestos as a contaminant of talc.[123]

These data incorporated light microscopy for assessing the larger markers of past asbestos exposure, ferruginous bodies. While determining ferruginous body content is a straightforward and fast way to screen samples for past exposure, it does not offer insight on chrysotile burden (because these fibers are often too short to form ferruginous bodies) or information about the longer fibers in samples from individuals who do not readily coat fibers.

A lavage study by Dodson and colleagues[128] used light and transmission electron microscopy techniques for screening digested material from controls and from patients occupationally exposed to asbestos (predominantly amphiboles). The level of sensitivity based on the presence of ferruginous bodies (by light microscopy) could be used to discriminate most of the occupationally exposed cases from controls as no ferruginous bodies were found in samples from the latter group. Ten of the 12 samples from exposed individuals were positive for ferruginous bodies (Fig. 28–28). Only one uncoated amphibole was found in a control patient while 10 of the 12 occupationally exposed individuals were positive for chrysotile and all were positive for amphiboles (Fig. 28–29).

A ferruginous body occasionally may be found in lavage material from controls (<1/ml).[125] De Vuyst[124] suggested that the presence of ferruginous bodies in lavage samples greater than 1 asbestos body/ml corre-

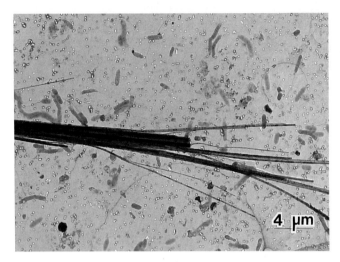

Fig. 28–29. Lavage material from occupationally exposed individuals such as seen in Fig. 28–28 also contained uncoated amosite fibers such as this. TEM.

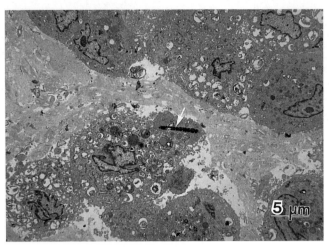

Fig. 28–30. Thin section of embedded sputum shows ferruginous body (*arrow*) with associated macrophages and mucous material. TEM.

lates with higher (occupational) levels of tissue burden. Ten of the occupationally exposed group would have been discriminated from control samples on the basis of more than 1 asbestos body/ml. However, samples from the remaining two patients were distinguished as being from the exposed group only after establishment of uncoated fiber burden.[128]

Work histories may provide adequate background for linking disease with past asbestos exposure. However, if the history is incomplete, if other causes of disease are suspected, or if the documentation of mixed dust exposures (including asbestos) poses special concerns about future health risks, a lung lavage analyzed by light microscopy, and when necessary supplemented by electron microscopy, can offer insight about past asbestos exposure. Such information may be useful to the diagnostician for present and future assessment of the individual's health.

Ferruginous Bodies and Fibers

Sputum

Another human material in which asbestos structures are found is sputum (Fig. 28–30). The mucous material and the macrophages, with phagocytized particles, are cleared via the mucociliary escalator to the back of the throat for elimination via this route. Large particles such as ferruginous bodies are carried to the escalator at a slower rate than short fibers or small particulates, in part because the latter can fit within the mobile macrophages. Some ferruginous bodies are present in sputa, as reported by Stewart and Haddow.[129]

The significance of asbestos bodies in sputa has been evaluated in a limited number of studies, most of which reported their presence secondarily during cytopathol-

ogy screening. McLarty et al.[130] have reported clinically significant correlations as related to the presence of ferruginous bodies in former amosite workers. Roggli et al.[131] also reported a correlation between asbestos body production in sputa and tissue burden. From sputa from a large cohort consisting of the general population[132] and in a study of a smaller population, Dodson et al.[133] concluded that although production of ferruginous bodies in sputa varies, when found they were highly specific markers of past occupational exposure. The variable presence of ferruginous bodies in sputa has been confirmed through serial samples collected from the same individuals who had been heavily exposed to amosite in the work force.[130,134] Further, light microscopy assessment of sputa reveals nothing about the numbers of uncoated fibers in a sample. A comparative study using sputa samples from former amosite workers consisted of analysis of random samples from a series of sputa previously collected for cytopathology assessment. The workers had documented exposures of 2–5 years in an amosite plant. For comparison, an additional series of sputa were collected from control volunteers.[133] By light microscopy, all samples from the exposed and control group were negative for asbestos bodies. However, when control samples were assessed by electron microscopy only one chrysotile fiber was found although 10 of the 12 occupationally exposed samples were positive for uncoated amosite fibers. These observations concerning ferruginous bodies were expected based on reported variability in the presence of asbestos bodies in sputa. However, it was surprising that following a mean latency period of 21.4 years from last exposure, small randomly collected samples would contain amosite fibers in 10 of the 12 samples from the exposed group. This sensitivity should improve as increased numbers of samples are pooled. The presence of ferruginous bodies in sputa therefore should alert the analyst that there was a likely substantial past exposure in that patient.

Uncoated Fibers: Small Samples

Transbronchial Biopsy Specimen

The question about the value of assessing small samples for asbestos content has been addressed by emphasizing the need to take multiple samples when possible. If, therefore, only a small sample is available, is it of no value for assessing past asbestos exposure? To begin to understand the answers to this question, one must review the qualifiers for establishing asbestos/asbestosis–disease relationships. The "minimal features that permit the diagnosis (of asbestosis) are the demonstration of discrete foci of fibrosis in the walls of respiratory bronchioles associated with the accumulations of asbestos bodies."[10] In theory, therefore, if a fine-needle aspiration biopsy or transbronchial biopsy specimen met these qualifiers, such a small sample would be considered highly sensitive. It would also be a rare occurrence because the concentration of both uncoated fibers (i.e., most asbestos fibers in the lung) and ferruginous bodies vary from site to site and lobe to lobe.[114,135,136]

The problem of detecting ferruginous bodies via small samples was emphasized in the study by Roggli and Pratt[37] in which small samples (tissue sections) from larger samples (tissue blocks) were screened for ferruginous bodies. Their calculation defined the lack of sensitivity in tissue sections and argues when possible for the use of larger sampling schemes and the use of procedures such as digestion techniques for increasing the volume sampled. Thus, ideally multiple subpleural areas of parenchyma should be sampled and pooled through digestion or other particulate-concentrating techniques to compensate for the random distribution in tissue of ferruginous bodies or fibers. As already discussed, even this approach, if used with light microscopy, offers information about a limited population of fibers, those longer than 8 μm that have become coated (ferruginous bodies). Most of the fiber burden is of the uncoated form in any sampled site, and information about this population requires analysis by transmission electron microscopy. Warnock and Wolery,[38] recognizing the limitations of tissue sections for determining past exposure, have suggested that higher levels of uncoated amphiboles from digested material may be adequate for defining asbestos-indicated disease.

Considering the weighted significance of the number of uncoated fibers rather than mandating that one find ferruginous bodies in tissue to establish cause and effect

also permits analysis in cases where the possibility of a heavy burden of chrysotile exists (a less likely stimulus for ferruginous body formation) or when high levels of amphiboles may exist and the individual simply may not form ferruginous bodies (similar to that which occurs in some animal species).

If one has only small samples available, the most information can be gained from applying digestion procedures and evaluating the collected digest for both ferruginous bodies (light microscopy) and uncoated fibers (transmission electron microscopy). This type of sample of necessity will usually yield data for wet weight only. To test what information can be gained from small samples, a simulated transbronchial procedure was carried out on autopsied lungs of 12 controls and 12 formerly amosite-exposed individuals.[137] The small samples were divided into those used for digestion procedures and those to be embedded for histopathological screening. The histopathological screen of tissue sections was the least sensitive method for distinguishing the amosite-exposed individuals because a ferruginous body was found in sections from only 4 occupationally exposed individuals. In contrast, at least one ferruginous body was found in the digests of 9 of the 12 occupational samples while none were found in those from control tissue.

When electron microscopy was carried out on the digests, 70 fibers were found in the control group. Sixty-five of these were nonasbestos, 4 were noncommercial amphiboles, and 1 was a chrysotile fiber. In the occupationally exposed individuals, 2242 fibers were found with 1886 being amosite, 157 chrysotile, and 199 nonasbestos fibers. Given that the test group had been heavily exposed, nevertheless the evaluation of their small samples could be best made when light and electron microscopy assessments were combined.

How does one, therefore, interpret the data from a small sample? While individual opinions vary, it seems logical based on the random distribution of fibers and ferruginous bodies to consider the following argument. Negative data from a small sample may or may not reflect lung burden because there are appreciable areas in an occupationally exposed lung with few particles. However, a positive finding may be a more reliable monitor because an area with ferruginous bodies or fibers samples in a small biopsy surely cannot reflect an isolated concentration that is unrepresentative of the existence of other similar areas.

Uncoated Fibers

Toxicity and Carcinogenicity

Inhaled fibrous dusts induce diseases through several mechanisms. Some are common to all dusts and others

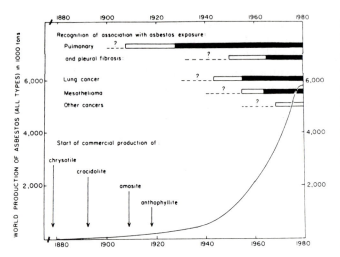

Fig. 28–31. World output of asbestos during past century in relationship to recognition of serious asbestos-related lung diseases; figure also indicates approximately when association with exposure was suspected (?), was considered probably causal (open bars), or was considered definitely causal (solid bars). (Reprinted with permission from Becklake MR. Clin Invest Med 1983;6:305–317.)

same phagocytes that attempt to isolate asbestos creates an abundant opportunity for such reactions to take place within the lung and thus affect these cells and adjacent epithelial components.

An illustration of the complexities associated with understanding toxicity of asbestos is shown in the preliminary data by Lund et al.[194] They observed that ferruginous bodies, previously considered by some to be inert, may act through the same Fenton reaction as iron to produce more radicals than equal amounts of uncoated iron-rich amphiboles such as amosite and crocidolite.

At present, the prevention of exposure to asbestos and potentially to a number of replacement fibers is the logical approach in avoiding the toxic responses possible following inhalation and, over time, the resultant pathologic events.

History of Asbestos Diseases

The incidence of various asbestos diseases can be correlated with the commercial production of asbestos, which began in the late 1800s.[195] As shown by the graph Fig. 28–31), there is a direct correlation between the incidence of various asbestos diseases and the amount of commercial production of asbestos. In the early years of the twentieth century, case reports appeared giving clinical descriptions of severe pulmonary fibrosis and pleural fibrosis of those who had been occupationally exposed to asbestos; general recognition of this problem, occurred by the 1920s. Two epidemiologic studies,

one in the United States[196] and one in the United Kingdom,[197] provided evidence of the assertion that disease was directly related to the severity of exposure to asbestos. Based on the conclusion reached in the U.S. study, it was decided that an exposure concentration of less than 5 million particles per cubic foot (mpcf) would not cause disease, even though that study had been heavily criticized, primarily on the basis that many people who had already died were not considered. Nevertheless, it was the asbestos standard of 5 mpcf that was initially adopted in the United States until more complete data became available.

Most scientists accepted the concept that there was a direct correlation between the incidence of asbestos-related diseases such as pulmonary fibrosis, pleural fibrosis, lung cancer, and mesothelioma and the concentration of asbestos exposure. However, it became quite obvious that there were significant differences in incidence of these disease between various worker cohorts. As reviewed by Becklake,[195] a number of hypotheses were proposed to explain this, although none was perfect, and there continue to be considerable gaps in our knowledge concerning the pathogenesis of most asbestos-related diseases.

Asbestos-Induced Pleural Effusion

In 1982, Epler et al.[198] reported on the prevalence and incidence of benign asbestos pleural effusion in a working population. They reported 34 benign effusions among 1135 asbestos-exposed workers, and compared them with otherwise unexplained effusions among 717 unexposed control subjects. The prevalence of benign asbestos-induced pleural effusions was dose related, with 7%, 3.7%, and 0.2% associated with severe, indirect, and peripheral asbestos exposure, respectively. They found that the latency period (time from first exposure to asbestos to the time of disease development) was shorter for asbestos-induced pleural effusions than it was for other asbestos-related disorders, and that benign asbestos pleural effusion was the most common asbestos-related abnormality during the first 20 years after exposure. Incidence studies showed 9.2 effusions for 100,000 person-years for level 3 exposure, 3.9 for level 2 exposure, and 0.7 for level 1 exposure. They also reported that most of these effusions were small and that the majority (66%) were asymptomatic. In 28.6% of the cases there was recurrence, and in 1 case, mesothelioma was reported 6 years after the first effusion appeared. Their final conclusion was that asbestos exposure should be carefully searched for in persons with "idiopathic" pleural effusion.

Eleven years earlier, Gaensler and Kaplan[199] reviewed their files of 4077 patients who had been evaluated in their laboratory between 1951 and 1969. In this population, 91 patients had pleural effusions. Of these 4077 patients, 57 had asbestosis or asbestos exposure, and 24 of these had pleural effusion. Of these they excluded 12, because the effusion possible occurred in association with mesothelioma, carcinoma of the lung, or congestive heart failure. The remaining 12 (21.1% of those with asbestosis or asbestos exposure) were thought to have an asbestos-induced pleural effusion.

Clinical Manifestations of Asbestos-Induced Pleural Effusions

In 1968, Collins[200] described 2 patients with pulmonary fibrosis who had effusion, and concluded that the changes were caused by inhalation of asbestos. Mattson and Ringqvist[201] reported 7 cases of exudative pleural effusion in patients without signs or symptoms of other disease, and 42 men with pleural plaques who had been exposed to asbestos. Mattson[202] later reported on 25 persons with monosymptomatic exudative pleurisy of unknown etiology, and found that 11 of the patients had been exposed to asbestos. No other cause of the pleural effusion was noted in these 11 men during an observation period of 4–8 years. Diffuse pleural fibrosis developed in 9 of these 11 patients during the 4- to 8-year period, and in 1 patient there was evidence of the development of asbestosis.

Eisenstadt[203] reported a case of an asbestos pleural effusion in a 54-year-old male insulator who had been suffering from acute left-hemithorax chest pain. The patient subsequently had similar symptoms and evidence of a pleural effusion on his right side, and over a period of time progressed to pleural thickening requiring decortication. Eisenstadt commented that benign asbestos pleurisy resembled tuberculosis in its appearance, and was apparently a self-limited disease, although could obviously progress to fibrosis. He thought that the correct diagnosis required pleuropulmonary biopsy for the demonstration of asbestos bodies.

In Gaensler and Kaplan's report,[199] all patients were symptomatic with pleuritic chest pain, sometimes recurrent, being the most frequent symptom. Several of the patients also had dyspnea, which may have been related to asbestosis. One patient presented with joint pains and lumps on the elbows, and another patient had fatigue. The effusions were bilateral in 10 of the 12 cases, and fluid was sanguineous or serosanguineous in 6 of the 12 patients, and clear or straw-colored in 5 patients (1 patient had no tap). This is in contrast to the report of Epler et al.[198] in which 66% of the patients were asymptomatic. In Hillerdal and Ozemi's series[204] of 60 patients with benign asbestos pleural effusions, 47% had no symptoms, 34% had chest pain, 6% had dyspnea, and the remainder had a variety of other symptoms.

Characteristics of the Pleural Fluid

The pleural fluid in benign asbestos-induced pleural effusion is characteristically an exudate that is either serous or serosanguineous. Pleural fluid generally has an elevated white blood cell count, reported to be as high as approximately 30,000/μl.[204] The differential white blood cell count usually shows either a predominant population of polys or lymphocytes. An increased number of eosinophils appears to be characteristic of asbestos pleural effusions, although this is not absolutely diagnostic. In the report by Mattson,[202] more than 50% of the white blood cells in the pleural fluid were eosinophils in 5 of the 11 effusions tested, and 15%–17% of the cells were eosinophils in an additional 2 effusions. These pleural fluids generally have a high protein content as well.

Pathology and Pathogenesis of Asbestos Pleural Effusion

If a "closed"-needle pleural biopsy or thoracotomy and an "open" pleural biopsy are performed at the time of pleural effusion, the pleura usually is abnormal and will show either an acute pleuritis with increase vascularity, an infiltrate of acute inflammatory cells, and a layer of fibrin on the outer surface of the pleura (Fig. 28–32), or will be markedly thickened with a predominantly chronic inflammatory cell infiltrate (Fig. 28–33). As time progresses, there is a tendency for more fibrosis to develop, which is used as one of the explanations of how pleural fibrosis develops in patients with asbestos exposure.

The pathogenesis of pleural effusion is not well understood, but probably relates to the presence of asbestos fibers in the pleural space or pleural tissue, which causes inflammation and irritation of the pleural surface. As previously discussed, asbestos has a variety of biologic properties and results in the release of various cytokines from inflammatory cells, which may be important in the generation of the fluid. Why there is a relatively long latent period in this condition is not well known, but perhaps it is related to the accumulation of a certain concentration of asbestos fibers in the pleural tissue before the resulting inflammation and biologic effects take place to produce the effusion.

Hyaline Pleural Plaques

Definition, Location, Incidence, and Morphologic Appearance

Hyaline pleural plaques are discrete, white to yellow-white, irregularly shaped, frequently calcified, raised structures involving the parietal pleura (Fig. 28–34). In

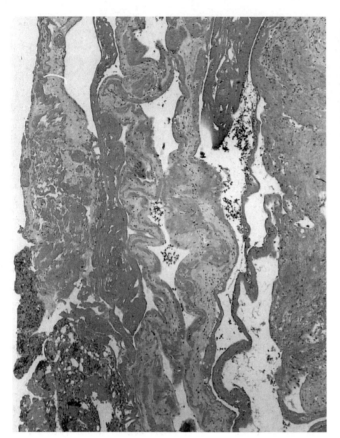

Fig. 28–32. Pleural biopsy from patient with benign acute asbestos-induced pleural effusion shows pleural thickening from fibrin deposition with mild acute inflammation. ×125.

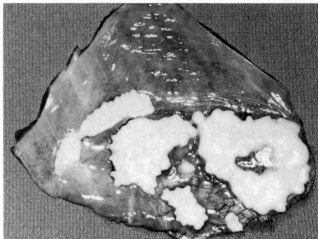

A

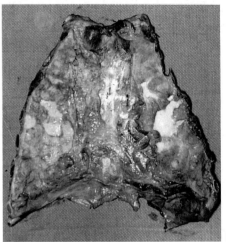

B

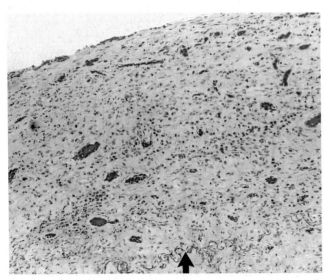

Fig. 28–33. Open lung biopsy from 78-year-old retired refinery worker who presented with bilateral pleural effusion; markedly thickened pleura with predominantly chronic inflammatory cell infiltrate. ×300.

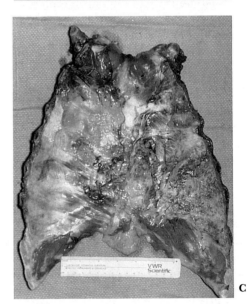

C

Fig. 28–34. A–C. Representative apperance of hyaline pleural plaques. **A.** Plaque on diaphragmatic surfaces. **B** and **C,** Plaques on parietal pleural surface of anterior chest wall, from patients with malignant mesotheliomas.

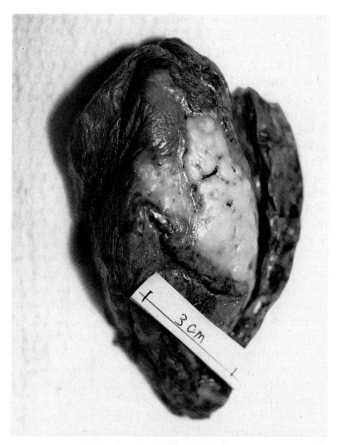

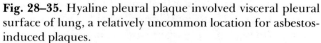

Fig. 28–35. Hyaline pleural plaque involved visceral pleural surface of lung, a relatively uncommon location for asbestos-induced plaques.

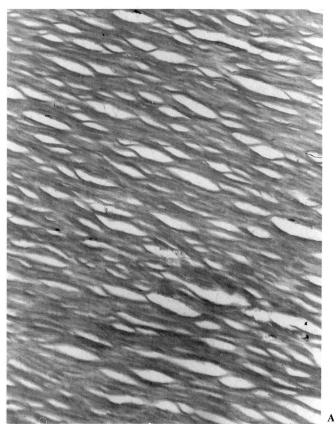

persons occupationally exposed to asbestos, they occur most frequently on the parietal pleural covering the diaphragm, and also commonly occur between the fifth and eighth ribs in the posterior and lateral portions of the chest, characteristically sparing the apices and costophrenic angles. Plaques are occasionally seen on the visceral pleural surface (Fig. 28–35), and may also be rarely seen on the visceral or parietal pericardium and occasionally even on the outer surface of the adventitia of the aorta. Rarely, pleural plaques have been identified on the peritoneal serosal surface.[205,208] Microscopically, hyaline plaques have a characteristic appearance, being composed of dense, relatively hypocellular connective tissue, often exhibiting a basket-weave pattern (Fig. 28–36). They are often associated with foci of chronic inflammation.

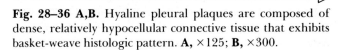

Fig. 28–36 A,B. Hyaline pleural plaques are composed of dense, relatively hypocellular connective tissue that exhibits basket-weave histologic pattern. **A,** ×125; **B,** ×300.

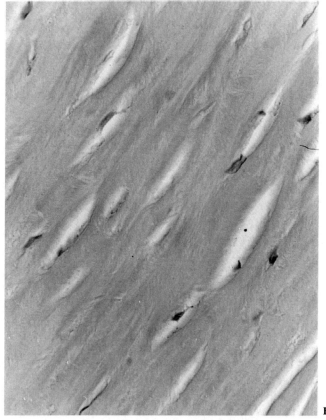

The exact incidence of pleural plaques is uncertain. Wain et al.[207] reported finding 25 cases of pleural plaques in 434 autopsies performed over a 2.5-year period. As summarized by Schwartz,[208] who reviewed 16 separate autopsy studies, pleural plaques were found in 857 of 7085 routine autopsies (12.2%; range, 0.5%–30.3%). In our experience, more than 80% of persons occupationally exposed to asbestos will have hyaline pleural plaques at autopsy, most frequently occurring on the diaphragmatic surfaces. In our experience all patients with plaques have had elevated numbers of asbestos bodies or fibers in their lung tissues.

Association of Plaques with Asbestos

As previously stated, hyaline pleural plaques are seen predominantly in persons who have been exposed to asbestos. In the study by Wain et al.,[207] asbestos bodies were identified in lung digests from all 25 patients with pleural plaques, and exceeded the normal range for their laboratory (20 asbestos bodies/g of wet lung tissue) in 14 cases. In their 25 patients with plaques, 3 had definite exposure to asbestos, 7 had probable exposure to asbestos, 9 had possible exposure to asbestos, and 6 were considered unlikely to have been exposed to asbestos. In the report by Hourihane et al.,[209] hyaline pleural plaques were seen in 4.2% of 381 autopsies (16 cases). However, the authors indicated they had not personally attended all the autopsies, and wondered if the incidence was lower than expected. During 1965, a more vigorous effort was made to evaluate all autopsies performed in the Department of Forensic Medicine, and between January and March, 15 of 134 necropsies (11.2%) showed hyaline pleural plaques, many of which were associated with metastatic lung neoplasms or primary diffuse mesothelioma. To analyze for asbestos bodies, the authors cut 30-μm-thick sections of unstained lung tissue and examined them for asbestos bodies. In 115 routine autopsies, classical asbestos bodies were found in 28 cases (24.3%). In contrast, asbestos bodies were found in all 56 cases of patients with hyaline pleural plaques. The authors stated that the association between plaques and asbestos bodies in the lungs was statistically significant ($p < .01$) when compared with the control series, whether asbestosis was present or not. The authors also stated that there was an attempt to identify asbestos bodies in plaques by incineration technique using phase-contrast microscopy, and in 12 cases examined, four incinerated plaques were found to contain asbestos bodies.

As reviewed by Warnock et al.,[210] epidemiological studies have shown that all types of asbestos are incriminated in the development of plaques. Likewise, some plaques develop in persons who are exposed to talc,[211] which may be due to asbestos fibers such as tremolite that are present in talc. Warnock et al.[210] found that plaques occur most frequently in persons 60–80 years old, and have a latency usually in the range of 20 years, although there have been some cases of plaques reported with a latency as short as 5–6 years after initial exposure.[212] In the Warnock et al.[210] study, lung tissue from 20 persons with pleural plaques identified at autopsy was analyzed for the presence of asbestos fibers, and the concentration and type of fibers in their lung tissue was compared to persons who had no plaques with little or no history of exposure to asbestos. Warnock et al. found that there was a significantly higher concentration of amosite and crocidolite fibers in the lung tissue of persons with plaques as compared to the control group. They also found focal minimal areas of asbestosis in 3 patients who had plaques, with the highest concentration of amosite in their lung tissue. In the control patients, they found the fibers to consist mostly of chrysotile, tremolite, actinolite, and anthophyllite, with relatively few amosite and crocidolite fibers. In the subjects with plaques, they found that most of the amosite and crocidolite fibers had high aspect ratios, and concluded that the fibers were of commercial origin.

Sebastien et al.[213] analyzed lung tissue from two groups of patients with pleural plaques, and found 10^7 fibers/cm^3 in those with asbestosis and 10^6 fibers/cm^3 in those without asbestosis. Whitwell et al.[214] also found a correlation between pleural plaques and asbestos fibers in lung tissue. Whitwell found that 55% of the subjects with more than 20,000 fibers/g of dry lung tissue had plaques, but only 5.5% of those with fewer than 20,000 fibers/g of dry lung tissue had pleural plaques. The studies by Sebastien et al.[213] and Whitwell et al.[214] did not provide any information concerning what type of asbestos fibers were identified in the lung tissue.

Churg[215] studied the total pulmonary asbestos burden in 29 patients identified as having pleural plaques at autopsy and compared the concentration of asbestos in this group with 25 persons who had no history of occupational exposure to asbestos. He found the average number of asbestos bodies in the plaque group was 1732 per gram of wet lung tissue, and, in the control group, 42 per gram of wet lung tissue. Fiber analysis showed that the plaque group had a concentration of asbestos fibers similar to that of the control group (114,000 versus 99,000/g of wet lung tissue), and similar numbers of chrysotile fibers (51,000 versus 68,000/g of wet lung tissue) and noncommercial amphiboles (13,000 versus 29,000/g of wet lung tissue). However, the number of commercial amphiboles identified in the plaque group was significantly higher (50,000/g of wet lung tissue) than in the control group (1000/g of wet lung tissue). Churg found a history of fairly certain asbestos exposure in 16 of 29 plaque patients, and concluded that about half the patients in the general autopsy population who developed plaques had a history of asbestos exposure, while the etiology of the plaques in the other half was unclear. He also concluded that the presence of pleural plaques correlated with an approximately 50-fold increase in the number of high-aspect-ratio commercial amphiboles in the lung tissue, but it was not correlated with the number of chrysotile fibers, noncommercial amphiboles, or the total number of asbestos fibers.

Churg and dePaoli[216] identified four men 70 years of age or older with pleural plaques who resided in or near the chrysotile mining town of Thetford Mines, Quebec, but who had never been employed in a chrysotile mining or milling industry (two men, farming only; one man, farming and construction; one man, road construction). Lung asbestos content of these persons was compared with nine persons living in the same vicinity who did not have pleural plaques. They found an equal concentration of chrysotile in the plaque persons versus the non-plaque persons, but a fourfold elevation in the median tremolite content of the plaque persons' lung tissue versus the lung tissue in persons without plaques. They concluded that environmental pleural plaques in this region of Quebec were possibly caused by tremolite derived from local soils/rocks, and were possibly also caused by titanium oxide of environmental origin.

Kishimoto et al.[217] determined the concentration of asbestos bodies in 400 autopsy lungs, and found 71 cases in which asbestos bodies were significantly elevated. In all 71 cases hyaline pleural plaques were identified. They correlated the number of asbestos bodies in the lung tissue with the presence of pleural plaques as identified radiographically [three classifications: (1) probable pleural plaque, 24 cases; (2) definite pleural plaque, 22 cases; and (3) definite pleural plaque with calcification, 25 cases]. They found that cases whose pleural plaques were definite radiographically had more asbestos bodies than the indefinite cases, and that those who had definite pleural plaques with calcification had a higher median and mean concentration of asbestos in their lung tissue than those who had definite pleural plaques without calcification and those whose radiographs showed probable pleural plaques.

Pathogenesis of Hyaline Pleural Plaques

The pathogenesis of pleural plaques remains uncertain. As mentioned earlier in this chapter, asbestos fibers that are not removed from the larger conducting airways and which reach the alveolar parenchyma are cleared primarily by the lung lymphatic channels.[97,218] Fibers that are present in the vicinity of the parenchymal lymphatic plexus drain to the mediastinal lymph nodes, whereas the fibers in the network of the pleural lymphatic plexus drain to the periphery of the lung and collect in the subvisceral pleural location. Most investigators have not been able to identify asbestos bodies in pleural plaques,[219] although Rosen et al.[53] and Roberts[220] have identified asbestos bodies in some pleural plaques, and Sebastien and colleagues[213] identified asbestos bodies in most plaques they examined. LeBouffant et al.[221] identified chrysotile fibers in plaques by electron microscopy, and concluded that chrysotile was the cause of the plaques. In the Warnock et al.[210] study, chrysotile was identified in several plaques, although no chrysotile was found in most of the plaques.

Kiviluoto[222] and Meurman[219] suggested that hyaline pleural plaques form as a direct result of local inflammation of the parietal pleura caused by asbestos fibers that protrude from the visceral pleura and directly "irritate" the parietal pleura. No pathologic evidence has been found to support this theory, and it has therefore not gained wide acceptance. Asbestos fibers have been identified in pleural effusions of persons occupationally exposed to asbestos,[116] and Wang[223] has described preformed lymphatic stoma on the surface mesothelium of the parietal pleura connecting the pleural cavity and the lymphatics of the parietal pleura. It is possible that fibers gain access to the parietal pleura via this route. A study concerning the pathogenesis of mesothelioma[224] showed that when fibers are directly injected into the pleural cavity, they accumulate around the lymphatic stoma where they cause an inflammatory reaction. Taskinen et al.[225] suggested that asbestos fibers can reach the parietal pleura via retrograde lymphatic flow from the mediastinal lymph nodes through the retrosternal and intercostal lymphatic channels.

Of potential importance with respect to which asbestos fiber type causes hyaline pleural plaques, it is important to remember the experimental study by Wagner et al.,[226] who exposed rats via inhalation to comparable daily doses of chrysotile and amphibole asbestos from 1 day to 24 months, and determined the concentration of asbestos as measured by silica content in the dust isolated from the lungs of the rats. They found a direct correlation between the concentrations of amphiboles in the lungs of the rats, but not of chrysotile, with the dose given. In the rats exposed to asbestos for 24 months, the weight of the amphiboles was 35 times that of the chrysotile. Despite this, asbestosis and tumors developed just as frequently in the animals exposed to chrysotile asbestos as in those exposed to amphiboles. Therefore, as stated by Warnock et al.,[210] one must be extremely careful in interpreting low concentrations of chrysotile in the lungs of persons occupationally exposed to asbestos, because it may not rule out the possibility that chrysotile was responsible for the disease.

Diffuse Pleural Fibrosis

Diffuse pleural fibrosis is relatively common in patients occupationally exposed to asbestos. The exact incidence of this condition is not well documented, although in our experience, it is less frequent than localized hyaline pleural plaques. This disease appears to have a latent period of about 15 years, and there is a dose–response relationship.

Morphology and Location of Diffuse Pleural Fibrosis

The morphology of pleural fibrosis is highly variable and depends on the severity of change. The process characteristically involves the visceral pleura, and frequently involves the costophrenic angles, although it may be relatively diffuse (Fig. 28–37). The condition may also involve the apical region of the upper lobes.[227] In some instances this condition can become severe, with fusion of the visceral and parietal layers of the pleura, sometimes producing a condition known as fibrothorax in which the pleural cavity is obliterated (Fig. 28–38). Microscopically, the fibrous tissue can show significant vascularity and inflammation, with the outer portion of the fused visceral and parietal pleura not infrequently having the appearance of hyaline pleural plaque tissue.

Pathogenesis of Diffuse Pleural Fibrosis

The pathogenesis of diffuse pleural fibrosis is poorly understood, and it is probable that factors involved in the formation of hyaline pleural plaques are also involved in the production of visceral pleural fibrosis. As reviewed by Schwartz,[208] visceral pleural fibrosis may be a direct extension of parenchymal fibrosis. Both may begin as inflammatory-type processes initiated by asbestos, with the progressive development of scarring from a variety of mechanisms, possibly the same mechanisms that cause asbestosis. Asbestos has been reported to be somewhat preferentially deposited in the periphery of the lung below the pleural surface.[213] We have observed several cases of diffuse visceral-parietal pleural fibrosis that have been diagnosed radiographically as asbestosis. However, many if not most of these cases show some degree of subpleural parenchymal fibrosis, which could be diagnosed as asbestosis. As recently discussed, this is

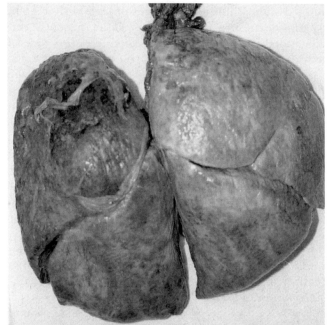

A

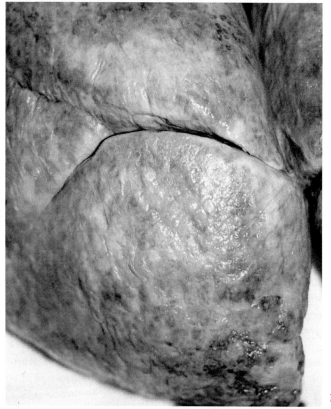

B

Fig. 28–37 A,B. Lungs from asbestos insulation worker show diffuse visceral pleural scarring. Normally transparent visceral pleura becomes opacified by scarring.

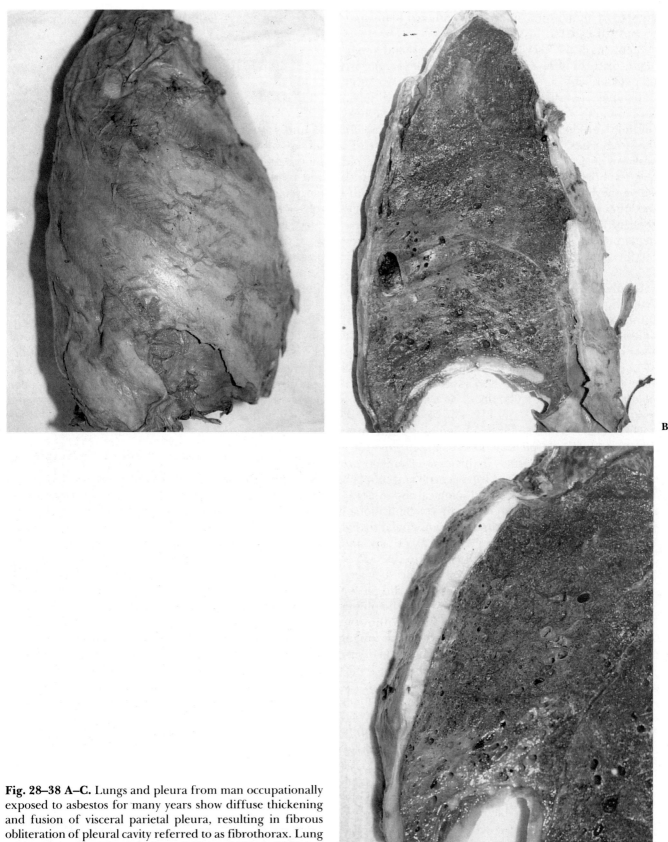

Fig. 28–38 A–C. Lungs and pleura from man occupationally exposed to asbestos for many years show diffuse thickening and fusion of visceral parietal pleura, resulting in fibrous obliteration of pleural cavity referred to as fibrothorax. Lung parenchyma shows focal regions of asbestosis. Note thick rind of fibrous tissue encasing lung on cut sections (**B** and **C**).

an area of controversy in asbestos-induced pleuropul-monary disease.[227]

Stephens et al.[228] reviewed the pathologic and miner-alogic features of seven cases of diffuse pleural fibrosis in persons with known asbestos exposure. All seven individuals described had a significant asbestos expo-sure ranging from 2 to 25 years, and the necropsy findings fulfilled criteria for compensable disease. In the seven cases, the histologic features were those of a basket-weave pattern of thickened pleural tissue and dense subpleural parenchymal interstitial fibrosis with fine honeycombing extending to a depth of 1 cm into the underlying lung tissue. Crocidolite and amosite concentrations were elevated in six of the seven pa-tients, and chrysotile counts were elevated in four cases. Stephens et al.[228] concluded that diffuse pleural fibrosis was a specific asbestos entity of uncertain pathogenesis, with lung tissue containing asbestos mineral fiber con-centrations between those found in plaques and those found in minimal asbestosis (2.4–28×10^6 fibers of amosite or crocidolite per gram of dry lung tissue). In their laboratory, they stated that nonexposed individu-als had light microscopic counts less than 20,000 fibers/g of dry lung tissue, whereas persons with pleural plaques had 10,000–50,000 fibers per gram of dry lung tissue.

Gibbs et al.[229] subsequently studied lung tissue from 13 cases of diffuse pleural fibrosis associated with a history of asbestos exposure. In this study, samples were taken from the visceral pleura and central and subpleu-ral zones of the lung for histopathological and mineral-ogic studies. They found an increased concentration of amphibole fiber counts in a concentration similar to that seen in cases of pleural plaques, mild asbestosis, and mesothelioma. They found a wide case-to-case varia-tion, and there was no significant difference between the central and subpleural zones, whereas the pleura had low asbestos counts, and the asbestos in the pleura consisted mostly of short chrysotile fibers. Within the lung tissue, more than 45% of the asbestos was longer (>4 μm) and thinner (<0.25 μm) amphibole fibers, which they interpreted to suggest that the longer, thin-ner fibers were important in the pathogenesis of asbes-tos-related disease, including pleural fibrosis. Once again, it is important to recall the experiment by Wag-ner et al.[226] concerning chrysotile asbestos inhaled in rats and the production of disease. The conclusion by Gibbs et al.[229] that amphiboles rather than chrysotile fibers are retained in the lungs appears correct, al-though whether or not that implies that amphiboles were necessarily responsible for the observed changes remains uncertain. As reviewed by Schwartz[208] and as reported by Kilburn and Warshaw,[230] diffuse pleural fibrosis is associated with signs and symptoms of respi-ratory disease and also with abnormal pulmonary func-tion tests.

Round Atelectasis

Description and History

Round atelectasis is a condition most frequently ob-served by radiologists in persons occupationally ex-posed to asbestos. These persons are usually asymptom-atic, and radiographically have a unilateral round peripheral density in the lower lobe of the lung (usually the right-lower or -middle lobe), with one or more curvilinear shadows that radiate from this density to-ward the hilum of the lung (Fig. 28–39) and which may be misinterpreted as a neoplasm.

In 1928, Loeschke[231] observed localized atelectasis due to pleural effusion, and Hanke[232] reported a simi-lar condition in 1971 that he called "round atelectasis." Blesovsky,[233] in 1966, described the condition in the English literature as "folded lung," and Dernevik et al.[234] reported on 28 patients with similar radio-graphic and histologic features they termed "shrinking pleuritis with atelectasis." This entity has also been reported as Blesovsky's syndrome,[235] pleuroma,[236] and pulmonary pseudotumor.[237]

Pathologic Features of Round Atelectasis

The pathologic features of round atelectasis have been described in the German literature by Schummel-feder[238] and Giese,[239] and in the English literature by Dernevik et al.,[239] Mark,[240] and, more recently, by Menzies and Frazier[241] and by Chung-Park et al.[242] Macroscopically, the visceral pleura shows localized irregular fibrosis and may be fused with a thickened parietal pleura. Below the area of pleural fibrosis there is an infolding of the pleura, causing one or more areas of invagination. Histologically the pleural fibrosis is superficial to the outer layer of visceral pleural elastic tissue, and the portion of the visceral pleura consisting of the internal and external layers of elastic tissue are thrown into variably sized and complex wrinkles that extend downward into the underlying lung tissue for a variable distance (Fig. 28–40). The lung tissue under the area of invagination of the visceral pleura may be normal or may show compressive atelectasis or intersti-tial fibrosis.

Etiology of Round Atelectasis

As reviewed by Chung-Park et al.,[242] of the 107 cases of round atelectasis reported in the literature 61 (57%) had a history of asbestos exposure. The remaining 46

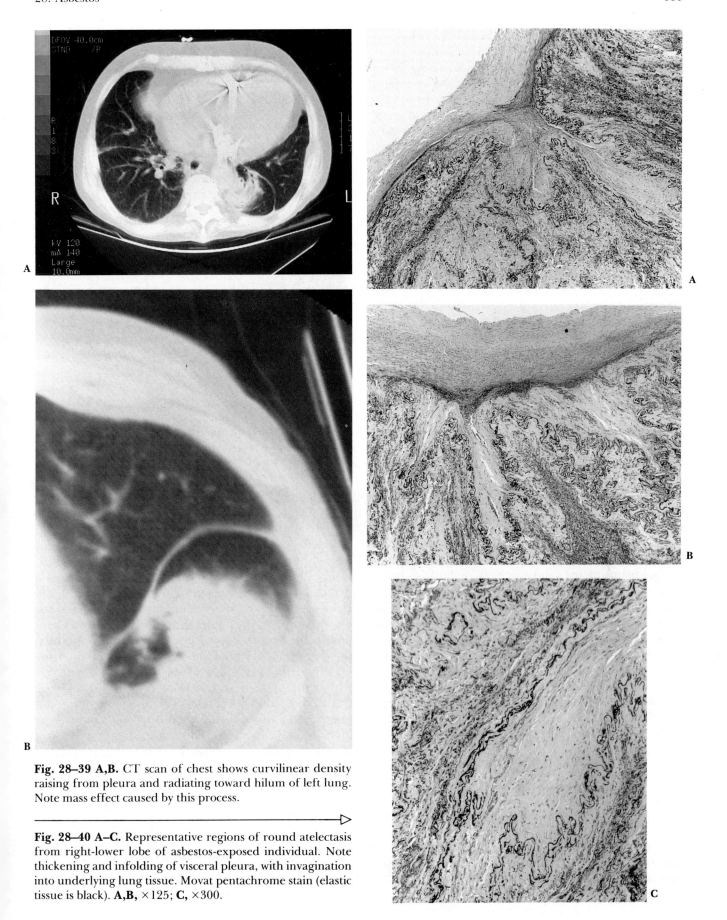

Fig. 28–39 A,B. CT scan of chest shows curvilinear density raising from pleura and radiating toward hilum of left lung. Note mass effect caused by this process.

——————————————————————————⟹

Fig. 28–40 A–C. Representative regions of round atelectasis from right-lower lobe of asbestos-exposed individual. Note thickening and infolding of visceral pleura, with invagination into underlying lung tissue. Movat pentachrome stain (elastic tissue is black). **A,B,** ×125; **C,** ×300.

had no history of exposure to asbestos or evidence of asbestosis, but developed localized atelectasis apparently because of other factors such as tuberculosis, exudative pleural infection, congestive heart failure, myocardial infarction, or trauma. Of the three cases reported by Chung-Park et al.,[242] 2 patients had recurrent or long-standing pleural effusion from congestive heart failure and chronic renal failure, and a third case had evidence of remote fibrocaseous tuberculosis. However, patients #2 and #3 were former coal miners, and had evidence of a mixed-dust exposure with elevated numbers of asbestos bodies in their lung tissue indicating the potential role of asbestos as a contributing factor to the pleural fibrosis.

Pathogenesis of Round Atelectasis

As discussed by Menzies and Frazier[241] concerning the pathogenesis of round atelectasis, Loeschke,[231] and later Hanke[232] and Kretzschmar,[237] proposed that round atelectasis began with the development of a pleural effusion large enough to result in a separation of the visceral pleural-covered lung from the parietal pleura. According to their theory, focal collapse of the lung parenchyma occurred because the effusion formed a groove or cleft in the lung tissue with folding of this lung tissue upon itself, causing an area of invagination (Fig. 28–41). Organization of the fibrinous exudate on the pleural surface resulted in mature fibrous tissue being formed, which then fixed the area of fold and maintained the underlying atelectasis. The alternative theory proposed by Blesovsky[233] and Dernevik et al.[234] is shown in Fig. 28–42, as illustrated by Menzies and Frazier.[241] According to this theory, the pleural fibrous tissue matures and contracts, pulling the underlying pleura with it. Because the pleura can only be minimally compressed, there is no alternative other than for it to buckle into the lung tissue in accordion fashion, which leads to collapse of the lung parenchyma with the associated thickened pleura. We have observed many cases similar to that described by Chung-Park et al.,[242] which they refer to as shrinking pleuritis, in patients exposed to asbestos, probably related both to the pleural fibrosis and the pleural effusion, with the understanding that the pleural fibrosis may be a consequence of organization of the pleural fluid.

Asbestosis

Historical Perspective

As reviewed by Selikoff and Lee,[243] cases of severe pulmonary fibrosis in association with asbestos were described in the early 1900s. In 1914, T. Fahr, a German pathologist, described the pathologic features of

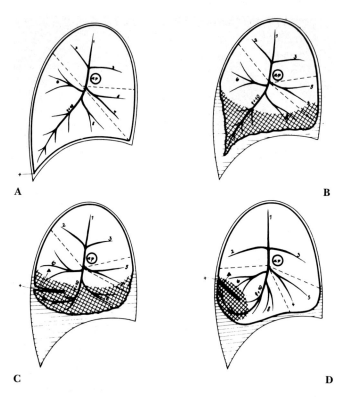

Fig. 28–41 A–D. "Folding" theory of pathogenesis of round atelectasis. **A.** Normal lung and pleura. Pleural effusion causes the lung to float, collapse (**B**), and eventually fold about itself (**C**). Because of adhesions within cleft, one region remains collapsed as the remainder of the lung reexpands (**D**). (Reprinted with permission from Am J Surg Pathol 1987;11:674–681.)

interstitial pulmonary fibrosis in a 35-year-old asbestos worker,[244] and attributed them to asbestos. In 1924, Cooke[245] coined the term asbestosis and published a detailed pathologic description of the disease. In 1938, Dresen et al.[246] reported the prevalence of ground-glass changes in chest radiographs of 440 South Carolina textile industry workers, and described the relationship of abnormalities to the duration and intensity of exposure to asbestos of each individual worker. Although their study has been criticized, they concluded that if the concentration of asbestos in the air did not exceed 5 mpcf, then no abnormalities would occur in the chest radiographs. This concentration of asbestos was thus adopted as the environmental standard at that time. A similar study was done by Merewether and Price,[197] who reported in 1930 on the effects of asbestos dust on the lungs and the issue of dust suppression in the asbestos industry.

Morphology

The most comprehensive pathologic description of asbestosis is that by Craighead.[10] More recent reviews

Fig. 28–42 A–C. "Fibrosing" theory of round atelectasis. **A.** Normal pleura. Fibrous tissue in superficial pleura contracts, causing wrinkling (**B**), and eventually folding (**C**) of pleura, associated with collapse of the underlying parenchyma. (Reprinted with permission from Am J Surg Pathol 1987;11:674–681.)

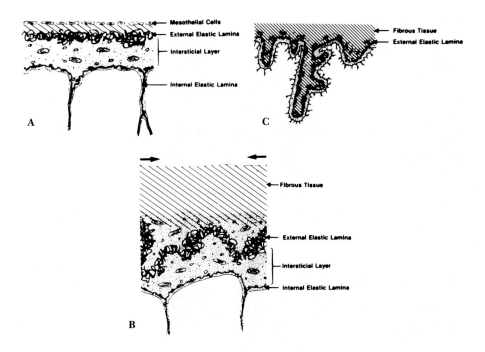

have also been published by Roggli[247,248] and by Roggli et al.[249] Becklake's review in 1976[115] is also superb. The simplest definition of asbestosis is that of pulmonary fibrosis caused by accumulation of airborne asbestos in the lungs. Although the term pleural asbestosis has sometimes been used to refer to scarring of the pleura caused by asbestos, it is our opinion that this term should be avoided because it adds confusion to an area that already lends itself to confusion with respect to terminology. Not infrequently medical scientists use the terms asbestos and asbestosis improperly. Asbestosis is a disease that has a dose–response relationship, but probably also relates as well to host factors. As discussed by Warnock and Isenberg[250] concerning the development of lung cancer and asbestosis, the degree of fibrosis in persons lung with the same concentrations of asbestos varies significantly. As is discussed later, cigarette smoke may influence the development of asbestosis, although the exact relationship between asbestosis and cigarette smoking is not clear.

The macroscopic appearance of asbestosis depends on the severity of the disease. Persons with histologic grade 1–2 asbestosis usually show no gross abnormalities. As the fibrosis becomes more severe, there are streaks and foci of greyish-white fibrous tissue in the parenchyma, usually in a subpleural location (Fig. 28–43). As the disease becomes more severe, there are additional deposits of greyish-white fibrous tissue in the peripheral parts of the lung, and honeycombing may occur (Fig. 28–44). Asbestosis is stated to begin in and be

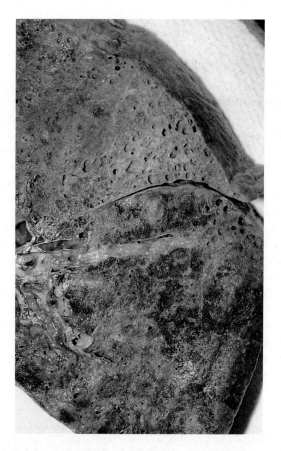

Fig. 28–43. Cross section of lung shows severe asbestos-induced pleural fibrosis and mild scarring in lower lobe, which had irregular streaks of gray-white fibrous tissue.

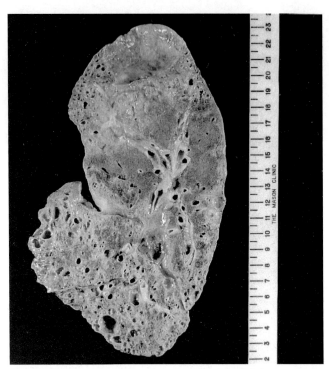

Fig. 28–44. "End-stage" pulmonary fibrosis with honeycombing caused by asbestos. Macroscopic features are identical to those seen in idiopathic pulmonary fibrosis.

most severe in the lower lobes, although this author is not convinced of that finding. The same has been said of idiopathic pulmonary fibrosis, and as published in 1978 in an open lung biopsy study of idiopathic pulmonary fibrosis,[251] fibrosis was just as severe in the upper lobes as in the lower lobes, even though chest radiographs suggested more severe disease in the lower lobes. Also, as reported by Churg et al.[252] and Dodson et al.,[50] the concentration of asbestos in the lungs of those occupationally exposed is just as great in the upper lobes as it is in the lower lobes.

The panel commissioned by the College of American Pathologists and the National Institutes for Occupational Safety and Health,[10] headed by Craighead, graded asbestos into four categories depending on the location of the fibrosis and its severity (see Table 28-9). They also developed a grading scheme for asbestosis that was intended for the semiquantitative estimation of the degree of asbestosis, and not as an aid in diagnosis. The grading scheme depended on the severity of asbestosis according to the four grades, and the extent of the

————————————————————————▷

Fig. 28–45 A,B. A. Grade 1 asbestosis characterized by peribronchiolar fibrosis in association with asbestos bodies and other dusts. **B.** Ferruginous body consistent with asbestos body. **A,** ×125; **B,** ×550.

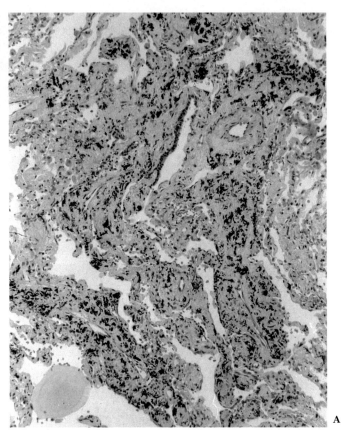

A

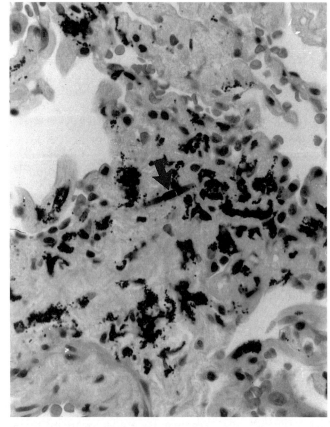

B

disease as determined by the proportion of respiratory bronchioles involved in a slide of lung tissue, and not the numbers involved by the maximum degree of fibrosis as determined by severity. Three grades of extent of disease were described, as follows: grade A (1), only occasional bronchioles are involved, most show no lesion; grade B (2), more than occasional involvement is seen, but less than half of all bronchioles in the section of lung tissue are involved; and grade C (3), more than half of all bronchioles are involved. The total score of any given slide of lung tissue was determined by multiplying the grade of the asbestosis by the extent, in which the letter is converted to a number. The authors indicated that it could be argued that this product could be inappropriate, because a relatively high score could be obtained by a focal area of severe fibrosis in a localized area (grade 4 × extent = 1) although this was not usually observed. They found that high scores were usually found when the disease was widespread in the tissue.

Histologic grade 1 asbestosis is described as peribronchiolar fibrosis, with possible extension into the septa of the adjacent layer of the alveoli, but with no fibrosis in the more distant alveoli (Fig. 28–45). Histologic grade 2 asbestosis is characterized by involvement of alveolar ducts, of two or more layers of adjacent alveoli, with a zone of nonfibrotic alveolar tissue between adjacent bronchioles (Fig. 28–46). Histologic grade 3 asbestosis is characterized by coalescence of the fibrotic change, with alveoli between at least two adjacent bronchioles showing interstitial fibrosis in addition to the peribronchiolar fibrosis (Fig. 28–47). Histologic grade 4 asbestosis is characterized by diffuse interstitial fibrosis with honeycombing in association with asbestos bodies. The morphology of grade 4 asbestosis is essentially identical to that of end-stage idiopathic pulmonary fibrosis, with the exception that asbestos bodies are observed (Fig. 28–48).

A variety of other changes are seen in some cases of asbestosis. Occasionally it can be difficult to find asbestos bodies in cases of diffuse fibrosis consistent with grade 4 asbestosis (Fig. 28–49), whereas in other cases, large numbers of asbestos bodies are present (Fig. 28–50) in persons with similar histories of occupational exposure to asbestos. This may be related to clearance of asbestos from the lung or to the "ability" to form asbestos bodies. Asbestos bodies are frequently seen in the cytoplasm of multinucleate histiocytic giant cells (Fig. 28–51), often being fragmented. Foci of ossification are not uncommonly seen in grade 4 asbes-

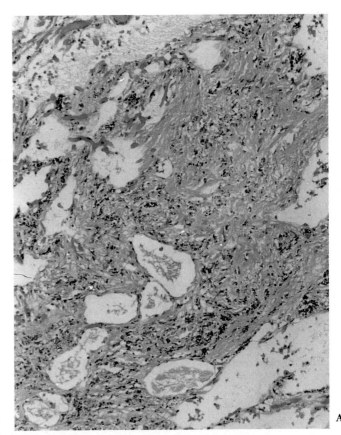

A

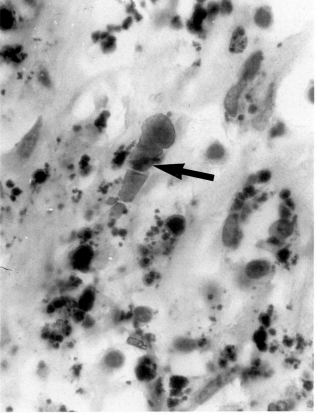

B

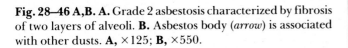

Fig. 28–46 A,B. A. Grade 2 asbestosis characterized by fibrosis of two layers of alveoli. **B.** Asbestos body (*arrow*) is associated with other dusts. **A,** ×125; **B,** ×550.

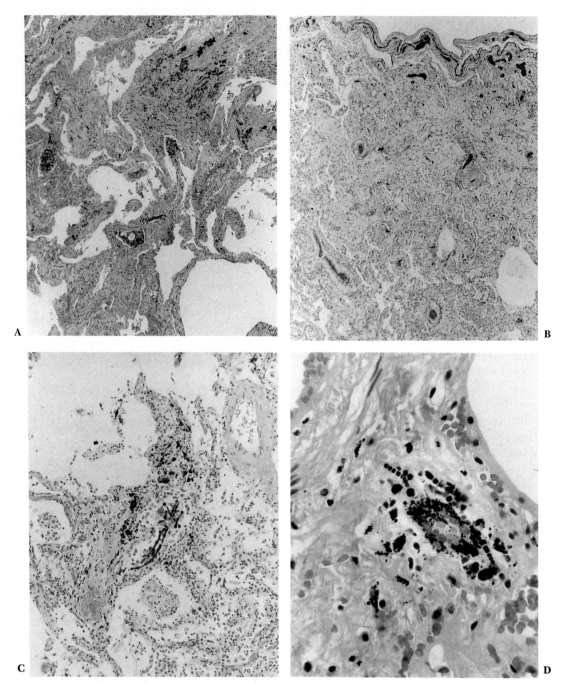

Fig. 28–47 A–D. A and **B,** Relatively low magnifications of lung tissue exhibiting changes of grade 3 asbestosis characterized by coalescence of fibrosis, with involvement of two adjacent alveoli. **B** and **C,** Several ferruginous bodies consistent with asbestos bodies present in fibrotic lung tissue. **A,** ×25; **B,** ×25; **C,** ×125; **D,** ×500.

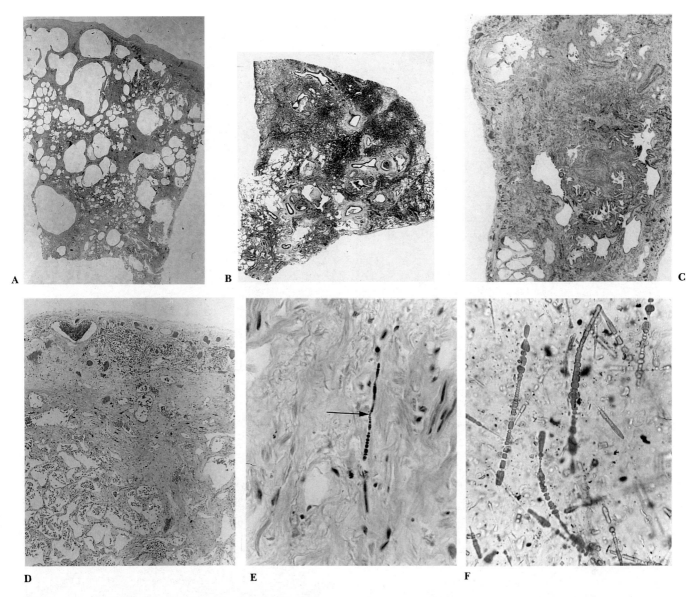

Fig. 28–48 A–F. Representative regions of grade 4 asbestosis. **A** and **B,** Low-magnification photographs show honeycombing and diffuse nature of disease. **C** and **D,** Fibrosis in subpleural location, the region of most severe fibrosis in grade 4 asbestosis. **E,** Asbestos body (*arrow*) in dense connective tissue; **F,** region of filter preparation made from case of grade 4 asbestosis. **A,B,** ×4; **C,D,** ×25; **E,** ×550.

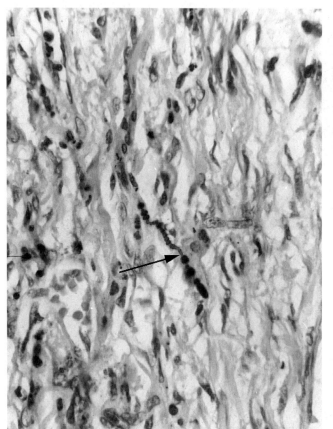

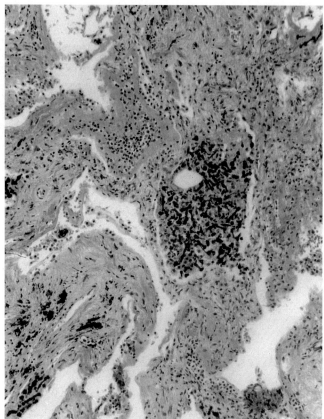

Fig. 28–49. In this case of grade 4 asbestosis, it was difficult to identify asbestos bodies (*arrow*); however, high concentrations of asbestos fibers were found in lung tissue. ×550.

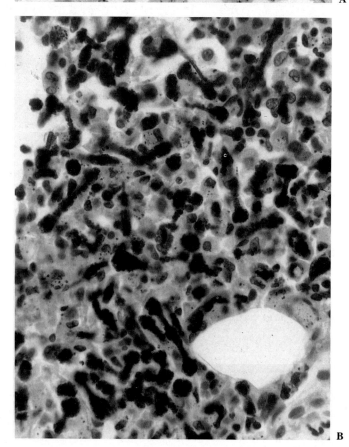

Fig. 28–50 A,B. In this case of grade 4 asbestosis, high numbers of asbestos bodies, many of them fragmented, were present. **A,** ×125; **B,** ×550.

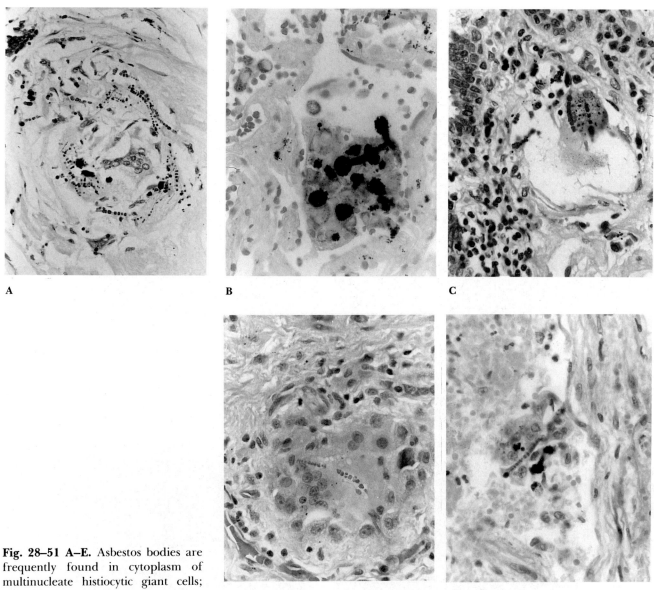

A   **B**   **C**

Fig. 28–51 A–E. Asbestos bodies are frequently found in cytoplasm of multinucleate histiocytic giant cells; they are often fragmented. **A–E,** ×550.

D   **E**

tosis (Fig. 28–52), as are blue bodies (Fig. 28–53). In rare cases, asteroid bodies are noted in multinucleate histiocytic giant cells, but these are nondiagnostic (Fig. 28–54). Roggli[248] has categorized the histiologic changes in 100 cases of asbestosis (Table 28–9).

Several controversies exist concerning the pathologic features and pathologic diagnosis of asbestosis.[227] For example, Churg[253] defined asbestosis as "bilateral diffuse interstitial fibrosis of the lungs caused by exposure to asbestos," and states that "diffuse interstitial fibrosis is the only process to which the term asbestosis should be applied." This definition in part may relate to his concept of whether the lesion referred to as grade 1 asbestosis (peribronchiolar fibrosis in association with

asbestos bodies) should be referred to as asbestosis. As discussed by Churg and Wright[254] and Wright et al.,[255] a variety of mineral dusts, including coal, talc, mica, silica, aluminum oxide, and iron oxide, as well as chrysotile and amphibole asbestos, can induce small airways disease consisting of fibrotic thickening of the walls of the membranous bronchioles and respiratory bronchioles. They have suggested that the generic term "mineral dust-induced airways disease" be used to describe such lesions. As reviewed by Wright et al.,[255] part of the problem in determining whether mineral dust induced such a change is the fact that many of the persons exposed to mineral dust are cigarette smokers, and cigarette smoking can cause a somewhat similar

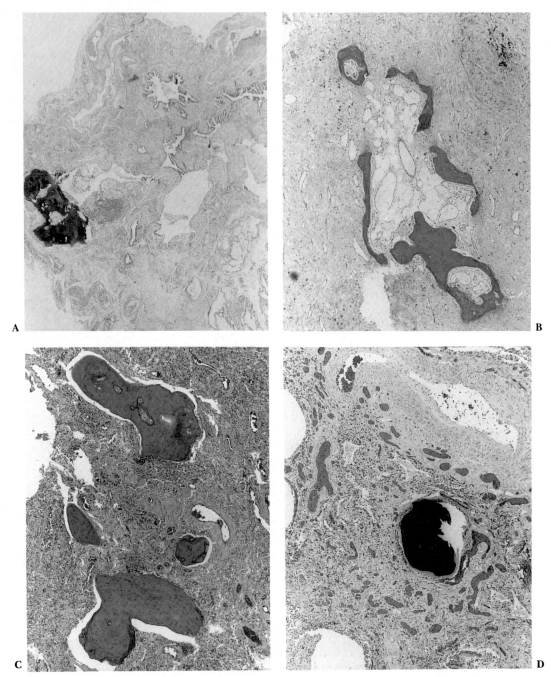

Fig. 28–52 A–D. These areas of grade 4 asbestosis show regions of ossification, a relatively frequent finding in severe asbestosis. **A,** ×25; **B–D,** ×125.

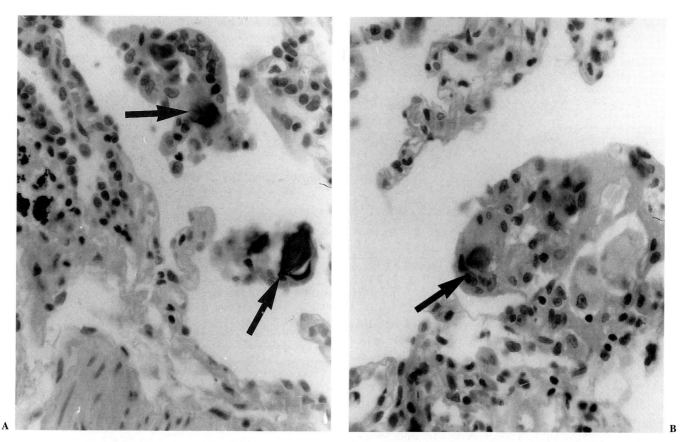

Fig. 28–53 A,B. In this case of asbestosis, blue bodies (calcium salts) (*arrows*) were commonly seen in macrophages.

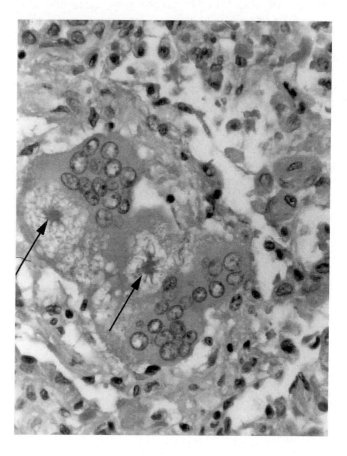

Fig. 28–54. In this case of asbestosis, asteroid bodies (*arrows*) were observed in several multinucleate histiocytic Langhan's-type giant cells. These have no diagnostic significance in this setting. ×550.

Table 28–9. Histologic features found in 100 cases of asbestosis.[a]

Histologic feature	Percent
Always present	
Asbestos bodies	100
Peribronchiolar fibrosis	100
Often present	
Alveolar septal fibrosis	82
Occasionally present	
Honeycomb changes	15
Foreign-body giant cells	15
Pulmonary adenomatosis	10
Cytoplasmic hyalin	7
Desquamative interstitial pneumonitis-like areas	6
Rarely present	
Osseous metaplasia (dendriform pulmonary ossification)	2
Pulmonary blue bodies	1

[a] Reprinted with permission from Roggli VL. Asbestosis: A critical review. Adv Pathol 1989;2:31–60.

type of lesion. The authors provided evidence that mineral dust appeared to cause membranous bronchial fibrosis above and beyond that caused by cigarette smoking alone. As indicated by Wright et al.,[255] only 4% of control (non-dust-exposed) smokers showed fibrosis in the region of respiratory bronchioles, whereas this was found in 48% of respiratory bronchioles from smoking workers with asbestos exposure, and 35% of the alveolar ducts from such workers. Similar type changes were seen in 31% of the respiratory bronchioles and 14% of the alveolar ducts from subjects with other types of dust exposure. These latter findings would suggest that asbestos is more potent than other dusts in inducing fibrosis.

Mineralogy of Asbestosis

Asbestosis is a disease that shows a dose–response relationship, and in general relatively high concentrations of asbestos are needed to cause asbestosis. Although a recent report[256] suggested that asbestosis does not occur in individual exposed only to chrysotile asbestos, several experimental studies show that all commercial types of asbestos cause asbestosis. A number of experimental studies have suggested that short-fiber chrysotile asbestos (<5 μm long) is nonfibrogenic.[154,257–263] However, there is no doubt that long-fiber chrysotile asbestos causes asbestosis in asbestos miners and millers and in asbestos textile workers.[36,264] As already discussed in this chapter, considerable investigation needs to be done in the area of short asbestos fibers with respect to their potential for injury.

Asbestos can be found in the lungs of most adults in industrialized nations, and therefore by itself is not a specific marker for asbestosis. In general, the concen-

Table 28–10. Asbestos content of lung tissue in reported series of patients with asbestosis[a]

Source	No. of cases	Method[b]	Asbestos bodies/g dried lung	Uncoated fibers/g dried lung
Whitwell et al.	23	PCLM	. . . .	8 (1.0–7.0)
Ashcroft and Heppleston	22	PCLM	12.2 (0.49–192)	32 (1.3–493)
Warnock et al.	22	TEM‡	0.123 (0.001–7.38)	5.68 (1.6–121)
Wagner et al.	100	PCLM	—	1.5 (0.001–31.6)
	170	TEM	—	372 (<1.0–10,000)
Roggli (present study)	76	SEM[c]	0.378§ (0.006–16)	3.3[d] (0.18–125)

[a] Values reported are the median counts for millions (10^6) of asbestos bodies or uncoated fibers per gram of dried lung tissue, with ranges indicated in parentheses, except for the study of Wagner et al., where only the mean value could be obtained from the data presented. Reprinted with permission from Roggli VL. Asbestosis: A critical review. Adv Pathol 1989;2:31–60.
[b] PCLM, phase contrast light microscopy; TEM, transmission electron microscopy; SEM, scanning electron microscopy.
[c] In these two studies, asbestos bodies were counted by conventional light microscopy.
[d] Values multiplied by a factor of 10 (approximate ratio of wet to dry lung weight) for purposes of comparison.

tration of asbestos in dry lung is 10 times that in wet lung, because the wet weight:dry weight ratio is usually about 1:10. There often is a significant variation in asbestos body/fiber concentration as determined by different laboratories.[265] Roggli[248] has reviewed the asbestos content of lung tissue in four reported series of patients with asbestosis (Table 28–10), and reported on the asbestos body count in the lung of 76 patients with histologically confirmed asbestosis (Fig. 28–55). The median asbestos body count for patients with asbestosis was 37,800 per gram of wet lung tissue, whereas the median values for patients with idiopathic pulmonary fibrosis was 16 asbestos bodies per gram of wet lung tissue, and for controls, 0.4 asbestos bodies per gram of wet lung tissue. He found that in 95% of the cases of asbestosis, the asbestos body count was 1700 asbestos bodies per gram of wet lung tissue or greater. As pointed out by Roggli, when this concentration of asbestos is present in the lung tissue, one can usually (but not always) see several asbestos bodies in a 2×2 cm iron-stained section. As illustrated by Roggli[248] (Fig. 28–56), asbestosis best correlates with the content of uncoated asbestos fibers in the lung tissue. Roggli found that very few patients with alveolar septal fibrosis (total score of 4 or higher) have uncoated fiber counts of less than 100,000 per gram of dry lung tissue. As reported by Churg[69] and by Bellis et al.,[266] it takes considerably less

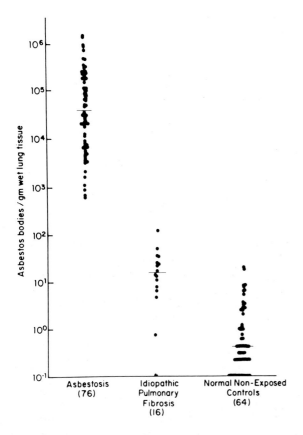

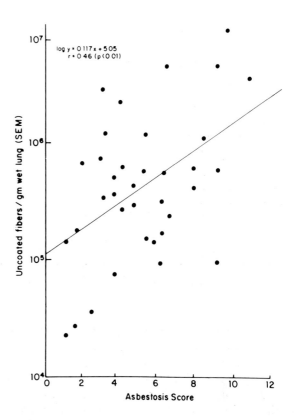

Fig. 28–55. Numbers of asbestos bodies in lung tissue in patients with asbestosis compared to patients with idiopathic pulmonary fibrosis and normal non-asbestos-exposed controls. (Reprinted with permission from Roggi VL. Asbestosis: A critical review. Adv Pathol 1989;2:31–60.)

Fig. 28–56. Correlation of asbestos score (asbestos grade × extent of disease), with concentration of uncoated fibers in lung tissue. (Reprinted with permission from Roggli VL. Asbestosis: A critical review. Adv Pathol 1989;2:31–60.)

asbestos to cause grade 1 asbestosis. Bellis et al.[266] found evidence of grade 1 asbestosis in some patients with fiber counts as low as 1,000 to 10,000/g of dry lung tissue, and in the 15 patients they reported with grade 1 asbestosis, 13 had fiber counts less than 100,000/g of dry lung tissue. Roggli[248] correlated the histologic grade of asbestosis with tissue asbestos content and other parameters (Table 28–11), and found only that the uncoated fibers (>5 μm long as determined by scanning electron microscopy) and the total fibers per gram of lung tissue (coated and uncoated) had the highest correlation coefficients, and were statistically significant. Asbestos bodies per gram of lung tissue, smoking history, age, and duration of exposure to asbestos had correlation coefficients between 0.26 and 0.06, and were not statistically significant.

Table 28–11. Correlation of histologic grade of asbestosis with tissue asbestos content and other parameters[a]

	Correlation coefficient (r)	p
Uncoated fibers/g (>5 μm) SEM	0.46	<.01
Total fibers/g (coated and uncoated), SEM	0.44	<.01
Asbestos bodies/g, LM	0.26	NS
Smoking history, pk-yr	0.22	NS
Age	0.12	NS
Duration of exposure, yr	0.06	NS

[a] SEM, scanning electron microscopy; LM, light microscopy; pk-yr, packs smoked daily × no. years smoked. NS, not significant. (Reprinted with permission from Roggli VL. Asbestosis: A critical review. Adv Pathol 1989;2:31–60.)

Pathogenesis of Asbestosis

The cellular and molecular basis of asbestosis has been recently reviewed by Rom et al.[267] As diagrammed by

these authors (Fig. 28–57), asbestos fibers are initially deposited in the region of the respiratory bronchioles and alveolar ducts. This is followed by a rapid accumulation in this area of pulmonary macrophages, which phagocytose the asbestos fibers. This causes activation of the macrophages that release certain cytoplasmic lysosomal enzymes and cytokines, resulting in an intense inflammatory response that eventually leads to fibrosis.[268–272] The alveolar macrophages produce a

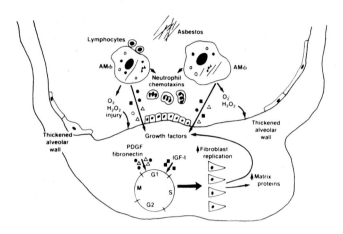

Fig. 28–57. Schematic diagram of pathogenesis of asbestosis. (Reprinted with permission from Rom WN, Travis WD, Brody AR. Cellular and molecular basis of asbestos-related diseases. Am Rev Respir Dis 1991;143:408–422.)

variety of substances, including fibroblast growth factor, that appear to stimulate fibroblasts to produce collagen, resulting in fibrosis.

With respect to the pathogenicity of asbestos in causing asbestosis, recent studies have suggested that the most important factor is the total surface area of the asbestos fibers, rather than their concentration in the lung tissue.[168,273]

In experimental animals such as sheep, whose pulmonary anatomy most closely resembles that of humans, the initial lesion caused by experimentally delivered asbestos involves the respiratory bronchioles and the alveolar ducts.[274] Bellis et al.[266] studied the minimal pathologic changes in the lungs of humans exposed to asbestos, and concluded that minimal bronchioalveolar fibrotic changes with concomitant asbestos bodies could be considered a mild pneumoconiotic lesion referred to as asbestosis grade 1, and that similar lesions referred to as "small airways lesions" in which no asbestos bodies were identified could also be regarded as an additional indicator of asbestos exposure, because the concentration of asbestos present in the lung tissue from these two groups was similar. It should also be mentioned that Harless et al.[275] reported relatively acute-onset obstructive airway disease in 17 of 23 construction workers after an intense 5-month exposure to chrysotile asbestos, and referred to a paper published by Jodoin et al.[276] that reported that asbestos could cause obstructive disease of small airways early after asbestos exposure. Harless et al.[275] reported that no possible cause other than asbestos could be identified in 6 of the men with described airway obstruction. That asbestos can cause larger airways disease, including cylindric bronchiectasis and fibrotic narrowing, was reported by Jacob et al.[277]

With respect to asbestos airways disease and parenchymal lung disease, one study suggested that the deposition of asbestos in the lung may be related to the length of the airway from the hilum to the periphery of the lung and to the degree of branching of the airways.[278] This theory has recently been challenged by Delfino et al.,[279] who studied 178 construction insulators and found no association of pleural abnormalities with airway geometry or length of the airways.

In many persons, asbestosis appears to be a progressive disease, even after removal from exposure to asbestos. Becklake[115] cited studies suggesting that autoimmune mechanisms may be responsible for the development of fibrosis in that there is a higher incidence of antinuclear antibodies in persons with asbestosis compared to the general population.

Asbestos/Asbestosis and Cigarette Smoking

A major problem in determining the exact relationship between cigarette smoke and asbestosis is that the vast majority of persons who have been occupationally exposed to asbestos and who have developed asbestosis have also been chronic cigarette smokers. Churg et al.[280] studied the effect of cigarette smoke on the retention of amosite fibers in the lungs of guinea pigs, and found that smoking caused a marked increase in the number of fibers found in macrophages in the lung, but did not appear to change the size of the fibers in the macrophage or the phagocytic capacity of the macrophages. Their data suggested that macrophage removal via the mucociliary escalator was decreased by cigarette smoke, and that macrophage mobility was impaired by cigarette smoke. McFadden et al.[281] found that cigarette smoke increased the penetration of UICC amosite asbestos fibers into airway walls in guinea pigs, resulting in an increased concentration of fibers in the interstitium.

Clinical studies evaluating the effect of cigarette smoke on the development of small opacities in chest radiographs of asbestos-exposed workers have recorded variable findings. These have been reviewed in the recently published reports by Barnhart et al.[282] and Blanc and Gamsu.[283] Barnhart et al.[282] concluded that the cumulative evidence supported that, in the setting of exposure to both asbestos and tobacco smoke, asbestos exposure and not cigarette smoke was the necessary risk factor for the development of roentgenographic small opacities. They also concluded that cigarette smoking appeared to add to the risk, particularly for lesser degrees of roentgenographic small opacities, and it was uncertain whether roentgenographic small opacities represented interstitial fibrosis. Blanc and Gamsu[283] found no correlation between high-resolution CT scan abnormalities and asbestosis and cigarette smoking. They concluded that high-resolution CT scan analysis of lung may be the best method for separating the radiographic abnormalities caused by asbestos and those caused by cigarette smoke. A somewhat different conclusion has been reached by Weiss[284] concerning cigarette smoking and small irregular opacities in the lungs. He concluded that the data in his study suggested that abnormalities observed in 181 workers not exposed to asbestos were directly related to age and smoking habits, among workers who were not exposed to any hazardous dusts. Weiss[285] had previously suggested that cigarette smoke may be responsible for the development of radiographically detected small irregular opacities in the lung, and has suggested that cigarette smoke caused pulmonary fibrosis.

Clinical Features of Asbestosis

The clinical feature of asbestosis depend on the severity of the disease. Those persons with pathologic grade 1–2 asbestosis may have no symptoms or radiographic abnormalities. Patients with grade 4 asbestosis (diffuse interstitial fibrosis with honeycombing) are usually symptomatic, with the most common symptom being dyspnea on exertion.[266,267] There is an increased incidence of clubbing of the fingers, although the diagnostic usefulness of this finding is minimal. Most patients with pathologic grade 4 asbestosis have basilar rales, frequently described as "velcro" rales. Pulmonary function tests show evidence of a restrictive lung disease with decrease in total lung capacity and forced vital capacity. Hypoxemia may be present at rest or may develop with exercise. The diffusing capacity is usually decreased. The American Thoracic Society proposed the following criteria for the clinical diagnosis of asbestosis:[287] (1) a reliable history of exposure to asbestos; (2) an appropriate latent interval between exposure and detection of disease; (3) chest roentgenographic evidence of type "s," "t," or "u" small, irregular opacifications of a profusion of 1:1 or greater; (4) a restrictive pattern of lung impairment with forced vital capacity below the lower limit of normal; (5) a diffusing capacity below the lower limit of normal; and (6) bilateral late or pan-inspiratory crackles at the posterior lung bases, not cleared by coughing.

In the report by Huuskonen[286] of 202 patients diagnosed as having asbestosis by the Institute of Occupational Health between 1934 and 1976, 88.7% had a symptom of breathlessness, 71.4% with persistent sputum production, crepitations in 58%, and finger clubbing in 32.3%. Of the 174 men registered as having asbestosis, 56 had died, whereas the expected number of deaths among men of the same age in the Finnish general population was 23.4. Of the 62 patients who had died before 1977, the cause of death was (1) asbestosis, 26 (41.9%); (2) lung cancer, 20 (32.2%); (3) other malignant diseases, 4 (6.5%); and (4) other causes, 12 (19.4%).

Approach to the Diagnosis, and Pathologic Differential Diagnosis

The pathologic criteria for diagnosing asbestosis have been previously reviewed. In general, the pathologic diagnosis is simply defined as the presence of fibrosis in association with asbestos bodies or fibers. The NIOSH-CAP Committee required the presence of two asbestos bodies in association with fibrosis. In our experience there are some cases of asbestosis in which asbestos bodies are not easily identified. In a situation in which there is a strong history of occupational history of exposure to asbestos in association with pulmonary fibrosis but no observable asbestos bodies in H and E-stained and iron-stained sections, one should attempt to perform asbestos fiber analysis on the tissue. Examples of asbestosis have been reported in which asbestos bodies have not been recognized in the lung tissue but in which asbestos fibers have been found in great enough concentrations to cause asbestosis.[38,39,288]

In the proper clinical context, specifically, the clinical features of asbestosis, analysis of bronchoalveolar lavage fluid can strongly suggest the diagnosis of asbestosis by containing an increased number of neutrophils and eosinophils in the fluid[289] (Fig. 28–58), and in some instances can be relatively specific by containing asbestos bodies (Fig. 28–59). Likewise, the identification of asbestos bodies in sputum (Fig. 28–60) or in transbronchial biopsy specimens (Fig. 28–61) can also strongly suggest the diagnosis, in the correct clinical setting.

The primary pathologic differential diagnosis of asbestosis is idiopathic pulmonary fibrosis. This differential diagnosis occurs in cases in which there is a history of exposure to asbestos, but in which the lung tissue sections show no asbestos bodies. As just indicated, one must always be aware of the cases in which bodies are present in lung tissue in low concentrations, but in which there is a significantly elevated fiber concentration; as already discussed, asbestosis correlates best with the total content of uncoated asbestos fibers. Gaensler et al.[290] reported on 176 asbestos-exposed persons in which lung tissue was available for analysis, and identified 9 cases in which the clinical features were consistent with asbestosis, but the histologic sections did not show asbestos bodies and there was no evidence of increased numbers of asbestos fibers. They concluded: (1) the American Thoracic Society criterion of "a reliable history of exposure" is sometimes difficult to define; (2)

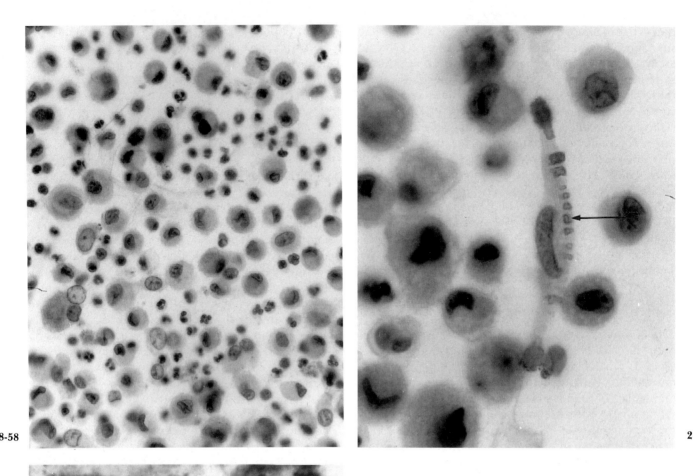

28-58

28-5

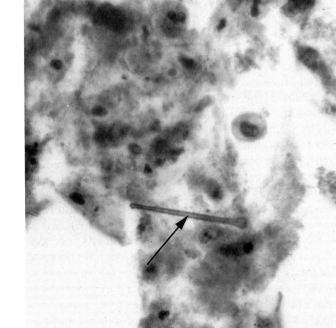

28-60

Fig. 28–58. Representative region of cytocentrifuge preparation of bronchoalveolar lavage fluid from a patient with clinical features of asbestosis. Note increased numbers of polys. ×550.

Fig. 28–59. Cellular component of bronchoalveolar lavage fluid shown in Fig. 28–58 also contained several asbestos bodies. One is shown within macrophage (*arrow*). ×1000.

Fig. 28–60. Cytologic preparation of sputum from patient with clinical features of asbestosis shows ferruginous body (*arrow*) consistent with asbestos body. ×550.

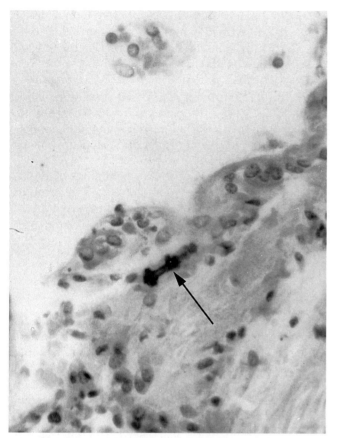

Fig. 28–61. Transbronchial biopsy specimen from patient with clinical features of asbestosis shows ferruginous body (*arrow*) consistent with an asbestos body. ×550.

asbestos bodies are seen in tissue sections only when exposure has been reasonably high, and given the proper clinical setting, the presence of diffuse fibrosis and asbestos bodies in tissue sections are sensitive and specific criteria for the diagnosis of asbestosis; and (3) the prevalence here of 5.1% non-asbestos-induced interstitial lung disease among asbestos-exposed persons is artefactually high because of atypical case selection. They further concluded that because asbestosis was a disappearing disease, cases of "idiopathic" pulmonary fibrosis in persons with a history of asbestos exposure will increase. Roggli[291] came to a somewhat similar conclusion in his study of 24 cases of diffuse pulmonary fibrosis of unknown cause. He found that patients with advanced pulmonary fibrosis whose tissue samples did not meet histologic criteria for asbestosis usually did not have asbestos-induced fibrosis. However, as discussed by Roggli,[291] there was concern whether cases #23 and #24 in his series represented idiopathic pulmonary fibrosis or asbestosis. In case #23 the asbestos mineral fiber content was below the 95% confidence limit for diffuse (grade 9 total score) asbestosis, although was well within the range of milder asbestosis, which may

have been obscured by superimposed radiation-associated fibrosis. Case #24 concerned an 85-year-old man who developed fatal pulmonary fibrosis 20 years after retirement from his occupation as a brakeline grinder. In that case, uncoated fiber content was low, although asbestos body content by light microscopy and scanning electron microscopy was within the range expected in cases of asbestosis. Monso et al.[292] evaluated 25 patients diagnosed as having idiopathic pulmonary fibrosis by standard examination, and in two cases found a high number of asbestos fibers (>100 fibers per scanning electron microscopy field) and concluded that standard pathologic techniques overdiagnosed idiopathic pulmonary fibrosis in a few cases in which asbestos bodies were not found with the optical microscope.

Persons who are occupationally exposed to asbestos are sometimes exposed to other dusts that can cause pulmonary fibrosis. These dusts include silica, talc, and welding fumes, all of which may cause fibrosis. In some instances the pattern of fibrosis, for example, silicosis, allows for the easy differentiation from asbestosis. Also, one can identify "pseudoasbestos" bodies in some lung tissue sections, which would suggest a nonasbestos cause for the fibrosis.

Localized and Unusual Pulmonary Diseases in Persons Occupationally Exposed to Asbestos

Organizing Pneumonia–Bronchiolitis Obliterans Type Change

Although asbestos is usually not thought of as producing localized parenchymal masses, Hillerdal and Hemmingson[293] reported 10 patients with localized visceral pleural fibrosis and fibrosis of the underlying lung parenchyma that caused a pseudotumor. Lynch et al.[294] identified 16 localized masses (9 intraparenchymal, 7 subpleural) in 260 asbestos-exposed individuals that were evaluated radiographically. A case reported as a clinicopathologic correlation in the *New England Journal of Medicine* in 1961 suggested that asbestos could cause a localized bronchiolitis obliterans—organizing pneumonia-like pulmonary lesion.[295] In that case, a 61-year-old man developed a localized consolidation in his left-upper lobe that histologically showed changes of an organizing pneumonia in which numerous asbestos bodies were identified. A secondary infection was suggested in that case, although was never proven. Saldana[296] in 1981 described 4 men whose chest radiograph showed localized infiltrates in the absence of diffuse changes. These masses exhibited the histologic changes of bronchiolitis obliterans with the presence of

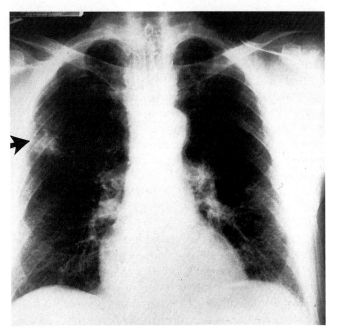

Fig. 28–62. Chest radiograph shows nodular mass in right-upper lobe that was interpreted radiographically as likely representing primary lung neoplasm (*arrow*).

asbestos bodies within the organizing masses of granulation-like tissue occluding the bronchi, obstructive pneumonia in which there were a large number of histiocytes and confluent giant cell graulomata, a lymphocytic angiitis and dense lymphoplasmacytic cellular infiltrate, and varying degrees of organizing pneumonia and fibrosis. Because he could find no other etiology for these changes, Saldana referred to them as localized asbestos pneumonia. Roggli[248] reported observing organizing pneumonia in several asbestos-exposed patients who underwent thoracotomy for suspected malignancy. Spencer[297] also described an organizing pneumonia as a primary pathologic feature of asbestosis. We[298] recently reported 4 cases of an organizing pneumonia with focal bronchiolitis obliterans in patients occupationally exposed to asbestos who had significantly elevated concentrations of asbestos in their lung tissue, and in which no other obvious cause was identified.

Keith et al.,[299] in studying asbestos in rats using intratracheally injected UICC Canadian chrysotile-B asbestos, observed alveolar and interstitial edema at 1, 3, and 6 months after treatment and found bronchiolitis obliterans in 33%–45% of the bronchioles examined.

In the cases of organizing pneumonitis that we reported,[298] patients usually were asymptomatic and presented with nodular masses identified radiographically (Fig. 28–62). Histologically the masses showed the pathologic features of bronchiolitis obliterans–organiz-

ing pneumonia. Nodular masses of moderately cellular, somewhat loose myxomatous granulation tissue filled the alveolar spaces and bronchioles (Fig.28–63) and were associated with frequent ferruginous bodies consistent with asbestos bodies (Fig. 28–64). In one case, a fairly distinct nodule was composed predominantly of edema fluid and proteinaceous material within the alveolar spaces, in association with many inflammatory cells, and showed foci of organization (Fig. 28–65). We wondered if the changes in this case may have represented the early phase of the bronchiolitis obliterans–organizing pneumonia. We also observed other nodular masses composed of randomly dispersed dense fibrous tissue with varying numbers of inflammatory cells and relatively frequent asbestos bodies (Fig. 28–66).

Desquamative Interstitial Pneumonitis-Like Change

Corrin and Price[300] reported a case of desquamative interstitial pneumonitis in a 53-year-old man who had smoked 10 cigarettes a day until 1 year before his illness. Asbestos bodies were associated with the intraalveolar macrophages. Freed et al.[301] reported a caseof desquamative interstitial pneumonitis in a man with a 32-year history of working in the drywall construction trade and a 3-pack/day cigarette-smoking history. A single asbestos body was identified in the frozen section of the lung tissue specimen, and asbestos digestion analysis showed 4666 asbestos bodies per gram of wet lung tissue, 819×10^6 chrysotile fibers per gram of dry lung tissue, and 20×10^6 tremolite fibers per gram of dry lung tissue. In our study,[298] we observed one patient who had a desquamative interstitial pneumonitis-like pathologic picture in which asbestos bodies were easily identified in the tissue, specifically in the macrophages that filled the alveolar spaces (Fig.28–67).

The exact significance of the desquamative interstitial pneumonitis-like pattern is uncertain, although in the case we described, it was localized. One has to be cautious in overinterpreting the DIP-like pattern, because desquamative interstitial pneumonitis is almost exclusively associated with cigarette smoking.

Aspergillus Infection in Asbestos-Exposed Individuals

Hillerdal and Hecksher[302] reported *Aspergillus* infection "in the lungs of four asbestos-exposed persons," two of whom reportedly had localized lung masses. Another case of an aspergilloma in association with asbestosis was reported, and the authors suggested that asbestos could cause cylindric bronchiectasis and fi-

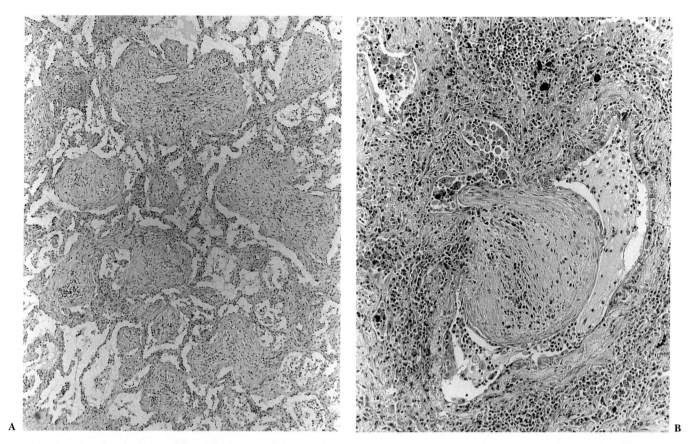

Fig. 28–63 A,B. Histologically, nodular mass seen in Fig. 28–62 shows organizing pneumonitis–bronchiolitis obliterans characterized by inflammation and fibrosis in distal airways. **A,** ×125; **B,** ×330.

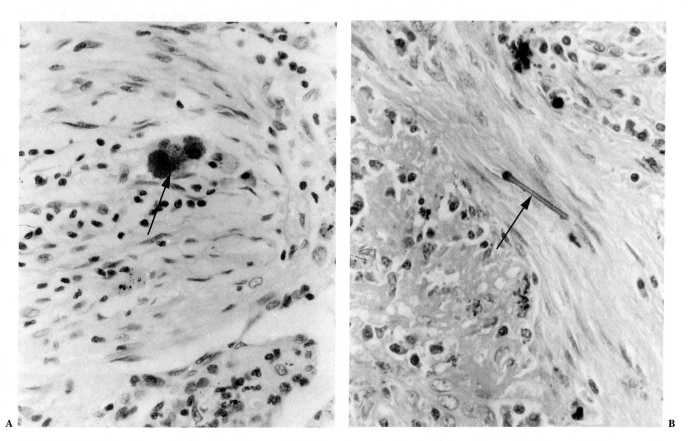

Fig. 28–64 A,B. Heavily coated (**B**) and lightly coated (**A**) ferruginous bodies (*arrows*) consistent with asbestos bodies present in organizing connective tissue. **A,B,** ×550.

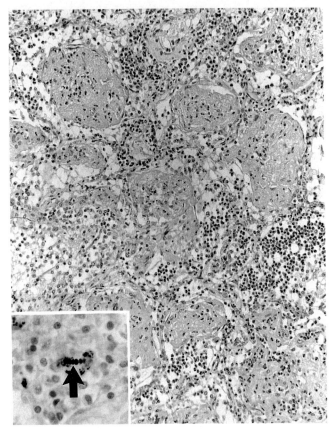

Fig. 28–65. Nodular mass was composed predominantly of edema fluid and active inflammatory cells, but showed regions of organization. Asbestos bodies were easily identified in this tissue (inset: *arrow*). ×330; inset, ×550.

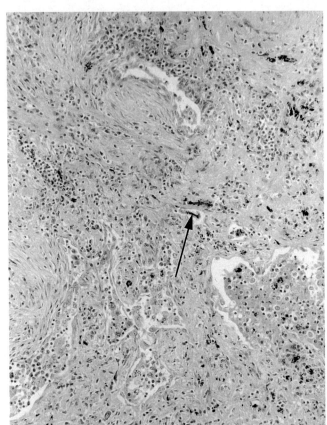

28-66A

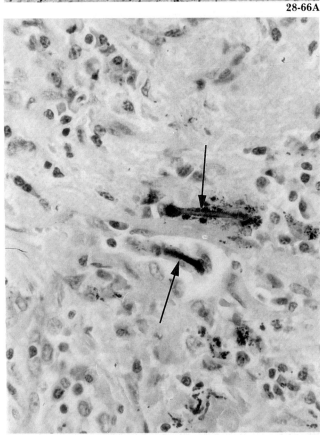

▷

Fig. 28–66 A,B. Nodular mass composed of dense disorganized connective tissue with scattering of inflammatory cells. Ferruginous bodies consistent with asbestos bodies (*arrow*) are easily identified in tissue. **A,** ×125; **B,** ×550.

28-66B

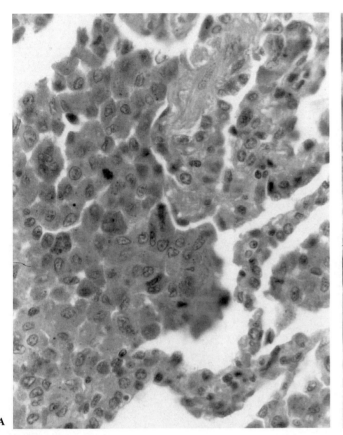
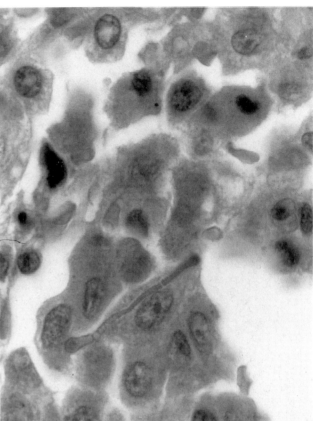

Fig. 28–67 A,B. Representative region of right-upper lobe mass shows desquamative-type infiltrate of macrophages. Ferruginous body consistent with asbestos body is noted in cytoplasm of macrophage. **A,** ×300; **B,** ×550.

brotic narrowing of the bronchi.[303] Hillerdal and Hecksher[302] suggested that asbestos can potentially lead to immune dysfunction and perhaps result in the opportunistic infection with *Aspergillus* fungal organisms. Roggli et al.[304] also mentioned five cases in which *Aspergillus* was identified in the lungs of persons occupationally exposed to asbestos.

In our study[298] of eight patients with localized masses, we found one in which there was a focal area of *Aspergillus* infection (Fig. 28–68) in association with a relatively localized nodular area of fibrosis (Fig. 28–69) in which ferruginous bodies were common. This patient had worked at the Puget Sound Naval Shipyard (Washington State) and had a history of occupational exposure to asbestos. In our case there was no evidence of allergic bronchopulmonary aspergillosis, and the patient was not asthmatic. We recently observed two additional cases of focal aspergillosis in association with asbestos-induced pulmonary fibrosis (unreported observations).

Granulomatous Inflammatory Changes

As previously illustrated, histiocytic giant cells containing asbestos bodies or fibers are not infrequently seen in

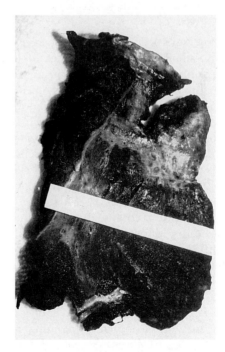

Fig. 28–68. In left-upper lobe was relatively well-demarcated region of nodular fibrosis. Radiographically area was thought to most likely represent neoplasm.

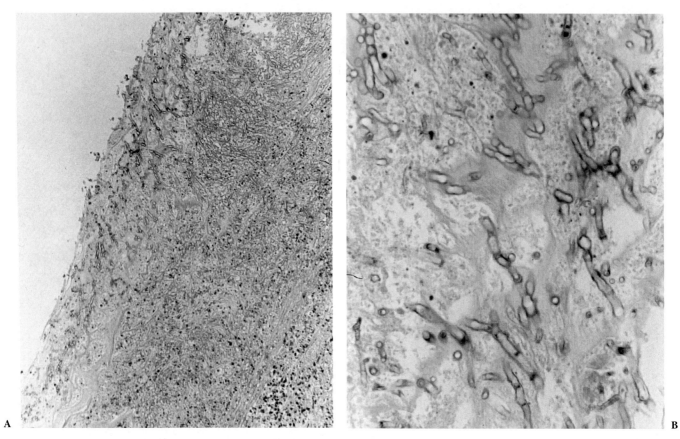

A   B

Fig. 28–69 A,B. Nodule shown in Fig. 28–68 was composed mostly of dense fibrous tissue that showed focal necrosis with Aspergillus organisms. ×550.

the lungs of persons occupationally exposed to asbestos. Occasionally, small nodular aggregates of histiocytes resembling nonnecrotizing granulomata are seen in the lungs of persons exposed to asbestos. In one of the cases we reported,[298] fairly striking granulomatous inflammation was localized in the lung, in which one could identify asbestos bodies in the giant cells forming some of the granulomata (Fig. 28–70). The patient in whom we observed these changes had a history of rheumatoid arthritis, although had a negative rheumatoid factor and had no clinical or laboratory evidence of sarcoidosis. With respect to granulomatous inflammation induced by asbestos, Monseur et al.[305] reported a granulomatous inflammatory reaction in the urinary bladder of a patient who had worked in an asbestos factory and in whom asbestos fibers were identified in tissue. De Vuyst et al.[306] reported granulomatous inflammation in the lung of a 32-year-old chemist who had worked for 8 years in a dusty environment containing aluminum powders. His report indicated that the pathologic changes observed in the lung biopsy of that patient were similar to those of berylliosis and sarcoidosis, but demonstrated that the patient had neither of those diseases.

We have reviewed pathology material from two patients who developed granulomatous inflammation proven by open lung biopsies and who had been occupationally exposed to aluminum dust. These observations suggest that asbestos, aluminum dust, and beryllium can cause a granulomatous inflammatory reaction in the lung that can be confused with sarcoidosis or an infectious process.

Lymphocytic Interstitial Pneumonitis

Rom and Travis[307] reported a lymphocyte-macrophage alveolitis in the open lung biopsy specimens from two nonsmoking patients who had been occupationally exposed to asbestos. The pathologic changes reported by Rom and Travis, in our opinion, are similar to those seen in hypersensitivity pneumonitis, although there is no proof that asbestos induces a hypersensitivity reaction. In our report,[298] we described a patient who was occupationally exposed to asbestos and who had high concentrations of asbestos fibers in his lung tissue and who developed a similar type of diffuse lymphoid interstitial infiltrate (Fig. 28–71). In that case, the patient

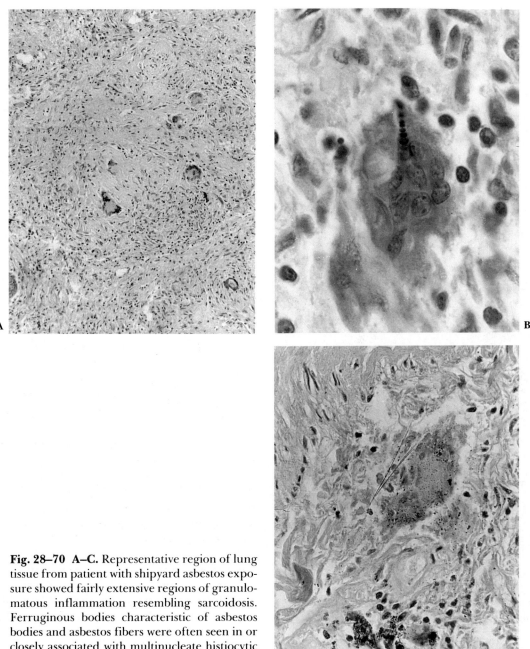

Fig. 28–70 A–C. Representative region of lung tissue from patient with shipyard asbestos exposure showed fairly extensive regions of granulomatous inflammation resembling sarcoidosis. Ferruginous bodies characteristic of asbestos bodies and asbestos fibers were often seen in or closely associated with multinucleate histiocytic giant cells. **A,** ×330; **B,** ×550; **C,** ×550.

developed what was described radiographically as diffuse interstitial fibrosis consistent with grade 4 asbestosis.

The mechanism by which asbestos causes these localized or unusual reactions is unclear, although with the numerous reports in the literature that asbestos can activate lymphocytes and macrophages, and cause the release of various cytokines and lymphokines, it is perhaps not surprising that localized or unusual inflammatory or fibrotic processes occur in areas of the lung in which asbestos is concentrated.

Asbestos and Lung Cancer

The potential association of asbestos and lung cancer can be traced to publications beginning in the mid-1930s.[308] Wood and Gloyne[309] reported 2 cases of carcinoma of the lung identified at autopsy in 43 cases of asbestosis. Gloyne[310] in 1935 reported two women, one aged 35 years and one aged 71 years, with asbestosis of moderate severity who developed squamous cell carcinoma of the lung. In the 35-year-old woman, the neoplasm developed in the base of the right-upper lobe

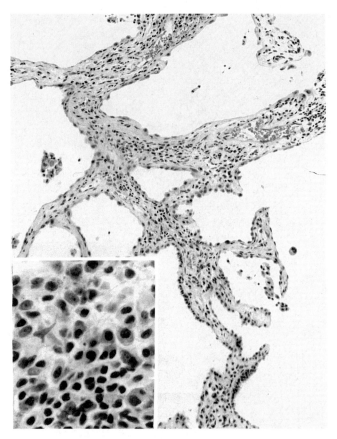

Fig. 28–71. Lung tissue shows diffuse mild thickening of alveolar septa with interstitial infiltrate of lymphocytes and plasma cells. Morphology of inflammatory cells is better seen in inset. ×125; inset, ×550.

and was centered around a small bronchus. In the 71-year-old woman, the neoplasm developed in the right-lower lobe. There was no evidence of metastases in either case. Asbestos bodies and fibers were described in the fibrotic lung tissue. In the discussion and summary of this paper, Gloyne remarked that: "The asbestosis, though fairly advanced, was not sufficiently advanced to cause death. The neoplasms also were small and had involved no vital parts (a small meningeal hemorrhage having terminated life in the first case). Indeed, compared with squamous carcinoma of the lung in general, as it reaches the postmortem room, the growths were unusually small. A tentative suggestion may be made that in asbestosis, a small tumor turns the scale, just as bronchitis with early bronchopneumonia will do, probably as a result of toxemia." Gloyne noted a similar occurrence in a case of oat cell carcinoma in association with asbestosis.

In 1936, Egbert and Geiger[311] reported a case of an acinar type of adenocarcinoma arising from the mainstem bronchus to the left-lower lobe in a 41-year-old Hungarian factory man who was found at autopsy to have extensive pleural adhesions with obliteration of the pleural cavities by fibrous adhesions, and diffuse pulmonary asbestosis. The tumor metastasized to tracheobronchial lymph nodes, periaortic lymph nodes, the right adrenal gland, the left external oblique abdominal muscle, and to the bones of the pelvis, vertebrae, and skull. Egbert and Geiger[311] cited a publication concerning asbestosis by Gloyne, who described a case of pulmonary asbestosis with carcinoma of the pleura, which we would interpret to possibly be a description of either pseudomesotheliomatous carcinoma or mesothelioma. Egbert and Geiger[311] reported that the relationship between exposure to irritating dusts and malignancies of the lung had aroused a great deal of interest, because various statistics showed that there was an increased incidence of pulmonary cancer in patients so exposed. They cited the publication by Hruby and Sweany,[312] who analyzed the incidence of cancer in the lungs of persons exposed to dust, and concluded that there had been an approximately 10-fold increase in the number of cases coming to autopsy in the last 40 years and a twofold increase that had occurred in the last 10 years; the report by Klotz and Simpson,[313] which indicated that lung cancer was frequent in other forms of pneumoconiosis; and the report by Obendorfer[314] of an increased incidence of lung cancer in tin miners in Schneeberg who came to autopsy. Egbert and Geiger[311] concluded that the irritating effects of inhaled asbestos particles may have been the significant factor in the development of the primary lung cancer that developed in the patient they described.

Lynch and Smith,[315] in the United States, reported one case, and Nordmann[316] in Germany reported two cases, of lung cancer in patients with asbestosis and suggested a cause-and-effect relationship. The association between lung cancer and asbestosis was accepted rapidly in Germany, in part on the basis of an experimental study in white mice that developed pulmonary cancers after the inhalation of asbestos dust.[317]

The association between lung cancer and asbestosis was further strengthened by Wedler[318] from Germany, who reviewed public records from several countries and found 14 cases of malignant neoplasms of the lung and pleura in 92 postmortem examinations (16%). This was found to be in excess of the proportion of lung cancers that occurred in a general autopsy population, which was between 2% and 6%. Wedler found that carcinoma as a complication of asbestosis was observed most frequently in males between ages 35 and 41 years of age, and was seen most frequently in the portion of the lung that was affected with asbestosis. The latent period in these cases was between 12 and 42 years, and there was often a long interval between cessation of exposure to asbestos and the development of cancer. Wedler suggested that the increased frequency of lung cancer in persons with asbestosis resulted from the mechanical and probable chemical reactions to asbestos, which caused proliferation of lung tissue, including epithelial desquamation and cell modification, macrophage response, giant foreign-body cell formation, and epithelial metaplasia of bronchial mucus membrane. Wedler concluded that development of cancer was attributed to metaplasia of the bronchial mucus membrane and the accompanying inflammatory reaction. He further concluded that cancer of the lung and asbestosis was a disease legally justified for insurance claims. In Wedler's report,[318] the exposure time ranged from 3 to 27 years (average, 15 years), and the ages in the 14 cases were 35–75 years (average, 50 years).

Merewether's[319] report in 1947 further suggested an association between asbestos exposure and lung cancer. In the Annual Report of the Chief Inspector of Factories in England in 1947, he reported that 235 deaths occurred between 1924 and 1946 that were either caused by asbestosis or occurred in persons in whom asbestosis was proven at autopsy. In these 235 cases, there were 31 (13.2%) recorded cases of carcinoma of the lungs or pleura. Of this group of 235, 22 of 128 male deaths (17.2%) were caused by carcinoma of the lung and pleura, and 9 of 107 female deaths (8.4%) were caused by cancer of the lung and pleura. The cases of asbestosis developing carcinoma of the lung/pleura had a mean exposure to asbestos of 16.5 years, compared to 13.4 years for those dying only of asbestosis and without cancer. Merewether's report[319] was significant because lung cancer among the adults examined at necropsy in England at that time was about 4%, and the male:female sex ratio in the general population was 5:1, whereas the ratio in persons exposed to asbestos who developed lung cancer was 2.4:1. The data in Merewether's report strongly suggested a causal association between asbestos, asbestosis, and lung cancer.

Enterline[320] published a provocative editorial in 1978 entitled "Asbestos and Cancer: The International Lag." This editorial contains many references concerning asbestos and lung cancer, but many conclusions reached by Enterline have been debated and challenged.[321–329]

The first epidemiologic study evaluating the association of lung cancer in asbestos workers was published by Doll in 1955.[330] He studied 113 men who had worked for at least 20 years in places where they were likely to be exposed to asbestos. They were followed, and the mortality among them was compared with that which would have been expected on the basis of mortality experienced for the entire male population. Thirty-nine deaths occurred in the group, whereas only 15.4 were expected. The excess deaths were from lung cancer (11

occurring, 0.8 expected) and from other respiratory diseases as well as cardiovascular diseases (22 observed, 7.6 expected). Doll concluded that lung cancer was a specific industrial hazard in asbestos workers, and that the average risk among men employed for 20 or more years was of the order of 10-fold that experienced in the general population.

In 1980, McDonald[331] published another epidemiologic study involving 17 cohorts, 1 of which represented the Doll[330] cohort. Many different occupations were represented in the various cohorts, and all revealed an increased proportion of deaths from lung cancer. Acheson and Gardner[332] came to a similar conclusion in their report published in 1979. The data presented in a conference held in New York City in 1964[333] left little doubt that asbestos was causally related to lung cancer.

Pathogenesis of Asbestos-Related Lung Cancer

Although some studies initially suggested that asbestos was only a tumor promoter,[334,335] more recent studies have, in our opinion, proven conclusively that asbestos is a complete carcinogen and is able to act both as a tumor initiator and a tumor promoter.[336–340] Asbestos can induce chromosomal changes consisting of aneuploidy, deletions, translocations, and other changes in a variety of different mammalian cells.[341–344] Asbestos was first regarded as a carcinogen in 1982.[345]

Walker et al.[346] recently reviewed the possible cellular and molecular mechanisms involved in asbestos carcinogenicity. Their hypothesis is shown in Fig. 28–72. Their excellent review discusses many of the basic mechanisms concerning the causation of lung cancer by asbestos, and also indicates where uncertainties exist.

The association between cigarette smoke and asbestos in causing lung cancer has been evaluated in several epidemiologic studies. Sadly, the majority of persons occupationally exposed to asbestos have also been cigarette smokers, and in many series, the number of persons in the asbestos-exposed, non-cigarette-smoking group has been few. Nevertheless, the majority of these studies have suggested a multiplicative synergistic interaction between cigarette smoke and asbestos. The study by Selikoff et al.[347] has been cited most often; it showed an approximately 5-fold increase in the incidence of lung cancer in asbestos-exposed persons compared to nonsmoking, non-asbestos-exposed workers, and an approximately 61-fold increase in the incidence of lung cancers in persons who were both cigarette smokers and occupationally exposed to asbestos.

Saracci[348] studied the interactions of tobacco smoking and other agents in the etiology of cancer. He listed 13 studies evaluating this subject, and came to the conclusion that in 10, there was evidence of multiplica-

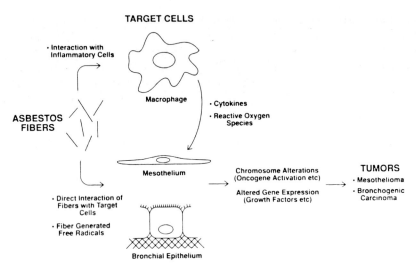

Fig. 28–72. Possible mechanism by which asbestos may cause cancer. (Reproduced by permission from Walker et al.[346])

tive synergism between cigarette smoke and asbestos in causing lung cancer (Table 28-12). The exact mechanism by which cigarette smoke interacts with asbestos is not known, although one theory is that carcinogens present in cigarette smoke are carried into cells by being attached to asbestos fibers. As previously stated in this chapter, studies by Churg and colleagues[280] demonstrated that cigarette smoke inhibits the clearance of asbestos, and also may have an effect on macrophages.

The relationship between lung cancer and asbestosis has been the subject of controversy. There is no doubt that there is a high incidence of lung cancer in persons with asbestosis.[349–356] Hughes and Weill[357] recently reviewed the issues of asbestosis and lung cancer, and published a prospective mortality study of 839 men employed in the manufacture of asbestos cement products since 1969. They stated that 20 or more years after hire, no excess lung cancer was found among workers without radiographically detectable lung fibrosis, even among long-term workers, nor was there a trend in risk by level of cumulative exposure to asbestos among such workers. By contrast, however, employees with small opacities (greater than 1/0 profusion according to I.L.O. classification) experienced a significantly raised risk of lung cancer, even though their exposures to asbestos were similar to the exposures of long-term workers without the small opacities in their chest radiographs. They concluded that asbestos was a lung carcinogen because of its ability to cause lung asbestosis, and that the practice of attributing lung cancer to exposure to asbestos should be done only if asbestosis was present. Browne,[358] in an editorial published in 1986, came to a similar conclusion. However, Warnock and Isenberg[250] came to a different conclusion in their study of 75 men with lung cancer, all but 8 of whom had some history of exposure to asbestos. They performed analytical determinations of the concentration of amosite and crocidolite in the lungs of the subjects, and divided them into three groups: low (less than 10^5), intermediate (10^5–10^6) and high (greater than 10^6) fibers of amosite and/or crocidolite per gram of dry lung tissue. Of 62 men evaluated, 0 of 14 in the low group, 7 of 29 in the intermediate group, and 5 of 19 in the high group had asbestosis. Thus, their study showed a marked variation in the presence of asbestosis in persons with the same concentrations of asbestos fibers in their lung tissue which, as previously stated,[248] has been shown to be the factor that best correlated with the presence of asbestosis. Warnock and Isenburg[250] concluded that the subjects in their intermediate- and high-concentration groups may have been at increased risk for cancer, even when they did not have asbestosis, and because large burdens of asbestos did not always cause pulmonary fibrosis, asbestosis may be a poor marker of asbestos fiber-caused lung cancer.

Our thoughts concerning the association of asbestos and lung cancer are similar to those of Warnock and Isenberg.[250] We would like to add the observation that (as is discussed in the subsection **Morphology of Asbestos-Related Lung Cancer**) the types of lung cancer that develop in persons who are occupationally exposed to asbestos are the same as those that occur in the non-asbestos-exposed poplation. Thus, in the neighborhood of 40%–60% of all lung cancers occurring in asbestos-exposed persons will be squamous cell carcinomas and small cell undifferentiated carcinomas, most of which arise in the hilar region (central area) of the lung. While we understand and accept the idea that some peripheral adenocarcinomas occur in a background of pulmonary fibrosis such as idiopathic pulmonary fibrosis (see Chapters 20 and 32), we canot accept the hypothesis that asbestosis is necessarily important in the development of centrally located squamous cell carcinomas and oat cell carcinomas unless there is some growth factor induced by asbestos, or some other mechanism by which asbestosis causes the development of these neoplasms.

Table 28–12. Studies on the interaction of tobacco smoking with asbestos in lung cancer causation[a]

Author(s), reference no., design, years of observation, exposure investigated	Exposure assessment to		No. of		Relative risk for asbestos[c]		Interaction magnitude	
	Smoking	Asbestos	Lung cancer cases	Controls or expected cases	Smokers	Nonsmokers	Absolute	Relative (PERDI)[d]
Liddell et al.,[348a] case control within cohort, 1950–1975, chrysotile mining and milling	O, P	D	223	715	*1.67*	*2.97*	~A	<25
Baker,[348b] historical cohort, 1944–1981, crocidolite mining and milling	D, O	D	62	29[f]	*4.98*	0.71	>M	≥75
Selikoff et al.,[348c] historical cohort, 1961–1977, amosite factory	P	D	50	9.8	*4.69*	25	I	25–49
Acheson et al.,[348d] historical cohort, 1947–1980, amosite factory	D	D	23	14.5	1.57[e]	*2.00*	~M	25–49
Berry et al.,[348e] historical cohort, 1960–1970, mixed asbestos factory	D, O	D	27 males / 15 females	12.0 / 2.1	2.25[e] / 7.36[e]	/ 5.00	>M / >M	50–74 / ≥75
Berry et al.,[348f] cohort, 1971–1980, mixed asbestos factory	P	D	53 males / 13 females	26.0 / 2.58	2.01[e] / 4.27[e]	6.25 / 12.50	A / I	0 / <25
Selikoff and Hammond,[348g] cohort, 1963–1974, chrysotile and amosite in insulation (New Jersey)	P	D	45	7.62	*6.0*	*0.0*	>M	≥75
Hammond et al.,[348h] cohort, 1967–1976, chrysotile and amosite in insulation (U.S. and Canada)	P	D	272	51.7	5.25	*5.71*	M	50–75
Blot et al.,[348i] case-control, 1970–1976, shipyard exposures	R, O	R, O	458	553	*1.61*	*1.28*	~M	<25
Blot et al.,[348j] case-control, 1972–1976, shipyard exposures	O	O	319	341	*1.57*	*1.88*	~M	25–49
Martischnig et al.,[348k] case-control, 1973–1974, any asbestos exposure	R	R	201	201	*3.19*	1.08	>M	≥75
Pastorino et al.,[348l] population case-control, 1976–1979, any asbestos exposure	R	R	204	211	*1.80*	*2.80*	I	25–49
Kjuus et al.,[348m] case control, 1979–1983, any asbestos exposure	R	R	176	176	*2.05*	*2.40*	~M	25–49

[a] Reprinted with permission from Saracci R. The interactions of tobacco smoking and other agents in cancer etiology. Epidemiol Rev 1987;9:175–193.

[b] Abbreviations used in this table: O, exposure information collected prospectively or retrospectively from informants other than the study subjects, for example, relatives; P, exposure information collected prospectively (i.e., before cancer occurrence) from study subjects; D, exposure information extracted from existing documents, e.g., medical records, company rolls, etc.; R, exposure information collected retrospectively from study subjects; A, additive; M, multiplicative; I, intermediate.

[c] Italicized numbers are estimates reconstructed from published data.

[d] PERDI, per cent of excess risk due to interaction.

[e] Excluding ex-smokers from both the category of smokers and that of nonsmokers.

[f] Lung cancers in control cohort.

In our opinion, a more logical conclusion is that asbestosis and lung cancer are dose-related diseases, and that each requires a significantly large burden of asbestos for causation. In both situations, it is probably the concentration of asbestos that is the most important factor, although not the only factor, in the development of these diseases.

Parietal Pleural Plaques and Lung Cancer

Because circumscribed parietal pleural plaques are considered a marker of asbestos exposure, although they do not necessarily indicate how much asbestos a person was exposed to, the potential association of hyaline pleural plaques and the development of lung cancer has arisen. Studies evaluating this relationship are summarized in Table 28–13.[207,359–365] In a study by Kiviluoto et al.,[359] 60 cases of neoplasm were noted among the plaque group and 53 cases among the controls. In the plaque group, there were 13 cases of lung cancer, and 14 cases occurred in the control group. The authors concluded that there was no association between pleural plaques and lung cancer. In a second study, they concluded that pleural plaques appeared to be linked to lung cancer only when accompanied by lung fibrosis. They reasoned that slight exposure to asbestos caused

Table 28–13. Studies evaluating association of lung cancer and hyaline pleural plaques

Reference	Number of persons with plaque	Number of persons in control group	Number of lung cancers in plaque group	Number of lung cancers in control group	Conclusion of study
Kivilvoto et al.[359]	700	700	13	14	No increased incidence of lung cancer in persons with plaques
Edge[360]	359	339	19	4	Approximately two times increased incidence of lung cancer in persons with plaques.
Mollo et al.[362]	199 men, 22 women	566 men, 310 women	Men and women combined, 14	Men and women combined, 26	Increased relative risk of 1.5 for lung cancer in men with pleural plaques.
Wain et al.[207]	25 (men)	409	4	55	No increased incidence of lung cancer in persons with plaques. Significant increase in risk for laryngeal cancer in persons with plaques.
Harber et al.[363]	Not given	Not given	×13	Not given	No association between pleural plaques and asbestos-associated malignancies that were independent of other causative factors such as duration of asbestos exposure, age, and cigarette smoking.
Hillerdal[364]	Not given	Not given	43	21	Increased incidence of lung cancer in persons with pleural plaques.
Partanen et al.[365]	604	604	28	25	Relative risk of 1.1 for lung cancer in persons with pleural plaques. Results inconclusive due to potential bias.

plaques, while heavy exposure led to plaques and fibrosis, for which there was a higher incidence of lung cancer. Edge[360] evaluated 429 men from the Barrow Shipyard workforce of 7000 men who had pleural plaques. A group of 429 men from the neighboring city of Carlisle, where there was no industrial exposure to asbestos, was used as the control group. It was not possible for Edge to obtain information concerning cigarette smoking, although the causes of death from two other smoking-related diseases (ischemic heart disease and chronic bronchitis) were similar in the two groups. In the plaque group, there was an excess of 53 deaths, of which 19 were due to carcinoma of the lung, whereas only 4 cases of lung cancer were noted in the control group. Edge[360] also found that there were no mesotheliomas in the Carlisle group, whereas 23 occurred in the Barrow group. On rescrutinizing the records, Edge found that 6 of the 19 persons dying of lung cancer already had symptoms or suggestive radiographic findings at the time of entry into the series. He thus excluded these patients, resulting in 13 lung cancer deaths in the persons with plaques compared with 4 in the control group, a finding still having statistical significance ($p < .05$). Edge[360] concluded that men with pleural plaques carried an approximately twofold increased risk of dying of lung cancer compared with the general population.

Hillerdal[361] reported on 761 cases of bilateral plaques

(739 men, 22 women) which had been identified by radiographic screening by the end of 1978. Of the men, 519 of 739 (82.6%) had been exposed to asbestos (see Hillerdal's Table 2), and 52 of 109 men who denied exposure to asbestos had occupations in which asbestos exposure was expected. The latency period of development of plaques ranged from 3 to 57 years, with a mean value of 32.7 years. An increased incidence of lung cancer was found in those with pleural plaques, compared to the control group with no plaques.

Mollo et al.[362] studied the occurrence of neoplastic disease and the presence of pleural plaques in a series of 1097 autopsies performed in Turin, Italy, from the adult general population. In that autopsy series, 199 men and 22 women were found to have hyaline pleural plaques, whereas 566 men and 310 women did not have plaques. A total of 14 cases of lung cancer (4.36%) were noted in the subjects with plaques, and 26 lung cancers (2.96%) were noted in the subjects without plaques. There was an increased relative risk of 1.5 for the presence of lung cancer in the plaque group. Only laryngeal carcinoma had a significant increased relative risk for cancer in the plaque group, which was 8.79 for men. The authors graded the severity of the pleural plaques according to their total area, and found no relationship between the severity and the presence of cancer.

Wain et al.[207] evaluated 434 consecutive autopsies

Table 28–14. Lung cancer cell type in eight series of patients with asbestos exposure[a]

Reported patient series, N	Cell types, no. (%)			
	Squamous carcinoma	Small-cell carcinoma	Adenocarcinoma	Large-cell carcinoma[b]
Asbestos-exposed				
Hourihane and McCaughey,[369a] 26	7 (27)	5 (19)	12 (46)	2 (8)
Whitwell et al.,[369b] 93	21 (23)	26 (28)	33 (35)	13 (14)
Hasan et al.,[369c] 12	4 (33)	2 (16)	6 (50)	0 (0)
Kannerstein and Churg,[369d] 39	11 (30)	11 (30)	11 (30)	6 (10)
Martischnig et al.,[369e] 49	26 (53)	22 (45)	1 (2)	0 (0)
Finkelstein,[369f] 23	9 (39)	7 (30)	6 (26)	1 (4)
Blot (cited by Ives et al.),[369g] 361	24 (67)	7 (19)	5 (14)	0 (0)
Auerbach et al.,[369h] 193	96 (50)	48 (25)	29 (15)	20 (10)
Total, 471	198 (42)	128 (27)	103 (22)	42 (9)
Nonexposed				
Cox and Yesner (1958–1967), 617[c]	213 (35)	143 (23)	158 (26)	103 (17)
Cox and Yesner (1968–1977), 400	123 (31)	82 (21)	129 (32)	66 (17)

[a] Reprinted with permission from Churg A. Lung cancer cell type and asbestos exposure. JAMA 1985;253:2984–1985. Copyright 1985 by the American Medical Association.

[b] Reports that do not use large-cell carcinoma have had this category counted as zero.

[c] Based on death certificates.

performed during a 2.5-year period, and found pleural plaques in 25 cases, but no gross evidence of pulmonary parenchymal fibrosis. In the 25 men with pleural plaques, 4 (16%) cases of lung cancer were identified, and 3 cases (12%) of laryngeal carcinoma were found. Of the 409 men who did not have pleural plaques, there were 55 cases of lung cancer (13.6%) and 3 cases (0.7%) of laryngeal carcinoma. The authors concluded that there was no increased incidence of lung cancer in persons with plaques, but there was a significant increase in laryngeal cancer in persons with hyaline pleural plaques.

Harber et al.[363] evaluated 1500 asbestos-exposed workers for the detection of asbestos-associated disease between 1979 and 1983. Each patient was individually matched to a control of the same race, smoking status, hospital examination, age, duration of asbestos exposure, and pack-years of smoking. The radiographs from patients and controls were obtained and read by two radiologists independently who were familiar with the I.L.O. system and one of whom was a certified B reader. A total of 16 cases of asbestos-associated malignancy were identified, of which 13 were lung cancer. The other 3 included carcinoma of the colon, carcinoma of the kidney, and carcinoma of the "throat." The authors found no significant association between pleural plaques and asbestos-associated malignancies that were independent of other causative factors, such as duration of asbestos exposure, age, and cigarette smoking. They concluded that if an asbestos worker were known to have significant asbestos exposure, it appeared unwise to deny them appropriate examinations that they might not otherwise receive simply because parietal pleural plaques were not detected.

Hillerdal,[364] in a follow-up of his previous study,[54]

evaluated 1596 asbestos-exposed men with pleural plaques for a total of 14,910 man-years, and observed 425 deaths. Forty-three lung cancers and 9 mesotheliomas occurred in the cohort, while only 21 and 1, respectively, were expected. Hillerdal concluded that the presence of pleural plaques was an indication of sufficient exposure to asbestos to increase the risk of lung cancer.

Partanen et al.[365] evaluated 7986 residents of three Finnish communities in 1979. The subjects ranged between 20 and 74 years old, with a mean age of 60 years; 604 subjects (7.6%) had pleural plaques but no other asbestos-related radiographic abnormalities. The persons with plaques were matched with persons of the same age, sex, and community who did not have plaques, and were followed to determine the incidence of lung cancer between 1972 and 1989. The authors found an increased relative risk of lung cancer in the plaque group of only 1.1, but concluded that the risk ratio estimate may be biased, and that the results were therefore inconclusive in predicting the assessment of lung cancer risk among carriers of pleural plaques.

Type and Morphology of Lung Cancer Associated with Asbestos Exposure

While several reports have suggested that adenocarcinoma is the most common type of lung cancer occurring in persons occupationally exposed to asbestos,[366–368] Churg[369] tabulated the incidence of the four major types of lung cancer in patients exposed to asbestos, to various control groups. As shown in Tables 28–14 and 28-15, only the study by Whitwell et al.[368] showed a preponderance of adenocarcinomas; the other studies showed no significant difference between the types of

Table 28–15. Lung cancer cell type in reports with asbestos-exposed workers and internal controls[a]

Reported series, N	Cell type, no. (%)			
	Squamous carcinoma	Small-cell carcinoma	Adenocarcinoma	Large-cell carcinoma*
Kannerstein and Churg[369d]				
Exposed, 39	11 (28)	11 (28)	11 (28)	6 (15)
Control, 43	12 (28)	14 (33)	9 (21)	8 (19)
Whitwell et al.[369b]				
Exposed, 93	21 (23)	26 (28)	33 (35)	13 (14)
Control, 96	17 (18)	38 (40)	29 (30)	12 (13)
Martischnig et al.[369e]				
Exposed, 49	26 (53)	22 (45)	1 (2)	9 (0)
Control, 112	77 (69)	27 (24)	8 (7)	0 (0)
Auerbach et al.[369h]				
Exposed, 193	96 (50)	48 (25)	29 (15)	20 (10)
Control, 648	335 (52)	102 (16)	122 (19)	89 (14)
Blot (cited by Ives et al.[369g])[c]				
Exposed, 36	24 (67)	7 (19)	5 (14)	0 (0)
Control, 161	103 (64)	27 (17)	31 (19)	0 (0)
Total				
Exposed, 410	178 (43)	114 (28)	79 (19)	39 (10)
Control, 1,060	544 (51)	208 (20)	199 (19)	109 (10)

[a] Reprinted with permission from Churg A. Lung cancer type and asbestos exposure. JAMA 1985;253:2984–2985.

[b] Reports that do not use large-cell carcinoma have had this category counted as zero.

[c] Based on death certificates.

lung cancers occurring in the asbestos-exposed group of individuals and the nonexposed group of individuals. The combined data showed that 43% of the total 410 tumors occurring in the asbestos group were squamous carcinomas, 28% small cell carcinomas, 19% adenocarcinomas, and 10% large cell undifferentiated carcinomas.

Several studies have suggested that asbestos-related lung cancers occur more commonly in the lower lobes than upper lobes,[370–373] while nonasbestos lung cancers have been reported to occur most frequently in the upper lobe.[374–377] With respect to the lobe of origin in the attribution of a lung cancer to asbestos, Weiss[378] concluded that the lobar site of origin of a lung carcinoma (upper lobe: cigarette-smoke-associated lung cancer; lower lobe: asbestos-associated lung cancer) was another factor that may help in the estimate of attribution, in addition to such other variables as the degree and duration of exposure to asbestos, the interval from onset of exposure to asbestos to disease, and the type of work done. Weiss[378] failed to cite the 1984 publication by Auerbach et al.,[379] who evaluated the histologic types and location of lung cancer in 855 patients (747 men, 107 women) from three hospitals of whom 196 had asbestos exposure. In the cases with asbestos exposure, the lung cancer was present in the upper lobes in 61.6% of cases, in the middle lobe in 1.9%, in the lower lobes in 32.1%, and multicentric in 4.4%. This observation is in contradiction to what Weiss[378] suggested. It is our experience that lung cancers causally related to asbestos are not predominant in the lower lobes. With respect to

concentration of asbestos, Dodson et al.[50] and Churg et al.[252] have found concentrations of asbestos as great in the upper lobes as in the lower lobes in persons occupationally exposed. If lung cancer is related to the carcinogenic effect of asbestos, a hypothesis we believe, then one would expect to find just as many cancers in the upper lobes as in the lower lobes. The Auerbach study[379] found a predominance of squamous carcinoma in persons exposed to asbestos (49%), which was no different than that found in persons who were not exposed to asbestos (50.8%). Auerbach et al.[379] did find an increased incidence of small cell undifferentiated carcinomas (24.5%) in the asbestos-exposed group compared to the non-asbestos-exposed group (15.5%). The percentages of adenocarcinomas were approximately the same in the two groups (14.8% in the asbestos-exposed group, 18.4% in the non-asbestos-exposed group), as were the number of large cell undifferentiated carcinomas (10.2% in the asbestos-exposed group, 13.5% in the non-asbestos-exposed group).

Figure 28-73 shows an 8-cm-diameter greyish-white tumor mass in the lower portion of the left-upper lobe. Histologically this tumor was a moderately well-differentiated squamous cell carcinoma (Fig. 28–74). The left- and right-lower lobes showed macroscopic honeycombing (Fig. 28–75), and histologically there was grade 3–4 asbestosis (Fig. 28–76). Asbestos digestion analysis showed greater than 100,000 asbestos bodies per gram of wet lung tissue. In a case such as this, there would be no dispute the asbestos was a causative factor in the development of the lung neoplasm.

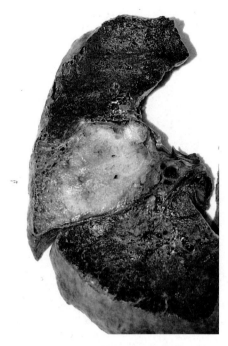

Fig. 28–73. Slice of left lung from asbestos insulator worker shows 8-cm-diameter, greyish-white lung neoplasm in lower portion of left-upper lobe. Note visceral pleural fibrosis.

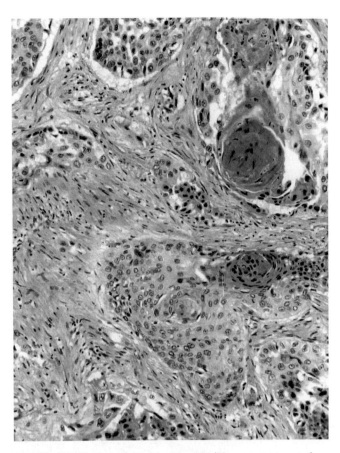

Fig. 28–74. Tumor shown in Fig. 28–73 represents moderately well-differentiated squamous cell carcinoma. ×300.

As one would expect, there are no histopathological features of a lung neoplasm that allow one to state with certainty that it is causally related to asbestos. However, in some cases one can find asbestos bodies intimately associated with the tumor (Fig. 28–77), and in such instances, we have found that the person will usually have a concentration of asbestos in their lung at least 3000 asbestos bodies per gram of wet lung tissue or greater, a concentration of asbestos more than enough to potentially cause asbestosis.

Pseudomesotheliomatous Lung Cancer

Mention should be made of a special form of lung cancer that we believe is related to occupational exposure to asbestos. This neoplasm is referred to as pseudomesotheliomatous carcinoma or adenocarcinoma, and was probably first described in 1940 by Babolini and Blasi[380] as a primary lung cancer of the pleura. Babolini and Blasi cited reports of similar tumors observed in Italy.[381–383] In 1976, Harwood et al.[384] described 6 cases of such a neoplasm, all of which were adenocarcinomas, and they referred to the

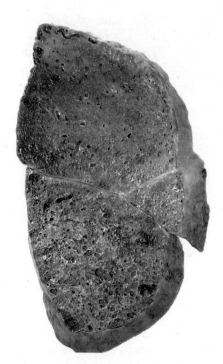

Fig. 28–75. Slice of right lung from asbestos insulator worker whose lung tumor is seen in Fig. 28–73 shows interstitial fibrosis with honeycombing that appears most severe in right-lower lobe but also involves right- and left-lower lobes.

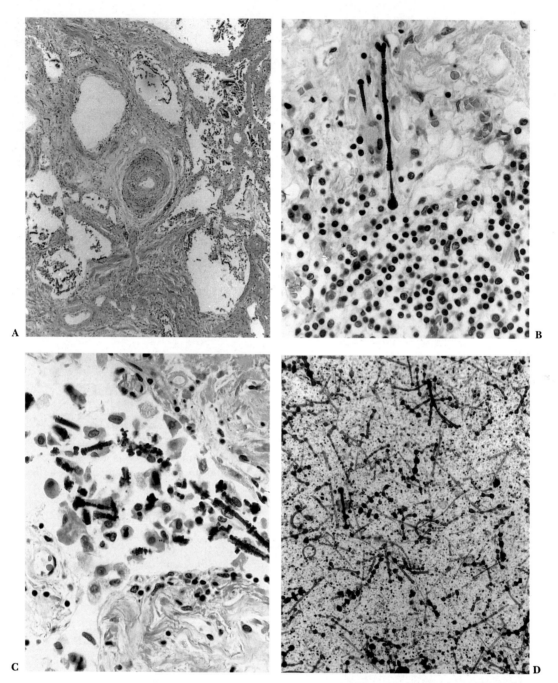

Fig. 28–76 A–D. Section of right- and left-lower lobes shows grade 4 asbestosis with numerous ferruginous bodies consistent with asbestos bodies. Asbestos filter preparation **(D)** was saturated with asbestos bodies of concentration greater than 100,000/g of wet lung tissue. **A,** ×125; **B,C,** ×500; **D,** x125.

neoplasm as pseudomesotheliomatous carcinomas. Their concept, to which we ascribe, was that these were peripheral lung neoplasms that for reasons unknown invaded into the pleural and grew like a mesothelioma. In 1992, Koss et al.[385] published a series of 30 cases of pseudomesotheliomatous carcinoma (15 from their own files and 15 from published literature), and found that 17% were associated with possible or definite asbes-

tos exposure. In the previously reported examples of this neoplasm,[384,386–391] 3 were reported to be associated with asbestos exposure. Subsequently, we[392] reported 27 cases of pseudomesotheliomatous lung carcinoma. An occupational history was available in 17 cases, of which 16 had a history of exposure to asbestos, and in 8 of 11, there was mineralogic evidence of increased concentrations of asbestos bodies in lung tissue. The

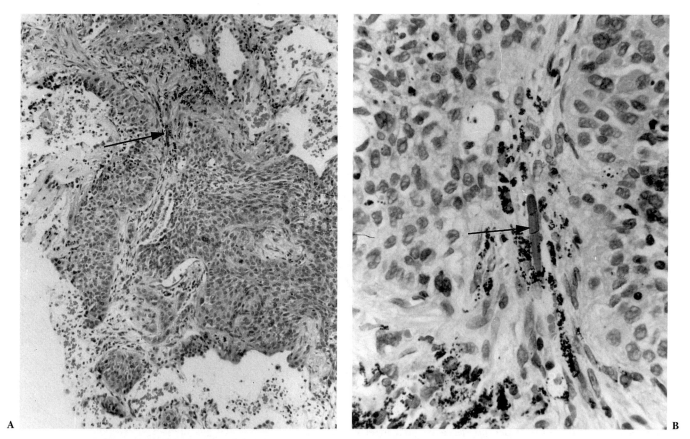

Fig. 28–77 A,B. Poorly differentiated squamous cell carcinoma from occupationally exposed individual contains asbestos body (*arrows*) closely associated with neoplastic cells. **A,** ×125; **B,** ×500.

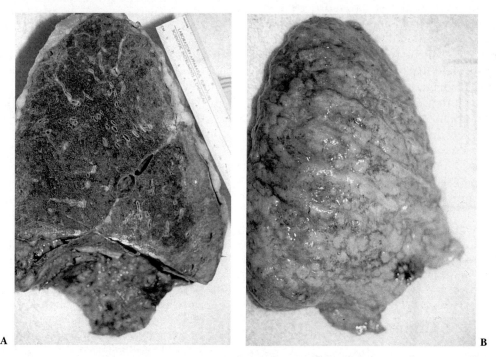

Fig. 28–78 A,B. Macroscopic appearance of pseudomesotheliomatous carcinoma. These neoplasms grow like mesotheliomas and encase the lung.

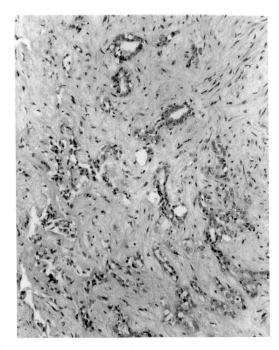

Fig. 28–79. Most frequent histologic type of pseudomesotheliomatous carcinoma is adenocarcinoma, which we refer to as tubular-desmoplastic adenocarcinoma. ×300.

existence of pseudomesotheliomatous lung cancer perhaps should have been expected, because Merewether's[319] and Wedler's[318] reports referred to tumors of the pleura, although it was not clear whether these were lung cancers or mesotheliomas. Kannerstein and Churg[339] also noted that there was more frequent severe pleural involvement by lung neoplasms occurring in those who were exposed to asbestos.

The morphology of pseudomesotheliomatous carcinomas is dramatic, and macroscopically are essentially indistinguishable from mesotheliomas. They encase the lung (Fig. 28–78), often in an irregular manner, and grow into the chest wall. At autopsy the lung and tumor are usually extremely difficult to remove from the chest cavity, just like a mesothelioma. Histopathologically, most are adenocarcinomas and most have a tubular desmoplastic type of histologic appearance (Fig. 28–79). A few have histologic features of squamous carcinoma, adenocarcinoma, large cell undifferentiated carcinoma, and small cell undifferentiated carcinoma. These neoplasms can be proven to be lung cancer rather than mesothelioma by a combination of histochemical, immunohistochemical and electron microscopic techniques.

Summary

This chapter has reviewed many basic biological features of asbestos, the morphogenesis and characteristics of asbestos and non-asbestos ferruginous bodies, and the pulmonary diseases caused by asbestos. Mesothelioma, which was not discussed in this chapter, is described in detail in Chapter 34. As we hope has been pointed out in this chapter, much is left to be learned concerning the basic properties of asbestos and the mechanisms by which asbestos causes pleuropulmonary disease.

References

1. Webster's medical dictionary. Springfield: Merriam-Webster, 1986:51.
2. Weill H, Abraham JL, Balmes JR, et al. Health effects of tremolite. Am Rev Respir Dis 1990;142:1453–1458.
3. Occupational exposure to asbestos, tremolite, anthophyllite and actinolite: Final rule. Department of Labor. Fed Reg 1992;57(110):24310–24331.
4. Henderson DW, Shilkin KB, Whitaker D. Introduction and historical aspects, with comments on mesothelioma registries. In: Henderson DW, Shilkin KB, Langlois SL, Whitaker D, eds. Malignant mesothelioma. New York: Hemisphere, 1992:1–22.
5. Pooley FD. Asbestos mineralogy. In: Antman K, Aisner J, eds. Asbestos-related malignancy. Orlando: Grune & Stratton, 1987:3–27.
6. Teta MJ, Lewinsohn HC, Meigs JW, Vidone RA, Mowad LZ, Flannery JT. Mesothelioma in Connecticut, 1955–1977. J Occup Med 1983;25:749–756.
7. Marchand F. Uber eigentumliche pigmentkristalle in den lungen. Verh Dtsch Ges Pathol 1906;17:223–228.
8. Cooke WE. Asbestos dust and the curious bodies found in pulmonary asbestosis. Br Med J 1929;2:578–580.
9. Gloyne SR. The formation of the asbestos body in the lung. Tubercle 1931;12:399–401.
10. Craighead JE, Abraham JL, Churg A, et al. Asbestos-associated diseases. Arch Pathol Lab Med 1982;106:542–596.
11. Barclay WR, Craighead JE, Cugell DW, et al. A physician's guide to asbestos-related diseases. JAMA 1984;252:2593–2597.
12. Gross P, deTreville RTP, Cralley LJ, Davis JMG. Pulmonary ferruginous bodies. Arch Pathol 1968;85:539–546.
13. Gross P, Tuma J, deTreville RTP. Unusual ferruginous bodies. Arch Environ Health 1971;22:534–537.
14. Timbrell V. The inhalation of fibrous dusts. Ann NY Acad Sci 1965;132:255–273.
15. Dodson RF, Williams MG, Hurst GA. Acute lung response to amosite asbestos: A morphological study. Environ Res 1983;32:80–90.
16. Davis JMG. Further observations on the ultrastructure and chemistry of the formation of asbestos bodies. Exp Mol Pathol 1970;13:346–358.
17. Suzuki Y. Interaction of asbestos with alveolar cells. Environ Health Perspect 1974;9:241–252.
18. Brody AR, Hill LH, Adkins B, O'Connor RW. Chrysotile asbestos inhalation in rats: Deposition pat-

tern and reaction of alveolar epithelium and pulmonary macrophages. Am Rev Respir Dis 1981;123:670–679.

19. Davis JMG. Electron microscope studies of asbestosis in man and animals. Ann NY Acad Sci 1965;132:98–111.

20. Suzuki Y, Churg J. Structure and development of the asbestos body. Am J Pathol 1969;55:79–107.

21. Pooley FD. Asbestos bodies, their formation, composition and character. Environ Res 1972;5:363–379.

22. Botham SK, Holt PF. The mechanism of formation of asbestos bodies. J Pathol Bacteriol 1968;96:443–453.

23. Davis JMG. The ultrastructure of asbestos bodies from human lung. Br J Exp Pathol 1964;45:642.

24. Holt PF, Mills J, Young DK. Experimental asbestosis in the guinea pig. J Pathol Bacteriol 1966;92:185–195.

25. Davis JMG. The ultra structure of asbestos from guinea pig lungs. Br J Exp Pathol 1964;45:634.

26. Godwin MC, Jagatic JJ. Asbestos and mesotheliomas. Environ Res 1970;3:391–416.

27. Holmes A, Morgan A, Davison W. Formation of pseudo-asbestos bodies on sized glass fibres in the hamster lung. Ann Occup Hyg 1983;27:301–313.

28. Churg A, Warnock ML. Analysis of the cores of ferruginous (asbestos) bodies from the general population. III. Patients with environmental exposure. Lab Invest 1979;40:622–626.

29. Churg A, Warnock ML. Analysis of the cores of ferruginous (asbestos) bodies from the general population. I. Patients with and without lung cancer. Lab Invest 1977;37:280–286.

30. Churg A, Warnock ML. Asbestos and other ferruginous bodies. Am J Pathol 1981;102:447–456.

31. Langer AM, Rubin IB, Selikoff IJ. Chemical characterization of asbestos body cores by electron microprobe analysis. J Histochem Cytochem 1972;20:723–734.

32. Gross P, deTreville RTP. Pulmonary ferruginous bodies in city dwellers. Arch Environ Health 1969;19:186–188.

33. Churg A, Warnock ML. Analysis of the cores of asbestos bodies from members of the general population: Patients with probable low-degree exposure to asbestos. Am Rev Respir Dis 1979;120:781–786.

34. Dodson RF, O'Sullivan MF, Williams MG, Hurst GA. Analysis of cores of ferruginous bodies from former asbestos workers. Environ Res 1982;28:171–178.

35. Warnock ML, Isenberg W. Asbestos burden and the pathology of lung cancer. Chest 1986;89:20–26.

36. Holden J, Churg A. Asbestos bodies and the diagnosis of asbestosis in chrysotile workers. Environ Res 1986;39:232–236.

37. Roggli VL, Pratt PC. Numbers of asbestos bodies on iron-stained tissue sections in relation to asbestos body counts in lung tissue digests. Hum Pathol 1983;14:355–361.

38. Warnock ML, Wolery G. Asbestos bodies or fibers and the diagnosis of asbestosis. Environ Res 1987;44:29–44.

39. Dodson RF, Williams MG, O'Sullivan MF, Corn CJ, Greenberg SD, Hurst GA. A comparison of the ferrug-inous body and uncoated fiber content in the lungs of former asbestos workers. Am Rev Respir Dis 1985;132:143–147.

40. Churg A, Warnock ML, Green N. Analysis of the cores of ferruginous (asbestos) bodies from the general population. Lab Invest 1979;40:31–38.

41. Mueller PK, Stanley RL. Asbestos fiber atlas. Washington, DC: U.S. Environmental Protection Agency, 1975:9–19.

42. Hendry NW. The geology occurrences and major uses of asbestos: In: Boland B, ed. Annals of the New York Academy of Sciences. 132d ed. New York: New York Academy of Sciences, 1965:12.

43. Clifton RA. Asbestos. In: Bureau of Mines, ed. Bureau of Mines mineral yearbook. Washington, DC: U.S. Department of the Interior, 1973:1–5.

44. Wagner JC. The significance of asbestos in tissue. Recent Results Cancer Res 1972;39:37–46.

45. Dodson RF, Williams MG, Hurst GA. Method for removing the ferruginous coating from asbestos bodies. J Toxicol Environ Health 1983;11:959–966.

46. Telischi M, Rubenstone AI. Pulmonary asbestosis. Arch Pathol 1961;72:116–125.

47. Langer AM. Inorganic particles in human tissues and their association with neoplastic disease. Environ Health Perspect 1974;9:229–233.

48. Auerbach O, Conston AS, Garfinkel L, Parks VR, Kaslow HD, Hammond EC. Presence of asbestos bodies in organs other than the lung. Chest 1980;77:133–137.

49. Keal EE. Asbestosis and abdominal neoplasms. Lancet 1960;ii:1211–1216.

50. Dodson RF, Williams MG, Corn CJ, Brollo A, Bianchi C. Asbestos content of lung tissue, lymph nodes and pleural plaques from former shipyard workers. Am Rev Respir Dis 1990;142:843–847.

51. Roggli VL, Benning TL. Asbestos bodies in pulmonary hilar lymph nodes. Mod Pathol 1990;3:513–517.

52. Szendroi M, Nemeth L, Vajta G. Asbestos bodies in a bile duct cancer after occupational exposure. Environ Res 1983;30:270–280.

53. Rosen P, Gordon P, Savino A, Melamed M. Ferruginous bodies in benign fibrous plural plaques. Am J Clin Pathol 1973;60:608–617.

54. Kobayashi H, Ming ZW, Watanabe H, Ohnishi Y. A quantitative study on the distribution of asbestos bodies in extrapulmonary organs. Acta Pathol Jpn 1987;37:375–383.

55. Kanazawa K, Birbeck MSC, Carter RL, Roe FJC. Migration of asbestos fibres from subcutaneous injection sites in mice. Br J Cancer 1970;24:96–106.

56. Koerten HK, de Bruijn JD, Daems WT. The formation of asbestos bodies by mouse peritoneal macrophages. Am J Pathol 1990;137:121–134.

57. Cook PM, Glass GE, Tucker JH. Asbestiform amphibole minerals: Detection and measurement of high concentrations in municipal water supplies. Science 1974;185:853–855.

58. Millette JR, Clark PJ, Stober J, Rosenthal M. Asbestos

in water supplies of the United States. Environ Health Perspect 1983;53:45–48.

59. Cotruvo JA. Asbestos in drinking water: A status report. Environ Health Perspect 1983;53:181–183.

60. Toft P, Meek ME. Asbestos in drinking water: A Canadian view. Environ Health Perspect 1983;53:177–180.

61. Biles B, Emerson TR. Examination of fibers in beer. Nature (London) 1968;219:93–94.

62. Gaudichet A, Bientz M, Sebastien P, et al. Asbestos fibers in wines: relation to filtration process. J Toxicol Environ Health 1978;4:853–860.

63. Selikoff IJ, Lee DHK. Historical background. In: Lee DHK, Hewson EW, Okun D, eds. Asbestos and disease. New York: Academic Press, 1978:3–8.

64. Churg A. The diagnosis of asbestosis. Hum Pathol 1989;20:97–99.

65. Williams E. "Curious bodies" found in the lungs of coal-workers. Lancet 1934;ii:541–542.

66. Masse S, Begin R, Cantin A. Pathology of silicon carbide pneumoconiosis. Mod Pathol 1988;1:104–108.

67. Dodson RF, O'Sullivan MF, Corn C, Williams MG, Hurst GA. Ferruginous body formation on a nonasbestos mineral. Arch Pathol Lab Med 1985;109:849–852.

68. Churg A, Wiggs B. Mineral particles, mineral fibers, and lung cancer. Environ Res 1985;37:364–372.

69. Churg A. Asbestos fiber content of the lungs in patients with and without asbestos airways disease. Am Rev Respir Dis 1983;127:470–473.

70. Dodson RF, Williams MG, Corn CJ, Brollo A, Bianchi C. Non-asbestos fibre burden in individuals exposed to asbestos. In: Brown RC, Hoskins JA, Johnson NF, eds. Mechanisms in fibre carcinogenesis. New York: Plenum, 1991:29–37.

71. Omenn GS, Merchant J, Boatman E, et al. Contribution of environmental fibers to respiratory cancer. Environ Health Perspect 1986;70:51–56.

72. Langer AM. Chrysotile asbestos in the lungs of persons in New York City. Arch Environ Health 1971;22:348–361.

73. Langer AM, Pooley FD. Identification of single asbestos fibres in human tissues. In: Biological effects of asbestos. Lyon: International Agency for Research on Cancer, 1973:119–125.

74. Dodson RF, Williams MG, Corn CJ, Brollo A, Bianchi C. A comparison of asbestos burden in lung parenchyma, lymph nodes, and plaques. Ann NY Acad Sci 1991;643:53–60.

75. Champness PE, Cliff G, Lorimer GW. The identification of asbestos. J Microsc 1976;108:231–249.

76. Millette JR, Twyman JD, Hansen EC, Clark PJ, Pansing MF. Chrysotile, palygorskite, and halloysite in drinking water. Scand Electron Microsc 1979;1:579–586.

77. Berkley C, Churg J, Selikoff IJ, Smith WE: The detection and localization of mineral fibers in tissue. In: Boland B, Hitchcock J, Kates S, eds. Biological effects of asbestos. 132d, New York: New York Academy of Sciences, 1965:48–63.

78. Carter RE, Taylor WF. Identification of a particular amphibole asbestos fiber in tissue of persons exposed to a high oral intake of the mineral. Environ Res 1980;24:85–93.

79. Pooley FD. Electron microscope characteristics of inhaled chrysotile asbestos fibers. Br J Ind Med 1972;29:146–153.

80. Chatfield EJ. Preparation and analysis of particulate samples by electron microscopy, with special reference to asbestos. Scanning Electron Microsc 1979;1:563–578.

81. Chatfield EJ, Dillon MJ. Some aspects of specimen preparation and limitations of precision in particulate analysis by SEM and TEM. Scanning Electron Microsc 1978;1:487–496.

82. Ashcroft T, Heppleston AG. The optical and electron microscopic determination of pulmonary asbestos fiber concentration and its relation to the human pathological reaction. J Clin Pathol 1973;26:224–234.

83. Churg A, Warnock ML. Asbestos fiber in the general population. Am Rev Respir Dis 1980;122:669–678.

84. Stasny JT, Husach C, Albright FR, Schumacher DV, Sweigart DW, Boyer K. Development of methods to isolate asbestos from spiked beverages and foods for SEM characterization. Scanning Electron Microsc 1979;1:587–595.

85. Sundius N, Bygden A. Isolation of the mineral dust in lungs and sputum. J Ind Hyg Toxicol 1938;20:351–359.

86. Vallyathan V, Green FHY. The role of analytical techniques in the diagnosis of asbestos-associated disease. CRC Crit Rev Clin Lab Sci 1985;22:1–42.

87. Gylseth B, Baunan RH, Bruun R. Analysis of inorganic fibre concentrations in biological samples by scanning electron microscopy. Scand J Work Environ Health 1981;7:101–108.

88. Gylseth B, Baunan RH. Topographic and size distribution of asbestos bodies in exposed human lungs. Scand J Work Environ Health 1981;7:190–195.

89. O'Sullivan MF, Corn CJ, Dodson RF. Comparative efficiency of Nuclepore filters of various pore sizes as used in digestion studies of tissue. Environ Res 1987;43:97–103.

90. Gloyne SR. The presence of the asbestos fibre in the lesions of asbestos workers. Tubercle 1929;10:404–407.

91. Sebastien P, Masse R, Bignon J. Recovery of ingested asbestos fibers from the gastrointestinal lymph in rats. Environ Res 1980;22:201–216.

92. Williams MG, Dodson RF, Corn C, Hurst GA. A procedure for the isolation of amosite asbestos and ferruginous bodies from lung tissue and sputum. J Toxicol Environ Health 1982;10:627–638.

93. Gross P, Detreville RT. The lung as an embattled domain against inanimate pollutants. Am Rev Respir Dis 1972;106:684–691.

94. Evans JC, Evans RJ, Holmes A, et al. Studies on the deposition of inhaled fibrous material in the respiratory tract of the rat and its subsequent clearance using radioactive tracer techniques. Environ Res 1973;6:180–201.

95. Pinkerton KE, Pratt PC, Brody AR, Crapo JD. Fiber

localization and its relationship to lung reaction in rats after chronic inhalation of chrysotile asbestos. Am J Pathol 1984;117:484–498.

96. Coin PG, Roggli VL, Brody AR. Deposition, clearance, and translocation of chrysotile asbestos from peripheral and central regions of the rat lung. Environ Res 1992;58:97–116.

97. Lauweryns JM, Baert JH. Alveolar clearance and the role of the pulmonary lymphatics. Am Rev Respir Dis 1977;115:625–683.

98. Spencer H. The anatomy of the lung. In: Pathology of the lung. 4th Ed. Oxford: Pergamon, 1985:417.

99. McMillan CH, Jones AD, Vincent JH, Johnston AM, Douglas AN, Cowie H. Accumulation of mixed mineral dusts in the lungs of rats during chronic inhalation exposure. Environ Res 1989;48:218–237.

100. Fishman AP. Pulmonary diseases and disorders. New York: McGraw-Hill, 1980:638.

101. Viallat JR, Raybuad F, Passarel M, Boutin C. Pleural migration of chrysotile fibers after intratracheal injection in rats. Arch Environ Health 1986;41:282–286.

102. Hallenbeck WH, Patel-Mandlik KJ. Presence of fibers in the urine of a baboon gavaged with chrysotile asbestos. Environ Res 1979;20:335–340.

103. Cook PM, Olson GF. Ingested mineral fibers: Elimination in human urine. Science 1979;204:195–198.

104. Haque AK, Mancuso MG, Williams MG, Dodson RF. Asbestos in organs and placenta of five stillborn infants suggests transplacental transfer. Environ Res 1992;58:163–175.

105. Dement JM. Overview: Workshop of fiber toxicology research needs. Environ Health Perspect 1990;88:261–268.

106. U.S. Environmental Protection Agency. Asbestos-containing materials in schools. Fed Reg 1991;40 CFR 763, Subpt. E, App. A, p. 494.

107. Morgan A, Holmes A. The distribution and characteristics of asbestos fibers in the lungs of Finnish anthophyllite mine-workers. Environ Res 1984;33:62–75.

107a. Case BW, Sebastien P, McDonald JC. Lung fiber analysis in accident victims: A biological assessment of general environmental exposures. Arch Environ Health 1988;43:178–179.

107b. Warnock ML, Wolery G. Asbestos bodies or fibers and the diagnosis of asbestosis. Environ Res 1987;44:29–44.

108. Dodson RF, O'Sullivan MF, Corn CJ. Technique dependent variations in asbestos burden as illustrated in a case of nonoccupational exposed mesothelioma. Am J Ind Med 1993;24:235–240.

109. Roggli VL, Pratt PC, Brody AR. Asbestos content of lung tissue in asbestos-associated diseases. A study of 110 cases. Br J Ind Med 1986;43:18–28.

110. Churg A. Fiber counting and analysis in the diagnosis of asbestos-related disease. Hum Pathol 1982;13:381–392.

111. Churg A, Wiggs B, Depaoli L, Kampe B, Stevens B. Lung asbestos content in chrysotile workers with mesothelioma. Am Rev Respir Dis 1984;130:1042–1045.

112. McDonald AD, McDonald JC, Pooley FD. Mineral fibre content of lung in mesothelial tumours in North America. Ann Occup Hyg 1982;26:417–422.

113. Breedin PH, Buss DH. Ferruginous (asbestos) bodies in the lungs of rural dwellers, urban dwellers and patients with pulmonary neoplasms. South Med J 1976;69:401–404.

114. Dodson RF, Greenberg SD, Williams MG, Corn CJ, O'Sullivan MF, Hurst GA. Asbestos content in lungs of occupationally and nonoccupationally exposed individuals. JAMA 1984;252:68–71.

115. Becklane MR. Asbestos-related diseases of the lung and other organs: Their epidemiology and implications for clinical practice. Am Rev Respir Dis 1976;114:187–227.

116. Hillerdal G. The pathogenesis of pleural plaques and pulmonary asbestosis: Possibilities and impossibilities. Eur J Respir Dis 1980;61:129–138.

117. Churg A, Green FHY. Pathology of occupational lung disease. New York: Igaku-Shoin, 1988:213–277.

118. Churg A. Nonasbestos pulmonary mineral fibers in the general population. Environ Res 1983;31:189–200.

119. Fulmer JD. Bronchoalveolar lavage. Am Rev Respir Dis 1982;126:961–962.

120. Crystal RG, Reynolds HY, Kalica AR. Bronchoalveolar lavage. The report of an international conference. Chest 1986;90:122–131.

121. Springmeyer SC. The clinical use of bronchoalveolar lavage. Chest 1987;92:771–772.

122. Craighead JE, Mossman BT. The pathogenesis of asbestos-associated diseases. N Engl J Med 1982;306:1446–1455.

123. De Vuyst P, Dumortier P, Leophonte P, Vande Weyer R, Yernault JC. Mineralogical analysis of bronchoalveolar lavage in talc pneumoconiosis. Eur J Respir Dis 1987;70:150–156.

124. De Vuyst P, Dumortier P, Moulin E, et al., Asbestos bodies in bronchoalveolar lavage reflect lung asbestos body concentration. Eur Respir J 1988;1:362–367.

125. De Vuyst P, Dumortier P, Moulin E, Yourassowsky N, Yernault JC. Diagnostic value of asbestos bodies in bronchoalveolar lavage fluid. Am Rev Respir Dis 1987;136:1219–1224.

126. De Vuyst P, Jedwab J, Dumortier P, Vandermoten G, Vande Weyer R, Yernault JC. Asbestos bodies in bronchoalveolar lavage. Am Rev Respir Dis 1982;126:972–976.

127. De Vuyst P, Mairesse M, Gaudichet A, Dumortier P, Jedwab J, Yernault JC. Mineralogical analysis of bronchoalveolar lavage fluid as an aid to diagnosis of "imported" pleural asbestosis. Thorax 1983;38:628–629.

128. Dodson RF, Garcia JGN, O'Sullivan M, et al. The usefulness of bronchoalveolar lavage in identifying past occupational exposure to asbestos: A light and electron microscopy study. Am J Ind Med 1991;19:619–628.

129. Stewart MJ, Haddow AC. Demonstration of the peculiar bodies of pulmonary asbestos in material obtained

by lung puncture and in the sputum. J Pathol Bacteriol 1929;32:1782.

130. McLarty JW, Greenberg SD, Hurst GA, et al. The clinical significance of ferruginous bodies in sputa. J Occup Med 1980;22:92–96.

131. Roggli VL, Greenberg SD, McLarty JW, et al. Comparison of sputa and lung asbestos body counts in former asbestos workers. Am Rev Respir Dis 1980;122:941.

132. Modin BE, Greenberg SD, Buffler PA, Lockhart JA, Seitzman LH, Awe RJ. Asbestos bodies in a general hospital/clinic population. Acta Cytol 1982;26:667–670.

133. Dodson RF, Williams MG, Corn CJ, Idell S, McLarty JW. Usefulness of combined light and electron microscopy evaluation of sputum samples for asbestos to determine past occupational exposure. Mod Pathol 1989;2:320–322.

134. Farley ML, Greenberg SD, Shuford EH, Hurst GA, Spivey CG, Christianson C. Ferruginous bodies in sputa of former asbestos workers. Acta Cytol 1977;21:693.

135. Churg A, Wood P. Observations on the distribution of asbestos fibers in human lungs. Environ Res 1983;31:374–380.

136. Churg A, Wiggs B. The distribution of amosite asbestos fibers in the lungs of workers with mesothelioma or carcinoma. Exp Lung Res 1989;15:771–783.

137. Dodson RF, Hurst GA, Williams MG, Corn CJ, Greenberg SD. Comparison of light and electron microscopy for defining occupational asbestos exposure in transbronchial lung biopsies. Chest 1988;94:366–370.

138. Pritchard JN. Dust overloading causes impairment of pulmonary clearance: Evidence from rats and humans. Exp Pathol 1989;37:39–42.

139. Cohen D, Arai SF, Brain JD. Smoking impairs long-term dust clearance from the lung. Science 1979;204:514–517.

140. McFadden D, Wright JL, Wiggins B, Churg A. Smoking inhibits asbestos clearance. Am Rev Respir Dis 1986;133:372–374.

141. McFadden D, Wright J, Wiggs B, Churg A. Cigarette smoke increases the penetration of asbestos fibers into airway walls. Am J Pathol 1986;123:95–99.

142. Stanton MF, Wrench C. Mechanisms of mesothelioma induction with asbestos and fibrous glass. J Natl Cancer Inst 1972;48:797–821.

143. Stanton MF, Layard M, Tegeris A, Miller E, May M, Kent E. Carcinogenicity of fibrous glass: Pleural response in the rat in relation to fiber dimension. J Natl Cancer Inst 1977;58:587–603.

144. Stanton MF, Layard M, Tegeris E, et al. Relation of particle dimension to carcinogenicity in amphibole asbestoses and other fibrous minerals. J Natl Cancer Inst 1981;67:965.

145. Selikoff IJ. Historical developments and perspectives in inorganic fiber toxicity in man. Environ Health Perspect 1990;88:269–276.

146. Wagner JC. Asbestos cancers. J Natl Cancer Inst 1979;52:41–46.

147. Wagner JC, Pooley FD, Berry G, et al. A pathological and mineralogical study of asbestos-related deaths in the United Kingdom in 1977. Ann Occup Hyg 1982;26:423–431.

148. Churg A. Chrysotile, tremolite, and malignant mesothelioma in man. Chest 1988;93:621–628.

149. Wagner JC. Mesothelioma and mineral fibers. Cancer (Philadelphia) 1986;57:1905–1911.

150. Merchant JA. Human epidemiology: A review of type and characteristics in the development of malignant and nonmalignant disease. Environ Health Perspect 1990;88:287–293.

151. Begin R, Gauthier JJ, Desmeules M, Ostiguy G. Work-related mesothelioma in Quebec, 1967–1990. Am J Ind Med 1992;22:531–542.

152. Sebastien P, McDonald JC, McDonald AD, Case B, Harley R. Respiratory cancer in chrysotile textile and mining industries: Exposure inferences from lung analysis. Br J Ind Med 1989;46:180–187.

153. Dement JM. Carcinogenicity of chrysotile asbestos: A case control study of textile workers. Cell Biol Toxicol 1991;7:59–65.

154. Davis JMG, Jones AD. Comparisons of the pathogenicity of long and short fibres of chrysotile asbestos in rats. Br J Exp Pathol 1988;69:717–737.

155. Pott F. Problems in defining carcinogenic fibres. Ann Occup Hyg 1987;31:799–802.

156. Pott F, Roller M, Ziem U, et al. Carcinogenicity studies on natural and man-made fibres with the intraperitoneal test in rats. In: Symposium on mineral fibres in the non-occupational environment, Lyon, September 8–10, 1987. 1988:1–4.

157. Pott F, Ziem U, Reiffer FJ, Huth F, Ernst H, Mohr U. Carcinogenicity studies on fibres, metal compounds, and some other dusts in rats. Exp Pathol 1987;32:129–152.

158. Lippmann M. Asbestos exposure indices. Environ Res 1988;46:86–106.

159. Churg A, Wright JL, Gilks B, Depaoli L. Rapid short-term clearance of chrysotile compared with amosite asbestos in the guinea pig. Am Rev Respir Dis 1989;139:885–890.

160. Churg A, Wright J, Wiggs B, Depaoli L. Mineralogic parameters related to amosite asbestos-induced fibrosis in humans. Am Rev Respir Dis 1990;142:1331–1336.

161. U.S. Environmental Protection Agency. Asbestos-containing materials in schools: Final rule and notice. 40 CFR Part 763, Fed. Reg. 1987;52:41826–41905.

162. Warheit DB, Overby LH, George G, Brody AR. Pulmonary macrophages are attracted to inhaled particles through complement activation. Exp Lung Res 1988;14:51–66.

163. Till GO, Ward PA. Systemic complement activation and acute lung injury. Fed Proc 1986;45:13–18.

164. Bowden DH. Macrophages, dust, and pulmonary diseases. Exp Lung Res 1987;12:89–107.

165. du Bois RM. Advances in our understanding of the pathogenesis of fibrotic lung disease. Respir Med 1990;84:185–187.

166. Shaw RJ, Benedict SH, Clark RAF, King TE. Pathogenesis of pulmonary fibrosis in interstitial lung disease. Am Rev Respir Dis 1991;143:167–173.

167. Case BW, Micheal PC, Padilla M, Kleinerman J. Asbestos effects on superoxide production. Environ Res 1986;39:299–306.

168. Hansen K, Mossman BT. Generation of superoxide from alveolar macrophages exposed to asbestiform and non-fibrous particles. Cancer Res 1987;47:1681–1686.

169. Hansen K, Mossman BT. Generation of superoxide from alveolar macrophages exposed to asbestiform and from alveolar macrophages exposed to asbestiform and non-fibrous particles. Cancer Res 1987;47:1681–1686.

170. Ward PA, Duque RE, Sulavik MC, Johnson KJ. In vitro and in vivo stimulation of rat neutrophils and alveolar macrophages by immune complexes. Am J Pathol 1983;110:297–309.

171. Rahman Q, Das B, Viswanathan PN. Biochemical mechanisms in asbestos toxicity. Environ Health Perspect 1983;51:299–303.

172. Jaurand MC, Gaudichet A, Atassi K, Sebastien P, Bignon J. Relationship between the number of asbestos fibres and the cellular and enzymatic content of bronchoalveolar fluid in asbestos exposed subjects. Bull Eur Physiopathol Respir 1980;16:595–606.

173. Brain JD. Macrophage damage in relation to the pathogenesis of lung diseases. Environ Health Perspect 1980;35:21–28.

174. Hahon N, Vallyathan V, Booth JA, Sepulveda MJ. In vitro biologic responses to native and surface-modified asbestos. Environ Res 1986;39:345–355.

175. Hayes AA, Rose AH, Musk AW, Robinson WS. Neutrophil chemotactic factor release and neutrophil alveolitis in asbestos-exposed individuals. Chest 1988;94:521–525.

176. Dubois CM, Bissonnette E, Rola-Pleszczynski M. Asbestos fibers and silica particles stimulate rat alveolar macrophages to release tumor necrosis factor. Am Rev Respir Dis 1989;139:1257–1264.

177. Donaldson K, Li XY, Dogra S, Miller BG, Brown GM. Asbestos-stimulated tumour necrosis factor release from alveolar macrophages depends on fibre length and opsonization. J Pathol 1992;168:243–248.

178. Zone JJ, Rom WN. Circulating immune complexes in asbestos workers. Environ Res 1985;37:383–389.

179. Huuskonen MS, Rasanen JA, Harkonen H, Asp S. Asbestos exposure as a cause of immunological stimulation. Scand J Resp Dis 1978;59:326–332.

180. Valerio F, Balducci D, Lazzarotto A. Adsorption of proteins by chrysotile and crocidolite: Role of molecular weight and charge density. Environ Res 1987;44:312–320.

181. Hamilton JA. Asbestos fibers, plasma and inflammation. Environ Health Perspect 1983;51:281–285.

182. Bonneau L, Malard C, Pezerat H. Studies on surface properties of asbestos II. Role of dimensional characteristics and surface properties of mineral fibers in the induction of pleural tumors. Environ Res 1986;41:268–275.

183. Jolicoeur C, Poisson D. Surface physico-chemical studies of chrysotile asbestos and related minerals. Drug Chem Toxicol 1987;10:1–47.

184. Bonneau L, Suquet H, Malard C, Pezerat H. Studies on surface properties of asbestos I. Active sites on surface of chrysotile and amphiboles. Environ Res 1986;41:251–267.

185. Eberhardt MK, Roman-Franco AA, Quiles MR. Asbestos-induced decomposition of hydrogen peroxide. Environ Res 1985;37:287–292.

186. Kennedy TP, Ky H, Rao NV, et al. Asbestos and kaolin cause red cell hemolysis by acting as fenton reagents. Am Rev Respir Dis 1987;135:A166.

187. Jaurand MC. Mechanisms of fibre genotoxicity. In: Brown RC, Hoskins JA, Johnson NF, eds. Mechanisms in fibre carcinogenesis. New York: Plenum, 1991:287–307.

188. MacDonald JL, Kane AB. Identification of asbestos fibers within single cells. Lab Invest 1986;55:177–185.

189. Brody AR, Hill LH, Stirewalt WS, Adler KB. Actin-containing microfilaments of pulmonary epithelial cells provide a mechanism for translocating asbestos to the interstitium. Chest 1983;83:11–12.

190. Somers ANA, Mason EA, Gerwin BI, Harris CC, Lechner JF. Effects of amosite asbestos fibers on the filaments present in the cytoskeleton of primary human mesothelial cells. In: Brown RC, Hoskins JA, Johnson NF, eds. Mechanisms in fibre carcinogenesis. New York: Plenum, 1991:481–490.

191. Aust AE, Lund LG. Iron mobilization from crocidolite results in enhanced iron-catalyzed oxygen consumption and hydroxyl radical generation in the presence of cysteine. In: Brown RC, Hoskins JA, Johnson NF, eds. Mechanisms in fibre carcinogenesis. New York: Plenum, 1991:397–405.

192. Lund LG, Aust AE. Iron mobilization from crocidolite asbestos greatly enhances crocidolite-dependent formation of DNA single-strand breaks in øX174 RFI DNA. Carcinogenesis 1992;13:637–642.

193. Leanderson P, Tagesson C. Hydrogen peroxide release and hydroxyl radical formation in mixtures containing mineral fibres and human neutrophils. Br J Ind Med 1992;49:745–749.

194. Lund LG, Williams MG, Dodson RF, Aust AE. Iron associated with asbestos bodies is responsible for the formation of single-strand breaks in øX174 RFI DNA. Br J Ind Med (in press).

195. Becklane MR. Occupational lung disease: Past record and future trend using the asbestos case as a model. Clin Invest Med 1983;6:305–317.

196. Dressen WC, Dallavalle JM, Edward TI, Miller JM, Sayers RR. The study of asbestos in the asbestos textile industry. Public Health Bulletin No. 241. Washington, DC: U.S. Treasury Department, 1938:1–126.

197. Merewether ERA, Price CW. Report on the effects of asbestos dust on the lungs and dust suppression in the asbestos industry. London: HM Stationery Office, 1930:1–34.

198. Epler GR, McCloud TC, Gaensler EA. Prevalence and incidence of benign asbestos pleural effusion in a working population. JAMA 1982;247:617–622.

199. Gaensler EA, Kaplan AI. Asbestos pleural effusion. Ann Intern Med 1971;74:178–191.

200. Collins TFB. Pleural reaction associated with asbestos exposure. Br J Radiol 1968;41:655–661.

201. Mattson S, Ringqvist T. Pleural plaques and exposure to asbestos. Scand J Respir Dis 1970;75(Suppl.):1–41.

202. Mattson S. Monosymptomatic exudative pleurisy in persons exposed to asbestos dust. Scand J Respir Dis 1975;56:263–272.

203. Eisenstadt HB. Asbestos pleurisy. Dis Chest 1964;46:78–81.

204. Hillerdal G, Ozesmi M. Benign asbestos pleural effusion: 73 exudates in 60 patients. Eur J Respir Dis 1987;71:113–121.

205. Fondimare A, Duwoos H, Desbordes J, et al. Plaques fibroyalines calcifiees du foie dans l'asbestose. Nouv Presse Med 1973;3:893.

206. Andrion A, Pira E, Mollo F. Peritoneal plaques and asbestos exposure. Arch Pathol Lab Med 1983;107:609–610.

207. Wain SL, Roggli VL, Foster WL, Jr. Parietal pleural plaques, asbestos bodies, and neoplasia: A clinical, pathologic and roentgenographic correlation of 25 consecutive cases. Chest 1985;86:707–713.

208. Schwartz DA. New developments in asbestos-induced pleural disease. Chest 1991;99:191–198.

209. Hourihane DO, Lessof L, Richardson PC. Hyaline and calcified pleural plaques as an index of exposure to asbestos: A study of radiological and pathological features of 100 cases with a consideration of epidemiology. Br Med J 1966;1:1069–1074.

210. Warnock ML, Prescott BT, Kuwahara TJ. Numbers and types of asbestos fibers in subjects with pleural plaques. Am J Pathol 1982;109:37–46.

211. Rohl AN. Asbestos in talc. Environ Health Perspect 1974;9:129–132.

212. Hillerdal G. Pleural plaques in a health survey material: Frequency, development and exposure to asbestos. Scand J Respir Dis 1978;59:257–263.

213. Sebastien P, Fondimare A, Bignon J, Monchaux G, Desbordes J, Bonnaud G. Topographic distribution of asbestos fibres in human lung in relation to occupational and non-occupational exposure. In: Walter WH, McGovern B, eds. Inhaled particles. New York: Pergamon Press, 1977;4(2):435–444.

214. Whitwell F, Scott J, Grimshaw M. Relationship between occupations and asbestos fibre content of the lungs in patients with pleural mesothelioma, lung cancer, and other diseases. Thorax 1977;32:377–386.

215. Churg A. Asbestos fibers and pleural plaques in a general autopsy population. Am J Pathol 1982;109:88–96.

216. Churg A, dePaoli L. Environmental pleural plaques in residents of a Quebec chrysotile mining town. Chest 1988;94:58–60.

217. Kishimoto T, Ono T, Okada K, Ito H. Relationship between numbers of asbestos bodies in autopsy lung and pleural plaques on chest x-ray film. Chest 1989;95:549–552.

218. Lee KP. Lung response to particles with emphasis on asbestos and other fibrous dusts. CRC Crit Rev Toxicol 1985;14:33–86.

219. Meurman L. Asbestos bodies and pleural plaques in a Finnish series of autopsy cases. Acta Pathol Microbiol Scand 1966;181(Suppl.):7–107.

220. Roberts GH. The pathology of parietal pleural plaques. J Clin Pathol 1961;24:348–353.

221. LeBouffant L, Martin JC, Durif S, Daniel H. Structure and composition of pleural plaques. In: Bogovski P, Gilson JC, Timbrell V, Wagner JC, eds. Biological effects of asbestos. Lyon, France: International Agency for Research on Cancer, 1973:249–257.

222. Kiviluoto R. Pleural calcification as a roentgenologic sign of nonoccupational endemic anthophyllite asbestosis. Acta Radiol 1960;194(Suppl.):1–67.

223. Wang NS. The preformed stomas connecting the pleural cavity and the lymphatics in the parietal pleura. Am Rev Respir Dis 1975;111:12–20.

224. Moalli PA, MacDonald JL, Goodglick LA, Kane AB. Acute injury and regeneration of the mesothelium in response to asbestos fibers. Am J Pathol 1987;128:426–445.

225. Taskinen E, Ahlmon K, Wiikeri M. A current hypothesis of the lymphatic transport of inspired dust to the parietal pleura. Chest 1973;64:193–196.

226. Wagner JC, Berry G, Skidmore JW, Timbrell V. The effects of the inhalation of asbestos in rats. Br J Cancer 1974;29:252–269.

227. Hammar SP. Controversies and uncertainties concerning the pathologic features and pathologic diagnosis of asbestosis. Semin Diagn Pathol 1992;9:102–109.

228. Stephens M, Gibbs AR, Pooley FD, Wagner JC. Asbestos-induced diffuse pleural fibrosis: Pathology and mineralogy. Thorax 1987;42:583–588.

229. Gibbs AR, Stephens M, Griffiths DM, Blight BJN, Pooley FD. Fiber distribution in the lungs and pleura of subjects with asbestos-related diffuse pleural fibrosis. Br J Ind Med 1991;48:762–770.

230. Kilburn KH, Warshaw R. Pulmonary functional impairment associated with pleural asbestos disease: Circumscribed and diffuse thickening. Chest 1990;98:965–972.

231. Loeschke H. Storungen des Lufgehalts der Lunge. In: Hanke-Lubarsch Hanbuch der Spezielleu pathologischen Anatomie und Histologie. 3. Bd, I. Teil. Berlin: Springer, 1928:599.

232. Hanke R. Rundatelektasen (Kugel and Walzenatelektasen): Ein bietrag zur differential diagnosis intrapulmonaler rundherde. Roefo 1971;114:164–183.

233. Blesovsky A. The folded lung. Br J Dis Chest 1966;60:19–22.

234. Dernevik L, Gatzinsky P, Hultman E, et al. Shrinking pleuritis with atelectasis. Thorax 1982;37:252–258.

235. Payne CR, Jaques P, Kerr IH. Lung folding simulating

peripheral pulmonary neoplasm (Blesovsky's syndrome). Thorax 1980;35:936–940.

236. Sinner WN. Pleuroma. A cancer-mimicking atelectactic pseudotumor of the lung. Roefo 1980;133:578–585.

237. Kretzschmar R. Uber atelaktatische pseudotumoren der Lunge. Roefo 1975;122:19–29.

238. Schummelfeder N. Umfaltungen und verwachsungen an freien Lungenradem. Beitr Pathol Anal Allg Pathol 1956;116:422–435.

239. Giese W. Pathologische anatomie der pleuaerkrankeungen. Prax Pneumol 1972;26:574–587.

240. Mark EJ. Case 24-1983. N Engl J Med 1983;308:1466–1472.

241. Menzies R, Fraser R. Round atelectasis: Pathologic and pathogenetic features. Am J Surg Pathol 1987;11:674–681.

242. Chung-Park M, Tomashefski JF, Jr., Cohen AM, El-Gazzar M, Cotes EE. Shrinking pleuritis with lobar atelectasis: A morphologic variant of "round atelectasis." Hum Pathol 1989;20:382–387.

243. Selikoff IJ, Lee DHK. Asbestos and disease. New York: Academic Press, 1978.

244. Craighead JE. Eyes for the epidemiologist: The pathologist's role in shaping our understanding of asbestos-associated diseases. Am J Clin Pathol 1988;89:281–287.

245. Cooke WE. Pulmonary asbestosis. Br Med J 1927;2:1024–1025.

246. Dresen WC, Dallavalle JM, Edward TI, Miller JM, Sayers RR. A study of asbestos in the asbestos textile industry. Public Health Bulletin #24. Washington, DC: U.S. Treasury Department, 1938:1–126.

247. Roggli VL, Shelburne JD. New concepts in the diagnosis of mineral pneumoconiosis. Semin Respir Med 1982;4:128–138.

248. Roggli VL. Pathology of human asbestosis: A critical review. Adv Pathol 1989;2:31–60.

249. Roggli VL. Asbestosis. In: Roggli VL, Greenberg SD, Pratt PC, eds. Pathology of asbestos-associated diseases. Boston: Little Brown, 1992:77–108.

250. Warnock ML, Isenberg W. Asbestos burden and the pathology of lung cancer. Chest 1986;89:20–26.

251. Winterbauer RH, Hammar SP, Hallman KO. Diffuse interstitial pneumonitis: Clinicopathologic correlations in 20 patients treated with prednisone/azathioprine. Am J Med 1977;65:661–672.

252. Churg A, Sakoda N, Warnock ML. A simple method of preparing ferruginous bodies for electron microscopic examination. Am J Clin Pathol 1976;68:513–517.

253. Churg A. Non-neoplastic diseases caused by asbestos. In: Churg A, Green FHY, eds. Pathology of occupational lung diseases. New York: Igaku-Shoin, 1988:253–277.

254. Churg A, Wright JL. Small airway lesions in patients exposed to nonasbestos mineral dusts. Hum Pathol 1983;14:688–693.

255. Wright JL, Cagle P, Churg A, Colby TV, Myers J. Diseases of the small airways. Am Rev Respir Dis 1992;146:240–262.

256. Wagner JC, Newhouse ML, Corrin B, et al. Correlation between fibre content of the lung and disease in East London asbestos factory workers. Br J Ind Med 1988;45:305–308.

257. Vorward AJ, Durkan TM, Pratt PC. Experimental studies of asbestosis. Arch Ind Hyg Occup Med 1951;3:1–43.

258. Wright GW, Kuschner M. The influence of varying length of glass and asbestos fibers on tissue response in guinea pigs. In: Walton WH, ed. Inhaled particles IV. Oxford: Pergamon Press, 1977:455–474.

259. Davis JMG, Beckett ST, Bolton RE, Collings P, Middleton AP. Mass and the number of fibers in the pathogenesis of asbestos-related lung disease in rats. Br J Cancer 1978;37:673–688.

260. Crapo JD, Barry BE, Brody AR, O'Neil JJ. Morphological, morphometric and x-ray microanalytical studies on lung tissue of rats exposed to chrysotile asbestos in inhalation chambers. In: Wagner JC, ed. Biological effects of mineral fibers. Lyon, France: IARC Scientific Publications, 1980:273–283.

261. Davis JMG, Addison J, Bolton RE, Donaldson K, Jones AD, Smith T. The pathogenicity of long versus short fibre samples of amosite asbestos administered to rats to inhalation and intraperitoneal injection. Br J Exp Pathol 1986;67:415–430.

262. Adamson IYR, Bowden DH. Response of mouse lungs to crocidolite asbestos. I. Mineral fibrotic reaction to short fibers. J Pathol 1987;152:99–107.

263. Adamson IYR, Bowden DH. Response of mouse lungs to crocidolite asbestos. II. Pulmonary fibrosis after long fibres. J Pathol 1987;152:109–117.

264. McDonald AD, Fry JS, Woolley AJ, McDonald JC. Dust exposure and mortality in an American chrysotile textile plant. Br J Ind Med 1983;40:361–367.

265. Gylseth B, Churg A, Davis JMG, et al. Analysis of asbestos fibers and asbestos bodies in tissue samples from human lung: An international interlaboratory trial. Scand J Work Environ Health 1985;11:107–110.

266. Bellis D, Andrion A, Desedime L, et al. Minimal pathologic changes of the lung and asbestos exposure. Hum Pathol 1989;20:102–106.

267. Rom WN, Travis WD, Brody AR. Cellular and molecular basis of asbestos-related diseases. Am Rev Respir Dis 1991;143:408–422.

268. Hartman DP. Immunological consequences of asbestos exposure. Immunol Rev 1985;4:65–68.

269. Kagan E. The alveolar macrophage: Immune derangement and asbestos-related malignancy. Semin Oncol 1980;8:258–267.

270. Spurzem JR, Saltini C, Rom W, et al. Mechanism of macrophage accumulation in the lungs of asbestos subjects. Am Rev Respir Dis 1987;136:276–280.

271. Dubois CM, Bissonnette E, Rola-Pleszycynski M. Asbestos fibers and silica particles stimulate rat alveolar macrophages to release tumor necrosis factor. Am Rev Respir Dis 1989;139:1257–1264.

272. Lemaire I, Beaudoin H, Masse S, et al. Alveolar macrophage stimulation of lung fibroblast growth in asbes-

tos-induced pulmonary fibrosis. Am J Pathol 1986; 122:205–211.

273. Timbrell V, Ashcroft T, Goldstein B, et al. Relationships between retained amphibole fibers and fibrosis in human lung tissue specimens. Ann Occup Hyg 1988; 32:323–340.

274. Begin R, Masse S, Bureau MA. Morphologic features and function of the airways in early asbestosis in the sheep model. Am Rev Respir Dis 1982;126:870–876.

275. Harless KW, Watanabe S, Renzetti AD. The acute effects of chrysotile asbestos exposure on lung function. Environ Res 1978;16:360–372.

276. Jodoin G, Gibbs GW, Macklem PT, McDonald JC, Becklake MR. Early effects of asbestos exposure on lung function. Am Rev Respir Dis 1971;104:525–535.

277. Jacob G, Bohling H. Das verhalten des bronchialbaumes bei der asbestaublunge. Arch Gewerbepathol Gewerbehyg 1960;18:247–257.

278. Pinkerton KE, Plopper GC, Mercer RR, et al. Airway branching patterns influence asbestos fiber location and the extent of tissue injury in the pulmonary parenchyma. Lab Invest 1986;55:688–695.

279. Delfino R, Ernst P, Bourbeau J. Relationship of lung geometry to the development of pleural abnormalities in insulation workers exposed to asbestos. Am J Ind Med 1989;15:417–425.

280. Churg A, Tron V, Wright JL. Effects of cigarette smoke exposure on retention of asbestos fibers in various morphologic compartments of the guinea pig lung. Am J Pathol 1987;129:385–393.

281. McFadden D, Wright J, Wiggs B, et al. Cigarette smoke increases the penetration of asbestos fibers into airway walls. Am J Pathol 1986;123:95–99.

282. Barnhart S, Thornquist M, Omen GS, et al. The degree of roentgenographic parenchymal opacities attributable to smoking among asbestos-exposed subjects. Am Rev Respir Dis 1990;141:1102–106.

283. Blanc PD, Gamsu G. The effect of cigarette smoking on the detection of small radiographic opacities in organic dust diseases. J Thorac Imag 1988;3:51–56.

284. Weiss W. Cigarette smoking and small irregular opacities. Br J Ind Med 1991;48:841–844.

285. Weiss W. Smoking and pulmonary fibrosis. J Occup Med 1988;30:33–39.

286. Huuskonen MS. The clinical features, mortality and survival of patients with asbestosis. Scand J Work Environ Health 1978;4:265–274.

287. Murphy RL, Becklake MR, Brooks SM, et al. The diagnosis of nonmalignant diseases related to asbestos. Am Rev Respir Dis 1986;134:363–368.

288. Becklake MR. Asbestosis criteria. Arch Pathol Lab Med 1984;108:93.

289. Robinson BWS, Rose AH, James A, Whitaker D, Musk AW. Alveolitis of pulmonary asbestosis: Bronchoalveolar lavage studies in crocidolite- and chrysotile-exposed individuals. Chest 1986;90:396–402.

290. Gaensler EA, Jederline PJ, Churg A. Idiopathic pulmonary fibrosis in asbestos-exposed workers. Am Rev Respir Dis 1991;144:689–696.

291. Roggli VL. Scanning electron microscopic analysis of mineral fiber content of lung tissues in the evaluation of diffuse pulmonary fibrosis. Scanning Microsc 1991; 5:71–83.

292. Monso E, Tura JM, Morell F, Ruiz J, Morera J. Lung dust content in idiopathic pulmonary fibrosis: A study with scanning electron microscopy and energy-dispersive x-ray analysis. Br J Ind Med 1991;48:327–331.

293. Hillerdal G, Hemmingson A. Pulmonary pseudotumors and asbestos. Acta Radiol Diagn 1980;21(Facs. 5):615–620.

294. Lynch DA, Gamsu G, Ray CS, Aberle DR. Asbestos-related focal lung masses: manifestations on conventional and high-resolution CT scans. Radiology 1988; 169:603–607.

295. Case Records of the Massachusetts General Hospital. Case 73-1961. N Engl J Med 1961;265:745–751.

296. Saldana MJ. Localized asbestos pneumonia. Lab Invest 1981;44:57A–58A (abstr.).

297. Spencer H. The pneumoconioses and other occupational lung diseases. In: Pathology of the lung. 3d Ed. Oxford: Pergamon Press, 1977:427–429.

298. Hammar SP, Hallman KO. Localized inflammatory pulmonary disease in persons occupationally exposed to asbestos. Chest 1993;103:1792–1799.

299. Keith I, Day R, Lemaire S, Lemaire I. Asbestos-induced fibrosis in rats: Increase in lung mast cells and autocoid contents. Exp Lung Res 1987;13:311–327.

300. Corrin B, Price AB. Electron microscopic studies in desquamative interstitial pneumonia associated with asbestos. Thorax 1972;27:324–331.

301. Freed JA, Miller A, Gordon RE, Fischbein A, Kleinerman J, Langer AM. Desquamative interstitial pneumonia associated with chrysotile asbestos fibers. Br J Ind Med 1991;48:332–337.

302. Hillerdal G, Heckscher T. Asbestos exposure and Aspergillus infection. Eur J Respir Dis 1982;63:420–424.

303. Hinson KFW, Moon AJ, Plummer NS. Bronchopulmonary aspergillosis. Thorax 1952;7:317–333.

304. Roggli VL, Johnson WW, Kaminsky DB. Asbestos bodies in fine needle aspirates of the lung. Acta Cytol 1984;28:493–498.

305. Monseur J, Leguene B, Lebouffant L, Tichoux G. Asbestose du col vesical et de la prostate. J Urol 1986;92:17–21.

306. De Vuyst P, Dumortier P, Schandene L, Esenne M, Verhest A, Yernault J. Sarcoid-like lung granulomatosis induced by aluminum dusts. Am Rev Respir Dis 1987;135:493–497.

307. Rom WN, Travis WD. Lymphocyte-macrophage alveolitis in non-smoking individuals occupationally exposed to asbestos. Chest 1992;101:779–786.

308. Greenberg SD, Roggli VL. Carcinoma of the lung. In: Roggli VL, Greenberg SD, Pratt PC, eds. Boston: Little Brown, 1992:189–210.

309. Wood WB, Gloyne SR. Pulmonary asbestosis: a review of one hundred cases. Lancet 1934;ii:1383–1385.

310. Gloyne SR. Two cases of squamous carcinoma of the lung occurring in asbestosis. Tubercle 1935;17:5–10.

311. Egbert DS, Geiger AJ. Pulmonary asbestosis and carcinoma: Report of a case with necropsy findings. Am Rev Tuberc 1936;34:143–150.

312. Hruby AJ, Sweany HC. Primary carcinoma of lung with special reference to incidence, early diagnosis and treatment. Arch Intern Med 1933;52:497–540.

313. Klotz O, Simpson W. Silicosis and carcinoma of lung. Libman Annu 1932;2:685–691.

314. Obendorfer S. Das lungenkarzinom. Munchen Med Wochenschr 1933;80:688–696.

315. Lynch KM, Smith WA. Pulmonary asbestosis. III. Carcinoma of the lung in asbestosis. Am J Cancer 1936;14:56–64.

316. Nordmann M. Der Berufskrebs der Asbestarbeiter. Z Krebsforsch 1938;47:288–302.

317. Nordmann M, Sorge A. Lungenkrebs durch Asbestaub im Tierversuch. Z Krebsforsch 1941;51:168–178.

318. Wedler HW. Uber den Lungenkrebs bei Asbestose. Dtsch Med Wochenschr 1943;69:575–576.

319. Merewether ERA. Annual Report of the Chief Inspector of Factories for the Year 1947. London: HM Stationery Office, 1949:78–81.

320. Enterline PE. Asbestos and cancer: The international lab. Am Rev Respir Dis 1978;118:975–978.

321. Berry G. Changing opinions and attitudes regarding asbestos and cancer. Am J Ind Med 1992;22:447–448.

322. Bignon J. How are we going to change our attitudes and opinions regarding asbestos and cancer in the next 20 years? Am J Ind Med 1992;22:443–446.

323. Egilman DS. Public health and epistemology. Am J Ind Med 1992;22:457–459.

324. Lerman Y. Asbestos and cancer 1943–1965. And what happened thereafter? Am J Ind Med 1992;22:455–456.

325. Levin SM. Prevention delayed is prevention denied. Am J Ind Med 1992;22:435–446.

326. Morgan RW. Attitudes about asbestos and lung cancer. Am J Ind Med 1992;22:437–441.

327. Schepers GWH. Changing attitudes and opinions: Asbestos and cancer, 1934–1965. Am J Ind Med 1992;22:461–466.

328. Wikeley NJ. Asbestos and cancer: An early warning to the British TVC. Am J Ind Med 1992;22:449–454.

329. Keane J. Changing attitudes and opinions regarding asbestos and cancer, 1934–1965. Am J Ind Med 1992;22:429–433.

330. Doll R. Mortality from lung cancer in asbestos workers. Br J Ind Med 1955;12:81–86.

331. McDonald JC. Asbestos and lung cancer: Has the case been proven? Chest 1980;67(Suppl.):374–376.

332. Acheson ED, Gardner MJ. The ill effects of asbestos on health. In: Health and Safety Commission. Asbestos. Final Report of the Advisory Committee, Vol. 2. London: HM Stationery Office, 1979:7–84.

333. Selikoff IJ, Churg J, Hammond EC. Asbestos exposure and neoplasia. JAMA 1964;188:22–26.

334. Browne K. Asbestos-related malignancy and the cairns hypothesis. Br J Ind Med 1991;48:73–76.

335. Boyland E. Tumour initiators, promoters and complete carcinogens. Br J Ind Med 1985;42:716–718.

336. Trosic I, Horvat D, Stilinovic L, Pisl Z. Cytotoxic, hemolytic and mutagenic issue caused by chyrsotile asbestos in vitro. In: Mossman BT, Begin RO, eds. Effect of mineral dusts on cells. New York: Springer-Verlag, 1988:423–437.

337. Barrett JC, Lamb PW, Wiseman RW. Multiple mechanisms for the carcinogenic effect of asbestos and other mineral fibers. Environ Health Perspect 1989;81:81–89.

338. Selikoff IJ, Leè DHK. Asbestos and disease. New York: Academic Press, 1982.

339. Kannerstein M, Churg J. Mesothelioma in man and experimental animals. Environ Health Perspect 1980;34:31–36.

340. Hesterberg TW, Barett JC. Induction by asbestos fibers of anaphase abnormalities: Mechanism for aneuploidy induction and possible carcinogenesis. 1985;6:473–475.

341. Craighead JE, Akley NJ, Gould LB, Libbus BNL. Characteristics of tumors and tumor cells cultured from experimental and asbestos-induced mesotheliomas in rats. Am J Pathol 1987;129:448–462.

342. Lechner JF, Tokiwa T, LaVeck MA, et al. Asbestos-associated chromosomal changes in human mesothelial cells. Proc Natl Acad Sci USA 1985;82:3884–3888.

343. Fatima N, Jain AK, Rahman Q. Frequency of sister chromatid exchange and chromosomal aberrations in asbestos cement workers. Br J Ind Med 1991;148:103–105.

344. Rom WN, Livingston GK, Casey KR, et al. Sister chromatid exchange frequency in asbestos workers. J Natl Cancer Inst 1983;70:45–48.

345. International Agency for Research on Cancer. Evaluation of the carcinogenic risk of chemicals to humans. IARC Monograph 1–29(4). Geneva: World Health Organizationa, 1982.

346. Walker C, Everett J, Barret JC. Possible cellular and molecular mechanisms for asbestos carcinogenicity. Am J Ind Med 1992;21:253–273.

347. Selikoff EJ, Hammond EC, Churg J. Asbestos exposure, smoking, and neoplasia. JAMA 1968;204:104–110.

348. Saracci R. The interactions of tobacco smoking and other agents in cancer etiology. Epidemiol Rev 1987;175–193.

348a. Liddell FDK, Thomas DC, Gibbs JW, et al. Fibre exposure and mortality from pneumoconiosis, respiratory and abdominal malignancies in chrysotile production in Quebec, 1926–75. Singapore Ann Acad Med 1984;13(Suppl 2):340–344.

348b. Baker JE. Lung cancer incidence amongst previous employees of an asbestos mine in relationship to crocidolite exposure and tobacco smoking. PhD thesis, University of Western Australia, Perth, 1985.

348c. Selikoff IJ, Seidman H, Hammond EC. Mortality effects of cigarette smoking among amosite asbestos factory workers. JNCI 1980;65:507–513.

348d. Acheson ED, Gardner MJ, Winter PD, et al. Cancer in a

factory using amosite asbestos. Int J Epidemiol 1984;
13:3–10.

348e. Berry G, Newhouse ML, Antonis P. Combined effect of
asbestos exposure and smoking on mortality from lung
cancer in factory workers. Lancet 1972;2:476–479.

348f. Berry G, Newhouse ML, Antonis P. Combined effect of
asbestos and smoking on mortality from lung cancer
and mesothelioma in factory workers. Lancet 1972;2:
476–479.

348g. Selikoff IJ, Hammond ED. Multiple risk factors in
environmental cancer. In: Fraumeni J, ed. Persons at
high risk of cancer. New York: Academic Press, 1975:
467–483.

348h. Hammond EC, Selikoff IJ, Seidman H. Asbestos exposure, cagarette smoking and death rates. Ann NY Acad
Sci 1979;330:473–490.

348i. Blot WJ, Harrington JM, Toledo A, et al. Lung cancer
after enployment in shipyards during World War II. N
Engl J Med 1978;299:620–624.

348j. Blot WJ, Morris LE, Stroube R, et al. Lung and laryngeal cancer in relation to shipyard employment in
coastal Virginia. JNCI 1980;65:571–575.

348k. Martischnig KM, Newell DJ, Barnsley WC, et al. Unsuspected exposure to asbestos and bronchogenic carcinoma. Br Med J 1977;1:746–749.

348l. Pastorino U, Berrino F, Gervasio A, et al. Proportion of
lung cancers due to occupational exposure. Int J Cancer 1984;33:231–237.

348m. Kijuus H, Skjaerven R, Langård S, et al. A case-referent
study of lung cancer, occupational exposure and smoking. 2. Role of asbestos exposure. Scand J Work Environ Health 1986;12:203–209.

349. Berry G. Mortality of workers certified by pneumoconiosis medical panels as having asbestosis. Br J Ind Med
1981;38:130–137.

350. Finkelstein M, Kusiak R, Suranyi G. Mortality among
workers receiving compensation for asbestosis in Ontario. Can Med Assoc J 1981;125:259–262.

351. Cookson WO, Most AW, Glancy JJ, et al. Compensation, radiographic changes, and survival in applicants
for asbestosis compensation. Br J Ind Med 1985;
42:461–468.

352. Coutts IJ, Gilson JC, Kerr IH, Parkes WR, Turner-
Warwick M. Mortality in cases of asbestosis diagnosed
by a pneumoconiosis medical panel. Thorax 1987;a42:
111–116.

353. Weill H. Asbestos. A summing up. In: Wagner JC, ed.
Biological effects of mineral fibers, Vol. 2. IARC Publication #30. Lyon: International Agency for Research
on Cancer, 1980:867–873.

354. Kipen HM, Lilis R, Suzuki V, Valciukas JA, Selikoff IJ.
Pulmonary fibrosis in asbestos insulation workers with
lung cancer: A radiological and histopathological evaluation. Br J Ind Med 1987;44:96–100.

355. Newhouse ML, Berry G, Wagner JC. Mortality of
factory workers in East London, 1933–1980. Br J Ind
Med 1985;42:4–11.

356. Sluis-Cremer GK, Bezuidenhout BN. Relation between

asbestosis and bronchial cancer in amphibole miners.
Br J Ind Med 1989;46:537–540.

357. Hughes HJM, Weill H. Asbestosis as a precursor of
asbestos-related lung cancer: Results of a prospective
mortality study. Br J Ind Med 1991;48:229–233.

358. Browne K. Is asbestos or asbestosis the cause of the
increased risk of lung cancer in asbestos workers? Br J
Ind Med 1986;43:145–149.

359. Kiviluoto R, Meurman LO, Hakama M. Pleural plaques
and neoplasia in Finland. Ann NY Acad Sci 1979;330:
31–33.

360. Edge JR. Incidence of bronchial carcinoma in shipyard
workers with pleural plaques. Ann NY Acad Sci 1979;
330:289–294.

361. Hillerdal G. Pleural plaques and risks for cancer in the
county of Uppsala. Eur J Resp Dis 1980;61(10):111–
117 (Suppl.).

362. Mollo F, Andrion A, Colombo A, Segnan N, Pira E.
Pleural plaques and risk of cancer in Turin, Northwestern Italy. Cancer (Philadelphia) 1984;54:1418–1422.

363. Harber P, Mohsenifar Z, Oren A, Lew M. Pleural
plaques and asbestos-associated malignancy. J Occup
Med 1987;29:641–644.

364. Hillerdal G. Risk and type of lung cancer and mesothelioma in patients with pleural plaques. Lung Cancer
1991;7(Suppl.):5.

365. Partanen T, Nurimen M, Zitting A, Koskinen H, Wiikeri M, Ahlman K. Localized pleural plaques and lung
cancer. Am J Ind Med 1992;22:185–192.

366. Parkes WR. Occupational Lung disorders. 2d Ed. London: Butterworths, 1982.

367. Medical Advisory Panel to the Asbestos International
Association. Criteria for the diagnosis of asbestosis and
considerations in the attribution of lung cancer and
mesothelioma to asbestos exposure. Int Arch Occup
Environ Health 1982;49:357–361.

368. Whitwell F, Newhouse MI, Bennett DR. A study of the
histological types of lung cancer in workers suffering
from asbestosis in the United Kingdom. Br J Ind Med
1974;31:298–303.

369. Churg A. Lung cancer cell type and asbestos exposure.
JAMA 1985;253:2984–2985.

369a. Hourihane DO'B, McCaughey WTE. Pathological aspects of asbestosis. Postgrad Med J 1966;42:613–622.

369b. Whitwell F, Newhouse ML, Bennett DR. A study of the
histological types of lung cancer in workers suffering
from asbestosis in the United Kingdom. Br J Ind Med
1974;31:298–303.

369c. Hasan FM, Nash G, Kazemi H. Asbestos exposure and
related neoplasia. Am J Med 1978;65:649–654.

369d. Kannerstein M, Churg J. Pathology of carcinoma of the
lung associated with asbestos exposure. Cancer 1972;
30:14–21.

369e. Martischnig KM, Newell DJ, Barnsley WC, et al. Unsuspected exposure to asbestos and bronchogenic carcinoma. Br Med J 1977;1:746–749.

369f. Finkelstein MM. Asbestosis in long-term employees of
an Ontario asbestos-cement factory. Am Rev Respir Dis
1982;125:496–501.

369g. Ives JC, Buffler PA, Greenberg D. Environmental associations and histopathologic patterns of carcinoma of the lung. Am Rev Respir Dis 1983;128:195–209.

369h. Auerbach O, Garfinkel L, Parks VR, et al. Histologic type of lung cancer and asbestos exposure. Cancer 1984;54:3017–3021.

370. Jacob G, Anspach M. Pulmonary neoplasia among Dresden asbestos workers. Ann NY Acad Sci 1965; 132:536–548.

371. Hueper WC. Occupational and environmental cancers of the respiratory system: New York: Springer-Verlag, 1966:43.

372. Kannerstein M, Churg J. Pathology of carcinoma of the lung associated with asbestos exposure. Cancer (Philadelphia) 1972;30:14–21.

373. Huuskonen MS. Clinical features, mortality and survival of patients with asbestosis. Scand J Work Environ Health 1978;265–274.

374. Garland LH, Beier RL, Coulson W, Heald JH, Stein RL. The apparent sites of origin of carcinomas of the lung. Radiology 1962;78:1–11.

375. Lulu DJ, Lawson LJ. Carcinoma of the lung. Arch Surg 1964;88:213–217.

376. Weiss W, Boucot KR. The Philadelphia pulmonary neoplasm research project: Early roentgenographic appearance of bronchogenic carcinoma. Arch Intern Med 1974;134:306–311.

377. Byers TE, Vena JE, Rzepka TF. Predilection of lung cancer for the upper lobes: An epidemiologic survey. J Natl Cancer Inst 1984;72:1271–1275.

378. Weiss W. Lobe of origin in the attribution of lung cancer to asbestos. Br J Ind Med 1988;45:544–547.

379. Auerbach O, Garfinkel L, Parks VR, Conston A, Galdi V, Joubert L. Histologic type of lung cancer and asbestos exposure. Cancer (Philadelphia) 1984;54:3017–3021.

380. Babolini G, Blasi A. The pleural form of primary cancer of the lung. Dis Chest 1956;29:314–323.

381. Verga P, Botteri G. Il carcinoma primitivo del polmone. Cappelli, ed. Bologne: 1931.

382. Liberti R, Stella G. Il cancro primitivo del polmone. E.A.T., Napoli, 1949.

383. Sival L. La neoplasia primitiva polmonare: Rapporti tra tipo istologico, sede e gli altri principali caratteri. Biol Lat 1951;4:212.

384. Harwood TR, Gracey Dr, Yokoo H. Pseudomesotheliomatous carcinoma of the lung: A variant of peripheral lung cancer. Am J Clin Pathol 1976;65:159–167.

385. Koss M, Travis W, Moran C, Hochholzer L. Pseudomesotheliomatous adenocarcinomas: A reappraisal. Semin Diagn Pathol 1992;9:117–123.

386. Simonsen J. Pseudomesotheliomatous carcinoma of the lung with asbestos exposure. Am J Forensic Med Pathol 1986;7:49–51.

387. Nishimoto Y, Ohno T, Saito K. Pseudomesotheliomatous carcinoma of the lung with histochemical and immunohistochemical study. Acta Pathol Jpn 1983;33: 415–423.

388. Lin JI, Tyy Seng CH, Tsung SH. Pseudomesotheliomatous carcinoma of the lung. South Med J 1980; 73:655–656.

389. Brganza JM, Butler EB, Fox H, et al. Ectopic production of salivary type amylase by a pseudomesotheliomatous carcinoma of the lung. Cancer (Philadelphia) 1978;41:1522–1525.

390. Broghamer WL, Jr., Collins WM, Mojsenjenko IK. The cytohistopathology of a speudomesotheliomatous carcinoma of the lung. Acta Cytol 1978;22:239–242.

391. Dessy E, Pietra GG. Pseudomesotheliomatous carcinoma of the lung: An immunohistochemical and ultrastructural study of three cases. Cancer (Philadelpha) 1991;68:1747–1753.

392. Robb JA, Hammar SP, Yokoo H. Pseudomesotheliomatous lung carcinoma: A rare asbestos-related malignancy readily separable from epithelial pleural mesothelioma. Hum Pathol (in press).

CHAPTER 29

Vascular Diseases

C.A. WAGENVOORT and W.J. MOOI

The blood vessels of the lung are unique in many respects. The pulmonary circulation accommodates the entire right-ventricular output, and its vasculature is particularly adapted to its primary function, gas exchange. The normal lung vessels are wide and thin walled, reflecting the high flow and low resistance within the pulmonary circulation. They are also vulnerable.

Acquired and congenital abnormalities of the heart or its great vessels expose the pulmonary vasculature to hemodynamic alterations such as increase or decrease of pulmonary blood flow, transmission of high pressure, and obstruction of venous outflow. Parenchymal diseases of the lung, including lung fibrosis and emphysema, may reduce the vascular bed by compression or destruction, or may elicit reactive fibrosis of vascular walls. The peripheral lung vessels in particular are in close contact with the respiratory air. Thus, changes in air composition, such as alveolar hypoxia, or contamination by toxic gases, or fumes, may have a direct effect on the vascular walls. Finally, the bloodstream itself may provide an entry for toxic agents that affect the lung vessels, or for particulate matter obstructing their lumina.

In view of the multitude of potential hazards, it is not surprising that the pathology of the pulmonary vasculature is extremely varied, far more so than that of the systemic vessels. Within this variety, several histologic patterns or combinations of vascular changes emerge. Each of these patterns is associated with a different pathogenesis; a pathogenesis rather than an etiology, because various unrelated etiologic agents may set into motion a process that eventually leads to a characteristic combination of lesions.

Pulmonary vascular disease is most often associated with pulmonary hypertension. Sometimes, however, prominent vascular alterations are observed when the pressure is normal. This is because the lesions provide less obstruction than their morphology suggests (e.g., recanalized thrombotic changes in tetralogy of Fallot), or because the lesions are not generalized. Severe medial and intimal vascular changes in lung fibrosis may be interpreted erroneously as a sign of pulmonary hypertension when a lung biopsy is studied and the focal occurrence of the changes is not appreciated. Generally, however, widespread and significant lesions in pulmonary arteries or veins suggest elevation of pulmonary arterial pressure.

Hypertensive pulmonary vascular disease is not an entity, neither etiologic nor pathogenetic nor morphologic. In fact, it is possible to classify its various forms according to histologic patterns that are called arteriopathies when the arterial tree is the only or the predominant structure affected or vasculopathies when the pulmonary veins are also involved. Of course, these terms should be used only if the lesions are sufficiently widespread and not when isolated changes occur in occasional vessels. The recognition of the different patterns and thereby of the type of vascular disease is an important task of the diagnostic pathologist when evaluating a lung biopsy specimen. In some cases of pulmonary hypertension, it may even be possible to indicate the cause of the elevated pulmonary arterial pressure.

In normal individuals the mean pulmonary arterial pressure is approximately 15 mm Hg, far lower than in the systemic circulation. The pulmonary arterial wedge pressure, representing the left atrial pressure, is normally about 8 mm Hg.

Pulmonary hypertension is usually defined as a mean pulmonary arterial pressure exceeding 18 mm Hg.

However, the pulmonary circulation is also abnormal when there is an elevated pressure gradient from pulmonary artery to vein or an increased pulmonary vascular resistance.[1] In some patients, pulmonary arterial pressures may equal or even exceed systemic pressures so that the relative increase in pressure is far greater than is ever encountered in the systemic circulation.

Changes in the pulmonary arterial pressure are reflected in the morphology of the lung vessels, particularly of the muscular pulmonary arteries, the most reactive part of the pulmonary circulation.[2] In normal adults these arteries are thin walled with a relatively wide lumen; the thickness of their muscular coat is about 5% of the external diameter. In pulmonary hypertension both media and intima often increase in thickness, sometimes to an extreme degree.

At birth, pulmonary arterial medial thickness is similar in the pulmonary and systemic circulations. After birth, the pulmonary arterial media decreases in thickness, rapidly during the first few weeks of life and more gradually during the remainder of the first year. Fibrotic intimal thickening occurs regularly in healthy adult individuals, particularly after the age of 40 years. These so-called age changes are usually mild. However, it is clear that the age of the patient has to be taken into account in evaluating the morphology of the lung vessels.

This chapter is concerned with the various forms of pulmonary vascular disease, with the exception of vasculitis and congenital malformations, which are discussed elsewhere (see Chapters 1, 7, and 30). Following a discussion of pulmonary edema, the pathology of pulmonary trunk and elastic arteries, pulmonary embolism, and the various vasculopathies affecting the more peripheral arteries and veins are discussed. A discussion of bronchial vascular pathology concludes this chapter.

Pulmonary Edema

Pulmonary edema can be defined as an abnormal accumulation of extravascular fluid within the lung. The excess fluid is initially located within the pulmonary interstitium but later spreads to the alveolar air spaces. Pulmonary edema greatly impedes the most vital function of the lung, gas exchange; as a consequence, it is a potentially life-threatening disorder.

Etiology and Pathogenesis

Fluid movements between the vascular lumina and the interstitium of the lung are largely dependent on the hydrostatic and colloid osmotic pressures of the intra-vascular and extravascular spaces (Starling forces). In the normal lung, these forces are in dynamic equilibrium; there is a constant net movement of fluid across the walls of small pulmonary blood vessels into the perivascular space, and from there it flows via the pulmonary lymphatics within the interlobular septa and peribronchial interstitial spaces to the systemic venous circulation. Imbalance of the Starling forces primarily results in alterations in volume of lymphatic drainage, which can increase about tenfold before a significant accumulation of liquid occurs within the pulmonary interstitium.[3] Rhythmic contractions of smooth muscle cells in the walls of lymph vessels are thought to contribute to the lymph flow;[4] ventilatory movements also assist.

Pulmonary edema develops, at first within the interstitial space, when the reserve capacity of the lymph vessels is overcome. A mild degree of interstitial edema does not impede gas exchange across the thin side of the alveolar wall because it accumulates primarily at the other, thick side (Chapter 2); it is the accumulation of fluid within alveolar lumina that constitutes the clinically important phase of the development of acute pulmonary edema.

Because fluid movement across vessel walls depends on intravascular and extravascular hydrostatic and colloid osmotic pressures, the pathogenesis of pulmonary edema can usually be understood in terms of changes in one or several of these parameters.[3,5] Accordingly, pulmonary edema can be roughly subdivided into *hemodynamic edema*, resulting from increased intravascular pressure at capillary level, and *permeability edema*, caused by microvascular damage and leakage of protein-rich fluid which in turn leads to an increased extravascular osmotic pressure, further stimulating fluid extravasation. Hemodynamic pulmonary edema is usually caused by pulmonary venous hypertension; permeability edema may be the result of a wide variety of exogenous or endogenous agents leading to damage of the pulmonary parenchyma. Insufficiency of the pulmonary lymphatics, which normally have a great reserve capacity for removal of excess fluid from the pulmonary interstitial space, may be a causal or contributing factor. Some forms of pulmonary edema have a poorly understood pathogenesis: *neurogenic pulmonary edema*, associated with central nervous system injury and raised intracranial pressure; *high-altitude pulmonary edema*, for which it has been hypothesized that nonhomogeneous severe arteriolar vasoconstriction causes increased pressure at the capillary level[6,7]; and *pulmonary edema associated with abuse of narcotics* (especially heroin). The main causes of pulmonary edema are summarized in Table 29–1.

It is important to realize that more than one pathoge-

Table 29–1. Causes of pulmonary edema[a]

Hemodynamic pulmonary edema
   Left-ventricular myocardial failure
   Mitral or aortic valve disease
   Congenital cardiac disease
   Overtransfusion
Permeability pulmonary edema
   Sepsis, septic shock syndrome
   Inhalation of toxic gases and fumes
   Aspiration of water (drowning)
   Cytostatic treatment
   Pulmonary irradiation
   Paraquat poisoning
   Uremia
   Oxygen treatment
   Allograft rejection after lung transplant
Pulmonary edema with poorly understood pathogenesis
   High-altitude pulmonary edema
   Parenteral and oral narcotic overdose (especially heroin)
   Neurogenic pulmonary edema (central nervous system trauma,
     increased intracranial pressure)

[a] Often more than one of these factors plays a role, especially in severe debilitating disease. *Hypoalbuminemia* and *pulmonary lymphatic insufficiency* (pulmonary and mediastinal tumors, lymphatic duct obstruction, pulmonary lymphangitis carcinomatosa, pulmonary fibrotic diseases, lung transplant) may be important contributing factors.

netic factor may be involved in pulmonary edema, especially when there is severe and debilitating disease. For instance, septic shock may precipitate acute myocardial infarction and hemodynamic pulmonary edema, while bacterial endotoxins cause direct damage to the pulmonary microvasculature and lead to permeability edema. In a critical phase, oxygen treatment and transfusions may be indispensable, but these can also lead to or aggravate pulmonary edema.

Because pulmonary edema often occurs in the context of life-threatening disorders with multiorgan malfunction, it is impossible to give reliable statistics regarding its prognosis; pulmonary edema is certainly a well-known direct cause of death.

Clinical and Radiologic Features

The earliest signs and symptoms of pulmonary edema consist of dyspnea on exertion and a dry cough. Mild tachypnea may also be present; it has been suggested that this may contribute to the ventilatory pumping of lymphatic vessels. A mild degree of systemic arterial hypoxemia may already be demonstrable at this phase. The chest radiograph exhibits perihilar infiltrates that have been likened to a butterfly (Fig. 29–1); there is some redistribution of blood flow to the upper parts of the lungs. Accumulation of fluid within the interstitial space is evidenced on the chest radiograph in the form of so-called Kerley B lines, which represent edematous interlobular septa (Fig. 29–2).

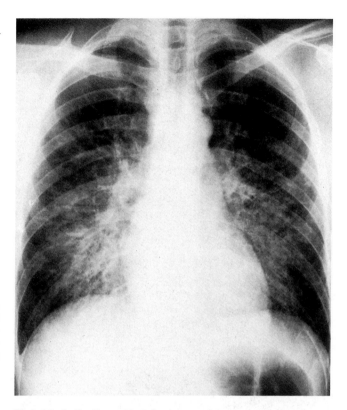

Fig. 29–1. Radiograph of acute pulmonary edema shows perihilar infiltrates and some redistribution of blood flow to upper lobes.

When the edema formation progresses and fluid starts to accumulate within alveolar air spaces, bilateral crepitations, wet rales, and rhonchi can be heard on auscultation, first in the basal regions of the lungs. There is often orthopnea, and frothy sputum, which may be blood tinged, is produced. The impairment of gas exchange is evidenced by a further decrease of systemic arterial oxygen tension, and arterial hypercapnia may arise. When treatment is ineffective, impaired gas exchange leads to the death of the patient.

Pathologic Features

At autopsy, acute pulmonary edema is evidenced by an increase in lung weight; when the lung is sectioned, frothy, blood-tinged fluid oozes from the cut surface.

Because the combined weight of normal lungs as measured in an autopsy series (about 700–800 g) is considerably greater than that measured immediately after death by execution,[8] it is apparent that an increase in lung weight caused by fluid accumulation generally occurs at the time of natural death or shortly thereafter and does not necessarily indicate that there has been pulmonary edema. Therefore, increased lung weight is a relatively insensitive technique to demonstrate pulmo-

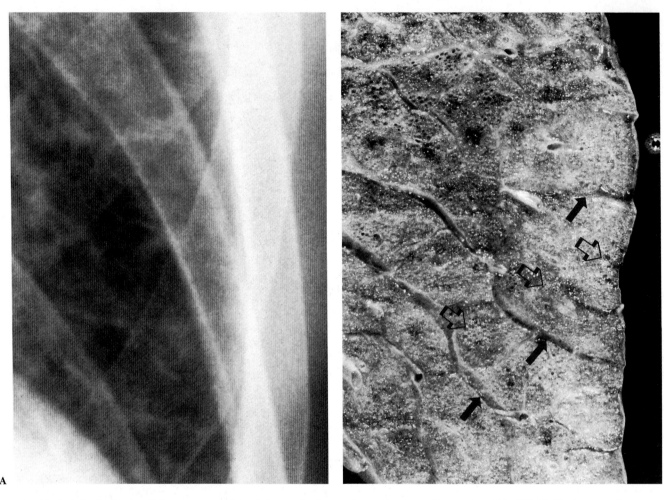

A   B

Fig. 29–2 A,B. A. Kerley B lines arranged at right angles from pleura (same radiograph as Fig. 29–1). **B.** Acute pulmonary edema. Foamy fluid has oozed from cut surface of lung (*open arrows*); interlobular septa are edematous (*solid arrows*).

nary edema. Indeed, it is often the clinician who is best informed whether there has been acute pulmonary edema in the terminal phase of the illness.

Severe acute pulmonary edema, which can be demonstrated as a marked increase in lung weight, is evidenced histologically by widening of interstitial spaces and distension of lymphatics in interlobular septa, peribronchial tissues, and pleura, and the presence of homogeneous or slightly fluffy and granular, pale eosinophilic material within alveolar spaces (Fig. 29–3).

After a few days, hyaline membranes may develop in those areas that are still aerogenated but also contain intraalveolar edema fluid. These hyaline membranes consist of edema fluid and cellular debris derived mainly from pneumocytes. Subsequently, hyaline membranes are resolved or overgrown by proliferating granular pneumocytes, resulting in thickening of alveolar septa. Some collapsed alveoli are also incorporated into these thickened alveolar septa, resulting in remodeling of the original delicate architecture of the pulmonary

parenchyma so that larger and more irregular air spaces are formed. These late changes result in a less effective gas exchange and shunting of blood because capillaries have been obliterated or are separated from the air space by fibrotic tissue. Further, the larger, abnormal air spaces are less efficiently ventilated. Together, these changes result in chronic respiratory insufficiency. The late changes of hemodynamic and permeability pulmonary edema are described more fully in the sections on pulmonary venous hypertension (p. 1010) and diffuse alveolar damage (Chapter 4), respectively.

Pulmonary Trunk and Elastic Arteries

Elastic pulmonary arteries are capacitance vessels, lacking the vasoreactivity of the muscular arteries. This is also reflected in the pathology: for example, there is a

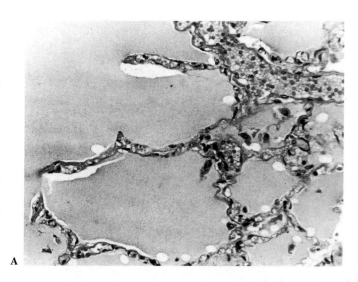

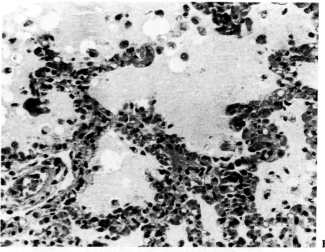

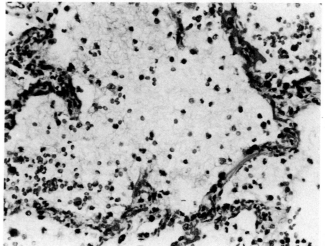

Fig. 29–3 A–C. Acute pulmonary edema. **A.** Alveoli filled with homogenous, eosinophilic edema fluid. **B.** Alveoli filled with pale, slightly granular edema fluid. Note marked congestion of alveolar capillaries. **C.** Fibrinous strands and some extravasated red cells are noted.

variety of histologic patterns of lesions in the peripheral lung vessels in various types of pulmonary hypertension, but the alterations observed in elastic arteries are essentially the same under these different circumstances.

Normal Structure

The caliber (diameter) of the pulmonary trunk is similar to that of the aorta, but the thickness of its wall is only approximately 60% of the aortic wall thickness. In contrast to the aorta, which exhibits a regular and dense arrangement of parallel elastic laminae, the adult pulmonary trunk has an irregular elastic configuration. The elastic laminae and fibers are unequal in thickness and generally disrupted and fragmented, with club-like terminations (Fig. 29–4).

In perinatal life, the pulmonary trunk has a pattern of elastic laminae closely resembling that of the aorta. The fibers forming these laminae are uniform in thick-

ness and follow a circumferential course. Within the first year of life, this fetal or "aortic" pattern gradually changes to the "adult" pattern.

These structural aspects apply also to left and right main pulmonary arteries. However, all other elastic arteries, from lobar and segmental down to a caliber of approximately 0.5 mm where the transition to muscular arteries takes place, retain their regular and intact elastic membranes.

The intima of pulmonary arteries is generally thin but mild intimal fibrosis may occur as an age change. In the main pulmonary arteries of adult patients in particular gross inspection may reveal small patches of atheroma with no demonstrable cause.

Structure in Pulmonary Hypertension

In the presence of acquired sustained pulmonary hypertension, as in mitral stenosis, the wall of the pulmonary trunk is usually increased to a thickness that may

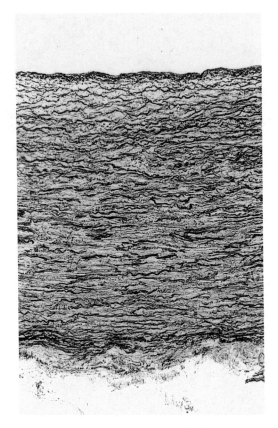

Fig. 29–4. Normal pulmonary trunk with discontinuous elastic membranes in 40-year-old man. ×90.

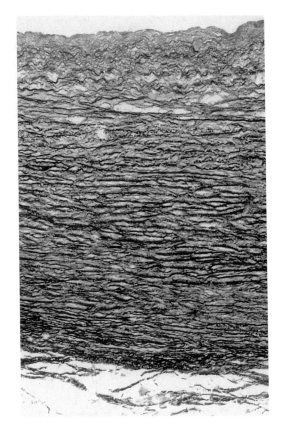

Fig. 29–5. Pulmonary trunk with thickened media and "aortic" configuration of elastic laminae in 12-year-old boy with ventricular septal defect and pulmonary hypertension. ×90.

equal that of the aorta. This thickening is mainly caused by increased collagen and smooth muscle. Although the total amount of elastic tissue is also increased, this has no effect on the elastic configuration, so that the "adult" pattern is maintained.[9]

When pulmonary hypertension is present from birth, as in congenital heart disease, the normal disintegration and disruption of elastic fibers in the early postnatal period do not occur (Fig. 29–5), so that the "aortic" pattern is maintained over the years.[10] As a diagnostic criterium, this difference in elastic pattern between congenital and acquired pulmonary hypertension should be applied with caution: in some patients with congenital heart disease there is some disruption of elastic laminae, while in normal individuals the degree of elastic fiber fragmentation varies considerably.

The intrapulmonary elastic arteries retain their "aortic" elastic pattern in pulmonary hypertension, but their walls may increase in thickness.

Intimal changes of the pulmonary trunk and main arteries are common in pulmonary hypertension; they range from mild intimal fibrosis to frank atherosclerosis. Atherosclerosis (Fig. 29–6) may occur in any form of

pulmonary hypertension[11] as well as in hypercholesterolemia and may already be present in young children. It rarely leads to marked calcification or to complicated lesions such as ulceration.

Bands and webs resulting from organized and recanalized thromboemoli, and found in extrapulmonary as well as intrapulmonary elastic arteries, are discussed in more detail in connection with pulmonary thromboembolism (p. 994).

Structure in Diminished Pulse Pressure

In patients with tetralogy of Fallot, the pulmonary stenosis results in a diminished pulse pressure and a pressure curve with relatively low systolic peaks. In these cases the wall of the pulmonary trunk tends to be abnormally thin. Also, the fragmentation of elastic laminae within the media is often even more pronounced than in the normal adult (Fig. 29–7).[10]

Aneurysms

Pulmonary hypertension is the most common cause of an aneurysm in the pulmonary trunk or its main

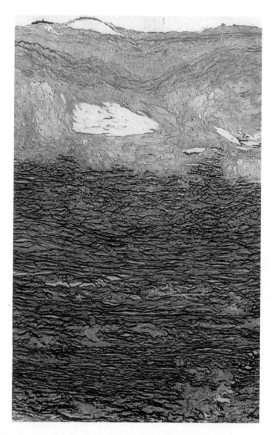

Fig. 29–6. Pulmonary trunk with atherosclerosis in 31-year-old man with ventricular septal defect and pulmonary hypertension. ×90.

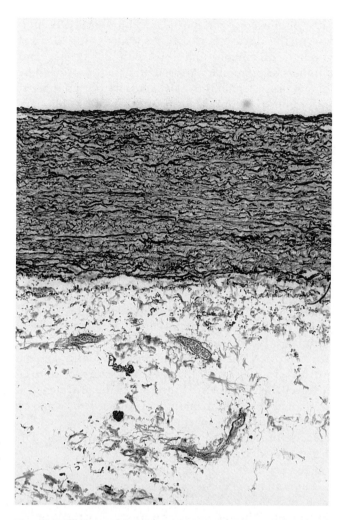

Fig. 29–7. Pulmonary trunk with thin media and prominent fragmentation of elastic laminae in 10-year-old boy with tetralogy of Fallot. ×90.

branches.[12] Saccular aneurysms are in particular observed in conjunction with patent ductus arteriosus,[13] especially when there is also mycotic infection.[14] They may also occur in other forms of congenital heart disease,[15] in acquired pulmonary hypertension,[16] and in primary pulmonary hypertension.[15] Aneurysms may be a complication of a Blalock's or Potts' anastomosis in patients with tetralogy of Fallot.[17,18] In normotensive patients, saccular aneurysms have been described in association with mycotic infections,[19] giant cell arteritis,[20] and trauma.[21] More than one pulmonary arterial aneurysm may occur in the same patient.

Dissecting aneurysms of pulmonary trunk or other major elastic arteries have been reported in various forms of pulmonary hypertension, including congenital heart disease,[22,23] mitral stenosis,[24] and primary pulmonary hypertension.[25]

Tumors

Tumors of the pulmonary trunk, which are rare, include fibrosarcomas, leiomyosarcomas, and rhabdomyosarcomas.[26–28] They may give rise to narrowing and obstruction of the lumen, leading to right-ventricular

failure and death. In some cases, pulmonary metastases come to clinical attention before the primary tumor is detected (see also Chapter 33).

Embolism and Infarction

An embolus is a corpuscle or mass carried by the bloodstream and subsequently impacted in a vessel, most commonly a vessel that is part of the pulmonary arterial tree. In fact, sieving out particles that have been formed in, or have entered, the venous side of the cardiovascular system is one of the functions of the pulmonary circulation. Particles or masses embolized to the lungs are generally thrombi but may consist of tissue or foreign material.

Pulmonary thromboembolism is not only common but is also, particularly in its acute form, an important cause of morbidity and mortality. The clinical presentation of the disease is closely associated with size and numbers of emboli, and thus with the caliber and numbers of pulmonary arterial branches obstructed by them. Massive embolism, in which an important part of the pulmonary trunk, main arteries, or intrapulmonary elastic arteries is occluded, forms a major health problem. Small thromboemboli, obstructing muscular pulmonary arteries, are more common but rarely symptomatic, although occasionally they may lead to pulmonary hypertension. This small-vessel embolism and its consequences are considered in connection with thrombotic arteriopathy (p. 1003).

Thromboembolism

Epidemiology and Risk Factors

Pulmonary thromboembolism appears to be particularly a disease of modern developed and industrialized countries. The incidence is believed to be much lower in African[29] and Asian[30] populations than in the Western world. Life-style rather than genetic factors seems to be involved, because in the United States the prevalence of pulmonary embolism among nonwhites is the same as, or even higher than, in whites.[31] It must be realized that because of diagnostic problems reliable statistical data for the incidence of pulmonary embolism are hard to obtain, certainly in developing countries.

Pulmonary embolism occurs somewhat more often in women than in men but is more often fatal in men than in women. The older age groups are particularly affected. It also does occur, but uncommonly, in children and adolescents. There is a distinct association of thromboembolism with orthopedic and gynecological surgery, cancer, and pregnancy. Other risk factors include immobility, obesity, and primary hypercoagulable states.[32,33]

In the United States, it is estimated that each year approximately 5 million patients suffer an episode of venous thrombosis with 500,000 (10%) having a pulmonary embolic event.[34] In 1 year, pulmonary embolism was responsible for an estimated 300,000 hospitalizations[35] and 50,000 deaths.[31] Here again, the accuracy of such estimates is hampered by the difficulty of the clinical diagnosis. Even though the diagnostic possibilities have improved in recent years, the condition is very often not recognized.[36–38] Therefore, in the absence of corroboration by autopsy, the incidence of pulmonary embolism may well be underestimated.

However, postmortem investigation also may not provide an unequivocal answer. If the patient survives for some time, emboli may disappear as a result of lysis. Also, primary and embolic thrombi cannot be distinguished morphologically. Far more important, however, is the way in which the search for emboli is carried out at autopsy and how embolism is defined.

Thromboembolism is recognized at gross inspection in 5%–28% of consecutive adult hospital autopsies. This variation is at least in part influenced by the way the pulmonary arterial branches are scrutinized. Moreover, when additional microscopic investigation is carried out and the number of thrombotic lesions in muscular pulmonary arteries is included in the count, the incidence increases to 51.7%[39] and 64%.[40] In our own experience, even these high figures are rather conservative when multiple blocks of tissue from various areas of both lungs are used for such a study. It is likely, however, that a considerable percentage of thrombotic lesions do not result from embolism but from primary thrombosis. The inevitable conclusion is that the incidence of pulmonary embolism in the general population is unknown.[41]

Origin

Pulmonary embolism has its origin in the systemic veins or in the right side of the heart. The deep veins of the legs are by far the most frequent source, and pulmonary thromboembolism is usually a complication of deep venous thrombosis.[34] The ileofemoral region is particularly important because thrombi detached from these veins are usually very large and therefore have more serious consequences. Less often, the pelvic veins are the site of origin for emboli, especially in the puerperium, in connection with gynecologic surgery or prostatectomy, and in cases of intravenous drug abuse. Also, any intravascular catheter constitutes a definite risk for thromboembolic events.

In the heart, emboli sources are right-auricular thrombosis caused by atrial fibrillation, right-ventricular thrombus at the site of myocardial infarction involving the ventricular septum or right-ventricular wall, or infectious valvular endocarditis of the right side of the heart.

Clinical Diagnosis, Prognosis, and Treatment

The clinical diagnosis of all forms of pulmonary thromboembolism is exceedingly difficult, including many cases of chronic pulmonary embolism, which is often asymptomatic (p. 1003), as well as the acute form in which symptoms are rarely absent. Although the introduction of lung scan and pulmonary angiography have improved the diagnostic possibilities, the clinical diagnostic accuracy remains very low.[42,43] Even when pulmonary embolism has contributed to the patient's death, autopsy studies have shown that a correct antemortem diagnosis was made in only approximately one of three cases.[36,38]

The most frequent symptoms in patients with the acute form of pulmonary thromboembolism are dyspnea and chest pain, symptoms that occur in a wide variety of heart and lung diseases. Deep venous thrombosis of the legs is almost always present in patients with pulmonary embolism, but in most instances it is nonsymptomatic so that it is not even suspected. Hemoptysis occurs in a minority of patients and may indicate pulmonary infarction.

Acute massive pulmonary thromboembolism may present in a dramatic way by acute increase in right-ventricular and pulmonary arterial pressure, a sharp decrease in cardiac output, and shock. Mortality is high in this group, but depends on prior embolic events, prior surgery, and underlying heart or lung disease. Death may be sudden or within hours or days. If the patient survives the embolic event and the immediate postembolic period, his fate depends on varying factors. Apart from underlying disease and surgical complications, these include the degree of obstruction of the pulmonary arterial tree and the development of shock, circulatory insufficiency, and cardiac arrest. However, thromboemboli may disappear completely by thrombolysis within a few weeks; it is believed that as much as 60% of the clots impacted in the lung vessels may resolve within 4 months.[44]

Therapeutic management of pulmonary embolism is aimed at resolution of emboli and prevention of recurrencies and includes anticoagulant and thrombolytic therapy. Surgical treatment generally is a last resort, but embolectomy may be indicated when more conventional therapy has failed and right-ventricular failure becomes life-threatening. Prevention of embolism by pharmacologic or nonpharmacologic prophylaxis, including intravenous interruption of the caval vein, is generally indicated in hospitalized patients.

Morphology of Thromboembolism

In case of sudden death from massive pulmonary embolism, thromboemboli are usually found in both main pulmonary arteries and pulmonary trunk, and may extend into the right side of the heart. Although vasoconstriction, either by reflex or in response to release of prostaglandins, has been implicated in the mechanism of sudden death, mechanical blockage of the pulmonary vasculature is most likely the predominant factor.[45] Embolic occlusion of one main pulmonary artery may also cause sudden death. Pulmonary emboli are generally multiple, and bilateral and acute massive or submassive pulmonary embolism is virtually always preceded by less dramatic and often asymptomatic embolic

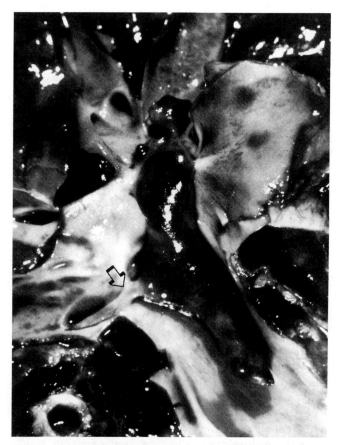

Fig. 29–8. Recent thromboembolus with blunt ends and dark color, lodging in right main pulmonary artery and overlying older organized embolus (*arrow*).

events. Thus, when a significant part of the pulmonary arterial tree is already occluded at a more peripheral level, a major unilateral embolization may well be fatal.

On the other hand, patients may survive massive pulmonary embolism for various periods or even permanently. This happens when a large thromboembolus is arrested while straddling the bifurcation of the pulmonary trunk. Such a "saddle embolus" usually permits some blood flow through both main pulmonary arteries. Similarly smaller thromboemboli may straddle more peripheral ramification points. Also, when emboli are impacted into pulmonary arterial branches, they are not always completely occlusive; in particular, larger thromboemboli are often coiled or folded or have a V or Y shape, as evidence of an origin from confluent veins. In all these instances a residual blood flow remains possible.

Morphologically, a thromboembolus does not differ essentially from a nondetached thrombus. It is roughly cylindrical, reflecting the shape and caliber of the vein or origin, with blunt ends and dark red in color (Fig. 29–8). Sometimes the impressions of venous valves, usually the site of initial thrombus formation, can be recognized on the surface of the embolus. A thromboembolus tends to be dry and brittle with pale lines on a cut surface. Microscopically, these so-called lines of Zahn appear to represent plate-like agglomerations of platelets and leukocytes, separating masses of erythrocytes and fibrin. In contrast, postmortem clots are moist, rubbery, soft, and structureless, without striations. They can often be extracted as a cast from the pulmonary vasculature.

Because there are no histologic differences between a thromboembolus and a thrombus formed within the pulmonary arterial tree, a problem exists when small thrombi, or their remnants in muscular pulmonary arteries, are concerned (p. 1004). For elastic pulmonary arteries, and certainly for the larger ones, it is generally safe to assume that thrombi contained in their lumen are embolic in nature, unless they are overlying a damaged area of the arterial wall, which is uncommon.

Thromboemboli generally favor the right over the left lung in a ratio of 3:2, which corresponds roughly with the ratio of blood flow through both lungs. Emboli are also found distinctly more often in the lower than in the upper lobes,[46] obviously also for reasons of flow distribution.

The fate of a pulmonary thromboembolus is essentially determined by four processes: fragmentation, thrombolysis, organization, and recanalization. *Fragmentation* of a thromboembolus may occur during its passage through the right ventricle and on impact in the pulmonary arteries, particularly at sites of bifurcation. The clot breaks up in smaller pieces that move to more peripheral branches before being arrested. Their downstream movement results in more and more arterial branches becoming available for the blood flow, thus lowering the resistance. In some cases of thromboembolic pulmonary hypertension, extensive thrombotic obstruction of muscular pulmonary arteries occurs, with one or more larger and more recent emboli in elastic pulmonary arteries. In such instances it is likely that it concerns neither primary thrombi nor emboli originating in very small veins, but fragments of larger thromboemboli.

As we have seen, pulmonary thromboemboli, just like thrombi or emboli in other sites, may be rapidly removed by *thrombolysis.* In this way, some emboli may disappear within days, while most are removed within 2–3 weeks. It is likely that lysis contributes to fragmentation when small parts become detached from an embolus to be swept away into peripheral branches.

When thrombolysis fails to remove the embolus, *organization* is the next process. At the sites of adhesion, fibroblasts, myofibroblasts, or smooth muscle cells grow into the clot. In early stages, the tissue replacing the

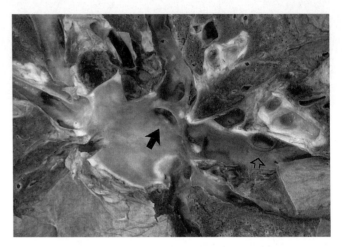

Fig. 29–9. "Bands and webs." Following organization and recanalization of thromboembolus, fibrous band (*open arrow*) and web-like structure (*solid arrow*) extend in lumen of right main pulmonary artery.

thromboembolus has a loose texture with few fibers. More and more collagen, and to a lesser extent elastic fibers, are gradually deposited, and ultimately the whole intravascular mass is converted into a patch of intimal thickening incorporated into the arterial wall. This patch is usually eccentric and irregular in form and may be completely occlusive. More often retraction and shrinkage of the organized clot produces widening of the remaining lumen.

Simultaneously with or immediately following the ingrowth of cells, endothelization and *recanalization* occur. Endothelial cells from the attachment point grow over the external surface of the thrombus to form a complete endothelial lining. From this lining and from the point of adherence, capillary buds invade the thrombus to form narrow channels, which anastomose and widen so that thoroughfares are produced traversing the embolus. To some extent the blood flow may be reestablished in this way.

Eventually macroscopic inspection may reveal the remnants of the organized, recanalized, and shrunken thromboembolus, standing out as the so-called bands and webs (Figs. 29–9 and 29–10), a term equivalent to the microscopic "intravascular septa" in muscular pulmonary arteries (p. 1004).

Infarction

Sudden and complete obstruction of an elastic pulmonary artery, almost always caused by a thromboembolus, has potential consequences for the area of lung tissue supplied by that artery. However, the lungs have a dual pathway for their blood supply, and thus bronchial arteries may take over and prevent serious damage

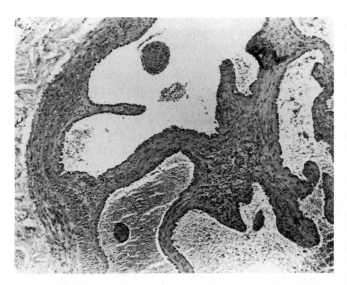

Fig. 29–10. "Bands and webs" in large elastic pulmonary artery. Multiple recanalization channels are separated by fibrotic strands.

to the tissue involved. Moreover, adjacent pulmonary arterial branches may provide some collateral flow so long as they are not separated from the ischemic area by interlobular septa. Anastomoses do not exist between adjacent pulmonary arteries and are very scarce and of small caliber between bronchial and pulmonary arteries, but at a capillary level there are extensive connections. Even so, bronchial arterial blood supply to the ischemic lung tissue is a borderline compensation and whether it will succeed in preventing damage depends not only on the size of the area involved but also on the quality of the bronchial circulation.

Occlusion of a small pulmonary arterial branch is likely to have no or little effect on the dependent lung tissue. When a major elastic artery is obstructed, the chance of infarction increases. Even then, infarction is unlikely to occur in the presence of a normal bronchial arterial blood supply and a normal pulmonary venous drainage. Thus, patients with decreased cardiac output or with pulmonary congestion are particularly at risk. In practice, however, only a very small percentage of pulmonary thromboemboli lead to pulmonary infarction. Infarcts are usually multiple and, like the emboli, most common in the lower lobes.

If ischemia of lung tissue develops, the alveolar capillaries and other small vessels dilate. The endothelium appears to be particularly susceptible, resulting in increased permeability and leakage of fluid and erythrocytes. Such an ischemic hemorrhage leaves the lung tissue viable and is essentially reversible (Fig. 29–11A). However, the next step may be infarction implying tissue necrosis (Fig. 29–11B). Because the capillaries are

destroyed, the whole area distal from the pulmonary arterial obstruction becomes filled with blood provided by the bronchial arteries. Pulmonary infarctions are almost always hemorrhagic.

The *gross appearance* of an ischemia-induced hemorrhage resembles that of a hemorrhagic infarct in many respects. Both are cone shaped or wedge shaped on cross section, with their base bordering the pleura and their apex pointing to the thromboembolus responsible for their development (see Fig. 29–11). Both are dark red and well demarcated. There are also differences. On cut section, the hemorrhage is firm, the infarction soft and friable. In a hemorrhagic area, the structure of the lung tissue is still vaguely recognizable, in contrast to an infarction where tissue structure is lost by coagulation necrosis. Infarcts occurring less than 24 h before the patient's death may not as yet have developed any demonstrable changes.

Microscopic examination confirms the gross findings. In hemorrhagic areas, the alveolar spaces are filled with blood but the original architecture is well preserved, although the capillaries are often greatly congested. In an infarct, only a ghost of alveolar walls, bronchi, and vessels can be recognized, while the cells have become acidophilic and opaque with loss of their nuclei. All spaces are engorged with blood, and some vessels may contain recent clots. In the outer zone of the infarction, the tissue is usually intact so that there is only hemorrhage (Fig. 29–12).

The thromboembolus initiating this process sometimes lies quite some distance proximal to the apex of the infarct, suggesting that a collateral supply from adjacent pulmonary arterial branches succeeded in keeping the outer zone preserved. Although embolus and infarct usually seem to be of approximately the same age, there are cases in which a recent hemorrhagic infarct is associated with an organized, occasionally calcified, thromboembolus. This happens after an embolic event when the bronchial circulation initally supplies the stricken area adequately, but later fails to do so because of general circulatory failure.

With the passage of time, in hemorrhagic areas erythrocytes disintegrate while macrophages containing iron pigment appear. Gradually, however, complete resolution occurs, so that in the long run nothing remains but the organized thromboembolus or its remnants.

In infarcts, progressive lysis of necrotic tissue is accompanied by a change in color, dark red becoming more brown because of hemosiderin production. The area becomes softer and the raised pleural surface becomes flat again. Subsequently, fibrosis begins in the periphery, often witnessed by a greyish-white marginal area. Gradually the entire infarct is converted to grey fibrous scar tissue with a dimple on the pleural surface.

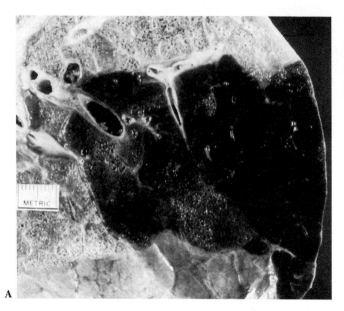

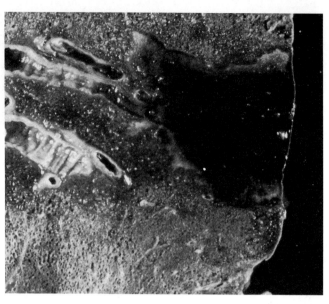

Fig. 29–11 A,B. Effects of emboli seen on surface of lung tissue. **A.** Well-demarcated, wedge-shaped area of hemorrhage in which lung structure is still recognizable. **B.** Wedge-shaped hemorrhagic infarct shows loss of structure. Lesions in **A** and **B** both border pleura; thromboembolic obstruction of pulmonary artery is seen near top of wedge.

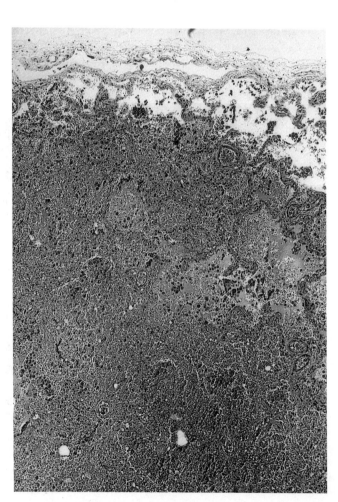

These scars are usually small and easily overlooked at autopsy, even when resulting from large infarcts. Inflation of the lungs is the best way to demonstrate them.

A *septic infarct* is usually the result of an infectious embolus, sometimes of sepsis and sometimes of an infectious process in the lungs. The vascular wall offers great resistance to spreading infection, but only so long as the blood flow through the vessel is uninterrupted. Thus, infection spreads immediately from a septic embolus that has stopped the local circulation so that a septic infarct is formed. If infarction takes place in an infected area of lung tissue, it will also become septic. In either situation a lung abscess may result (Chapter 5). Accumulation of granulocytes with simultaneous lysis of erythrocytes may turn the color of an infected infarct from red to greyish-white.

Nonthrombotic Embolism

Nonthrombotic emboli are uncommon, and their clinical manifestations are even more rare. Such emboli consist of either body constituents or foreign material. Tissue and cell embolism refers to pieces of tissue, groups of cells, or isolated cells large enough to lodge in pulmonary arterial branches or capillaries. Further, fat

Fig. 29–12. Hemorrhagic infarction. Congested alveolar walls stand out in outer zone but become ghost like and indistinct in necrotic central area.

and bile may form microglobules that can be arrested in the pulmonary vasculature. Most of these emboli enter the circulation as a result of trauma, including surgery and delivery. In some instances invasion of vessels (tumor emboli) or developmental disturbances (brain emboli) are responsible.

A wide variety of foreign material, including air, may be embolized to the lungs, most often as a result of surgery or invasive procedures such as injection, infusion, or cardiac catheterization. Thus, a large proportion of foreign-body emboli are iatrogenic, introduced either accidentally or purposefully.

Tissue and Cell Embolism

Bone Marrow. Bone marrow embolism is the only common form of tissue embolism. It is found very commonly in autopsy material, even in 80 of 507 (16%) consecutive autopsies.[47] The clinical importance is limited; fatal bone marrow embolism has been reported in multiple myeloma,[48] but concurrent fat embolism may have been important. Fragments of bone marrow, large enough to lodge in muscular pulmonary arteries, are almost always associated with fractures of bones.

Fractures may be traumatic, spontaneous, or iatrogenic. Following an accidental bone fracture, fat and pieces of bone marrow may be released and be sucked into the circulation. Spontaneous fractures resulting from osteoporosis[49] or metastatic tumors have caused bone marrow embolism. In a case of multiple myeloma, the abnormal composition of the bone marrow could be recognized in an embolus lodged in a pulmonary artery.[50] Rarely, epileptic attacks[51] or eclampsia are the cause of bone marrow embolism.

Among a variety of medical interventions associated with bone marrow embolism, cardiac resuscitation causing fractures of the ribs stands out particularly.[52,53] Bone marrow emboli are also often found following cardiac surgery with cleavage of the sternum.[54]

Occasionally bone marrow embolism occurs in the absence of fractures, from bone metastases of a carcinoma,[55] or in crises of sickle cell anemia with infarction of bone marrow.[56,57]

Histologically, bone marrow emboli are recognized as groups of fat cells alternating with hemopoietic tissue (Fig. 29–13). Sometimes there are also bone fragments. With time, the emboli show degeneration and may be converted into patches of intimal fibrosis.

Megakaryocytes. Megakaryocytes, which have entered venules within the bone marrow and subsequently lodged in the alveolar capillaries, can be found in most routine hospital autopsies,[58,59] even in infants. Because these cells are compressed within the capillary lumen, their nuclei have a pycnotic appearance (Fig. 29–14),

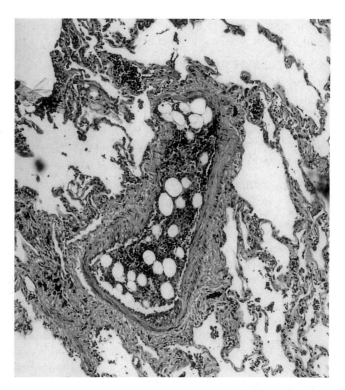

Fig. 29–13. Bone marrow embolus in muscular pulmonary artery. Hemopoietic cells and fat cells are recognizable.

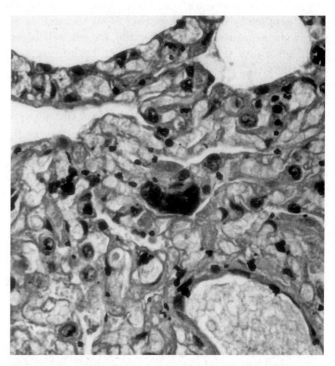

Fig. 29–14. Megakaryocyte with compressed nuclei lodging in alveolar capillary.

and it may seem as if they are devoid of cytoplasm. In some cases they are extremely numerous.[60]

Adipose Tissue and Muscle. Following extensive contusion of adipose tissue, small pieces of fatty tissue or isolated fat cells may be embolized to the lungs.[50] It is sometimes difficult to distinguish them from bone marrow emboli when the latter are very rich in fat cells. Laceration of muscle may result in fragments ending up in the pulmonary circulation.

Bone. As mentioned earlier, bone spicules are occasionally associated with bone marrow emboli. There are, however, rare cases in which massive embolization of bone fragments occurs after orthopedic surgical procedures such as hip replacement. Small bone fragments are also a regular finding in pulmonary arteries of patients subjected to bone marrow transplantation.[61]

Skin and Hairs. During intravenous injection or comparable procedures, minute pieces of skin may be introduced into the bloodstream and end up in the lung vessels.[62,63] Hairs may meet a similar fate. It is likely that such events are not very uncommon, but the chance of finding these small emboli in the lungs is remote.

Liver. Pulmonary emboli composed of hepatic tissue are very rare, but have been reported occasionally after laceration of the liver[64] or in case of hepatic necrosis due to viral hepatitis.[65]

Brain. Emboli consisting of cerebral tissue may occur in two completely different settings. One possibility is severe head injury, either traumatic, particularly after gunshot wounds, or surgical, in patients who survived cerebral laceration for at least a short interval.[66–68] In Oppenheimer's case,[69] there was a massive embolization.

A completely different cause of cerebral embolism is malformations of the brain in newborn infants, including frontal meningocoele and anencephaly.[70,71] It is believed that these fragments of tissue gained access to cerebral veins in early intrauterine life. Occasionally, however, brain injury sustained during delivery is responsible.[72,73] Brain tissue lodged in small pulmonary arteries may retain its viability and may even show some growth.

Trophoblast. During pregnancy and delivery, uterine contractions may dislodge fragments of placental tissue that subsequently reach the lungs as emboli. This occurs almost always during the powerful contractions of eclampsia but also very commonly in normal delivery and during abortion.[74,75] Placental emboli, almost always consisting of multinucleated trophoblast cells, are lodged in arterioles and capillaries. Their nuclei may show degeneration and their cytoplasm is sometimes seemingly absent when the cellular mass is squeezed in a capillary, but confusion with megakaryocytes is not often likely.

Hydatidiform moles may be responsible for embolism of trophoblast and sometimes of chorionic villi. In some instances, trophoblast embolism caused thrombosis of pulmonary arteries and infarction, eventually leading to cor pulmonale and death.[76,77] Aneurysmatic dilatation and rupture of pulmonary arteries has also been reported.[78.]

Decidua. On very rare occasions, small pieces of decidua have been found embolized to pulmonary arteries. The decidual cells may remain vital and even proliferate so as to grow outside the vessel,[79] although such deciduosis may be difficult to diagnose. Decidual embolism may occur in association with trophoblast embolism.[50,80]

Amniotic Fluid. During labor, powerful spastic uterine contractions, generally following rupture of the membranes, may force amniotic fluid into the maternal circulation, usually in the presence of a partial detachment of the placenta or a rupture of the myometrium. When minimal quantities are involved, such an event is probably not uncommon but asymptomatic. Massive amniotic fluid injection into the circulation causes dyspnea, cyanosis, and shock, and often death within 1 h.

The term amniotic fluid embolism is regularly used, although it actually concerns infusion of the fluid, and only embolism of particulate constituents that are arrested in the pulmonary vasculature. These are epithelial squames, lanugo hairs and fat, and mucus and bile from meconium (Fig. 29–15). Special staining methods may be necessary to demonstrate these emboli, because most of them are small and lodging in capillaries.

Mechanical obstruction of the lung vessels by the amniotic fluid contents may be responsible for the clinical findings of acute cor pulmonale. Other factors, however, are probably involved. In amniotic fluid embolism the lung vessels regularly contain thrombi and aggregates of leucocytes or platelets. It is likely that these contribute to vascular obstruction.

Cor pulmonale, however, is not the only hazard associated with amniotic fluid embolism. If the patient survives the initial episode, some thromboplastic substances may induce disseminated intravascular coagulation and fibrinogen depletion, resulting in severe hemorrhagic diathesis often with a fatal outcome.

Fat. Microglobules of fat enter the circulation following long bone fractures or contusion of subcutaneous adipose tissue. The fat droplets lodge in pulmonary capillaries (Fig. 29–16) and sometimes also in arterial branches. Microscopically they can be demonstrated with specific fat stains. In severe cases, gross inspection of the cut surface of the lung may reveal an oily shine.

Fig. 29–15 A,B. Amniotic fluid emboli. **A.** Keratinizing squamous cells are trapped in a small pulmonary vessel. Atwood stain ×400. **B.** Mucin fills this small pulmonary vessel, allowing room for only a few red cells. Atwood stain ×200.

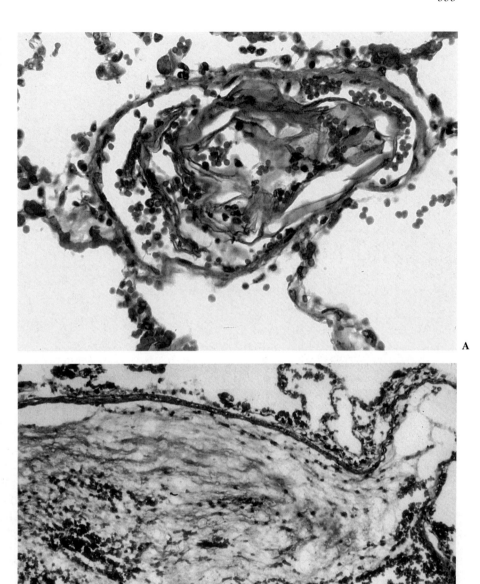

Fat embolism is very common. Sometimes fat droplets may be identified in alveolar capillaries even in nontraumatic patients with varying diseases, particularly diabetes, pancreatitis, sickle cell anemia, and fatty liver caused by alcoholism, and occasionally in individuals without any seemingly predisposing disorders. In general, such findings are completely without clinical significance.[81] In battle casualties, microglobules were observed in the pulmonary vasculature in approximately 90%[82] and in 100%[83] of patients following routine surgery. Even then, significant clinical consequences are uncommon.

In a minority of these patients, particularly with serious injuries and multiple fractures,[84] the fat embolism syndrome develops. This is a variant of the adult respiratory distress syndrome (ARDS), which is marked by progressive respiratory insufficiency, bilateral pulmonary infiltrates, thrombocytopenia, petechiae, and mental confusion.[85,86] Cells recovered by bronchoalveolar lavage often contain intracellular fat droplets.[87]

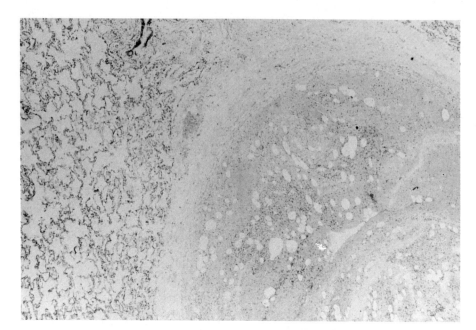

Fig. 29–16. Fat embolus. As versus bone marrow emboli, fat emboli are often hard to recognize unless suspected. This one has some fat necrosis with it aiding its detection. This is from a case of massive soft tissue trauma to the leg during an auto accident. H and E ×50.

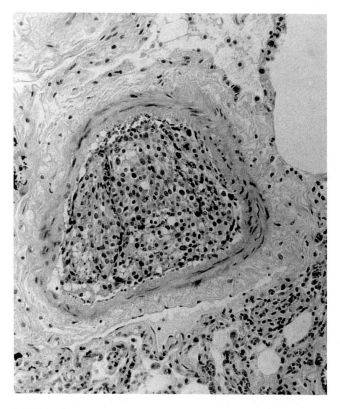

Fig. 29–17. Muscular pulmonary artery completely occluded by tumor embolus in 67-year-old man with undifferentiated carcinoma of the esophagus.

Traumatic lipemia may be caused by instability of emulsion; the elevated levels of fatty acids and chylomicrons agglomerate to further increase damage to capillary walls. The resulting diffuse leakage is likely to play an important part in the production of ARDS.

Bile. Embolism of bile thrombi to alveolar capillaries is a rare event in patients suffering from cholestasis and jaundice.[88] The nature of the golden-yellow pigment should be identified by the Fouchet stain.

Tumor

By invasion of vascular walls, malignant tumors release small pieces or clumps of tumor cells that end up in pulmonary arterial branches (Fig. 29–17). Although, in principle any malignant neoplasm may cause pulmonary tumor embolism, there are some known to produce such widespread obstruction of pulmonary arteries by tumor cells that the pulmonary vascular resistance becomes greatly increased. This applies particularly to adenocarcinomas of the stomach and mammary gland and to a lesser extent to hepatocellular carcinoma and choriocarcinoma.[89–91]

In some of these instances, the primary tumor had been unsuspected as it was asymptomatic, so that tumor embolism caused unexplained pulmonary hypertension (p. 1018). In patients with pulmonary hypertension from tumor embolism, there is sometimes widespread carcinomatosis of the lungs,[89,92] but this is not necessarily so. When tumor cells within the pulmonary arteries fail to invade the lung tissue, they will gradually show degeneration. Occasionally they remain vital, forming a lining over the inner arterial wall for a considerable extent (Fig. 29–18).

Obstruction of pulmonary arteries by tumor emboli alone may occasionally cause pulmonary hypertension; more often there is associated thrombosis,[93,94] because tumor cells may induce thrombosis.[95] Benign tumors

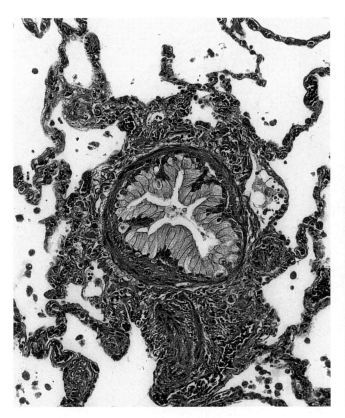

Fig. 29–18. Muscular pulmonary artery with tumor embolus causing single-cell lining over inner arterial surface in 39-year-old man with adenocarcinoma of bile duct.

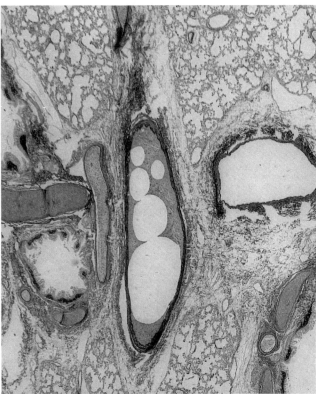

Fig. 29–19. Accidental air embolism during surgery in 68-year-old woman. Elastic pulmonary artery contains large air bubbles.

rarely cause pulmonary embolism, but it has been reported in right-atrial myxoma.[96]

Air

Air may enter the circulation by being sucked into large veins, particularly in the head and neck area, during the negative pressure phase of inspiration or by being forcefully introduced into systemic veins. Apart from accidental trauma, a wide variety of surgical, diagnostic, and therapeutic procedures may accidentally result in air embolism. These include operations in the region of head and neck with injury to large veins, intravenous injections and infusions, intrauterine injection of soap solution intended to procure abortion, insufflation of fallopian tubes, and forced positive pressure ventilation in newborn infants with respiratory distress. Rapid decompression may result in embolism of gas bubbles in two different ways: air that expands but cannot escape the lung may damage the lung tissue and be forced into the vessels, and gas dissolved in the blood will be released in the form of small bubbles. In the latter situation, known as *caisson disease,* the presence of these

bubbles in the systemic circulation has far greater consequences than their embolization to the pulmonary capillaries.

The clinical symptoms of air embolism depend on the amount of air that has entered the circulation. Minor quantities of air, less than 80 ml, produce no or few symptoms while the air is gradually absorbed. Massive pulmonary air embolism causes acute respiratory distress, shock, and neurologic disturbances. When large air bubbles occlude the pulmonary trunk or main arteries, sudden death is usually the result.

If air embolism is suspected, the pathologist should open the right-cardiac ventricle under water to demonstrate the presence of air. Another indication is dilatation of the right side of the heart and of the pulmonary vasculature, containing blood with a frothy appearance, while the contracted left ventricle is empty. Microscopically, the presence of air bubbles in pulmonary arteries can be recognized by their outlines within the blood (Fig. 29–19). Experimental work suggests that air embolism in surviving patients eventually may result in thickening of the pulmonary arterial intima and the formation of intravascular septa.[97–99]

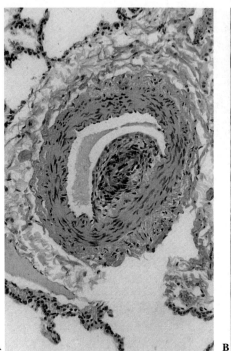
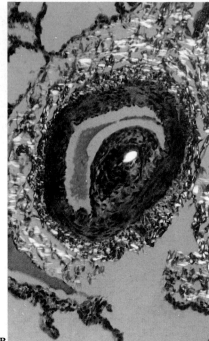
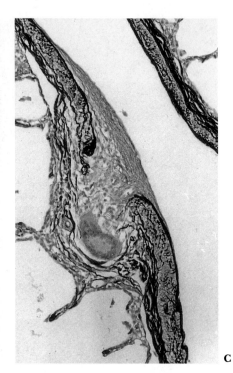

Fig. 29–20 A–C. Cotton wool fiber embolism in muscular pulmonary artery caused eccentric intimal thickening. **A.** Fiber is not easily recognized without use of polarized light **(B). C.** cotton wool fiber caused rupture of arterial wall with granulomatous reaction.

Foreign Bodies

Any object introduced into the venous side of the systemic circulation may be carried to and become impacted in the pulmonary vasculature. Foreign bodies embolized to the lung include relatively large items such as bullets,[100] lead pellets,[101] intravascular catheters,[102] and a variety of other objects.

Far more common are small foreign-body emboli, particularly fibers of cotton wool or gauze pads. Dimmick et al.[103] found them in pulmonary arteries in 8 of 173 patients who died after cardiac surgery or catheterization. In our own experience they are fairly common even in lung biopsies taken during operations for congenital or acquired heart disease; occasionally they are present in multiple arterial branches. The birefringency of these emboli is helpful in locating them, but foreign-body granulomas produced by them also will not be easily overlooked. The fibers may pierce the vascular wall to elicit an extravascular inflammatory reaction (Fig. 29–20).

Accidental introduction into the circulation of a wide variety of foreign material such as gel foam, Teflon fragments,[104] and barium sulfate crystals following an enema[105] has been reported.

A special form of foreign-body embolism is the injection of plastic particles into bronchial or collateral systemic arteries in an attempt to arrest hemoptysis in patients with an extensive collateral circulation. Through anastomoses, these corpuscles will eventually lodge in pulmonary arterial branches where they cause a granulomatous reaction (Fig. 29–21).

Another far more dramatic form of embolism is caused by a variety of foreign materials in drug addicts. Drug-containing tablets intended for oral use are crushed, brought into an aqueous suspension, and injected intravenously. These tablets contain filler material, usually talc, starch, or cellulose, which causes widespread granulomatous arteritis and pulmonary hypertension.[106–111] The condition may be confused with granulomatosis of the lung caused by cocaine sniffing.[112]

Parasites

A variety of parasitic worm species may be embolized to the human lung in the form of eggs, larvae, or adults, either as part of their life cycle or accidentally. In the lungs they may gain access to air passages and be coughed up, or they may cause a granulomatous reaction or even infarcts.

Among the nematodes, species such as *Wuchereria bancrofti* and *Brugia malayi* are known to cause ischemic

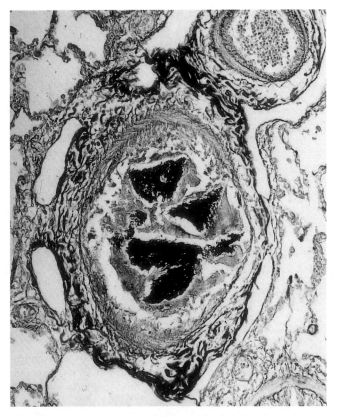

Fig. 29–21. Polyvinyl granules were injected into bronchial artery to arrest hemoptysis in 5-year-old girl with pulmonic atresia and extensive collateral circulation and lodged in pulmonary artery.

infarcts.[113,114] *Dirofilaria immitis* has been increasingly identified in man as a cause of pulmonary coin lesions[115,116] or ischemic infarcts.[117,118] The larvae of *Ascaris lumbricoides*, a very common human parasite, penetrate the walls of alveolar capillaries to reach the air spaces, but the damage to the lung tissue is usually limited although a granulomatous reaction may occur, even with ossification.[119] Rarely, adult worms cause thrombosis of lung vessels and infarction.[120]

Of the trematodes, species of *Schistosoma* in particular are associated with pulmonary vascular changes. Schistosomiasis is a widespread and very common tropical disease. In a high percentage of the cases, ova can be found in lung tissue and lung vessels, usually without important consequences, but pulmonary hypertension and plexogenic pulmonary arteriopathy often develop in the presence of pipestem cirrhosis of the liver (p. 1006). Occasionally the adult flukes embolize to the pulmonary vasculature; they elicit little reaction as long as they are alive but cause thrombosis and necrosis of surrounding tissue as soon as they die.[121] Among the cestodes, larval stages of *Echinococcus granulosus* may be transported from the intestines to the lungs where they may cause hydatid cysts.

Thrombotic Arteriopathy

The long-term effect of thrombosis or thromboembolism in pulmonary arteries is referred to as thrombotic arteriopathy. Obviously, the term should not be used for isolated lesions, which are very common, but only when there is widespread involvement of the pulmonary arterial tree. In practice it can be equated with thrombotic or thromboembolic pulmonary hypertension.

Clinical Presentation

Thrombotic or thromboembolic pulmonary hypertension is usually preceded by signs and symptoms of episodes of embolism and infarction (p. 992), which often are not diagnosed as such because these events may be subtle. The development of embolic pulmonary hypertension is usually insidious, particularly in the silent form in which symptoms are completely absent until the signs of severe and irreversible pulmonary hypertension appear. In these instances the condition is generally indistinguishable clinically from primary plexogenic arteriopathy and some other forms of pulmonary hypertension (p. 1018). Under such circumstances, a firm diagnosis can be made only on the basis of a lung biopsy.[122,123] Women are somewhat more often affected than men, and those over the age of 30 years more often than young individuals, although the young are not immune.

Pathogenesis

Thrombi and their sequelae are far more common in muscular than in major elastic pulmonary arteries. In large arteries, thrombi are generally considered to be embolic in origin unless there is an apparent underlying cause such as damage to the arterial wall. In muscular pulmonary arteries the situation is different. Thrombotic lesions here are either the result of embolism or of primary thrombosis, and it is generally impossible to distinguish between these two options or to give an estimate of their relative frequency. There is little doubt, however, that both modes of development can occur. In unquestionable cases of chronic thromboembolism, in addition to embolic alterations in major arteries such as bands and webs, the peripheral muscular arteries often show numerous old thrombotic lesions; this suggests a common source of development rather than two different mechanisms operating simul-

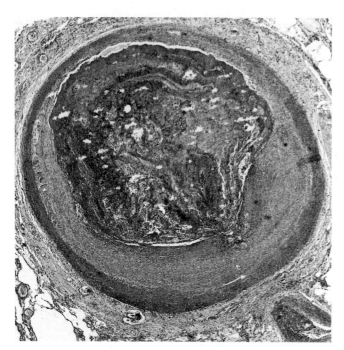

Fig. 29–22. Recent thrombus on top of eccentric intimal fibrosis in pulmonary artery in 59-year-old man with recurrent silent thromboembolism.

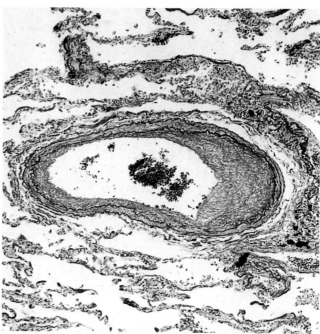

Fig. 29–23. Eccentric intimal fibrosis resulted from organization of thromboembolus in muscular pulmonary artery in 66-year-old woman with recurrent silent thromboembolism.

taneously. The source of such small emboli may be a venous plexus, for instance, in the pelvis. However, it is likely that fragmentation of larger thromboemboli is also involved in this peripheral distribution. Primary thrombosis of muscular pulmonary arteries is clearly involved when not only small arterial branches but also veins are affected, or when, as in tetralogy of Fallot, there is a strong tendency to thrombosis in the lungs.

As has been discussed (p. 992), small numbers of thrombotic lesions are found in the majority of routine autopsies in adult patients.[39,40] Muscular pulmonary arteries may be occluded without a significant effect on the pulmonary arterial pressure, so long as a large proportion of the arterial bed is not occluded. The mechanism of this arterial obstruction is mechanical rather than vasoconstrictive.[41,124] The majority of patients with chronic pulmonary hypertension caused by thrombotic arteriopathy do not have an increased amount of arterial smooth muscle, as would be expected if prolonged vasoconstriction was an important contributing factor to increased vascular resistance. However, it is possible (see p. 1005) that vasoconstriction plays a part in some cases in which there is prominent medial hypertrophy of muscular pulmonary arteries.

Pulmonary Vascular Changes

Although the vascular changes in thrombotic arteriopathy are essentially based on thrombosis, recent (Fig. 29–22) or early-organizing thrombi, easily recognizable

as such, are uncommon even in fatal silent embolic pulmonary hypertension.[123] Thrombi often are lodged or formed in the pulmonary circulation over a long period, and because their organization occurs fairly rapidly, few recent thrombi are to be found at any given moment. The thrombi are incorporated into the arterial wall and transformed in irregular patches of intimal thickening. This eccentric intimal fibrosis (Fig. 29–23) lacks the concentric-laminar arrangement of the intimal thickening in plexogenic arteriopathy. In the early stages it sometimes suggests cellular proliferation of the intima, as seen in that disease (p. 1007). Thrombotic intimal thickening often leads to severe narrowing or obliteration of the arterial lumen (Fig. 29–24). However, it tends to occur over short spans so that in a random histologic section many arteries look patent and normal.[125,126]

Recanalization of these obliterating lesions usually begins with formation of capillary-like channels, in part traversing the arterial media. As these channels widen, their lumina are separated only by intravascular fibrous septa (Fig. 29–25), which are the counterparts of the "bands and webs" in the major pulmonary arteries. These septa have sometimes been confused with plexiform lesions. Indeed, this confusion has fueled in part controversies regarding the distinction between plexogenic and thrombotic arteriopathies. Arteritis is uncommon in thrombotic arteriopathy and almost always caused by septic emboli.

Occasionally, a thromboembolus fails to become or-

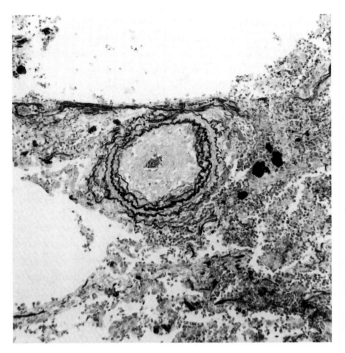

Fig. 29–24. Almost complete obliteration of muscular pulmonary artery (same patient as in Fig. 29–23).

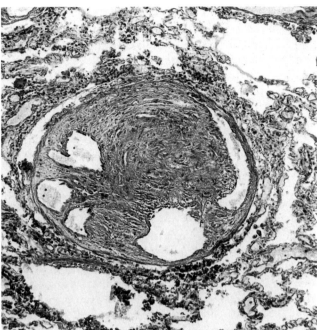

Fig. 29–25. Intravascular fibrous septa caused by recanalization of organized thromboembolus in 25-year-old woman with recurrent silent thromboembolism.

ganized. In these instances there is usually no close contact with the arterial wall, although an endothelial layer may cover the thrombus which may show degeneration and uncommonly calcification (Fig. 29–26).

The media of the pulmonary arteries in most instances is normal or only mildly thickened, usually with no muscularization of arterioles. In approximately 20% of cases of thrombotic or embolic pulmonary hypertension, however, prominent medial hypertrophy suggests that vasoconstriction plays a contributing role in a minority of the cases.

Reversibility and Prognostic Significance

In its silent form in particular, embolic pulmonary hypertension has a poor prognosis because symptoms of the increased pressure will not appear until the lesions have progressed to an irreversible stage. Obliteration of arteries is essentially irreversible; recanalization and shrinkage of the lesions may restore some patency, but the effect in terms of hemodynamics is probably very limited.

Plexogenic Arteriopathy

The term plexogenic arteriopathy has been proposed for a characteristic pattern of morphologic alterations in the lung vessels.[127] Because the most specific of these,

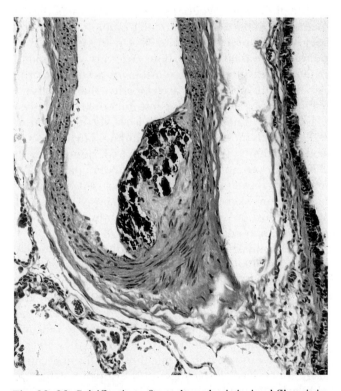

Fig. 29–26. Calcification of postthrombotic intimal fibrosis in 32-year-old woman with embolic pulmonary hypertension.

the plexiform lesion, is found only in the terminal stage, the term plexogenic is appropriate for the entire condition. It is not always appreciated that plexiform lesions need not be present to use the name plexogenic arteriopathy or to diagnose it with confidence.[128] Plexogenic arteriopathy is a morphologic entity with a definite sequence of increasingly severe vascular changes, but in its earliest stage there may be medial hypertrophy only, although this rarely suffices for a diagnosis.

Etiology and Pathogenesis

Plexogenic arteriopathy is not an etiologic entity; there is a wide spectrum of causal factors. The pattern is found in congenital heart disease with a left-to-right shunt such as atrial and ventricular septal defects, patent ductus arteriosus, or persistent truncus arteriosus.[129,130] Plexogenic arteriopathy may also occur in acquired shunts, as has been demonstrated in experimental animals following the creation of a shunt between systemic and pulmonary circulations.[131,132] The pattern has also been found in patients with tetralogy of Fallot in whom too large a surgical shunt was established between the two circulations.[133,134]

Plexogenic arteriopathy is sometimes associated with portal hypertension from hepatic disease or prehepatic block.[135–138] Although this association is uncommon, it is too predominant to be attributed to coincidence.[139]

Patients with severe hepatic disease without demonstrable pulmonary hypertension may have an increased medial thickness of their muscular pulmonary arteries, suggesting a preclinical state.[140] On the other hand, pulmonary vascular alterations are very complex in patients with portal hypertension. In addition to the patients with plexogenic arteriopathy, there is also a group with so-called hepatogenic pulmonary angiodysplasia[141] in whom the lung vessels are dilated and thin walled; this is indeed a common finding. Further, occasional patients combine portal hypertension with thrombotic pulmonary arteriopathy. Pulmonary hypertension in these patients is possibly caused by thromboembolism from portal vein thrombosis by way of spontaneous or surgical portacaval shunts[142,143] or from thrombosed small hepatic veins.[144]

Schistosomiasis may be associated with pulmonary hypertension, which occurs in a small percentage of the cases. Schistosomiasis is so widespread and common in tropical and subtropical countries, however, that the absolute number of patients suffering from this combination is very large. The ova of the parasite become lodged in small pulmonary arteries where they elicit a granulomatous reaction. While these lesions may cause arterial obstruction, plexogenic arteriopathy, which is regularly observed in these cases, is more important for the development of pulmonary hypertension. Ova may be found within plexiform lesions, but there is no reason to assume a direct causal relationship because ova are regularly released in the circulation and the plexiform lesions act as sieves. Moreover, most vessels with plexiform lesions or other alterations of plexogenic arteriopathy do not contain ova.[145,146] Because schistosomiasis patients with pulmonary hypertension almost always have pipestem fibrosis of the liver, it is likely that the association of schistosomiasis with plexogenic arteriopathy is in fact hepatogenic in nature.

A widespread epidemic of plexogenic arteriopathy, observed in central Europe between 1967 and 1970, appeared to have been caused by ingestion of the anorectic drug Aminorex.[147,148] The epidemic abated after the drug was taken off the market.

Finally, there is a group of patients in whom plexogenic arteriopathy develops without identifiable cause (p. 1018). This form of primary pulmonary hypertension particularly affects children and young adults; in adults, it is more common in women than in men.[149] Primary plexogenic arteriopathy usually runs a fatal course within 1–3 years; a minority of the patients survive for up to 20 years.

In spite of the heterogeneity of these etiologic factors, it is likely that the pathogenesis of this type of hypertensive pulmonary vascular disease is the same in all instances. Intense spastic vasoconstriction probably is a central factor in the development of the various lesions,[125] although this may well be in interplay with sheer stress, endothelial damage, platelet reactivity, etc.

Another, at least as important, factor is likely to be hyperreactivity of muscular pulmonary arteries. Variations in vascular reactivity would explain why some patients with a large ventricular septal defect have only minimal pulmonary vascular disease, while others with a small defect but more reactive lung vessels develop severe and rapidly progressive plexogenic arteriopathy. Similarly, only a very small percentage of individuals using the appetite suppressant Aminorex and of patients with hepatic disease or systemic schistosomiasis develop sustained pulmonary hypertension. It is a reasonable assumption that there are important individual differences in pulmonary arterial reactivity in response to vasoconstrictive stimuli. In primary plexogenic arteriopathy, it probably concerns extreme hyperreactivity.

Clinical Presentation

The clinical presentation of plexogenic arteriopathy depends to a large extent on the underlying condition. The greatest problems arise in the primary form because signs and symptoms often appear in a terminal and irreversible stage at which no adequate therapy

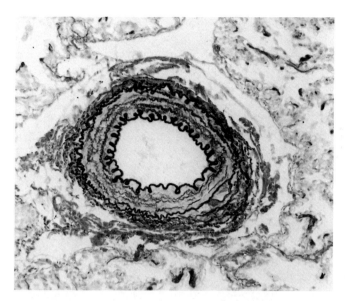

Fig. 29–27. Medial hypertrophy of muscular pulmonary artery in 2.5-year-old girl with ventricular septal defect.

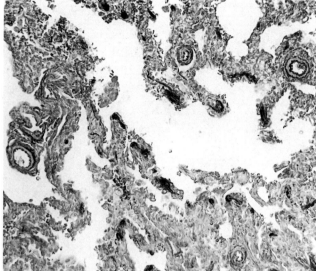

Fig. 29–28. Muscularization of pulmonary arterioles in 1-year-old girl with atrioventricular septal defect.

short of lung or heart-lung transplantation is available. Moreover, clinical distinction between primary plexogenic arteriopathy and other forms of "unexplained pulmonary hypertension" (p. 1017) is usually impossible.

Pulmonary Vascular Changes

In plexogenic arteriopathy, the arterial lesions, which form a considerable variety, tend to develop in a sequence.

As in most forms of hypertensive pulmonary vascular disease, *medial hypertrophy* (Fig. 29–27) is the first and most widespread lesion. The thickening of the media is caused by an increase in size as well as in numbers of smooth muscle cells.[125] Both collapse and constriction of vessels may contribute to thickening of the vascular wall including the muscular coat. Expansion of lung tissue abolishes vascular collapse and the resulting medial thickening; comparison of arteries in areas of lung tissue with and without collapse will also usually clarify the presence or absence of medial hypertrophy. The effect of vasoconstriction, however, is not removed by expansion of the lungs so that confusion with mild-to-moderate medial hypertrophy certainly remains possible.

An increase in the number of arterial smooth muscle cells is particularly apparent in small peripheral arteries. Smooth muscle cells appear along distal segments of previously nonmuscular intraacinar branches, a process known as muscularization of arterioles (Fig. 29–28 and 29–29).

The earliest change of the intima consists of a *cellular*

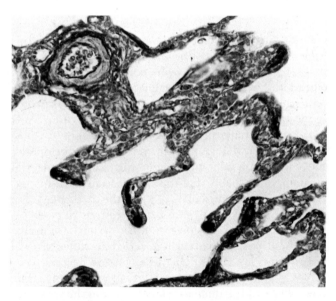

Fig. 29–29. Muscularization of arteriole (from Fig. 29–28 at higher magnification).

proliferation. It is very likely that the medial smooth muscle cell is the provenance of these newly formed intimal cells.[150–151a] The ultrastructural features of these intimal cells are those of myofibroblasts or well-differentiated smooth muscle cells. In this stage, there are few or no collagen or elastic fibers within the thickened intima, but cellular proliferation may cause considerable narrowing of arterial branches (Figs. 29–30 and 29–31).

With the subsequent gradual deposition of collagen and elastic fibers, this cellular layer is transformed into a

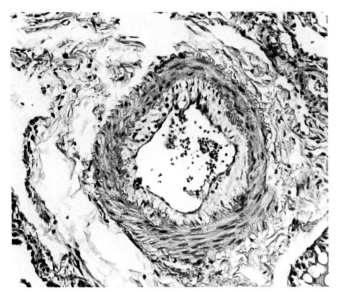

Fig. 29–30. Cellular intimal proliferation in muscular pulmonary artery with narrowing of lumen in 18-year-old girl with ventricular septal defect.

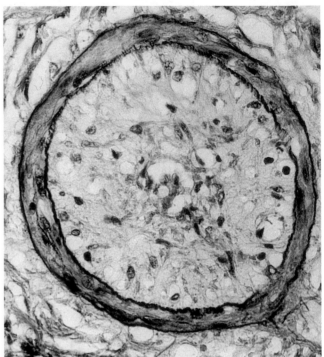

Fig. 29–31. Cellular intimal proliferation in muscular pulmonary artery with prominent narrowing of lumen in 6-year-old boy with ventricular septal defect.

layer of intimal fibrosis with a peculiar onion-skin configuration. This *concentric-laminar intimal fibrosis* (Fig. 29–32) usually occurs over considerable distances within the arteries.[125] Often it consists of an outer paucicellular layer with an inner layer of cellular proliferation. Concentric-laminar intimal fibrosis often leads to complete obliteration of the arterial lumen.

Certain arterial changes in plexogenic arteriopathy have in common a prominent dilatation of arterial segments. It is likely that this is caused by local incompetence of the muscular coat in the presence of a severely elevated intraluminal pressure. These so-called dilatation lesions[152] vary from "vein-like branches" to clusters of dilated, very thin-walled arterial segments (Fig. 29–33). If these clusters become very large, the term angiomatoid lesion may apply. The exact place of the dilatation lesions within the sequence of vascular alterations is not entirely clear, but it seems likely that they may develop at various stages, although only in the presence of severe pulmonary hypertension.

One of the most advanced arterial lesions, *fibrinoid necrosis* (Fig. 29–34), is found particularly in branches shortly after their ramification from a larger parent artery. A short stretch of the vascular wall becomes swollen with fibrin, followed by disintegration of the medial smooth muscle cells and often also of the elastic laminae. A clot of fibrin and platelets usually is formed within the lumen. There is much evidence suggesting that fibrinoid necrosis results from intense, spastic vasoconstriction and that the clot is caused by damage of the arterial wall.

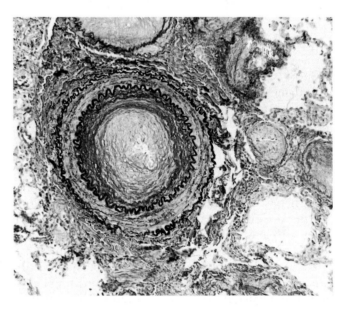

Fig. 29–32. Concentric-laminar intimal fibrosis in muscular pulmonary artery in 9-year-old girl with atrial septal defect.

Fibrinoid necrosis may or may not be accompanied by an inflammatory exudate that is usually mild to moderate and most commonly consists of lymphocytes. Sometiems, however, particularly in patients with congenital cardiac shunts, plexogenic arteriopathy is dominated by

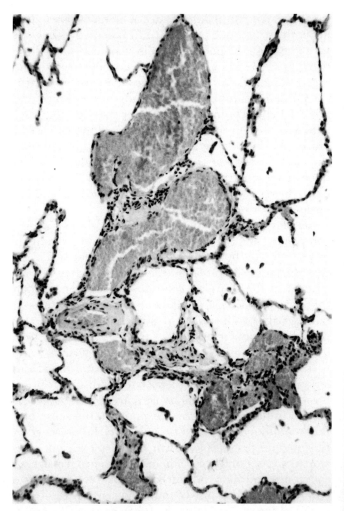

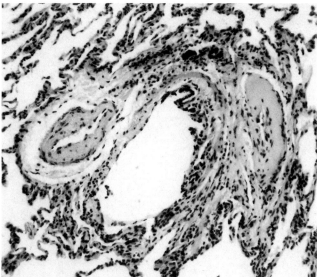

Fig. 29–34. Fibrinoid necrosis in muscular pulmonary artery (from case in Fig. 29.33).

Fig. 29–33. Dilatation lesions (vein-like branches) in 10-year-old boy with complete transposition of the great arteries and ventricular septal defect.

pulmonary arteritis with a very extensive exudate of polymorphonuclear cells extending well into the adjacent lung tissue (Fig. 29–35); the picture resembles that of polyarteritis nodosa. In these instances, the necrosis of the arterial wall varies in severity. The elastic laminae sometimes are intact, even in the presence of a pronounced inflammatory reaction. Arterial branches affected by this prominent form of arteritis are generally of larger caliber than those with mere fibrinoid necrosis, and the vascular segment involved bears no special relationship with points of ramification. It is therefore unlikely that fibrinoid necrosis and arteritis have a similar pathogenesis.

The last alteration in the sequence of changes in plexogenic arteriopathy is the *plexiform lesion* (Fig. 29–36), which probably develops in segments affected by fibrinoid necrosis.[125] Plexiform lesions are found especially in supernumerary arteries[153] and in a loca-

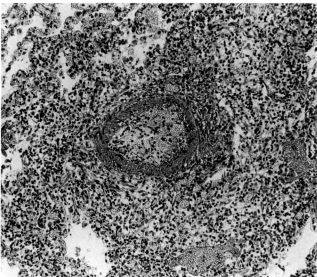

Fig. 29–35. Pulmonary arteritis with fibrinoid necrosis in 13-year-old girl with primary plexogenic arteriopathy.

tion similar to that of fibrinoid necrosis, that is, immediately distal to a site of ramification. Here there is a focal destruction of the arterial wall in which fibrinoid necrosis is often still recognizable. The plexiform lesion consists of local dilatation of the artery; the arterial lumen is filled by a plexus of capillary-like channels separated by strands of cells with hyperchromatic nuclei. This plexus is apparently formed by organization and recanalization of the fibrin clot. The channels of the plexus open up into dilated, thin-walled distal branches

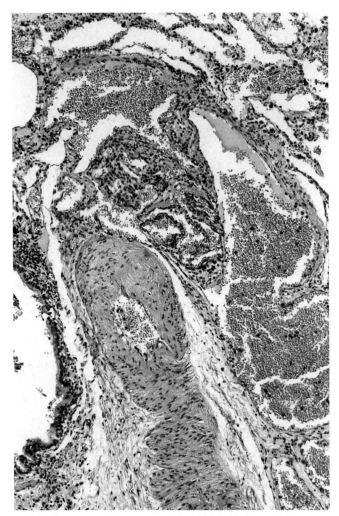

Fig. 29–36. Plexiform lesion in 32-year-old man with plexogenic arteriopathy associated with hepatic cirrhosis. Afferent part of artery shows fibrinoid necrosis; distal to plexus, artery is dilated and thin walled.

of the artery containing the plexiform lesion (see Fig. 29–36).

Some other vascular lesions may be found in association with plexogenic arteriopathy, although they do not strictly belong to that pattern but rather complicate it. These include pulmonary venous changes, in the presence of cardiac failure or mitral incompetence (p. 1012), thrombotic changes, particularly in primary plexogenic arteriopathy and in complete transposition of the great arteries (p. 1004), and longitudinal smooth muscle bundles in the intima of arterioles.[154]

Reversibility and Prognostic Significance

In patients with congenital cardiac disease and pulmonary hypertension who undergo pulmonary artery banding and, a few years later, correction of their

cardiac defect, lung biopsies are sometimes taken during both the banding procedure and corrective surgery. By comparing the pulmonary vascular changes in these two biopsy specimens, it has been possible to study the regression of lesions following the creation of the artificial pulmonic stenosis.[155] Such studies have shown that medial hypertrophy of pulmonary arteries regresses either completely or to a great extent. In the absence of more advanced lesions at the time of corrective surgery, such cases carry a good prognosis. Very severe medial hypertrophy, particularly in infants, may cause problems during or shortly after surgery because of sudden episodes of severe vasoconstriction.[156]

Cellular intimal proliferation may regress almost completely, and the same applies to concentric-laminar intimal fibrosis but only so long as it is mild. It is likely that dilatation lesions may regress when they are restricted to the so-called vein-like branches and when these are few. Large numbers of dilatation lesions and particularly of clusters and angiomatoid lesions are probably always irreversible, and in any event such lesions carry a far more unfavorable prognosis.

In our experience, fibrinoid necrosis and plexiform lesions are virtually always associated with a poor prognosis, even when such lesions are scarce or when there is a good initial postoperative response in the sense of a fall in pulmonary arterial pressure. In the presence of fibrinoid necrosis or plexiform lesions, plexogenic arteriopathy is not only irreversible but also progressive, so that more and more advanced lesions develop despite elimination of the cause of pulmonary hypertension by repair of the cardiac anomaly. It becomes a self-perpetuating vascular disease, usually with a gradual deterioration leading to death within a few years but sometimes with a protracted course for as long as 20 years or more.

It is clear, therefore, that in plexogenic arteriopathy there is a point of no return; histologically, this is represented somewhere between moderate and severe concentric-laminar intimal fibrosis with medial hypertrophy and cellular intimal proliferation on the favorable side and fibrinoid necrosis and plexiform lesions on the unfavorable side.[157]

Plexogenic arteriopathy is particularly progressive and thus has an especially bleak prognosis in patients with Down's syndrome and complete atrioventricular canal.[158]

Congestive Vasculopathy

The term congestive vasculopathy is used for a combination of pulmonary vascular lesions occurring in cases of chronic congestion of the lungs. The lesions are not limited to the pulmonary arteries but are often also prominent in the pulmonary veins, so that it is preferable to speak of vasculopathy. Significant changes of this pattern are virtually always associated with pulmonary venous hypertension, although they form no reliable basis for estimating the magnitude of the increase in pulmonary arterial pressure.

Clinical Presentation

The clinical manifestations associated with congestive vasculopathy depend largely on the underlying condition. The signs and symptoms of congestive failure include dyspnea, edema, cough, and chest pain. Right-ventricular hypertrophy and failure may occur; the right-atrial pressure may be elevated. In some patients extrasystoles or atrial fibrillation may be observed.

Etiology and Pathogenesis

Any impediment to the pulmonary venous outflow may result in pulmonary venous hypertension and congestive vasculopathy. Obstruction of major veins, as in congenital stenosis, is rare. In *cor triatriatum*, where a membranous septum divides the left atrium into two chambers, and in *left-atrial myxoma* the impediment to venous return is at atrial level. In virtually all other instances, the impediment is at or distal to the mitral valve. These conditions include congenital mitral stenosis or atresia, acquired rheumatic mitral stenosis, mitral or aortic valve incompetence, and chronic left-ventricular failure from any cause. Processes outside the heart such as mediastinal fibrosis may also lead to secondary compression of pulmonary venous trunks and thus to pulmonary venous hypertension. Independent of the cause of pulmonary venous hypertension, the pattern of pulmonary vascular lesions in which arteries, veins, lymphatics, and even the lung parenchyma participate is the same.

The pathogenesis of congestive vasculopathy is incompletely understood. Elevated pressure in the pulmonary veins is transmitted through the alveolar capillaries to the pulmonary arteries. However, for unknown reasons the pressure in the arteries is disproportionally increased, and may become equal to or exceed the systemic pressure. Possibly the initial mild elevation transmitted from the pulmonary veins results in a slight dilatation of the arteries, which in turn may be a stimulus for vasoconstriction. Individual differences in reactivity of the lung vessels are also likely to influence arterial contraction.[159]

Pulmonary Arterial Changes

In all muscular arteries there is a definite tendency to *medial hypertrophy*, which may be very pronounced (Fig. 29–37); it is usually associated with muscularization of

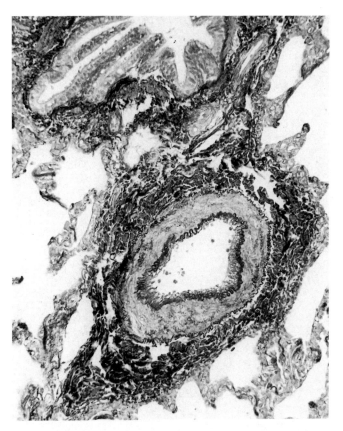

Fig. 29–37. Severe medial hypertrophy in muscular pulmonary artery in 39-year-old woman with rheumatic mitral stenosis.

arterioles. In contrast to plexogenic arteriopathy, there is generally a poor correlation between medial thickness on the one hand and pulmonary arterial pressure and resistance on the other.[125,160] Strikingly, a very thick media is often associated with only a mild or moderate increase in pressure. In part this may be explained by interstitial edema and deposition of collagen and ground substance, resulting in an increase of medial thickness but a decrease of relative muscularity.[161] The increase in medial thickness tends to be more severe in the lower parts of the lungs.

Intimal fibrosis is common, often severe, and involves long stretches of the arteries. However, it does not lead to obliteration of the lumen. It is usually eccentric (Fig. 29–38), but even when circumferential it does not have an onion-skin appearance. The degree of intimal thickening does not correlate closely with pressure and resistance.[162] In contrast to medial hypertrophy, intimal fibrosis is usually more severe in the upper parts of the lungs.

The *adventitia* is also increased in thickness.[163] Pulmonary arteritis, usually with fibrinoid necrosis, is occasionally observed but dilatation lesions and plexiform lesions are absent.

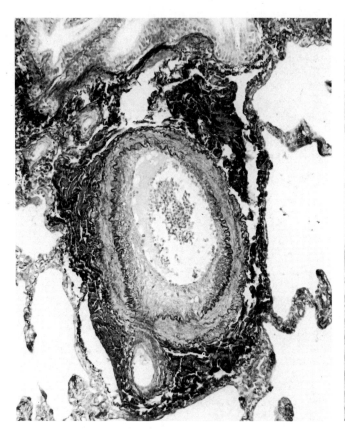

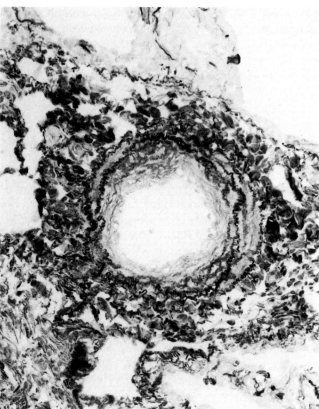

Fig. 29–38. Medial hypertrophy and intimal fibrosis in muscular pulmonary artery (from case in Fig. 29.37).

Fig. 29–39. Medial thickening and arterialization of pulmonary vein in 49-year-old woman with rheumatic mitral stenosis.

Pulmonary Venous Changes

In contrast to thrombotic and plexogenic arteriopathy, in congestive vasculopathy the pulmonary veins are also affected. Usually there is *medial hypertrophy* of the venous wall, which may become very prominent. The elastic configuration also changes in such a way that distinct internal and external elastic laminae are formed, just as in a muscular pulmonary artery (Fig. 29–39).[164,165] This *arterialization* sometimes makes it difficult to distinguish between arteries and veins, so that their location next to bronchi and in interlobular septa, respectively, becomes the only criterion. Intimal fibrosis of veins is common but is usually mild.

Pulmonary Parenchymal Changes

Interstitial edema causes widening not only of interlobular septa but, in many instances, also of alveolar walls, resulting in *interstitial fibrosis*. When iron pigment from extravasated erythrocytes accumulates in alveolar macrophages or within the interstitium, this *hemosiderosis* (Fig. 29–40) in combination with the interstitial fibrosis

produces the gross picture of brown induration of the lung. *Corpora amylacea*, concentrically ringed rounded bodies consisting of glycoproteins, and somewhat similar but calcified bodies, the *microliths*, are relatively often found in the alveolar spaces although neither is specific for congestive vasculopathy. Trabeculated *osseous nodules* are occasionally observed in pulmonary venous hypertension (see Chapter 22). The pulmonary lymphatics are usually dilated.

Reversibility

Data on the reversibility of congestive vasculopathy are scarce. Following commissurotomy in patients with rheumatic mitral stenosis, there is usually a distinct fall of pressure in the pulmonary circulation. This fall is sometimes surprisingly abrupt, not only in the presence of pronounced medial hypertrophy but also in that of severe intimal fibrosis, suggesting that elimination of interstitial edema from the vascular wall results in a rapid decrease of vascular resistance. Long-term and virtually complete regression of extensive and severe

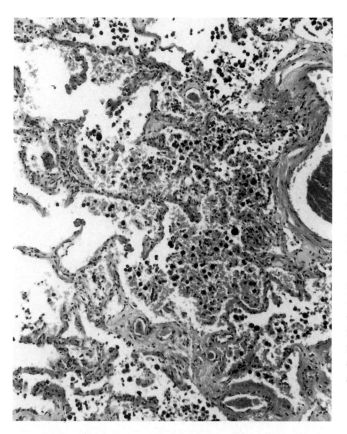

Fig. 29–40. Prominent hemosiderosis and focal interstitial fibrosis of lung tissue (from case in Fig. 29–39).

medial hypertrophy and intimal fibrosis has also occasionally been demonstrated.[125] In some patients with similar pulmonary vascular changes, pulmonary hypertension persisted following mitral valve surgery[166]; others, despite a marked decrease in pulmonary arterial pressure, did poorly, probably as a result of extensive alterations in the lung tissue.[167]

Pulmonary Veno-Occlusive Disease

The term pulmonary veno-occlusive disease[168] is used for a form of hypertensive pulmonary vascular disease in which the pulmonary veins and venules are particularly involved. The name has retained its general use, even after it became clear that in many cases the pulmonary arteries are also affected.

Clinical Presentation

As in primary plexogenic arteriopathy and silent embolic pulmonary hypertension, the development of pulmonary veno-occlusive disease is insidious, the clinical diagnosis exceedingly difficult, and the prognosis very

unfavorable. The course of the disease is sometimes very rapid, but more often protracted and gradually downhill; very rare reports mention improvement. Hemoptysis is one of the risks.[169]

Etiology and Pathogenesis

There is little doubt that the causes of pulmonary veno-occlusive disease are extremely varied. Viral infections, toxic agents, and chemotherapy are among the suspected eliciting factors.[170] However, the pathogenesis is likely to be the same in all instances. The nature of the vascular lesions suggests that thrombosis of pulmonary veins and, to a lesser extent, of arteries is basic to their development.

Pulmonary veno-occlusive disease particularly affects children and young adults, although no age is exempt. As in primary plexogenic arteriopathy, the sex ratio in children is equal, but in contrast to the latter condition, in adulthood men are more often affected.[171] Clinically these two forms of pulmonary hypertension are very difficult to distinguish, and the prognosis of both is equally poor.

Pulmonary Venous Changes

In pulmonary veno-occlusive disease the small veins and venules are particularly affected, although large veins even close to the hilum may occasionally be involved. The lumens of the vessels are narrowed or occluded by intimal fibrosis, which usually is of loose texture (Fig. 29–41) but sometimes is dense and rich in collagen. Recanalization of intimal fibrosis and intravascular septa, indicating a thrombotic origin of the lesions, are common in pulmonary veno-occlusive disease. The media of the pulmonary veins is often thickened with distinct arterialization.

Pulmonary Arterial and Parenchymal Changes

The pulmonary arteries exhibit varying degrees of medial hypertrophy. In approximately half of the cases there is intimal fibrosis as well, although often less severe in arteries (Fig. 29–42) than in veins.[171,172] This has often been taken as a change secondary to pulmonary venous obstruction, but the loose type of intimal fibrosis suggests that its pathogenesis is the same as in the veins. Recanalization and septa formation frequently occur, and sometimes an artery is completely obliterated, alterations that are uncommon in pulmonary venous hypertension. In many cases, the arterial lesions are suggestive as being of later date than the venous lesions; in particular, recent thrombi are un-

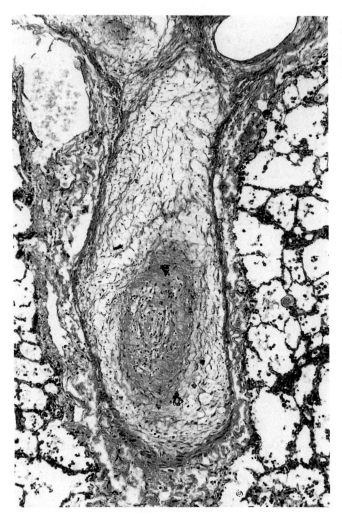

Fig. 29–41. Pulmonary vein completely obliterated by loose connective tissue in 16-year-old boy with pulmonary veno-occlusive disease.

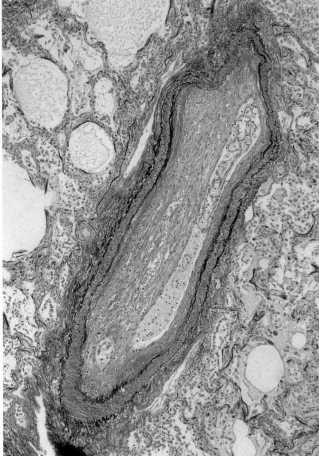

Fig. 29–42. Muscular pulmonary artery with prominent intimal fibrosis in 39-year-old woman with pulmonary veno-occlusive disease.

common in veins but are commonly observed in arteries.[171]

In most patients with pulmonary veno-occlusive disease, scattered small nodular areas of congestion or interstitial fibrosis are associated with prominent hemosiderosis (Fig. 29–43); this is a useful diagnostic sign. Lymphatics are often dilated, sometimes to an extraordinary extent.

Reversibility

Little is known about the reversibility of the vascular lesions of pulmonary veno-occlusive disease. Regression of obliterative intimal fibrosis of veins is unlikely, and restoration of flow as the result of recanalization is probably very limited. This is in keeping with the clinical experience that it is a progressive disease; with

rare exceptions, the results of therapy are disappointing.

Hypoxic Arteriopathy

Acute alveolar hypoxia acts as a potent vasconstrictor on the pulmonary arterial tree, causing an immediate elevation of pulmonary arterial pressure. Chronic alveolar hypoxia may produce persistent pulmonary hypertension and vascular alterations. Although the lesions are not confined to the pulmonary arteries but may be found in the veins, the latter changes are often minimal and not readily detectable without morphometric methods. Therefore, this pattern of pulmonary vascular changes is known as hypoxic arteriopathy.

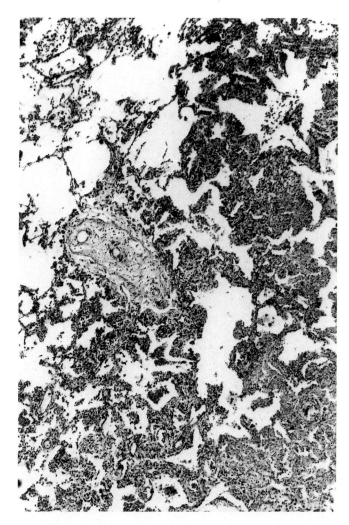

Fig. 29–43. Part of nodular area of congestion with some interstitial fibrosis of lung tissue and one obliterated vein (from case in Fig. 29–41).

Clinical Presentation

To a large extent, the clinical course and the prognosis of chronic hypoxic pulmonary hypertension are determined by the condition that caused the hypoxia and therefore may vary greatly. However, as compared to several other forms of pulmonary hypertension, and considering the usually mild or moderate elevation of pulmonary arterial pressure in many patients with hypoxic lung disease, the incidence of right-ventricular failure is disproportionally high. If the cause of the hypoxia can be eliminated, the pulmonary hypertension appears to be reversible. A good example is seen following adenoidectomy in children with upper-airway obstruction caused by enlarged adenoids.[173]

Etiology and Pathogenesis

Alveolar hypoxia produces pulmonary vasoconstriction and thereby in the long run persistent pulmonary hypertension, right-ventricular hypertrophy, and pulmonary vascular lesions. This happens regardless the cause of the hypoxia. Any chronic obstruction of the airways may produce hypoxic pulmonary hypertension. In children, obstruction by enlarged adenoid tonsils may have this effect. In adults, the most common cause of airway obstruction is chronic obstructive lung disease. Alveolar hypoxia may also result from impaired respiration, as occurs in Pickwickian syndrome, kyphoscoliosis, or thoracic muscular atrophy.

A mild-to-moderate degree of pulmonary hypertension occurs in healthy people living at high altitudes, particularly in the Andes and the Himalayas. At the prevailing low barometric pressures, the oxygen pressure of the atmospheric air is decreased. Rarely, residents of this altitude suffer from chronic mountain sickness and severe pulmonary hypertension. Another hazard of high altitudes is high-altitude pulmonary edema (p. 986), particularly following a too rapid ascent in combination with severe physical exercise. Young healthy people and mountain residents returning to their homes after spending some time at sea level are especially at risk.

An individual variation in pulmonary vascular reactivity explains why some people are far more affected by hypoxia than others. Experimentally, it has been shown that hyperreactivity as well as hyporeactivity of the lung vessels is genetically determined.[174] There are also racial differences in vascular response to hypoxia.[175] Although the morphologic vascular alterations are clearly initiated by vasoconstriction, the way in which contraction is mediated has not yet been satisfactorily solved.[176,177] The search for a mediator is still going on, and it has not even been determined whether there is a mediator or whether arterial constriction is caused by a direct effect on the muscular coat. In this respect, it is important to note that the changes are predominantly to be found in the small-caliber intraacinar lung vessels that are in close contact with the alveolar air.

Pulmonary Arterial Changes

The most striking finding in hypoxic pulmonary hypertension is usually the discrepancy between the lesions in large and medium-sized muscular pulmonary arteries on the one hand, and those in small, particularly intraacinar, arteries on the other. The larger vessels may be completely normal. If there is medial hypertrophy, it is generally mild. In contrast, small arteries show distinct medial hypertrophy, while previously nonmuscular branches become muscularized (Fig. 29–44).[178,179]

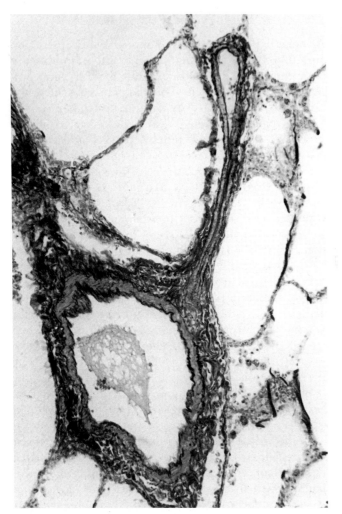

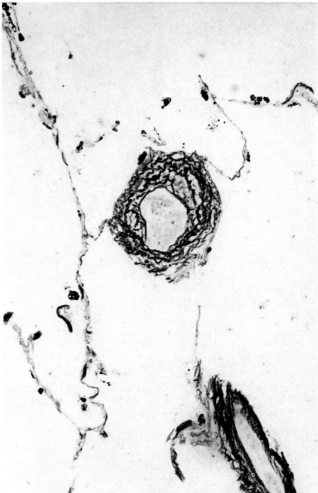

Fig. 29–44. Muscular pulmonary artery with normal media gives rise to pulmonary arteriole with distinct muscularization in 37-year-old man with Pickwickian syndrome and hypoxic pulmonary hypertension.

Fig. 29–45. Pulmonary arteriole with development of longitudinal smooth muscle fibers in 50-year-old man with chronic bronchitis and emphysema.

A second alteration, also limited to small arteries although not as widely distributed, is the development of longitudinal smooth muscle bundles or layers within the intima (Fig. 29–45). Intimal fibrosis is not a feature of hypoxic arteriopathy. In chronic obstructive lung disease, however, it is commonly found, but then it is either a reaction to the accompanying inflammation and peribronchial fibrosis or the result of thromboembolic events.

Pulmonary Venous Changes

In experimental hypoxia, it can be demonstrated that there is a reaction not only of small arteries but also of small veins; the smooth muscle cells within the venous media show the ultrastructural signs of intense contrac-

tion.[180] In humans, morphologic assessment of the pulmonary venous walls has shown that the thickness of the media is also increased in the veins. Moreover, intimal bundles of longitudinal smooth muscle may be found in occasional small veins.[181]

Reversibility

An opportunity to study regression of morphologic vascular changes after elimination of the cause of hypoxic pulmonary hypertension almost never occurs. Such a regression is sometimes suggested from clinical data. In experimental animals it has been demonstrated that hypoxic arteriopathy is essentially reversible, although it takes more time for the arterial muscularity to decrease than to develop.

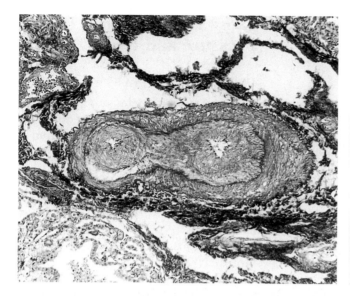

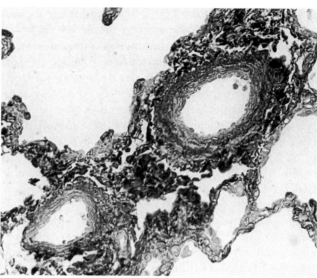

Fig. 29–46. Muscular pulmonary artery with severe medial hypertrophy and intimal fibrosis lying within area of lung fibrosis in 61-year-old man.

Fig. 29–47. Pulmonary vein with medial thickening and intimal fibrosis lying close to area of lung fibrosis (from case in Fig. 29–46).

Pulmonary Vasculopathy in Lung Fibrosis

Etiology and Pathogenesis

Various forms of focal or interstitial lung fibrosis and granulomatosis are regularly accompanied by alterations in the lung vessels. These changes, which usually are very pronounced although nonspecific, occur in pulmonary arteries as well as in veins and in media as well as in intima.[125] The importance of these lesions lies in the danger of misinterpretation; they may easily be confused with those of congestive vasculopathy. Moreover, it is often not realized that, despite the severity of the alterations, the pulmonary arterial pressure is not necessarily elevated. In fact, severe pulmonary hypertension is uncommon in most forms of lung fibrosis. The exact cause of the vascular alterations is not well understood.

Pulmonary Vascular Changes

Both muscular pulmonary arteries and pulmonary veins of comparable size exhibit pronounced thickening of the media. In the veins, this is usually accompanied by arterialization. Severe intimal fibrosis, which is eccentric and nonlaminar, also occurs in these vessels (Figs. 29–46 and 29–47). Although such changes would strongly suggest pulmonary hypertension when found in a lung biopsy specimen from a fibrotic area, the pulmonary arterial pressure may be completely normal because the changes are limited to arteries and veins within or adjacent to fibrotic areas. In areas of normal lung tissue, the vessels are also normal. The chance of mistaking these vascular lesions for those of congestive vasculopathy, thus suggesting pulmonary venous hypertension, is enhanced by the presence of interstitial fibrosis, because interstitial fibrosis is commonly found when there is an impediment to the pulmonary venous flow (p. 1012).

Reversibility

Because fibrosis and scarring of lung tissue do not revert to normal, it must be assumed that the reactive vascular lesions are irreversible.

Unexplained Pulmonary Hypertension

In 1975 a Committee of the World Health Organization[127] suggested using the term primary pulmonary hypertension as an equivalent of clinically unexplained pulmonary hypertension. In their report, it was pointed out that patients suffering from pulmonary hypertension for which no cause could be identified clinically usually belong to one of three morphologically completely different categories.[149,182,183] These were listed as silent recurrent thromboembolism, pulmonary veno-occlusive disease, and primary plexogenic arteriopathy.

In the past, the latter condition was often referred to as "primary pulmonary hypertension," but because this is a clinical hemodynamic term by definition, substitution by a designation on the basis of morphology was deemed advisable. While this is certainly true, in practice the present terminology has led to some confusion because the term primary pulmonary hypertension is often used as a diagnosis, which it is not, and because it is also often used in the old sense of the plexogenic variety. The morphology of the primary form of plexogenic arteriopathy is essentially the same as that in secondary forms.[149,184,185] However, progression to more advanced changes such as plexiform lesions is apparently rapid because these are found in the great majority of cases. Thrombotic changes complicating the histologic pattern of primary plexogenic arteriopathy are particularly common in adult patients.[185a]

Any form of pulmonary hypertension, as well as the three conditions mentioned, may remain clinically unexplained for various reasons. Some very rare forms of hypertensive pulmonary vascular disease are not recognized because the clinician is not familiar with them. Examples are multiple *medial defects of muscular pulmonary arteries,* resulting in a peculiar type of intimal fibrosis that gradually obliterates the arterial tree,[186] and *capillary hemangiomatosis,* an active proliferation of capillary-like channels invading pleura and interlobular septa and the walls of bronchi and vessels.[187] In infants and young children, a rare syndrome consisting of persistent fetal pulmonary circulation, underdevelopment of alveoli, interstitial fibrosis, and *misalignment of lung vessels,* has been recognized.[188] In these instances the pulmonary veins are in abnormal position, being located next to the pulmonary arteries instead of within interlobular septa.

For various reasons, more common forms of pulmonary hypertension sometimes remain unexplained. This may happen in patients with hypoxic pulmonary hypertension as there is occasionally a great discrepancy between a mild form of chronic obstructive lung disease and a very severe pulmonary hypertension.[149] Pulmonary venous hypertension also is sometimes not recognized when technical problems during catheterization prevent detection of an acquired or congenital valvular abnormality. Finally, an underlying condition responsible for the elevation of pulmonary arterial pressure may remain asymptomatic so that it escapes recognition. Tumor embolism, particularly from a gastric or mammary carcinoma, may in this way be the cause of unexplained pulmonary hypertension.[91,93] In all these situations an open lung biopsy is the only reliable method to establish the diagnosis.[122]

Vasculopathy in Diminished Pulse Pressure and Flow

Etiology and Pathogenesis

A diminished pulse pressure in the pulmonary circulation occurs particularly when there is an impediment to the pulmonary arterial flow. It is observed most often in congenital heart disease with pulmonary or tricuspid stenosis. In tetralogy of Fallot, it is associated with a diminished pulmonary flow and usually with an increased hematocrit. Rarely, acquired obstruction of the pulmonary trunk or one of its larger branches may produce similar lesions. As a rule, the mean pulmonary arterial pressure in these instances is only slightly below normal. Therefore, it is clear that the absence of prominent systolic peaks from the pressure curve, which may become almost completely flat, is an important factor in producing these sometimes pronounced pulmonary arterial alterations. Other lesions, particularly in tetralogy of Fallot, are based on an increased tendency to thrombosis.

Pulmonary Vascular Lesions

The most constant pulmonary arterial change in the presence of a pulmonary or tricuspid stenosis is thinning of the media.[189] This is not always immediately recognized, because the difference compared to normal thin-walled arteries is often not striking and may require morphometric assessment. There are, however, many cases, particularly of tetralogy of Fallot, in which the media becomes extremely atrophic (Fig. 29–48). In these instances, even medium-sized muscular pulmonary arteries are sometimes completely devoid of smooth muscle. Both arteries and veins are usually dilated.

Recent or organized thrombi are common, particularly in tetralogy of Fallot. In our experience they are virtually limited to pulmonary arteries and are very uncommon in veins. There is a marked tendency to recanalization, and the channels formed in this way usually become very wide so that delicate intravascular fibrous septa, separating the lumen into multiple compartments, develop (Fig. 29–49).[190] Bronchopulmonary anastomoses are increased in size and numbers, as are the collateral arteries within the pleura.

Reversibility: Effects of Cardiac Surgery

Correction of the cardiac anomaly will result in some increase in medial thickness. It is doubtful whether the postthrombotic lesions, including the intravascular septa, will regress. However, postoperative pulmonary

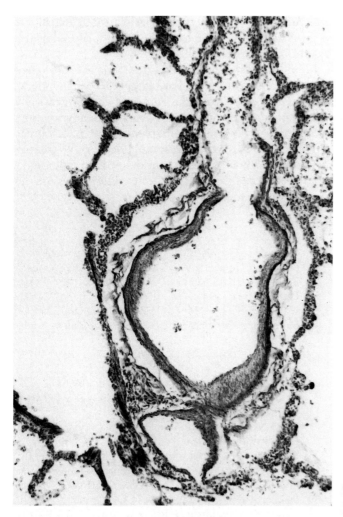

Fig. 29–48. Severe medial atrophy with complete absence of vascular smooth muscle in 5-year-old boy with tetralogy of Fallot. Note layer of intimal fibrosis.

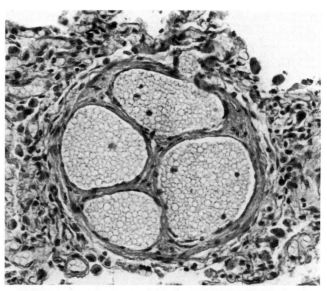

Fig. 29–49. Delicate intravascular fibrous septa caused by recanalization of organized thrombus in muscular pulmonary artery in 19-year-old woman with tetralogy of Fallot. Note also medial atrophy.

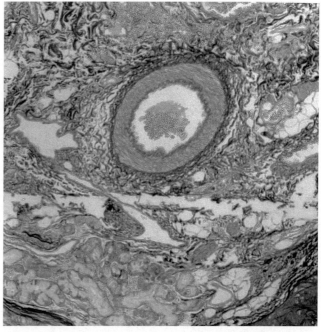

Fig. 29–50. Bronchial artery with increased medial thickness in 32-year-old man with systemic hypertension.

hypertension as a result of such postthrombotic lesions is very uncommon. Plexogenic arteriopathy with severe pulmonary hypertension is a well-documented complication of palliative operations when too large a shunt between systemic and pulmonary circulations has been created (see p. 1006).

Bronchial Vessels and Pulmonary Lymphatics

In only a few situations do conspicuous alterations occur in the bronchial vessels, which tend to be normal in pulmonary hypertension but may show some medial hypertrophy in systemic hypertension, in the same way as other systemic arteries (Fig. 29–50). Bundles or layers of longitudinal smooth muscle cells are often found within the intima of bronchial arteries in normal persons, particularly older individuals; these may narrow or even occlude the lumens of these arteries. Such changes are even more common in patients with pulmonary venous hypertension or lung fibrosis. Similar

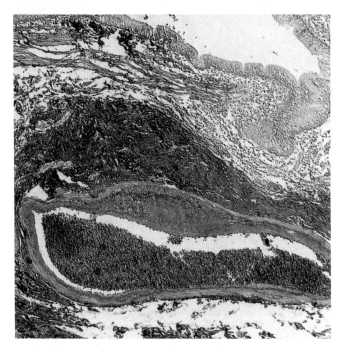

Fig. 29–51. Greatly enlarged bronchial arteries with some eccentric intimal fibrosis in wall of dilated bronchus in 14-year-old boy with bronchiectasis.

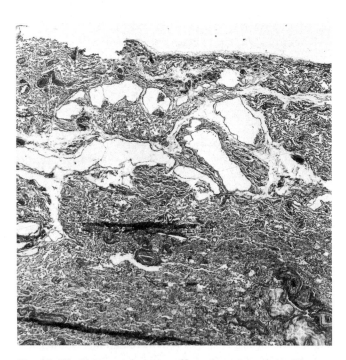

Fig. 29–52. Circumscript area of lymphangiectasis in 45-year-old man with rheumatic mitral stenosis.

smooth muscle bundles are common in collateral arteries in diminished pulmonary flow.

In bronchiectasis the flow through the bronchial arteries increases manyfold (see Chapter 5). Accord-ingly, the caliber of these arteries is usually extremely large, although the lumen may be secondarily narrowed by intimal fibrosis (Fig. 29–51).

In pulmonary venous hypertension, the bronchial veins and the pulmonary lymphatics are usually mark-edly dilated. The bronchial veins are characteristically located around the bronchi, whereas dilated lymphatics are observed particularly in pleura and interlobular septa. Clusters of dilated lymphatics or lymphang-iectases (Fig. 29–52) are sometimes found in pulmonary venous hypertension. They occur only rarely in the absence of an elevated pressure.

References

1. Reeves JT, Groves BM. Approach to the patient with pulmonary hypertension. In: EK Weir, JT Reeves, eds. Pulmonary hypertension. Mount Kisco, New York: Futura, 1984:1–44.
2. Wagenvoort CA, Mooi WJ. Biopsy pathology of the pulmonary vasculature. London: Chapman & Hall, 1989.
3. Staub NC. Pulmonary edema. Physiol Rev 1974; 54:678–811.
4. Hall JG, Morris B, Woolley G. Intrinsic rhythmic pro-pulsion of lymph in the unanesthesized sheep. J Physiol 1965;180:336–349.
5. Staub NC. The pathophysiology of pulmonary edema. Hum Pathol 1970;1:419–432.
6. Hultgren HN. High altitude pulmonary edema. In: Staub, NC, ed. Lung water and solute exchange. Lung biology in health and disease, Vol. 7. New York: Marcel Dekker, 1978:437–469.
7. Bärtsch P, Maggiorini M, Ritter M, Noti C, Vock P, Oelz O. Prevention of high-altitude pulmonary edema by nifedipine. N Engl J Med 1991;325:1284–1289.
8. Sandritter W, Thomas C. Makropathologie. Lehrbuch und Atlas für Studierende und Ärzte. Stuttgart: Schat-tauer Verlag, 1977:4.
9. Plank L, James J, Wagenvoort CA. Caliber and elastin content of the pulmonary trunk. Arch Pathol Lab Med 1980;104:238–241.
10. Heath D, Wood EH, DuShane JW, Edwards JE. The structure of the pulmonary trunk at different ages and in cases of pulmonary hypertension and pulmonary stenosis. J Pathol Bacteriol 1959;77:443–456.
11. Heath D, Wood EH, DuShane JW, Edwards JE. The relation of age and blood pressure to atheroma in the pulmonary arteries and thoracic aorta in congenital heart disease. Lab Invest 1960;9:259–272.
12. Bartter T, Irwin RS, Nash G. Aneurysms of the pulmo-nary arteries. Chest 1988;94:1065–1075.
13. Shull WK, Kapadia SB, Zuberbuhler JR. Aneurysm of the main pulmonary artery. Association with patent ductus arteriosus and ostium secundum defect. Am J Dis Child 1970;119:507–509.
14. Goh TH. Mycotic aneurysm of the pulmonary artery; a report of 2 cases. Br Heart J 1974;36:387–390.

15. Butto F, Lucas RV, Edwards JE. Pulmonary arterial aneurysm. A pathologic study of five cases. Chest 1987;91:237–241.

16. Barbour DJ, Roberts WC. Aneurysm of the pulmonary trunk unassociated with intracardiac or great vessel left-to-right shunting. Am J Cardiol 1987;59:192–194.

17. Epstein S, Naji AF. Pulmonary artery aneurysm with dissection after Blalock operation for tetralogy of Fallot. Am J Cardiol 1960;5:560–563.

18. Lakhani ZM, McGarry KM, Taylor RF, Fortune RL, Juglutt BI. Two-dimensional echocardiographic detection of left pulmonary artery aneurysm following Potts' anastomosis. Chest 1983;84:782–783.

19. Charlton RW, Du Plessis LA. Multiple pulmonary artery aneurysms. Thorax 1961;16:364–371.

20. Dennison AR, Watkins RM, Gunning AJ. Simultaneous aortic and pulmonary artery aneurysms due to giant cell arteritis. Thorax 1985;40:156–157.

21. Symbas PN, Scott HW. Traumatic aneurysm of the pulmonary artery. J Thorac Cardiovasc Surg 1963; 45:645–649.

22. Nguien GK, Dowling GP. Dissecting aneurysm of the pulmonary trunk. Arch Pathol Lab Med 1989; 113:1178–1179.

23. Sardesai SH, Marshall RJ, Farrow R, Mourant AJ. Dissecting aneurysm of the pulmonary artery in a case of unoperated patient ductus arteriosus. Eur Heart J 1990;11:670–673.

24. Rosenson RS, Sutton MSJ. Dissecting aneurysm of the pulmonary trunk in mitral stenosis. Am J Cardiol 1986;58:1140–1141.

25. Steurer J, Jenni R, Medici TC, Vollrath T, Hess OM, Siegenthaler W. Dissecting aneurysm of the pulmonary artery with pulmonary hypertension. Am Rev Respir Dis 1990;142:1219–1221.

26. Hayes WL, Farha SJ, Brown RL. Primary leiomyosarcoma of the pulmonary artery. Am J Cardiol 1974; 34:615–617.

27. Bleisch VR, Kraus FT. Polypoid sarcoma of the pulmonary trunk: analysis of the literature and report of a case with leptomeric organelles and ultrastructural features of rhabdomyosarcoma. Cancer 1980;46:314–324.

28. Baker PB, Goodwin RA. Pulmonary artery sarcomas: A review and report of a case. Arch Pathol Lab Med 1985;109:35–39.

29. Thomas WA, Davies JNP, O'Neal RM, Dimakulangan AA. Incidence of myocardial infarction correlated with venous and pulmonary thrombosis and embolism. A geographic study based on autopsies in Uganda, East Africa and St. Louis, U.S.A. Am J Cardiol 1960;5: 41–47.

30. Woo KS, Tse LKK, Tse CY, Metreweli C, Vallance-Owen J. The prevalence and patterns of pulmonary thromboembolism in the Chinese in Hong Kong. Int J Cardiol 1988;20:373–380.

31. Lilienfeld DE, Chan E, Ehland J, Godbold JH, Landrigan PJ, Marsh G. Mortality from pulmonary embolism in the United States: 1962 to 1984. Chest 1990; 98:1067–1072.

32. Fleming HA, Bailey SM. Massive pulmonary embolism in healthy people. Br Med J 1966;1:1322–1327.

33. Goldhaber SZ, Savage DD, Garrison RJ, et al. Risk factors for pulmonary embolism. The Framingham Study. Am J Med 1983;74:1023–1028.

34. Moser KM. Venous thromboembolism. Am Rev Respir Dis 1990;141:235–249.

35. Gillum RF. Pulmonary embolism and thrombophlebitis in the United States, 1970–1985. Am Heart J 1987; 114:1262–1264.

36. Goldhaber SZ, Hennekens CH, Evans DA, Newton EC, Godleski JJ. Factors associated with correct antemortem diagnosis of major pulmonary embolism. Am J Med 1982;73:822–826.

37. Gross JS, Neufeld RR, Libow LS, Gerber I, Rodstein M. Autopsy study of the elderly institutionalized patient. Review of 234 autopsies. Arch Intern Med 1988; 148:173–176.

38. Rubinstein I, Murray D, Hoffstein V. Fatal pulmonary emboli in hospitalized patients. An autopsy study. Arch Intern Med 1988;148:1425–1426.

39. Morrell T, Dunnill MS. The post-mortem incidence of pulmonary embolism in a hospital population. Br J Surg 1968;55:347–352.

40. Freiman DG, Suyemoto J, Wessler S. Frequency of pulmonary thromboembolism in man. N Engl J Med 1965;272:1278–1280.

41. Messer JV. Thromboembolic pulmonary hypertension. In: EK Weir, JT Reeves, eds. Pulmonary hypertension. Mount Kisco, New York: Futura, 1984:169–249.

42. Karwinski B, Svendsen E. Comparison of clinical and postmortem diagnosis of pulmonary embolism. J Clin Pathol 1989;42:135–139.

43. PIOPED Investigators. Value of the ventilation/perfusion scan in acute pulmonary embolism: Results of the prospective investigation of pulmonary embolism diagnosis (PIOPED). JAMA 1990;263:2753–2796.

44. Fowler EF, Bollinger JA. Pulmonary embolism. Surgery (St. Louis) 1954;36:650–63.

45. Knisely WH, Wallace JM, Mahaley MS, Satterwhite WM. Evidence, including in vivo observations, suggesting mechanical blockage rather than reflex vasospasm as the cause of death in pulmonary embolization. Am Heart J 1957;54:483–497.

46. Pryce DM, Heard B. The distribution of experimental pulmonary emboli in the rabbit. J Pathol Bacteriol 1956;71:15–25.

47. Havig O, Grumer OPN. Pulmonary bone marrow embolism. A histological study of a non-selected autopsy material. Arch Pathol Microbiol Scand 1973;81:276–280.

48. McCarty PJ, Shmookler BM, Pierce LE. Fatal bone marrow pulmonary emboli in multiple myeloma. Ann Intern Med 1977;86:317–318.

49. Pyun KS, Katzenstein RE. Widespread bone marrow

embolism with myocardial involvement. Arch Pathol 1970;89:378–381.

50. Wagenvoort CA, Heath D, Edwards JE. The pathology of the pulmonary vasculature. Springfield: Thomas, 1964:302–304.

51. Rappaport H, Raum M, Horrell JB. Bone marrow embolism. Am J Pathol 1951;27:407–432.

52. Yanoff M. Incidence of bone marrow embolism due to closed-chest cardiac massage. N Engl J Med 1963;269: 837–839.

53. Garvey JW, Zak FG. Pulmonary bone marrow emboli in patients receiving external cardiac massage. JAMA 1964;187:59–60.

54. Evans EA, Wellington JS. Emboli associated with cardiopulmonary bypass. J Thorac Cardiovasc Surg 1964;48:323–330.

55. Deland FH, Bennett WA. Death due to bone-marrow and tumor embolization in the absence of fracture. Arch Pathol 1957;63:13–16.

56. Shelley WM, Curtis EM. Bone marrow and fat embolism in sickle cell anemia and sickle cell-hemoglobin C disease. Bull Johns Hopkins Hosp 1958;103:8–26.

57. Diggs LW. Sickle cell crises. Am J Clin Pathol 1965; 44:1–19.

58. Sharnoff JG, Kim ES. Evaluation of pulmonary megakaryocytes. Arch Pathol 1958;66:176–182.

59. Aabo K, Hansen KB. Megakaryocytes in pulmonary blood vessels. Incidence at autopsy, clinicopathological relations especially to disseminated intravascular coagulation. Acta Pathol Microbiol Scand 1978;86A:285–291.

60. Bettendorf U, Meyer-Breiting E. Massive megakaryozytenembolie der Lungen. Dtsch Med Wochenschr 1974;99:1918–1922.

61. Abrahams C, Catchatourian R. Bone fragment emboli in the lungs of patients undergoing bone marrow transplantation. Am J Clin Pathol 1983;79:360–363.

62. Nosanchuk JS, Littler ER. Skin embolus to lung. Arch Pathol 1969;87:542–543.

63. Andrew JH. Pulmonary skin embolism: A case report. Pathology 1976;8:185–187.

64. Straus R. Pulmonary emboli caused by liver tissue. Arch Pathol 1942;33:69–71.

65. Dunnill MS. The pathology of pulmonary embolism. Br J Surg 1968;55:790–794.

66. McMillan JB. Emboli of cerebral tissue in the lungs following severe head injury. Am J Pathol 1956; 32:405–415.

67. Tackett LB. Brain tissue pulmonary emboli. Arch Pathol 1964;78:292–294.

68. Levine SB. Embolism of cerebral tissue to lungs. Arch Pathol Lab Med 1973;96:183–185.

69. Oppenheimer EH. Massive pulmonary embolization by cerebral cortical tissue. Bull Johns Hopkins Hosp 1954;94:86–93.

70. Potter EL, Young RL. Heterotopic brain tissue in the lungs of two anencephalic monsters. Arch Pathol 1942; 34:1009–1015.

71. Campo E, Bombi JA. Central nervous system heteroto-

pia in the lung of a fetus with cranial malformation. Virchows Arch A 1981;391:117–122.

72. Valdes-Dapena MA, Arey JB. Pulmonary emboli of cerebral origin in the newborn. Arch Pathol 1967;84: 643–646.

73. Bohm N, Keller KM, Kloke WD. Pulmonary and systemic cerebellar tissue embolism due to birth injury. Virchows Arch A 1982;398:229–235.

74. Attwood HD, Park WW. Embolism to the lungs by trophoblast. J Obstet Gynecol 1961;68:611–617.

75. Tanimura A, Natsuyama H, Kawano M, Tanimura Y, Tanaka T, Kitazono M. Primary choriocarcinoma of the lung. Hum Pathol 1985;16:1281–1284.

76. Arnold HA, Bainborough AR. Subacute cor pulmonale following trophoblastic pulmonary emboli. Can Med Assoc J 1957;76:478–482.

77. Roffman BY, Simons M. Syncytial trophoblastic embolism associated with placenta increta and preeclampsia. Am J Obstet Gynecol 1969;104:1218–1219.

78. Schmid KO. Mola hydatidosa intravasalis et destruens uteri et pulmonum. Beitr Pathol Anat 1960;123:453–472.

79. Park WW. The occurrence of decidual tissue within the lung: Report of a case. J Pathol Bacteriol 1954;67:563–570.

80. Pope TL Jr, Paling MR, Anderson WA, Nunley WC, Jr. Acute bilateral diffuse pulmonary shadowing after evacuation of hydatid mole. South Med J 1989;82:377–379.

81. Sevitt S. The significance and classification of fat embolism. Lancet 1960;ii:825–828.

82. Scully RE. Fat embolism in Korean battle casualties: Its incidence, clinical significance and pathologic aspects. Am J Pathol 1956;32:379–404.

83. Whiteley HJ. The relation between tissue injury and the manifestations of pulmonary fat embolism. J Pathol Bacteriol 1954;67:521–530.

84. Chan KM, Tham KT, Chiu HS, Chow YN, Leung PC. Posttraumatic fat embolism. Its clinical and subclinical presentations. J Trauma 1984;24:45–49.

85. Gurd AR, Wilson RI. The fat embolism syndrome. J Bone Jt Surg 1974;56B:408–415.

86. Ten Duis HJ, Nijsten MWN, Klasen HJ, Binnendijk B. Fat embolism in patients with an isolated fracture of the femoral shaft. J Trauma 1988;28:383–390.

87. Chastre J, Fagon JY, Soler P, et al. Bronchoalveolar lavage for rapid diagnosis of the fat embolism syndrome, in trauma patients. Ann Intern Med 1990; 113:583–588.

88. Mehta S, Rubenstone AI. Pulmonary bile thromboemboli. Am J Clin Pathol 1967;47:491–496.

89. Altemus LR, Lee RE. Carcinomatosis of the lung with pulmonary hypertension. Arch Intern Med 1967;119: 32–38.

90. Kupari M, Laitinen L, Hekali P, Luomanmaki K. Cor pulmonale due to tumor cell embolization. Report of a case and a brief review of the literature. Acta Med Scand 1981;210:507–510.

91. Schriner RW, Ryu RH, Edwards WD. Microscopic pulmonary tumor embolism causing subacute cor pul-

monale: A difficult antemortem diagnosis. Mayo Clin Proc 1991;66:143–148.

92. Morgan AD. The pathology of subacute cor pulmonale in diffuse carcinomatosis of the lungs. J Pathol Bacteriol 1949;61:75–84.

93. Roglan A, Artigas A, Sole J. Severe pulmonary artery hypertension. Clinico-pathological conference. Intensive Care Med 1988;14:510–518.

94. Demarchi-Aiello V, Mansur AJ, Lopes EA, Bellotti G, Pileggi F. Severe pulmonary hypertension due to carcinomatous lymphangitis of the lungs associated with unsuspected gastric cancer. Am Heart J 1988;116:197–198.

95. Dvorak H. Thrombosis and cancer. Hum Pathol 1987; 18:275–284.

96. Heath D, Mackinnon J. Pulmonary hypertension due to myxoma of the right atrium. Am Heart J 1964; 68:227–235.

97. Boerema B. Appearance and regression of pulmonary arterial lesions after repeated intravenous injection of gas. J Pathol Bacteriol 1965;89:741–744.

98. Balk AG, Mooi WJ, Dingemans KP, Wagenvoort CA. Development and regression of pulmonary arterial lesions after experimental air embolism. A light and electronmicroscopic study. Virchows Arch A 1985;406:203–212.

99. Perkett EA, Brigham KL, Meyrick B. Continuous air embolization into sheep causes sustained pulmonary hypertension and increased vasoreactivity. Am J Pathol 1988;132:444–454.

100. Stephenson WL, Workman RB, Aldrete JS, Karp RB. Bullet emboli to the pulmonary artery. A report of 2 patients and review of the literature. Ann Thorac Surg 1976;21:333–336.

101. Moulinier A. Un cas d'embolies pulmonaires par plombs de chasse. Arch Mal Coeur Vaiss 1960;53: 1415–1417.

102. Saylam A, Yurdakul Y, Bertan V, Aytac A. Foreign body in the right pulmonary artery. An unusual complication of Pudenz shunt. J Cardiovasc Surg 1975; 16:538–540.

103. Dimmick JE, Bove KE, McAdams AJ, Bensing G. Fiber embolization: A hazard of cardiac surgery and catheterization. N Engl J Med 1975;292:685–687.

104. Mittleman RE, Marraccini JV. Pulmonary teflon granulomas following periurethral teflon injection for urinary incontinence. Arch Pathol Lab Med 1983;107:611–612.

105. Truemner KM, White S, Vanlandingham H. Fatal embolization of pulmonary capillaries. Report of case associated with routine barium enema. JAMA 1960; 173:1089–1092.

106. Lamb D, Roberts G. Starch and talc emboli in drug addicts' lungs. J Clin Pathol 1972;25:876–881.

107. Siegel H. Human pulmonary pathology associated with narcotic and other addictive drugs. Hum Pathol 1972; 3:55–66.

108. Arnett EN, Battlo WE, Russo JV, Roberts WC. Intravenous injection of talc containing drugs intended for oral use. A cause of pulmonary granulomatosis and pulmonary hypertension. Am J Med 1976;60:711–718.

109. Tomashefski JF, Hirsch CS. The pulmonary vascular lesions of intravenous drug abuse. Hum Pathol 1980; 11:133–145.

110. Zeltner TB, Nussbauer U, Rudin O, Zimmermann A. Unusual vascular lesions after intravenous injections of microcrystalline cellulose. A complication of pentazocine tablet use. Virchows Arch A 1982;395:207–216.

111. Crougch ED, Churg A. Progressive massive fibrosis of the lung secondary to intravenous injection of talc. A pathologic and mineralogic analysis. Am J Clin Pathol 1983;80:520–526.

112. Cooper CB, Bai TR, Heyderman E, Corrin B. Cellulose granulomas in the lungs of a cocaine sniffer. Br Med J 1983;286:2021–2022.

113. Beaver PC, Fallon M, Smith GH. Pulmonary nodule caused by a living *Brugia malayi*-like filaria in an artery. Am J Trop Med Hyg 1971;20:661–666.

114. Beaver PC, Cran IR. Wuchereria like filaria in an artery associated with pulmonary infarction. Am J Trop Med Hyg 1974;23:869–876.

115. Larrieu AJ, Wiener I, Gomez LG, Williams EH. Human pulmonary dirofilariasis presenting as a solitary pulmonary nodule. Chest 1979;75:511–512.

116. Kochar AS. Human pulmonary dirofiliariasis. Report of three cases and brief review of the literature. Am J Clin Pathol 1985;84:19–23.

117. Goodman ML, Gore I. Pulmonary infarct secondary to dirofilaria larvae. Arch Intern Med 1964;113:702–705.

118. Harrison EG, Thompson JH. Dirofilariasis of human lung. Am J Clin Pathol 1965;43:224–234.

119. Baar HS, Galindo J. Ossifying pulmonary granulomatosis due to larvae of ascaris. J Clin Pathol 1965;18:737–742.

120. Stermer E, Bassan H, Oliven A, Grishkau A, Boss Y. Massive thrombosis as a result of triple infestation of the pulmonary arterial circulation by *Ascaris*, *Candida* and mucor. Hum Pathol 1984;15:996–998.

121. Spencer H. Pathology of the lung, 4th Ed. Oxford: Pergamon Press 1985;382–389.

122. Wagenvoort CA. Lung biopsy specimens in the evaluation of pulmonary vascular disease. Chest 1980;77: 614–625.

123. Wagenvoort CA. Lung biopsies in the differential diagnosis of thromboembolic versus primary pulmonary hypertension. Prog Respir Res 1980;13:16–21.

124. Rosenow EC, Osmundson PJ, Brown ML. Pulmonary embolism. Mayo Clinic Proc 1981;56:161–178.

125. Wagenvoort CA, Wagenvoort N. Pathology of pulmonary hypertension. New York: Wiley, 1977.

126. Wagenvoort CA, Mooi WJ. Controversies and potential errors in the histological evaluation of pulmonary vascular diseases. In: CA Wagenvoort, H Denolin, eds. Pulmonary circulation, advances and controversies. Amsterdam: Elsevier, 1989:7–26.

127. Hatano S, Strasser T, eds. Primary pulmonary hypertension. Report of committee. Geneva: World Health Organization, 1975.

128. Wagenvoort CA. The terminology of primary pulmonary hypertension. In: CA Wagenvoort, H Denolin, eds. Pulmonary circulation, advances and controversies. Amsterdam: Elsevier, 1989:191–197.

129. Wagenvoort CA. Open lung biopsies in congenital heart disease for evaluation of hypertensive pulmonary vascular disease. Predictive value with regard to corrective operability. Histopathology 1985;9:417–436.

130. Haworth SG. Pulmonary vascular disease in ventricular septal defect: Structural and functional correlations in lung biopsies from 85 patients, with outcome of intracardiac repair. J Pathol 1987;152:157–168.

131. Downing SE, Vidone RA, Brandt HM, Liebow AA. The pathogenesis of vascular lesions in experimental hyperkinetic pulmonary hypertension. Am J Pathol 1963;43: 739–756.

132. Saldana ME, Harley RA, Liebow AA, Carrington CB. Experimental extreme pulmonary hypertension and vascular disease in relation to polycythemia. Am J Pathol 1968;52:935–981.

133. Wagenvoort CA, DuShane JW, Edwards JE. Hypertensive pulmonary arterial lesions as a late result of anastomosis of systemic and pulmonary circulations. Proc Mayo Clinic 1960;35:186–191.

134. Newfeld EA, Waldman JD, Paul MH, et al. Pulmonary vascular disease after systemic-pulmonary arterial shunt operations. Am J Cardiol 1977;39:715–720.

135. Molden D, Abraham JL. Pulmonary hypertension. Its association with hepatic cirrhosis and iron accumulation. Arch Pathol Lab Med 1982;106:328–331.

136. Cohen MD, Rubin LJ, Taylor WE, Cuthbert JA. Primary pulmonary hypertension: An unusual case associated with extrahepatic portal hypertension. Hepatology 1983;3:588–592.

137. Edwards BS, Weir EK, Edwards WD, Ludwig J, Dykoski RK, Edwards JE. Coexistent pulmonary and portal hypertension: morphologic and clinical features. J Am Coll Cardiol 1987;10:1233–1238.

138. Groves BM, Brundage BH, Elliott CG, et al. Pulmonary hypertension associated with hepatic cirrhosis. In: AP Fishman. The pulmonary circulation: Normal and abnormal. Philadelphia: University of Pennsylvania Press, 1990:359–369.

139. McDonnell PJ, Toye PA, Hutchins GM. Primary pulmonary hypertension and cirrhosis: Are they related? Am Rev Respir Dis 1983;127:437–441.

140. Matsubara O, Nakamura T, Uehara T, Kasuga T. Histometrical investigation of the pulmonary artery in severe hepatic disease. J Pathol 1984;143:31–37.

141. Felt RW, Kozak BE, Rosch J, Duell BP, Barker AF. Hepatogenic pulmonary angiodysplasia treated with coil-spring embolization. Chest 1987;91:920–922.

142. Mantz FA, Craige E. Portal axis thrombosis with spontaneous portacaval shunt and resultant cor pulmonale. Arch Pathol 1951;52:91–97.

143. Naeye RL. "Primary" pulmonary hypertension with coexisting portal hypertension. A retrospective study of six cases. Circulation 1960;22:376–384.

144. Lal KS, McFadzean AJS, Yeung R. Microembolic pulmonary hypertension in pyogenic cholangitis. Br Med J 1968;1:22–24.

145. Naeye RL. Advanced pulmonary vascular changes in schistosomal cor pulmonale. Am J Trop Med Hyg 1961;10:191–199.

146. Al-Naaman YD, Shamma AH, Damluji SF, El-Sayed HM. Angiologic manifestations of cardiopulmonary schistosomiasis "Bilharziasis." Angiology 1967;17: 40–45.

147. Gurtner HP. Chronische pulmonale Hypertonie vaskulären Ursprungs, plexogene pulmonale Arteriopathie und der Appetitzügler Aminorex: Nachlese zu einer Epidemie. Schweiz Med Wochenschr 1985; 115:782–789, 818–827.

148. Gurtner HP. Aminorex pulmonary hypertension. In: AP Fishman, ed. The pulmonary circulation: Normal and abnormal. Philadelphia: University of Pennsylvania Press, 1990:397–411.

149. Wagenvoort CA, Wagenvoort N. Primary pulmonary hypertension: A pathologic study of the lung vessels in 156 clinically diagnosed cases. Circulation 1970;42: 1163–1184.

150. Esterly JA, Glagov S, Ferguson DJ. Morphogenesis of intimal obliterative hyperplasia of small arteries in experimental pulmonary hypertension. An ultrastructural study of the role of smooth muscle cells. Am J Pathol 1968;52:325–348.

151. Balk AG, Mooi WJ, Dingemans KP, Wagenvoort CA. Development and regression of pulmonary arterial lesions after experimental air embolism. A light and electronmicroscopic study. Virchows Arch A 1985;406:203–212.

151a. Smith P, Heath D, Yacoub M, et al. The ultrastructure of plexogenic arteriopathy. J Pathol 1990;160:111–121.

152. Heath D, Edwards JE. The pathology of hypertensive pulmonary vascular disease. A description of six grades of structural changes in the pulmonary arteries with special reference to congenital cardiac septal defects. Circulation 1958;18:533–547.

153. Yaginuma G, Mohri H, Takahashi T. Distribution of arterial lesions and collateral pathways in the pulmonary hypertension of congenital heart disease: A computer-aided reconstruction study. Thorax 1990; 45:586–590.

154. Wagenvoort CA, Keutel J, Mooi WJ, Wagenvoort N. Longitudinal smooth muscle in pulmonary arteries. Occurrence in congenital heart disease. Virchows Arch A 1984;404:265–274.

155. Wagenvoort CA, Wagenvoort N, Draulans-Noe Y. Reversibility of plexogenic pulmonary arteriopathy following banding of the pulmonary artery. J Thorac Cardiovasc Surg 1984;87:876–886.

156. Del Nido PJ, Williams WG, Villamater J, et al. Changes in pericardial surface pressure during pulmonary hypertensive crises after cardiac surgery. Circulation 1987;76(Suppl.):93–101.

157. Wagenvoort CA. Open lung biopsies in congenital heart disease for evaluation of pulmonary vascular

disease. Predictive value with regard to corrective operability. Histopathology 1985;9:417–436.

158. Clapp S, Perry BL, Farooki ZQ, et al. Down's syndrome, complete atrioventricular canal and pulmonary vascular obstructive disease. J Thorac Cardiovasc Surg 1990; 100:115–121.

159. Harris P, Heath D. The human pulmonary circulation. 3d Ed. Edinburgh: Churchill Livingstone, 1986.

160. Jordan SC, Hicken P, Watson DA, Heath D, Whitaker W. Pathology of the lungs in mitral stenosis in relation to respiratory function and pulmonary haemodynamics. Br Heart J 1966;28:101–107.

161. Wagenvoort CA, Wagenvoort N. Smooth muscle content of pulmonary arterial media in pulmonary venous hypertension compared with other forms of pulmonary hypertension. Chest 1982;81:581–585.

162. Wagenvoort CA. Pathology of congestive pulmonary hypertension. Prog Respir Res 1975;9:195–202.

163. Olsen EGJ. Perivascular fibrosis in lungs in mitral valve disease. A possible mechanism of production. Br J Dis Chest 1966;60:129–136.

164. Heath D, Edwards JE. Histological changes in the lung in diseases associated with pulmonary venous hypertension. Br J Dis Chest 1959;53:8–18.

165. Wagenvoort CA. Morphologic changes in intrapulmonary veins. Hum Pathol 1970;1:205–213.

166. Tryka AF, Godleski JJ, Schoen FJ, Vandevanter H. Pulmonary vascular disease and hypertension after valve surgery for mitral stenosis. Hum Pathol 1985; 16:65–71.

167. Ohno K, Nakahara K, Hirose H, Kawashima Y. Effects of valvular surgery on overall and regional lung function in patients with mitral stenosis. Chest 1987; 92:224–228.

168. Heath D, Segel N, Bishop J. Pulmonary venoocclusive disease. Circulation 1966;34:242–248.

169. Cohn RC, Wong R, Spohn WA, Komer M. Death due to diffuse alveolar hemorrhage in a child with pulmonary venoocclusive disease. Chest 1991;100:1456–1458.

170. Wagenvoort CA. Pulmonary veno-occlusive disease. Entity or syndrome? Chest 1976;69:82–86.

171. Wagenvoort CA, Wagenvoort N, Takahashi T. Pulmonary veno-occlusive disease. Involvement of pulmonary arteries and review of the literature. Hum Pathol 1985;16:1033–1041.

172. Hasleton PS, Ironside JW, Whittaker JS, Kelly W, Ward C. Pulmonary veno-occlusive disease. A report of four cases. Histopathology 1986;10:933–944.

173. Sofer S, Weinhouse E, Tal A, Wanderman KL, Margulis G, Leiberman A, Gueron M. Cor pulmonale due to adenoidal or tonsillar hypertrophy or both in children. Non-invasive diagnosis and follow-up. Chest 1988 ;93:119–122.

174. Weir EK, Ticker A, Reeves JT, Will DH, Grover RF. The genetic factor influencing pulmonary hypertension in cattle at high altitude. Cardiovasc Res 1974; 8:745–749.

175. Grover RF. Chronic hypoxic pulmonary hypertension. In: Fishman AP, ed. The pulmonary circulation: Normal and abnormal. Philadelphia: University of Pennsylvania Press, 1990:283–299.

176. Cutaia M, Rounds S. Hypoxic pulmonary vasoconstriction. Physiological significance, mechanism, and clinical relevance. Chest 1990;97:706–718.

177. Fishman AP. The enigma of hypoxic pulmonary vasoconstriction. In: Fishman AP, ed. The pulmonary circulation: Normal and abnormal. Philadelphia: University of Pennsylvania Press, 1990:109–129.

178. Arias-Stella J, Saldana M. The terminal portion of the pulmonary arterial tree in people native to high altitudes. Circulation 1963;28:915–925.

179. Heath D, Williams DR. Man at high altitude. 2d Ed. Edinburgh: Churchill-Livingstone, 1981.

180. Dingemans KP, Wagenvoort CA. Pulmonary arteries and veins in experimental hypoxia. Am J Pathol 1978;93:353–368.

181. Wagenvoort CA, Wagenvoort N. Pulmonary venous changes in chronic hypoxia. Virchows Arch A 1976; 372:51–56.

182. Edwards WD, Edwards JE. Clinical primary pulmonary hypertension. Three pathologic types. Circulation 1977;56:884–888.

183. Bjornsson J, Edwards WD. Primary pulmonary hypertension: A histopathologic study of 80 cases. Mayo Clin Proc 1985;60:16–26.

184. Palevsky HI, Schloo BL, Pietra GG, et al. Primary pulmonary hypertension. Vascular structure, morphometry, and responsiveness to vasodilator agents. Circulation 1989;80:1207–1221.

185. Pietra GG, Edwards WD, Kay JM, et al. Histopathology of primary pulmonary hypertension. A qualitative and quantitative study of pulmonary blood vessels from 58 patients in the National Heart, Lung and Blood Institute, primary pulmonary hypertension registry. Circulation 1989;80:1198–1206.

185a. Wagenvoort CA, Mulder PGH. Thrombotic lesions in primary plexogenic arteriopathy. Similar pathogenesis or complication? Chest 1993;103:844–849.

186. Wagenvoort CA. Medial defects of lung vessels. A new cause for pulmonary hypertension. Hum Pathol 1986; 17:722–726.

187. Wagenvoort CA, Beetstra A, Spijker J. Capillary haemangiomatosis of the lungs. Histopathology 1978;2: 401–406.

188. Wagenvoort CA, Misalignment of lung vessels: A syndrome causing persistent neonatal pulmonary hypertension. Hum Pathol 1986;17:727–730.

189. Wagenvoort CA, Nauta J, Van der Schaar PJ, Weeda HWH, Wagenvoort N. Vascular changes in pulmonic stenosis and tetralogy of Fallot studied in lung biopsies. Circulation 1967;36:924–932.

190. Rich AR. A hitherto unrecognized tendency to the development of widespread pulmonary vascular obstruction in patients with congenital pulmonary stenosis (tetralogy of Fallot). Bull Johns Hopkins Hosp 1948;82:389–401.

CHAPTER 30
Vasculitis

WILLIAM D. TRAVIS and MICHAEL N. KOSS

The pathology of pulmonary vasculitis is a complex and confusing subject for several reasons: (1) in virtually all the idiopathic vasculitis syndromes, accurate diagnosis requires careful correlation with clinical and laboratory data and cannot be based on histopathologic findings alone. (2) The histopathologic manifestations of idiopathic vasculitis syndromes vary depending when in the course of disease a biopsy specimen is obtained; lung biopsies may therefore have atypical pathologic manifestations that do not meet the traditional diagnostic criteria. (3) The differential diagnosis is complex and includes rare systemic diseases with which few pathologists have much experience. (4) Because necrotizing granulomatous inflammation is a frequent feature of the pulmonary idiopathic vasculitis syndromes, the pathologic manifestations can be mimicked by granulomatous infections. Thus, it is important to distinguish idiopathic vasculitis syndromes from infectious processes because the former are often treated with immunosuppressive agents. (5) The pathogenesis of these disorders varies greatly and is poorly understood. (6) Proper subclassification of these disorders is essential since many of the idiopathic pulmonary vasculitis syndromes can be life threatening without effective therapy.

By definition, vasculitis means inflammation of a blood vessel wall. In the lung, vasculitis can occur in a broad spectrum of settings including idiopathic vasculitis syndromes, miscellaneous systemic disorders, and pulmonary hemorrhage syndromes. It may also occur as a phenomenon secondary to diseases localized to the lung (Table 30–1). During the past several decades, most reviews of the pathology of pulmonary vasculitis have focused attention on the idiopathic vasculitis syndromes that commonly involve the lung, including Wegener's granulomatosis, Churg–Strauss syndrome (allergic angiitis and granulomatosis), and necrotizing sarcoid granulomatosis.[1-10] However, few reviews have dealt fully with idiopathic vasculitis syndromes which uncommonly affect the lung such as polyarteritis nodosa, small vessel vasculitis, Takayasu's arteritis, Henoch-Schönlein purpura, and Behçet's syndrome (see Table 30–1).[7] Secondary or localized pulmonary vasculitis can also occur in a heterogeneous group of conditions including pulmonary infections, bronchocentric granulomatosis, pulmonary hypertension, interstitial lung diseases, inflammatory pseudotumors, pseudolymphomas, and extralobar sequestrations, or in association with embolic material, drug or toxic substances, organ transplantation, and radiation.

Understanding of the pathology of pulmonary vasculitis is aided by knowledge of the history of the subject. In 1973, Averill Liebow[10] reviewed pulmonary angiitis and granulomatosis and included the entities of Wegener's granulomatosis, limited Wegener's granulomatosis, necrotizing sarcoid granulomatosis, bronchocentric granulomatosis, and lymphomatoid granulomatosis. In this comprehensive review, each of these entities was addressed as a distinct vasculitis syndrome. During the past two decades there has been considerable evolution and progress in our understanding of these disorders. For example, it is now known that limited Wegener's granulomatosis simply represents one potential presentation of Wegener's granulomatosis rather than a distinct disease. Necrotizing sarcoid granulomatosis remains controversial in that some regard it to be a nodular variant of classical sarcoidosis,[6] while others interpret it as a distinct form of vasculitis.[11] Bronchocentric granulomatosis, once viewed as a distinctive entity, is now regarded as a morphologic lesion that can

Table 30–1. Pulmonary vasculitis syndromes

Idiopathic vasculitis syndromes that commonly affect the lung
  Wegener's granulomatosis
  Churg–Strauss angiitis and granulomatosis
  Necrotizing sarcoid granulomatosis
  Vasculitis overlap syndromes
Idiopathic vasculitis syndromes that uncommonly affect the lung
  Polyarteritis nodosa
  Small vessel vasculitis
  Takayasu's arteritis
  Henoch–Shönlein purpura
  Behçet's syndrome
  Cryoglobulinemic vasculitis
  Hypocomplementemic vasculitis
  Idiopathic granulomatous arteritis
    Giant cell arteritis
    Disseminated visceral giant-cell angiitis
Miscellaneous systemic disorders
  Classical sarcoid
  Collagen vascular disease
    Rheumatoid arthritis
      Rheumatoid nodules
      Rheumatoid vasculitis
    Systemic lupus erythematosus
    Sjögren's syndrome
    Scleroderma
    Idiopathic inflammatory myopathy
    Mixed connective tissue disease
  Inflammatory bowel disease
  Malignancy
Diffuse pulmonary hemorrhage syndromes
Secondary or localized vasculitis
  Pulmonary infection
  Bronchocentric granulomatosis
  Pulmonary hypertension
  Interstitial lung diseases
    Chronic eosinophilic pneumonia
    Histiocytosis X
  Inflammatory pseudotumors and pseudolymphomas
  Sequestration
  Embolic material (intravenous drug abuse)
  Drug or toxic substances
  Transplantation
  Radiation
Vascular involvement in lymphoproliferative disorders
  Angiocentric immunoproliferative lesion
    (lymphomatoid granulomatosis)
  Non-Hodgkin's lymphoma
  Intravascular malignant lymphoma

occur in association with a wide variety of infectious and noninfectious pulmonary granulomatous disorders as well as in an idiopathic form. Finally, lymphomatoid granulomatosis (LYG) is now viewed as neither a type of vasculitis nor a form of granulomatosis; rather it appears to be an immunoproliferative disorder closely related to T-cell lymphoma. Some authors therefore propose the term angiocentric immunoproliferative lesion (AIL) to replace LYG (AIL/LYG).[3–5,12]

The discovery and characterization of antineutrophil cytoplasmic antibodies (ANCA) over the past decade has had a tremendous impact on diagnosis and understanding of the pathogenesis of the idiopathic vasculitis syndromes.[13–21] It may be that Wegener's granulomatosis, polyarteritis nodosa, Churg–Strauss syndrome, small vessel vasculitis, and idiopathic crescentic glomerulonephritis are related processes, with ANCA as a shared serologic marker.[13] In these vasculitis disorders, ANCA may play an important role in the pathogenesis of vascular injury.[13,22] The nature of this role remains to be elucidated.

Major Idiopathic Vasculitis Syndromes

Wegener's Granulomatosis

Wegener's granulomatosis is a multisystem disorder characterized by aseptic necrotizing granulomatous inflammation and vasculitis that affects the upper and lower respiratory tracts and the kidneys. Accurate diagnosis of Wegener's granulomatosis has become imperative since the discovery of effective therapy using the combination of cyclophosphamide and prednisone. This has dramatically reduced mortality and led to prolonged remission for many patients.[23,24] Because the diagnosis must be confirmed pathologically, the surgical pathologist plays a critical role in the diagnosis and the treatment of this disorder.[23,25,26]

Clinical Features

Wegener's granulomatosis most commonly affects the head and neck region, followed by the lung, kidney, and eye (Fig. 30–1A).[1,23,27–29] Respiratory manifestations include infiltrates or nodules seen on chest radiograph, followed by cough, hemoptysis, and pleuritis (Fig. 30–1B).[29] Chest radiographic infiltrates or nodules can be found in asymptomatic patients in 34% of cases.[29] Head and neck manifestations consist of sinusitis, nasal disease, otitis media, hearing loss, subglottic stenosis, ear pain, cough, and oral lesions (Table 30–2).[29,30] Other systemic manifestations include arthralgias, fever, skin lesions, weight loss, peripheral neuropathy, central nervous system abnormalities, and pericarditis (Table 30–3).[29] Skin lesions may take the form of purpura and petechiae, nodules, hemorrhagic bullae, and pyoderma gangrenosum-like lesions.[31] Unusual sites of involvement include the breast,[29] salivary gland,[32] colon,[33] prostate,[34] urethra,[35] cervix,[29] vagina,[29] and perianal region.[36]

Laboratory abnormalities frequently found in Wegener's granulomatosis include active urinary sediment, as well as elevated erythrocyte sedimentation rate

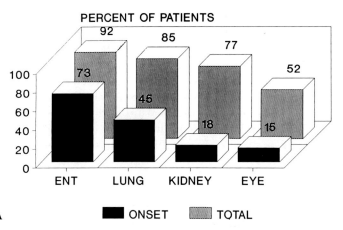

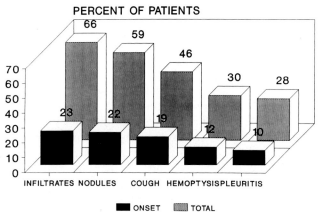

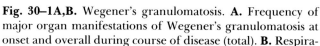

A   B

Fig. 30–1A,B. Wegener's granulomatosis. **A.** Frequency of major organ manifestations of Wegener's granulomatosis at onset and overall during course of disease (total). **B.** Respira-tory symptoms in Wegener's granulomatosis patients at onset and overall during the course of disease (total). Modified from Hoffman et al.,[29] with permission.

Table 30–2. Wegener's granulomatosis: Head and neck manifestations[a]

Disease	Percent of patients
Sinusitis	85
Nasal disease	68
Otitis media	44
Hearing loss	42
Subglottic stenosis	16
Ear pain	14
Oral lesions	10

[a] From Hoffman et al.[29] and Lebovics et al.[30]

Table 30–3. Wegener's granulomatosis: Systemic manifestations[a]

Manifestation	Percent of patients
Arthralgias	67
Fever	50
Skin lesions	46
Weight loss	35
Peripheral neuropathy	15
Central nervous system abnormalities	8
Pericarditis	6

[a] From Hoffman et al.[29]

(ESR), anemia, and elevated rheumatoid factor ti-ters.[23,28] ANCA produce two major immunofluores-cence patterns with ethanol-fixed neutrophils: cytoplas-mic or classical (C-ANCA) and perinuclear (P-ANCA). The pattern of staining correlates with the specificity of the ANCA. For example, ANCAs with specificity for granule proteins that remain localized in neutrophil granules after alcohol fixation give cytoplasmic (C-ANCA) staining. By contrast, ANCAs directed against granule proteins that artifactually redistribute to the nucleus during alcohol fixation give a perinuclear (P-ANCA) staining pattern.[13,14] ANCA can be detected using indirect immunofluorescence or by solid-phase techniques such as ^{125}I-labeled or enzyme-linked im-munosorbent assays (ELISAs).[22,37]

Approximately 95% of C-ANCAs react with protein-ase 3 (PR3 or myeloblastin), a 29-kdalton serine pro-tease found in lysosomal granules and on plasma mem-branes of neutrophils and monocytes.[13,15–17,38] In patients with Wegener's granulomatosis, C-ANCA is most common, although P-ANCA can also be encoun-tered.* C-ANCA with PR3 specificity can be found in 84%–99% of patients with active generalized Wegener's granulomatosis, in 50%–71% of patients in partial re-mission, and in 30%–40% of patients in complete remis-sion.[46] However, in patients with limited Wegener's granulomatosis, C-ANCA can be found in 67% of patients with active disease, in 54% of patients in partial remission, and 32% of patients in complete remission.[45] It is possible that C-ANCA-positive patients with disease limited to episcleritis, subglottic stricture, or diffuse pulmonary hemorrhage may represent part of the spectrum of Wegener's granulomatosis, even though traditional histopathologic criteria are not fulfilled.[39–41]

For patients with Wegener's granulomatosis compli-cated by infection, ANCA must be interpreted with caution.[46] In patients who present with apparent clini-cal reactivation of disease, negative ANCA titers may heighten concern of a possible opportunistic infection.

*References: 14, 18, 22, 38–44.

On the other hand a positive ANCA does not exclude the possibility of opportunistic infection.[43,46] Carder and Harrison reported three Wegener's granulomatosis patients who had opportunistic infections. Two had negative ANCA, but the third had a strongly positive ANCA and at open lung biopsy was found to have *Legionella pneumophila* pneumonia.[46]

C-ANCA is not entirely specific for Wegener's granulomatosis.[46A] It has been detected in a variety of other conditions including Kawasaki disease,[47] small vessel vasculitis associated with cystic fibrosis,[48] and atrial myxoma.[49] C-ANCA has also been observed in occasional patients with rheumatoid arthritis,[20] but may not be detectable in paients with rheumatoid vasculitis.[50]

Approximately 90% of P-ANCAs have specificity for myeloperoxidase (MPO).[17] P-ANCA may also be directed against elastase and lactoferrin, which are found in the primary and secondary neutrophil granules, respectively.[13,16,20] P-ANCAs are found most commonly in patients with idiopathic necrotizing and crescentic glomerulonephritis, regardless of the presence or absence of associated systemic vasculitis.* Elevated P-ANCA titers mostly with MPO specificity can be found in Churg–Strauss syndrome, systemic polyarteritis nodosa, and small vessel vasculitis (microscopic polyarteritis), although C-ANCA can also occur.** P-ANCA has also been found in 11% of patients with giant cell arteritis.[38] P-ANCA can also be found in a few diseases generally regarded as nonvasculitic disorders, such as Felty's syndrome,[38] antiglomerular basement membrane antibody disease,[20] atypical pneumonia and Legionnaire's disease,[20] poststreptococcal glomerulonephritis,[20] systemic lupus erythematosus (SLE),[20,38] mixed connective tissue disease,[20] and inflammatory bowel disease.[13,44]

Therapy and Prognosis

The combination of cyclophosphamide and prednisone is effective treatment for Wegener's granulomatosis, achieving a high rate of remission.[23,27] However, recognition of the complications of cytoxan and prednisone has led to investigation of other forms of therapy including bactrim, pulse cyclophosphamide, and methotrexate.[29,54,55]

Morbidity in patients with Wegener's granulomatosis can be attributed to disease or therapy only and to disease plus therapy. Permanent disease-related morbidity can occur in up to 86% of patients and includes

---

*References: 3, 17, 42, 51, 52.
**References: 13–16, 18, 20, 40, 41, 45, 53.

chronic renal insufficiency (42%), hearing loss (35%), cosmetic and functional nasal deformities (28%), tracheal stenosis (13%), and visual loss (8%).[29] Complications due to disease plus therapy include chronic sinus dysfunction (47%) and pulmonary insufficiency (17%). Morbidity caused by therapy alone includes temporary hair loss (17%), glucocorticoid-induced diabetes mellitus (8%), cyclophosphamide-induced cystitis (43%), bladder carcinoma (3%), myelodysplasia (2%), cataracts (21%), pathologic fractures from osteoporosis (11%), and aseptic necrosis (3%).[29]

Approximately 20% of patients followed at the National Institute of Health (NIH) for a mean of 8 years died.[29] In 13% of patients, death was attributed to Wegener's granulomatosis or therapeutic complications. Specific causes included renal disease (3%), pulmonary disease (3%), concomitant renal and pulmonary disease (1%), infection (3%) and malignancy (2.5%).[29]

Pathologic Features

The pathologic features of Wegener's granulomatosis vary depending on the site of involvement, the type of pathologic specimen, and whether the biopsy is obtained early or late in the course of disease. The original descriptions of Wegener's granulomatosis were based on autopsy specimens of patients who died before the discovery of effective therapy; for this reason these early studies emphasized the full-blown pathologic manifestations.[56–58] However, with the discovery of effective forms of therapy and the greater reliance on open lung biopsies for diagnosis early in the course of disease, a broader spectrum of pathologic manifestations is now observed.[25,26]

Open lung biopsies are the optimal tissue specimens for the premortem diagnosis of pulmonary Wegener's granulomatosis.[25] Due to the small sample size, transbronchial biopsies rarely yield a definitive diagnosis; however, on occasion, the clinical diagnosis of Wegener's granulomatosis can be supported on the basis of a transbronchial biopsy specimen.[59] Transthoracic needle biopsies may also rarely show features suggestive of Wegener's granulomatosis.[60,60a] Review of 59 transbronchial biopsy specimens from 48 NIH patients revealed vasculitis in 4 (7%) and granulomas in 3 (5%).[29]

Gross Pathologic Features

The most common gross appearance is that of multiple bilateral nodular masses with an average diameter of 2.4 cm (median, 2.0 cm; range, 0.3–8 cm). The nodule often has an irregular border with a tan-brown cut surface and it may be either solid and firm or centrally

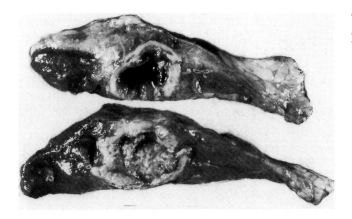

Fig. 30–2. Wegener's granulomatosis. Gross photograph of segmental resection of right-lower lobe demonstrates 5 × 4 × 3.5 cm subpleural cavitating mass with peripheral consolidation and central brown-red necrotic center. (From Travis et al.,[25] with permission.)

cavitated (Fig. 30–2). Dark yellow or red areas of necrosis are commonly visible in the center of the lesion. The surrounding parenchyma is usually grossly unremarkable; but it may be red and hemorrhagic or yellow and consolidated.

Discrete gross nodules may be absent in the minority of lung specimens. Such specimens can show several types of pathology: (1) diffuse pulmonary hemorrhage with patchy or diffusely red, hemorrhagic parenchyma; (2) interstitial fibrosis with firm, tan fibrotic parenchyma; and (3) lipoid pneumonia with diffuse yellow consolidation. Rarely, bronchopneumonia may be encountered with small, 1- to 2-mm nodules of consolidation centered on bronchi and bronchioles. Bronchial stenosis may also occur and appears as dense, firm, white fibrous tissue causing marked narrowing or obliteration of the bronchial lumen.

Histologic Features

The pathologic manifestations of pulmonary Wegener's granulomatosis can be divided into major and minor features (Tables 30–4 and 30–5). The major histopathologic features of Wegener's granulomatosis are those generally regarded as diagnostic criteria: (1) parenchymal necrosis, (2) vasculitis, and (3) granulomatous inflammation accompanied by a mixed infiltrate of neutrophils, lymphocytes, plasma cells, macrophages, giant cells, and eosinophils (Table 30–4). Most lung biopsies show a varying mixture of these three features. Vasculitis and necrosis combined can be found in 89% of open lung biopsy specimens, granulomas and necrosis in 90%, and the combination of vasculitis, necrosis, and granulomatous inflammation in 91% of specimens.[25] The inflammatory and nodular lesions of We-

Table 30–4. Major pathologic manifestations (diagnostic criteria) of Wegener's granulomatosis

I. Vasculitis
    A. Arteritis, venulitis, capillaritis[a]
    B. Six types: Acute, chronic, necrotizing granulomatous, nonnecrotizing granulomatous, fibrinoid necrosis, cicatricial changes[b]
II. Parenchymal necrosis
    A. Microabscess
    B. Geographic necrosis
III. Granulomatous inflammation (& mixed inflammatory infiltrate)
    A. Microabscess surrounded by granulomatous inflammation
    B. Palisading histiocytes
    C. Scattered giant cells
    D. Poorly formed granulomas
    E. Sarcoid-like granulomas (rare)

[a] Capillaritis was characterized primarily be acute inflammation. Veins and arteries demonstrated all the types of inflammation listed in IB.
[b] Cicatricial vascular changes are nonspecific and should not be used as a diagnostic criteria.

Table 30–5. Minor pathologic manifestations of Wegener's granulomatosis[a]

I. Parenchymal
    A. Nodular interstitial fibrosis
    B. Endogenous lipoid pneumonia
    C. Alveolar hemorrhage
    D. Organizing intraluminal fibrosis
    E. Lymphoid aggregates
    F. Tissue eosinophils
    G. Xanthogranulomatous lesions
    H. Alveolar macrophage accumulation
II. Bronchial/bronchiolar lesions
    A. Chronic bronchiolitis
    B. Acute bronchiolitis/bronchopneumonia
    C. Bronchiolitis obliterans or BOOP[b]
    D. Bronchocentric granulomatosis
    E. Follicular bronchiolitis
    F. Bronchial stenosis

[a] May uncommonly represent a dominant pathologic feature.
[b] BOOP, Bronchiolitis obliterans with organizing pneumonia.

gener's granulomatosis can involve and destroy virtually any component of the lung architecture including blood vessels, bronchi/bronchioles, alveolar parenchyma, and pleura.

Vasculitis is most commonly found in blood vessels situated within the nodular inflammatory lesions of Wegener's granulomatosis. Vascular changes can be found in up to 96% of lung biopsy specimens. Arteries and veins of all sizes less than 5 mm and capillaries can be affected, and more than one type of vascular change is often present in a single specimen. Chronic inflammation of arteries and veins is most common, followed

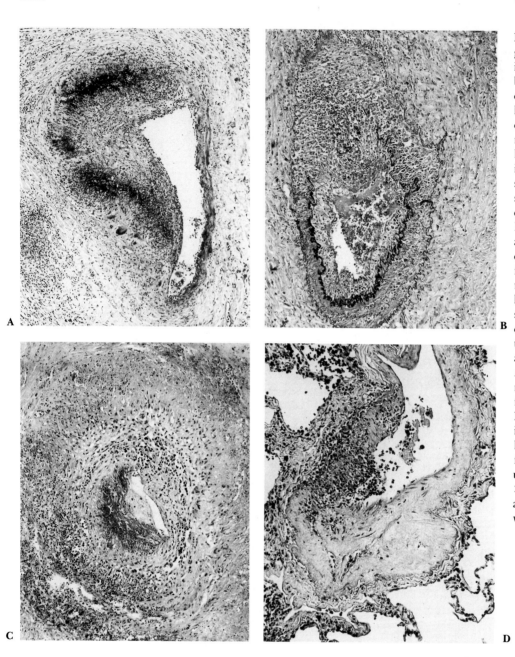

Fig. 30–3A–D. Wegener's granulomatosis. **A.** Vasculitis in this artery is characterized by necrotizing granuloma centered on one side of vascular wall. Multinucleated giant cells are located at edge of this necrotizing granuloma, which has peripheral rim of palisading histiocytes. Parenchyma surrounding blood vessel shows extensive acute and chronic inflammation. H and E, ×60. **B.** Vasculitis in this artery is characterized by eccentric transmural chronic inflammatory infiltrate that disrupts inner and outer elastic lamellae. Van Gieson elastic stain, ×125. **C.** Fibrinoid necrosis is present in artery infiltrated by numerous chronic and acute inflammatory cells. Artery is also surrounded by necrotizing granulomatous inflammation. H and E, ×125. **D.** Focal, eccentric transmural infiltration of lymphocytes and histiocytes in vein situated far from nodular Wegener's granulomatosis lesions. H and E, ×125. (A,C,D: from Travis et al.,[25] B: from Hoffman et al.,[29] with permission.)

by acute inflammation, necrotizing granulomatous inflammation, nonnecrotizing granulomatous inflammation, and fibrinoid necrosis (Fig. 30–3A–D). Cicatricial vascular changes occur in the form of medial scarring or intimal proliferation. They often result in narrowing or obliteration of vascular lumens. Only about 10% of open lung biopsy specimens show vasculitis apart from the major inflammatory lesions of Wegener's granulomatosis (Fig. 30–3D). Neutrophilic infiltration of alveolar septa (capillaritis) can be seen in up to 43% of cases; it is encountered most often in the presence of alveolar hemorrhage.

Arteritis and venulitis may be absent in approximately 10% of open lung biopsy specimens. They are often not seen in specimens showing predominantly nodular interstitial fibrosis or diffuse pulmonary hemorrhage associated with capillaritis. Rarely, vasculitis may be absent in specimens where geographic necrosis, microabscesses, and scattered giant cells are present. Vascular thromboses can be seen in about 5% of cases.

Although Wegener's granulomatosis is regarded as a vasculitis, the parenchymal changes usually overshadow the vasculitis. They typically consist of nodular areas of consolidation showing (1) parenchymal necrosis, (2) granulomatous inflammation accompanied by a mixed inflammatory infiltrate composed of lympho-

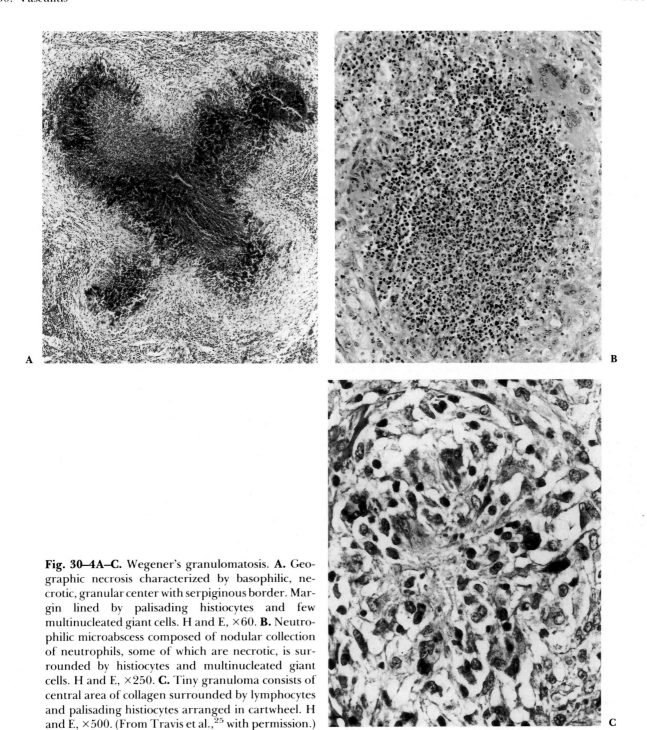

Fig. 30–4A–C. Wegener's granulomatosis. **A.** Geographic necrosis characterized by basophilic, necrotic, granular center with serpiginous border. Margin lined by palisading histiocytes and few multinucleated giant cells. H and E, ×60. **B.** Neutrophilic microabscess composed of nodular collection of neutrophils, some of which are necrotic, is surrounded by histiocytes and multinucleated giant cells. H and E, ×250. **C.** Tiny granuloma consists of central area of collagen surrounded by lymphocytes and palisading histiocytes arranged in cartwheel. H and E, ×500. (From Travis et al.,[25] with permission.)

cytes, plasma cells, neutrophils, eosinophils, macrophages and giant cells, and (3) fibrosis.

Parenchymal necrosis, in the form of neutrophilic microabscesses or areas of geographic necrosis, can be found in 84% of biopsy specimens. Punctate neutrophilic microabscesses are encountered in 65% of biopsy specimens and probably represent an early form of parenchymal necrosis. Geographic necrosis is present in 69% of lung biopsy specimens and is characterized by a basophilic, granular center with a serpentine border, often lined by a peripheral rim of palisading histiocytes and multinucleated giant cells (Fig. 30–4A). Other types of granulomatous inflammation include microabscesses surrounded by giant cells and epithelioid cells (Fig. 30–4B), poorly formed granulomas composed of loose clusters of multinucleated giant cells, scattered giant cells, and small foci consisting of palisading histiocytes arranged in a cartwheel pattern (Fig. 30–4C).

Occasionally vasculitis or geographic necrosis is absent in open lung biopsies from patients with otherwise classical Wegener's granulomatosis. If a biopsy demonstrates classical geographic necrosis, microabscesses, and granulomatous inflammation, the absence of vasculitis does not exclude the diagnosis of Wegener's granulomatosis. Geographic necrosis is the type of necrosis traditionally emphasized; however, the presence of neutrophilic microabscesses can be a helpful morphologic clue to the diagnosis when geographic necrosis is absent.

Minor pulmonary pathologic features of Wegener's granulomatosis are frequently present in lung biopsy specimens, but these are usually inconspicuous and do not represent diagnostic criteria (see Table 30–5). These minor lesions are often found at the periphery of typical nodules of Wegener's granulomatosis that demonstrate major pathologic manifestations (vasculitis, necrosis, and granulomas). They are the dominant manifestation in up to 18% of lung biopsy specimens from Wegener's granulomatosis patients.[25] Dense interstitial fibrosis (7%) and diffuse pulmonary hemorrhage (7%) are most common.[25] Rarely, lipoid pneumonia (1%) or acute bronchopneumonia (1%) may be the dominant pathologic finding.[25] Awareness that these nonspecific features can occasionally predominate is important; one should not exclude a diagnosis of Wegener's granulomatosis in these instances.

Diffuse pulmonary hemorrhage is an acute, potentially life-threatening complication of Wegener's granulomatosis.[45,61–64] Lung biopsies from such patients display acute or chronic hemorrhage, often associated with capillaritis. Microscopic foci of alveolar hemorrhage are a frequent incidental finding in lung biopsies showing typical Wegener's granulomatosis. The problem of vasculitis and diffuse pulmonary hemorrhage is discussed in detail later.

Two major types of interstitial fibrosis can be seen: dense fibrosis and loose, intraluminal fibrosis.[25] Dense interstitial fibrosis in the form of a localized nodular scar (Fig. 30–5) or diffuse interstitial fibrosis is found in as many as 26% of biopsy specimens but is the dominant finding in only about 5% of cases.[26] Localized nodular interstitial fibrosis probably represents scarring of inflammatory lesions of Wegener's granulomatosis. Progression to diffuse interstitial fibrosis with the pattern of idiopathic pulmonary fibrosis is uncommon and may be a complication of cyclophosphamide therapy,[25] although this is difficult to prove conclusively. By contrast, loose intraluminal fibrosis is a relatively common and nonspecific finding at the edge of inflammatory lesions.[25]

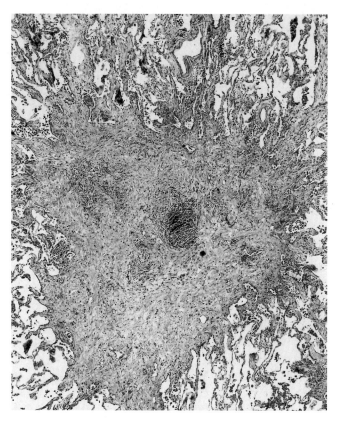

Fig. 30–5. Wegener's granulomatosis. Large area of nodular fibrosis in biopsy that also contained active lesions of Wegener's granulomatosis. Fibrotic nodule has stellate border at periphery. Scattered foci of chronic inflammation include lymphoid aggregate. H and E, ×36. (From Travis et al.,[25] with permission.)

A spectrum of bronchial or bronchiolar lesions can occur (see Table 30–5). Bronchiolitis obliterans or bronchitis obliterans with organizing pneumonia (BOOP) is usually inconspicuous and probably is a nonspecific localized response to bronchiolar damage induced by Wegener's granulomatosis. They should not be confused with the clinical forms of lung diseases that bear these names. Bronchial chondritis is not a lesion specific to Wegener's granulomatosis because it can occur in any destructive inflammatory process involving bronchi (Fig. 30–6A). In approximately 1% of cases, lesions of Wegener's granulomatosis are centered on bronchi or bronchioles (Fig. 30–6B).[25,65,66] Because Wegener's granulomatosis has traditionally been classified as an angiocentric rather than a bronchocentric process,[10,67,68] these cases may be misdiagnosed as bronchocentric granulomatosis.[25,65,69,70] Bronchial stenosis caused by dense fibrotic scarring is a complication that may be treated by lobectomy, or excision or dilatation of the stenotic portion of the bronchus.

Xanthomatous lesions consist of foamy macrophages

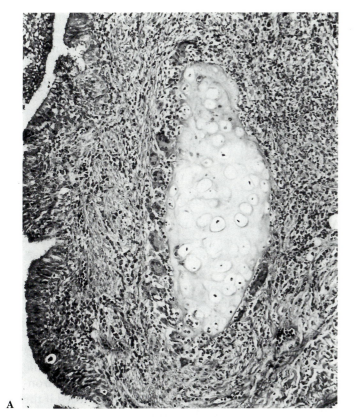

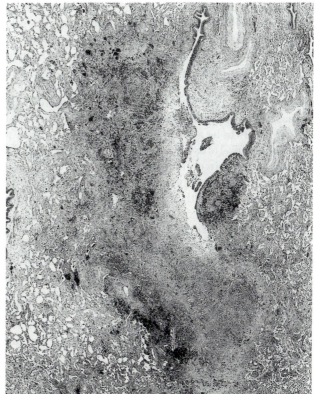

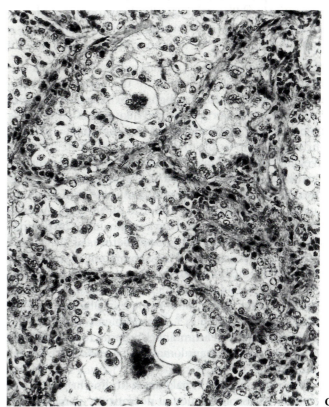

Fig. 30–6A–C. Wegener's granulomatosis. **A.** Chondritis characterized by numerous multinucleated giant cells surrounding and focally eroding bronchial cartilage. Biopsy was characterized primarily by bronchocentric inflammation. H and E, ×125. **B.** Necrotizing granulomatous inflammation centered on bronchiole with pattern of bronchocentric granulomatosis. H and E, ×16. **C.** Endogenous lipoid pneumonia illustrated by numerous macrophages with foamy cytoplasm filling alveolar spaces. Several foam cells are multinucleated. H and E, ×250. (**A** and **C:** from Travis et al.,[25] with permission.)

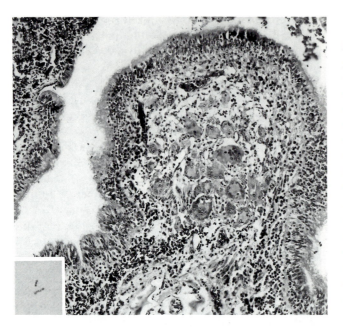

Fig. 30–8. Mycobacterium-avium-intracellulare infection in patient with Wegener's granulomatosis. Sarcoid-like granuloma situated beneath bronchiolar mucosa was found in association with necrotizing granulomatous inflammation. H and E, ×125. Inset: Rare acid-fast bacilli were present within necrotizing granulomas. Ziehl–Neelsen, ×1000.

important complication of the immunosuppressive therapy administered to patients with Wegener's granulomatosis (see Fig. 30–8).

Secondary vasculitis may be seen adjacent to the necrotizing granulomas of rheumatoid nodules and occasionally may histologically resemble Wegener's granulomatosis.[6] However, the two entities are rarely confused clinically because most patients who develop pulmonary rheumatoid nodules also have rheumatoid arthritis and do not demonstrate the upper airway and renal disease.

Although it has been referred to as a distinct clinical entity, bronchocentric granulomatosis is a morphologic lesion that can occur in a variety of clinical settings, as discussed next.[6,106] Wegener's granulomatosis has been traditionally classified as an angiocentric process; however, it has recently been recognized that bronchocentric granulomatosis can represent the primary pathologic manifestation of Wegener's granulomatosis in at least 1% of cases.[25,65,66]

Although the pathologic features can be distinctive, the diagnosis of Wegener's granulomatosis should be established only after correlation with the clinical features. This is particularly true when atypical histologic features are found or the patient has limited disease. In such cases C-ANCA determinations may be helpful in supporting the diagnosis of Wegener's granulomatosis.

Pathogenesis

Little is known about the pathogenesis of Wegener's granulomatosis. The frequency of ANCA as well as neutrophilic microabscesses in upper and lower respiratory tract biopsy specimens suggest that neutrophils may play an important role in pathogenesis.* The morphologic resemblance of the necrotizing granulomas of Wegener's granulomatosis to infectious granulomas and the clinical response in some cases to Bactrim have been used to argue that the etiology may be related to an inhaled infectious agent.[54] Cellular immunity appears to be more important than humoral immunity in the pathogenesis. The parenchymal and vascular infiltrates are composed primarily of T cells and monocytes,[109] and neither IgG, IgA, IgM, or C3, nor electron-dense deposits, can be found in pulmonary vessels or alveolar septa. On the other hand, the potentially important role of ANCA needs to be explored.

Churg–Strauss Angiitis and Granulomatosis

Churg–Strauss syndrome is an allergic disorder characterized by asthma, peripheral blood eosinophilia, and systemic vasculitis.** Before recognition of Churg–Strauss syndrome as a distinct entity, these cases were probably classified as polyarteritis nodosa with asthma.*** In 1939, Rackemann and Greene[113] first suggested that polyarteritis nodosa with allergic features was a distinct variant of vasculitis.

The original description of this syndrome was made by Drs. J. Churg and L. Strauss in 1951, based on 23 patients with polyarteritis nodosa-like vasculitides who had histories of asthma and peripheral eosinophilia.[88] Because their paper concentrated on the details of 13 autopsy cases, for many years pathologic features were considered essential diagnostic criteria. However, during the past few decades several studies have indicated that the classic histopathologic features of necrotizing vasculitis, eosinophilic tissue infiltration, and extravascular granulomas are not found in all cases of Churg–Strauss syndrome.[87,91] Churg–Strauss syndrome evolves through several phases, and because the tissue infiltrates are often fleeting, the pathology varies depending on when biopsy specimens are obtained; thus, diagnostic pathologic features may not always be present. Moreover, the pathologic findings typical of Churg–Strauss syndrome are not specific and can be induced by medications[114] and parasitic infection.[115,116] As a result, there has been a shift toward a

---

*References: 25, 26, 74, 107, 108.
**References: 9, 87–89, 91, 103, 104, 110.
***References: 2, 88, 91, 92, 103, 111, 112, 112a.

clinical approach to the diagnosis, and in 1984 Lanham et al. proposed the following criteria for the diagnosis of Churg–Strauss syndrome: asthma, peripheral blood eosinophilia ($>1.5 \times 10^9$/liter), and systemic vasculitis involving two or more extrapulmonary organs.[91]

More recently, a subcommittee of the American College of Rheumatology proposed two approaches to the diagnosis of Churg–Strauss syndrome (known as the ACR 1990 Criteria): a *traditional format classification* and a *classification tree*.[117,118] According to the traditional format classification, six criteria are identified: (1) asthma, (2) eosinophils greater than 10% of the white blood cell differential count, (3) mononeuropathy (including multiplex) or polyneuropathy, (4) nonfixed radiographic pulmonary infiltrates, (5) paranasal sinus abnormalities, and (6) a biopsy containing a blood vessel with extravascular eosinophils.[117] If four of six of these criteria are identified, the diagnosis can be established with a sensitivity of 85% and a specificity of 99.7%.[117] The major criteria used in the *classification tree* include: asthma, eosinophilia greater than 10%, and a history of allergy.[117] According to this method, patients with well-documented systemic vasculitis who do not have a history of asthma can be diagnosed as having Churg–Strauss syndrome if they have peripheral eosinophilia greater than 10% and a history of allergy other than drug sensitivity.[117] This seems appropriate, because patients without asthma but with a history of allergic disease can develop Churg–Strauss syndrome.[119–121] Both classification methods appear to be useful in the diagnosis of Churg–Strauss syndrome with greater sensitivity provided by the *classification tree* and more specificity by the traditional approach.[117]

It is important to keep in mind that pathologic findings do not play an essential role in the diagnostic criteria established by Lanham et al. or the ACR 1990 Criteria.[91,117] In fact, the most characteristic pathologic lesion of Churg–Strauss syndrome, allergic granuloma, is observed in only 10%–20% of patients with the syndrome.[117] The most useful criteria for pathologic specimens proposed in the ACR 1990 criteria was the presence of extravascular eosinophils in a biopsy specimen that includes an artery, arteriole, or venule; this finding had a sensitivity of 81% and a specificity of 16%.[117] Thus, during the past four decades since the original description of Churg–Strauss syndrome,[88] the diagnosis has shifted from a primarily pathologic approach to a clinical one.

Clinical Features

Churg–Strauss syndrome has its most profound effect on the lungs, heart, and peripheral nerves.[87,91,103] It typically evolves through three clinical phases. The first is a prodrome characterized by one or more of the following: allergic rhinitis, asthma, peripheral eosinophilia, and eosinophilic infiltrative disease.* Allergic rhinitis can be found in 70%–90% of patients; it is frequently accompanied by nasal polyposis and is the most common initial manifestation of Churg–Strauss syndrome.[91,103,122] The mean age at onset of asthma is 35 years. The mean duration of asthma before onset of vasculitis varies from 3 to 8 years but it may range to 30 years.[87,88,91] In one study, a short interval between onset of asthma and onset of vasculitis was a poor prognostic sign with only a 3-year mean duration of asthma for those patients who died.[87] Peripheral eosinophilia can occur at any phase of Churg–Strauss syndrome, but it frequently occurs in the prodrome.[103] Eosinophilic infiltrative disease often involves the lungs, causing Löffler's syndrome and chronic eosinophilic pneumonia, or the gastrointestinal tract, causing eosinophilic gastroenteritis. The prodromal phase may last for years with multiple exacerbations of these manifestations.

The next phase is characterized by systemic vasculitis. During this phase all features of Churg–Strauss syndrome are present; thus, only during this phase can the diagnosis be established.[103] Rare cases are reported in which the vasculitic phase appeared to be precipitated by hypoallergen injections[123–125] or exposure to inhaled antigens such as *Actinomycetes thermophilus*.[126] Hypersensitivity to aspergillus was also suggested as a possible precipitating agent, based on one case in which Churg–Strauss syndrome developed after a 17-year history of allergic bronchopulmonary aspergillosis.[127]

In the postvasculitic phase, patients may continue to have asthma and allergic rhinitis; however, they may suffer from sequelae of neuropathy and hypertension.[91,103] These phases do not necessarily follow an orderly sequence. In 20% of cases, asthma, eosinophilia, and vasculitis present simultaneously.[87]

The term limited Churg–Strauss syndrome has been suggested for cases in which one of the primary diagnostic features, such as asthma or eosinophilia, is lacking. In some cases the vasculitis may not be systemic, and pathologic changes are restricted to a single organ such as the conjunctiva,[128] the prostate,[129] or the gallbladder.[130]

Other than asthma, the most common pulmonary abnormalities of Churg–Strauss syndrome include chest radiograph infiltrates, which are sometimes transient and migratory, resembling Löffler's syndrome, and pleural effusions (Fig. 30–9A).[91,103] Analysis of pleural effusions may reveal acidotic exudates with

---

*References: 7, 9, 87, 91, 103, 104.

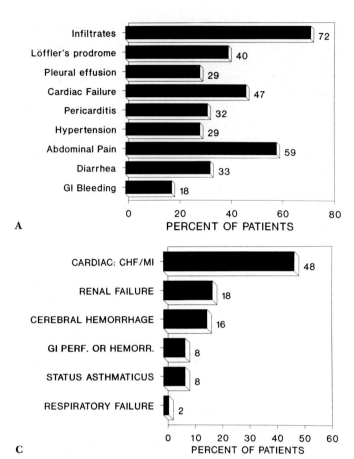

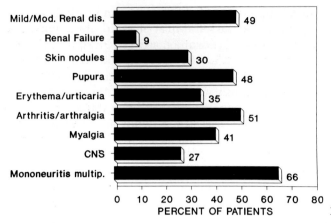

Fig. 30–9A–C. Churg–Strauss granulomatosis. **A.** Pulmonary, cardiovascular, and gastrointestinal manifestations. Infiltrates, chest radiographic infiltrates; Gl, gastrointestinal. **B.** Renal, cutaneous, musculoskeletal, and neurologic manifestations. Mod., moderate; Dis., disease; CNS, central nervous system; Multip., multiplex. **C.** Causes of death. CHF, congestive heart failure; MI, myocardial infarction; Gl Perf. or Hemorr., gastrointestinal perforation or hemorrhage. (Modified from Lanham et al.[91])

marked eosinophilia and markedly low glucose.[131] Severe, life-threatening pulmonary hemorrhage is an uncommon complication.[132] High-resolution computerized tomographs of the lung may show enlarged, irregular, and stellate-shaped arteries, and small patchy opacities.[133] Head and neck manifestations include nasal obstruction or rhinorrhea (69%), nasal polyps (34%), thick crusts (25%), both nasal polyps and crusting (12.5%), abnormal sinus roentgenograms (47%), septal perforations (6%), and subcutaneous nodules involving the skin from the head and neck region.[122] Conjunctival involvement has also been reported.[128,134]

The heart is frequently affected. The most common cardiac manifestations are cardiac failure followed by pericarditis and hypertension (Fig. 30–9A); however, restrictive cardiomyopathy, acute myocardial infarction, and arrhythmias may also occur.* Mitral regurgitation was reported in 33% of patients who underwent cardiac echocardiography; in two patients it was severe enough to require valve replacement.[135]

The most common gastrointestinal finding is abdominal pain followed by diarrhea and gastrointestinal

_____
*References: 87, 88, 91, 135–137.

bleeding (see Fig. 30–9A).[87,91,103] Eosinophilic enteritis most commonly affects the small intestine, followed by the stomach and colon.[138] Mucosal ulceration is uncommon, although it appears to be more frequent in Japanese cases, and may resemble ulcerative colitis.[87,91,103,138] Perforation is an infrequent, but potentially life-threatening, complication.[87,138] Rarely, Churg–Strauss syndrome may present as acalculous cholecystitis.[139]

Renal disease occurs in 33%–58% of patients (Fig. 30–9B)[87,91]; it is usually mild or moderate with renal failure occurring in less than 10% of cases.[87,103] A recent review suggests that renal failure is more common and severe than previously thought.[140] Ureteral stenosis can occasionally occur following inflammatory involvement of the urinary tract.[103,141] The prostate and penis may also be affected.[87,129,142]

Cutaneous nodules, purpura, and erythema or urticaria are common (see Fig. 30–9B).[31,143] Arthritis or arthralgias and myalgias occur in 40–50% of patients (Fig. 30–9B).[91,103] Peripheral neuropathy in the form of mononeuritis multiplex occurs in two-thirds of patients, and central nervous system abnormalities occur in about one-quarter (Fig. 30–9B).[91,103]

During the vasculitic phase, laboratory abnormalities

include peripheral eosinophilia, anemia, leukocytosis, and thrombocytosis as well as elevated ESR erythrocyte sedimentation rate and C-reactive protein.[87,91,103] Although C-ANCA has been reported in Churg–Strauss syndrome,[144] antimyeloperoxidase antibodies (P-ANCA) appear to be more common; this contrasts with the C-ANCA (proteinese 3 antibodies) that are characteristic of Wegener's granulomatosis.[18,65] Serum rheumatoid factor may be weakly positive, complement may be increased, and most patients have elevated IgE levels.[87,90,91,103] Titers of circulating immune complexes have been shown to be significantly higher in Churg–Strauss syndrome than in hepatitis B-related polyarteritis nodosa.[91,103,145] In contrast to polyarteritis nodosa, hepatitis B infection is remarkably uncommon in Churg–Strauss syndrome with only one reported case in a patient infected with the human immunodeficiency virus.[146] Churg–Strauss syndrome has been reported in association with antecedent primary biliary cirrhosis[147] and malignant melanoma.[148]

Therapy and Prognosis

Most patients with Churg–Strauss syndrome respond well to corticosteroid therapy. In the past, therefore, cyclophosphamide has been reserved for those patients who do not respond to corticosteroids. However, because a significant number of patients may rapidly develop irreversible organ injury, it is currently recommended that immunosuppressive medication such as cyclophosphamide, azathioprine, or chlorambucil be given from the beginning.[103] Data from the Cooperative Study Group for Polyarteritis Nodosa suggest that plasma exchange, if used during the acute phase of disease in conjunction with medication, may reduce the incidence of relapses and improve the quality of the clinical response.[149,150] However steroids plus plasma exchange may not be superior to steroids alone.[150a] Pulse cyclophosphamide[151] and pulse steroids[152] have also been effective in some cases. Renal[103,140] and heart[136] transplantation have been performed in a few patients who have developed end-stage renal or cardiac disease. The most common cause of death is cardiac complication (congestive heart failure or myocardial infarction), followed by renal failure, cerebral hemorrhage, gastrointestinal perforation or hemorrhage, status asthmaticus, and respiratory failure (see Fig. 30–9C).

Pathologic Features

The three major pathologic features of Churg–Strauss syndrome are necrotizing vasculitis predominantly affecting medium-sized arteries and veins, tissue infiltration by eosinophils, and extravascular granulomas. However, it is rare to obtain biopsy specimens that exhibit all the classic pathologic features.

In the lung, the principal microscopic findings include asthmatic bronchitis, eosinophilic pneumonia, extravascular granulomas, and vasculitis.[88,103,153] Asthmatic bronchitis is characterized by mucus plugging, hypertrophy of submucosal glands, thickening of the subepithelial basement membrane, edema and inflammation involving the bronchial wall with numerous eosinophils, and hypertrophy of the smooth muscle wall of the airways (see Chapter 16). Eosinophilic pneumonia consists of intraalveolar accumulations of eosinophils (Fig. 30–10A), which may be accompanied by varying degress of organizing intraluminal fibrosis. The extravascular granulomas, also known as "allergic" granulomas, are composed of palisading histiocytes and multinucleated giant cells surrounding a central core of necrotic eosinophils (eosinophilic abscess) (Figs. 30–10B,C). Healed allergic granulomas can be fibrotic or calcified.

Necrotizing vasculitis primarily affects medium-sized muscular arteries or veins. The vascular inflammation consists of transmural infiltrates of chronic inflammatory cells, eosinophils, epithelioid cells, multinucleated giant cells, or neutrophils (Figs. 30–11A,B). Fibrinoid necrosis can be seen, and allergic granulomas may rarely be centered on blood vessels (Fig. 30–11C). Healed vasculitis in the form of cicatricial vascular changes may also be encountered, but such changes are nonspecific. Ischemia and infarction are potential complications of vascular narrowing or occlusion by inflammation. Aneurysms may also result from inflammatory destruction of the wall. Occasionally the inflammatory lesions of Churg–Strauss syndrome primarily involve the pleura, interlobular septa, and bronchovascular bundles with minimal spread to the alveolar parenchyma.

Biopsies from the nasal region may demonstrate allergic polyps, allergic granulomas, and eosinophilic submucosal infiltrates accompanied by chronic inflammation, sometimes with giant cells. Vasculitis can be difficult to demonstrate.[122]

The heart is a frequent site of significant damage,* and cardiac involvement accounts for as many as 48% of deaths (see Fig. 30–9C).[103] Acute fibrinous pericarditis and pericardial fibrosis are common. Eosinophilic and granulomatous myocarditis frequently lead to interstitial myocardial fibrosis. Coronary arteritis may be complicated by thrombosis and acute myocardial infarction; endocarditis with mural thrombi is uncommon.[103] En-

---

*References: 88, 103, 121, 135, 136.

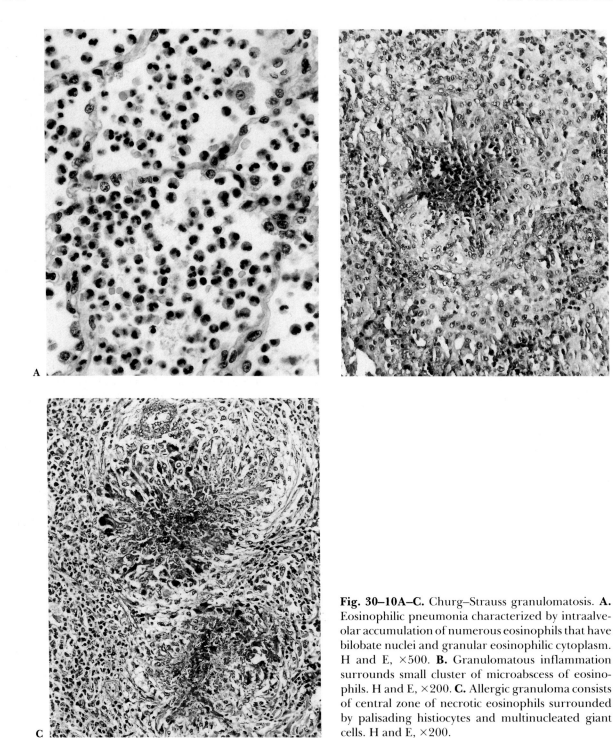

Fig. 30–10A–C. Churg–Strauss granulomatosis. **A.** Eosinophilic pneumonia characterized by intraalveolar accumulation of numerous eosinophils that have bilobate nuclei and granular eosinophilic cytoplasm. H and E, ×500. **B.** Granulomatous inflammation surrounds small cluster of microabscess of eosinophils. H and E, ×200. **C.** Allergic granuloma consists of central zone of necrotic eosinophils surrounded by palisading histiocytes and multinucleated giant cells. H and E, ×200.

domyocardial biopsy may reveal myocarditis or fibrosis, depending on the phase during which the biopsy is performed.[136,154] Eosinophilic infiltrates, vasculitis, and allergic granulomas may also affect other organs such as the liver, kidney, gastrointestinal tract, and skin. In skin, the vasculitis may be of the leukocytoclastic type.[103,143]

Differential Diagnosis

The differential diagnosis of Churg–Strauss syndrome includes Wegener's granulomatosis,[25] eosinophilic pneumonia,[155] allergic bronchopulmonary fungal disease (ABPFD),[156] parasitic infection,[115] drug-induced vasculitis,[114,157] necrotizing sarcoid,[6,11,93] and bron-

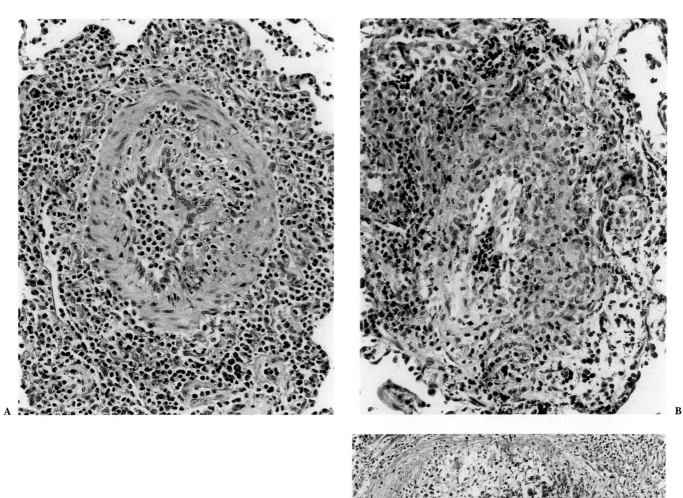

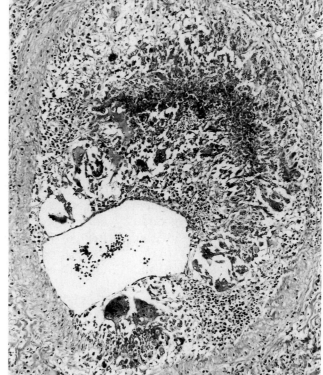

Fig. 30–11A–C. Churg–Strauss granulomatosis. **A.** Vasculitis characterized by cicatricial changes and inflammation of lymphocytes and eosinophils. H and E, ×200. **B.** Granulomatous vasculitis in this vessel consists of numerous epithelioid histiocytes. H and E, ×200. **C.** Allergic granuloma is centered on arteriole. H and E, ×100.

chocentric granulomatosis.[6,95,158] The differential diagnosis with Wegener's granulomatosis has been discussed. Eosinophilic diseases, such as eosinophilic pneumonia, ABPFD, and bronchocentric granulomatosis, differ from Churg–Strauss syndrome clinically in that systemic vasculitis is absent. In chronic eosinophilic pneumonia, lung biopsies may show mild nonnecrotizing vasculitis and allergic granulomas. Secondary vasculitis may also be seen in arteries adjacent to bronchi or bronchioles in bronchocentric granulomatosis or ABPFD; however, necrotizing vasculitis is not a characteristic feature of these diseases. Parasitic infection, particularly that caused by *Strongyloides stercoralis*[116] and *Toxocara canis*,[115] can cause asthma and a systemic illness that may clinically resemble Churg–Strauss syndrome. Visceral larva migrans has been reported to cause allergic granulomas similar to those seen in Churg–Strauss syndrome as well as necrotizing venulitis.[115] However, *Toxocara* larva were also found within the lumen of blood vessels in this case.[115] Thus, the diagnosis of Churg–Strauss syndrome should be made only after careful exclusion of parasites in stool, sputum, and/or pleural fluid specimens, and in tissue biopsies. A careful history of drug exposure should also be obtained, because drug-induced eosinophilic granulomatous vasculitis characterized by cutaneous and renal involvement has been described with carbamazepine.[114]

In the past, the term allergic or Churg–Strauss granuloma has mistakenly been used to describe cutaneous necrotizing granulomas found in a wide variety of conditions including Wegener's granulomatosis, polyarteritis nodosa, connective tissue diseases, lymphoproliferative disease, subacute bacterial endocarditis, chronic active hepatitis, and chronic ulcerative colitis.[159,160] However, the cutaneous necrotizing granulomas in these diseases do not have the necrotic microabscesses of eosinophils characteristic of allergic granulomas seen in Churg–Strauss syndrome.

Patients with Churg–Strauss syndrome occasionally have clinical or pathologic features of a second type of idiopathic vasculitis syndrome, producing a vasculitis overlap syndrome. Churg–Strauss syndrome has been observed in association with giant cell (temporal) arteritis[147,161] and Takayasu's arteritis.[7,162] Overlap between Wegener's granulomatosis and Churg–Strauss syndrome can be more difficult to establish; in Wegener's granulomatosis, peripheral blood eosinophilia greater than 5% can be found in up to 12% of patients, and striking tissue eosinophilia can be observed in lung biopsy specimens in up to 6% of cases.[25,54] Rarely, peripheral eosinophilia greater than 10% is found in Wegener's granulomatosis patients. This may cause confusion with the diagnosis of Churg–Strauss syndrome, even using the ACR 1990 criteria.[117] Wegener's

granulomatosis should be considered if such a patient does not have a history of asthma and the peripheral eosinophilia is less than either 10% of the white blood cell count or 1,000 eosinophils/mm^3.[163]

Necrotizing Sarcoid Granulomatosis

Necrotizing sarcoid granulomatosis was originally described by A.A. Liebow in 1973.[10] Necrotizing sarcoid granulomatosis primarily affects the lung, and histologically consists of confluent sarcoid-like or epithelioid granulomas with areas of necrosis and vasculitis.[10] Including Liebow's initial 11 patients, there are approximately 95 published cases of necrotizing sarcoid granulomatosis in the English literature.[6,11,93,164–170] Review of this literature confirms the rarity of necrotizing sarcoid granulomatosis, its variable radiographic appearance, and its benign clinical behavior. Whether necrotizing sarcoid granulomatosis represents a form of sarcoidosis or a distinct entity remains controversial.[6,11,170]

Clinical Features

The clinical features of necrotizing sarcoid granulomatosis are summarized in Figs. 30–12A,B and Table 30–6. Unlike other pulmonary vasculitides (such as Wegener's granulomatosis) in which men predominate, women outnumber men by a ratio of 2.2:1. The mean age of patients with necrotizing sarcoid granulomatosis is 49 years, with a range from 11 to 75 years old and a peak incidence in the third and seventh decades (Fig. 30–12A). Only two cases have been reported in children (11 and 12 years old).[167,168]

Fifteen to 25% of patients are asymptomatic at presentation (Fig. 30–12B). The most common presenting symptom is cough, followed by fever, chest pain, dyspnea, malaise, and weight loss (Fig. 30–12B).* Symptoms usually occur in the setting of extensive bilateral infiltrates or nodules.[11]

Extrapulmonary symptoms and signs have been reported for up to 13% of patients,[6] but they are rare in most series. Leg weakness and numbness can arise from spinal cord involvement.[167,168] Diabetes insipidus can occur from hypothalamic insufficiency.[6] There may be ocular abnormalities, including iritis,[11*] uveitis,[6] and unilateral loss of vision from retinal involvement.[168] Ulcerative colitis has been reported in one patient[170]; glomerulonephritis has not been observed. Physical examination is typically nondiagnostic; however, on

_____
*References: 93, 164–166, 168, 169, 171.

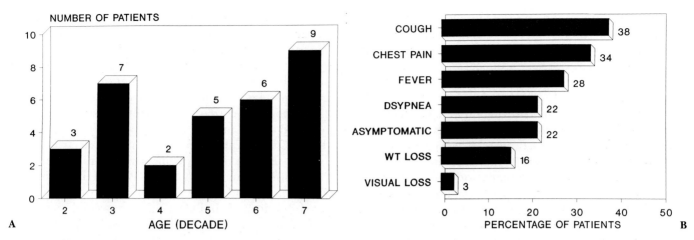

Fig. 30–12A,B. Necrotizing sarcoid granulomatosis. **A.** Age of patients. **B.** Presenting symptoms. (Compiled from References 11,93,164–169,171.)

Table 30–6. Clinical and roentgenographic features of patients with necrotizing sarcoid granulomatosis[a]

	Liebow[10]	Saldana[170]	Churg[93]	Koss[11]	Case reports[b]
Number of cases	11	30	32	13	8
Men:Women	Approximately 1:1	12:18	1:4	3:10	3:5
Bilateral (%)	82	12	72	62	50
Solitary (%)	18[a]	88	22	15	25
Hilar Adenopathy (%)	9	7	65	8	25
Cavitation (%)	NA	3	0	23	13
Patients with recurrence (%)	25	11	12	15	13
Died (%)	0	0	4[c]	0	13[d]

[a] Described as "localized, unilateral disease."
[b] Case reports.[164–169,171]
[c] One patient died of pneumonia several months postresection of a solitary nodule.
[d] Patient died of oat cell carcinoma.
NA, not available.

auscultation rales may be detected when patients have extensive bilateral pulmonary infiltrates.[11]

Chest radiographic patterns that can occur in necrotizing sarcoid granulomatosis include diffuse bilateral nodules, unilateral nodules, nodular infiltrates, or infiltrates (see Table 30–6).[10,11,93] The most common pattern appears to be multiple nodules or nodular infiltrates. The size of the nodules can range from several millimeters to 5 cm in diameter.[93,169] They tend to involve lower lobes[6]; they can disappear spontaneously, and they show cavitation in nearly one-quarter of cases (Table 30–6). Cavitation of poorly defined infiltrates may also occur.[11] Pleural effusion often occurs in the setting of diffuse lung disease.[11] The incidence of unilateral and solitary or localized lesions is 18%–33% in most series (see Table 30–6), but 88% of the 24 patients reported by Saldana et al.[170] had unilateral,

localized lesions. These localized lesions may mimic carcinoma or infectious granulomatous disease.[165] Bilateral hilar lymphadenopathy is uncommon in most series, being observed in only 7%–9% of patients (Table 30–6).[10,11,170] However, it was observed in 65% of the patients reported by Churg[6] and has been seen by others as well.[166,167]

Pulmonary function test abnormalities include decreased forced vital capacity (FVC) and forced expiratory volume (FEV_1) and reduced arterial oxygen saturation and diffusion constants.[164] Other reported laboratory abnormalities findings include a moderately elevated ESR,[11,168] and hypergammaglobulinemia.[11] These findings, although not specific, may be seen in sarcoidosis. However, only one of three patients tested showed elevation in the serum angiotensin-converting enzyme (ACE) level.[164,166,167] One other patient had elevated serum alkaline phosphatase levels (suggesting hepatic involvement) that returned to normal following treatment.

Pathologic Features

In gross appearance, necrotizing sarcoid granulomatosis typically shows nodular lesions that are less widespread and necrotic than those seen in Wegener's granulomatosis.[6] Microscopically, there are three elements: (1) granulomatous pneumonitis with many "sarcoid-like" granulomas; (2) necrosis of variable extent; and (3) vasculitis of several histologic types. Sarcoid-like granulomas consist of discrete clusters of epithelioid histiocytes, Langhans' giant cells, and admixed lymphocytes (Fig. 30–13A). Similar to sarcoidosis, the granulomas are frequently located along the pleura, bronchovascular bundles, and interlobular septa; submucosal involvement of the bronchi or bronchioles is also common (Fig. 30–13B).[11,93,167] The granulomas frequently become confluent, and they may appear poorly defined.[10] Alveolar involvement may produce a granulomatous pneumonia.[11] Hyalinizing granulomas may also be seen, similar to sarcoidosis.[93]

Small central foci of coagulative necrosis can be present within granulomas; there also can be larger geographic zones of infarct-like necrosis (Fig. 30–13C).[11] Rolfes et al.[166] reported suppurative necrosis in one case, but the presence of this type of necrosis is most unusual and should suggest alternate possibilities, such as Wegener's granulomatosis. Churg[6] suggested that necrosis need not be considered a prerequisite for the diagnosis of necrotizing sarcoid granulomatosis; in particular, 6 of his 32 cases did not show it. However, this concept is debatable.

The vasculitis in necrotizing sarcoid granulomatosis affects muscular pulmonary arteries and veins. Three types of vascular inflammation can be seen: necrotizing granulomas (Fig. 30–14A), giant cell vasculitis (Fig. 30–14B), and infiltration by mononuclear cells including lymphocytes and macrophages (Fig. 30–14C).[10] Necrotic epithelioid granulomas within arteries may be a distinctive feature.[11] Giant cell vasculitis was found in 23% of cases in one series.[11] In giant cell vasculitis, there are many giant cells arrayed circumferentially within the walls of larger arteries. Elastic stains show the giant cells apposed to fragmented external elastic lamellae.

A variety of secondary changes can also be seen in necrotizing sarcoid granulomatosis. Bronchiolitis obliterans, sometimes granulomatous in appearance, can be present and may be associated with intraalveolar accumulation of foamy macrophages (postobstructive pneumonia).

There are few cases of histologically confirmed extra-pulmonary granulomas in necrotizing sarcoid granulomatosis. Nonnecrotizing granulomas have been seen most commonly in hilar and peribronchial lymph nodes.[6,11] Sarcoid-like granulomatous inflammation has been found in the liver in one other case.[6] Necrotizing granulomas without vasculitis were found in the dura of the spinal cord of one patient who subsequently developed typical pulmonary lesions.[167]

Reports of the immunopathologic and electron microscopic features of necrotizing sarcoid granulomatosis are both few and inconclusive. Periarterial staining for IgG, IgA, and, minimally, for IgM was demonstrated in one case, and electron micrographs showed small extracellular osmiophilic deposits.[167] In contrast, neither staining for immunoglobulins and complement nor obvious electron-dense deposits could be demonstrated in another case.[168]

Clinical Course and Differential Diagnosis

The prognosis for patients with necrotizing sarcoid granulomatosis is excellent (see Table 30–6).[166,167] No deaths directly attributable to the disease have been reported. Patients with diffuse bilateral infiltrates typically respond well to corticosteroids with clearing or diminution of infiltrates 1 week to 10 months after starting therapy. Radiographic infiltrates persist in the minority of cases,[6,93] and relapse can occur in 11%–25% of patients (Table 30–6).[10,11,164] Low-dose chlorambucil has been effective, particularly after relapse.[11,170] However, immunosuppressive therapy should be used with caution because it may be complicated by fatal opportunistic infections.[93] For localized lesions, resection is both diagnostic and usually curative.[10,170]

The diagnosis of necrotizing sarcoid granulomatosis requires exclusion of an infectious etiology with cultures or special stains for microorganisms. Similar histopathologic features including vasculitis and sarcoid-like granulomas can be seen in granulomatous infections.[25,94] Even though fungi or mycobacteria may not be found with special stains, cultures may be positive. For example, Churg et al.[93] excluded three otherwise typical cases of necrotizing sarcoid granulomatosis from their series because cultures of the biopsy yielded mycobacteria or fungi. Exclusion of infection by cultures of the tissue, and/or careful examination of methenamine silver and acid-fast stains, are therefore mandatory before making a diagnosis of necrotizing sarcoid granulomatosis.

The origin and pathogenesis of necrotizing sarcoid granulomatosis remains unknown. It may be that this disease, which was initially defined primarily by pathologic (primarily light microscopic) criteria, has more than one etiology. Because the pathology can be mim-

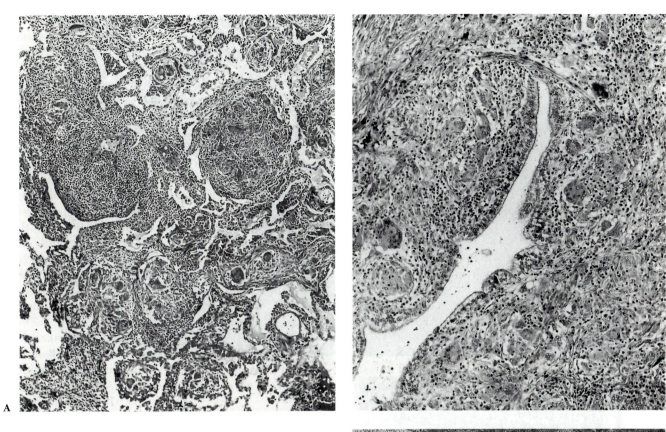

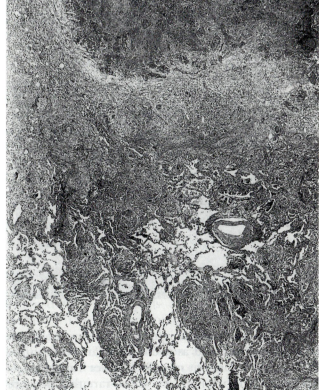

Fig. 30–13A–C. Necrotizing sarcoid granulomatosis. **A.** Multiple sarcoid-like granulomas consisting of clusters of epithelioid histiocytes and multinucleated giant cells infiltrate interstitium adjacent to necrotizing lesions. H and E, ×75. **B.** Granulomatous inflammation extends into bronchiolar submucosa. H and E, ×100. **C.** Nodular mass of confluent sarcoid-like granulomas has central large zone of necrosis. H and E, ×30.

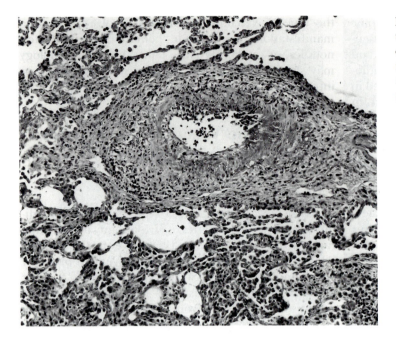

Fig. 30–15. Polyarteritis nodosa. Transmural necrotizing acute inflammation in pulmonary arteriole in open lung biopsy from patient with polyarteritis nodosa. Neither venular involvement nor parenchymal inflammatory or granulomatous lesions are present. H and E, ×100.

Table 30–7. Conditions associated with small vessel vasculitis[2,92,178,179]

Small vessel vasculitis associated with known conditions
  Hypersensitivity vasculitis (drug-induced)[48]
    Penicillin
    Sulfonamides
    Diuretics
    Nonsteroidal antiinflammatory agents
    Anticonvulsants
  Infection[9,179]
    Hepatitis B
    Upper respiratory tract streptococcal infections
  Other diseases
    Collagen vascular diseases[2,92]
    Malignancy[204,291–297]
    Henoch–Schönlein purpura[182,190,197]
    Mixed cryoglobulinemia[199,200,204]
    Pulmonary interstitial fibrosis in elderly patients[489]
    Cystic fibrosis[48]
  Bone marrow transplantation[376]
Idiopathic small vessel vasculitis[a]
  Systemic
  Localized pulmonary small vessel vasculitis

[a] The term hypersensitivity vasculitis has been used for idiopathic small vessel vasculitis syndromes.[178]

yielded the lowest sensitivity and specificity among the different vasculitis syndromes evaluated by the 1990 American College of Rheumatology subcommittee on vasculitis.

The concept of small vessel vasculitis encompasses not only hypersensitivity vasculitis but also a spectrum of other vasculitides, several of which are not caused by hypersensitivity reactions to drugs or other agents (Table 30–7).[2,92,179] Many forms of small vessel vasculitis

affect the skin, but renal, joint, pulmonary, gastrointestinal tract, and neurologic involvement can also occur.

The frequency of lung disease is difficult to determine precisely; however, it has been described in up to 24% of cases of hypersensitivity vasculitis.[9,159] Vasculitis is seldom demonstrated in lung biopsy material from these patients, because the pulmonary disease is often transient and biopsies are rarely obtained; as a result, there is little information about the lung pathology. Although leukocytoclastic vasculitis may be the classical histology for hypersensitivity vasculitis, pulmonary involvement by other small vessel vasculitis syndromes may demonstrate primarily lymphocytic (Fig. 30–16) or eosinophilic vasculitis. Pulmonary venular involvement has been demonstrated in one patient with urticarial vasculitis.[180]

Active small vessel vasculitis is usually responsive to steroids. If a specific precipitating agent can be identified, the patient's exposure should be discontinued. Patients with chronic small vessel vasculitis may not respond to steroids.[9]

Henoch–Schönlein Purpura

Henoch–Schönlein purpura is a distinct form of small vessel vasculitis characterized by palpable purpura, abdominal pain, gastrointestinal hemorrhage, arthralgias, and renal disease.[181–184] The *traditional format* criteria proposed by the American College of Rheumatology include: (1) age equal to or less than 20 years at onset of disease; (2) palpable purpura; (3) acute abdominal pain; and (4) biopsy showing granulocytes in the walls of

Fig. 30–16. Small vessel vasculitis. Venule is involved by intense transmural lymphocytic infiltrate with few eosinophils. H and E, ×200.

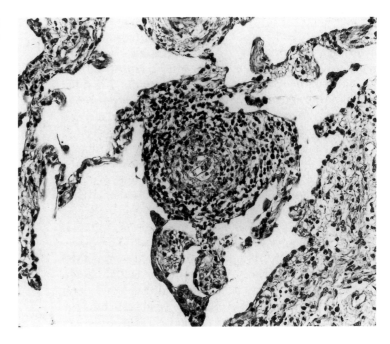

small arterioles or venules.[183] The presence of two or more of these criteria yields a sensitivity of 87.1% and a specificity of 87.7%.[183] The disease occurs mostly in children between 2 and 10 years old, but it can also occur in adults.[181,182,184] Immunofluorescence reveals IgA and complement deposits, with or without IgG, in both dermal vessels and renal mesangium.[184] IgA deposits have also been identified in pulmonary alveolar septal vessels.[185] Renal glomeruli may show a spectrum of changes including normal findings and mesangial hypercellularity as well as focal and diffuse glomerulonephritis. Henoch–Schönlein purpura can also occur as a paraneoplastic syndrome that coincides with presentation or relapse of lung carcinoma.[186–189]

Pulmonary involvement is uncommon but has been reported in as many as 6.5% of adult cases.[181] Pulmonary symptoms include hemoptysis, dyspnea, and pleuritic chest pain.[181,190] The most serious pulmonary complication is severe intraalveolar hemorrhage, which can be fatal.[181,185,191–196] Patients who develop severe pulmonary hemorrhage often also have acute renal failure. Pathologic changes in the lung may include pulmonary edema,[190,197] perivascular inflammatory infiltrates,[197] and capillaritis in cases of pulmonary hemorrhage.[191]

Cryoglobulinemic Vasculitis

Cryoglobulinemia can be idiopathic (essential) or it can occur in association with lymphoproliferative disorders, collagen vascular diseases, or infections.[198] Patients with cryoglobulinemia have serum immunoglobulins that precipitate reversibly in cold temperatures.[199] Clin-

ically, they show cutaneous purpura, arthralgias, hypocomplementemia, and glomerulonephritis with or without vasculitis. Pulmonary involvement is common with radiographic signs of interstitial lung involvement in up to 78% of patients.[200] Pulmonary symptoms consist of dyspnea (39%), cough (13%), asthma (9%), pleurisy (4%), and hemoptysis (4%).[200,201] One report suggested that patients with essential mixed cryoglobulinemia following hepatitis B infection are more likely to have pronounced pulmonary disease.[200] However, there are few published data about the lung pathology in cryoglobulinemia.[9,199,200,202] The vasculitis of cryoglobulinemia is usually leukocytoclastic, but vasculitis involving medium-sized arteries has also been described. In the lung, histologic sections may show infiltration of alveolar septa and small vessel walls by a mixture of neutrophils, lymphocytes, and plasma cells.[199] In addition, one may encounter pulmonary hemorrhage and interstitial fibrosis.[202–205]

Takayasu's Arteritis

Takayasu's arteritis is a large vessel vasculitis that affects primarily the aorta and its branches. It occurs most commonly in women less than 40 years of age.[206] Pulmonary arterial involvement can be detected angiographically in 12%–86% of cases,[207–211] but it is rarely suspected clinically.[208,209] Pulmonary involvement is more common in patients with the HLA Bw52/Dw12 haplotype.[212] In 1990, the American College of Rheumatology proposed six criteria for the diagnosis, including: (1) onset at age less than 40 years; (2) claudication of an extremity; (3) decreased brachial artery pulse; (4)

greater than 10 mm Hg difference in systolic blood pressure between arms; (5) a bruit over the subclavian arteries or the aorta; and (6) arteriographic evidence of narrowing or occlusion of the entire aorta and its primary branches or large arteries in the proximal upper or lower extremities.[206] The presence of three of these six criteria has a sensitivity of 90.5% and a specificity of 97.8%.[206]

Takayasu's arteritis progresses through three phases, beginning with an inflammatory phase characterized by fever, malaise, weight loss, arthralgias, and elevated ESR.[213] The second phase consists of vascular inflammation, which can present as localized pain, vascular stenosis, or formation of aneurysms. The third phase is characterized by ischemia caused by vascular narrowing or occlusion; the resulting ischemia has led to use of the term pulseless disease. The diagnosis is usually established by angiography because it is difficult to obtain tissue biopsy specimens from large vessels such as the aorta or pulmonary artery. Takayasu's arteritis can have cerebrovascular manifestations and can cause aortic insufficiency, aortic aneurysms, or renovascular hypertension.

Pulmonary artery angiography can demonstrate vessel stenosis, irregular narrowing, and occlusion.* Abnormal ventilation perfusion scans, seen in as many as 76% of cases,[216] typically show multiple, bilateral,[217] or unilateral defects.[216,218] Fistulas may develop between the pulmonary arteries and bronchial or coronary arteries as well as systemic arteries.[211,219,220] Bronchial artery to coronary artery fistula has also been reported.[220] Respiratory symptoms are uncommon, but can consist of dyspnea and pleuritic chest pain. Pulmonary hypertension can also occur.[215]

The large elastic pulmonary arteries are affected. Histologically, the arteritis consists of lymphocytes, macrophages, and giant cells affecting adventitia, media, and intima, sometimes associated with thrombus formation. This can progress to diffuse or nodular fibrosis of the artery wall and disintegration or loss of elastic fibers.[221-223] The fibrosis can result in stenosis or obliteration of the vascular lumen and cause aneurysm formation or dilatation of the artery.[221] Interstitial lung disease and glomerulonephritis have been reported in one case.[224]

Corticosteroid therapy is often successful, but cyclophosphamide may be necessary in some cases. Vascular surgery is sometimes necessary to reverse ischemia.[214,225,226]

---

*References: 207, 209, 210, 213–216.

Behçet's Syndrome

Behçet's syndrome is a systemic vasculitic syndrome characterized by oral and genital ulcers and iridocyclitis. The majority of cases occur in the Mediterranean basin, the Middle East, and Japan, although the distribution is worldwide.[227-232] The diagnosis is based primarily on clinical criteria. It requires the presence of recurrent oral aphthosis and at least two of the following five clinical manifestations: recurrent genital aphthosis, uveitis, synovitis, cutaneous vasculitis, meningoencephalitis and the absence of inflammatory bowel disease or other collagen vascular diseases.[231] Pulmonary symptoms include dyspnea, cough, chest pain, and hemoptysis.[228] Males are more likely to have pulmonary involvement and hemoptysis.[228,229] Demonstration of circulating immune complexes in association with active pulmonary disease suggests that immune complexes may be important in the pathogenesis of pulmonary involvement.[229,233] The clinical and pathologic features of the Hughes–Stoven syndrome are remarkably similar to those of Behçet's syndrome suggesting that it represents a forme fruste of Behçet's syndrome. It has even been recently suggested that bilateral pulmonary artery aneurysms may represent the first appearance of Behçet's syndrome.[234]

The major pulmonary pathologic finding in Behçet's syndrome is that of lymphocytic and necrotizing vasculitis involving pulmonary arteries of all sizes, veins, and alveolar septal capillaries (Fig. 30–17A). Complications of the vasculitis include aneurysms of elastic pulmonary arteries (Fig. 30–17B), arterial and venous thromboses, pulmonary infarcts, bronchial erosion by pulmonary artery aneurysms, and arteriobronchial fistulas.[228,235,236] Perivascular adventitial fibrosis can be prominent. Newly formed collateral vessels lacking elastic lamellae an derived from smooth muscle metaplasia around arterioles can be found in the periadventitial fibrous tissues around thrombosed arteries and aneurysms (Fig. 30–17C). Pulmonary angiography may be useful in demonstrating aneurysms and thromboses.[228,230] Pulmonary hemorrhage[237] and acute interstitial pneumonia[238] represent potential life-threatening complications. Bronchial obstruction has also been reported.[239]

Medical therapy, including corticosteroids, may be used to try to control the vasculitis. Anticoagulation may benefit patients who develop thromboses.[229] Cyclosporine has been attempted in a patient with rapidly progressive thromboembolic disease.[240] Corticosteroid therapy may be complicated by opportunistic infections such as mucormycosis.[241] Surgical intervention with lobectomy may be necessary for life-threatening hemoptysis.[237]

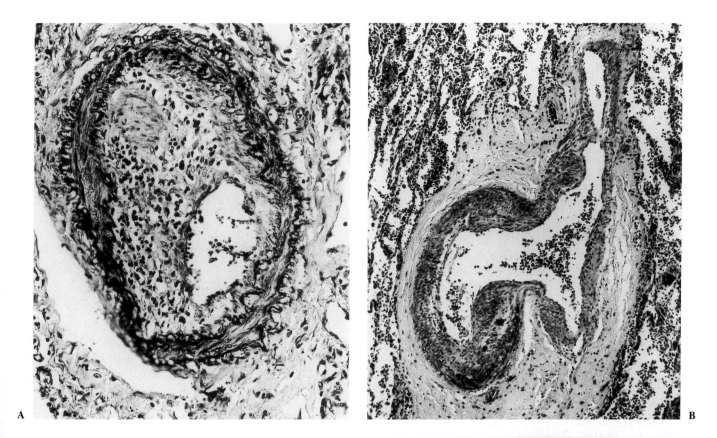

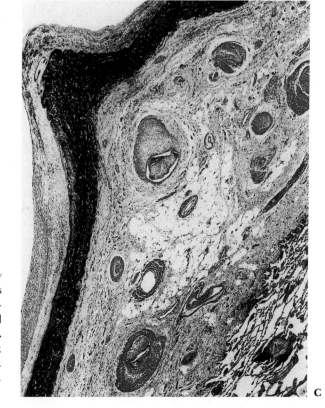

Fig. 30–17. Behçet's syndrome. **A.** Venulitis is characterized by lymphocytic medial chronic inflammatory infiltrate with fibrosis and narrowing of the vascular lumen. Movat, ×200. **B.** Aneurysmal dilatation of arteriole with marked thinning of muscular wall and eccentric expansion of vascular lumen. H and E, ×100. **C.** Marked periadventitial fibrosis surrounds pulmonary artery; within fibrotic zone are newly formed collateral vessels with thick musclar walls but not elastic lamellae. Movat, ×27. (Courtesy of Dr. Richard E. Slavin and Dr. Ramon Sanchez, Galveston, Texas.[236])

Hypocomplementemic Vasculitis

Hypocomplementemic vasculitis was defined by McDuffie in 1973 as a syndrome characterized by hypocomplementemia, cutaneous vasculitis, and arthritis.[242] Subsequently, the following criteria were proposed: (1) chronic urticaria of more than 6 months duration; (2) hypocomplementemia; and (3) two of the following: biopsy-confirmed dermal venulitis, arthralgias, or arthritis; glomerulonephritis, uveitis, or episcleritis; recurrent abdominal pain; and a positive C1q precipitin test.[243] The diagnosis requires exclusion of the presence of significant cryoglobulinemia, elevated anti-DNA titers ($>1:32$), hepatitis B antigenemia, decreased blood c1-esterase inhibitor, or a hereditary complement deficiency.[243] Pulmonary involvement is uncommon, but pleuritic chest pain and transient lung infiltrates have been observed.[243] Patients often have asthmatic symptoms; however, this is usually caused by laryngeal edema.[243] Chronic obstructive pulmonary disease may be seen in up to 50% of patients.[244] Although vasculitis involving small vessels of the lung has been postulated, histologic confirmation has not been documented. A close relationship between hypocomplementemic vasculitis and systemic lupus erythematosus (SLE) has been observed, and this type of vasculitis may represent a manifestation of collagen vascular disease.[245-247] Conservative management with low-dose steroids may be effective.[244] For patients with renal disease, cyclophosphamide or azathioprine may be required.[245]

Idiopathic Granulomatous Vasculitis

Giant Cell Arteritis

As many as 9% of patients with giant cell (temporal) arteritis can have respiratory tract symptoms; however, these symptoms are primarily caused by upper respiratory tract involvement and consist of cough, sore throat, hoarseness, and, less often, chest pain.[248] Giant cell arteritis most commonly affects the cranial arteries, but large extracranial arteries such as the aorta may be involved in 10%–15% of cases.[249] Pulmonary arterial involvement by giant cell arteritis is rare.[250] Reported radiographic findings include lung nodules,[251,252] interstitial infiltrates,[253] and unilateral pleural effusions.[248] The pulmonary trunk and main pulmonary arteries may be affected in addition to large and medium-sized intrapulmonary elastic arteries.[250] Vascular histologic changes consist of medial and adventitial mononuclear inflammation with giant cells and disruption of the elastic laminae; focal fibrinoid necrosis of the media may be seen.[250] Mural thrombi can also be present.[250] Bronchoscopic biopsies can reveal granulo-

matous inflammation of pulmonary arteries with fragmented elastic fibers.[250,251] The absence of extravascular granulomas separates pulmonary giant cell arteritis from other granulomatous pulmonary vasculitides such as Wegener's granulomatosis, necrotizing sarcoid granulomatosis, Churg–Strauss syndrome, and granulomatous infections.[250] Thus published cases of giant cell arteritis characterized by necrotizing granulomas in one case[252] and interstitial infiltrates with poorly defined granulomas in the peribronchial and alveolar interstitium in two others,[253] may actually be Wegener's granulomatosis[252] or sarcoidosis,[253] respectively. Distinction from Takayasu's arteritis is based on the prominent involvement of the temporal artery (in addition to other large arteries such as the aorta) and the older age of the patients with giant cell arteritis, as well as on the histologic features.[250]

Giant cell arteritis rarely is isolated to the pulmonary arteries.[254-256] In such cases of "idiopathic isolated pulmonary giant cell arteritis," patients may present with dyspnea on exertion but they generally do not have hemoptysis, fever, or elevated ESR. Two such patients were treated effectively with lobectomy or pneumonectomy.[254,255] One patient with cor pulmonale underwent successful vascular surgery to relieve a severe stenosis of the right main pulmonary artery.[256] Histologic vascular changes in these cases also demonstrate organized thrombi with recanalization and narrowing of large pulmonary arteries associated with a destructive inflammatory infiltrate in the vessel wall. The vascular inflammation consists of giant cells, histiocytes, and lymphocytes (Fig. 30–18); fragmentation of elastic laminae is frequent.[254-256] Infarcts in the distal lung may be present.

Disseminated Visceral Giant Cell Angiitis

Pulmonary involvement has been observed in three of the five reported cases of disseminated visceral giant cell arteritis.[257,258] All patients were male, and disseminated visceral giant cell arteritis was clinically unsuspected with discovery of the diagnosis as an incidental autopsy finding.[257] Arteritis primarily affects extracranial small arteries and arterioles, and typically involves at least three of the following organs: heart, lung, kidneys, liver, pancreas, and stomach. None of these patients had evidence of sarcoid, collagen vascular disease, hepatitis, or other infection. The arterial inflammation consists predominantly of histiocytes, lymphocytes, and plasma cells; multinucleated giant cells of both the foreign-body type and Langhans' types can be seen in large numbers. Eosinophils are uncommon. Cases of combined sarcoidosis and disseminated visceral giant cell arteritis may exist, although such cases

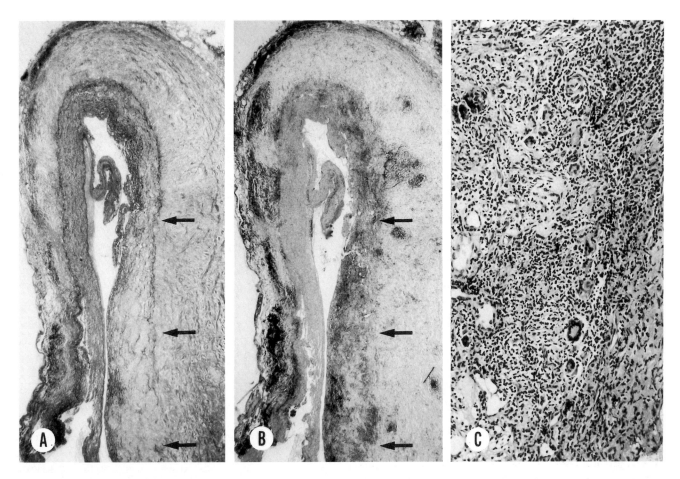

Fig. 30–18A–C. Isolated giant cell arteritis of pulmonary artery. **A.** Elastic stain, ×40. **B.** H and E-stained sections of pulmonary artery giant cell arteritis. Note segmental disruption of medial elastic lamellae and diffuse lymphoplasmacytic infiltrate with giant cells (*arrows*). H and E, ×40. **C.** Higher power close-up view of inflammatory cell infiltrate with multiple multinucleated giant cells. H and E, ×160. (From case reported in Reference 264. Courtesy of Dr. J.T. Lie, Rochester, Minnesota.)

are difficult to classify and may be very controversial.[259–261]

Miscellaneous Systemic Disorders That Can Affect the Lung

Classical Sarcoidosis

Vasculitis can be seen in up to 69% of open lung biopsy specimens[174–176] and 53% of transbronchial biopsy specimens[262] from patients with classical sarcoidosis (see also Chapter 19). The vasculitis may be granulomatous, consisting of epithelioid histiocytes or giant cells (Fig. 30–19A), or it may consist of lymphocytes and plasma cells (Fig. 30–19B). Venous involvement (61%) is more common than combined venous and arterial or arterial involvement.[176] In sarcoidosis, pulmonary hypertension with cor pulmonale can result from granulomatous vasculitis,[263,264] interstitial fibrosis,[265] or mechanical compression of pulmonary artery by enlarged hilar lymph nodes.[266,267] If detected early enough, the pulmonary hypertension may be reversible with corticosteroid therapy.[268] Rarely, granulomatous venulitis in sarcoidosis can lead to veno-occlusive disease and result in pulmonary hypertension.[269,270] Patients with pulmonary sarcoid may also develop a systemic vasculitis.[271]

Collagen Vascular Disorders

Pulmonary vasculitis is one of the many manifestations of collagen vascular diseases. It often occurs in the setting of systemic vasculitis and can take several forms, including vasculitis of medium-size vessels (sometimes having the pattern of polyarteritis nodosa),[272] pulmonary hypertension, and capillaritis with pulmonary hemorrhage.[98] Vasculitis can also be seen as a localized

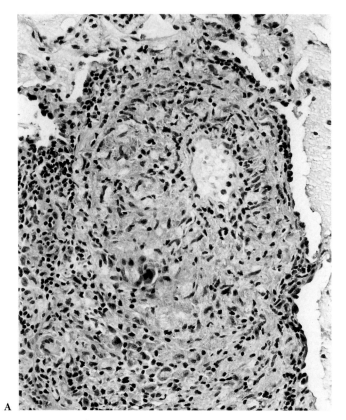

A

Fig. 30–19A,B. Sarcoid. A. Granulomatous arteritis consists of numerous epithelioid histiocytes infiltrating through wall of arteriole. H and E, ×250. B. Chronic venulitis with numer-

B

ous lymphocytes and plasma cells infiltrate wall of venule. H and E, × 250.

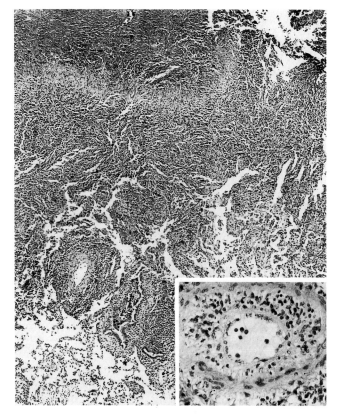

phenomenon adjacent to rheumatoid nodules (Fig. 30–20).[273] Pulmonary vasculitis can occur in virtually any of the collagen vascular diseases, including rheumatoid arthritis (Fig. 30–21A),[272,274,275] SLE (Fig. 30–21B),[276] scleroderma,[277] idiopathic inflammatory myopathy (dermatomyositis or polymyositis),[278] and mixed connective tissue disease.[279]

Certain types of vasculitis are more common in specific collagen vascular diseases. For example, in scleroderma, vascular changes associated with pulmonary hypertension are the most common type of blood vessel abnormality; these may be accompanied by a focal endothelialitis, consisting of lymphocytes and plasma cells, within the arterial intimal proliferation.[277] The pulmonary vasculitis in scleroderma is usually nonnecrotizing, and fibrinoid necrosis and acute vasculitis are uncommon.[280,281] The most common type of pulmonary vasculitis in rheumatoid arthritis is the localized

◁————————————————————————

Fig. 30–20. Rheumatoid nodule. Necrotizing granuloma consists of necrotic zone surrounded by palisading histiocytes. Chronic inflammation with secondary vasculitis is present in surrounding lung parenchyma. Inset: Wall of arteriole is infiltrated by lymphocytes and plasma cells. H and E, ×200.

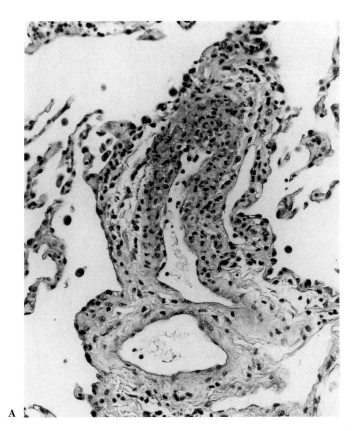

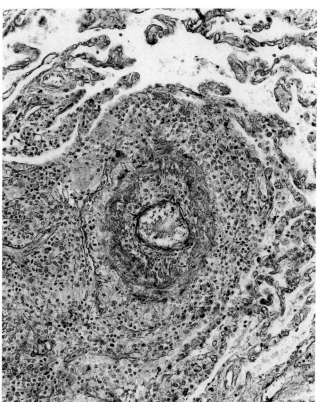

Fig. 30–21A,B. A. Rheumatoid arthritis. Venulitis characterized by focal, transmural infiltrate of mononuclear cells consisting of histiocytes and lymphocytes. H and E, ×200. **B.** Systemic lupus erythematosus. Chronic arteritis characterized by infiltration of arteriolar wall by lymphocytes and associated with chronic interstitial pneumonitis. H and E, ×200.

vasculitis found adjacent to rheumatoid nodules. Vasculitis affecting medium-sized vessels can occur,[272] but it is uncommon and it was conspicuously absent in two series reporting open lung biopsy findings from patients with rheumatoid arthritis.[273,282] Pulmonary vasculitis was seen in 17% of patients with polymyositis and 2% of patients with dermatomyositis in one autopsy study[278]; interstitial lung disease was present in each of these cases. Pathologic changes in the blood vessels included necrotizing vasculitis and chronic or healed proliferative lesions.

Diffuse pulmonary hemorrhage has been reported in SLE, rheumatoid arthritis, and juvenile rheumatoid arthritis, but can probably occur in any of the collagen vascular diseases.[98] Similar to pulmonary hemorrhage syndromes associated with other conditions, it is often associated with a fulminant clinical presentation and acute renal failure.

Pulmonary hypertension can also occur in SLE,[276,283–287] rheumatoid arthritis,[273,282,288–290] and idiopathic inflammatory myopathy.[278] In some cases it appears to be a complication of pulmonary vasculitis.[288] In patients with rheumatoid arthritis, pulmonary hypertension should be considered, especially when Raynaud's phenomenon is present.[289,290]

Malignancy, Vasculitis, and the Lung

Rarely malignancy may result in vasculitis affecting the lung. Most patients present with a cutaneous small vessel vasculitis, and the lung is only one of several sites involved.[204,291–297] Vasculitis as a paraneoplastic syndrome occurs most often in association with lympho- or myeloproliferative disorders.[204,291–297] Pulmonary involvement by a polyarteritis nodosa-like syndrome can occur in hairy cell leukemia.[296,298] Churg–Strauss syndrome has also been reported in a patient with malignant melanoma.[148] Pulmonary vasculitis has been reported in a patient with cholangiocarcinoma.[293] In addition, lung cancer may be associated with systemic vasculitis[294] in the form of a microvasculitis of the vasa nervorum[294,295,299] or Henoch–Shönlein purpura.[186–189]

Vasculitis can also occur as a local phenomenon when there is prominent intraarterial or lymphangitic spread of metastatic tumor (Fig. 30–22).

Inflammatory Bowel Disease

Pulmonary vasculitis has been reported in patients with inflammatory bowel disease, especially ulcerative colitis.[300,301] Because these patients are frequently treated

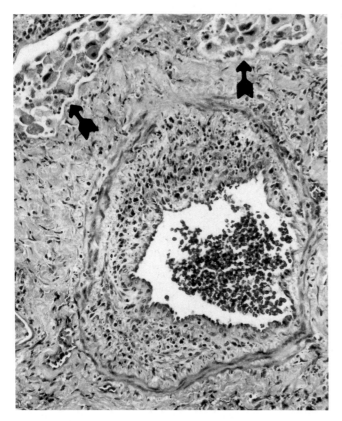

Fig. 30–22. Metastatic renal cell carcinoma. Wall of arteriole has marked chronic inflammatory infiltrate. Metastatic tumor cells fill surrounding lymphatics (*arrows*). H and E, ×200.

with sulfonamides, a known cause of pulmonary vasculitis,[302] a drug reaction must be carefully excluded before attributing pulmonary vasculitis to inflammatory bowel disease. Although P-ANCA can be found in patients with inflammatory bowel disease, in particular in ulcerative colitis, it does not correlate with activity of disease or evidence of systemic or pulmonary vasculitis.[44]

Diffuse Pulmonary Hemorrhage Syndrome

Diffuse pulmonary hemorrhage is one of the most fulminant, life-threatening pulmonary manifestations of the vasculitis syndromes. Many patients with diffuse pulmonary hemorrhage also present with renal failure, which may be rapidly progressive and irreversible. Management of these patients requires an aggressive approach to therapy and careful follow-up because these disorders can have a relapsing course.[303–307] Diffuse pulmonary hemorrhage can occur in a variety of vasculitic as well as nonvasculitic disorders (see also

Table 30–8. Vasculitic disorders associated with diffuse pulmonary hemorrhage[a]

Wegener's granulomatosis[98]
Churg–Strauss angiitis and granulomatosis[132]
Collagen vascular diseases[98]
Systemic lupus erythematosus[490–494]
Rheumatoid arthritis[98]
Juvenile rheumatoid arthritis[98]
Henoch–Schönlein purpura[185,191–196]
Mixed cryoglobulinemia[203,495]
Behçet's syndrome[228,236,237]
Small vessel vasculitis associated with bone marrow transplantation[376]
Systemic sarcoid-like granulomatous vasculitis[22,496]
Systemic necrotizing vasculitis (± hepatitis B infection)[98,497,498]
Anti-basement membrane antibody disease[98]
Idiopathic pulmonary hemorrhage[98]
IgA nephropathy[98]
Idiopathic glomerulonephritis (with and without immune complexes)[13,29,52,98]
Circulating IgM antineutrophil antibody (P-ANCA pattern) associated with glomerulonephritis[22,496]

[a]Although several of these conditions are not considered to be primary vasculitides, histologic evidence of capillaritis in lung biopsy specimens and/or elevated serum ANCA titers suggest that vasculitis may play a role in the pathogenesis of the pulmonary hemorrhage.

Chapter 4). The vasculitides, the largest category of disorders associated with diffuse pulmonary hemorrhage, are summarized in Table 30–8.[98] Accurate subclassification is necessary, because the therapy may differ for individual diseases and several of the therapeutic options carry significant toxicity. Histologic confirmation of the diagnosis often requires open lung biopsy and is almost always necessary before initiation of therapy.[304]

In the majority of cases, the disease producing diffuse pulmonary hemorrhage cannot be precisely determined on the basis of light microscopic examination of lung biopsy specimens alone.[98] Capillaritis consisting of neutrophilic infiltration of alveolar septal walls is the typical finding in diffuse pulmonary hemorrhage syndromes, present in 88% of lung biopsies (Fig. 30–23A).[98] In Wegener's granulomatosis, capillaritis may rarely consist of epithelioid histiocytes, giving a granulomatous appearance (Fig. 30–23B). Wegener's granulomatosis is probably the only diagnosis that can be suggested from light microscopic review of the lung biopsy. Clues to the diagnosis of Wegener's granulomatosis also include foci of necrosis, granulomatous inflammation, and vasculitis involving arterioles or venules. These may be subtle findings, requiring careful search and in some cases deeper sections. The absence of histologic features of Wegener's granulomatosis does not exclude the diagnosis, because lung biopsy specimens showing only pulmonary hemorrhage and capillaritis may precede[308] or follow[64] development

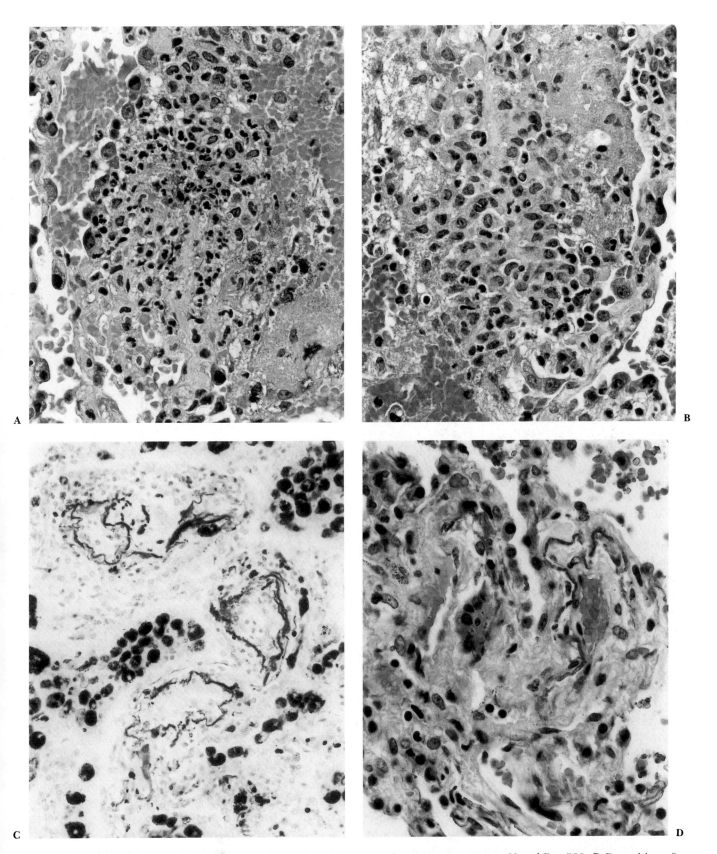

Fig. 30–23A–D. Diffuse alveolar hemorrhage in patient with Wegener's granulomatosis. **A.** Capillaritis characterized by neutrophilic infiltration and necrosis of the wall of alveolar septa with neutrophils and fibrin spilling into adjacent alveolar spaces that also contain numerous red blood cells consistent with intraalveolar hemorrhage. H and E, ×500. **B.** In this case, capillaritis consists primarily of epithelioid cells giving granulomatous appearance. H and E, ×500. **C.** Deposition of iron on vascular elastic fibers is highlighted by Prussian blue stain. In addition to positive staining for iron, elastic fibers show fragmentation. Prussian blue, ×250. **D.** Multinucleated giant cells in wall of small venule are associated with fragmented and iron-coated elastic fibers. H and E, ×500. (**A,C,D**: from Travis et al.,[25] with permission.)

of classic pathologic features of the disease.[98] Rarely, Wegener's granulomatosis and antibasement membrane antibody disease may coexist.[309]

For patients who do not already have a diagnosis such as Wegener's granulomatosis or collagen vascular disease, classification of diffuse pulmonary hemorrhage syndrome requires correlation with a variety of other findings, including the clinical history, laboratory tests for serum antibasement membrane antibody (ABMA) or ANCA, and data from immunofluorescence or electron microscopy, as well as results of biopsies of the kidney, nasal sinus, or skin prompted by clinical abnormalities detected at these sites. Immunofluorescence and electron microscopy of renal biopsy specimens can be helpful in the subclassification of diffuse pulmonary hemorrhage syndromes such as ABMA-mediated diffuse pulmonary hemorrhage, IgA nephropathy, and SLE. Less often, immunofluorescence or electron microscopy on lung biopsy specimens can be useful in identifying immune complexes, linear IgG staining in ABMA-mediated diffuse pulmonary hemorrhage, or electron-dense deposits in immune complex disease such as SLE. Thus, it may be useful to snap-freeze a small piece of unfixed lung tissue and save a small piece of lung in glutaraldehyde for electron microscopy if a diffuse pulmonary hemorrhage syndrome is suspected clinically or on a frozen section.

In some patients with diffuse pulmonary hemorrhage syndromes it is difficult to fit the spectrum of clinical, laboratory, and pathologic findings into a specific disease entity. For patients with pulmonary renal syndromes who have features suggestive of Wegener's granulomatosis but who do not meet traditional clinical or pathologic criteria, the term probable Wegener's granulomatosis can be used. The term unclassified pulmonary renal syndrome can be used for cases in which the clinical, laboratory, and pathologic data do not permit classification into a specific diffuse pulmonary hemorrhage syndrome.

In biopsies demonstrating diffuse pulmonary hemorrhage with marked hemosiderosis, the elastic layers of the arteriolar and venular walls are occasionally encrusted by a dark basophilic material that stains strongly for iron with Prussian blue stain (Fig. 30–23C). These basophilic elastic fibers are frequently fragmented and are sometimes associated with a giant cell reaction (Fig. 30–23D), a finding that has been wrongly termed endogenous pneumoconiosis in the past (see also Chapter 22). These giant cells should not be mistaken for granulomatous vascular lesions of Wegener's granulomatosis because they actually represent a foreign-body giant cell reaction to the iron-encrusted elastica produced by chronic hemorrhage.

The importance of recognizing an associated vasculitis syndrome in a patient presenting with diffuse pulmonary hemorrhage is underscored by the finding of Sanchez-Masiques et al.,[305] who reported 50% mortality for patients with alveolar hemorrhage associated with Wegener's granulomatosis on the basis of literature review. All survivors had been treated with cytotoxic agents; those who died had either no specific therapy or were treated with corticosteroids alone, or died before cytotoxic therapy could be expected to be effective. An aggressive diagnostic approach and the earliest possible administration of cytotoxic drugs in combination with corticosteroids offer the best chance of survival in this fulminant condition. Sanchez-Masiques et al. also found that patients with alveolar hemorrhage had more evidence of systemic vasculitis and glomerulonephritis and less evidence of upper airway disease when compared with patients with more "typical" Wegener's granulomatosis.[305]

Secondary or Localized Vasculitis

Pulmonary Infection

Pulmonary vasculitis can occur in association with a variety of infections in the lung. Invasion and necrosis of blood vessel walls is a characteristic feature of certain bacterial pneumonias, particularly *Pseudomonas aeruginosa*,[310,311] and *Legionella pneumophila*.[312] Vasculitis can also occur in association with necrotizing granulomas caused by fungal (Figs. 30–24A,B) or mycobacterial organisms,[94] and on occasion can mimic Wegener's granulomatosis pathologically. *Malassezia furfur*, a fungus of low pathogenicity that usually infects the skin, has been reported to cause vasculitis in infants who developed pulmonary artery lipid deposits associated with Intralipid therapy.[313] In immunocompromised patients, pneumonias caused by certain fungi such as *Aspergillus* and *Mucor* are notorious for causing angioinvasion associated with pulmonary infarction.[314]

Vasculitis can also be seen in association with pulmonary infection by certain parasites such as *Dirofilaria immitis*,[315] *Schistosoma*,[316–318] and *Wuchereria*.[49,319,320] In pulmonary dirofilariasis the adult worm embolizes a pulmonary artery, occluding the lumen and resulting in an infarct that may be surrounded by granulomatous reaction and eosinophilia. The affected pulmonary artery is often situated in the center of the infarct and may have inflammatory changes in the wall with infiltration by chronic inflammatory cells or eosinophils.[315]

Vasculitis has also recently been described as a rare complication of *Pneumocystis carinii* pneumonia in HIV-infected patients.[321] *P. carinii* can invade blood vessels in the lung and cause vasculitis (Figs. 30–25A,B,C).

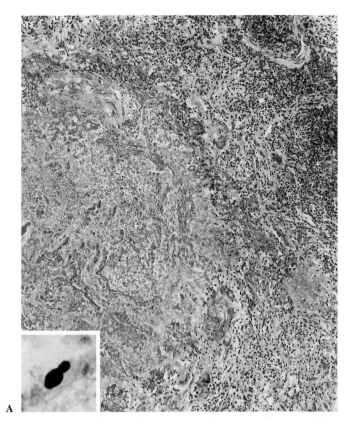

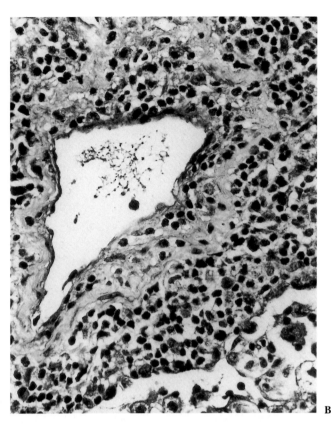

Fig. 30–24A,B. *Histoplasma capsulatum* infection in a patient with Wegener's granulomatosis. **A.** Necrotizing granulomatous inflammation with palisading histiocytes surrounds central necrotic zone. H and E, ×50. Inset: Budding yeast with morphology consistent with *Histoplasma capsulatum*. Gomori methenamine silver ×1650. **B.** Secondry venulitis in lung parenchyma adjacent to necrotizing granuloma. H and E, ×400.

Sometimes this may be observed adjacent to cavitary nodular lesions in lung[322] or in association with disseminated extrapulmonary infection by *P. carinii*.[323]

Bronchocentric Granulomatosis

The term bronchocentric granulomatosis was introduced by Liebow in 1973 to describe a new type of idiopathic pulmonary granulomatosis in which necrotizing granulomas were centered on bronchi or bronchioles.[10] Subsequently it was shown that two clinicopathologic forms of bronchocentric granulomatosis exist, depending on the presence or absence of asthma, and that most cases in asthmatics are associated with allergic bronchopulmonary aspergillosis (ABPA).[95,158,324–326] In recent years, it has become apparent that bronchocentric granulomatosis actually represents a nonspecific histologic reaction of the lung that can occur in a wide variety of conditions, most prominently allergic bronchopulmonary fungal disease (ABPFD), but also with rheumatoid arthritis, ankylosing spondylitis, Wegener's granulomatosis (see Fig. 30–

6B), and a number of mycobacterial, fungal, and parasitic infections (Table 30–9). When none of these conditions can be identified, the patient is considered to have an idiopathic form of bronchocentric granulomatosis (see also Chapter 16). Still, it is possible that some of these cases actually represent granulomatous infections in which the organisms are not detectable by cultures or light microscopic examination of special stains.[95]

As many as 50% of cases of bronchocentric granulomatosis are associated with ABPFD.[95,158,326] While ABPA associated with *Aspergillus fumigatus* is the most common form of ABPFD, other fungi may also rarely be involved (see Table 30–9).[156] Virtually all these patients are asthmatics, although ABPFD can occur rarely in nonasthmatics.[156,327] The age at presentation for patients with ABPA varies widely from 9 to 71 years, but most patients are in the second and third decades of life (Fig. 30–26A).[158] Men outnumber women by a ratio of 3 : 2 (Table 30–10). Patients typically have a combination of cough, wheezing, dyspnea, chest pain, and fever (Fig. 30–26B).[95] The symptom complex often suggests an exacerbation or recurrence of asthma.[158]

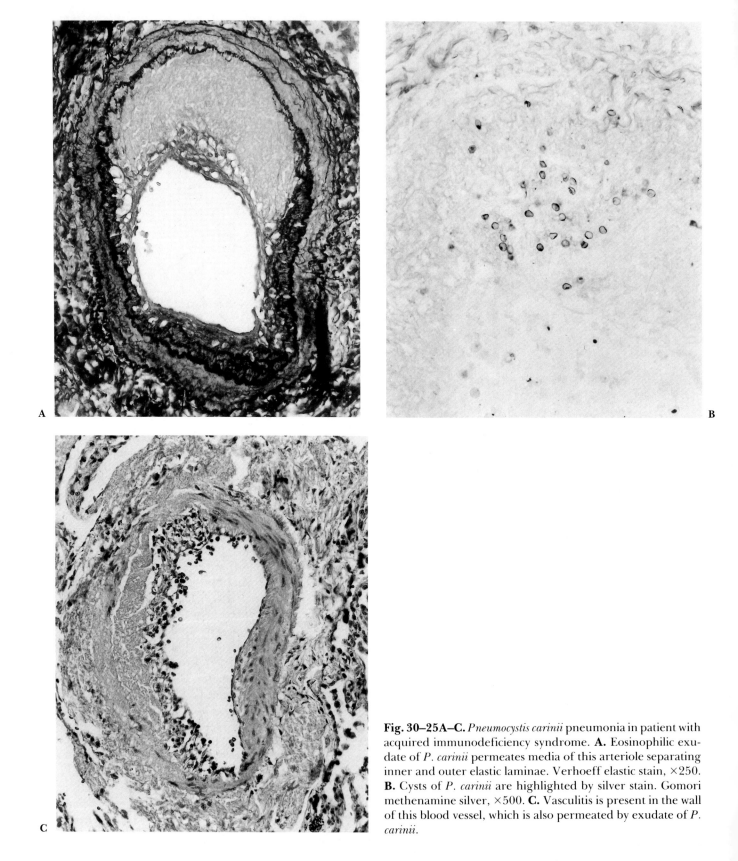

Fig. 30–25A–C. *Pneumocystis carinii* pneumonia in patient with acquired immunodeficiency syndrome. **A.** Eosinophilic exudate of *P. carinii* permeates media of this arteriole separating inner and outer elastic laminae. Verhoeff elastic stain, ×250. **B.** Cysts of *P. carinii* are highlighted by silver stain. Gomori methenamine silver, ×500. **C.** Vasculitis is present in the wall of this blood vessel, which is also permeated by exudate of *P. carinii*.

Table 30–9. Bronchocentric granulomatosis: Associated conditions

History of asthma?	Associated condition	Infectious agent
Asthmatics[a]	Allergic bronchopulmonary fungal disease (ABPFD)[156,158,324]	Aspergillus sp.[156,158,163,324] Curvularia sp.[163] Bipolaris sp.[163] Geotrichum[163] Stemphylium lanuginosum[163] Penicillium rubrum[163] Candida albicans[163]
Nonasthmatics	Infection	Mycobacterium sp.[108,499] Histoplasma capsulatum[106] Blastomyces dermatidis Aspergillus sp. (Nagata)[500–502] Echinococcus sp.[503]
	Rheumatoid arthritis[504,505] Wegener's granulomatosis[65,66] Ankylosing spondylitis[506] Idiopathic bronchocentric granulomatosis[95,158,507]	

[a] Rarely, ABPFD can occur in nonasthmatics.[327]

Table 30–10. Clinical and pathologic findings in bronchocentric granulomatosis with tissue eosinophilia

	Katzenstein et al.[158]	Koss et al.[95]	Jelihovsky[325]
Number of patients	10	5	10
Males:Females	7:3	5:0	3:7
Age			
Range (years)	11–43	17–68	22–71
Mean (median) (years)	22 (22)	33 (28)	43 (39)
Asthma (%)	100	60	50
Blood eosinophilia (% patients)	90	40	NA
+ Serum fungal precipitins	4 of 7	NA	
+ Cultures Aspergillus[a]	1 of 10	1 of 6[b]	5 of 7
Mucoid impaction (%)	30	40	100
+ Tissue Aspergillus (%)	90	20	80
Treatment with steroids (%)	50	60	NA
Recurrence (%)	20	0	NA
Mortality (%)	0	0	NA

[a] Either sputum or resected tissue.
[b] All patients, including those without tissue eosinophilia. NA, Not available.

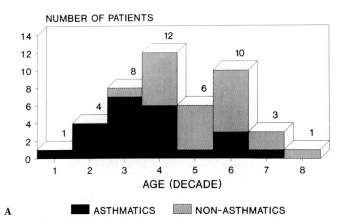
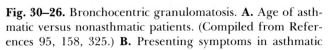
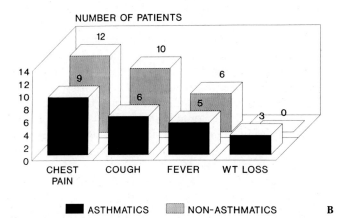

Fig. 30–26. Bronchocentric granulomatosis. **A.** Age of asthmatic versus nonasthmatic patients. (Compiled from References 95, 158, 325.) **B.** Presenting symptoms in asthmatic versus nonasthmatic patients. (Compiled from References 95, 158.)

Laboratory abnormalities include leukocytosis and, in 40%–90% of patients, peripheral blood eosinophilia (see Table 30-10). The white blood cell count can reach 25,000/mm³; more typically, the leukocytosis is mild. Most patients have peripheral blood eosinophilia that ranges between 5% and 69% of the white blood cell count.[95,158] The ESR is characteristically elevated, ranging from 22 to 120 mm per hour. Skin tests for aspergillus antigens may be positive.[328] In about one-half of cases, serum precipitin titers to fungal antigens are elevated, with *Aspergillus* being the most common fungus.[158] Serum IgE levels, including specific antibody directed against *Aspergillus*, were elevated in the few patients tested.[328] Typically, fungi are cultured in only 10%–50% of cases, about as often as they are seen in histologic sections of either lung or impacted intrabronchial mucus.[95,158,325]

When bronchocentric granulomatosis is not associated with asthma, a careful clinical and pathologic search must be made to exclude known associated conditions before diagnosing idiopathic bronchocentric granulomatosis. Patients with idiopathic bronchocentric granulomatosis tend to be older (see Fig. 30–26A) and are more likely to be female (Table 30–11). While asthmatic symptoms are typically absent, these patients often have chest symptoms, particularly cough (see Fig. 30–26B).[158] Other symptoms, such as hemoptysis, pleuritic chest pain, and fever can occur.[95,158,326] In nonasthmatics, marked blood eosinophilia is infrequent (see Table 30–11).[95,158] In most cases aspergillus is not detected by serum precipitins or cultures of sputum, or tissue (see Table 30–11). ESR may be elevated.

The radiologic manifestations of bronchocentric granulomatosis with and without asthma are similar.* Solitary or multiple nodules or masses resembling primary or metastatic cancer can be found in 20%–60% of patients. Solitary lesions are most common. Some of these masses arise from consolidation or atelectasis of entire lobes or segments of lobes.[158] Multiple small nodules or a fine reticulonodular pattern and alveolar or pneumonic infiltrates can be seen. A branching pattern of nodular lesions resembling mucoid impaction can be observed in up to 10% of cases,[95,158] and cavitated infiltrates or air-filled spaces occur in 6%–27% of cases.[95,158] Some patients show more than one type of lesion. The only feature that asthmatics show more frequently than nonasthmatics is sublobar atelectasis or consolidation.[158]

Histologically, bronchocentric granulomatosis is characterized by necrotizing granulomas involving small bronchi and bronchioles. The granulomatous

---

*References: 95, 156, 326, 328, 329.

Table 30–11. Clinical and pathologic findings in bronchocentric granulomatosis without tissue eosinophilia

	Katzenstein et al.[158]	Koss[95]
Number of patients	13[a]	10
Males:Females	6:7	3:7
Age		
Range (years)	32–76	29–60
Mean (median) (years)	50 (47)	47 (52)
Asthma (%)	0	0
+ Serum fungal precipitins	0 of 4	NA
+ Cultures *Aspergillus*[a]	0 of 11	1 of 6[b]
Mucoid impaction (%)	10	0
+ Tissue *Aspergillus* (%)	0	0
Treatment with steroids (%)	20	10
Recurrence (%)	0	0
Mortality (%)	12.5	10

[a] Either sputum or resected tissue.
[b] All patients, including those without tissue eosinophilia. NA, Not available.

inflammation is composed of giant cells and epithelioid histiocytes arrayed in a radial or palisading fashion in the bronchial wall (Fig. 30–27A). Identifying the bronchocentric location of the granulomas and showing that they are localized to the airways are critical to the diagnosis. The necrotizing granulomas may focally or completely destroy the bronchus or bronchiole. If the airway is completely destroyed, it can be difficult to be sure the granulomas are situated around bronchioles. In such cases one can use elastic stains to demonstrate residual elastica of the airway or the adjacent pulmonary artery (Fig. 30–27B). Small necrotizing or nonnecrotizing granulomas may involve the walls of larger cartilage-bearing bronchi, and severe chondritis may be present, but the mucosal linings are only infrequently involved by granulomatous inflammation.[158] A mild arteritis is not uncommon; however, it is caused by secondary extension of the airway inflammation to the adjacent arteries (Fig. 30–27B).

Microscopically, bronchocentric granulomatosis has been divided into two types on the basis of the presence or absence of eosinophilia.[96] Most cases associated with tissue eosinophilia are found in asthmatic patients with ABPA.[158,324,325] In addition to bronchocentric granulomatosis, ABPA is often associated with mucoid impaction of bronchi with allergic mucin (Figs. 30–28A,B), eosinophilic pneumonia, exudative bronchiolitis, and chronic bronchiolitis.[324] Large proximal bronchi show mucoid impaction in 30%–100% of specimens.[168,324,325] Allergic mucin is characterized by inspissated bronchial mucus plugs containing aggregates of eosinophils arrayed in layers parallel to the circumference of the plug and sometimes showing a characteristic wedge-shaped or fir-tree outline (Fig. 30–

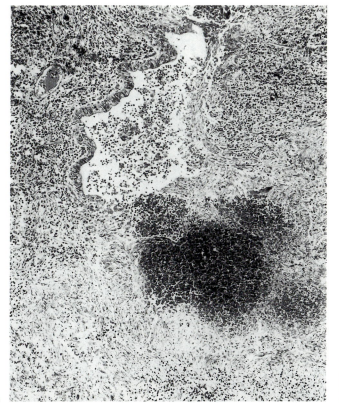

A

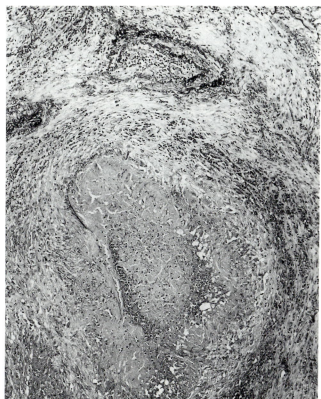

B

Fig. 30–27 A,B. Bronchocentric granulomatosis. **A.** Biopsy from patient with allergic bronchopulmonary fungal disease shows necrotic granulomatous inflammation centered on bronchiole, causing ulceration of bronchiolar epithelium. Necrotic area contains numerous necrotic eosinophils and is surrounded by palisading histiocytes. H and E, ×75. **B.** Biopsy from nonasthmatic patient shows necrotic granulomatous inflammation that has destroyed the bronchiole; adjacent arteriole highlighted by elastic stain helps identify the location where bronchiole used to be. Vasculitis in this arteriole is secondary to spillover of bronchiolar inflammation. Vessel wall is permeated by lymphocytes; elastic lamellae are disrupted. Verhoff elastic stain ×75.

28B).[324,325] Dense infiltrates of eosinophils that are often partially or totally necrotic can be seen not only within the intrabronchial mucus but also within the bronchial wall, within the centers of the granulomas, and in the surrounding alveoli, causing eosinophilic pneumonia. Charcot–Leyden crystals may be present in association with necrotic eosinophils (Fig. 30–28B); a foreign-body giant cell reaction to the necrotic debris can be seen in 40% of cases. Prominent tissue eosinophilia is not limited to patients with asthma; it can also be seen in Wegener's granulomatosis with a bronchocentric pattern of lung involvement.[66]

In 20%–90% of cases of ABPA, silver stains reveal septate fungal hyphae within the mucus of the dilated airways, or, occasionally, they are found within areas of central necrosis.[95,156,158,324] The fungi often appear dilated or varicose with fragmentation of the hyphae. Usually morphology typical of *Aspergillus* can be discerned; however, the hyphae may occasionally suggest other unusual fungi (Fig. 30–28C), and sometimes the organisms are too degenerated to classify. Rarely the hyphae may be surrounded by a radial arrangement of eosinophilic club-like structures, typical of the Splendore–Hoeppli phenomenon.[330] Importantly, invasion of the bronchial wall or of surrounding tissues by the fungi is not seen.

Bronchocentric granulomatosis without tissue eosinophilia is usually found in nonasthmatics and is characterized histologically by necrotic, bronchocentric granulomas containing many neutrophils or acellular necrotic material. These cases differ from those with prominent tissue eosinophilia in that Charcot–Leyden crystals, mucoid impaction of larger bronchi, and eosinophilic pneumonia are not seen. Notably, fungi and other organisms are also absent. In nonasthmatics, careful examination of histologic sections must be performed to exclude the possibility of infection (Fig. 30–29). Subtle features suggestive of Wegener's granu-

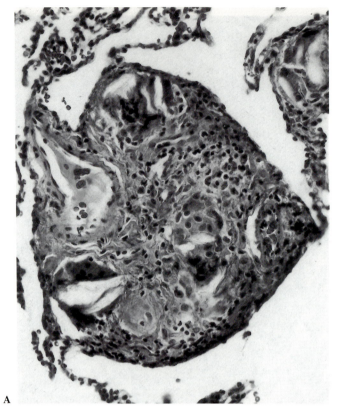

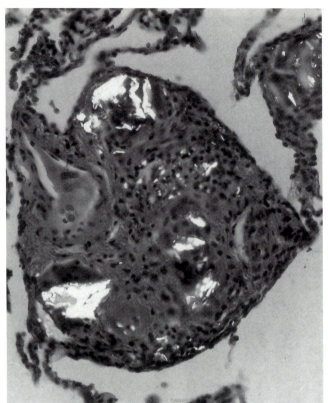

Fig. 30–33A,B. Embolic foreign material in intravenous drug abuser. **A.** Perivascular granulomas consist of foreign body giant cells and refractile material. H and E, ×200. **B.** Foreign material is birefringent with polarized light. H and E, ×200, polarized light.

a vasculitis characterized by mural infiltration by eosinophils and lymphocytes and by intimal fibrosis (Fig. 30–34A).[355–357] Interestingly, pulmonary disease in patients taking L-tryptophan was not always associated with full-blown manifestations of the EMS.[355,356] The etiology of the EMS was subsequently traced to a single manufacturer in Japan, the Showa Denko K.K., who had temporarily modified their manufacturing technique, resulting in contamination by a substance identified by high-performance liquid chromatography as peak E.[359–362]

A similar epidemic, known as the Spanish toxic oil syndrome, occurred in Spain in the early 1980s. Patients developed a scleroderma-like illness that passed through several phases. The disease began with a febrile pneumonia (early phase), followed by eosinophilia, gastrointestinal abnormalities (intermediate phase), and neuromuscular manifestations, including severe myalgias (late phase).[337,338] Pulmonary symptoms included nonproductive cough, dyspnea, pleuritic chest pain, and bilateral pulmonary infiltrates.[338] Patients developed pulmonary hypertension, and histologic evidence of pulmonary vasculitis was found.[363] The cause of this syndrome was traced to ingestion of denatured rapeseed oil.[337,338]

Pulmonary vasculitis induced by drugs is uncommon. It may reflect a localized pulmonary reaction or be a part of a systemic vasculitis. Information regarding the pathology is often poorly documented and available only in isolated case reports. Because patients with drug-induced vasculitis often have a complex clinical picture, it can be difficult to prove that a given drug was the sole cause of the vasculitis. Careful correlation with the history of drug intake, the clinical presentation, and the response to withdrawal of the drug is essential before implicating the drug as the cause. It is reported to occur in association with a variety of drugs including alpha-adrenergic nasal sprays,[364] carbamazepine,[114,365] diphenylhydantoin,[365,366] allopurinol,[367,368] cromoglycate,[364] penicillin,[369] nitrofurantoin,[372,372a] propylthiouracil,[370–372] sulfonamides,[302,364] and experimental anti-Tac antibodies for the treatment of adult T-cell leukemia/lymphoma (Fig. 30–34B).

A spectrum of histologic changes may be seen with pulmonary vasculitis associated with drugs or toxic substances. Depending on the particular reaction, the vasculitis may affect medium-sized or small arteries, veins, or capillaries. The inflammatory cells infiltrating the blood vessel walls may be primarily mononuclear

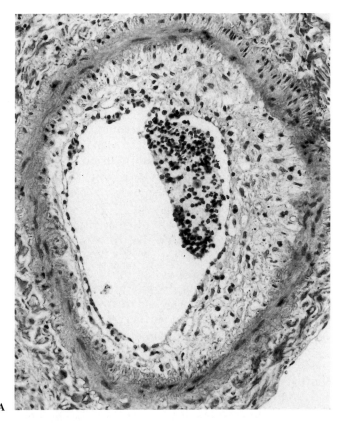

A

B

Fig. 30–34A,B. Toxic or drug-induced vasculitis. **A.** Pulmonary arteriole shows intimal fibrosis and focal subendothelial eosinophils from patient who had been taking L-tryptophan. H and E, ×125. **B.** Small vessel vasculitis in lung biopsy from patient who developed hypersensitivity reaction associated with anti-Tac therapy for adult T-cell leukemia/lymphoma. H and E, ×400.

cells, giant cells, or eosinophils. The surrounding lung may show an interstitial pneumonitis consisting of chronic inflammatory cells, lymphoid aggregates, granulomas, cavitary lung nodules[365,370,371] or eosinophils. Thus, a variety of histologic patterns of vasculitis may be encountered including those resembling polyarteritis nodosa, small vessel vasculitis,[367] Churg–Strauss syndrome,[114] and giant cell arteritis.

Transplantation

The pulmonary vascular changes seen in heart-lung transplant recipients consist primarily of periarteriolar and perivenular mononuclear inflammation with intimal hyperplasia and mild muscular hypertrophy (see Chapter 24).[373] Perivascular lymphocytic cuffing is a morphologic marker for acute rejection.[373,374] Arteriosclerosis of pulmonary arteries can occur in long-term survivors of heart-lung transplantation.[375]

A long-term survivor of bone marrow transplantation has recently been reported to have developed a vasculitis with recurrent pulmonary hemorrhage, clinical and pathologic evidence of a cutaneous and pulmonary leukocytoclastic vasculitis, and an elevated serum ANCA.[376] It is not certain whether this pulmonary vasculitis syndrome was a coincidental phenomenon or whether it represents a newly recognized complication of bone marrow transplantation.[376] The vasculitis in this patient responded to treatment with cyclophosphamide and prednisone.

Radiation

Vasculitis may also be seen as a complication of radiation exposure.[314,377] Early vascular injury in radiation damage to the lungs consists of edema of the walls of small arteries and arterioles followed by intimal proliferation and medial injury. Fibrinoid necrosis can affect small arteries, and hyaline thickening can occur in vessel walls. Foam cell plaques, highly suggestive of radiation vasculitis, consist of subintimal deposition of macrophages with foamy cytoplasm in arterial walls.[314,377]

Vascular Involvement in Lymphoproliferative Disorders

Angiocentric Immunoproliferative Lesion (Lymphomatoid Granulomatosis)

Angiocentric immunoproliferative lesion (AIL) was first described by Liebow and co-workers in 1972 under the name "lymphomatoid granulomatosis" (LYG). AIL/LYG was defined as an atypical lymphoproliferative process characterized by histologic features of angioinvasion and necrosis[12] (see also Chapter 31). Its curious name reflected Liebow's uncertainty whether it was a variant of Wegener's granulomatosis or an unusual form of lymphoma. In the nasal region a similar type of lymphoid lesion consisting of a polymorphous cell population and vascular infiltration had been described several years previously under the name polymorphic reticulosis.[379] During the next decade, it became apparent that not only was there considerable overlap in both the histologic and clinical features of AIL/LYG and polymorphic reticulosis[378-383] but that these entities shared features with malignant lymphomas of the lung[384,386] and nasal region,[386] respectively. In the past decade, a number of studies have led to the conclusion that many cases of AIL/LYG[84,387-391] and lethal midline granuloma[386,392-396] are malignant lymphomas of T-cell origin. An alternative view, that AIL/LYG is an aberrant immune reaction that can progress to malignant lymphoma, led Jaffe and colleagues to propose the more conservative term angiocentric immunoproliferative lesion (AIL).[84,102,391,397]

Clinical Features

AIL/LYG is more common in men than in women with a ratio of approximately 2 : 1. Most patients are 40 to 60 years old. The mean age is in the fifth decade, but children as young as 13 months[398-400] and adults as old as 76 years can be affected (Table 30–12).[12]

Symptoms associated with pulmonary AIL/LYG include cough, chest pain, or dyspnea (Fig. 30–35). Patients may also present with constitutional symptoms such as fever, anemia and weight loss (Fig. 30–35).[401,402] Clubbing[402,403] and polyarthritis[404,405] may be presenting findings. Rare individuals are asymptomatic, presenting with lung nodules found in a routine chest x ray.[85,99] The chest radiograph most frequently shows bilateral peripheral lung nodules that usually spare the apices, range in size from 1 to 9 cm, and tend to wax and wane spontaneously.[406,407] Cavitation occurs in up to 25% of cases.[12,86,99,408] Diffuse reticulonodular infiltrates, localized masses or infiltrates, and pleural effusions also occur.[407,409-411] Rarely AIL/LYG can present with the adult respiratory distress syndrome.[412] Hilar lymphadenopathy is very infrequent; it occurred in only 2% of cases in one series.[99] Palpable lymphadenopathy is present in less than 10% of cases.

Skin lesions represent the most common extrapulmonary site of involvement and may be seen in up to 54% of patients (see Table 30–12). Subcutaneous or dermal nodules are seen most often, followed by erythematous maculopapular rashes or ulceration.[413] Necrobiosis-lipoidica-like lesions can also occur.[414] The skin lesions are frequently widespread and often are found on the extremities or occasionally on the trunk or head and neck.[411,414A]

Neurologic symptoms occur in up to 30% of cases and can be the presenting finding in as many as 21% (Table 30–12).[415] AIL/LYG may involve the central nervous system (CNS), cranial nerves, or peripheral nerves.[411,415-420,420A] Symptoms include spinal cord or cranial nerve deficits,[416,418] diplopia, blindness,[420] ataxia, paresthesias, peripheral neuropathy, central neurogenic hypoventilation,[421] parkinsonism,[419] vertigo, and headache or seizures.[411] Neurologic involvement tends to correlate with a less favorable prognosis.[415]

Genitourinary involvement is common. Renal involvement can occur in 45% of cases and usually consists of nodular infiltrates. AIL/LYG presenting with a large renal mass and multiple pulmonary masses may mimic metastatic renal cell carcinoma.[422] Rarely, AIL/LYG presents with bladder outlet obstruction from prostatic involvement.[423] It may also cause ureteral obstruction and hydronephrosis.[423A]

Ear nose and throat involvement may occur in perhaps one-third of patients.[411,424,425] Oral ulceration and odynophagia may also occur.[426] Ocular[427,428] and conjunctival[429] involvement can occur, and presentation with sudden blindness has been reported.[420] Gastrointestinal involvement, a rare presenting manifestation of AIL/LYG, may cause gastric ulceration and intestinal perforation.[426,430,431]

AIL/LYG-like lesions can arise in immunocompromised patients, such as those with malignancies,[399] myeloproliferative disorders,[432] retroperitoneal fibrosis,[433] renal transplants,[425,434,435] Sjögren's syndrome,[436,437] and immunodeficiency syndromes[433,438] including the Wiskott–Aldrich syndrome[439] and the acquired immunodeficiency syndrome (AIDS).[417,426,433,440] While some of these may be lymphomas or Epstein–Barr virus-induced B-cell lymphoproliferations simulating AIL/LYG, others appear to be bona fide cases.[440]

Table 30–12. Clinical features in patients with lymphomatoid granulomatosis

	Liebow et al. 1972[12]	Fauci et al. 1982[86]	Katzenstein et al. 1979[99]	Israel et al.[b] 1977[408]	Koss et al.[a] 1986[85]	Pisani and DeRemee 1990[111]
Number of patients	40	15	152	43	42	28
Men:Women	5:3	6.5:1	1.7:1	5:4	3:1	17:11
Age						
Mean (years)	45	34	48	43	47	51
Range (years)	8.5–76		16–65	7–85	20–68	24–79
Clinical organ involvement (% patients)						
Lung	90	67	56	16	55	100
Skin	43	20	39	5	33	54
Neurologic	23	33	30	2	29	21
Other						
Fever	63	60	58	NA	33	50
Asymptomatic	NA	0	3	0	10	0
Adenopathy	NA	7	8	NA	0	11
Upper airways	0	0**	NA	2	0	29

[a] At clinical presentation only.
[b] Two patients had eye involvement.

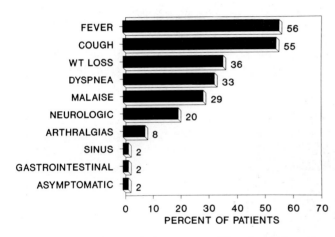

Fig. 30–35. Angiocentric immunoproliferative lesion. Presenting clinical manifestations. (Compiled from References 99, 411.)

Patients with AIL/LYG may have profound immunologic dysfunction with severe impairment of cellular immune function.[441,442] Rarely occurring endocrine abnormalities include hypoadrenalism, hypercalcemia, hypothyroidism, diabetes insipidus, and hypogonadism.[443,444]

Pathologic Features

Grossly, the cut surface of the lung in AIL/LYG typically shows white or yellow, circumscribed, nonencapsulated masses. Similar masses can be seen in the kidneys, brain, and skin; lymph node involvement is rare.

Microscopically, there are three major histologic features: (1) an atypical, polymorphous, lymphoreticular infiltrate; (2) vascular invasion by the infiltrate (Fig. 30–36A); and (3) coagulative necrosis (Fig. 30–36B).[12] The lymphoid infiltrate consists of small round lymphocytes, lymphocytes with elongate nuclei, plasma cells, and variable numbers of atypical large mononuclear lymphoid cells that are probably immunoblasts. These immunoblasts have one to three nucleoli and ample cytoplasm. On occasion, the nuclei of these atypical lymphoid cells are bilobed and may superficially resemble Reed–Sternberg cells.[388] Macrophages with eosinophilic cytoplasm may be admixed with the lymphoid cells. When prominent, these may vaguely suggest a granulomatous appearance; however, true granulomatous inflammation in the form of Langhans' giant cells and epithelioid granulomas is characteristically absent.[12]

The smallest lesions consist of a mixed lymphoid and histiocytic infiltrate centered on vessels, that is, along the lymphatic pathways (Fig. 30–36C). The lymphohistiocytic cells frequently permeate walls of small arteries and veins, producing a vasculitic appearance. Yet, fibrinoid necrosis is rare, and the vascular invasion does not represent a true inflammatory vasculitis.

Jaffe and colleagues suggested a histologic grading system for AIL/LYG[84,390,391,397] that is based on the degree of cytologic atypia, presence of necrosis, and retention of a polymorphous character in the cellular infiltrate (Figs. 30–37A–C). Grade 1 lesions are polymorphous but consist primarily of small lymphocytes admixed with many histiocytes (Fig. 30–37A). The

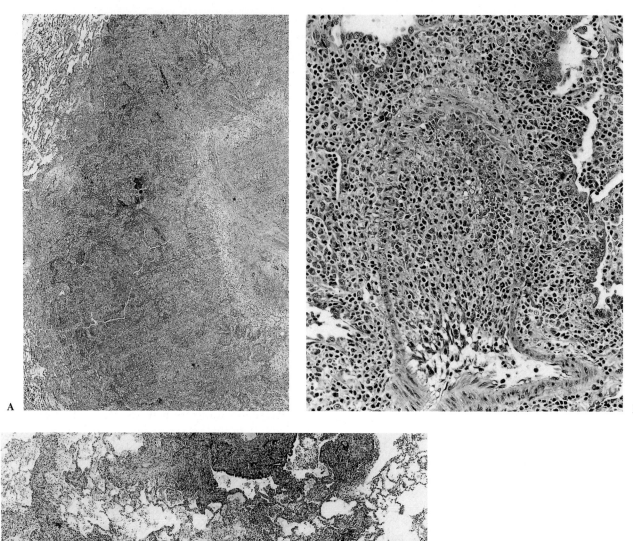

Fig. 30–36A–C. Angiocentric immunoproliferative lesion. **A.** Grade 3 AIL. Arteriole shows extensive infiltration of wall with narrowing of vascular lumen by polymorphous atypical lymphoid infiltrate. H and E, ×200. **B.** Grade 3 AIL. Nodular lymphoid infiltrate with central necrosis and peripheral rim of uninvolved lung. H and E, ×23. **C.** Grade 1 AIL. Interstitial angiocentric infiltrate without discrete nodules or necrosis. H and E, ×50.

small lymphoid cells show minimal cytologic atypia; large lymphoid cells and mitoses are rare. Grade 2 lesions are composed of a mixture of small lymphocytes and histiocytes, but the small lymphocytes may have more irregular nuclear contours than seen in grade 1 lesions (Fig. 30–37B). Large lymphoid cells may be seen, but represent less than 5% of the total cell population and usually less than 1%. Scattered mitoses are seen. Coagulative necrosis may be present, but is usually not extensive. In grade 3 lesions, the small lymphoid cells show a greater degree of atypia with irregular nuclear contours, and large atypical lymphoid cells are more numerous (Fig. 30–37C). The large lymphoid cells show coarse nuclear chromatin and occasionally prominent nucleoli. Mitoses are easily identified, but are usually not numerous. Coagulative necrosis may be extensive. Grade 3 lesions probably correspond to "angiocentric lymphomas."

In 1977, Saldana and others described a polymorphous lymphoid infiltrate that was angiocentric and occasionally angiodestructive and which they termed benign lymphocytic angiitis and granulomatosis (BLAG).[408,445] The disease usually involved only lung and had fewer atypical cells or immunoblasts than classical AIL/LYG. Therapy with chlorambucil and cyclophosphamide was effective, and the disease had a better prognosis than AIL/LYG.[393,408,445] Some cases progressed to LYG[408] or large cell lymphoma[84,397] and others involved extrapulmonary sites.[446] Although there has been skepticism regarding the existence of benign lymphocytic angiitis and granulomatosis as a distinct entity, Jaffe recently proposed that it may represent grade 1 AIL.[84,397]

When the disease involves extrapulmonary organs such as the nasopharynx, the cellular infiltrate is microscopically similar to that seen in the lung. In the CNS, AIL/LYG is often multicentric and angiocentric, with extensive necrosis. Unfortunately, other lymphomas involving the brain can produce a similar pattern; it can therefore be difficult to diagnose AIL/LYG on purely histologic grounds when the lesion is in the brain.[385,417,447] Peripheral neuropathy is characterized by demyelination and lymphoid cell infiltration.[415]

Nodular masses similar to those seen in the lungs can occur in the kidney in 33%–45% of cases.[12,99] Early lesions consist of perivascular and interstitial infiltrates.[448] With extensive or advanced disease, large renal masses with central necrosis can occur.[86] Unlike Wegener's granulomatosis, glomerulonephritis is not seen.[12]

Skin lesions are characterized by an infiltrate of atypical lymphocytes and plasmacytoid cells around dermal appendages, nerves, and vessels, generally without involvement of the epidermis or papillary dermis.* Recognition of the pathologic diagnosis may be difficult, and lesions of AIL/LYG may be mistaken for necrotizing vasculitis[452] and necrobiosis lipoidica.[423] Skin biopsy yields a diagnosis in about 45% of cases.[411] Other sites of reported involvement by AIL/LYG include the liver and spleen and, uncommonly, the adrenals, heart, prostate, gall bladder, parotid,[453] pancreas, gastrointestinal tract, and skeletal muscle.[99,424,431] Lymph node involvement is uncommon and occurs in the setting of outright large cell lymphoma.[84,86,431]

Prognosis and Therapy

There are several indicators of poor prognosis, including CNS involvement, increased numbers of atypical large lymphoid cells (immunoblasts),[99] anergy, fever, and leukopenia.[86] According to the grading system proposed by Jaffe et al., higher grade lesions have a worse prognosis.[84,390,397] Grade 2 and 3 lesions can have an "aggressive" clinical course.[84,390,397]

AIL/LYG can be treated with a variety of approaches. Long-term remission may be obtained in some patients with cyclophosphamide and steroids, but up to 50% of patients eventually die of lymphoma (Table 30–13).[86] Recent studies advocate early use of aggressive combination chemotherapy,[84,454] sometimes supplemented by radiation therapy.[455] Bone marrow transplantation has been successfully attempted.[456] Radiation therapy can be effective for AIL/LYG patients presenting with nasal involvement.[457]

Pathogenesis

Immunophenotypic studies suggest that most cases of AIL/LYG are a proliferation of T cells,** although a B-cell origin has also been suggested.[462,463] The cells are most often of helper-inducer[387,458,460] or a mixture of helper-inducer and suppressor T-cell phenotypes.[84,397] Suppressor T cells can occasionally dominate the lymphoid infiltrate in the setting of AIDS or in lymphomas arising in AIL/LYG.[392,440]

At least 12% of patients with AIL/LYG develop large cell lymphoma in lymph nodes, although lymph node involvement at presentation is uncommon.[99] It is currently debated whether AIL/LYG is a lymphoma de novo or whether it is an aberrant immune reaction that can progress to malignant lymphoma. The extranodal

---

*References: 12, 99, 413, 449–451.
**References: 84, 387–389, 397, 458–461.

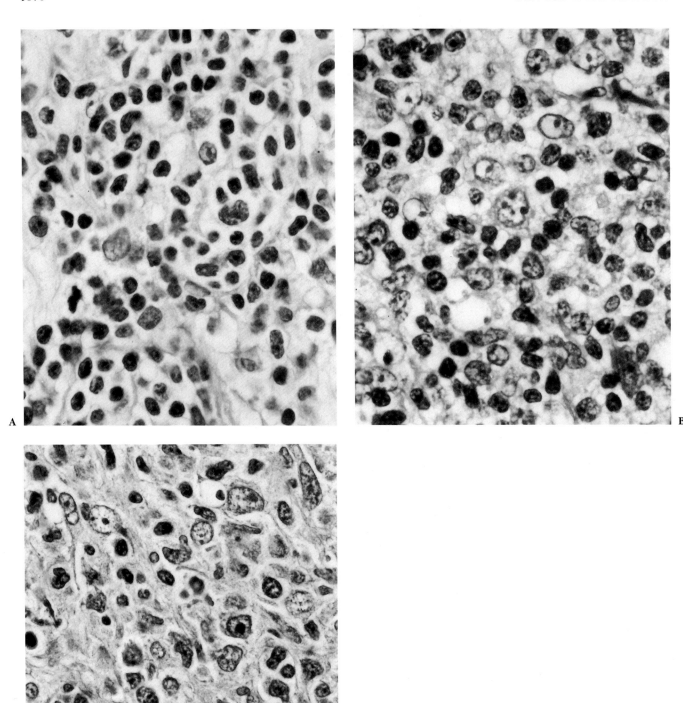

Fig. 30–37A–C. Angiocentric immunoproliferative lesion. **A.** Grade 1 AIL. Polymorphous lymphoid infiltrate consists of small lymphocytes, histiocytes, and rare large lymphoid cells. H and E, ×1000. **B.** Grade 2 AIL. Small lymphocytes have slightly more irregular nuclei than those in Grade 1 AIL and are mixed with histiocytes; large atypical cells are slightly more numerous. H and E, ×1000. **C.** Grade 3 AIL. Large atypical lymphoid cells are prominent and admixed with small lymphocytes that also show atypia. H and E, ×1000.

Table 30–13. Therapy and prognosis in AIL/LYG

Initial treatment	Number of patients	Died (%)	Mean follow-up
Katzenstein et al. (1979)[99]			
Steroids	67	64	13.8
Steroids/chemotherapy	42	64	10.4
Fauci et al. (1982)[86]			
Steroids/cytoxan	15	53	43
Koss et al. (1986)[85]	36	38	50
Lipford et al. (1988)[84]			
Steroids/cytoxan	15	53	43
Combination chemotherapy	8	13	70
Pisani/DeRemee (1990)[411]			
Steroids/cytoxan or			
Combination chemotherapy	28	43	72 (median)

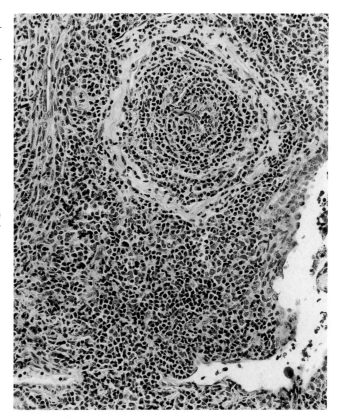

Fig. 30–38. Non-Hodgkin's lymphoma. Interstitial infiltration by large lymphoma with prominent vascular involvement. H and E, ×200.

location of disease in AIL/LYG and its mixed cell pattern originally suggested a reactive process. It is now known that these features can be seen in peripheral T-cell lymphomas.[460,464] Indeed, Weis and associates[40] classified AIL/LYG as a subcategory of peripheral T-cell lymphoma, along with Lennert's lymphoma, angioimmunoblastic lymphadenopathy, and Hodgkin's-like disease. According to this concept, AIL/LYG is a lymphoma with a broad range of morphologic expression, from low-grade lesions in which small lymphocytes predominate (e.g., "benign lymphocytic angiitis and granulomatosis") to high-grade variants that resemble diffuse large cell lymphoma or immunoblastic sarcoma. DNA analysis has shown clonal rearrangement of the T-cell receptor gene in a few cases, supporting a clonal or neoplastic T-cell proliferation.[102,458,461] Cytogenetically abnormal (neoplastic) clones can also occur in AIL/LYG without immunophenotypic or T-cell receptor gene abnormalities.[387] On the other hand, only a small subset of cases show the gene rearrangements or immunophenotypic abnormalities expected in T-cell lymphomas.[84,391,397] For example, Medeiros et al.[391] could not demonstrate gene rearrangements of either the T-cell receptor or immunoglobulin genes by Southern blot hybridization in 7 of 8 cases. These results suggest that at least some cases of AIL/LYG are a part of a spectrum of premalignant lymphoproliferative disease rather than frank malignant lymphoma from the beginning.[465] These interesting questions need additional study.

The role of Epstein–Barr virus (EBV) infection in AIL/LYG is receiving increasing attention.[391,440,466,467] EBV-induced B-cell lymphoproliferations can occur in the setting of immunodeficiency, but an association with T-cell lymphoid proliferations was not previously known. Veltri et al.[467] reported a case of AIL/LYG presenting as a reactivated EBV infection and proposed that EBV may have played a role in impairing the immune system, thereby predisposing the patient to developing AIL/LYG. Subsequently, Katzenstein and Peiper[466] used polymerase chain reaction to identify EBV DNA in 72% of 21 AIL/LYG cases. In situ hybridization demonstrated EBV RNA in large T cells in five cases of grade 3 AIL although seven other cases of grade 1 or 2 AIL were negative or had only few positive cells.[468] On the basis of this finding it was suggested that EBV may play a role in transformation of low-grade AIL/LYG to high-grade lesions or angiocentric malignant lymphoma.[468] EBV-containing clones of B-cell lymphocytes have also been detected in AIL/LYG in an AIDS patient.[440] It is still unclear however whether EBV is a passenger or plays a more significant role in the pathogenesis of AIL/LYG.

Non-Hodgkin's Lymphoma

Vascular permeation is a frequent finding in pulmonary non-Hodgkin's lymphomas that can be mistaken for vasculitis (Fig. 30–38). The non-Hodgkin's pulmo-

Table 30–14. Clinical features of patients with pulmonary intravascular lymphomatosis

Author	Age/race/sex	Symptoms	Laboratory findings	Chest radiograph	Treatment	Follow-up
Tan et al.[483]	56 W F	Fever, dyspnea, cough, malaise	Negative bone marrow Restrictive PFT	Bilateral interstitial infiltrates	Chemotherapy	10 months, NED[a]
Yousem and Colby[182]	60 W M	Cough, fever weight loss	Circulating atypical cells	Bilateral reticulonodular infiltrates	Chemotherapy	9 months, DOD[b]
	48 W F	Fever, dyspnea, headache, unilateral papilledema	Hypoxemia	Bilateral reticulonodular infiltrates	Chemotherapy and steroids	8 months, ANED[c]
	40 W F	Fever, obtunded, dyspnea	Hypercalcemia	Bilateral reticulonodular infiltrates	Chemotherapy	6 months, DOD[b]
	59 W F	Dyspnea, fever		Bilateral reticulonodular infiltrates	Chemotherapy	8 years, ANED[c]
Snyder et al.[480]	79 M	Dyspnea, fatigue, fever	Hypoxemia, +ANA, hemolytic anemia, pulmonary hypertension	Right apical pleural thickening, bilateral pleural effusion, enlarged central pulmonary artery	None	DOD[b]
Curtis et al.[484]	76 W M	Dyspnea, confusion, weight loss, fatigue, anorexia, headache	Hypercalcemia Atypical lymphocytosis Positive bone marrow	Right apical pleural thickening	None	1 month, DOD[b]

[a] NED, No evidence of disease.
[b] DOD, Dead of disease.
[c] ANED, Alive with no evidence of disease.

nary lymphomas can be divided into two major groups: low-grade tumors composed of cytologically bland, small lymphoid cells (including small lymphocytic and plasmacytoid lymphocytic lymphomas and lymphomas composed of small centrocyte-like cells); and high-grade tumors such as large cell immunoblastic sarcomas and small noncleaved cell lymphomas.[390] The percentage of low-grade lymphomas varies from 35% to 78% of lung lymphomas, depending on the series.[348] Most of these tumors are of B-cell or presumed B-cell lineage, and have been termed low-grade B-cell lymphomas of bronchus-associated lymphoid tissue (BALT)[469] (see also Chapter 31).

Low-grade B-cell lymphomas of BALT typically grow as solid masses, obliterating the normal lung architecture in their centers. At the periphery of these lesions, the lymphoid infiltrate may insinuate around airways and vessels, that is, along lymphatic pathways, producing a nodular interstitial pattern. These lymphomas often invade the walls of small veins[348,470,471] but involvement of large muscular arteries and necrosis is rare.[348]

High-grade lymphomas of B-cell origin range from 2% to 19% of primary lymphomas of lung.[348,469,470,472]

Large cell pleomorphic lymphomas of T-cell origin can also occur. They develop as an outgrowth of AIL/LYG in up to 50% of those cases[86] or as apparently de novo lesions.[469,473] High-grade pulmonary lymphomas show tumoral "pneumonias" produced by intraalveolar infiltration by malignant cells. The neoplastic cells invade the walls of muscular arteries and veins in more than 55% of cases, and more than 60% of cases show areas of infarct-like necrosis, possibly because of vascular involvement.[469] Unlike a vasculitis, there is no fibrinoid necrosis of blood vessel walls; rather, there is infiltration of vessels by malignant cells or by mixtures of reactive and malignant cells.[385] Vascular involvement in these cases may be caused by secondary extension from adjacent infiltrates along the lymphatic pathways.[385] Li et al.[469] pointed out that the vascular infiltration and necrosis is more likely caused by the high grade of the tumors than by the specific immunophenotype.

Intravascular Lymphomatosis

Intravascular (angiotrophic) lymphomatosis is a rare lesion in which neoplastic lymphoid cells aggregate within small vessels, leading to thrombosis and subse-

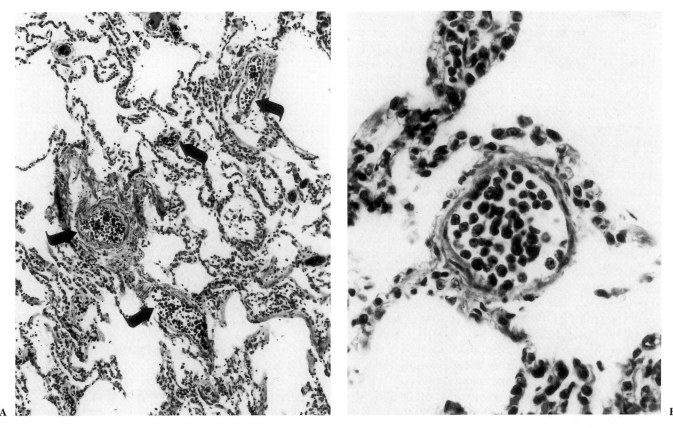

Fig. 30–39A,B. Intravascular lymphoma. **A.** Arterioles, venules, and lymphatics distended by atypical lymphoid cells (*arrows*). H and E, ×100. **B.** Numerous atypical lymphoid cells within distended venule. H and E, ×400.

quent organ injury. The CNS is the initial site of disease in 47% of cases.[474] This involvement produces symptoms such as fever, headache, dementia, multifocal sensorimotor deficits, seizure, and obtundation. The neoplasm also involves the skin in perhaps one-third of cases,[474] producing indurated, violaceous, and sometimes ulcerated plaques that occur slightly more frequently over the trunk than the face or extremities.[475–479] Disease can also involve the heart and pancreas, liver and spleen (producing hepatosplenomegaly), kidneys, genital tract, bone marrow, adrenal, and nasopharynx.[475–479]

The lungs can show microscopic foci of tumor in up to 60% of cases at autopsy.[480] However, pulmonary symptoms are rarely the initial presenting manifestation of the disease (Table 30–14). When pulmonary symptoms do occur, they are most frequently dyspnea or shortness of breath, followed by fever, cough, fatigue, and headache.[480–482] Yousem and Colby[482] suggested that dyspnea is caused by patchy intravascular aggregates of tumor cells that lead to ventilation-perfusion mismatching with secondary hypoxemia. The chest radiograph typically shows bilateral interstitial or reticulonodular infiltrates,[482,483] but the lung fields can also

appear unremarkable.[484] One patient had enlarged central pulmonary arteries due to pulmonary hypertension.[480]

Patients can show several abnormal laboratory values, including positive antinuclear antibody titers,[480] hemolytic anemia[480] that may be due to antierythrocyte autoantibodies,[478,479] and atypical lymphocytosis. Abnormalities specifically related to the lung include arterial hypoxemia, evidence of pulmonary hypertension,[480] and pulmonary function tests showing a restrictive defect.[483] Two patients had hypercalcemia[482,484]; one of them had normal parathormone levels. As noted previously, there are also patients who have Addisonian electrolyte disturbances or elevated rheumatoid factor titers.[479]

Intravascular lymphomatosis is a tumor with a poor prognosis. The disease typically kills the untreated patient within 24 months; however, use of combination chemotherapy early in the clinical course can lead to prolonged survival.[479,483] The mortality in 73 cases was greater than 80%.[483] Pulmonary symptomatology does not appear to affect adversely survival; 2 of 7 patients were alive after 8 months and 8 years, respectively (see Table 30–14).

Microscopically, the lungs typically show patchy congestion and hemorrhage, and at low magnification the appearance can superficially mimic interstitial pneumonitis. Atypical lymphoid cells distend alveolar septal capillaries, venules, small pulmonary arteries, and lymphatics (Figs. 30–39A,B).[480–483] At high magnification, the neoplastic cells have large vesicular, sometimes prominently convoluted nuclei, one or two eosinophilic nucleoli, and moderate cytoplasm. Perivascular and intramural chronic inflammatory cells, including lymphocytes, plasma cells, and macrophages, can produce an appearance resembling angiitis.[484] Pulmonary arteries can show not only muscular hypertrophy but also intraluminal thrombi and eccentric and concentric intimal fibrous scars.[480] Some authors have noted sparse numbers of tumor cells admixed with the perivascular reactive inflammatory infiltrate.[482] In other organs, extensive extravascular spread of the tumor has been reported.[485]

Intravascular lymphomatosis was initially viewed as a neoplastic endothelial disorder and therefore was called by different terms including angioendotheliomatosis proliferans systemisista, neoplastic angioendotheliosis, and malignant angioendotheliosis.[479] However, several studies subsequently identified the immunophenotype of the neoplastic cells to be lymphoid. The tumor cells express common leukocyte antigen (CD45),[482,484] LN1, LN2, and MB$_2$;[480] LN3, L26;[484,486] monotypic IgM, and Leu-14.[479] Most cases therefore appear to exhibit a B-cell immunophenotype,[481] but occasional cases may show a T-cell immunophenotype.[487] Endothelial markers, including attachment sites for Ulex Europaeus I lectin and the antigens that bind monoclonal antibodies B15 and Factor VIII, are absent.[479,486]

Gene rearrangement studies in a few cases showed clonal rearrangements of the immunoglobulin heavy chain gene.[474,488] One case showed a translocation and other chromosomal aberrations.[486]

It is unclear why this lymphoma localizes within vascular lumens. Because the neoplastic cells appear to circulate in the peripheral blood,[486] the malignant cells may lack receptors, as yet unknown, that allow adhesion to endothelium. Alternatively, there may be a molecular defect that impairs lymphocyte egress from the vascular lumens following adhesion.[484]

References

1. Leavitt RY, Fauci AS. Wegener's granulomatosis. Curr Opin Rheumatol 1991;3:8–14.

1a. Leavitt RY, Fauci AS. Less common manifestations and presentations of Wegener's granulomatosis. Curr Opin Rheumatol 1992;4:16–22.

2. Churg J, Churg A. Idiopathic and secondary vasculitis: A review. Mod Pathol 1989;2:144–160.

3. Weisbrod GL. Pulmonary angiitis and granulomatosis: A review. Can Assoc Radiol J 1989;40:127–134.

4. Staples CA. Pulmonary angiitis and granulomatosis. Radiol Clin North Am 1991;29:973–982.

5. Feigin DS. Vasculitis in the lung. J Thorac Imaging 1988;3:33–48.

6. Churg A. Pulmonary angiitis and granulomatosis revisited. Hum Pathol 1983;14:868–883.

7. Leavitt RY, Fauci AS. Pulmonary vasculitis. Am Rev Respir Dis 1986;134:149–166.

8. DeRemee RA, Weiland LH, McDonald TJ. Respiratory vasculitis. Mayo Clin Proc 1980;55:492–498.

9. Leavitt RY, Travis WD, Fauci AS. Vasculitis. In: Shelhamer J, Pizzo PA, Parrillo JE, Masur H, eds. Respiratory disease in the immunosuppressed host. Philadelphia: JB Lippincott, 1991;703–727.

10. Liebow AA. The J. Burns Amberson lecture—pulmonary angiitis and granulomatosis. Am Rev Respir Dis 1973;108:1–18.

11. Koss MN, Hochholzer L, Feigin DS, Garancis JC, Ward PA. Necrotizing sarcoid-like granulomatosis: clinical, pathologic, and immunopathologic findings. Hum Pathol 1980;11S:510–519.

12. Liebow AA, Carrington CR, Friedman PJ. Lymphomatoid granulomatosis. Hum Pathol 1972;3:457–558.

13. Jennette JC, Charles LA, Falk RJ. Antineutrophil cytoplasmic autoantibodies: Disease associations, molecular biology, and pathophysiology. Int Rev Exp Pathol 1991;32:193–221.

13a. Hagen EC, Ballieux BE, Daha MR, van Es LA, van der Woude FJ. Fundamental and clinical aspects of anti neutrophil cytoplasmic antibodies (ANCA). Autoimmunity 1992;11:199–207.

13b. Roberts DE. Antineutrophil cytoplasmic autoantibodies. Clin Lab Med 1992;12:85–98.

14. Jennette JC. Antineutrophil cytoplasmic autoantibody-associated diseases: A pathologist's perspective. Am J Kidney Dis 1991;18:164–170.

15. Calafat J, Goldschmeding R, Ringeling PL, Janssen H, van der Schoot CE. In situ localization of double-labeling immunoelectron microscopy of anti-neutrophil cytoplasmic autoantibodies in neutrophils and monocytes. Blood 1990;75:242–250.

16. Goldschmeding R, van der Schoot CE, Ten Bokkel Huinink D, et al. Wegener's granulomatosis autoantibodies identify a novel diisopropylfluorophosphate-binding protein in the lysosomes of normal human neutrophils. J Clin Invest 1989;84:1577–1587.

17. Jennette JC, Falk RJ. Antineutrophil cytoplasmic autoantibodies and associated diseases: a review. Am J Kidney Dis 1990;15:517–529.

18. Cohen Tervaert JW, Limburg PC, Elema JD, et al. Detection of autoantibodies against myeloid lysosomal enzymes: A useful adjunct to classification of patients with biopsy-proven necrotizing arteritis. Am J Med 1991;91:59–66.

19. Savage CO, Lockwood CM. Autoantibodies in primary

systemic vasculitis. Adv Intern Med 1990;35:73–92.

20. Gallicchio MC, Savige JA. Detection of anti-myeloperoxidase and anti-elastase antibodies in vasculitides and infections. Clin Exp Immunol 1991;84:232–237.

21. Cohen Tervaert JW, Goldschmeding R, Elema JD, et al. Association of autoantibodies to myeloperoxidase with different forms of vasculitis. Arthritis Rheum 1990;33:1264–1272.

22. Savage CO, Lockwood CM. Antineutrophil antibodies in vasculitis. Adv Nephrol 1990;19:225–236.

23. Fauci AS, Haynes BF, Katz P, Wolff SM. Wegener's granulomatosis: Prospective clinical and therapeutic experience with 85 patients over 21 years. Ann Intern Med 1983;98:76–85.

24. Wolff SM, Fauci AS, Horn RG, Dale DC. Wegener's granulomatosis. Ann Intern Med 1974;81:513–525.

25. Travis WD, Hoffman GS, Leavitt RY, Pass HI, Fauci AS. Surgical pathology of the lung in Wegener's granulomatosis. Review of 87 open lung biopsies from 67 patients. Am J Surg Pathol 1991;15:315–333.

26. Mark EJ, Matsubara O, Tan-Liu NS, Feinberg R. The pulmonary biopsy in the early diagnosis of Wegener's (pathergic) granulomatosis: a study based on 35 open lung biopsies. Hum Pathol 1988;19:1065–1071.

27. Fauci AS, Haynes BF, Katz P. Wegener's granulomatosis: studies in eighteen patients and a review of the literature. Medicine 1973;52:535–561.

28. DeRemee RA, McDonald TJ, Harrison EG, Coles DT. Wegener's granulomatosis. Anatomic correlates, a proposed classification. Mayo Clin Proc 1976;51:777–781.

29. Hoffman GS, Kerr GS, Leavitt RY, et al. Wegener's granulomatosis: A prospective analysis of 158 patients. Ann Intern Med 1992;116:488–498.

30. Lebovics RS, Hoffman GS, Leavitt RY, et al. The management of subglottic stenosis in patients with Wegener's granulomatosis. Laryngoscope 1992;102:1341–1345.

31. Gibson LE. Granulomatous vasculitides and the skin. Dermatol Clin 1990;8:335–345.

32. Specks U, Colby TV, Olsen KD, DeRemee RA. Salivary gland involvement in Wegener's granulomatosis. Arch Otolaryngol Head Neck Surg 1991;117:218–223.

33. Tupler RH, McCuskey WH. Wegener granulomatosis of the colon: CT and histologic correlation. J Comput Assist Tomogr 1991;15:314–316.

34. Bray VJ, Hasbargen JA. Prostatic involvement in Wegener's granulomatosis. Am J Kidney Dis 1991;17:578–580.

35. Fowler M, Martin SA, Bowles WT, Packman R, Katzenstein AL. Wegener granulomatosis. Unusual cause of necrotizing urethritis. Urology 1979;14:66–69.

36. Aymard B, Bigard MA, Thompson H, Schmutz JL, Finet JF, Borrelly J. Perianal ulcer: An unusual presentation of Wegener's granulomatosis. Report of a case. Dis Colon Rectum 1990;33:427–430.

37. Wieslander J. How are antineutrophil cytoplasmic antibodies detected? Am J Kidney Dis 1991;18:154–158.

38. Gross WL, Schmitt WH, Csernok E. Antineutrophil cytoplasmic autoantibody-associated diseases: A rheu-

matologist's perspective. Am J Kidney Dis 1991;18:175–179.

39. DeRemee RA. Antineutrophil cytoplasmic autoantibody-associated diseases: A pulmonologist's perspective. Am J Kidney Dis 1991;18:180–183.

40. Specks U, DeRemee RA. Do anticytoplasmic autoantibodies (ACPA) extend our understanding of the spectrum of Wegener's granulomatosis? Pneumologie 1990;44(Suppl)1:424–425.

41. Specks U, Wheatley CL, McDonald TJ, Rohrbach MS, DeRemee RA. Anticytoplasmic autoantibodies in the diagnosis and follow-up of Wegener's granulomatosis. Mayo Clin Proc 1989;64:28–36.

42. Jayne DRW, Marshall PD, Jones SJ, Lockwood CM. Autoantibodies to GBM and neutrophil cytoplasm in rapidly progressive glomerulonephritis. Kidney Int 1990;37:965–970.

43. De Clerck LS, Van Offel JF, Smolders WA, et al. Pitfalls with anti-neutrophil cytoplasmic antibodies (ANCA). Clin Rheumatol 1989;8:512–516.

44. Saxon A, Shanahan F, Landers C, Ganz T, Targan S. A distinct subset of antineutrophil cytoplasmic antibodies is associated with inflammatory bowel disease. J Allergy Clin Immunol 1990;86:202–210.

45. Nölle B, Specks U, Lüdemann J, Rohrbach MS, DeRemee RA, Gross WL. Anticytoplasmic autoantibodies: Their immunodiagnostic value in Wegener's granulomatosis. Ann Intern Med 1989;111:28–40.

46. Carder PJ, Harrison DJ. Opportunistic infection and antineutrophil cytoplasm antibodies in Wegener's granulomatosis. Respir Med 1989;83:421–424.

46a. Davenport A. "False positive: perinuclear and cytoplasmic anti-neutrophil cytoplasmic antibody results leading to misdiagnosis of Wegener's granulomatosis and/or microscopic polyarteritis. Clin Nephrol 1992;37:124–130.

47. Savage CO, Tizard J, Jayne D, Lockwood CM, Dillon MJ. Antineutrophil cytoplasm antibodies in Kawasaki disease. Arch Dis Child 1989;64:360–363.

48. Finnegan MJ, Hinchcliffe J, Russell-Jones D, et al. Vasculitis complicating cystic fibrosis. Q J Med 1989;72:609–621.

49. Faust EC, Agosin M, Garcia-Laverde A, Sayad WY, Johnson VM, Murray NA. Unusual findings of filarial infections of man. Am J Trop Med Hyg 1952;1:239–249.

50. Nässberger L, Sjöholm AG, Sturfelt G. Absence of circulating antineutrophil cytoplasm antibodies (ANCA) in severe vasculitis associated with rheumatoid arthritis. Scand J Rheumatol 1990;19:189–192.

51. Cohen Tervaert JW, Goldschmeding R, Elema JD, et al. Autoantibodies against myeloid lysosomal enzymes in crescentic glomerulonephritis. Kidney Int 1991;37:799–806.

52. Falk RJ, Jennette JC. Anti-neutrophil cytoplasmic autoantibodies with specificity for myeloperoxidase in patients with systemic vasculitis and idiopathic necrotizing and crescentic glomerulonephritis. N Engl J Med 1988;318:1651–1657.

53. Cohen Tervaert JW, Goldschmeding R, Elema JD, von dem Borne AE, Kallenberg CG. Antimyeloperoxidase antibodies in the Churt–Strauss syndrome. Thorax 1991;46:70–71.

54. DeRemee RA, McDonald TJ, Weiland LH. Wegener's granulomatosis: Observations on treatment with antimicrobial agents. Mayo Clin Proc 1985;60:27–32.

55. Hoffman GS, Leavitt RY, Fleisher TA, Minor JR, Fauci AS. Treatment of Wegener's granulomatosis with intermittent high-dose intravenous cyclophosphamide. Am J Med 1990;89:403–410.

56. Wegener F. A unique rhinogenic granulomatosis with especial involvement of the arterial system and kidneys (Translation). Beitr Pathol Anat 1939;102:36–68.

57. Wegener F. Generalized septic vascular diseases (Translation). Verh Dtsch Ges Pathol 1936;29:202–210.

58. Walton EW. Giant-cell granuloma of the respiratory tract (Wegener's granulomatosis). Br Med J 1958;2:265–270.

59. Lombard CM, Duncan SR, Rizk NW, Colby TV. The diagnosis of Wegener's granulomatosis from transbronchial biopsy specimens. Hum Pathol 1990;21:838–842.

60. Fekete PS, Campbell WG, Jr., Bernardino ME. Transthoracic needle aspiration biopsy in Wegener's granulomatosis. Morphologic findings in five cases. Acta Cytol 1990;34:155–160.

60a. Pitman MB, Szyfelbein WM, Niles J, Fienberg R. Clinical utility of fine needle aspiration biopsy in the diagnosis of Wegener's granulomatosis. A report of two cases. Acta Cytol 1992;36:222–229.

61. Colby TV. Diffuse pulmonary hemorrhage in Wegener's granulomatosis. Semin Respir Med 1989;10:136–140.

62. Kjellstrand CM, Simmons RL, Uranga VM, Buselmeier TJ, Najarian JS. Acute fulminant Wegener granulomatosis. Therapy with immunosuppression, hemodialysis, and renal transplantation. Arch Intern Med 1974;134:40–43.

63. Leatherman JW, Davies SF, Hoidal JR. Alveolar hemorrhage syndromes: Diffuse microvascular lung hemorrhage in immune and idiopathic disorders. Medicine (Baltimore) 1984;63:343–361.

64. Travis WD, Carpenter HA, Lie JT. Diffuse pulmonary hemorrhage. An uncommon manifestation of Wegener's granulomatosis. Am J Surg Pathol 1987;11:702–708.

65. Yousem SA. Bronchocentric injury in Wegener's granulomatosis: A report of five cases. Hum Pathol 1991;22:535–540.

66. Travis WD, Colby TV, Koss MN. Pulmonary Wegener's granulomatosis with prominent bronchocentric involvement (in manuscript).

67. Katzenstein AL. Necrotizing granulomas of the lung. Hum Pathol 1980;11:596–597.

68. Katzenstein AL, Askin FB. Surgical pathology of nonneoplastic lung disease. Major Probl Pathol 1982;13:1–430.

69. Sitara D, Hoffbrand BI. Chronic bronchial suppuration and antineutrophil cytoplasmic antibody (ANCA) positive systemic vasculitis. Postgrad Med J 1990;66:669–671.

70. Foo SS, Weisbrod GL, Herman SJ, Chamberlain DW. Wegener granulomatosis presenting on CT with atypical bronchovasocentric distribution. J Comput Assist Tomogr 1990;14:1004–1006.

71. Fienberg R. Necrotizing granulomatosis and angiitis of the lungs and its relationship to chronic pneumonitis of the cholesterol type. Am J Pathol 1953;29:913–931.

72. Yoshikawa Y, Watanabe T. Pulmonary lesions in Wegener's granulomatosis: A clinicopathologic study of 22 autopsy cases. Hum Pathol 1986;17:401–410.

73. Yousem SA, Lombard CM. The eosinophilic variant of Wegener's granulomatosis. Hum Pathol 1988;19:682–688.

74. Devaney KO, Travis WD, Hoffman GS, Leavitt RY, Lebovics R, Fauci AS. Interpretation of head and neck biopsies in Wegener's granulomatosis. A pathologic study of 126 biopsies in 70 patients. Am J Surg Pathol 1990;14:555–564.

75. Del Buono EA, Flint A. Diagnostic usefulness of nasal biopsy in Wegener's granulomatosis. Hum Pathol 1991;22:107–110.

76. Colby TV, Tazelaar HD, Specks U, DeRemee RA. Nasal biopsy in Wegener's granulomatosis (Editorial). Hum Pathol 1991;22:101–104.

76a. Kalina PH, Lie JT, Campbell RJ, Garrity JA. Diagnostic value and limitations of orbital biopsy in Wegener's granulomatosis. Ophthalmology 1992;99:120–124.

77. Antonovych T, Sabnis SG, Tuur SM, Sesterhenn IA, Balow JE. Morphologic differences between polyarteritis and Wegener's granulomatosis using light, electron and immunohistochemical techniques. Mod Pathol 1989;2:349–359.

78. Weiss MA, Crissman JD. Renal biopsy findings in Wegener's granulomatosis: Segmental necrotizing glomerulonephritis with glomerular thrombosis. Hum Pathol 1984;15:943–956.

79. Novak RF, Christiansen RG, Sorensen ET. The acute vasculitis of Wegener's granulomatosis in renal biopsies. Am J Clin Pathol 1982;78:367–371.

80. Watanabe T, Nagafuci Y, Yoshikawa Y, Toyoshima H. Renal papillary necrosis associated with Wegener's granulomatosis. Hum Pathol 1983;14:551–557.

81. Watanabe T, Yoshikawa Y, Toyoshima H. Morphological and clinical features of the kidney in Wegener's granulomatosis. A survey of 28 autopsies in Japan. Jpn J Nephrol 1981;23:921–930.

82. Hu CH, O'Loughlin S, Winkelmann RK. Cutaneous manifestations of Wegener's granulomatosis. Arch Dermatol 1977;113:175–182.

83. Chyu JYH, Hagstrom WJ, Soltani K, Faibisoff B, Whitney DH. Wegener's granulomatosis in childhood: Cutaneous manifestations as the presenting signs. J Am Acad Dermatol 1984;10:341–346.

84. Lipford EH, Jr., Margolick JB, Longo DL, Fauci AS, Jaffe ES. Angiocentric immunoproliferative lesions: A

clinicopathologic spectrum of post-thymic T-cell proliferations. Blood 1988;72:1674–1681.

85. Koss MN, Hochholzer L, Langloss JM, Wehunt WD, Lazarus AA, Nichols PW. Lymphomatoid granulomatosis: A clinicopathologic study of 42 patients. Pathology 1986;18:283–288.

86. Fauci AS, Haynes BF, Costa J, Katz P, Wolff SM. Lymphomatoid granulomatosis. Prospective clinical and therapeutic experience over 10 years. N Engl J Med 1982;306:68–74.

87. Chumbley LC, Harrison EG, Jr., DeRemee RA. Allergic granulomatosis and angiitis (Churg–Strauss syndrome). Report and analysis of 30 cases. Mayo Clin Proc 1977;52:477–484.

87a. Case records of the Massachusetts General Hospital. Weekly clinicopathological exercises. Case 18--1992. Asthma, peripheral neuropathy, and eosinophilia in a 52-year-old man. N Engl J Med 1992; 326:1204-1212.

88. Churg J, Strauss L. Allergic granulomatosis, allergic angiitis and periarteritis nodosa. Am J Pathol 1951;27:277–294.

89. Churg J. Allergic granulomatosis and granulomatous-vascular syndromes. Ann Allergy 1963;21:619–628.

90. Koss MN, Antonovych T, Hochholzer L. Allergic granulomatosis (Churg–Strauss syndrome). Am J Surg Pathol 1981;5:21–28.

91. Lanham JG, Elkon KB, Pusey CD, Hughes GR. Systemic vasculitis with asthma and eosinophilia: A clinical approach to the Churg–Strauss syndrome. Medicine (Baltimore) 1984;63:65–81.

92. Churg J. Nomenclature of vasculitic syndromes: A historical perspective. Am J Kidney Dis 1991;18:148–153.

93. Churg A, Carrington CB, Gupta R. Necrotizing sarcoid granulomatosis. Chest 1979;76:406–413.

94. Ulbright TM, Katzenstein AL. Solitary necrotizing granulomas of the lung: Differentiating features and etiology. Am J Surg Pathol 1980;4:13–28.

95. Koss MN, Robinson RG, Hochholzer L. Bronchocentric granulomatosis. Hum Pathol 1981;12:632–638.

96. Leatherman JW, Sibley RK, Davies SF. Diffuse intrapulmonary hemorrhage and glomerulonephritis unrelated to antiglomerular basement membrane antibody. Am J Med 1982;72:401–410.

97. Mark EJ, Ramirez JF. Pulmonary capillaritis and hemorrhage in patients with systemic vasculitis. Arch Pathol Lab Med 1985;109:413–418.

98. Travis WD, Colby TV, Lombard CM, Carpenter HA. A clinicopathologic study of 34 cases of diffuse pulmonary hemorrhage with lung biopsy confirmation. Am J Surg Pathol 1990;14:1112–1125.

99. Katzenstein AL, Carrington CB, Liebow AA. Lymphomatoid granulomatosis: A clinicopathologic study of 152 cases. Cancer 1979;43:360–373.

100. Colby TV, Carrington CB. Pulmonary lymphomas: Current concepts. Hum Pathol 1983;14:884–887.

101. Colby TV, Carrington CB. Lymphoreticular tumors and infiltrates of the lung. Pathol Annu 1983;18(Part 1):27–70.

102. Jaffe ES. Pathologic and clinical spectrum of post-thymic T-cell malignancies. Cancer Invest 1984;2:413–426.

103. Lanham JG, Churg J. Churg–Strauss syndrome. In: Churg A, Churg J, eds. Systemic vasculitides. New York: Igaku-Shoin, 1991;101–120.

104. Specks U, DeRemee RA. Granulomatous vasculitis. Wegener's granulomatosis and Churg–Strauss syndrome. Rheum Dis Clin NorthAm 1990;16:377–397.

105. Carrington CB, Liewbow AA. Limited forms of antiitis and granulomatosis of Wegener's type. Am J Med 1966;41:497–527.

106. Myers JL. Bronchocentric granulomatosis. Disease or diagnosis? (editorial). Chest 1989;96:3–4.

107. Baltaro RJ, Hoffman GS, Sechler JM, et al. Immunoglobulin G antineutrophil cytoplasmic antibodies are produced in the respiratory tract of patients with Wegener's granulomatosis. Am Rev Respir Dis 1991;143:275–278.

108. Hoffman GS, Sechler JM, Gallin JI, et al. Bronchoalveolar lavage analysis in Wegener's granulomatosis. A method to study disease pathogenesis. Am Rev Respir Dis 1991;143:401–407.

109. Gephardt GN, Shah LF, Tubbs RR, Ahmad M. Wegener's granulomatosis. Immunomicroscopic and ultrastructural study of four cases. Arch Pathol Lab Med 1990;114:961–965.

110. Desgys GE, Mintzer RA, Vira RF. Allergic granulomatosis: Churg–Strauss syndrome. Am J Radiol 1980;135:1821–1882.

111. Zeek PM. Periarteris nodosa: A critical review. Am J Clin Pathol 1952;22:777–790.

112. Rosen S, Falk RJ, Jennette JC. Polyarteritis nodosa, including microscopic form and renal vasculitis. In: Churg A, Churg J, eds. Systemic vasculitides. New York: Igaku-Shoin, 1991;57–77.

112a. Rose GA, Spencer H. Polyarteritis nodosa. Q J Med 1957;26:43–81.

113. Rackemann FM, Greene EJ. Periarteritis nodosa and asthma. Trans Assoc Am Physicians 1939;54:112–118.

114. Imai H, Nakamoto Y, Hirokawa M, Akihama T, Miura AB. Carbamazepine-induced granulomatous necrotizing angiitis with acute renal failure. Nephron 1989;51:405–408.

115. Brill R, Churg J, Beaver PC. Allergic granulomatosis associated with visceral larva migrans. Am J Clin Pathol 1953;23:1208–1215.

116. Strazzella WD, Safirstein BH. Asthma due to parasitic infestation. N J Med 1989;89:947–949.

117. Masi AT, Hunder GG, Lie JT, et al. The American College of Rheumatology 1990 criteria for the classification of Churg–Strauss syndrome (allergic granulomatosis and angiitis). Arthritis Rheum 1990;33:1094–1100.

118. Lie JT. Illustrated histopathologic classification criteria for selected vasculitis syndromes. American College of Rheumatology Subcommittee on Classification of Vasculitis. Arthritis Rheum 1990;33:1074–1087.

119. Lipworth BJ, Slater DN, Corrin B, Kesseler ME, Haste

AR. Allergic granulomatosis without asthma: A rare 'forme fruste' of the Churg–Strauss syndrome. Respir Med 1989;83:249–250.

120. Gambari PF, Ostuni PA, Lazzarin P, Fassina A, Todesco S. Eosinophilic granuloma and necrotizing vasculitis (Churg–Strauss syndrome?) involving a parotid gland, lymph nodes, liver and spleen. Scand J Rheumatol 1989;18:171–175.

121. Sasaki A, Hasegawa M, Nakazato Y, Ishida Y, Saitoh S. Allergic granulomatosis and angiitis (Churg–Strauss syndrome). Report of an autopsy case in a nonasthmatic patient. Acta Pathol Jpn 1988;38:761–768.

122. Olsen KD, Neel HB, DeRemee RA, Weiland LH. Nasal manifestations of allergic granulomatosis and angiitis (Churg–Strauss syndrome). Otolaryngol Head Neck Surg 1980;88:85–89.

123. Phanuphak P, Kohler PF. Onset of polyarteritis nodosa during allergic hyposensitization treatment. Am J Med 1980;68:479–485.

124. Case Records of the Massachusetts General Hospital. Case 18-1987. N Engl J Med 1987;316:1139–1147.

125. Guillevin L, Guittard TH, Bletry O, Godeau P, Rosenthal P. Systemic necrotizing angiitis with asthma: Causes and precipitating factors in 43 cases. Lung 1987;165:165–172.

126. Guillevin L, Amouroux J, Arbeille B, Boura R. Churg–Strauss angiitis. Arguments favoring the responsibility of inhaled antigens. Chest 1991;100:1472–1473.

127. Stephens M, Reynolds S, Biggs AR, Davies B. Allergic bronchopulmonary aspergillosis progressing to allergic granulomatosis and angiitis (Churg–Strauss Syndrome). Am Rev Respir Dis 1988;137:1226–1228.

128. Nissim F, Von der Valde J, Czernobilsky B. A limited form of Churg–Strauss syndrome. Ocular and cutaneous manifestations. Arch Pathol Lab Med 1982;106:305–307.

129. Kelalis PP, Harrison EG, Greene LF. Allergic granulomas of the prostate in asthmatics. JAMA 1964;188:963–967.

130. Lasser A, Ghofrany S. Necrotizing granulomatous vasculitis (allergic granulomatosis) of the gallbladder. Gastroenterology 1976;71:660–662.

131. Erzurum SC, Underwood GA, Hamilos DL, Waldron JA. Pleural effusion in Churg–Strauss syndrome. Chest 1989;95:1357–1359.

132. Clutterbuck EJ, Pusey CD. Severe alveolar hemorrhage in Churg–Strauss syndrome. Eur J Respir Dis 1987;71:158–163.

133. Buschman DL, Waldron JA, Jr., King TE, Jr. Churg–Strauss pulmonary vasculitis. High-resolution computed tomography scanning and pathologic findings. Am Rev Respir Dis 1990;142:458–461.

134. Lally Shields C, Shields JA, Rozanski TI. Conjunctival involvement in Churg–Strauss syndrome. J Ophthalmol 1986;102:601–605.

135. Morgan JM, Raposo L, Gibson DG. Cardiac involvement in Churg–Strauss syndrome shown by echocardiography. Br Heart J 1989;62:462–466.

136. Thomson D, Chamsi-Pasha H, Hasleton P. Heart transplantation for Churg–Strauss syndrome. Br Heart J 1989;62:409–410.

136a. Balestrieri GP, Valentini U, Cerudelli B, Spandrio S, Renaldini E. Reversible myocardial impairment in the Churg–Strauss syndrome: report of a case. Clin Exp Rheumatol 1992;10:75–77.

137. Lanham JG, Cooke S, Davies J, et al. Endomyocardial complications of the Churg–Strauss syndrome. Postgrad Med J 1985;61:341–344.

138. Shimamoto C, Hirata I, Ohshiba S, Fujiwara S, Nishio M. Churg–Strauss syndrome (allergic granulomatous angiitis) with peculiar multiple colonic ulcers. Am J Gastroenterol 1990;85:316–319.

139. Imai H, Nakamoto Y, Nakajima Y, Sugawara T, Miura AB. Allergic granulomatosis and angiitis (Churg–Strauss syndrome) presenting as acute acalculous cholecystitis. J Rheumatol 1990;17:247–249.

140. Clutterbuck EJ, Evans DJ, Pusey CD. Renal involvement in Churg–Strauss syndrome. Nephrol Dial Transplant 1990;5:161–167.

141. Cortellini P, Manganelli P, Poletti F, Sacchini P, Ambanelli U, Bezzi E. Ureteral involvement in the Churg–Strauss syndrome. J Urol 1988;140:1016–1018.

142. Kelalis PP, Harrison EG, Utz DC. Allergic granulomas of the prostate: treatment with steroids. J Urol 1966;96:573–577.

143. Strauss L, Churg J, Zak FG. Cutaneous lesions of allergic granulomatosis. A histopathologic study. J Invest Dermatol 1951;17:349–359.

144. Harrison DJ, Simpson R, Kharbanda R, Abernethy VE, Nimmo G. Antibodies to neutrophil cytoplasmic antigens in Wegener's granulomatosis and other conditions. Thorax 1989;44:373–377.

145. Guillevin L, Ronco P, Verroust P. Circulating immune complexes in systemic necrotizing vasculitis of the polyarteritis nodosa group. Comparison of HBV-related polyarteritis nodosa and Churg–Strauss angiitis. J Autoimmun 1990;3:789–792.

146. Cooper LM, Patterson JA. Allergic granulomatosis and angiitis of Churg–Strauss. Case report in a patient with antibodies to human immunodeficiency virus and hepatitis B virus. Int J Dermatol 1989;28:597–599.

147. Conn DL, Dickson ER, Carpenter HA. The association of Churg–Strauss syndrome with temporal artery involvement, primary biliary cirrhosis, and polychondritis in a single patient. J Rheumatol 1982;9:744–748.

148. Cupps TR, Fauci AS. Neoplasm and systemic vasculitis: a case report. Arthritis Rheum 1982;25:475–477.

149. Guillevin L, Jarrousse B, Lok C, et al. Longterm followup after treatment of polyarteritis nodosa and Churg–Strauss angiitis with comparison of steroids, plasma exchange and cyclophosphamide to steroids and plasma exchange. A prospective randomized trial of 71 patients. The Cooperative Study Group for Polyarteritis Nodosa. J Rheumatol 1991;18:567–574.

150. Guillevin L. Treatment of polyarteritis nodosa and Churg–Strauss angiitis: Indications of plasma exchange. Results of three prospective trials in 162 patients. The Cooperative Study Group for the Study of

Polyarteritis Nodosa. Prog Clin Biol Res 1990; 337:309–317.

150a. Guillevin L, Fain O, Lhote F, et al. Lack of superiority of steroids plus plasma exchange to steroids alone in the treatment of polyarteritis nodosa and Churg–Strauss syndrome. A prospective, randomized trial in 78 patients. Arthritis Rheum 1992;35:208–215.

151. Chow CC, Li EK, Lai FM. Allergic granulomatosis and angiitis (Churg–Strauss syndrome): Response to 'pulse' intravenous cyclophosphamide. Ann Rheum Dis 1989;48:605–608.

152. MacFayden R, Tron V, Keshmiri M, Road JD. Allergic angiitis of Churg and Strauss syndrome. Response to pulse methylprednisolone. Chest 1987;91:629–631.

153. Travis WD, Koss MN, Colby TV, Churg A, Churg J. Pulmonary pathologic findings in Churg–Strauss syndrome (in manuscript).

154. Leung WH, Wong KK, Lau CP, Wong CK, Cheng CH, So KF. Myocardial involvement in Churg–Strauss syndrome: the role of endomyocardial biopsy. J Rheumatol 1989;16:828–831.

155. Liewbow AA, Carrington CB. The eosinophilic pneumonias. Medicine (Baltimore) 1969;48:251–285.

156. Travis WD, Kwon-Chung KJ, Kleiner DE, et al. Unusual aspects of allergic bronchopulmonary fungal disease: Report of two cases due to *Curvularia* organisms associated with allergic fungal sinusitis. Hum Pathol 1991;22:1240–1248.

157. Tolmie J, Steer CR, Edmunds AT. Pulmonary eosinophilia associated with carbamazepine. Arch Dis Child 1983;58:833–834.

158. Katzenstein AL, Liebow AA, Friedman PJ. Bronchocentric granulomatosis, mucoid impaction, and hypersensitivity reactions to fungi. Am Rev Respir Dis 1975;111:497–537.

159. Winkelmann RK, Ditro WB. Cutaneous and visceral syndromes of necrotizing or "allergic" angiitis: A study of 38 cases. Medicine (Baltimore) 1964;43:59–89.

160. Finan MC, Winkelmann RK. The cutaneous extravascular necrotizing granuloma (Churg–Strauss granuloma) and systemic disease: A review of 27 cases. Medicine (Baltimore) 1983;62:142–158.

161. Amato MB, Barbas CS, Delmonte VC, Carvalho CR. Concurrent Churg–Strauss syndrome and temporal arteritis in a young patient with pulmonary nodules. Am Rev Respir Dis 1989;139:1539–1542.

162. Leavitt RY, Fauci AS. Polyangiitis overlap syndrome. Classification and prospective clinical experience. Am J Med 1986;81:79–85.

163. Henochowicz S, Eggensperger D, Pierce L, Barth WF. Necrotizing systemic vasculitis with features of both Wegener's granulomatosis and Churg–Strauss vasculitis. Arthritis Rheum 1982;29:565–569.

164. Spiteri MA, Gledhill A, Campbell D, Clarke SW. Necrotizing sarcoid granulomatosis. Br J Dis Chest 1987;81:70–75.

165. Chabalko JJ. Solitary lung lesion with cavitation due to necrotizing sarcoid granulomatosis. Del Med J 1986;58:15–16.

166. Rolfes DB, Weiss MA, Sanders MA. Necrotizing sarcoid granulomatosis with suppurative features. Am J Clin Pathol 1984;82:602–607.

167. Singh N, Cole S, Krause PJ, Conway M, Garcia L. Necrotizing sarcoid granulomatosis with extrapulmonary involvement. Clinical, pathologic, ultrastructural, and immunologic features. Am Rev Respir Dis 1981;124:189–192.

168. Beach RC, Corrin B, Scopes JW, Graham E. Necrotizing sarcoid granulomatosis with neurologic lesions in a child. J Pediatr 1980;97:950–953.

169. Stephen JG, Braimbridge MV, Corrin B, Wilkinson SP, Day D, Whimster WF. Necrotizing 'sarcoidal' angiitis and granulomatosis of the lung. Thorax 1976;31:356–360.

170. Saldana MJ. Necrotizing sarcoid granulomatosis: Clinicopathologic observations in 24 patients (abstract). Lab Invest 1978;38:364.

171. Fisher MR, Christ ML, Bernstein JR. Necrotizing sarcoid-like granulomatosis: radiologic-pathologic correlation. J Can Assoc Radiol 1984;35:313–315.

172. Sharma OP, Hewlett R, Gordonson RH. Nodular sarcoidosis: An unusual radiographic appearance. Chest 1973;64:189–192.

173. Onal E, Lopata M, Lourenco RV. Nodular pulmonary sarcoidosis. Clinical, roentgenographic and physiologic course in five patients. Chest 1977;72:296–300.

174. Carrington CB, Gaensler EA, Mikus JP, Schachter AW, Burke GW, Goff AM. Structure and function in sarcoidosis. Ann NY Acad Sci 1976;278:265–283.

175. Rosen Y, Vuletin JC, Pertschuk LP, Silverstein E. Sarcoidosis from the pathologist's vantage point. Pathol Annu 1979;14(Part I):405–439.

176. Rosen Y, Moon S, Huang C, Gourin A, Lyons HA. Granulomatous pulmonary angiitis in sarcoidosis. Arch Pathol Lab Med 1977;101:170–174.

177. Zeek PM, Smith CC, Weeter JC. Studies on periarteritis nodosa. III. The differentiation between the vascular lesions of periarteritis nodosa and of hypersensitivity. Am J Pathol 1948;24:889–917.

178. Calabrese LH, Michel BA, Bloch DA, et al. The American College of Rheumatology 1990 criteria for the classification of hypersensitivity vasculitis. Arthritis Rheum 1990;33:1108–1113.

179. Swerlick RA, Lawley TJ. Small-vessel vasculitis and cutaneous vasculitis. In: Churg A, Churg J, eds. Systemic vasculitides. New York: Igaku-Shoin, 1991;193–201.

180. Falk DK. Pulmonary disease in idiopathic urticarial vasculitis. J Am Acad Dermatol 1984;1:346–352.

181. Cream JJ, Gumpel JM, Peachey RDG. Schönlein-Henoch purpura in the adult. Q J Med 1970;39:461–484.

182. White RHR. Henoch-Schönlein purpura. In: Churg A, Churg J, eds. Systemic vasculitides. New York: Igaku-Shoin, 1991;203–217.

183. Mills JA, Michel BA, Bloch DA, et al. The American College of Rheumatology 1990 criteria for the classification of Henoch-Schönlein purpura. Arthritis Rheum 1990;33:1114–1121.

184. Roth DA, Wilz DR, Theil GB. Schönlein-Henoch syndrome in adults. Q J Med 1985;55:145–152.

185. Kathuria S, Cheifec G. Fatal pulmonary Henoch-Schönlein syndrome. Chest 1982;82:654–656.

186. Mitchell DM, Hoffbrand BI. Relapse of Henoch-Schönlein disease associated with lung carcinoma. J R Soc Med 1979;72:614–615.

187. Cairns SA, Mallick NP, Lawler W, Williams G. Squamous cell carcinoma of bronchus presenting with Henoch-Schönlein purpura. Br Med J 1978;2:474–475.

188. Maurice TR. Carcinoma of bronchus presenting with Henoch-Schönlein purpura. Br Med J 1978;2:831.

189. Pfitzenmeyer P, Besancenot JF, Brichon P, Gonzalez G, Andrë F. The association of bronchial carcinoma and rheumatoid purpura (letter). Ann Med Interne (Paris) 1989;140:423–424.

190. Marandian MH, Ezzati M, Behvad A, Moazzami P, Rakhchan M. Pulmonary involvement in Schönlein-Henoch's purpura. Arch Fr Pediatr 1982;39:255–257.

191. Markus HS, Clark JV. Pulmonary haemorrhage in Henoch-Schönlein purpura. Thorax 1989;44:525–526.

192. Veale D, Venning MC, Quinn A. Pulmonary haemorrhage in Henoch-Schönlein purpura (Letter). Thorax 1990;45:496.

193. Shichiri M, Tsutsumi K, Yamamoto I, Ida T, Iwamoto H. Diffuse intrapulmonary hemorrhage and renal failure in adult Henoch-Schönlein purpura. Am J Neprhol 1987;7:140–142.

194. Payton CD, Allison ME, Boulton-Jones JM. Henoch Schönlein purpura presenting with pulmonary haemorrhage. Scott Med J 1987;32:26–27.

195. Weiss VF, Naidu S. Fatal pulmonary hemorrhage in Henoch-Schönlein purpura. Cutis 1979;23:687–688.

196. Jacome AF. Pulmonary hemorrhage and death complicating anaphylactoid purpura. South Med J 1967;60:1003–1004.

197. Fiegler W. Siemoneit KD. Pulmonary manifestations in anaphylactoid purpura (Henoch-Schönlein Syndrome). ROFO Fortschr Geb Rontgenstr Nuklearmed 1981;134:269–272.

198. Gorevic PD, Kassab HJ, Levo Y, et al. Mixed cryoglobulinemia: Clinical aspects and long-term follow-up of 40 patients. Am J Med 1980;69:287–308.

199. Churg J. Cryoglobulinemic vasculitis. In: Churg A, Churg J, eds. Systemic vasculitides. New York: Igaku-Shoin, 1991;293–298.

200. Bombardieri S, Paoletti P, Ferri C, Di Munno O, Fornai E, Giutini C. Lung involvement in essential mixed cryoglobulinemia. Am J Med 1979;66:748–756.

201. Viegi G, Fornai E, Ferri C, et al. Lung function in essential mixed cryoglobulinemia: A short-term follow-up. Clin Rheumatol 1989;8:331–338.

202. Chejfec G, Lichtenberg L, Lertratanakul Y, Lange C, Baerwaldt M, Gould VE. Respiratory insufficiency in a patient with mixed cryoglobulinemia. Ultrastruct Pathol 1981;2:295–302.

203. Madrenas J, Vallës M, Ruiz Marcellan MC, Fort J,

Garcia Bragado F, Pelegri A. Pulmonary hemorrhage and glomerulonephritis associated with essential mixed cryoglobulinemia. Med Clin (Barc) 1989;93:262–264.

204. MontiG, Galli M, Cereda UG, Cannatelli G, Invernizzi F. Mycosis fungoides with mixed cryoglobulinemia and pulmonary vasculitis. A case report. Boll Ist Sieroter Milan 1987;66:324–328.

205. Clinicopathologic Conference: Mixed cryoglobulinemia. Am J Med 1975;61:95.

206. Arend WP, Michel BA, Bloch DA, et al. The American College of Rheumatology 1990 criteria for the classification of Takayasu arteritis. Arthritis Rheum 1990;33:1129–1134.

207. He NS, Liu F, Wu EH, et al. Pulmonary artery involvement in aorto-arteritis. An analysis of DSA. Chin Med J (Engl Ed) 1990;103:666–672.

208. Sharma S, Rajani M, Shrivastava S, et al. Non-specific aorto-arteritis (Takayasu's disease) in children. Br J Radiol 1991;64:690–698.

209. Sharma S, Kamalakar T, Rajani M, Talwar KK, Shrivastava S. The incidence and patterns of pulmonary artery involvement in Takayasu's arteritis. Clin Radiol 1990;42:177–181.

210. Yamato M, Lecky JW, Hiramatsu K, Kohda E. Takayasu arteritis: Radiographic and angiographic findings in 59 patients. Radiology 1986;161:329–334.

211. Ishikawa T. Systemic artery–pulmonary artery communication in Takayasu's arteritis. AJR 1977;128:389–393.

212. Numano F, Ohta N, Sasazuki T. HLA and clinical manifestations in Takayasu disease. Jpn Circ J 1982;46:184–189.

213. Lie JT. Takayasu's Arteritis. In: Churg A, Churg J, eds. Systemic vasculitides. New York: Igaku-Shoin, 1991:159–179.

214. Chauvaud S, Mace L, Brunewald P, Tricot JL, Camilleri JP, Carpentier A. Takayasu's arteritis with bilateral pulmonary artery stenosis. Successful surgical correction. J Thorac Cardiovasc Surg 1987;94:246–250.

215. Haas A, Stiehm ER. Takayasu's arteritis presenting as pulmonary hypertension. Am J Dis Child 1986;140:472–374.

216. Umehara I, Shibuya H, Nakagawa T, Numano F. Comprehensive analysis of perfusion scintigraphy in Takayasu's arteritis. Clin Nucl Med 1991;16:352–357.

217. Reinig JW, Simmons JT, Bielory L, Lewallen C. Multiple lung perfusion defects in a patient with Takayasu's arteritis. Clin Nucl Med 1985;10:893–894.

218. Suzuki Y. Ventilation/perfusion mismatch of one lung in a patient with Takayasu's arteritis. Clin Nucl Med 1986;11:733–734.

219. Horimoto M, Igarashi K, Aoi K, Okamoto K, Takenaka T. Unilateral diffuse pulmonary artery involvement in Takayasu's arteritis associated with coronary-pulmonary artery fistula and bronchial-pulmonary artery fistula: A case report. Angiology 1991;42:73–80.

220. Halon DA, Turgeman Y, Merdler A, Hardoff R, Sharir T. Coronary artery to bronchial artery anastomosis in Takayasu's arteritis. Cardiology 1987;74:387–391.

221. Nasu T. Takayasu's truncoarteritis. Pulseless disease or aortitis syndrome. Acta Pathol Jpn 1982; 32(Suppl)1:117–131.

222. Rose AG, Sinclair-Smith CC. Takayasu's arteritis. A study of 16 autopsy cases. Arch Pathol Lab Med 1980;104:231–237.

223. Lie JT. Diagnostic histopathology of major systemic and pulmonary vasculitic syndromes. Rheum Dis Clin North Am 1990;16:269–292.

224. Greene NB, Baughman RP, Kim CK. Takayasu's arteritis associated with interstitial lung disease and glomerulonephritis. Chest 1986;89:605–606.

225. Jakob H, Volb R, Stangl G, Reifart N, Rumpelt HJ, Olert H. Surgical correction of a severely obstructed pulmonary artery bifurcation in Takayasu's arteritis. Eur J Cardiothorac Surg 1990;4:456–458.

226. Moore JW, Reardon MJ, Cooley DA, Vargo TA. Severe Takaysu's arteritis of the pulmonary arteries: Report of a case with successful surgical treatment. J Am Coll Cardiol 1985;5:369–373.

227. Fairley C, Wilson JW, Barraclough D. Pulmonary involvement in Behçet's syndrome. Chest 1989;96:1428–1429.

228. Raz I, Okon E, Chajek-Shaul T. Pulmonary manifestations in Behçet's syndrome. Chest 1989;95:585–589.

229. Efthimiou J, Johnston C, Spiro SG, Turner-Warwick M. Pulmonary disease in Behçet's syndrome. Q J Med 1986;58:259–280.

230. Grenier P, Bletry O, Cornud F, Godeau P, Nahum H. Pulmonary involvement in Behçet disease. AJR 1981;137:565–569.

231. Chajek T, Fainaru M. Behçet's disease. Report of 41 cases and a review of the literature. Medicine (Baltimore) 1975;54:179–196.

232. Cadman EC, Lundberg WB, Mitchell MS. Pulmonary manifestations of Behçet syndrome. Arch Intern Med 1976;136:944–947.

233. Gamble CN, Wiesner KB, Shapiro RF, Boyer WJ. The immune complex pathogenesis of glomerulonephritis and pulmonary vasculitis in Behçet's disease. Am J Med 1979;66:1031–1039.

234. Jerray M, Benzarti M, Rouatbi N. Possible Behçet's disease revealed by pulmonary aneurysms. Chest 1991;99:1282–1284.

235. Lakhanpal S, Tani K, Lie JT, Katoh K, Ishigatsubo Y, Ohokubo T. Pathologic features of Behçet's syndrome: A review of Japanese autopsy registry data. Hum Pathol 1985;16:790–795.

236. Slavin RE, de Groot WJ. Pathology of the lung in Behçet's disease. Case report and review of the literature. Am J Surg Pathol 1981;5:779–788.

237. Salamon F, Weinberger A, Nili M, et al. Massive hemoptysis complicating Behçet's syndrome: The importance of early pulmonary angiography and operation. Ann Thorac Surg 1988;45:566–567.

238. Corren J. Acute interstitial pneumonia in a patient with Behçet's syndrome and common variable immunodeficiency [clinical conference]. Ann Allergy 1990;64:15–20.

239. Gibson JM, O'Hara MD, Beare JM, Stanford CF. Bronchial obstruction in a patient with Behçet's disease. Eur J Respir Dis 1982;63:356–360.

240. Vansteenkiste JF, Peene P, Verschakelen JA, van de Woestijne KP. Cyclosporin treatment in rapidly progressive pulmonary thromboembolic Behçet's disease. Thorax 1990;45:295–296.

241. Santo M, Levy A, Levy MJ, et al. Pneumonectomy in pulmonary mucormycosis complicating Behçet's disease. Postgrad Med J 1986;62:485–486.

242. McDuffie FC, Sams WM, Maldonado JE, Andreini PH, Conn DL, Samayoa EA. Hypocomplementemia with cutaneous vasculitis and arthritis. Mayo Clin Proc 1973;48:340–348.

243. Zeiss CR, Burch FX, Marde RJ, Furey NL, Gewurz H. A hypocomplementemic vasculitis urticarial syndrome. Report of four new cases and definition of the disease. Am J Med 1980;68:867–875.

244. Schwartz HR, McDuffie FC, Black LF, Schroeter AL, Conn DL. Hypocomplementemic urticarial vasculitis. Association with chronic obstructive pulmonary disease. Mayo Clin Proc 1982;57:231–238.

245. Grishman E, Spiera H. Vasculitis in connective tissue diseases, including hypcomplementemic vasculitis. In: Churg A, Churg J, eds. Systemic vasculitides. New York: Igaku-Shoin, 1991:273–292.

246. Angello V, Ruddy S, Winchester RJ, Christian CL, Kunkel HG. Hereditary C2 deficiency in systemic lupus erythematosus and acquired complement abnormalities in an unusual SLE-related syndrome. Birth Defects 1975;11:312–317.

247. Feig PU, Soter NA, Yager HM, Caplan L, Rosen S. Vasculitis with urticaria, hypocomplementemia, and multiple systems involvement. JAMA 1976;236:2065–2068.

248. Larson TS, Hall S, Hepper NGG, Hunder GG. Respiratory tract symptoms as a clue to giant cell arteritis. Ann Intern Med 1984;101:594–597.

249. Klein RG, Hunder GG, Stanson AW, Sheps SG. Large artery involvement in giant cell (temporal) arteritis. Ann Intern Med 1975;83:806–812.

250. Ladanyi M, Fraser RS. Pulmonary involvement in giant cell arteritis. Arch Pathol Lab Med 1987;11:1178–1180.

251. Rodat O, Buzelin F, Weber M, et al. Manifestations broncho-pulmonaires de la maladie de Horton: A propos d'une observation. Rev Med Interne 1983;4:225–230.

252. Bradley JD, Pinals RS, Blumenfeld HB, Poston WM. Giant cell arteritis with pulmonary nodules. Am J Med 1984;77:135–140.

253. Karam GH, Fulmer JD. Giant cell arteritis presenting as interstitial lung disease. Chest 1982;82:781–789.

254. Wagenaar SS, van den Bosch JMM, Westermann CJJ, Bosman HG, Lie JT. Isolated granulomatous giant cell vasculitis of the pulmonary elastic arteries. Arch Pathol Lab Med 1986;110:962–964.

255. Wagenaar SSC, Westermann CJJ, Corrin B. Giant cell

arteritis limited to large elastic pulmonary arteries. Thorax 1981;36:876–877.

256. Okubo S, Kuneida T, Ando M, Nakajima N, Yutani C. Idiopathic isolated pulmonary arteritis with chronic cor pulmonale. Chest 1988;94:665–666.

257. Lie JT. Disseminated visceral giant cell arteritis. Histopathologic description and differentiation from other granulomatous vasculitides. Am J Clin Pathol 1978;69:299–305.

258. Morita T, Kamimura A, Koizumi F. Disseminated visceral giant cell arteritis. Acta Pathol Jpn 1987;37:863–870.

259. Lie JT. Combined sarcoidosis and disseminated visceral giant cell angiitis: A third opinion (Letter). Arch Pathol Lab Med 1991;115:210–211.

260. Marcussen N, Lung C. Combined sarcoidosis and disseminated visceral giant cell vasculitis. Path Res Pract 1989;184:325–330.

261. Shintaku M, Mase K, Ohtsuki H, Yasumizu R, Yasunaga K, Ikehara S. Generalized sarcoidlike granulomas with systemic angiitis, crescentic glomerulonephritis, and pulmonary hemorrhage. Report of an autopsy case. Arch Pathol Lab Med 1989;113:1295–1298.

262. Takemura T, Matsui Y, Oritsu M, Akiyama O, et al. Pulmonary vascular involvement in sarcoidosis: Granulomatosis angiitis and microangiopathy in transbronchial lung biopsies. Virchows Arch[A] 1991;418:361–368.

263. Smith LJ, Lawrence JB, Katzenstein AL. Vascular sarcoidosis: A rare cause of pulmonary hypertension. Am J Med Sci 1983;285:38–44.

264. Levine BW, Saldana MJ, Hutter AM. Pulmonary hypertension in sarcoidosis. A case report of a rare but potentially treatable cause. Am Rev Respir Dis 1971;103:413–417.

265. Battesti JP, Georges R, Basset F, Saumon G. Chronic cor pulmonale in pulmonary sarcoidosis. Thorax 1978;33:76–84.

266. Martin JME, Dowling GP. Sudden death associated with compression of pulmonary arteries in sarcoidosis. Can Med Assoc J 1985;133:423–424.

267. Damuth TE, Bower JS, Cho K, Dantzker DR. Major pulmonary artery stenosis causing pulmonary hypertension in sarcoidosis. Chest 1980;78:888–891.

268. Davies J, Goodwin JF, Nellen M. Reversible pulmonary hypertension in sarcoidosis. Postgrad Med J 1982;58:282–285.

269. Hoffstein V, Ranganathan N, Mullen JBM. Sarcoidosis simulating pulmonary veno-occlusive disease. Am Rev Respir Dis 1986;134:809–811.

270. Crissman JD, Koss MN, Carson RP. Pulmonary veno-occlusive disease secondary to granulomatous venulitis. Am J Surg Pathol 1980;4:93–99.

271. Petri M, Barr E, Cho K, Farmer E. Overlap of granulomatous vasculitis and sarcoidosis: presentation with uveitis, eosinophilia, leg ulcers, sinusitis, and past foot drop. J Rheumatol 1988;15:1171–1173.

272. Lakhanpal S, Conn DL, Lie JT. Clinical and prognostic significance of vasculitis as an early manifestation of connective tissue disease syndromes. Ann Intern Med 1984;101:743–748.

273. Yousem SA, Colby TV, Carrington CB. Lung biopsy in rheumatoid arthritis. Am Rev Respir Dis 1985; 131:770–777.

274. Kay JM, Banik S. Unexplained pulmonary hypertension with pulmonary arteritis in rheumatoid disease. Br J Dis Chest 1977;7:53–59.

275. Baydur A, Mongan ES, Slager UT. Acute respiratory failure and pulmonary arteritis without parenchymal involvement. Demonstration in a patient with rheumatoid arthritis. Chest 1979;75:518–520.

276. Fayemi AO. Pulmonary vascular disease in systemic lupus erythematosus. Am J Clin Pathol 1976;65:284–290.

277. Yousem SA. The pulmonary pathologic manifestations of the CREST syndrome. Hum Pathol 1990;21:467–474.

278. Lakhanpal S, Lie JT, Conn DL, Martin WJ. Pulmonary disease in polymyositis/dermatomyositis: A clinicopathological analysis of 65 autopsy cases. Ann Rheum Dis 1986;46:23–29.

279. Prakash UBS, Luthra HS, Divertie MB. Intrathoracic manifestations in mixed connective tissue disease. Mayo Clin Proc 1985;60:813–821.

280. Young RH, Mark EJ. Pulmonary vascular changes in scleroderma. Am J Med 1978;64:998–1004.

281. Naeye RL. Pulmonary vascular lesions in systemic scleroderma. Dis Chest 1963;44:374–380.

282. Hakala M, Pääkkö P, Huhti E, Tarkka M, Sutinen S. Open lung biopsy of patients with rheumatoid arthritis. Clin Rheumatol 1990;9:452–460.

283. Sivaramkrishnan S, Askari AD, Popelka CG, Kleinerman JF. Pulmonary hypertension and systemic lupus erythematosus. Arch Intern Med 1980;140:109–111.

284. Marchesoni A, Messina K, Carrieri P, Sinigaglia L, Tosi S. Pulmonary hypertension and systemic lupus erythematosus. Clin Exp Rheumatol 1983;1:247–250.

285. Haupt HM, Moore GW, Hutchins GM. The lung in systemic lupus erythematosus. Analysis of the pathologic changes in 120 patients. Am J Med 1981;71:791–798.

286. Simonson JS, Schiller NB, Petri M, et al. Pulmonary hypertension in systemic lupus erythematosus. J Rheumatol 1989;16:918–925.

287. Quismorio FP, Sharma O, Koss MN, et al. Immunopathologic and clinical studies in pulmonary hypertension associated with systemic lupus erythematosis. Semin Arthritis Rheum 1984;13:349–359.

288. Young ID, Ford SE, Ford PM. The association of pulmonary hypertension with rheumatoid arthritis. J Rheumatol 1989;16:1266–1269.

289. Walker WC, Wright V. Pulmonary lesions and rheumatoid arthritis. Medicine (Baltimore) 1968;47:501–520.

290. Gardner DL, Duthie JJR, Macleod J, Allan WSA. Pulmonary hypertension in rheumatoid arthritis: report of a case with intimal sclerosis of the pulmonary and digital arteries. Scott Med J 1957;2:183–188.

291. Caldwell DS, McCallum RM. Rheumatologic manifes-

tations of cancer. Med Clin North Am 1986;70:385–417.

292. Greer JM, Longley S, Edwards NL, Elfenbein GJ, Panusch RS. Vasculitis associated with malignancy. Experience with 13 patients and literature review. Medicine (Baltimore) 1988;67:220–230.

293. Ong EL, Evans S, Hanley SP. Pulmonary vasculitis associated with cholangiocarcinoma liver. Postgrad Med J 1989;65:791–793.

294. Johnson PC, Rolak LA, Hamilton RH, Laguna JF. Paraneoplastic vasculitis of nerve: A remote effect of cancer. Ann Neurol 1979;5:437–445.

295. Fortin PR, Esdaile JM. Vasculitis and malignancy. In: Churg A, Churg J, eds. Systemic vasculitides. New York: Igaku-Shoin, 1991:327–341.

296. Komadina KH, Houch RW. Polyarteritis nodosa presenting as recurrent pneumonia following splenectomy for hairy-cell leukemia. Semin Arthritis Rheum 1989;18:252–257.

297. Krol T, Robinson J, Bekeris L, Messmore H. Hairy cell leukemia and a fatal periarteritis nodosa-like syndrome. Arch Pathol Lab Med 1983;107:583–585.

298. Westbrook CA, Golde DW. Autoimmune disease in hairy cell leukemia: Clinical syndromes and treatment. Br J Haematol 1985;61:346–356.

299. Vincent D, Dubas F, Hauw JJ, et al. Nerve and muscle microvasculitis in peripheral neuropathy: A remote effect of cancer? J Neurol Neurosurg Psychiatry 1986;49:1007–1010.

300. Forrest JAH, Shearman DJC. Pulmonary vasculitis and ulcerative colitis. Digest Dis 1975;20:482–486.

301. Isenberg JI, Goldstein H, Korn AR, Ozeran RS, Rosen V. Pulmonary vasculitis—an uncommon complication of ulcerative colitis. Report of a case. N Engl J Med 1968;279:1376–1377.

302. French AJ. Hypersensitivity in pathogenesis of histopathologic changes associated with sulfonamide chemotherapy. Am J Pathol 1946;22:679–701.

303. Misset B, Glotz D, Escudier B, et al. Wegener's granulomatosis presenting as diffuse pulmonary hemorrhage. Intensive Care Med 1991;17:118–120.

304. Young KR, Jr. Pulmonary-renal syndromes. Clin Chest Med 1989;10:655–675.

305. Sanchez-Masiques J, Ettensohn DB. Alveolar hemorrhage in Wegener's granulomatosis. Am J Med Sci 1989;297:390–393.

306. Cordier JF, Valeyre D, Guillevin L, Loire R, Brechot JM. Pulmonary Wegener's granulomatosis. A clinical and imaging study of 77 cases. Chest 1990;97:906–912.

307. Leatherman JW, Davies SF, Hoidal JR. Alveolar hemorrhage syndromes: Diffuse microvascular lung hemorrhage in immune and idiopathic disorders. Medicine (Baltimore) 1984;63:343–361.

308. Myers JL, Katzenstein AL. Wegener's granulomatosis presenting with massive pulmonary hemorrhage and capillaritis. Am J Surg Pathol 1987;11:895–898.

309. Wahls TL, Bonsib SM, Schuster VL. Coexistent Wegener's granulomatosis and anti-glomerular basement membrane disease. Hum Pathol 1987;18:202–205.

310. Soave R, Murray HW, Litrenta MM. Bacterial invasion of pulmonary vessels. *Pseudomonas* bacteremia mimicking pulmonary thromboembolism with infarction. Am J Med 1978;65:864–867.

311. Teplitz C. Pathogenesis of *Pseudomonas vasculitis* and septic lesions. Arch Pathol Lab Med 1965;80:297–307.

312. Winn WC, Myerowitz RL. The pathology of the *Legionella* pneumonias. A review of 74 cases and the literature. Hum Pathol 1981;12:401–422.

313. Redline RW, Dahms BB. Malassezia pulmonary vasculitis in an infant on long-term intralipid therapy. N Engl J Med 1981;305:1395–1398.

314. Travis WD, Roth DB. Histopathologic evaluation of lung biopsy specimens. In: Shelhamer J, Pizzo PA, Parrillo JE, Masur H, eds. Respiratory disease in the immunosuppressed host. Philadelphia: JB Lippincott, 1991:182–217.

315. Ro JY, Tsakalakis PJ, White VA, et al. Pulmonary dirofilariasis: The great imitator of primary or metastatic lung tumor. A clinicopathologic analysis of seven cases and a review of the literature. Hum Pathol 1989;20:69–76.

316. Jawahiry KL, Karpas CM. Pulmonary schistosomiasis: A detailed clinicopathologic study. Am Rev Respir Dis 1963;88:517–527.

317. Sadigursky M, Andrade ZA. Pulmonary changes in schistosomal cor pulmonale. Am J Trop Med Hyg 1982;31:779–784.

318. McCully RM, Barron CN, Cheever AW. Schistosomiasis. In: Binford CH, Connor DH, eds. Pathology of tropical and extraordinary diseases. Washington, DC: Armed Forces Institute of Pathology, 1976;402–508.

319. Beaver PC, Cran IR. *Wuchereria*-like filaria in an artery associated with pulmonary infarction. Am J Trop Med Hyg 1974;23:869–876.

320. Beaver PC, Fallon M, Smith GH. Pulmonary nodule caused by a living *Brugia-malayi*-like filaria in an artery. Am J Trop Med Hyg 1971;20:661–666.

321. Travis WD, Pittaluga S, Lipschik GY, et al. Atypical pathologic manifestations of *Pneumocystis carinii* pneumonia in the acquired immune deficiency syndrome. Review of 123 lung biopsies from 76 patients with emphasis on cysts, vascular invasion, vasculitis, and granulomas. Am J Surg Pathol 1990;14:615–625.

322. Liu YC, Tomashefski JF, Tomford JW, Green H. Necrotizing *Pneumocystis carinii* vasculitis associated with lung necrosis. Arch Pathol Lab Med 1989;113:494–497.

323. Davey RT, Jr., Margolis D, Kleiner D, Deyton L, Travis WD. Digital necrosis and disseminated *Pneumocystis carinii* infection after aerosolized pentamidine prophylaxis. Ann Intern Med 1989;111:681–682.

324. Bosken CH, Myers JL, Greenberger PA, Katzenstein AL. Pathologic features of allergic bronchopulmonary aspergillosis. Am J Surg Pathol 1988;12:216–222.

325. Jelihovsky T. The structure of bronchial plugs in mucoid impaction, bronchocentric granulomatosis and asthma. Histopathology 1983;7:153–167.

326. Saldana MJ. Bronchocentric granulomatosis: Clinico-

pathologic observations in 17 patients (Abstract). Lab Invest 1979;40:281–282.

327. Glancy JJ, Elder JL, McAleer R. Allergic bronchopulmonary fungal disease without clinical asthma. Thorax 1981;36:345–349.

328. Clee MD, Lamb D, Clark RA. Bronchocentric granulomatosis: A review and thoughts on pathogenesis. Br J Dis Chest 1983;77:227–234.

329. RobinsonRG, Wehunt WD, Tsou E, Koss MN, Hochholzer L. Bronchocentric granulomatosis: Roentgenographic manifestations. Am Rev Respir Dis 1982;125:751–756.

330. Yoshikawa Y, Truong LD, Watanabe T. Splendore–Hoeppli phenomenon in bronchocentric granulomatosis. Thorax 1988;43:157–158.

331. Warren J, Pitchenik AE, Saldana MJ. Bronchocentric granulomatosis with glomerulonephritis. Chest 1985;87:832–834.

332. Goldstein MH, Wright JL, Churg J. Vasculitis and hypertension. In: Churg A, Churg J, eds. Systemic vasculitides. New York: Igaku-Shoin, 1991:359–372.

333. Heath D, Edwards JE. The pathology of hypertensive pulmonary vascular disease. A description of six grades of structural changes in the pulmonary arteries with special reference to congenital cardiac septal defects. Circulation 1958;18:533–547.

334. World Health Organization. Primary pulmonary hypertension. In: Morphology of primary pulmonary hypertension. Geneva: World Health Organization, 1975:14–17.

335. Wagenvoort CA, Wagenvoort N. Primary pulmonary hypertension: A pathologic study of the lung vessels in 156 clinically diagnosed cases. Circulation 1970; 42:1163–1184.

336. Gurtner HP. Pulmonary hypertension, plexogenic pulmonary arteriopathy: and the appetite depressant drug aminorex: Post or propter? Bull Physiopathol Respir 1979;15:897–923.

337. Rigau-Peréz JGT, Pérez-Alvarez L, Dueñas-Castro S, et al. Epidemiologic investigation of an oil-associated pneumonic paralytic eosinophilic syndrome in Spain. Am J Epidemiol 1984;119:250–260.

338. Kilbourne EM, Rigau-Perez JH, Heath CW, et al. Clinical epidemiology of toxic oil syndrome. Manifestations of a new illness. N Engl J Med 1983;309:1408–1414.

339. O'Neill D, Ferrari R, Ceconi C, et al. Pulmonary peptides, norepinephrine and endocrine cells in monocrotaline pulmonary hypertension. Cardioscience 1991;2:27–33.

340. Heath D, Shaba J, Williams A, Smith P, Kombe A. A pulmonary hypertension-producing plant from Tanzania. Thorax 1975;30:399–404.

341. Heath D. Dietary pulmonary hypertension. Br Heart J 1971;33:616.

342. Kay JM, Smith P, Heath D. Aminorex and the pulmonary circulation. Thorax 1971;26:262–270.

343. Kay JM, Heath D, Smith P, Bras G, Summerell J.

344. Smith P, Kay JM, Heath D. Hypertensive pulmonary vascular disease in rats after prolonged feeding with *Crotalaria spectabilis* seeds. J Pathol 1970;102:97–106.

345. Wagenvoort CA, Wagenvoort N, Takahashi T. Pulmonary veno-occlusive disease: Involvement of pulmonary arteries and review of the literature. Hum Pathol 1985;16:1033–1041.

346. Travis WD, Borok Z, Rom J, et al. Pulmonary Langerhans' cell granulomatosis (PLCG): A clinicopathologic study of 48 cases (in manuscript).

347. Warter A, Satge D, Roeslin N. Angioinvasive plasma cell granulomas of the lung. Cancer 1987;59:435–443.

348. Koss MN, Hochholzer L, Nichols PW, Wehunt WD, Lazarus AA. Primary non-Hodgkin's lymphoma and pseudolymphoma of lung: a study of 161 patients. Hum Pathol 1983;14:1024–1038.

349. Heath D, Watts GT. The significance of vascular changes in an accessory lung presenting as a diaphragmatic cyst. Thorax 1957;12:142–147.

350. Mahadevia PS. Necrotizing vasculitis in an extralobar sequestered lung (Letter). Arch Pathol Lab Med 1980;104:115.

351. Ostrow PT, Salyer WR, White JJ, et al. Hypertensive pulmonary vascular disease in intralobar sequestration (Abstract). Am J Pathol 1973;70:33A–34A.

352. Yang YM, Wheeler VR, Mankad VN. Pulmonary lipid nodules after intralipid infusion in a child with rhabdomyosarcoma and *Staphylococcus* epidermidis sepsis. Am J Pediatr Hematol Oncol 1990;12:231–236.

353. Klotz SA, Huppert M, Drutz DJ. Pulmonary vasculitis on intralipid therapy (letter). N Engl J Med 1982;306:994–995.

354. Tomashefski JF, Jr., Hirsch CS. The pulmonary vascular lesions of intravenous drug abuse. Hum Pathol 1980;11:133–145.

355. Banner AS, Borochovitz D. Acute respiratory failure caused by pulmonary vasculitis after L-tryptophan ingestion. Am Rev Respir Dis 1991;143:661–664.

356. Tazelaar HD, Myers JL, Drage CW, King TE, Jr., Aguayo S, Colby TV. Pulmonary disease associated with L-tryptophan-induced eosinophilic myalgia syndrome. Clinical and pathologic features. Chest 1990;97:1032–1036.

357. Travis WD, Kalafer ME, Robin HS, Luibel FJ. Hypersensitivity pneumonitis and pulmonary vasculitis with eosinophilia in a patient taking an L-tryptophan preparation. Ann Intern Med 1990;112:301–303.

358. Swygert LA, Maes EF, Sewell LE, Miller L, Falk H, Kilbourne EM. Eosinophilia-myalgia syndrome. Results of national surveillance. JAMA 1990;264:1698–1703.

359. Belongia EA, Hedberg CW, Gleich GJ, et al. An investigation of the cause of the eosinophilia-myalgia syndrome associated with tryptophan use. N Engl J Med 1990;323:357–365.

360. Slutsker L, Hoesly FC, Miller L, Williams LP, Watson JC, Fleming DW. Eosinophilia-myalgia syndrome asso-

Fulvine and the pulmonary circulation. Thorax 1971;26:249–261.

ciated with exposure to tryptophan from a single manufacturer. JAMA 1990;264:213–217.

361. Sakimoto K. The cause of the eosinophilia-myalgia syndrome associated with tryptophan use (Letter). N Engl J Med 1990;323:992–993.

362. Varga J, Uitto J, Jimenez SA. The cause and pathogenesis of the eosinophilia-myalgia syndrome. Ann Intern Med 1992;116:140–147.

363. Toxic Epidemic Syndrome Study Group. Toxic epidemic syndrome, Spain, 1981. Lancet 1982;ii:697–702.

364. Demeter SL, Ahmad M, Tomashefski JF. Drug-induced pulmonary disease. Part I. Patterns of response. Clevel Clin Q 1979;46:89–99.

365. Muren C, Strandberg O. Cavitary pulmonary nodules in atypical collagen disease and lupoid drug reaction. Report of two cases. Acta Radiol 1989;30:281–284.

366. Yermakov VM, Hitti IF, Sutton AL. Necrotizing vasculitis associated with diphenylhydantoin: Two fatal cases. Hum Pathol 1983;13:182–184.

367. Jarzobski J, Ferry J, Wombolt D, Fitch DM, Egan JD. Vasculitis with allopurinol therapy. Am Heart J 1970;79:116–121.

368. Bailey RR, Neale TJ, Lynn KL. Allopurinol-associated arteritis (letter). Lancet 1976;ii:907.

369. Schrier RW, Bulger RJ, Van Arsdel PP. Nephropathy associated with penicillin and homologues. Arch Intern Med 1966;64:116–127.

370. Cassorla FG, Finegold DN, Parks JS, Tenore A, Thawerani H, Baker L. Vasculitis, pulmonary cavitation, and anemia during antithyroid drug therapy. Am J Dis Child 1983;137:118–122.

371. Houston BD, Crouch ME, Brick JE, DiBartolomeo AG. Apparent vasculitis associated with propylthiouracil use. Arthritis Rheum 1979;22:925–928.

372. Cooper JAD, White DA, Matthay RA. Drug-induced pulmonary disease. Part 2: Noncytotoxic drugs. Am Rev Respir Dis 1986;133:488–505.

372a. Taskinen E, Tukiainen P, Sovijärvi ARA: Nitrofurantoin-induced alterations in pulmonary tissue. Acta Path Microbiol Scand [A] 85:713–20, 1977.

373. Tazelaar HD, Yousem SA. The pathology of combined heart-lung transplantation: An autopsy study. Hum Pathol 1988;19:1403–1416.

374. Yousem SA, Burke CM, Billingham ME. Pathologic pulmonary alterations in long-term human heart-lung transplantation. Hum Pathol 1985;16:911–923.

375. Yousem SA, Paradis IL, Dauber JH, et al. Pulmonary arteriosclerosis in long-term human heart-lung transplant recipients. Transplantation 1989;47:564–569.

376. Seiden MV, O'Donnell WJ, Weinblatt M, Licht J. Vasculitis with recurrent pulmonary hemorrhage in a long-term survivor after autologous bone marrow transplantation. Bone Marrow Transplant 1990; 6:345–347.

377. Bennett DE, Million RR, Ackerman LV. Bilateral radiation pneumonitis, a complication of the radiotherapy of bronchogenic carcinoma (Report and analysis of seven cases with autopsy). Cancer 1969;23:1001–1018.

378. Eichel BS, Harrison EG, Devine KD, Scanlon PW, Brown HA. Primary lymphoma of the nose including a relationship to lethal midline granuloma. Am J Surg 1966;112:597–605.

379. Crissman JD, Weiss MA, Gluckman J. Midline granuloma syndrome: A clinicopathologic study of 13 patients. Am J Surg Pathol 1982;6:335–346.

380. Stamenkovic I, Toccanier MF, Kapanci Y. Polymorphic reticulosis (lethal midline granuloma) and lymphomatoid granulomatosis: Identical or distinct entities? Virchows Arch [A] 1981;390:81–91.

381. Crissman JD. Midline malignant reticulosis and lymphomatoid granulomatosis. A case report. Arch Pathol Lab Med 1979;103:561–564.

382. DeRemee RA, Weiland LH, McDonald TJ. Polymorphic reticulosis, lymphomatoid granulomatosis. Two diseases or one? Mayo Clin Proc 1978;53:634–640.

383. McDonald TJ, DeRemee RA, Harrison EG, Facer GW, Devine KD. The protean clinical features of polymorphic reticulosis (lethal midline granuloma). Laryngoscope 1976;86:936–945.

384. Nonomura A, Ohta G. Lymphomatoid granulomatosis-like lesions in malignant lymphoma. Acta Pathol Jpn 1986;36:1617–1626.

385. Colby TV, Carrington CB. Pulmonary lymphomas simulating lymphomatoid granulomatosis. Am J Surg Pathol 1982;6:19–32.

386. Ishii Y, Yamanaka N, Ogawa K, et al. Nasal T-cell lymphoma as a type of so-called "lethal midline granuloma." Cancer 1982;50:2336–2344.

387. Donner LR, Dobin S, Harrington D, Bassion S, Rappaport ES, Peterson RF. Angiocentric immunoproliferative lesion (lymphomatoid granulomatosis). A cytogenetic, immunophenotypic, and genotypic study. Cancer 1990;65:249–254.

388. Nichols PW, Koss MN, Levine AM, Lukes RJ. Lymphomatoid granulomatosis: A T-cell disorder? Am J Med 1982;72:467–471.

389. Petras RE, Tubbs RR, Gephardt GN, Sebek BA, Golish JA, Weick JK. T lymphocyte proliferation in lymphomatoid granulomatosis. Clevel Clin J Med 1985;52:137–146.

390. Jaffe ES, Travis WD. Lymphomatoid granulomatosis and lymphoproliferative disorders of the lung. In: Lynch JP, DeRemee RA, eds. Immunologically mediated pulmonary diseases. Philadelphia: JB Lippincott, 1991:274–301.

391. Medeiros LJ, Peiper SC, Elwood L, Yano T, Raffeld M, Jaffe ES. Angiocentric immunoproliferative lesions: A molecular analysis of eight cases. Hum Pathol 1991;22:1150–1157.

392. Whittaker S, Foroni L, Luzzatto L, et al. Lymphomatoid granulomatosis—evidence of a clonal T-cell origin and an association with lethal midline granuloma. Q J Med 1988;68:645–655.

393. Gracey DR. DeRemee RA, Colby TV, Unni KK, Weiland LH. Benign lymphocytic angiitis and granulomatosis: experience with three cases. Mayo Clin Proc 1988;63:323–331.

394. Lippman SM, Grogan TM, Spier CM, et al. Lethal

midline granuloma with a T-cell phenotype as found in peripheral T-cell lymphoma. Cancer 1987;59:936–939.

395. Chan JKC, Ng CS, Lau WH, Lo STH. Most nasal/nasopharyngeal lymphomas are peripheral T-cell neoplasms. Am J Surg Pathol 1987;11:418–429.

396. Chott A, Rappersberger K, Schlossarek W, Radaskiewicz T. Peripheral T cell lymphoma presenting primarily as lethal midline granuloma. Hum Pathol 1988;19:1093–1101.

397. Jaffe ES. Pulmonary lymphocytic angiitis: A nosologic quandary. Mayo Clin Proc 1988;63:411–413.

398. Lehman TJ, Church JA, Isaacs H. Lymphomatoid granulomatosis in a 13-month-old infant. J Rheumatol 1989;16:235–238.

399. Bëkassy AN, Cameron R, Garwicz S, Laurin S, Wiebe T. Lymphomatoid granulomatosis during treatment of acute lymphoblastic leukemia in a 6-year old girl. Am J Pediatr Hematol Oncol 1985;7:377–380.

400. Pearson AD, Kirpalani H, Ashcroft T, Bain H, Craft AW. Lymphomatoid granulomatosis in a 10 year old boy. Br Med J 1983;286:1313–1314.

401. Patton WF, Lynch JP. Lymphomatoid granulomatosis. Clinicopathologic study of four cases and literature review. Medicine (Baltimore) 1982;61:1–12.

402. Prabhu R, Berger HW, Subietas A, Lee M. Lymphomatoid granulomatosis. Report of a patient with severe anemia and clubbing. Chest 1980;78:883–885.

403. Lalloo UG, Cooper K, Irusen EM, le Roux BT, Jogessar VB. Lymphomatoid granulomatosis. A report of 4 cases. S Afr Med J 1991;79:274–278.

404. Ralston SH, McVicar R, Finlay AY, Morton R, Pitkeathly DA. Lymphomatoid granulomatosis presenting with polyarthritis. Scott Med J 1988;33:373–374.

405. Bergin C, Stein HB, Boyko W, Hogg J, Schlappner O. Lymphomatoid granulomatosis presenting as polyarthritis. J Rheumatol 1984;11:537–539.

406. Glickstein M, Kornstein MJ, Pietra GG, et al. Nonlymphomatous lymphoid disorders of the lung. AJR 1986;147:227–237.

407. Hicken P, Dobie JC, Frew E. The radiology of lymphomatoid granulomatosis in the lung. Clin Radiol 1979;30:661–664.

408. Israel HL, Patchefsky AS, Saldana MJ. Wegener's granulomatosis, lymphomatoid granulomatosis, and benign lymphocyic angiitis and granulomatosis of lung: recognition and treatment. Ann Intern Med 1977;87:691–699.

409. Prénovault JM, Weisbrod GL, Herman SJ. Lymphomatoid granulomatosis: A review of 12 cases. Can Assoc Radiol J 1988;39:263–266.

410. Wechsler RJ, Steiner RM, Israel HL, Patchefsky AS. Chest radiograph in lymphomatoid granulomatosis: comparison with Wegener granulomatosis. AJR 1984;142:79–83.

411. Pisani RJ, DeRemee RA. Clinical implications of the histopathologic diagnosis of pulmonary lymphomatoid granulomatosis. Mayo Clin Proc 1990;65:151–163.

412. Da Silva AM, Weiner J, Dean P, Kerwin DM. Lym-

phomatoid granulomatosis beginning as adult respiratory distress syndrome and rapidly progressing to lymphoma. South Med J 1983;76:805–808.

413. James WD, Odom RB, Katzenstein AL. Cutaneous manifestations of lymphomatoid granulomatosis. Report of 44 cases and a review of the literature. Arch Dermatol 1981;117:196–202.

414. Akagi M, Taniguchi S, Ozaki M, et al. Necrobiosis-lipoidica-like skin manifestation in lymphomatoid granulomatosis (Liewbow). Dermatologica 1987;174:84–92.

414a. Carlson KC, Gibson LE. Cutaneous signs of lymphomatoid granulomatosis. Arch Dermatol 1991;127:1693–1698.

415. Hogan PJ, Greenberg MK, McCarty GE. Neurologic complications of lymphomatoid granulomatosis. Neurology 1981;31:619–620.

416. Collins S, Helme RD. Lymphomatoid granulomatosis presenting as a progressive cervical cord lesion. Aust N Z J Med 1989;19:144–146.

417. Anders KH, Latta H, Chang BS, Tomiyasu U, Quddusi AS, Vinters HV. Lymphomatoid granulomatosis and malignant lymphoma of the central nervous system in the acquired immunodeficiency syndrome. Hum Pathol 1989;20:326–334.

418. Herderscheë D, Troost D, de Visser M, Neve AJ. Lymphomatoid granulomatosis: clinical and histopathological report of a patient presenting with spinal cord involvement. J Neurol 1988;235:432–434.

419. Oliveras C, D'Olhaberriague L, Garcia J, Matias-Guiu X. Parkinsonism as first manifestation of lymphomatoid granulomatosis (letter). J Neurol Neurosurg Psychiatry 1988;51:999–1001.

420. McKay D, Ell J, Williams R, Taylor F. Lymphomatoid granulomatosis presenting as sudden blindness. Aust N Z J Ophthalmol 1990;18:215–219.

420a. Kleinschmidt-DeMasters BK, Filley CM, Bitter MA. Central nervous system angiocentric, angiodestructive T-cell lymphoma (lymphomatoid granulomatosis). Surg Neurol 1992;37:130–137.

421. Sunderrajan EV, Passamonte PM. Lymphomtoid granulomatosis presenting as central neurogenic hyperventilation. Chest 1984;86:634–636.

422. Klein FA, Koontz WW, Jr., Schneider V. Lymphomatoid granulomatosis masquerading as hypernephroma with lung metastases. J Urol 1984;131:942–944.

423. Feinberg SM, Leslie KO, Colby TV. Bladder outlet obstruction by so-called lymphomatoid granulomatosis (angiocentric lymphoma). J Urol 1987;137:989–990.

423a. Feddersen RM, Smith AY. Ureteral obstruction and hydronephrosis as a complication of lymphomatoid granulomatosis: a case report and literature review. J Urol 1992;147:118–119.

424. Schmalzl F, Gasser RW, Weiser G, Zur Nedden D. Lymphomatoid granulomatosis with primary manifestation in the skeletal muscular system. Klin Wochenschr 1982;60:311–316.

425. Gardiner GW. Lymphomatoid granulomatosis of the

larynx in a renal transplant recipient. J Otolaryngol 1979;8:549–555.

426. Lin-Greenberg A, Villacin A, Moussa G. Lymphomatoid granulomatosis presenting as ulcerodestructive gastrointestinal tract lesions in patients with human immunodeficiency virus infection. A new association. Arch Intern Med 1990;150:2581–2583.

427. Robin JB, Schanzlin DJ, Meisler DM, deLuise VP, Clough JD. Ocular involvement in the respiratory vasculitides. Surv Ophthalmol 1985;30:127–140.

428. Tse DT, Mandelbaum S, Chuck DA, Nichols PW, Smith RE. Lymphomatoid granulomatosis with ocular involvement. Retina 1985;5:94–97.

429. Chung YM, Yeh TS, Tsai YY, Chiang H, Liu JH. Conjunctival involvement of lymphomatoid granulomatosis. Ophthalmologica 1988;196:161–166.

430. Rubin LA, Little AH, Kolin A, Keystone EC. Lymphomatoid granulomatosis involving the gastrointestinal tract. Two case reports and a review of the literature. Gstroenterology 1983;84:829–833.

431. Rattinger MD, Dunn TL, Christian CD, Jr., et al. Gastrointestinal involvement in lymphomatoid granulomatosis. Report of a case review of the literature. Cancer 1983;51:694–700.

432. Naschitz JE, Yeshurun D, Grishkan A, Boss JH. Lymphomatoid granulomatosis of the lung in a patient with agnogenic myeloid metaplasia. Report of a case. Respiration 1984;45:316–320.

433. Hammar SP, Gortner D, Sumida S, Bockus D. Lymphomatoid granulomatosis: Association with retroperitoneal fibrosis and evidence of impaired cell-mediated immunity. Am Rev Respir Dis 1977;115:1045–1050.

434. Walter M, Thomson NM, Dowling J, Fox R, Atkins RC. Lymphomatoid granulomatosis in a renal transplant recipient. Aust N Z J Med 1979;9:434–436.

435. Hammar S, Mennemeyer R. Lymphomatoid granulomatosis in a renal transplant recipient. Hum Pathol 1976;7:111–116.

436. Capron F, Audouin J, Diebold J, Ameille J, Lebeau B, Rochemaure J. Pulmonary polymorphic centroblastic type malignant lymphoma in a patient with lymphomatoid granulomatosis. Sjögren syndrome and other manifestations of a dysimmune state. Pathol Res Pract 1985;179:656–665.

437. Weisbrot IM. Lymphomatoid granulomatosis of the lung, associated with a long history of benign lymphoepithelial lesions of the salivary glands and lymphoid interstitial pneumonitis. Report of a case. Am J Clin Pathol 1976;66:792–801.

438. Cohen ML, Dawkins RL, Henderson DW, Sterrett GF, Papadimitriou JM. Pulmonary lymphomatoid granulomatosis with immunodeficiency terminating as malignant lymphoma. Pathology 1979;11:537–550.

439. Ilowite NT, Fligner CL, Ochs HD, et al. Pulmonary angiitis with atypical lymphoreticular infiltrates in Wiskott–Aldrich syndrome: Possible relationship of lymphomatoid granulomatosis and EBV infection. Clin Immunol Immunopathol 1986;41:479–484.

440. Mittal K, Neri A, Feiner H, Schinella R, Alfonso F. Lymphomatoid granulomatosis in the acquired immunodeficiency syndrome. Evidence of Epstein–Barr virus infection and B-cell clonal selection without *myc* rearrangement. Cancer 1990;65:1345–1349.

441. Sordillo PP, Epremian B, Koziner B, Lacher M, Lieberman P. Lymphomatoid granulomatosis: An analysis of clinical and immunologic characteristics. Cancer 1982;49:2070–2076.

442. Firstater E, Yust I, Topilsky M, Tartakowsky B, Segal S, Abramov A. Lymphomatoid granulomatosis with impaired cellular immunity. Eight year survival without treatment. Chest 1983;84:777–779.

443. Scheinman SJ, Kelberman MW, Tatum AH, Zamkoff KW. Hypercalcemia with excess serum 1,25-dihydroxyvitamin D in lymphomatoid granulomatosis/angiocentric lymphoma. Am J Med Sci 1991;301:178–181.

444. Leedman PJ, Matz LR, Pullan P. Endocrine dysfunction in lymphomatoid granulomatosis. Aust N Z J Med 1989;19:97–102.

445. Saldana MJ, Patchefsky AS, Israel HI, Atkinson GW. Pulmonary angiitis and granulomatosis. The relationship between histological features, organ involvement, and response to treatment. Hum Pathol 1977;8:391–409.

446. Weiss MA, Rolfes DB, Alvira MA, Cohen LJ. Benign lymphocytic angiitis and granulomatosis: A case report with evidence of an autoimmune etiology. Am J Clin Pathol 1984;81:110–116.

447. Ioachim HL. Lymphomatoid granulomatosis versus lymphoma of the brain and central nervous system in the acquired immunodeficiency syndrome (Letter). Hum Pathol 1989;20:1222–1224.

448. Lee SC, Roth LM, Brashear RE. Lymphomatoid granulomatosis: A clinicopathologic study of four cases. Cancer 1976;38:846–853.

449. Cohen Tervaert JW, Goldschmeding R, Elema JD, et al. Association of autoantibodies to myeloperoxidase with different forms of vasculitis. Arthritis Rheum 1990;33:1264–1272.

450. Jambrosic J, From L, Assaad DA, Lipa M, Sibbald RG, Walter JB. Lymphomatoid granulomatosis. J Am Acad Dermatol 1987;17:621–631.

451. Kessler S, Lund HZ, Leonard DD. Cutaneous lesions of lymphomatoid granulomatosis. Comparison with lymphomatoid papulosis. Am J Dermatopathol 1981;3:115–127.

452. Foley JF, Linder J, Koh J, Severson G, Purtilo DT. Cutaneous necrotizing granulomatous vasculitis with evolution to T cell lymphoma. Am J Med 1987;82:839–844.

453. Jensen JK, Lund C, Schlichting J. Lymphomatoid granulomatosis presenting primarily in a parotid gland. J Laryngol Otol 1982;96:961–964.

454. Letendre L. Treatment of lymphomatoid granulomatosis: Old and new perspectives. Semin Respir Med 1989;10:178–181.

455. Atkinson CH, Davis AL, Colls BM, Wolever THS, Burry AF, Hart DNJ. Sequential half-body irradiation

in lymphomatoid granulomatosis. Report of a case and an immunohistologic study. Cancer 1989;63:652–656.

456. Bernstein ML, Reece ER, de Chadarëvian JP, Koch PA. Bone marrow transplantation in lymphomatoid granulomatosis. Report of a case. Cancer 1986;58:969–972.

457. Halperin EC, Dosoretz DE, Goodman M, Wang CC. Radiotherapy of polymorphic reticulosis. Br J Radiol 1982;55:645–649.

458. Gaulard P, Henni T, Marolleau JP, et al. Lethal midline granuloma (polymorphic reticulosis) and lymphomatoid granulomatosis. Evidence for a monoclonal T-cell lymphoproliferative disorder. Cancer 1988;62:705–710.

459. Minase T, Ogasawara M, Kikuchi T, et al. Lymphomatoid granulomatosis. Light microscopic, electron microscopic and immunohistochemical study. Acta Pathol Jpn 1985;35:711–721.

460. Weis JW, Winter MW, Phyliky RL, Banks PM. Peripheral T-cell lymphomas: histologic, immunohistologic, and clinical characterization. Mayo Clin Proc 1986;61:411–426.

461. Troussard X, Galateau F, Gaulard P, et al. Lymphomatoid granulomatosis in a patient with acute myeloblastic leukemia in remission. Cancer 1990;65:107–111.

462. Bender BL, Jaffe R. Immunoglobulin production in lymphomatoid granulomatosis and relation to other benign: lymphoproliferative disorders. Am J Clin Pathol 1980;73:41–47.

463. Kapanci Y, Toccanier MF. Lymphomatoid granulomatosis of the lung. An immunohistochemical study. Appl Pathol 1983;1:97–114.

464. Weisenburger DD, Linder J, Armitage JO. Peripheral T-cell lymphoma: A clinicopathologic study of 42 cases. Hematol Oncol 1987;5:175–187.

465. Bleiweiss IJ, Strauchen JA. Lymphomatoid granulomatosis of the lung: Report of a case and gene rearrangement studies. Hum Pathol 1988;19:1109–1112.

456. Katzenstein AL, Peiper SC. Detection of Epstein–Barr virus genomes in lymphomatoid granulomatosis: Analysis of 29 cases by the polymerase chain reaction technique. Mod Pathol 1990;3:435–441.

467. Veltri RW, Raich PC, McClung JE, Shah SH, Sprinkle PM. Lymphomatoid granulomatosis and Epstein–Barr virus. Cancer 1982;50:1513–1517.

468. Medeiros LJ, Jaffe ES, Chen Y-Y, Weiss LM. Localization of Epstein–Barr viral genomes in angiocentric immunoproliferative lesions. Mod Pathol 1992;5:83A (Abstract).

469. Li G, Hansmann ML, Zwingers T, Lennert K. Primary lymphomas of the lung: Morphological, immunohistochemical and clinical features. Histopathology (Oxf) 1990;16:519–531.

470. Addis BJ, Hyjek E, Isaacson PG. Primary pulmonary lymphoma: a re-appraisal of its histogenesis and its relationship to pseudolymphoma and lymphoid interstitial pneumonia. Histopathology (Oxf) 1988;13:1–17.

471. Herbert A, Wright DH, Isaacson PG, Smith JL. Primary malignant lymphoma of the lung: histopatho-

logic and immunologic evaluation of nine cases. Hum Pathol 1984;15:415–422.

472. L'Hoste RJ, Jr., Filippa DA, Lieberman PH, Bretsky S. Primary pulmonary lymphomas. A clinicopathologic analysis of 36 cases. Cancer 1984;54:1397–1406.

473. Harrison NK, Twelves C, Addis BJ, Taylor AJ, Souhami RL, Isaacson PG. Peripheral T-cell lymphoma presenting with angioedema and diffuse pulmonary infiltrates. Am Rev Respir Dis 1988;138:976–980.

474. Domizio P, Hall PA, Cotter F, et al. Angiotropic large cell lymphoma (ALCL): Morphological, immunohistohemical and genotypic studies with analysis of previous reports. Hematol Oncol 1989;7:195–206.

475. Bhawan J. Angioendotheliomatosis proliferans systemisata: An angiotropic neoplasm of lymphoid origin. Semin Diagn Pathol 1987;4:18–27.

476. Bhawan J, Wolff SM, Ucci AA, Bhan AK. Malignant lymphoma and maligant angioendotheliomatosis: one disease. Cancer 1985;55:570–576.

477. Ansell J, Bhawan J, Cohen S, Sullivan J, Sherman D. Histiocytic lymphoma and malignant angioendotheliomatosis: One disease or two? Cancer 1982;50:1506–1512.

478. Wick MR, Mills SE, Scheithauer BW, Cooper PH, Davitz MA, Parkinson K. Reassessment of malignant angioendotheliomatosis: Evidence in favor of its reclassification as intravascular lymphomatosis. Am J Surg Pathol 1986;10:112–123.

479. Wick MR, Mills SE. Intravascular lymphomatosis: Clinicopathologic features and differential diagnosis. Semin Diagn Pathol 1991;8:91–101.

480. Snyder LS, Harmon KR, Estensen RD. Intravascular lymphomatosis (malignant angioendotheliomatosis) presenting as pulmonary hypertension. Chest 1989;96:1199–1200.

481. Kamesaki H, Matsui Y, Ohno Y, et al. Angiocentric lymphoma with histologic features of neoplastic angioendotheliomatosis presenting with predominant respiratory and hematologic manifestations. Report of a case and review of the literature. Am J Clin Pathol 1990;94:768–772.

482. Yousem SA, Colby TV. Intravascular lymphomatosis presenting in the lung. Cancer 1990;65:349–353.

483. Tan TB, Spaander PJ, Blaisse M, Gerritzen FM. Angiotropic large cell lymphoma presenting as interstitial lung disease. Thorax 1988;43:578–579.

484. Curtis JL, Warnock ML, Conrad DJ, Helfend LK, Boushey HA. Intravascular (angiotropic) large-cell lymphoma ('malignant angioendotheliomatosis') with small vessel pulmonary vascular obstruction and hypercalcemia. West J Med 1991;155:72–76.

485. Elner VM, Hidayat AA, Charles NC, et al. Neoplastic angioendotheliomatosis: A variant of malignant lymphoma. Immunohistochemical and ultrastructural observations of three cases. Ophthalmology 1986; 93:1237–1245.

486. Molina A, Lombard CM, Donlon T, Bangs CD, Dorfman RF. Immunohistochemical and cytogentic studies indicate that malignant angioendotheliomatosis is a

primary intravascular (angiotropic) lymphoma. Cancer 1990;66:474–479.

487. Stroup RM, Sheibani K, Moncada A, Purdy LJ, Battifora H. Angiotropic (intravascular large cell lymphoma. A clinicopathologic study of seven cases with unique clinical presentations. Cancer 1990;66:1781–1788.

488. Ostrakji CL, Voigt W, Amador A, Nadji M, Gregorios JB. Malignant angioendotheliomatosis—a true lymphoma: A case of intravascular malignant lymphomatosis studied by southern blot hybridization analysis. Hum Pathol 1988;19:475–478.

489. Nada AK, Torres VE, Ryu JH, Lie JT, Holley KE. Pulmonary fibrosis as an unusual clinical manifestation of a pulmonary-renal vasculitis in elderly patients. Mayo Clin Proc 1990;65:847–856.

490. Churg A, Franklin W, Chan KL, Kopp E, Carrington CB. Pulmonary hemorrhage and immune-complex deposition in the lung. Complications in a patient with systemic lupus erythematosus. Arch Pathol Lab Med 1980;104:388–391.

491. Eagen JW, Memoli VA, Roberts JL, Matthew GR, Schwartz MM, Lewis EJ. Pulmonary hemorrhage in systemic lupus erythematosus. Medicine (Baltimore) 1978;57:545–560.

492. Marino CT, Pertschuk LP. Pulmonary hemorrhage in systemic lupus erythematosus. Arch Intern Med 1981;141:201–203.

493. Myers JL, Katzenstein AL. Microangiitis in lupus-induced pulmonary hemorrhage. Am J Clin Pathol 1986;85:552–556.

494. Mintz G, Galindo LF, Fernandez-Diez J, Jimënez FJ, Robles-Saavedra E, Enriquez-Casillas RD. Acute massive pulmonary hemorrhage in systemic lupus erythematosus. J Rheumatol 1978;5:39–50.

495. Martinez JS, Kohler PF. Variant "Goodpasture's syndrome"? Ann Intern Med 1971;75:67–76.

496. Jayne DRW, Jones SJ, Lockwood CM. Severe pulmonary hemorrhage and systemic vasculitis in association with isolated circulating IgM antineutrophil antibody (Abstract). Kidney Int 1988;33:3–28.

497. Imoto EM, Lombard CM, Sachs DPL. Pulmonary capillaritis and hemorrhage. A clue to the diagnosis of systemic necrotizing vasculitis. Chest 1989;96:927–928.

498. Bocanegra TS, Espinoza LR, Vasey F, Germain BF. Pulmonary hemorrhage in systemic necrotizing vasculitis associated with hepatitis B. Chest 1981;81:102–103.

499. Maguire GP, Lee M, Rosen Y, Lyons HA. Pulmonary tuberculosis and bronchocentric granulomatosis. Chest 1986;89:606–608.

500. Tazelaar HD, Baird AM, Mill M, Grimes MM, Schulman LL, Smith CR. Bronchocentric mycosis occurring in transplant recipients. Chest 1989;96:92–95.

501. Tron V, Churg A. Chronic necrotizing pulmonary aspergillosis mimicking bronchocentric granulomatosis. Pathol Res Pract 1986;181:621–626.

502. Dikman SH. Asbestosis, endobronchial *Aspergillus* infection, and bronchocentric granulomatosis presenting with hemoptysis. Lung 1991;169:25–30.

503. Den Hertog RW, Wagenaar SS, Wastermann CJ. Bronchocentric granulomatosis and pulmonary echinococcosis. Am Rev Respir Dis 1982;126:344–347.

504. Bonafede RP, Benatar SR. Bronchocentric granulomatosis and rheumatoid arthritis. Br J Dis Chest 1987;81:197–201.

505. Hellems SO, Kanner RE, Renzetti AD, Jr. Bronchocentric granulomatosis associated with rheumatoid arthritis. Chest 1983;83:831–832.

506. Rohatgi PK, Turrisi BC. Bronchocentric granulomatosis and ankylosing spondylitis. Thorax 1984;93:317–318.

507. Myers JL, Katzenstein AL. Granulomatous infection mimicking bronchocentric granulomatosis. Am J Surg Pathol 1986;10:317–322.

CHAPTER 31

Lymphoproliferative Diseases

THOMAS V. COLBY

Lymphoreticular diseases affecting the lung include primary and secondary lymphomas and related disorders, leukemias, and a number of lesions that are generally considered benign and hyperplastic processes. Pseudolymphoma, lymphocytic interstitial pneumonia, small (well-differentiated) lymphocytic lymphomas, and lymphomatoid granulomatosis have long been difficult lesions for pathologists.[1-5] Lymphomatoid granulomatosis, with its synonyms,[6-8] has been considered by some to be a peculiar vasculitis and by others a lymphoproliferative disorder, with the latter being the prevailing view.[8]

Classically, lymphomas comprise a monomorphous population of atypical lymphoid cells manifesting as clinically aggressive neoplasms. An immunologic definition of a lymphoma has recently been accepted: a clonal proliferation of lymphoid cells that in many cases can be identified with immunologic marker studies and subclassified as T or B lymphocytic or true histiocytic in origin.[9] The clinical and histologic spectrum of lymphomas has broadened considerably to include lesions that pursue a very indolent clinical course and those with a polymorphous cellular composition.

Normal Lymphoid Tissue and Lymphatic Routes of the Lung

Understanding the histology of lymphoreticular infiltrates in the lungs requires knowledge of the normal lymphatic routes and lymphoid tissue of the lung. The lymphatic routes are found along the bronchovascular bundles, the pulmonary veins, and in the septa and pleura.[10,11] The lymphatics themselves are barely discernible in normal lungs but are easily recognized in pathologic states such as pulmonary edema and passive congestion. Lesions that tend to show a distribution along the lymphatic routes include lymphoreticular infiltrates, lymphangitic carcinoma, sarcoidosis, and some pneumoconioses, the last reflecting lymphatic drainage of the inhaled dust.

Hilar and peribronchial lymph nodes are present in all individuals, but intrapulmonary lymph nodes are uncommon. *Intrapulmonary lymph nodes* are usually incidental findings in lobectomy specimens or at autopsy. In one study of 10 clinically recognized cases, all were adult, all were smokers, and 80% were men.[12] Intrapulmonary lymph nodes are usually below the level of the carina, well circumscribed, and less than 2 cm in diameter, and are located close to the pleura or a septum; they may be multiple, are usually anthracotic, and may contain or coexist with silicotic nodules.[12]

Bienenstock and others[13-16] have drawn attention to a relatively extensive system of pulmonary lymphoid tissue termed bronchus-associated lymphoid tissue (BALT). BALT represents lymphoid aggregates found along airways, particularly at bifurcations, as well as those along other lymphatic routes of the lung, and is thought to be part of a more generalized mucosa-associated lymphoid tissue (MALT) that is distinguished from the peripheral somatic (nodal) lymphoid tissue.[15,16] MALT synthesizes IgA and other immunoglobulins in response to mucosal surface antigens, and lymphocytes in this system have the ability to circulate and "home" to other MALT organs. The lymphoid tissue of MALT is intimately associated with the adjacent epithelium (Fig. 31–1), and lymphomas of MALT show a tendency to invade adjacent epithelium.[17-19] Lymphomas of MALT in general are indolent, low

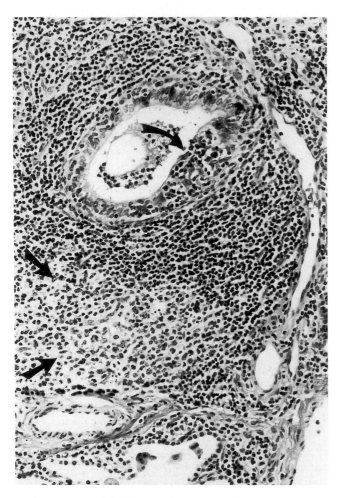

Fig. 31–1. Bronchus-associated lymphoid tissue (BALT) adjacent to bronchiole. There is a somewhat pale staining germinal center (*arrows*) with a cuff of small lymphocytes which show prominent infiltration of the epithelium of the adjacent bronchiole (*curved arrows*). H and E, ×100.

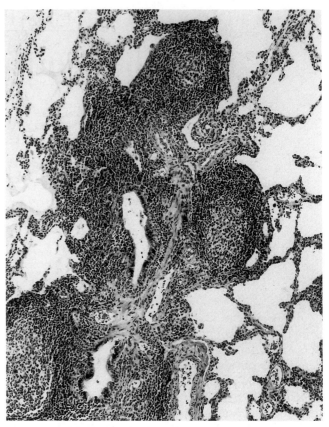

Fig. 31–2. Follicular bronchiolitis with germinal centers along a small airway from a child with an uncharacterized immunodeficiency state. H and E, ×40.

grade, and tend to remain localized for long periods of time.[14–18,20–22] In addition to the lung, other organs in the MALT system include salivary gland, intestinal tract, thyroid, cervix, endometrium, and breast.*

The radiologic manifestations of lymphoreticular infiltrates include a broad and nonspecific spectrum of changes.[24–26] The radiographic patterns of disease can often be correlated with the histologic findings: lesions that are characterized histologically by diffuse infiltrates along lymphatic routes without extensive nodular expansions produce a diffuse interstitial pattern radiographically, whereas mixed interstitial and nodular or frankly nodular patterns are associated with progressively larger nodules along the lymphatic distribution.

Massive infiltration with spillover into air spaces produces a pneumonic or alveolar pattern. Combinations of these patterns are common.[24–26]

Lymphoid Hyperplasias, Benign Lymphoid Infiltrates, and Related Lesions

Hyperplasia of lymphoid tissue in the lung is similar to lymphoid hyperplasia of other sites, with the production of germinal centers distributed along the normal locations of lymphatic tissue, specifically the pulmonary lymphatic routes. Exuberant lymphoid hyperplasia along the airways is termed follicular bronchitis or follicular bronchiolitis (Fig. 31–2), depending on the size of airway involved.[27] Lymphoid hyperplasia may also involve the septa and pleura.

In healthy children one may see a few lymphocytes and a rare germinal center in the lung, but in normal adults one generally does not see any significant quantity of lymphoid tissue in histologic sections[16]; when

---

*References: 13–15,17,18,20–23.

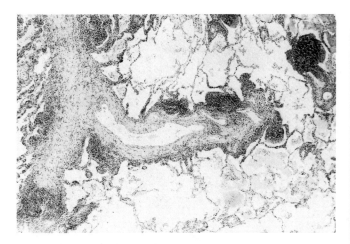

Fig. 31–3. Lymphoid hyperplasia adjacent to active tuberculosis. Septal and perivascular lymphoid follicles represent lymphoid reaction to nearby tuberculous granulomas. H and E, ×25.

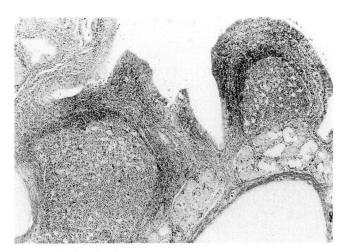

Fig. 31–4. Submucosal lymphoid hyperplasia (follicular bronchitis) in bronchiectasis. H and E, ×40.

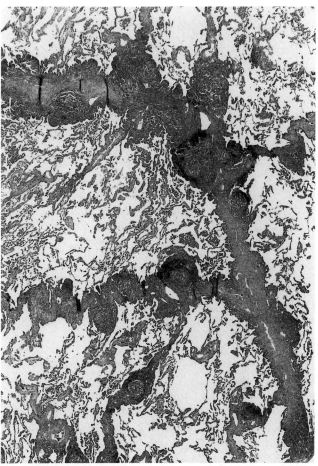

Fig. 31–5. Lymphoid hyperplasia in rheumatoid lung disease with germinal centers following septa and bronchovascular structures. The adjacent parenchyma has minor changes, and this patient's radiographic infiltrates were due to lymphoid hyperplasia. Such a lesion has also been referred to as lymphocytic interstitial pneumonia. H and E, ×10.

lymphoid tissue is prominent, a pathologic condition is usually present. Hyperplasia of lymphoid tissue in the lung is most commonly a manifestation of chronic infections, chronic bronchitis, bronchiectasis, or cystic fibrosis, or is a reaction around chronic inflammatory processess such as granulomatous infections or abscesses[28] (Figs. 31–3 and 31–4). Primary and secondary tumors can also have an associated lymphoid reaction including germinal centers, sheets of plasma cells, or granulomas, especially in foci of obstructive pneumonia. Metastases from the lymphoepithelial variant of nasopharyngeal carcinoma and primary lymphoepithelioma-like carcinomas of the lung represent particularly florid examples.

Diffuse lymphoid hyperplasia (Fig. 31–5) producing bi-lateral pulmonary infiltrates on chest radiographs may sometimes be the only histologic finding, particularly in collagen vascular diseases (e.g., rheumatoid arthritis, Sjögren's syndrome), congenital and acquired immunodeficiency states, and systemic hypersensitivity reactions,[27,29,30] and there is histologic overlap with lymphocytic interstitial pneumonia (see following). In collagen vascular diseases the proliferation in the lung is probably analogous to the exuberant lymphoid hyperplasia seen in lymph nodes of some of these patients.[31] The lymphoid hyperplasia may at times be most prominent along airways (follicular bronchitis/bronchiolitis) and may be associated with clinical evidence of interstitial *or* airflow obstructive disease.[27]

When first described, *angioimmunoblastic lymphadenop-*

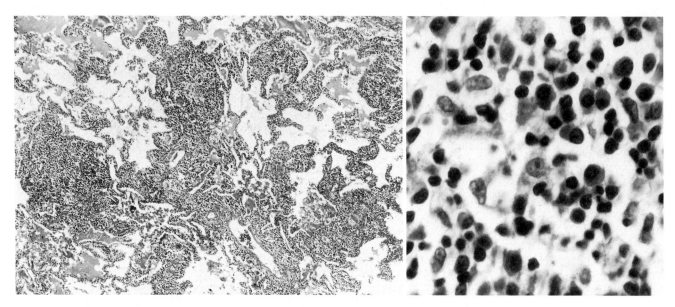

Fig. 31–6. Lymphocytic interstitial pneumonia. Note the dense diffuse polymorphous interstitial infiltrate with lymphocytes, plasma cells, and histiocytes. H and E: Left, ×40; right, ×630.

athy was thought to represent a peculiar autoimmune reaction,[32] but a significant number of cases are now recognized as T-cell lymphomas.[33] Pulmonary involvement may be a conspicuous feature of the syndrome,[32,34–36] which usually includes generalized lymphadenopathy, hepatosplenomegaly, Coombs-positive hemolytic anemia, skin rash, polyclonal hypergammaglobulinemia, and anemia.[32] Histologically, a polymorphous proliferation of immunoblasts, plasma cells, and occasionally histiocytes are found along the lymphatic routes of the lung.

Lymphocytic (lymphoid) interstitial pneumonia (LIP) is a chronic interstitial pneumonia characterized by a dense and diffuse interstitial infiltrate of cells that are histologically benign, polymorphous, and polyclonal.* These histologically diffuse interstitial lymphoid infiltrates can be distinguished from diffuse lymphoid hyperplasia, which is primarily related to the lymphatic routes, although in the literature both patterns have often been called lymphocytic interstitial pneumonia. Also, unlike lymphomas, LIP is usually more diffuse in its involvement of alveolar walls. Lymphoid follicles with or without germinal centers distributed along the lymphatic routes may be found, and when they are the dominant feature (Fig. 31–5), the term diffuse lymphoid hyperplasia is appropriately descriptive.[30]

The majority of patients are adults and have symptoms similar to other chronic interstitial pneumonias including cough, dyspnea, weight loss, and progressive shortness of breath.[1,37,38] Children may also be affected.[39] Chest radiographs show bibasilar infiltrates. Pulmonary functions reflect infiltrative lung disease with restriction and abnormal gas exchange. Dysproteinemias are a common laboratory finding, and either hyper- or hypogammaglobulinemia may be identified. A number of patients with LIP have associated conditions including collagen vascular diseases, autoimmune diseases, bone marrow transplantation, intestinal lymphoid hyperplasia, and immunodeficiency states including congenital and acquired immunodeficiency syndromes.[37–46] These associated conditions should be excluded before considering a diagnosis of idiopathic LIP.

The histology of LIP is characterized by a marked interstitial infiltrate of lymphocytes, plasma cells, and histiocytes (Fig. 31–6). Some cases have giant cells, granulomas, or reactive lymphoid follicles (Figs. 31–7 and 31–8. Interstitial fibrosis and honeycombing may be present. In contrast to lymphomas, LIP lacks large monomorphous foci of small lymphocytes or plasmacytoid lymphocytes and fails to show an overwhelming lymphatic distribution. A number of cases previously reported as LIP represented examples of diffuse bilateral small (well-differentiated) lymphocytic lymphomas presenting in the lung.[19,47,48] Immunophenotypic studies of LIP fail to show a clonal population of lymphoid cells.[38] T or B lymphocytes may predominate.[38,46]

The differential diagnosis of LIP includes nonspecific reactive changes; extrinsic allergic alveolitis, and small lymphocytic and lymphoplasmacytic lymphomas. In immunosuppressed patients, pneumocytis should be

*References: 1,4,30,37,38.

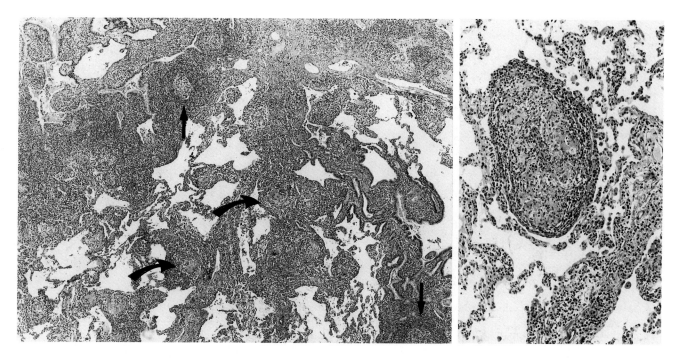

Fig. 31–7. Lymphocytic interstitial pneumonia from case of Sjögren's syndrome. Note dense diffuse lymphoid infiltrate with germinal centers (*straight arrows*) and granulomas (*curved arrows, and right*). H and E: left, ×25; right, ×100.

excluded. The treatment of lymphocytic interstitial pneumonia is not resolved, but a number of patients, even those with immunodeficiency states, respond to steroids.[37,49]

A *pseudolymphoma* represents a localized lymphoid proliferation in the lung that usually presents as a single nodule confined to one lobe.[30,47,50] Many of the lesions that had been called pulmonary pseudolymphoma (nodular lymphoid hyperplasia[30]) have been reinterpreted as small lymphocytic lymphomas[19,47–55] and the category of pseudolymphoma has shrunk considerably in size. Of all cases with massive accumulations of lymphocytes in the lung, roughly four of five (80%) were previously interpreted as pseudolymphomas,[56] whereas roughtly four of five (80%) are now interpreted as small lymphocytic lymphomas.[50]

Most patients are adults, and a few have a history of a prior pneumonia at the site. The majority of patients are asymptomatic and have a localized mass or infiltrate on routine chest radiography. Laboratory studies are generally noncontributory, but four cases in the series

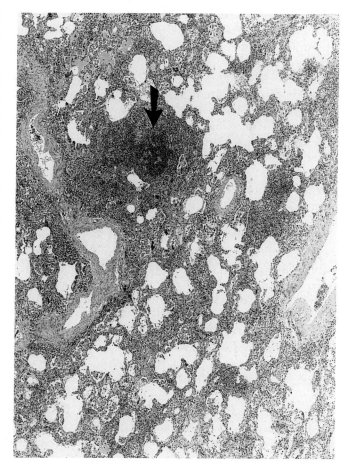

Fig. 31–8. Lymphocytic interstitial pneumonia in acquired immunodeficiency syndrome (AIDS). The moderately dense diffuse interstitial infiltrate of lymphocytes and plasma cells has occasional reactive germinal center (*arrow*). H and E, ×25.

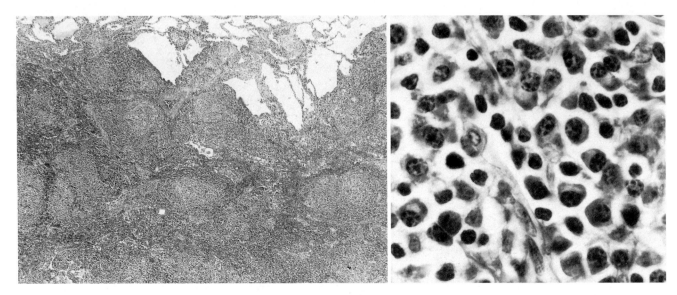

Fig. 31–9. Pseudolymphoma (localized lymphoid hyerplasia). This localized circumscribed mass of hyperplastic lymphoid tissue has numerous germinal centers and an associated mixed cellular population with lymphocytes and mature plasma cells. H and E: left, ×25; right, ×630.

of Koss et al.[50] had a polyclonal hypergammaglobulinemia.

Grossly, pseudolymphomas are tan and well circumscribed from the surrounding tissue.[30] Fibrosis within the lesion may cause retraction of tissue toward the center of the mass. The key microscopic feature in pseudolymphoma is the heterogeneity in cellular composition and variation from field to field (Fig. 31–9). Russell bodies and germinal centers may be prominent. The cellular infiltrate is mixed and generally includes lymphocytes, plasma cells, and occasional histiocytes that may form nonnecrotizing granulomas. Giant cells are seen in approximately one-third of cases. There is a variable amount of scarring that may be cellular and fibroblastic or acellular and hyaline in appearance. When fibroblastic proliferation is marked, focal or chronic organizing pneumonia may be more appropriate terms.[57] Confusion with the entity pulmonary hyalinizing granuloma should not occur. See Chapter 33 (p. 1336). Amyloid-like material may be present in pseudolymphomas. At the edge of the lesion, one does not see lymphatic tracking of a monomorphous population of cells, which characterizes lymphomas. Necrosis was found in one case reported by Koss et al.[50] Immunologic marker studies of pseudolymphomas fail to show a clonal population of cells.[50]

Castleman's disease (giant lymph node hyperplasia), particularly the hyaline vascular type, may involve nodes that are partially or completely intrapulmonary in location.[58]

In summary, much is made of distinguishing small lymphocytic lymphomas from either pseudolymphoma or lymphocytic interstitial pneumonia. In the case of pseudolymphoma, the distinction is often academic because both these lesions are usually resected for diagnosis, and solitary small lymphocytic lymphomas managed in this way rarely recur and often lack extrapulmonary involvement. It is reasonable to do noninvasive lymphoma staging procedures, but most patients will not require further therapy.

Malignant Lymphomas Presenting in the Lung

Definitions of a "primary" lymphoma occurring in an extranodal site, including the lung,[59] are somewhat arbitrary and cases that have evidence of disseminated disease are generally excluded. From a practical point of view, it is useful to divide pulmonary lymphomas into those in which the lung is the major site of involvement at presentation and those in which the lymphoma has presented at another site before secondary pulmonary involvement has occurred.[60]

A lymphatic distribution of involvement can be recognized in the majority of pulmonary lymphomas whether presenting in the lung or involving it secondarily.[47,48,60] A spectrum is encountered from diffuse infiltrates along lymphatic routes without mass formation to large necrotic masses with no discernible distribution. The lymphatic distribution is best appreciated at low power or even with naked-eye examination of the glass slide. (Fig. 31–10).

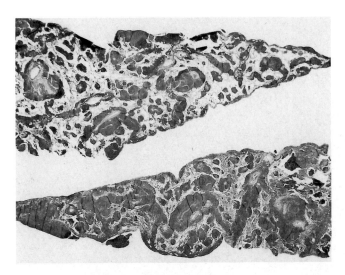

Fig. 31–10. Small lymphocytic lymphoma of lung shows diffuse involvement of lymphatic routes in pleura, septa, and along bronchovascular bundles. H and E, ×6.

Although the absence of involvement of hilar lymph nodes has been used as evidence against a diagnosis of lymphoma when evaluating a pulmonary lesion,[2,56] recent studies have emphasized that absence of hilar lymph node involvement is a frequent occurrence.[48,50,51]

If a pulmonary lymphoid lesion is suspected at the time of frozen section, the surgeon should be asked to sample hilar nodes as they may be helpful in both diagnosis and staging. Some tumor tissue should be appropriately saved (usually frozen) for immunologic marker studies, which may be helpful in confirming a light microscopic impression.[51]

Pulmonary Lymphomas Composed Predominantly of Small Lymphocytes

This category includes small (well-differentiated) lymphocytic lymphomas with or without plasmacytoid features, lymphocytic lymphomas of intermediate differentiation, and small cleaved cell lymphomas. Some cases are difficult to classify, a feature not uncommon in lymphomas of mucosa-associated lymphoid tissue.[17]

The following description is a summary of six series.[48,50,52–55] Most patients are older than 20 (mean age, approximately 55 years), although patients as young as 12 have been observed. Slightly more than half are asymptomatic with the lesion being discovered on chest radiographs. Those with symptoms describe cough, dyspnea, hemoptysis, weight loss, chest pain, and systemic complaints such as malaise. The male to female ratio is approximately 1:1.

Laboratory findings are generally nonspecific. Some-

thing less than a third of the patients are found to have a monoclonal serum protein spike either at presentation or subsequently. This finding is probably more common in patients with lymphoplasmacytic lymphomas.[54] An IgM monoclonal gammopathy is seen in cases of Waldenstrom's macroglobulinemia with lung involvement.[61–63] Cryoglobulinemia has also been reported.[64] Pulmonary function studies are rarely recorded because the majority of patients have radiographically localized disease. In the minority of patients that have diffuse bilateral disease radiographically, pulmonary function abnormalities of restriction and decreased diffusing capacity may be present.

The chest radiographic findings are quite variable, and any combination of the following may be seen: single or multiple nodules; unilateral or bilateral disease; localized alveolar and/or interstitial infiltrates; or diffuse bilateral alveolar and/or interstitial infiltrates. The most common presentation is a solitary, noncalcified nodule that may be 20 cm or more in diameter. Cavitation and hilar adenopathy are rarely observed.

Histologically, there is a monomorphous (or homogeneous) population of lymphocytes or plasmacytoid lymphocytes following lymphatic routes (see Fig. 31–10) with consolidation to masses (Figs. 31–11 and 31–12). The distribution may not be readily discernible in large masses, but tracking of the lymphoid infiltrate along lymphatic routes may be seen at their edge, and smaller satellite lesions may be found distributed along lymphatic routes. Cytologically, most cases are small lymphocytic lymphomas or lymphoplasmacytic lymphomas; lymphocytic lymphomas of intermediate differentiation and small cleaved cell lymphomas are less frequent.[48,50,52,53] Plasmacytoid differentiation is usually appreciated in patients with Waldenstrom's macroglobulinemia.[61–63] As in lymphomas of MALT at other sites, some cases show considerable cellular heterogeneity including the small lymphocytes, atypical small lymphocytes, plasmacytoid cells, plasma cells, and immunoblasts, and the term polymorphous immunocytoma is descriptively appropriate;[17,18,55] germinal centers may be numerous and be infiltrated by the neoplastic cell population.[65] Epithelial infiltration with the formation of lymphoepithelial lesions is also common (Fig. 31–13).

Pseudofollicular proliferation centers and true germinal centers are often scattered through the lesions (Fig. 31–14).[48,50–54,66] At the edge of masses one may find admixed plasma cells and histiocytes or a nonspecific intraalveolar accumulation of inflammatory cells. These foci may show a polyclonal immunostaining pattern. Granulomas, giant cells, dense sclerosis, and hyalinized material (which may or may not stain positively for amyloid) are sometimes seen. A few cases mimick nodular amyloidosis. A relatively common ap-

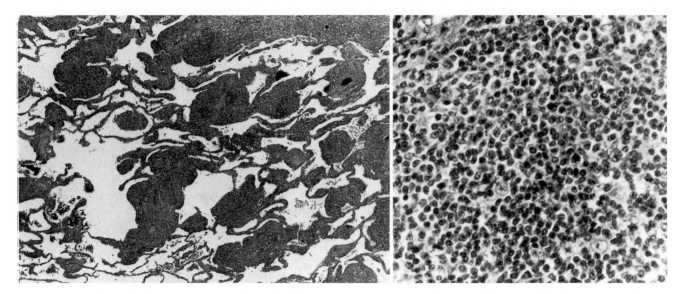

Fig. 31–11. Small lymphocytic lymphoma presenting as diffuse radiographic infiltrates. Biopsy shows pleural and perivascular monomorphous infiltrates of small lymphocytes. Involvement of alveolar walls is relatively inconspicuous compared to marked perivascular infiltrates. H and E: left, ×25; right, ×250.

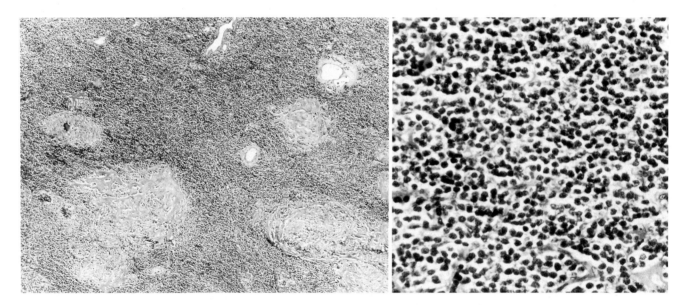

Fig. 31–12. Small lymphocytic lymphoma presenting as solitary mass. Between islands of sclerotic connective tissue are sheets of monomorphous small lymphocytes. In such cases there may be either monoclonal or polyclonal plasma cells in sclerotic regions. H and E: left, ×40; right, ×250.

pearance is bands of dense sclerosis surrounding islands of small lymphocytes with occasional plasma cells (See Fig. 31–12).

The differential diagnosis includes LIP, diffuse lymphoid hyperplasia, pseudolymphoma, other lymphomas, and chronic lymphocytic leukemia affecting the lung.

Immunologically, most small lymphocytic lymphomas are B-cell tumors.[17–19,55] A cytogenetic study of one case revealed karyotypic abnormalities with a translocation.[67]

The vast majority of these neoplasms are indolent and may be cured by surgery alone if they are localized.* Those that recur may do so within months or up to decades after initial recognition. At presentation, a

_____

*References: 18,21,22,30,48,50,52–55.

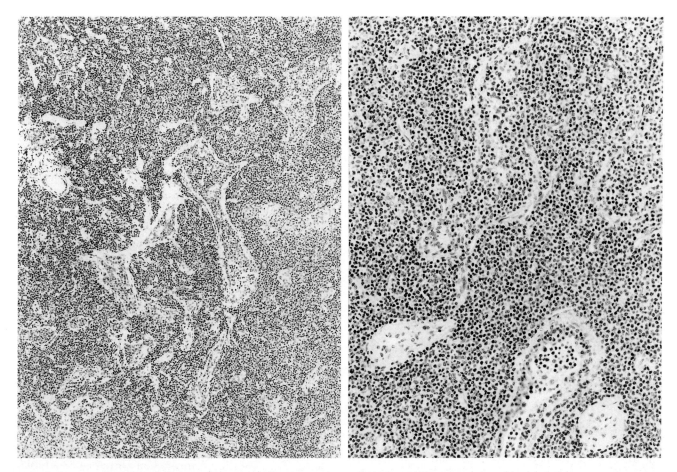

Fig. 31–13. Lymphoepithelial lesions from case of small lymphocytic lymphoma of the lung. A monomorphous population of small lymphocytes surrounds irregular-shaped islands, which represent epithelium infiltrated by lymphocytes. H and E: left, ×40; right, ×100.

minority, probably less than one-fourth, are found to have evidence of extrapulmonary lymphoma.[48] Transformation into a large-cell lymphoma, analogous to Richter's syndrome, may occur.[47,55]

Therapy and staging procedures should be tempered by the indolent nature of these lesions. Because resection alone may cure a significant number of patients, initial staging procedures should be noninvasive. The indolent behavior of these lymphomas is thought to reflect lymphomas of MALT in general.** Similarly, these lung lymphomas may be associated with gastrointestinal lymphomas or lymphomas of other MALT sites, before, after, or concurrently with the pulmonary lesions.***

Other Non-Hodgkin's Pulmonary Lymphomas

This heterogeneous group includes cases that would most often be classified as diffuse mixed-cell or large

cell lymphomas if encountered in lymph nodes. It also includes a majority, if not all, of the angiocentric immunoproliferative lesions discussed separately next. As a group they are about one-fourth as common as small lymphocytic lymphomas. Both T-cell and B-cell types occur.[55] Follicular lymphomas, diffuse small noncleaved cell lymphomas, and lymphoblastic lymphomas rarely involve the lung.

The clinical and radiographic findings are summarized from two series.[50,60] Although most patients are adults, there is a wide age range and children may be affected, particularly in immunodeficiency states. Occasional patients are asymptomatic, but the majority have cough, shortness of breath, fever, and a variety of other systemic complaints. The laboratory findings are noncontributory. Either at presentation or during the course, patients may develop a variety of extrapulmonary lesions, including paraneoplastic syndromes and involvement of multiple other organ systems. Involvement of the nervous system, skin, and subcutaneous tissues is not uncommon.

Radiographically, the patients show any combination

**References: 17,18,20–22,55.
***References: 22,48,50,55,68.

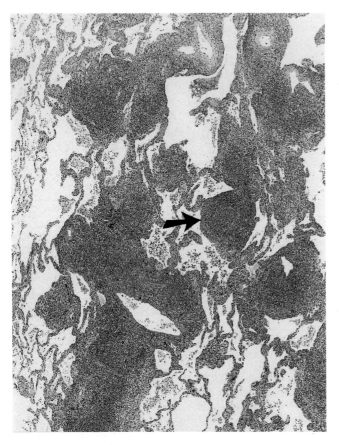

Fig. 31–14. Small lymphocytic lymphoma involving lung. An occasional germinal center (*arrow*), is seen, but elsewhere a dense monomorphous population of small lymphocytes expands septa and shows a perivascular distribution. H and E, ×40.

of nodule(s) or infiltrate(s) that may involve one or multiple lobes. Cavitation is relatively frequent, and a single cavitating mass mimicking tuberculosis may be seen. The development of infiltrates may be so rapid as to suggest an accute infection.[26,69,70]

Grossly, the lungs are consolidated by gray-tan, nodular infiltrates that may show necrosis and cavitation. When the infiltrates are not so massive, a lymphangitic pattern may be appreciated grossly. These lymphomas tend to show the broadest histologic spectrum, reflective both of the inherent heterogeneity of such a large subgroup and the frequent secondary changes in the adjacent lung parenchyma (Figs. 31–15 through 31–17). Subclassification of the lymphoma is based on identifying the neoplastic cell population: large lymphoid cells in the case of large-cell lymphoma, and a mixture of atypical small lymphocytes and large cells in the case of mixed-cell lymphomas. In the latter group there may be interspersed plasma cells and histiocytes.[33,51] Extensively necrotic lesions often have a rim of viable cytologically benign cells, and one may need to search several blocks to find foci of recognizable lymphoma. In cases that present as diffuse infiltrates along lymphatic routes without mass formation, the cellular heterogeneity may be so great that one is extremely reluctant to make a diagnosis of lymphoma. In such cases, cytologic atypia should be sought in infiltrates along pulmonary veins and in plaques of tumor in the pleura, because the peribronchial and peribronchiolar infiltrates tend to be the most polymorphous (see Fig. 31–10).

Vascular infiltration (Fig. 31–16) is common in this

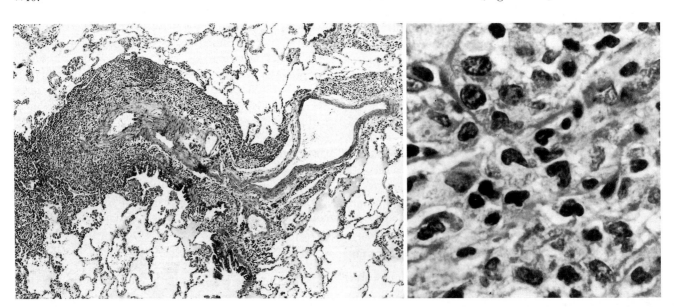

Fig. 31–15. Mixed-cell lymphoma presenting as diffuse radiograph infiltrates. The process surrounds airways and vessels and infiltrates the vessels. The mixed-cell population suggests a T-cell lymphoma with numerous atypical small lymphocytic forms. H and E: left, ×40; right, ×630.

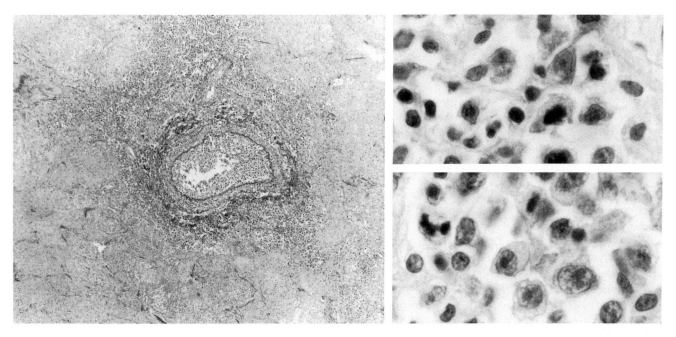

Fig. 31–16. Large cell lymphoma presenting as multiple nodules on chest radiograph. Prominent vascular infiltration is surrounded by tumor necrosis (left). The vascular infiltrate (upper right) is mixed in composition but includes atypical large cell similar to those seen among viable lymphoma (lower right). Such a case might also be interpreted as high-grade angiocentric lymphoma. H and E: left, ×40; right, upper and lower, ×630.

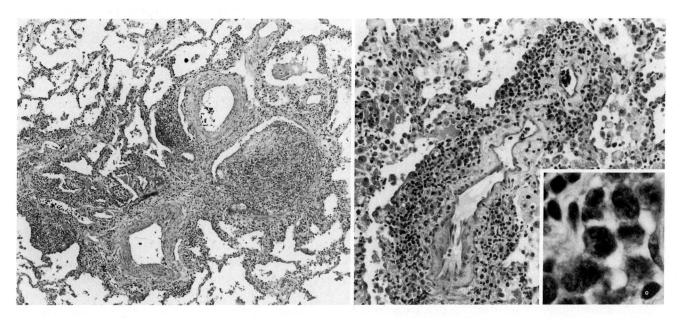

Fig. 31–17. Malignant lymphoma simulating airway inflammatory disease in patient with bilateral lower lobe infiltrates on chest radiograph, cough, and dyspnea. Small airways are surrounded by polymorphous infiltrates with some bronchiolitis obliterans (left). The neoplastic population (right inset) is most easily demonstrated along pulmonary veins (right). H and E: left, ×40; right, ×100; inset, ×630.

subgroup, although necrosis *limited to* vessel walls is unusual. When a necrotic vessel is seen, it is usually in the midst or at the edge of a large zone of tissue necrosis. Vascular infiltration may be by malignant cells, cytologically benign cells, or a mixture.

Invasion of airways (Fig. 31–17) also occurs and may produce a secondary bronchiolitis or bronchiolitis obliterans with more distal obstructive changes, including foamy macrophages in alveoli and inflammatory infiltrates in alveolar walls. An intraalveolar exudate and hyperplasia of type II pneumocytes is also common in the parenchyma adjacent to lymphomatous infiltrates. Less common secondary changes include organizing pneumonia and infarcts.

Like lymphomas presenting at other extranodal sites,[71,72] lymphomas presenting in the lung may have an associated cytologically benign infiltrate, usually at the periphery.[47,60] It is quite remarkable how extensive this infiltrate may be relative to the foci recognizable as lymphoma.

As with small lymphocytic lymphomas, a localized lymphoma in this group that is entirely resected may be cured.[54] However, the majority of patients have extensive bilateral disease, are clinically ill, and require aggressive chemotherapy that may result in either temporary or long-term remissions.[51,60]

Angiocentric Immunoproliferative Lesions (Lymphomatoid Granulomatosis)

Lymphomatoid granulomatosis was originally described as an angiocentric and angiodestructive process composed of lymphoreticular cells that showed a propensity to infiltrate blood vessels.[5] It was not clear whether it was primarily a disease of the lymphoid system, a peculiar vasculitis, or a hybrid.[5] Since the initial report, several sizable series have been published.[73,74] Other labels have also been applied to this condition, including polymorphic reticulosis,[6] benign and malignant angiitis and granulomatosis,[7] and most recently angiocentric immunoproliferative lesions.[8] This group of conditions shows considerable overlap with mixed-cell lymphomas as discussed previously.

As the histologic spectrum of lesions that are accepted as lymphomas has broadened, particularly since the recognition of T-cell lymphomas, it has become apparent that many if not most cases of lymphomatoid granulomatosis represent lymphoproliferative processes. It is acknowledged that these are somewhat different from the classical lymphomas presenting in lymph nodes.* In addition to lymphomas of T- and B-cell type,[75,76] some other lesions previously included with cases of lymphomatoid granulomatosis are pulmonary Hodgkin's disease and angioimmunoblastic lymphadenopathy involving the lung. The presence of vascular invasion, although characteristic of lymphomatoid granulomatosis, is common in many lymphoid lesions at a variety of sites,[77] most notably in primary brain lymphomas. The term vasculitis has often been used in this context but vascular invasion or infiltration is more appropriate.

This subset of lymphoproliferative diseases involving the lung is distinct and has recognizable differences from more conventional lymphomas. There are frequently infiltrates of the skin or nervous system, both central and peripheral. While one may simply call these mixed-cell lymphomas, the concept of angiocentric immunoproliferative lesions,[8] divided into low-grade and high-grade types, is appealing and preferable to continued use of the term lymphomatoid granulomatosis. Most angiocentric immunoproliferative lesions have been shown immunophenotypically to be postthymic T-cell lymphoproliferations, and the high-grade lesions, which represent the majority of cases, are designated angiocentric lymphomas.[8] Molecular studies show clonal gene rearrangements in a minority of cases, which is further evidence to segregate this group of lesions from more conventional lymphomas.[78]

The histologic features of angiocentric immunoproliferative lesions are distinctive (Figs. 31–18 through 31–20). Most commonly, there are nodular infiltrates of lymphoid cells which, when small, are seen to center on or be adjacent to vascular structures (Fig. 31–18). Less commonly, there are more diffuse infiltrates along vascular structures and within septa. As the nodular lesions enlarge, there is a central fibrinous exudation into air spaces (Fig. 31–19) and eventually central necrosis with a rim of viable tissue (Fig. 31–20A). Extremely large nodules can develop. The lymphoid infiltrate constituting the nodules is heterogeneous and includes lymphoid cells, histiocytes that may form small epithelioid clusters, plasma cells, and rarely giant cells. Variable numbers of large lymphoid cells and small and intermediate-sized lymphoid cells with atypical nuclear membranes and mitotic figures are seen in increasing numbers from low-grade to high-grade lesions. There are associated changes in the air spaces including accumulation of pulmonary alveolar macrophages that may be foamy and prominent type II cells. Vascular infiltration by the lymphoid infiltrate is a distinctive feature

---

*References: 6,8,30,50,60.

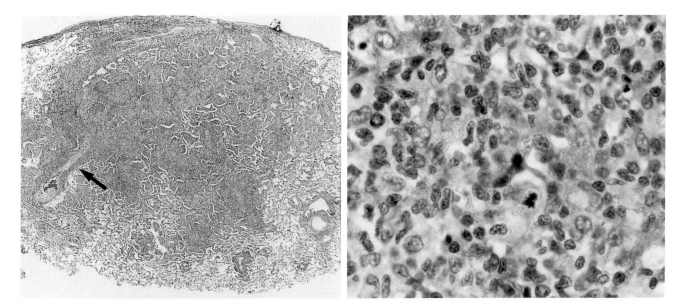

Fig. 31–18. Angiocentric lymphoma. Note the nodular infiltrate with interstitial, air space, and vessel (*arrow*) involvement. The infiltrate is composed of a mixed population of lymphoid cells (right) with relatively numerous atypical small lymphoid forms and moderate numbers of large lymphoid cells; a few histiocytes are present. The features are those of an intermediate to high-grade angiocentric immunoproliferative lesion (angiocentric lymphoma). H and E: left, ×20; right, ×250.

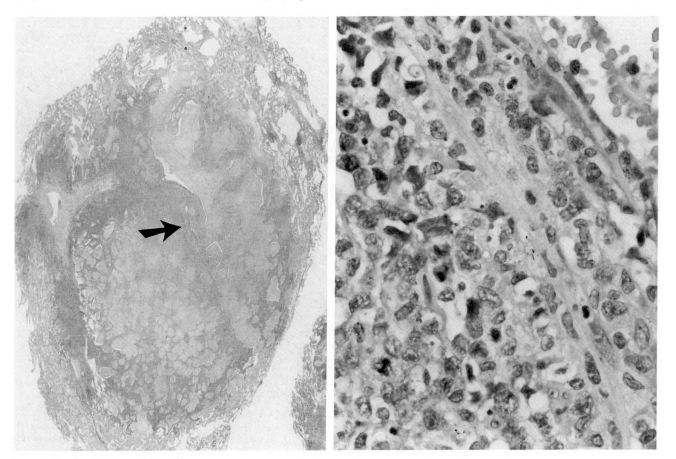

Fig. 31–19. Angiocentric lymphoma. This nodular infiltrate has central exudation into air spaces that precedes central necrosis in such cases. The neoplastic infiltrate (right) is composed of a monomorphous population of large cells. The field at the right is from an involved vessel wall (*arrow*) with the lumen at upper right. The pattern here is that of a high-grade angiocentric immunoproliferative lesion (angiocentric lymphoma). H and E: left, ×10; right, ×250.

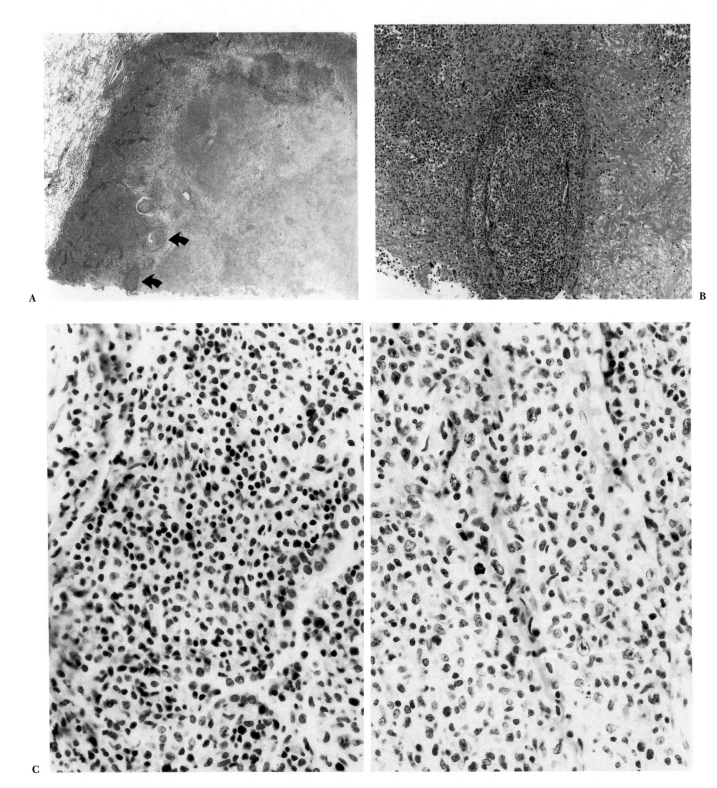

Fig. 31–20A–C. Angiocentric lymphoma. Note the large nodule with central necrosis (**A**) and vascular infiltration (**B**). The viable lymphoid infiltrate varied from a relatively bland cytologic appearance with small round small lymphocytes and modest numbers of intermediately sized cells lacking atypia (**C,** left) to a pattern characteristic of mixed-cell lymphoma with atypical small lymphocytes and large lymphoid forms (**C,** right). Based on the cytologic features (**C**), this would be classified as intermediate to high-grade angiocentric immunoproliferative lesion (angiocentric lymphoma). H and E. **A,** ×20; **B,** ×100; **C,** ×250.

(Fig. 31–20B), but is not seen in all sites of involvement and may not involve all vessels. The vascular infiltrate may be by cytologically benign cells, cytologically malignant cells, or a mixture of the two. The number of atypical cells varies from field to field (Fig. 31–20C), and one should search out the most atypical field in order to classify a given case. Not uncommonly, biopsies that show several nodules may reveal monomorphous foci of atypical large cells in only one of the nodules.

While initially a three-grade scheme for angiocentric immunoproliferative lesions was devised, a two-grade system with low-grade and high-grade categories has proved most practical.[8] At the low-grade end, one has difficulty convincing oneself of a neoplastic lymphoproliferative process. Because perivascular infiltrates are common in many conditions, a key feature is the density and mass-like character of the process; expansile nodules, central necrosis, and vascular infiltration are less common in benign lesions. At the high-grade end of the spectrum, recognition of the lymphomatous process is easy.

Early series of lymphomatoid granulomatosis suggested a poor prognosis despite chemotherapy,[5,73] with less than half of the patients living 2 years. This prognosis is similar to earlier series of large cell and mixed-cell lymphomas presenting in the lung.[60,73] More recent studies have suggested a more favorable prognosis with aggressive chemotherapy for high-grade lesions, with more than 50% long-term remissions.[8]

Lymphomatoid granulomatosis has been described in a number of clinical settings including immunodeficiency states.[60,73,79,80] Such a process in an immunocompetent individual should probably not be equated with a histologically similar process in an immunodeficient individual, but a common theme may be Epstein–Barr virus (EBV). Epstein–Barr virus has been found in a significant number of cases of lymphomatoid granulomatosis,[78,81] and it is also associated with lymphoproliferations in the acquired autoimmune deficiency syndrome and organ transplantation.[80,82–84] The significance of these findings in relationship to classical lymphomas remains to be clarified.

Pulmonary Lymphomas and Lymphoproliferations in the Setting of Transplantation and the Acquired Immunodeficiency Syndrome

Patients who have undergone transplantation are at increased risk to develop lymphoid proliferations.[82,83] Initially these were considered lymphomas; however, many have been found to be associated with EBV,

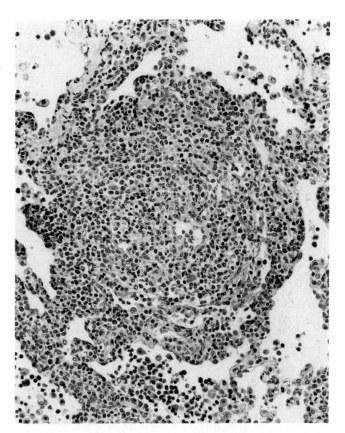

Fig. 31–21. EBV-associated lymphoproliferative lesion. This histologically polymorphous lesion composed predominantly of small lymphocytes shows marked propensity for vascular infiltration. The lesion regressed with decreased immunosuppression. H and E, ×150. (Courtesy of S.A. Yousem, M.D., University of Pittsburgh.)

usually a primary infection by the virus after transplantation.[82,83] Clinically these patients may present with nonspecific signs and symptoms or those similar to pulmonary lymphomas, and histologically they show a spectrum from a polymorphous infiltrate of plasma cells, small lymphocytes, and histiocytes to an appearance identical to diffuse large cell lymphoma (Figs. 31–21 and 31–22). Necrosis and vascular infiltration may be prominent. Immunophenotypically, they may be polyclonal or monoclonal, with the latter usually associated with a monotonous population of immunoblasts and large lymphoid cells. In one case the proliferating cells in the allograft were shown to be recipient lymphoid cells containing the EBV genome.[83] Many of these lymphoproliferations can be directly attributed to the immunosuppressive therapy, because they often resolve when immunosuppressive therapy is decreased. Such behavior may even be seen with lesions that are proven to be monoclonal. Molecular study of these lymphoproliferations shows the EBV genome to be

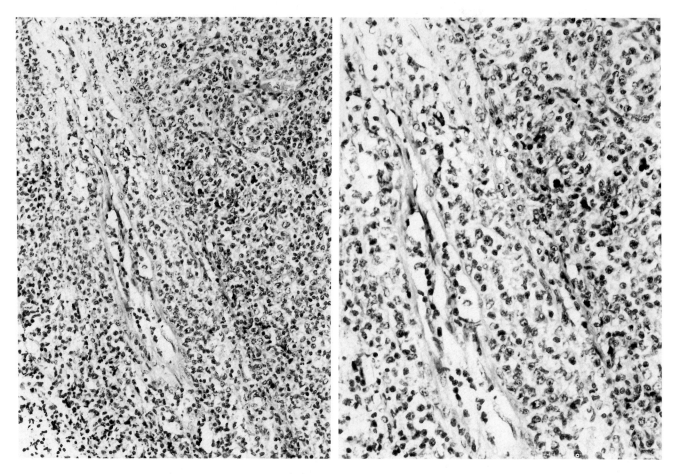

Fig. 31–22. EBV-associated lymphoproliferative lesion. There is marked vascular infiltration by cytologically malignant cells which have features of diffuse large cell lymphoma. This lesion regressed when immunosuppression was decreased. H and E: left, ×150; right, ×250. (Courtesy of S.A. Yousem, M.D., University of Pittsburgh.)

present in the neoplastic cells, although only serologic studies can determine if the infection is primary or secondary (i.e., reactivation).

Practically speaking, transplant-associated EBV lymphoproliferations often cannot be distinguished from lymphomas on morphologic or immunophenotypical grounds. Prognostication is difficult, and one often must wait for the follow-up to determine the behavior of a given lesion.

A number of pulmonary lymphoid proliferations are seen in the setting of acquired immunodeficiency syndrome (AIDS),[85,86] and EBV has been associated with a significant proportion.[60,61] Lymphocytic interstitial pneumonia (LIP) (see Fig. 30–8) may be encountered either as diffuse dense infiltration of alveolar septa by a mixed population of inflammatory cells or diffuse lymphoid hyperplasia. LIP in AIDS is more common in children than in adults. Kaposi's sarcoma of the lung is sometimes an associated lesion (see Chapter 33, p. 1400).

The lung is one of the less common sites of de novo lymphomas developing in patients with AIDS.[86]

Intravascular Lymphomatosis Presenting in the Lung

Intravascular lymphomatosis, also known as angiotropic lymphoma and malignant angioendotheliomatosis, is an uncommon form of lymphoma that has a marked propensity for intravascular growth.[87] The condition most commonly involves the central nervous system and the skin, but primary pulmonary presentation is also well described.[88,89] Patients have shortness of breath, fever, and diffuse interstitial infiltrates on chest radiographs. Histologically, there is a proliferation within vessels of atypical large lymphoid cells that at low power may mimic an interstitial pneumonia (Fig. 31–23). Cytologic evaluation reveals these cells to be distinct from endothelial cells, and immunophenotypically most cases are B cell,[87] in contrast to the angiocentric immu-

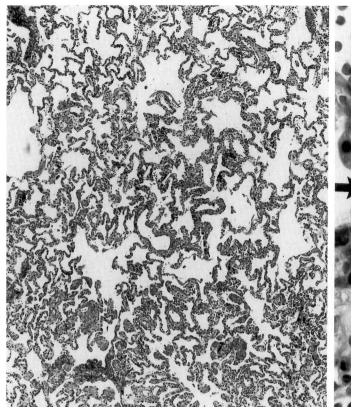 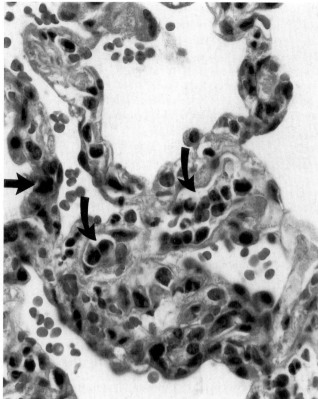

Fig. 31–23. Intravascular lymphomatosis presenting in lung. Low-power pattern (left) suggests diffuse interstitial pneumonia; however, the cytologic features (right) are those of neoplastic large lymphoid cells with intravascular location (*arrows*). H and E: left, ×40; right, ×500.

noproliferation lesions. Involved vessels are usually capillaries, although clusters of cells in larger vessels may be seen.

Because relatively few cases have been described, assessment of therapeutic intervention is difficult to analyze; some cases do show a response to chemotherapy.[89]

Hodgkin's Disease Presenting in the Lung

Primary pulmonary Hodgkin's disease is considered rare, and some have disputed its existence. Relapse of Hodgkin's disease in the lung or pleura is much more common. Nevertheless, case reports and small series of primary pulmonary Hodgkin's disease have appeared for many years,[90,91] and 61 cases in the literature were recently reviewed.[92]

Primary pulmonary Hodgkin's disease occurs more frequently in women (2:1), and patients are older than those with primary nodal Hodgkin's disease; the average age is 33 years for men and 51 years for women.[91] The majority had the following symptoms in decreasing

order of frequency: cough, fever, weight loss, dyspnea, fatigue, anorexia, chest pain, and pruritis.[91] Radiographically, reticulonodular infiltrates and single or multiple nodules are described.[91,92] Cavitation is not uncommon.[92]

The histologic findings of pulmonary Hodgkin's disease are identical to those in lymph nodes: Reed–Sternberg cells in the appropriate cellular milieu are needed for the diagnosis. In small nodules and diffuse infiltrates, a lymphatic distribution of infiltration can be discerned; vascular infiltration occurs. Other patterns include a pneumonic growth pattern (in which the infiltrate fills alveoli in a consolidative fashion), endobronchial lesions, and extensive subpleural or pleural involvement.[90,91,93] Some cases may show a dramatic sarcoid-like granulomatous reaction.[94]

The patients in Yousem's series were treated with conventional chemotherapeutic protocols for Hodgkin's disease.[91] Approximately half showed a favorable response to combination chemotherapy with long-term remissions. Unfavorable prognosis was linked to "B" symptoms, age greater than 60 years, and bilateral disease.

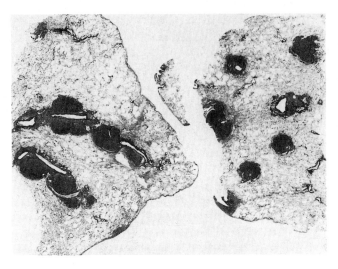

Fig. 31–24. Pulmonary relapse of large cell lymphoma presenting radiographically as a localized infiltrate. Small lymphomatous nodules are distributed along bronchovascular bundles and in the pleura. H and E, ×5.

Secondary Lymphomas Involving the Lung

Histologically, secondary pulmonary lymphomas in the lung cannot be distinguished from those presenting in the lung.[47,60] (Figs. 31–24 and 31–25). The knowledge of prior lymphoma is critical in making the diagnosis because the cytologic features may then be compared with the initial lesion. There may be transformation to a more unfavorable histology, with an increase of large cells in the case of non-Hodgkin's lymphomas and a relative increase in large cells and decrease in small lymphocytes and other inflammatory cells in Hodgkin's disease.[60]

Chronic lymphocytic leukemia involving the lung cannot be distinguished from primary or secondary small lymphocytic lymphomas. Among secondary mixed-cell and large cell lymphomas, necrosis and vascular infiltration are common findings. When Hodgkin's disease relapses in the lung, histologically diffuse infiltrates along lymphatic routes tend to be relatively frequent, and central fibrinoid necrosis with viable cells rimming vessels is quite common.

Leukemic Infiltrates in the Lung

Clinically significant leukemic pulmonary infiltrates recognized during life are quite rare, and infections, hemorrhage, heart failure, the effects of chemotherapy or radiotherapy, alveolar proteinosis, and opportunistic neoplasms should first be excluded.[95–97] Even when an unequivocal leukemic infiltrate is histologically identified in the lung, it may be incidental (although still significant) to a coexisting lesion, especially infection, that is the cause of the patient's immediate lung problem. The incidence of leukemic infiltration of the lung found histologically at autopsy, which varies from 25% to 64%,[95] is much greater than clinically significant infiltrates found during life, which occur in less than 7% percent of leukemic patients.[95,98,99] Any histologic subtype may be seen, but in the author's experience chronic lymphocytic leukemia is the type most often encountered in biopsy material. An interesting but quite rare

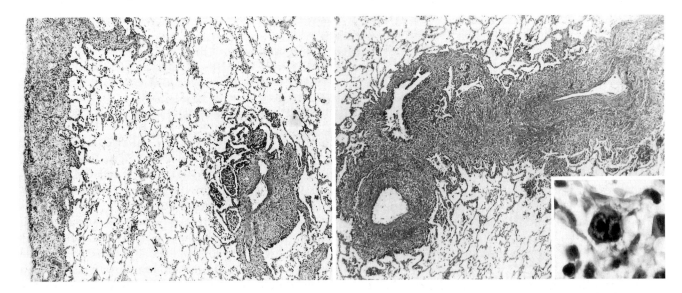

Fig. 31–25. Pulmonary relapse of Hodgkin's disease. Infiltrates are present in the pleura and along pulmonary veins and bronchovascular rays. H and E: left and right, ×25; inset, ×630.

manifestation of chronic lymphocytic leukemia is diffuse infiltration of bronchioles producing airway obstructive disease.[100].

Among acute leukemias, pulmonary infiltration is more common with nonlymphocytic leukemias,[95,101] and severe pulmonary disease may be a major initial manifestation, especially in patients with high (40% or greater) blast counts.[95]

Three unusual reactions that appear unique to leukemia are leukostasis, leukemic cell lysis pneumopathy, and hyperleukocytic reaction.[97,102,103] In leukostasis, there is vascular occlusion by aggregates of blasts in patients with peripheral leukocyte counts greater than 200,000/μl. Leukemic cell lysis pneumopathy is associated with severe hypoxemia and diffuse pulmonary infiltrates developing within 48 h after the onset of chemotherapy in patients with high leukocyte counts, generally greater than 200,000/μl. The high blast count combined with the effects of the chemotherapy on the leukemic cells is associated with aggregates of blasts within capillaries, small infarcts, hemorrhage, interstitial edema, and subsequent diffuse alveolar damage. In the hyperleukocytic reaction, a rapid increase in the peripheral blast count (generally greater than 245,000/μl) is associated with acute respiratory distress and accumulations of blast cells in small vessels with microhemorrhages and alveolar edema.

In both acute and chronic adult T-cell leukemias, clinically evident pulmonary leukemic infiltrates appear to be relatively common and were seen in 13 of 29 patients reported by Yoshioka et al. (Fig. 31–26).[104] In 6 of the 13 cases, a diagnosis of "chronic lung disease" had been carried for 2 to 6 years before this diagnosis of leukemia, and 4 of the 6 were histologically confirmed as having leukemic infiltrates, often associated with interstitial fibrosis.

Radiographically, leukemic involvement of the lung may present as localized or diffuse infiltrates, nodule(s), pleural disease, or recurrent "pneumonias."[97–100,105–108]

Histologically, leukemic infiltrates of the lung follow the lymphatic routes (Fig. 31–27). Formation of nodules is unusual.[105] The leukemic cells may be so sparse that they are easily overlooked. Special stains, such as chloroacetate esterase, may be helpful in confirming their presence and in identifying a phenotype. Both lymphoid and myeloid leukemias may involve the lung or pleura.[100,105,106]

Agnogenic myeloid metaplasia and acute myelosclerosis are occasionally associated with pulmonary involvement.[109] Infiltrates along the lymphatic routes are seen with variable amounts of fibrous tissue production. The amount of fibrous tissue may overshadow the hematopoietic cells (Fig. 31–28).

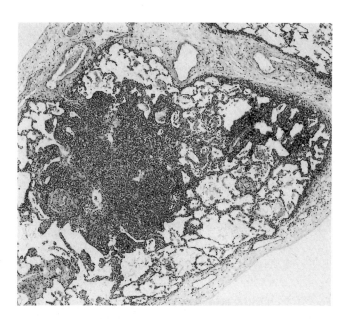

Fig. 31–26. Adult T-cell leukemia/lymphoma. Dense peribronchiolar and alveolar septal lymphoid infiltrates are seen in this biopsy from a patient who had a chronic pulmonary infiltrate. The cytological features of the cells were identical to those of the patient's lymphoreticular malignancy. H and E, ×25. (Courtesy of M. Kitaichi, M.D., Kyoto.)

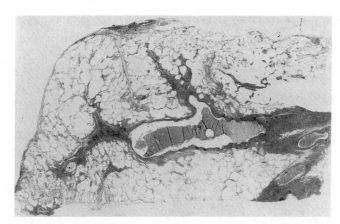

Fig. 31–27. Pulmonary infiltration by chronic myelogenous leukemia at autopsy. The infiltrate is restricted to a distribution along airways and vessels. H and E, ×4.

Malignant Histiocytosis

Malignant histiocytosis is a rare lymphoreticular malignancy caused by a systemic proliferation of neoplastic cells that resemble histiocytes,[110–113] although many cases classified as malignant histiocytosis have been reinterpreted as T-cell[114] or Ki-1 lymphomas.[115] Pulmonary involvement was described before the recognition of these latter two groups of lymphomas, and the

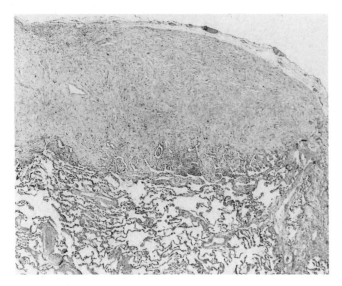

Fig. 31–28. Pleural involvement by agnogenic myeloid metaplasia. A thick pleural plaque is composed predominantly of fibrous tissue. Within this, a few islands of hematopoietic cells including megakaryocytes can be identified. This patient had a long history of agnogenic myeloid metaplasia and evidence of extramedullary myelofibrotic lesions at other sites including the pulmonary parenchyma. H and E, ×25.

features of lung involvement in malignant histiocytosis, as presently defined, are not well characterized. Pulmonary symptoms include cough, fever, and shortness of breath.[110,111,113] Pulmonary functions may show a severe restrictive deficit, and even respiratory failure.[110,111,113] Chest radiographs show bilateral interstitial infiltrates or, rarely, multiple nodules.[110]

Histologically, an infiltrate of atypical lymphoid cells (sometimes with features recognizable as histiocytic) involves lymphatic routes. There may be a variable amount of septal widening and fibrous tissue proliferation, and the cells may occur singly or in clusters. The infiltrates may expand to form nodules.

Mycosis Fungoides/ Sezary's Syndrome

The lung is the second most frequently involved extracutaneous site, after lymph nodes, in mycosis fungoides (cutaneous T-cell lymphoma)[116,117] (Fig. 31–29). Localized, diffuse, or sometimes nodular radiographic infiltrates are seen. The infiltrates are distributed along lymphatic routes, and the cytologic spectrum is similar to that seen in mycosis fungoides at other sites. Vascular infiltration and necrosis may be present.

Plasma Cell Tumors and Multiple Myeloma

Plasma cell tumors in the lung are extremely rare.[118] Pure plasmacytomas should be distinguished from other lesions with numerous plasma cells, including lymphoplasmacytoid small lymphocytic lymphomas and plasma cell granulomas. The number of cases of pulmonary plasmacytomas that have been reported is too small to make any firm statements about their behavior. Amin[119] has reported three cases that all

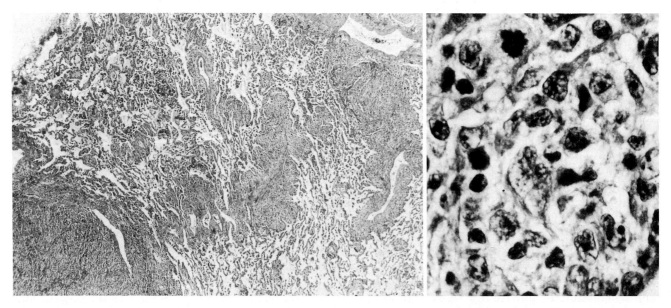

Fig. 31–29. Disseminated mycosis fungoides involving the lung shows both discrete nodules (low left) and diffuse perivascular infiltrates. A mixed cytologic composition includes cells with convoluted nuclei. H and E: left, ×25; right, ×630.

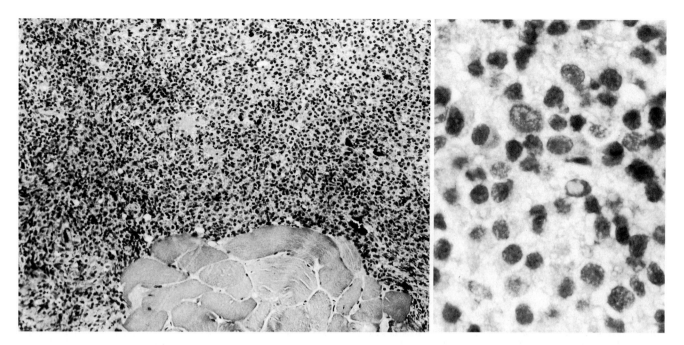

Fig. 31–30. Waldenstrom's macroglobulinemia presenting as recurrent pleural effusions. A closed pleural biopsy shows a dense infiltrate of lymphocytes and plasmacytoid lymphocytes, some with Dutcher bodies. H and E: left, ×100; right, ×630.

showed systemic dissemination within 3 years of presenting with localized or only regional lung disease. Roikjaer and Thomsen[120] described a patient with two separate pulmonary plasmacytomas occurring during a 5-year period. Both were resected, and there was no evidence of dissemination during the next 4 years.

Pulmonary involvement in patients with multiple myeloma is more frequent than is primary pulmonary plasmacytoma, although it still is not common. Most of the patients have clinically obvious disseminated myeloma, and pulmonary involvement is part of the systemic disease.[121,122] Pulmonary presentation with infiltrates resembling pneumonia has also been described.[123] Multiple nodules are more frequent than diffuse infiltrates.[123] Also in this setting, diffuse alveolar septal amyloid deposition or other forms of amyloidosis secondary to the myeloma may also be a cause of lung disease.[123] Kijner and Yousem[124] reported a case of systemic light chain disease presenting as bilateral nodular infiltrates on chest radiographs. Light chain deposition was distinguished from amyloid by electron microscopy.

phocytic lymphomas is the fact that extrapleural plaques of infiltrate strongly favor a lymphoma over a benign process.[50] Elastic tissue stains may be necessary to identify the exact location of the visceral pleura in the case of massive infiltrates. Lymphomas, including Waldenstrom's macroglobulinemia, rarely present as pleural disease (Fig. 31–30). In these cases, the extensive and predominately visceral pleural infiltration is out of proportion to the relatively scant infiltration of the underlying pulmonary parenchyma.

Immunologic marker studies may be helpful ancillary aids in recognizing a clonal population of cells in effusions. Pleural effusions found at presentation in patients with Hodgkin's disease and (less commonly) non-Hodgkin's lymphomas are usually caused by lymphomatous involvement of mediastinal lymph nodes and secondary lymphatic obstruction.[125] In cases that require biopsy, the visceral pleura should be biopsied in preference to the parietal pleura, as the extent of infiltrate is usually much more severe in the visceral pleura. Widespread myeloma may cause pleural effusions.[121,122]

Pleural Lymphoma/Leukemia

Pleural involvement by lymphomas and leukemias is not unexpected, because the pleura represents one of the lymphatic routes that these lesions generally affect. Indeed, one of the helpful features in identifying lym-

Practical Considerations

Overall, the majority of pulmonary lymphomas and leukemias are diagnosed on the basis of open lung biopsy or a resection specimen. Primary diagnosis by transbronchial biopsy is feasible in selected situations,

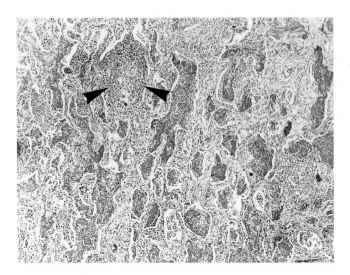

Fig. 31–31. Pulmonary parenchymal reaction adjacent to primary pulmonary Hodgkin's disease. There is extensive nonspecific interstitial widening with granulomas (*arrowheads*) and dense intraalveolar exudate; these nonspecific and apparently inflammatory changes were quantitively much more extensive than the Hodgkin's disease in this case. H and E ×40.

particularly with support of immunohistochemical studies.[126] Endobronchial involvement may be seen with both leukemias and lymphomas.[127–130] These cases are particularly amenable to biopsies through the bronchoscope. Techniques such as bronchial washings and bronchoalveolar lavage are occasionally useful in the primary diagnosis of lymphoma, but their role is probably greater in patients who already carry a histologic diagnosis and for whom a pulmonary relapse needs to be confirmed. Confirmation of pulmonary involvement by these techniques has been shown with all varieties of lymphoreticular infiltrates.[96,131–135]

A trap in the evaluation of many lung lymphomas is the presence of an associated benign or reactive-appearing infiltrate that may obscure the neoplasm population (Fig. 31–31).

References

1. Liebow AA, Carrington CB. Diffuse pulmonary lymphoreticular infiltrations associated with dysproteinemia. Med Clin North Am 1973;57:809–843.
2. Saltzstein SL. Extranodal malignant lymphomas and pseudolymphomas. Pathol Annu 1969;4:159–184.
3. Greenberg SD, Heisler JG, Gyorkey F, Jenkins DE: Pulmonary lymphomas versus pseudolymphoma: a perplexing problem. South Med J 1972;65:775–784.
4. Julsrud PR, Brown LR, Li Cy, Rosenow EC, Crowe JK. Pulmonary processes of mature-appearing lymphocytes: Pseudolymphoma, well-differentiated lympho-cytic lymphoma, and lymphocytic interstitial pneumonitis. Radiology 1978;127:289–296.
5. Liebow AA, Carrington CB, Friedman PJ. Lymphomatoid granulomatosis. Hum Pathol 1972;3:457–558.
6. DeRemee RA, Weiland LH, McDonald TJ. Polymorphic reticulosis, lymphomatoid granulomatosis. Two diseases or one? Mayo Clinic Proc 1978;53:634–640.
7. Saldana MJ, Patchefsky AS, Israel HI, Atkinson GW. Pulmonary angiitis and granulomatosis. Hum Pathol 1977;8:391–409.
8. Lipford EH, Jr., Margolick JB, Longo DL, Fauci AS, Jaffe ES. Angiocentric immunoproliferative lesions: A clinicopathologic spectrum of post-thymic T-cell prolif-erations. Blood 1988;72:1674–1681.
9. Berard CW, Greene MH, Jaffe ES, Magrath I, Ziegler J. A multidisciplinary approach to non-Hodgkin's lymphomas. Ann Intern Med 1981;94:218–235.
10. Nagaishi C. Functional anatomy and histology of the lung. Baltimore: University Park, 1972.
11. Okada Y. Lymphatic system of the human lung. Kyoto: Kinpodo, 1989.
12. Kradin RL, Spirn PW, Mark EJ. Intrapulmonary lymph nodes. Chest 1985;87:662–667.
13. Bienenstock J, Johnston N, Perey DYE. Bronchial lymphoid tissue. I. Morphologic characteristics. Lab Invest 1973;28:686–692.
14. Bienenstock J, Johnston N, Perey DYE. Bronchial lymphoid tissue. II. Functional characteristics. Lab Invest 1973;28:693–698.
15. Bienenstock J, Befus AD. Gut- and bronchus-associated lymphoid tissue. Am J Anat 1984;170:437–445.
16. Pabst R, Gehrke I. Is the bronchus-associated lymphoid tissue (BALT) an integral structure of the lung in normal mammals, including humans? Am J Respir Cell Mol Biol 1990;3:131–135.
17. Harris NL. Extranodal lymphoid infiltrates and mucosa-associated lymphoid tissue (MALT): A unifying concept. Am J Surg Pathol 1991;16:879–883.
18. Isaacson PG, Spencer J. Malignant lymphoma of mucosa-associated lymphoid tissue. Histopathology (Oxf) 1987;11:445–462.
19. Addis BJ, Hyjek E, Isaacson PG. Primary pulmonary lymphoma: A re-appraisal of its histogenesis and its relationship to pseudolymphoma and lymphoid interstitial pneumonia. Histopathology (Oxf) 1988;13:1–17.
20. Isaacson P, Wright DH. Malignant lymphoma of mucosa-associated lymphoid tissue. Cancer 1983;52:1410–1416.
21. Isaacson P, Wright DH. Extranodal malignant lymphoma arising from mucosa-associated lymphoid tissue. Cancer 1984;53:2515–2524.
22. Hernandez JA, Sheehan WW. Lymphomas of the mucosa-associated lymphoid tissue. Cancer 1985;55:592–597.
23. Morris H, Edwards J, Tiltman A, Emms M: Endometrial lymphoid tissue: An immunohistological study. J Clin Pathol 1985;38:644–652.
24. Bragg DG. The clinical, pathologic, and radiologic spectrum of the intrathoracic lymphomas. Invest Radiol 1978;13:2–11.

25. Balikian JP, Herman PG. Non-Hodgkin's lymphoma of the lungs. Radiology 1979;132:569–576.

26. Blank N, Castellino RA. The intrathoracic manifestations of the malignant lymphomas and the leukemias. Semin Roentgenol 1980;15:227–245.

27. Yousem SA, Colby TV, Carrington CB. Follicular bronchitis/bronchiolitis. Hum Pathol 1985;16:700–706.

28. Meuwissen HJ, Hussian M. Bronchus-associated lymphoid tissue in human lung: Correlation of hyperplasia with chronic pulmonary disease. Clin Immunol Immunopathol 1982;23:548–561.

29. Yousem SA, Colby TV, Carrington CB. Lung biopsy in rheumatoid arthritis. Am Rev Respir Dis 1985;131:770–777.

30. Kradin RL, Mark EJ. Benign lymphoid disorders of the lung with a theory regarding their development. Hum Pathol 1983;14:857–867.

31. Dorfman RF, Warnke RA. Lymphadenopathy simulating malignant lymphomas. Hum Pathol 1974;5:519–550.

32. Frizzera G, Moran EM, Rappaport H. Angioimmunoblastic lymphadenopathy with dysproteinemia. Am J Med 1975;59:803–818.

33. Watanabe S, Shimosato Y, Shimoyama M. Lymphoma and leukemia of T-lymphocytes. Pathol Annu 1981;16(Part 2):155–204.

34. Iseman MD, Schwarz MI, Stanford RE. Interstitial pneumonia in angioimmunoblastic lymphadenopathy with dysproteinemia. Ann Intern Med 1976;85:752–755.

35. Zylak CJ, Banerjee R, Galbraith PA, McCarthy DS. Lung involvement in angioimmunoblastic lymphadenopathy. Radiology 1976;121:513–519.

36. Weisenburger D, Armitage L, Dick F. Immunoblastic lymphadenopathy with pulmonary infiltrates, hypocomplementemia and vasculitis. Am J Med 1977;63:849–854.

37. Strimlan CV, Rosenow EC, III, Weiland LH, Brown LR. Lymphocytic interstitial pneumonitis. Ann Intern Med 1978;88:616–621.

38. Koss MN, Hochholzer L, Langloss JM, Wehunt WD, Lazarus AA. Lymphoid interstitial pneumonia: Clinicopathological and immunopathological findings in 18 cases. Pathology 1987;19:178–185.

39. Church JA, Isaacs H, Saxon A, Keens TG, Richards W. Lymphoid interstitial pneumonitis and hypogammaglobulinemia in children. Am Rev Respir Dis 1981;124:491–496.

40. Dukes RJ, Rosenow EC, Hermans PE. Pulmonary manifestations of hypogammaglobulinemia. Thorax 1978;33:603–607.

41. Yoshizawa Y, Ohdama S, Ikeda A, Ohtsuka M, Masuda S, Tanaka M. Lymphoid interstitial pneumonia associated with depressed cellular immunity and polyclonal gammopathy. Am Rev Respir Dis 1984;130:507–509.

42. Solal-Celigny P, Couderc LJ, Herman D, et al. Lymphoid interstitial pneumonitis in acquired immunodeficiency syndrome-related complex. Am Rev Respir Dis 1985;131:956–960.

43. Greico MH, Chinoy-Acharya P. Lymphocytic interstitial pneumonia associated with the acquired immune deficiency syndrome. Am Rev Respir Dis 1985;131:952–955.

44. Perreault C, Cousineau S, D'Angelo G, et al. Lymphoid interstitial pneumonia after allogeneic bone marrow transplantation. Cancer 1985;55:1–9.

45. Khardori R, Eagleton LE, Soler NG, McConnachie PR. Lymphocytic interstitial pneumonitis in autoimmune thyroid disease. Am J Med 1991;90:649–654.

46. Kohler PF, Cook RD, Brown WR, Manguso RL. Common variable hypogammaglobulinemia with T-cell nodular lymphoid interstitial pneumonitis and B-cell nodular lymphoid hyperplasia: Different lymphocyte populations with a similar response to prednisone therapy. J Allergy Clin Immunol 1982;70:299–305.

47. Colby TV, Carrington CB. Lymphoreticular tumors and infiltrates of the lung. Pathol Annu 1983;18:27–70.

48. Turner RR, Colby TV, Doggett RS. Well-differentiated lymphocytic lymphoma: A study of 47 cases with primary manifestation of the lung. Cancer 1984;54:2088–2096.

49. Kohler PF, Cook RD, Brown WR, Manguso RL. Common variable hypogammaglobulinemia with T-cell nodular lymphoid interstitial pneumonitis and B-cell nodular lymphoid hyperplasia: Different lymphocyte populations with a similar response to prednisone therapy. J Allergy Clin Immunol 1982;70:299–305.

50. Koss MN, Hochholzer L, Nichols PW, Wehunt WD, Lazarus AA. Primary non-Hodgkin's lymphoma and pseudolymphoma of the lung: A study of 161 patients. Hum Pathol 1983;14:1024–1038.

51. Weiss LM, Yousem SA, Warnke RA. Non-Hodgkin's lymphomas of the lung. Am J Surg Pathol 1985;9:480–490.

52. L'Hoste RJ, Filippa DA, Lieberman PH, Bretsky S. Primary pulmonary lymphomas. Cancer 1984;54:1397–1406.

53. Herbert A, Wright DH, Isaacson PG. Primary malignant lymphoma of the lung: Histopathologic and immunologic evaluation of nine cases. Hum Pathol 1984;15:415–422.

54. Kennedy JL, Nathwani BN, Burke JS, Hill LR, Rappaport H. Pulmonary lymphomas and other lymphoid lesions. Cancer 1985;56:539–552.

55. Li G, Hansmann M-L, Zwingers T, Lennert K. Primary lymphomas of the lung: Morphological, immunohistochemical, and clinical features. Histopathology (Oxf) 1990;16:519–531.

56. Saltzstein SL. Pulmonary malignant lymphomas and pseudolymphomas: Classification, therapy, and prognosis. Cancer 1963;16:928–955.

57. Colby TV, Lombard C, Yousem SA, Kitaichi M. Atlas of pulmonary surgical pathology. Philadelphia: WB Saunders, 1991.

58. Keller AR, Hochholzer L, Castleman B. Hyaline-vascular and plasma-cell types of giant lymph node hyperplasia of the mediastinum and other locations. Cancer 1972;29:670–683.

59. Papaioannou AN, Watson WL. Primary lymphoma of the lung: An appraisal of its natural history and a

comparison with other localized lymphoma. J Thorac Cardiovasc Surg 1965;47:373–387.

60. Colby TV, Carrington CB. Malignant lymphoma simulating lymphomatoid granulomatosis. Am J Surg Pathol 1982;6:19–32.

61. Essig LJ, Timms ES, Hancock DE, Sharp GC. Plasma cell interstitial pneumonia and macroglobulinemia. Am J Med 1974;56:398–405.

62. Winterbauer RH, Riggins RCK, Griesman FA, Bauermeister DE: Pleuropulmonary manifestations of Waldenstrom's macroglobulinemia. Chest 1974;66:368–375.

63. Case records of the Massachusetts General Hospital, Case 43-1982. N Engl J Med 1982;307:1065–1073.

64. Case records of the Massachusetts General Hospital, Case 41-1984. N Engl J Med 1984;311:969–978.

65. Isaacson PG, Wotherspoon AC, Diss T, Pan L. Follicular colonization in B-cell lymphoma of mucosa-associated lymphoid tissue. Am J Surg Pathol 1991;15:819–828.

66. Nichols PW, Koss MN, Taylor CR, Hochholzer L. Immunoperoxidase studies in the diagnosis of 51 primary pulmonary lymphoid lesions. Lab Invest 1980;44:48A.

67. Wotherspoon AC, Soosay GN, Diss TC, Isaacson PG. Low-grade primary B-cell lymphoma of the lung. Am J Clin Pathol 1990;94:655–660.

68. Gaulard PH, Couderc LJ, Post C, et al. Primary pulmonary lymphoma with gastric involvement in four cases. Am Rev Respir Dis 1985;131:A117.

69. Cathcart-Rake W, Bone RC, Sabonya RE, Stephens RL. Rapid development of diffuse pulmonary infiltrates in histiocytic lymphoma. Am Rev Respir Dis 1978;117:587–593.

70. Chechani V, Allam AA, Kamholz SL. Pulmonary non-Hodgkin's lymphoma mimicking infection. Respir Med 1990;84:401–405.

71. Colby TV, Dorfman RF. Malignant lymphomas involving the salivary glands. Pathol Annu 1979;14:307–324.

72. Lewin KJ, Ranchod M, Dorfman RF. Lymphomas of the gastrointestinal tract. Cancer 1978;42:693–707.

73. Katzenstein ALA, Carrington CB, Liebow AA. Lymphomatoid granulomatosis. A clinicopathologic study of 152 cases. Cancer 1979;43:360–373.

74. Koss MN, Hochholzer L, Langloss JM, Wehunt WD, Lazarus AA, Nichols PW. Lymphomatoid granulomatosis: A clinicopathologic study of 42 patients. Pathology 1986;18:283–288.

75. Petras RE, Sebek BA, Tubbs RR. Immunomorphology of lymphomatoid granulomatosis. Am J Clin Pathol 1981;74:354 (Abstract).

76. Nichols PW, Koss M, Levine AM, Lukes RJ. Lymphomatoid granulomatosis: A T-cell disorder? Am J Med 1982;72:467–471.

77. Nonomura A, Ohta G. Lymphomatoid granulomatosis-like lesions in malignant lymphoma. Acta Pathol Jpn 1986;36:1617–1626.

78. Medeiros LJ, Peiper SC, Elwood L, Yano T, Raffeld M, Jaffe ES. Angiocentric immunoproliferative lesions: A molecular analysis of eight cases. Hum Pathol 1991; 21:1150–1157.

79. Mittal K, Neri A, Feiner H, Schinella R, Alfonso F. Lymphomatoid granulomatosis in the acquired immunodeficiency syndrome. Cancer 1990;65:1345–1349.

80. Ilowite NT, Fligner CL, Ochs HD, et al. Pulmonary angiitis with atypical lymphoreticular infiltrates in Wiskott-Aldrich syndrome: Possible relationship of lymphomatoid granulomatosis and EBV infection. Clin Immunol Immunopathol 1986;41:479–484.

81. Katzeinstein ALA, Peiper SC. Detection of Epstein–Barr virus geromas in lymphomatoid granulomatosis: Analysis of 29 cases by the polymerase chain reaction technique. Mod Pathol 1990;3:435–441.

82. Randhawa PS, Yousem SA, Paradis IL, Dauber JA, Griffith DP, Locker J. The clinical spectrum, pathology, and clonal analysis of Epstein–Barr virus-associated lymphoproliferative disorders in heart-lung transplant recipients. Am J Clin Pathol 1989;92:177–185.

83. Randhawa PS, Yousem SA. Epstein–Barr virus-associated lymphoproliferative disease in a heart-lung allograft. Transplantation 1990;49:126–130.

84. Andiman WA, Martin K, Rubinstein A, Paliwa S, Eastman R, Katz BZ, Pitt J, Miller G. Opportunistic lymphoproliferations associated with Epstein–Barr viral DNA in infants and children with AIDS. Lancet 1985; ii:1390–1391.

85. Teirstein AS, Rosen MJ. Lymphocytic interstitial pneumonia. Clin Chest Med 1988;9:467–471.

86. Heitzman ER. Pulmonary neoplastic and lymphoproliferative disease in AIDS: A review. Radiology 1990; 177:347–351.

87. Stroup RM, Shebani K, Moncada A, Purdy LJ, Battifora H. Angiotropic (intravascular) large cell lymphoma. Cancer 1990;66:1781–1788.

88. Tan TB, Spaander PJ, Blaisse M, Gerritzen FM. Angiotropic large cell lymphoma presenting as interstitial lung disease. Thorax 1988;43:578–579.

89. Yousem SA, Colby TV. Intravascular lymphomatosis presenting in the lung. Cancer 1990;65:349–353.

90. Kern WH, Crepeau AG, Jones JC. Primary Hodgkin's disease of the lung. Cancer 1961;14:1151–1165.

91. Yousem SA, Weiss LM, Colby TV. Primary pulmonary Hodgkin's disease: A clinicopathologic study of 15 cases. Cancer 1986;57:1217–1224.

92. Radin AI. Primary pulmonary Hodgkin's disease. Cancer 1990;65:550–563.

93. Harper PG, Fisher C, McLennan K, Souhami RL. Presentation of Hodgkin's disease as an endobronchial lesion. Cancer 1984;53:147–150.

94. Daly PA, O'Briain D, Robinson I, Guckian M, Prichard JS. Hodgkin's disease with a granulomatous pulmonary presentation mimicking sarcoidosis. Thorax 1988;43:407–409.

95. Rosenow EC, Wilson WR, Cockerill FR. Pulmonary disease in the immunocompromised host. Mayo Clin Proc 1985;60:473–487.

96. Rossi GA, Balbi B, Risso M, Repetto M, Ravazzoni C. Acute myelomonocytic leukemia: Demonstration of pulmonary involvement by bronchoalveolar lavage. Chest 1985;87:259–260.

97. Hildebrand FL, Rosenow EC III, Habermann TM, Tazelaar HD. Pulmonary complications of leukemia. Chest 1990;98:1233–1239.

98. Green RA, Nichols NJ. Pulmonary involvement in leukemia. Am Rev Respir Dis 1959;80:833–844.

99. Klatte EC, Yardley J, Smith EB, Rohn R, Campbell JA. The pulmonary manifestations and complications of leukemia. AJR 1963;89:598–609.

100. Palosaari D, Colby TV. Bronchiolocentric chronic lymphocytic leukemia. Cancer 1986;58:1695–1698.

101. McCabe RE, Brooks RG, Mark JBD, Remington JS. Open lung biopsy in patients with acute leukemia. Am J Med 1985;78:609–616.

102. Myers TJ, Solon RC, Klatsky AU, Hild DH. Respiratory failure due to pulmonary leukostasis following chemotherapy of acute nonlymphocytic leukemia. Cancer 1983;51:1808–1813.

103. Lester RJ, Johnson JW, Cuttner J. Pulmonary leukostasis is the single worst prognostic factor in patients with acute myelocytic leukemia and hyperleukocytosis. Am J Med 1985;79:43–48.

104. Yoshioka R, Yamaguchi K, Yoshinaga T, Takatsuki K. Pulmonary complications in patients with adult T-cell leukemia. Cancer 1985;55:2491–2494.

105. Callahan M, Wall S, Askin F, Delaney D, Koller C, Orringer EP. Granulocytic sarcoma presenting as pulmonary nodules and lymphadenopathy. Cancer 1987;60:1902–1904.

106. Hicklin GA, Drevyanko TF. Primary granulocytic sarcoma presenting with pleural and pulmonary involvement. Chest 1988;94:655–656.

107. Desjardins A, Ostiguy G, Cousineau S, Gyger M. Recurrent localised pneumonia due to bronchial infiltration in a patient with chronic lymphocytic leukaemia. Thorax 1990;45:570.

108. Kovalski R, Hansen-Flaschen H, Lodato RF, Pietra GG. Localized leukemic pulmonary infiltrates: Diagnosis by bronchoscopy and resolution with therapy. Chest 1990;17:674–678.

109. Beckman EN, Oehrle JS. Fibrous hematopoietic tumors arising in angiogenic myeloid metaplasia. Hum Pathol 1982;13:804–810.

110. Colby TV, Carrington CB, Mark GJ. Pulmonary involvement in malignant histiocytosis: A clinicopathologic spectrum. Am J Surg Pathol 1981;5:61–73.

111. Wongchaowart B, Kennealy JA, Crissman J, Hawkins H. Respiratory in malignant histiocytosis. Am Rev Respir Dis 1981;124:640–642.

112. Van Heerde P, Feltkamp CA, Hart AAM, Somers R. Malignant histiocytosis and related tumors: A clinicopathologic study of 42 cases using cytological, histochemical, and ultrastructural parameters. Hematol Oncol 1984;2:13–32.

113. Aozasa K, Tsujimoto M, Inoue A. Malignant histiocytosis: Report of 25 cases with pulmonary, renal, and/or gastrointestinal involvement. Histopathology (Oxf) 1985;9:39–49.

114. Kadin ME. T Gamma cells: A missing link between malignant histiocytosis and T cell leukemia-lymphoma. Hum Pathol 1981;12:771–772.

115. Delsol G, Saati TA, Gatter KC, et al. Coexpression of epithelial membrane (EMA), Ki-1, and interleukin-2 receptor by anaplastic large cell lymphomas: Diagnostic value in so-called malignant histiocytosis. Am J Pathol 1988;130:59–70.

116. Marglin SI, Soulen RL, Blank N, Castellino RA: Mycosis fungoides: Radiographic manifestations of extracutaneous intrathoracic involvement. Radiology 1979;130:35–37.

117. Wolfe JD, Trevor ED, Kjeldsberg CR. Pulmonary manifestations of mycosis fungoides. Cancer 1980;46:2648–2653.

118. Carter D, Eggleston JC. Tumors of the lower respiratory tract. Atlas of tumor pathology, Ser. II, Fasc. 17. Washington DC: Armed Forces Institute of Pathology, 1980:270–272.

119. Amin R. Extramedullary plasmacytoma of the lung. Cancer 1985;56:152–156.

120. Roikjaer O, Thomsen JK. Plasmacytoma of the lung. A case report describing two tumors of different immunologic type in a single patient. Cancer 1986;58:2671–2674.

121. Garewal H, Durie BGM. Aggressive phase of multiple myeloma with pulmonary plasma cell infiltrates. Case reports. JAMA 1982;248:1875–1876.

122. Case records of the Massachusetts General Hospital, Case 17-1984. N Engl J Med 1984;310:1103–1112.

123. Gabriel S. Multiple myeloma presenting as pulmonary infiltration. Dis Chest 1965;47:123–126.

124. Kijner CH, Yousem SA. Systemic light chain deposition disease presenting as multiple pulmonary nodules. Am J Surg Pathol 1988;12:405–413.

125. Kaplan HS. Hodgkin's disease. Cambridge: Harvard, 1972.

126. Bellotti M, Elsner B, Esteva H, Mackinlay TA. Fiberoptic bronchoscopy in the diagnosis of pulmonary lymphomas. Respiration 1987;52:201–204.

127. Rose RM, Grigas D, Strattemeier E, Harris NL, Linggood RM. Endobronchial involvement with non-Hogkin's lymphoma. Cancer 1986;57:1750–1755.

128. Dugdale DC, Salness TA, Knight L, Charan NB. Endobronchial granulocytic sarcoma causing acute respiratory failure in acute myelogenous leukemia. Am Rev Respir Dis 1987;136:1248–1250.

129. Snyder LS, Cherwitz DL, Dykoski RK, Rice KL. Endobronchial Richter's syndrome. A rare manifestation of chronic lymphocytic leukemia. Am Rev Respir Dis 1988;136:980–983.

130. Ieki R, Goto J, Kouzai Y, Morisaki T, Asano S, Shimada K, Takaku F. Endobronchial non-Hodgkin's lymphoma. Respir Med 1989;83:87–89.

131. Kilgore TL, Chasen MH. Endobronchial non-Hodgkin's lymphoma. Chest 1983;84:58–61.

132. Miller KS, Sahn SA. Mycosis fungoides presenting as ARDS and diagnosed by bronchoalveolar lavage. Radio-

graphic and pathologic pulmonary manifestations. Chest 1986;89:312–314.

133. Oka M, Kawano K, Kanda T, Hara K. Bronchoalveolar lavage in primary pulmonary lymphoma with monoclonal gammopathy. Am Rev Respir Dis 1988;137:957–959.

134. Riazmontazer N, Bedayat G. Cytology of plasma cell myeloma in bronchial washing. Acta Cytol 1989;33:519–522.

135. Wisecarver J, Ness MJ, Rennard SI, Thompson AB, Armitage JO, Linder J. Bronchoalveolar lavage in the assessment of pulmonary Hodgkin's disease. Acta Cytol 1989;33:527–532.

CHAPTER 32

Common Neoplasms

SAMUEL P. HAMMAR

Lung cancer remains the most frequently diagnosed malignant neoplasm throughout the world and is the number one cause of cancer death in the American male and female. It is responsible for about 25% of all cancer deaths[1] and about 6% of all deaths in the United States.[2] Since 1930, more people have died from lung cancer than all other types of cancer combined.[3] An estimated 161,000 will be diagnosed in the United States in 1991 with an approximate 143,000 deaths.[4]

The four main histopathologic types of lung neoplasms—adenocarcinoma, squamous carcinoma, large cell undifferentiated carcinoma, and small cell undifferentiated carcinoma—account for more than 95% of diagnosed cases[5-7] and are discussed in this chapter. The spectrum of neuroendocrine lung neoplasms is also discussed in this chapter.

Incidence

In the United States, age-adjusted lung cancer death rates in men have risen from 11 per 100,000 population in 1940 to 73 per 100,000 population in 1982. The death rate has recently leveled off and in 1987 was 74 per 100,000 population.[8] In women the lung cancer death rate began rising in the early 1960s from 6 per 100,000 population to 28 per 100,000 population in 1987. Fortunately, lung cancer rates started to decline in men aged 35–44 years in 1970 and in men aged 45–54 years in the early 1980s, with a leveling-off of the mortality rate in men aged 55–64 years.[8-10] In women, the rate of lung cancer in those 55 years old and greater continues to increase although there has been a decrease incidence rate in the 35- to 44-year-old group beginning in the 1980s and a leveling-off in the 45- to

54-year-old group.[8-10] Even if all cigarette smokers were to quit smoking in 1992, it would be 20 years before the resulting decrease in mortality from lung cancer would be completely evident. Age-adjusted death rates for lung cancer in other countries in years 1975 and 1980–1981 are shown in Tables 32–1 through 32–3 and Fig. 32–1.[11-13] In 1975, stomach cancer was estimated to be the most common global malignancy with lung cancer in second place. Lung cancer has now surpassed stomach cancer as the most frequent malignant neoplasm worldwide. In the former Soviet Union, for example, a 55% increase in lung cancer was reported between 1970 and 1980.[14]

Lung Cancer in Women

Lung cancer rates in women have risen dramatically worldwide, including the United States.[15-22] The increase began in about 1935, and the age-adjusted death rate doubled between 1965 and 1974.[23] This contrasts with most other cancers in which there has been minimal or no increase in death rates.[24] In the state of Washington (United States), the incidence of breast cancer deaths between 1972 and 1981 stayed stable at a rate of 28.1 to 27.3 deaths per 100,000 women whereas the lung cancer death rate increased from 13.5 to 29.5 deaths per 100,000 women.[25] The incidence of lung cancer deaths in males in Washington State has been relatively stable since 1974 at approximately 61 deaths per 100,000 men.[25] Andrews and colleagues[26] reported the Lahey Clinic experience of lung cancer in women between 1957 and 1980. The incidence increased from 13% in 1957, with a male-to-female ratio of 6.8:1, to 35% in 1977–1980, with a male-female ratio of 1.8:1.

Lung cancer has now surpassed breast cancer as the

Table 32–1. Worldwide incidence of lung cancer, 1975[a]

	Male	Female
1. Northern Europe	93 (1)	23 (1)
2. Western Europe	87 (2)	11 (5)
3. North America	68 (3)	21 (2)
4. Southern Europe	62 (4)	13 (3)
5. Australia/New Zealand	57 (6)	12 (4)
6. Eastern Europe	59 (5)	8.5 (8)
7. U.S.S.R.	43 (7)	10 (6)
8. Carribean	35 (9)	12 (4)
9. Temperate South America	39 (8)	7 (9)
10. Japan	24 (10)	9 (7)
11. Eastern South Asia	17 (12)	6 (10)
12. Southern Africa	19 (11)	3 (12)
13. Other East Asia	13 (13)	5 (11)
14. China	11 (14)	5 (11)
15. Tropical South America	11 (15)	3 (13)
16. Western South Asia	11 (15)	2.5 (15)
17. Middle America	7.5 (17)	3 (14)
18. Micronesia/Polynesia	8 (16)	2 (16)
19. Middle South Asia	6 (18)	1.5 (17)
20. Melanesia	4 (19)	1 (18)
21. Middle Africa	2.5 (20)	1 (18)
22. Northern Africa	2.5 (20)	0.6 (19)
23. East Africa	2 (21)	0.4 (21)
24. Western Africa	0.9 (22)	0.5 (20)

[a] Incidence per 100,000 population, listed in decreasing order of incidence. Numbers in parentheses indicate relative rank.

Table 32–2. Worldwide incidence of lung cancer, 1980–1981[a]

	Male	Female
1. Scotland	109.6 (1)	28.1 (2)
2. England and Wales	92.5 (3)	21.9 (5)
3. Netherlands	103.2 (2)	7.9 (26)
4. Hong Kong	71.9 (8)	29.7 (1)
5. Luxembourg	89.7 (4)	9.8 (16)
6. Singapore	72.5 (7)	23.4 (4)
7. Finland	86.9 (5)	8.1 (24)
8. United States	71.6 (9)	21.4 (6)
9. Denmark	70.6 (11)	18.7 (7)
10. Hungary	76.1 (6)	12.8 (12)
11. Northern Ireland	71.6 (9)	17.3 (9)
12. Canada	68.4 (12)	16.6 (11)
13. New Zealand	65.9 (15)	17.2 (10)
14. Australia	65.1 (17)	12.2 (13)
15. Poland	68.4 (12)	8.9 (21)
16. Ireland	58.5 (21)	18.7 (7)
17. Austria	65.9 (15)	9.7 (17)
18. Italy	67 (14)	7.6 (28)
19. Germany, F.R.	65 (18)	7.6 (28)
20. Malta and Gozo	63.7 (19)	8.4 (22)
21. Switzerland	62 (20)	6.8 (34)
22. Greece	56.4 (22)	7.7 (27)
23. France	53.7 (23)	5 (36)
24. Iceland	30.7 (31)	27.1 (3)
25. Yugoslavia	48.7 (24)	8.1 (24)
26. Bulgaria	42.9 (25)	7.3 (31)
27. Romania	38.7 (26)	7.6 (28)
28. Israel	34.8 (27)	11.1 (15)
29. Japan	33.7 (29)	9.5 (20)
30. Kuwait	30.6 (32)	12.6 (14)
31. Sweden	32.5 (30)	9.7 (17)
32. Norway	34.7 (28)	7.2 (32)
33. Chile	26.6 (35)	7.1 (33)
34. Mauritius	27.1 (33)	4.0 (39)
35. Puerto Rico	19.4 (38)	9.7 (17)
36. Panama	23.7 (36)	6.1 (35)
37. Bahamas	27.1 (33)	1.4 (45)
38. Barbados	22 (37)	4.3 (38)
39. Costa Rica	17.9 (39)	8.2 (23)
40. Suriname	16.7 (40)	2.8 (41)
41. Paraguay	12.5 (41)	4.5 (37)
42. Cape Verde	6.7 (44)	4 (39)
43. Thailand	8 (42)	2.4 (42)
44. Brazil	7.5 (43)	2.2 (43)
45. El Salvador	2.6 (46)	2.2 (44)
46. Guatemala	3.1 (45)	1.3 (46)
47. Syrian Arab Republic	2.2 (27)	0.7 (47)

[a] Incidence per 100,000 population, listed in decreasing order of incidence. Numbers in parentheses indicate relative rank.

Reprinted with permission of The American Cancer Society. From S. Werbeg et al. Cancer Statistics 1987. Ca-A Cancer Journal for Clinicians 1987;37:2–19.

leading cause of cancer death in women in several states in the United States.[21,27–28]

McDuffie et al.[29] studied differences between female and male patients with primary lung cancer using a mailed questionnaire and data from the Saskatchewan Cancer Foundation Tumour Registry. In their evaluation of 730 men and 197 women, women were more frequently diagnosed with lung cancer before age 60 years (42%) than were men (25.6%) (p = .001) and were significantly more likely to be lifetime nonsmokers of cigarettes than men (23% vs. 3.7%; p = .05). They also found that women developed lung cancer after fewer years of smoking than men.

Osann,[30] using a case control type study, evaluated the importance of cigarette smoking, family history of lung cancer, and a medical history of repiratory disease in 217 women diagnosed with primary carcinoma of the lung between 1969 and 1977 at northern California Kaiser hospitals. As observed in other studies of female lung cancer, adenocarcinoma was the cell type most frequently diagnosed in the cigarette smokers (33%) and nonsmokers (67%). Osann also found an increased risk of developing lung cancer in those women with a family history of cancer and evidence of chronic ob-

Table 32–3. Classification by cell type of 230 primary lung tumors in children[a]

Type of tumor	Number of patients
Benign (n = 79)	
Inflammatory pseudotumor	45
Harmartoma	15
Neurogenic tumor	9
Leiomyoma	6
Mucous gland adenoma	2
Myoblastoma	2
Malignant (n = 151)	
Bronchial "adenoma"	65
Bronchogenic carcinoma	47
Pulmonary blastoma	14
Leiomyosarcoma	9
Rhabdomyosarcoma	6
Hemangiopericytoma	3
Lymphoma	3
Teratoma	2
Plasmacytoma	1
Myxosarcoma	1

[a] Reproduced with permission of publisher. From Hartman GE, Shochat SJ. Primary pulmonary neoplasms of childhood: a review. Ann Thorac Surg 1983;36:108–119.

structive pulmonary disease (chronic bronchitis and emphysema).

Lung Cancer in Young Adults

Lung cancer in young adults has been well documented.[31–42] More than 300 cases have been reported in persons less than 45 years old, ranging from 11 to 45 years of age. Roviaro et al.[42] reviewed their records of 1,514 cases of lung cancer between 1967 and 1980 and found 155 cases (10%) in persons less than 45 years old. They concluded that there had been no percentage increase in lung cancer in the young and no significant difference in survival rates in those less than 45 years old versus those older than 45 years. In several of these reports documenting carcinoma of the lung in young patients, a relatively greater proportion of females, when compared to the general population with lung cancer, was noted.[32,36–39]

McDuffie et al.[43] evaluated 2,800 patients registered as having primary carcinoma of the lung (2,129 men and 671 women) and divided the group into those who were diagnosed with lung cancer at younger than 50 or older than 50 years of age; 187 patients (101 men and 86 women) were 50 years old or less. The male-to-female ratio was lower (1.7) in the younger age group compared to the older age group (3.47). Adenocarcinoma was the most frequent cell type in the younger age group and squamous carcinoma was most frequent in

the older age group. In the younger age group, 85% were current or ex-smokers compared to 78% in the older age group. A positive family history of lung cancer or other types of lung cancer had no effect of presentation of lung cancer at a younger age, nor did the presence of other conditions affecting the lungs.

Jubelirer and Wilson[44] reviewed the features of 52 patients less than 40 years old with primary lung cancer diagnosed between 1965 and 1985. The ages of the patients ranged between 20 to 39 years with a median age of 36 years. There were 35 men and 17 women in the group, which indicated a significantly lower male:female ratio than in the over-40 age group with lung cancer. Like McDuffie et al.[43] these authors found an increased number of women, a preponderance of adenocarcinomas, and a similar resectability rate of those patients aged over 40 years. They found no significant difference in survival rates in the younger versus the older age group.

Bourke et al.[45] performed a study to characterize the clinical and pathologic features of carcinoma of the lung in patients 45 years old or less; to compare and contrast these features in patients with lung cancer older than 45 years; and to determine if the clinical and pathologic features and prognosis of lung cancer in those less than 45 years old was similar in different parts of the world. Medical centers in Chicago, northern Israel, and northern Italy were involved in the study, which consisted of identifying patients less than 45 years old from tumor registry records, pathology reports, and hospital charts and comparing them with patients older than 45 years having primary lung cancer.

In Chicago, 102 patients less than 45 years with lung cancer, 8% of the total of 1,327 patients with lung cancer, were identified between 1977 and 1988. Nineteen of the 102 patients were rejected for various reasons. No differences were found between the younger and the older patients with regard to gender, race, smoking history, and family history of cancer, although there was a trend of more male subjects in the younger group. More than 90% of the patients in both groups were cigarette smokers. There were slight differences in presenting symptoms between the younger and the older groups, and the youger patients had a longer duration of symptoms before a diagnosis of lung cancer was made; also, fewer younger patients were asymptomatic at the time of diagnosis. As determined by chest radiographs, the younger patients had more lower-lobe lesions, and also had more advanced disease at presentation with only 14% having stage I or II disease and 46% having metastatic disease (stage IV) at presentation. Adenocarcinoma was the leading cell type in both age groups, but adenocarcinoma occurred in

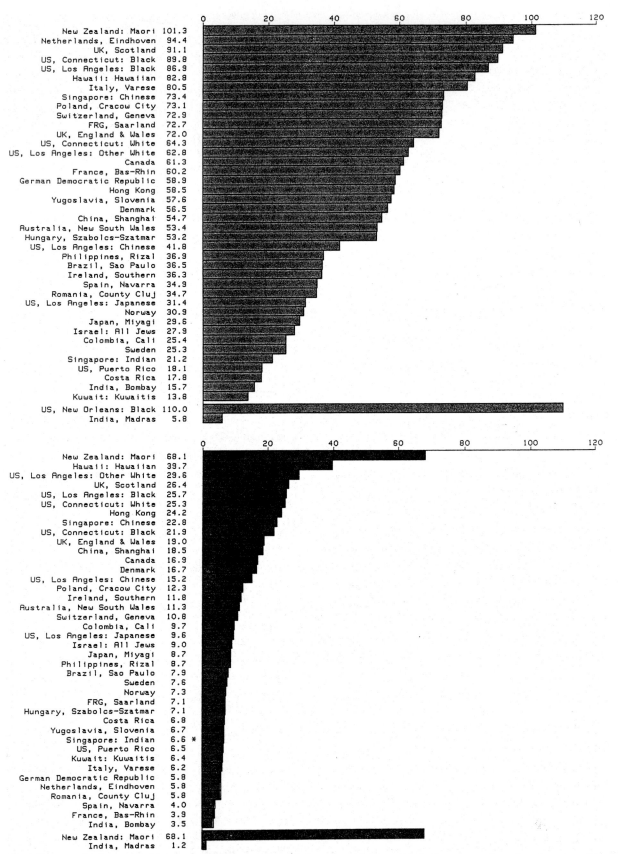

Fig. 32–1. Bar graph shows relative rates of lung cancer throughout world. (Asterisk indicates rate based on less than 10 cases. Reprinted by permission from Whelan SL, Parkin DM, Masuyer E (eds). Patterns of cancer incidence in five continents: a picture book. IARC Scientific Publications, #102, World Health Organization, Lyon, 1990.)

69% of the younger age group and 44% in the older patients. Survival was lower in the younger patients; only 8% were alive after 5 years versus 25% for the older age group.

In northern Israel, 43 younger and 476 older patients were available for review between 1977 and 1988. Approximately 75% of the patients in both groups were male, and 81% of the younger and 84% of the older patients were chronic cigarette smokers. Local and systemic symptoms were similar in both age groups, and most of the neoplasms were in the upper lobes (59% in younger, 52% in older patients). Of the younger patients, 56% had adenocarcinoma and only 18% had squamous carcinoma, whereas 39% of the older patients had squamous carcinoma and 32% adenocarcinoma. In both groups, 81% of the patients had either stage III or IV disease although there were more younger patients with stage I disease. In contrast to the Chicago groups, 26% of the younger patients and 8% of the older patients were alive at the end of 5 years after diagnosis.

In northern Italy, only limited data were available so a full comparison could not be made, but 52 patients less than 45 years old were identified, of which 90% were males and 81% cigarette smokers. Symptoms were present for a longer time in the younger age group from Italy compared to those of northern Israel and Chicago. Squamous carcinoma was the most common neoplasm in the younger Italian patients and 32% were diagnosed as having stage I or II disease. Survival rate was poor, with a median survival of 5 months for those with stage III and IV disease. Of the 17 patients with stage I or II disease, only 2 survived 2 or more years with 1 patient alive more than 5 years after diagnosis.

The authors concluded that differences exist in the clinical characteristics, pathologic features, and prognosis of younger and older patients with primary carcinoma of the lung from the same region and of younger patients from different geographical regions. As would be expected, stage of disease was the most important prognostic factor.

Lung Cancer in Children

Lung cancer in children is rare. In a review of 4,000 cases of carcinoma of the lung, Fontenelle[46] reported and incidence of 0.16% in the first decade of life and 0.7% in the second decade of life. Hartman and Shochat[47] reviewed 230 lung tumors in children and found that two thirds of these were bronchial adenomas (carcinoid, mucoepidermoid carcinoma, adenoid cystic carcinoma), plasma cell granulomas (inflammatory pseudotumors), or primary carcinoma of the lung (see Table 32–3). Of these three groups, primary carcinoma of the lung is second in frequency to the "bronchial adenoma" group and makes up about one-third of primary malignant neoplasms in children. There is an equal sex distribution in childhood lung cancer, and the etiology of these neoplasms is unknown. In the review by Hartman and Shochat,[47] adenocarcinoma and small cell undifferentiated carcinoma represented 80% of the primary lung cancers whereas squamous carcinoma made up only 12%. The majority of children with primary lung cancers are symptomatic and, in general, have a poor prognosis related primarily to the stage of the disease.[48–52]

Etiology—Epidemiology

Cigarette Smoke

Cigarette smoking is the single most important factor in the causes of lung cancer. Tobacco exposure is such an important health issue that Chapter 25 has been devoted to this subject. Between 80% and 85% of deaths from lung cancer are directly attributable to cigarette smoking.[53] In a recently published study in which smoking habits in 2,668 patients diagnosed as having lung cancer were examined, only 1.9% of men and 13.0% of women were nonsmokers.[54] As early as 1941, Ochsner and DeBakey[55] drew attention to the rising prevalence of lung cancer and increased consumption of cigarettes. In 1950 Wynder and Graham[56] published their now-classic article correlating tobacco smoking and carcinoma of the lung. They performed an accurate retrospective study of the smoking habits of 684 patients with proven cases of carcinoma of lung from many different locations in the United States, and found that 96.5% of 605 patients with lung cancer (excluding adenocarcinoma) were heavy cigarette smokers, usually of 20 or more years duration. Their findings suggested the currently recognized latent period of 20 to 25 years, which explains the highest incidence of lung cancer in persons between ages 45 and 70. Their report also referenced the substantial evidence before this time suggesting a link between cigarette smoking and lung cancer.

E. Cuyler Hammond and Daniel Horn[57] published a now-famous prospective study concerning smoking and death rates in 187,783 men aged 50 to 69 years who were followed between May 31, 1952 and October 31, 1955 in which they reported a startling association between excess death rate and cigarette smoking. They found a total of 7,316 deaths among cigarette smokers, which represented an excess of 2,665 deaths compared to the nonsmokers. Lung cancer accounted for 13.5% (988) of the deaths, and the ratio of the observed versus

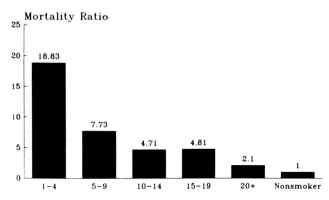

Number of Years Stopped Smoking

Fig. 32–2. Lung cancer mortality ratio for male former smokers. (From "Reducing the health consequences of smoking: 25 years of progress. A report of the Surgeon General. U.S. Department of Health and Human Services. DSHS Publication Number (CDC) 89-8411, 1989.)

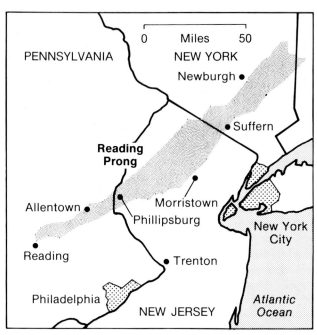

Fig. 32–3. Dotted region is referred to as the Reading Prong, a naturally occurring radiation "hot spot" in the United States of America. (Copyright 1985 by Consumers Union of United States, Inc., Mount Vernon, NY 10553. Reprinted by permission from CONSUMER REPORTS, October 1985.)

the expected death rates in men smoking one pack of cigarettes per day was between 23 and 88. Rogot and Murray[58] found a mortality ratio (observed/expected) of 11.29 in cigarette-smoking United States veterans studied for 16 years. As recently pointed out by Pollin and Ravenholt,[59] cigarette smoking, when measured by morbidity and mortality, is the most serious and widespread drug addiction in the world.

Guyatt and Newhouse[60] have also reviewed the evidence showing a causal relationship between cigarette smoking and lung cancer. As reported by these authors, a dose–response correlation between smoking and lung cancer has been shown in eight prospective studies. This report elucidates some of the weaknesses and inconsistencies in the reported prospective studies. In the reports of persons with lung cancer who were less than 45 years old and whose smoking habits were documented, 87%–100% were cigarette smokers.[31,33,37–48]

Shopland et al.[61] reviewed and analyzed the American Cancer Society prospective study of 1.2 million men and women and found that mortality risk among smokers increased for most of the eight major cancer sites associated with cigarette smoking. Lung cancer risk for male smokers was found to double and for female smokers to increase fourfold. Despite the evidence indicating a decline in the incidence of lung cancer, the carcinogens in cigarette smoke were projected to contribute to approximately 157,000 of the 514,000 total cancer deaths expected to occur in the United States in 1991. The data suggested that cigarette smoking contributed to 21.5% of cancer deaths in women and 45% in men. The data also indicated that lung cancer displaced coronary heart disease as the single leading cause of excess mortality in the United States.

One note of good news is found in the study of Peto

and Doll.[52] Although there were many variables that were difficult to control, they found that a steady decrease in lung cancer mortality ratios of British doctors who stopped smoking; 15 years after stopping, the mortality ratio was 2 compared to 15.8 in active smokers. The surgeon general's report[63] has reviewed the beneficial effect of stopping the smoking of cigarettes (Fig. 32–2).

Involuntary or passive smoking has now been proven as a cause of lung cancer in nonsmokers.[64–66] The Surgeon General's Report concluded that passive smoke exposure (defined as exposure to tobacco combustion products in the indoor environment) was related to respiratory symptoms and illnesses in young children, a modest but real reduction in lung function in children, and an increase in lung cancer in nonsmoking adults. The report further indicated that separation of smokers from nonsmokers in the work environment did not completely reduce the risk of exposure because the environments often shared ventilatory systems that used processes which recirculated the air. Janerich et al.[67] evaluated whether lung cancer was associated with exposure to tobacco smoke within the household by conducting a population-based study of 191 patients with histologically proven lung cancer who had never smoked. They found that household exposure to 25 or more smoker-years during childhood and adolescence doubled the risk of lung cancer. They concluded that approximately 17% of lung cancer among nonsmokers could be attributed to high levels of exposure to cigarette smoke during childhood and adolescence.

The effect, if any, on lung cancer mortality rates of low tar–low nicotine cigarettes is also uncertain. Cigarette-smoking machines measure tar and nicotine concentrations in cigarettes in a manner that does not accurately reflect actual concentrations of these substances as delivered to the lungs and blood of persons when smoking cigarettes. In real life, the number of puffs and volume of inhaled smoke per puff greatly vary the tar and nicotine yield of cigarettes.[68] Benowitz et al.[69] measured the nicotine content in commercial cigarettes with different reported yields of nicotine intake in cigarette smokers as indicated by their blood concentration of the nicotine metabolite cotinine. They found an inverse relationship between the nicotine content of cigarette tobacco and the nicotine yield in smoke as measured by a smoking machine. Blood cotinine concentration correlated with number of cigarettes smoked per day, but not with nicotine yield as measured by smoking machines.[69]

Despite these data, information has been published suggesting that low tar–low nicotine cigarettes are safer with respect to the development of lung cancer than cigarettes with higher concentrations of tar and nicotine. Auerbach et al.[70] compared the histologic changes (basal cell hyperplasia, loss of cilia, degree of dysplasia) in bronchial epithelium of cigarette smokers who died between 1955 and 1960 versus those dying between 1970 and 1977 (low tar–low nicotine cigarettes were introduced in the late 1960s and early 1970s). They found abnormal histologic changes in 0 nonsmokers, in 2.6% of those smoking 1–19 cigarettes per day, in 13.2% of those smoking 20–39 cigarettes per day, and in 22.5% of those smoking more than 40 cigarettes per day in persons dying between 1955 and 1960. In contrast, in those dying between 1970 and 1977, the percentages of abnormal changes in the same group were 0, 0.1%, 0.8%, and 2.2%, respectively. Auerbach et al.[70] suggested these significant differences resulted from the new generation of cigarettes that contained less tar and nicotine. More pertinent was a large study that followed more than 1 million smokers for 12 years.[71] Those who smoked low tar–low nicotine cigarettes (17.6–25.8 mg tar) had a 26% reduction in lung cancer mortality rates as compared to those who smoked high tar–high nicotine (25.8–35.7 mg tar) cigarettes.

Zang and Wynder[72] evaluated 1,274 patients with Kreyberg type I lung cancers (squamous carcinoma, small and large cell undifferentiated carcinomas) and 1,022 patients with Kreyberg type II (adenocarcinoma) lung cancers for lifetime exposure to tar from cigarette smoking by determining the different brands of cigarettes smoked, the number of days each brand of cigarette was smoked, the number of cigarettes of each brand consumed per day, and the concentration of tar of each cigarette as defined as that portion of the mainstream smoke of a machine-smoked cigarette that was retained on a glass fiber filter, minus nicotine and water. They found that cigarette smokers had a more than 20-fold increase in the frequency of Kreyberg type I lung cancers and a 6- to 7-fold increase in Kreyberg type II lung cancer compared to those who had never smoked. They also found a direct correlation between Kreyberg type I and II lung neoplasms and the lifetime tar exposure, although the association was much greater for the Keyberg type I tumors than for type II tumors. Based on their estimates of odds ratios associated with tar exposure, the authors projected an approximate 15%–20% decrease in Kreyberg type I lung cancer risk among long-term smokers who smoked heavily for every 10-mg decrease in tar in the cigarettes they smoked.

In 1982, Winters and DiFranza[73] published a letter to the editor of the New England Journal of Medicine entitled "Radioactivity in cigarette smoke" citing evidence the alpha-emitters polonium-210 and lead-210 were highly concentrated on tobacco trichomes and insolute particles in cigarette smoke. The radioactive particles accumulate at regions of bifurcation of segmental bronchi, a common site for the origin of squamous cell carcinomas. In a person smoking 1.5 packs of cigarettes per day, the radiation dose to the bronchial epithelium would be approximately 8,000 mrem per year, which is equivalent to the dose to the skin of 300 chest radiographs per year. They concluded that the radioactivity of cigarette smoke could be an effective carcinogen if a multiple mutation mechanism were operative. This short letter was greeted with a variety of responses, most of which supported the conclusions of Winter and DiFranza and concisely reviewed the literature relating lung cancer and other neoplasms to radiation exposure.[74–80]

This brief interchange focused attention on radiation as a possible important cause of lung cancer. Of further interest concerning the possible carcinogenic effect of radiation was the report of lung cancer in Navajo uranium miners.[81] In a total of 17 Navajo men diagnosed as having lung cancer between February 1965 and May 1979, 16 were uranium miners and only 2 of the uranium miners were cigarette smokers. Interestingly, 62.5% of these neoplasms were small cell undifferentiated carcinomas. This was followed by the report by Samet et al.[82] of 32 lung cancers in Navajo men between 1962 and 1982. Of the 32 patients, 23 (72%) had been employed as uranium miners. Of these, only 8 were nonsmokers, but the median cigarette consumption of the smokers was only one to three cigarettes daily.

Other reports confirmed the apparent excess risk of lung cancer in persons exposed to radon, the gaseous product of radium decay.[83–85] Radon has a half-life of 3.8 days and decays into two solid alpha-emitting particles or radon daughters that are deposited on dust and other particles inhaled into the bronchial tree. Radon is being suggested as the most likely causative agent for the 10%–15% of lung cancers that occur in nonsmokers. Well-insulated, airtight homes, for example, apparently trap radon that would ordinarily disperse into the atmosphere. There are certain radon hot spots in the United States and probably throughout the world. In the United States, the most publicized radon hot spot is a subterranean rock formation referred to as Reading Prong (Fig. 32–3). Information concerning radon has reached lay publications,[86,87] and devices for detecting radon are being sold commercially.

The causal association between radon and lung cancer has been well documented.[88] Epidemiologic and animal studies show an increase risk of lung cancer with increasing exposure to radon or its decay products, and the epidemiologic data suggest synergism between radon decay products and cigarette smoke.[88] In September 1988, the administrator of the U.S. Environmental Protection Agency (E.P.A.) and the assistant surgeon general of the U.S. Public Health Service suggested that most houses in the United States be tested for radon. They characterized radon as the second major cause of lung cancer, contributing up to 20,000 deaths per year. In a survey of homes in seven states by the E.P.A., nearly one in three that were monitored with a short-term screening test had a radon level that exceeded 4 pCi per liter, the E.P.A.'s highest acceptable annual average concentration according to its publication "A Citizen's Guide to Radon."[89] However, Samet and Nero[90] concluded that the E.P.A. estimate that one in three homes had an unacceptable radon level reflected a bias in the test protocol. They also indicated that the quantitative relation between exposure to radon or its decay products and the risk of developing lung cancer had not been described precisely, and there was continued uncertainty about how age, sex, cigarette smoke, and other factors affected the risk. They also questioned the validity of extrapolating risk estimates to the general public from studies of miners and concluded that any standard for an acceptable radon concentration in indoor air was subject to question.

Occupational Factors

There are several other etiologic factors important in the development of lung cancer. Most of these are occupation-related factors, and, as correctly pointed out by Vena et al.,[91] multiple factors are frequently operable. For example, cigarette smoking and asbestos exposure, and exposures to noxious agents, can be highly variable within a group of workers with the same occupation. Of all these occupational factors, more has been written about asbestos exposure and lung cancer than any other. (See Chapter 28). This in part is because there are numerous possible asbestos-related lung cancer cases under litigation, the most controversial of which are lung carcinomas in heavy cigarette smokers with a poorly documented or short history of exposure to asbestos.

Most of the studies examining the interactions between asbestos exposure and cigarette smoking have shown a synergistic-multiplicative effect between cigarette smoking and asbestos exposure.[92,93] Unfortunately, persons with a history of occupational asbestos exposure are also usually cigarette smokers and it has been difficult to find large groups of nonsmoking persons with occupational asbestos exposure. Even the frequently quoted study of Hammond et al.,[94] found the ratio of observed to expected deaths in nonsmoking persons with 20+ years of occupational asbestos exposure was 5.33, but that increased relative risk was based on only four cases. The initial article published by Selikoff et al.[95] and a subsequent editorial by Selikof[96] stressed that most of lung cancer deaths in those occupationally exposed to asbestos will occur in cigarette smokers.

While some authors suggest that lung cancer cannot be designated as asbestos related without a diagnosis of asbestosis,[97,98] other have found an increased incidence of lung cancer in persons exposed to asbestos who do not have asbestosis.[99–101] In an experimental animal study using rats, a dose–response relationship was found for asbestos exposure and lung cancer[102]; a similar situation has been reported to occur in humans.[103] Cigarette smoke may exert its synergistic effect with asbestos by interfering with the clearance of asbestos[104] or causing increased penetration of asbestos fibers into airway walls.[105] (See Chapter 28.)

Occupational exposure to other agents has also been associated with carcinoma of the lung. Exposure to nickel compounds is usually associated with squamous cell carcinoma,[106] exposure to copper is associated with adenocarcinoma and small cell undifferentiated carcinoma,[107] exposure to beryllium is associated with adenocarcinoma and small cell undifferentiated carcinoma,[108] and exposure to arsenic and chromate is not associated with a specific cell type.[109,110] Among those exposed to various chemicals, small cell undifferentiated carcinoma occurs in those exposed to chloromethyl ether,[111] adenocarcinoma and large cell undifferentiated carcinoma in vinyl chloride workers,[112] and small cell undifferentiated carcinoma in those exposed to benzene[113] and in those working with mustard gas.[114] Benzene appears to be a potent carcinogen that principally causes hematopoietic neoplasms and primary lung cancer.[115–117]

In 1983, Dubrow and Wegman[118] published a review of epidemiologic studies relating occupation to various malignant neoplasms and identified 34 occupations with an excess risk of lung cancer, most of which were in the manufacturing and construction trades. Their study did not adequately control for cigarette smoking, which caused some concern about their results. Morabia et al.[119] reviewed 13 additional case-control studies that examined occupational risk factors for lung cancer, some of which confirmed the conclusions of Dubrow and Wegman.[118] According to Morabia et al.,[119] these additional studies were often limited by sample size and by distribution of occupations in the geographical area under study. Therefore, Morabia et al.[119] performed a multicenter case-control study of 24 hospitals in nine metropolitan areas in the United States. They matched 1,793 male lung cancer cases for race, age, hospital, year of interview, and cigarette smoking with two types of controls, cancer and noncancer hospital patients. They found that sheet metal workers and tinsmiths; cranemen, derrickmen and hoistmen; heated metal workers, construction laborers, and electricians; and bookbinders and related printing trade workers had a significant increase in risk of lung cancer that was independent of cigarette smoking. In all these occupations, the workers were exposed to confirmed or suspected carcinogens including asbestos, nickel, chromium, polycyclic aromatic hydrocarbons, and diesel exhaust.

Burns and Swanson[120] analyzed 5,935 incident lung cancer cases and 3,956 incident colon and rectum cancer referents. Their analysis included 43 usual occupational groups and 48 usual industry groups. The strengths of their study included outcome data from hospital abstracts of incident cancer cases rather than death certificates, a lifetime history of occupation obtained by interview rather than a single entry from death certificates, and a large number of lung cancer cases. They found a significantly elevated risk of lung cancer among excavating and mining workers, furnace workers, armed services personnel, agricultural workers, mechanics, painters, and drivers. Industries with a significant elevated risk of lung cancer included farming, mining, and primary ferrous metals manufacturing. Of interest was the finding that 5 of the occupations observed more often among lung cancer cases had probable exposure to diesel exhaust. With respect to diesel exhaust exposure, Guberan et al.[121] found an excess risk of lung cancer, stomach cancer, and rectal cancer among Geneva professional drivers and suggested that the excess risk of lung cancer was related to prolonged exposure to diesel or other petroleum exhaust emissions.

Viruses

Yousem et al.[122] studied the occurence of human papilloma virus (HPV) DNA in primary lung carcinomas and in squamous metaplasia of the bronchus using in situ hybridization techniques and commercially available biotyinylated DNA probes to HPV subtypes 6/11, 16/18, and 31/33/35. They reported HPV DNA in 6 of 20 cases of squamous cell carcinoma and 1 of 6 cases of large cell undifferentiated carcinoma. No HPV DNA was identified in 12 cases of adenocarcinoma or 16 cases of bronchioloalveolar cell carcinoma and 4 cases of small cell undifferentiated carcinoma. In the positive cases, they found 2 cases each of the 6/11 and 16/18 serotypes and 3 cases of the 31/33/35 serotypes. They also observed HPV DNA in regions of squamous metaplasia in 15% of positive tumor cases, especially in those that showed condylomatous atypia, and reported that 5.8% of random bronchial biopsies showing squamous metaplasia were positive for HPV DNA. The authors reviewed some of the literature concerning cancer causation by HPV, and suggested that their findings accentuated the possibility that HPV played a significant role in the development of carcinoma of the lung.

Lung cancer in persons with human immunodeficiency virus (HIV) infection has emerged as a concern because of reports of a variety of solid tumors in HIV-infected patients including multiple myeloma, breast carcinoma, colon carcinoma, testicular cancer, carcinoma of the pancreas, and brain cancer.[123–126] Sridhar et al.[127] performed a retrospective case-control study to determine if there were differences in age, sex, stage distribution, and in survival between HIV-positive and HIV-indeterminate lung cancer patients. They compared 19 HIV-positive men who had carcinoma of the lung (8 adenocarcinomas, 6 squamous carcinomas, 2 large cell undifferentiated carcinomas, 1 small cell undifferentiated carcinoma, and 1 adenosquamous carcinoma) with 1,335 HIV-indeterminate (presumably negative) lung cancer patients who were identified between 1977 and 1986. Each HIV-positive lung cancer patient was matched with 2 control lung cancer patients of the same race and stage of disease, and within 5 years (±) in age. Sixteen of the HIV-positive lung cancer patients were cigarette smokers, 1 was a nonsmoker, and for 2 HIV-positive patients the smoking history was not available; the HIV-positive patients had a median smoking history of 60 pack-years. The HIV-positive patients were significantly younger than the HIV-indeterminate patients (48 versus 61 years) but the histologic type of lung cancer and smoking history were similar in both groups. Survival data were available for 16 of the HIV-positive lung cancer patients, and these were compared with the 32 HIV-indeterminate matched control subjects. The median survival in the HIV-positive group was 3 months versus 10 months in the HIV-indeterminate group, which was statistically significant at $p = .002$.

This article was commented on in an editorial[128] that raised some interesting points. Even though there was no statistically significant difference in lung cancer cell type between the HIV-positive patients and the HIV-indeterminate controls, only 1 case of small cell undifferentiated carcinoma was reported in the HIV-positive group whereas in most larger series of lung cancer, small cell undifferentiated carcinoma constitutes about 25% of all lung cancers. This difference suggests that lung cancer cell type in HIV-positive patients should be followed carefully to see if this difference persists. Nine of the 19 HIV-positive lung cancer patients had no HIV-related opportunistic infections and as a group had a median CD4 lymphocyte count of $301/\mu$ liter, suggesting that immunodeficiency was not a cofactor in the pathogenesis of lung cancer; this finding further suggests that lung cancer, in contrast to other neoplasms that commonly occur in HIV-infected persons, occurs earlier in the course of the HIV infection. Additional studies are needed to evaluate the exact risk of lung cancer in HIV-positive individuals.

Genetic Factors

Because relatively few people who develop lung cancer are exposed to an occupation-associated carcinogen and since only about 10% of cigarette smokers develop lung cancer, other unknown factors appear operative. One such factor may be genetics. Do certain people have a genetic predisposition to cancer? Markman et al.[129] found that 52% of patients with small cell undifferentiated lung cancer possessed histocompatibility antigen type HLA-BW 44 (HLA-B12) compared to 26.1% of controls ($p < .001$). They suggested that the genetic material linked to the BW 44 allele could contribute to the establishment of a chromosomal abnormality (deletion 3p3), which has been identified in tumor cell lines established from patients with small cell undifferentiated carcinoma.[130]

Other investigations have also suggested that genetic factors may be important in lung cancer etiology. Several studies have shown an increased familial risk for cancer, and specifically lung cancer, among relatives of lung cancer patients.[131–137] One study[138] suggested an increased familial occurrence for small cell undifferentiated carcinoma.

Vitamin A (Retinol) and Beta-Carotene

Vitamin A and beta-carotene have received attention as possible cancer prevention agents.[139–143] In retrospective epidemiologic studies, persons with low serum concentrations or low dietary intake of beta-carotene and vitamin A have had an increased incidence of cancer compared to matched controls with high-to-normal serum concentrations of these substances. The administration of vitamin A and beta-carotene has prevented chemically induced cancers in animals, and has reversed preneoplastic changes in humans.[144–146] Several prospective intervention studies in human, using vitamin A and beta carotene to prevent cancer, are under way.[140,147]

Screening for Lung Cancer

The high incidence of lung cancer among chronic cigarette smokers raises the question as to whether some type of screening program of this high-risk group would reduce the mortality rate of lung cancer. Four studies begun in the 1950s and early 1960s, only two of which were controlled, attempted to determine if screening chest radiographs would reduce the mortality rate of lung cancer.[148–151] Each study differed in various ways, and not all patients enrolled were cigarette smokers. Only one study[149] showed a reduction in mortality rate from lung cancer. Three separate controlled screening programs sponsored by the National Cancer Institute (USA), all involving cigarette-smoking males 45 years or older, have subsequently been conducted.[152–154] The objectives of the screening programs were to determine whether the detection of lung cancer could be improved by combining modern sputum cytologic screening techniques with the examination of regularly taken chest radiographs, and to determine whether the mortality of lung cancer could be reduced by this screening program in conjunction with appropriate therapy.

In the Johns Hopkins Lung Project, 10,387 men were evaluated; in the Memorial Sloan-Kettering Study, 10,933 men, and in the Mayo Clinic Study, 10,933 men. The Johns Hopkins Lung Project and the Memorial Sloan Kettering project differed from the Mayo Clinic study in that the men were divided into a dual screen group (cytology plus chest radiograph) and a control group (chest radiograph only); all men in the Mayo Clinic Study were initially screened by both modalities and then divided into two groups, of which one was screened by chest radiograph and sputum cytology and the other was advised but not required to have annual radiography and sputum tests. A total of 223 prevalance cases were detected in the three programs. In the dual-screened group, 160 lung cancers were detected; 123 were detected radiographically (30 in this group were also detected cytologically) and 37 were identified by cytologic screening. Of the 10,233 men who had only chest radiographs for screening, 63 cases of lung cancer were found, which was nearly the same number detected by radiographs in the dual screened group. Thirty-five of the 37 cases of lung cancer detected by sputum cytology alone were squamous cell carcinomas. More than 50% of the lung cancers detected by radiographic examination of the chest were adenocarcinomas or large cell undifferentiated carcinomas, with the majority of these being peripheral. Approximately 40% of those tumors detected by chest radiograph examination were stage 1 whereas 81% of those detected by the cytology screen were stage 1. However, 95% of those detected by sputum cytology alone represented central squamous carcinomas.

The effect of screening program on the mortality of lung cancer is still uncertain and requires additional incidence data and long-term follow-up. Only the Memorial Sloan-Kettering study reported incidence findings after the initial prevalence data were collected. In the dual-screened group that had annual chest radiographs and 4-month sputum cytology examinations, 114 cases of lung cancer were detected in 8+ years (3.7 cases/1000 man-years); in those receiving annual chest radiographs, 121 new cases were found (3.8 cases/1000 man-years). Many problems inherent in these screening programs, such as cost and true benefit, have been raised.[155,156] Of particular interest was the finding of the Sloan-Kettering radiologists that 20%–30% of positive chest radiographs were missed if only one radiologist examined the films.[157] As a result, three radiologists currently read their screening chest radiographs.

The number-one question in all screening programs is whether they reduce mortality rates. The data presented to date suggest they do not. On the basis of lack of reduction in mortality and cost of screening, the American Cancer Society does not recommend annual screening chest radiographs. Fontana et al.[158] recently reviewed the Mayo Lung Cancer Screening Project. The Mayo Clinic trial compared offering chest radiography and sputum cytology every 4 months to offering advice that these two tests could be obtained once a year. This screening study demonstrated a significantly increased lung cancer detection, resectability, and survivorship in the group offered the screening every 4 months compared with the control group, although there was no significant difference in lung cancer mortality rates between the two groups. Based on the lack of difference in mortality rates, the authors concluded that the results did not justify recommending large-scale radiologic or cytologic screening for detecting early lung cancer at this time. A more practical approach has been advised by Dreis,[159] who suggested a yearly PA radiograph for any person over 50 who smokes one pack of cigarettes per day.

Staging of Lung Cancer

Of all the factors evaluated to date concerning lung cancer survival, tumor stage is most important.[160] This applies to small cell undifferentiated neuroendocrine carcinomas as well as non-small cell lung cancers.[161] Lung neoplasms, like other malignancies, are staged according to size (T designation), nodal metastases (N designation), and distant metastases (M designation) as follows (Table 32–4).[162]

The location of N1 and N2 are shown diagramatically in Fig. 32–4. This is referred to as the Naruke map.[163] Typically, the surgeon supplies the pathologist with paratracheal (numbers 2, 3, 4) and subcarinal nodes (number 7) that may be obtained via mediastinoscopy before thoracotomy. The resected lobe or lung usually contains hilar and bronchopulmonary nodes (numbers 10, 11, 12) that must be dissected from the specimen and submitted separately for accurate identification and evaluation.

Numerical values are also used in staging lung cancer (Table 32–5). A tumor with a numerical value of 2 or less is stage 1. A tumor with a numerical value of 3 is stage 2 (T2 N1 is the only combination for stage 2), and a lung neoplasm with a numerical value of 4 or greater is stage 3.

In 1986 Mountain[164] published a new international staging system for lung cancer based on the TNM system (Table 32–6). This new system is based on survival data of 3,753 patients with lung cancer that had been accurately staged according to the previously used TNM system. Because of the variation in survival rates, changes were made in the T and N descriptors as shown in Table 32–6 (compare to Table 32–4). This author is in agreement with this proposed new staging system, and it is his opinion that pathologists performing pathologic analysis of resected lung specimens containing neoplasms should provide, in the diagnosis or in a comment to the diagnosis, the TN designation of the tumor and the appropriate stage according to the new staging scheme. It should be mentioned that the M designation may be based on clinical and radiologic studies. Mountain et al.[165] provided an update on

Table 32–4. AJC definitions of TNM categories[a]

Primary Tumors

T Primary tumor.

TO No evidence of primary tumor.

TX Tumor proven by presence of malignant cells in bronchopulmonary secretions but not visualized roentgenographically or bronchoscopically

TIS Carcinoma in situ.

T1 Tumor that is 3.0 cm or less in greatest diameter, surrounded by lung or visceral pleura and without evidence of invasion proximal to a lobar bronchus at bronchoscopy.

T2 Tumor more than 3.0 cm in greatest diameter, or tumor of any size that invades the visceral pleura or is associated with atelectasis or obstructive pneumonitis and extends to the hilar region. At bronchoscopy, the proximal extent of demonstrable tumor must be within a lobar bronchus or at least 2.0 cm distal to the carnia. Any associated atelectasis or obstructive pneumonitis must involve less than an entire lung, and there must be no pleural effusion.

T3 Tumor of any size with direct extension into an adjacent structure, such as chest wall, diaphragm, or mediastinum and its contents, or tumor demonstrated bronchoscopically to involve a main bronchus less than 2.0 cm distal to the carina; any tumor associated with atelectasis or obstructive pneumonitis of an entire lung or pleural effusion.

Regional Lymph Nodes

N Regional lymph nodes

N0 No demonstrable metastasis to regional lymph nodes.

N1 Metastasis to lymph nodes in peribronchial and/or ipsilateral hilar region (including direct extension).

N2 Metastasis to lymph nodes in the mediastinum.

Distant Metastasis

M Distant metastasis.

M0 No distant metastasis.

M1 Distant metastasis, such as scalene, cervical, or contralateral hilar lymph nodes, brain, bones, lung, liver.

These categories of T, N, and M may be combined into the following groups or stages:

Occult Carcinoma

TX N0 M0 Occult carcinoma with bronchopulmonary secretions containing malignant cells but without other evidence of the primary tumor or evidence of metastasis.

Stage I

TIS N0 M0 Carcinoma in situ.

T1 N0 M0 Tumor that can be classified T1 without any metastasis to the regional lymph nodes.

T1 N1 M0 Tumor that can be classified T1 with metastasis to the lymph nodes in the ipsilateral hilar region only.

T2 N0 M0 Tumor that can be classified T2 without any metastasis to nodes or distant metastasis.

Note: TX N1 M0 and T0 N1 M0 are also theoretically possible, but such a clinical diagnosis would be difficult if not impossible to make. If such a diagnosis is made, it should be included in stage 1.

Stage II

T2 N1 M0 Tumor classified as T2 with metastasis to the lymph nodes in the ipsilateral hilar region only.

Stage III

T3 with any N or M Any tumor more extensive than T2.

N2 with any T or M Any tumor with metastasis to the lymph nodes in the mediastinum.

M1 with any T or N Any tumor with distant metastasis.

[a] Reprinted with permission from Seminars in Respiratory Medicine 1982; 3:154–163, Thieme Medical Publishers, Inc.

N2 Nodes

● Superior Mediastinal Nodes
  1. Highest Mediastinal
  2. Upper Paratracheal
  3. Pre- and Retrotracheal
  4. Lower Paratracheal
     (including Azygos Nodes)

● Aortic Nodes
  5. Subaortic (aortic window)
  6. Para-aortic (ascending aorta or phrenic)

● Inferior Mediastinal Nodes
  7. Subcarinal
  8. Paraesophageal (below carina)
  9. Pulmonary Ligament

N1 Nodes

10. Hilar
11. Interlobar
12. Lobar
13. Segmental

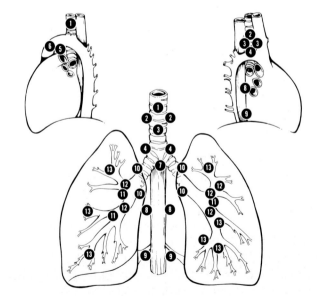

Fig. 32–4. Naruke lymph node map used by American Joint Commission for staging of primary carcinomas of the lung. Note locations of N1 and N2 lymph nodes. (Reprinted with permission.[168])

Table 32–5. Numerical values in the staging of lung cancer

Stage	Numerical value [a]
1	1–2
2	3
3	4 or greater

[a] Equivalents: T1–1 N0–0 M1–4
T2–2 N1–1
T3–4 N2–4

non-small cell carcinoma of the lung staging, more graphically illustrating the various stages (Fig. 32–5). Fernando and Goldstraw[166] compared the clinical stage with surgical/pathologic stage in 103 patients undergoing thoracotomy for carcinoma of the lung between 1985 and 1988. The T subsets were identical in 81.6% of patients, and the nodal status remained unchanged in 55.3% of patients. Preoperative evaluation underestimated more commonly than it overestimated anatomic stage. Bulzebruck et al.[167] performed a similar

study that evaluated 3,823 lung cancer patients prospectively for concordance between clinical and pathologic staging. They found an identical T designation in 63% of cases and 47% agreement in lymph node involvement, with an overall agreement in stage of 56%.

Several situations arise that can create confusion in staging lung cancers. These are as follows:

1. Designation of lymph nodes: Nodal map. The Naruke map as shown in Fig. 32–4 is the standard used in identifying the various lymph nodes in the previously used American Joint Commission (AJC) staging system and the new international staging system proposed by Mountain.[164] In 1983 Tisi et al.[168] drew attention to the fact that several studies had shown that a small but significant group of patients with stage 3 disease based on N2 nodes survived 5 years. They suggested that these reports raised the question as to whether there should be refinement of the location of the various lymph nodes based on computed tomography scanning of

Table 32–6. TNM definition[a]

Stage Grouping

Occult Carcinoma	TX	N0	M0
Stage 0	TIS	Carcinoma in situ	
Stage I	T1	N0	M0
	T2	N0	M0
Stage II	T1	N1	M0
	T2	N1	M0
Stage IIIa	T3	N0	M0
	T3	N1	M0
	T1–3	N2	M0
Stage IIIb	Any T	N3	M0
	T4	Any N	M0
Stage IV	Any T	Any N	M1

Nodal Involvement (N)

N0 No demonstrable metastasis to regional lymph nodes.

N1 Metastasis to lymph nodes in the peribronchial or the ipsilateral hilar region, or both, including direct extension.

N2 Metastasis to ipsilateral mediastinal lymph nodes and subcarinal lymph nodes.

N3 Metastasis to contralateral mediastinal lymph nodes, contralateral hilar lymph nodes, ipsilateral or contralateral scalene or supraclavicular lymph nodes.

Primary Tumor (T)

TX Tumor proven by the presence of malignant cells in bronchopulmonary secretions but not visualized

roentgenographically or bronchoscopically, or any tumor that cannot be assessed as in a retreatment staging.

TO No evidence of primary tumor

TIS Carcinoma in situ

T1 A tumor that is 3.0 cm or less in greatest dimension, surrounded by lung or visceral pleura, and without evidence of invasion proximal to a lobar bronchus at bronchoscopy.[b]

T2 A tumor more than 3.0 cm in greatest dimension, or a tumor of any size that either invades the visceral pleura or has associated atelectasis or obstructive pneumonitis extending to the hilar region. At bronchoscopy, the proximal extent of demonstrable tumor must be within a lobar bronchus or at least 2.0 cm distal to the carina. Any associated atelectasis or obstructive pneumonitis must involve less than an entire lung.

T3 A tumor of any size with direct extension into the chest wall (including superior sulcus tumors), diaphragm, or the mediastinal pleura or pericardium without involving the heart, great vessels, trachea, esophagus or vetebral body, or a tumor in the main bronchus within 2 cm of the carina without involving the carina.

T4 A tumor of any size with invasion of the mediastinum or involving heart, great vessels, trachea, esophagus, vetebral body or carina or presence of malignant pleural effusion.[c]

[a] Reprinted with permission.[164]

[b] T1. The uncommon superficial tumor of any size with its invasive component limited to the bronchial wall which may extend proximal to the main bronchus is classified as T1.

[c] T4. Most pleural effusions associated with lung cancer are due to tumor. There are, however, some few patients in whom cytopathologic examination of pleural fluid (on more than one specimen) is negative for tumor, the fluid is nonbloody and is not an exudate. In such cases where these elements and clinical judgment dictate that the effusion is not related to the tumor, the patients should be staged T1, T2 or T3, excluding effusion as a staging element.

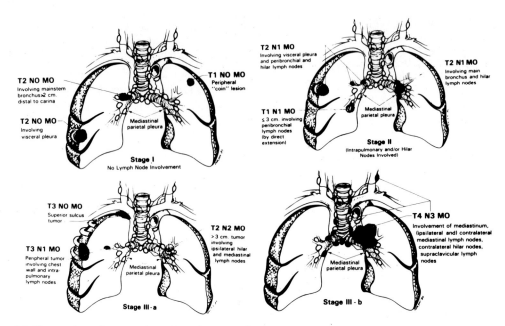

Fig. 32–5. Graphic illustration of currently accepted stages of lung cancer. (Reprinted with permission from Chest 1991; 99:1258–1260.)

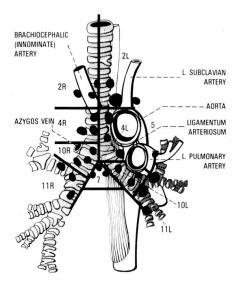

Fig. 32–6. Lymph node map proposed by American Thoracic Society committee for staging of primary lung cancers. Nodal areas 4 and 10 are thought to represent critical nodal areas in predicting resectability and survivorship. (Reprinted with permission.[168])

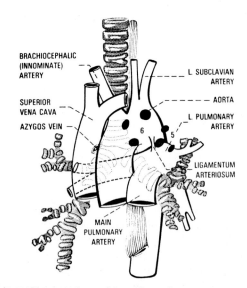

Fig. 32–7. Different view of lymph node map proposed by American Thoracic Society committee for staging of primary lung cancers. (Reprinted with permission.[168])

Table 32–7. Proposed definitions of regional nodal stations for prethoracotomy staging[a]

X	Supraclavicular nodes.
2R	Right-upper paratracheal (suprainnominate) nodes: nodes to the right of the midline of the trachea between the intersection of the caudal margin of the innominate artery with the trachea, and the apex of the lung. (Includes highest R mediastinal node). (Radiologists may use the same caudal margin as in 2L.)
2L	Left-upper paratracheal (supraaortic) nodes: nodes to the left of the midline of the trachea between the top of the aortic arch and the apex of the lung. (Includes highest L mediastinal node.)
4R	Right-lower paratracheal nodes: nodes to the right of the midline of the trachea between the cephalic border of the azygos vein and the intersection of the caudal margin of the brachiocephalic artery with the right side of the trachea. (Includes some pretracheal and paracaval nodes.) (Radiologists may use the same cephalic margin as in 4L.)
4L	Left-lower paratracheal nodes: nodes to the left of the midline of the trachea between the top of the aortic arch and the level of the carina, medial to the ligamentum arteriosum. (Includes some pretracheal nodes.)
5	Aortopulmonary nodes: subaortic and paraaortic nodes, lateral to the ligamentum arteriosum or the aorta or left pulmonary artery, proximal to the first branch of the LPA.
6	Anterior mediastinal nodes: nodes anterior to the ascending aorta or the innomin artery (Includes some pretracheal and preaortic nodes.)
7	Subcarinal nodes: nodes arising caudal to the carina of the trachea but not associated with the lower lobe bronchi or arteries within the lung.
8	Paraesophageal nodes: nodes dorsal to the posterior wall of the trachea and to the right or left of the midline of the esophagus. (Includes retrotracheal, but not subcarinal nodes.)
9	Right or left pulmonary ligament nodes: nodes within the right or left pulmonary ligament.
10R	Right tracheobronchial nodes: nodes to the right of the midline of the trachea from the level of the cephalic border of the azygos vein to the origin of the right upper-lobe bronchus.
10L	Left peribronchial nodes: nodes to the left of the midline of the trachea between the carina and the left upper lobe bronchus, medial to the ligamentum arteriosum.
11	Intrapulmonary nodes: nodes removed in the right or left lung specimen plus those distal to the mainstem bronchi or secondary carina. (Includes interlobar, lobar, and segmental nodes.)[b]

[a] Reprinted with permission.[168]
[b] Postthoracotomy staging: nodes could be divided into stations 11, 12, 13 according to the AJC classification.

the mediastinum and mediastinoscopy. They proposed a new map (Figs. 32–6 and 32–7) based on data obtained from mediastinoscopy and CT scanning of the mediastinum. They recommended new nodal mapping criteria based on recognizeable CT and mediastinoscopy landmarks (Table 32–7; Figs. 32–8 and 32–9). They proposed that nodal stations 2, 5, 6, 7, 8 and 9 (in Figs. 32–6 and 32–7) be considered N2 nodes and that nodal station 11 be considered an N1 node (same as used by AJC). They indicated that nodal station 4 and 10 represented critical areas in predicting resectability and survivorship and suggested that prospective data be collected to determine survivorship when such nodes were positive before they were assigned as either N1 or N2 status.

2. Pleural involvement by tumor (Figure 32–10) shows the various possible ways a lung neoplasm may involve the visceral and parietal pleural. The morphologic landmark used for the visceral pleura is the elastic lamina and the outer surface layer of mesothelial cells, which may be quite inconspicuous. The morphologic landmark for parietal pleural invasion is adipose tissue. Occasionally the visceral and parietal pleura will be fused and significantly thick-

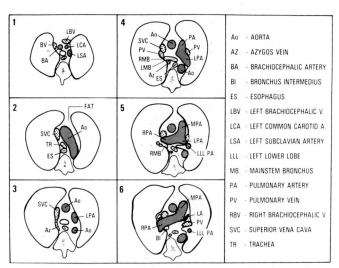

Fig. 32–8. Six representative transverse sections through area of regional pulmonary lymph nodes as obtained by CT scanning: (1) level of brachiocephalic vessels (innominate artery); (2) level of arch of aorta; (3) level of top of left main pulmonary artery; (4) level of bifurcation of left and right mainstem bronchi; (5) level of carina of trachea and bifurcation of right-upper-lobe bronchus; (6) level of bifurcation of bronchus intermedius. (Major anatomic structures identified in legend.) (Reprinted with permission.[168])

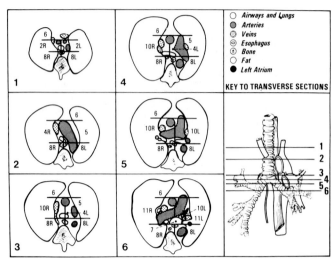

Fig. 32–9. Designation of nodal stations at each of six transverse sections of CT scan (key to level of transverse sections is presented in figure insert; symbols representing major anatomic structures also in figure insert). (Reprinted with permission.[168])

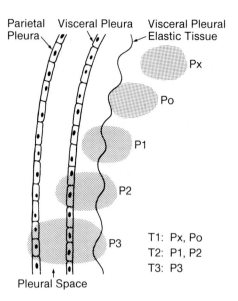

Fig. 32–10. Diagram shows possible types of pleural involvement by primary lung neoplasm. Note that Px and Po are designated T1; P1 and P2 are designated T2; P3 is T3 tumor.

ened; even in this situation one can still usually identify the parietal pleura by the presence of fat.

3. Pleural effusion with a negative pleural fluid cytology especially in the situation of an obstructive pneumonitis and pleural effusion caused by a proximal neoplasm; how is such a tumor staged? Decker et al.[169] reported on 73 patients with lung cancer and no prior therapy who had a cytologically negative ipsalateral pleural effusion by thoracentesis. Sixty-six patients were explored and all except 4 patients (94.5%) had surgically unresectable disease, indicating that even a pleural effusion negative for malignant cells was a poor prognostic sign.

4. A lung neoplasm less than 2 cm from the carina but with a bronchial margin of resection showing normal respiratory mucosa; how is this tumor staged? In years past, a tumor this close to the carina was considered unresectable although recent reports have shown that such neoplasms are resectable.[170–172] Such neoplasms frequently show direct nodal invasion, and survival rates are in the neighborhood of 20% although these tumors are still considered T3 lesions.

5. How are synchronous primary tumors of the lung designated with respect to T status? Synchronous primary tumors of the lung of different cell types are considered separate primary lung cancers and are staged independently. If the neoplasms are of the same cell type they are generally designated T2 or as T2 N1 if one neoplasm was considered to be metastatic from the other. Some pathologists designate

multiple tumors of the same cell type as TX, indicating that the T designation cannot be assessed.

Histologic Classification of Lung Cancer

The chronology and evolution of the histologic classification of lung cancer is shown in Fig. 32–11. The second edition of the World Health Organization's (WHO) histologic typing of lung tumors was published in 1982.[173] This classification is shown in association with that used by the Lung Cancer Study Group in Table 32–8. The numbers associated with the WHO classification correspond to the morphology codes of the International Classification of Disease for Oncology (ICD-O, 1976) and the Systematized Nomenclature of Medicine (SNOMED). The numbers in association with the Lung Cancer Study Group diagnoses were developed by the Working Party for the Study of Lung Cancer that was operative in the 1960s and 1970s; these numbers are occasionally still seen in publications concerning the pathologic features of lung neoplasms, for example, 22–40 (intermediate small cell–large cell undifferentiated carcinoma).

The histologic criteria used by the pathology section of the Lung Cancer Study Group for diagnosing common lung neoplasms are shown in Table 32–9; these are similar to those used by the World Health Organization. As a general rule common lung neoplasms are classified by the best-differentiated region of the tumor and are

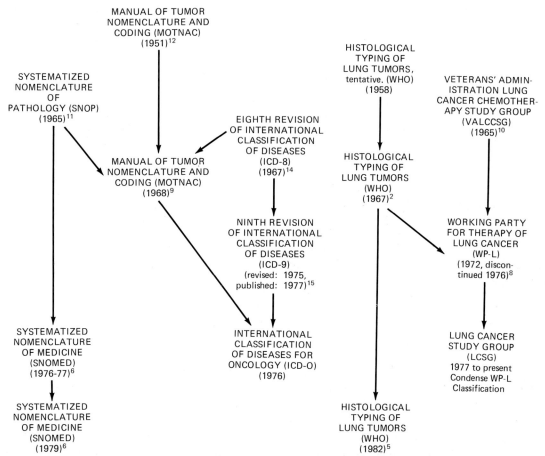

Fig. 32–11. Chronology and relationships among histologic classifications of carcinoma of the lung. The Manual of Tumor Nomenclature (MOTNAC) was first compiled and published in 1951 and revised in 1968 with the addition of the histologic code from Sections 8 and 9 of The Systematized Nomenclature of Pathology (SNOP, 1965) and the topographic code from Sections 140–99 in the Eighth Revision of the International Classification of Diseases (ICD-8, 1967). The SNOP was the first histologic code designed for computerization and used a 4-field organizational system, i.e., topography, morphology, etiology, and function. The SNOP was restructured and expanded into The Systematized Nomenclature of Medicine (SNOMED, 1976–77) with the addition of 2 fields: disease and procedures. The SNOMED was revised in 1979, and the morphology section dealing with neoplasms is identical to The International Classification of Diseases for Oncology (ICD-0, 1976), except that the ICD-0 provides for more subtypes. The ICD-0 represents an extension of Chapter 11 (Neoplasms) of The Ninth Revision of the International Classification of Diseases (ICD-9, 1975, 1977) and permits coding by topography, histology (morphology), and behavior as well as histologic grading and differentiation. Particular effort was made in developing the ICD-0 to use compatible terms for neoplasms listed in The International Histologic Classification of Tumours series also published by WHO. The Histological Typing of Lung Tumours (tentative version, 1958; published 1967) is the first of a series of "blue books" published by the World Health Organization (WHO) entitled The International Histological Classification of Tumours. The first revision of the WHO classification of lung tumors was published in 1982. The Veterans' Administration Lung Cancer Chemotherapy Study Group (VALCCSG) modified the WHO tentative (1958) histological classification in 1965. The Pathology Panel of the International Workshop for Therapy of Lung Cancer devised a classification in 1972, The Working Party for Therapy of Lung Cancer (WP-L), which was compatible both with the WHO Histological Typing of Lung Tumours (1967) and the VALCCSG classifications. The WP-L was discontinued in 1976 because chemotherapy was determined to be of little value (13) and the Lung Cancer Study Group (LCSG) replaced it in 1977. The LCSG uses a modified and condensed version of the WP-L. (Reprinted with permission from Ives JC, Buffler PA, Greenberg SD. Environmental association and histopathologic patterns of carcinoma of the lung: The challenge and dilemma in epidemiologic studies. Am Rev Respir Dis 1983;128:195–209.

Table 32–8. Histologic classification of lung tumors[a]

WHO[b]	WPL–LCSG[c]
	01—Carcinoma in situ
1. Squamous cell carcinoma (epidermoid carcinoma)	10—Squamous cell carcinoma
Variant:	11—Well-differentiated
a. Spindle cell (squamous carcinoma	12—Moderately differentiated
	13—Poorly differentiated
2. Small cell carcinoma	20—Small cell
a. Oat cell carcinoma	21—Lymphocyte-like/oat cell
b. Intermediate cell type	22—Intermediate
c. Combined oat cell carcinoma	
3. Adenocarcinoma	30—Adenocarcinoma
a. Acinar adenocarcinoma	31—Well-differentiated
b. Papillary adenocarcinoma	32—Moderately differentiated
c. Bronchioloalveolar carcinoma	33—Poorly differentiated
d. Solid carcinoma with mucus formation	34—Bronchiolar/alveolar
4. Large cell carcinoma	40—Large cell undifferentiated
Variants:	41—Giant cell
a. Giant cell carcinoma	
b. Clear cell carcinoma	
5. Adenosquamous carcinoma	50—Poorly differentiated carcinoma
6. Carcinoid	60—Bi/Multicomponent or Multidifferentiated
7. Bronchial gland carcinomas	70—Carcinoid
a. Adenoid cystic	
b. Mucoepidermoid carcinoma	
c. Others	
8. Others	80—Bronchial gland tumors
	81—Adenoid cystic
	82—Mucoepidermoid
	83—Mixed tumors

[a] Reprinted with permission.[173,453]
[b] WHO, World Health Organization. Adapted from Histological Typing of Lung Tumours. *Tumori* 67:253–272, 1981 (with permission). (1–3)
[c] WPL-LCSG, Working Party for the Study of Lung Cancer. Modified by Lung Cancer Study Group, National Cancer Institute.

Table 32–9. Histologic criteria used for diagnosing common lung neoplasms[a]

Squamous cell carcinoma
Keratin formation, keratin pearl formation, intercellular junctions (bridges, processes) located between adjacent cells. These junctions are referred to as "prickles" or "spines"

Adenocarcinoma
Definite gland formation or the presence of mucus production in a solid tumor, as determined by a mucosubstance special stain, e.g., PAS-D, mucicarmine

Undifferentiated large cell carcinoma
Large cells with vesicular nuclei and prominent eosinophilic nucleoli; no evidence of squamous or glandular differentiation; negative for mucin stain

Multicomponent tumor, e.g., mixed squamous cell and adenocarcinoma
Tumors composed of more than one histologic type according to criteria as defined above.

[a] Developed by the pathology section of the Lung Cancer Study Group.

Table 32–10. Frequency of histologic cell types from two large screening projects[a,b]

Cell types	Memorial Sloan–Kettering (%)	Mayo Clinic	
		Prevalence (%)	Incidence (%)
Adenocarcinoma	45	27	24
Squamous cell carcinoma	33	43	30
Undifferentiated carcinoma			
Small cell	16	13	26
Large cell	6	17	19

[a] Based on results from 20,000 screened patients.
[b] Reprinted by permission from Western Journal of Medicine 1986; 145:52–64.

graded by its most poorly differentiated portion. For example, a neoplasm showing obvious squamous differentiation as defined by the presence of keratin production and/or intercellular junctions in which most of the tumor was composed of cells lacking these features would be classified as a poorly differentiated squamous cell carcinoma and not as a combined squamous carcinoma–large cell undifferentiated carcinoma. Although usually not done, it may be more accurate to give the percentage of tumor showing well, moderate, and poor differentiation.

Most neoplasms classified as bicomponent or multicomponent tumors are adenosquamous carcinomas that show a well-defined squamous and glandular component. In such tumors the dominant histologic type should be indicated for treatment protocol purposes, and the neoplasm is usually assigned to that treatment protocol corresponding to the major histologic pattern.

As is discussed, there are problem areas in the histologic classification of common lung neoplasms, especially in the small cell undifferentiated carcinoma group. In addition, electron microscopic and immunohistochemical examination of common lung neoplasms have provided new insights into the exact nature of these tumors as have cell culture studies. It should be mentioned that the World Health Organization uses light microscopic criteria for the classification of lung neoplasms. The frequencies of the common lung neoplasms in two large screening studies[153,154] are shown in Table 32–10.

Table 32–11. Distribution of World Health Organization[a]

Period and Place of Study	Type of Study[b]	Number of Cases	Distribution of WHO Subtypes (%)[c]			
			I	II	III	IV
64–73 Bombay	P	691	34	3	16	(46)[g]
68–71 Finland	P	405	47	27	11	4
73–76 U.S.A.	P	1179	48	22	20	8
76–80 W. Europe	P	7804	51	18	12	(9)[e]
74–81 U.S.A.	P	8897	30	17	29	7
35–84 U.S.A.	P	613	30	19	30	16
50–59 England	H	2364	45	27	6	(16)[f]
55–72 U.S.A.	H	662	35	25	25	14
60–72 Hong Kong	H	853	37	23	22	16
62–75 U.S.A.	H	1682	38	19	24	19
63–76 U.S.A.	H	219	26	16	39	11
U.S.A.[d]	H	476	37	28	19	13
55–78 U.S.A.	H	6686	47	(28)[h]	19	—
73–82 Hong Kong	H	1055	30	18	41	6
81–84 Scotland	H	2117	48	24	13	10
		Mean (%)	39	20	22	11
		S.D.	8	6	10	8
		Range	26–51	3–28	6–41	4–19

[a] Reprinted with permission from Watkin SW. Temporal demographic and epidemiologic variation in histologic subtypes of lung cancer: a literature review. Lung Cancer 1989;5:69–81.
[b] P, Population-based series; H, hospital- or institution-band series.
[c] Figures may not reach 100% due to presence of other sub-types not further classified.
[d] Published 1981; period of study not specified.
[e] Miscellaneous group not classified as I, II or III.
[f] Carcinoma simplex.
[g] Carcinoma bronchus, N.O.S. (not otherwise specified).
[h] Combined anaplastic group comprising types II and IV.

Changes and Variations in the Histologic Subtypes of Lung Cancer

Watkin[174] reviewed the various factors that influence distribution of lung cancer among the four major histologic subtypes. His review was published in 1989, and the reader is referred to this paper for a relatively complete list of references until 1989. The significance of the distribution of histologic subtypes of lung cancer is that selection of treatment is specifically related to the histologic type of lung cancer in many instances, and the differences in patterns of various studies and various geographic locations may imply a different etiology for the different histologic subtypes of lung cancer. As pointed out by Watkin,[174] Kung et al.[175] were the first to suggest that certain types of lung cancer (Kreyberg group 1, squamous cell carcinoma and small cell undifferentiated carcinoma) were related to smoking, while adenocarcinoma and other subtypes (Kreyberg group 2) were not. This suggestion, however, has been disputed, and an excess of all major types of lung cancer that can be attributed to cigarette smoking.

Watkin[174] categorized the differences in histologic distribution of lung cancer subtypes between institutions and also in population base series (Table 32–11).

As one can see, there are differences in the incidence of the World Health Organization subtypes (W.H.O. subtype I, squamous cell carcinoma; II, small cell undifferentiated carcinoma; III, adenocarcinoma; IV, large cell undifferentiated carcinoma). As discussed by Watkin,[174] these differences may in part be artefactual and depend on the use of different systems of histopathological classification, differences in the methods by which the material for diagnosis was obtained, and intra- and interobserver variability in histologic subtyping. As the 1981 W.H.O. revised classification of lung cancer came into use, the percentage of large cell undifferentiated carcinomas in one study, which typed 1,055 cases according to both the 1967 and the 1981 W.H.O. classifications, showed a decrease in percentage from 13% to 6% because solid large cell tumors with mucin secretion were included in the adenocarcinoma category. As reported by Whitwell in 1961,[176] there was a significant difference in the histologic distribution of lung cancers based on the type of specimen obtained. In 1,329 bronchial biopsies, 907 surgical resection specimens, and 128 postmortem cases, the proportion of adenocarcinomas rose from 2% in the biopsy series to 10% in the resections and 28% in the postmortem group. Squamous cell carcinoma occurred most com-

Table 32–12. Effect of histopathologic review on lung cancer subtype distributon (see text)[a,b]

Period of study	Type of study	Number of cases reviewed	Change in histology (%)	Main effects on WHO groups	WHO cell type distribution following review (%)			
					I	II	III	IV
1962–1975	H	289	35	IV→I/II/III (III from 17% to 33%)	38	19	24	19
1963–1976	H	219	29	IV→III	26	16	39	11
1981	H	476	21	IV→I/III	37	28	19	13
1973–1976	P	1179	36	IV→I/III (IV confirmed in 16%; 84% of 'others' were reviewed as I–IV)	male 54	20	17	7
					female 28	28	31	9

[a] Reprinted by permission from Watkin SW. Temporal demographic and epidemiologic variation in histologic subtypes of lung cancer: a literature review. Lung Cancer 1989;5:69–81.

[b] WHO sub-types: I = squamous carcinoma; II = small cell carcinoma; III-adenocarcinoma; IV = large cell/undifferentiated carcinoma; P = population-based study; H = hospital or institution-based study.

monly in the biopsy and resection series specimens, 42% and 54% of cases, respectively, whereas small cell undifferentiated carcinoma was found most frequently in the postmortem series.

Feinstein et al.[177] addressed the factor of intraobserver variability by pairing two separate readings of 50 lung neoplasms by five pathologists, and found a difference between the first and second reading of the same slide by the same pathologist in 2%–20% of the cases. Watkin[174] tabulated the studies dealing with interobserver variability (Table 32–12). Stanley and Matthews[178] evaluated the rates of agreement and patterns of disagreement in the classification of 476 lung cancers reviewed by three pathologists. Diagnoses were made in accordance with the working party–lung cancers classification system. In 67% of the cases, there was unanimous agreement in the histologic type of lung cancer, and in 27%, two of the three panel members gave the same diagnosis. The highest rate of agreement was for squamous cell carcinoma and for small cell undifferentiated carcinoma, and the lowest rate of agreement was for large cell undifferentiated carcinoma. Vincent et al.[179] found a relatively high rate of reclassification from undifferentiated small cell and large cell carcinomas, and an increase in the rate of adenocarcinomas. They found an increase in the diagnosis of adenocarcinoma from 17% of the cases between 1962 to 1968, to 33% of the cases between 1973 and 1975. Larsson[180] found agreement between his diagnosis and the original pathologic diagnosis in 77% of squamous cell carcinomas, and 79% of adenocarcinomas, but only 46% of small cell and large cell undifferentiated carcinomas, of which 33% were reclassified as either squamous cell carcinoma or adenocarcinoma.

Watkin[174] also reviewed the geographical differences in distribution of histopathologic types of lung cancer (Table 32–13). Age-related changes in the distribution of lung cancer subtypes is also reviewed,[174] and in general, there appears to be an increased proportion of squamous cell carcinomas in the older age group and an increased percentage of adenocarcinomas in the younger age group. The issue of smoking versus nonsmoking and histologic subtypes of lung cancer was also addressed. In general, there is a higher proportion of women with lung cancer who are nonsmokers than men. The majority of tumors in non-smoking women are adenocarcinomas.

There have been several more recent studies along the same lines as those reviewed by Watkin. For example, El-Torky et al.[181] reviewed 4,928 cases of primary lung cancer between 1964 and 1985, and found an increasing incidence of adenocarcinoma, particularly in men, and also found that adenocarcinoma was the most common type in women. Somewhat surprisingly, they found that small cell undifferentiated carcinoma was the second most frequent histologic type in women, having steadily increased over the last several years, and probably correlating the cigarette smoking. Auerbach and Garfinkel[182] evaluated 505 cases of lung carcinoma during a time period in which there was a significant

Table 32–13. Geographical variation in distribution of lung cancer subtypes[a]

Population	Period	Number of cases	WHO Grouping (%)			
			I	II	III	IV
Iceland	1931–64	136	17	34	23	17
Finland	1968–71	175	54	30	9	1
Singapore	1968–72	522	37	26	20	14
Switzerland	1974–76	223	56	19	13	12
Western Europe	1976–80	7804	51	18	12	9
Eastern U.S.A.	1974–81	8897	30	17	29	7
Hong Kong	1973–82	1055	37	22	22	16
Scotland	1981–84	2117	48	24	13	10

[a] Reproduced by permission of publisher. From Watkin SW. Temporal demographic and epidemiologic variation in histologic subtypes of lung cancer: a literature review. Lung Cancer 1989;5:69–81.

change in tobacco-smoking habits. They found that peripheral tumors increased from 30.7% of the total in 1978 to 42% of the total between 1986 to 1989, and that centrally originating bronchial carcinomas decreased from 69.3% to 57.3% in the same time period. The incidence of bronchioloalveolar cell carcinoma more than doubled, from 9.3% in the earlier time period to 20.3% between 1986 to 1989. They believed that these changes in incidence resulted from a decrease in lung cancers related to cigarette smoking, and raised the possibility that other etiologies, such as viral oncogenes, may be important in the development of some lung neoplasms.

Morabia and Wynder[183] performed a case control-type study evaluating 507 women and 851 men with lung cancer. They found that cigarette smoking was associated with each of the different cell types, and that the differences in smoking habits according to cell type were relatively small. However, they found that an increased risk of lung cancer, according to the number of cigarettes smoked per day, was correlated more strongly with small cell undifferentiated carcinoma than for adenocarcinoma. They suggested that cigarette smoking was perhaps related to lung cancer location, with the central squamous cell carcinomas and small cell undifferentiated carcinomas having a stronger association with cigarette smoking than do the peripheral adenocarcinomas.

Lung Tumor Heterogeneity

All lung tumors show histologic heterogeneity. That is not to say that all lung tumors are bicomponent or multicomponent. It simply means that in any given neoplasm, each tumor cell does not have exactly the same cytologic appearance. For example, pulmonary adenocarcinomas may be composed of cells forming well-defined glands in some areas while in other regions may have a bronchioloalveolar cell pattern or be composed of solid nests of cells with no obvious glandular differentiation (Fig. 32–12).

In 1976, Yesner[184] reported that 2% of 10,000 lung cancers showed more than one histologic type, the most common combination being differentiated squamous carcinoma and mucin-producing adenocarcinoma. Adelstein et al.[185] reported that 10% of 176 small cell carcinomas had a nonsmall cell component. Roggli et al.[186] reported that 45% of 100 consecutive cases of lung cancer in which the entire tumor or 10 tissue blocks were examined showed major heterogeneity (as defined by one slide showing a major histologic type different than that seen in one other slide). One might question whether this degree of heterogeneity would exist if these tumors were adequately examined by electron microscopy. As illustrated, some adenocarcinomas and squamous carcinomas show regions of small cell and large cell undifferentiated carcinoma but when examined ultrastructurally these undifferentiated areas show obvious glandular or squamous features. The same is true for neuroendocrine carcinomas of the lung, which can show a divergence of histologic appearance in the same neoplasm.

Synchronous and Metachronous Lung Neoplasms

Synchronous or metachronous lung neoplasms of the same or different histologic types have been reported. Synchronous tumors are defined as those found at the same time, while metachronous tumors are defined as a second neoplasm occurring at some time after resection of an initial tumor. Approximately 1% of common lung neoplasms are multiple[187–189] when using the criteria of Warren and Gates.[190] In an autopsy study of 258 patients dying from lung cancer in which the entire tracheobronchial tree was serially sectioned, Auerbach et al.[191] reported second primary invasive carcinomas in 3.5% of cases. Most of the second primary tumors reported are either squamous or adenocarcinomas.[1,85,191,192] Jung-Legg and colleagues[193] recently reported synchronous triple malignant tumors of the lung (bronchial carcinoid, small cell carcinoma, adenocarcinoma) in a 49-year-old male with a 60-pack-year history of cigarette smoking. In their review of the literature, their report was the fourth well-documented case of triple synchronous lung cancer in the English literature.

Wu et al.[194] reported 30 cases of multiple primary lung tumors observed at the Shanghai Hospital between November 1957 and June 1984, of which 10 were synchronous and 20 were metachronous. Seventeen cases were unilateral, and thirteen cases were bilateral. Among the 10 synchronous cases, 4 cases of multiple primary lung cancers were diagnosed before surgery by either chest radiography or fiberoptic bronchoscopy. Among the 20 metachronous tumors, 11 neoplasms were diagnosed as a second primary lesion by chest radiograph during periodic followups after the initial resection, and 9 cases were proven by thoracotomy. The average postoperative survival in the 10 synchronous cases was 29 months, and in the 20 metachronous cases, 26.2 months. Deschamps et al.[195] reported on 80 cases of multiple primary lung neoplasms they observed in a 13-year period; of these, 44 were metachronous. The actuarial 5- and 10-year survival rates after the first pulmonary resection for stage 1 disease were 55.2% and 27%, respectively; 5- and 10-year survival rates for stage 1 disease after the second pulmonary resection were

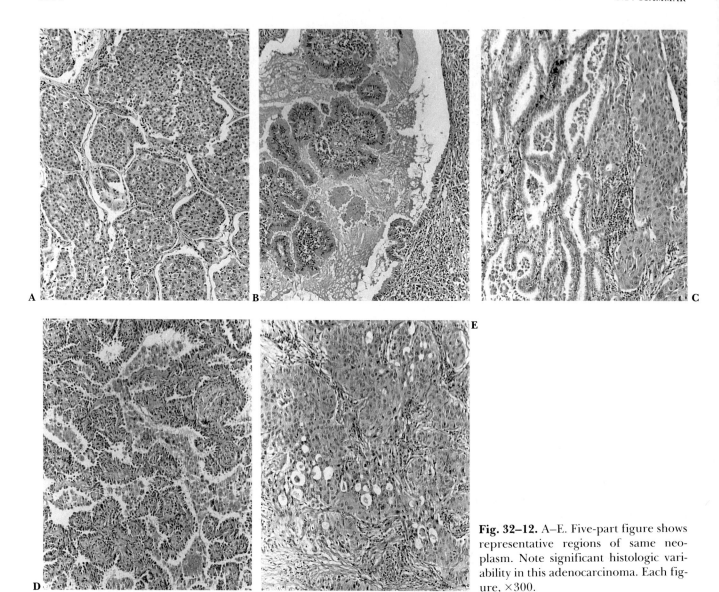

Fig. 32–12. A–E. Five-part figure shows representative regions of same neoplasm. Note significant histologic variability in this adenocarcinoma. Each figure, ×300.

41% and 31.5%, respectively. In the 36 patients with synchronous primary lung cancers, pulmonary resection consisted of lobectomy in 18 patients, bilobectomy in 3 patients, pneumonectomy in 10 patients, and wedge resection or segmentectomy in 8 patients. The 5- and 10-year survival rates after pulmonary resection were 15.7% and 13.8%, respectively. The authors concluded that an aggressive surgical approach was warranted in most patients with multiple primary lung cancers, and that synchronous primary cancers of the lung had a poor prognosis.

Histogenesis of Common Lung Neoplasms

The histogenesis of common lung neoplasms is poorly understood and is undergoing an evolution with increasing knowledge. The histogenesis of squamous carcinoma is most completely understood on the basis of

animal and human studies. Over many years, metaplastic squamous epithelium is thought to become dysplastic (neoplastic), eventually progressing into carcinoma in situ and invasive squamous carcinoma.[41,196] According to Auerbach,[197] all lung neoplasms develop from progressive transformation of normal respiratory epithelial cells into atypical cells that eventually become neoplastic. Based primarily on lung tumor heterogeneity, Yesner[184] believes that various histologic types of common lung neoplasms develop from a small cell type of neoplasm (oat cell carcinoma) that undergoes a transition to an intermediate or polygonal cell cancer, which then may develop into a large cell undifferentiated carcinoma. The large cell carcinomas are the precursors of adenocarcinomas and squamous carcinomas. This is shown diagramatically in Fig. 32–13.

Ultrastructural and immunohistochemical analysis of common lung neoplasms has shown that many of these

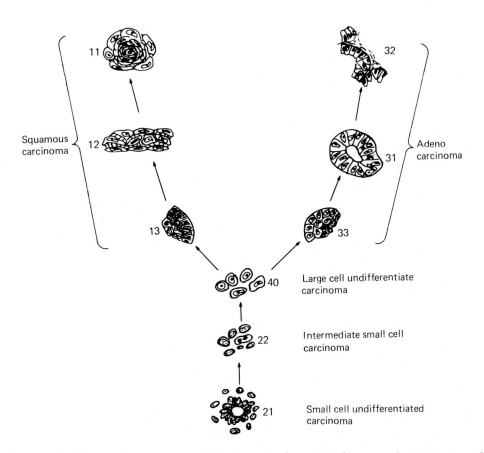

Fig. 32–13. Dr. R. Yesner's diagram shows proposed histogenesis of common lung neoplasms (see text for explanation). (Reprinted with permission.[184])

neoplasms are composed of cells that have morphologic features similar to normal mature cells of the lung. For example, many bronchioloalveolar cell carcinomas are composed of cells that resemble mature Clara cells, type II pneumocytes, or mucous goblet cells. Similarly (as illustrated), neuroendocrine tumors such as carcinoids are composed of cells that resemble normal bronchial mucosal neuroendocrine cells. This author's view on the histogenesis of common lung neoplasms is similar to that of Auerbach[197]; any respiratory epithelial cell can undergo a neoplastic transformation developing into a carcinoma. From a practical point of view, the histogenesis of common lung neoplasms is of relative minor importance compared to their morphologic features and clinical behavior.

Growth Factors, Growth Factor Receptors, Oncogenes, Anti-Oncogenes, and Human Lung Cancer

Oncogenes are genes of either cellular of viral origin that are frequently amplified in malignant conditions and which are capable of transforming cells in vitro into a malignant phenotype.[198–201] Many oncogenes appear to be amplified (replicated) in malignant cells. More than 50 different well-characterized oncogene sequences have been recognized to date, and in physiologic conditions they serve as growth factor-related, tyrosine kinase-like, G-protein-related, or serine-threonine kinase-like functions, or are involved in the regulation of nucleoprotein synthesis.[202] Involvement of the *ras* and *myc* families of genes has been best described in lung cancer, and Damstrup et al.[201] have listed the majority of the various growth factors that seem to be operative in lung cancer. Tumor suppressor genes (anti-oncogenes), namely the retinoblastoma gene and p53, exert a normalizing or negative regulatory role on growth, and inactivation through deletions or mutations of the anti-oncogenes is thought to allow for the emergence of a malignant phenotype. The major oncogenes and tumor suppressor genes involved in lung cancer are listed in Table 32–14.

Doubling Time of Lung Neoplasms

The doubling time of a human lung neoplasm can be calculated on the basis of the hypothesis, first suggested

Table 32–14. Major dominant oncogenes and tumor suppressor genes involved in lung cancer[a]

Gene	Function	Frequency[b]
Dominant *ras* family (H-, N-, and Ki-)	p21 membrane-associated protein. Signal transduction? Activated by point mutations.	15 of 77 NSCLC. SCLC?
myc family	Nuclear phosphoproteins. Function unknown. *c-myc* expression coupled to cell cycle. All can cooperate with *ras* in transforming primary cells. Activated by increased expression.	SCLC: amplified in 30 to 50% of cell lines (47, 51) and 11 to 24% of tumors. Overexpressed in 89% of cell lines and 83% of tumors. NSCLC: amplified in 8% of tumors.
Tumor suppressor		
3p	Putative tumor suppressor genes not yet identified.	92 to 100% of SCLC and 25 to 50% of NSCLC.
rb	Nuclear phosphoprotein. Cell cycle regulation?	Inactivated in >90% SCLC and 10 to 20% NSCLC.
p53	Nuclear protein. Function unknown.	Inactivated in >50% SCLC and NSCLC.

[a] Reprinted with permission from Viallet J, Minna JD. Dominant oncogenes and tumor suppressor genes in the pathogenesis of lung cancer. Am J Respir Cell Mol Biol 1990;2:225–232.

by Collins et al.[203] in 1956, that a solid neoplasm starts as a single cell and divides exponentially at a constant rate. As reviewed by Geddes,[204] a cell 10 μm in diameter will have a diameter of 1 mm after 20 doublings, which would represent a total of 10^6 cells. The tumor reaches a size of 1 cm after 30 doublings, which would be a total of 10^9 cells. Most tumors are diagnosed radiographically at 35 doublings, or $10^{10.5}$ cells, at which time they are about 3 cm in diameter. Figure 32–14 shows this schematically, and illustrates the potential misconception that a tumor appears to be small and slow-growing for the majority of its life until it reaches the size where it is diagnosable, at which time it grows very rapidly. Although lung cancers are usually not perfectly spherical, calculation of doubling times is determined using the formula for the volume of a cube (4/3 πr^3). Variations in the size of the tumors over time are usually determined radiographically. Charts such as that published by Geddes have also been devised to measure tumor doubling times (Fig. 32–15); and some of the variables that have entered into the calculations of

doubling time have been discussed in some detail by Chahinian and Israel.[205,206] Nathan et al.[207] collected 177 cases of measurable primary or metastatic lung neoplasms, and assessed the maximum doubling time range, which was from 7 to 465 days. They indicated that this range defined a "malignant zone." If the doubling time of the lung mass was between these values, a malignant tumor was to be expected. However, if doubling time was less than 7 days, then an infectious or inflammatory lesion was to be expected, and if the doubling time exceeded 465 days, a benign tumor was to be suspected.

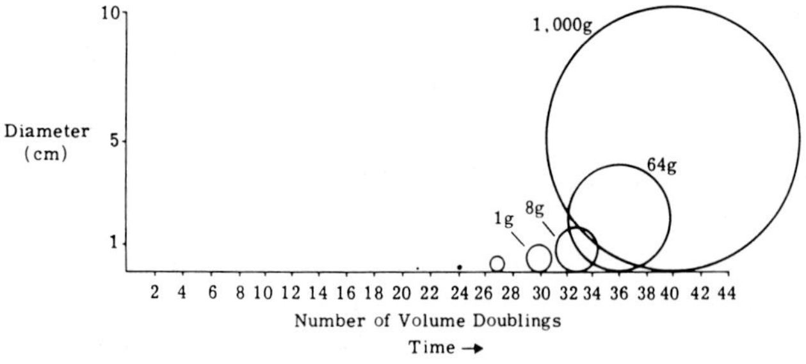

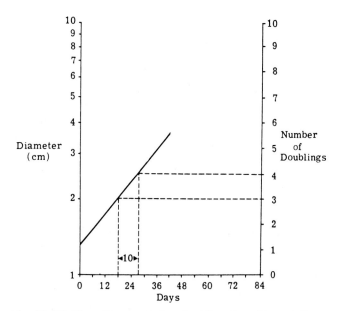

Fig. 32–15. Chart for measuring doubling time. Tumor diameter is plotted on logarithmic scale against time: Using right-hand scale, one volume doubling can be marked on growth curve and doubling time read from time scale. (Reproduced by permission of publisher. From Geddes DM. The natural history of lung cancer: A review based on rates of tumour growth. Br J Dis Chest 1979;73:1–17.

Fig. 32–14. Life of solid tumor. Time is expressed as volume doublings. Tumor with doubling time of 1 month requires 40 months to reach 10 cm in diameter, while another with doubling time of 1 year requires 40 years. (Reprinted by permission from Geddes DM. The natural history of lung cancer: A review based on rates of tumour growth. Br J Dis Chest 1979;73:1–17.)

Table 32–15. Reports of doubling times of primary lung cancer[a,b]

	Squamous	Adeno	Undifferentiated	Oat	Other	Total
Brenner et al. 1967[204a]	3		1			4
Breur 1966[204b]	2					2
Chahinian 1972[204c]	21	3		3		27
Garland et al. 1963[204d] and Garland 1966[204e]	36	12	9		3	60
Meyer 1973[204f]	11	7	1	2	1	22
Schwartz 1961[204g]	10	2				12
Steele and Buell 1973[204h]	16	24	23		4	67
Weiss et al. 1966[204i] and Weiss 1974[204j]	12	12	8		2	34
Total	111	60	42	5	10	228
Log mean T_2	4.476 ± 0.725	5.084 ± 0.815	4.456 ± 0.596	3.362 ± 0.540	—	4.621 ± 0.791
Mean T_2 (days)	88	161	86	29		102

[a] Reprinted with permission from Geddes DM. The natural history of lung cancer: a review based on rates of tumour growth. Br J Dis Chest 1979:1–17.
[b] Figures represent the number of tumors measured.

Table 32–16. Comparison of data on doubling times of primary carcinoma of lung[a]

Histopathologic type	Mean DTact days	Range	Number of cases	Mean[a] DTact days	Range[a]	Number of cases[a]
Squamous	146	20–382	7	101	7–381	115
Adeno-	72	23–110	4	179	17–590	66
Small cell	66	24–94	4	33	17–71	5
Large cell	111	37–260	7	113	112–114	2
"Undifferentiated"				100	34–480	33

[a] Left column is from study by Kerr and Lamb[208]; right column is compilation from the literature. (Reproduced by permission from Kerr and Lamb.[208])

The mean doubling times of primary lung cancers have been tabulated by Geddes[204] (Table 32–15) and by Kerr and Lamb[208] (Table 32–16). As can be seen, the mean doubling time for squamous cell carcinomas in the Geddes tabulation was 88 days; adenocarcinoma, 161 days; large cell undifferentiated carcinoma, 86 days; and small cell undifferentiated carcinoma, 29 days. Obviously, there is a range in the doubling time of all neoplasms. Using doubling times, a number of different investigators have predicted survival, and have drawn survival curves, based on the size of the tumor at the time of detection.

Greengard et al.[209] argued that the location or irregular shape of a primary pulmonary neoplasm precluded accurate radiologic measurement of volume in most cases. They also argued that to determine the doubling time, there must be a long enough time for appreciable growth to have occurred to make the necessary calculations. As an alternative, they introduced the concept of biochemical doubling time based on the existence of enzymes that bear close quantitative relationships to the volume growth rate of neoplasms. This was first observed in experimental animals. Specifically,

they found that there was an inverse correlation between the doubling time of a pulmonary neoplasm to the thymidine kinase and uridine kinase concentration of the biopsy tumor sample measured per gram of wet weight of tumor or milligram of DNA. They correlated the concentrations of the enzymes in the tumors with the radiographically measured doubling time, hoping to create a nomogram on which one could read off the unknown doubling times of a given tumor based on the enzyme analysis. They indicated that the regression lines they had produced to date were not good enough for practical routine use, and that additional studies were needed.

Pathologic Features of Common Lung Neoplasms

Squamous Carcinoma

Squamous carcinomas comprise approximately 30%–40% of common lung neoplasms. Most squamous cell carcinomas of the lung occur "centrally" in cigarette-

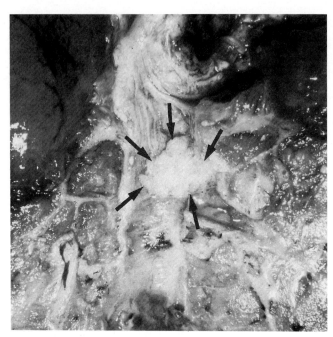

Fig. 32–16. Right-upper lobe shows 1.5 × 1.5 cm squamous carcinoma in lobar bronchus *(arrows)*. This tumor caused obstruction of bronchus, resulting in postobstructive pneumonitis.

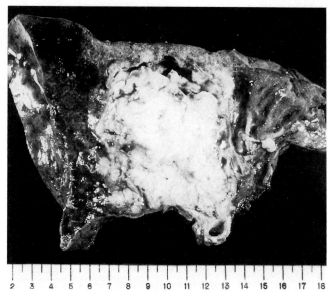

Fig. 32–18. Very large squamous carcinoma, also probably arising in lobar bronchus, shows focal necrosis and cavitation.

smoking males and arise in mainstem, lobar, or segmental bronchi (Figs. 32–16 through 32–18). However, approximately one-third arise in small bronchi in peripheral lung tissue, occasionally in association with a scar.[210,211] Most superior sulcus tumors (Pancoast tumors)[210,211] are squamous carcinomas. Squamous carcinomas frequently obstruct bronchi causing postobstructive pneumonia that may cause a large area of consolidated lung parenchyma, which may appear as a mass in a chest radiograph giving the appearance of a tumor much larger than actually present (Fig. 32–19). As squamous carcinomas become larger they have a

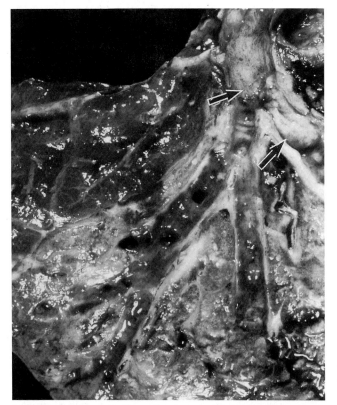

Fig. 32–17. Sausage-shaped squamous carcinoma occludes major bronchus *(arrow)* and is associated with obstructive pneumonitis.

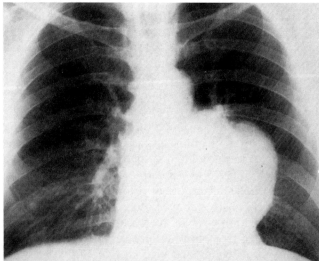

Fig. 32–19. Chest radiograph of tumor shown in Fig. 32–16. Large size of mass is caused by obstructive pneumonitis.

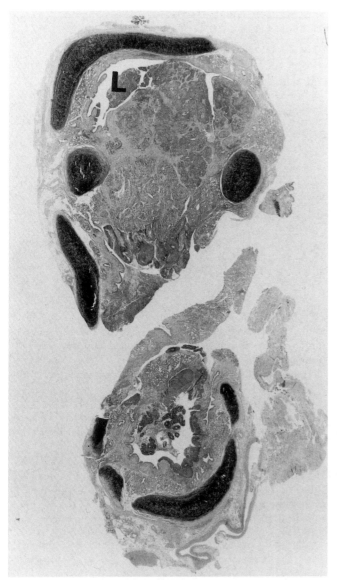

Fig. 32–20. Low-power magnification through segmental bronchi involved by squamous cell carcinoma. Lumen (L) of one bronchus is nearly completely occluded by tumor. ×4.

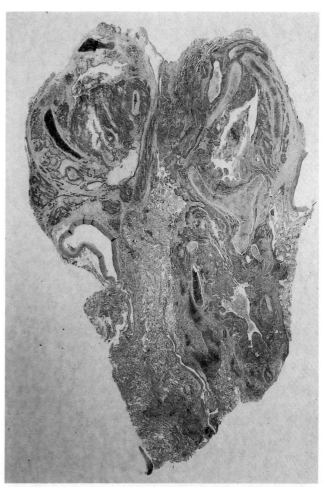

Fig. 32–21. Section through lobar bronchus as it divides into three smaller bronchi, all of which are involved by squamous carcinoma. Note that tumor infiltrates through wall of bronchus. ×6.

tendency to become necrotic and show central cavitation.[212]

As would be expected from gross examination of squamous lung carcinomas, the bronchial lumen may be partially or near totally occluded by the tumor (Figs. 32–20 and 32–21). The neoplasm also usually invades into the underlying lamina propria and peripheral lung tissue. As described by Dulmet-Brender et al.,[213] squamous carcinomas of the bronchus may be entirely exophytic although their prognosis is no better than other stage 1 lung cancers.

The histologic diagnosis of squamous carcinoma is based on identifying intercellular junctions (prickles) between the tumor cells (Fig. 32–22) and/or keratinization (Fig. 32–23). Ultrastructurally, squamous cancer cells have short filopodial processes that inderdigitate with processes of neighboring cells (Fig. 32–24) with desmosomes connecting the processes to each other (Fig. 32–25); these correspond to the "prickles" noted by light microscopy. Squamous cancer cells that are well to moderately differentiated by light microscopy typically contain numerous cytoplasmic tonofilaments (Fig. 32–26), with the remainder of the cytoplasm being relatively unspecialized. The tonofilaments are responsible for the eosinophilic appearance of the cytoplasm in hematoxylin and eosin-stained sections. The majority of invasive squamous lung cancers show a chronically inflamed desmoplastic stroma associated with the nests of tumor cells (see Fig. 32–23).

Most squamous carcinomas show a significant degree

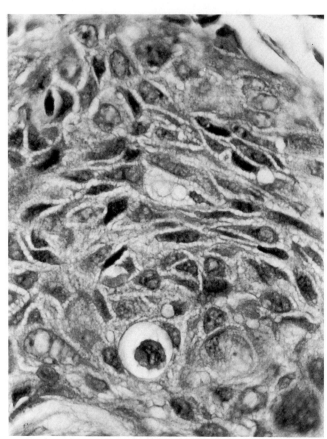

Fig. 32–22. Representative region of moderately well-differentiated squamous carcinoma shows "prickles" between cells. ×550.

Fig. 32–24. Ultrastructural appearance of squamous carcinoma. Note filopodial processes (FP) of tumor cells and numerous desmosomes interconnecting processes. Also note numerous tonofilaments in cytoplasm of tumor cells and electron-dense material representing keratohyaline granules *(arrows).* ×16,000.

Fig. 32–25. Greatly magnified region of filopodial processes interconnected by desmosomes. Tonofilaments insert into desmosomal plaques. ×51,500.

Fig. 32–26. Part of well-differentiated squamous cancer cell shows numerous tonofilaments in cytoplasm. Number of tonofilaments is roughly directly proportional to degree of squamous differentiation noted in tumor by light microscopy. ×10,500.

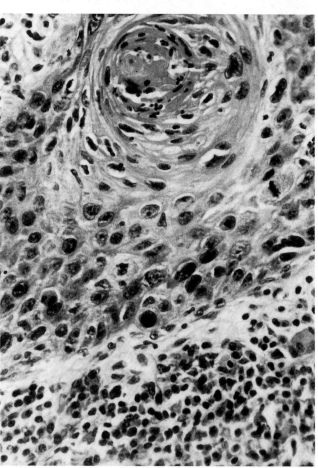

Fig. 32–23. Distinct keratinization of tumor cells in this area of squamous carcinoma. Also note fibroinflammatory stroma associated with tumor. ×330.

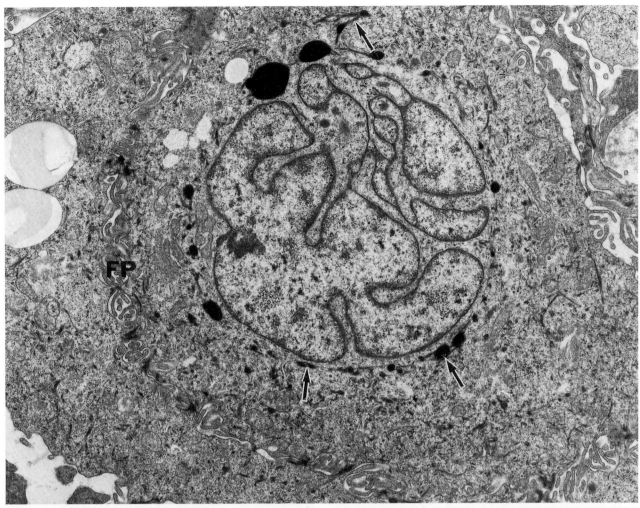

FP

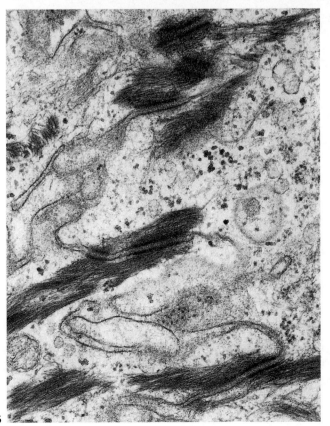

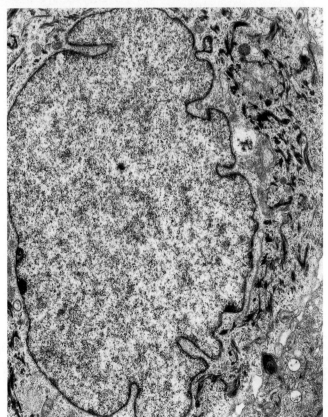

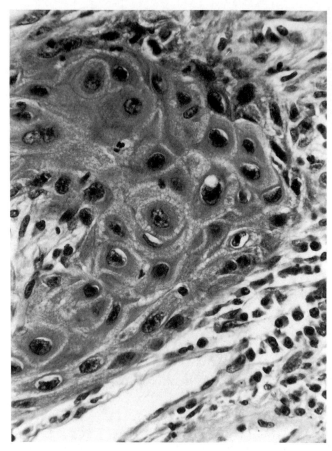

Fig. 32–27. Region of well-differentiated squamous carcinoma shows obvious "prickles" between cells. ×550.

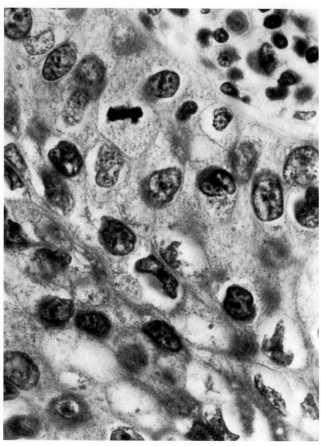

Fig. 32–28. Different region of tumor shown in Fig. 32–27. Tumor cells show no features of squamous differentiation. ×775.

of histologic heterogeneity. In some areas they are composed of nest and cords of differentiated neoplastic squamous cells (Fig. 32–27), while in other areas they are composed of cells that do not show obvious keratinization or intercellular junctions (Fig. 32–28). By electron microscopy, the areas that are poorly differentiated by light microscopy are formed by cells that usually lack filopodial processes, have fewer desmosomes connecting them to each other, and contain fewer cytoplasmic tonofilaments (Fig. 32–29). In many squamous lung carcinomas tumor giant cells are present (Fig. 32–30).

Other histologic patterns of squamous carcinoma exist. Some squamous lung cancers will be composed predominantly of spindle-shaped cells (Fig. 32–31). Intercellular junctions and keratinization are often difficult to identify in such neoplasms. Ultrastructurally

these cells have obvious squamous features with filopodial processes, desmosomes, and cytoplasmic tonofilaments (Fig. 32–32). Other squamous neoplasms will be composed of large oncocytic-appearing cells (Fig. 32–33) that correlate with numerous mitochondria ultrastructurally (Fig. 32–34); these cells still retain some squamous features. Occasionally well-differentiated squamous carcinomas coexist with small cell undifferentiated carcinomas (Fig. 32–35), and in some instances they are in direct apposition or even may show an apparent transition from a malignant squamous cell to an undifferentiated small cell (Fig. 32–36). Tumors such as this could be correctly classified as combined small cell undifferentiated carcinoma-squamous carcinomas although, in this author's experience, the small component of such neoplasms usually have "primitive" squamous features and lack neuroendocrine differenti-

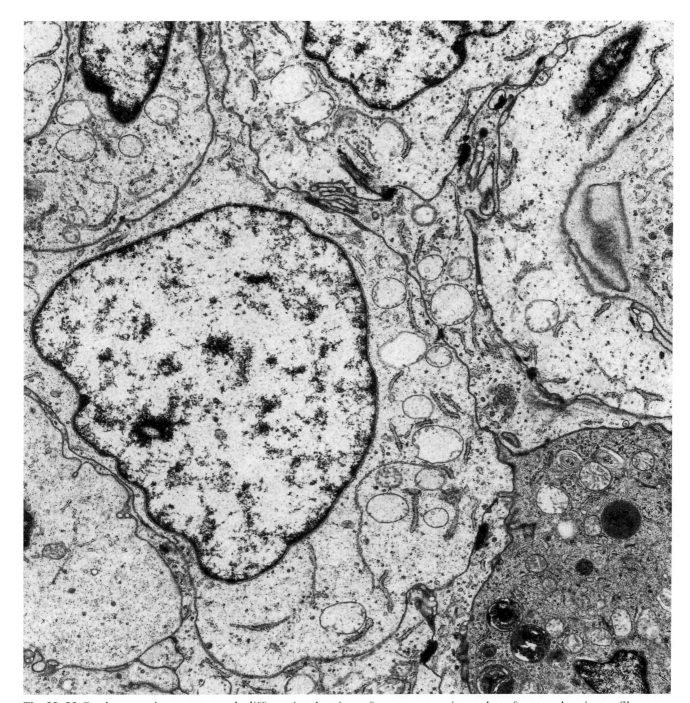

Fig. 32–29. By electron microscopy, poorly differentiated regions of squamous carcinoma have few cytoplasmic tonofilaments, lack filopodial processes, and have fewer desmosomes interconnecting cells. ×16,000.

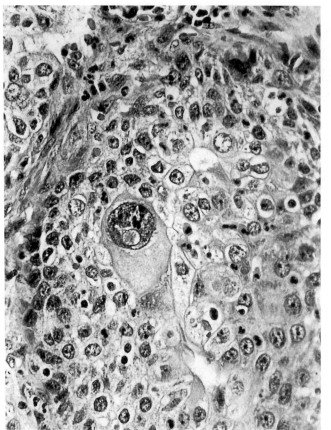

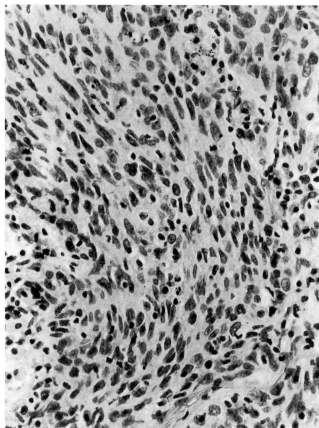

Fig. 32–30. Another region of tumor shown in Fig. 32–27. In this region, tumor is much more poorly differentiated with obvious tumor giant cell. ×550.

Fig. 32–31. Some squamous carcinomas are composed predominantly of spindle cells. ×330.

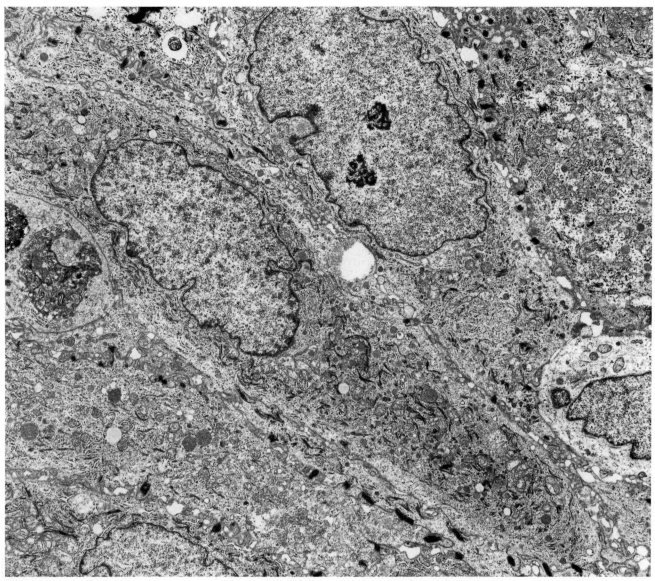

Fig. 32–32. Ultrastructural appearance of tumor shown in Fig. 32–31. Spindle-shaped cells are interconnected by numerous desmosomes, and moderate number of tonofilaments appear in cytoplasm of tumor cells. ×10,500.

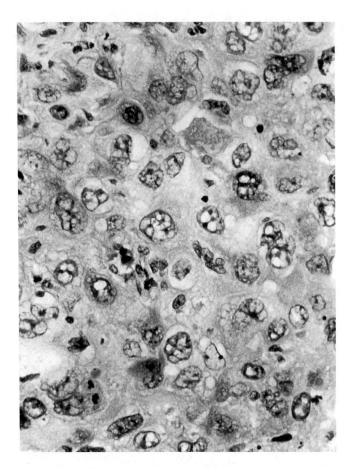

Fig. 32–33. Some squamous carcinomas are composed of large cells that do not show definite keratinization but have oncocytic cytoplasm. ×550.

ation when examined by electron microscopy (Fig. 32–37).

Finally, the cells of an occasional squamous cell carcinoma of lung will be composed of cells with clear cytoplasm (Fig. 32–38). These cells usually show periodic acid–Schiff-positive cytoplasm (Fig. 32–39) that is negative if pretreated with diastase. Ultrastructurally the clear cytoplasm is caused by the accumulation of glycogen in the cell (Fig. 32–40), and this most likely represents a degenerative change. Any lung cancer cell can degenerate an accumulate glycogen in its cytoplasm giving it a "clear" appearance in hematoxylin and eosin-stained sections. (See discussion in Chapter 33.)

Many of the immunohistochemical features of squamous carcinoma and other common lung neoplasms are shown in Table 32–17. Squamous lung cancers characteristically contain several different molecular weight keratins (Figs. 32–41 and 32–42). They can be differentiated from squamous carcinomas of skin by their cytokeratin profile in that squamous carcinomas of epidermal origin usually only express high molecular weight cytokeratin. Squamous lung carcino-

mas usually express carcinoembryonic antigen (Fig. 32–43) and epithelial membrane antigen (Fig. 32–44); the immunostaining for carcinoembryonic antigen is most intense in areas of keratinization. They may also focally express LeuM1 (CD15), B72.3, and BerEP4, often in a cell membrane distribution.

Squamous carcinoma of the lung is thought to arise from a progressive dysplasia of metaplastic squamous epithelium eventually leading to squamous cell carcinoma in situ and invasive carcinoma[214] (Figs. 32–45 through 32–47). Controversy exists with respect to the origin of the metaplastic squamous epithelium. Most standard pathology reference textbooks indicate the process results from the proliferation of basal reserve cells that differentiate into squamous epithelial cells. Trump et al.,[215] however, suggested that it resulted from a metaplasia of mucous columnar epithelial cells into squamous epithelial cells. In 1987, Yamamoto et al.[216] studied squamous metaplasia by immunoelectron microscopy using peroxidase-tagged antibodies against secretory component. They found that both processes—mucous cell metaplasia and basal cell hyper-

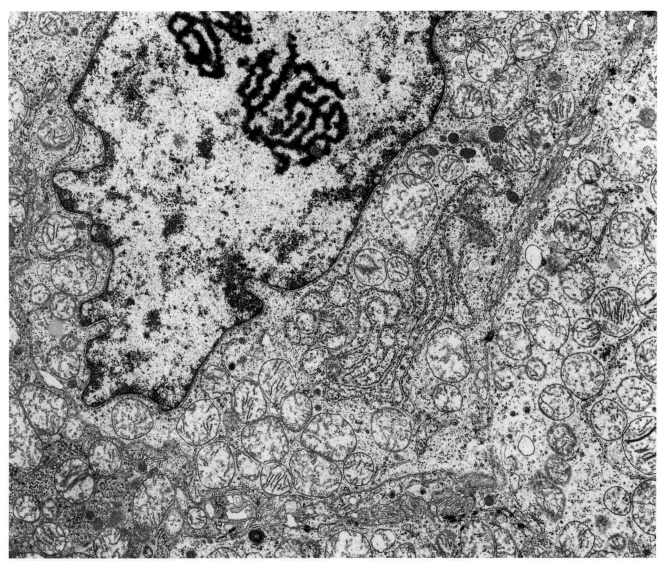

Fig. 32–34. Ultrastructural appearance of tumor shown in Fig. 32–33. The neoplastic cells contain large numbers of mitochondria which probably explains their eosinophilic appearance in the H&E stained sections. ×42,000.

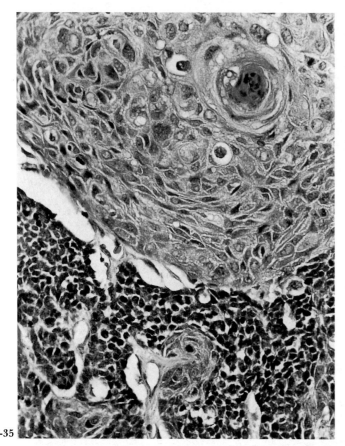

32-35

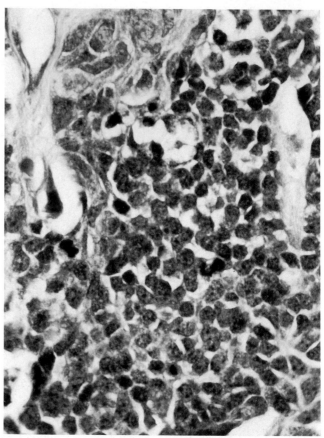

32-36

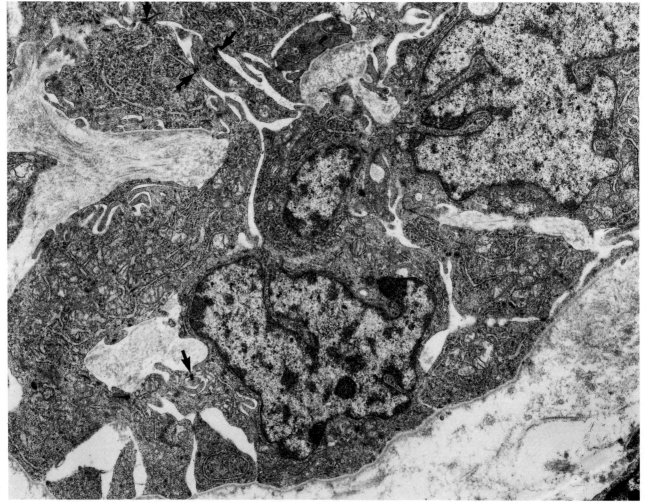

32-37

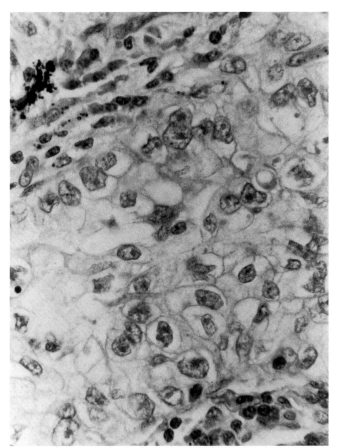

Fig. 32–38. Squamous carcinoma shows, "clear" cytoplasm of tumor cells. ×550.

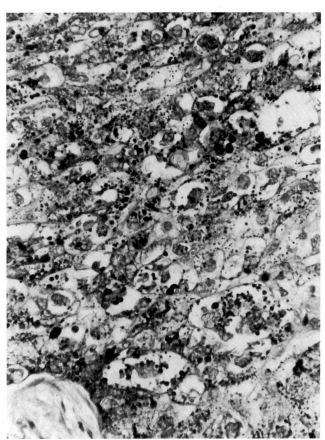

Fig. 32–39. "Clear" cytoplasm of tumor cells contains numerous periodic acid–Schiff-positive granules that can be removed with pretreatment of tissue section with diastase, suggesting "clear" cytoplasm is caused by glycogen accumulation within cell. ×550.

◁ ――――――――――――――――――

Fig. 32–35. Region of primary lung tumor shows obvious squamous carcinoma in association with small cell undifferentiated carcinoma. ×330.

Fig. 32–36. Tumor shown in Fig. 32–35; in this region it is composed mostly of small undifferentiated cells with few larger squamous-appearing cells in one area. ×550.

Fig. 32–37. Ultrastructural features of small cell component of tumor shown in Figs. 32–35 and 32–36. Cells are small and relatively unspecialized, but lack neuroendocrine features and are interconnected by fairly frequent desmosomes *(arrows)*. ×16,000.

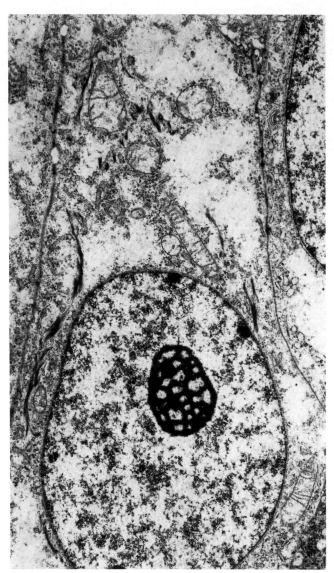

Fig. 32–40. By electron microscopy, tumor cells shown in Figs. 32–38 and 32–39 contain cytoplasmic glycogen. Note tonofilaments in cytoplasm and small desmosomes interconnecting portions of tumor cells. ×16,000.

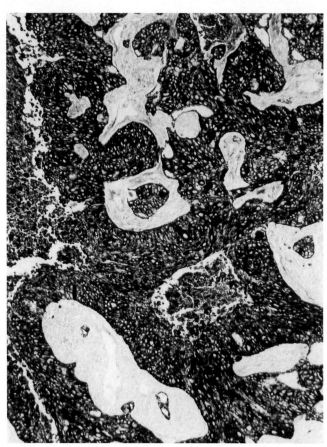

32-4

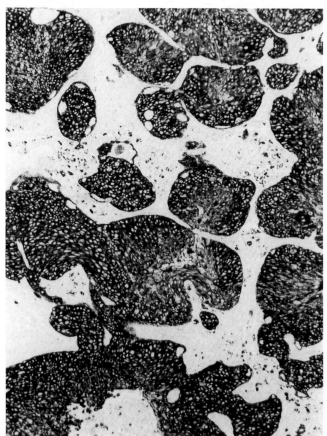

32-4

Fig. 32–41. Cords of squamous carcinoma show intense immunostaining *(black)* for high molecular weight cytokeratin. ×75.

Fig. 32–42. Squamous carcinoma also shows intense immunostaining *(black)* for low molecular weight cytokeratin. ×75.

Table 32–17. Immunohistochemical features of common lung neoplasms

Type of neoplasm	Low MW cytokeratin[a]	High MW cytokeratin[a]	Carcino-embryonic antigen[a]	Human milk fat globule protein[a]	Neuron-specific enolase[a]	Chromogranin[a]	Leu MI	B72.3	BerEPA
Squamous carcinoma	+[b]	+	±[c]	±	−	−	±[d]	±[d]	±[d]
Adenocarcinoma	+	+	+	+	±	−	±[e]	±[e]	±[e]
Large cell undifferentiated carcinoma	+	±	±	±	±	−	±[f]	±[f]	±[f]
Small cell undifferentiated carcinoma	+	±	±	±	±	±	−[g]	−[g]	−[g]
Mature carcinoid	+	±	±	±	+	+	−[g]	−[g]	−[g]
Atypical carcinoid	+	±	±	±	+	±	−[g]	−[g]	−[g]
Large cell neuroendocrine carcinoma	+	±	±	±	+	±	−[g]	−[g]	−[g]

[a] Antigens tested for.
[b] Plus = positive reaction, minus = negative.
[c] Some report positive, others negative results.
[d] Most frequently negative. If positive, it is usually foral and often in cell membrane distribution.
[e] Positive in 30%–50% of cases in this author's experience.
[f] Positive in 20%–30% of cases in this author's experience.
[g] Information inadequate to state results.

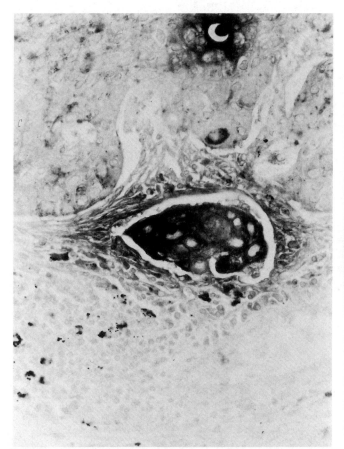

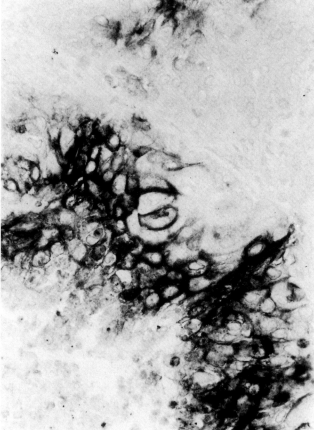

Fig. 32–43. Some squamous carcinomas display focal areas of immunostaining for carcinoembryonic antigen that is often most intense in regions of keratinization. ×330.

Fig. 32–44. Focal immunostaining *(black)* for epithelial membrane antigen is seen in many squamous carcinomas. ×330.

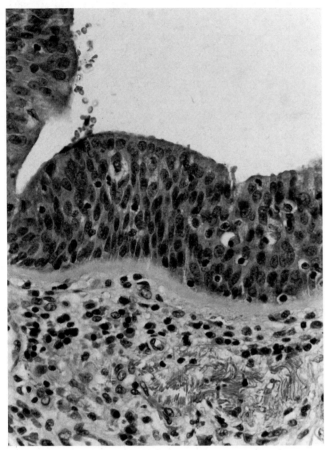

Fig. 32–45. Region of squamous metaplasia of respiratory mucosal epithelium. Cells are uniform and have somewhat basaloid appearance. ×330.

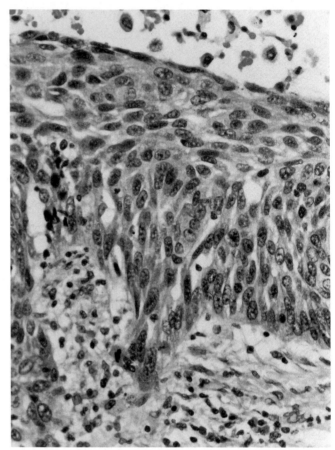

Fig. 32–46. Region of respiratory mucosal epithelium shows variation in cellular morphology and slight nuclear enlargement characteristic of squamous dysplasia. ×330.

plasia and metaplasia—occur, but that the basal cell change was most important in forming the metaplastic squamous epithelium.

Adenocarcinoma

Adenocarcinoma of the lung is the most morphologically heterogeneous major type of lung cancer and in some series has replaced squamous carcinoma as the most frequently diagnosed lung neoplasm.[179,217] A re-evaluation of previously diagnosed large cell undifferentiated carcinomas with the aid of a mucosubstance stain, such as periodic acid–Schiff diastase or Mayer's mucicarmine stain, has shown that many large cell undifferentiated carcinomas are in fact poorly differentiated adenocarcinomas as demonstrated by the pres-

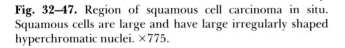

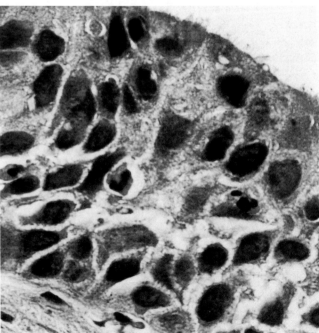

Fig. 32–47. Region of squamous cell carcinoma in situ. Squamous cells are large and have large irregularly shaped hyperchromatic nuclei. ×775.

ence of mucosubstance.[217] Adenocarcinoma is the most common type of lung cancer in women[217] and also is the most common form of lung cancer in nonsmokers,[218,219] although most patients with lung adenocarcinoma are cigarette smokers.[218]

Most adenocarcinomas arise in the periphery of the lung,[211,220,221] and in this author's experience the most commonly seen lung tumor by the practicing surgical pathologist today is a peripheral adenocarcinoma that was usually identified on a routine chest radiograph in an asymptomatic patient. This type of tumor frequently causes pleural "puckering" (Figs. 32–48 and 32–49). Other adenocarcinomas of the lung are located within the midzone region of the lung (Fig. 32–50) or may be cystic, especially when they produce mucus (Fig. 32–51).

The histologic criteria for diagnosing adenocarcinoma include gland formation by tumor cells or the demonstration of a mucosubstance within the cells. Adenocarcinomas are classified histologically by the World Health Organization into four categories: (1) acinar adenocarcinomas in which the tumor cells form acini or glands (Fig. 32–52); (2) papillary adenocarcinomas in which there is a predominance of papillary structures (Fig. 32–53); (3) bronchioloalveolar cell carcinoma (discussed following), and (4) solid adenocarcinoma (Fig. 32–54), in which mucosubstance is identified by a mucosubstance stain.

In this author's experience the majority of pulmonary adenocarcinomas are associated with scarring. The more recent literature suggests that the scarring represents a desmoplastic reaction to the tumor rather than the tumor arising in a scar; this information is summarized here. The association of lung cancer and scarring can be traced to the reports of Raeburn and Spencer,[222,223] who described adenocarcinomas, squamous carcinomas, and large cell undifferentiated carcinomas in association with scarring. In 1962, Carroll[224] reported that the presence of elastic fibers and anthracotic pigment in scars suggested that they had been present prior to the origin of the tumor.

In 1979, Auerbach et al.[225] reported on 82 lung cancers (59 adenocarcinomas, 15 squamous carcinomas, and 8 large cell undifferentiated carcinomas) thought to have been associated with scars. They tried to determine the cause of the scar in which the tumor had arisen and reported that 46 of the tumors occurred in scars resulting from pulmonary infarcts and 19 in scarring caused by tubeculomas. Scannell[226] introduced the term "bleb" carcinoma when he reported 4 carcinomas (2 adenocarcinomas and 2 squamous carcinomas) that were associated with emphysematous blebs, which are characteristically associated with some degree of scarring. This author has observed 3 squamous carcino-

mas arising in apices of upper lobes associated with regions of emphysema (unreported observations). In addition, in 1952, Konwaler and Reingold[227] described a squamous carcinoma arising in a region of bronchiectasis.

Several reports[228–232] have suggested that in almost all localized "scar carcinomas" the scarring is a desmoplastic reaction to the neoplasm rather than representing a preexisting scar. Shimosato et al.[228] analyzed 58 cases of peripheral lung cancer (48 adenocarcinomas, 8 squamous carcinomas, 2 large cell undifferentiated carcinomas) and demonstrated that the degree of pleural invasion and incidence of lymph node metastases and blood vessel invasion was greater and the prognosis of the patient worse in those patients whose tumors showed increase in collagenization or hyalinization versus those whose tumors did not show fibrosis. They suggested that those tumors that showed significant fibrosis had been present longer than those that did not show fibrosis, and that scar formation occurred in association with tumor development rather than preceding it.

Madri and Carter[229] examined 69 peripheral adenocarcinomas for the type and degree of fibrosis and related these factors to survival. In addition, they studied 7 lung carcinomas with affinity-purified antibodies specific for types I, III, IV, and V collagen. They found no association with the type and degree of fibrosis and survival but did demonstrate that scar cancers had increased amounts of type III collagen, suggesting that the scarring was a host response to the tumor. Kung and colleagues[230] evaluated 22 lung cancers that fit the description for scar carcinomas. They concluded that pleural puckering and scarring characteristic of some peripheral and central lung cancers was caused by collapse of alveolar spaces (atelectasis) rather than fibrosis. They found tuberculosis in 10 of the lung specimens examined but in only 1 specimen was the tuberculosis associated with a neoplasm. Cagle et al.[231] studied 22 pulmonary scar cancers in which 10-year or longer follow-up information was available. They found that patients whose tumors had the greatest degree of scarring were more likely to die of their cancer, and concluded that the "scar" in these neoplasms develops secondary to the cancer. In 1986, Barsky et al.[232] compared the nature of the "fibrous tissue" in lung carcinomas with scarring versus that seen in apical scars. They found a marked difference in cellular composition and biochemical composition of scar carcinomas and apical scars. More than 90% of the stromal cells identified ultrastructurally and immunohistochemically in scar carcinomas were myofibroblasts, whereas only 0–10% of the stromal cells in apical scars were myofibroblasts. They concluded that pulmonary scar carcinomas were

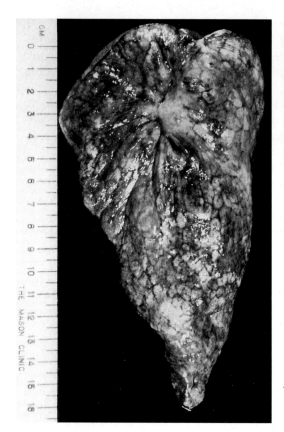

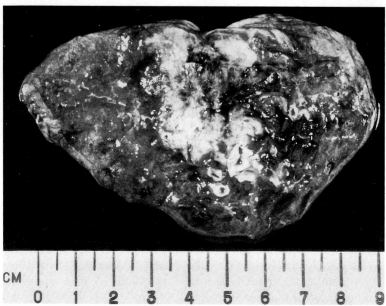

Fig. 32–48. Lateral pleural surface of resected lobe of lung shows region of pleural puckering.

Fig. 32–49. Slice through lobe shown in Fig. 32–48. Large, focally necrotic tumor causes retraction of pleura.

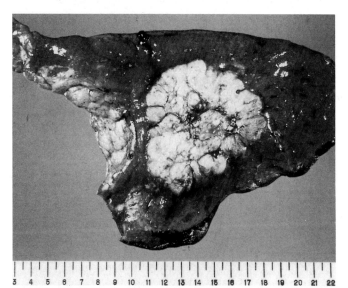

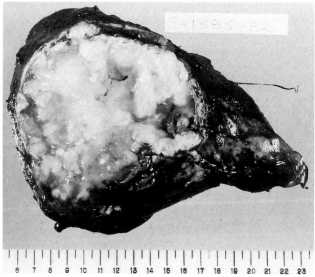

Fig. 32–50. Large, centrally necrotic adenocarcinoma is in midlung field.

Fig. 32–51. Mucus-producing adenocarcinoma appears cystic; cyst is filled with thick mucous material.

desmoplastic carcinomas and were analagous to breast carcinomas (Fig. 32–55).

A typical example of a peripheral pulmonary adenocarcinoma associated with significant scarring is shown in Fig. 32–56. It should also be mentioned that pulmonary adenocarcinoma (frequently the bronchioloalveolar variety) may be associated with diffuse interstitial pulmonary fibrosis. In 1965, Meyer and Liebow[233]

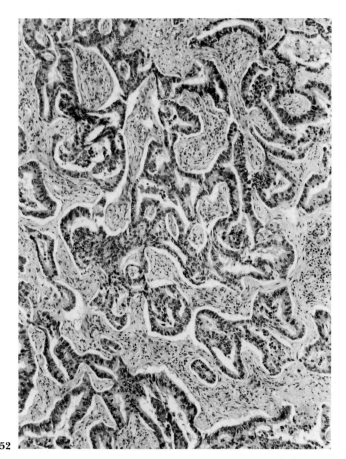

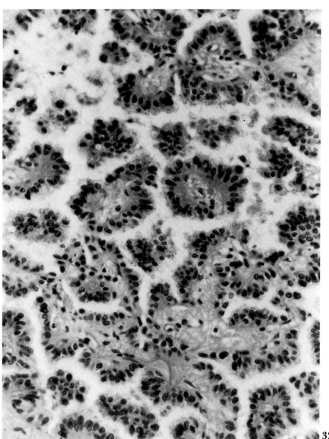

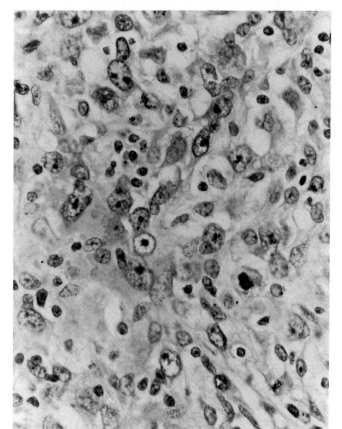

Fig. 32–52. Adenocarcinoma exhibits acinar pattern. Desmoplastic stroma is associated with tumor. ×75.

Fig. 32–53. Adenocarcinoma shows distinct papillary histologic appearance. ×75.

Fig. 32–54. Adenocarcinoma exhibits solid growth pattern. This tumor was focally mucin positive. ×550.

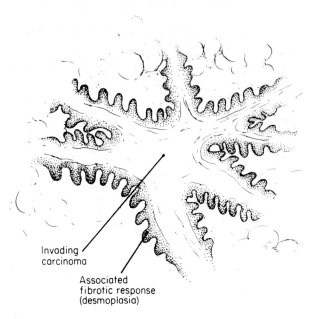

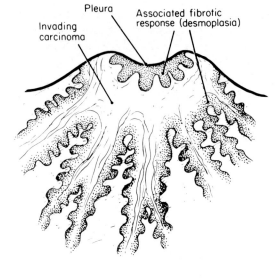

Fig. 32–55. Hypothesis that "scar" associated with pulmonary scar carcinoma represents desmoplastic response to tumor invasion and not a preexisting scar. In breast carcinoma, tumor cells invade in all directions and evoke a stellate, fibrous response. In pulmonary scar carcinoma, tumor cells are free to invade adjacent lung parenchyma but are limited in one direction by overlying pleura. The desmoplastic response accumulates along this direction and condenses, giving appearance of dense subpleural scar. Myofibroblast nature of this subpleural desmoplastic response, in turn, retracts the pleura. (Reprinted with permission from Barsky SH, Huang SJ, Bhuta S. The extracellular matrix of pulmonary scar cacinomas is suggestive of a desmoplastic origin. Am J Pathol 1986;124:412–419.)

drew attention to the frequent occurrence of atypical bronchiolar and alveolar cell proliferation in cases of interstitial pneumonia. (This is illustrated in Chapter 20). Subsequent reports confirmed the association of diffuse fibrosis with pulmonary adenocarcinoma.[234–237] In addition, adenocarcinoma, usually bronchioloalveolar cell carcinoma, is well recognized as occurring in the background of pulmonary fibrosis associated with scleroderma.[238–241]

Bronchioloalveolar cell carcinoma is a type of pulmonary adenocarcinoma that has been written about widely in recent years mainly because of ultrastructural studies showing that many of these neoplasms are composed of cells that resemble normal Clara cells or alveolar type II cells. In 1960, Liebow[242] published an extensive review article on the gross and histologic features of bronchiolo-alveolar cell carcinoma. He defined this tumor as a "well-differentiated adenocarcinoma primary in the periphery of the lung beyond a grossly recognizable bronchus, with a tendency to

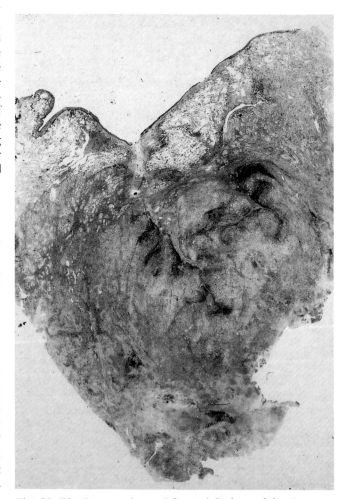

Fig. 32–56. "Scar carcinoma" from right-lower lobe. In some instances, most of tumor mass is composed of dense fibrous tissue and some elastic tissue. Note pleural retraction. ×6.

spread chiefly within the confines of the lung by aerogenous and lymphatic routes, the walls of the distal air spaces often acting as supporting stroma for the neoplastic cells." Dr. Liebow admitted that in 1960 an absolute distinction could not be made between a bronchioloalveolar cell carcinoma and an "ordinary" pulmonary adenocarcinoma but emphasized the "very peripheral origin" of the tumor, the "good cytologic differentiation," and the "tendency to spread within the lungs" as features characteristic of bronchioloalveolar cell carcinoma. Liebow further commented on another area of controversy concerning bronchioloalveolar cell carcinomas when he said "to insist that tumors to be called bronchioloalveolar grow on the unaltered walls of alveoli or without destruction of pulmonary architecture is to add confusion, because some of the illustrations presented usually show both of these changes in varying degree." As Liebow also emphasized, it must be recognized that many types of metastatic carcinoma can "grow" in a manner indistinguishable from a primary bronchioloalveolar cell carcinoma. Metastatic tumors resembling primary bronchioloalveolar cell carcinomas were nicely illustrated and tabulated (Table 32–18) by Rosenblatt et al.[243]

The exact incidence of bronchioloalveolar cell carcinoma is uncertain. In this author's experience, they make up a significant percentage of peripheral lung carcinomas. Clayton[244,245] reviewed the features of bronchioloalveolar cell carcinomas in 1988, and divided them into three histologic subtypes: mucinous, nonmucinous, and sclerosing. The sclerosing variety is similar to the nonmucinous type, and has a central area of dense sclerosis with small entrapped glands. In this author's experience, the majority of the nonmucinous bronchioloalveolar cell carcinomas show some degree of central scarring and more often than not show a fair amount of histologic variability. Macroscopically they may occur as an isolated nodule, as multiple nodules, or as a relatively diffuse "pneumonic" tumor (Figs. 32–57 and 32–58). They may be associated with central scarring (Fig. 32–59) and usually show some degree of histologic variability (Figs. 32–60 through 32–64). Two common histologic patterns are shown in Figs. 32–65 and 32–66. In Fig. 32–65, neoplastic cuboidal, columnar, or hobnail-shaped cells with apical nuclei grow in an alveolar pattern. In Fig. 32–66, the tumor is composed of tall columnar cells with basally located nuclei and abundant apical cytoplasm. Bronchioloalveolar carcinomas frequently disseminate aerogenously within the lung and appear to attach to normal alveolar septa (Fig. 32–67). Numerous ultrastructural studies have shown that many bronchioloalveolar cell carcinomas are composed of cells that closely resemble nonneoplastic type II pneumocytes and Clara cells.[246–258]

Table 32–18. Distribution of bronchioloalveolar metastases in 416 extrathoracic carcinomas[a,b]

Primary site	Number of cases	Pulmonary metastases (%)	Bronchioloalveolar metastases (%)
Colon	101	41 (41)	6 (6)
Breast	64	46 (72)	6 (9.4)
Pancreas	54	30 (55.5)	8 (14.8)
Stomach	38	17 (47.4)	4 (10.5)
Ovary	31	9 (29)	0
Bilary tract	21	7 (33.3)	1 (4.7)
Skin and melanoma	18	14 (77.7)	0
Prostate	16	8 (50)	1 (6.3)
Uterus	16	7 (43.7)	0
Kidney	12	11 (91.6)	3 (25)
Urinary bladder	11	5 (44.4)	0
Esophagus	10	6 (60)	0
Thyroid	7	4 (57.1)	1 (14.3)
Adrenal	5	4 (80)	1 (20)
Larynx	5	2 (40)	0
Nasopharynx	3	2 (66.6)	1 (33.3)
Duodenum	2	1 (50)	1 (50)
Jejunum	1	1 (100)	1 (100)
Total	416	215 (51.7)	34 (8.1)

[a] Relationship of bronchioloalveolar metastases to total pulmonary metastases = 15.8%.
[b] Reprinted with permission from Rosenblatt MB, Lisa JR, Collier F. Primary and metastatic broncho-alveolar carcinoma. *Dis Chest* 1967; 52:147–152.

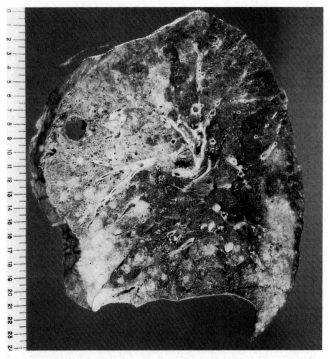

Fig. 32–57. Bronchioloalveolar carcinoma shows "pneumonic consolidation" by tumor.

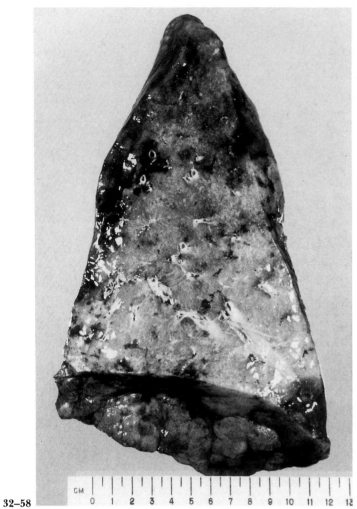

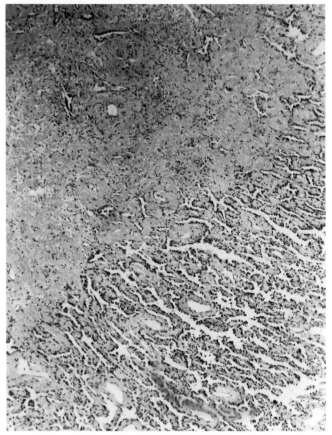

32-5

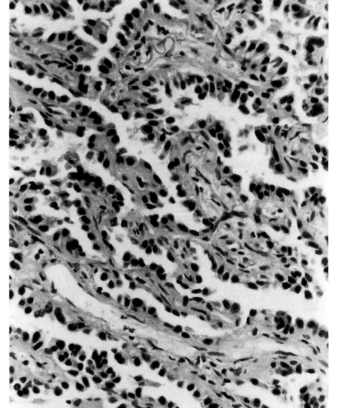

32-6

Fig. 32–58. Bronchioloalveolar carcinoma composed of firm mucoid grayish-white tissue causes consolidation of most of lobe.

Fig. 32–59. Bronchioloalveolar carcinoma shows dense central region of scarring. This form of bronchioloalveolar cell carcinoma is referred to as a sclerosing bronchioloalveolar cell carcinoma. ×75.

Fig. 32–60. Bronchioloalveolar carcinoma composed of relatively small cuboidal-to-columnar cells grows in alveolar pattern. ×330.

1168

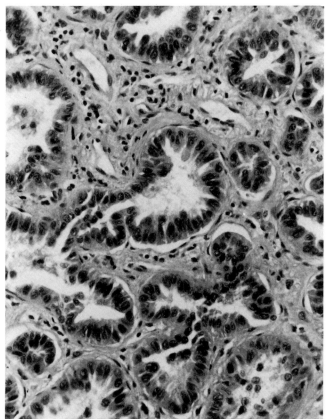

32-61

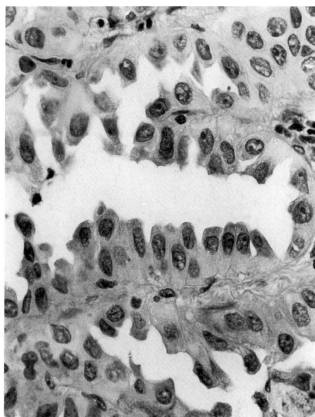

32-63

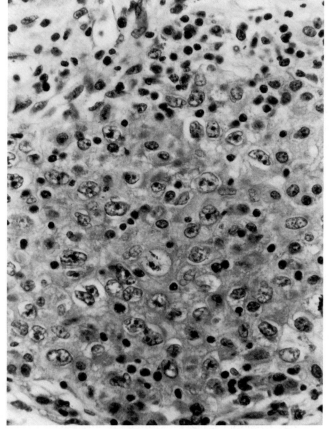

2-62

Fig. 32–61. Another region of tumor shown in Fig. 32–60 has obvious acinar appearance. ×330.

Fig. 32–62. In this region of tumor shown in Figs. 32–60 and 32–61, cells are large and poorly differentiated; this area of tumor would be classified as large cell undifferentiated carcinoma. Figures 32–60 through 32–62 show the heterogeneity that exists in many lung tumors. ×330.

Fig. 32–63. Bronchioloalveolar cell carcinoma composed of tall columnar and hobnail cells with apical located nuclei. ×550.

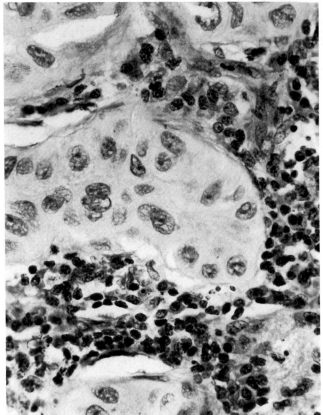

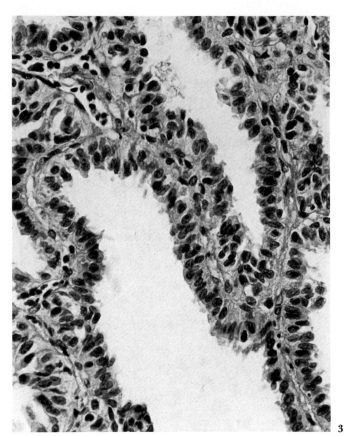

32-64

32-65

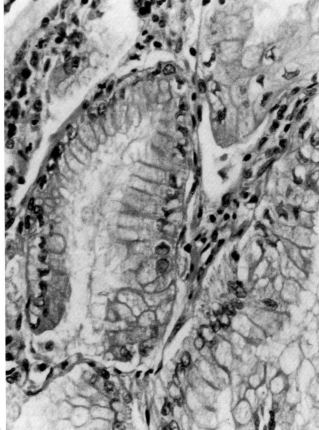

32-66

Fig. 32–64. Another region of tumor shown in Fig. 32–63 displays obvious heterogeneity. ×550.

Fig. 32–65. Typical nonmucinous type of bronchioloalveolar carcinoma composed of columnar and hobnail cells growing in alveolar pattern. ×330.

Fig. 32–66. Mucinous type of bronchioloalveolar carcinoma composed of tall columnar cells with basally located nuclei and abundant apical mucinous cytoplasm. ×330.

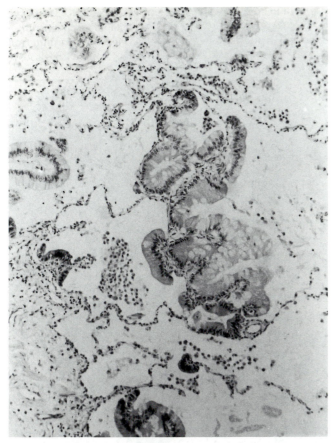

Fig. 32–67. Bronchioloalveolar carcinomas, especially mucinous variety, have tendency to spread within lung aerogenously. Note aggregates of tumor cells in association with normal alveolar septa. ×75.

As might be expected from the light microscopic appearance of bronchioloalveolar cell carcinomas, these neoplasms exhibit significant ultrastructural heterogeneity. Ultrastructurally, the mucus-producing bronchioloalveolar cell carcinomas are composed of tall cells with basally located nuclei and aggregates of mucous granules in the apical cytoplasm (Fig. 32–68). These cells usually have short, uniform microvilli associated with prominent rootlets and a fuzzy glycocalyx and glycocalyceal bodies (Fig. 32–69). The nonmucus-secreting bronchioloalveolar cell carcinomas are similar to each other; the nuclei are usually in the center of the cell with varying numbers of relatively large "granules" in the apical cytoplasm; some of these are amorphous and electron dense, and others represent multivesicular and lamellar bodies (Figs. 32–70 through 32–72). The ultrastructural spectrum of these apical bodies is shown in Fig. 32–73. Other bronchioloalveolar carcinomas will show extensive smooth and rough endoplasmic reticulum, which is frequently seen in nonneoplastic Clara cells, in the apical cytoplasm (Figs. 32–74 and 32–75). A rare bronchioloalveolar cell carcinoma contains

lamellar-glycogen bodies in the cytoplasm of the tumor cells (Fig. 32–76). Dekmezian et al.[259] described a unique bronchioloalveolar cell carcinoma characterized by glandular spaces formed by a lumina layer of cells with the ultrastructural features of Clara cells and type II pneumocytes, with a basal layer of myoepithelial cells (Fig. 32–77).

As extensively described by Singh and others,[260–264] many bronchioloalveolar cell carcinomas contain intranuclear tubular inclusions thought to arise from the inner nuclear membrane (Fig. 32–78). These correlate with eosinophilic intranuclear inclusions by light microscopy (Fig. 32–79) that frequently stain positive with periodic acid–Schiff stain. The same type of inclusions can also be seen in metastatic bronchioloalveolar cell carcinomas[265] (Figs. 32–80 and 32–81). Immunohistochemically these inclusions immunostain for the apoprotein portion of surfactant,[262] indicating their relationship to alveolar type II cells. Many bronchioloalveolar cell carcinomas contain Langerhans' cells, an observation first made by Basset et al.[266] and later expanded upon by this author and colleagues.[267,268] Langerhans' cells are easiest identified in these tumors using an immunoperoxidase procedure for S-100 protein (Figs. 32–82 and 32–83) and can always be demonstrated by electron microscopy (Fig. 32–84). Takakura et al.[269] and Furukawa et al.[270] have provided evidence that bronchioloalveolar cell carcinomas with many Langerhans' cells in them have a better prognosis than those that do not. This author is uncertain about this association because we have frequently seen numerous Langerhans' cells in metastatic bronchioloalveolar cell carcinomas (Figs. 32–85 and 32–86).

A morphologic feature that we have observed most frequently in bronchioloalveolar cell carcinomas, usually ones that are relatively pleomorphic, is eosinophilic hyaline globules in the cytoplasm of the tumor cells (Figs. 32–87 and 32–88). As shown, these are usually round and vary considerably in size with some being as large as an erythrocyte. Ultrastructurally, these are electron dense (Figs. 32–89 and 32–90), and the larger ones may resemble red blood cells; they probably represent lysosomes. They were reported by Nakanishi et al.[271] in adenocarcinomas, squamous carcinomas, and large cell undifferentiated carcinomas, and were considered to possibly represent a variant of Clara cell granules. Scroggs et al.,[272] in a review of 100 consecutive cases of lung carcinoma, identified intracytoplasmic eosinophilic globules ranging in size from less than 1 μm to 20 μm in diameter in six cases of mucin-positive adenocarcinomas. They described the globules as being similar to Russell bodies in plasma cells, to be intensely PAS positive, brick red with Masson trichrome stain, and to show variable staining with phosphotungstic acid–hematoxylin and Ziehl–Neelsen stains. By immunohistochemistry, they found some globules to show

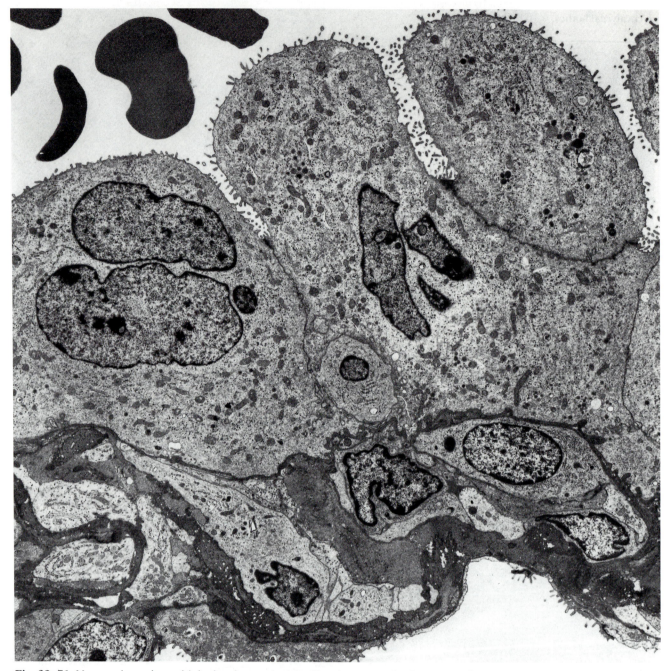

Fig. 32–71. Nonmucinous bronchioloalveolar carcinoma. Note large neoplastic tumor cells on one side of alveolar septum and benign alveolar lining cells on other side. ×4,100.

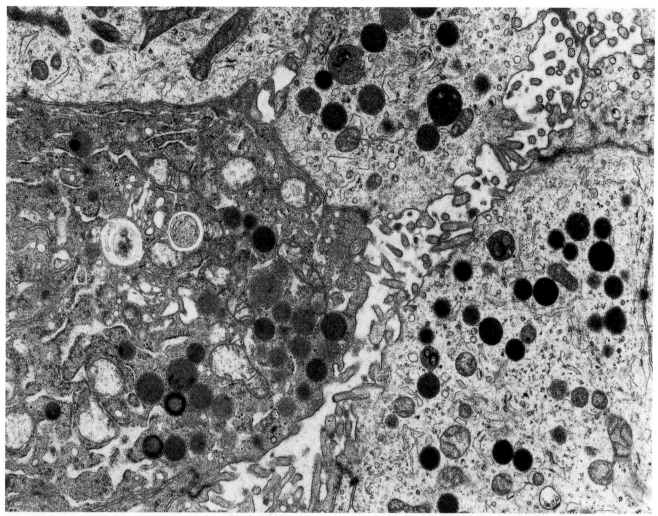

Fig. 32–72. Most nonmucinous bronchioloalveolar carcinomas contain varying numbers variable electron-dense "bodies" 500–1500 nm in diameter in their apical cytoplasm. Some have appearance of lamellar bodies and others have appearance of dense bodies and multivesicular bodies. ×26,500.

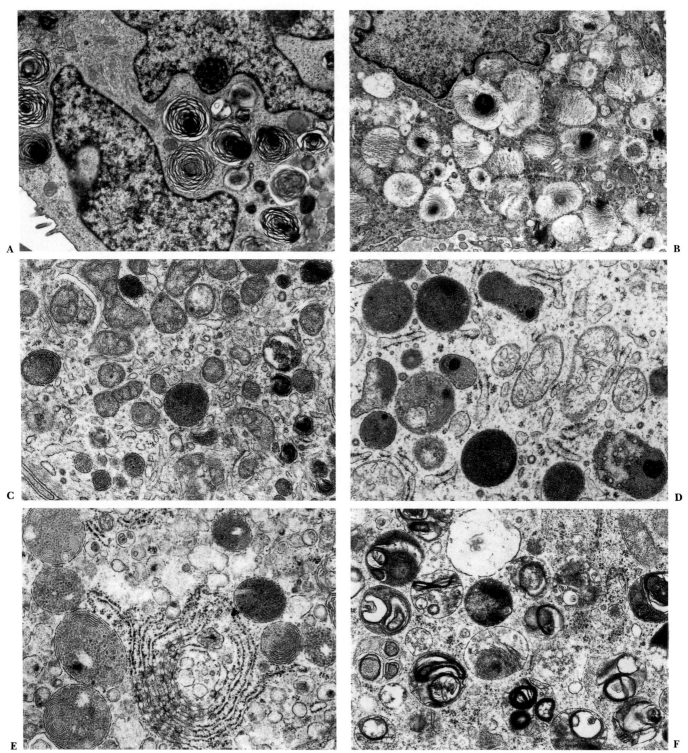

Fig. 32–73. A–F. Variable appearance of cytoplasmic "bodies" in apical portion of cytoplasm of nonmucinous bronchioloalveolar carcinomas. Care must be taken to not "overinterpret" such "bodies" because they can be found in other adenocarcinomas; Fig. 32–73F, for example, represents "lamellar-like bodies" found in prostatic adenocarcinoma. ×26,500.

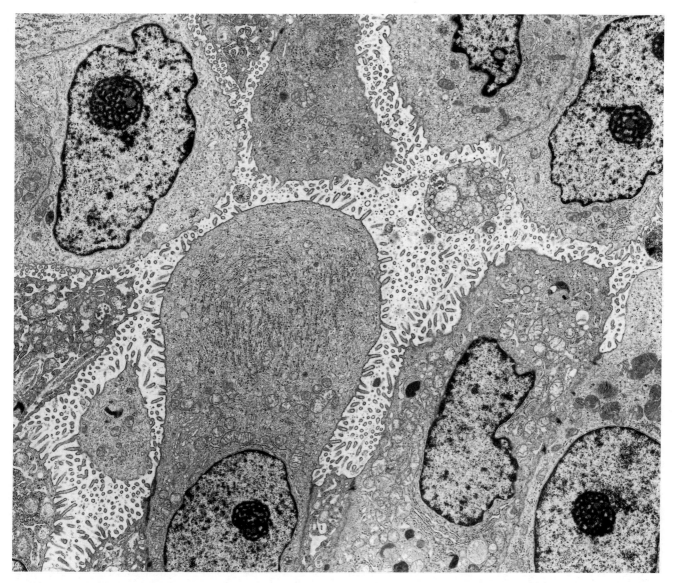

Fig. 32–74. Bronchioloalveolar carcinoma has ultrastructural appearance suggesting Clara cell origin of tumor. Note prominent endoplasmic reticulum in apical cytoplasm. ×10,500.

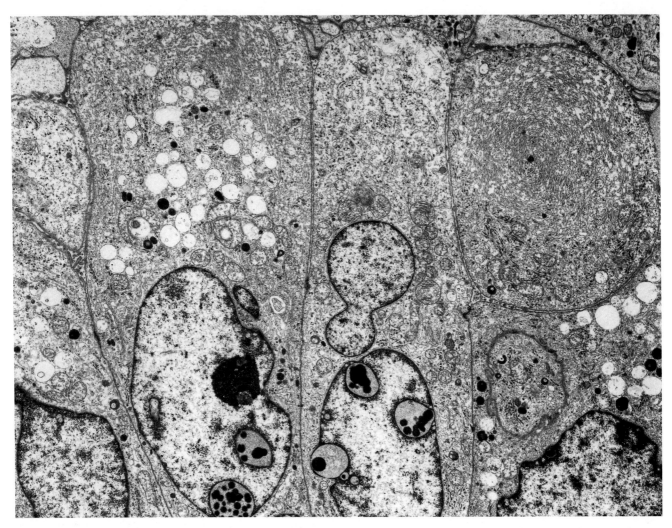

Fig. 32–75. Another bronchioloalveolar carcinoma of probable Clara cell origin. Prominent smooth endoplasmic reticulum in apical cytoplasm of tumor cells is commonly found in normal Clara cells. Also note electron-dense nuclear inclusions. ×6,400.

Fig. 32–76. Bronchioloalveolar carcinoma cell contains lamellar-glycogen body in apical cytoplasm *(arrows)*. This structure is not specific for bronchioloalveolar cell carcinoma although some of these neoplasms contain glycogen as do normal Clara cells. ×16,000.

Fig. 32–77. Unusual bronchioloalveolar cell carcinoma composed of neoplastic type II pneumocytes surrounded by myoepithelial cells *(arrows)*. (Reprinted by permission from Dekmezian R, Ordonez NG, Mackay B. Bronchioloalveolar adenocarcinoma with myoepithelial cells. Cancer 1991;67: 2356–2360.)

Fig. 32–78. Intranuclear tubular inclusion in this bronchioloalveolar carcinoma cell corresponds to that seen by light microscopy in Fig. 32–79. These inclusions immunostain for the apoprotein portion of surfactant and are considered to be specific markers for cells of type II pneumocyte origin; they are seen in benign and neoplastic cells. ×26,500.

Fig. 32–79. Region of poorly differentiated adenocarcinoma; tumor cells contain frequent intranuclear inclusions *(arrow)*. When examined by electron microscopy these had the same appearance as shown in Fig. 32–78. Nuclear inclusions suggest tumor is type II pneumocyte in origin. ×775.

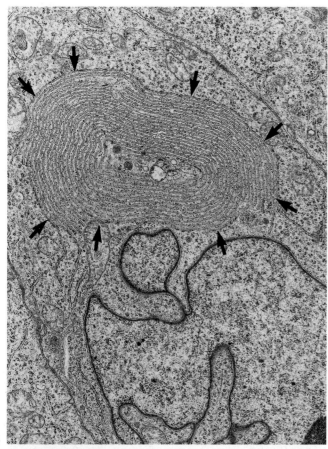

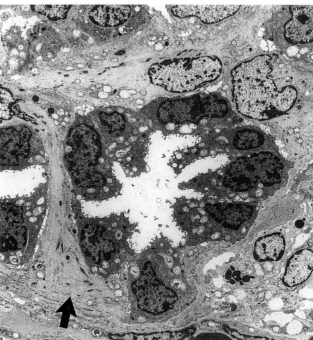

32-76

32-77

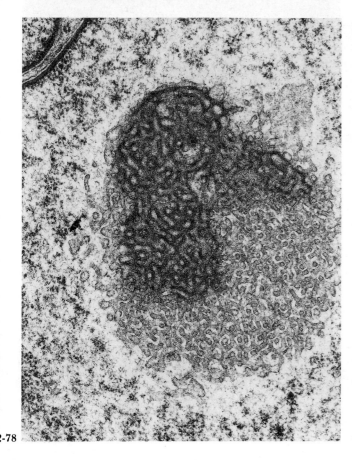

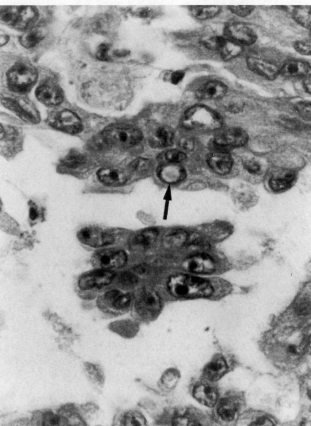

2-78

32-79

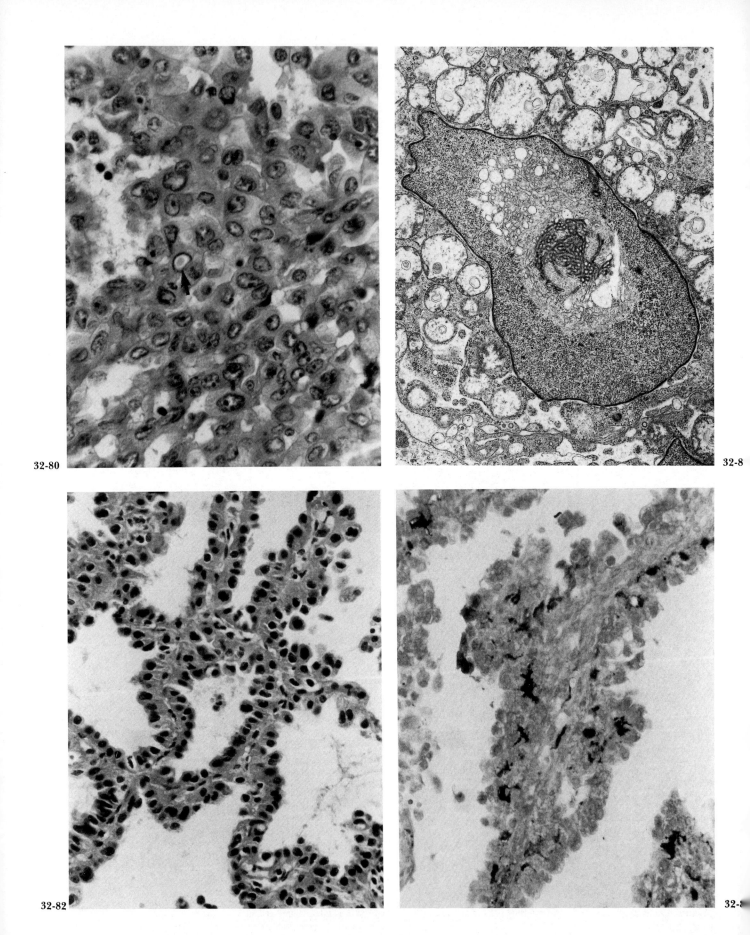

32-80

32-8

32-82

32-8

1180

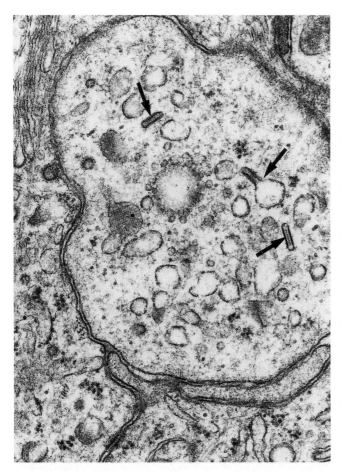

Fig. 32–84. When examined ultrastructurally, tumor shown in Figs. 32–82 and 32–83 contained processes of Langerhans' cells with Langerhans' cell granules *(arrows)*. ×51,500.

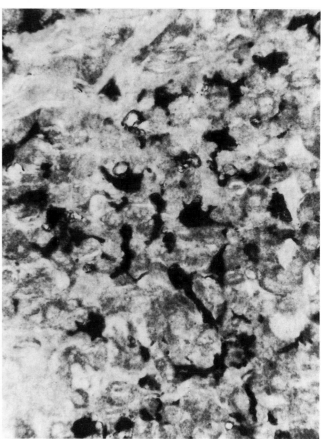

Fig. 32–85. Section of metastatic tumor shown in Fig. 32–80 immunostained for S-100 protein. Note numerous positive *(black)* Langerhans' cells mixed with tumor cells. ×330.

◁

Fig. 32–80. Nuclear inclusions *(arrow)* can also be seen in metastatic adenocarcinomas, which indicates such neoplasms are of pulmonary origin. ×775.

Fig. 32–81. Ultrastructural appearance of tumor cell with intranuclear inclusion shown in Fig. 32–80 is identical to that in Fig. 32–78. ×16,000.

Fig. 32–82. Nonmucinous type of bronchioloalveolar carcinoma that was immunostained for S-100 protein as shown in Fig. 32–83. ×330.

Fig. 32–83. When immunostained for S-100 protein, numerous dendritic S-100-positive *(black)* cells correspond to Langerhans' cells. ×330.

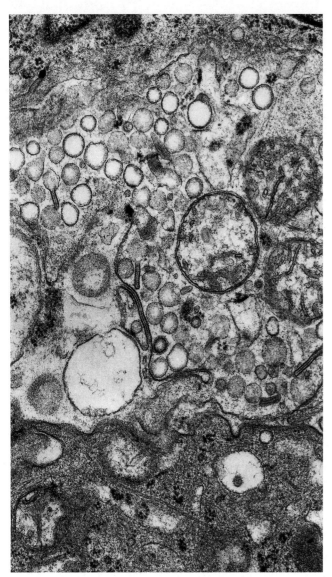

Fig. 32–86. Part of Langerhans' cell seen in association with tumor cell. ×43,000.

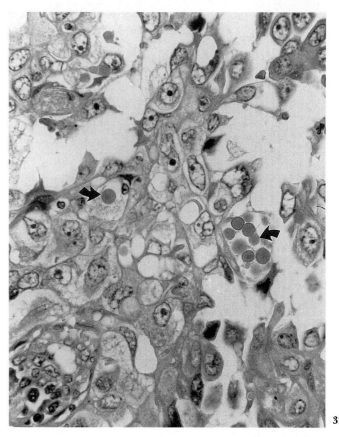

32-8

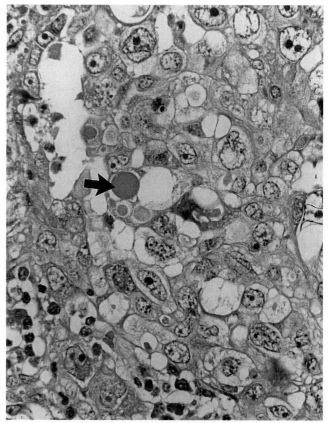

32-8

Fig. 32–87. In many degenerating carcinomas of lung, eosinophilic bodies are found in cytoplasm of tumor cells *(arrow)*. These resemble Russell bodies in plasma cells. ×330.

Fig. 32–88. Eosinophilic bodies noted in some degenerating tumor cells are large and round and resemble red blood cells *(arrow)*. ×550.

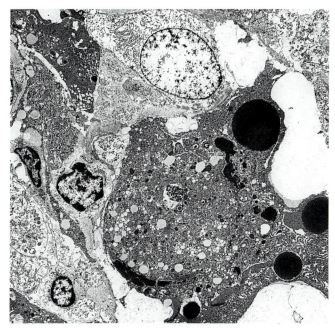

Fig. 32–89. Ultrastructurally, eosinophilic bodies occur in degenerating cells and have same electron density as red blood cells. ×8,200.

slight staining for albumin, IgG, IgA, and alpha-1 antitrypsin. Scroggs et al.[272] suggested that the globules represented secretory glycoprotein that accumulated in the cytoplasm of injured tumor cells.

Another somewhat uncommon pattern of bronchioloalveolar cell carcinoma is the presence of an intense lymphocyte-plasma cell interstitial infiltrate in some mucinous bronchioloalveolar cell carcinomas (Figs. 32–91 and 32–92). As might be expected, and as is discussed by Axiotis and Jennings,[273] most of the lymphocytes are B cells.

Another unusual morphologic pattern of bronchioloalveolar cell carcinoma is the presence of varyingly sized but often relatively large, intensely PAS-positive, and mucicarmine-negative extracellular globules (Figs. 32–93 and 32–94). By electron microscopy the neoplastic cells show type II pneumocyte differentiation (Fig. 32–95), and the extracellular globules represent surfactant material, including lamellar bodies and tubular myelin (Fig. 32–96).

In 1988, Miller et al.[274] reported on 62 consecutive resections for adenocarcinoma of the lung, and found a high incidence of multiple pulmonary adenocarcino-

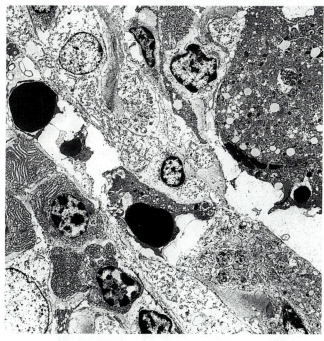

Fig. 32–90. Two large electron-dense bodies in cytoplasm of degenerating tumor cells. ×8,200.

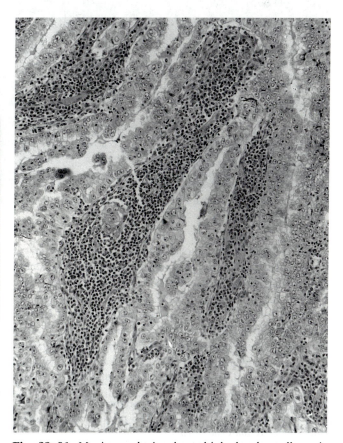

Fig. 32–91. Mucin-producing bronchioloalveolar cell carcinoma is associated with heavy infiltrate of lymphocytes and plasma cells. ×75.

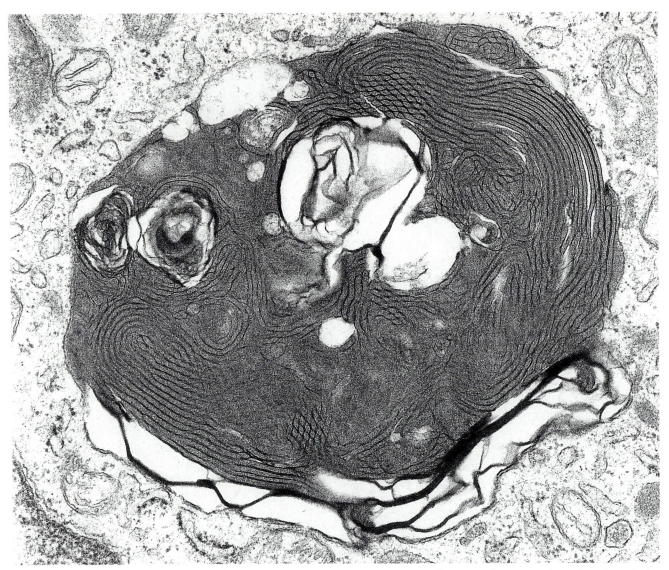

Fig. 32–96. Extracellular material shown in Figs. 32–93 and 32–94 represented surfactant and was sometimes found as tubular myelin inside tumor cells. ×63,800.

observed represented separate primary tumors or resulted from aerogenous dissemination. She concluded these adenomas did not represent aerogenous dissemination of a nonmucinous bronchioloalveolar cell carcinoma, but were multiple tumors analogous to colonic polyposis.

This author has observed several examples of bronchioloalveolar adenomas, most frequently in lobectomy or pneumonectomy specimens removed for bronchioloalveolar carcinomas. In formalin-fixed (inflated) lungs these are difficult to see macroscopically, and it should be recalled that Miller inflated her lung specimens with Bouin solution, which results in more contrast between the normal parenchyma and the small white nodules. Histologically, bronchioloalveolar ade-

nomas are exactly as Miller described, showing a proliferation of atypical alveolar lining cells growing in a lepidic fashion (Figs. 32–97 and 32–98). In our experience and as described by Miller, these cells usually show type II pneumocyte differentiation (Figs. 32–99).

Along the same line, Yousem and Hochholzer[276] reported six cases of a lesion they referred to as alveolar adenoma, which were described as solitary, well-demarcated nodules, 1.2 to 2.5 cm in diameter, with a prominent cellular component. Travis et al.[277] reported two cases of small pulmonary nodules resembling bronchioloalveolar carcinoma in adolescent cancer patients. The patient in the first case was a 16-year-old male who was diagnosed as having Ewing sarcoma of the left tibia with pulmonary metastases at age 9. He was initially

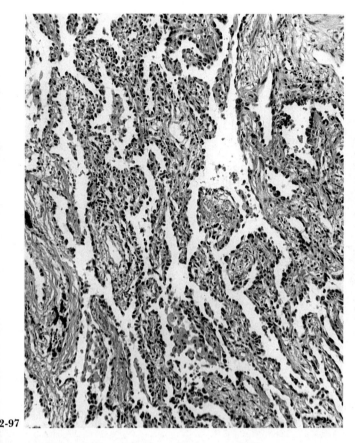

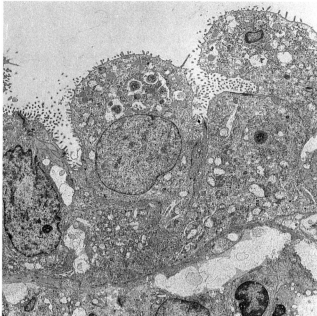

Fig. 32–99. Ultrastructurally, cells forming bronchioloalveolar adenoma have features of type II pneumocytes. ×4,100.

treated with vincristine, doxorubicin, cyclophosphamide, and dicarbazine, had a recurrence 5 years later treated with etoposide and ifosfamide, and then 20 months later was found to have a right-lower-lobe, 1-cm nodule that was resected. Histologically, it had the appearance of a bronchioloalveolar cell carcinoma and by DNA analysis contained an aneuploid population of cells. It was different than the nodules illustrated by Miller[275] in that there was significantly more stroma. The other case concerned a 19-year-old male with a testicular teratocarcinoma who developed retroperitoneal and pulmonary metastases. After being treated with three cycles of etoposide, ifosfamide, and cisplatin, a thoracotomy was done with multiple wedge resections of nodules present in the right-upper, right-middle, and right-lower lobes. Nine of the 10 resected nodules represented metastatic testicular neoplasm; the tenth nodule had the appearance of a nonmucinous bronchioloalveolar cell carcinoma. The authors raised the possibility of these being chemically induced neoplasms. Noguchi et al.[278] reported a 1.5-cm-diameter papillary neoplasm referred to as an adenoma of type II pneu-

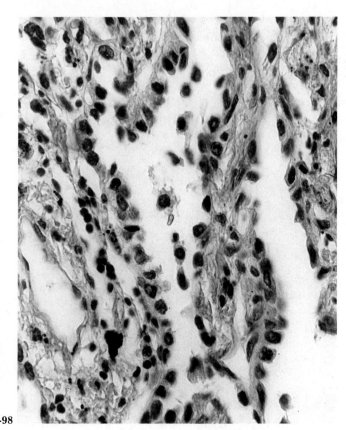

Fig. 32–97. This region of lung tissue shows mildly atypical alveolar lining cell hypertrophy and hyperplasia, referred to as bronchioloalveolar adenoma. ×125.

Fig. 32–98. At higher magnification, cellular features of bronchioloalveolar adenoma are more easily seen. ×550.

mocytes, and Hegg et al.[279] described three cases of well-demarcated, partially encapsulated papillary neoplasms 1.2–2.5 cm in diameter that ultrastructurally showed evidence of type II pneumocyte or Clara cell differentiation.

Other histologic types of pulmonary adenocarcinomas occur.[280] Some primary pulmonary adenocarcinomas closely resemble colonic adenocarcinomas and in this author's opinion cannot be definitely differentiated from metastatic colon tumors by light microscopy, electron microscopy, or immunohistochemistry. They are analagous to the intestinal type of adenocarcinomas that occur in the nasal cavity and paranasal sinuses.[281] They may originate from the mucous cells that are part of the bronchial epithelium, which may closely resemble intestinal mucous cells ultrastructurally.[282] An example of such a tumor is shown in Figs. 32–100 and 32–101. Ultrastructurally these cells closely resemble neoplastic colonic adenocarcinoma cells, showing short uniform microvill, glycocalyceal bodies, and prominent rootlets in the apical cytoplasm as well as mucous granules (Fig. 32–102). With respect to mucous granules in pulmonary adenocarcinomas, they also show a great deal of ultrastructural heterogeneity (Fig. 32–103). Rarely, some pulmonary adenocarcinomas will have a signet ring appearance (Figs. 32–104 through 32–106).

Several reports have been published since the first edition of *Pulmonary Pathology* concerning primary "mucinous" adenocarcinomas of the lung. Kish et al.[283] reported five cases of primary adenocarcinoma of the lung with a prominent component of signet ring cells essentially identical to those shown in Figs. 32–104 through 32–106. In their cases, the percentage of signet ring cells ranged from 10% to 50%, with a mean of 22% and a median of 20%. They performed a detailed histochemical evaluation using various mucosubstance stains and were unable to demonstrate a quantitative or qualitative difference between mucopolysaccharides produced by lung, stomach, or colon tumors. In their series, three of five patients died of their disease within 9 months, and two patients showed no evidence of disease 5 months after presentation. Two of the five tumors reported were anatomic stage IV, and two were at least anatomic stage II.

Graeme-Cook and Mark[284] reported data on 11 patients who had solitary pulmonary nodules resected in which mucus was the major histologic component. The neoplasms were composed of cystic spaces lined by mucus-producing columnar epithelial cells with cyto-

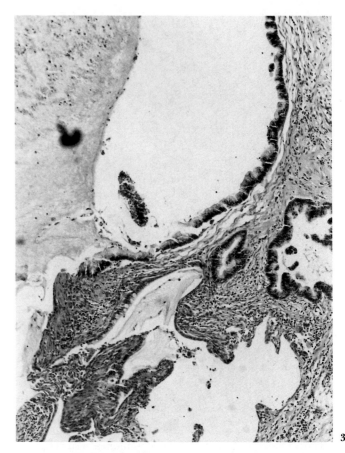

32-1

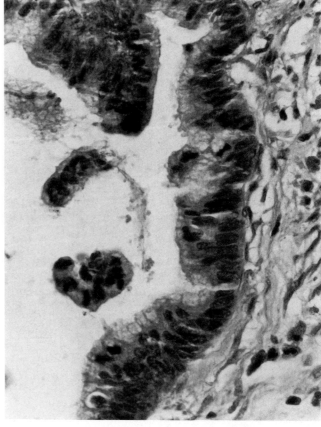

32-1

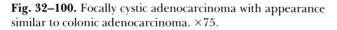

Fig. 32–100. Focally cystic adenocarcinoma with appearance similar to colonic adenocarcinoma. ×75.

Fig. 32–101. Greater magnification of tumor shown in Fig. 32–100. Note similarity to colon adenocarcinoma. ×550.

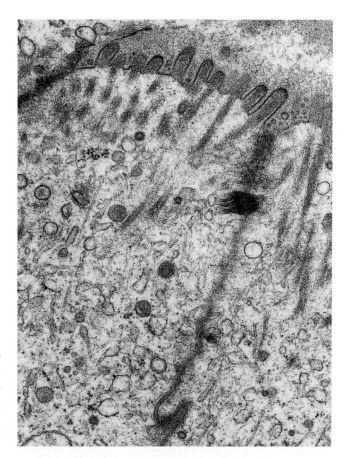

Fig. 32–102. Ultrastructurally, tumor shown in Figs. 32–100 and 32–101 closely resembles colonic adenocarcinoma. Tumor cells have short uniform microvilli covered by glycocalyx and associated with glycocalyceal bodies plus numerous filaments in apical cytoplasm. Histologically, immunohistochemically, and ultrastructurally, this tumor cannot be differentiated from metastatic colonic adenocarcinoma. ×26,500.

logic and architectural atypia, varying from minimal to microscopic foci of carcinoma. In their series, there was no evidence of local recurrence or metastatic spread of tumor in a followup between 1 to 9.5 years (mean, 4.7 years). Graeme-Cook and Mark concluded that histologic and clinical findings were consistent with a mucinous cystic tumor of low or borderline malignant potential. Two of the cases in their series were contributed by this author, and the macroscopic appearance of one is shown in Fig. 32–51. We have encountered another interesting example of such a neoplasm in an asbestos-exposed shipyard worker, who was treated with a left-lower lobectomy in May 1971. He was well until 1985, when he developed central nervous system symptoms and was found to have an isolated mass in his brain. This was resected, and proved to have an histologic appearance identical to the primary tumor. He subsequently developed metastases in his right lung and regional lymph nodes, and at autopsy the tumor had the same histologic appearance (Figs. 32–107 and 32–108). Two similar cases of cystic-mucus variants of primary lung adenocarcinoma were described by Higashiyama et al.[285] These authors stated that because the neoplasms contained very few cancer cells, and those present were at the periphery, it was impossible to

diagnose them as malignant preoperatively via cytologic examination. Moran et al.[286] reported 24 cases of a neoplasm they referred to as primary mucinous or colloid carcinoma of the lung. The tumors were described as measuring 5 mm to 10.9 cm in greatest dimension, and macroscopically were poorly circumscribed, soft tan-to-grey mucoid lesions. They did not observe cystic structures in any of the cases reported. Histologically, small clusters of atypical cells were observed in intraalveolar pools of mucin, and foci of neoplastic columnar epithelium lined some alveoli. Seven cases were stated to show solid, well-differentiated malignant glands adjacent to pools of mucin. Nineteen patients were available for follow-up from 6 days to 16 years later. Two patients died postoperatively, and 11 of 17 patients were alive between 2 and 192 months (median, 97 months), with 9 having no evidence of tumor and 2 alive with tumors. The authors concluded that these neoplasms probably represented a variant of bronchioloalveolar cell carcinoma and because of their bland cytologic appearance and paucity of malignant cells, could be difficult to diagnose.

Tsao and Fraser[287] reported a primary lung neoplasm that showed small intestinal differentiation. The tumor was in the right-upper lobe and described as a

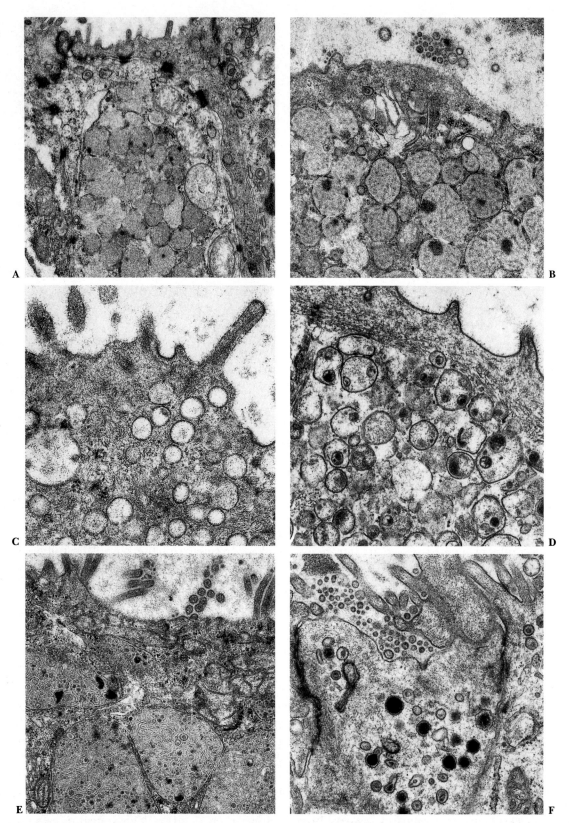

Fig. 32–103. A–F. Mucous granules of pulmonary adenocarcinomas show wide range in ultrastructural appearance. Mucous granules in Fig. 28–83F have appearance of neuroendocrine glands. ×26,500.

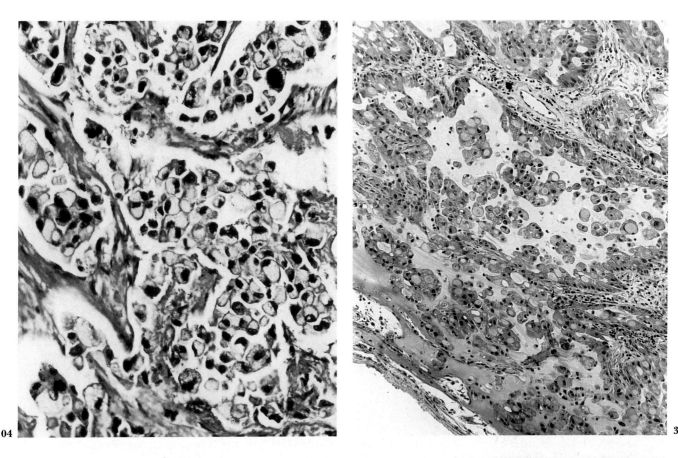

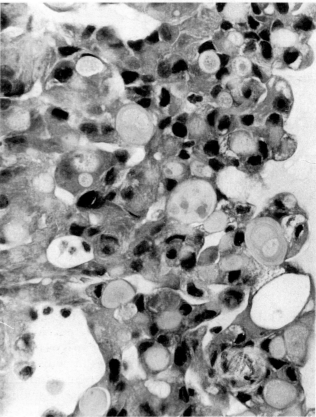

Fig. 32–104. This pulmonary adenocarcinoma is composed of signet ring cells and closely resembles some gastric adenocarcinomas. ×330.

Fig. 32–105. Mucin-producing adenocarcinoma composed predominantly of signet ring-type cells. ×125.

Fig. 32–106. Greater magnification of tumor shown in Fig. 32–105. Signet ring cells are filled with mucus. ×550.

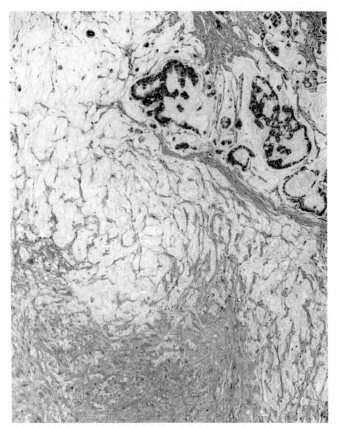

Fig. 32–107. Mucinous adenocarcinoma is cystic and composed predominantly of lakes of mucin. ×75.

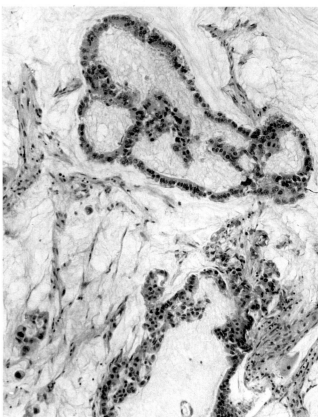

Fig. 32–108. Nests of glandular mucus-producing tumor cells present in some regions of tumor. ×330.

well-circumscribed but unencapsulated nodule 2 cm in diameter and containing large quantities of mucus. Histologically, it was composed of columnar absorptive cells, goblet cells, Paneth cells, and some cells showing neuroendocrine differentiation. The authors reasoned that it was a primary lung neoplasm, because a follow-up of 4 years had not revealed a primary neoplasm elsewhere. They concluded that such a neoplasm provided evidence for the existence of a common stem cell in the lower respiratory and gastrointestinal tract mucosa.

Also uncommon are what this author refers to as small cell adenocarcinomas, which may closely resemble small cell undifferentiated neuroendocrine carcinomas (see neuroendocrine tumors later in this chapter). Small cell adenocarcinomas are composed of nests and cords of relatively small cells with high nuclear cytoplasmic ratios (Figs. 32–109 through 32–111). They frequently show necrosis and a high mitotic rate. They are diagnosed as adenocarcinomas primarily by electron microscopy in which definite gland formation is seen (Figs. 32–112 and 32–113) and by their lack of neuroendocrine features. In addition, they are negative for neuron-specific enolase and chromogranin when studied immunohistochemically, and usually express low and

high molecular weight cytokeratin, a feature not usually seen in small cell neuroendocrine carcinomas, which express only simple epithelial cytokeratin of low molecular weight. In many respects, this small cell adenocarcinoma resembles the neoplasm recently described by Brambilla et al.[288] as basal cell or basaloid carcinoma of the lung.

Two other uncommon glandular pulmonary neoplasms have been described. Kodama et al.[289] described an endobronchial polypoid adenocarcinoma of the lung composed of cells showing bronchiolar and mucus differentiation. Despite the intrabronchial nature of the tumor, three of five cases had regional lymph node metastases. Cagle et al.[290] recently reported two cases of a neoplasm they considered unique which they referred to as a peripheral biphasic adenocarcinoma. The two patients, a 79-year-old man and a 64-year-old woman, had peripheral neoplasms composed of a definite glandular component and a sarcomatoid stromal component that showed immunostaining for keratin, epithelial membrane antigen and in one case, carcinoembryonic antigen. The stromal component showed no expression of vimentin, B72.3, LeuM1, muscle-specific actin, S100 protein, or desmin. We have observed a

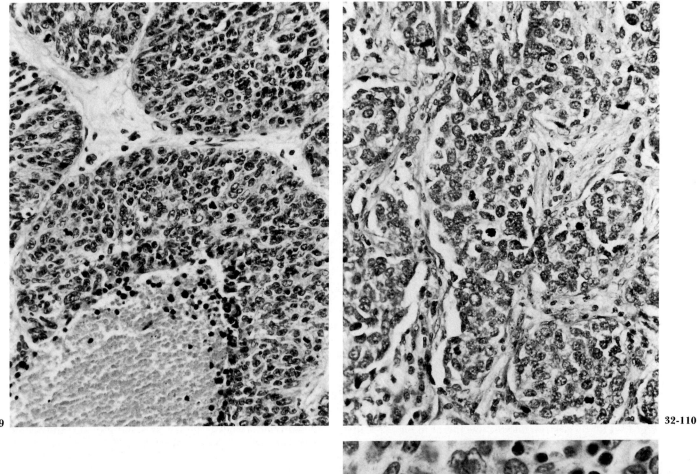

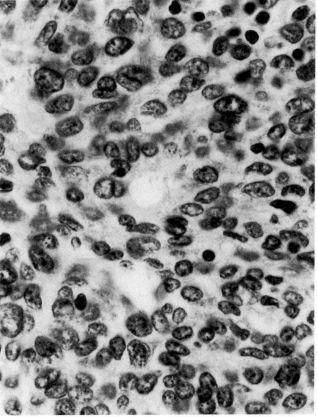

Fig. 32–109. Poorly differentiated tumor best classified as an intermediate small cell undifferentiated carcinoma. When studied by electron microscopy, this tumor lacked neuroendocrine features and showed definite gland formation by tumor cells. ×330.

Fig. 32–110. Another poorly differentiated carcinoma that showed glandular differentiation by electron microscopy.

Fig. 32–111. Rudimentary glands are seen occasionally in such small cell tumors, but this does not necessarily exclude possibility of neuroendocrine carcinoma. ×550.

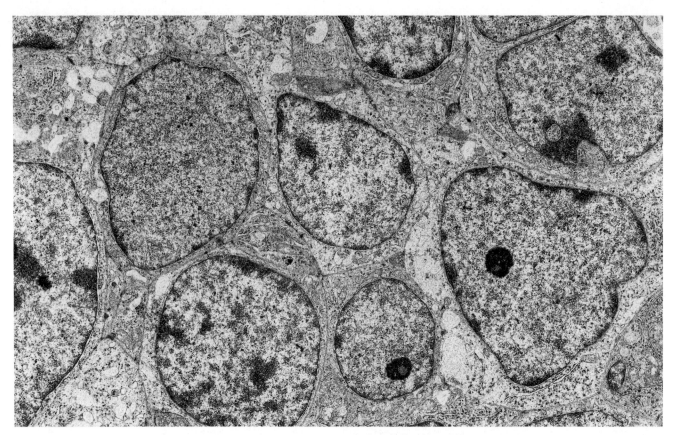

Fig. 32–112. By electron microscopy, tumor in Fig. 32–110 is composed of small round cells with high nuclear-toxcytoplasmic ratios. Cytoplasm has more organelles than typical small cell neuroendocrine carcinomas, and there are no cytoplasmic neuroendocrine granules. ×6,400.

somewhat similar neoplasm in which there appeared to be a transition between the glandular component of the neoplasm and a spindle cell component (Figs. 32–114 and 32–115).

Pulmonary adenocarcinomas of all histologic types show similar immunohistochemical features (see Table 32–17). They usually express low and high molecular weight cytokeratin, carcinoembryonic antigen, epithelial membrane antigen, and human milk fat globule protein (Fig. 32–116).[169,280]

Most pulmonary adenocarcinomas show a cytoplasmic distribution of immunostaining with antibodies against epithelial membrane antigen and human milk fat globule protein-2. However, this author has seen several cases of nonmucinous bronchioloalveolar cell carcinomas that have shown a cell membrane pattern of immunostaining for epithelial membrane antigen and human milk fat globule proteins. This is of some significance in that most well- and moderately well differentiated epithelial mesotheliomas show cell membrane immunostaining for human milk fat globule protein-2, and epithelial membrane antigen. Therefore, the cell membrane pattern of immunostaining for these two

antibodies is not specific. In addition, in this author's experience, only about 50% of pulmonary adenocarcinomas immunostain for LeuM1 and BerEP4, and fewer (approximately 30%) immunostain for B72.3. Some reports[291,292] have indicated that a significant percentage of adenocarcinomas express vimentin; this has not been this author's experience when using three different commercially available antibodies against vimentin. Another report indicated that some lung carcinomas express S-100 protein.[293]

Linnoila et al.[294] examined immunohistochemically 247 primary and metastatic non-small cell lung carcinomas, the corresponding nonneoplastic lung tissue, and 75 nonpulmonary neoplasms for the presence of peripheral airway cell surfactant-associated proteins (two antibodies against surfactant protein: SAM, SP-2), and 10-kdalton Clara cell protein. Sixty-two percent of the pulmonary adenocarcinomas, 17% of the squamous cell carcinomas, and 15% of large cell undifferentiated carcinomas showed positive immunostaining, which was usually focal and discordant among the three antibodies. Only 1 breast neoplasm and 1 papillary carcinoma of the thyroid were positive for surfactant pro-

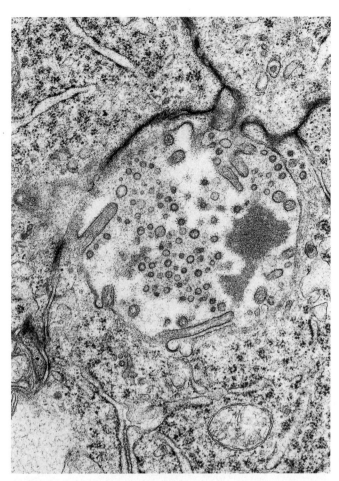

Fig. 32–113. In several regions of tumor shown in Fig. 32–111, tumor cells were forming distinct small glands. ×43,000.

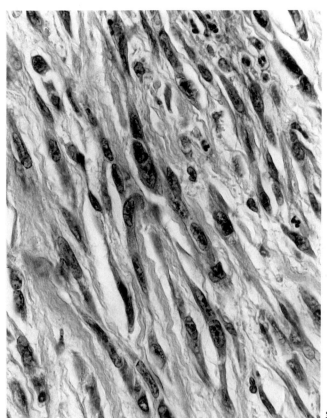

32-114

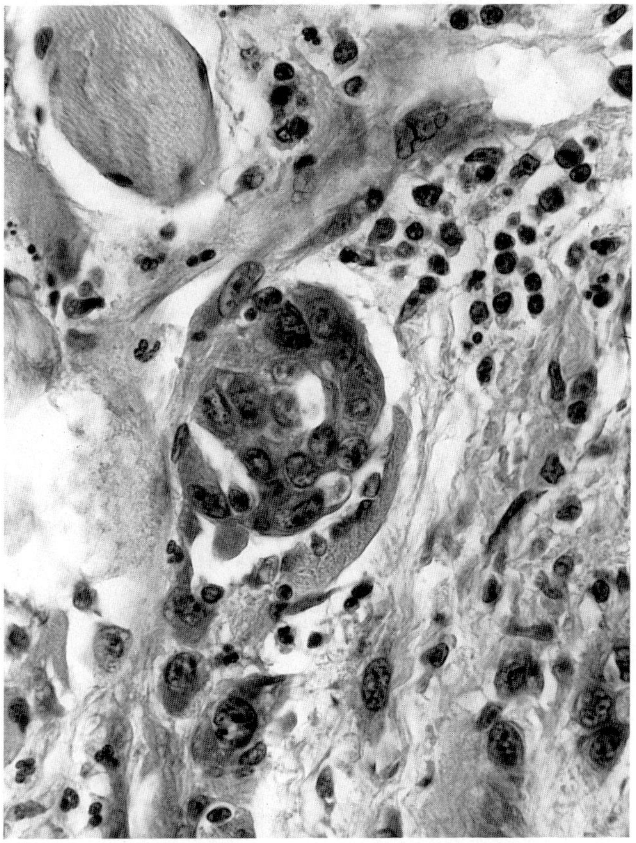

32-115

Fig. 32–114. Upper-lobe mass composed predominantly of spindle-shaped cells. ×500.

Fig. 32–115. In many areas of tumor shown in Fig. 32–114 were transitions between spindle cell component and a glandular component. ×550.

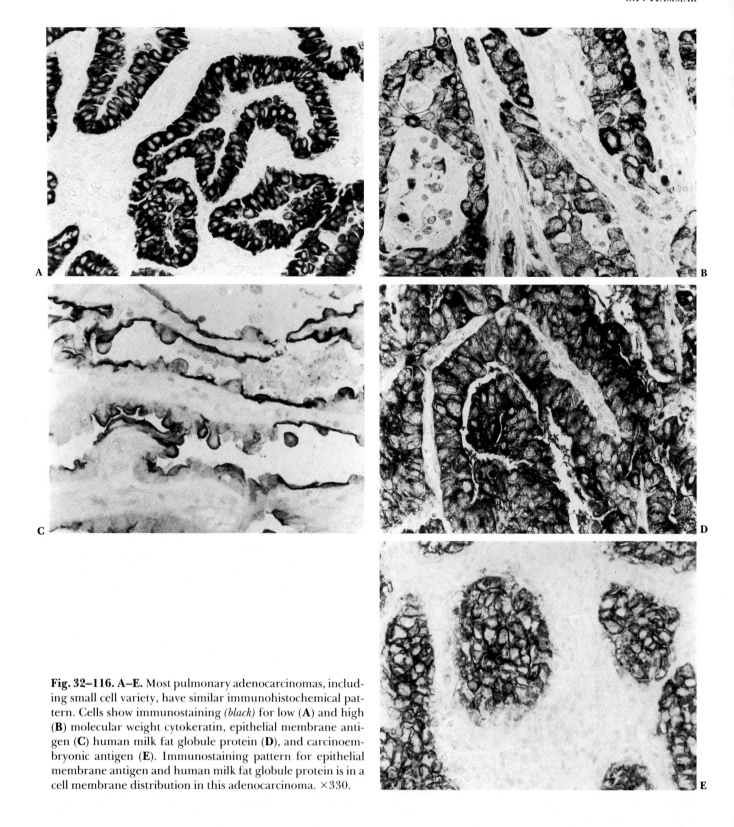

Fig. 32–116. A–E. Most pulmonary adenocarcinomas, including small cell variety, have similar immunohistochemical pattern. Cells show immunostaining *(black)* for low (**A**) and high (**B**) molecular weight cytokeratin, epithelial membrane antigen (**C**) human milk fat globule protein (**D**), and carcinoembryonic antigen (**E**). Immunostaining pattern for epithelial membrane antigen and human milk fat globule protein is in a cell membrane distribution in this adenocarcinoma. ×330.

tein-A antibody, and 4 of 9 prostate adenocarcinomas were positive with the antibody against the 10-kdalton Clara cell antigen. The authors concluded that the surfactant-associated and 10-kdalton Clara cell protein were specific markers for non-small cell lung carcinomas showing peripheral airway cell differentiation.

Large Cell Undifferentiated Carcinomas

Large cell undifferentiated carcinoma is defined by the World Health Organization's classification of lung neoplasms[173] as a malignant epithelial tumor with large nuclei, prominent nucleoli, and usually well-defined cell borders, without the characteristic features of squamous cell carcinoma, small cell carcinoma, or adenocarcinomas. This description is somewhat of a "wastebasket" diagnosis and, as reviewed by Delmonte et al.,[295] has been criticized by several authors. When these neoplasms are studied by electron microscopy the majority show evidence of squamous or glandular differentiation.[256,280,295-299] In our experience,[256,280] approximately 80% of light microscopically diagnosed

large cell undifferentiated carcinomas show evidence of glandular differentiation (adenocarcinoma) (Figs. 32–117 and 32–118), 10% show evidence of squamous differentiation (squamous carcinoma) (Figs. 32–119 through 32–121), and 10% show features of other types of neoplasms (Table 32–19). Included in this "other" category are large cell lymphocytic lymphoma that ultrastructurally may have microvillous processes[300] (Figs. 32–122 through 32–124), metastatic melanoma (Figs. 32–125 through 32–127), large cell neuroendocrine carcinomas (see section on neuroendocrine tumors), and truly undifferentiated carcinomas that lack obvious glandular, squamous, or neuroendocrine differentiation (Figs. 32–128 and 32–129) and characteristically express cytokeratin and frequently vimentin[291] (Figs. 32–130 and 32–131).

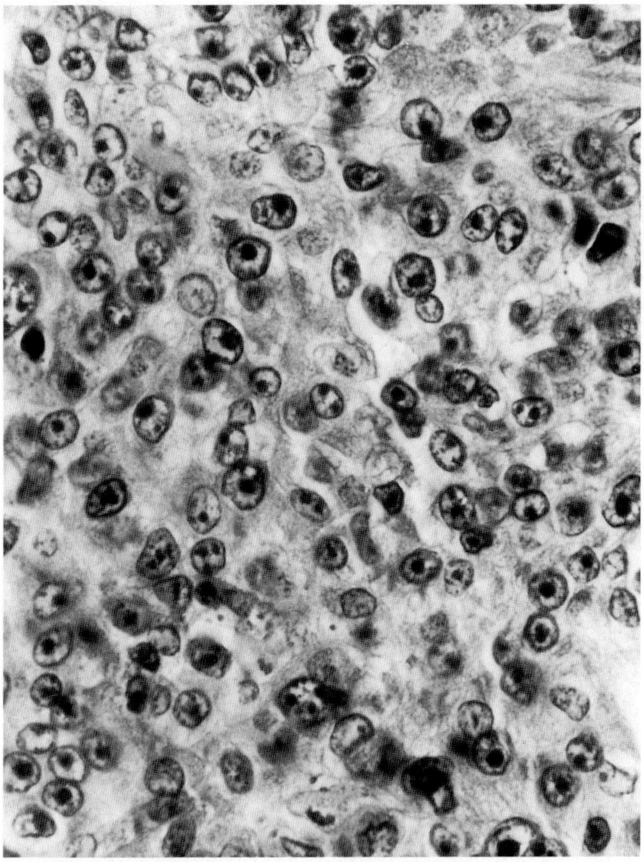

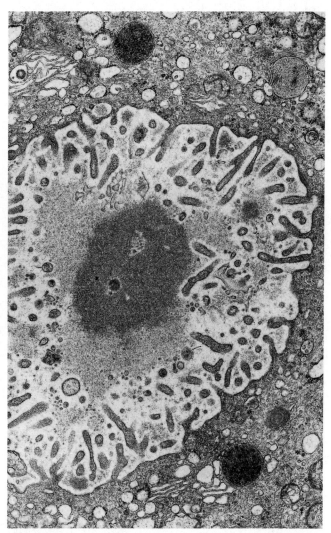

Fig. 32–117. Typical histologic appearance of large cell undifferentiated carcinoma composed of large cells with large vesicular nuclei and prominent nucleoli. ×550.

Fig. 32–118. When examined ultrastructurally, the tumor shown in Fig. 32–117 showed glandular differentiation. ×26,500.

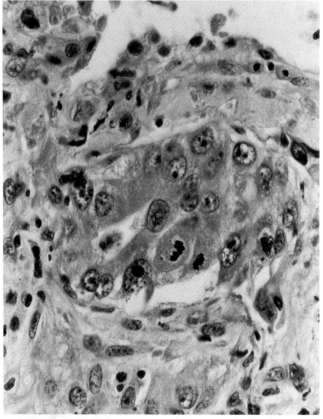

32-119

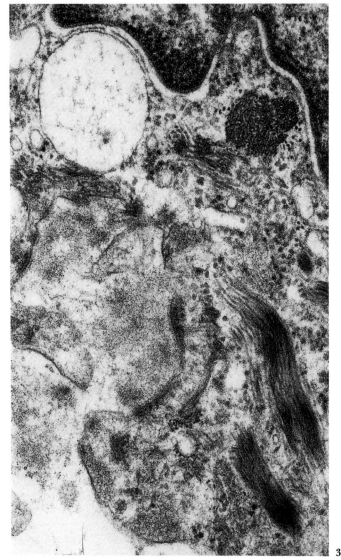

32-12

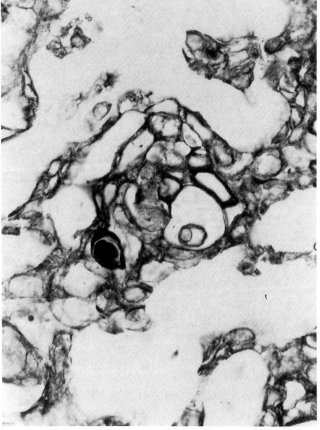

32-121

Fig. 32–119. Large cell undifferentiated carcinoma shows no areas of glandular or squamous differentiation. ×550.

Fig. 32–120. By electron microscopy, most tumor cells shown in Fig. 32–119 contained tonofilaments and were united by desmosomes, characteristic features of squamous differentiation. ×43,000.

Fig. 32–121. Tumor shown in Fig. 32–119 immunostained for high molecular weight cytokeratin, a nonspecific finding consistent with squamous carcinoma. ×330.

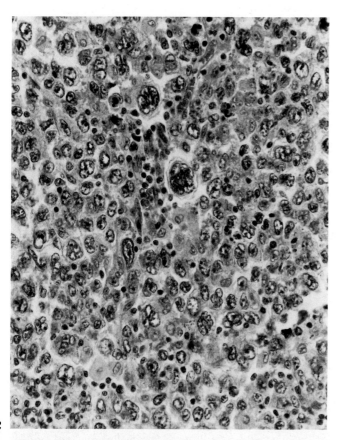

Fig. 32–122. Large cell undifferentiated neoplasm of lung containing few tumor giant cells. ×75.

Table 32–19. Ultrastructural diagnosis of lung neoplasms diagnosed by light microscopy as large cell undifferentiated carcinoma

Number of cases	Adenocarcinoma	Squamous carcinoma	Other[a]
100	79	8	12

[a] Large cell lymphocytic lymphoma, 3 cases; large cell neuroendocrine carcinoma, 2 cases; metastatic melanoma, 2 cases; large cell undifferentiated carcinoma, not otherwise specified (cytokeratin and vimentin positive), 3 cases; not able to classify, 2 cases.

Fig. 32–123. Tumor cells shown in Fig. 32–122 lacked ultrastuctural features of epithelial differentiation but had relatively long, microvillus-like processes. ×16,000.

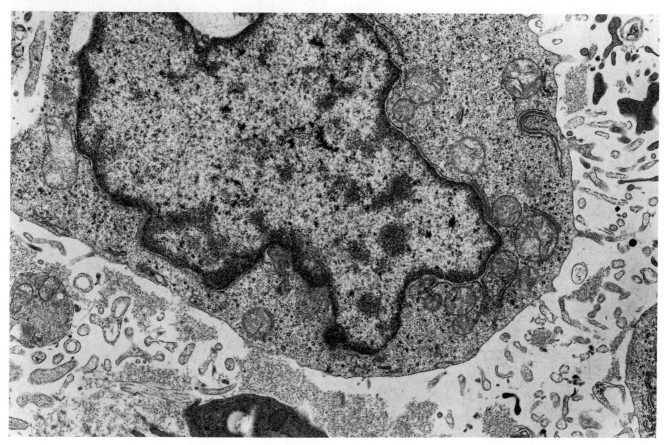

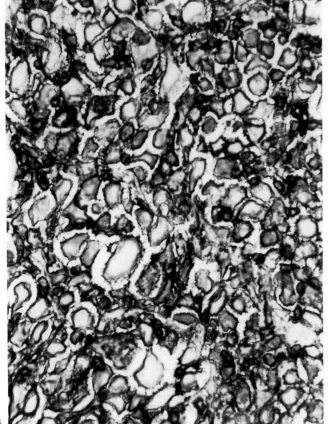

32-124

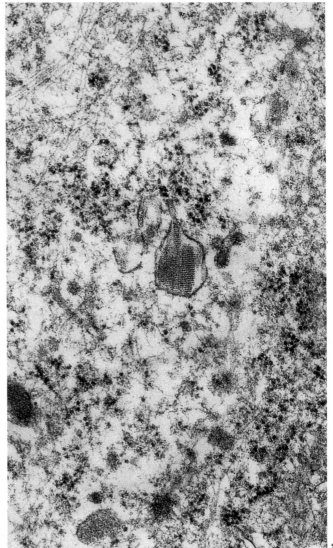

32-12

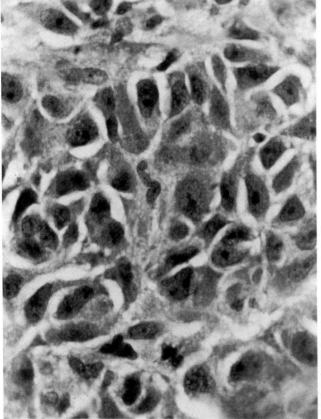

32-125

Fig. 32–124. Tumor cells shown in Fig. 32–122 showed intense cell membrane immunostaining *(black)* for leukocyte common antigen, strongly suggesting diagnosis of lymphoma. ×75.

Fig. 32–125. Large cell undifferentiated neoplasm of lung. ×775.

Fig. 32–126. When examined ultrastructurally, tumor cells shown in Fig. 32–125 contained melanosomes, indicative of diagnosis of malignant melanoma. ×51,500.

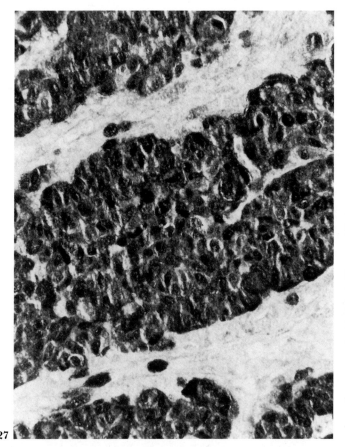

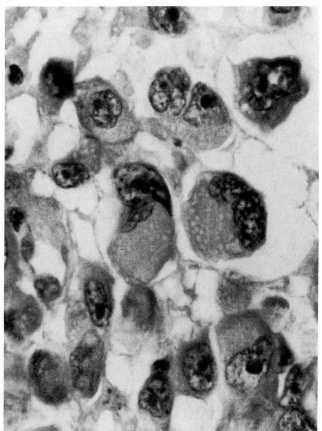

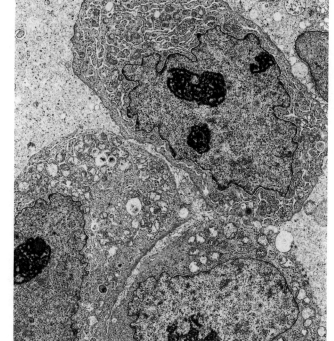

Fig. 32–127. Tumor shown in Fig. 32–125 showed intense immunostaining for S-100 protein, a finding highly characteristic of melanoma. ×330.

Fig. 32–128. Pleomorphic large cell undifferentiated neoplasm showed no obvious squamous or glandular differentiation. ×775.

Fig. 32–129. Ultrastructurally, tumor cells shown in Fig. 32–128 appear epithelial but show no intercellular junctions and lack microvilli. ×6,400.

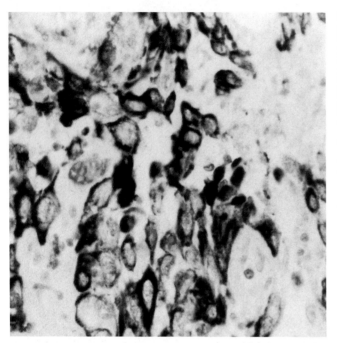

Fig. 32–130. Tumor cells shown in Fig. 32–128 immunostain *(black)* for low molecular weight cytokeratin, suggesting this neoplasm is a carcinoma. ×550.

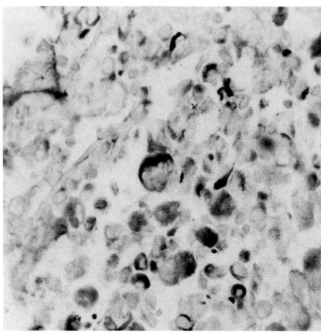

Fig. 32–131. Tumor cells shown in Fig. 32–128 also immunostain for vimentin; finding is nonspecific but consistent with anaplastic carcinoma. ×550.

Butler et al.[301] recently described a lymphoepithelioma-like primary carcinoma of the lung. Like lymphoepithelioma–carcinomas described in other locations, this neoplasm is composed of large anaplastic cells with an associated intense inflammatory cell infiltrate (Figs. 32–132 and 32–133). This type of neoplasm could be considered as a large cell undifferentiated carcinoma, although ultrastructurally has some features that could be considered squamous (Fig. 32–134), including well-formed desmosomes and intracellular tonofilaments.

Giant Cell Carcinoma

Giant cell carcinoma is classified as a subtype of large cell undifferentiated carcinoma by the World Health Organization[173] and is composed of highly pleomorphic, frequently multinucleated, tumor giant cells (Figs. 32–135 and 32–136) that frequently contain polymorphonuclear leukocytes in their cytoplasm (Figs. 32–137 and 32–138). This category of tumor does not include obvious adenocarcinomas and squamous carcinomas that contain occasional tumor giant cells. To be considered a giant cell carcinoma, the tumor must be composed of at least 40% giant cells that are greater than 40 μm in diameter.

Nash and Stout[302] in 1958 described five cases of giant cell carcinoma of the lung, based on autopsy observations. The five patients had survival times be-

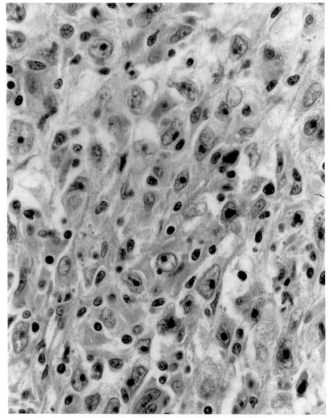

Fig. 32–132. Neoplasm composed of large anaplastic cells with large nuclei and prominent nucleoli. Heavy infiltrate of lymphocytes present throughout neoplasm. ×330.

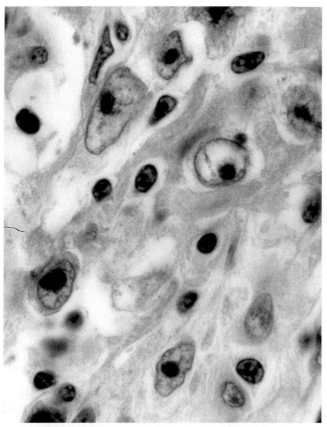

Fig. 32–133. Higher magnification of tumor shown in Fig. 32–132. Note large undifferentiated-appearing tumor cells in association with lymphocytes. ×1,000.

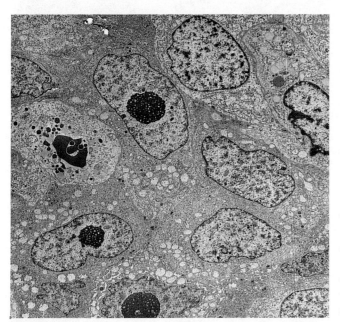

Fig. 32–134. Electron micrograph of tumor seen in Figs. 32–132 and 32–133 shows epithelial features consisting of intercellular junctions and intracellular tonofilaments. ×10,400.

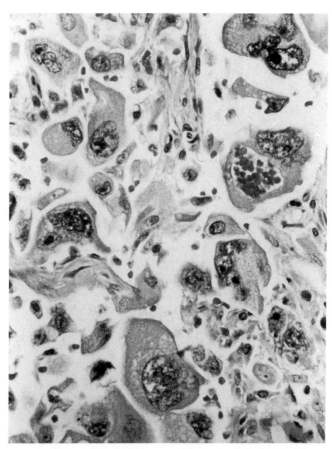

Fig. 32–135. Characteristic histologic appearance of giant cell carcinoma. One tumor cell appears to contain red blood cells in cytoplasm. ×550.

tween 5 days and 7 months, and the neoplasm had extensively metastasized to the liver, adrenal glands, kidneys, gastrointestinal tract, and mesentery. Other studies also described this neoplasm as having a poor prognosis.[303–306] Ozzello and Stout[307] demonstrated the epithelial nature of giant cell carcinoma by tissue culture techniques, and in this author's experience these neoplasms usually express cytokeratin and carcinoembryonic antigen by immunohistochemistry (Figs. 32–139 and 32–140). Wang et al.[308] studied giant cell carcinoma by electron microscopy and indicated the polymorphonuclear leukocytes entered the tumor giant cells by emperipolesis rather than being phagocytosed.

Ginsberg et al.[309] retrospectively evaluated 16 cases of giant cell carcinoma of lung. Nine of their 16 cases were anatomic stage I or II neoplasms, and their data suggested that the distribution of stage of disease at time of presentation was similar to that seen in other non-small cell lung carcinomas. Like other series of giant cell carcinoma of lung, there was an increased frequency of metastases to the gastrointestinal tract (2

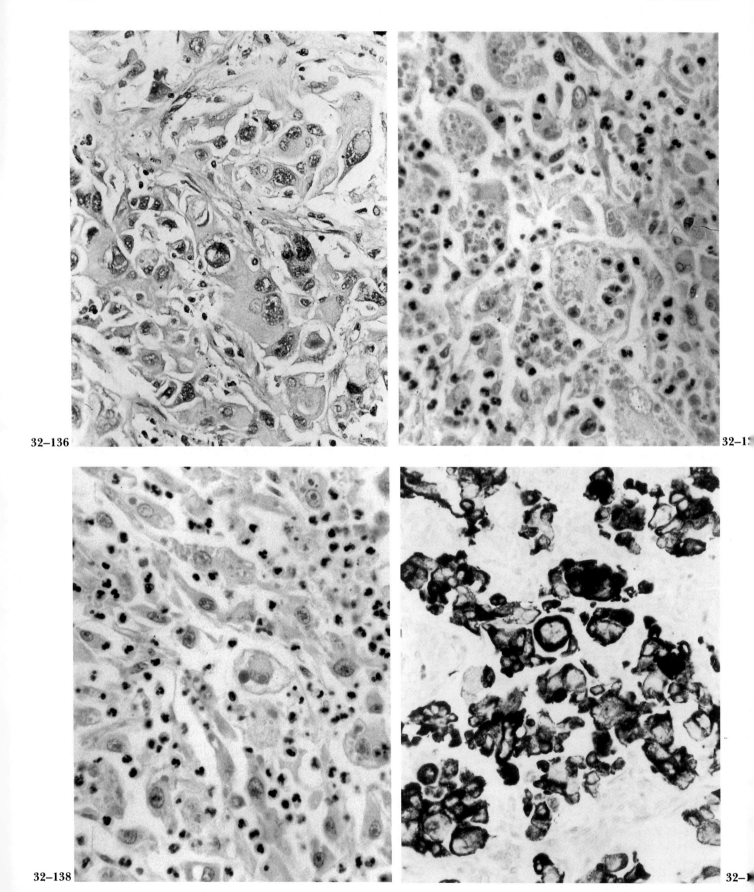

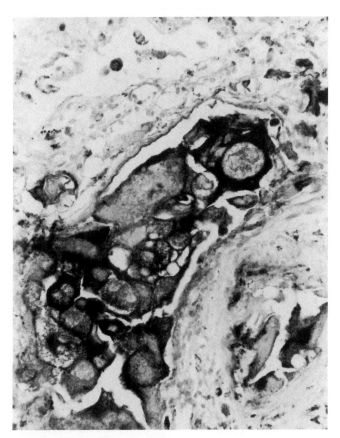

Fig. 32–140. Many giant cell carcinomas also immunostain *(black)* for carcinoembryonic antigen. ×330.

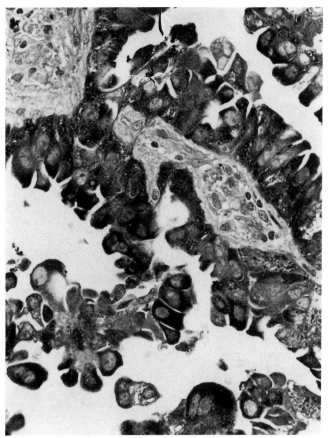

Fig. 32–141. Representative region of lung neoplasm shows pattern suggestive of bronchiolo-alveolar cell carcinoma. ×330.

of 16 cases, 12.5%). Survival data in their series did not support the characterization of giant cell carcinoma of the lung being more aggressive than other histologic types of non-small cell carcinoma of lung.

Adenosquamous Carcinoma

Adenosquamous carcinoma is defined by the World Health Organization[173] as a malignant lung neoplasm showing malignant squamous and glandular compo-

---

◁ ———————————————————————————————————

Fig. 32–136. Another example of giant cell carcinoma. ×550.

Fig. 32–137. Giant cell carcinoma of lung composed of cells as large as 100 μm in diameter. Note neutrophils in cytoplasm of tumor cells. ×300.

Fig. 32–138. Higher magnification of tumor shown in Fig. 32–137. Note polys in cytoplasm of tumor cells. ×550.

Fig. 32–139. Most giant cell carcinomas of lung immunostain *(black)* for low molecular weight cytokeratin. ×330.

nents. The incidence of this neoplasm as identified by light microscopy is between 0.4 and 4.0%.[310–314] When lung tumors are examined ultrastructurally there may be a higher frequency of this tumor,* although this author disagrees with the interpretation of some of these studies. Adenosquamous carcinomas are usually located in the periphery of the lung and usually associated with early metastases and a poor prognosis.[313] Adenosquamous carcinoma may show glandular differentiation in one region (Fig. 32–141) and squamous differentiation in another (Fig. 32–142), or show glandular and squamous differentiation in the same nest of tumor cells (Figs. 32–143 through 32–145).

Takamori et al.[317] evaluated 56 surgically resected adenosquamous carcinoma of the lung. They defined such neoplasms by light microscopy as having both adenocarcinoma and squamous cell carcinoma components with each component occupying at least 5% of the tumor area examined. Adenosquamous carcinomas

---

*References: 296, 297, 312, 315, 316.

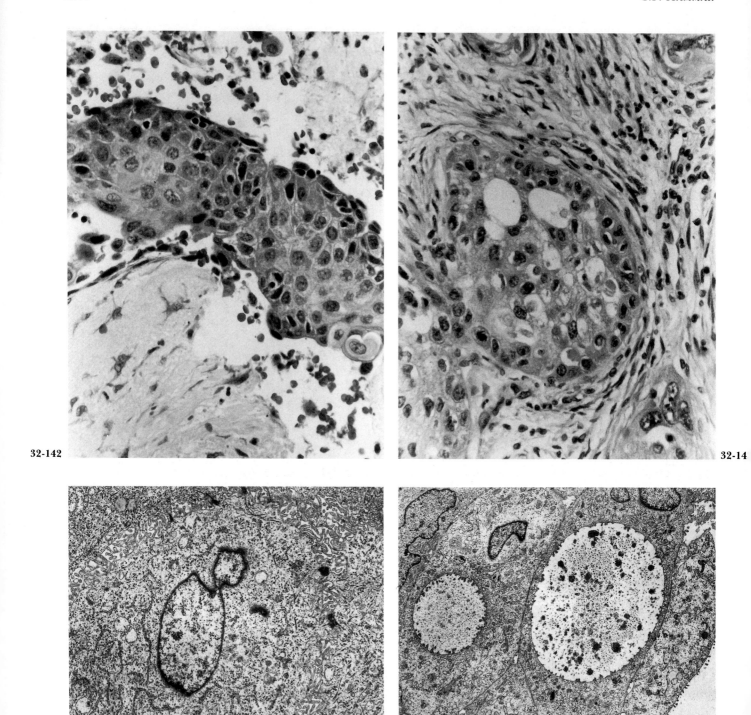

32-142

32-14

32-144

32-1

had a frequency of 2.6% (56 of 2160) and were found to have a shorter survival rate than adenocarcinomas and squamous carcinomas, especially in anatomic stage I and II neoplasms.

Ishida et al.[318] evaluated 11 patients with adenosquamous carcinoma of the lung, in their series representing 1.8% of the total resected lung neoplasms. In their cases, the amount of the squamous component of the tumors was 20% compared to 80% for the adenocarcinoma. They found a 5-year survival rate of 35%, which was similar for other non-small cell lung carcinomas.

In 1989, Yousem[319] described two unusual adenosquamous lung carcinomas that were associated with extracellular eosinophilic material resembling amyloid that was deposited in the basement membrane region of the tumor cells. These neoplasms were unusual in that they coexpressed keratin and vimentin, and also showed nuclear and cytoplasmic staining for S-100 protein, as well as luminal surface staining for carcinoembryonic antigen and epithelial membrane antigen. Amyloid was not identified ultrastructurally.

This author has observed a similar neoplasm to the two cases described by Yousem.[319] The patient was a 31-year-old man with a peripheral tumor 5 cm in maximum dimension that extended through the visceral pleura. Histologically it was composed of round, polygonal, and spindle-shaped cells that showed squamous and glandular differentiation (Figs. 32–146 and 32–147). In many regions of the neoplasm the tumor cells were surrounded by an eosinophilic material that resembled amyloid although did not have the ultrastructural features of amyloid. The neoplastic cells coexpressed keratin (Fig. 32–148) and vimentin (Fig. 32–149), and were focally positive for S-100 protein (Fig. 32–150).

◁————————————————————

Fig. 32–142. Another region of tumor shown in Fig. 32–141 has characteristic appearance of moderately well-differentiated squamous carcinoma. Tumor shown in Figs. 32–141 and 32–142 therefore fulfills criteria of adenosquamous carcinoma. ×330.

Fig. 32–143. Some adenosquamous carcinomas show both glandular and squamous differentiation in same nests of tumor cells. ×330.

Fig. 32–144. Ultrastructurally, tumor shown in Fig. 32–143 exhibits regions of obvious squamous differentiation with filopodial cell processes and well-formed desmosomes connecting cells. ×10,500.

Fig. 32–145. In another region of tumor shown in Fig. 32–143, there is obvious ultrastructural evidence of gland formation. ×10,500.

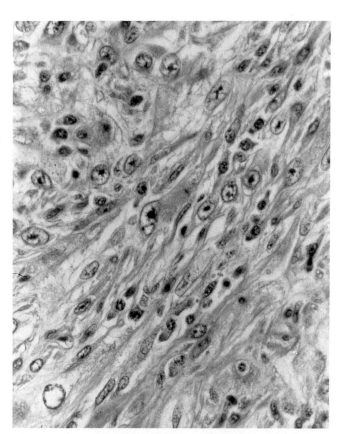

Fig. 32–146. Spindle cell neoplasm shows definite squamous and glandular differentiation in areas and is surrounded by eosmophilic amyloid-like material. ×330.

Neuroendocrine Neoplasms of the Lung

Of all the neoplasms that occur in the body, few have been studied or written about as much as neuroendocrine lung tumors. Neuroendocrine lung neoplasms exhibit a wide variety of morphologic appearances ranging from the mature carcinoid tumor to the small cell undifferentiated carcinoma. A conceptual understanding of these neoplasms is based on a knowledge of the neuroendocrine cell system and the evolution of the amine precursor uptake and decarboxylase (APUD) concept.

There exists in many tissues and organs in the body a population of cells, initially conceptualized by Feyrter in 1938[320] and referred to as "epithelial clear cells" and as part of a "diffuse epithelial endocrine system," that have similar morphologic and biochemical features. These cells were designated APUD cells on the basis of their capability to take up and decarboxylate amine precursors, including 3,4-dihydroxyphenylalanine (L-dopa) and 5-hydroxytryptophan (5-HTP). Because of this property, the cells could be identified histochem-

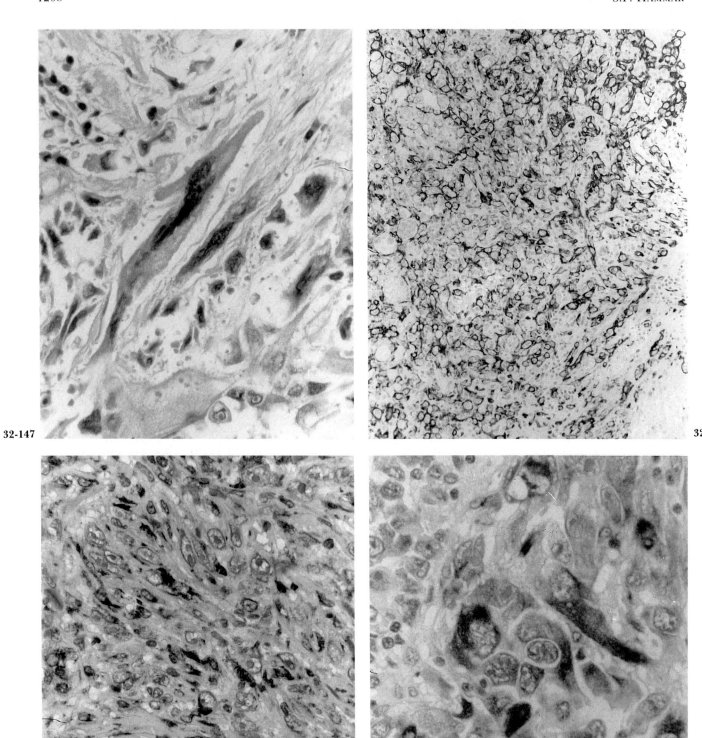

32-147

32-14

32-149

32-1

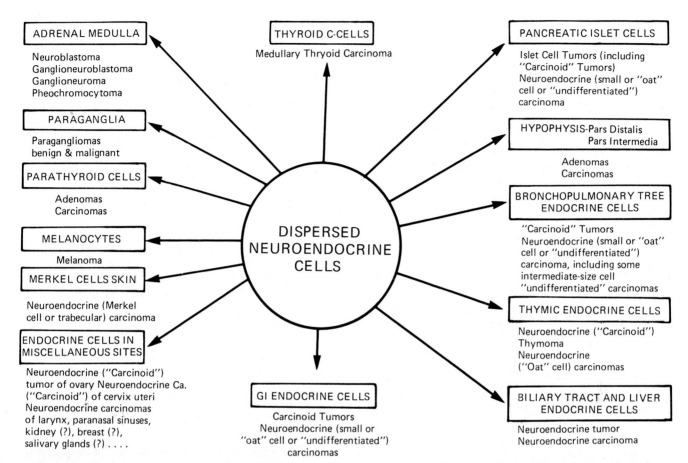

Fig. 32–151. Diagrammatic representation of dispersed neuroendocrine system. (From Gould VE, DeLellis RA. The neuroendocrine cell system: Its tumors, hyperplasias, and dysplasias. In: Silverberg SG, ed. Principles and practice of surgical pathology. New York: Wiley, 1983:1488–1501. Copyright © 1983 by Churchill Livingstone.)

ically as decarboxylated amines form highly fluorescent derivatives with formaldehyde vapor. Pearse[321] initially thought that all these cells were of neural crest origin, although numerous studies proved this to be incorrect. Pearse and Takor[322] now suggest that neuroendocrine cells have three derivations: (1) derivatives of neural crest, which include the adrenal medulla, all paraganglia, perifollicular-C cells of the thyroid, melanocytes, and possibly Merkel cells of the skin; (2) neural tube-

◁ ─────────────────────────────

Fig. 32–147. In some regions the tumor cells were quite pleomorphic. ×550.

Fig. 32–148. Neoplastic cells show expression of keratin *(dark areas)*. ×125.

Fig. 32–149. Neoplastic cells also expressed vimentin *(dark areas)*. ×330.

Fig. 32–150. Focal S-100 protein immunostaining noted in cytoplasm of some tumor cells *(dark areas)*. ×550.

and ridge-derived cells, which include those in the epiphysis, the hypophysis, and the hypothalamic neuroendocrine cells; and (3) derivatives of the neuroendocrine-programmed ectoblast, which include the neuroendocrine cells in the gastroenteropancreatic system, the bronchopulmonary tree, parathyroid chief cells, placental endocrine cells, and various other related cells. Pearse[323] introduced the term "diffuse neuroendocrine system" to refer to this group of cells.

Gould and DeLellis[324] and Gould et al.[325,326] extensively reviewed the cellular components and neoplasms of this system and suggested the term "dispersed neuroendocrine system" to refer to these cells (Figs. 32–151). As summarized and quoted by Gould et al.[327] in 1987, "the dispersed neuroendocrine system, as currently understood, encompasses elements of the central and peripheral nervous systems; a number of traditional neuroendocrine organs such as the hypophysis; assemblies of endocrine cells such as the pancreatic islets and the pulmonary neuroepithelial bodies; and a large number of widely distributed single endocrine cells demonstrable in numerous organs and tissues, including the thyroid, gastrointestinal and bronchopulmonary tract, and the skin." Not surprising, many of these cells have similar biochemical features and contain a variety of biogenic amines, peptide hormones, neurotransmitters, etc. that can be identified biochemically or immunohistochemically.[328] The location of neuropeptides within the autonomic nervous system of the lung and function of these neuropeptides has recently been reviewed.[329]

Identification of Neuroendocrine Cells and Neuroendocrine Neoplasms

Normal neuroendocrine cells and neoplasms of neuroendocrine cells can be identified as follows.

1. Histochemical identification. Neuroendocrine cells are argyrophilic, which can be demonstrated with a Grimelius or Sevier–Munger silver nitrate stain or by the property of argentaffinity. The cells also exhibit masked metachromasia with toluidine blue or coriophosphine O after acid hydrolysis.
2. Immunohistochemical-biochemical identification. (a) Neuron-specific enolase (2-phospho-D-glycerate hydrolase) catalyzes the interconversion of 2-phosphoglycerate and phosphoenolpyruvate in the glycolytic pathway. Enolases are dimers composed of three distinct subunits; alpha, beta, and gamma. The gamma subunit is in the highest concentration in the central and peripheral nervous system as alpha–gamma and gamma-gamma dimers. Neuron-specific enolase refers to gamma enolase, which can be identified biochemically or immunohistochemically in high concentrations in neuronal and neuroendocrine cells. Unfortunately, neuron-specific enolase is not found only in neurons or neuroendocrine cells. Haimoto et al.[330] reported the immunohistochemical localization of gamma enolase in many different normal nonneural and nonneuroendocrine cells (see their Table 1) such as smooth muscle cells, renal epithelial cells, lymphocytes, myoepithelial cells, megakaryocytes, and plasma cells. Pahlman et al.[331] measured neuron-specific enolase enzymatically and by radioimmunoassay in several different tumors and cell lines, and found that the enzyme was present in a variety of nonneuroendocrine neoplasms as well as neuroendocrine tumors. Vinores et al.[332] reported similar findings, identifying neuron-specific enolase in breast carcinoma, chordoma, and renal cell carcinoma. Bergh et al.[333] reported that 14 of 21 non-small cell lung carcinomas showed immunocytochemical staining for neuron-specific enolase, and Said et al.[334] found that 57% of nonneu-

roendocrine lung tumors showed immunostaining for the enzyme. Schmechel[335] reviewed the specificity of neuron-specific enolase and stated that the gamma subunit of enolase was neither nonspecific nor neuron specific. (b) Chromogranins are a family of acidic proteins containing high concentrations of glutamic acid and are located within the matrix of neuroendocrine granules in many normal neuroendocrine cells and in the cells of a variety of neuroendocrine neoplasms.[336–341] Chromogranins are subdivided into three classes: A, B, and C. Chromogranin-A was discovered by Banks and Helle[342] in 1965. Chromogranins B and C are also referred to as secretogranin 1 and 2. Angiletti[343] updated our knowledge on chromogranins and has discussed the controversy concerning these glycoproteins. Chromogranin A has been identified in normal neuroendocrine cells of the bronchopulmonary tract.[344,345] This author agrees with Said et al.[334] that the intensity of immunostaining with chromogranin A usually correlates with the density of the neuroendocrine granules as determined by electron microscopy. (c) Neurofilaments are one of five major classes of intermediate 7- to 10-nm-thick filaments that in vertebrates are composed of three polypeptides designated NF-H, NF-M, and NF-L having molecular weights of 200, 160, and 68 kdaltons, respectively. Neurons and some normal and neoplastic neuroendocrine cells contain neurofilaments, although they may be difficult or impossible to demonstrate in conventional formalin fixed processed tissue. They are often difficult to identify immunohistochemically in neuroendocrine neoplasms.[346] In a study of 112 neuroendocrine tumors, Shah et al.[347] were unable to demonstrate immunoreactivity for NF-H or NF-L in any of the neoplasms. Leoncini et al.[348] has reported that the ability to demonstrate neurofilaments in neuroendocrine lung neoplasms depends on whether the neurofilament epitopes were phosphorylated. Immunoreactivity for NF-M and NF-H was much more frequent when phosphorylation of the neurofilament subunit was present. Leoncini et al.[348] have suggested the lack of phosphorylation could explain the reported low rate of neurofilament expression. (d) Synaptophysin is a 38-kdalton glycoprotein component of presynaptic vesicle that was originally isolated from bovine neurons.[349] Using immunofluorescence microscopy on frozen sections, it can be demonstrated in neurons and neuroendocrine cells and in a variety of neuroendocrine neoplasms including neuroendocrine tumors of the lung.[327,350] (e) Leu7, initially used as a monoclonal antibody to identify natural killer cells, was observed to immunostain neuroendocrine tumor cells, including those of small cell undifferentiated carcinoma.[351,352] Leu7 has been demonstrated to react with a 75-82 kD protein within the matrix of some neuroendocrine granules.[353] (f) Monoclonal antibody 735, directed against the long-chain form of polysialic acid, which is part of the neural cell adhesion molecule (N-CAM), immunostains small cell undifferentiated carcinomas but shows minimal or no reaction against mature bronchopulmonary carcinoids and atypical carcinoids.[354,355] This and other similar antibodies directed against N-CAM antibody have also been reported to rarely show reactivity towards non-small cell lung neoplasms.[356] (g) Other immunocytochemical markers of neuroendocrine cells and neoplasms including various neuropeptides can be identified in normal and neoplastic neuroendocrine cells (Table 32–20). For example, clcitonin, vasoactive intestinal polypeptide, and adrenocorticotrophic hormone can be identified in neuroendocrine tumors of the skin and lung.[325,326] These substances are not present in every tumor cell and are not specific for any given neuroendocrine neoplasm. It should also be stressed that a significant number of nonneuroendocrine lung neoplasms contain one or more of these substances.[184] Although initially controversial,[357–362] all neuroendocrine tumors of "epithelial" origin such as neuroendocrine neoplasms of the lung contain keratin[363–366] and desmoplakin proteins.[367] Funa et al.[368] reported in 1986 that small undifferentiated carcinomas of lung and some other neuroendocrine neoplasms lacked beta-2 microglobulin, whereas non-small cell lung carcinomas strongly expressed this antigen. They suggested that the demonstration of this antigen could be used to differentiate neuroendocrine lung tumors from nonneuroendocrine lung neoplasms.

3. Ultrastructural identification. In 1984, Payne et al.[369] described a specific ultrastructural cytochemical stain, called the urnaffin stain, which distinguishes true neuroendocrine granules from neuroendocrine-like granules found in a variety of nonneuroendocrine neoplasms. Nagle et al.[370] studied 41 neuroendocrine tumors by an avidin-biotin immunoperoxidase technique for neuron-specific enolase, bombesin, adrenocorticotrophic hormone, calcitonin, and serotonin. In addition, they studied the tumors by transmission electron microscopy and with the uranaffin stain. All tumors contained neuroendocrine granules by electron microscopy and the uranaffin stain, but 7 of 16 poorly differentiated neuroendocrine neoplasms were negative with all antisera tested. They suggested that the uranaffin reaction and transmission electron microscopy was more specific for diagnosing poorly differentiated neuroendocrine tumors. Ultrastructurally, the most distinctive feature of all neuroendocrine neoplasms of lung is the dense-core, membrane-bound, neuroendocrine granule, which is also called a neurosecretory granule. The number and size of these granules may vary considerably from one neuroendocrine tumor to the next.[328] For example (and as is shown), neuroendocrine granules are numerous in most mature carcinoids of lung but are rare in small cell neuroendocrine lung neoplasms. It should be emphasized that ultrastructurally there are dense-core granules in some cells that resemble neuroendocrine granules.[371,372] Another ultrastructural feature common to most neoplastic neuroendocrine cells are processes that usually contain microtubules and intermediate filaments.

4. Molecular biology techniques. The study of gene expression has been useful in identifying some neuroendocrine lung neoplasms and requires molecular biology techniques, including Northern and Southern blotting, polymerase chain reaction, and in situ hybridization. Using cRNA probes and in situ hybridization, gastrin-releasing polypeptide gene expression was identified in most mature bronchopulmonary carcinoids but only in a few small cell and large cell undifferentiated carcinoma.[373] Chromogranin A is infrequently identified by immunohistochemistry in small cell undifferentiated carcinomas because of the relatively low concentration of neuroendocrine granules, whereas using molecular biology techniques, messenger RNA for chromogranin A can be identified in most small cell undifferentiated carcinoma of lung.[374]

Table 32–20. Neuropeptides and neuroamines commonly found in neuroendocrine lung neoplasms

Bombesin
Calcitonin
Adenocorticotrophic hormone
Leu-enkephalin
Gastrin
Somatostatin
Vasoactive intestinal polypeptide
Neurotensin
Arginine vasopressin
Serotonin

Normal Neuroendocrine Cells of the Lung

In 1949, Frohlich[375] described solitary and nodular aggregates of neuroendocrine cells in the bronchi. He

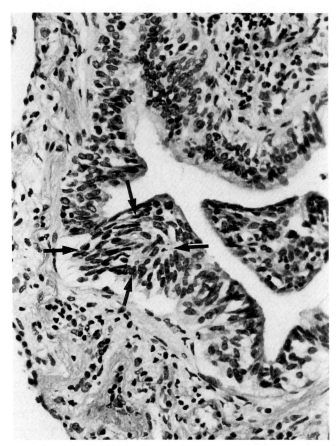

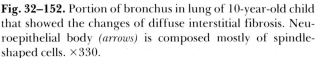

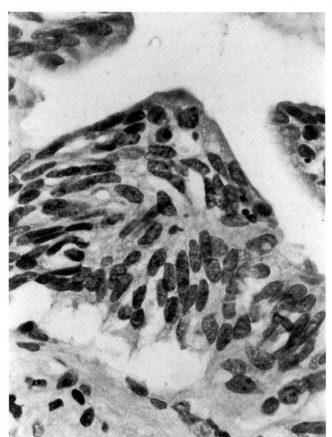

Fig. 32–152. Portion of bronchus in lung of 10-year-old child that showed the changes of diffuse interstitial fibrosis. Neuroepithelial body *(arrows)* is composed mostly of spindle-shaped cells. ×330.

Fig. 32–153. Neuroepithelial body at greater magnification. ×775.

thought these cells had a chemoreceptive or neurosecretory function. The presence of these cells was confirmed by Feyrter,[376] who suggested that bronchial carcinoids originated from them. In the mid-1960s, Bensch and colleagues[377,378] and Gmelich and Bensch[379] described the ultrastructural appearance of neuroendocrine cells and related these cells to bronchial carcinoids as well as oat cell carcinomas that were found to contain the same type of neuroendocrine granules. In 1972 and 1973, Lauweryns et al.[380] and Lauweryns and Goddeeris[381] reemphasized the morphology of neuroepithelial bodies (Figs. 32–152 and 32–153) as clusters of eosinophilic cells in hematoxylin and eosin-stained sections that extended from basement membrane of the bronchial mucosa to the lumen, displayed argyrophilia, and contained neuroendocrine granules when examined ultrastructurally (Figs. 32–154 and 32–155). Neuroepithelial bodies appear to be innervated and are frequently in association with vessels, which suggests that they have a neurosecretory or chemoreceptive function. Pulmonary neuroendocrine

cells are increased in persons living at high altitude, and are seen in increased numbers in children with bronchopulmonary dysplasia, cystic fibrosis, and bronchiectasis.[382,383] Their prominence in fetal tissue has suggested they produce growth factors such as gastrin-releasing peptide that might contribute to the morphogenesis and maturation of the lung.[384–386] They are also increased (? -induced) in cigarette smoke-associated pulmonary diseases in adults.[387–389] Aguayo et al.[390] reported increased concentrations of peptides of bombesin-like immunoreactivity in bronchoalveolar lavage fluid from "normal" cigarette smokers, and Tabassian et al.[391] found that subchronic cigarette-smoke exposure caused increased pulmonary concentrations of immunoreactive calcitonin and mammalian bombesin in hamster lungs. A recent intriguing report[392] found diffuse idiopathic hyperplasia of pulmonary neuroendocrine cells in six nonsmokers with obliterating small airways disease and suggested the product(s) produced by these neuroendocrine cells, for example, bombesin, the cause of the fibrotic airway disease. A summary of

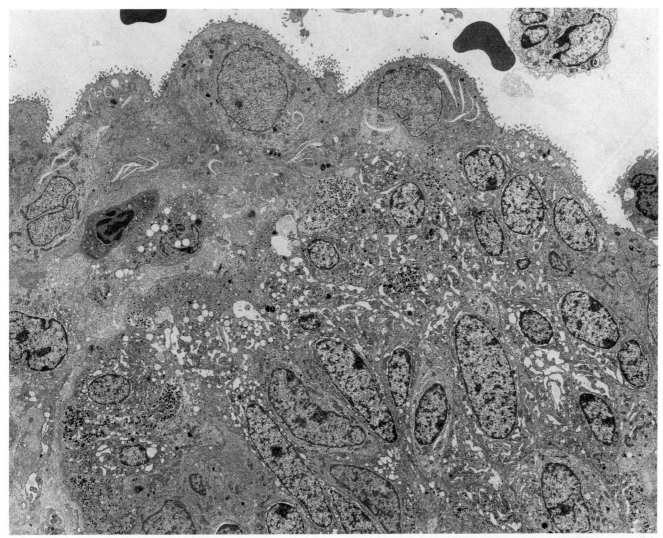

Fig. 32–154. Ultrastructural appearance of neuroepithelial body. Note surface epithelial cells and underlying neuroendocrine cells containing cytoplasmic electron-dense granules. ×2,700.

the reactions of normal neuroendocrine cells to stimuli is provided by Gould et al.[325] Neuroepithelial bodies are easily identified immunohistochemically with antibodies against neuron-specific enolase, chromogranin, or synaptophysin (Figs. 32–156 through 32–158).

Nomenclature of Neuroendocrine Neoplasms of Lung

The nomenclature of neuroendocrine neoplasms (Table 32–21) has undergone an evolution that somewhat parallels our increased understanding of normal neuroendocrine cells. As shown, some of these neoplasms are referred to by several different names. Controversy still exists concerning the nomenclature and nature of neuroendocrine lung neoplasms.[393]

Tumorlet

Tumorlet is a name designated by Whitwell[394] in 1955 who described 24 cases of localized proliferation of bronchial epithelium in lobes resected for bronchiectasis or lung abscess. Tumorlets represent localized regions of neuroendocrine cell proliferation, often in association with pulmonary fibrosis and bronchiectasis (Fig. 32–159). However, in the Churg and Warnock[395] autopsy study of 20 tumorlets, only one-third occurred in diseased lungs.

Tumorlets are often discovered incidentally at autopsy, in open biopsies that show pulmonary fibrosis, or in lobes that are resected for bronchiectasis or other "chronic" conditions. Ultrastructurally the cells of tumorlets closely resemble those forming neuroepithelial

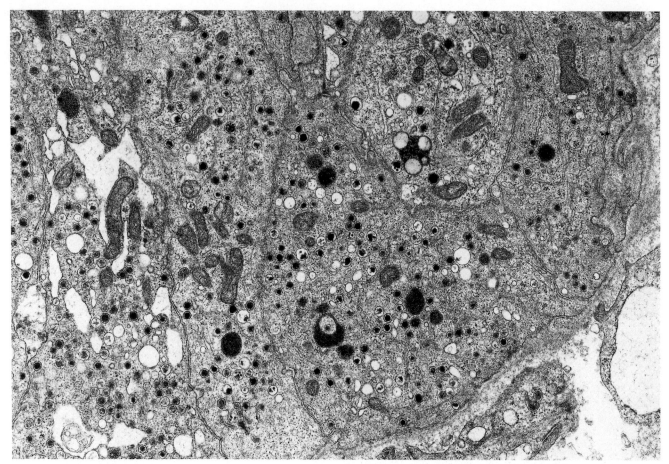

Fig. 32–155. At greater magnification, ultrastructural features of neuroendocrine cells forming neuroepithelial bodies are better seen. Note obvious dense-core granules and prominent lysosomes (residual bodies-ceroid pigment). ×16,000.

bodies and mature carcinoid tumors. Conceptually, tumorlets can be thought of as large neuroepithelial bodies or small carcinoids. An unusual case of multiple tumorlets and mature carcinoid tumors was reported in a 53-year-old woman with a 25-year history of non-productive hacking cough and occasional traces of he-moptysis.[396] These "tumors" were thought to be re-sponsible for the observed pulmonary function test abnormalities of mild restrictive and obstructive de-fects.

Pelosi et al.[397] reported hundreds of neuroendocrine tumorlets occurring in the sequestered right-lower lobe of a 49-year-old nonsmoking man. The tumorlets were located around distorted bronchioles or embedded in fibrotic pulmonary parenchyma with a distinctive infil-trative appearance. The cells forming the tumorlets were strongly argyrophilic, and by immunohistochem-istry, expressed calcitonin, serotonin, gastrin-releasing polypeptide, and vasoactive intestinal polypeptide. One case of lymph node metastasis has been reported in a person whose lung contained tumorlets.[398]

Mature Carcinoid

In 1882, Mueller[399] described a bronchial carcinoid observed at autopsy. In 1930, Kramer[400] described clinically a bronchial carcinoid under the designation "adenoma of the bronchus." It was Hamperl,[401] in 1937, who recognized the similarities between bron-chial carcinoids and gastrointestinal carcinoids that had been described by Oberndorfer[402] in 1907, who coined the term "carcinoid" to mean a carcinoma-like neo-plasm.

Most mature carcinoids occur in the large bronchi and are surfaced by intact bronchial epithelium. Rarely, they occur in the trachea,[403] and may occur in the peripheral airways or parenchyma[404] as well as being multiple.[405,406] Abdi et al.[407] reported an incidence of 21.1% (11/52) for peripheral carcinoid tumors of the lung.

Macroscopically they are yellow tan, well demarcated, and often invade into the adjacent pulmonary paren-chyma. When they occur centrally within the bronchi,

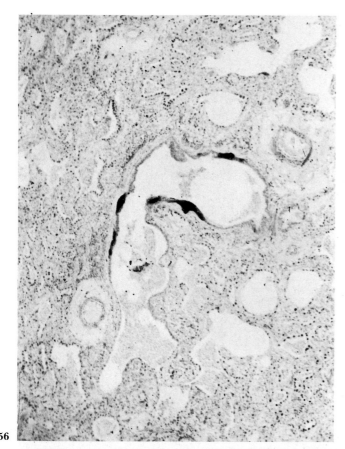

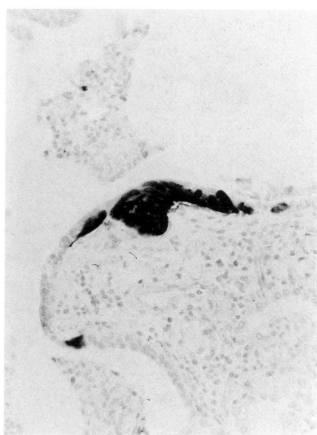

-156

32-157

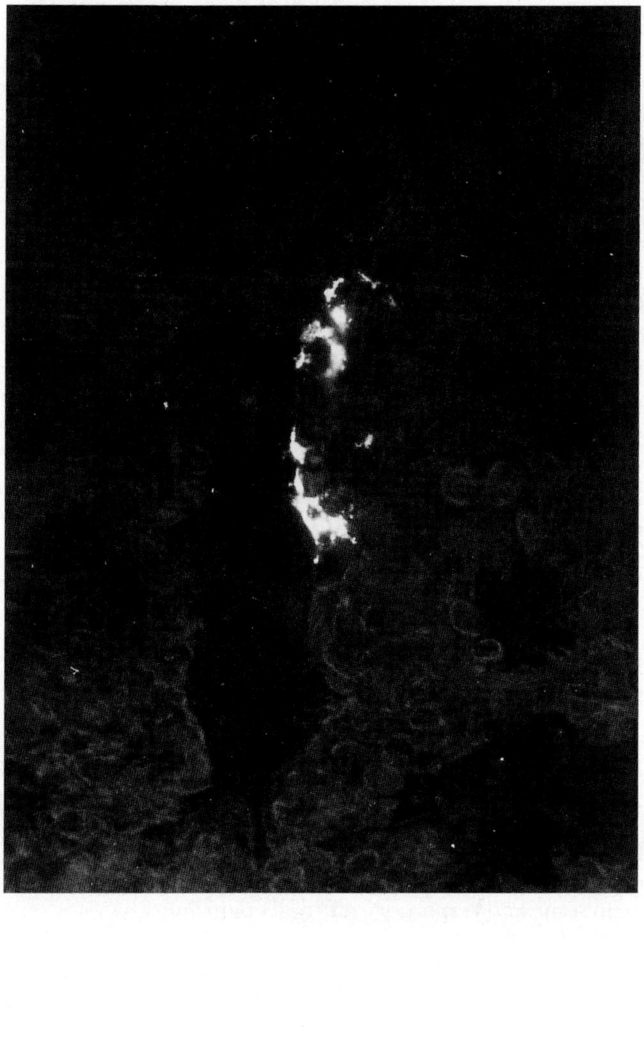

Table 32–21. Nomenclature of neuroendocrine lung neoplasms

Tumorlet
Mature carcinoid
Atypical carcinoid
  Malignant carcinoid
  Well-differentiated neuroendocrine carcinoma
  Kulchitsky cell carcinoma-II
  Peripheral small cell carcinoma of the lung resembling carcinoid tumor
Large cell neuroendocrine carcinoma
  Atypical endocrine tumor of the lung
  Neuroendocrine carcinoma of intermediate cell type
Small cell undifferentiated carcinoma
  Small cell neuroendocrine carcinoma
  Neuroendocrine carcinoma of small cell type
  Oat cell carcinoma

Fig. 32–156. Lung tissue shown in Fig. 32–152 immunostained for neuron-specific enolase, which highlights *(black)* neuroepithelial bodies. ×75.

Fig. 32–157. Neuroepithelial body in lung tissue shows intense immunostaining *(black)* for chromogranin. ×330.

Fig. 32–158. Neuroepithelial body also expresses synaptophysin using direct immunofluorescent technique. ×800. (Photograph courtesy of V. E. Gould, M.D.)

-158

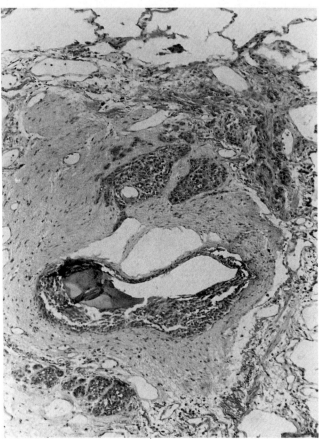

32-159

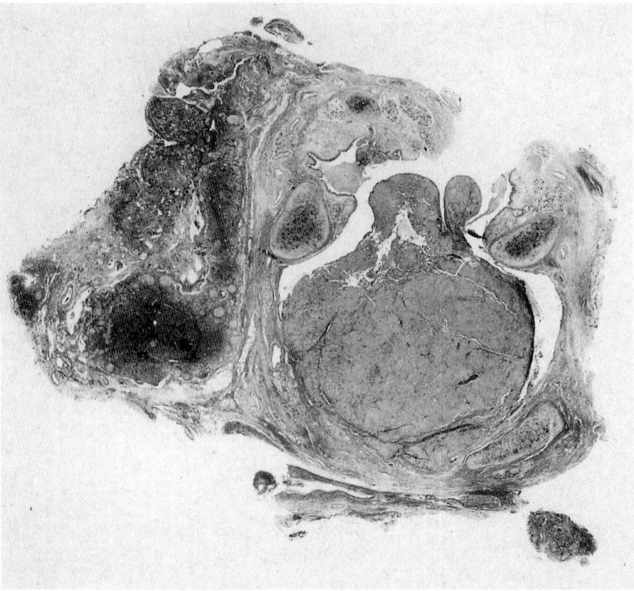

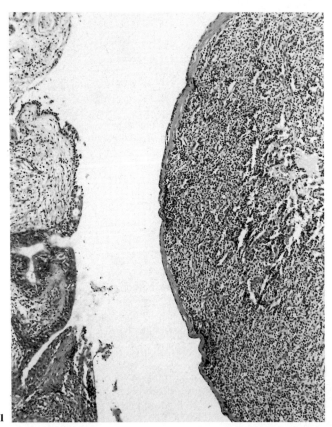

32-161

32-16

they are surfaced by respiratory epithelium or metaplastic squamous epithelium (Figs. 32–160 and 32–
161). They show a wide variety of histologic growth
patterns[408,409] including trabecular, insular, papillary,
"interstitial,"[408,409] solid, and spindle (Figs. 32–162
through 32–165). Ranchod and Levine[410] reported a
clinicopathologic evaluation of 35 cases of spindle cell
carcinoid tumors of lung. Of interest was the finding of
a disproportionate number (10/35) in the right-middle
lobe. The tumors ranged from 7 mm to 4 cm in greatest
dimension, and 29 of 35 (83%) were less than 2 cm in
diameter. Most were in a subpleural location, and the
spindle cells were sometimes arranged in an organoid
pattern. An oncocytic variety of carcinoid was reported
by Sklar et al.[411] in 1978; since then several reports of
oncocytic bronchial carcinoids have appeared in the
literature.[412–414] These are in contrast to a bronchial
oncocytoma[415] in that they are composed of neuroendocrine cells and often show a transition from a typical
carcinoid into a oncocytic variety (Figs. 32–166 and
32–167). Rare melanocytic carcinoids have also been
described in which the tumor cells contain melanosomes and neurosecretory granules.[416,417] Carlson and

Fig. 32–159. Proliferation of neuroendocrine cells in region
of distorted small airways is characteristic of this tumorlet.
×75.

Fig. 32–160. "Intrabronchial" carcinoid tumor almost completely obliterates lumen of bronchus. ×2.5.

Fig. 32–161. At greater magnification, "intrabronchial" carcinoid seen in Fig. 32–160 is covered by thickened basement
membrane and respiratory mucosal epithelium. ×75.

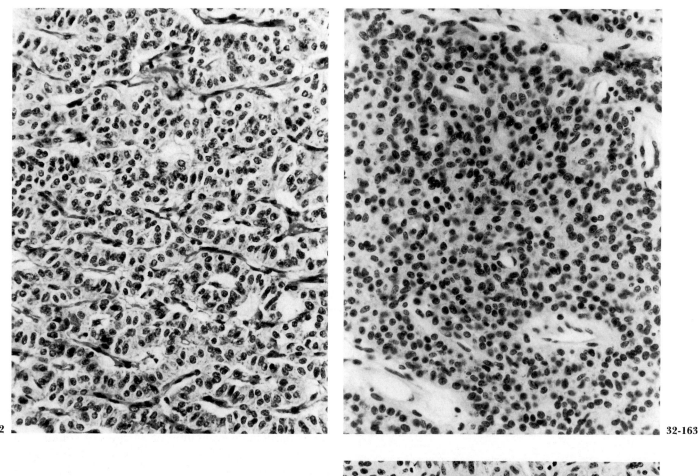

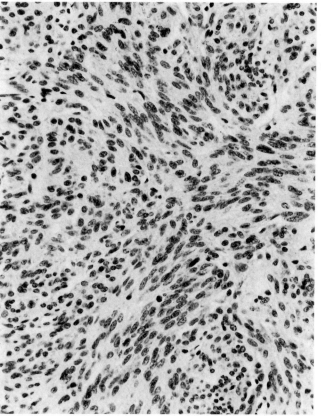

Fig. 32–162. Uniform cellular appearance of bronchopulmonary carcinoid. Cells arranged in somewhat trabecular pattern. ×330.

Fig. 32–163. Carcinoid tumor of bronchus in which tumor cells are somewhat haphazardly arranged in solid growth pattern. ×330.

Fig. 32–164. Peripheral carcinoid composed of spindle-shaped cells. ×330.

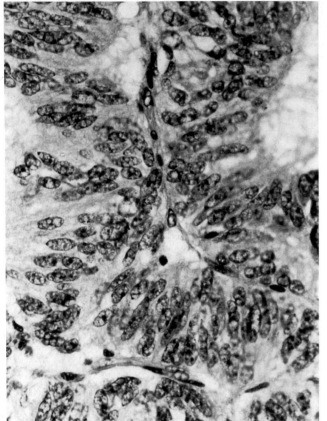

32-165

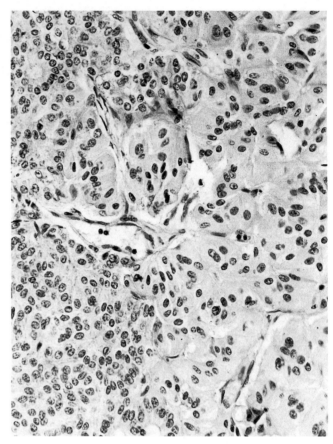

32-1[

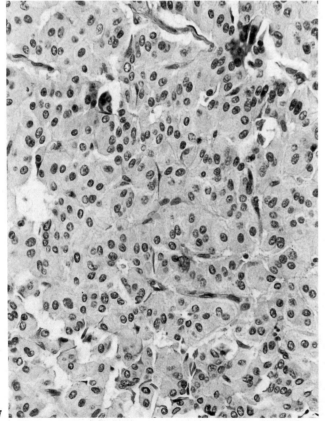

32-167

Fig. 32–165. Carcinoid tumor composed of tall columnar cells. As in all mature carcinoids, note uniformity of cells. ×550.

Fig. 32–166. Region of bronchopulmonary carcinoid shows transition from typical carcinoid (left) into oncocytic variety (right). ×330.

Fig. 32–167. Oncocytic carcinoid composed of relatively large cells with abundant cytoplasm. ×330.

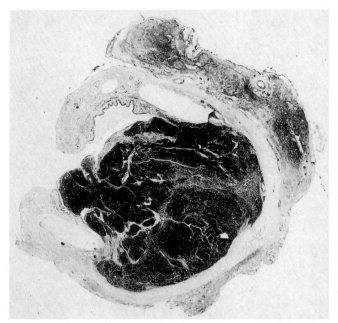

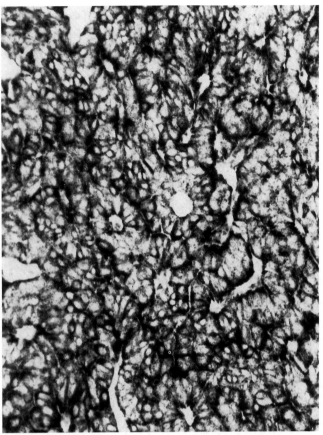

Fig. 32–168. Intrabronchial carcinoid shown in Fig. 32–162 displays intense immunostaining *(black)* for neuron-specific enolase. ×2.5.

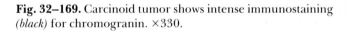

Fig. 32–169. Carcinoid tumor shows intense immunostaining *(black)* for chromogranin. ×330.

Dickersin[418] reported an intriguing case of a "melanotic paraganglioid carcinoid tumor." They thoroughly reviewed the well known fact that melanin production occurs in a wide variety of neuroendocrine neoplasms, and suggested that coexistent melanocytic and neuroendocrine differentiation was not surprising, because melanocytes are functional elements of the dispersed neuroendocrine system. They cited the observation of Barbareschi et al.[419] that 36% of bronchial carcinoids contained S100 protein-positive sustentacular cells, and suggested that these sustentacular cells (Schwann cells) were neoplastic and therefore suggested that such neoplasms be named paraganglioid carcinoid tumors, a name previously proposed by Capella et al.[420] In their case, Carlson and Dickersin[418] demonstrated that sustentacular cells showed melanocytic differentiation and reviewed literature showing such cells can show neuroendocrine differentiation.

Immunohistochemically, bronchial carcinoids express neuron-specific enolase (Fig. 32–168) and chromogranin (Fig. 32–169). The intensity of the chromogranin reaction varies from one bronchial carcinoid to another and roughly correlates with the number of neuroendocrine granules demonstrated by electron microscopy in the cytoplasm of the tumor cells. In this author's experience, nearly all bronchial carcinoids express low molecular weight cytokeratin (Figs. 32–170 through 32–172) and may occasionally express high molecular weight keratin. This author has also observed several bronchial carcinoids that contain vimentin, as demonstrated by immunohistochemistry, which may occur as punctate staining (Fig. 32–173). In some instances, vimentin has been the only intermediate filament identified in the neoplastic cells, although most coexpress vimentin and keratin. Although carcinoid tumors have been reported to contain neurofilament protein, this author has been unable to demonstrate this intermediate filament in formalin- or alcohol-based (methacarn-) fixed tissue. As previously discussed, this may be related to whether the neurofilament epitope is phosphorylated. Approximately 50% of bronchial carcinoids express carcinoembryonic antigen and epithelial membrane antigen or human milk fat globule protein. They may express any of the neuropeptides or other substances shown in Table 32–20. Approximately 25%–50% of carcinoids show S-100 protein-positive cells admixed with the tumor cells (Fig. 32–174). These are called sustentacular cells and ultrastructurally have the appearance of Schwann cells (Fig. 32–175).

Ultrastructurally, bronchial carcinoids are composed

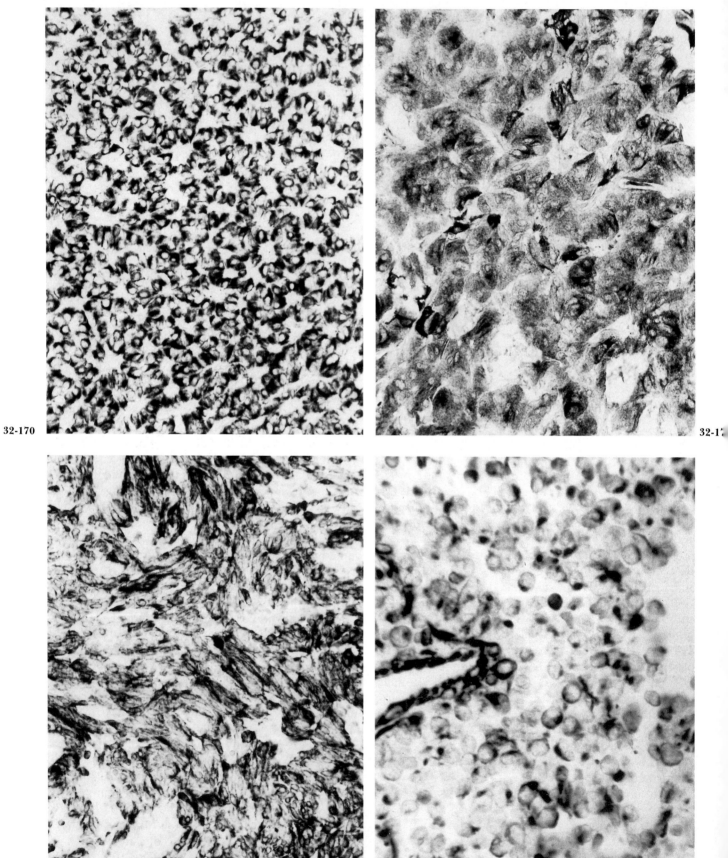

32-170

32-17

32-172

32-1

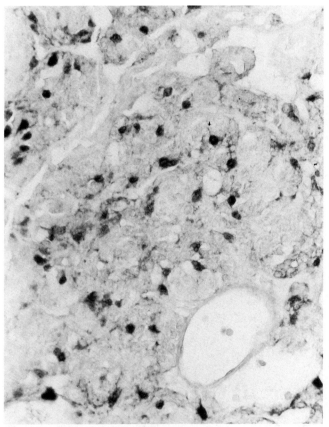

Fig. 32–174. Many bronchopulmonary carcinoids contain focal S-100-positive (black-staining) cells. ×330.

of uniform cells, the shape of which corresponds relatively well with their histologic appearance. The tumor cells resemble the cells forming neuroepithelial bodies, containing numerous, although variable numbers, of dense-core neuroendocrine granules and frequent lysosomes (Figs. 32–176 and 32–177). The nuclei of the tumor cells are relatively uniform, are composed of varying amounts of euchromatin and heterochromatin, and have inconspicuous or absent nucleoli. The tumor cells show processes that may be more pronounced in the spindle variant and which contain microtubules and

◁——————————————————————

Fig. 32–170. Nearly all bronchopulmonary carcinoids show immunostaining *(black)* for low molecular weight, simple epithelial cytokeratin. ×75.

Fig. 32–171. Oncocytic carcinoid shows different pattern of immunostaining *(black)* for cytokeratin. ×330.

Fig. 32–172. Spindle cell carcinoid shows immunostaining *(black)* pattern for cytokeratin. ×330.

Fig. 32–173. Bronchial carcinoid tumor shows focal, somewhat punctate immunostaining for vimentin *(black)*. ×330.

intermediate filaments. The cytoplasm of the cells also contains a moderate number of mitochondria, short profiles of rough endoplasmic reticulum that may be arranged in parallel stacks (Fig. 32–178), and prominent, often paranuclear, aggregates of intermediate filaments[421] (Fig. 32–179). Many carcinoids form distinct glands (Fig. 32–180) and may show multidirectional differentiation with mucous granules in their apical cytoplasm.

Atypical Carcinoid–Well-Differentiated Neuroendocrine Carcinoma

In 1972, Arrigoni et al.[422] described 23 neoplasms they referred to as "atypical carcinoids," identified in a review of lesions that had been categorized in their files as bronchial carcinoids. Subsequent reports of these neoplasms have appeared in the literature, and they have been variously termed malignant carcinoids,[423] well-differentiated neuroendocrine carcinoma,[424] peripheral small cell carcinoma of lung resembling carcinoid tumor,[425] and Kulchitsky cell carcinoma II.[426] The descriptions of this neoplasm have been remarkably similar. In contrast to mature bronchial carcinoids, atypical carcinoids occur in the periphery of the lung in more than 60% of cases. Like mature carcinoids, they are usually yellow tan and often well demarcated. Histologically, atypical carcinoids usually have an organoid appearance, especially at their periphery (Figs. 32–181 and 32–182). The organoid nests are usually separated by fibrous bands that can be quite prominent (Fig. 32–183). The organoid nests of cells frequently show palisading of their peripheral cell layer (Fig. 32–184), and compared to a mature carcinoid show more pleomorphism and mitoses as well as focal necrosis (Figs. 32–185 through 32–187). They may show focal gland formation (Fig. 32–188) and may be mucin positive.

Immunohistochemically, atypical carcinoids show essentially identical results of mature carcinoids. Immunostaining for neuron-specific enolase frequently outlines them rather vividly (Fig. 32–189). They immunostain for low molecular weight cytokeratin (Fig. 32–190) and may focally express high molecular weight cytokeratin (Fig. 32–191) as well as carcinoembryonic antigen (Fig. 32–192) and epithelial membrane antigen (Fig. 32–193).

Ultrastructurally, malignant carcinoids display more variability in cell size and shape than mature carcinoids and have fewer neuroendocrine granules than mature carcinoids (Figs. 32–194 and 32–195) and may have highly convoluted nuclei (Fig. 32–196).

Tsutsumi et al.[427] described a lung neoplasm they diagnosed as an atypical carcinoid, in which they de-

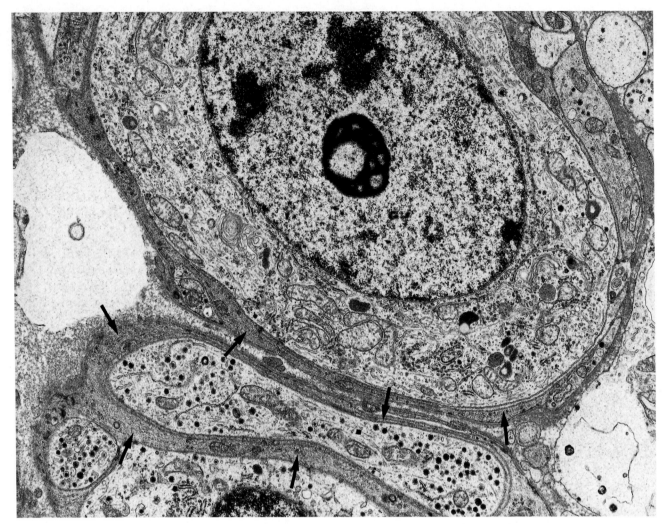

Fig. 32–175. S-100-positive cells shown in Fig. 32–174 correspond to Schwann cells that wrap around tumor cells *(arrows)*. ×16,000.

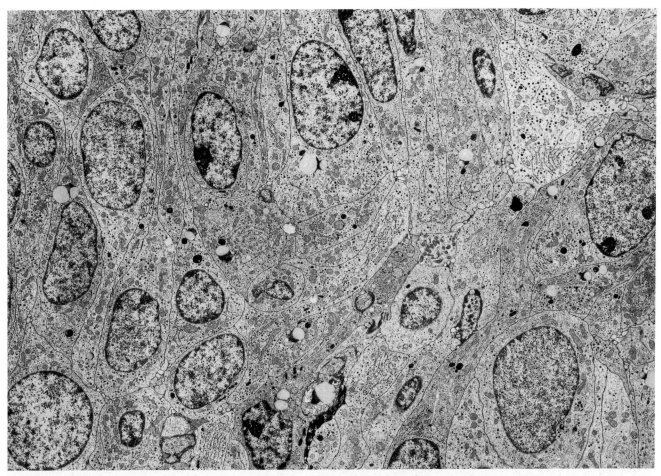

Fig. 32–176. Spindle cell carcinoid composed of uniform spindle-shaped cells contain numerous neuroendocrine granules in cytoplasm. Note numerous lysosomes (ceroid pigment) in cytoplasm of tumor cells. ×4,100.

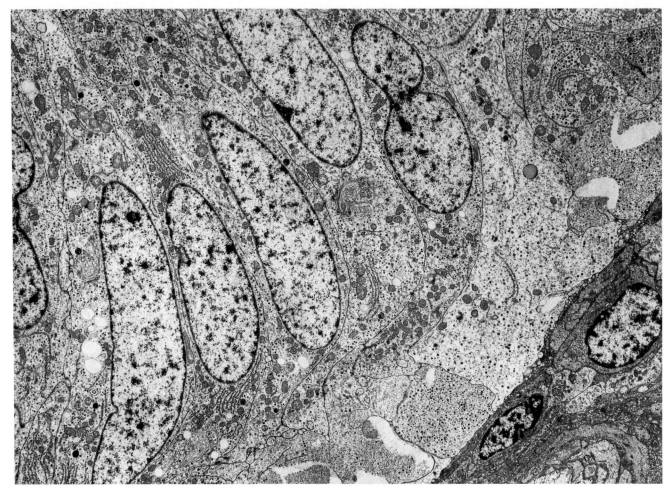

Fig. 32–177. Ultrastructural appearance of carcinoid shown in Fig. 32–165. Note density of neuroendocrine granules in cytoplasm. ×4,100.

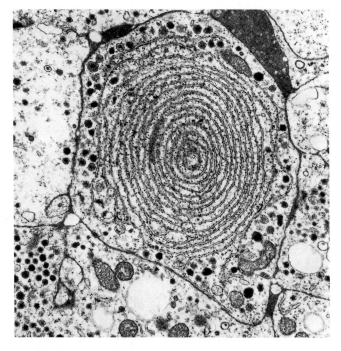

Fig. 32–178. Many carcinoids contain parallel arrays of rough endoplasmic reticulum in their cytoplasm. ×26,500.

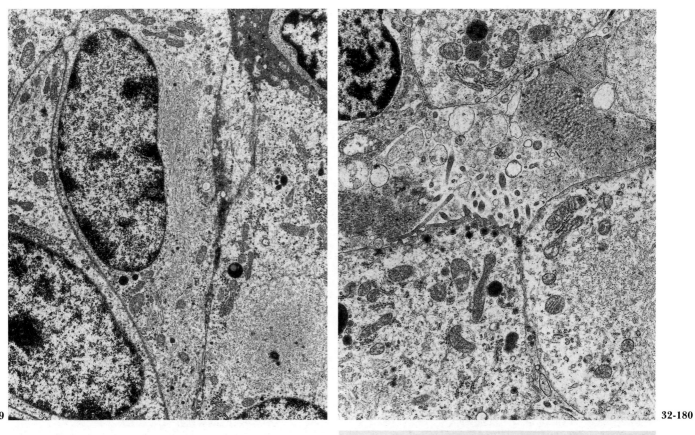

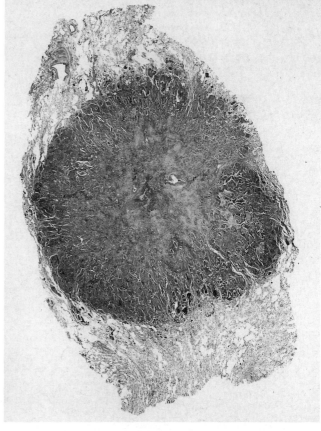

Fig. 32–179. As in other neuroendocrine tumors, paranuclear aggregates of intermediate filaments, probably corresponding to keratin and/or neurofilament, may be present. ×16,000.

Fig. 32–180. Some carcinoids form distinct glands with microvilli projecting into gland lumens. ×26,500.

Fig. 32–181. Well-demarcated, peripherally located, atypical carcinoid. ×4.

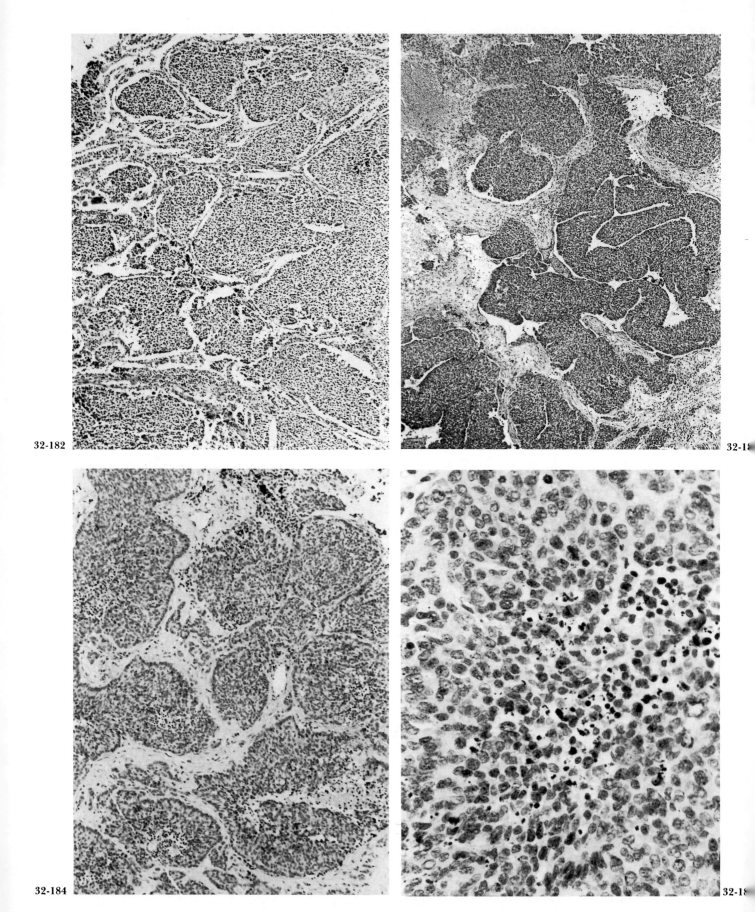

32-182

32-1[

32-184

32-18

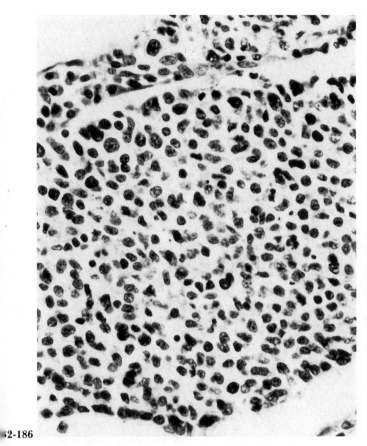

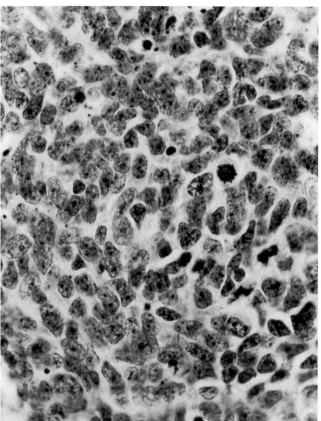

Fig. 32–186. Cellular pleomorphism, not seen in mature carcinoids, is characteristic feature of malignant carcinoids. ×330.

Fig. 32–187. Most atypical carcinoids show significant mitotic activity. ×550.

Fig. 32–188. Focal gland formation and mucin production are features of some atypical carcinoids. ×550.

⟶

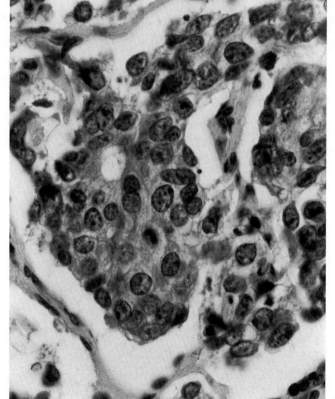

⟵

Fig. 32–182. Atypical carcinoids usually have organoid pattern especially at periphery. ×75.

Fig. 32–183. Organoid nests of tumor cells form atypical carcinoid, frequently separated by fibrous tissue bands. ×75.

Fig. 32–184. Palisading of peripheral cell layer is frequent feature of atypical carcinoids. ×75.

Fig. 32–185. Atypical carcinoids frequently show focal necrosis. ×330.

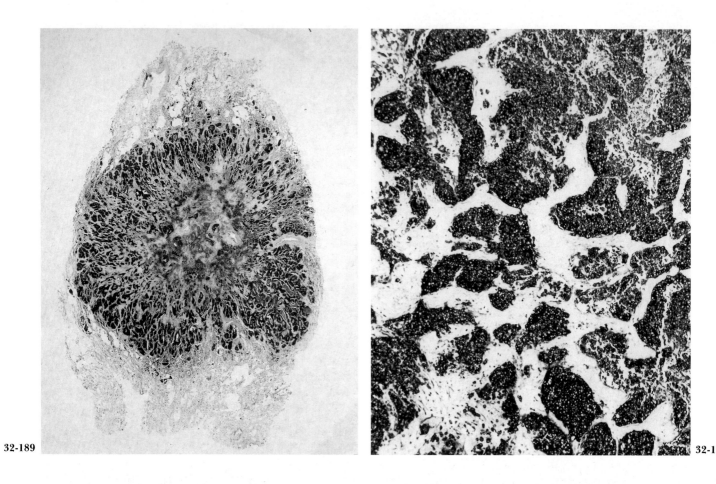

32-189   32-19

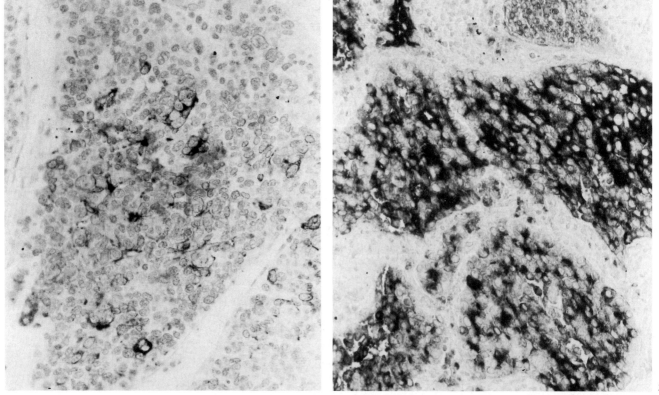

32-191   32-1

Fig. 32–189. Similar to other bronchopulmonary neuroendocrine neoplasms, atypical carcinoids show intense immunostaining *(black)* for neuron-specific enolase. ×4.

Fig. 32–190. Nests of tumor cells forming this atypical carcinoid show intense immunostaining *(black)* for low molecular weight cytokeratin. ×75.

Fig. 32–191. Some atypical carcinoids may show focal immunostaining *(black)* for high molecular weight cytokeratin. ×330.

Fig. 32–192. Approximately 50% of all neuroendocrine lung tumors, including this atypical carcinoid, show immunostaining *(black)* for carcinoembryonic antigen. ×330.

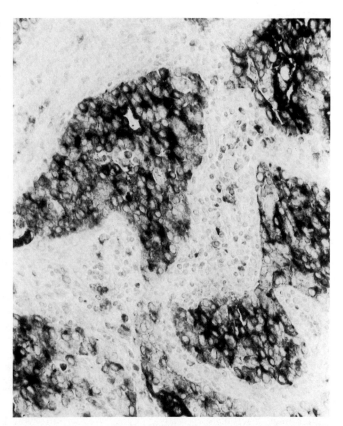

Fig. 32–193. Many carcinoids and atypical carcinoids express epithelial membrane antigen *(black)*. ×330.

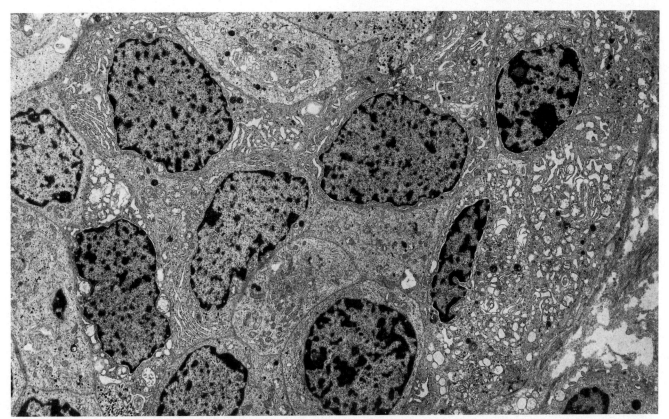

Fig. 32–194. In contrast to mature carcinoids, atypical carcinoids usually contain fewer neuroendocrine granules in their cytoplasm when examined ultrastructurally. ×4,100.

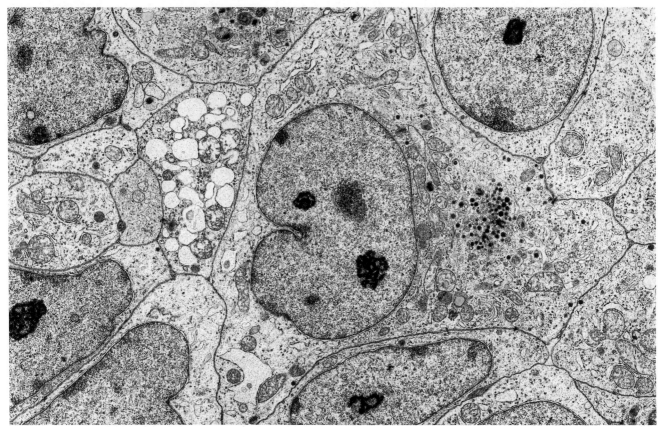

Fig. 32–195. Some atypical carcinoids have small but distinct nucleoli, a feature usually not seen in small cell neuroendocrine carcinomas. ×4,100.

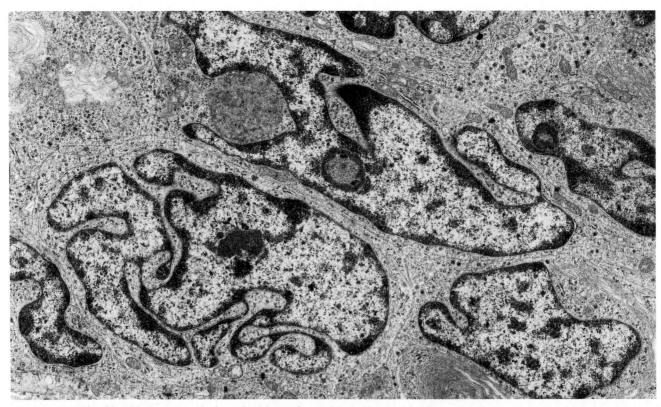

Fig. 32–196. Some atypical carcinoids are formed by cells with highly convoluted nuclei. ×16,000.

scribed the primary neoplasm as showing carcinoid-like histology and "large cell transformation" in bone metastases. We have observed "giant" neuroendocrine tumor cells in several primary lung neoplasms fulfilling the criteria of atypical carcinoids.[428] We have also observed significant interobserver variability in diagnosing atypical carcinoids. The primary difference in opinion in most of these cases has been between atypical carcinoid and small cell undifferentiated carcinoma. In this author's experience, atypical carcinoid usually shows a more organoid appearance, and by immunohistochemistry is usually positive for chromogranin, whereas in small cell undifferentiated carcinoma an organoid pattern is not present, and the chromogranin is almost always negative.

Large Cell Neuroendocrine Carcinoma–Atypical Endocrine Tumor of Lung

In 1978, Gould and Chejfec[429] demonstrated ultrastructurally and biochemically that some tumors diagnosed histologically as large cell undifferentiated carcinoma represented neuroendocrine carcinomas. In 1981 McDowell et al.[430] reported seven cases that had been diagnosed as squamous carcinoma, adenocarcinoma, or large cell undifferentiated carcinoma that contained neuroendocrine granules when examined by electron microscopy and contained serotonin when examined biochemically. In 1985, Hammond and Sause[431] reported on eight large cell neuroendocrine carcinomas, seven of which had been diagnosed histologically as large cell undifferentiated carcinomas. Their report was followed by that of Neal et al.,[432] who described 19 atypical endocrine tumors of the lung, which represented 9% of the 247 tumors they studied. Four had been diagnosed histologically as poorly differentiated carcinoma, 5 as poorly differentiated adenocarcinoma, 2 as undifferentiated nonsmall cell, non-large cell carcinoma, 6 as large cell undifferentiated carcinoma, and 1 each as adenocarcinoma and poorly differentiated adenosquamous carcinoma.

In 1989, Barbareschi et al.[433] reported a case of large cell neuroendocrine carcinoma of the lung in a 70-year-old man who was found on a routine chest radiograph to have a "coin" lesion in the left-upper lobe. The neoplasm was extensively necrotic and was initially diagnosed as a large cell undifferentiated carcinoma. The primary tumor and metastatic tumor in bone showed immunostaining for chromogranin, keratin, synaptophysin, and calcitonin. The tumor was also described as being composed in part of frequent giant anaplastic cells.

Travis et al.[434] reported on 35 primary neuroendo-crine neoplasms of the lung, including 20 typical carcinoids, 6 atypical carcinoids, 5 large cell neuroendocrine carcinomas, and 4 small cell undifferentiated carcinomas. The patients with large cell neuroendocrine carcinomas of the lung were between 35 and 75 years old, with a mean age of 59 years and a median age of 64 years; all were heavy cigarette smokers. The large cell neuroendocrine carcinomas ranged between 2.4 to 4 cm in diameter; 3 neoplasms were stage I and 2 were stage III-B. The criteria Travis et al.[434] used to diagnose large cell neuroendocrine carcinoma were as follows: (1) A tumor with a neuroendocrine appearance by light microscopy that included an organoid, trabecular, palisading, or rosette pattern; (2) large cells with most cells greater than the nuclear diameter of three small resting lymphocytes, a low nuclear-to-cytoplasmic ratio, polygonal-shaped cells, finely granular eosinophilic cytoplasm with an eosinophilic hue, coarse nuclear chromatin, and frequent nucleoli; (3) a mitotic rate greater than 10 per ten high power fields; (4) necrosis; and (5) neuroendocrine features by immunohistochemistry or electron microscopy or both.

Travis et al.[434] indicated that compared to small cell undifferentiated carcinoma, the tumor cells were larger and had abundant eosinophilic cytoplasm. The mitotic rate averaged 66 per 10 high power fields, which was considerably higher than that seen in atypical carcinoids. Nucleoli were stated to be prominent in two cases, and faint or focal in three cases. DNA encrustation of vascular elastic tissue was not observed. Ultrastructurally, neuroendocrine granules were observed in the four cases examined, by electron microscopy and varied between 100 to 270 nm in diameter. Glandular differentiation was prominent by electron microscopy in one case, and numerous desmosomes, which the authors interpreted to represent squamous differentiation, were seen in one case. By immunohistochemistry, five of five cases immunostained for neuron-specific enolase and carcinoembryonic antigen, and four of four cases were positive for keratin. Two of five tumors expressed synaptophysin and bombesin, whereas one of five neoplasms was positive for ACTH and one of four neoplasms expressed calcitonin and "big" ACTH.

Wick et al.[435] compared 12 primary large cell carcinomas of the lung, showing neuroendocrine differentiation, with 15 large cell undifferentiated carcinomas that lacked neuroendocrine differentiation. Large cell neuroendocrine carcinomas were defined by immunostaining for neuron-specific enolase, Leu7, synaptophysin and chromogranin-A, and by the presence of neurosecretory granules identified ultrastructurally. Wick et al.[435] found the large cell carcinomas with neuroendocrine features to have a significantly worse prognosis than the large cell carcinomas without neuroendocrine features, and suggested that the large cell neuroendocrine carcinomas were probably underdiagnosed.

Mooi et al.[436] reported 11 cases of resected primary carcinoma of the lung that histologically were stated to show bronchial carcinoid or small cell undifferentiated carcinoma features. Immunohistochemically, all tumors were positive for neuron-specific enolase and protein gene product 9.5, and ultrastructurally, 6 of 7 cases examined contained dense-core neuroendocrine type granules, these findings indicating neuroendocrine differentiation. The authors suggested that the histologic appearance of the tumors suggested neuroendocrine differentiation, which could perhaps be valuable in treatment and prognosis. In this series, all neoplasms were in the upper lobes and all but 1 patient expired within 15 months after surgery.

Large cell neuroendocrine tumors are most commonly located peripherally or in the midlung field and often are greater than 3 cm in diameter. Before proceeding with the description and illustration of large cell neuroendocrine carcinomas of the lung, a word of caution is in order. As perhaps best exemplified when classifying non-Hodgkin's malignant lymphoma, there is often considerable variation in opinion among trained, experienced pathologists as to what is a large cell and what is a small cell. With respect to lung neoplasms, this is best illustrated by a case report published several years ago.[437] The case concerned a 47-year-old male with a 4-cm mass in the hilum of the left lung, a 1.5-cm nodule at the left heart border, and right inguinal and axillary masses. The right axillary mass was biopsied and was diagnosed as showing metastatic large cell undifferentiated carcinoma. The patient was treated with lomustine at 130 mg/m^2 in 6-week cycles for 2 years. His tumor completely disappeared and he was free of disease 4 years after diagnosis and treatment. Several weeks after this article appeared in publication, a Letter to the Editor[438] of the journal in which the report appeared, raised concern that the neoplasm reported as a metastatic large cell undifferentiated carcinoma was a malignant lymphoma, probably a diffuse "histiocytic" lymphoma. The author of the report sent the slides of the biopsied tumor to three experts who offered their opinions as to the correct histologic diagnosis of the tumor. Dr. Mary Matthews[439] opined that the neoplasm was a small cell undifferentiated carcinoma, intermediate cell type. Dr. Raymond Yesner[439] stated: "The overall impression is that of an intermediate small cell carcinoma which is showing some large cell characteristic—i.e., 22/40" (22 refers to intermediate small undifferentiated carcinoma, and 40 to large cell undifferentiated carcinoma). Dr. Juan Rosai[438] stated: "It is a very undifferentiated tumor, and the differential diagnosis is between oat cell carci-

noma and large cell undifferentiated carcinoma. Although I admit there is room for disagreement, I definitely favor the diagnosis of oat cell carcinoma, because of the architectural pattern and nuclear shape."

To this author, this case report strongly suggests that even among experienced pathologists the size of neoplastic cells is to a certain extent "in the eyes of the beholder," which can cause problems in classification of lung neoplasms, especially neuroendocrine lung neoplasms. In the 9 cases we published in 1989[428] concerning neuroendocrine lung neoplasms, a considerable difference of opinion occurred in classification, even with a knowledge of the ultrastructural and immunohistochemical features of the tumor cells.

Histologically, large cell neuroendocrine carcinomas may have an organoid or trabecular pattern and at low magnification, resemble a carcinoid or an atypical carcinoid (Figs. 32–197 and 32–198). As described by Travis et al.,[434] large cell carcinomas have a variable cytologic appearance. As shown in Figs. 32–199 and 32–200, many are composed of large cells with large vesicular nuclei and prominent nucleoli. Neoplasms with this appearance are easily confused with nonneu-

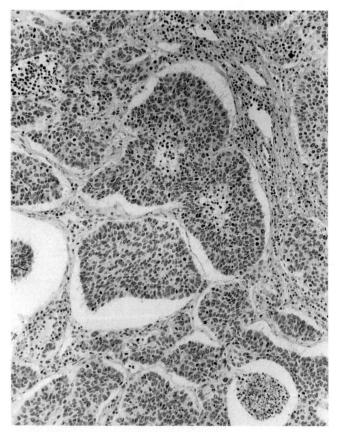

Fig. 32–197. Large cell neuroendocrine carcinoma exhibits organoid pattern at low magnification. ×75.

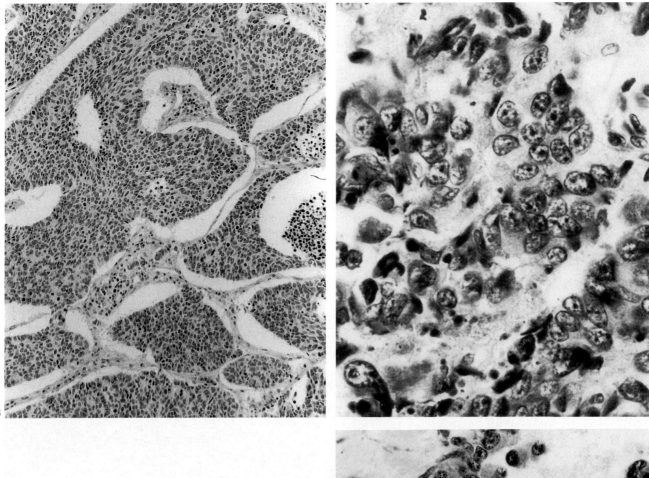

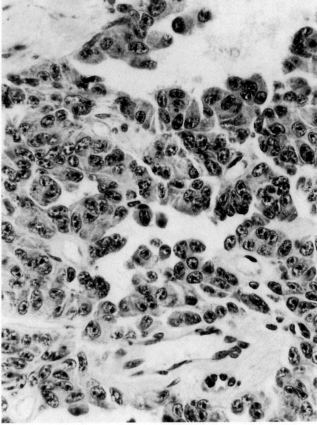

Fig. 32–198. Large cell neuroendocrine carcinoma shows organoid and trabecular pattern. ×75.

Fig. 32–199. Histologic appearance of large cell bronchopulmonary neuroendocrine carcinoma (atypical endocrine tumor of lung). ×550.

Fig. 32–200. Large cell neuroendocrine carcinoma. Note large vesicular nuclei and prominent nucleoli. ×550.

roendocrine large cell undifferentiated carcinomas. Other large cell neuroendocrine carcinomas are composed of cells that are large but have nuclear cytologic features resembling a small cell neuroendocrine carcinoma with small clumps of chromatin and absent or small nucleoli. The ultrastructural appearance of large cell neuroendocrine neoplasms usually correlates with their cytologic features. Those with large nucleoli cytologically have large nucleoli ultrastructurally (Figs. 32–201 and 32–202). They typically have a few cellular processes and variable numbers of dense-core neuroendocrine granules (Fig. 32–201). Those whose nuclei lack prominent nucleoli cytologically resemble "large" small cell undifferentiated carcinomas ultrastructurally, except that they have fewer processes and usually have more cytoplasmic organelles, including neuroendocrine granules (Fig. 32–203). We evaluated one large

cell neuroendocrine carcinoma that contained perinuclear aggregates of intermediate filaments similar to those in mature carcinoids (Fig. 32–204). They usually show a few processes by electron microscopy and have a variable number of neuroendocrine granules. They usually express low and high molecular weight cytokeratin as well as neuron-specific enolase, carcinoembryonic antigen and occasionally chromogranin and some of the substances shown in Table 32–20.

Small Cell Undifferentiated Carcinoma

Small cell undifferentiated carcinoma constitutes approximately 20%–25% of common lung neoplasms and is frequently called oat cell carcinoma or neuroendocrine carcinoma of small cell type. This neoplasm was initially thought to represent a sarcoma or lymphoma

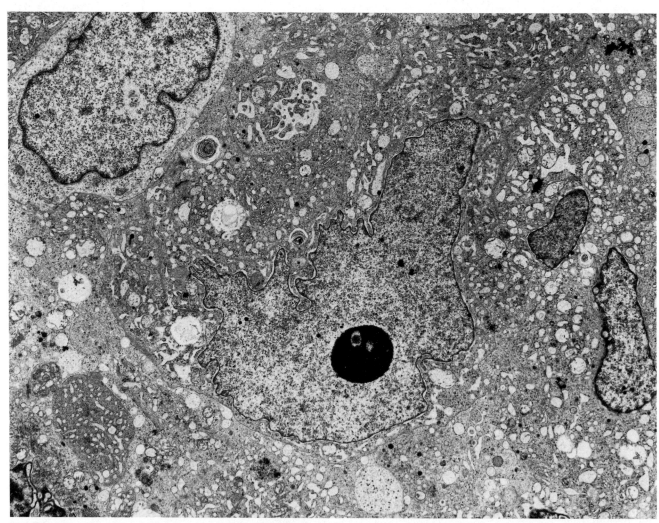

Fig. 32–201. Ultrastructural appearance of large cell neuroendocrine carcinoma. Note large irregularly shaped nucleus and prominent nucleolus. Tumor cells contain more neuroendocrine granules than small cell neuroendocrine carcinomas. ×16,000.

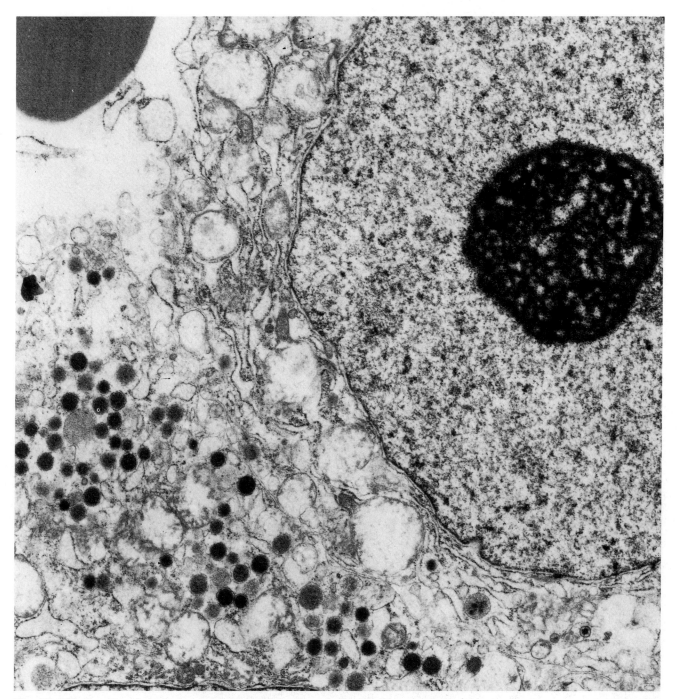

Fig. 32–202. Portion of single large cell neuroendocrine tumor cell. Note huge nucleolus and numerous neuroendocrine granules in cytoplasm. ×43,000.

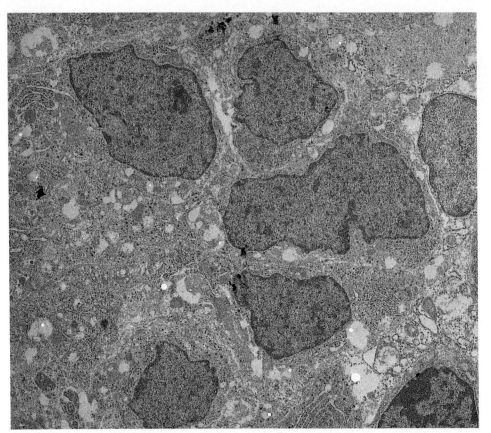

Fig. 32–203. Large cell neuroendocrine carcinoma composed of large cells with large nuclei with absent or small nucleoli. These neoplastic cells resemble those of a "large" small cell neuroendocrine carcinoma. ×10,400.

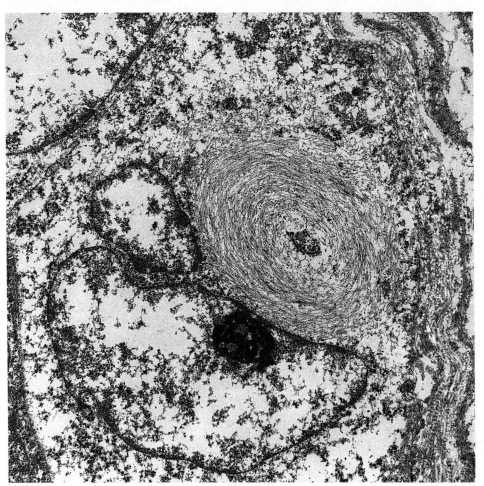

Fig. 32–204. Ultrastructurally, large cell neuroendocrine carcinoma contains perinuclear aggregates of intermediate filaments, an occasional finding in neuroendocrine carcinomas. ×26,000.

and it was not until 1926 that it was recognized as an epithelial neoplasm.[440] It was initially classified with large cell carcinoma of the lung as an "anaplastic carcinoma."[441] The most recent World Health Organization's classification of lung cancer[173] divides this neoplasm into three categories: (1) oat cell carcinoma, which was referred to as a lymphocyte-like type of small cell carcinoma in the 1967 World Health Organization classification of lung tumors and was characterized by a tumor composed of small round uniform cells approximately 1.5–3 fold larger than a lymphocyte with dense round oval nuclei and sparse cytoplasm; (2) small cell carcinoma, intermediate cell type, which was characterized as being composed of polygonal or fusiform cells less regular in appearance than oat cell carcinoma and having more cytoplasm than oat cell carcinoma; and (3) combined oat cell carcinoma, characterized by a combination of a definite oat cell carcinoma and squamous cell carcinoma or adenocarcinoma.

Azzopardi's[442] 1959 light microscopic description of oat cell carcinoma remains excellent. This neoplasm was reviewed in detail in 1983 by Yesner[443] and by Carter.[444] In 1985 Yesner[445] and the other members of the pathology committee of the International Association for the Study of Lung Cancer indicated that there was no significant biologic difference between the oat cell subtype and intermediate subtype of small cell undifferentiated carcinoma. They suggested that the terms "oat-cell," "lymphocyte-like," and "intermediate" be discarded and be replaced with the term "small cell carcinoma" to refer to such undifferentiated tumors that have no significant nonsmall cell elements. They also suggested that two variants of small cell lung carcinoma be recognized: (1) mixed small cell–large cell carcinoma, which is a neoplasm composed of small cells with a significant population of large cells that are arranged in nests or diffusely throughout the tumor, and (2) combined small cell carcinoma, composed of a combination of small cell carcinoma and neoplastic squamous or adenocarcinoma.

Stuart-Harris et al.[446] applied this new classification scheme to 124 cases of small cell lung cancer. A specimen for histologic examination was available in 59 cases, a specimen for cytological correlation in 91 cases, and a specimen for ultrastructural examination in 60 cases. Of the 124 cases, 120 were classified as small cell carcinoma, 2 as mixed small cell–large cell carcinoma, and 2 as combined small cell carcinoma. There was concordance by the three pathologists who reviewed the slides in all cases except one. The authors concluded that their study confirmed that small cell carcinoma accounted for more than 90% of untreated cases of small cell lung cancer, and that mixed small cell–large cell carcinoma was perhaps less common that previously proposed.

Yesner[443] indicated that small cell carcinomas may show transitions into large cell carcinomas, adenocarcinomas, squamous carcinomas, or all of them. In his study of 205 tumors diagnosed at biopsy as small cell carcinoma, approximately 20% of treated and untreated patients' tumors showed a different histology at autopsy, representing either a combined small cell tumor or a nonsmall cell tumor (see their Table 1). This is in keeping with the cell culture work of Gazdar et al.[447] who found that small cell carcinomas converted into large cell carcinomas without neuroendocrine features after 2 years in continuous culture.

Macroscopically, small cell undifferentiated carcinomas are centrally located in more than 90% of cases and have a tendency to directly invade and metastasize to regional lymph nodes (Fig. 32–205), although they may present as relatively small bronchial associated tumors (Figs. 32–206 and 32–207). Small cell undifferentiated

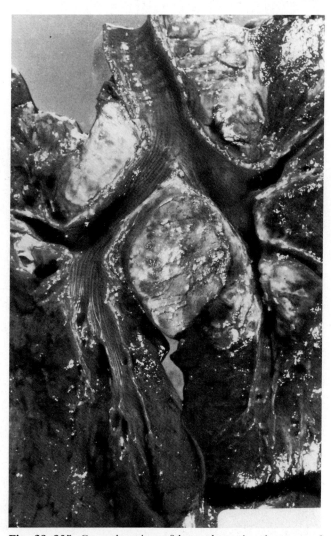

Fig. 32–205. Central region of lung shows involvement of regional lymph nodes by small cell undifferentiated carcinoma. Note lack of bronchial involvement.

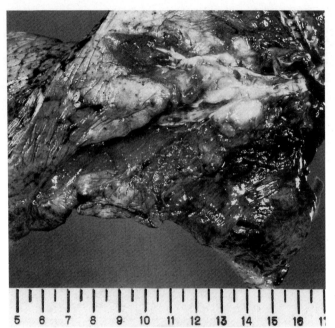

Fig. 32–206. Left-upper lobe shows relatively small tumor in parabronchial distribution but without occlusion of lumen of bronchus.

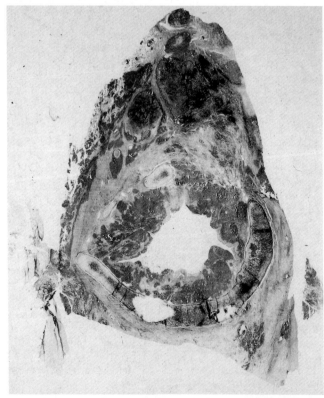

Fig. 32–207. Small cell undifferentiated carcinoma invades directly into bronchial wall. ×8.

carcinomas frequently metastasize and may present as liver failure secondary to metastatic tumor (Fig. 32–208), or occasionally be associated with Cushing's syndrome, because of ACTH production by the tumor (Fig. 32–209).

Microscopically, small cell carcinomas have round, or fusiform nuclei with a ground-glass or stippled chromatin pattern with small and usually indistinct nucleoli (Figs. 32–210 through 32–213). Some small cell tumors are composed of slightly larger cells with larger nuclei, occasional nucleoli, and more abundant cytoplasm; these correspond to those categorized as intermediate small cell carcinomas by the World Health Organization (Figs. 32–214 through 32–217), although some might classify these neoplasms as large cell neuroendocrine carcinomas. Small cell undifferentiated neuroendocrine lung carcinomas frequently show large areas of necrosis (Fig. 32–218) with nuclear encrustation of elastic tissue of vessels (Figs. 32–219 and 32–220). As shown in Figs. 32–212 and 32–213, the tumor cells show a high mitotic rate. Some small cell neuroendocrine carcinomas have a tendency to aggregate around small blood vessels (Fig. 32–221) and frequently show perineural space invasion (Fig. 32–222). An occasional small cell undifferentiated carcinoma will contain tumor giant cells (Fig. 32–223).

In transbronchial biopsies, the tumor cells can be relatively well preserved (Figs. 32–224 and 32–225) or often shown a great deal of artifactual distortion including crush artifact (Figs. 32–226). When the biopsy shows crush artifact and well-preserved cells are not present, this author is cautious in making an absolute diagnosis; in such specimens examined by electron microscopy, however, an accurate, unequivocal diagnosis is often possible on the basis of the presence of membrane-bound, dense-core neuroendocrine granules.

Immunohistochemically, most small cell neuroendocrine carcinomas express low molecular weight cytokeratin, which is frequently distributed in a streaky pattern within the cells (Fig. 32–227). In this author's experience these carcinomas usually do not express high molecular weight cytokeratin. They routinely express neuron-specific enolase (Fig. 32–228) and, like other types of neuroendocrine lung neoplasms, may show immunostaining for carcinoembryonic antigen (Fig. 32–229) and epithelial membrane antigen (Fig. 32–230). These neoplasms usually do not show immunostaining for chromogranin, which reflects the small number of neuroendocrine granules in their cytoplasm. Small cell neuroendocrine carcinomas may also contain any of the substances listed in Table 32–20.

Ultrastructurally, small cell neuroendocrine carcinomas are composed of small, round, unspecialized cells

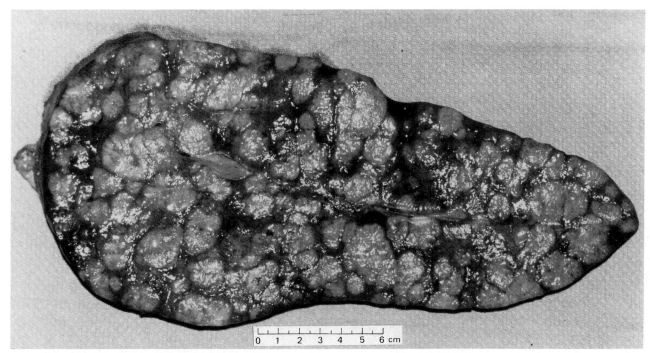

Fig. 32–208. Some patients with small cell undifferentiated carcinoma present with liver failure caused by massive metastases to liver.

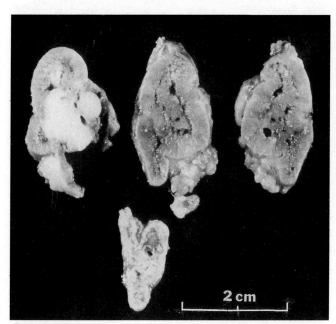

Fig. 32–209. Some small cell undifferentiated carcinomas produce adrenocorticotrophic hormone. ACTH-producing small cell neuroendocrine carcinoma has metastasized to adrenal and caused adrenal cortical hyperplasia secondary to ACTH production. Normal adrenal gland at bottom. (Photograph courtesy of Dr. John Bolen.)

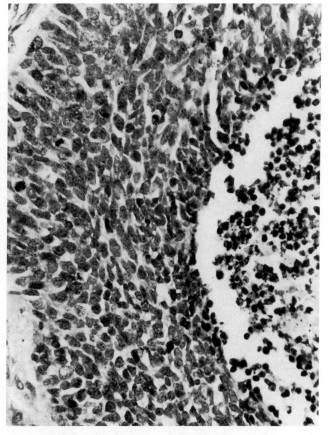

Fig. 32–210. Small cell undifferentiated carcinoma composed predominantly of fusiform cells. Note necrosis and frequent mitoses. ×330.

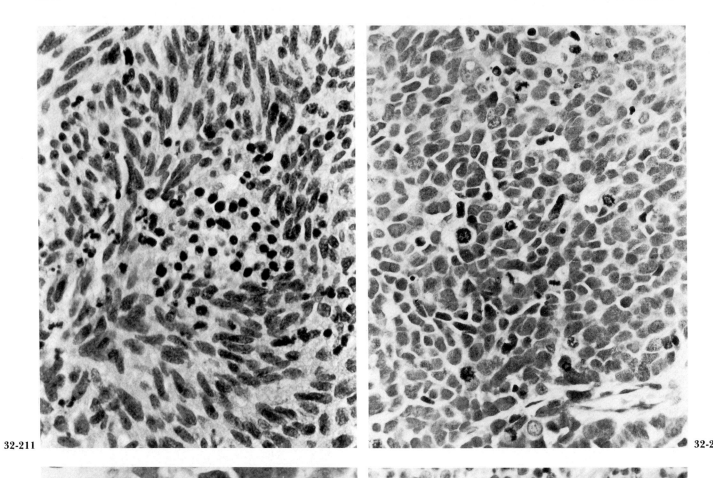

32-211   32-2

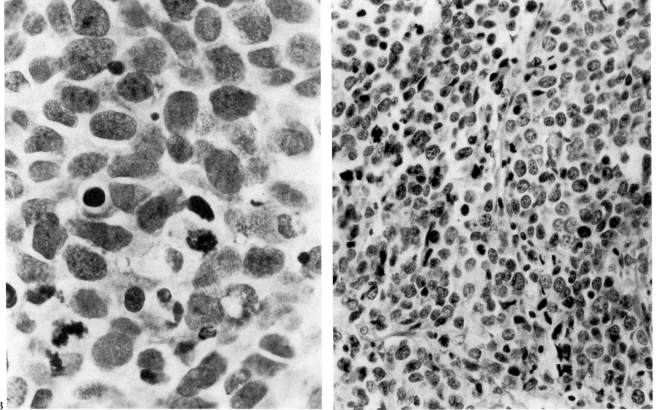

32-213   32-2

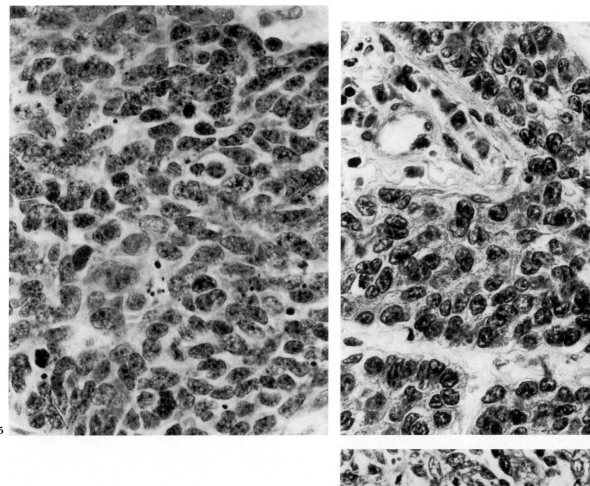

2-215

32-216

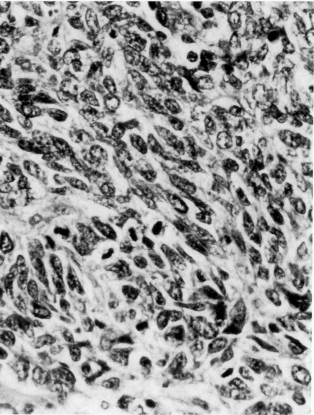

Fig. 32–211. Another example of small cell neuroendocrine carcinoma composed mostly of spindle cells. ×550.

Fig. 32–212. Small cell undifferentiated carcinoma cells show high nuclear cytoplasmic ratio, nuclear molding, and high mitotic rate. ×550.

Fig. 32–213. Greatly magnified small cell neuroendocrine tumor. Note large nuclei, inconspicuous cytoplasm; finely granular chromatin pattern; and absent nucleoli. ×775.

Figs. 32–214–217. Examples of small cell undifferentiated carcinomas that would be classified as intermediate type in World Health Organization Category. Note slightly larger size of cells and larger nuclei, occasionally having small nucleoli. All figures, ×550.

32-217

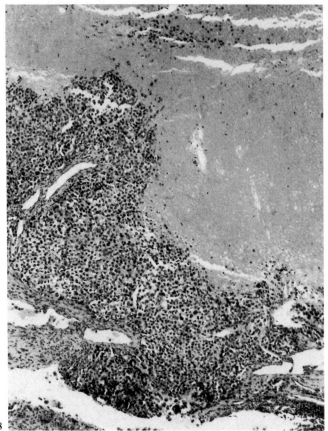

32-218

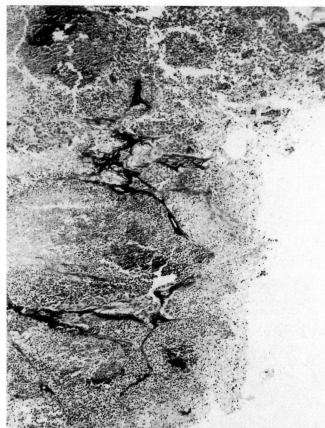

32-219

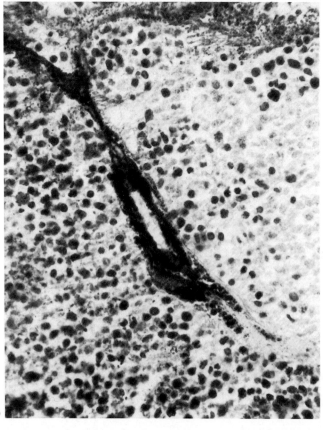

32-220

Fig. 32–218. Many small cell neuroendocrine carcinomas are mostly necrotic. ×75.

Fig. 32–219. Mostly necrotic small cell undifferentiated carcinoma shows prominent nuclear encrustation of elastic tissue of small blood vessels. ×75.

Fig. 32–220. Greater magnification of tumor shown in Fig. 32–219 shows nuclear encrustation of elastic tissue of small blood vessel. ×330.

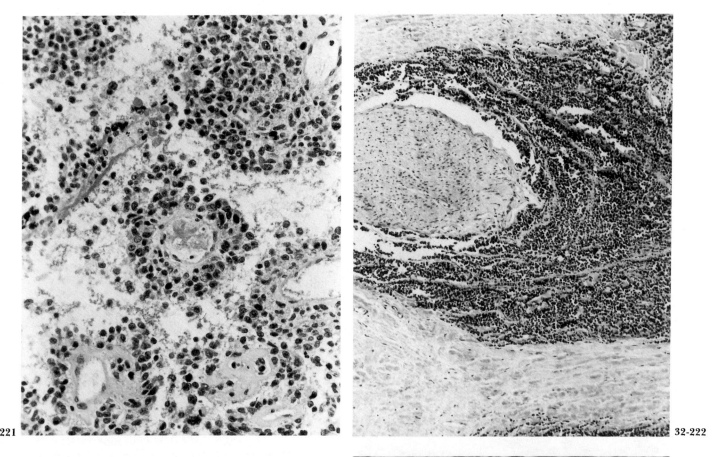

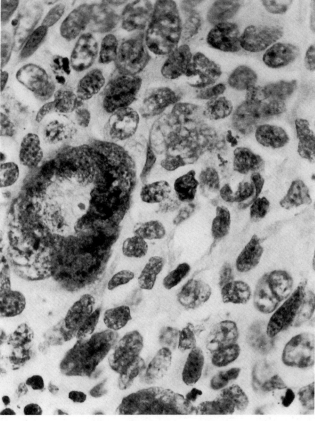

Fig. 32–221. Some small cell undifferentiated carcinomas show aggregation of tumor cells around small blood vessels. ×330.

Fig. 32–222. Perineural space invasion by small cell undifferentiated carcinoma is frequent. ×75.

Fig. 32–223. Some small undifferentiated neuroendocrine carcinomas contain occasional tumor giant cells. ×775.

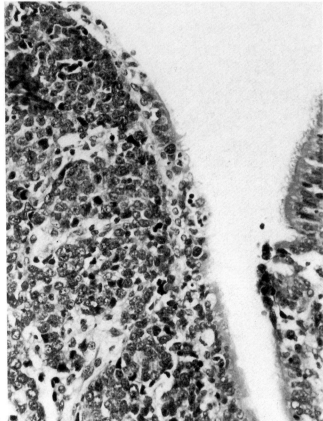

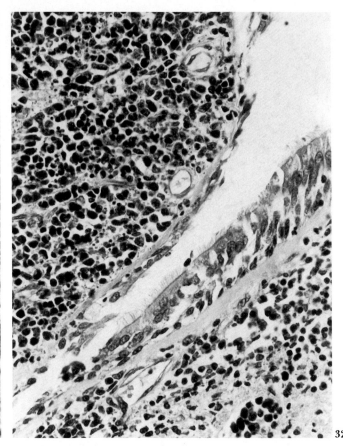

32-224

32-22

32-226

Fig. 32–224. Transbronchial biopsy of small cell undifferentiated carcinoma. Tumor cells frequently appose respiratory mucosal epithelium and may induce squamous metaplasia, but do not usually invade through the surface epithelium. ×550.

Fig. 32–225. Transbronchial biopsy shows infiltrating small cell undifferentiated carcinoma. Tumor cells are dying and have degenerated hyperchromatic nuclei. ×550.

Fig. 32–226. Crush artifact is common finding when small cell undifferentiated carcinomas are biopsied endoscopically. An absolute diagnosis frequently cannot be made. ×550.

Fig. 32–227. Low molecular weight cytokeratin is present in nearly all small cell neuroendocrine carcinomas examined using avidin-biotin immunoperoxidase technique (black staining). ×330.

Fig. 32–228. Small cell neuroendocrine carcinomas typically express neuron-specific enolase immunohistochemically (black staining). ×330.

Fig. 32–229. Approximately one-half of small cell undifferentiated carcinomas immunostain *(black)* for carcinoembryonic antigen. ×550.

Fig. 32–230. Immunostaining *(black)* for epithelial membrane antigen may also be seen by some small cell neuroendocrine carcinomas. ×550.

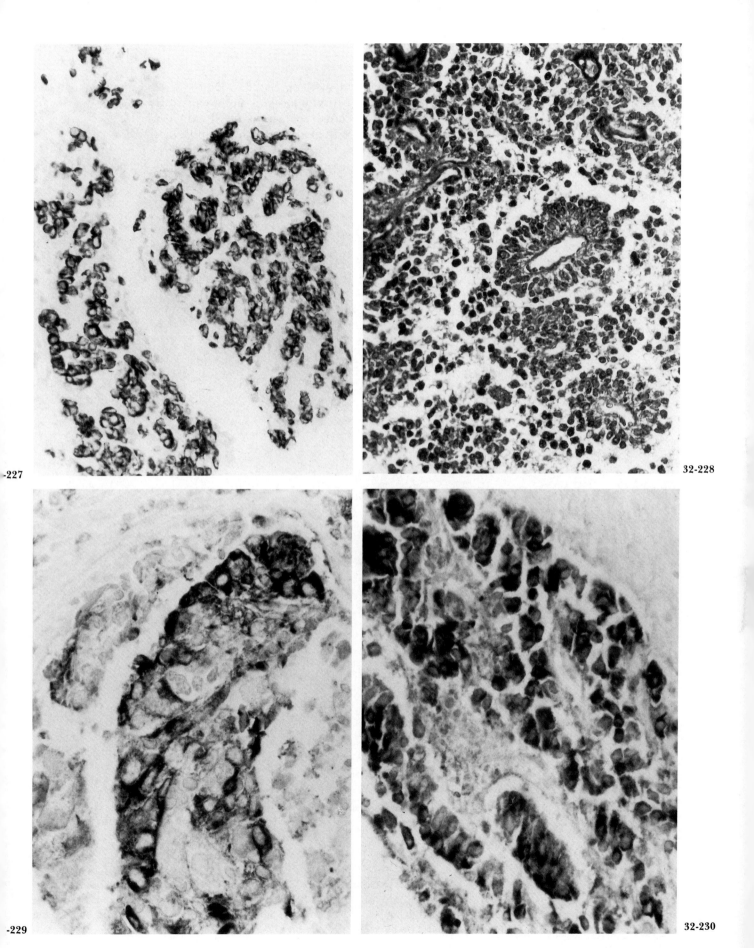

with high nuclear cytoplasmic ratios (Figs. 32–231 and 32–232). The tumor cells characteristically show processes that frequently contain microtubules and neuroendocrine granules (Fig. 32–233). Some small cell neuroendocrine carcinomas show desmosomes connecting the cells (Fig. 32–234) and occasional tonofila-ments (Fig. 32–235). Figure 32–236 shows a small cell neuroendocrine carcinoma with a slight degree of "crush artifact." Even with this distortion, cell processes with neuroendocrine granules are obvious.

Occasionally combined small cell tumors are encountered that are composed of a small cell neuroendocrine

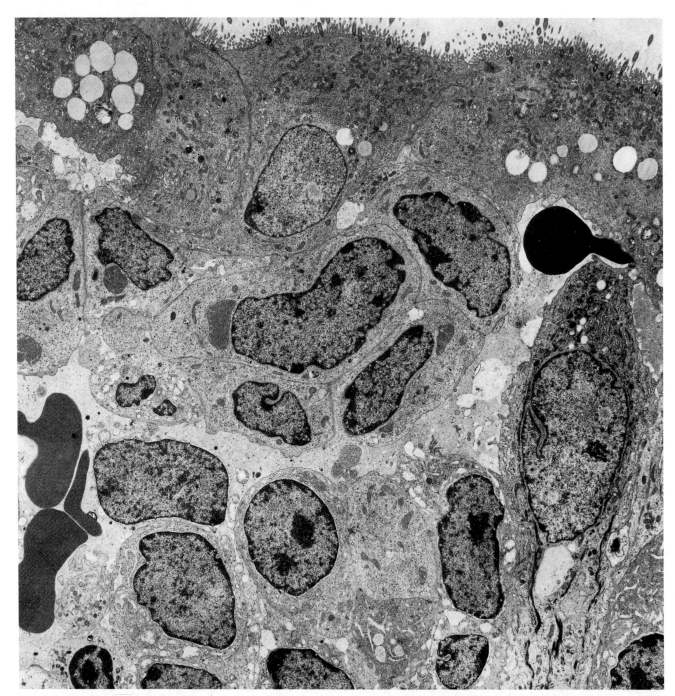

Figs. 32–231, 32–232. Typical ultrastructural appearance of small cell neuroendocrine carcinomas. Cells have high nuclear cytoplasmic ratios with small amount of unspecialized cyto-plasm. Nuclei generally lack nucleoli. Note mitoses in Fig. 32–232. Fig. 32–231. ×4,100; Fig. 32–232, ×6,400. *(See p. 1247 for Fig. 32–232.)*

carcinoma and either a squamous carcinoma or an adenocarcinoma. As previously shown in this chapter, this author recognizes small cell squamous carcinomas and small cell adenocarcinomas that frequently show regions of more mature squamous or glandular differentiation, but whose small cell component does not show neuroendocrine differentiation by electron microscopy or immunohistochemistry.

Combined small cell-large cell neuroendocrine carcinomas exist, and are composed of small undifferentiated cells admixed with large cells scattered among the smaller cells or in distinct nests. This author is still unclear as to the exact nature of the neoplasms referred to as small cell–large cell neuroendocrine neoplasms. Fushimi et al.[448] performed a retrospective evaluation of pathologic specimens from 430 patients with small

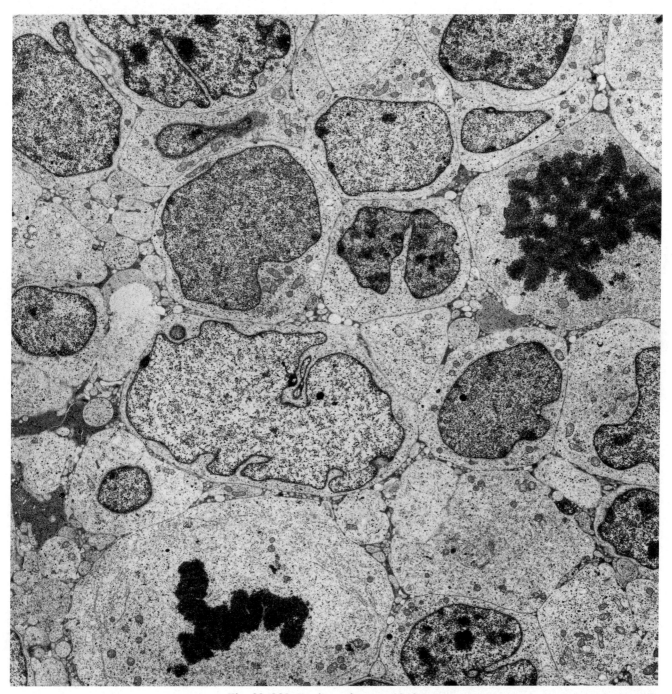

Fig. 32–232. For legend, see p. 1246.

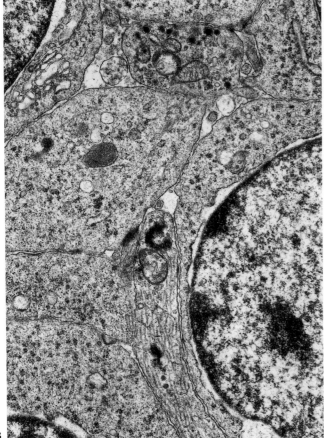

32-233

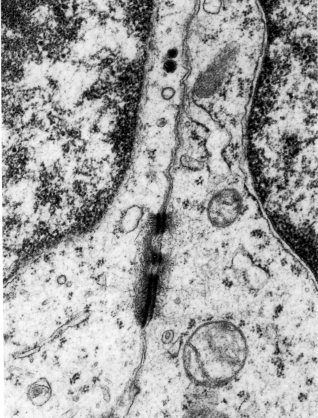

32-234

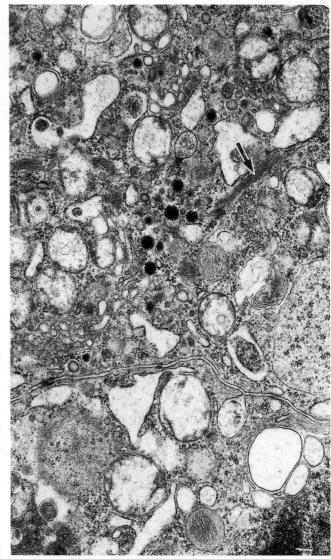

Fig. 32–235. Some small cell neuroendocrine carcinomas contain tonofilaments in cytoplasm *(arrow)*. ×26,500.

◁

Fig. 32–233. Tumor cells usually have processes containing microtubules and neuroendocrine granules. ×16,000.

Fig. 32–234. Small cell undifferentiated carcinoma cells are occasionally interconnected by desmosomes. Note neuroendocrine granule in cytoplasm. ×26,500.

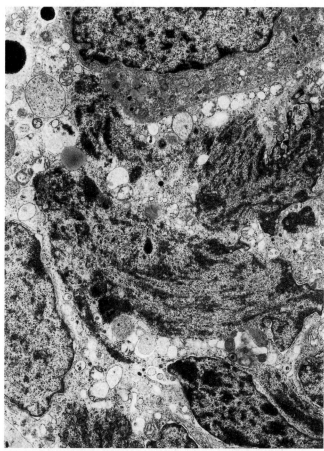

Fig. 32–236. Ultrastructural appearance of tumor cells showing a slight degree of crush artifact. ×6,400.

cell carcinoma of the lung. They defined mixed small cell–large cell carcinoma as neoplasms containing aggregates of, or single large cells, interspersed among tumor cells with the characteristic features of a small cell undifferentiated carcinoma. The large cells were defined histologically as having varying amounts of slightly eosinophilic cytoplasm showing distinct margins, and having large vesicular nuclei with distinct nucleoli. In cytologic specimens obtained by brushings or aspiration, the large cells occurred singly or in groups, and were described as having cyanophilic or amphophilic cytoplasm, and round vesicular nuclei and prominent nucleoli. In sputum cytologic specimens, the large cells were observed singly or in a loose cluster among the small cells, and were stated to show condensation of nuclear chromatin and shrinkage of cytoplasm, because of degenerative changes. In a review of the 430 cases, Fushimi et al. observed a frequency of mixed small cell–large cell carcinoma in 25 of 299 (8.4%) biopsy specimens, 75 of 400 (18.8%) cytologic specimens obtained by brushings or fine-needle aspiration biopsy, and in 8 of 232 (3.4%) sputum cytology

specimens. Fushimi et al.[448] reported that, whatever the diagnostic method, patients with mixed small cell–large cell carcinoma showed a worse response to therapy and had a worse prognosis than those with pure small cell lung carcinoma.

Neuroendocrine Differentiation in Non-Small Cell Lung Carcinomas

Visscher et al.[449] evaluated frozen unfixed tissue sections from 56 poorly differentiated non-small cell primary lung neoplasms with monoclonal antibodies against chromogranin-A, synaptophysin, S-100 protein, keratin, vimentin, and neurofilament antigens. Histologically, neuroendocrine features were stated to not be present in these neoplasms. Immunostaining for chromogranin-A or synaptophysin was identified in 5 of 17 (29%) large cell undifferentiated carcinomas and in 4 of 19 (21%) poorly differentiated adenocarcinomas. Diffuse intense immunostaining for synaptophysin was present in two large cell undifferentiated carcinomas and one poorly differentiated adenocarcinoma. Vimentin or neurofilament immunostaining was observed in 10 of 17 (59%) large cell undifferentiated carcinomas, 10 of 19 (53%) poorly differentiated adenocarcinomas, and accompanied neuroendocrine markers in 8 of 9 (89%) cases. Synaptophysin was expressed in only 1 of 20 (5%) of poorly differentiated squamous carcinomas and intermediate filaments other than keratin, that is, vimentin, was observed in 2 of 20 (10%) squamous cell carcinomas. The authors concluded that (1) immunohistologic evidence of neuroendocrine differentiation was present in a significant number of large cell undifferentiated carcinomas and poorly differentiated adenocarcinomas, and was rare in poorly differentiated squamous carcinomas; (2) neuroendocrine differentiation was often accompanied by heterogenous intermediate filament expression; and (3) divergent neuroendocrine differentiation was not necessarily reflected in the histologic features of the tumor.

Linnoila et al.[450] evaluated paraffin-embedded sections from 113 surgically resected primary lung neoplasms with antibodies against chromogranin-A, Leu7, neuron-specific enolase, serotonin, bombesin, calcitonin, ACTH, vasopressin, neurotensin, carcinoembryonic antigen, keratin, vimentin, and neurofilaments. They found that (1) the majority of carcinoids and small cell lung carcinomas expressed multiple neuroendocrine markers in a high percentage of tumor cells; (2) approximately 50% of non-small cell lung carcinomas contained subpopulations of tumor cells expressing neuroendocrine markers; and (3) occasional non-small cell lung carcinomas showed immunostaining patterns indistinguishable from small cell lung carcinomas. Neuroendocrine markers were more commonly expressed in large cell undifferentiated carcinomas and adenocarcinomas than in squamous carcinomas.

The question immediately rises as to whether the large cell lung carcinomas and poorly differentiated adenocarcinomas showing neuroendocrine features by immunohistochemistry should be classified as large cell neuroendocrine carcinomas. This is not an easy question to answer, but perhaps they should classify these neoplasms as large cell neuroendocrine carcinomas, especially if they showed the histologic features as outlined by Travis et al.[434] However, Travis et al.[434] referred to these neoplasms as non-small cell carcinomas with neuroendocrine features and indicated that they represented 10%–15% of non-small cell carcinomas but did not have the histologic/cytologic features of neuroendocrine neoplasms.

Approach to the Diagnosis of Primary and Metastatic Lung Cancer

In most cases in which an adequate sample of tumor is available for histologic examination, the diagnosis of common lung tumors is straightforward. Pathologists should use definite histologic criteria in diagnosing the various types of common lung neoplasms rather than making a diagnosis on the basis of "suspicions." In this author's opinion, one section of lung tumor should be taken for every 1 cm of tumor diameter in surgically resected specimens. If the tumor is close to the visceral pleura, causes pleural puckering, or results in adhesions between the visceral and parietal pleura, the entire region of pleural involvement should be carefully sectioned so that accurate staging can be done. It is also this author's opinion that all lymph nodes received with the resected specimen or submitted separately by the surgeon should be sliced into 1-mm-thick pieces and submitted entirely and examined for metastatic tumor, again to ensure accurate staging. If a frozen section is done on the lung neoplasm and the neoplasm is poorly differentiated or looks unusual, it is wise to prepare the tumor for possible ultrastructural and/or immunohistochemical examination. In some cases tumor should be snap-frozen for potential biochemical analysis or cell-surface markers to evaluate for potential lymphomas.

In today's medical environment, more "less invasive" procedures are being done, and the pathologist is faced with making accurate diagnoses on small tissue samples. As discussed in Chapter 1, it is often helpful to have tissue available for immunohistochemical and ultrastructural examination. In our experience this has been most useful in evaluating transbronchial biopsy speci-

mens, fine-needle aspiration biopsy specimens, and malignant cells in pleural fluid.

Figure 32–237 shows a transbronchial biopsy composed of bronchial mucosa with a small cell infiltrate in the lamina propria. When immunostained for low molecular weight cytokeratin, the tumor cells showed no immunostaining (Fig. 32–238) but were intensely positive for common leukocyte antigen (Fig. 32–239), strongly suggesting the diagnosis of lymphoma. This is in contrast to a small cell neuroendocrine carcinoma in which the tumor cells usually show immunostaining for low molecular weight cytokeratin (Fig. 32–240).

Figure 32–241 is a transbronchial biopsy specimen that shows a small collection of large neoplastic cells admixed with inflammatory cells. Often the clinician only wishes to know if the tumor is a small cell undifferentiated carcinoma versus a non-small cell lung cancer, and in most instances this is possible to say. However, if a more precise diagnosis is wished, such as large cell neuroendocrine carcinoma, ultrastructural and/or immunohistochemical examination of such small specimens is frequently helpful. Figure 32–242 shows the ultrastructural appearance of the tumor shown in Fig. 32–240). The tumor is an obvious adenocarcinoma with features suggestive of a bronchioloalveolar cell carcinoma.

It also is relatively easy to examine malignant cells in

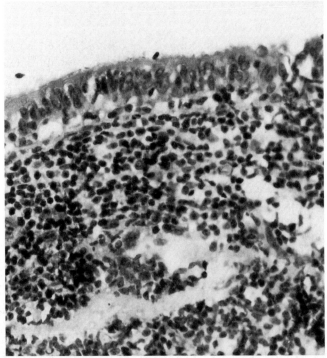

Fig. 32–237. Transbronchial biopsy shows cellular infiltrate in lamina propria. ×330.

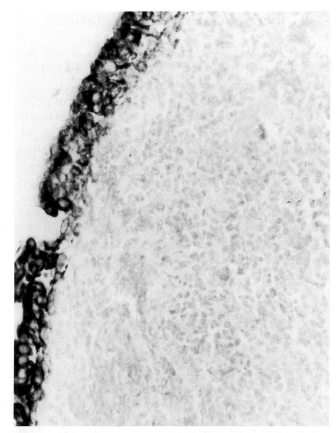

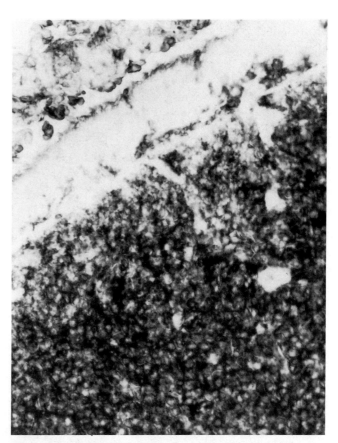

Fig. 32–238. When immunostained for low molecular weight cytokeratin, surface epithelium is positive *(black)* but cellular infiltrate in lamina propria is negative. ×330.

Fig. 32–239. Cells in lamina propria express common leukocyte antigen *(black)*, suggesting cells are lymphocytes and infiltrate probably represent lymphoma. ×330.

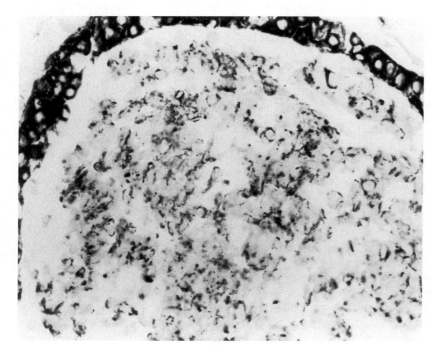

Fig. 32–240. In contrast to small cells in Fig. 32–239, these small cells immunostain *(black)* for low molecular weight cytokeratin, strongly suggesting diagnosis of small cell neuroendocrine carcinoma. ×330.

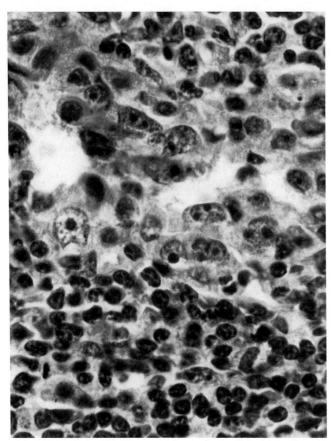

Fig. 32–241. Transbronchial biopsy specimen shows small collection of large malignant cells admixed with inflammatory cells. ×550.

pleural fluid and fine-needle aspiration biopsies by electron microscopy and immunohistochemistry.

Metastatic carcinoma should always be considered in the differential diagnosis of any lung cancer. As previously indicated, most common primary lung tumors occur as single masses in the lung with the exception of some bronchioloalveolar cell carcinomas and epithelioid hemangioendotheliomas (see Chapter 33). In small specimens it may be impossible to distinguish between primary and metastatic tumors, especially adenocarcinoma, even if electron microscopy and immunohistochemistry is done on available tissue specimens.[451]

Neuroendocrine tumors of the lung are the most diverse morphologically. Even these can be approached in a logical manner if considered in the differential diagnosis. Most mature carcinoids are diagnosed with ease. Atypical (malignant) carcinoids are often misdiagnosed as small cell undifferentiated carcinomas. In this author's opinion this is not a serious problem because these tumors act in an aggressive manner in more than half of cases.

Clinicopathologic Correlations

Patients with lung cancer usually present with nonspecific symptoms and signs. Chute et al.[451] studied the presenting symptoms of 1,539 lung cancer patients according to their cell type and stage. They found that the most common presenting symptoms were weight loss (46% of patients), cough (45%), dyspnea (37%), weakness (34%), chest pain (27%), and hemoptysis (27%). They found that the presence of symptoms was directly related to the stage of the disease, with patients at a more advanced stage more likely to have symptoms. They found no relationship between symptomatology and the histologic type of lung cancer.

Patients with lung cancer can present with a variety of extrathoracic signs and symptoms.[452] Many of the neurologic and metabolic manifestations of lung cancer are caused by neuroendocrine lung neoplasms. However, as reviewed by Yesner,[184] nonneuroendocrine tumors also frequently produce ectopic hormones. Squamous cell carcinoma, for example, frequently produces a parathyroid hormone-like substance that may cause hypercalcemia. Some carcinomas of the lung, especially large cell undifferentiated carcinoma, produce human chorionic gonadotropin, which can be demonstrated biochemically in the patient's serum and immunohistochemically in the tumor cells.

Carcinoma of the lung may frequently present as metastatic disease, with the brain, bone, and liver being frequent sites for metastatic tumor. It is not uncommon for patients to present with primary signs and symptoms referable to metastases in these organs. such as a patient presenting with liver failure resulting from extensive metastatic small cell undifferentiated carcinoma in the liver.

The most important factor in predicting the outcome of a patient with a malignant common lung neoplasm is the stage of the tumor.[160,453] Even in small cell neuroendocrine carcinoma of the lung, the stage of the disease is the most important factor in predicting survival.[161]

Neuroendocrine Lung Neoplasms

The biologic behavior of the neuroendocrine tumors of the lung is somewhat variable, and somewhat confusing because of the various ways these neoplasms have been classified. An overview of the clinicopathologic correlates of neuroendocrine tumors of the lung is shown in Table 32–22.

Mature bronchopulmonary carcinoids generally occur in a younger age group than atypical carcinoids, small cell neuroendocrine carcinomas or large cell neuroendocrine carcinomas. Approximately 5%–10% of bronchial carcinoids metastasize to regional lymph

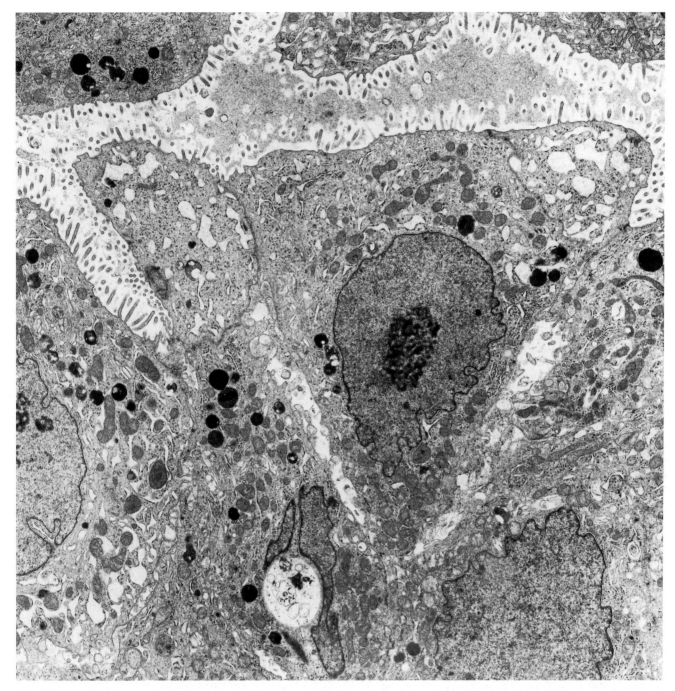

Fig. 32–242. When examined ultrastructurally, tumor cells show obvious glandular differentiation with features suggesting bronchioloalveolar cell carcinoma. ×16,000.

nodes.[454–456] Five-year survival rates in patients with bronchial carcinoids are between 90% and 95%.[454,455] Even the presence of lymph node metastases does not necessarily imply a bad prognosis, although Mc-Caughan et al.[456] found that disease-free survival at 5 and 10 years in 19 patients who had regional lymph node metastases was 74% and 53%, respectively, compared to 96% and 84%, respectively, in those patients with bronchopulmonary carcinoid tumors who did not have lymph node metastases.

Thunnissen et al.[457] found that nodal metastases in mature bronchopulmonary carcinoids were directly related to tumor size and mean nuclear area of the neoplastic cells. The mean diameter of bronchopulmonary carcinoids that did not metastasize was 1.9 cm (standard deviation, 1.1 cm), and 4.7 cm (standard

Table 32–22. Clinicopathologic features of neuroendocrine neoplasms of lung

Type of NE neoplasm [a]	Relative frequency	Location in lung	Histology-cytology	Necrosis	Mitotic rate	Metastases
Carcinoid	Rare	Central	Uniform cells; variable patterns	None	Low	Uncommon
Atypical carcinoid	Uncommon	Peripheral in 60% of cases	Organoid; cellular pleomorphism	Common	High	Common
Large cell NE carcinoma	Uncertain	Midzone or peripheral	Large undifferentiated cells; vesicular nuclei with large nucleoli	Variable	High	Variable incidence
Small cell NE carcinoma	Frequent; 20% of common lung neoplasms	Central	Small ovoid, fusiform, or polygonal cells; nucleoli inconspicuous	Common	High	Common

[a] NE, neuroendocrine.

deviation, 2.0 cm) in those that did metastasize. The mean nuclear area in the nonmetastasizing carcinoids was 34.7 μ^2 (standard deviation, 9.8 μ^2) and 38.2 μ^2 (standard deviation, 7.7 μ^2) in the metastasizing carcinoids.

Warren and Gould[458] reported the long-term followup of 27 cases of classical bronchial carcinoid for at least 10 years after curative resection. They found lymph node metastases in 2 patients at the time of surgery. Distant metastases were found in 2 patients at 5 and 10 years after surgery. Bone metastases involving the humerus were observed in both patients, and were treated with radiotherapy in both patients and chemotherapy in one. One patient died of an unrelated cause 10 years after surgery, and the other was alive 19 years after surgery. The demonstration of ACTH and related opiopeptides was not associated with a more aggressive course and was not associated with nodal metastases. Warren and Gould concluded that long-term survival was the rule even in cases of mature carcinoids with distant metastases.

In their study of spindle cell carcinoid tumors of the lung, Ranchod and Levine[410] found lymph node metastases in 7 patients (in 2 cases the metastases were observed only microscopically) and bony metastases in 1 patient. Follow-up information was available in 22 of 35 patients for 1 to 13 years, and no other sites of metastases were observed. None of the 22 patients that were followed died of their tumors.

Of the 35 neuroendocrine neoplasms reported by Travis et al.,[434] 20 were mature carcinoids. The patients had a mean age of 46.4 years and a median age of 46 years. Thirteen of the 20 carcinoids were associated with Cushing syndrome, and hilar lymph node metastases were present in 4 cases. Of the 20 patients, death occurred in a patient with ACTH production by

the tumor because of a cardiac arrhythmia in the immediate postoperative period. The remaining 19 patients were alive with a mean follow-up of 2.16 years (range, 0.33–13 years).

In their clinicopathologic analysis of 52 patients with mature carcinoid tumors of lung, Abdi et al.[407] reported that 11 were located peripherally in the lung. The mean age of the patients with peripheral carcinoid tumors was 60.2 years, and 9 of 10 patients were female. The mean tumor size of the peripheral carcinoids was 2.39 cm (range, 1.0–5.0 cm), and there were regional lymph node metastases in 3 of 11 cases. Except for the cases of peripheral carcinoid tumors diagnosed incidentally at autopsy, all patients were alive and disease free 1 to 6 years after surgery.

El-Naggar et al.[459] performed a clinicopathologic and flow cytometric evaluation of 33 typical carcinoids and 14 atypical carcinoids. The mean age of the patients with mature carcinoids was 52.3 years. Of the 33 typical carcinoids, 32 were centrally located and 1 was peripheral. Lymph node metastases occurred in 3 cases. Twenty-six of the carcinoids were less than 3 cm in diameter and 7 were greater than 3 cm in diameter. Only one patient with a histologically typical carcinoid, showing diploid DNA and a proliferative index of 5.0%, died of disease.

In the Yousem and Taylor[460] clinicopathologic and DNA analysis of 12 typical carcinoids and 7 atypical carcinoids, all the patients with typical carcinoids were alive with no evidence of disease between 1 and 46 months after diagnosis, except one patient who was lost to followup.

Bernstein et al.[461] described a case of a mature bronchial carcinoid originating in the right-mainstem bronchus of a 35-year-old nonsmoking woman. The right lung was resected, and the bronchial margin of resection showed no evidence of tumor; no metastases were noted in the hilar lymph nodes. The patient presented 18 years later with superior vena cava obstruction and carcinoid syndrome from a recurrence of the tumor. She was treated with radiotherapy and had a dramatic response, with resolution of her symptoms from superior vena caval obstruction and a drop in her 5-hydroxy indole acetic acid (HIAA) to normal levels.

Greengard et al.[462] evaluated 10 pulmonary carcinoid tumors for a variety of enzymes to determine the growth rate of these neoplasms. Uridine kinase to thymidine ratios were five times higher in the mature carcinoids than in pulmonary carcinomas, and the concentration of alpha glutamyl transpeptidase was lower in the 10 pulmonary carcinoids than in 35 pulmonary adenocarcinomas and 11 squamous carcinomas. Thymidine kinase, which bears a quantitative inverse correlation to volume doubling time, was present in lower titers in 9 mature carcinoids than in 6 small cell carcinomas of lung. The authors concluded that because of relatively long doubling times most carcinoids required a longer time (40.5 years) to reach a clinically detectable size than did carcinomas (17.8 years). The data also suggested that mature carcinoids had a prenatal or early childhood inception.

The biologic behavior of atypical carcinoids (malignant carcinoids) is significantly different than that of mature carcinoids.

Several papers have been published concerning the pathologic and clinical features of atypical carcinoids (well-differentiated neuroendocrine carcinomas) since the first edition of *Pulmonary Pathology*. Most of these have discussed the clinicopathologic features of these neoplasms, specifically how they differ from mature carcinoids and small cell undifferentiated carcinomas of the lung. Many studies have reported on the flow cytometric analysis of these neoplasms. An excellent editorial overview of atypical carcinoid neoplasms of the lung was published by Yousem[463] in 1991.

Warren et al.[464] reevaluated the clinicopathologic features of 50 cases of surgically resected small cell carcinomas. Thirty-four cases were confirmed to be correctly diagnosed as small cell carcinomas but in 12 cases the diagnosis was changed to well-differentiated carcinoma (atypical carcinoid). They found that 7 of 11 (64%) of patients with T1NO, T2NO well-differentiated neuroendocrine carcinomas survived more than 1 year, and 6 of 8 patients (75%) survived more than 2 years. They concluded that well-differentiated neuroendocrine carcinoma was distinctly less aggressive, and had a much better prognosis, than small cell undifferentiated carcinoma of the lung.

Several investigators have evaluated the DNA index and 5 phase of neuroendocrine neoplasms with an emphasis on atypical carcinoids. Larsimont et al.[465]

analyzed 18 mature carcinoids, 6 atypical carcinoids and 11 small cell undifferentiated carcinoma with a cell image processor. They found a significant increase in DNA content from typical carcinoids to small cell lung carcinomas, with atypical carcinoids showing an intermediate value. They found the nuclei of atypical carcinoids significantly larger than those of atypical carcinoids and similar to small cell lung carcinomas. They found an increased chromatin condensation in atypical carcinoids versus typical carcinoids, and less condensation than in small cell carcinomas of the lung. This correlated with the observation of a progressive increase in hyperchromatism of nuclei from typical carcinoid to small cell carcinoma.

Yousem and Taylor[460] compared the DNA index and S phase of 12 typical carcinoids to 8 atypical carcinoids (see their Table 1) using a cell image analyzer. They found that the patients with atypical carcinoids were older (mean age, 52.2 years). Three of 12 typical carcinoids had an abnormal DNA content: 1 diploid/tetraploid, 1 tetraploid, and 1 aneuploid. All 3 of these neoplasms had a benign behavior and were not different in any way from the other typical carcinoids. Four of 8 atypical carcinoids had aneuploid DNA indices and 1 a hypodiploid DNA index. Aneuploid tumors were found to commonly show vascular invasion. Typical carcinoids had generally low proliferation indices, except for 2 cases that were slightly elevated (12.5% and 27.6%). In contrast, the atypical carcinoids showed a higher proliferative index range, 7.5%–45.3%; mean 19.3%). The percentage of cells in S-G$_2$M phase generally correlated with mitotic rate identified in histologic sections. Yousem and Taylor[460] concluded that although atypical carcinoids were more frequently aneuploid, DNA ploidy could not be used independently to assess malignant potential.

Lequaglie et al.[466] evaluated 19 patients diagnosed as well-differentiated neuroendocrine carcinoma (atypical carcinoid). The patients were between 50 and 77 years old, and 83% were cigarette smokers. Sixteen of 19 resected tumors were stage I, 3 were stage II, and 1 was stage IIIa. Five patients were treated with adjuvant chemotherapy and 1 was given regional radiotherapy. The tumor recurred in 10 patients, including 4 who had been given adjuvant treatment and 6 with stage I disease. The presence of metastases did not correlate with pathologic stage; the brain was the first site of metastases in 7 cases. Sixty-eight percent of patients with stage I disease were alive after 100 months, and surgery was stated to be curative in more than half of patients with localized disease. Memoli[467] discussed the findings of Lequaglie et al.[466] and reviewed the entity of well-differentiated neuroendocrine carcinoma, indicating it had "come of age" and was a distinct clinicopathologic entity that should be recognized by pathologists.

Jackson-York et al.[468] evaluated the DNA content of nuclei from 53 primary and locally metastic pulmonary neuroendocrine neoplasms. Nine of 22 (41%) of well-differentiated neuroendocrine carcinomas (atypical carcinoids) were aneuploid; in contrast, 17 of 20 (85%) small cell neuroendocrine carcinomas and 8 of 11 (73%) large cell neuroendocrine carcinomas (intermediate cell neuroendocrine carcinomas) were aneuploid. When evaluated as a single group, tumors with a diploid DNA index had a longer survival than those neoplasms with an aneuploid DNA index. However, the DNA index was not a statistically significant indicator of survival when cases with limited-stage disease were analyzed. Patients with well-differentiated neuroendocrine carcinoma had a significantly longer survival than those with small cell neuroendocrine carcinoma or large cell neuroendocrine carcinoma (see their Table 1).

El-Naggar et al.[459] analyzed 47 bronchopulmonary carcinoids, of which 33 (70.2%) were typical carcinoids and 14 (29.8%) were atypical carcinoids, by flow cytometry. Thirty-three neoplasms (63.8%) had a diploid DNA content; of these, 27 (90%) were typical carcinoids and 3 (10%) were atypical carcinoids. Of the 17 neoplasms (36.2%) that had an aneupolid DNA index, 6 (35.3%) were typical carcinoids and 11 (64.7%) were atypical carcinoids. The DNA indices of the aneuploid neoplasms ranged from 1.15 to 1.98 (mean, 1.35) and 39 (83%) of the carcinoids had an S-phase percentage less than 7, and 8 (17%) had an S-phase percentage equal to or greater than 7. The proliferative index (S phase) was higher among the aneuploid neoplasms (7.5 ± 3.6 S.D.) than the diploid neoplasms (5.1 ± 1.3 S.D.). Only 1 patient with a typical carcinoid and a diploid DNA index and an S-phase fraction of 5.0% died of disease. All 3 patients with atypical carcinoids who had a diploid DNA index were alive at last follow-up; 8 of 11 patients with an aneuploid, histologically atypical carcinoid were dead of disease. Multifactorial regression analysis revealed that histologic category (typical versus atypical) and DNA content were equally important, independent pronostic factors. Additional significant prognostic factors included the size of the neoplasm and the presence of vascular invasion.

Travis et al.[434] performed flow cytometric analysis on 20 typical carcinoids, 6 atypical carcinoids, 5 large cell neuroendocrine carcinomas, and 4 small cell undifferentiated carcinomas. Eighteen of 20 typical carcinoids were diploid, 1 was aneuploid, and 1 was tetraploid. Of the atypical carinoids, 5 were diploid and 1 was aneuploid. Three of 5 large cell neuroendocrine carcinomas were aneuploid, 1 was diploid, and the data in 1 case were not interpretable. Three of 4 small cell undifferentiated carcinomas were aneuploid, and one was dip-

loid. The proliferative index (S phase) for 14 diploid typical carcinoids ranged between 3.5% and 9.97% (average, 6.9%). In the other 4 diploid typical carcinoid tumors, the S-phase fraction was 10.36%, 11.59%, 12.71%, and 18.36%. Interestingly, the proliferative index in the aneuploid and tetraploid typical carcinoids was 2.40% and 3.75%, respectively. In 2 diploid atypical carcinoids, the proliferative index was slightly greater than 10%, but in 3 diploid atypical carcinoids the proliferative index was less than or equal to 6%. In three aneuploid large cell neuroendocrine carcinomas, the proliferative index was 30.09%, 25.10%, and 5.15%. In the 1 diploid large cell neuroendocrine carcinoma, the S phase was 26.30%. The S phase was 9.76% and 29% in 2 aneuploid small cell undifferentiated neuroendocrine carcinomas and 26.30% in 1 diploid small cell carcinoma. Travis et al.[434] did not find any ancillary techniques (Immunohistochemistry, electron microscopy, DNA index–S- phase percentage) that provided an advantage over light microscopy for the classification or prognosis of pulmonary neuroendocrine neoplasms.

As already briefly discussed, large cell neuroendocrine neoplasms seem to pursue a more aggressive course than large cell undifferentiated carcinomas that do not have neuroendocrine features.

Small cell undifferentiated carcinoma of the lung is the most aggressive neuroendocrine tumor, and perhaps the most aggressive common lung tumor, although approximately 20% of patients with small cell undifferentiated carcinoma of the lung limited to the thorax are alive at 2 years. Small cell carcinoma of the lung is usually a neoplasm that arises in the hilar region of the lung, although it may present as a solitary pulmonary nodule. Quoix et al.[469] reviewed the cases of 408 individuals that were diagnosed as small cell carcinoma of the lung and identified 25 cases in which the neoplasm radiographically was a solitary pulmonary nodule. Pathologic review of these 25 cases confirmed 15 (60%) as small cell carcinoma (10 intermediate cell type, 4 oat cell, and 1 indeterminate). Of the 15 solitary pulmonary nodules, 10 were resected and 5 were treated with chemotherapy/radiotherapy; postoperative chemotherapy was also given to most of the resected patients. The median survival of patients whose small cell lung cancer presented as a solitary pulmonary nodule was 24 months, compared to 11 months for small cell lung cancer with limited disease and 3 months for those with extensive disease. Kreisman et al.[470] recently reviewed the subject of small cell lung cancer presenting as a solitary pulmonary nodule. They defined a solitary pulmonary nodule as a single spherical or oval intrapulmonary density not exceeding 6 cm in greatest diameter. Patients with radiographic or pathologic evidence of hilar or mediastinal adenopathy were excluded. As reviewed, 4%–12% of all solitary pulmonary nodules were small cell undifferentiated carcinomas. The therapy currently recommended for a small cell carcinoma presenting as a solitary pulmonary nodule is surgery followed by adjuvant chemotherapy and/or radiation therapy.

Shepherd et al.[471] reported that patients with small cell carcinoma who had "very limited disease," defined by a negative mediastinoscopy or negative chest radiograph for mediastinal tumor, had a significantly better survival than those with other limited small cell lung cancer.

Gephardt et al.[472] described the clinicopathologic features of 17 cases of surgically resected peripheral small cell undifferentiated carcinoma. The tumors were between 0.9 and 3.5 cm in diameter (mean, 2.1 cm) and histologically were predominantly mixed intermediate cell type with foci of oat cell carcinoma in 1 cases. Seven (41%) of the patients died of intrathoracic carcinoma and/or metastatic carcinoma involving the brain, with an average survival of 1.7 years. Of the patients whose tumor was stated to have an oat cell component histologically, five (71%) died of metastatic or recurrent disease. Of the 10 patients without definite foci of oat cell carcinoma, 2 (20%) patients died of recurrent or metastatic disease. This report is somewhat confusing in that Gephardt et al.[472] referred to these neoplasms as atypical carcinoids.

Fraire et al.[473] reviewed 147 cases of patients with primary lung neoplasms with recorded diagnoses of small cell lung cancer (114 cases) and undifferentiated carcinoma (35 cases). Part of this study was to test the new classification scheme for small cell undifferentiated carcinoma as proposed by the Pathology Section of the International Association for the Study of Lung Cancer. The neoplasms were classified into the three categories (classic, pure small cell; mixed small cell, large cell, combined small cell; adenocarcinoma or small cell, squamous carcinoma) and were clinically staged as local, regional, or distant. Consensus diagnosis was achieved in 144 (96.6%) of 149 cases. Of these 144 cases, 124 were classified as small cell lung carcinoma, 115 (92.8%) as pure small cell, 5 (4.0%) as mixed small cell, and 4 (3.2%) as combined. Twenty cases were reclassified as non-small cell carcinomas. Adequate staging data were available for 123 of 124 cases, of which 27 (21.9%) were local, 22 (17.9%) were regional, and 74 (60.2%) were distant. The median length of survival based on histologic subtype was 225, 110, and 203 days for the small, mixed, and combined subtypes, respectively. For stage, the median length of survival was 428 days for local disease, 251 days for regional disease, and 111 days for distant disease. Fraire et al.[473] concluded that stage was the major determinant in survival in small cell

lung cancer. The mixed histologic type had significantly longer survival times than small or combined subtypes.

Bepler et al.[474] also evaluated the relevance of histologic subtyping in small cell lung cancer. They evaluated pathologic specimens from 249 patients with small cell lung cancer that were classified into oat cell type, pure intermediate cell type, and small cell–large cell type; 170 specimens (68%) were classified as oat cell carcinoma, including 30 (18%) with mixed oat cell/ intermediate cell features, 66 (39%) with intermediate cell features, and 13 (5%) with mixed small cell–large cell features. Two year survival rates were 7%, 11%, and 15% for pure small cell, mixed small cell, and combined small cell, respectively. Bepler et al.[474] concluded that histologic subtypes of small cell lung cancer were not distinct entities of clinical relevance and that prognostic and therapeutic decisions could not be based on histologic subtypes.

Crown et al.[475] performed a retrospective analysis of 81 small cell lung cancer patients to determine what factors had prognostic significance for long-term survival, which was defined as disease-free survival for at least 5 years from the initiation of therapy. Six patients, 5 females (16.7%) and 1 male (2%), 4 with limited disease and 2 with extensive disease, were long-term survivors (73 to 96+ months from onset of therapy). Female gender and occurrence of herpes zoster were the only variables that were statistically significantly related to 5-year survival. Herpes zoster infection occurred at a median of 10 months from the inception of therapy, which would support the contention that herpes zoster acted as an immune stimulant or as a marker for intensity of treatment.

Albain et al.[476] analyzed 2,501 patients consecutively enrolled in small cell lung cancer trials since 1976 to determine the predictors of 2-year and 5-year survival in limited-stage disease and 1-year and 2-year survival in extensive-stage disease. Sixty-three patients with limited disease survived at least 5 years. Of these, there were 33 asymptomatic patients with no recurrent disease; 6 with recurrent small cell lung cancer, 3 of whom died; 7 who died of non-cancer-related causes or unknown causes; 3 who died of second primary lung cancer; and 14 alive with persistent central nervous system symptoms and signs, possibly caused by prophylactic brain radiation. Fifty-one patients with extensive disease survived for 2 years or longer. Of these, 25 died of recurrent small cell lung cancer. The majority of the long-term survivors had either a single metastatic site or metastases limited to the opposite side of the chest or regional lymph nodes. Multivariate analysis supported the conclusion that aggressive combined modality, concurrent induction therapy, and favorable prognostic variables independently contributed to improved long-term survival in patients with limited disease.

Oud et al.[477] performed image and flow DNA cytometry on isolated nuclei from paraffin-embedded tumor tissue of patients with small cell carcinoma of the lung. Tissue was obtained from 14 patients, and in 2 patients tissue was obtained by both surgery and at autopsy. They found that image cytometry was more reliable than flow cytometry in identifying different cell populations. More important, they found that ploidy determination was not useful in predicting survival.

Funa et al.[478] performed in situ hybridization on primary biopsies from 15 untreated patients with primary lung cancer for the expression of c-myc and N-myc oncogenes. The increased expression of N-myc oncogenes in small cell lung cancer was strongly associated with a poor response to chemotherapy, rapid tumor growth, and short survival.

Copple et al.[479] examined ultrastructurally tumors from 33 patients who had been diagnosed by light microscopy as small cell undifferentiated carcinomas of lung. They separated the tumors into four major groups based on ultrastructural criteria, such as whether or not they had neuroendocrine features, for example, neuroendocrine granules. They found that the complete and partial response rates to systemic chemotherapy, with or without radiation, was not significantly different in any of the four groups on the basis of ultrastructural findings. However, Vollmer et al.[480] studied 52 cases of oat cell carcinoma by electron microscopy, and related the ultrastructural findings to tumor stage in patient survival. They found that only the type of cell junction between the tumor cells was of prognostic importance with respect to survival. Patients whose tumors showed intermediate junctions, and especially those with desmosomes, had a significantly greater chance to have more localized disease and a potentially resectable tumor, and subsequently a longer survival, than those without these types of junctions. They found that the median survival periods for those with no identifiable junctions, intermediate junctions, or desmosomes was 6.4, 8.2, and 11.3 months, respectively. They indicated, however, that the ultrastructural subclassification was not as important as that obtained from careful clinical staging, a conclusion that we had previously reached.[161]

Non-Neuroendocrine/Non-Small Cell Carcinoma

As previously stated and as reviewed in the clinicopatholgic discussion on neuroendocrine neoplasms, anatomic stage of disease is the most important factor in predicting the prognosis of patients with lung cancer (Table 32–23).

Using the "old" three-stage scheme, patients with T1N0 squamous carcinomas and adenocarcinomas survive longer than those patients with stage I, T1N1, and T2N0 disease.[453] These observations were in part responsible for developing the current four-tier staging system.

Stage for stage, the survival rate for squamous carcinoma is significantly better than for adenocarcinoma.[453] Approximately 80% of patients with resected stage I, T1N0 squamous carcinoma are alive at 5 years after diagnosis whereas only 70% of similarly staged adenocarcinomas are alive at five years.[453] There also is a significant difference in survival rate for stage II squamous carcinoma versus stage II adenocarcinoma, with patients having squamous carcinoma surviving longer than those with adenocarcinoma. In general, patients with large cell undifferentiated carcinoma or

Table 32–23. New stage database: cumulative percentage surviving 5 years and median survival by clinical and surgical TNM subsets[a]

TNM subset	Number	Clinical Surviving (%)	Clinical Median survival (months)	Number	Surgical Surviving (%)	Surgical Median survival (months)
T1 N0 M0	591	61.9	60+	429	68.5	60+
T2 N0 M0	1,012	35.8	26	436	59.0	60+
T1 N1 M0	19	33.6	20	67	54.1	60+
T2 N1 M0	176	22.7	17	250	40.0	29
T3 N0 M0	221	7.6	8	57	44.2	26
T3 N1 M0	71	7.7	8	29	17.6	16
Any N2 M0	497	4.9	11	168	28.8	22
Any M1	1,166	1.7	6	—	—	—
Total	3,753			1,436		

[a] Reprinted with permission from Mountain CF. Chest 1986;89(Suppl.):225S–233S.

adenosquamous carcinoma have survival rates similar to those patients with adenocarcinoma.

Elson et al.[481] had previously reported that anatomic tumor stage was the only significant predictor of survival in primary carcinoma of the lung, with all patients surviving 5 years or longer who had stage I disease. They further evaluated the histologic features of 47 stage I lung caracinomas to determine if any features were predictive of prolonged survival. Ten slides made of each neoplasm were reviewed independently by three pathologists for vascular/lymphatic invasion, mitotic rate, anaplasia, inflammatory host response, presence or absence of necrosis, tumor giant cell reaction, a central scar, and the presence of desmoplasia. These histologic features were correlated with the patient's age, sex, tumor and nodal status, histologic type of tumor, and histologic heterogeneity. One pathologist found tumor giant cells to be an adverse factor, another pathologist found scar carcinoma to predict a worse survival, and a third pathologist found lymphocytic inflammatory host response to be a positive predictor of survival and venous invasion a negative predictor of survival. All three pathologists found the extent of tumor necosis to be an adverse factor. The fact that some parameters were significant predictors of survival in one pathologist's evaluation and not another's suggests that studies of histologic indicators of prognosis by a single observer may not be valid for another person evaluating the same neoplasm.

The same group of investigators[482] subsequently quantitated the degree of tumor necrosis in 28 cases of surgically resected stage I non-small cell carcinoma by morphometry. Fouteen of the patients were long-term survivors (mean survival after diagnosis of 92 months) and 14 had shorter survival (up to 62 months). Their quantitiative evaluation reaffirmed their previous findings that tumor necrosis was a useful factor in predicting prognosis of stage I lung carcinoma with those patients' neoplasms that showed little necrosis having a longer survival. Their study found no relationship between survival and the mitotic rate of the neoplasm or the degree of nuclear atypia.

Cagle et al.[483] evaluated nuclear morphometry in 46 cases of surgically resected, non-small cell carcinoma. The cases were divided into two groups: group I, alive with no evidence of disease; and group II, dead of disease or recurrent disease. The investigators were unable to demonstrate a correlation between nuclear morphometric parameters and prognosis in stage I non-small cell lung cancer.

Gallagher and Urbanski[484] studied the significance of 23 peripheral $T_2 N_0 M_0$ carcinomas with microscopic invasion of the visceral pleura as determined by elastic tissue stains and compared them to a matched control in which there was no visceral pleural invasion. In 19 of 23 cases examined with visceral pleural invasion, a distinction could not be made between invasion of the internal and external elastic lamina of the pleura. Considering all cases, there was a significant difference in survival between the involved and univolved visceral pleural groups, and the longest survival was in the squamous cell carcinoma group with uninvolved visceral pleura.

The clinical significance of minor pleural effusions in patients with potentially operable lung cancer was evaluated by Ratto et al.[485] in 20 patients, 10 of which had left-sided effusions and 10 right-sided effusions. Histologically there were 9 cases of squamous carcinoma, 8 cases of adenocarcinoma, and 3 cases of large cell undifferentiated carcinoma. The resectability rate was significantly lower in patients with carcinoma of the lung and minor pleural effusions than in control patients with no pleural effusions. Nine patients with cytologically negative and "non-bloody" pleural effusions had unresectable tumors. A cytologically positive pleural effusion was found in only 1 patient. Median survival was 14 months for the entire group, more than 37 months for the completely resected group, 11 months for stage III patients with minor pleural effusions, and 19 months for control stage III patients with no pleural effusion. The authors concluded that while minor pleural effusions that were nonbloody and cytologically benign did not preclude resectability, patients with primary lung neoplasms associated with minor pleural effusions should be "suspiciously" considered for operability.

Several studies have reported uncommon or novel immunhohistochemical features of primary lung neoplasms, a few of which have suggested a prognostic significance. Yoshimoto et al.[486] reported a case of a poorly differentiated mucin-producing adenocarcinoma with tumor cells showing immunostaining for carcinoembryonic antigen, alpha-fetoprotein, and human chorionic-gonadotropin. Evaluation of autopsy tissue showed these substances in different tumor cells, which the authors interpreted to suggest that the lung cancer consisted of at least three clones of cancer cells with different phenotypes.

Kuida et al.[487] evaluated 11 primary lung carcinomas for human chorionic gonadotropin expression using an avidin-biotin immunohistochemical technique and found that 4 of 11 (36%) tumors showed occasional cells immunostaining for human chorionic-gonadotropin. These investigators reviewed the published studies of human chorionic-gonadotropin poistive lung cancer and cited several reasons for differences in results.

This author has seen several cases of large cell undifferentiated carcinoma showing immunostaining for human chorionic-gonadotropin and a lesser number of cases expressing alpha-fetoprotein. In most cases, the positive cells have been the tumor giant cells. No prognostic significance of this immunostaining pattern has been made by this author.

Estrogen and androgens have been identified in a variety of benign and malignant neoplasms. Beattie et al.[488] performed a biochemical study to determine the presence of androgen, estrogen, and glucocorticoid receptors in 55 primary carcinomas of the lung, of which 30 (56%) were squamous cell carcinomas, 21 (38%) adenocarcinomas, and 4 (7%) large cell undifferentiated carcinomas. These authors reported some variations between the concentration of the various receptors in the different types of tumors and some differences in concentration based on stage of the neoplasm. Their study suggested that there was a significant incidence of specific, high-affinity receptors for estrogen, androgen and glucocoritcoids in non-small cell lung carcinoma which could be used as a starting point to determine if these neoplasms responded to hormonal therapy.

This author has evaluated several primary lung cancers for estrogen and progesterone receptor proteins by an avidin-biotin immunohistochemical technique and to date has observed no positive cases.

Battifora et al.[489] evaluated 231 primary carcinomas of lung (130 squamous carcinomas, 64 adenocarcinomas, 10 small cell carcinomas, 16 large cell carcinomas, and 11 adenosquamous carcinomas) immunohistochemically with monoclonal antibody 43-9F for the presence of a novel tumor-associated carhohydrate epitope. They found that patients with 43-9F epitope-positive squamous carcinomas had a significantly better prognosis than patients with epitope-negative squamous carcinomas. They further found that this association was prognostically superior to nodal classification. No association was found in cases of adenocarcinomas.

Poulakis et al.[490] investigated the serum concentrations of interleukin-2-receptors, carcinoembryonic antigen, alpha-fetoprotein, beta-human chorionic-gonadotropin, pregnancy-specific glycoprotein, and beta-2-micoglobulin in 92 patients with primary lung carcinomas (34 squamous carcinomas, 29 small cell carcinomas, 16 adenocarcinomas, 13 large cell undifferentiated carcinomas) by various enzyme immunoassay techniques. The mean value of interleukin-2-receptors was twice as high in the cancer group than in the control group and was highest in the patients with small cell carcinoma. Of the cancer patients, 51.1% had carcinoembryonic antigen levels greater than 5 ng/ml and, as might be expected, patients with advanced disease had higher serum carcinembryonic antigen levels. No differences were found between tumor type and the other

markers. The authors concluded that interleukin-2-receptor and carcinoembryonic antigen may be useful in monitoring the extent of lung neoplasms and potentially indicate histologic subtype, thus having a bearing on treatment and prognosis.

Based on the observation that H/Le-y/Le-b antigens are expressed in various histologic types of lung cancer, Miyake et al.[491] evaluated 149 patients with primary lung cancer as to whether monoclonal antibody MIA-15-5, a marker of H/Le-y/Le-b antigen and an inhibitor of tumor cell motility and metastasis, was of prognostic value. Among the 149 patients studied, 5-year survival rates for 91 patients with MIA-15-5-positive tumors was significantly lower than survival in 58 patients with MIA-15-5-negative tumors. The difference in survival between patients with MIA-15-5-positive versus -negative tumors was significant among patients with blood groups A and AB but not blood groups 0 or B.

Buccheri and Ferrigno[492] studied the prognostic significance of tissue polypeptide antigen, a single-chain polypeptide isolated from cell membranes and smooth endoplasmic reticulum of malignant cells, in 553 patients with primary lung cancers. The median value for tissue polypeptide antigen uas 130 μ/liter and the range was 30 to 5,203 μ/liter. Patients whose tissue polypetide antigen was less than 130 μ/liters had a longer survival than those with higher tissue polypeptide antigen values (median survival, 10.41 versus 5.57 months). However, tissue polypetide antigen was less important than stage of disease, performance status, and weight loss in predicting survival.

Oncogenes and anti-oncogenes have been evaluated with respect to their relationship to lung cancer. About 50 oncogenes or proto-oncogenes have been identified and, as previously reviewed, serve important functions in cellular metabolism and growth. Cline and Battifora[493] studied 27 non-small cell lung cancers by in situ hybridization for alterations in protooncogenes and found that 10 of 16 adenocarcinomas, 3 of 9 squamous carinomas, and 2 of 2 large cell carinomas (total of 56%) showed abnormalities. Five protooncogenes, c-myc, c-myb, c-ras-Ha, c-erb-B-1, and c-erb-B-2, were found to be altered in frequencies between 12% to 60%. Alterations in c-erb-B-1 and c-erb-B-2 were observed more common in advanced cases. Allelic deletions of c-ras-Ha or c-myb were frequently observed in primary tumors that recurred or progressed after surgery. The authors suggested that evaluation of proto-oncogenes could possibly provide insights into the pathogenesis of lung cancer and in predicting its clinical behavior.

Harada et al.[494] evaluated the clinical significance of the expression of ras oncogene product in 116 surgically resected non-small cell lung cancers using an immunohistochemical technique with anti-ras p21 monoclonal antibody rp-35. Positive immunostaining was observed in 72.5% of adenocarcinomas and 55.6% of squamous carcinomas. The higher stage tumors were more frequently positive than the lower stage tumors. Survival studies demonstrated that 64.1% of patients with p21-negative tumors had a 5-year survival rate whereas 11.5%–38% of patients with positive tumors survived 5 years.

Anti-onocgene p53 is located in the short arm of chromosome 17, a frequent site of abnormality in a variety of human tumors. Caamano et al.[495] evaluated 50 primary non-small cell primary lung carcinomas and 8 lung carcinoma cell lines by immunohistochemistry for p53 using two monoclonal antibodies. Sixteen of 35 (45.7%) adenocarcinomas and 7 of 15 (46.6%) squamous carcinomas showed moderate to marked immunoreactivity of the neoplastic cells. The exact biologic significance of the expression remains uncertain, although p53 can be detected immunohistochemically in a significant percentage of primary lung neoplasms and more advanced adenocarcinomas tend to be p53 positive.

Porter et al.[496] evaluated nuclear phosphoprotein p53 by immunohistochemistry using a monoclonal antibody on deparaffiniaed tissue sections of methacarn-fixed tissue. They studied 255 tumors of which 34 were primary lung neoplasms (10 small cell carcinomas, 13 adenocarcinomas, 7 squamous carcinomas, 3 mesotheliomas, and 1 carcinoid tumor). Positive immunostaining was noted in 17 of 34 lung neoplasms (50%), with approximately equal percentage of adenocarcinomas, squamous carcinomas, and small cell carcinomas being positive. No information was given concerning the prognostic significance of the expression of p53 in these malignant lung neoplasms. The authors did not find p53 in benign lung tumors.

Slebos et al.[497] evaluated the significance of K-*ras* oncogene activation in 69 patients with primary, surgically resected, pulmonary adenocarcinomas. Nineteen of 69 (65.5%) of the adenocarcinomas had a point mutation in codon 12 of the K-*ras* oncogene. Tumors positive for K-*ras* point mutations were found to be smaller and less differentiated than those without mutations. Twelve of 19 patients with K-*ras* point-mutation-positive tumors died during the follow-up period as compared with 16 of 50 patients with no K-*ras* oncogene mutation. The authors concluded that the presence of K-*ras* point mutations defined a subgroup of patients with primary pulmonary adenocarcinoma in whom prognosis was poor and disease-free survival short, despite radical resection and often a small tumor burden.

ten Velde et al.[498] evaluated 68 patients with stage I or II squamous cell carcinoma for the presence of base-ment membrane using polyclonal antibodies to human type IV collagen. In 27 of 62 patients, extensive (more than 75% immunoreactivity) basement membrane and in 35 of 62, moderate-to-limited basement membrane was found. Deposition of an appreciable amount of basement membrane in the center of a squamous cell carcinomas was a prognostically favorable sign, independent of tumor stage.

Nagamoto et al.[499] studied the relationship of primary tumor size and microscopic appearance to the presence of lymph node metatases in 103 roentgenographically occult lung cancers, of which 102 were squamous carcinomas. All patients were treated surgically, and the neoplasms were evaluated for bronchial invasion and the length of longitudinal extension, which was defined as the product of the thickness of the tumor and the length of its extension as determined by histologic examination of serial sections. No nodal metastases were found in 59 cancers when the length of longitudinal extension was less than 20 mm. Of 25 cancers with length of longitudinal extension 20 mm or more, 6 showed nodal involvement. The authors also found that 11 in situ carcinomas and 4 cancers designated as "suspicious for invasion" showed no lymph node involvement. The investigators concluded that no lymph node dissection was required when pulmonary resection was performed on roentgenographically occult squamous carcinomas when the length of longitudinal extension was less than 20 mm or when the tumor was in situ or designated as being "suspicious for invasion." While the Nagamoto et al.[499] observations are probably correct, the exact nature of the neoplasm could probably not be determined until after surgery was completed and "permanent" sections were obtained, unless extensive frozen sections were done at the time of surgery. Therefore the surgeon would not know if the tumor was in situ or had a length of longitudinal extension less than 20 mm until after surgery was completed and would not know if lymph nodes should be resected.

Atsushi et al.[500] evaluated the histologic prognostic factors of pulmonary adenocarcinomas less than 2 cm in diameter in 75 patients who had undergone surgical resection. The pathologic stage was the primary determinant of prognosis. A number of other histologic factors, such as standard deviation of nuclear area, infiltration of Langerhans' cells, mitotic index, vascular invasion, and degree of histologic differentiation were also statistically independent factors in predicting survival. Patients whose lung neoplasm had a small standard deviation of nuclear area, an increased number of infiltrating Langerhans' cells, a lack of vascular invasion, and a low mitotic intex had a significantly better survival.

Ohori et al.[501] evaluated the mucinous, nonmucinous and sclerosing types of bronchioloalveolar cell carcinoma by immunohistochemistry for laminin, collagen IV, fibronectin, and collagen III. In contrast to the mucinous and nonmucinous bronchioloalveolar cell carcinomas, the sclerosing neoplasms showed disruption or complete loss of laminin and collagen IV. An increase concentration of type IV collagenase activity was also noted in the sclerosing bronchioloalveolar cell carcinomas. These observations may explain the observed more aggressive behavior of sclerosing bronchioloalveolar cell carcinoma.

Delmomte et al.[502] studied a series of large cell undifferentiated carcinomas of the lung by electron microscopy and immunohistochemistry. These investigators found that all large cell undifferentiated carcinomas, despite their ultrastructural and immunohistochemical characteristics, behaved in a similar manner. Albain et al.[503] came to a similar conclusion in their evaluation of 48 patients with large cell undifferentiated carcinoma histologically although a previous electron microscopic study showed that large cell undifferentiated carcinomas that showed squamous differentiation ultrastructurally had a better prognosis than those that showed glandular differentiation.

Fairly extensive reports have been published in the last 3 years concerning the significance of nuclear DNA content and proliferative phase of primary lung neoplasms. Review articles have been published concerning the technical and interpretive aspects of flow cytometry[504] and a call for improvement in methodology, data analysis, and quality control.[505,506] Zimmerman et al.[507] evaluated archival paraffin sections of 100 surgically resected lung neoplasms (40 adenomas, 48 squamous, 12 adenosquamous) of which 45% were aneuploid and 55% diploid; specifically, 40% of adenocarcinomas, 46% of squamous carcinomas, and 58% of adenosquamous carcinomas were aneuploid. The patients with aneuploid tumors had a significantly shorter survival than those with diploid tumors. Patients with diploid tumors and no nodal metastases had the best survival; 41 of 45 (91%) were alive at 2 years compared with 16 of 29 (55%) of aneuploid neoplasms. The authors concluded that ploidy should be considered in planning management, estimating prognosis, and stratification for treatment trials.

Tirindelli-Danesi et al.[508] studied flow cytometric features of lung neoplasms from 101 patients (40 squamous carcinomas, 22 adenocarcinomas, 21 large cell carcinomas, 11 small cell carcinomas, and 7 undifferentiated carcinomas); 98 of 102 (96%) cases had at least one cytometrically aneuploid cell population and 55 of 102 (54%) cases showed more than one aneuploid stem cell line. The 77 surgically resected cases were

classified into group A tumors, as defined by one or more stem lines with DNA index between 1 to 2, and group B tumors, defined as tumors with at least one stem line with a DNA index less than 1 or greater than 2. Group B tumors were found to be fast growing and to exhibit a doubling time less than 90 days. A statistically better 12-month survival rate was observed in group A tumors (88%) than group B neoplasms (47%). The authors concluded that flow cytometric data could contribute to lung cancer prognosis determination, provided that cellular material was collected by multiple site sampling.

Asamura et al.[509] studied 72 surgically resected primary pulmonary adenocarcinoma by flow cytometry and by morphometry to determine nuclear area. The mean nuclear DNA content of poorly differentiated adenocarcinomas was larger than that of well-differentiated adenocarcinomas in stage I and II and in III and IV. As might be expected there were positive correlations between the mean nuclear DNA content and the mean nuclear area, and between the mean nuclear DNA content and the standard deviation of the mean nuclear area. The authors concluded that nuclear DNA content increased in less differentiated and more advanced adenocarcinomas and that nuclear atypia was reflected in abnormal nuclear DNA content (aneuploidy).

Salvati et al.[510] investigated 64 cases of primary carcinoma of the lung (4 small cell lung cancers, 57 non-small cell lung cancers, and 5 miscellaneous nonepithelial tumors) by flow cytometry and compared the findings to nonneoplastic lung tissue. Most nonneoplastic lung tissue was diploid. At least one aneuploid cell subpopulation was observed in 91% of non-small cell lung cancers and 50% of small cell lung cancers. When multiple sites of the tumor were analyzed, a high incidence of multiclonality was observed. Diploid tumors were associated with a higher survival rate than aneuploid monoclonal and multiclonal neoplasms. The authors concluded that cellular DNA content of lung neoplasms may be useful in prognostic evaluation.

One of the most interesting studies concerning flow cytometric analysis of lung neoplasms was that done by Carey et al.[511] who evaluated intratumoral heterogeneity of DNA content in primary lung carcinomas by flow cytometry. The 208 samples from 20 resected lung neoplasms (10 squamous carcinomas, 7 adenocarcinomas, 1 atypical carcinoid, 1 adenosquamous carcinoma, and 1 large cell carcinoma). Only 1 carcinoma (squamous cell type) was homogeneously diploid, with 18 neoplasms showing varying degrees of heterogeneity of DNA content. More than half of the tumors could have been labeled diploid if not widely sampled. The degree of tumor cell DNA heterogeneity is not surprising given the degree of histologic heterogeneity of most lung carcinomas.

Schmidt et al.[512] performed a retrospective flow cytometric analysis of 102 primary, accurately staged, T_1N_0 non-small cell carcinomas. They compared 51 recurrent primary lung neoplasms with 51 matched control cases in which the lung neoplasm did not recur. Sixty-two percent of the T_1N_0 tumors were aneuploid (67% recurrent group and 57% controls); 53 of the 61 aneuploid tumors had DNA indexes between 1 and 2. The authors concluded that (1) the majority of lung neoplasms, including small tumors, had at least one detectable abnormal stem cell population; (2) the presence of ploidy abnormalities had some prognostic significance; and (3) proliferative rates of tumor did not predict tumor recurrences.

Filderman et al.[513] determined DNA content and proliferative fraction on 44 surgically resected stage I non-small cell lung carcinomas (27 adenocarcinomas, 15 squamous carcinomas, and 2 large cell carcinomas); 32 (73%) were T1 N0 M0 lesions and 12 (27%) were T2 N0 M0 neoplasms. Patients with T1 N0 M0 lesions had a 5-year survival of 81%, and T2 N0 M0 tumor cases had a 5-year survival of 42%. Thirty-five tumors (79%) had a diploid DNA content and 9 (21%) had an aneuploid DNA content. The 5-year survival for diploid tumors was 77%, compared to 44% in aneuploid neoplasms. All patients with an S-phase percentage of 6% or less survived 5 years whereas only 41% of those with an S-phase percentage greater than 6% survived 5 years. The authors concluded that tumor proliferative fraction and, to a lesser extent DNA content, were significant prognostic factors in stage I non-small cell carcinoma.

Regional lymph node metastases are a significant negative prognostic indicator in primary lung cancer. Regional lymph nodes may also be the source of immunocompetent cells that react against lung cancers. Ogawa et al.[514] studied the relationship of ploidy in 74 primary lung cancers to regional lymph node metastases and to the morphology of regional nodes and the proportion of killer T lymphocytes in these nodes. They found the frequencies of diploid, peridiploid, and aneuploid tumors were 21 (28%), 18 (24%), and 35 (48%), respectively. In general there was an increase in advanced disease as the tumor ploidy pattern changed from diploid to peridiploid and aneuploid. Aneuploidy was found in higher frequency in adenocarcinomas, in tumors whose maximal dimension was greater than 6 cm, in cases with lymphatic invasion, and in cases with involvement of four or more regional lymph nodes by metastases. Aneuploid neoplasms were associated with significantly less lymph node paracortical hyperplasia and fewer killer T lymphocytes than diploid or peridip-

loid tumors in lymph nodes not involved by metastases in N_0 and N_1 disease. These findings were interpreted to suggest a decline in antitumor competence of these lymph nodes, which could make them susceptible to metastases. The authors found the recurrence rate to be 19% in diploid, 33% in peridiploid, and 54% in aneuploid tumors. Two-year survival rates in tumors classified this way were 87%, 78%, and 44%, respectively. Their findings suggested that ploidy status correlated with the biologic behavior of primary lung neoplasms.

As observed by pathologists, many malignant cells have large nuclei and nucleoli. The nucleolar organizing regions play an important role in organizing the nucleolus and can be visualized by a silver staining technique that stains acidic proteins associated with ribosomal genes. The number of nucleolar organizing regions may reflect proliferative activity of tumor cells. Ogura et al.[515] correlated the number of nucleolar organizing regions in 58 primary pulmonary adenocarcinomas and correlated this information with the tumor growth rate as determined by doubling time according to changes in the size of tumors over time. They found the number of nucleolar organizing regions ranged from 1.8 to 6.3 (mean ± S.D., 4.0 + 0.8). The degree of histologic differentiation and pathologic staging did not correlate with the number of nucleolar organizing regions. The doubling times of 13 neoplasms ranged from 80 to 760 days, and the authors found an inverse correlation between the number of nucleolar organizing regions and doubling time (see their figures). They concluded that the mean number of nucleolar organizing regions could be used as an index of proliferative activity of the neoplasm.

Summary

This chapter has presented a detailed pathologic description and clinicopathologic correlation of the most common neoplasms that occur in the lung. As indicated, it is most important for the pathologist to adequately sample and to accurately stage these tumors. The stage of the neoplasm and the histologic type are both important factors in determining survival.

References

1. Jett JR, Cortese DA, Fonatana RS. Lung cancer: Current concepts. Ca-A Cancer J Clin 1983;33:74–86.
2. Silverberg E, Lubera JA. Cancer statistics. Ca-A Cancer J Clin Bull Cancer Prog 1989;39:3–20.
3. Silverberg E, Lubera J. Cancer statistics, 1987. Ca-A Cancer J Clin 1987;37:2–19.
4. American Cancer Society. Cancer facts and figures, 1991 Atlanta: American Cancer Society, 1991:8.

5. Robbins SL. The respiratory system. In: Pathologic basis of disease. Philadelphia: Saunders, 1974:833–840.

6. Galofre M, Payne WS, Woolner LB, Claggett OT, Gage RP. Pathologic classification and surgical treatment of bronchogenic carcinoma. Surg Gynecol Obstet 1964;119:51–61.

7. Selawry OS, Hansen HH. Lung cancer. In: Holland JF, Frei E, eds. Cancer medicine. Part 2. Philadelphia: Lea and Febiger, 1973:1473–1518.

8. Garfinkel L, Silverberg E. Lung cancer smoking trends in the United States over the past 25 years. Ca-A Cancer J Clin 1991;41:137–165.

9. Devesa SS, Blot WJ, Fraumeni JF, Jr. Declining lung cancer rates among young men and women in the United States: a cohort analysis. J Natl Cancer Inst 1989;81:1568–1571.

10. Glass A. Declining rates of lung cancer in the United States in young men and women. J Natl Cancer Inst 1991;83:368–369.

11. Parkin DM, Sternsward J, Muir CS. Estimates of twelve major cancers. Inst WHO 1984;62:163–182.

12. Cancer Incidence in Five Continents. NYS Med 1989;92:432–433.

13. Patterns of cancer incidence in five continents: A picture book. Whelan SL, Parkin DM, Masuyer E, eds. IARC Sci Publ #102, Lyon; IARC, 1990:25.

14. Napalkov NP. Incidence of malignant tumors in the USSR between 1970 and 1980. Voprosky Onkologii 1982;28:26–27.

15. Doll R, Gray R, Hafner B, Peto R. Mortality in relation to smoking: Twenty two years' observations on female British doctors. Br Med J 1980;280:428–429.

16. Pollack ES, Horm JW. Trends in cancer incidence and mortality in the United States 1969–1976. J Natl Cancer Inst 1980;64:1091–1103.

17. Holck SE, Warren CW, Rochat RW, Smith JC. Lung cancer mortality and smoking habits: Mexican–American women. Am J Public Health 1982;72:38–42.

18. Lam Wk, So SY, Yu DYC. Clinical features of bronchogenic carcinoma in Hong Kong: Review of 480 patients. Cancer (Philadelphia) 1983;52:369–376.

19. Stolley PD. Lung cancer in women: Five years later, situation worse. N Engl J Med 1983;309:428–429.

20. L'Able KA, Hoey JR. Cigarette smoking, lung cancer and Canadian women. Can Med Assoc J 1984;130:1539–1540.

21. Harris J. Lung cancer among women: Tennessee. Morb Mortal Wkly Rep 1984;33:586–588.

22. Wu AH, Henderson BE, Pike MC, Yu MC. Smoking and other risk factors for lung cancer in women. J Natl Cancer Inst 1985;74:747–751.

23. Stolley PD. Lung cancer: unwanted equality for women. N Engl J Med 1977;297:886–887.

24. Lung cancer among women. JAMA 1984;252:2806–2811.

25. Staryzk PM. Lung-cancer deaths: Equality by 2000? N Engl J Med 1983;309:1289–1290.

26. Andrews JL, Bloom S, Balogh K, Beamis JF. Lung cancer in women: Lahey clinic experience 1957–1980. Cancer (Philadelphia) 1985;55:2894–2898.

27. Guinee V, Giocco G, Suarez L, et al. Lung cancer and breast cancer among women: Texas. JAMA 1984;251:2915–2916.

28. Chen VW. Lung cancer: Leading cause of cancer death in Louisiana white females. J Natl Cancer Inst 1984;73:1–2.

29. McDuffie HH, Klaassen DJ, Dosman JA. Female–male differences in patients with primary lung cancer. Cancer (Philadelphia) 1987;59:1825–1830.

30. Osann KE. Lung cancer in women: The importance of smoking, family history of cancer, and medical history of respiratory disease. Cancer Res 1991;51:4893–4897.

31. Anderson AE, Buechner HA, Yoger I, Ziskind MM. Bronchogenic carcinoma in young men. Am J Med 1954;16:404–415.

32. Neuman HW, Ellis FH, McDonald JR. Bronchogenic carcinoma in persons under forty years of age. N Engl J Med 1956;254:502–507.

33. Rivkin LM, Salyer JM. Bronchogenic carcinoma in men under 40 years of age. Chest 1958;34:521–524.

34. Hanbury WJ. Bronchogenic carcinoma in young persons. Br J Cancer 1958;12:202–206.

35. Large SE, Morgan WKC. Bronchial carcinoma in young adults. Br J Tuberc 1958;52:185–189.

36. Hood RH, Campbell DC, Dooley BN. Bronchogenic carcinoma in young people. Dis Chest 1965;48:469–470.

37. Kennedy A. Lung cancer in young adults. Br J Dis Chest 1972;66:147–154.

38. Kyniakos M, Webber B. Cancer of the lung in young men. J Thorac Cardiovasc Surg 1974;67:634–648.

39. Putnam JS. Lung carcinoma in young adults. JAMA 1977;238:35–36.

40. Ganz PA, Vernon SE, Preston D, Coulson WF. Lung cancer in younger patients. West J Med 1980;133:373–378.

41. DeCaro L, Benfield JR. Lung cancer in young persons. J Thorac Cardiovasc Surg 1982;83:372–376.

42. Roviaro GC, Varoli F, Zannini P, Fascianella A, Pezzuoli G. Lung cancer in the young. Chest 1985;87:456–459.

43. McDuffie HH, Klaassen DJ, Dosman JA. Characteristics of patients with primary lung cancer diagnosed at age 50 years or younger. Chest 1989;96:1298–1301.

44. Jubelirer SJ, Wilson RA. Lung cancer in patients younger than 40 years of age. Cancer (Philadelphia) 1991;67:1436–1438.

45. Bourke W, Milstein D, Giura R, et al. Lung cancer in young adults. Chest 1992;102:1723–1729.

46. Fontenelle LJ. Primary adenocarcinoma of the lung in a child: Review of the literature. Am Surg 1976;42:296–299.

47. Hartman GE, Shochat SJ. Primary pulmonary neoplasms of childhood: A review. Ann Thorac Surg 1983;36:108–119.

48. Cayley Ck, Caez HJ, Mersheimer W. Primary bronchogenic carcinoma of the lung in children. Am J Dis

Child 1951;82:49–60.

49. Niitu Y, Kubota H, Hasegawa S, et al. Lung cancer (squamous cell carcinoma) in adolescence. Am J Dis Child 1974;127:108–110.

50. LaSalle RJ, Andrassy RJ, Stanford W. Bronchogenic squamous carcinoma in childhood: A case report. J Pediatr Surg 1977;12:519–521.

51. Epstein DM, Aronchick JM. Lung cancer in childhood. Med Pediatr Oncol 1989;17:510–513.

52. McAldowie AM. Primary cancer of the lungs in a child five and a half months old. Lancet 1876;ii:570–571.

53. Fielding JE. Smoking: health effects and control. N Engl J Med 1985;313:491–498, 555–561.

54. Kabat GC, Wynder EL. Lung cancer in nonsmokers. Cancer (Philadelphia) 1984;53:1214–1221.

55. Ochsner A, DeBakey M. Carcinoma of the lung. Arch Surg 1941;42:209–258.

56. Wynder EL, Graham EA. Tobacco smoking as a possible etiologic factor in bronchogenic carcinoma. A study of six hundred and eight four proved cases. JAMA 1950;143:329–336.

57. Hammond EC, Horn D. Smoking and death rates: report on forty-four months of follow-up of 187,783 men. JAMA 1958;166:1294–1308.

58. Rogot E, Murray JL. Smoking and cause of death among American veterans: 16 years of observation. Public Health Rep 1980;3:213–222.

59. Pollin W, Ravenholt RT. Tobacco addiction and tobacco mortality. JAMA 1984;252:2849–2854.

60. Guyatt GH, Newhouse MT. Are active and passive smoking harmful? Determining causation. Chest 1985;88:445–451.

61. Shopland DR, Eyre HJ, Pechacek TF. Smoking-attributable cancer mortality in 1991: Is lung cancer now the leading cause of death among smokers in the United States? J Natl Cancer Inst 1991;83:1142–1148.

62. Peto R, Doll R. Mortality in relation to smoking: 20 years' observations on male British doctors. Br Med J 1976;1525–1536.

63. U.S. Department of Health and Human Services. *Reducing the Health Consequences of Smoking: 25 years of Progress. A Report of the Surgeon General.* U.S. Department of Health and Human Services, Public Health Service, Centers for Disease Control, Center for Chronic Disease Prevention and Health Promotion, Office on Smoking and Health. OHSH Publication No. (CDC) 89-8411, 1989:

64. Center for Disease Control, Public Health Service, U.S. Department of Health and Human Services. The Health consequences of involuntary smoking. A report of the Surgeon General. DHHS Publ. No. 87-8398. Washington, DC: U.S. Govt. Print Office, 1986.

65. National Academy of Sciences. Environmental tobacco smoke: Measuring exposures and assessing health effects. Washington, DC: National Academy Press, 1986.

66. U.S. Environmental Protection Agency. Health effects of passive smoking: Assessment of lung cancer in adults and respiratory disorders in children. Washington, DC: U.S. Environmental Protection Agency, 1990.

67. Janerich DT, Thompson D, Varela LR, et al. Lung cancer and exposure to tobacco smoke in the household. N Engl J Med 1990;323:632–636.

68. Kozlowski LT. Tar and nicotine delivery of cigarettes. What a difference a puff makes. JAMA 1981;245:158–159.

69. Benowitz NL, Hall SM, Herning RI, Jacobs P III, Jones RT, Osman AL. Smokers of low-yield cigarettes do not consume less nicotine. N Engl J Med 1983; 309:139–142.

70. Auerbach O, Hammond EC, Garfinkel L. Changes in bronchial epithelium in relation to cigarette smoking, 1955–1960 vs. 1970–1977. N Engl J Med 1979;300:381–386.

71. Lee PN, Garfinkel L. Mortality and type of cigarette smoked. J Epidemiol Community Health 1981;35:16–22.

72. Zang EA, Wynder EL. Cumulative tar exposure: A new index for estimating lung cancer risk among cigarette smokers. Cancer (Philadelphia) 1992;70:69–76.

73. Winters TH, DiFranza JR. Radioactivity in cigarette smoke. N Engl J Med 1982;306:364–365.

74. Martell EA. Radioactivity in cigarette smoke. N Engl J Med 1982;307:309–310.

75. Cohen JI. Radioactivity in cigarette smoke. N Engl J Med 1982;307:310.

76. Cohen BS, Harley NH. Radioactivity in cigarette smoke. N Engl J Med 1982;307:309–310.

77. Hill CR. Radioactivity in cigarette smoke. N Engl J Med 1982;307:311.

78. Wagner WL. Radioactivity in cigarette smoke. N Engl J Med 1982;307:311.

79. Ravenholt RT. Radioactivity in cigarette smoke. N Engl J Med 1982;307:312.

80. Hoffman D. Wynder EL. Radioactivity in cigarette smoke. N Engl J Med 1982;307:312.

81. Gottlieb LS, Husen LA. Lung cancer among Navajo uranium miners. Chest 1982;81:449–452.

82. Samet JM, Kutvirt DM, Waxweiler RJ, Key CR. Uranium mining and lung cancer in Navajo men. N Engl J Med 1984;310:1481–1484.

83. Radford EP, St. Clair Renard KG. Lung cancer in Swedish iron miners exposed to low doses of radon daughters. N Engl J Med 1984;310:1485–1494.

84. Radford EP. Radon daughters in the induction of lung cancer in underground miners. In: Peto R, Schneiderman M, eds. Quantification of occupational cancer. Cold Spring Harbor, New York: Cold Spring Laboratory, 1981:151–163.

85. Thomas DC, McNeill KG. Risk estimates for the health effects of alpha radiation. Ottawa: Report to the Canadian Atomic Energy Control Board, 1982.

86. The Seattle Times, Sunday, Sept 8, 1985.

87. Indoor air pollution. If you think your home is a bastion of clean air in a polluted world, think again. Consumer Reports 1985;50:600–603.

88. Committee on the Biological Effects of Ionizing Radiation, National Research Council. Health risks of radon and other internally deposited alpha emitters. BEIR

IV. Washington, DC: National Academy Press, 1988.

89. U.S. Environmental Protection Agency. A citizen's guide to radon: What it is and what to do about it. Washington, DC: Govt Printing Office, 1986.

90. Samet JM, Nero AV. Sounding board: Indoor radon and lung cancer. N Engl J Med 1989;320:591–593.

91. Vena JE, Byers TE, Cookfair D, Swanson M. Occupation and lung cancer risk. An analysis by histologic subtypes. Cancer (Philadelphia) 1985;56:910–917.

92. Saracci R. Asbestos and lung cancer: An analysis of the epidemiological evidence on the asbestos-smoking interaction. Int J Cancer 1977;20:323–331.

93. Saracci R. The interactions of tobacco smoking and other agents in cancer etiology. Epidemiol Rev 1987; 9:175–193.

94. Hammond EC, Selikoff IJ, Seidman H. Asbestos exposure, cigarette smoking and death rates. Ann NY Acad Sci 1979;330:473–490.

95. Selikoff IJ, Hammond EC, Churg J. Asbestos exposure, smoking and neoplasia. JAMA 1968;204:106–112.

96. Selikoff IJ. Asbestos and smoking. JAMA 1979;242:458–459.

97. Sluis-Cremer GK. The relationship between asbestosis and bronchial cancer. Chest 1980;78(Suppl.):380–381.

98. Browne K. Is asbestos or asbestosis the cause of the increased risk of lung cancer in asbestos workers? Br J Ind Med 1986;43:145–149.

99. Warnock ML, Churg AM. Association of asbestos and bronchogenic carcinoma in a population with low asbestos exposure. Cancer (Philadelphia) 1975;35:1236–1242.

100. Warnock ML, Kuwahara TJ, Wolery G. The relation of asbestos burden to asbestosis and lung cancer. Pathol Annu 1983;18(Part 2):109–145.

101. Warnock ML, Isenberg W. Asbestos burden and the pathology of lung cancer. Chest 1986;89:20–26.

102. Wagner JC, Berry G, Skidmore JW, Timbrell V. The effects of the inhalation of asbestos in rats. Br J Cancer 1974;29:252–269.

103. Browne K. A threshold for asbestos-related lung cancer. Br J Ind Med 1986;43:556–558.

104. McFadden D, Wright JL, Wiggs B, Churg A. Smoking inhibits asbestos clearance. Am Rev Respir Dis 1986;133:372–374.

105. McFadden D, Wright J. Wiggs B, Churg A. Cigarette smoke increases the penetration of asbestos fibers into airway walls. Am J Pathol 1986;123:95–99.

106. Barton RTH, Hogetveit ACH. Nickel-related cancers of the respiratory tract Cancer (Philadelphia) 1980;45:3061–3064.

107. Wicks MH, Archer VE, Auerbach O, Kuschner M. Arsenic exposure in a copper smelter as related to histological type of lung cancer. Am J Ind Med 1981;2:25–31.

108. Smith AB, Zuzuki Y. Histopathologic classification of bronchogenic carcinomas among a cohort of workers occupationally exposed to beryllium. Environ Res 1980;21:10–14.

109. Osburn HS. Lung cancer in a mining district in Rhodesia. S Afr Med J 1969;43:1307–1312.

110. National Academy of Sciences. Committee on biologic effects of atmospheric pollutants. Chromium. Washington DC: Division of Medical Sciences. National Research Council, 1974:58.

111. Figueroa WG, Raszkowki R, Weiss W. Lung cancer in chloromethyl methyl ether workers. N Engl J Med 1973;288:1096–1097.

112. Wasweiler RJ, Smith AH, Falk H, Tyroler HA. Excess lung cancer risk in a synthetic chemicals plant. Environ Health Perspect 1981;41:159–165.

113. Aksoy M. Different types of malignancies due to occupational exposure to benzene: A review of recent observations in Turkey. Environ Res 1980;23:181–190.

114. Yamada A. On the late injuries following occupational inhalation of the mustard gas with special references to carcinoma of the respiratory tract. Acta Pathol Jpn 1963;13:131–155.

115. Aksoy M. Hematotoxicity and carcinogenicity of benzene. Environ Health Perspect 1989;82:193–197.

116. Yin SN, Li GL, Tain FD, et al. A retrospective cohort study of leukemia and other cancers in benzene workers. Environ Health Perspect 1989;82:207–213.

117. Maltoni C, Ciiberti A, Cotti G, Conti B, Belpoggi F. Benzene, an experiment multipotential carcinogen: Results of the long-term bioassays performed at the Bologna Institute of Oncology. Environ Health Perspect 1989;82:109–124.

118. Dubrow R, Wegman D. Setting priorities for occupational cancer research and control: Synthesis of the results of occupational disease surveillance studies. J Natl Cancer Inst 1983;71:1123–1142.

119. Morabia A, Markowitz S, Garibaldi K. Wynder EL. Lung cancer and occupation: Results of a multicentre case-control study. Br J Ind Med 1992;49:721–727.

120. Burns PB, Swanson GM. The occupational cancer incidence surveillance sutdy (OCISS): Risk of lung cancer by usual occupation and industry in the Detroit metropolitan area. Am J Ind Med 1991;19:655–671.

121. Guberan E, Usel M, Raymond L, Bolay J, Fioretta G, Puissant J. Increased risk for lung cancer and for cancer of the gastrointestinal tract among Geneva professional drivers. Br J Ind Med 1992;49:337–344.

122. Yousem SA, Ohori P, Sonmez-Alpan E. Occurrence of human papilloma virus DNA in primary lung neoplasms. Cancer (Philadelphia) 1992;69:693–697.

123. Kaplan MH, Susan M, Pahwa SG, et al. Neoplastic complications of HTLV-III infection: Lymphomas and solid tumors. Am J Med 1987;82:389–396.

124. Monfardini S, Vaccher E, Pizzacaro G, et al. Unusual malignant tumors in 49 patients with HIV infection. AIDS 1989;3:449–452.

125. Braun MA, Killan DA, Remick SC, Ruckdeschel JC. Lung cancer in HIV seropositive patients. Radiology 1990:175:341–343.

126. Remick SC, Harper GR, Abdullah MA, McSharry JJ, Ross JS, Ruckdeschel JC. Metastatic breast cancer in a

young seropositive patient. J Natl Cancer Inst 1991;83:447–448.

127. Sridhar KS, Flores MR, Raub WA, Jr., Saldana M. Lung cancer in patients with human immunodeficiency virus infection compared with historic control subjects. Chest 1992;102:1704–1708.

128. Remick SC. Lung cancer: An HIV-related neoplasm or a coincidental finding? Chest 1992;106:1643–1644.

129. Markman M, Braine HG, Abeloff MD. Histocompatibility antigens in small cell carcinoma of the lung. Cancer (Philadelphia) 1984;54:2943–2945.

130. Whang-Peng J, Kao-Shan CS, Bunn PA, Carney DN, Gazdar AF, Minna JD. Specific chromosome defect association with human small-cell lung cancer: Deletion 3p(14–23). Science 1982;215:181–182.

131. Tokuhata GK, Lilienfeld AM. Familial aggregation of lung cancer in humans. J Natl Cancer Inst 1963; 30:289–312.

132. Ooi WL, Elston Rch Chen VW, Bailey-Wilson JE, Rothschild H. Increased familial risk for lung cancer. J Natl Cancer Inst 1986;76:217–222.

133. Sellers TA, Ooi WL, Elston RC, Chen VW, Bailey-Wilson JE, Rothschild H. Increased familial risk for non-lung cancer among relatives of lung cancer patients. Am J Epidemiol 1987;126:237–246.

134. Lynch HT, Kimberling WJ, Markvicka SE, et al. Genetics and smoking-associated cancers. Cancer (Philadelphia) 1986;57:1640–1644.

135. Samet JM, Humble CG, Pathak DR. Personal and family history of respiratory disease and lung cancer risk. Am Rev Respir Dis 1986;134:466–470.

136. McDuffie HH. Clustering of cancer in families of patients with primary lung cancer. J Clin Epidemiol 1991;44:69–76.

137. Shaw GL, Falk RT, Pickle LW, Mason TJ, Buffler PA. Lung cancer risk associated with cancer in relatives. J Clin Epidemiol 1991;44:429–437.

138. Sellers TA, Elston RC, Atwood LD, Rothschild H. Lung cancer histologic type and family history of cancer. Cancer (Philadelphia) 1992;69:86–91.

139. Peto R, Doll R, Buckley JD, et al. Can dietary beta-carotene materially reduce human cancer rates? Nature (London) 1981;290:201–208.

140. Goodman GE, Omenn GS, Feigel P, et al. Chemoprevention of lung cancer with retinol/beta-carotene. In: Meyskens FL, Prasad KN, eds. Vitamins and cancer: Human cancer prevention by vitamins and micronutrients. Clifton, NJ: Humana Press, 1985:341–350.

141. Menkes MS, Comstock GW, Vuillenmier JP, et al. Serum beta carotene, vitamins A and E, selenium, and risk of lung cancer. N Engl J Med 1986;315:1250–1254.

142. Ziegler RG, Mason TJ, Stemhagen A, et al. Carotenoid intake, vegetables, and the risk of lung cancer among white men in New Jersey. Am J Epidemiol 1986; 123:1080.

143. Mathews-Roth MM. Carotenoids and cancer prevention—experimental and epidemiologic studies. Pure Appl Chem 1985;57:717–722.

144. Kroes R, Beems RB, Bosland MC, et al. Nutritional factors in lung, colon, and prostate carcinogenesis in animal models. Fed Proc 1986;45:136–1451.

145. Stich H, Rosin M, Vallejera M. Reduction with vitamin A and beta-carotene administration of proportion of micronucleate buccal mucosal cells in Asian betel nut and tobacco chewers. Lancet 1984;i:1204–1206.

146. Bertram JS, Pung A, Churley M, Kappock TJ, Wilkins LR, Cooney RY. Diverse carotenoids protect against chemically induced neoplastic transformation. Carcinogenesis 1991;12:671–678.

147. Sestili MA. Chemoprevention clinical trials: Problems and Solutions. Publ. 85-2715. Bethesda: National Institutes of Health, 1984.

148. Weiss W, Seidman H, Boucot K. The Philadelphia pulmonary neoplasm research project: thwarting factors in periodic screening for lung cancer. Am Rev. Respir Dis 1975;111:289–297.

149. Nash FA, Morgan JM, Tomkins JG. South London cancer study. Br Med J 1968;2:715–721.

150. ACS report on the cancer-related checkup: cancer of the lung; Appendix B: Experimental biases. CA Bull Cancer Prog 1980;30:199–207.

151. Brett GZ. Earlier diagnosis and survival in lung cancer. Br Med J 1969;4:260–262.

152. Frost JK, Ball WC, Levin ML, et al. Early lung cancer detection: Results of the initial (prevalence) radiologic and cytologic screening in the Johns Hopkins study. Am Rev Respir Dis 1984;130:549–554.

153. Flehinger BJ, Melamed MR, Zaman MB, Heelan RT, Perchick WB, Martini N. Early lung cancer detection: Results of the initial (prevalence) radiologic and cytologic screening in the Memorial Sloan-Kettering study. Am Rev Respir Dis 1984;130:555–560.

154. Fontana RS, Sanderson DR, Taylor WF, et al. Early lung cancer detection: Results of the initial (prevlance) radiologic and cytologic screening in the Mayo Clinic study. Am Rev Respir Dis 1984;130:561–565.

155. Bailar JC, Screening for lung cancer—where are we now? Am Rev Respir Dis 1984;130:541–542.

156. Weiss W. Screening for lung cancer. Chest 1985; 87:273–274.

157. Merz B. Is screening for early lung cancer worthwhile? JAMA 1983;249:1537–1538.

158. Fontana RS, Sanderson DR, Woolner LB, et al. Screening for lung cancer: A critique of the Mayo Lung Project. Cancer (Philadelphia) 1991;67:1155–1164.

159. Dreis DF. Screening for lung cancer: Do chest x-rays save lives or waste money? Bull Mason Clin 1985; 39:113–121.

160. Feld R, Rubinstein LV, Weisenberger TH, and the Lung Cancer Study Group. Sites of recurrence in resected stage 1 non-small cell lung cancer: A guide for future studies. J Clin Oncol 1984;2:1352–1358.

161. Li W, Hammar SP, Jolly PC, Hill LD, Anderson RP. Unpredictable course of small cell undifferentiated lung carcinoma. J Thorac Cardiovasc Surg 1981;81:34–43.

162. Carr DT, Mountain CF. Staging of lung cancer. Semin

Respir Med 1982;3:154–163.

163. Naruke T, Suemasu K, Ishikawa S. Lymph node mapping and curability at various levels of metastatis in resected lung cancer. J Thorac Cardiovasc Surg 1978;76:832–839.

164. Mountain CF. A new international staging system for lung cancer. Chest 1986;89(Suppl):225S–233S.

165. Mountain CF, Greenberg SD, Fraire AE. Tumor stage in non-small cell carcinoma of the lung. Chest 1991;99:1258–1260.

166. Fernando HC, Goldstraw P. The accuracy of clinical evaluative intrathoracic staging in lung cancer as assessed by post-surgical pathologic staging. Cancer (Philadelphia) 1990;65:2503–2506.

167. Bulzebruck H, Bopp R, Drings P, et al. New aspects in the staging of lung cancer: Prospective validation on the international union against cancer TNM classification. Cancer (Philadelphia) 1992;70:1102–1110.

168. Tisi GM, Friedman PJ, Peters RM, et al. Clinical staging of primary lung cancer. Am Rev Respir Dis 1983;127:659–664.

169. Decker DA, Dines DE, Payne WS, et al. The significance of a cytologically negative pleural effusion in bronchogenic carcinoma. Chest 1978;74:640–642.

170. Grillo HC. Carinal reconstruction. Ann Thorac Surg 1982;34:356–373.

171. Sartori F. Right upper tracheal sleeve lobectomy for carcinoma of the lung. Reconstruction of tracheal bifurcation. Minerva Chir 1984;39:209–212.

172. Gilbert A, Deslauriers J, McLish A, Piraux M. Tracheal sleeve pneumonectomy for carcinoma of the proximal left main bronchus. Can J Surg 1984;27:583–585.

173. The World Health Organization histological typing of lung tumors. 2d Ed. Am J Clin Pathol 1982;77:123–136.

174. Watkin SW. Temporal demographic and epidemiologic variation in histologic subtypes of lung cancer: A literature review. Lung Cancer 1989;5:69–81.

175. Kung ITM, So KF, Lum TH. Lung cancer in Hong Kong Chinese: Mortality and histologic types 1973–1982. Br J Cancer 1984;50:381–388.

176. Whitwell F. The histopathology of lung cancer in Liverpool: The specificity of the histological cell types of lung cancer. Br J Cancer 1961;15:440–459.

177. Feinstein AR, Gelfman NA, Yesner R. Observer variability in the histopathologic diagnosis of lung cancer. Am Rev Respir Dis 1970;101:671–684.

178. Stanley KE, Matthews MJ. Analysis of a pathology review of patients with lung tumours. J Natl Cancer Inst 1981;66:989–992.

179. Vincent RG, Pickren JW, Lane WW, et al. The changing histopathology of lung cancer: A review of 1682 cases. Cancer (Philadelphia) 1977;39:1647–1565.

180. Larsson S. Completeness and reliability of lung cancer registration in the Swedish Cancer Registry. Acta Pathol Microbiol Scand A Pathol 1971;79:389–398.

181. El-Torky M, El-Zeky F, Hall JC. Significant changes in the distribution of histologic types of lung cancer: A review of 4928 cases. Cancer (Philadelphia) 1990; 65:2361–2367.

182. Auerbach O, Garfinkel L. The changing pattern of lung carcinoma. Cancer (Philadelphia) 1991;68:1973–1977.

183. Morabia A, Wynder EL. Cigarette smoking and lung cancer cell types. Cancer (Philadelphia) 1991;68:2074–2078.

184. Yesner R. Spectrum of lung cancer and ectopic hormones. Pathol Annu 1978;13(Part 1):217–240.

185. Adelstein DJ, Tomahefski JF, Snow NJ, Horrigan JP, Hines JD. Mixed small cell and non-small cell lung cancer. Chest 1986;89:699–704.

186. Roggli VL, Volmer RT, Greenberg SD, McGavran MH, Spjut HJ, Yesner R. Lung cancer heterogeneity: A blinded and randomized study of 100 consecutive cases. Hum Pathol 1985;16:569–579.

187. Martini N, Melamed MR. Multiple primary lung cancers. J Thorac Cardiovasc Surg 1975;70:606–612.

188. Razzuk MA, Pockey M. Urschel HC, Paulson DL. Dual primary bronchogenic carcinoma. Ann Thorac Surg 1974;17:425–433.

189. Rohwedder JJ, Weatherbee L. Multiple primary bronchogenic carcinoma. Ann Thorac Surg 1974; 17:425–433.

190. Warren S, Gates O. Multiple primary malignant tumors: a survey of the literature and a statistical study. Am J Cancer (Philadelphia) 1932;16:1358–1414.

191. Auerbach O, Stout AP, Hammond EC, Garfinkel L. Multiple primary bronchial carcinomas. Cancer (Philadelphia) 1967;20:699–705.

192. Struve-Christensen E. Diagnosis and treatment of bilateral primary bronchogenic carcinoma. J Thorac Cardiovasc Surg 1971;61:501–513.

193. Jung-Legg Y, McGowan SF, Sweeney KG, Zitzman JL, Pugntch RP. Synchronous triple malignant tumors of the lung: A case report of bronchial carcinoid, small cell carcinoma, and adenocarcinoma of the right lung. Am J Clin Pathol 1986;85:96–101.

194. Wu S, Lin Z, Xu C, Koo K, Huang O, Xie D. Multiple primary lung cancers. Chest 1987;92:892–896.

195. Deschamps C, Pairolero PC, Trastek VF, Payne WS. Multiple primary lung cancers: results of surgical treatment. J Thorac Cardiovasc Surg 1990;99:769–778.

196. Seydel HG, Chait A, Gmelich JT. The natural history of cancer of the lung. In: Seydel HG, Chait A, Gmelich JT, eds. Cancer of the lung. New York: Wiley, 1975:52–63.

197. Auerbach O. Natural history of carcinoma of the lung. In: Fishman AP, ed. Pulmonary diseases and disorders. New York: McGraw-Hill, 1980;1388–1396.

198. Miller YE. Growth factors, oncogenes and lung cancer. Am Rev Respir Dis 1985;132:178–179.

199. Wick MR. Oncogene analysis in diagnostic pathology: A current perspective. Am J Clin Pathol 1992; 97(Suppl.1):S1–S3.

200. Viallet J, Minna JD. Dominant oncogenes and tumor suppressor genes in the pathogenesis of lung cancer. Am J Respir Cell Mol Biol 1990;2:225–232.

201. Damstrup L, Rorth M, Poulsen HS. Growth factors and growth factor receptors in human malignancies with special reference to lung cancer: a review. Lung Cancer 1989;5:49–68.

202. Paul J. Oncogenesis. In: Anthony PP, MacSween RNM, eds. Recent advances in histopathology. London: Churchill-Livingstone, 1987:13–31.

203. Collins VP, Loeffler RK, Tivey H. Observations on growth rates of human tumors. Am J Roentgenol Radium Ther Nucl Med 1956;76:988–1000.

204. Geddes DM. The natural history of lung cancer: A review based on rates of tumour growth. Br J Dis Chest 1979;73:1–17.

204a. Brenner MW, Holsti LR, Pertolla Y. The study of graphical analysis of the growth of human tumours and metastases of the lung Br J Cancer 1967;1–13.

204b. Breuer K. Growth rate and radiosensitivity of human tumours. Europ J Cancer 1966;2:157–171.

204c. Chahinian P. Relationship between tumour doubling time and anatomoclinical features in 50 measurable pulmonary cancers. Chest 1972;61:340–345.

204d. Garland LH, Coulson W, Wollin E. The rate of growth and apparent duration of untreated primary bronchial carcinoma. Cancer, N.Y., 1963;16:694–707.

204e. Garland LH. The rate of growth and apparent duration of primary bronchial cancer. Am J Roent Rad Ther 1966;96:604–611.

204f. Meyer JA. Growth rate versus prognosis in resected primary bronchogenic cancer. Cancer, N.Y., 1973; 31:1468–1472.

204g. Schwartz M. A biomathematical approach to clinical tumour growth. Cancer, N.Y., 1961;14:1272–1294.

204h. Steele JD, Buell P. A symptomatic solitary pulmonary nodules. J Thorac Cardiovasc Surg 1973;65:140–151.

204i. Weiss W, Boucot KR, Cooper DA. Growth rate in the detection and prognosis of bronchogenic carcinoma. JAMA 1966;198:1246–1256.

204j. Weiss W. Tumour doubling time and survival of men with bronchogenic carcinoma. Chest 1974;65:3–8.

205. Chahinian P, Israel L. Rates and patterns of growth of lung cancer. In: Israel L, Chahinian P, eds. Lung cancer: Natural history, prognosis and therapy. New York: Academic Press, 1976:63–79.

206. Chahinian P, Israel L. Prognostic value of doubling times and related factors in lung cancer. In: Israel L, Chahinian P, eds, Lung cancer: Natural history, prognosis and therapy. New York: Academic Press, 1976:95–106.

207. Nathan MH, Collins VP, Adams RA. Differentiation of benign and malignant pulmonary nodules by growth rates. Radiology 1962;79:221–231.

208. Kerr KM, Lamb D. Actual growth rate and tumour cell proliferation in human pulmonary neoplasms. Br J Cancer 1984;50:343–349.

209. Greengard O, Head JF, Goldberg SL, Kirschner PA. Biochemical measure of the volume doubling time of human pulmonary neoplasms. Cancer (Philadelphia) 1985;55:1530–1535.

210. Byrd RB, Miller WE, Carr DT. The roentgenographic appearance of squamous cell carcinoma of the bronchus. Mayo Clin Proc 1968;43:327–332.

211. Walter JB, Pryce DM. The site of origin of lung cancer and its relation to histological type. Thorax 1955;10:117–126.

212. Chaudhuri MR. Primary pulmonary cavitating carcinomas. Thorax 1973;28:354–366.

213. Dulmet-Brender E. Jaubert F, Huchon G. Exophytic endobronchial epidermoid carcinoma. Cancer (Philadelphia 1986;57:1358–1364.

214. Carter D, Eggleston JC. Squamous cell carcinoma. In: Tumors of the lower respiratory tract (Atlas of tumor pathology, 2d Ser., Fasc. 17). Washington DC: Armed Forces Institute of Pathology 1980;70–94.

215. Trump BF, McDowell EM, Glavin F, et al. The respiratory epithelium. III. Histogenesis of epidermoid metaplasia and carcinoma in situ in the human. J Natl Cancer Inst 1978;61:563–575.

216. Yamamoto M, Shimokata K, Nagura H. Immunoelectron microscopic study on the histogenesis of epidermoid metaplasia in respiratory epithelium. Am Rev Respir Dis 1987;135:713–718.

217. Valaitis J, Warren S, Gamble D. Increasing incidence of adenocarcinoma of the lung. Cancer (Philadelphia) 1981;47:1042–1046.

218. Taylor AB, Shinton NH, Waterhouse JAH. Histology of bronchial carcinoma in relation to prognosis. Thorax 1963;18:178–181.

219. Weiss W, Boucot KR, Cooper DA. The histopathology of bronchogenic carcinoma and its relation to growth rate, metastasis, and prognosis. Cancer (Philadelphia) 1970;26:965–970.

220. Ashley DJB, Davies HD. Cancer of the lung: Histology and biological behaviour. Cancer (Philadelphia) 1967; 20:165–174.

221. Bennett DE, Sasser WR, Ferguson TB. Adenocarcinoma of the lung in men: A clinicopathologic study of 100 cases. Cancer (Philadelphia) 1969;23:431–439.

222. Raeburn C, Spencer H. A study of the origin and development of lung cancer. Thorax 1953;8:1–10.

223. Raeburn C, Spencer H. Lung scar cancers. Br J Tuberc Dis Chest 1957;51:237–245.

224. Carroll R. Influence of lung scars on primary lung cancer. J Pathol Bacteriol 1962;83:293–297.

225. Auerbach O, Garfinkel L, Parks VR. Scar cancer of the lung: Increase over a 21-year period. Cancer (Philadelphia) 1979;43:636–642.

226. Scannell JG. "Bleb" carcinoma of the lung. J Thorac Cardiovasc Surg 1980;80:904–908.

227. Konwaler BE, Reingold IM. Carcinoma arising in bronchiectatic cavities. Cancer (Philadelphia) 1952; 5:525–529.

228. Shimosato Y, Hashimoto T, Kodama T, et al. Prognostic implications of fibrotic focus (scar) in small peripheral lung cancers. Am J Surg Pathol 1980;4:365–373.

229. Madri JA, Carter D. Scar cancers of the lung: Origin and significance. Hum Pathol 1984;15:625–631.

230. Kung ITM, Lui IOL, Loke SL, et al. Pulmonary scar cancer: A pathologic reappraisal. Am J Surg Pathol

1985;9:391–400.

231. Cagle PT, Cohle SD, Greenberg SD. Natural history of pulmonary scar cancers: Clinical and pathologic implications. Cancer (Philadelphia) 1985;56:2031–2035.

232. Barsky SH, Huang SJ, Bhuta S. The extracellular matrix of pulmonary scar carcinomas is suggestive of a desmoplastic origin. Am J Pathol 1986;124:412–419.

233. Meyer EC, Liebow AA. Relationship of interstitial pneumonia honeycombing and atypical epithelial proliferation to cancer of the lung. Cancer (Philadelphia) 1965;218:322–351.

234. Fox B, Ridson RA. Carcinoma of the lung and diffuse interstitial pulmonary fibrosis. J Clin Pathol 1968;21:486–491.

235. Haddad R, Massaro D. Idiopathic diffuse interstitial pulmonary fibrosis (fibrosing alveolitis), atypical epithelial proliferation and lung cancer. Am J Med 1968;45:211–219.

236. Fraire AE, Greenberg SD. Carcinoma and diffuse interstitial fibrosis of lung. Cancer 1973;31:1078–1086.

237. Turner-Warwick M, Lebowitz M. Burrows B, Johnson A. Cryptogenic fibrosing alveolitis and lung cancer. Thorax 1980;35:496–499.

238. Zatuchni J, Campbell WN, Zarafonetis CJD. Pulmonary fibrosis and terminal bronchiolar ('alveolar cell') carcinoma in scleroderma. Cancer (Philadelphia) 1953;6:1147–1158.

239. Collins DH, Darke CS, Dodge OG. Scleroderma with honeycomb lung and bronchiolar carcinoma. J Pathol Bacteriol 1958;76:531–540.

240. Caplan H. Honeycomb lungs and malignant pulmonary adenomatosis in scleroderma. Thorax 1959;14:89–96.

241. Montgomery RD, Stirling GA, Hamer NAJ. Bronchiolar carcinoma in progressive systemic sclerosis. Lancet 1962;iii:693–695.

242. Liebow AA. Bronchiolo-alveolar carcinoma. Adv Intern Med 1960;10:329–358.

243. Rosenblatt MB, Lisa JR, Collier F. Primary and metastatic bronchiolo-alveolar carcinoma. Dis Chest 1967;52;147–152.

244. Clayton F. Bronchioloalveolar carcinomas: cell types, patterns of growth, and prognostic correlates. Cancer (Philadelphia) 1986;57:1555–1564.

245. Clayton F. The spectrum and significance of bronchioloalveolar carcinomas. Pathol Annu 1988;23:361–394.

246. Adamson JS, Senior RM, Merrill T. Alveolar cell carcinoma: an electron microscopic study. Am Rev Respir Dis 1969;100:550–557.

247. Coalson JJ, Mohr JA, Pirtle JK, Dee AL, Rhoades ER. Electron microscopy of neoplasms in the lung with special emphasis on the alveolar cell carcinoma. Am Rev Respir Dis 1970;101:181–197.

248. Kuhn C. Fine structure of bronchiolo-alveolar cell carcinoma. Cancer (Philadelphia) 1972;30:1107–1118.

249. Nash G, Langlinais PC, Greenwald KA. Alveolar cell carcinoma: Does it exist? Cancer (Philadelphia) 1972;29:322–326.

250. Bedrossian CWM, Weilbaecher DG, Bentinck DC,

Greenberg SD. Ultrastructure of human bronchioloalveolar cell carcinoma. Cancer (Philadelphia) 1975;36:1399–1413.

251. Bonikos DS, Hendrickson M, Bensch KG. Pulmonary alveolar cell carcinoma. Fine structural and in vitro study of a case and critical review of this entity. Am J Surg Pathol 1977;1:93–108.

252. Sidhu GS, Forrester EM. Glycogen-rich Clara cell-type bronchiolo-alveolar cell carcinoma. Light and electron microscopic study. Cancer (Philadelphia) 1977;40:2209–2215.

253. Kimula Y. A histochemical and ultrastructural study of adenocarcinoma of the lung. Am J Surg Pathol 1978;2:253–264.

254. Morningstar WA, Hassan MO. Bronchiolo-alveolar cell carcinoma with nodal metastases Am J Surg Pathol 1979;3:273–278.

255. Carter D, Eggleston JC. Bronchioloalveolar carcinoma. In: Tumors of the lower respiratory tract (Atlas of tumor pathology, 2d Ser., Fasc. 17). Washington, DC: Armed Forces Institute of Pathology, 1980:127–147.

256. Hammar SP, Bolen JW, Bockus D, Remington F, Friedman S. Ultrastructural and immunohistochemical features of common lung tumors: An overview. Ultrastruct Pathol 1985;9:283–318.

257. Clayton F. Bronchioloalveolar carcinomas: cell types, patterns of growth, and prognostic correlates. Cancer (Philadelphia) 1986;57:1555–1564.

258. Herrera GA, Alexander CB, deMoraes HP. Ultrastructural subtypes of pulmonary adenocarcinoma. Correlation with patient survival. Chest 1983;84:581–586.

259. Dekmezian R, Ordonez NG, Mackay B. Bronchioloalveolar adenocarcinoma with myoepithelial cells. Cancer (Philadelphia) 1991;67:2356–2360.

260. Torikata C, Ishiwata K. Intranuclear tubular structures observed in the cells of alveolar cell carcinomas of the lung. Cancer (Philadelphia) 1977;40:1194–1201.

261. Singh G, Katyal SL, Torikata C. Carcinoma of type II pneumocytes: Immunodiagnosis of a subtype of bronchioloalveolar carcinoma. Am J Pathol 1981;102:195–208.

262. Singh G, Katyal SL, Torikata C. Carcinoma of type II pneumocytes: PAS staining as a screening test for nuclear inclusions of surfactant-specific appoprotein. Cancer (Philadelphia) 1982;50:946–948.

263. Ghadially FN, Harawi S, Khan W. Diagnostic ultrastructural markers in alveolar cell carcinoma. J Submicrosc Cytol 1985;17:269–278.

264. Singh G, Scheithauer BW, Katyal S. The pathobiologic features of carcinomas of type II penumocytes. Cancer (Philadelphia) 1986;57:994–999.

265. Hammar S, Bockus D, Remington F. Metastatic tumor of unknown origin. Ultrastruct Pathol 1986;10:281–288.

266. Basset F, Soler P, Wyllie L, et al. Langerhans cells in a bronchioloalveolar tumor of lung. Virchow Arch [Pathol Anat] 1974;362:315–330.

267. Hammar SP, Bockus D, Remington F, et al. Langerhans cells and serum precipitating antibodies against

fungal antigen in bronchioloalveolar cell carcinomas; possible association with eosinophilic granuloma. Ultrastruct Pathol 1980;1:19–37.

268. Hammar SP, Bockus D, Remington F, Bartha M. The widespread distribution of Langerhans cells in pathologic tissues: An ultrastructural and immunohistochemical study. Hum Pathol 1986;17:894–905.

269. Takakura H, Hirohashi S, Shimosato Y, et al. Immunomorphologic responses of regional lymph nodes and prognosis in patients with stage I-A peripheral bronchial adenocarcinoma. Jpn J Cancer Clin 1983;29:777–785.

270. Furukawa T, Watanabe S, Kodoma T, Sato Y, Shimosato Y, Suemasu K. T-zone histiocytes in adenocarcinoma of lung in relation to postoperative prognosis. Cancer (Philadelphia) 1985;56:2651–2656.

271. Nakanishi K, Kawai T, Suzuki M. Large intracytoplasmic body in lung cancer compared with Clara cell granule. Am J Clin Pathol 1987;88:472–477.

272. Scroggs MW, Roggli VL, Fraire AE, Sanfilippo F. Eosinophilic intracytoplasmic globules in pulmonary adenocarcinomas: A histochemical, immunohistochemical and ultrastructural study of six cases. Hum Pathol 1989;20:845–849.

273. Axiotis A, Jennings TA. Observations on bronchioloalveolar carcinomas with special emphasis on localized lesions: A clinicopathologic, ultrastructural and immunohistochemical study of 11 cases. Am J Surg Pathol 1988;12:918–931.

274. Miller RR, Nelems B, Evans KG, Muller NL, Ostrow DN. Glandular neoplasia of the lung: A proposed analogy to colonic tumors. Cancer (Philadelphia) 1988;61:1009–1014.

275. Miller RR. Bronchioloalveolar cell adenomas. Am J Surg Pathol 1990;14:904–912.

276. Yousem SA, Hochholzer L. Alveolar adenoma. Hum Pathol 1986;17:1066–1071.

277. Travis WD, Linnoila RI, Horowitz M, et al. Pulmonary nodules resembling bronchioloalveolar carcinoma in adolescent cancer patients. Mod Pathl 1988;5:372–377.

278. Noguchi M, Kodama T, Shimosato Y, et al. Papillary adenoma of type II pneumocytes. Am J Surg Pathol 1986;10:134–139.

279. Hegg CA, Flint A, Sing G. papillary adenoma of the lung. Am J Clin Pathol 1992;97:393–397.

280. Hammar S. Adenocarcinoma and large cell undifferentiated carcinoma of the lung. Ultrastruct Pathol 1987;11:251–274.

281. Barnes L. Intestinal-type adenocarcinoma of the nasal cavity and paranasal sinuses. Am J Surg Pathol 1986;20:192–202.

282. Afzelius BA. Glycocalyx and glycocalyceal bodies in the respiratory epithelium of nose and bronchi. Ultrastruct Pathol 1984;7:1–8.

283. Kish JK, Ro JY, Ayala AG, McMurtrey MJ. Primary mucinous adenocarcinoma of the lung with signet-ring cells: A histochemical comparison with signet-ring cell carcinomas of other sites. Hum Pathol 1989;20:1097–1102.

284. Graeme-Cook F, Mark EJ. Pulmonary mucinous tumors of borderline malignancy. Hum Pathol 1991;22:185–190.

285. Higashiyama M, Doi O, Kodama K. Yokouchi H, Tateishi R. Cystic mucinous adenocarcinomas of the lung: Two cases of cystic variant of mucus-producing lung adenocarcinoma. Chest 1992;101:763–766.

286. Moran CA, Hochholzer L, Fishback N, Travis WD, Koss MN. Mucinous (so-called colloid) carcinomas of lung. Mod Pathol 1992;5:634–638.

287. Tsao M, Fraser RS. Primary pulmonary adenocarcinoma with enteric differentiation. Cancer (Philadelphia) 1991;68:1754–1757.

288. Brambilla E, Moro D, Veale D, et al. Basal cell (basaloid) carcinoma of the lung: A new morphologic and phenotypic entity with separate prognostic significance. Hum Pathol 1992;23:993–1003.

289. Kodama T, Shimosato Y, Koide T, Watanabe S, Yoneyama T. Endobronchial polypoid adenocarcinoma of the lung: Histologic and ultrastructural studies of five cases. Am J Surg Pathol 1984;8:845–854.

290. Cagle PT, Alpert LC, Carmona PA. Peripheral biphasic adenocarcinoma of the lung: light microscopic and immunohistochemical findings. Hum Pathol 1992;23:197–200.

291. Upton MP, Hirohashi S, Tome Y, Miyazawa N, Suemasu K, Shimosato Y. Expression of vimentin in surgically resected adenocarcinomas and large cell carcinomas of lung. Am J Surg Pathol 1986;10:560–567.

292. Jasani B, Edwards RE, Thomas ND, Gibbs AR. The use of vimentin antibodies in the diagnosis of malignant mesothelioma. Virchows Arch [Pathol Anat] 1985;406:441–448.

293. Cherwitz D, Swanson, P, Drier J, Wick M. S100-protein reactivity in poorly differentiated carcinomas: An immunohistochemical comparison with malignant melanoma. Lab Invest 1987;56:13A.

294. Linnoila R, Jensen SM, Steinberg SM, Mulshine JL, Eggelston JC, Gazdar AF. Peripheral airway cell marker expression in non-small cell lung carcinoma. Am J Clin Pathol 1992;97:233–243.

295. Delmonte VC, Alberti O, Saldiva PHN. Large cell carcinoma of the lung: Ultrastructural and immunohistochemical features. Chest 1986;90:524–527.

296. Churg A. The fine structure of large cell undifferentiated carcinoma of the lung: Evidence for its relation to squamous cell carcinomas and adenocarcinomas. Hum Pathol 1978;9:143–156.

297. Horie A, Ohta M. Ultrastructural features of large cell carcinoma of the lung with reference to the prognosis in patients. Hum Pathol 1981;12:423–432.

298. Leong AS. The relevance of ultrastructural examination in the classification of primary lung tumors. Pathology 1982;14:37–46.

299. Albain KS, True LD, Golomb HM. Hoffman PC, Little AG. Large cell carcinoma of the lung: ultrastructural differentiation and clinicopathologic correlations.

Cancer (Philadelphia) 1985;56:1618–1623.

300. Osborne BM, Mackay B. Butler JJ, Ordonez NG. Large cell lymphoma with microvilluslike projections: an ultrastructural study. Am J Clin Pathol 1983;79:443–450.

301. Butler AE, Colby TV, Weiss L, Lombard C. Lymphoepithelioma-like carcinoma of the lung. Am J Surg Pathol 1989;13:632–639.

302. Nash G, Stout AP. Giant cell carcinoma of the lung: report of 5 cases. Cancer (Philadelphia) 1958;11:369–376.

303. Hellstrom HR, Fisher ER. Giant cell carcinoma of lung. Cancer (Philadelphia) 1963;16:1080–1088.

304. Flanagan P, Roeckel IE. Giant cell carcinoma of the lung: Anatomic and clinical correlation. Am J Med 1964;36:214–222.

305. Kallenberg F, Jaque J. Giant cell carcinoma of the lung: Clinical and pathologic assessment; comparison with other large-cell anaplastic bronchogenic carcinomas. Scand J Thorac Cardiovasc Surg 1979;13:343–346.

306. Shin MS, Jackson LK, Shelton RW, Greene RE. Giant cell carcinoma of the lung: Clinical and roentgenographic manifestations. Chest 1986;89:366–369.

307. Ozzello L, Stout AP. The epithelial origin of giant cell carcinoma of the lung confirmed by tissue culture; report of a case. Cancer (Philadelphia) 1961;14:1052–1056.

308. Wang NS, Seemayer TA, Ahmed MN, Knaack J. Giant cell carcinoma of the lung: A light and electron microscopic study. Hum Pathol 1976;7:3–16.

309. Ginsberg SS, Buzaid AC, Stern H, Carter D. Giant cell carcinoma of the lung. Cancer (Philadelphia) 1992;70:606–610.

310. Yesner R, Gerstl B, Auerbach O. Application of World Health Organization classification of lung carcinoma to biopsy material. Ann Thorac Surg 1965;1:33–49.

311. Kern WH, Jones JC, Chapman ND. Pathology of bronchogenic carcinoma in long-term survivors. Cancer (Philadelphia) 1968;21:772–780.

312. Auerbach O, Frasca JM, Parks VR, et al. A comparison of World Health Organization (WHO) classification of lung tumors by light and electron microscopy. Cancer (Philadelphia) 1982;50:2079–2088.

313. Ashley DJ, Davies HD. Mixed glandular and squamous-cell carcinoma of the bronchus. Thorax 1967;22:431–436.

314. Fitzgibbons PL, Kern WH. Adenosquamous carcinoma of the lung: A clinical and pathologic study of seven cases. Hum Pathol 1985;16:463–466.

315. McDowell EM, McLaughlin JS, Merenyl DK, et al. The respiratory epithelium. V. Histogenesis of lung carcinomas in the human. J Natl Cancer Inst 1978;61:587–606.

316. Wilson TS, McDowell EM, Trump BF. Immunohistochemical studies of keratinization in human lung tumors. J Cell Biol 1981;91:299a.

317. Takamori S, Noguchi M, Moringa S, Goya T, Tsugane S, Kakegawa T, Shimosato Y. Clinicopathologic characteristics of adenosquamous carcinoma of the lung.

Cancer (Philadelphia) 1991;67:649–654.

318. Ishida T, Kaneko S, Yokoyama H, Inoue T, Sugio K, Sugimachi K. Adenosquamous carcinoma of the lung: Clinicopathologic and immunohistochemical features. Am J Clin Pathol 1992;97:678–685.

319. Yousem SA. Pulmonary adenosquamous carcinomas with amyloid-like stroma. Mod Pathol 1989;2:420–426.

320. Feyrter F. Ueber diffuse endokrine epitheliate organe. Zentralbl Inn Med 1938;59:545–561.

321. Pearse AGE. The cytochemistry and ultrastructure of polypeptide hormone-producing cells of the APUD series and the embryologic, physiologic and pathologic implications of this concept. J Histochem Cytochem 1969;17:303–313.

322. Pearse AGE, Takor Takor T. Embryology of the diffuse neuroendocrine system and its relationship to the common peptides. Fed Proc 1979;38:2288–2294.

323. Pearse AGE. The diffuse neuroendocrine system: an extension of the APUD concept. In: Taylor S, ed. Endocrinology. London: Heinemann, 1972:145.

324. Gould VE, DeLellis RA. The neuroendocrine cell system: its tumors, hyperplasias, and dysplasias. In: Silverberg SG, ed. Principles and practice of surgical pathology. New York: Wiley, 1983:1488–1501.

325. Gould VE, Moll R, Moll I, Lee I, Franke WW. Neuroendocrine (Merkel) cells of the skin: hyperplasias dysplasias and neoplasms. Lab Invest 1985;52:334–353.

326. Gould VE, Linnoila RI, Memoli VA, Warren WH. Neuroendocrine components of the bronchopulmonary tract: Hyperplasias, dysplasias, and neoplasms. Lab Invest 1983;49:519–537.

327. Gould VE, Wiedenmann B, Lee I, et al. Synaptophysin expression in neuroendocrine neoplasms as determined by immunocytochemistry. Am J Pathol 1987;126:243–257.

328. Hammar S, Gould VE. Neuroendocrine neoplasms. In: Azar HA, ed. Pathology of human neoplasms: an atlas of diagnostic electron microscopy and immunohistochemistry. New York: Raven Press, 1988: 333–404.

329. Barnes PJ, Baranivk JN, Belvisi MG. Neuropeptides in the respiratory tract. Am Rev Respir Dis 1991; 144(1):1187–1198; (2):1391–1399.

330. Haimoto H, Takahashi Y, Koshikawa T, Nagura H, Kato K. Immunohistochemical localization of γ-enolase in normal human tissues other than nervous and neuroendocrine tissues. Lab Invest 1985;52:257–263.

331. Pahlman S, Esscher T, Nilsson K. Expression of γ-subunit of enolase, neuron-specific enolase in human non-neuroendocrine tumors and derived cell lines. Lab Invest 1986;54:554–560.

332. Vinores SA, Bonnin JM, Rubinstein LJ, Marangos PJ. Immunohistochemical demonstration of neuron-specific enolase in neoplasms of the CNS and other tissues. Arch Pathol Lab Med 1984;120:186–192.

333. Bergh J, Escher T, Steinholtz L, Nilsson K, Pahlman S. Immunocytochemical demonstration of neuron-specific enolase (NSE) in human lung cancers. Am J Clin Pathol 1985;84:1–7.

334. Said JW, Vimadalal S, Nash G, et al. Immunoreactive neuron-specific enolase, bombesin, and chromogranin as markers for neuroendocrine lung tumors. Hum Pathol 1985;16:236–240.

335. Schmechel DE. γ-subunit of the glycolytic enzyme enolase: nonspecific or neuron specific? Lab Invest 1985; 52:239–242.

336. O'Connor DT, Burton D, Deftos LJ. Immunoreactive human chromogranin A in diverse polypeptide hormone producing human tumors and normal endocrine tissues. J Clin Endocrinol Metab 1983;57:1084–1086.

337. Lloyd RV, Wilson BS, Kovacs K, Ryan N. Immunohistochemical localization of chromogranin in human hypophyses and pituitary adenomas. Arch Pathol Lab Med 1985;109:515–517.

338. McNutt MA, Bolen JW. Adenomatous tumor of the middle ear. Am J Clin Pathol 1985;84:541–547.

339. Bussolati G, Gugliotta P. Sapino A, Eusebi V, Lloyd R. Chromogranin-reactive endocrine cells in argyrophilic carcinomas ("carcinoids") from normal tissue of the breast. Am J Pathol 1985;120:186–192.

340. O'Connor DT, Deftos LJ. ecretion of chromogranin A by peptide-producing endocrine neoplasms. N Engl J Med 1986;314:1145–1151.

341. Lloyd RV, Sisson JC, Shapiro B, Verhofstad AAJ. Immunohistochemical localization of epinephrine, norepinephrine, catecholamine-synthesizing enzymes and chromogranin in neuroendocrine cells and tumors. Am J Pathol 1986;125:45–54.

342. Banks P, Helle K. The release of protein from the stimulated adrenal medulla. Biochem J 1965;97:40C–41C.

343. Angeletti RH. Chromogranins and neuroendocrine secretion. Lab Invest 1986;55:387–390.

344. Wilson BS, Lloyd RV. Detection of chromogranin in neuroendocrine cells with a monoclonal antibody. Am J Pathol 1984;115:458–468.

345. Lauweryns JM, vanRanst K, Lloyd RV, et al. Chromogranin in bronchopulmonary neuroendocrine cells: Immunohistochemical detection in human, monkey and pig respiratory mucosa. J Histochem Cytochem 1987;35:113–118.

346. Mukai M, Torikata C, Iri H, et al. Expression of neurofilament triplet proteins in human neural tumor: An immunohistochemical study of paraganglioma, ganglioneuroma, ganglioneuroblastoma and neuroblastoma. Am J Pathol 1986;122:28–36.

347. Shah IA, Schlageter M, Netto D. Immunoreactivity of neurofilament proteins in neuroendocrine neoplasms. Mod Pathol 1991;4:215–219.

348. Leoncini P, DeMarco EB, Bugnoli M. Mencarelli C, Vindigni C, Cintorino M. Expression of phosphorylated and non-phosphorylated neurofilament subunits and cytokeratins in neuroendocrine lung tumors. Pathol Res Pract 1989;185:848–855.

349. Jahn B, Schibler W, Ouimet C, et al. A 38,000 dalton membrane protein (p38) present in synaptic vesicles. Proc Natl Acad Sci USA 1985;82:4137–4141.

350. Gould VE, Lee I, Wiedenmann B, Moll R, Chejfec G, Franke WW. Synaptophysin: A novel marker for neurons, certain neuroendocrine cells and their neoplasms. Hum Pathol 1986;17:979–983.

351. Bunn P, Linnoila I, Minna J, Carney D, Gazdar AF. Small cell cancer, endocrine cells of the fetal bronchus, and other neuroendocrine cells express Leu7 antigenic determinant present on natural killer cells. Blood 1985;65:764–768.

352. Tsutsumi Y. Leu7 immunoreactivity as a histochemical marker for paraffin-embedded neuroendocrine tumors. Acta Histochem Cytochem 1984;17:15.

353. Tischler AS, Mobtaker H, Mann K, et al. Anti-lymphocyte monoclonal antibody HNK-1 (Leu7) recognizes a constituent of neuroendocrine matrix. Lab Invest 1986;54:64A.

354. Komminoth P, Roth J, Lackie PM, Bitter-Suermann D, Heitz PU. Polysialic acid of the neural cell adhesion molecule distinguishes small cell lung carcinoma from carcinoids. Am J Pathol 1991;139:297–304.

355. Kibbelaar RE, Moolenaar CEC, Michalides RJAM, Bitter-Suermann D, Addis BJ, Mooi WJ. Expression of the embryonal neural cell adhesion molecular N-CAM in lung carcinoma. Diagnostic usefulness of monoclonal antibody 735 for the distinction between small cell lung cancer and non-small cell lung cancer. J Pathol 1989;159:23–28.

356. Moolenaar CE, Muller EJ, Schol DJ, Expression of neural cell adhesion molecule-related sialoglycoprotein in small cell lung cancer, and neuroblastoma cell lines H69 and CHP-212. Cancer Res 1990;50:1102–1106.

357. Kahn HJ, Garrido A, Huang S-N, Baumal R. Intermediate filaments and tumor diagnosis. Lab Invest 1983;49:509.

358. Lehto V-P, Stenman S, Miettinen M, Dahl D, Virtanen I. Expression of a neural type of intermediate filament as a distinguishing feature between oat cell carcinoma and other lung cancers. Am J Pathol 1983;110:113–118.

359. VanMuijen GNP, Ruiter DJ, Leeuwen CV, Prins FA, Rietsema K, Warnaar SO. Cytokeratin and neurofilament in lung carcinomas. Am J Pathol 1984;116:363–369.

360. Lehto V-P, Miettinen M, Dahl D, Virtanen I. Bronchial carcinoid cells contain neural-type intermediate filaments. Cancer (Philadelphia) 1984;54:624–628.

361. Clark RK, Miettinen M, Leij L, Damjanov I. Terminally differentiated derivatives of pulmonary small cell carcinomas may contain neurofilaments. Lab Invest 1985; 53:243–244.

362. Broers J, Huysmans A, Moesker O, Vooijs P, Ramaekers F, Wagenaar S. Small cell lung cancer contains intermediate filaments of the cytokeratin type. Lab Invest 1985;52:113–114.

363. Moll R, Franke WW, Schiller DL, et al. The catalogue of human cytokeratins. Patterns of expression in normal epithelia, tumors and cultured cells. Cell 1982;31:11–24.

364. Cooper D, Schermer A, Sun T-T. Classification of

human epithelia and their neoplasms using monoclonal antibodies to keratins: Strategies, applications
and limitations. Lab Invest 1985;52:243–256.

365. Gown AM, Gabbiani G. Intermediate-sized (10-nm)
filaments in human tumors. In: DeLellis, RA, ed.
Advances in immunohistochemistry. New York: Masson, 1984:89–109.

366. Miettinen M, Lehto V-P, Virtanen I. Antibodies to
intermediate filament proteins in the diagnosis and
classification of human tumors. Ultrastruct Pathol
1984;7:83–107.

367. Moll R, Cowin P, Kapprell H-P, Franke WW. Desmosomal proteins: New markers for identification and
classification of tumors. Lab Invest 1986;54:4–25.

368. Funa K, Gazdar AF, Minna JD, Linnoila RI. Paucity of
B2-microglobulin expression on small cell lung cancer,
bronchial carcinoids, and certain other neuroendocrine tumors. Lab Invest 1986;55:186–192.

369. Payne CM, Nagle RB, Borduin V. Methods in laboratory investigation: an ultrastructural cytochemical stain
specific for neuroendocrine neoplasms. Lab Invest
1984;51:350–365.

370. Nagle RB, Payne CM, Clark VA. Comparison of the
usefulness of histochemistry and ultrastructural cytochemistry in the identification of neuroendocrine
neoplasms. Am J Clin Pathol 1986;85:289–296.

371. Gould VE, Benditt EP. Ultrastructural and functional
relationships of some human endocrine tumors. Pathol
Annu 1973;8:205–230.

372. Gould VE. Neuroendocrinomas and neuroendocrine
carcinomas: APUD-cell system neoplasms and their
aberrant secretory activities. Pathol Annu 1977;12
(Part 2):33–62.

373. Sunday ME, Choi N, Spindel ER, Chin WW, Mark EJ.
Gastrin-releasing peptide gene expression in small cell
and large cell undifferentiated carcinomas. Hum
pathol 1991;22:1030–1039.

374. Hamid Q, Corrin B, Sheppard MN, Polak JM. Localization of chromogranin mRNA in small cell carcinoma
of the lung. J Pathol 1991;163:293–297.

375. Frohlich F. Die 'Helle Zelle' der Bronchialschleimhaut
und ihre Beziehungen zum Problem der Chemorecep-
toren. Frankfurt Ztschr Z Pathol 1949;60:517–559.

376. Feyrter F. Zur Pathologie des argyrophilen Helle-Zell-
Organes im Bronchialbaum des Menschen. Virchows
Arch 1954;325:723–732.

377. Bensch KG, Gordon GB, Miller LR. Studies on the
bronchial counterpart of the Kultschitzky (argentaffin)
cell and innervation of bronchial glands. J Ultrastruct
Res 1965;12:668–686.

378. Bensch KG, Gordon GB, Miller LR. Electron microscopic and biochemical studies on the bronchial carcinoid tumor. Cancer 1965;18:592–602.

379. Gmelich JT, Bensch KG, Liebow AA. Cells of Kultch-
itzky type in bronchioles and their relation to the origin
of peripheral carcinoid tumor. Lab Invest 1967;17:
88–98.

380. Lauweryns JM, Cokelaere M. Theunynck PK. Neuroepithelial bodies in the respiratory mucosa of various

mammals: a light optical, histochemical, and ultrastructural investigation. Z Zellforsch Mikrosk Anat 1972;
135:569–592.

381. Lauweryns JM, Goddeeris P. Neuroepithelial bodies in
the human child and adult lung. Am Rev Respir Dis
1975;111:469–476.

382. Johnson DE, Loch JE, Elde RP, Thompson TR. Pulmonary neuroendocrine cells in bronchopulmonary dysplasia and hyaline membrane disease. Pediatr Res
1982;16:446–454.

383. Johnson DE, Wobken JD, Landrum BG. Changes in
bombesin, calcitonin and serotonin immunoreactive
pulmonary neuroendocrine cells in cystic fibrosis and
after prolonged mechanical ventilation. Am Rev Respir
Dis 1988;137:123–131.

384. Stahlman MT, Gray ME. Ontogeny of neuroendocrine
cells in human fetal lung. I. An electron microscopic
study. Lab Invest 1984;51:449–463.

385. Stahlman MT, Kasselberg AG, Orth DN, Gray ME.
Ontogeny of neuroendocrine cells in human feta lung.
II. An immunohistochemical study. Lab Invest
1985;52:52–60.

386. Spindel ER, Sunday ME, Hofler H, Wolfe HJ, Habener
JF, Chin WW. Transient elevation of messenger RNA
encoding gastrin releasing peptide, a putative pulmonary growth factor in human fetal lung. J Clin Invest
1987;80:1172–1179.

387. Sobol RE, O'Connor DT, Addison J, Suchocki K, Roys-
ton I, Deftos LJ. Elevated serum chromogranin A levels
in small cell lung carcinoma. Ann Intern Med
1986;1095:698–700.

388. Gosney JR, Sissons MCJ, Allibone RO, Blakely AF.
Pulmonary endocrine cells in chronic bronchitis and
emphysema. J Pathol 1989;157:127–133.

389. Aguayo SM, King TE, Jr., Waldron JA, Jr., Sherritt
KM, Kane MA, Miller YE. Increased pulmonary neuroendocrine cells with bombesin-like immunoreactivity
in adults with eosinophilic granuloma. J Clin Invest
1989;86:838–844.

390. Aguayo SM, Kane MA, King TE, Jr., Schwarz MI,
Graver L, Miller YE. Increased levels of bombesin-like
peptides in the lower respiratory tract of asymptomatic
cigarette smokers. J Clin Invest 1989;84:1105–1113.

391. Tabassian AR, Nylen ES, Linnoila RI, Snider RH,
Cassidy MM, Becker KL. Stimulation of hamster pulmonary neuroendocrine cells and associated peptides
by repeated exposure to cigarette smoke. Am Rev
Respir Dis 1989;140:436–440.

392. Aguayo SM, Miller YE, Waldron JA, Jr., et al. Brief
report: Idiopathic diffuse hyperplasia of pulmonary
neuroendocrine cells and airways disease. N Engl J
Med 1992;327:1285–1288.

393. Benfield JR. Neuroendocrine neoplasms of the lung. J
Thorac Cardiovasc Surg 1990;100:628–629.

394. Whitwell F. Tumorlets of the lung. J Pathol Bacteriol
1955;70:529–541.

395. Churg A, Warnock ML. Pulmonary tumorlet: A form
of peripheral carcinoid. Cancer (Philadelphia) 1976;
37:1469–1477.

396. Miller MA, Mark J, Kanarek D. Multiple peripheral pulmonary carcinoids and tumorlets of carcinoid type, with restrictive and obstructive lung disease. Am J Med 1978;65:373–378.

397. Pelosi G, Zancanaro C, Sbubo L, Bresaola E, Martignoni G, Bontempini L. Development of innumerable neuroendocrine tumorlets in pulmonary lobe scarred by intralobular sequestration: Immunohistochemical and ultrastructural study of an unusual case. Arch Pathol Lab Med 1992;116:1167–1174.

398. D'Aggti VD, Perzin KH. Carcinoid tumorlets of the lung with metastasis to a peribronchial lymph node: report of a case and review of the literature. Cancer (Philadelphia) 1985;55:2472–2476.

399. Mueller H. Zur Untersuchungsgeschichte der bronchialen Weiterungen. Inaug Diss Halle, 1882.

400. Kramer R. Adenoma of bronchus. Ann Otol Rhinol Laryngol 1930;39:689–695.

401. Hamperl H. Über gutartige Bronchialtumoren. Virchows Arch [Pathol Anat] 1937;300:1937:46–88.

402. Oberndorfer S. Karzinoide Tumoren des Diinndarms. Frankfurt Zeitschr Pathol 1907;1:426–432.

403. Briselli M, Mark GJ, Grillo HC. Tracheal carcinoids. Cancer (Philadelphia) 1978;42:2870–2879.

404. Bonikos DS, Bensch KG, Jamplis RW. Peripheral pulmonary carcoinoid tumors. Cancer (Philadelphia) 1976;37:1977–1998.

405. Felton WL, Liebow AA, Lindskog GE. Peripheral and multiple bronchial adenomas. Cancer (Philadelphia) 1953;6:555–567.

406. Skinner C, Ewen SWB. Carcinoid lung: diffuse pulmonary infiltration by a multifocal bronchial carcinoid. Thorax 1976;31:212–219.

407. Abdi EA, Goel R, Bishop S, Bain GO. Peripheral carcinoid tumours of the lung: A clinicopathological study. J Surg Oncol 1988;39:190–196.

408. Carter D, Eggleston JC, Carcinoid tumors. In: Tumors of the lower respiratory tract. Atlas of tumor pathology, 2d Ser., Fasc. 17. Washington, DC: Armed Forces Institute of Pathology, 1980:162–188.

409. Mark EJ, Quay SC, Dickensin GR. Papillary carcinoid tumor of the lung. Cancer (Philadelphia) 1981;48:316–324.

410. Ranchod M, Levine GD. Spindle cell carcinoid tumors of the lung: A clinicopathologic study of 35 cases. Am J Surg Pathol 1980;4:315–331.

411. Sklar JL, Churg A, Bensch KG. Oncocytic carcinoid tumor of the lung. Am J Surg Pathol 1980;4:287–292.

412. Sajjad SM, Mackay B, Lukeman JM. Oncocytic carcinoid tumor of the lung. Ultrastruct Pathol 1980;1:171–176.

413. Scharifker D, Marchevsky A. Oncocytic carcinoid of lung: an ultrastructural analysis. Cancer (Philadelphia) 1981;47:530–532.

414. Ghadially FN, Block HJ. Oncocytic carcinoid of the lung. J Submicrosc Cytol 1985;17:435–442.

415. Santos-Briz, Terron J, Sastre R, Romero L, Valle A. Oncocytoma of the lung. Cancer 1977;40:1330–1336.

416. Cebelin MS. Melanocytic bronchial carcinoid tumor. Cancer (Philadelphia) 1980;46:1843–1848.

417. Grazer R, Cohen SM, Jacobs JB, Lucas P. Melanin-containing peripheral carcinoid of the lung. Am J Surg Pathol 1982;6:73–78.

418. Carlson JA, Dickersin GR. Melanocytic paraganglioid carcinoid tumor: A case report and review of the literature. Ultrapathol (in press).

419. Barbareschi M, Frigo B, Mosca L, et al. Bronchial carcinoids with S100 positive sustenatacular cells. Pathol Res Pract 1990;186:212–217.

420. Capella C, Gabrielli M, Polak JM, Buffa R, Solcia E. Ultrastructural and histological study of 11 bronchial carcinoids. Virchows Arch Pathol Anat [A] 1979;381:313–329.

421. Barbareschi M, Frigo B, Cristina S, Valentini L, Leonardi E, Mosca L. Bronchial carcinoid with paranuclear fibrillary inclusions related to cytokeratins and vimentin. Virchows Arch [A] Pathol Anat 1989;415:31–36.

422. Arrigoni MG, Woolner LB, Bernatz PE. Atypical carcinoid tumors of the lung. J Thorac Cardiovasc Surg 1972;64:413–421.

423. Leschke H. Über nur regionär bösartige und über krebsig entartete Bronchusadenome bzw. Carcinoide. Virchows Arch [Path Anat] 1956;328:635–657.

424. Warren WH, Memoli VA, Gould VE. Immunohistochemical and ultrastructural analysis of bronchopulmonary neuroendocrine neoplasms. II. Well-differentiated neuroendocrine carcinomas. Ultrastruct Pathol 1984;7:185–199.

425. Mark EJ, Ramirez JF. Peripheral small-cell carcinoma of the lung resembling carcinoid tumor: A clinical and pathologic study of 14 cases. Arch Pathol Lab Med 1985;109:263–269.

426. Paladugu RR, Benfield JR, Pak HY, Ross RK, Teplitz RL. Bronchopulmonary kulchitzky cell carcinomas. Cancer (Philadelphia) 1985;55:1303–1311.

427. Tsutsumi Y, Yazaki K, Yoshioka K. Atypical carcinoid tumor of the lung, associated with giant cell transformation in bone metastases.

428. Hammar S, Bockus D, Remington F, Cooper L. The unusual spectrum of neuroendocrine lung neoplasms. Ultra Pathol 1989;13(5,6):515–560.

429. Gould VE, Chejfec G. Ultrastructural and biochemical analysis of pulmonary "undifferentiated" carcinomas. Hum Pathol 1978;9:377–384.

430. McDowell EM, Wilson TS, Trump BF. Atypical endocrine tumors of the lung. Arch Pathol Lab Med 1981;105:20–28.

431. Hammond ME, Sause WT. Large cell neuroendocrine tumors of the lung: Clinical significance and histopathologic definition. Cancer (Philadelphia) 1985;56:1624–1629.

432. Neal MH, Kosinki R, Cohen P, Orenstein JM. Atypical endocrine tumors of the lung: a histologic, ultrastructural and clinical study of 19 cases. Hum Pathol 1986;17:1264–1277.

433. Barbareschi M, Mariscotti C, Barberis M, Frigo B, Mosca L. Large cell neuroendocrine carcinoma of the lung. Tumori 1989;75:583–588.

434. Travis WD, Linnoila I, Tsokos MG, et al. Neuroendo-crine tumors of the lung with proposed criteria for large cell neuroendocrine carcinoma: An ultrastruc-tural, immunohistochemical and flow cytometric study of 35 cases. Am J Surg Pathol 1991;15:529–533.

435. Wick MR, Berg LC, Hertz MI. Large cell carcinoma of the lung with neuroendocrine differentiation; a com-parison with large cell "undifferentiated" pulmonary tumors. Am J Clin Pathol 1992;987:796–805.

436. Mooi WJ, Dewar A, Springall D, Polak JM, Addis BJ. Non-small cell lung carcinomas with neuroendocrine features: A light microscopic, immunohistochemical and ultrastructural study of 11 cases. Histopathology 1988;13:329–337.

437. Vosika GJ. Large cell bronchogenic carcinoma: Pro-longed disease-free survival following chemotherapy. JAMA 1979;241:594–595.

438. Gibbs FA. Lymphoma versus carcinoma. JAMA 1979;242:514.

439. Vosika GJ. Large cell—small cell bronchogenic carci-noma. JAMA 1979;242:1259–1260.

440. Bernard WG. The nature of the "oat-celled sarcoma" of the mediastinum. J Pathol Bacteriol 1926;29:241–244.

441. Gibbon JH Jr, Nealon TF Jr. Neoplasms of the lungs and trachea. In: Gibbon JH Jr, ed. Surgery of the chest. Philadelphia: Saunders, 1962:484.

442. Azzopardi JG. Oat-cell carcinoma of the bronchus. J Pathol Bacteriol 1959;78:513–519.

443. Yesner R. Small cell tumors of the lung. Am J Surg Pathol 1983;7:775–785.

444. Carter D. Small-cell carcinoma of the lung. Am J Surg Pathol 1983;7:787–795.

445. Yesner R. Classification of long-cancer histology. N Engl J Med 1985;312:652–653.

446. Stuart-Harris R, Boyer M, Greenberg M, Stevens S, Yung T. The histopathological classification of small cell lung cancer: Application of the IASLC classifica-tion in 124 cases. Lung Cancer 1992;8:63–70.

447. Gazdar AF, Carney DN, Baylin SB, et al. Small cell carcinoma of the lung. Altered morphological, biolog-ical and biochemical characteristics in long term cul-tures and heterotransplanted tumors. Proc Am Assoc Cancer Res 1980;21:51.

448. Fushimi H, Kihui M, Morino H, et al. Detection of large cell component in small cell lung carcinoma by com-bined cytologic and histologic examinations and its clinical implications. Cancer (Philadelphia) 1992;70:599–605.

449. Visscher DW, Zarbo RJ, Trojanowski JQ, Sakr W, Crissman JD. Neuroendocrine differentiation in poor-ly-differentiated lung carcinomas: a light microscopic and immunohistologic study. Mod Pathol 1990;3:508–512.

450. Linnoila RI, Mulshine JL, Steinberg SM, et al. Neu-roendocrine differentiation in endocrine and nonen-docrine lung carcinomas. Am J Clin Pathol 1988;90:641–652.

451. Chute CG, Greenberg ER, Baron J, Korson R, Baker J,

452. Yates J. Presenting conditions of 1539 population-based lung cancer patients by cell type and stage in New Hampshire and Vermont. Cancer (Philadelphia) 1985;56:2107–2111.

452. Andersen HA, Bernatz PE. Extrathoracic manifesta-tions of bronchogenic carcinoma. Med Clin N Am 1964;48:921–931.

453. Mountain CF, Lukeman JM, Hammar S, et al. Lung cancer classification: The relationship of disease extent and cell type to survival in a trial population. J Surg Oncol 1987;35:147–156.

454. Okike N, Bernatz PE, Woolner LB. Carcinoid tumors of the lung. Ann Thorac Surg 1976;22:270–275.

455. Brandt B, Heintz SE, Rose EF, Ehrenhaft JL. Bronchial carcinoid tumors. Ann Thorac Surg 1984;38:63–65.

456. McCaughan BC, Martini N, Bains MS. Bronchial carci-noids: Review of 124 cases. J Thorac Cardiovasc Surg 1985;89:8–17.

457. Thunnissen FBJM, van Eijk J, Baak JPA, Schipper NW, Uyterlinde AM, Breederveld RS, Meijer S. Bron-chopulmonary carcinoids and regional node me-tastases: a quantitative pathologic investigation. Am J Pathol 1988;132:119–122.

458. Warren WH, Gould VE. Long-term follow-up of clas-sical bronchial carcinoid tumors. Scan J Thor Cardio-vasc Surg 1990;24:125–130.

459. El-Naggar A, Ballance W, Abdu Karim FW, Ordonez NG, McLemore D, Giacco GG, Batsakis JG. Typical and atypical bronchopulmonary carcinoids: A clinico-pathologic and flow cytometric study. Am J Clin Pathol 1991;95:828–834.

460. Yousem SA, Taylor SR. Typical and atypical carcinoid tumors of lung: A clinicopathologic and DNA analysis of 20 tumors. Mod Pathol 1990;3:502–507.

461. Bernstein C, McGoey J, Lertzman M. Recurrent bron-chial carcinoid tumor. Chest 1989;95:693–694.

462. Greengard O, Head JF, Goldberg SL, Kirschner PA. Pulmonary carcinoid tumors: Enzymic discriminants, growth rate and early age of inception. Cancer Res 1986;46:2600–2605.

463. Yousem SA. Pulmonary carcinoid tumors and well differentiated neuroendocrine carcinomas: Is there room for atypical carcinoid? Am J Cln Pathol 1991;95:828–834.

464. Warren WH, Memoli VA, Jordan AG, Gould VE., Reevaluation of pulmonary neoplasms as small cell neuroendocrine carcinomas. Cancer 1990;65:1003–1010.

465. Larsimont D, Kiss R, deLaunoit Y, Melamed MR. Characterization of the morphonuclear features and DNA ploidy of typical and atypical carcinoids and small cell cell carcinomas of the lung. Am J Clin Pathol 1990; 94:378–373.

466. Lequaglie C, Patriarca C, Cataldo I, Muscolino G, Preda F, Ravasi G. Prognosis of resected well-differen-tiated neuroendocrine carcinoma of the lung. Chest 1991;100:1053–1056.

467. Memoli VA. Well-differentiated neuroendocrine carci-

noma: A designation comes of age. Chest 1991; 100:892.

468. Jackson-York GL, Davis GH, Warren WH, Gould VE, Memoli VA. Flow cytometric DNA content analysis in neuroendocrine carcinoma of the lung: Correlation with survival and histologic subtype. Cancer (Philadelphia) 1991;68:374–379.

469. Quoix E, Fraser R, Wolkove N, Finkelstein H, Kreisman H. Small cell lung cancer presenting as a solitary pulmonary nodule. Cancer (Philadelphia) 1990;66:577–582.

470. Kreisman H, Wolkove N, Quoix E. Small cell lung cancer presenting as a solitary pulmonary nodule. Chest 1992;101:225–229.

471. Shepherd FA, Ginsberg R, Evans WK, Haddad R, Feld R, DeBoer G. "Very limited" small cell lung cancer: Results of nonsurgical treatment. Proc Am Soc Clin Oncol 1984;3:223–228.

472. Gephardt GN, Grady KJ, Ahmad M, Tubbs RR, Mehta ACl, Shepard KV. Peripheral small cell undifferentiated carcinoma of the lung: Clinicopathologic features of 17 cases. Cancer (Philadelphia) 1988;61:1002–1008.

473. Fraire AE, Johnson EH, Yesner R, Zhang XB, Spjut HJ, Greenberg SD. Prognostic significance of histopathologic subtype and stage in small cell lung cancer. Hum Pathol 1992;23:520–528.

474. Bepler G, Neumann K, Holle R, Havemann K, Kalbfleisch H. Clinical relevance of histologic subtyping in small cell lung cancer. Cancer (Philadelphia) 1989; 64:74–79.

475. Crown JPA, Chahinian AP, Jaffrey IS, Glidewell OJ, Kaneko M, Holland JR. Predictors of 5-year survival and curability in small cell lung cancer. Cancer (Philadelphia) 1990;66:382–386.

476. Albain KS, Crowley JJ, Livingston RB. Long-term survival and toxicity in small cell lung cancer: Expanded Southwest Oncology Group experience. Chest 1991;99:1425–1432.

477. Oud PS, Pahlplatz MM, Beck LM, Wiersma-Van Tilburg A, Wagenaar SJ, Vooijs GP. Cancer (Philadelphia) 1989;64:1304–1309.

478. Funa K, Steinholtz L, Nov E, Bergh J. Increased expression of N-myc in human small cell lung cancer biopsies predicts lack of response to chemotherapy. Am J Clin Pathol 1987;88:216–220.

479. Copple B, Wright SE, Moatamed F. Electron microscopy in small cell lung carcinomas: Clinical correlation. J Clin Oncol 1984;2:910–916.

480. Vollmer RT, Shelburne JD, Iglehart JD. Intercellular junctions and tumor stage in small cell carcinoma of the lung. Hum Pathol 1986;18:22–27.

481. Elson CE, Roggli VL, Vollmer RT, Greenberg SD, Fraire AE, Spjut HJ, Yesner R. Prognostic indicators for survival in stage I carcinoma of the lung: A histologic study of 47 surgically resected cases. Mod Pathol 1988;1:288–291.

482. Shahab I, Fraire AE, Greenberg SD, Johnson EH, Langston C, Roggli VL. Morphometric quantitation of tumor necrosis in stage I non-small cell carcinoma of

lung: Prognostic implications. Mod Pathol 1992; 5:521–524.

483. Cagle PT, Langston C, Fraire AE, Roggli VL, Greenberg SD. Absence of correlation between nuclear morphometry and survival in stage I non-small cell lung carcinoma. Cancer (Philadelphia) 1992;69:2454–2457.

484. Gallagher B, Urbanski SJ. The significance of pleural elastica invasion by lung carcinomas. Hum Pathol 1990;21:512–517.

485. Ratto GB, Frola C, Sacco G, Motta G. The prognostic significance of minor pleural effusions in patients with potentially operable bronchogenic carcinoma. Lung Cancer 1987;3:117–122.

486. Yoshimoto T, Higashino K, Hada T, et al. A primary lung carcinoma producing alpha-fetoprotein, carcinoembryonic antigen and human chorionic-gonadotropin. Cancer (Philadelphia) 1987;60:2744–2750.

487. Kuida CA, Braunstein GD, Shintaku P, Said JW. Human chorionic-gonadotropin expression in lung, breast, and renal carcinomas. Arch Pathol Lab Med 1988;112:282–285.

488. Beattie CW, Hansen NW, Thomas PA. Steroid receptors in human lung cancer. Cancer Res 1985;45:4206–4214.

489. Baltifora H, Sorensen HR, Mehta P, et al. Tumor-associated antigen 43-9F is of prognostic value in squamous cell carcinoma of the lung. Cancer 1992;70:1867–1872.

490. Poulakis N. Sarandakou S, Rizos D, Phocas I, Kontozoglou T, Polyzogopoulos D. Soluble interleukin-2-receptors and other markers in primary lung cancer. Cancer (Philadelphia) 1991;68:1045–1049.

491. Miyake M, Taki T, Hitomi S, Hakomori S. Correlation of expression of H/Le-y/Le-b antigens with survival in patients with carcinoma of the lung. N Engl J Med 1992;327:14–18.

492. Buccheri G, Ferrigno D. Prognostic value of the tissue polypetide antigen in lung cancer. Chest 1992; 101:1287–1292.

493. Cline MJ, Battifora H. Abnormalities of protooncogenes in non-small cell lung cancer: Correlations with tumor type and clinical characteristics. Cancer (Philadelphia) 1987;60:2669–2674.

494. Harada M, Dosaka-Akita H, Miyamoto H, Kuzumaki N, Kawakami Y. Prognostic significance of the expression of ras oncogene product in non-small cell lung cancer. Cancer 1992;69:72–77.

495. Caamano J, Ruggeri B, Momiki S, Sickler A, Zhang SY, Klein-Szanto AJP. Detection of p53 in primary lung tumors and non-small cell lung carcinoma cell lines. Am J Pathol 1991;139:839–845.

496. Porter PL, Gown AM, Kramp SG, Coltrea MD. Widespread p53 overexpression in human malignant tumors: An immunohistochemical study using methacarn-fixed, embedded tissue. Am J Pathol 1992; 140:145–152.

497. Slebos RJC, Kibbelaar RE, Dalesio O, et al. K-ras oncogene activation as a prognostic marker in adenocarcinoma of the lung. N Engl J Med 1990;323:561–565.

498. ten Velde GPM, Havenith MG. Volovics A, Bosman FT. Prognostic significance of basement membrane deposition in operable squamous cell carcinomas of the lung. Cancer (Philadelphia) 1991;67:3001–3005.

499. Nagamoto N, Saito Y, Ohta S. Relationship of lymph node metastasis to primary tumor size and microscopic appearance of roentgenographically occult lung cancer. Am J Surg Pathol 1989;13:1009–1013.

500. Atsushi T, Kodama T, Shimosato Y, Watanabe S, Suemasu K. Histopathologic prognostic factors in adenocarcinomas of the peripheral lung less than 2 cm in diameter. Cancer (Philadelphia) 1988;61:2083–2088.

501. Ohori NP, Yousem SA, Griffin J, et al. Comparison of extracellular matrix antigens in subtypes of bronchioloalveolar carcinoma and conventional pulmonary adenocarcinoma: An immunohistochemical study. Am J Surg Pathol 1992;16:675–686.

502. Delmomte VC, Alberti O, Saldiva PHN. Large cell carcinoma of the lung-ultrastructural and immunohistochemical features. Chest 1986;90:524–527.

503. Albain KS, True LD, Golomb HM, Hoffman PC, Little AG. Large cell carcinoma of the lung: Ultrastructural differentiation and clinicopathologic correlations. Cancer (Philadelphia) 1985;56:1618–1623.

504. Coon JS, Landay AL, Weinstein RS. Biology of disease: Advances in flow cytometry for diagnostic pathology. Lab Invest 1987;57:453–479.

505. Wersto RP, Liblit RL, Koss LG. Flow cyctometric DNA analysis of human solid tumors: A review of the interpretation of DNA histograms. Hum Pathol 1991; 22:1085–1098.

506. Frierson HF, Jr. The need for improvement in flow cytometric analysis of ploidy and S-phase fraction. Am J Clin Pathol 1991;96:439–441.

507. Zimmerman PV, Bint MH, Hawson GAT, Parsons PG. Ploidy as a prognostic determinant in surgically treated lung cancer. Lancet 1987;ii:530–533.

508. Tirindelli-Danesi D, Teodori L, Mauro F, et al. Prognostic significance of flow cytometry in lung cancer: A 5-year study. Cancer (Philadelphia) 1987;60:844–851.

509. Asamura H, Nakajima T, Mukai K, Noguchi M, Shimosato Y. DNA cytofluorometric and nuclear morphometric analyses of lung adenocarcinoma. Cancer (Philadephia) 1989;64:1657–1664.

510. Salvati F, Teodori L, Gagliiardi L, Signora M, Aquilini M, Storniello G. DNA flow cytometric studies of 66 human lung tumors analyzed before treatment: Prognostic implications. Chest 1989;96:1092–1098.

511. Carey FA, Lamb B, Bird CC. Intramural heterogeneity of DNA content in lung cancer. Cancer (Philadelphia) 1991;64:2266–2269.

512. Schmidt RA, Rusch VW, Piantadosi S. A flow cytometric study of non-small cell lung cancer classified as T_1N_0. Cancer (Philadelphia) 1992;69:78–85.

513. Filderman AE, Silvestri GA, Gatsonis C, Lithringer DJ, Honig J, Flynn SD. Prognostic significance of tumor proliferative fraction and DNA content in stage I non-small cell lung cancer. Am Rev Respir Dis 1992; 146:707–710.

514. Ogawa J, Tsurmi T, Inove H, Shohtsu A. Relationship between tumor DNA ploidy and regional lymph node changes in lung cancer. Cancer (Philadelphia) 1992; 69:1688–1695.

515. Ogura S, Abe S, Sukoh N, Kunikane H, Nakajima I, Inoue K, Kawakami Y. Correlation between nucleolar organizer regions visualized by silver staining and the growth rate in lung adenocarcinoma. Cancer (Philadelphia) 1992;70:63–68.

CHAPTER 33

Uncommon Tumors

DAVID H. DAIL

With the exception of hamartomas, most of the tumors described in this chapter occur so infrequently that the average pathologist may only remember seeing one of these a few years ago or be aware they occur without ever having seen a case of his or her own. Within the different groups, the frequency of occurrence varies. A few are rare lesions with only one or two case reports. Nearly 300 cases of some other lesions, such as the plasma cell granuloma—histiocytoma complex, have been described in the lung. Perhaps it is because these tumors are infrequent and yet create reproducibly distinct patterns of tumor growth that they arouse curiosity as if each "has a story to tell." They cause the pathologist to search for books and articles describing their distinctive characteristics, knowing each is, or should be, characteristic of something with a name.

Most lesions described in this chapter are tumor masses. Of the entire group, hamartomas are the most frequent; they accounted for 100 of 130 (77%) benign tumors in the lung summarized in a 10-year experience from Mayo Clinic by Arrigoni et al.[1] in 1970. As "common" as they may sound, in absolute terms even hamartomas sadly trail far behind, by my estimate, by a factor of 20:1 or so, the large volume of common malignancies that are covered in Chapter 32.

Benign glandular spaces are present in several of the tumors that will be considered in this chapter. They are considered by some to be inherent components of such tumors, and it is important at the start of this discussion to clarify this misconception. Some have used these spaces to try to distinguish central chondromas from peripheral hamartomas, and fibroleiomyomatous hamartomas from mestatasizing leiomyomas. They have also been used to suggest a glandular origin for sclerosing hemangiomas. These inclusions represent en-trapped bronchiolar lining cells or metaplastic alveolar lining cells, are incidental in the lesions listed in Table 33–1, and are not part of the neoplastic process. These benign entrapped linings should be separated from truly neoplastic glandular spaces, such as in adenocarcinomas (Chapter 32), or as further discussed in this chapter with pulmonary blastomas or bronchial gland tumors.

The cell or origin of some of these lesions is well defined, while in others it is quite obscure. Better names may be formulated for some tumors as their cells of origin are identified. Examples of those remaining enigmas include sclerosing hemangioma and alveolar adenomas; the tumor cells of benign sugar tumors, chemodectoma-like bodies, and plasma cell granulomas are becoming better characterized.

Several other monographs or texts discuss uncommon lung tumors,[2–15] and several of these are most helpful.[9,12–15] The historical aspects are emphasized by some.[2,3,6]

This chapter covers epithelial and mesenchymal lesions, beginning in the trachea and then continuing to bronchi and lung parenchyma. Common and uncommon pleural tumors are discussed separately in Chapter 34.

Tracheal Tumors

The trachea is such a natural introduction to the lower respiratory tract that it seems appropriate to introduce this chapter with tumors of this region. The trachea is subject to many of the same tumors of the lungs and bronchi that are discussed, and cross reference is given in those sections to similar tumors in the trachea. How-

be more frequent in other locations where salivary glands exist; instead, they are most frequent in the gastrointestinal tract. Most of these tumors in the lung are within reach of the flexible bronchoscope, but biopsy may be hazardous because of their extensive vascular supply. These tumors are discussed more thoroughly in Chapter 32.

In the series of "mucous gland" tumors by Payne et al.[44] in 1964, 124 carcinoid tumors (91% of all), 4 adenoid cystic carcinomas (5% of all and 58% of noncarcinoid tumors), 4 mucoepidermoid tumors (3% of all and 33% of noncarcinoid tumors), and 1 mixed tumor of salivary gland type (0.7% of all and 8% of noncarcinoid tumors) were present. In the 50-year Mayo Clinic experience reviewed by Conlan et al.[45] in 1978, during which time 236 typical carcinoid and 30 atypical carcinoid tumors were seen in lung, bronchi, and trachea, 20 adenoid cystic and 12 mucoepidermoid tumors occurred in these locations. In the series by Spencer[46] based on consultations collected to 1979, he reported on 10 adenoid cystic carcinomas (38% of all), 8 mucoepidermoid tumors (31% of all), 5 cystadenomas (19% of all), 2 mixed tumors of salivary gland type (8% of all), and 1 oxyphil adenoma (4% of all). Several authors[46–48] have estimated that these tumors as a group account for about 0.2%–0.5% of all primary lung tumors. The individual types are discussed, and the reader is also referred to the section on tracheal tumors that precedes this section.

Adenoid Cystic Carcinoma

Adenoid cystic carcinomas were originally called "cylindromas," a term now discarded. Within the tracheobronchial system these are the most common bronchial gland tumor in the trachea and account for some 20%–35% of all tracheal tumors,[21,25,49–51] and 75%–80% of tracheobronchial gland tumors.[19] A 1988 series of 12 of these lesions, 9 in the trachea and 3 in mainstem bronchi, was presented by Nomori et al.[52] When in the lung, they are usually in the central bronchi and are infrequent more distally,[53,54] unless they represent metastases from another site. They may present as nodules within, or a generalized constriction of, the major airways. They have a tendency to grow in linear fashion along the tracheobronchial walls.[44,46,55] This tendency is in contrast to carcinoid tumors and mucoepidermoid tumors, which have a tendency to be nodular.[44]

Symptoms, usually resulting from partial airway obstruction, include wheezing, progressive shortness of breath, and hemoptysis. Hemoptysis is caused by surface ulceration, but may also be related to effects of more distal obstruction (see Chapter 5). These obstructive symptoms may include chronic cough, which becomes more productive, fever, and general cachexia. As in the trachea, radiographs may miss the centrally placed tumors but may detect the effects of distal obstruction. Computerized tomography and magnetic resonance scans work well in the central areas to distinguish solid masses from air-containing structures.[25] These patients range in age from 18 to 82 years, with an average in most series of 45-47 years. Men and women are about equally represented, and tobacco exposure is not a risk factor in this tumor.[25]

Grossly, the tumor masses are rubbery to quite firm and pink-tan to gray-white. Although the masses are always infiltrative, Nomori et al.[52] have divided these into three groups: those that are grossly polypoid with minimum infiltration of walls, these usually being less aggressive; those both polypoid and infiltrative, intermediate in behavior; and those predominantly infiltrative and extralumenal, the most aggressive group. Sometimes it is difficult to identify remnant lumens (Fig. 33–1). Direct extension in adjacent structures, including nodes, may occur, usually in higher grade solid tumors (see following). This same group of high-grade tumors has a greater tendency toward radial spread to adjacent lung than linear spread along the bronchi and trachea.[52]. This lung tumor usually infiltrates the adjacent lung in continuity with the edge of infiltration, but may have lymphatic extension away from the main tumor mass. Because of the late detection of many of these tumors, spread may be more extensive than at first anticipated.

Histologically, these tumors may infiltrate bronchi in a radial fashion and encase vessels (Fig. 33–2). They appear identical to those in the salivary gland tissue, with compact nuclei, relatively high nuclear/cytoplasmic ratio, cysts rather evenly contoured but of varying caliber within larger tubules of tumor (Figs. 33–3 and 33–4), and a stroma that is often hyalinized. Mitoses and necrosis are uncommon. The larger cystic spaces contain hyaluronidase-sensitive, alcian-blue-positive mucin, while the small rather indistinct true glandular spaces contain periodic acid–Schiff- (PAS-) positive, diastase-resistant, neutral to weakly acidic mucin. A combined alcian blue/PAS stain nicely highlights these characteristics. Duplicated and thickened PAS-positive basal lamina often surrounds the columns of tumor cells. Three different microscopic patterns are recognized here[52] as in the salivary glands,[56–58] and include tubular-trabecular, the most typical intermediate cribriform-microcystic, with no more than 20% solid component, and a poorly differentiated category with greater than 20% solid component. In general the histological grades compare with the three gross appearance described. As noted in the Nomori et al.[52] series, normal tracheobronchial glands have serous, but

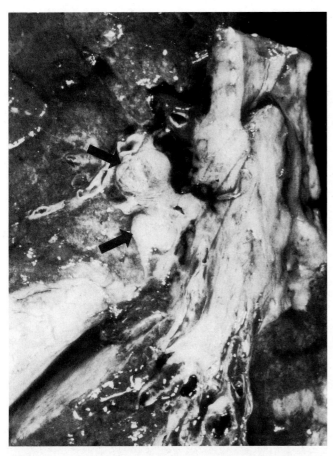

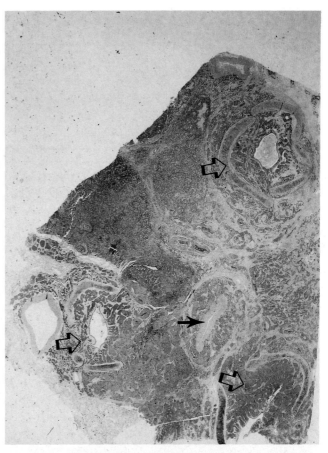

Fig. 33–1. Adenoid cystic carcinoma. A very firm tumor mass extends into lower lobe from mainstem bronchus. Extensions into upper lobe (*arrows*) show dense cores of tumor with minimal evidence of remaining bronchial lumens. Note polypoid nature of tumor proximally yet thickening of adjacent proximal bronchial wall by tumor.

Fig. 33–2. Adenoid cystic carcinoma. Low-power view shows three bronchi with radial involvement by tumor (*open arrows*), along with one artery (*solid arrow*) with perivascular cuffing. H and E, ×10.

not much mucous, cell stain with secretory component (SC), S100 protein, lactoferrin, and cytokeratin, and myoepithelial cells of the acini and epithelial cells of the ducts stain intensely with cytokeratins. The tubular and cribriform components of adenoid cystic carcinoma stain positively but variably for SC, S100 lactoferrin, and cytokeratin. The solid components did not stain with these antigens. A similar immunoperoxidase study of five tracheobronchial adenoid cystic carcinomas by Ishida et al.[59] generally confirmed these findings. These tumors are occasionally diagnosed by aspiration cytology, but the material is usually submucosal so an abrasive or extractive technique must be used.[60]

These tumors have an interesting tendency to form in linear strands around nerves (Fig. 33–5), as is characteristic of these tumors elsewhere. The cartilage may be easily circumvented by the tumor, but cartilaginous erosion also occurs. Lymphatic spaces may be infil-

trated, and the nodes may be directly infiltrated eccentrically toward the side of the tumor mass.

Occasional metastases have been described to regional nodes,[61] and rare extrathoracic spread may be to liver, bone, adrenal glands,[46] and kidney. One very aggressive tracheal case with widespread metastases has already been discussed.[41] When the tumor is resectable long survival may result, but recurrences in the local region are a problem, and have occurred up to 17 years later[62] in the bronchi and 25 and 30 years later in the trachea.[21] Radiotherapy may cause some shrinkage of the tumor mass, but nonsurgical cure is difficult, if possible at all. Obtaining clear surgical margins may be difficult at attempted resection, because the tumor tends to spread along the course of the bronchus and/or trachea, often well beyond that grossly visible, and even CT scans tend to underestimate the extent of intramural spread.[23] Perhaps some of the newer treatment

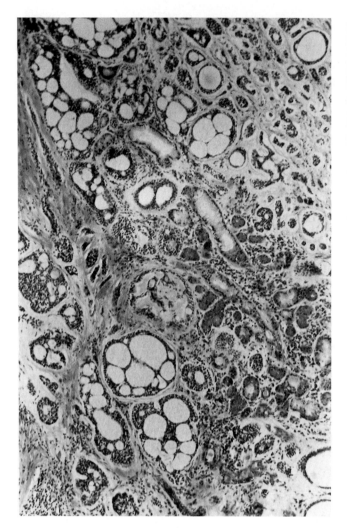

Fig. 33–3. Adenoid cystic carcinoma. Typical-appearing well-differentiated tumor is infiltrating submucosal gland in center. H and E, ×100.

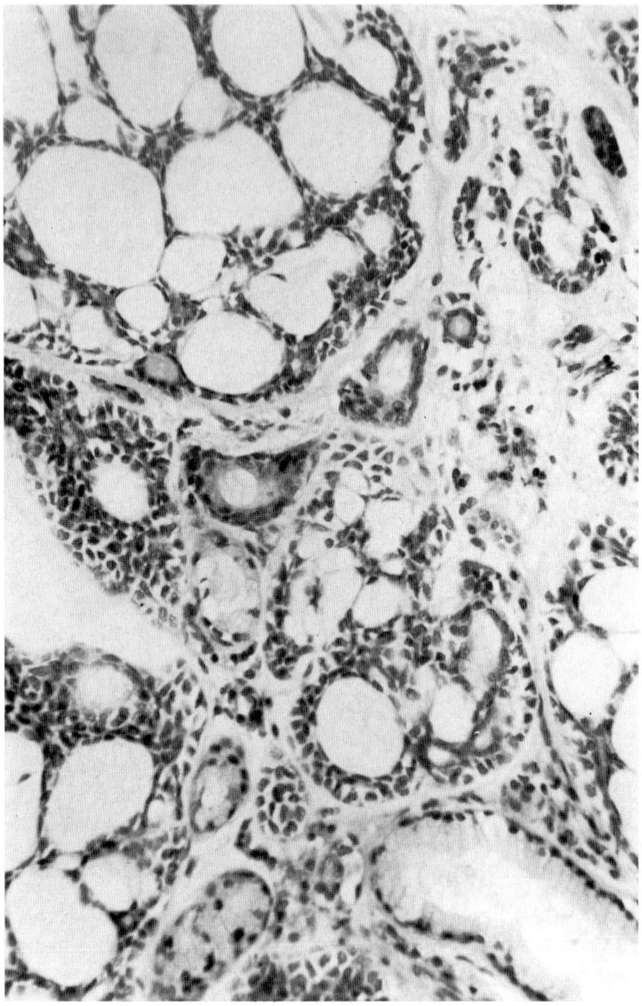

Fig. 33–4. Adenoid cystic carcinoma. High-power view of top left of Fig. 29–3 shows typical intermediate cells and cysts of adenoid cystic carcinoma. H and E. ×400.

protocols with neutron beam therapy or combined radiotherapy and chemotherapy may be helpful. YAG laser therapy may help preserve luminal patency in unresectable cases.[63]

The differential diagnosis of this tumor often includes other carcinomas, mostly adenocarcinomas. The monotony of the tumor cells and their generally stiff-appearing mucinous spaces and separation of often hylanized stroma are helpful indicators of adenoid cystic carcinoma when they are present. Some poorly differentiated carcinomas suggest they may have been adenoid cystic carcinomas, but I prefer calling these poorly differentiated adenocarcinomas with focal adenoid cystic areas. When more solid sheets of tumor cells are seen they may be mistaken for possible oat cell carcinoma, but their chromatin pattern is not as homogeneous and there is more euchromatin evident than in

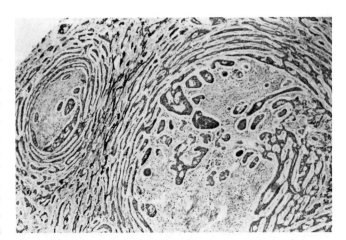

Fig. 33–5. Adenoid cystic carcinoma. Typical peri- and intra-neural tumor infiltration of this tumor occurs in lung as elsewhere. H and E, ×75.

oat cell carcinoma. Also, they do not have as much nuclear crowding or molding, and individually infiltrating cells are not as predominant in adenoid cystic carcinomas as in oat cell carcinomas. Finding focal areas of typical adenoid cystic carcinoma will help in difficult cases as these are required for an adenoid cystic carcinoma diagnosis, and are not seen in oat cell carcinoma. Differentiation should also be made with metastatic adenoid cystic carcinomas, which in contrast to primary lesions are usually peripheral, small, and multiple. Metastatic adenoid cystic carcinomas may be some of the more slowly growing metastases to lung (see Chapter 35)[64] and rarely have spontaneous regression.[65]

Mucoepidermoid Tumors

Mucoepidermoid tumors represent the second most frequent group of bronchial gland tumors. By 1979,[47] about 80 in the bronchi but only a few in the trachea had been reported.[66–68] Those in the trachea are usually located in the lower trachea-supercharinal position.[9] Several larger series of those in bronchi have more recently been described, including 18 cases by Heitmiller et al.[69] and 58 cases by Yousem and Hochholzer.[70] They are more common in the central bronchi than in the trachea, in contrast to adenoid cystic carcinomas. They are commonly referred to as "tumors" as many (perhaps some 80% or more) are very low grade and cured with local excision.

Mucoepidermoid tumors occur in the age group 4 to 78 years, with about two-thirds in the age range 45 to 70[49] and about 14% in children under the age of 14.[71] Of interest, Spencer[46] described seven of eight of his patients under the age of 21, even though his consultation practice was not biased toward the pediatric population. Also of interest, the other patient in Spencer's series[46] who had a malignant mucoepidermoid tumor was 68 years old. There is about an equal sex incidence,

although some series show a slight male and some a slight female predominance.

These were originally described in the lung by Smetana et al. in 1952[72] In that same year this lesion was also illustrated as a peculiar variant of adenoid cystic carcinoma by Liebow[2] In relationship to primary lung tumors, they accounted for 12 of 5,500 (0.22%),[48] 5 of 2,200 (0.23%),[73] and 4 in 2,500 (0.16%)[74] in different series.

In the past these lesions have been considered by some[44,50,62,75] to be so low grade as to be called "benign." Reichle and Rosemond[76] reviewed 29 cases in 1966. Metastases of this tumor from the lung were not described until 1961, by Ozlu et al.,[77] and in 1962 by Dowling et al.[78] Healey et al.[79] described criteria for low-grade and high-grade mucoepidermoid tumors in the salivary gland system, and in the next year Turnbill and associates[48] published 12 cases occurring in the lung, all high-grade mucoepidermoid tumors; 5 of these presented with metastases by the time of diagnosis, and 7 developed metastases shortly thereafter. The average duration of symptoms to death in these patients varied from 6 to 18 months, and the average survival was 9.8 months. These might be better considered adenosquamous carcinomas.[70]

These lesions in children are almost all benign in their behavior, and it was not until 1984 that a 4-year-old child was reported with a metastatic regional node lesion.[71] Two other low-grade-appearing lesions have metastasized in younger individuals; one in a 26-year-old man had multiple metastases to skin,[80] and the other in a 32-year-old woman had spread to skin, subcutaneous tissue, bones, and pericardium.[81] Both died within 3 months of original bronchial excision. Others have confirmed metastases in low-grade lesions.[45,67,70,78]

The criteria for low-grade and high-grade mucoepidermoid tumors in the lung have been defined by

Table 33–2. Diagnostic criteria of low-grade mucoepidermoid lesions of the bronchus[a]

	Low-grade	High-grade
Gross	Exophytic mass confined mainly to the bronchus with minimal extension into underlying parenchyma	Mass in association with bronchus but less polypoid and more invasive, extending into muscularis and lung parenchyma
Microscopic	Sheets of monomorphic cells with no or few mitosis; numerous well-formed mucus glands; absence of necrosis	Sheets of more atypical, pleomorphic cells with numerous mitoses; fewer well-formed mucus glands; presence of necrosis; metastases often more undifferentiated
Ultrastructural	Numerous globlet cells	Rare goblet cells
	Abundant mitochondria and glycogen-rich cells with well-formed microvilli	Infrequent mitochondria and glycogen-rich cells with poorly formed microvilli
	Prominent glandular lumen formation	Infrequent glandular lumen formation
	Common undifferentiated cells	Common undifferentiated cells
	Rare transitional cells	Abundant transitional cells
	Rare squamous cells	Rare squamous cells

[a] The gross and microscopic criteria,[4] and the ultrastructural criteria.[47] Reprinted with permission from Reference 81.

Klacsmann et al.[47] and Carter and Eggleston,[4] and have been summarized by Barsky et al. (Table 33–2).

In 1987, Yousem and Hochholzer[70] published the largest series to date of mucoepidermoid tumors in the lung. This series, which included 45 low-grade and 13 high-grade lesions, is worthy of discussing in some detail and further reference by the interested reader. Their low-grade group contained 27 women and 18 men, despite the male predominance of their Armed Forces Institute of Pathology (AFIP) database. The group age range was 9–78 years, averaging 34.8 years; 7 (16%) were younger than 20 and 25 (56%) younger than 30 years of age and only 4 persons over 60 at the time of resection. Of interest, 89% were symptomatic, usually with cough, "pneumonia," fever, or hemoptysis. Tobacco was smoked by 41%. Chest radiographs showed a solitary mass in 29 (64%), focal pneumonic consolidation in 15 (33%), and in 1 (3%) the chest radiograph was normal. Upper-lobe bronchi were more often involved (59%) than lower lobes. Some 60% were predominantly glandular, 36% were of equal admixture, and 4% were predominantly solid. There was only mild nuclear pleomorphism; mitoses were rare, fewer than 1 per 20 high power fields, and no necrosis was seen. Calcification of extracellular mucin was noted in 10 (22%) and ossification in 4 (9%); no invasion was identified in 3 (7%). The bronchial wall was infiltrated in 40 (89%), but lung invasion occurred in only 2 (4%) and 1 (2%) had nodal spread. The 1 with nodal spread was lost to follow-up, and the significance of the case remains undetermined.

In contrast, the Yousem and Hochholzer[70] high-grade group included 13 patients, with an age range of 13–67 years (average, 44.5), and 4 persons were less than 30 years and 5 more than 60 years of age. Ten were symptomatic. Of interest, there were fewer symptoms in this group than in the low-grade mucoepidermoid group, probably related to the prominent endobronchial polypoid protrusion of the low-grade group with less wall invasion. This prospect is supported by the findings of obstructive pneumonia in only 1 (8%), and lung infiltration in 6 (46%), of these high-grade cases. Tumor size varied from 1.5 to 4 cm, averaging 2.75 cm. Histologically, a solid appearance predominated in 7, mixed in 3, and predominantly glandular in 3. There was moderate to marked cytological atypia, and mitotic activity averaged 4 per 10 high-power fields; necrosis was present in almost half and spread to hilar nodes was seen in 2. Those that recurred in this group were all 58 years of age or older, and death from this tumor occurred in about one-third of this age group. There were no histological criteria within the high-grade group that distinguished those that did poorly. Attention was drawn in this series[70] to some less common

cellular patterns, as described in mucoepidermoid tumors of the salivary glands elsewhere, including oncocytic change,[82] clear cell change,[83], focally dense hyaline sclerosis,[84] and the colloid quality to some of the intracystic mucin.[85]

Another series by Heitmiller et al.[69] in 1989 described 18 patients, 15 low grade and 3 high grade. This series confirmed the foregoing findings except that 2 of their 3 high-grade cases could not be resected and the 1 who could had extensive hilar and mediastinal lymph node spread; all 3 (100%) in this group died of their tumors. Also, 5 of their 18 (28%) chest radiographs were normal because of the central location of the tumor. Grossly, as noted, these tumors, especially the lower grade ones, are usually polypoid in the bronchi (Fig. 33–6) and the higher grade lesions are less polypoid (Fig. 33–7) than the low-grade lesions. They do not extend in as linear a fashion along the wall as those adenoid cystic carcinomas discussed in the preceding section.

Microscopically, the low-grade lesion shows significant heritage to bronchial glands, with abundant mucinous cysts staining with acidic, weakly acidic, and neutral mucosubstance stains. These cystlike spaces and/or goblet cells may be predominant within the tumor (Figs. 33–8 and 33–9). The mucoepidermoid nature is determined by more solid collections of nonkeratinizing squamoid or transitional cells or bland pale cells adjacent to these cysts, sometimes occurring as small nests or larger sheets. Some of these cells appear intermediate between glandular and true squamous cells. Some accept small sites of keratinization, others not.[70] Rare mitoses are present in the low-grade lesions, and some of these tumors overlap with those described as mucous gland adenomas in the following section. The high-grade lesions have an abundance of solid sheets of intermediate cells. Clear or oncocytic cells are seen in low- and high-grade lesions. Rarely, giant cells are seen in high grade ones.[86] Increasing pleomorphism and mitotic rate are seen in higher grade lesions, along with necrosis. Cytology is diagnostic or suggestive in some cases.[60]

The different diagnosis in the higher grade lesions is with poorly differentiated squamous carcinoma, especially when the few mucin pools are missed and when the intermediate character of these cells is not readily apparent. Significant keratinization should make one consider squamous or adenosquamous carcinoma a more likely diagnosis.

Adenosquamous carcinomas are in the differential diagnosis of both low- and high-grade lesions. These are aggressive tumors that usually do not center on bronchi, and usually are large and without the sheetlike transitional cells of mucoepidermoid tumors. Some tumors overlap, however. Even the high-grade mu-

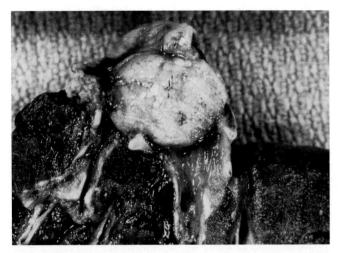

Fig. 33–6. Mucoepidermoid tumor. Gross appearance of low-grade tumor may be spherical tumor mass in major bronchi. (Courtesy of A.A. Liebow Pulmonary Collection, La Jolla, California)

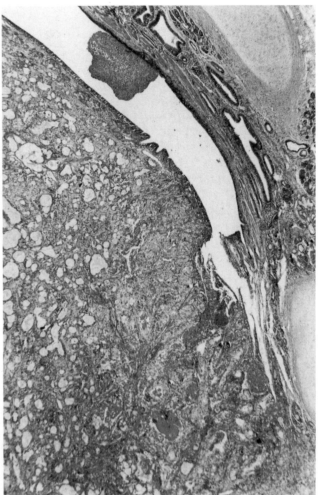

Fig. 33–8. Mucoepidermoid tumor. Endobronchial tumor mass correlates with gross appearance in Fig. 33–6. H and E. ×25.

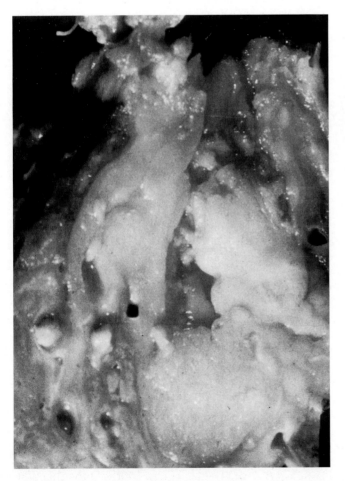

Fig. 33–7. Mucoepidermoid tumor. Gross appearance of higher grade tumor shows more infiltration of wall. (Courtesy of A.A. Liebow Pulmonary Collection, La Jolla, California.)

coepidermoid tumors tend to fare better than the more routine types of lung cancer, so attempts at differentiation are helpful if possible. Heitmiller et al.[69] suggested adenosquamous carcinomas and mucoepidermoid tumors were part of a continuum. One peripheral mucoepidermoid tumor has been described[87] but is perhaps better considered adenosquamous carcinoma.

Mucous Gland Adenomas

As noted in the previous section, some bronchial gland tumors retain distinct heritage with the bronchial glands themselves, and in a certain group that is so distinct as to be called "bronchial gland adenoma" in the true sense of the word. Only rarely have these been described in the lower trachea[88] or more peripheral than the major bronchi,[89] as reviewed by Allen et al.[90] These have variously been referred to as adenomatous

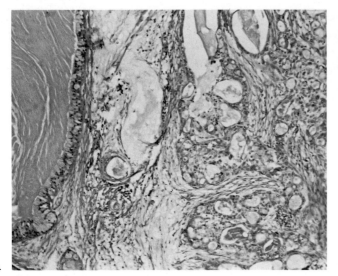

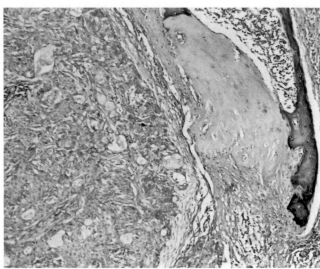

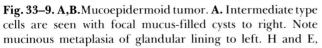

A

B

Fig. 33–9. A,B. Mucoepidermoid tumor. **A.** Intermediate type cells are seen with focal mucus-filled cysts to right. Note mucinous metaplasia of glandular lining to left. H and E,

×250. **B.** More solid mucoepidermoid tumor with fewer mucinous cysts shows focal bronchial cartilage reaction to right. H and E, ×250.

polyps, adenomas of mucous gland type, bronchial cystadenomas, or papillary cystadenomas, again as reviewed by Allen et al.[90] One study of seven cases concentrated on electron microscopic appearances.[91] To me, these cases seem to fall into three distinct histological patterns. The first group consists of fairly orderly tubular glands lined by single columnar mucous cells, often surrounded by some chronic inflammatory reaction separating the tubules. They do not appear histologically complex or aggressive, and I think of these as mucinous tubular adenomas. Examples of this type are the cases of Ramsey and Reimann,[92] Weinberger et al.,[89] Gilman et al.,[93] and Kroe and Pitcock.[94] Whether some of the larger mucinous cystadenomas/cystadenocarcinomas described later in this chapter belong in this category is unclear. They are separated because of their distinct appearance. It is also unclear whether an occasional case described as pulmonary blastoma might qualify for this category.

The second group is composed of papillary and cystic adenomas, sometimes with a predominance of one pattern over another, but at least cystic in some parts (Fig. 33–10) The papillary components tend to favor the luminal borders, and the cystic component is preserved toward the cartilage side of these submucosal tumor masses. The cells lining both areas are usually columnar (Fig. 33–11), cuboidal, and rather monotonous, or may be more squamoid or flattened in appearance, particularly those lining enlarging cysts. Fluid filling these cysts is usually homogeneous and appears dense and eosinophilic, sometimes like colloid. Exam-

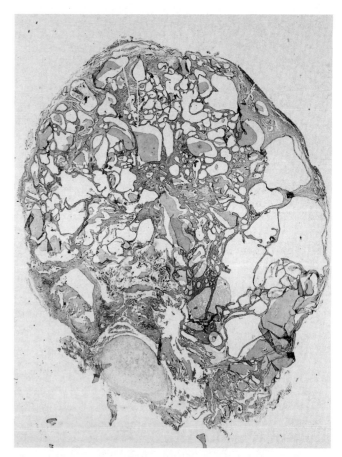

Fig. 33–10. Mucous gland adenoma. Multiple colloid-filled cysts of varying diameter in polypoid lesion. Note bronchial cartilage at bottom. H and E. ×10.

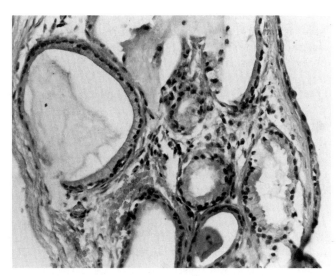

Fig. 33–11. Mucous gland adenoma. Goblet cells in single layer line variously sized cysts. Portion of larger cyst at right with only one wall illustrated. H and E, ×600.

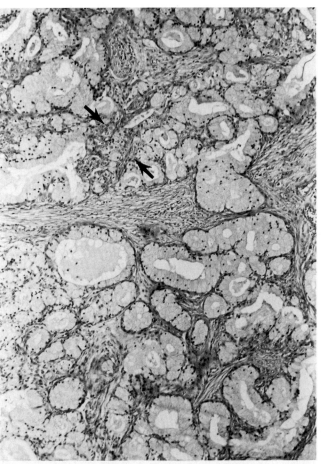

Fig. 33–13. Very low-grade mucoepidermoid tumor (? adenoma). Well-differentiated. Excess goblet cell production may line many cysts with only focal areas still indicating tumor is mucoepidermoid (*arrows*). H and E, ×250.

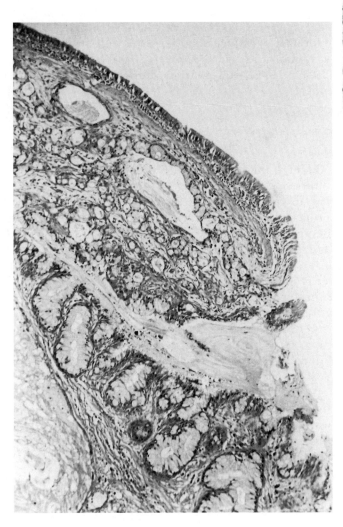

ples of these in the literature are the cases of Allen et al.[90] and several reported by Spencer et al.[46] The Clara or alveolar cell papillomas described below mostly arise in and grow on lung parenchyma and generally do not have cystic spaces, although some overlap may occur.[95]

The third group is close to or composed of the lowest grade mucoepidermoid tumors (Figs. 33–12 and 33–13), as reported by Rosenblum and Klein,[96] Arrigoni and associates,[1] and Emory et al.[97] These contain small mucinous spaces with some "intermediate" cell types, possibly intercalated duct-type cells. In one case, tumor was expectorated during suctioning.[96] These are so low

◁——————————————————

Fig. 33–12. Low-grade mucoepidermoid tumor (? adenoma). Well-differentiated character seen in mucinous change at bottom and true nature of tumor identified just below ciliated mucosa. H and E, ×100.

grade in histological appearance as to suggest an adenoma designation. Heard et al.[91] published a study of seven such tumors with emphasis on ultrastructure. Perhaps some members of the next several groups should also be considered as further variants.

Oncocytomas

Nonneoplastic oncocytic change has been described by Matsuba et al.[98] in 30 of 33 lungs examined (Fig. 33–14). This change is usually in the mucous membrane, and most particularly in the bronchial glands. This change is not present in patients under age 33 years, and increases in incidence with age beyond that time. As in other locations, these are oxyphilic because of greatly increased numbers of mitochondria. This change most likely represents a curious form of degeneration within cells. Oncocytic change has also been described with some carcinoid tumors (see Chapter

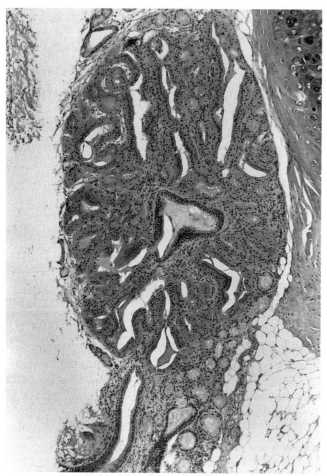

Fig. 33–14. Oncocytoma. Small, 3-mm focus of oncocytic change in bronchial gland surrounds intercalated duct in submucosa of bronchus. Note cartilage to the right. Mucosa is missing to left over this nodule. H and E, ×35.

32),[99–103] glomus tumors of the trachea,[104] and some bronchial gland adenomas.[91] It is also seen in mucoepidermoid tumors,[70,105] and, in one series, oncocytic change was described as significant in 9 of 53 (20%).[70] It has also been noted in an adenoma of type II pneumocyte derivation,[106] and in a bronchial adenoma with pleomorphic features,[107] which are discussed separately next. Very thorough sampling and special procedures help separate these. The term, as used here, should be limited to those with only oncocytes throughout, and, on electron microscopy, with abundant mitochondria and no neurosecretory features. Although oncocytomas of salivary gland account for some 0.8% to 1%–2% of all salivary gland tumors, they are very rare in the lung according to this ultramicroscopic definition.

Fechner and Bentinck[108] in 1973 were the first to describe an acceptable case in the lung studied by electron microscopy. Black[109] had described a case under this name in 1969, but Black illustrated larger serous-appearing granules in the cytoplasm, and perhaps this tumor is better thought of as a variant of acinic cell carcinoma.[108] These have been reported in the lung and confirmed ultrastructurally by other authors.[46,110–115] One case of bronchial oncocytoma with bronchial wall invasion and nodal spread was described by Nielson in 1983.[114] Most are associated with bronchi, but some are not.[110]

Acinic Cell Tumors

Although the mucinous quality of bronchial glands is most evident in some diseases, the acinic cells may give rise to rare tumors. As in the original definition of bronchial oncocytoma in lung,[108] again Fechner and Bentinck, this time with the addition of Askew,[116] described the first such case of acinic cell tumor in lung, in an incidental 1.2-cm pale-tan tumor in the right-lower lobe of a 63-year-old man. It was not grossly connected with bronchus, and the cells were indistinguishable from acinic cell tumors of salivary gland, either by special histochemical stain or electron microscopy. Other cases have been reported by Katz and Bubis,[117] Gharpure et al.,[118] Heard et al.,[119] and Yoshido et al.[120]

Moran et al.[121] in 1992 described the largest series, fine cases of acinic cell carcinoma of lung. Together with those described in the literature, the age range for this tumor is 12–75, averaging 38 years. So far, 60% are in women and most are asymptomatic, with a rare case presenting with persistent cough. These carcinomas are usually discrete and may be found either centrally or peripherally.

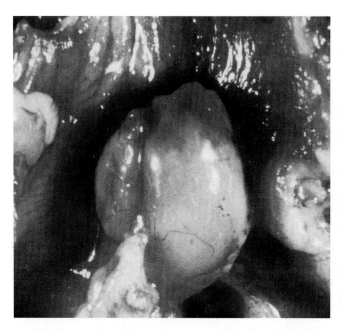

Fig. 33–15. Acinic cell tumor. Gross picture of nodular acinic cell tumor at bifurcation of bronchi. (Courtesy A.A. Liebow Pulmonary Pathology Collection, San Diego, California; original contributor, J.R. Henneford, MD, Columbus Hospital, Great Falls, Montana.

Grossly, such tumors are well circumscribed but lack a capsule. They are tan-white or yellow, nonnecrotic and nonhemorraghic, and soft to rubbery. Some are endobronchial and polypoid (Fig. 33–15). Microscopically they are composed of sheets of medium to large cohesive granular cells with varying degrees of stromal fibrosis-fibrosepta. Septa sometimes divide islands of tumor cells, and this pattern suggests an almost organoid appearance. There is the same variation within the lung as seen in the salivary glands,[122–126] and there may be more clear cell change (Fig. 33–16), variation of cell size, or tubular or papular formation.

Of interest only one of five cases in the series of Moran et al.[121] stained vividly with PAS–PASD, and the tumors had a lower content of amylase than normal acinar cells. Electron microscopy showed the typical serous-type cytoplasmic zymogen granules. These tumors are strongly cytokeratin and epithelial membrane-antigen positive while being negative with vimentin, S100 protein, and chromagranin.[121]

In the differential diagnosis of these lesions are clear to granular cell PAS-positive lesions, including benign clear cell "sugar" tumors, primary clear cell carcinoma of lung, glycogen-rich bronchioloalveolar carcinoma (BAC), metastatic acinic cell salivary gland-derived tumors, and metastatic renal cell carcinomas. History is helpful in excluding metastases from salivary gland lesions as pulmonary metastases usually occur after

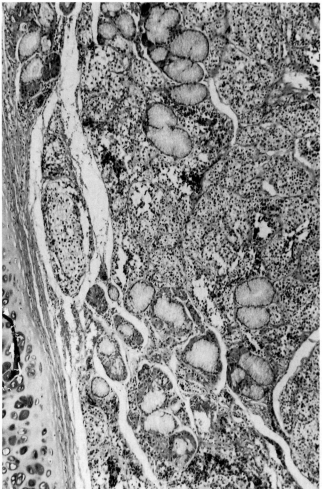

Fig. 33–16. Acinic cell tumor. Clear cells are infiltrating submucosal gland. H and E, ×100.

discovery of the primary malignancy. With head and neck primaries, however, metastases can occur many years later despite a noninvasive and benign-appearing primary sources.[124–126] Renal cell carcinoma has coexistent lipid and glycogen, the latter digests with diastase, and these tumors are more often focally necrotic and invasive than acinic carcinomas. Benign clear cell "sugar" tumors of lung do not usually stain with epithelial markers, and their PAS-positivity digests with diastase. They also have a sinusoidal vascular pattern and are more typically clear than granular. Primary clear cell carcinomas of lung have mitoses, usually more pleomorphic large cells, may have glycogen but no postdiastase PAS-positivity, and these same characteristics apply to the entity of glycogen-rich bronchioloalveolar carcinomas. Electron microscopy may help in difficult cases. Other more remote possibilities in the differential diagnosis mentioned by Moran et al.[121] are oncocytic lesions such as carcinoid tumors and other (see forego-

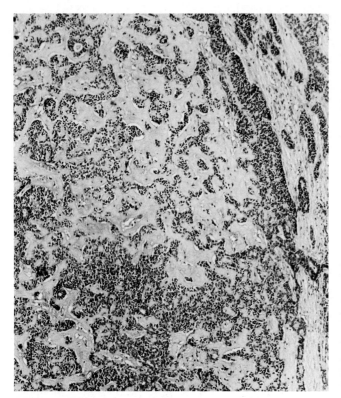

Fig. 33–17. Pleomorphic mixed tumor of salivary gland type. Low-power view of hyalinized stroma and tumor cells. H and E, ×100.

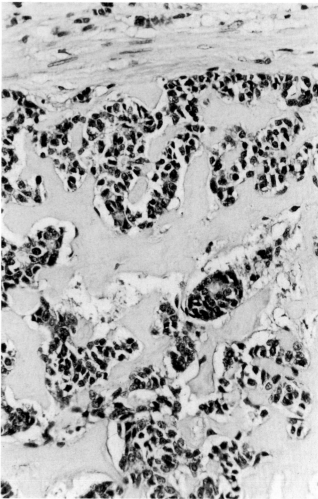

Fig. 33–18. Pleomorphic mixed tumor of salivary gland type. High-power view of nests of cells admixed with densely hyalinized stroma. On H and E stain alone, differential diagnosis includes thyroid-type medullary carcinoma. H and E, ×400.

ing) metastatic clear and papillary carcinomas from thyroid, parathyroid, adrenal, or liver primaries.

One case that was described by Miura et al.[127] had cytoplasmic granules larger than 600 nm in diameter, but was argyrophilic and seratonin positive, and is most likely, therefore, a carcinoid tumor. Peculiarities of classification also apply to the tumor described by Black et al.[109]

Pleomorphic Mixed Tumors of Bronchial Gland Type

This tumor is very uncommon in the lung. Payne et al.[128] first described 2 cases in 1965, and by 1991 a total of 12 cases had been reported in bronchi and lungs[46,128–136] while by 1988[135] 16 had been described in the trachea.[137–140] An additional case is shown here. These tumors occur in patients 47–74 years old (average, 68.1 years), and occur equally in men and women. Some are extrabronchial,[46,135] and several recurred 4–11 years later, one at the line of excision[128] and another in the opposite lung 9 years later with no other lesions during an additional 3-year follow-up.[135] One has recurred in a lumbar vertebra[46]; one other was reported to show malignant behavior,[130] but so far no

deaths are attributable to this tumor. As with other tracheobronchial gland-derived tumors, those reported outside the trachea and bronchi raise the possibility of metastases to the lung, as have been described from the major salivary glands.[141,142] The lung is relatively infrequently the destination for such metastasizing mixed tumors; in the series by Wenig et al.,[141] only 2 of 11 spreading from the main salivary glands had pulmonary metastases.

As noted, although still rare, these tumors are slightly more frequent in the trachea. Ma et al.[138] in an extensive review of the literature from 1922 to 1978 documented 14 cases in this location and 4 more were added by 1988.[140] In this location this tumor occurs in more men than women by a factor of 2:1; these have occurred in the age range 26–76, with a mean age of 50, and some have acted in a malignant fashion. In whatever location, they should appear similar to those occurring more frequently in the head and neck and be similar by immunoperoxidase, being S100, cytokeratin, glial fibrillary acid protein, actin, and vimentin positive.

Microscopically these tumors appear in the assorted patterns seen in the benign mixed tumors of salivary glands (Figs. 33–17 and 33–18). All have both abundant epithelial and abundant stromal components, with varying degrees of differentiation of the stroma into other elements such as cartilage. The epithelial cells are usually in tubules or cell clusters, and have an angulated form and sometimes line-flattened smaller ducts. Mitoses and necrosis are infrequent, other than the case of the metastasizing lesion reported by Spencer.[46] Recognizing monomorphic adenomas in this location has been an even rarer event (Fig. 33–19).

The differential diagnosis includes carcinosarcomas, unclassifiable bronchial gland tumors, polymorphous low-grade adenocarcinomas, and occasional poorly de-

fined peculiar variants with mucoepidermoid or adenoid cystic characteristics.

Myoepithelioma

One case was described in the lung by Strickler et al.[143] in 1987, with typical electron microscopy and light microscopy appearances; this was extrabronchial and composed of sheets of spindle cells that were S100 positive.

Low-Grade Adenocarcinomas with Polymorphous Features

These lesions were described in the major and minor salivary glands by Evans and Batsakis.[144] In the head and neck, this is usually an oral lesion, favoring the palate, and when it arises in major salivary glands, it is only found in association with carcinomas arising in mixed tumors.[145,146] Although this lesion has not been described in the lung so far, I have seen several cases

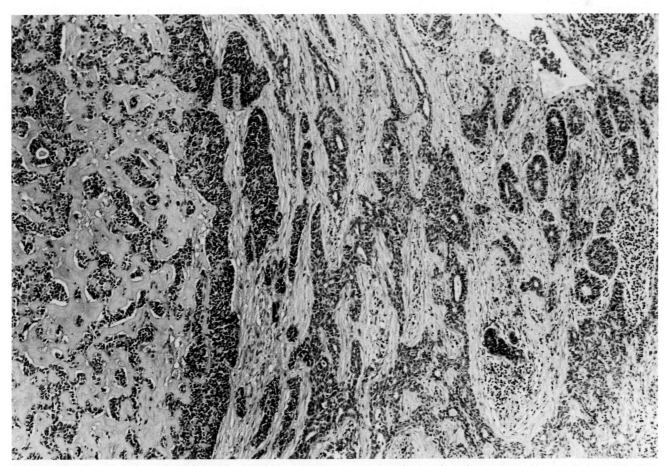

Fig. 33–19. Mixed tumor with additional component. Same focus shown in Figs. 33–17 and 33–18 shows area adjacent to apparent benign mixed tumor, either monomorphic adenoma or polymorphous low-grade adenocarcinoma. H and E, ×100.

that possibly qualify as this entity. One tumor contained elements of benign mixed tumor, a bland tubular element almost monomorphic or adenoid cystic in nature (Fig. 33–19), along with a solid variant of adenocarcinoma. This awaits substantiation.

In a series of four of these tumors in salivary glands, Gnepp et al.[145] found more than 90% of the tumor cells stained diffusely with S100 protein and epithelial membrane antigen (EMA), while 75%–95% stained with cytokeratin and some stained variably with smooth muscle actin and carcinoembryonic antigen (CEA). This was in contrast to adenoid cystic carcinoma where EMA and CEA positivity was localized to ductal lumens and the S100 stain was less diffusely positive than in polymorphous low grade adenocarcinomas. Distant metastases from primaries in the oral cavity have so far not been reported.[145]

Akhtar et al.[107] in 1974 reported a "bronchial adenoma with polymorphous features" from the right-upper lobe of a 35-year-old man. The tumor had a maximum dimension of 2.5 cm and contained a variety of patterns, mostly papillary and ciliated, but also mucinous with goblet cells and a significant oncocytic change. There were clear cells, both sheet like and similar to mucoepidermoid tumors, and tall columnar, similar to pulmonary blastomas.

Other Adenocarcinomas of Bronchial Glands

Although the major group of more common adenocarcinomas in the lung discussed in Chapter 32 has been referred to as bronchogenic carcinomas, many of these occur more distally and their origin from bronchi is in doubt. There is no reason, however, that adenocarcinomas cannot arise in bronchial glands. Schinella and Fazzini[147] in 1978 published criteria for these tumors in abstract form. The tumors are centrally located in the lung, oriented toward the lumen with much of the tumor in a submucosal location, and with "striking similarity" to adjacent submucosal glands. These have a prominent acinar pattern and abundant mucin production. Most occur in men, who present with obstructive symptoms. The survival is poor, with median survival of only 4 months, and cautioning the clinicians of this poor survival may be warranted.

Hirata et al.[148] in 1990 published 23 cases of bronchial gland-type adenocarcinomas of lung, with the basic characteristics of histologic and cytologic differentiation toward bronchial glands. These occurred on an average 10 years younger than the usual adenocarcinomas, having a mean age of 50.5 compared to 60.1 years for general carcinomas. One of the authors in this review, Dr. Y. Shimosato, has authored several other

papers addressing this problem, including several in Japanese in 1973,[149] updated in English in 1982.[150,151] These tumors occurred most often in large bronchi, especially in the second- to fourth-order bronchi,[149–151] and were endobronchial in almost half, often causing occlusion. The tumors reported by Hirata et al. were positive with immunoperoxidase stains with CEA in 50% of the cases, with surfactant apoprotein in 68%, and with secretory component in 64%; these findings were similar to peripheral adenocarcinomas. These authors proposed the high percentage (68%) of positivity of the central tumors with surfactant apoprotein may reflect "traces of differentiation toward peripheral airway epithelium." This field is evolving, and the interested reader is also referred to the work of Kimula[152] on use of mucin stains and other characteristics to better define bronchial gland-derived tumor cells.

Those adenocarcinoms truly derived from bronchial glands fulfill the criteria of "bronchogenic carcinoma," a term that has been misused in medical school teaching and textbooks. Most adenocarcinomas, of course, are peripheral and are not associated with a bronchus, and invasion of bronchi from metastases may recreate many of the H and E appearances of primary bronchial gland adenocarcinomas (Fig. 33–20); also see endobronchial metastases in Chapter 35). Some primary adenocarcinomas of surface bronchial mucosa are also possible but appear rare. It seems most of the bronchial surface lesions betray their glandular origins and undergo squamous metaplasia, dysplasia, and squamous carcinoma.

In considering low-grade papillary and cystic lesions in the lung, one must always be cautious of metastatic low-grade malignancies, such as tumors from salivary gland or thyroid. Some of these metastasize adjacent to, or in continuity with, bronchial surface, and one case (Fig. 33–21) was a challenging case of a 52-year-old man, which was considered possibly as a primary lesion until it was realized that two separate nodules had appeared 1 and 4 years previously and another 1 year after the biopsy was taken. Given this multifocal spread, the patient was presumed to have metastases from a parotid gland excision, interpreted as low-grade adenocarcinoma, that he had some 21 years previously. The original slides from the parotid carcinoma were not found despite extensive search. An almost identical case in a 58-year-old man with an unusual submandibular carcinoma excised 10 years previously was presented in a mystery slide seminar in 1980 by P. Conen (Dalhousie University, Halifax, Canada); this case bore similarity to a case published by Sidhu and Forrester.[126] These cases also may be related to the types of carcinoma described in salivary gland tissue by Mills et al.[153] and Corio et al.,[154] or variants of polymorphous low-grade adeno-

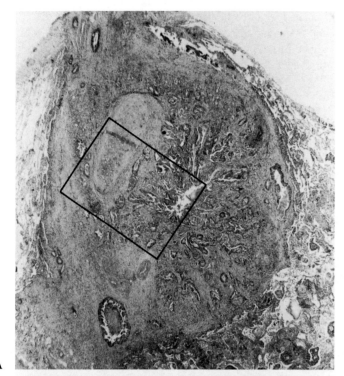

A

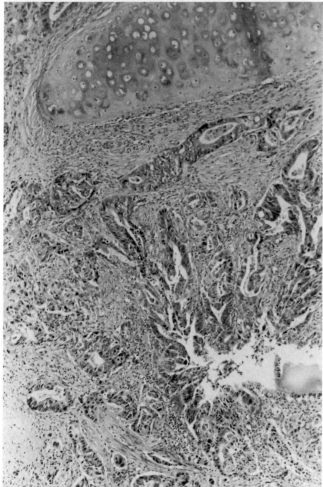

B

carcinoma, as described in the previous section on **Tracheobronchial Gland Tumors**.

Paget's Disease

An interesting case of extramammary Paget's disease of bronchial wall with a focal infiltration of bronchial submucosa and adjacent lung parenchyma was described by Higashiyama et al.[155] This case involved a 69-year-old man who had one year history of positive sputum cytologies. The lesion was identified after selective cytology sampling. These authors noted one other case proposed to bronchial origin for Paget's disease, this being in a retroperitoneal teratoma with bronchial epithelium, but without sweat glands.[156] However, this remains a hypothesis as no direct transition was noted. Melanomas, either primary or secondary, can also have Pagetoid spread (see **Melanoma** discussion, this chapter) as can more common primary and secondary lung tumors. However, these are usually associated with tumor masses.

Uncommon Surface Tumors

Squamous Papillomas

Benign viral-induced squamous papillomas of the larynx occur most often in children and teenagers and are usually self-limited. The most probable theory for their origin is that the papilloma virus is spread transvaginally through the birth canal at the time of birth, infecting the oropharyngeal secretions of the child. The nasosinal membranes seem immune to such early growths.[157] In children, multiple papillomas in the bronchi and lung are always associated with multiple papillomas of trachea or larynx. In a compilation of four series of juvenile laryngeal papillomas by Singer and associates,[158] 9 of 430 (2.1%) cases had spread beyond the larynx, and this spread was usually limited to the trachea. Lukens,[159] in his series from a single institution, found 3 tracheal papillomas in 310 (1%) cases of laryngeal papillomas. Kramer et al.[160] estimated that 5% spread to the trachea and proximal bronchi, but less than 1% spread to the lung. Majoros et al.[161] found, in 101 cases of laryngeal papillomatosis seen at a referral center, 8 (8%) extended to trachea, and 4 (4%) extended to bronchi. Al-Saleem et al.[162]

◁ ———————————————————————

Fig. 33–20. A,B. Metastatic colon cancer to endobronchus appears like primary adenocarcinoma of bronchus. Note orientation of tumor toward lumen, and radial infiltration of wall, from metastasis from proven metastatic colon cancer. Area in box in **A** is enlarged as **B**. A. Low power. H and E, ×50. **B.** High power. H and E, ×250.

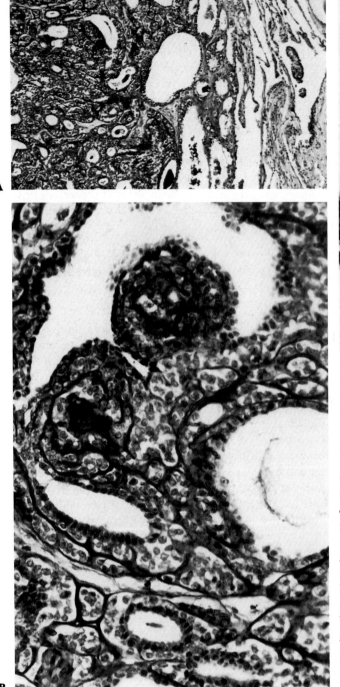

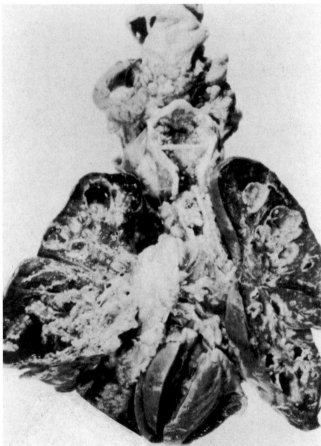

Fig. 33–22. Squamous papillomatosis. Extensive spread of laryngeal, tracheal, bronchial, and pulmonary papillomatosis caused death in this 9-year-old child. (Used with permission of Laryngoscope 1951;61:1022–1029.[167])

others do not. The vascular stalks are narrow but have some focal chronic inflammation. Spread to adjacent reported on 11 cases of lower respiratory tract papillomatosis from one institution, and thought an incidence of 2%–3% compared to all laryngeal papillomas was more accurate.

True spread more distally into the bronchial system and lung carries a poor prognosis, and is associated with fulminant disease, usually starting at an early age, often before age 5 and even by age 1–2 years, with a rare case noted at age 48 days.[163] These lesions are characterized by multiple recurrences requiring multiple excisions, and several cases had up to 100 excisions.[164,165] These patients required persistent tracheostomies 14 months

Fig. 33–21. A,B. Metastatic low-grade salivary gland tumor. **A.** Low power shows one of several cystic and tubular, and focally solid, lesions occurring 21 years after parotid gland adenocarcinoma was excised (see text). Some similarity exists with primary bronchial gland tumors of lung. PAS, ×100. **B.** High-power view of top left of Fig. 33–21A shows clear cells and distinctly smaller lining cells; basal lamina-like material well illustrated. PAS, ×400.

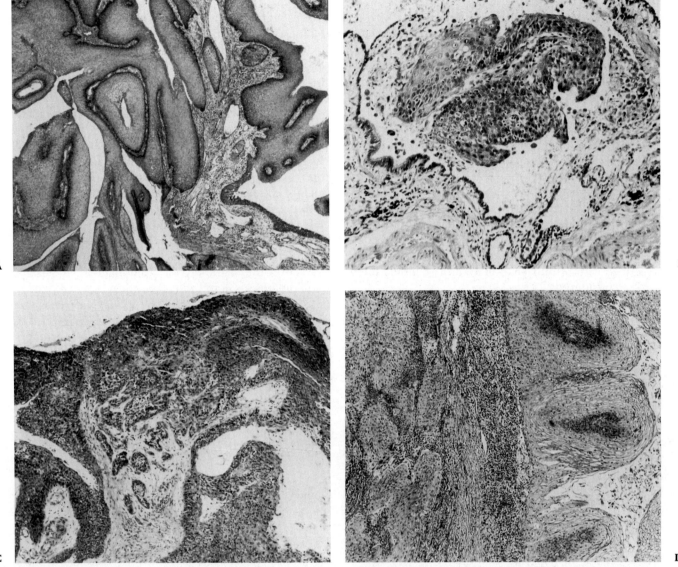

Fig. 33–23. A–D. Variations in squamous papillomas-cancer. **A.** Bland acanthosis and papillomatosis of usual papilloma type. H and E, ×50. **B.** Transition from less dysplatic squamous epithelium at top left to carcinoma in situ is shown centrally. H and E, ×250. **C.** Focally infiltrating squamous cell carcinoma in center of atypical-appearing lining. H and E, ×250. **D.** Better differentiated "bland" papillomatous lining to right, but extensive spread to parenchyma is seen on left. H and E, ×250.

to 24 years before tracheobronchial spread was noted. Majoros et al.[161] found 56% of their patients with tracheostomies had distal spread, compared to only 10% of those not requiring tracheostomy. Some[4] have wondered whether the tracheostomy itself is responsible for spread more distally, but it is difficult to distinguish this event from the fact that tracheostomies are only required in patients with severe laryngeal papillomatosis. Most appear related to human papilloma virus (HPV), and viral spread helps account for their contiguous spread along mucous membranes, eventually extending throughout the respiratory system.

With bronchopulmonary spread of multiple papillomas, obstructive changes and symptoms are frequent, with cough, fever, and weight loss. Multiple cavities are seen on chest radiography, and have been interpreted as bronchiectasis. Kramer et al.[160] reported seven cases of cavitary pulmonary papillomatosis. Sometimes these cavities are missed and are only appreciated retrospectively. Rarely, pseudoepitheliomatous hyperplasia-papillomatous change occurs around impacted foreign bodies in bronchi.[166]

Grossly the papillomas are exophytic from the wall and endophytic into the air canals of the trachea and bronchial system and there is bronchiectasis in the bronchi, both around the lesions and distally with peripheral atelectasis, abscess formation, and obstructive pneumonia. The case illustrated in Fig. 33–22 is that of Kirchner,[167] who noted the "autopsy revealed an almost unbelievable extensive involvement of the trachea, bronchi and lung by various sized nodules and cavities."

Microscopically these are usually composed of bland nonkeratinizing or minimally keratinizing squamous cells that are multilayered, forming papillomatous projections, perhaps with a little parakeratosis on the surface (Fig. 33–23A). Some have HPV koilocytic change; alveoli through terminal ducts shows small squamous nodules on the alveolar septa, and the differential diagnosis of this spread may include viral-induced squamous metaplasia, such as seen in influenzae pneumonia, or perhaps a drug reaction such as has been described with bleomycin. Squamous carcinoma might also be considered.

Malignancy has been described in bronchopulmonary papillomatosis and tracheal papillomatosis (Fig. 33–23), both in children,[165,168–181] as reviewed by Runckel and Kessler,[165] and in adults.[168,169,173,181] As in the larynx, radiation or chemotherapy are contraindicated and tobacco and other cocarcinogen effects should be avoided. Helmuth and Strate[173] described squamous carcinoma rising in the setting of papillomatosis, including three cases in the larynx and 7 in the lung. In nonsmoking nonirradiated cases of juvenile

papillomatosis, these occurred in their series in the age group 6–28 years at the time of diagnosis; five were diagnosed during life and two at autopsy. These tumors had often extended to the regional node, chest wall, and diaphragm, and a few had spread more distally. Five of the seven in the lung were well differentiated, the other two poorly differentiated, squamous carcinomas.

In all ages, evidence of invasion may be noted by lymphangitic spread (Fig. 33–24) and reactive tumor desmoplasia at their bases, with individual or small clusters of atypical squamous cells appearing to elicit this reaction, or obvious invasion of adjacent structures. Surface extension of benign squamous mucosa into submucosal glands should not be mistaken for invasion (Fig. 33–25). At times carcinoma may develop many years later, and in one particular case it became more and more dysplastic, eventually developing to cancer 34 years after the beginning of papillomatosis.[170] Usually papillomatosis is noted with symptoms by age 3 years in these cases.[165] A mortality of 37.5% is associated with papillomatous spread to the lungs; some of this is caused by the cyst formation, obstructive recurrent pneumonias, and other nonmalignant effects.[162]

Solitary papillomas are rare,[172,181] usually occur in adults, and have a higher incidence of cancer. Perhaps some of these were well-differentiated cancers even before they were recognized. However, some papillomas in adults are multiple, and some in children are solitary. Those that are multiple in adults rarely ap-

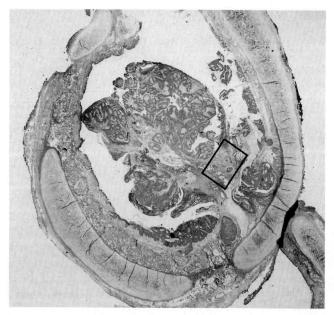

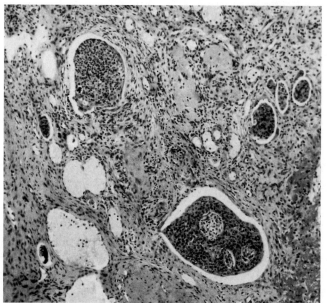

A   **B**

Fig. 33–24. A, B. Rather bland-appearing solitary papilloma in adult. **A.** Low power of entire bronchus intermedius, with area in box shown in **B**. H and E, ×15. **B.** Area in box in **A** in high-power view shows apparent lymphatic space invasion at base. This tumor has now recurred in this position and spread in upward fashion (see text). H and E, ×250. (Original contributor, J. Bolen, Virginia Mason Clinic, Seattle, Washington.)

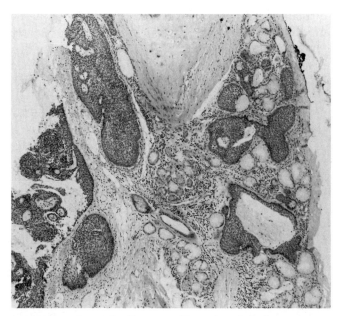

Fig. 33–25. Base of solitary papilloma in adult shows extension into gland necks through bronchial wall. This represents part of contiguous surface spread and is not indicative of invasion. H and E. ×100.

proach the large numbers seen in children and do not usually extend to lung parenchyma. Most of the older patients who have solitary squamous papilloma are heavy smokers, as are those that develop cancer as young adults.[165] Some 90% of solitary papillomas in adults occur in men, usually in the age group of mid-fifties to mid-seventies, with an average age of 60 years.[172]

I have seen a case of benign laryngeal and tracheal papillomas in a patient aged 16; by age 28 years, this woman had invasive squamous carcinoma of the lung. She was a smoker and it appears that smoking, as with radiotherapy, is an additive force in driving these proliferations to malignancy. Certainly such patients should be discouraged from smoking. As with verrucous carcinomas, accurate diagnosis of the malignant potential of some of these lesions is quite challenging.

Most cases of papillomas spread from the larynx down to involve the pulmonary system. The case illustrated in Fig. 33–24 is interesting because it first presented in 1983 in a 49-year-old man in the bronchus intermedius. Despite bland histology, lymphangitic invasion was suggested. In 1985 and again in 1988, squamous papillomas were documented in the midtrachea, and by 1990 papillomas were documented in the nasopharynx and nose, and by 1991 and again in 1992 in the larynx, mastoid region, middle ear, jugular foramen, nasopharynx, and nose, and additional recurrence has been seen in the right-middle lobe where it

was originally detected in 1983. The histology has not changed much, but represents an interesting case of spread that is the reverse of the usual downward pattern.

Human papilloma virus (HPV) serotypes have been applied to these lesions. These have been summarized by Béju-Thivolet et al.,[182] who described 10 cases with serotype evaluation in pulmonary squamous metaplasias or papillomas and 33 cases of squamous carcinoma of lung. They found that serotypes 6 and 11 usually occurred in the benign lesions and serotypes 16 and 18 in the malignant ones, as previously proven in uterine cervix. Benign laryngeal papillomatosis in youth is thought to be caused by cervical and vaginal secretion contamination of the oral pharynx of infants during birth and is usually of serotypes 6 and 11. As serotypes 16 and 18 are also present in the same sites in the vaginal canal in some women, it is curious why they are not more frequent.

As noted, some reactive benign squamous proliferations in bronchi have been initiated by retained foreign bodies[166] and have been called papillomas; however, these are not as organized as the typical squamous papillomas just described. Likewise, some polyps have been called inverted polyps or inverted papillomas of the bronchus[4] (Fig. 33–26) and it is difficult to know whether these are similarly reactive. (See basal cell-transitional cell-surface tumors in the following section.) Some cysts in the lung, although rarely, have accumulated keratin in them, similar to epidermal cysts; and these have been called "keratinizing cysts of bronchus."[183]

Evaluating transbronchial biopsies in patients with squamous papillomas, especially the solitary ones, can be hazardous. One must be cautious not to under- or overextrapolate findings based on the limited tissue provided by these procedures. Poorly differentiated and well-differentiated squamous carcinomas can both appear bland in select areas, and squamous papillomas can appear atypical. It is best to diagnose some biopsies as atypical, while discussing both these possibilities, and indicate that a limited excision should be done for endotracheal and endobronchial lesions and that all the tissue should be submitted for examination in a manner similar to villous adenoma of colon. If the mass is an obvious large solitary tumor mass in lung, a more aggressive approach may be taken based on clinical judgment of obvious malignancy.

Inverted Polyps and Basal Cell Adenomas/Carcinomas

As just noted, some polyps have been called inverted polyps or papillomas of bronchus[14] (Fig. 33–26). It is

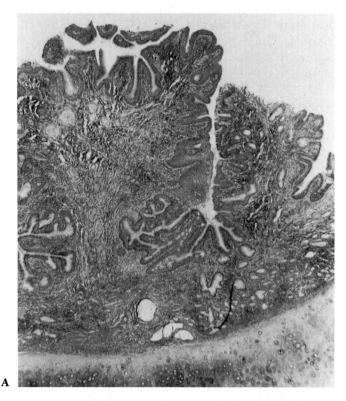

A

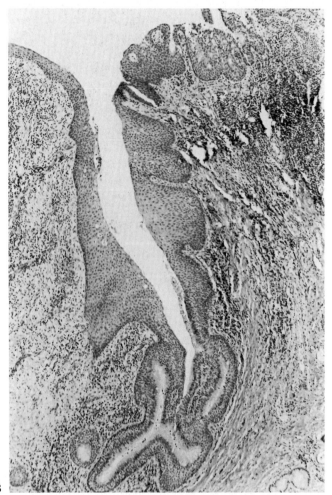

B

difficult to know whether these are reactive to underlying thickened stroma or are neoplastic in themselves. Some papillomas are lined by nonkeratinized lining that is not so squamous in quality and has been termed transitional cell, or basal cell, papillomas (Fig. 33–26).[184–186]

Similar histology has been seen in carcinomas of the lung, termed basal cell, basaloid, or transitional cell carcinoma[187,188] (Fig. 33–27). Spencer[6] originally described this entity, and his few cases had a very favorable prognosis. In a case presented by Daroca and Robichaux,[167] this was a small, 2-cm, tumor without nodal spread, and the patient died during the postpneumonectomy recovery period.

The series by Brambilla et al.[188] is the largest available, and in their study of 671 lung tumors, 115 were poorly or undifferentiated; 38 of those they classified as basaloid carcinoma. This number represent 6% of the total or 33% of the 115 poorly or undifferentiated tumors. Their criteria were lobular growth pattern with small cells surrounded by rims of perpendicular oriented, slightly enlarged basal cells, with nuclei with moderate hyperchromasia and no prominent nuclei, and scant cytoplasm but a high mitotic rate. Half those cases were pure and half were mixed with squamous carcinoma, large cell carcinoma, or adenocarcinoma. Brambilla et al. required at least 60% of the tumor to be basaloid before so classifying it. Of interest, all these patients were men in the age range 36–79 years, median 60 years. In 36 of their 38 (95%) cases, the tumor was in the lobar segmental bronchi, and in the other 2 more distally. Therefore, it does not appear to be a tumor of mainstem bronchi. The authors emphasized the differential diagnosis of a non-small cell neuroendocrine tumor, poorly differentiated squamous carcinoma, and adenoid cystic carcinoma, solid variant. Survival of their patients was poor, worse than for the usual bronchogenic squamous carcinoma, perhaps because these tumors were less differentiated. There was no difference in the pure and mixed basaloid carcinomas in their group.

Lower Grade Glandular Surface Tumors

In addition to adenomas and adenocarcinomas of tracheobronchial mucous gland origin (salivary gland

◁———————————————————

Fig. 33–26. A,B. Almost inverted and mixed benign squamous and glandular papilloma. **A.** Low-power view shows thickening of inflamed and fibrous submucosa that throws surface into projections into lumen. Note overall mucosal thickening and protrusion compared to more normal thickness at right edge. H and E, ×50. **B.** High power shows inflamed stroma and squamous replacement and some basal cell hyperplasia of lining underneath areas of preserved glandular lining. H and E, ×250.

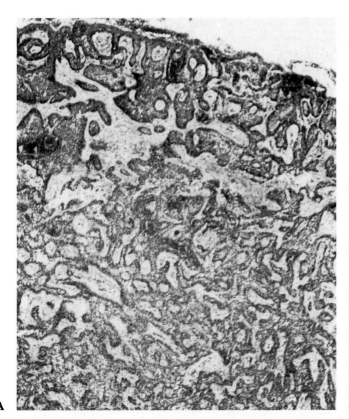

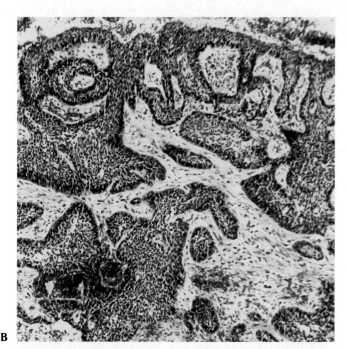

Fig. 33–27. A,B. Basal cell adenoma/carcinoma. **A.** Basal cell type proliferation has replaced nodular protrusion of bronchial mucosa. H and E, ×50. **B.** Higher power view shows basilar orientation of nuclei near stroma in multifocal origin from surface. H and E, ×150. (Courtesy of H. Spencer, St. Thomas Hospital, London, England)

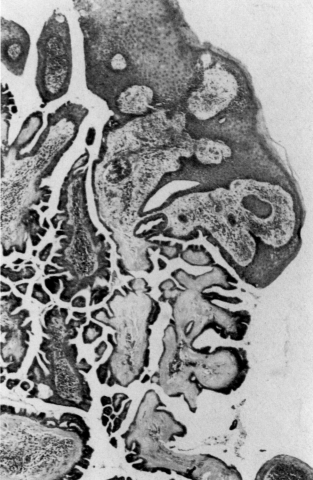

Fig. 33–28. Mixed squamous and glandular papilloma with more active glandular component than in Fig. 33-26. Note focal hyalinized stroma. H and E ×50.

type), surface-oriented papillomatous and otherwise glandular lesions have been described in several cases. In 1980, in our review of 19 cases of noninvasive bronchial papillary tumors,[171] glandular differentiation was present or certainly suggested in three of eight solitary lesions. Some of these may represent in situ neoplasia of adjacent mucous glands, as sometimes seen in the endocervix adjacent to areas of squamous dysplasia (Fig. 33–28).

Assorted discrete epithelial proliferations on peripheral lung architecture have been described as adenomas (Figs. 33–29 through 33–31). Some have been described with Clara cell lining, some with alveolar type II cell lining,* and some are described with features of both. Clara cell lining has also been described covering a peculiar tumor with some neurosecretory features.[193]

---

*References 46, 95, 106, 189–192.

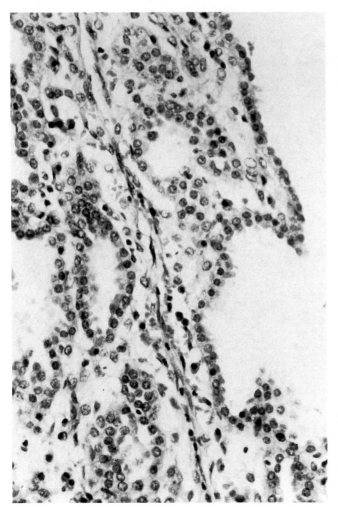

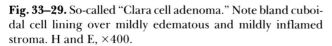

Fig. 33–29. So-called "Clara cell adenoma." Note bland cuboidal cell lining over mildly edematous and mildly inflamed stroma. H and E, ×400.

Fig. 33–30. Acinar atypical proliferation. Atypical cells line slightly thickened interstitium. There is a subtle but definite difference in degree of atypia and pleomorphism of lining cells here as compared to Fig. 33–29. H and E, ×400.

Clara cell adenomas have also been chemically induced in mice.[194,195]

The smaller adenomas need to be distinguished from early sclerosing hemangiomas and small mesenchymal cystic hamartomas of lung. Each of these entities is separately described in this chapter. Of note, some people believe that even the larger sclerosing hemangiomas of lung are epithelial adenomas, whereas I happen to think these are mesenchymal, as discussed in that section. Likewise, the entity of "alveolar adenoma" is discussed separately, and I believe that is likewise mesenchymal.

Early epithelial proliferations growing on alveolar septa have been described associated with adenocarcinomas, particularly bronchioloalveolar carcinoma (Fig. 33–30). They were found in two adolescents by Travis et al.[196] Miller et al.[197–199] studied small glandular

parenchymal lesions in lung tissues of adults resected for carcinomas in the lung. These areas were called acinar atypical proliferations by Dr. A. A. Liebow in the 1960s and 1970s. They have also been called alveolar epithelial hyperplasias,[200] bronchioloalveolar tumors of uncertain malignant potential, and bronchioloalveolar adenomas.[199] They were found in 15 of 70 (21%) resection of specimens by Nakanishi[200] and in 23 of 247 (9.3%) of Miller's 1990 series.[199] In both series they were only several millimeters in maximum dimension, but Miller[197] noted these are apparent after Bouin's inflation of gross lung specimens but are not easily seen with other fixatives such as formalin. They are certainly observed microscopically with greater frequency in lungs excised for adenocarcinomas, but not all cancers were adenocarcinomas, at least in one series.[200] Cytological atypia increased with lesion size, being mild in

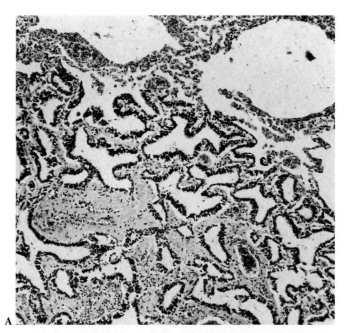
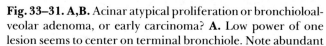
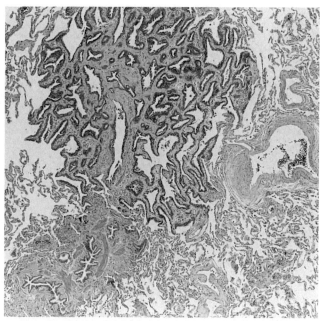

Fig. 33–31. A,B. Acinar atypical proliferation or bronchioloalveolar adenoma, or early carcinoma? **A.** Low power of one lesion seems to center on terminal bronchiole. Note abundant and rather regular stromal hyalinization. H and E, ×20. **B.** Slightly higher power of isolated 3-mm nodule in separate case shows relationship similar to that in A. H and E, ×50.

76% of those 3 mm or less in diameter, and moderate to markedly atypical in 67% of those 4 mm or larger.[199] These may represent multifocal origin or perhaps aerogenous spread, and perhaps most, if observed long enough, may "grow up" to become adenocarcinomas; when observed early, however, they appear to have some limited growth potential. Malignancies may of course start with a single cell, but not be recognizable for a certain number of duplications.

A variant of this problem with dense sclerosis is illustrated in Fig. 33–31. As noted in Chapter 32, in the section under **Bronchioloalveolar Carcinomas**, in the entity of "scar carcinoma," the tumor cells induce the fibrosis and not the reverse, as was originally thought. The same mechanism would appear to be functioning here, and these proliferations are typically around terminal bronchioles and may be multifocal, each being accompanied by dense sclerosis. These proliferations sometimes grow larger, and I believe that even they are precursors or early variants of bronchioloalveolar carcinoma, with the interstitial sclerosis perhaps indicating a slower growth pattern. This, however, awaits scientific study.

Mucinous Cystadenomas/Cystadenocarcinomas

An entity well described in other organs, particularly in the ovary, pancreas, appendix, and peritoneal cavity, and more recently in breast,[201] this tumor consists of tall columnar mucinous cells whose presence is noted mostly by a large amount of mucus. In the abdominal cavity, this has been called pseudomyxoma peritonei, and elsewhere they are mucinous tumors of low grade or indeterminate malignant potential. This entity has more recently been described in the lungs; the original description has been credited to Eck in Germany in 1969[202] and the next case to Sambrook-Gowar in England in 1978.[203] As of 1991, about 26 cases had been described[202–210]; 5 of these lack sufficient clinical detail, and the single largest series is 11 cases by Graeme-Cook and Mark in 1991.[210] This has been referred to by various names including mucinous cyst adenoma, mucinous cyst adenocarcinoma, mucinous cystic tumor borderline malignancy, mucinous multilocular cyst carcinoma, mucocele-like tumor, ususual mucous cyst, Schleimbildende cystische bronchial adenoma, pseudomyxomatous pulmonary adenocarcinoma, and mucinous or colloid carcinoma.

The age range is 41–78 years, averaging 62 years. The tumors are solitary, ranging from 0.8 to 15 cm in maximum diameter and averaging 4.7 cm. Two-thirds are right sided, especially in the right-lower lobe, which accounts for 38% of all. The gross appearance is usually gray, tan, or white or some combination, semitranslucent, gelatinous, rubbery, sticky, or slippery (Fig. 33–32) Their cystic quality is due to abundant mucin. Sometimes they are friable, breaking apart from the surrounding lung tissue, and even breaking apart of

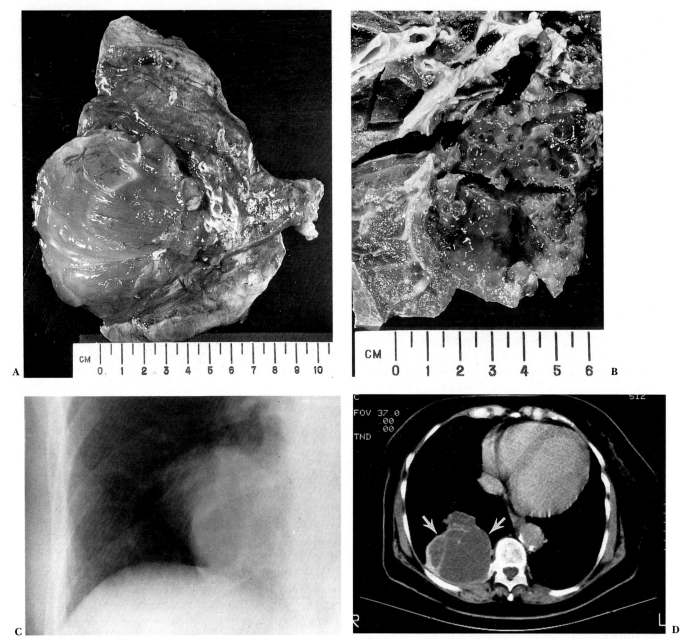

Fig. 33–32. A–D. Mucinous cystadenoma/cystade-nocarcinoma. **A.** Large, semitranslucent gelatinous periph-eral bulging cyst full of tenacious mucus is seen, appearing almost as one cyst. **B.** Different example shows multiple smaller cysts composing this case. **C.** Plain film of right-lower lung of example in **A.. D.** CT scan shows large right-posterior lung field tumor, representing that shown in **A..** (B is courtesy of Dr. Terrance Gleason, Providence Medical Center, Seattle, Washington.)

themselves on handling (Fig. 33–32). They usually have smooth contours with only slight irregularities of the borders. Microscopically there are pools of mucus that appears very dense, filling alveoli, with an irregular distribution of tumor cells in small rows on remnant lung architecture (Fig. 33–33). Free-floating tumor cells are not a feature (see following).

How these tumors relate to mucinous or so-called colloid carcinomas of the lung is unclear. A series of 24 of these cases thought to be primary in the lung was published by Moran et al.[211] This series included pa-tients 33–81 years old, with a median age of 57 years, 15 men and 9 women; the lesions presented as poorly defined peripheral nodules, sometimes large, varying in size from 0.5 to 10 cm. In this series 2 cases had lymph node metastases, 1 had bony metastases, while another

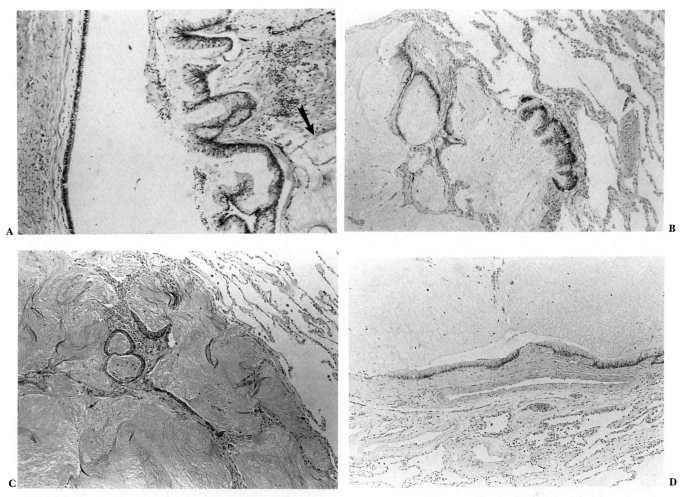

Fig. 33–33. A–D. Mucinous cystadenoma/cystadenocarcinoma. **A.** Example shown in 33–32A shows normal bronchial lining to left and neoplastic lining to right. Notice mucous pools spilling into adjacent lung parenchyma (*arrow*). **B** and **C.** Lesion from Fig. 33–32B. Note focal areas of tall columnar mucinous cohesive cells lining existent structures. Skip areas without tumor cells are present Dense mucus is best seen in **C.** No capsule is present in this example. **D.** Rarely compressed fibrous rim is seen as capsule in some of these tumors. H and E, ×50.

had intrapulmonary recurrences during a follow-up period of 2–192 months. The median survival was 48 months, and 8 patients died with or of their tumors. These tumors differ in three ways from mucinous cystodenomas/cystadenocarcinomas: (1) They are not cystic; (2) they consistently have individual or small nests of free-floating tumor cells in mucin pools, similar to typical colloid carcinomas elsewhere; and (3) they are more aggressive.[211] Some overlap in these entities seems probable, however, and may represent the spectrum implied in the name cystodenoma/cystadenocarcinoma.[211]

Moran et al.[211] proposed that their cases were a variant of bronchioloalveolar carcinoma (BAC). Several cases published under the BAC designation appear to better represent this tumor.[212,213] Whether they are truly mucinous variants of BAC is open to discussion. In contrast to the usual spectrum of BAC tumors, these are usually solitary and are not multifocal, nor do they present with the mucinous-unresolved pneumonia pattern of BAC. The total volume of tumor cells appear less than in BAC. Also, the sticky tenacious mucin in this tumor differs from the wetter, slimy type in the mucinous-unresolved pneumonia pattern of BAC, and they are not as malignant, especially considering their sizes. Therefore, I think they should be considered as a tumor separate from the entity BAC.

A few probably act aggressively,[211,214] and therefore the same dilemma in naming exists as for similar tumors in other organs. Some may prefer mucinous tumor of low or undetermined malignant potential, and assorted names are given here. Mucinous cystadenoma was originally suggested by Kragel et al.[209] and I have been now chosen mucinous cystadenomas/cystadenocarcinomas to try to recognize this spectrum. Most, however, are benign and can be cured by excision, and I believe calling all these carcinoma would be unfair, even detrimental, to many patients.

In the differential diagnosis are metastases from excess mucin-producing tumors elsewhere, one from a colloid carcinoma of breast, more difficult to distinguish, is shown in Fig. 33–34A, and one from a more easily distinguished mucinous tumor of colon in (Fig. 33–34B).

Malignant Mixed Tumors of Lung

The tumors to be discussed in this section are rare primary pulmonary tumors that have malignant epithelial and mesenchymal or mesenchymal-appearing components. Classically these have been called pulmonary carcinosarcomas and blastomas, and recently interest has been directed toward spindle cell carcinomas (or carcinomas with spindle cell stroma) in lung and elsewhere and to more monomorphic adenocarcinomas with endodermal or fetal-type linings similar to those seen in blastomas.

Stromal changes seen in association with carcinomas in lung may be reactive or neoplastic. The reactive ones cover a variety of reaction patterns from the usual modestly to moderately cellular desmoplasias to dense hyalinization; the latter is further discussed in Chapter 32 in the section on **Bronchioloalveolar Carcinoma**,

and early lesions, perhaps precursors to the same, are discussed in this chapter under **Surface Adenomas**. Those with malignant stroma may have stromal characteristics that are classified as spindle cell, both with longer tapering fibrosarcomatous type cells, and another of more plump epithelioid cells, which may be primitive (see **Blastomas**), or the tumor may differentiate into one of the soft-tissue type of sarcomas such as osteosarcoma or chondrosarcoma. Spindle cell carcinomas are discussed with carcinosarcomas, as they have some characteristics in common. Sometimes these spindle cells appear epithelioid and have more of the spindle component of carcinoma, which is sometimes confirmed by electron microscopy or immunoperoxidase. Differentiated soft-tissue sarcomatous patterns can occur in either carcinosarcomas or blastomas, and this characteristic has been used to separate out carcinosarcoma from spindle cell carcinoma.[215] The typical blastoma has a primitive smaller cell and somewhat edematous appearing stroma without fascicles of spindle cells, with a typical glandular lining, the combination that recapitulates the fetal growth period of 10–16 weeks in the human embryo. Greater stromal cellularity is present in some (see following). Ashworth[216] noted that a blastoma reproduces, in a disorderly fashion, the embryonal structure of the organ in which it arose. The World Health Organization classification of lung tumors refers to this group as "carcinoma of the embryonal type (blastoma)."[217] As discussed in that section, at times more typical adenocarcinoma, and at times the

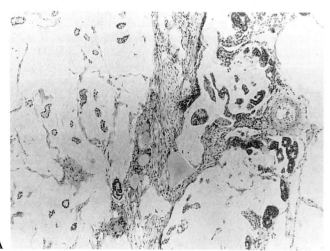

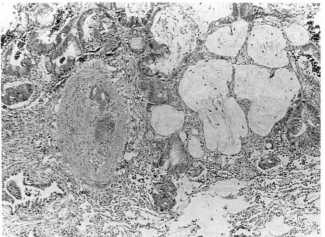

A   B

Fig. 33–34. A,B. Mucinous tumor metastases to lung. In the differential diagnosis of mucinous cystadenoma/cystadenocarcinoma are metastases from mucinous or colloid carcinomas. **A.** Example of metastasis from colloid carcinoma of known breast primary, with positive estrogen and progesterone receptor analysis on lung tissue, can present a problem. Note cells are more individual, loosely cohesive, and smaller and more cuboidal than tall and columnar ones in the mucinous cystadenomas/cystadenocarcinoma. H and E, ×100. **B.** Metastatic colon cancer. Note tumor in thrombosed vessel; this higher grade lesion with more abundant tumor cells should not be difficult to distinguish from low-grade or well-differentiated patchy-paucicellular one of mucinous cystadenomas/cystadenocarcinoma. H and E, ×100.

typical fetal lung type adenocarcinomas, predominate to the exclusion of the stromal component.

Sometimes the word mixed tumor is used in referring to benign salivary gland or bronchial gland tumors, as noted in that section in this chapter. Occasionally carcinoma arises in these bronchial gland mixed-type tumors; it is usually epithelial, is mentioned briefly in that section, and is further discussed here. Also, some carcinomas undergo such complete sarcomatous metaplasia that they are considered metaplastic carcinomas, and these are mentioned in the lung in the osteosarcoma section to follow. In humans, this is seen most frequently in the breast. The multiple differentiation capacity within the epithelial line is discussed in adenocarcinomas and other mixed epithelial tumors in Chapter 32, **Common Neoplasms**, and adenosquamous carcinomas are contrasted with mucoepidermoid carcinomas in this section. Two or more differentiated soft-tissue sarcomas components in a sarcoma can occur, fulfilling the criteria of mesenchymoma, and this occurs more commonly than would be implied by the frequency of the use of that term. At times higher grade epithelial tumors have a benign osteoclast-like giant cell response; this is discussed separately in this chapter.

The usual type of epithelium in carcinosarcoma and spindle cell carcinomas is squamous cell, although some adenocarcinomas can elicit or be associated with a similar reaction.[218-220] Even a small cell polypoid endobronchial neuroendocrine tumor has been associated with spindle cell actin and epithelial marker positive stroma.[221] Glandular epithelium is always the type associated with pulmonary blastomas, and it is usually of embryonal type; occasionally however is of the more typical adenocarcinoma type, as is noted in that section. Some tumors appear to have crossover features between these descriptions, and at times a descriptive diagnosis is best.

Malignant tumors with both carcinomatous and intimately admixed sarcomatous components have been subject to much speculation in the lung and elsewhere. The proposed mechanisms are discussed. In way of introduction, there are some excellent large series and reviews available that should be highlighted for the interested reader; these include 48 cases of pulmonary carcinosarcoma by Cabarcos and associates in 1985,[222] 83 cases of pulmonary blastoma, most from the literature, reviewed by Francis and Jacobsen in 1983,[223] and 52 new cases of pulmonary blastoma from the Armed Forces Institute of Pathology published by Koss et al. in 1991.[224] These serve as excellent sources for reviewing the tumors in this section. Koss et al.[224] also elaborated on the epithelial predominant variant of blastoma. Although all the variants discussed in this section are described separately, it should be emphasized that

parenchymal carcinomas and biphasic blastomas are usually as malignant as common lung carcinoma, and their subdivisions arise more from histological curiosity than any prognostic significance.

Carcinosarcomas

Intimately admixed carcinomas and sarcomas have been described in other organs, particularly where associated with glandular neoplasms in the uterus, and squamous neoplasms in the upper airway and esophagus, among other sites.[222]

The first reported case of carcinosarcoma in the lung is attributed to Kika in 1909, as noted by Herxheimer and Reinke in 1912.[225] No details of this first case are available. Early cases from 1908 to 1951 have been reviewed by Bergmann et al.[226] Cabarcos and associates[222] offered tabulation of many of the details of the other cases in their fine review. By 1961, Moore[226] had reviewed 13 cases reported in the lung, and noted that pulmonary carcinosarcomas appear in two forms: smaller more central ones with a high degree of endobronchial spread, and larger more peripheral ones with less endobronchial spread. Those with endobronchial spread produce bronchial obstruction with distal atelectasis, bronchiectasis, abscess formation, and signs of acute and chronic suppuration (see Chapter 5). Such endobronchial spread is also seen with spindle cell carcinomas, as discussed next. They presumably come to attention earlier and therefore are detected at a smaller size than the peripheral ones, which provides a better prognosis than either the larger more peripheral carcinosarcomas, spindle cell carcinomas, or biphasic pulmonary blastomas. Despite an earlier suggestion of better survival, as noted, parenchymal carcinosarcoma and biphasic blastoma patients have poor survival, quite similar to that of general primary lung cancers. Of interest, tobacco use has been documented in 83% of pulmonary blastomas[224] and 93% of both carcinosarcomas[226] and spindle cell carcinomas[229] incidences that are similar to more common forms of lung cancer.

Pulmonary carcinosarcomas account for some 0.2%–0.3% of all pulmonary neoplasms.[230,231] These are basically a tumor of older people, especially men, and 40 of 48 cases reported by 1985[222] were in men (male-to-female = 5:1). The youngest patient was 21, another was 35, 4 were in their forties, and 42 of 48 (87.5%) were 50 years or older. Therefore only 4% were less than 40 and 12.5% less than 50 years of age. In the review by Carbarcos et al.,[222] these tumors have a propensity for occurring in the upper lobes, with 28 of 46 (61%) with described locations in the upper lobes, 2 each in the right-middle lobe and lingula of the left-upper lobe, and 7 each in the lower lobes. Also in one review from

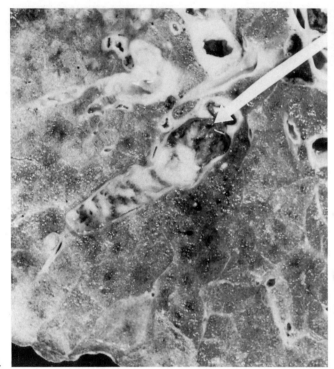

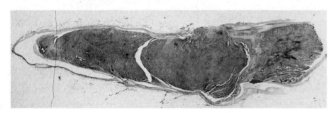

Fig. 33–35. A,B. Central carcinosarcoma and spindle cell carcinomas each can have endobronchial extension. **A.** Tongue of tumor fills (*arrow*). **B.** Low-power view; much of this tongue toward left is free of bronchial wall attachment, tears to occur on right edge. H and E, ×10.

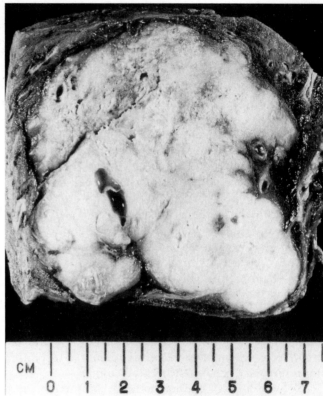

Fig. 33–36. Peripheral carcinosarcoma. Larger tumor mass without prominent endobronchial spread was predominantly sarcomatous until multiple sections showed transition to in situ squamous cell carcinoma (see text).

the Mayo Clinic, Davis et al.[238] noted upper-lobe occurrence in 10 of their 17 cases (59%). Only 14% were less than 2 cm in diameter, and many approached a large size.

Of those reported as having died as a result of the tumor, 73% did so within the first 6 months of diagnosis. Metastases are often present at initial diagnosis, and direct invasion may occur through the pleura into the chest wall or mediastinum, either before attempted excision or in recurrent form. The tumor spreads in a metastatic pattern quite similar to primary lung cancers, and involves hilar lymph nodes with regularity.

Grossly, the tumors may present as either a relatively homogeneous grey-pink mass or with a fair degree of variegation (Figs. 33–35 and 33–36). The peripheral larger tumors show frequent necrosis and hemorrhage. Those with endobronchial spread are usually smaller,

rubbery, grey-pink, and tubular, distending the bronchi in which they occur (see Fig. 33–35). Sometimes adjacent bronchi are involved with fingers of tumor. Obvious hemorrhage and necrosis are not as frequent in the endobronchial lesion as in their generally large peripheral counterpart. About half or slightly more of all carcinosarcomas present with a predominant endobronchial spread pattern. The sites of tumor attachment are usually focal, and there may be adjacent extension into the parenchyma. Endobronchial spread is not usually very prevalent grossly in those arising in the periphery, perhaps because of the lack of bronchi of adequate size to shape their spreading pattern.

Histologically,[222] the most common epithelial component is squamous carcinoma (69%) (Fig. 33–37); adenocarcinoma is represented in 20% (Fig. 33–38) and undifferentiated large cell carcinoma in 11%. With one exception,[221] small cell carcinoma is usually not a component, but at times an almost neuroendocrine appearance is suggested (Fig. 33–39). Several articles have addressed adenocarcinomas with sarcomatous or sarcomatoid stromal change,[218–220,232] two of which describe

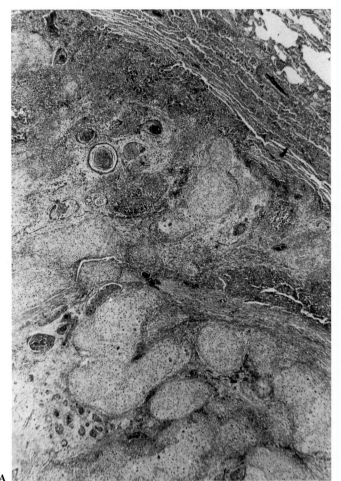

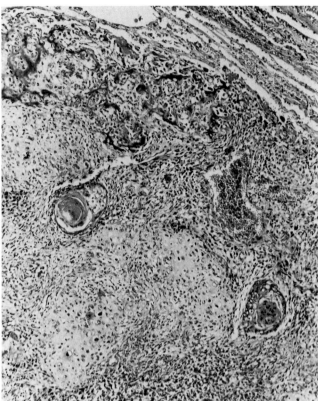

Fig. 33–37. A,B. Carcinosarcoma. **A.** Low power shows nests of squamous cells and hint of chondroid material. H and E, ×50. **B.** Higher power confirms these impressions, plus some possible osteoid at top. Keratin nests are present in both **A** and **B.** H and E, ×400.

polypoid endobronchial tumors.[218,232] The most frequent stromal component is spindle cell type, classically referred to as "fibrosarcoma" and present in 43% of cases. The stroma is usually looser and more pleomorphic than that accepted by current criteria for fibrosarcoma, so this term is used loosely. Close behind this is a category called "undifferentiated appearing sarcoma," accounting for 39% of the tumors. Osteoid differentiation has been mentioned in 18%, and chondroid and rhabdoid differentiation are present in lesser degrees. Usually the sarcomatous-appearing component is the dominant component. (See section to follow on spindle cell-sarcomatoid carcinoma.)

With endobronchial spread (Fig. 33–40), the carcinomatous component is usually a nonkeratinizing squamous carcinoma composed of small basilar or peribasilar type cells covering the tongues of tumor, focally seen within its substance and focally replacing adjacent bronchial mucosa (Fig. 33–41A). Transition between epithelial and spindle cells may be seen (Fig. 33–41B). Sometimes focal keratinization (Fig. 33–37) or less frequently atypical glands (Fig. 33–38) are seen in

epithelial nests in the midst of the tumor stroma. In the peripheral tumors and focally in some of the endobronchial tumors, the cellular stroma can become quite pleomorphic and show differentiated mesenchyme (Figs. 33–37 and 33–38).

At least some of the tumors classically thought to be primary sarcomas in the lung, even with adult differentiation of stroma, on further sectioning show a carcinomatous component. Colby et al.[233] have seen this in two of their five osteosarcomas thought primary in lung. We have seen this in another 11-cm tumor thought to be a fibrosarcoma of lung, which when further sectioned for similar purposes showed a transition to squamous carcinoma. A similar case thought to be primary osteosarcoma was found on examination of spread to mediastinum to contain an epithelial component.[234] Therefore, any tumor in lung now, even those with an adult sarcomatous component, may eventually be seen to have an epithelial component, and their origin therefore is presumably in a carcinosarcomatous setting. This may also apply to some of the tumors described next as malignant fibrous histiocytomas.

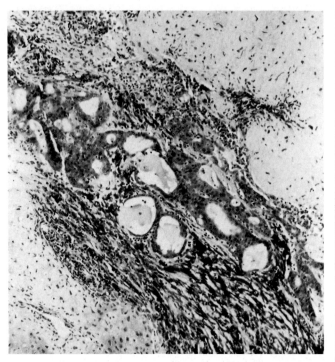

Fig. 33–38. Carcinosarcoma. Immature cartilage on both sides of malignant glands. Note pleomorphic stromal cells. H and E, ×100.

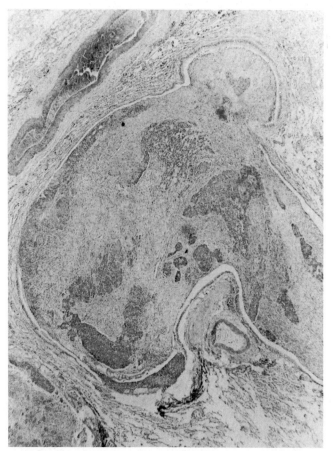

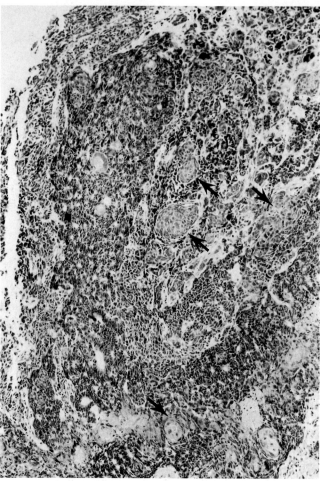

Fig. 33–39. Carcinosarcoma. Focal squamous component is throughout (*arrows*) areas of otherwise primitive, mostly spindled, almost neuroendocrine-like, rosette-forming epithelial cells. H and E, ×250.

Spindle Cell or Sarcomatoid Carcinoma

As the most common stroma in carcinosarcoma is spindle cell, distinction of carcinosarcomas from carcinoma with spindle cell or sarcomatoid change can be challenging. The nomenclature in the lung has not followed similar nomenclature in the endometrium, that of carcinosarcoma or mixed Müllerian sarcomas with homologous or heterologous elements. Spindle cell or sarcomatoid stromal change most often occurs with squamous carcinomas (Figs. 33–40 and 33–41), but as noted has also been described in the lung with adenocarcinomas and neuroendocrine tumors. I wonder if some lung cancers will eventually also have desmoplastic characteristics, as have been described in pleural

◁ ─────────────────────────

Fig. 33–40. Central spindle cell carcinoma with endobronchial extension. Refer to Fig. 33–35. H and E, ×50.

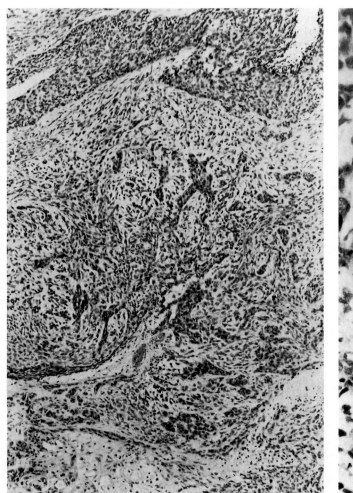 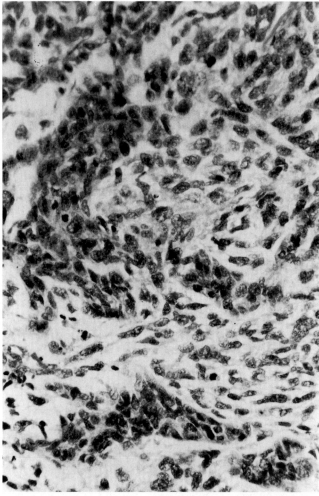

Fig. 33–41. A,B. Spindle cell carcinoma. **A.** Dysplastic lining cells at top and bottom left give way to infiltrating prongs and spindle cell forms of tumor. H and E, ×100. **B.** High-power view of **A** shows transition between more epithelial- and more mesenchymal-appearing components. Note similarity of nuclei in these two compartments. H and E. ×400.

mesotheliomas and cutaneous melanomas. Addis and Corrin[232] in 1985 performed immunoperoxidase on five spindle cell carcinomas, four blastomas, and nine carcinosarcomas, and confirmed at least focally the epithelial nature of the spindle cell areas in all the tumors called spindle cell carcinoma and in four of the nine called carcinosarcomas, but not in the other five carcinosarcomas or in any of the four pulmonary blastomas. Further immunoperoxidase studies on biphasic lung tumors were done by Ishida et al.[215] and IP and EM studies by Humphrey et al.[235] and Ro et al.[229] Each addresses this problem. Humphrey et al.[235] suggested that those pulmonary carcinomas with epithelial differentiation by any technique be termed spindle cell carcinomas and those lacking such differentiation, or with adult-type sarcomatous differentiation, be classified as carcinosarcomas. However, these authors admit that

these tumors may act equally aggressively and that this distinction may not be necessary. After eliminating endobronchial carcinosarcomas, pulmonary blastomas, and lesions thought as primary sarcoma of lung, 12 of the 14 cases studied by Ro et al.[229] had an identifiable epithelial carcinomatous component being adenocarcinoma in 4, squamous carcinoma in 3, adenosquamous carcinoma in 2, and large cell undifferentiated in 3.

The subsets of both carcinosarcomas and spindle cell carcinomas with predominant endobronchial spread do need to be considered separately as both have better prognoses than their peripheral counterparts. Probably many of the tumors classified as endobronchial carcinosarcomas in the past better fit the endobronchial spindle cell carcinoma designation today, as they are usually poorly differentiated squamous carcinoma with a spindle cell component.

Conclusion

These findings challenge our original concepts of the three-cell theory of development, but with improved techniques seem irrefutable. The logical conclusion is that a cell once it becomes tumorous can dip into its heritage pool of totipotentiality and do several things, even within a single tumor. It may be that more cases of differentiated sarcoma will be proven to have epithelial components, and, by deduction, perhaps be derived from carcinomas. Therefore, the attempts by past authors at making sense of these tumors, developed within the confines of the three- germ-cell layer theory, such as epithelial carcinoma eliciting an pseudosarcomatous component, or a collision of true malignant epithelial and sarcomatous components, are no longer necessary once we accept this totipotentiality. It seems an easy next step is to presume that even in those tumors with spindle cell or differentiated sarcoma stroma, but without epithelial differentiation markers, that they likewise may have arisen through similar neoplastic evolution and originated from one cell, only losing, or never gaining, their epithelial characteristics along the way.

Pulmonary Blastoma

This tumor was first described in 1945 by Barnett and Barnard[236] as a mixed carcinoma and sarcoma of lung among a group of unusual thoracic tumors. In this report one of the original pathologists (presumably Barnard) was quoted as noting that the glandular component closely resembled immature bronchus and that the connective tissue relationship suggested that seen both in "embryomata of kidney" and "embryonic lung." It was further suggested by the same pathologist that the tumor may have arisen from a part of the lung that remained dormant or underdeveloped, or perhaps the tumor was "recapitulating its own life history." The latter idea has gained more favor than the former, except perhaps in those cases described in infants.

This original tumor was 12 × 7 × 7 cm when removed from the middle of the right lung of a 40-year-old woman. She had previously coughed up a bronchial cast about the size of her forefinger, which on microscopic examination contained malignant cells. This case was again reported by Barnard[237] in 1952 as a single case report, with the suggestion that it be called "embryoma of lung."

Spencer[238] in 1961 reviewed Barnard's case and noted by then the patient was free of tumor 15 years. He added three additional cases and elaborated on some of the similarities to embryologic lung and kidney previously mentioned. He noted in Barnard's case and in two additional cases that "the differentiation of the stroma in some parts was poor enough to justify a diagnosis of carcinosarcoma." He also noted "In the more immature parts, the stromal cells condense to form a sheath of elongated cells surrounding each tubule." Spencer[238] proposed the term "blastoma" in comparison with the appearance of a nephroblastoma (Wilms' tumor) in the kidney, and used the embryologic work of Waddell[239] in 1949, who thought the periphery of the lung, like the kidney, was solely mesodermal in its derivation and that the peripheral air spaces derived from mesoderm and joined the more central endodermal outpouchings. Spencer[6] continues to support this theory while others, as reviewed by Fung et al.,[240] believe that the lung is formed in its entirety from two germ layers, with the endodermal outpouchings stimulating surrounding mesenchyme.

These tumors classically had a biphasic age distribution, with the first peak in the first decade, some drop in the second decade, and a steady rise beginning thereafter with maximum incidence in the seventh decade.[223] The age spectrum would be similar to carcinosarcomas except for those occurring at an earlier age. An extensive and carefully studied 1991 series of 52 cases of pulmonary blastoma by Koss et al.[224] from the Armed Forces Institute of Pathology noted only a unimodal age curve, peaking in the thirties. Manivel et al.[241] wondered if there is truly a biphasic pulmonary blastoma in youth, but others[224,242] believe there are. As with thoracoblastoma as described by Askin et al.[243] I wonder if some, or many, of these tumors would fit into the more newly described entity of primitive neuroectodermal tumor (PNET). In the first decade several cases occurred in the early months of life, including one that was documented soon after birth.[216] These are presumably congenital in origin. In the large review by Francis and Jacobsen[223] the mean age for all cases was 43 years (48.2 years for men, 29.2 years for women). Twenty percent occurred before age 20, and 40% before age 40. The oldest patient was 80 years old at the time of diagnosis. In this literature review,[223] there was a male predominance of 2.1:1 when all cases were considered; in a series solely of pediatric blastomas, this ratio approached 1.1.[244] (The reader is referred to a discussion of this tumor in the pediatric age group in Chapter 8 of this book.) The Koss et al. series[224] contained 28 women and 24 men (54% women) and only 2 patients were younger than 10 years. There was no significant age difference between men and women. A high percentage (83%) of patients were smokers, and asymptomatic (41%). No particular lobe was favored. The tumors were more often peripheral than central, and when large, they were both. Some endobronchial tumor spread was noted in 21% of these cases. Blastomas account for 0.25%–0.5% of primary lung tumors in several large series.[223,245,246] This, too, is an aggressive tumor; only 16% survived for 5 years in the largest series, documented by Francis and Jacobsen.[223]

This group of tumors is distinctive because of its suggested recapitulation of early embryologic lung development. If one retains this pattern of "recapitulation," with glycogen-rich, clear, rather orderly glandular cells in a primitive but bland stroma as being the basis for classification of the tumor, it also appears distinctive from carcinosarcomas. The reader must be aware of different authors' use of the word "immature," and think of this word more as "embryonal," which would indicate at least a certain degree of maturity or blandness without the alternate connotation of pleomorphic anaplasia.

In the review by Francis and Jacobsen,[223] many of their tumors so accepted as blastoma do conform to this definition, but other components or parts of the tumor in other regions vary significantly into areas of poorly and well-differentiated squamous differentiation. Certainly tumors can have aspects that have been classically described as both blastoma and carcinosarcoma.[247-251] Survival rates between the two tumors are similar. A few of these patients have had prolonged survival, up to 24 years in the longest known cases;[244,252] however, again similar to carcinosarcomas, in Francis and Jacobsen's review[223] about 75%–80% of patients were dead at the first anniversary of the diagnosis of the tumor. However, survival is affected by differentiation and several other features.

Using data from the large Koss et al. series[224] (Table 33–3), grossly pulmonary blastoma have a mean diameter of 7.4 cm with 36% less than 5 cm, 45% in the range of 5 to 10 cm (therefore, 81% are less than 10 cm), and 19% more than 10 cm. They are usually peripheral or midlung in location with 27% involving bronchi, 10% involving only wall, and 17% of the total having an endobronchial polypoid component. The peripheral ones are typically rounded with fairly even contours, but some have some peripheral lobulations. Their color is typically variegated with mixtures of white, tan, gray, hemorrhagic red or brown, yellow, or pink. They are often soft and pliable but sometimes rubbery. Some 50% have necrosis, usually focal and central; necrosis involves more than 25% of the tumor volume in only 4%. Macroscopic pulmonary vessel invasion was seen in only 7% and one had bilateral iliac artery embolization (see Chapter 35). Cavitation, atelectasis, lymphadenopathy by chest radiographic, nodal disease pathologically, or pleural effusion were infrequent findings.

Microscopically, the glandular component consists of branching tubules lined by clear stratifying glycogen-rich columnar cells with relatively little hyperchromasia or pleomorphism or mitotic rate (Figs. 33–42 through

Table 33–3. Comparative pathologic features of pulmonary blastomas by histologic subtype[a]

Subtype	WDFA No. (%)[b]	Biphasic blastoma No. (%)
No. of cases	28	24
Mean size (range) (cm)	4.5 (1–10)	10.2 (2–27)
Solitary/multiple	26/0	20/4
Subpleural	24 (86)	16 (67)
Intrabronchial	6 (21)	7 (29)
Well-circumscribed	21 (86)	14 (67)
Endometrioid (≥75% of epithelium)	17 (61)	5 (21)
Solid cords of cells	2 (7)	16 (67)
Adenocarcinoma (>0%[c] of epithelium)	9 (32)	10 (36)
Undifferentiated sheets of cells	0	13 (54)
Morules	24 (86)	12 (43)
Necrosis (≥25% of tumor)	2 (7)	12 (50)
No. of mitoses/10 HPF	20	24
Tumor giant cells	1 (4)	6 (21)
Embryonic stroma (≥1+)†	0	20 (83)
Adult sarcoma (≤1+)†	0	20 (83)
Striated muscle present	0	6 (25)
Cartilage present	3[d]	6 (25)
Bone present	0	3 (13)
Lymph node metastasis	3	3
Pathologic stage		
=1	20	19
>1	4	3

[a] Used with permission from Koss MN, Hochholzer L, O'Leary T. Pulmonary balstomas. Cancer 1991; 67:2368–2381.
[b] WDFA: well-differentiated fetal adenocarcinoma; HPF: high-power field.
[c] >0% correct as verified with original author.
[d] Two cases may be residual bronchial cartilage.

33–44). They often have bland-appearing squamous morula at the base of the glands (Fig. 42–43). Koss et al.[224] refers to this pattern as endometrioid (Table 33–4), and one-third of their cases had a more typical adenocarcinoma with glands lined by single cells, with minimal marked atypia. Mucin is usually stained along luminal border and only rarely presents as goblet cells. The stroma may represent either adult-type sarcoma, or most often has somewhat edematous stroma with small cells or spindle cells without other differentiation. A small cell aggressive component sometimes evolves from cellular stroma, in which it is difficult to distinguish primitive epithelial origin from stromal origin by light microscopy alone (Fig. 33–45). The adult sarcomatous types may have benign or malignant specialized differentiation,[223] including cartilage in 24% (Fig. 33–45C), and muscle in 20% including cross striations in 5% or bone in 5%. Stroma is scant and bland in the well-differentiated group (Fig. 33–34). Yolk sac carcinoma[253] and melanoma differentiation[254] have been noted in these tumors. I have seen one large mediastinal

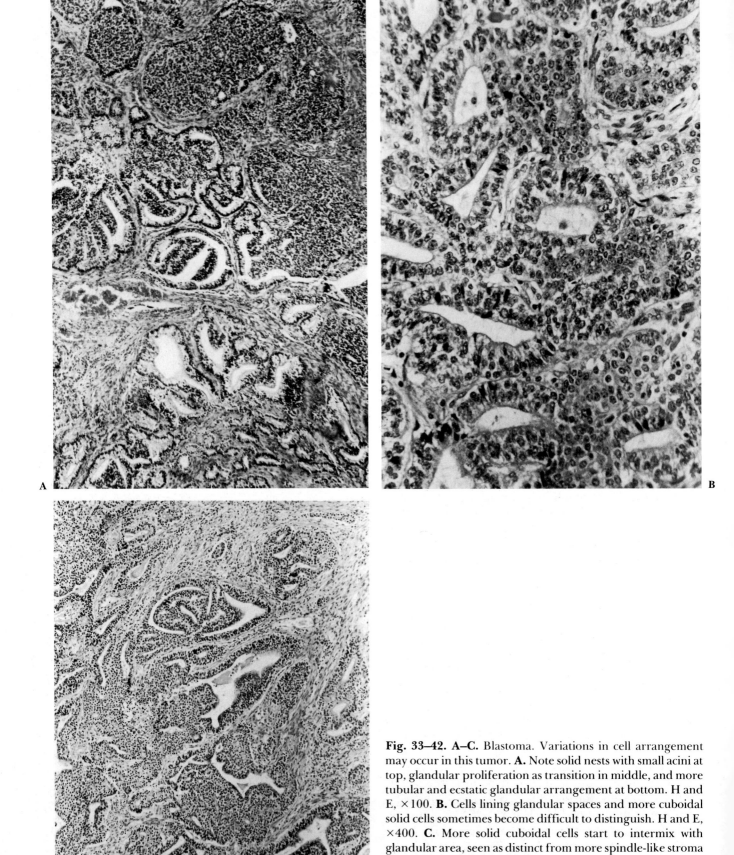

Fig. 33–42. A–C. Blastoma. Variations in cell arrangement may occur in this tumor. **A.** Note solid nests with small acini at top, glandular proliferation as transition in middle, and more tubular and ecstatic glandular arrangement at bottom. H and E, ×100. **B.** Cells lining glandular spaces and more cuboidal solid cells sometimes become difficult to distinguish. H and E, ×400. **C.** More solid cuboidal cells start to intermix with glandular area, seen as distinct from more spindle-like stroma at top. H and E, ×100.

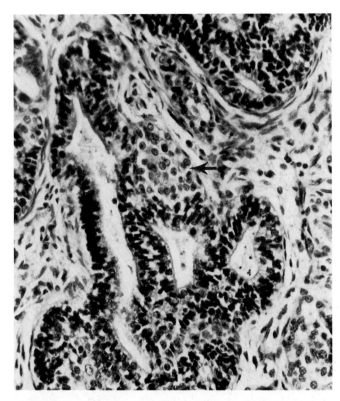

Fig. 33–43. Blastoma. Glands may contain one or two layers of elongated nuclei; discrete focal nests, sometimes appearing as morula, may be seen (*arrow*). H and E, ×400.

Table 33–4. Pulmonary blastomas immunostaining cumulative data[224,232,256–263]

	No. positive no. tested	Positive (%)
Keratin	56/58	97
CEA	35/44	80
Milk fat globule	13/15	87
B72.3	0/3	0
Clara cell antigen	5/9	56
Surfactant apoprotein	8/14	57
Vimentin	19/20	95
Desmin	10/30	33
Actin	28/30	93
Myoglobulin	2/4	50
S-100	2/12	17
NSE	11/16	69
Chromogranin	32/45	71

yolk sac tumor that invaded the lung and caused some confusion for the entity of pulmonary blastoma. Of note, yolk sac tumors have been described with spindle cell stroma in both primary locations and in their pulmonary metatases.[255] The interested reader is referred to the excellent series by Koss et al.[224] for more detail.

There may be focal argyrophilia in scattered individual cells lining the glands. Immunoperoxidase studies up to 1990[224,232,256–263] have been summarized by Yousem et al.[262] These findings, and the large series by Koss et al.[224] in 1991, are summarized in Table 33–4 as follows: the epithelial markers of cytokeratin, CEA and EMA stain the epithelial tubules and morules, while vimentin and, to a somewhat lesser extent, actin and desmin, stain stromal cells. With rare exception,[232,262] epithelial markers are usually limited to the epithelium and do not stain stroma, and vice versa. Chromogranin is focally positive in most cases, and is seen in select cells in epithelial tubules. Of interest, B72.3 has been negative in all those stained,[224] in contrast to more routine types of adenocarcinomas (see Table 33–4). The interested reader is referred to more recent immunoperoxidase studies on spindle cell carcinomas.[264–266]

Prognosis is related to differentiation, as noted in the series by Koss et al.[224] Mark[267] also considered those predominantly glandular as well differentiated, those with about equal glandular and mesenchymal components as intermediate, and those that were predominantly mesenchymal as poorly differentiated. Other prognostic factors noted by Koss et al.[224] were presence of metastases at presentation, recurrences, tumor size,

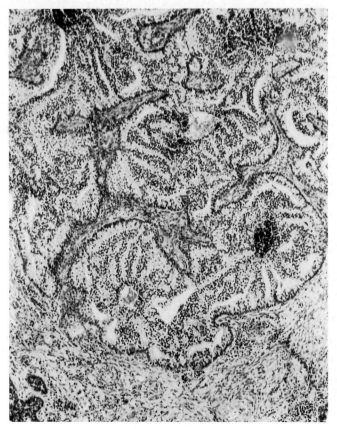

◁ ─────────────────────────────

Fig. 33–44. Blastoma. Low-power view of predominantly glandular arrangement toward top; some spindle cell stroma at bottom. H and E, ×100.

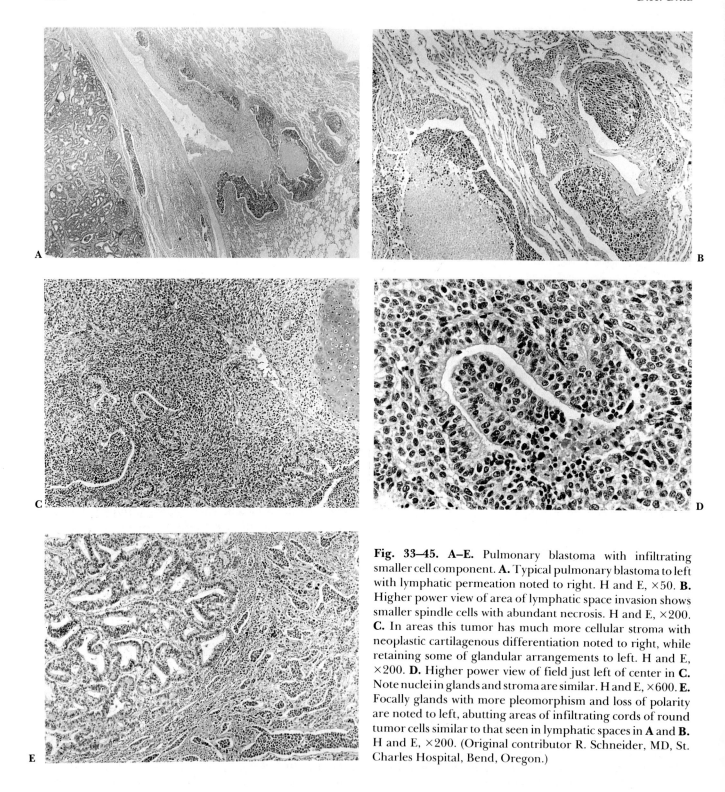

Fig. 33–45. A–E. Pulmonary blastoma with infiltrating smaller cell component. **A.** Typical pulmonary blastoma to left with lymphatic permeation noted to right. H and E, ×50. **B.** Higher power view of area of lymphatic space invasion shows smaller spindle cells with abundant necrosis. H and E, ×200. **C.** In areas this tumor has much more cellular stroma with neoplastic cartilagenous differentiation noted to right, while retaining some of glandular arrangements to left. H and E, ×200. **D.** Higher power view of field just left of center in **C.** Note nuclei in glands and stroma are similar. H and E, ×600. **E.** Focally glands with more pleomorphism and loss of polarity are noted to left, abutting areas of infiltrating cords of round tumor cells similar to that seen in lymphatic spaces in **A** and **B.** H and E, ×200. (Original contributor R. Schneider, MD, St. Charles Hospital, Bend, Oregon.)

thoracic lymphadenopathy by chest radiographs, nodal metastases pathologically, pathological stage, stromal nuclear pleomorphism, and presence of an adult sarcoma type stroma. In the well-differentiated predominantly glandular subgroup, survival was affected by tumor size and recurrence more so than in the biphasic group.

Predominantly Glandular/Endodermal-Type Tumors

Mark[267] described "better differentiated" areas of pulmonary blastomas as predominantly orderly glandular clear cell proliferations, with or without morulae, in associated solid more epithelial areas (Fig. 33–44). These areas can be seen among cellular stroma in more typical blastomas, or can be seen without the associated stroma typical of blastomas. More recently some solely glandular tumors have been described with special emphasis on their focal neurosecretory features. Kradin and associates[268] described the first such case in a 35-year-old woman. The argyrophilic-staining cells were singular in the glandular mucosa. Kradin et al.[268] confirmed neurosecretory granules by transmission electron microscopy and also confirmed the glandular and glycogen-rich characteristics in these same areas of cells adjacent to the neurosecretory cells. See discussion of immunoperoxidase neuroendocrine markers. They proposed the somewhat lengthy term of "pulmonary endodermal tumor resembling fetal lung," while noting the tumor's similarity to the epithelium of blastoma.

Kodama and associates[256] described six cases of similar clear cell well-differentiated tubular adenocarcinomas without sarcomatous components, and compared these to three more typical cases of blastoma. Focal argyrophilia was noted on special stains in one case of the adenocarcinoma and in two of three blastomas. Abundant glycogen was present in all, and cilia and mucin were absent in most. Four of the six predominantly glandular tumors and one of the three blastomas had isolated cells that stained positively by anticalcitonin and antigastrin-releasing peptide stains by immunohistochemistry. Two of the six adenocarcinomas had neurosecretory features confirmed by electron microscopy. These tumors, whether they were monomorphic and glandular or biphasic and blastomatous, were large and had an equally poor prognosis.

Manning et al.[257] described a similar tumor in a 12-year-old boy. Müller-Hermelink and Kaiserling[258] described an additional case in 1986 and found argyrophilic qualities in the solid morulae in their case. Some of their cells had larger inclusions on electron microscopy, suggesting those seen in Clara cells, but also had some concentric laminated bodies suggesting the type seen in alveolar type II cells. Tamai and associates[269]

transplanted typical pulmonary blastoma with epithelial and mesenchymal components into athymic nude mice, and on repeated passage, the stromal elements of the tumor disappeared and the epithelial elements showed squamous metaplasia and focal mucus production; neuroendocrine granules were observed in a few cells, although these granules were not identified in the original tumor. A few retained their glycogen-rich quality and occasionally developed microvilli after their fourth passage: These authors also noted 2 cases of tumors similar to that just described of well-differentiated adenocarcinoma among 380 cases in their files of lung adenocarcinoma, for an incidence of 0.5%.[269] Nakatani et al.[263] described five similar cases using the term "pulmonary endodermal tumor resembling fetal lung," and Koss et al.[224] described 28 of their 52 cases (54%) as this type, using the name well-differentiated fetal adenocarcinoma. Their patients had a better survival with only 29% recurring and 14% dying of their tumor, with a mean follow-up of 97 months (8.1 years) in the well-differentiated category, compared to their other category, the more classical biphasic blastoma, in which 24 patients had a 43% recurrence and a 52% death from tumor and a mean follow-up of 49 months (4.1 years); this follow-up was about half of that in the well-differentiated group.

Sclerosing Hemangioma

The entity of so-called sclerosing hemangioma of lung was separated from the general group of histiocytomas by Liebow and Hubbell[270] in 1956. They described 7 cases, 1 of which had been separately published as a capillary hemangioma of lung.[271] A very careful description of this entity was given in this original series, and little can be added to it as far as the descriptive light microscopy. Katzenstein et al.[272] in 1980 described 51 cases seen in consultation by Liebow during the 17 years (1957–1974) following his 1956 review.[270] By 1982, Chan et al.[273] described 14 cases from Hong Kong collected from 1974 to 1980, 10 of these coming from one hospital. These authors wondered whether there was some environmental factor(s) involved, such as herbs. In 1986, Spencer and Namba[274] also noted an increase in Asian patients, and in that same year, Thomas and Lee[274,275] described 11 cases in Singapore. Indeed this appears to be valid. Much of the recent work on this entity has come from the Orient, especially Japan, and the 196 cases published in Japan by 1988 were reviewed by Kimura et al.[275] and most likely incorporate some of the other Japanese series described

Table 33–5. Major series of sclerosing hemagiomas

Investigators	Liebow and Hubbell[270]	Katzenstein et al.[272]	Chan et al.[273]	Katzenstein et al.[277]	Haimoto et al.[278]	Nagata et al.[279,280]	Spencer and Nambu[274]	Yousem et al.[281]	Sugio et al.[282]	Kimura et al.[276d]	All[e] (average)
Number of cases	7	51	14	9	7	16	29	8	10	196	300
Sex (F:M ratio)	6:1	42:8	14:0	7:2	7:0	11.5	12:7[a]	7:1	8:2	142:26	216:47
Female (%)	86	84	100	78	100	77	63	88	80	85	82
Age range	15–59	15–69	16–78	22–65	34–59	15–54	22–83	26–63	15–77	7–76	7–83
(average)	(40)	(42)	(51)	(47)	(46)	(—)	(—)	(43)	(42)	(46)	(45)
Maximum size	1.5–7.5	0.4–8.0	1.3–3.5	1.2–7.0	1.0–5.0	(—)	(—)	0.8–3.0	1.3–8.2	0.4–8.2	
(average)	(—)	(3)	(2.3)	(2.7)	(—)	(—)	(—)	(2.1)	(3.1)		(2.8)
Location											
RUL	0	5	0	1	2	3	2	0	1	16	22 (9%)
RML	1	11	2	1	0	3	5	2	2	24	46 (20%)
RLL	4	13	5	2	2	3	7	3	0	37	66 (28%)
RILF[b]	1	0	0	1	0	0	0	0	0	3	5 (2%)
LUL	0	7	5	1	2	2	1	1	3	14	24 (10%)
LLL	1	13	1	2	0	5	2	2	7	47	67 (29%)
LILF[c]	0	0	1	1	1	0	0	0	0	2	3 (1%)

[a] Sex accounted for in only 19 of the series of 29.

[b] Right interlobar fissue.

[c] Left interlobar fissure.

[d] Probably includes other series (references 272, 278–280, 282).

[e] Best estimate of total excluding overlap in series.

in Table 33–5. The largest series are summarized in Table 33–5.*

A review of 34 cases from the literature, possibly conforming to this entity, was conducted by Arean and Wheat in 1962,[283] but unfortunately a large number of these cases probably better fit into other "histiocytoma" groups and true postinflammatory reactions such as organizing pneumonias. It is difficult to select out the pertinent individual cases, both from the early literature and from this 1962 summary, that would be representative of sclerosing hemangioma of lung as defined in 1956. The same problem is present with acceptance of 24 cases in the literature review in 1968 by Mori.[284] Limited descriptions and limited photographic fields prevent distinction of this entity from others in many of these earlier articles. Even more recently, some published cases have been misclassified.

Sclerosing hemangiomas are benign lesions, often presenting as round-to-oval masses (Figs. 33–46 and 33–47). They are usually solitary and subpleural, but in 5% of cases[285,286] are multiple, usually with one dominant mass and smaller lesions nearby.[272,274,285–288] The case described by Noguchi et al.[288] had two larger lesions, to 3.7 cm, and "innumerable" smaller ones in the right-lower lobe, somewhat appearing as tumor aspiration spread with none in the attached middle lobe. Another case by Lee et al.[285] had four separate lesions, two in the left-lower lobe in different basilar

segments and one each in the right-middle and right-lower lobes. Several are bilateral,[285,287] one of which is probably one of the two multiple lesions referred to in the series of 51 cases by Katzenstein et al.[272] Another case is illustrated here. Spencer and Nambu[274] noted that they have seen spread to regional nodes in two cases, the significance of which is unclear, and one of the two, separately published cases looks suspiciously like a clear cell adenocarcinoma.[289]

In Table 33–5, each series contains a majority of women with an overall average of 82% of the cases

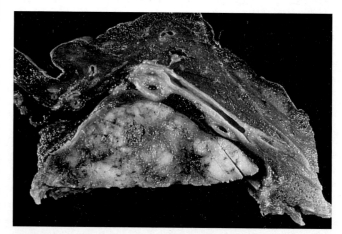

Fig. 33–46. Sclerosing hemangioma. Note variegation of texture and color in this gross specimen, reflecting varieties of histologic appearances. (Refer to Fig. 33–47.)

*References: 270, 272–274, 276–282.

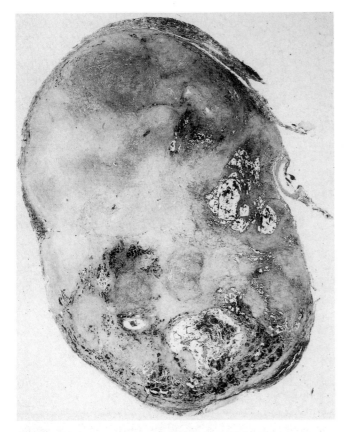

Fig. 33–47. Sclerosing hemangioma. Tuberous appearance at low power shows dense sclerosis in middle, some fine papillary folds toward top, and some hemangiomatous areas at right and bottom. H and E, ×10.

occurring in women. The reason for this predominance in women may relate to recently described estrogen and progesterone positivity in these tumors.[290] The average age at diagnosis is 45 years. Cases have been described from ages 15 to 83, and most are in the fifth decade.

These lesions average 2.8 cm in maximum size, with a range of 0.4 to 8.2 cm with even smaller minute ones described in those with multiple lesions.[288] Some 90% of lesions are less than 5 cm. Their distribution somewhat favors the lower lobes in about half (right-lower lobe, 26%; left-lower lobe, 21%; right-middle lobe, 21%; upper lobes or interlobar fissures, remaining 32%. Considering the volume of lung tissue in each lobe, this would indicate some preference for the right-middle lobe. Chan et al.[273] have emphasized the subpleural location of many. Sometimes these cross over fissures[273] or may bulge the pleural surface, almost as a polyp,[273] or rarely may be adherent to adjacent structures, such as the pericardium.[270] These are benign, and there have been no instances of spread outside the

rarely involved adjacent lymph nodes, or of recurrence after excision, and the prognosis is uniformly good to this date.

The number of patients presenting without symptoms is large, and was 50%,[273] 63%,[281] 67%,[270] 78%,[272] and 90%[282] in different series. Those patients with symptoms usually have hemoptysis or vague chest pain. Where previous radiographs are available, these nodules have often been demonstrated to grow slowly or to show no growth at all. In the large series by Katzenstein et al.,[272] 14 patients had past radiographs demonstrating the lesion from 1 to 14 years previously, with an average of 5 years. In one of the cases in the original Liebow and Hubbel[270] series, the lesion was followed for 12 years with little change. In another case,[291] a lesion had been present for some 15 years, but no comment as to whether it had changed or not was noted in the report.

Grossly, these lesions are well circumscribed and free up ("shell out") from the adjacent lung parenchyma easily (Figs. 33–46 and 33–47). They vary in color depending on the amount of fresh and old blood within them. They may be grey-white or tan-yellow when relatively bloodless, with some being a stronger color of yellow, with increased fatty histiocytes and iron, or even dark red in those with abundant blood. Focal variegation of lighter colored tumor with zones of blood and possibly focal yellow flecks is frequently observed. The cut surface shows some clefts, often defined as fine or slight clefts. Sometimes these lesions have a spongy appearance, which usually coincides with blood-filled lesions that are dark red (Fig. 33–47). In other cases the cut surface is granular or rubbery. The nearby lung parenchyma is compressed but does not have a true capsule, and sometimes there is a rim of red or brown discoloration near the tumor. In these cases the tumor is often also a darker color. Further away from the tumor the surrounding lung parenchyma is usually normal. In a multiple lesion case with two nodules larger than 2 cm, and "innumerable" smaller ones, red color and corresponding histologic angiomatous pattern was seen only in the two more than 2 cm, and all those that were less than 1 cm were described as gray-white and lacked histologic angiomatous change.

Microscopically, these tumors are quite variegated (Figs. 33–48 through 33–55); this is a consistent and diagnostic part of the tumor proliferation, and is of importance when considering the differential diagnosis. There are some more cellular solid zones, others that are more papillary, or both cellular and sclerotic, while others have more confluent sclerotic zones and some have an angiomatous or hemorrhagic type pattern. Often these patterns are mixed, usually consisting of at least three types. Focal sclerosis of some part is

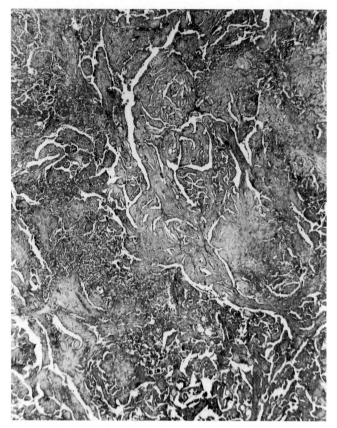

Fig. 33–48. Sclerosing hemangioma. Note various proliferations, some papillary and more delicate, some more broadly based and sclerotic. H and E, ×50.

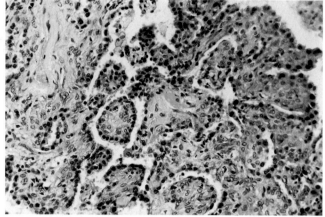

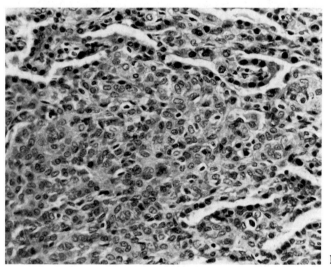

Fig. 33–49. A,B. Sclerosing hemangioma. **A.** Papillary fronds; some are cellular, some fibrous stalks. Note distinctly different cells lining surface. H and E, ×250. **B.** More solid cellular variant. Again note difference in cells lining spaces. H and E, ×400.

common but is not dominant. The other patterns described may be dominant. I have seen one case with a dominant angiomatous component misinterpreted as an angiosarcoma. Occasionally, in a more solid cellular one, entrapped bronchioles are present (Fig. 33–53).

These tumors usually also have a slight admixture of lymphocytes, plasma cells, and mast cells (Figs. 33–53 and 33–54). These are often scattered among the tumor cells and are confirmed by electron microscopy and special stains (Fig. 33–54). Rarely, a tumor designated as solitary mast cell tumor is probably a solid type sclerosing hemangioma.[292] Sometimes some lymphocytes, plasma cells, and histiocytes are common in the rim of interface with more normal lung tissue. Iron-stained and foamy macrophages (Figs. 33–52 and 33–55) are also seen with some regularity, and are increased in the lesions that contain bloody cysts.

The typical variegation of this tumor and its mixed inflammatory reaction has caused some confusion in diagnosis. The key to recognizing the true neoplastic nature of this lesion is to identify the bland and rather monotonous underlying tumor cells. These cells are of

medium size, have round to oval to slightly convoluted nuclei, finely reticular chromatin with moderate euchromatin, and slight to moderate condensation of chromatin in the subnuclear membrane region of the nucleus (Figs. 33–49, 33–55, and 33–56). These contain small centrally placed inconspicuous nucleoli, and have a moderate amount of eosinophilic cytoplasm. Some of the cells have a greater degree of clear cytoplasm. Cytoplasmic borders are often indistinct. Mitoses are rare or nonexistent. The tumor cells are most easily identified in the solid or sheet-like zones. Also, the tumor cells form most of some papillae, and are in the septa between the larger blood lakes in the hemangiomatous regions. Some of these cells are gradually replaced by dense collagen, as is described here.

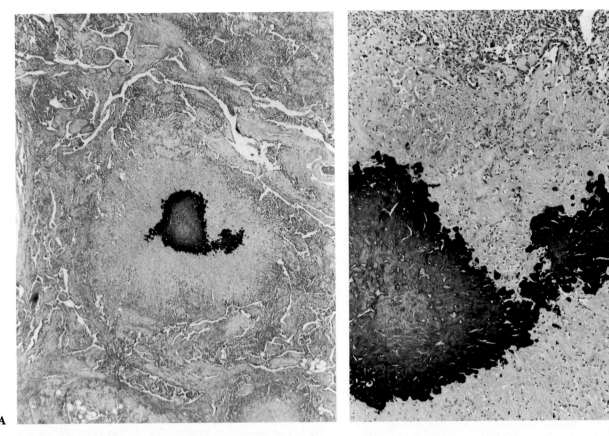

A

B

Fig. 33–50. A,B. Sclerosing hemangioma. **A.** Calcification in center of sclerotic area is surrounded by papillary folds. H and E, ×75. **B.** Fig. 29–50A shown at higher power. H and E, ×250.

The tumor cells in the interstitium are sometimes covered by a single layer of slightly darker squamoid-to-cuboidal cells (Figs. 33–49 and 33–55). At times smaller collections of cuboidal cells appear in cystic spaces and probably represent hyperplastic lining cells. Hyalinized areas may evolve from the solid, (Fig. 33–47), papillary (Fig. 33–50), and hemangiomatous zones (Fig. 33–47). These hyalinized areas may be more confluent and spherical with short radiating arms corresponding to adjacent papillae or connections to other tumor or adjacent lung (Fig. 33–50). Longer arms of sclerosis may cause a "Medusa-head" appearance. Occasional discoid plaques of lamellar fibrosis are seen adjacent to foci of cholesterol clefts. Central dystrophic calcification may be present in the spherical type of hyalinization (Fig. 33–50).

Corresponding to the red areas seen grossly, hematogenous areas contain blood lakes that vary in size (Fig. 33–51). Foamy and iron-stained macrophages may be in some of the blood pools, and sometimes are in the interstitium of the tumor admixed with the tumor cells, sometimes in a zonal arrangement (Fig. 33–55). There may be cholesterol clefts with focal giant cells around

them in some areas, and often these are associated with discoid areas of lamellar fibrosis as mentioned previously. Many of the red cells appear viable, but focally they are undergoing necrosis with adjacent foamy, fat-filled, or iron-stained histocytes and the cholesterol clefts just mentioned. When considering this lesion as an angioma, Liebow and Hubbell[270] thought perhaps these breakdown products were occurring inside bays of the mainstream viable red cells seen in the nearby vascular pools.

Other inclusions have been described in these tumors. Small collections of mature fat cells are sometimes identified in the middle of sheets of solid tumor cells (Fig. 33–57). Bronchiolar inclusions have already been noted (Fig. 33–53). Delicately whorled eosinophilic to slightly basophilic and somewhat cleared bodies have been described (Fig. 33–55B; and description and Fig. 22–47 in Chapter 22). These were seen in 12 of 51 cases (24%) in the Katzenstein et al. large review.[272] They seem to be formed in spaces from excess lipid in foamy macrophages in somewhat a similar fashion as cholesterol clefts, and presumably come from blood and other cell breakdown products or possibly from accumulated

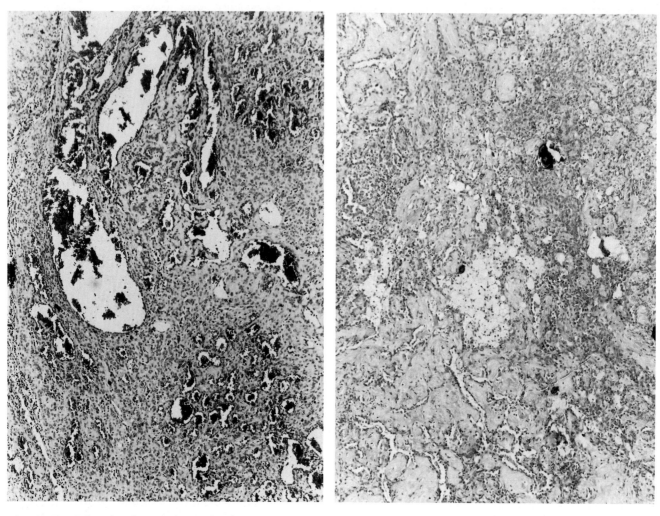

Fig. 33–51. Sclerosing hemangioma. Angiomatous component is seen as blood-filled cystic spaces of varying caliber. H and E, ×150.

Fig. 33–52. Sclerosing hemangioma. Sclerotic papillary component at bottom, cellular component toward top, dystrophic calcification in several sites, and foamy cells in middle. H and E, ×100.

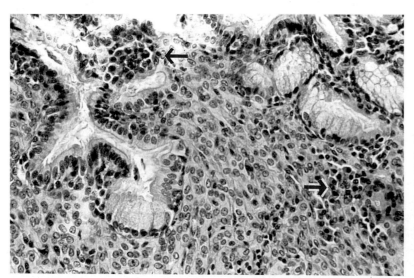

Fig. 33–53. Sclerosing hemangioma. More solid and cellular example with entrapped bronchiole(s) shows focal mucinous metaplasia among ciliated mucosa. Note clusters of plasma cells (*arrows*) in several sites. Also note bland appearance of tumor cells with distinct cytoplasmic borders and homogeneous cytoplasm. H and E, ×100. (Original contributor: Dr. E. Cassell, Pennock Hospital, Hastings, Michigan.)

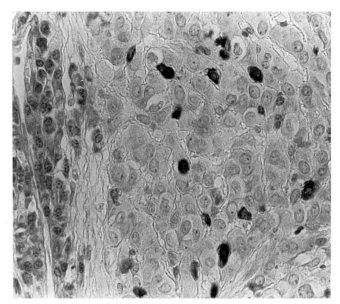

Fig. 33–54. Sclerosing hemangioma. Same case as Fig. 33–53. Giemsa stain shows scattered numerous mast cells. Note cluster plasma cells to left. Giemsa, ×400.

surfactant or other secretions. Why they are more spherical than the cholesterol clefts is unclear. Why they are seen in this tumor most often is also unclear. Rarely, I have seen them in plasma cell granulomas. Perhaps this is related to trapping of surfactant-type products with formation of giant myelin figures. After processing, most of this lipid matrix is removed from these bodies and only a few delicate spherical or partially circumferential lines remain.

The borders of the tumor nodules compress the adjacent lung parenchyma without true capsule formation (Fig. 33–58). There may be focal interstitial spread, and there may be a focal interface of inflammatory cells separating the nearby lung parenchyma from the tumor infiltrated zone. One often has the impression that progressive thickening of the interstitium is entrapping airspaces, but because of profuse but irregular overexpansion of the interstitial compartment with papillary protrusions and other convolutions, these entrapped air spaces quickly become irregular and more difficult to recognize. Although best seen as the periphery, this complexity makes directly tracing these spaces further into and through the tumor more difficult than the other lesions mentioned in Table 33–1. (See later,

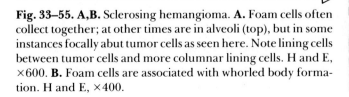

Fig. 33–55. A,B. Sclerosing hemangioma. A. Foam cells often collect together; at other times are in alveoli (top), but in some instances focally abut tumor cells as seen here. Note lining cells between tumor cells and more columnar lining cells. H and E, ×600. B. Foam cells are associated with whorled body formation. H and E, ×400.

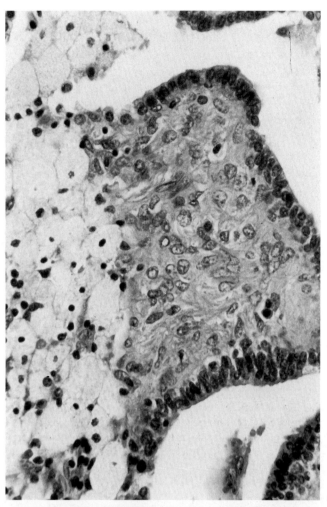

A

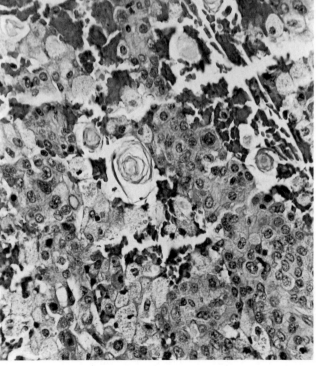

B

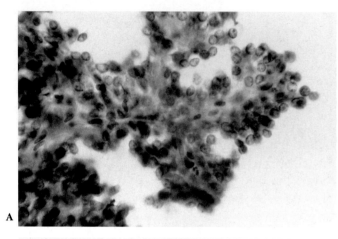

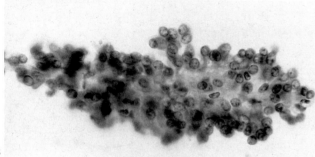

Fig. 33–56. A,B. Sclerosing hemangioma by fine-needle aspiration (FNA). **A.** Complex papillary arrangement. **B.** Single papillar or portion of solid area highlights bland cytology. It is difficult to tell whether nuclei seen are stromal or lining cells (see text). Papanicolaou, ×400. (Courtesy of Drs. R. K. Nieberg and S. E. Wang, UCLA Medical Center, Los Angeles, California.)

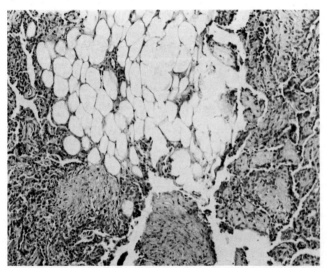

Fig. 33–57. Sclerosing hemangioma. Focally mature fat is occasionally identified. H and E, ×100.

immunoperoxidase staining of lining cells.) Background lung architecture is destroyed within the tumor nodules.

On the lung side of this transition zone there may be heavily pigmented hemosiderin-laden macrophages, and rarely an occasional small focus of iron encrustation of vascular elastica (see this entity in Chapter 22). Bronchioles may occasionally be traced into these tumors and appear to become distorted by nodules of proliferating tumor and papillary fronds. Sometimes edges of bronchiolar mucosa with cilia are seen in the midst of the tumor, as are entrapped pulmonary arteries, which appear otherwise intact. There is no evidence of endothelial proliferation in these vessels or evidence of similar change in the adjacent lung parenchyma.

There is no capillary hemangiomatosis or Kaposi's sarcoma-like areas of cleftlike small vessels, but there are some of the smaller cystic spaces that can become more angulate and slitlike. These are larger than the Kaposi-type changes, and are lined by cuboidal cells instead of endothelial cells. Remnant bronchial cartilage is usually not seen, perhaps relating to the peripheral origin of many of these lesions. Neither neoplastic nor metastatic cartilage or bone is seen. In four cases in the literature, small areas of incidental carcinoid atypical proliferations or tumorlets have been described.[272,280,288] No chemodectoma-like structures have been described in the vicinity of these lesions. One more typical mucinous glandular proliferation was noted between multiple nodules,[274] and one bronchiolar-like mucosal complexity was described within a solitary lesion.[274] I am aware so far of only one case report of fine-needle cytologic description of this tumor[293] (Fig. 33–56).

Some presumably related small adjacent lesions have been described, and are illustrated by Katzenstein et al.[272] and Noguchi et al.[288] These appear as slight cellular interstitial thickenings, focally seen adjacent to terminal bronchioles with cuboidal metaplastic-appearing lining cells. The cells in the interstitium are smaller than the basic tumor cells and are difficult to identify as tumor cells. The significance of these lesions is unknown. Are they precursors to sclerosing hemangioma or are they somehow caused by but incidental to the nearby tumor mass? In contrast, the case of multiple sclerosing hemangiomas shown in Fig. 33–58 has more characteristic sclerotic and papillary lesions, even though many of the lesions are small. This illustrated case is apparently similar to that of Noguchi and associates.[288]

Special Procedures and Theories of Cell Origin

The nature of the basic tumor cell of this lesion remains elusive. By evidence from light microscopy, Liebow and

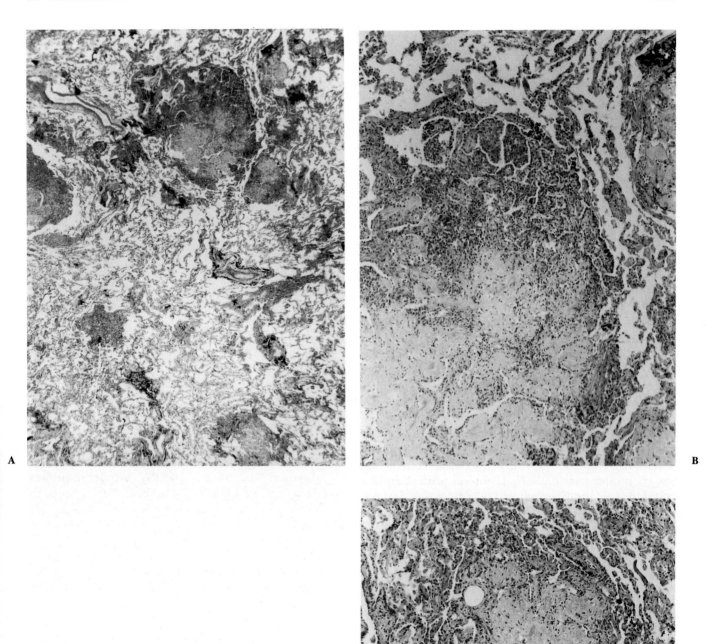

Fig. 33–58. A–C. Multiple sclerosing hemangiomas. **A.** At least five nodules are seen at low power. H and E, ×50. **B.** Higher power view of largest nodule shows sclerosis and cellular component and papillary arrangement. H and E, ×200. **C.** Separate small nodule with predominant sclerosis. H and E, ×200.

Hubbell[270] believed this lesion to be endothelial. The vascular lakes, the papillary fronds of varying caliber, of which some are fibrotic with small central capillaries, blood breakdown products, and the history of hemoptysis in some patients all suggested a vascular lesion to these authors. Also compatible with this is the subtle presentation of many of these tumor. A bronchial angiogram study of this lesion showed a characteristic vascular network wrapped around the tumor, but the tumor itself was not hypervascular.[294] Judging by the ease with which these separate from the adjacent lung parenchyma, and the fact that three cases now have had air meniscus signs,[272,295] representing spontaneous separation from surrounding tissue, the fact that histologically there are no identified feeding or draining vessels at the borders, the fact that the tumors are relatively hypovascular and are supplied by delicate capillary network, and that the tumor cells are negative by EM and IP for endothelial cell markers puts to rest the idea that this is a hemangioma. One point of persistent interest is the viability of the red cells seen in the hemangiomatous pattern, and this has yet to be explained. Certainly there is some hemosiderin around some of these. Some favor hamartomatous etiology.[274,296] The odd but bland admixture of cells, appearing both epithelial and stromal, the blood filled spaces in some, mature fat in others, and lack of a proven single cell type are used to support this theory. The role and relationship of the fairly frequent mast cells is unclear. These tumors do not have ultrastructural or immunoperoxidase markers of histiocytomas. The search continues to identify the cell of origin.

Although everyone agrees the lining cells are epithelial, and particularly have markers of alveolar type II cells with surfactant production or clear cell characteristics, this is where the agreement stops. The solid, over-to-round tumor cells in the interstitium between these glandular linings are the true tumor cells to me and deserve particular attention in studying histogenesis of this tumor.

Most of the electron microscopic examinations show a very similar appearance (Fig. 33–59).* The tumor cells are generally composed of three types, presumed to be variations of the same type, with the darker cells having the greatest degree of internal contents, with abundant rough endoplasmic reticulum, free ribosomes, and mitochondria. In these cells there are osmiophilic laminar bodies similar to the surfactant-like bodies seen in alveolar type II cells. The cell surfaces, however, are unlike alveolar type II cells or other known epithelial cells in the periphery of the lung; their microvilli vary between being long and slender and more blunted, and are not as universally long as those in mesothelial cells. There are no true cilia. When the cells are adjacent to each other there is an interdigitation of the cell membranes, and focal primitive desmosomes are seen without tonofilaments. The other two cells represent the opposite end of the spectrum; there are lighter cells with less cytoplasmic inclusions and a transition cell between the dark and light cells.

*References: 273, 274, 277, 289–308.

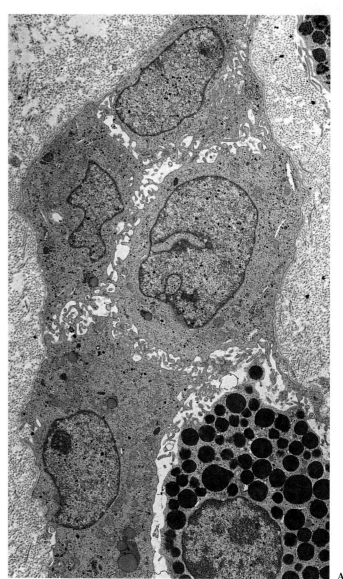

A

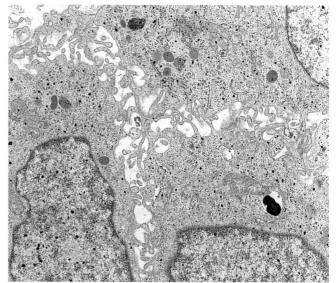

B

Fig. 33–59. A,B. Ultrastructure of sclerosing hemangioma. **A.** Cluster of tumor cells in midst of sclerosing collagen of this lesion shows typical finger-like cell processes extending into shared common space between cells. Note mast cell at bottom. (Refer to Figs. 33–53 and 33–54). TEM, ×2500. **B.** Cell processes are better shown at higher power. TEM, ×6300.

Katzenstein et al.[277] studied well-fixed tissue of five cases by electron microscopy. Non-membrane-bound glycogen was present in a moderate number of cases. Pinocytosis was not prevalent, and there was no abundance of intermediate filaments. Discontinuous basement membrane was described around individual cells and around some groups of cells and adjacent to some of the blood lakes. Many of these spaces were lined by more cuboidal and clearer cells than the nearby tumor clear cells; however, some of these spaces were lined by tumor cells with microvilli projecting into the vascular-like spaces. Lymphocytes, plasma cells, and mast cells were confirmed scattered among the tumor cells. Sometimes mast cells were more dominant than expected by light microscopy[299] (Fig. 33–54). The sclerotic zones were composed of dense collagen with entrapped and somewhat distorted tumor cells that were similar to those in the more cellular parts of the tumor. Slender microvilli and discontinuous basement membrane were still evident. The authors concluded that their findings were strong evidence against an endothelial origin but did not completely exclude an epithelial origin. Other authors have favored these findings as indicating epithelial cell characteristics. Katzenstein et al.[277] concluded these cells were unlike any normal ones described so far in peripheral lung.

Immunoperoxidase studies are interesting and somewhat conflicting. In 1983, both Katzenstein et al.[277] and Dail et al.[307] confirmed that these tumor cells were negative for Factor VIII-related antigens. This work has been confirmed by others* and with *Ulex europa* antigen.[280,312] Recently, CD34 done in our laboratory, is also negative, and adenosine triphosphatase[304] enzyme stain also is negative. The tumor cells are positive with vimatin in most studies,† but not all agree.[278,281] The lining cells coexpressed vimentin and cytokeratin in several larger series.[278,281] Epithelial membrane antigen stained not only lining cells but most of the tumor cells in several series,[278,281,306] only focally in some,[280,306,312] and in a few this stain has been negative.[288] In one study,[278] the lining cells stained both with a membranous and cytoplasmic EMA positivity while the tumor cells stained with only membranous pattern. Another study showed very intense staining of both compartments in the tumor cells.[281] In one study,[306] EMA was found only in association with lumen formation. Cytokeratins,[278,280,306,312,313] surfactin apoprotein,[280,289,311] and its variant PE10,[307] Clara cell antigen and secretory component[278,280] have been positive in some series. These along with CEA may monotonously

or focally stain lining cells but generally not stromal cells, with a few exceptions.[280,281,307]

I have personally studied two cases, one in fixed Carnoy's and the other in formalin. The staining procedure seemed to be clean, with good external and internal controls; the lining cells in both cases were vividly positive with cytokeratin, moderately positive with EMA, and focally positive with CEA, while negative for vimentin, and the tumor cells were vividly positive with vimentin only (Fig. 33–60). Both compartments were negative with S100, human melanin black (HMB 45), actin, desmin, Ulex Factor VIII-related antigen, CD34, and panhematopoetic antigen. My experience with cytokeratin only in the lining cells and vimentin only in the tumor cells confirms the frozen section immunofluorescent marker studies in the case presented by Huszar et al.[313]

One immunoperoxidase study of eight cases by Yousem et al.[281] reported in 1988 deserves special mention. These authors studied their cases for an extensive group of antigens. They obtained more positive results than any other series. In all their cases, lining cells stained positive with cytokeratin, EMA, and surfactant apoprotein, while five of the eight cases showed coexpression of vimentin, and Clara cell antigen was positive in six of eight cases. The tumor cells stained positive for surfactant apoprotein in all eight for cytokeratin and EMA in seven of eight, and Clara cell antigen in five of eight. Vimentin stained lining cells and tumor cells in seven of eight cases, Ulex was positive in seven of eight tumor cells, and placental alkaline phosphatase (PLAP) was positive in six of eight lining cells and seven of eight lining cells. CEA was positive in five of eight lining cells, and Ulex was positive in six of eight lining cells. There was no positivity with S100, B72.3, or leu M1 staining in either the lining cells or the tumor cells. The extensive staining of many of these markers in this series remains to be confirmed. These investigators are certainly experienced, and whether they are exposing true antigens with their rather excessive antigen retrieval system or perhaps causing some staining beyond that usually accepted is unclear.

Other techniques have been applied to this tumor. One case was studied by cell culture,[304] and these authors noted the cells had characteristics that "lack any similarity to other epithelial or mesenchymal tumors, including blood vascular neoplasms." They also noted their culture results showed no similarity to any cultured normal peripheral lung cells. This is reminiscent of the conclusion by EM studies by Katzenstein et al.,[277] that these cells were unlike any respiratory epithelial cells by light or electron microscopy. Katzenstein et al.[277] used hyaluronidase and dissolved any mucin positive areas. They used glycosaminoglycan electro-

---

*References: 278, 280, 288, 306, 310–313.
†References: 280–281, 282, 288, 291, 313.

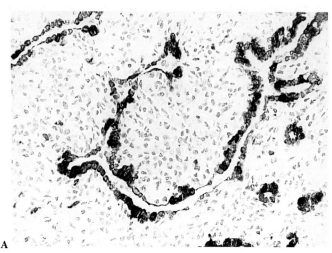

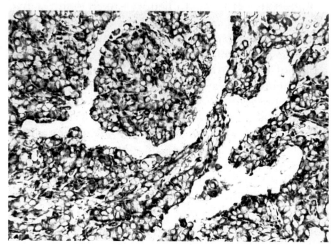

Fig. 33–60. A,B. Immunoperoxidase of sclerosing hemangioma. **A.** Stained with low molecular weight cytokeratin, lining cells are positive and tumor cells are unstained. Note smaller cross-cut portions appearing as tubules in right-lower portion. ×200. Field in **B** is similar to that in **A**. Stained with vimentin, tumor cells stain vividly while lining cells represent cleftlike ghost spaces without nuclear counterstain. ×100

phoresis and though there was some similarity of mesotheliomas, but this conclusion has been questioned by others.[310]

The complexity of this tumor has led to confusion, and it is unclear from some studies whether the cells examined were truly tumor cells or en face section of some of the lining cells. The dark cells, by electron microscopy, appear to be in continuity with the light cells and to contain bodies that have been interpreted as lamellar bodies of surfactant. This, together with epithelial markers, including EMA, CEA, apoprotein, and Clara cell antigen and secretory components in some of the tumor cells, is as yet unclarified, but perhaps, like the EM findings, relates to some epithelial inclusions or, in the case of antigens, some leakage artifact. The complexity of the tumor may lead to en face sectioning in some instances.

Some[273,288,296,302] believe the lining cells are neoplastic, perhaps representing an extremely well-differentiated epithelial component. Chan et al.[273] believe this is a biphasic epithelial tumor and has suggested the name benign sclerosing pneumocytoma. Ng and Ma wondered if it were an alveolar mixed tumor.[313a] Others* believe the lining cells are reactive entrapped metaplastic cells. I favor the metaplastic theory.

As with the cell of origin of chemodectoma-like bodies, pulmonary meningiomas, and benign sugar tumors, the cells of origin of some tumors in the lung remain undermined. In each they proliferate consistently in their own distinct forms, and therefore appear to be derived from one cell. In these cases a tumorous proliferation may eventually lead us to discover one or more normal cells that can account for these lesions.

Differential Diagnosis

The differential diagnosis for this tumor includes benign and malignant lesions, as shown by the broad spectrum of suggested diagnoses in each category in the series of 51 cases described by Katzenstein et al.[272] Because of the papillary nature of these lesions, adenocarcinomas, especially the rare papillary noninvasive ones, are often considered. The papillary fronds in sclerosing hemangiomas usually vary in diameter and composition from each other more than those seen with adenocarcinomas. There are tumor cells within the papillary fronds and in more solid areas of sclerosing hemangiomas. In the less differentiated adenocarcinomas with more solid areas, the cell pleomorphism, mitotic rate, and invasive capacities, without the multiple histologic patterns of sclerosing hemangioma, helped distinguish this. Focal mucin production in adenocarcinoma cells is also helpful. The bland-appearing cell monotony in some tumor areas of sclerosing hemangioma and blood-filled spaces brings in the differential carcinoid tumors. Usually carcinoid tumors are less papillary, although a rare exception occurs,[193] and neurosecretory stains are easy to do. Another monotonous tumor is lobular carcinoma of breast, but this rarely metastases to lung as a nodule and much more frequently metastasizes as lymphangitic spread or serosal surface spread.[314] Keep in mind that sclerosing hemangiomas are ERA/PRA positive.

---

*References: 270, 272, 277, 279, 297, 298.

Pulmonary blastomas, benign sugar cell tumors, plasma cell granulomas, and metastases from other sites such as thyroid or kidney are not usually a problem to distinguish. Of interest, 3 benign epithelial localized mesotheliomas were reported in the classic series of 18 localized mesotheliomas; all 3 were found on slide review to be sclerosing hemangiomas.[277]

Epithelioid hemangioendotheliomas have sometimes been confused with this lesion. The cells of epithelioid hemangioendothelioma usually appear bland, can be rather monotonous, and have abundant cytoplasm. Epithelioid hemangioendotheliomas tend to infiltrate the lung in a different pattern, being respective of the background alveolar architecture, while extending from one alveolus to another in a micropolypoid fashion. They are not as papillomatous as the sclerosing hemangioma. In some cells in the epithelioid hemangioendothelioma there are primitive vascular lumens. These tumor cells stain positively for factor VIII-related and Ulex antigens, and by electron microscopy have endothelial characteristics, including Weibel–Palade bodies. I have seen one case of this entity misidentified as multiple sclerosing hemangiomas.

I wonder if several lesions represent variations of sclerosing hemangioma. One was presented in poster form entitled "Placental Transmogrification of Lung"[315] (Fig. 33–61). An additional three cases of this (two in men ages 24 and 27; one 33-year-old woman) were presented in 1993 in abstract form.[315a] I agree with Semeraro and Gibbs[316] that the cell of origin of the entity of "alveolar adenoma" is yet unclear and appears mesenchymal and cystic, with some characteristics of that described in the current entity. I suspect it will be unique. An occasional case may be confused with mes-

enchymal cystic hamartoma (see discussion in separate section).

Histiocytomas may sometimes be papillary and have the admixture of inflammatory cells as seen in sclerosing hemangiomas, including the foam cells and cholesterol clefts. One must be sure to identify the tumor cell type of proliferation before making a diagnosis of sclerosing hemangioma.

Plasma Cell Granuloma–Histiocytoma Complex

Various names have been proposed for this group of lesions, including inflammatory pseudotumor, histiocytoma, xanthoma, fibroxanthoma, mast cell granuloma, and plasma cell granuloma, and an occasional case has even been identified as a solitary plasmocytoma. The terms post inflammatory (pseudo)tumor have been used for the entities of plasma cell granuloma, sclerosing hemangiomas, and pseudolymphomas, plus a broad spectrum of organizing pneumonias and other reactive and inflammatory or fibrotic reactions. Most often the term, however, has been applied to plasma cell granulomas. Because this term is vague, it should not be used when identifying specific entities, but its descriptive qualities are a temptation to some. Bahadori and Liebow[317] published the largest series of 40 cases in 1973, and chose the term "plasma cell granuloma," or PCG, as they thought it most closely characterized the disease entity. It appears, when reactive and other inflammatory reactions are eliminated (see following), that about 90%–95% of these lesions in the lung conform to their description, and the other names apply to various com-

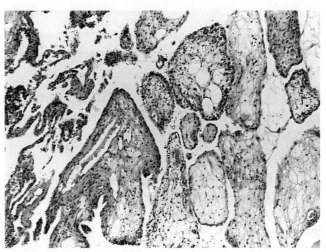

Fig. 33–61. A,B. Unusual entity labeled placental "transmogrification" of lung. **A.** Low power view shows discrete cluster of papillary excrescences of varying caliber and varying density. H and E, ×50. **B.** High power shows cystic spaces within some papilla with possible remnant of normal lung to left of smaller fragments. H and E, ×200. (Courtesy of Dr. Thomas Chesney, Memphis, Tennessee.[315])

ponents and/or true histiocytic lesions, as is discussed in the following two sections. Therefore, the term "plasma cell granuloma" (PCG) will be used for this prototypical lesion, but, acknowledging a spectrum, the heading for this section is a compound name, as suggested by Spencer[318] in his 1984 series of 27 cases. In addition to the series by Bahadori and Liebow,[317] Berardi et al.[319] in 1983 did a very thorough review of the clinical details of 180 cases. Warter et al.[320] in 1987 added 8 well-studied histologic cases to the 300 or so cases identified and reported to date. Pettinato et al.[321] in 1990 presented 20 cases, half in the age group 2–17 years, with accompanying electron microscopic and immunoperoxidase studies. These authors noted about 350 cases in the lung were reported by 1989. These reviews should save the reader well for additional details. One more recent large additional review of 32 cases by Matsubara et al.[322] covers a broad spectrum of inflammatory pseudotumors and is separately discussed next.

The reader is alerted early in this discussion to some ambiguity as to what should be included under the term, "granuloma" in lung. This term is used loosely here to mean a mass of inflammatory-appearing tissue, in a way similar to its use in Wegener's and lymphomatoid granulomatoses. Used in this way it does not imply discrete epithelioid granulomas as would be seen in infections or sarcoid. The generic term of "tumor" to imply a mass effect is used in discussing this lesion, but does not by itself necessarily imply a neoplastic growth.

Part of the problem in naming these tumors is to try to decide the cell of origin that caused such a mixed reaction and what, if any, is the major stimulus. Is it inflammatory, postinflammatory, altered immune response, or neoplastic? Most investigators believe these are reactive lesions, but admit their unusual characteristics. Approximately 30%–50% of adults have a history of pulmonary infections,[319] or at least of past respiratory symptoms, while some 20% of children have a similar history. A less significant number have evidence of preceding normal chest radiographs, infiltrates at the time of respiratory symptoms, and residual in the same area eventually diagnosed as plasma cell granulomas. Previous pulmonary disease occurred from 1 month to 34 years earlier, 41% within 1 year, but 23% from 6 to 34 years before.[319] It seems prior infection and/or other pulmonary disease is not as significant a factor as once thought.

Although the lung is the major area in which these types of reaction and tumor masses have been described, they have also been described in the trachea, thyroid, heart, stomach, liver, pancreas, spleen, lymph nodes, kidney, retroperitoneum, mesentery, bladder, pelvic soft tissue, breast, spinal cord meninges, posterior cranial fossa, and orbit. Studies in these extrapul-

monary sites have offered little additional insight into their mechanisms. Although one should be concerned about possible malignancy in any mass growing in any location without explanation, these lesions are generally benign and cause difficulties only when they occur in or spread to vital structures.

As noted, separating out this tumor in the lung from organizing pneumonia and other benign inflammatory reactions is not always clear in the literature. Matsubara et al.,[322] in a study of 32 cases, proposed a sequence and overlapping categories of organizing pneumonia, fibrous histiocytoma, and lymphoplasmocytic subsets. I believe organizing pneumonia can certainly be confused with plasma cell granuloma as defined here, but should be separated and is not a proven precursor lesion. The fibrous histiocytoma subsets includes some lesions that are perhaps better classified as true fibrous histiocytomas with storiform stroma (see following section), and their third group contains lesions that they and I would agree by classical terminology have been called the pseudolymphomas of lung. I am unclear whether any of the cases in this large series belong to the entity of plasma cell granuloma as defined herein. Other recent series should be critically reviewed for some of the same classification problems.[323] I am cautious in accepting published cases unless typical areas of plump myofibroblastic cells with some plasma cells are illustrated. Sometimes no illustrations are given, making such judgments impossible. The discussion to follow focuses on that part of the spectrum which may be neoplastic and for which the term inflammatory myofibroblastic tumor has been proposed.[324] The hallmark of this tumor so defined is a large number of plump myofibroblastic cells, with a scattering of plasma cells.

It was partially a result of ambiguities of nomenclature, that it has been difficult to obtain good incidence figures for this lesion. As noted by Bahadori and Liebow,[317] Golbert and Pletnev[324] in 1967 had reported a 0.7% incidence of these lesions in 1,075 lung and tracheal tumors seen at the P.A. Herzen's Moscow Oncological Institute. In the comprehensive review of childhood pulmonary neoplasms by Hartman and Shochat,[325] these accounted for 45 of 79 benign tumors in lung (57%), and in their whole series including malignant lesions, these represented 20% of all primary lung tumors in children. It may be that part of this significant incidence in children is that children do not have the multitude of other lung tumors seen in adults. As they are important in the pediatric age group, this is also discussed in Chapter 8, and the reader is referred to this discussion.

Data from the very nice reviews by Berardi et al.[319] and Pettinato et al.[321] are summarized. These lesions occur in individuals from age 1 to 77 years, with an

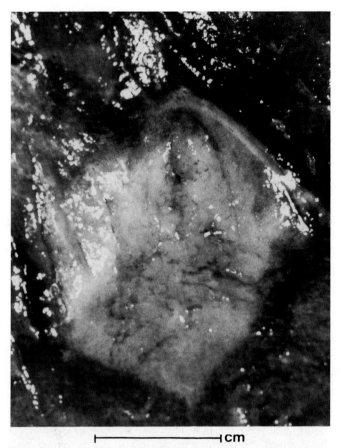

Fig. 33–62. Plasma cell granuloma. A 2-cm nodule appeared in right-lower lobe in 63-year-old woman with documented negative chest radiograph 2 years previously when bladder cancer was diagnosed.

average of 29.6 years. About 59% were less than 40 years old, and 8% were in their first decade. The highest incidence rates were in persons in their thirties, followed by those in their seventies. These lesions occurred 61% of the time on the right side and 39% on the left side. Six of 180 (3.3%) were multiple in the same lung; an additional 3 (1.7%) were bilateral, and 2 (1.1%) were confined to the trachea.

Other details from the Berardi et al.[319] series of 181 cases include the fact that 74% of the patients were asymptomatic. Radiographically most lesions (77) were well defined, but some (11) were poorly defined. Calcification was sometimes present (in 8), as was cavitation (in 7). Others rarely report osseous metaplasia, and PMNs or eosinophils are rare. Mitoses are occasionally seen, but fewer than 10% showed any growth when follow-up films were available. One case that did show growth is illustrated in Fig. 33–62. There was no pleural effusion.

CT findings are nonspecific in most series. Finding calcifications and an enhancing border-rim was suggested as distinctive, but are unusual findings.[326] Laboratory tests were normal in 94% of their series, with minor white blood cell elevations in some and/or elevated erythrocyte sedimentation rates (ESR) in others. A series of three children with elevated serum immunoglobulins and ESR was studied by Monzon et al.[327] Tests of their serum returned to normal after excision of their lung tumors. Cultures were negative for bacteria, fungi, and acid-fast bacilli. Skin tests showed the usual background positivity, with 5 of 32 tested for tuberculosis being positive, 1 of 28 positive for histoplasmosis, and 1 of 19 for blastomyocosis.[319] One correlative cytology case report is available.[328]

Grossly, these tumors vary from 0.5 to 36 cm in diameter, with 70% in the range 0.5–6.0 cm, 20% in the range 6–10 cm, and 10% larger than 10 cm. They usually have well-defined margins without true encapsulation (Fig. 33–62). Their color and texture vary depending on the predominant cell population. Those with more myofibroblasts are firmer and grey-white, those with an increased number of plasma cells are tan and rubbery, and those with abundant fat-filled macrophages assume a more brilliant yellow-orange color and are softer and more friable. Central necrosis may be found focally, and grossly identified calcification and/or hemorrhage have been reported but are infrequent.

Microscopically, these tumor masses eradicate most of the fine architecture of the lung background, although an occasional invaded vessel and/or entrapped bronchus or bronchiole can be identified. The alveolar septal network is usually lost, although some remnant entrapped metaplastic cuboidal cell-lined air spaces often persist (Fig. 33–63). The borders are rather sharp, with only focal interstitial spread. There may be minor reactions of inflammatory infiltrate or macrophage response nearby.

The cellular composition of the tumor is composed predominantly of plump spindle cells and plasma cells (Figs. 33–63 and 33–64). The spindle cells have large vesicular nuclei and generally run in the same direction as their neighbors, but can form some intertwining fascicles and occasionally a storiform pattern. The storiform pattern is much more evident when the spindle cells become thinner, and the inflammatory cell reaction is less prominent. This is discussed later in reference to fibrous histiocytomas. Immunoperoxidase stains detail the length of some of these cells. The stromal cells can also become more hyalinized and have a cytoplasmic appearance between fibrillar and waxy.

The plasma cells are seen scattered among the spindle cells, often in small clumps, but sometimes number up to 100. Russell bodies are easily identified. There is a

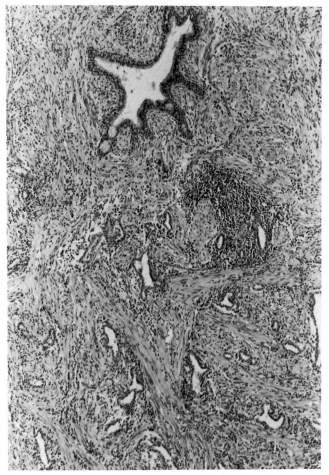

A

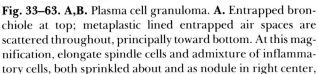

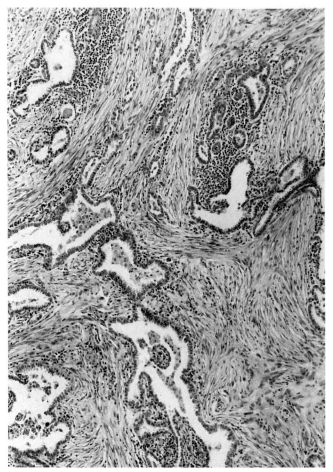

B

Fig. 33–63. A,B. Plasma cell granuloma. **A.** Entrapped bronchiole at top; metaplastic lined entrapped air spaces are scattered throughout, principally toward bottom. At this magnification, elongate spindle cells and admixture of inflammatory cells, both sprinkled about and as nodule in right center, are seen. H and E, ×100. **B.** Another example with many metaplastic cuboidal cell-lined spaces. Note long spindle myofibroblasts. Most of plasma cells and lymphocytes are around metaplastic-lined spaces. H and E, ×100.

scattering of lymphocytes with these plasma cells, but the lymphocytes are usually not as prevalent except at the edges of the lesion where the lymphocytes form a greater percentage of the inflammatory cell reaction. There is also a scattering of other inflammatory cells, most prominently histiocytes, which sometimes clump together and phagocytize fat and appear as foamy histiocytes. Mast cells are sometimes present, their identity often aided by special stains and/or electron microscopy, and these sometimes are prevalent enough to suggest the term "mast cell granuloma"[329] or mast cell tumor[292] (see **Sclerosing Hemangioma** discussion). (See also section on Other Histiocytomas.) PMNs and eosinophils are sometimes seen but are never very prevalent, and do not form abscesses. Rarely, small multinucleate giant cells are seen, but these are never very frequent, and true granulomas with epithelioid histiocytes are not a part of this lesion, and are not seen in adjacent lung parenchyma. Other or dual diseases should be considered if true granulomas are present. Cholesterol clefts may form from degenerating fat products, and focal flecks of dystrophic calcification or quite rarely small areas of dystrophic ossification may occur. Necrosis, when present, is focal, and usually toward the center of these lesions.

Entrapped air spaces may be seen with metaplastic cuboidal somewhat cleared lining cells. (see Fig. 33–63). These are best seen as transitions from nearby air spaces at the periphery and are similar to those seen in other low-grade lesions (see Table 33–1). Sometimes they are so prevalent as to be misinterpreted as adenocarcinomas. One needs to pay attention to the intervening stroma with its spindle cells and scattering of plasma cells in these cases, however. Plasma cells alone may be a part of a very cellular reaction to adenocarcinomas in the more usual sense, so they have to be in an appropri-

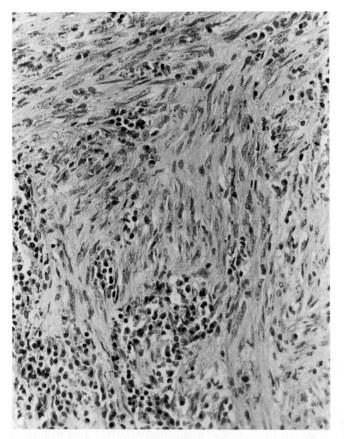

Fig. 33–64. Plasma cell granuloma. Elongated spindle cells in collections of plasma cells are easily identified. H and E, ×400.

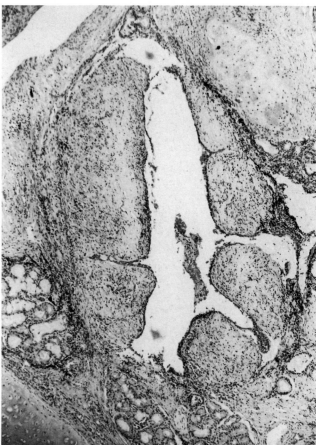

Fig. 33–65. Plasma cell granuloma. Sometimes this reaction stimulates polyp formation in bronchial mucosa. H and E, ×50.

ate spindle cell setting. There is no evidence of capsule formation.

Within the tumor masses, bronchi and/or bronchioles can sometimes be seen to be invaded by this type of reaction, and it is estimated about 5%–10% have endobronchial spread (Fig. 33–65) although one series[330] demonstrated that four of their five patients had endobronchial spread. Vessels are often identified with identical polymorphous cellular reactions inside as well as outside their walls (Fig. 33–66). The review by Warter et al.[320] in 1987 emphasized this vascular invasion. These vessels may be highlighted with elastic stains. Remnant bronchioles may also be detailed with elastic stains, but very little of the surrounding lung architecture is identified with either elastic or reticulin stains. Rarely these masses extend to the pleura and cause a fibrous adhesion. Sometimes this is cellular and causes trouble with residual or unresectable tumor in the pleura, diaphragm, or mediastinum. Regional nodes are sometimes enlarged and reactive, but do not show the type of cellular reaction or spindle cell component as seen in the lung nodules themselves. These nodes also do not show granulomatous inflammation.

Cultures and special stains for infective organisms have been unrevealing. However, some cases of organizing pneumonia seen with Aspergillus,[331] Q fever,[332] or *Rhodococcus equi*[333] are thought by some to have an overlap appearance with the type of infiltrate in plasma cell granuloma. Again, organizing pneumonia always comes into the differential diagnosis.

Electron microscopy has shown the spindle cells to have features of fibroblasts and myofibroblasts, and has confirmed the presence of assorted inflammatory cells, including plasma cells and mast cells.[320,321,334–340]

Histiocytes when present appear reactive. No virus particles or other peculiar structures have been identified in these lesions to suggest persistent organisms that can be identified. Immunoperoxidase stains the stromal cells heavily for vimentin, moderately for actin, and focally for desmin, and is negative for Factor VIII-related antigen. Cytokeratins and epithelial membrane antigen are limited to the entrapped epithelial lining cells, and S100 and leu 7 are negative.[321,340]

Lipid analysis of the tumors has been conducted by

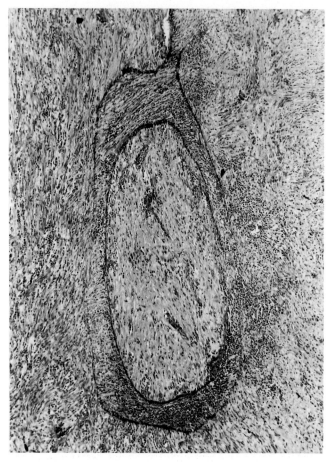

Fig. 33–66. Plasma cell granuloma. Same spindle cell and inflammatory reaction extends into vessel wall and fills intima, as is seen about vessel. H and E, ×100.

several authors[341,342] who found lipids that are consistent with the serum and cell breakdown products, and possibly surfactant. When the spindle cell component is prevalent and the inflammatory component is not appreciated, the differential diagnosis is with other spindle cell lesions of lung, including most mesenchymal neoplasms. Adenocarcinomas have been considered when the entrapped metaplastic glandular spaces are frequent, as noted previously. Plasmocytomas have been described in lung, but should consist of sheets of moderately well-differentiated plasma cells without the admixture of other inflammatory cells and without the spindle cell component. Some cases of organizing pneumonia may have mixed inflammatory cell infiltrate and spindle cells, but the lung architecture is more intact and the density of reaction is generally less than with PCGs. In Hodgkin's disease, more eosinophils, fewer myofibroblasts, and atypical mononuclear or classical Reed–Sternberg cells should be present to confirm this diagnosis. Sclerosing hemangiomas and pseudolymphomas have been discussed in the setting of (post)

inflammatory (pseudo) tumors, but are distinct entities that should not be confused, and each is separately discussed. Confusion with pulmonary hyalinizing granuloma should not occur.

Tissue sections have been examined for monoclonality, and in all the published series* so far, there is a polyclonal cellular infiltrate. I have seen one case of a dominant lambda light chain marking, but the significance of this is unknown, as it was in an otherwise perfectly acceptable sample of plasma cell granuloma. T-lymphocyte gene rearrangement studies have not been reported, but lymphocytes are such a minor component that it is doubted whether they will add much information. It is hoped this will be done at some time in the future.

These lesions have caused trouble when the reaction extends transpleurally into the diaphragm or extends into the mediastinum, making them unresectable. In cases in which these have been resected, the patients have done quite well with no evidence of metastasis to other organs, and only a rare case has recurred when there was a limited excision, such as an endobronchial resection of a predominantly endobronchial tumor, or when the tumor has been "shelled out" without adequate margins of normal tissue. Higher grade lesions are discussed later. Radiotherapy or steroids have been used, in some cases with minimal effect and in others with more beneficial effect when vital structures are involved. Confusion with organizing pneumonia is a problem at times but less so when the reaction extends into the chest wall, mediastinum, or other vital structures. Sometimes with unresectable cases associated with hypergammaglobulinemia, treatment cures both the tumor and the hypergammaglobulinemia.[346]

The polymorphous inflammatory appearance, the bland spindle cell proliferations, the polyclonality, and the cell culture and electron micrographic appearances comparing these cells to granulation tissue myofibroblasts have all suggested reactive changes. However, the tumor's true nature is still in doubt. It would be unusual for an inflammation, even though it were ongoing, to cause such an often large, persistent, growing, usually solitary tumor mass without other symptoms. Although pulmonary infection and upper respiratory tract disease may precede some of these, they are probably not occurring much out of proportion to their incidence in the general population, or perhaps are partially caused by the tumor itself. In general, these lung nodules occur quite infrequently in relationship to all the infections that have occurred in people's lungs. Perhaps we are identifying the host response predominantly, as is seen

References: 320, 321, 323, 327, 338, 340, 343–345.

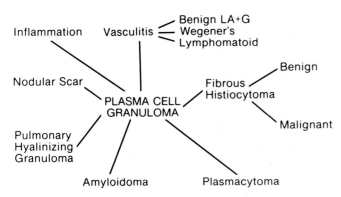

Fig. 33–67. Plasma cell granuloma. This entity has components of many diseases as illustrated here. Benign LAG, benign lymphocytic angiitis and granulomatosis.

in many cases of Hodgkin's disease. I believe these are neoplasms with the proliferating cell being a myofibroblast. Some[347] believe these are in the spectrum of fibrous and other histiocytomas, to be discussed. Those who consider them reactive may perhaps compare them to nodular fasciitis or its variant of intravascular fasciitis.[348,349] Its histologic aspects have components that overlap with many diseases (Fig. 33–67), but it is recognizable as a distinct entity from all of these.

Other Histiocytomas

Histiocytes have been the predominant cell in many pulmonary reactions. Sometimes these are reactive, such as in exogenous and endogenous lipid pneumonias (see Chapter 5), and as seen in sclerosing hemangiomas, where they are apparently phagocytizing lipid debris. They can be induced by drugs (Chapters 22 and 23). At the other end of the spectrum, there have been cases of true malignant histiocytosis involving the lung, discussed under **Sarcomas** in this chapter, but these appear distinctly different.

Rare tumor masses described in the lung are composed almost entirely of finely vacuolated cells (Fig. 33–68). At least some of these appear to represent true benign histiocytomas. Several cases have been published. One such case in a 48-year-old man was described by Katzenstein and Maurer[350] in 1979: abundant round-to-polygonal cells with granular, foamy or vacuolated cytoplasm, abundant fat, fine PAS particles, and negative mucin, argyrophil, and argentaffin stains were present. Electron microscopy showed some histiocyte differentiation. There was only a very low mitotic rate. Two cases that appear somewhat similar have been described in children,[351,352] and one other in an adult[329] appeared similar. Another case is illustrated as Fig. 33–68). As noted by Katzenstein and Maurer,[350] many of the other cases reported as pulmonary histiocytomas, xanthomas, or xanthogranulomas actually contained increased numbers of spindle cells, and probably fit better in plasma cell granuloma or fibrous histiocytoma categories. The differential diagnosis of these more histiocytic-appearing tumors includes metastases from adenocarcinoma of kidney, adrenal carcinoma, balloon cell type of malignant melanoma, or hepatoma. Consideration of primary lesions includes benign clear cell (sugar) tumors of lung, oncocytomas, and oncocytic carcinoids. Absence of fat would exclude most of these primary lesions. Inflammatory reactions of malakoplakia, xanthogranulomas, Whipple's dis-

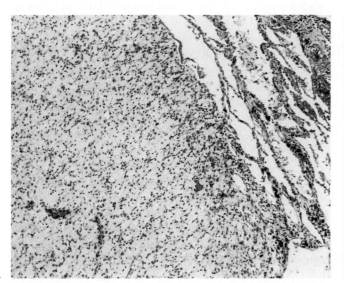
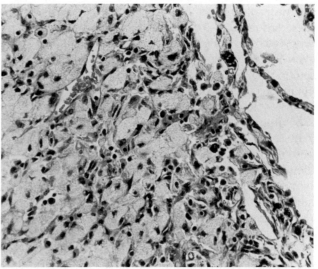

Fig. 33–68. A,B. True histiocytoma. Nodule is composed solely of finely vacuolated bland-appearing cells. **A.** Low power. H and E, ×100. **B.** High power. H and E, ×400.

ease, or *Mycobacterium avium intracellulare* should be considered, but are usually in a more inflammatory setting. See respective sections for details on each of these entities.

Fibrous histiocytomas and osteoclastic tumors are each separately described later in the chapter.

Pulmonary Hyalinizing Granuloma

This entity was defined in consultation by Dr. A.A. Liebow. His series of cases, summarized in 1977 by Engleman et al.,[353] consisted of 20 cases. Additional cases have been reported.[354–365] In 1986 Yousem and Hochholzer[365] summarized 24 cases derived from both the consultation files of the Armed Forces Institute of Pathology and those of C.B. Carrington. Between this series and the series by Engleman et al.[353] there is probably some overlap from dual consultations, but it is not possible to further separate these cases for a total count. These will be referred to as tumors, meaning masses, and as their true nature is undetermined, reactive or neoplastic, this is not intended to imply neoplasia.

Although gender is not indicated in the large series of 24 cases,[365] in the others there are an equal number of men and women. Their age range is 24–77 years at the time of diagnosis, with a mean age of 42.3 years. Tumors vary from several millimeters to 15 cm in greatest dimension, and in the Yousem and Hochholzer series[365] the average was 2.8 cm. One case had only multiple 2–4 mm nodules.[355] Seventy-three percent had multiple lesions, with most being bilateral (Fig. 33–69). Some pulmonary lesions are accompanied by a similar mediastinal involvement, which may lead to tracheal compression.[353,360,363] When occurring as isolated lesions, the right side is favored in 10 of 14 reported cases (71%) with no single lobe excluded from involvement. Cavitation rarely occurs. In a few cases finely speckled calcification was noted. Hilar nodes are not involved, even though in some cases the hilar region itself was described as being involved with tumor.

Symptoms varied from minimal to mild in the Engleman et al.[353] series, while in the Yousem and Hochholzer series,[365] multiple symptoms were reported but their severity was not quantitated. Of the 24 cases with symptoms, 8 had cough, 7 had shortness of breath, 6 had chest pain, 4 had weight loss, and 5 were reported as being asymptomatic. This tabulation accounts for more than 30 reported symptoms in 19 patients, and it is unclear how many symptoms were present in how many patients.

Solitary lesions usually are resected, with good follow-up and good long-term survival. In the cases with

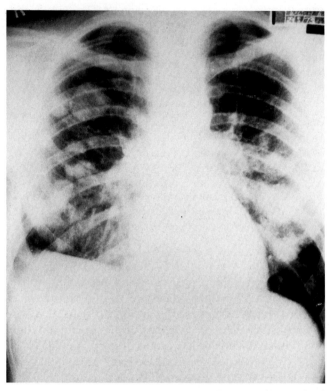

Fig. 33–69. Pulmonary hyalinizing granuloma. Radiograph of 28-year-old woman shows multiple bilateral nodules.

multiple lesions (see Fig. 33–69), approximately half experienced progressive enlargement of the tumor and progressive shortness of breath.[353,357] However, so far no deaths have been directly related to this tumor.

Four patients in each of the two large series[353,365] also had sclerosing mediastinitis (8 of these 44, or 18%). One patient had tuberculosis and 7 years later sclerosing mediastinitis was diagnosed, followed 9 years after that diagnosis by fibrosing retroperitonitis. Two additional cases of sclerosing mediastinitis were separately reported.[357,364] In one case the kidneys were involved bilaterally with lesions appearing very similar to those in the lung, and grossly described as infarcts. In this case four lesions were present in the left kidney and two on the right. No gross or microscopic pictures were included in this report.[357] In one case reported by Patel et al.,[364] multiple lung lesions were calcified and cavitary, but hilar and mediastinal nodes were also calcified and there were multiple splenic granulomas; also the patient had a positive skin test for histoplasma. This case therefore most likely represents histoplasmosis with overlap histology. I have seen one other case with histoplasma organisms in a typical hyalizing granuloma.[366]

One case occurred in an unusual setting, well described by the title of the article as "Pulmonary hyalinizing granuloma in a patient with malignant lymphoma, with development nine years later of multiple myeloma and systemic amyloidosis."[354] In this case report the authors concluded these events were probably independent occurrences. Amyloid was seen in this case in a widespread interstitial distribution, favoring vessels, and amyloid has been reported in extrathoracic sites in two other cases.[355]

The gross appearance of these lesions is either sharply outlined or with mild irregularity, correlating with a radiographic appearance sometimes described as "cotton ball-like." They are homogeneous, white-tan, and usually firm to like hard rubber (Fig. 33–70). They may be near to but usually do not infiltrate into pleura. Many may be in the midst of the lung, and a few are perihilar, the latter position bringing up the potential for vascular construction. Most are quite solid and only very rarely cavitary.

Microscopically, these nodules are composed of a dominant central mass that is quite characteristic, containing dense lamellar collagen strands in a somewhat irregular parallel arrangement, concentrically around larger vessels (Fig. 33–71), and in adjacent zones in a serpentine pattern (Fig. 33–71B). Often a larger vessel is involved in the midst of the lesion (Fig. 33–71A). Between the denser lamella there may be less dense stroma (Figs. 33–71B and 33–72) or a few inflammatory cells and sometimes a retraction-like artefactual space. These lamella vary in width and direction within the same lesion.

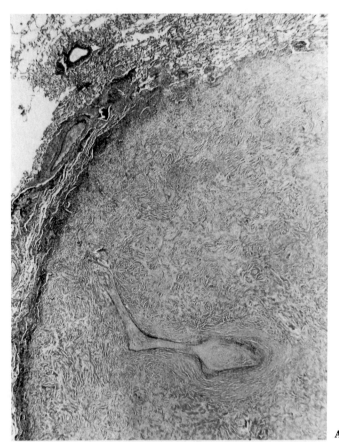

A

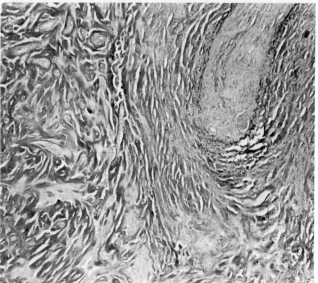

B

Fig. 33–71. A,B. Pulmonary hyalinizing granuloma. **A.** Narrow rim of inflammation at border surrounds dense area of fibrous tissue and scarred vessel. Elastic van Gieson, ×50. **B.** Higher power view of sclerosed vessel, with circumferential lamellar hyalinization around vessel but serpentine hyalinization in adjacent area. Elastic van Gieson, ×400.

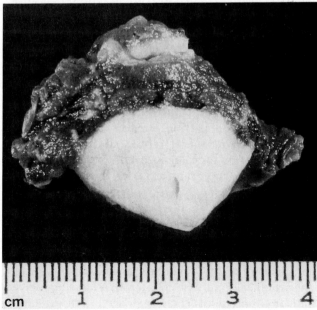

Fig. 33–70. Pulmonary hyalinizing granuloma. Gross view of one lesion shows very firm tumor mass. Note sharp borders of acute angle quadrisecting this nodule.

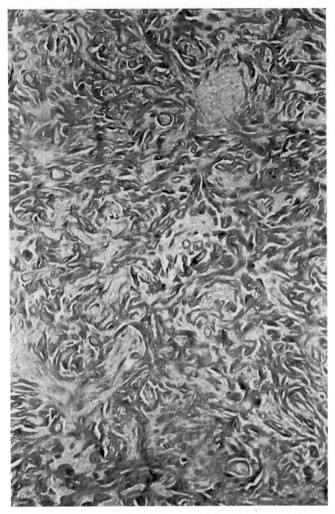

Fig. 33–72. Pulmonary hyalinizing granuloma. Serpentine type of hyalinization is better seen in this view. Sometimes small lumens suggest remnant capillaries. Notice less dense areas between more sclerotic zones.

In looking at the hyalinized substance of this lesion, I have wondered if the distinct lamella could represent collapsed structure of the lung with scarring. For example, could hyalinization occur in alveolar septa, encasing some vessels, and as the lesions collapse and coalesce, the airspaces are obliterated and epithelial cells disappear, leaving behind this interesting arrangement? A very similar appearance with eosinophilic nonamyloid deposits in ring forms occurs outside the lung in lymph nodes in assorted lymphoproliferations and as an isolated finding, the latter was referred to as "proteinaceous lymphadenopathy" in 1979 by Osborne et al.[367] Also, this entity in lung histologically has been described as being identical to sclerosing mediastinitis[357,368] and in neither case would there be background lung. Perhaps small blood vessels or other stroma in any location can be involved in a similar manner, as in the lung.

Elastic stains do not help distinguish a scarred lung background, as they stain only in larger vessels in this setting. Small lumens are often present, suggesting small vascular spaces (Fig. 33–72). Bronchioles are sometimes trapped in the center. The arteries nearby show some intimal and medial thickening, probably as a response to the constriction more distally. There has been no evidence of independent granulomas in nearby lung parenchyma or of distinct epithelioid granuloma in or about the tumor masses. Occasionally multinucleate foreign body-type cells are seen, and these are usually small.

Fibroblasts are usually most evident at the periphery, but probably also represent a few of the cells between the hyalinized lamellae. The peripheries of these nodules are surrounded by a rim of more intense chronic inflammation with lymphocytes (Fig. 33–73), and sometimes lymphoid follicles, some plasma cells, and occasionally eosinophils. The peripheral portion of the tumor appears to be the reactive or growing component, with a central portion representing a scar. Many cases have light deposits of speckled dystrophic calcification on some of the lamella, but no ossification or chondroid metaplasia is seen. There may be focal areas of coagulative necrosis, which are not central but scattered around and may relate to focal ischemia from vascular occlusion. Sometimes the lamella appear waxy (Fig. 33–73), and in a variable number of cases Congo red stains show positive staining with polarization (8 of 11 tested in the Engleman et al.[353] series, but none so tested in the series of Yousem and Hochholzer[365]). It would not be surprising if this should represent nonspecific Congo red positivity, as the hyalinized lamella appear so dense and therefore are prime candidates for this artifact.

Several cases have been studied by electron microscopy, and in the evaluation of Guccion et al.[355] the dense material is amorphous and electron dense, with no suggestion of amyloid. Their suggestion was that perhaps this material represented immune deposits. Another electron micrographic study by Chalaoui et al.[357] reported only collagen with 640 Å periodicity, with no evidence of granular background like immune deposits, but also no evidence of fibrillar material like amyloid.

The differential diagnosis includes other causes of hyalinizing masses. Occasionally sclerosing mediastinitis can extend into the hilar aspect of the lung, where it may obstruct vessels.[369] Pulmonary hyalinizing granulomas do have some association with sclerosing mediastinitis (8 of a total of 52 cases, or 15%), but most cases (85%) do not. Although the histology is identical, the spherical intrapulmonary lesions should be considered distinct at the current level of understanding. This type

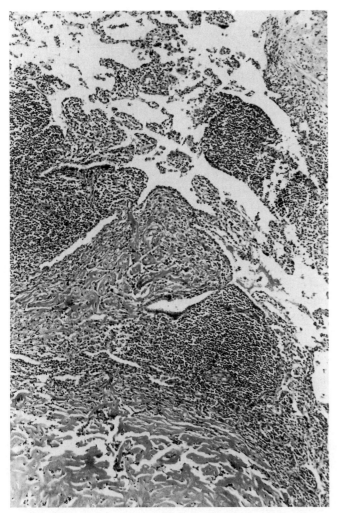

Fig. 33–73. Pulmonary hyalinizing granuloma. Rim of sclerotic mass shows moderate amount of lymphoid infiltrate. H and E, ×250.

of hyalinization and cellularity is different from that seen with neoplastic tumor growths of carcinoid tumors, sclerosing hemangiomas, or epithelioid hemangioendotheliomas in lung. Amyloid is deposited in the lung in three forms (see Chapter 22). Histologically, in the nodular form, amyloid may be deposited as plaques or clumps of homogeneous dense material without the lamellar conformation. There are multinucleate giant cells in both diseases, and only in amyloid are ossification and chondrification seen. There are more plasma cells in amyloid. A Congo red stain may not help distinguish these two diseases, as noted previously, but no ultrastructural characteristics of amyloid have been described in pulmonary hyalinizing granulomata. Of interest, I have recently studied a typical case of nodular amyloid by light microscopy that by electron microscopy had only electron-dense amorphous material in it and was without more typical amyloid. Its appearance

was similar to that described by Guccion et al.,[355] as noted, and may perhaps relate to light chain disease. Perhaps this appearance is of unorganized immune complexes.

Histoplasmosis and sometimes tuberculosis can cause granulomas, described as "old hyalinized granulomas." The hyalinization is often confluent and concentric on the epicenter of the lesions, and the dystrophic calcification may be orderly in rings, or more irregular and geographic (see Chapter 11). Certainly tuberculosis and histoplasmosis have been associated with sclerosing mediastinitis,[370,371] either remotely by involvement of the same areas by infective granuloma and later sclerosing mediastinitis, or by documenting coexistent organisms when abundant tissue is available.[368] No infective organisms have been found by special stains or cultures so far in pulmonary hyalinizing granulomas. In the group of pulmonary hyalinizing granulomas, there are some patients with skin test positivity, and several in the past has been documented with fungal and mycobacterial diseases. In a study of 86 solitary necrotizing granulomata by Ulbright and Katzenstein,[372] 2 of 86 cases were diagnostic of pulmonary hyalinizing granulomata. Probably other cases have been coded as scars, nodular fibrosis, old granulomas, or amyloid.

Nodular sarcoid and/or necrotizing sarcoid granulomatosis (see Chapter 19) might scar in this fashion, but the lack of remnant granulomata anywhere in the lesion, and the lack of scarring in adjacent lung parenchyma and/or involvement of nodes by either, would be against this lesion representing a form of sarcoid. Some nodules in the lung are excised as "burned-out sarcoid" and consist of dense scarring, often entrapping a muscular artery, with some remnant granulomata in the center of the collapsed vessel. These probably do represent residual lesions of nodular sarcoid. These do not have the lamellar arrangement going in all directions as is present in the current lesion. Whatever causes this must entrap and fill fairly good-sized vessels without apparent collapse of the vessels and/or "scarring down" of involved lung.

The natural history of plasma cell granulomas is unknown. No lesions have been followed with recurrent biopsies, and only a rare one appears to become smaller or to disappear following biopsy. The active plasma cell granuloma lesions have abundant elongated fibroblasts and abundant plasma cells. Sometimes these are arranged in storiform pattern and may have trapped benign background lung and invaded vessels. A lamellar arrangement may be focally suggested in the area of scarring, but this is not prevalent. Plasma cell granuloma is most often solitary, may cause larger nodules, and some of these lesions occur at an earlier age than has been reported for pulmonary hyalinizing granuloma. In the early lesion of pulmonary hyalinizing granuloma, the characteristic hyalinization begins in the center of a focus with a relatively large band of chronic inflammation. Experience with small or early lesions is limited, but so far there is no evidence of a preexisting plasma cell granuloma or other associated lesions.

Skin tests for fungal or mycobacterial infections were positive in 5 of 20 cases in the series of Engleman et al.[353] and 4 of 11 cases in the series of Yousem and Hochholzer.[365] Histoplasmin skin test was positive in 2 patients reported by Engleman et al.,[353] and in 2 of 12 (17%) of the other series.[365] One of the 12 tested in the latter series was positive for coccidioidin. A separately reported case[364] with calcified cavitary pulmonary lesions, probably caused by histoplasmosis, was described previously. As noted, cultures have been negative, and in fact positive organisms on stain or culture eliminated these lesions from consideration in the large series by Yousem and Hochholzer.[365] With the exception of two cases of possible histoplasma already noted, it does not appear that documented infection in the lung has given this exact appearance.

Immunologic abnormalities have been detected in a fair number of cases. Six of 10 so tested (perhaps a preselected group with a suspicion of some abnormalities) had some abnormalities in Yousem and Hochholzer's series.[365] These included 4 of 6 positive for antinuclear natibodies, 1 of 8 positive for rheumatoid factor, and 3 cases of hemolytic anemia. Schlosnagle et al.[356] published 2 cases with autoantibodies of some type, and both had circulating immune complexes. As already noted, in their 1 case studied by electron microscopy, they proposed the electron-dense amorphous deposits might be immune complexes.

It may be that several instigating causes can stimulate a similar-appearing lesion. Certainly in sclerosing mediastinitis it is known that histoplasmosis and tuberculosis are important instigating causes, although they are infrequently or rarely diagnosed as containing these organisms. The active cellular reaction is centered at the periphery, and perhaps the mass of the lesion represents old scarring of a peculiar type. Although there is some striking overlap histologically with the entity of proteinaceous lymphadenopathy, this does not seem to represent a plasma cell dyscrasia, and it is not amyloid. These lesions may remain stable for years, and occasionally show some sudden increase in size, raising concern of possible malignancy. In one series,[365] three were rebiopsied for this reason, one at 10, another at 17, and another at 28 years after the first biopsy: each had an appearance identical to the original biopsy. Another patient had sclerosing mediastinitis with histoplasmosis, with lung nodules thought to be related to this infection.

Fourteen years later the nodules increased significantly in size and were biopsied, with the diagnosis of pulmonary hyalinizing granuloma.[357] Whether this is a neoplastic or inflammatory reaction is unclear, but most favor this as being inflammatory/postinflammatory reaction to an unknown stimulus.

Benign Clear Cell "Sugar" Tumor of Lung

The entity of benign clear cell "sugar" tumor of lung was first described in 4 cases in abstract form by Liebow and Castleman[373] in 1963. A well-detailed series of 12 cases was published by the same authors in 1971.[374] These were also reviewed by Andrion et al. in 1985,[375] Gaffey et al. in 1990,[376] and Gaffey et al. in 1991[377] and Gal et al. in 1991.[378] As of 1992, about 50 cases had been published. The literature is carefully detailed up to about 1990 by Gal et al.[378] There may be some overlap in the total number of cases published. This must still be considered a very rare lung tumor.

The patients with benign clear cell "sugar" tumor are asymptomatic and the tumors are usually found incidentally. They vary in age at the time of diagnosis from 8 to 70 years, with about 66% in the age range of 45–69 years. The tumors occur about equally in each sex and have an even distribution in the lung. These are always solitary, usually more peripheral, with even contours radiographically and grossly, and most measure in the range of 1.5–3.0 cm although one in the original larger series[374] measured a maximum of 6.5 cm. The largest one was lost to follow-up,[374] and the next largest[379] one was 4.5 cm and had several atypical features at the time of diagnosis, including necrosis, and later metastasized, as noted below. One case of fine-needle aspiration of this tumor has been published by Ngyuen.[380] One case also has been described in the trachea[381] that seems to be identical.

Grossly, they are usually semitranslucent pale pink-tan grey, dark tan brown, or dark red. The usual tumor shows no necrosis, but there have been several exceptions. Grossly identified necrosis and multiple lesions would make one think of more aggressive lesions, including metastatic hypernephromas. Sugar tumors are usually described as away from bronchi or arteries, and are dislodged easily from lung parenchyma. One case of mine surrounds a nerve in the peripheral portion of lung parenchyma (see following), but no other association with nerve, artery, or bronchiole has been noted. They usually occur within 2 cm of the pleura but do not involve the pleura. Grossly identified bronchial or arterial spread has not been seen. There is no pleural spread, pleural effusion, or hilar node involvement.

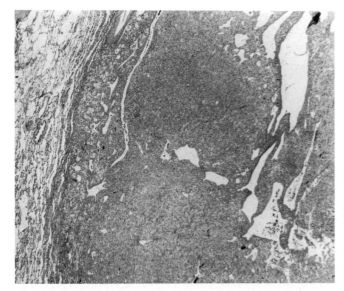

Fig. 33–74. Benign clear cell sugar tumor. Lower power view shows even contour to border with normal lung and no encapsulation. Ectatic sinusoidal vascular spaces are variably sized. H and E, ×50.

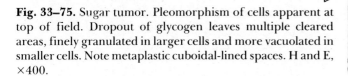

Fig. 33–75. Sugar tumor. Pleomorphism of cells apparent at top of field. Dropout of glycogen leaves multiple cleared areas, finely granulated in larger cells and more vacuolated in smaller cells. Note metaplastic cuboidal-lined spaces. H and E, ×400.

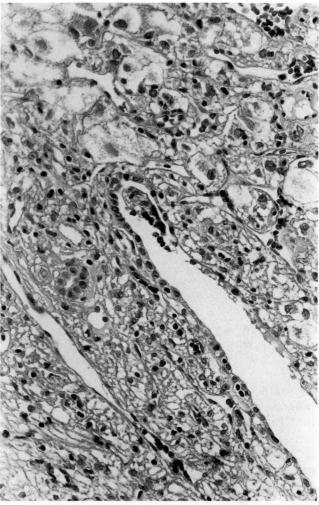

The nodules are sharply circumscribed from the adjacent lung parenchyma, with no true encapsulation (Fig. 33–74). The tumor cells themselves can be moderately pleomorphic (Fig. 33–75), in the fashion of a benign endocrine tumor, and the cytoplasm varies from eosinophilic and granular to lightly granular to clear. Cytoplasmic borders are distinct, and this is particularly noted when there is some clearing of the cell cytoplasm (Fig. 33–76). The nuclei are round to oval to slightly indented, with inconspicuous nucleoli, and mitoses are quite infrequent. Occasionally there are multinucleate cells. Some light-yellow pigment may be present, representing lipochrome. Cytoplasmic inclusions in the nuclei of some cells produce a granular red eccentric-to-central intranuclear mass. Reticulin stains surround some individual cells, but also surround some clumps of cells.

Within the substance of the tumor, there may be a few entrapped bronchioles evident at the edge, but these are usually not present throughout the tumor or in the middle of its substance. Toward the periphery there

may be some small spaces with cuboidal cells that presumably are metaplastic alveolar lining cells (Fig. 33–75). True acini and papillary configurations are not present in most of the tumors. Characteristically, there are dilated sinusoidal-like vascular spaces (Figs. 33–74, 33–76 and 33–77). with varying degrees of hyalinization around some (Fig. 33–77). Where the spaces are hyalinized, a separate discrete endothelial cell lining is seen by light microscopy, but where tumor cells are quite close to the lining, no distinction can be made between the edge of the tumor mass and the lining itself. These sinusoidal vessels have no muscle coat. Rarely, these vessel walls may serve as sites of small calcification. When hyalinization is present it may be more diffuse, or it may be zonal in certain regions of the tumor, with sheets of more monotonous tumor cells without this change immediately adjacent.

This tumor is so named because its cells are rich in glycogen. The PAS stain before diastase is usually quite intense, but this completely digests with diastase pretreatment. Mayer's mucicarmine and Best's carmine

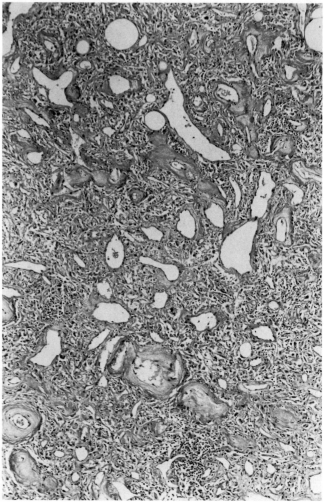

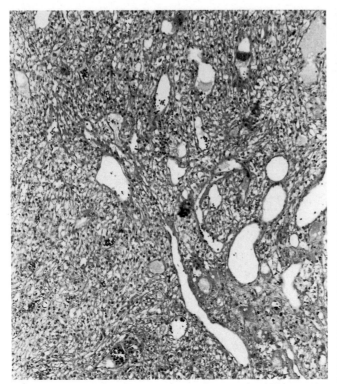

Fig. 33–76. Sugar tumor. Vascular spaces and clear cells with distinct cytoplasmic borders are apparent even at this lower magnification. H and E, ×100.

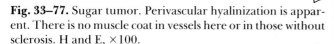

Fig. 33–77. Sugar tumor. Perivascular hyalinization is apparent. There is no muscle coat in vessels here or in those without sclerosis. H and E, ×100.

stain for glycogen show a similar reaction.[374] There is a trace alcian blue reaction and a moderate colloidal iron reaction.[374] Analysis of one of these tumors was reported by Gerstl and associates[382] to contain 10,656.5 μmol hexos/100 g wet tissue. Several other benign and maligant lung lesions and control normal lung had values up to 27.5 μmol of hexos/100 g wet tissue. No analysis was available for hypernephromas, either primary or secondary in the lung, to contrast with this. Such a measurement would be interesting, but the degree of sugar in hypernephromas is reported by light microscopy to be less than in the sugar tumors.

In 1970, Becker and Soifer[383] separately reported case #10 of the 1971 series[374] with accompanying electron microscopy. They characterized the ultrastructure of these cells well, with abundant free and membrane-bound glycogen. The membrane-bound glycogen appears unique to this lung tumor (Fig. 33–78), although it is typically described in Pompe's disease (type II glycogenesis). In Pompe's disease, glycogen

usually accumulates mainly in lysosomes, principally in the liver, because of a deficiency of acid glucosidase (acid maltase) necessary to further break down glycogen in these lysosomes. There is no evidence that sugar tumor of lung has ever occurred in a background of Pompe's disease. The only independent tumor was in the case described in the trachea[381] with a 1-cm mixed follicular and papillary thyroid carcinoma without vascular invasion.

These electron micrographic findings have been confirmed in several additional studies.[384–386] Necrosis has been seen in three lesions, including one seen in consultation by A.A. Liebow, but apparently has been unreported, as noted by Sale and Kulander.[385] There was apparently a thrombus in one of the vessels near the necrotic lesion in the case not reported, but in the 4.5-cm case of Sale and Kulander[385] that eventually metastasized, there was no evidence of thrombi near the tumor. Finding adjacent thrombi may, of course, depend on the plane of section. A 1.5-cm tumor cavity was

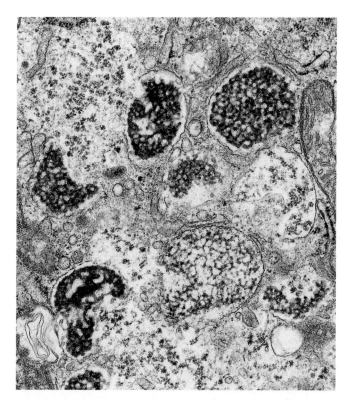

Fig. 33–78. Sugar tumor. Membrane-bound glycogen is typical. TEM, ×10,000.

present in the lesion reported by Zolliker et al.[387] Electron microscopy of their lesion failed to show the membrane-bound glycogen, but this is found by electron microscopy only in 60% of the tumors. Fukuda et al.[388] described a similar lesion in an 8-year-old girl; their material was poorly fixed, and on retrieval from the paraffin block it was not possible to confirm membrane-bound glycogen or the rosette forms of glycogen, which have been associated with sugar tumors. The case reported in the trachea[381] also demonstrated what was thought to be membrane-bound glycogen.

The case reported by Ozdemir et al.[389] probably cannot be accepted as a sugar cell tumor because of the highly papillary acinar configuration and abundant inflammatory cells. Their tumor may represent a primary clear cell carcinoma of lung, such as glycogen-rich bronchioloalveolar tumor[390] and an almost identical lesion has been reported as a metastasizing sclerosing hemangioma. Both of these would appear to me to be other than benign clear cell tumors. The case of Sale and Kulander originally reported in 1976[385] was larger than most, had necrosis, was composed of taller, more columnar cells than the usual benign sugar tumors, and recurred 10 years later as an 18-cm liver mass; the patient died 17 years after original diagnosis with recurrent tumor in liver and peritoneum, and at autopsy had

uninvolved kidneys.[391] Some caution about this case is necessary[392] until more is known about the full spectrum of this disease,[393] I agree with Gaffey et al.[376] that clear cell tumors of the lung larger than 2.5 cm and with necrosis and/or presenting with symptoms should be considered potentially malignant and that this group needs to be more carefully studied.

The cell of origin of clear cell tumor of lung has been and still is in debate. Liebow and Castleman[374] discussed the possibilities of this being myoid or neuroid. They noted that the clear cell leiomyomas that might be in the differential diagnosis did not contain glycogen. Smooth muscle tumors would be expected to arise in association with bronchioles or pulmonary vessels, neither of which seemed to be true in this case. Liebow continued to wonder about some smooth muscle-derived origin, as the muscle of some shellfish is rich in glycogen. Becker and Soifer[383] saw electron-dense small granules in 2%–5% of cells, and proposed that perhaps these are variants of Kulchitsky cells. Hoch et al.[384] were more struck with the possibility of a smooth muscle or pericyte derivation. I have had the opportunity to stain one such tumor with S-100 protein, which vividly stained a nerve in the center of the tumor, but the tumor cells themselves did not stain with S-100 protein (Fig. 33–79).

These lesions have been studied more recently by others with immunoperoxidase techniques with some potentially exciting and perhaps confusing results. Andrion et al.[375] found negative staining with neuronal specific enolase, actin, and multiple neuropeptides. Nakanishi et al.[393] found S100 staining positivity. Gaffey et al. in 1990[376] found S100 and nonspecific enolase (NSE) positivity. Pea et al.[394] in 1991 first documented HMB-45 positivity. Gaffey et al.[377] and Gal et al.[378] found S100 and HMB-45 positivity, and Gaffey et al.[377] illustrated a full spectrum of premelanosome differentiation in three of nine cases studied by electron microscopy. Cytokeratins, carcinoembryonic antigen, chromogranin, neurofilament, actin, and specialized neuropeptides have all been negative when examined.

The apparent melanosomic differentiation with S100 and human melanin black (HMB) is intriguing and warrants further discussion. Nakanishi et al.[393] reported S100 positivity in 10% of the cells. Gaffey et al.[376] found S100 focally positive in three of eight cases, and in the same three of eight reported positivity for NSE. In 1991, Gaffey et al.[377] found increased staining characteristics after strong trypsin predigestion, and found S100 positivity in all nine of the cases examined by them, while only three till retained their NSE positivity. When Pea et al.[394] described HMB-45 positivity, Gaffey et al.[395] reexamined their material and reported all five of the cases so tested were positive

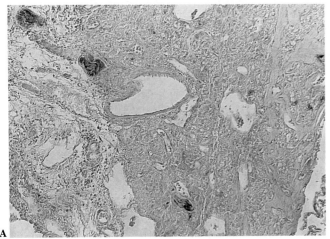

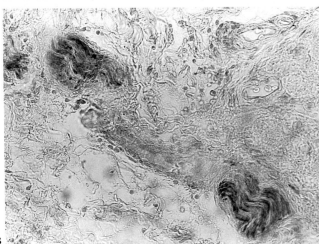

Fig. 33–79. A,B. Benign "sugar" tumor. **A.** Peripherally placed tumor nodule has been stained with S100 protein; three portions of one nerve are seen extending into and along upper border of tumor. Tumor cells however, are not stained in this preparation. ×100 **B.** Higher power view shows positive staining of nerve with negative staining of cells immediately adjacent. ×400.

for HMB. In this expanded 1991[377] series after predigestion, seven of nine cases were reported as strongly positive HMB-45, and six of eight stained HMB-50 positive. One case[377] was positive on frozen section for the melanacytic marker NKI/BETEV. Gal et al.[378] concurred that four of five of their cases were diffusely positive with HMB-45 and added that five of their five were cathepsin B positive, the latter perhaps indicating lysosomal activity in this tumor. Gal et al.[378] reported four of their five cases were vimentin positive, a finding not originally present in the Nakanishi cases, but originally found by Termeer et al.[396] and confirmed by others.[376–378,394]

To complement these findings, Pea et al.[397] reported

that the clear perivascular myoblastic-type cells in renal angiomyolipoma[394,397] and lymphangioleiomyomatosis[398] stained HMB-45 positive with purified antigen. These cells accounted for only about 5% of the tumor cells in their angiomyolipoma study.[394,397] Unger et al.[399] in 1992 reported HMB-45 positivity in the granular polygonal chief cells of adrenal pheochromocytoma in 4 of 12 cases examined, staining a minority (5%) in 3 and a majority (50%) of the chief cells in the others. It has also been noted in assorted tumors of the central nervous system,[400] and cardiac rhabdomyomas.[401] I have found focal positivity in only about 2%–4% of the cells in 1 case of benign sugar cell tumor I stained, these cells representing the larger cells scattered at the periphery. Some HMB-45 commercial preparations were impure and led to false epithelial positives.[402]

These immunoperoxidase findings warrant further evaluation. What does it mean to have vimentin positivity in only one of eight cases in one series? What antigens are being stained with strong trypsin predigestion that usually are not easily stained with routine procedures? Is HMB-45 staining the same type of cells in these lung tumors as the smooth muscle cells of angiomyolipoma and lymphangioleiomyomatosis or presumed neurosecretory cells in pheochromocytoma? The cases presented with premelanosomes-melanosomes appear convincing, but many other cases in that series and the other series and the individual cases studied by electron microscopy have failed to confirm these; however, perhaps they will be observed more carefully now that they have been described. Melanosomes have also been found in pulmonary carcinoid tumors (see **Melanoma,** following), soft-tissue pigmented dermatofibrosarcoma protuberans,[403] and pigmented nerve sheath tumors. Are the tumor cells surrounding a nerve in Fig. 33–79 a suggestion of perineural origin or is this relationship in this one case incidental? Even Gaffey et al.[377,404] have been cautious in defining this tumor as melanocytic. Dense core granules are also present, and even actin has been shown to coexist in some of the HMB-45-positive cells.[405] I agree with others[378,404,405] that the final answer as to the exact cell that forms this tumor may not be yet found. These findings are certainly intriguing and offer direction for further study.

The differential diagnosis principally involves metastatic hypernephromas and primary clear cell carcinomas of lung. Also to be considered are clear cell oncocytic carcinoid tumors,[99,102,406] acinic cell tumors, and at times oncocytomas and other granular cell tumors. All of these lack the typical sinusoidal vascularity in the blood and glycogen of benign clear cell tumors, and each has its own distinctive characteristics. Other entities and some of their characteristics are listed in Table 33–6.

Metastatic hypernephromas can be solitary and can present before, during, or after diagnosis of hypernephromas, and may even be present many years after primary excision. Katzenstein et al.[407] nicely described a series of 44 metastatic hypernephromas to lung. In their study, 27 occurred after hypernephroma was resected, 19 had the lung lesions before a kidney tumor was known, and 5 cases were added for interest from the A.A. Liebow Pulmonary Pathology Collection, which represented metastases occurring a long time after initial resection (9-28 years, with an average of 15.75 years). Men represented 85% of the first group and 79% of the second, but only 40% of the third group. Multinodular pulmonary spread or spread to regional pulmonary nodes were bad prognostic indicators, while necrosis greater than 10% carried a favorable prognosis. Hypernephroma is one of the "typical" tumors that may metastasize to the endobronchus (see Metastases, Chapter 35). I have seen a case present with expectorated tumor, and a similar case was described by Katzenstein et al.[407] Discovery of lesion(s) in the lung after discovery of hypernephroma carried a better prognosis than discovery of metastasis as the first presentation. In the group with discovery of hypernephromas first with metastases later, 12 of 17 were solitary in the lung.[407] Solitary metastases to any location from hypernephromas is estimated to be about 2% at the time of diagnosis.[408]

Many of these cases of sugar tumor have had renal evaluations, and this may still be warranted, because of the rarity of sugar tumors and the possibility of confusion with metastatic lesions. However, there are histologic differences, including rare or no necrosis, no mitoses, no fat, little iron, and a differential reticulin pattern, that separate sugar tumors from metastatic renal cell carcinomas (Fig. 33–80, and Table 33–6). The sinusoidal thin-walled nonmuscular vessels in sugar cell tumor are also distinct from the muscular arteries supplying metastatic hypernephroma (Fig. 33–80). Immunoperoxidase stains help with metastatic renal cell carcinomas, these being more vimentin, cytokeratin, and epithelial membrane antigen positive than clear cell tumors, and in reverse, if S100 and HMB-45 are positive, this is more typical of benign clear cell tumor.

Primary clear cell carcinomas of lung were mentioned by Liebow in 1952[409] and by Walter and Pryce in 1955.[410] Morgan and Mackenzie[411] described 13 cases of clear cell carcinomas of lung. In 1980, Katzenstein et al.[412] studied 348 consecutive cases of lung carcinoma to determine the incidence of clear cell carcinomas, and found that clear cells were common in all types except small cell carcinoma. Of these, 14 of 348 (4%) contained more than 50% clear cells, and of these 10 showed foci of epidermoid differentiation and 4 showed gland formation by light microscopy. The tumors with more than 50% clear cell change behaved no differently than their nonclear cell variants. These authors suggested this characteristic should be considered a variation only within lung cancer proper.

Edwards and Carlile[413] in 1985 studied six tumors considered primary clear cell carcinomas of lung by electron microscopy, and found adenocarcinoma differentiation in three and squamous differentiation in two. The other was considered a large cell anaplastic carcinoma. Edwards and Carlile[413] found no membrane-bound glycogen in their six cancer cases. They reached the same conclusion as Katzenstein et al.,[412] namely, that this is only a change within primary lung cancer of the more usual type.

Chemodectoma-Like Bodies and Similar Tumors

This section is divided into two parts. The first covers the incidental, small, hyperplastic-appearing chemodectoma-like bodies and the second the larger tumors that are possibly related to these bodies.

Table 33–6. Differential diagnoses and staining reactions for benign sugar tumors[a]

Lesion/feature	PAS	Fe	Fat	Reticulum[b]	Vessels[c]	Necrosis
Benign clear cell	4+	0	0	i	S	0
Metastatic renal canal	+−2+	0−3+	+−3+	g	A	+−4+
Chemodectoma	0	0	0	g	S	0
Carcinoid tumor	0	0		g	S	0
Sclerosing hemangioma	0−+	+−3+	2+−4+	g	S,A	0
Alveolar soft parts tumor	0−+	0	0	g	A	0
Hemangiopericytoma	0	0	0	i	S	0−+

[a] Reprinted with permission of Yale J Biol Med 1971; 43:213–222.[374]

[b] Retuculin: i, individual cells surrounded; g, cell groups surrounded.

[c] Vessels: S, large, thin-walled, or sinusoidal vessels; A, thick-walled arterioles.

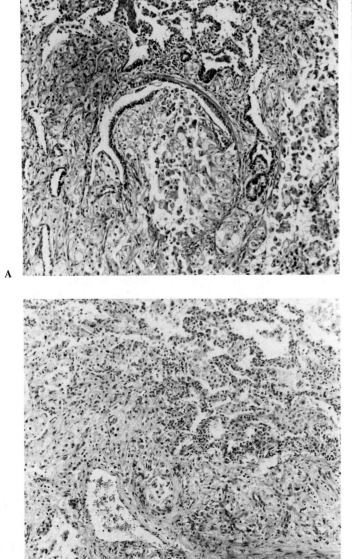

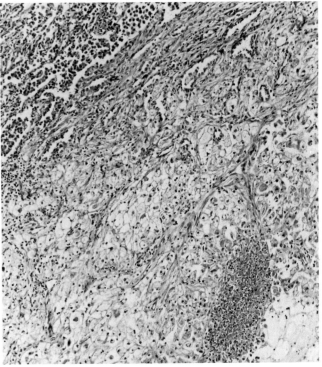

Fig. 33–80. A–C. Metastatic hypernephroma. A. Loosely cohesive clear cells infiltrate lung and submucosa of centrally placed bronchiole. H and E, ×100. B. Metastatic hypernephroma. Focal necrosis is seen. H and E, ×100. C. Metastatic hypernephroma. This tumor derives its blood supply from thick-walled muscular arteries in center. H and E, ×100.

Small Chemodectoma-Like Bodies

These incidental small or minute bodies were first described by Korn and associates in 1960.[414] These authors described 19 cases, including 14 in women and 4 in men, in whom these bodies were detected incidentally in the lung tissue. In only 1 case were they observed grossly; in the other 18, they were incidental findings on microscopic exam. These authors did serial sections and attempted injection techniques to further study the character of these cell collections. The injection techniques (see Chapter 1) did not penetrate the small-caliber vessels in the center of the lesions, probably because of a technical problem, and did not show arteriovenous anastomoses elsewhere. Their serial sections confirmed that these bodies were centered on veins, without a significant arterial supply, and without significant capillary plexus arrangement.

These bodies were noted in 12 of 3,635 (about 1 in every 300) unselected autopsy cases.[414] The original authors pointed out that no systematic search or study of these bodies had been done, and it was probable that if such were done the incidence would be higher Korn et al.[414] titled their article "Multiple minute pulmonary tumors resembling chemodectomas," and the term used here is "small chemodectoma-like bodies in lung." Because of the similarity of these bodies in appearance to paraganglionic tissue, the original authors[414] wondered about their possible chemoreceptor function. The nesting of some of the cells suggested the cell balls ("Zellballen") arrangement around veins, which also suggested some type of oxygenated blood monitoring function.

In 1962, Spencer[415] suggested that these might be reactive or possibly hamartomatous. Zak and Chabes[416] in 1963 studied six cases, all in women, and called them "chemodectomatosis." Using some delicate silver staining techniques, in the 1960s Barroso-Moguel and Costero[416,417] published several articles in which some nervelike filaments were shown that extended into the center of some cell balls (Fig. 33–81). They stained some structure that was quite distinct, while some of the silver-staining filaments appear to be entrapped elastic fibers. Some appear almost neuroid in arrangement, and it is unclear on the basis of follow-up studies (reviewed later) what the fine filaments and cell ball arrangement (Fig. 33–81B) really were. They also found some nonspecific argentaffin-positive reaction in these cells, endothelial cells, and pleural cells, but this finding remains unconfirmed by others. Follow-up by Costero et al.[419] with electron microscopy data in 1972 seemed to reverse this earlier suggestion, because no nerves, nervelike features, or secretory granules could be identified. They wondered if they could be pleural-derived rests or hamartomas in the lung. Spain[420] published 15 cases in 1967, and was the first to draw attention to the high rate of associated acute and organizing pulmonary emboli with these bodies. Ichinose et al.[421] added 10 cases, and carefully itemized the associated conditions in these 10 and in the 46 cases reported in the literature by 1971. Of these, 29 of 56 (52%) were associated with pulmonary emboli, 30 of 56 (54%) had cardiovascular disease, 17 of 56 (30%) had malignancy, and of those, only 2 were primary malignancies in the chest. Some patients had more than one of the these findings Some 91% of these patients had conditions predisposing them to thromboemboli. On

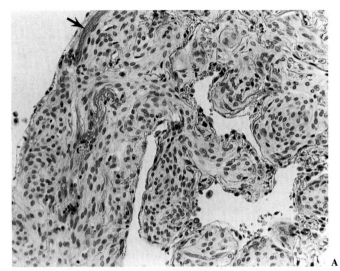

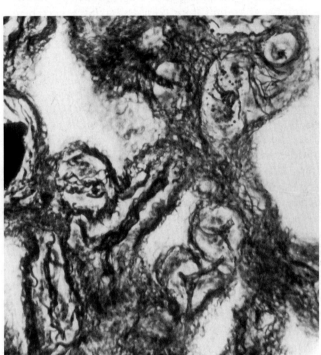

Fig. 33–81. A,B. Small chemodectoma-like body. **A.** Cells may be more organoid appearing with varying cell nests (Zellballen). Vessel at left has thick band of connective tissue at to (*arrow*). H and E, ×100. **B.** Small chemodectoma-like bodies with silver stain by Costero and Barroso–Miguel show similar thick fibers as in **A**; several nearby collections of cells suggest of fibers going into these bodies, but may only be thick fibers from **A** cut on end. Hortega silver stain, ×400.

histologic review, 6 of the 10 new cases had changes compatible with old pulmonary emboli.

Although Korn et al.[414] had not identified any recognized coexistent factors and had not noted emboli, most of their cases had pulmonary congestion, some had emphysema, and a rare case had cancer. Costero et al.[419] noted "the only common circumstance (of the occurrence of these lesions) was the special interest in the microscopic study of the lungs," but 4 of their 5 cases were in young women (ages 12–29) who died of fulminant heart or lung disease. Spain[420] noted that ischemia from whatever cause was the probable stimulus for their formation. In 1976, Churg and Warnock[422] carefully studied 26 new cases, and found most were associated with pulmonary injury; 23% were associated with thromboemboli (compared with their recent autopsy rate for pulmonary emboli of 8.2%) and heart failure, with more than half their patients having severe heart disease, ephysema, chronic bronchitis, and malignancies. They proposed that lung damage could also stimulate the formation of these small tumors.

Small chemodectoma-like bodies in the lung have been found in people aged from 12 to 91 years, mostly in the seventh decade. This may well reflect the age of autopsy series used to collect most of the data on these cases, and they are also found in surgical excisions of middle- to older aged individuals. They are multiple in some 30% to 50% and grossly have been seen in only a few cases. In one case of Korn et al.,[414] literally hundreds were seen on the pleural surface. Ichinose[421] went back to the paraffin-embedded blocks and found grey specks in 2 of the 10 cases detected, and when he cut more tissue in 5 of his cases, no more bodies were found nearby. I have found 1 grossly in the adjacent cut of a sample from a lobectomy specimen, but this was only detected after it was seen microscopically on the opposing face. Eighty-four percent of all cases to date have occurred in women. These bodies were thought to be more frequent toward the pleural surface,[414] but more recently were found in the deep parenchyma.[422] In a series by Churg and Warnock[422] in which location was identified, the bodies seemed to follow lung volume, being most frequent in the lower lobes (6 of 13, or 46%) and next most common in the upper lobes (5 of 13, or 38%), and least common in the middle lobe and lingula (2 of 13, 15%). Although the sample number was small, it is interesting that in the cases described by Churg and Warnock[422] these lesions were three times more common on the right side than on the left. Those with multiple lesions were most often in adjacent lung, as a single location was given. The 1 case described as multiple in the series by Korn et al.[414] grossly identified multiple lesions in all lobes.

The frequency of occurrence varies in different series. As noted by Korn et al.,[414] they occurred in 12 of 3,635 (0.3%), or at a frequency of about 1 in 300 of routine autopsies. Ichinose et al.[421] found them in 9 of 1828 autopsies, or about 1 in 200. The rate was 1 in 360 (0.3%) in selected autopsies in the retrospective review by Churg and Warnock,[422] but when prosectors were made aware of these lesions and asked to be alert for them, the rate was 6 in 200 (3%), or about 1 in 33. Considering their higher incidence in women, Churg and Warnock[422] estimated they occurred in about 1 in every 20 women in their autopsy series. Spain[420] found a rate of 15 in 303 autopsies, or about 1 in 20. Half of his cases were selected for ischemic conditions, and the other half were a series of all autopsies followed in his hospital for 1 year. The incidence in each of these groups is not specified. Once one is aware of these lesions, my experience suggests that they occur in about 1 of 40 well-sampled lung specimens, whether they be autopsies or resections handled through surgical pathology. I have seen one on transbronchial biopsies.

As most of these lesions are incidental and microscopic in size, they are not grossly identified. However, one good description was given by Korn et al.[414] of multiple lesions up to 1–2 mm. Korn et al. described them, particularly on the pleura surface, as being small, grey-pink, translucent, slightly raised, round to slightly irregular nodules often occurring near interlobular septa. They have been described as resembling miliary disease. About 1–2 mm is their maximum diameter, but one report[419] described them up to 4 mm. Small lymphoid nodules may also be in the gross differential diagnosis, but these are usually more translucent and associated directly with lymphatic pathways. Cases of miliary disease might also be considered. Grossly, small metastatic tumor nodules might also be considered.

Microscopically, these lesions vary and may be delicate or thick (Fig. 33–82). As they surround veins, they are usually in the middle or peripheral portions of the acini or lobules of the lung, but occasionally are seen to outline an alveolar duct (Fig. 33–82). At low power these bodies often have a somewhat stellate shape, usually with central thickening and with retraction of nearby airspaces giving a focal emphysema effect. These bodies may also be contained in a more linear fashion within the interstitium. Occasionally they abut the pleura or interlobular septa, but they do not extend into either of these structures. They are not seen in bronchi or in branches of pulmonary or bronchial arteries.

Microscopically, the cells making up these proliferations have bland-looking, oval to slightly indented nuclei with finely granular chromatin and inconspicuous nucleoli. These cells have no mitoses. The cytoplasm is usually abundant, granular, light pink, and homoge-

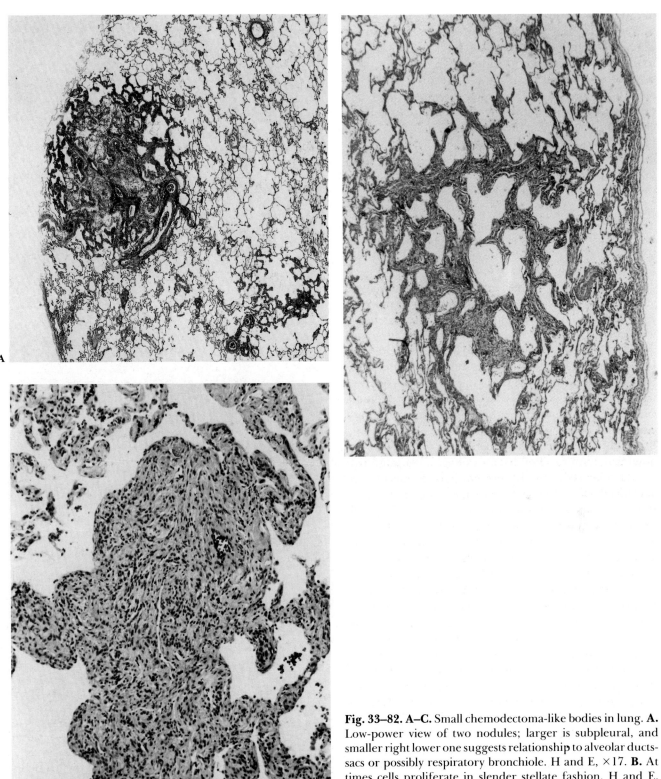

Fig. 33–82. A–C. Small chemodectoma-like bodies in lung. **A.** Low-power view of two nodules; larger is subpleural, and smaller right lower one suggests relationship to alveolar ducts-sacs or possibly respiratory bronchiole. H and E, ×17. **B.** At times cells proliferate in slender stellate fashion. H and E, ×50. **C.** At other times they are more nodular yet still are in interstitium. Note small cleftlike vessel in center. H and E, ×200.

neous throughout. They have poorly defined cytoplasmic borders, and the cells measure about 30 μm in
diameter. At times they are more elongated, and appear
to either form nodules or to be cut in different directions of orientation, giving some variation to the pattern. In about 20% of cases, some hemosiderin is associated with the cells in the interstitium. Tumor cells are
always separated from the alveolus by a delicate crown
of capillaries, and the alveolar type II cells are only
minimally reactive (Fig. 33–83). Perhaps the juxtaposi-
tion of capillaries prevents the usual alveolar type II cell
thickening seen in most interstitial thickenings.

The tendency toward formation of cell nests has
suggested to one group of authors[421] that these appear
like nevus cells. There is no suggestion of this ultrastructurally or by S-100 protein staining by immunoperoxidase techniques. (See following.)

The tissue changes in the surrounding parenchyma
vary. As noted already, there is a history of pulmonary
emboli, including acute, subacute, or chronic emboli,
with corresponding histologic changes in pulmonary
arteries. There may be edema and interstitial widening,
but sometimes the lung appears remarkably normal. I
have seen some 40–50 of these in routine practice, and
in one case there was associated aspiration pneumonia,
causing the more diffuse and linear type of proliferation noted above. In another the small chemodectoma-
like body was associated with a scar at the center of an
adenocarcinoma. They have not been associated with
the vascular changes of pulmonary hypertension, and
specifically have not been seen adjacent to angiomatoid
or other dilatational lesions of this disease. They stain
negative with argyrophil and argentaffin stains in almost all cases (note exception in the beginning of this
section). They may contain a scant amount of PAS
material, and hemosiderin, when present, stains positive with iron. Focally collagen and elastic fibers extend
between the tumor cells, but appear to be native to the
alveolar septal structure and to be passively incorporated by the proliferating cells (again see Fig. 33–81).
These fibers sometimes appear quite stout.

Three electron microscopic studies are available, and
we have studied one case. In the first, Costero and
Barroso-Moguel[419] commented on the lack of nerve or
neurosecretory granule features and noted the presence of well-developed desmosomes (Fig. 33–84A,B).
Two more recent studies, done almost concurrently,
have shown similar architecture, and the authors of

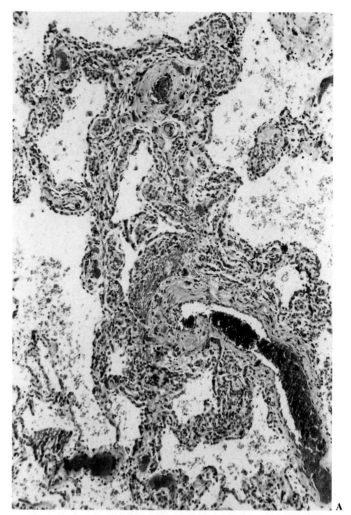

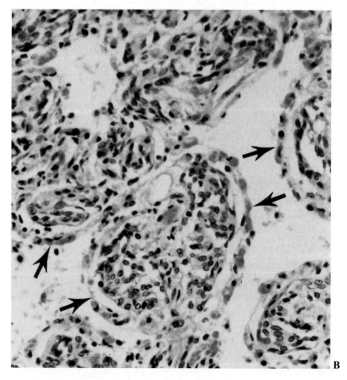

Fig. 33–83. A,B. Small chemodectoma-like body in lung. A.
Thick-walled vessel occurs in many; proliferating nests of cells
in interstitium are seen even at this magnification. H and E,
×100. B. Higher power view shows interstitial nests of cells,
usually separated from air spaces by rim of capillaries (arrows).
H and E, ×400.

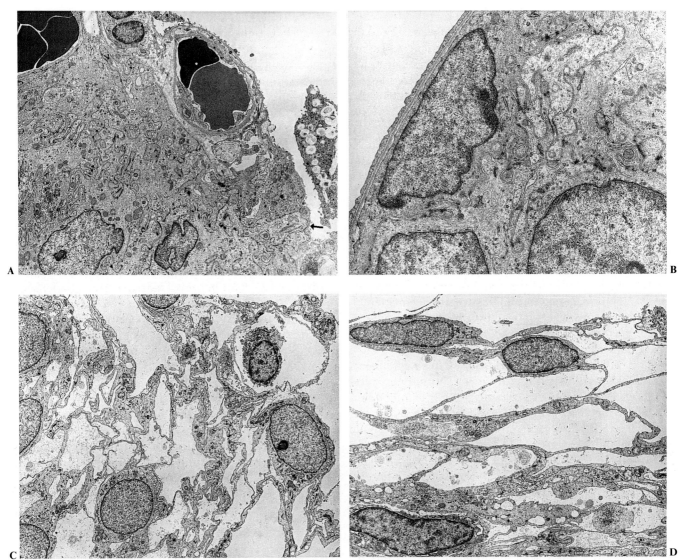

Fig. 33–84 A–D. Ultrastructure of small chemodectoma-like bodies. **A.** Cluster of cells with highly convoluted cell membranes and well-developed desmosomes seen beneath basement lamina of endothelium. Note focal proximity to alveolus (*arrow*). TEM, ×3000. **B.** Higher power view highlights complex interdigitation of cell membranes and well-developed desmosomes. TEM, ×8000. **C.** Cystic spaces are well developed in portion of proliferation. TEM, ×2000. **D.** Sometimes cystic spaces appear dominant, similar to those seen in meningiomas. TEM, ×3000. (Courtesy of D. Bockus and F. Remington, Diagnostic Specialties Laboratory, Bremerton, Washington.)

both studies have reached almost identical conclusions. The first was published in 1975 by Kuhn and Askin[423] and the other in 1976 by Churg and Warnock.[422] Both studies showed broad irregular cytoplasmic membrane processes (Fig. 33–84) that were closely opposed ("in a jigsaw fashion") and generally separated by 200 Å or so, occasionally opening to some 800 Å for short distances. There were numerous well-formed desmosomes. Most of the cytoplasm was filled with 60- to 100-Å filaments oriented toward the longer axis of the cells (Fig. 33–84). Our case concurred and also showed some remarkably generous cystic spaces (Fig. 33–84C,D). The Golgi ap-

paratus was usually prominent but other organelles, including mitochondria, were scant.

A few lipid or lipofuscin granules and occasional glycogen granules were seen. Some pinocytotic vesicles were seen along the cell membranes, but there was no basement membrane material around the cells and none encapsulating the group of cells. Collagen and elastic tissue were confirmed as radiating between the tumor cells, were extracellular, and did not appear to be produced by the tumor cells themselves. The more peripheral cells in the nodules were more elongated and spread around the more central tumor cells in a circumferential manner. No tumor cells infiltrated capillaries or alveolar lining cells. No nerves were seen in or near these nodules. Confirming the earlier study, no neurosecretory granules were identified. Also, there was no intracytoplasmic lumen formation to suggest angioblasts, and no Weibel–Palade bodies, but the cystic spaces shown in Fig. 33–84 were noted. These cells look most like pia arachnoid cells of meningiomas.[422,423] They are distinct from the ultramicroscopic appearance of both mesothelial cells and submesothelial fibroblasts. (Also, see meningiomas in lung, following).

I have used immunoperoxidase on several of these cases, and the tumor cells stain vividly with vimentin and are negative for cytokeratins, S-100 protein, and chromogranin. Desmoplakin would be interesting to run, as this antigen is positive in meningeal cells but is unusual in other mesenchymal cells. Unfortunately, with current techniques this test requires frozen tissue, and as chemodectoma-like bodies are usually incidental findings, so far it has not been possible to do this test. I am unaware of other immunoperoxidase studies on these bodies.

The differential diagnosis includes several entities. Carcinoid atypical proliferation, or "tumorlets," are collections of neurosecretory cells, usually in and about smaller bronchioles and terminal bronchioles, that are associated with distortion of the architecture with some scarring in these areas. These clusters of cells are neuroendocrine with appropriate stains and electron microscopy, may be multiple, and invade the adjacent airspaces. There is a higher nuclear-to-cytoplasmic ratio, and a moderate degree of hyperchromasia with thicker chromatin and more elongated cell arrangement than in the small chemodectoma-like bodies.

One might wonder what would be the appearance of small hemangiopericytomas or glomus tumors. These have usually been described as larger nodules, and have not been seen in their minute states. However, no proliferations of these chemodectoma bodies have been found nearby in the well-developed tumors of both types. Other entities in the differential diagnosis include benign clear cell (sugar) tumors, epithelioid hemangioendothelioma, small sclerosing hemangioma, metastatic paraganglioma, and small primary or metastatic meningiomas. The benign sugar tumors have larger cells that are more polygonal, glycogen rich, and permeated by ectatic sinusoids with some collagen in their vascular walls. Sugar tumors form consolidated nodules destroying the background lung architecture. Epithelioid hemangioendotheliomas can be epithelioid-appearing bland cells with granular cytoplasm filled with filaments, but these tumors proliferate predominantly in alveolar spaces, with some protrusion in a retrograde fashion in terminal bronchioles. They are

also seen in vessels and have a tendency to become more spindle like. Only rarely can interstitial tumor spread be identified, quite unlike the findings of small chemodectoma-like bodies. Small sclerosing hemangiomas have caused interstitial thickening, and even when these tumors are small they begin to have central sclerosis. Their tumor cells are more cuboidal, their cytoplasm more granular, and they stimulate the overlying alveolar type II cells more than the small chemodectoma-like bodies.

A case of multiple miliary metastatic chemodectomas from a left carotid body tumor was reported by Tu and Bottomley.[424] There were multiple lesions in the lung; none was greater than 2 mm, being the size of minute chemodectoma-like bodies. They even illustrated some centering of veins, but there was more obvious pleomorphism and larger round cells, with a moderate infiltrate of lymphocytes, particularly condensed around the periphery. The patient was symptomatic, versus the usual case with chemodectoma-like bodies, and he had a primary paraganglioma elsewhere. Another case in a 20-year-old woman, reported by Pinkser et al.,[425] included a carotid body tumor and multiple bilateral 0.05- to 1-cm lung nodules. Another such case of metastatic paraganglioma to lung is shown in Fig. 33–85. These tumors should have neurosecretory features not present in chemodectoma-like bodies. They may also have a more sinusoidal vascular pattern recapitulating that seen in the primary tumor. Most of the other reported cases of metastatic chemodectomas reviewed by Tu and Bottomley[424] showed larger metastases of paragangliomas.

Discussion

It is now clear that the small chemodectoma-like bodies are not chemoreceptors in the usual sense, despite some superficial light microscopic similarities. They are not nerve- or otherwise neurosecretory related. Blessing and Hora[426] have described paraganglia in serial sections of fetal lungs, usually near major bifurcation points of pulmonary arteries and bronchi, but these have not been well described in adult lungs. Their cell characteristics, when described, will probably be similar to paraganglioma elsewhere and be quite unlike bodies discussed in this section. The small chemodectoma-like bodies in lung apparently respond to ischemia and have limited growth potential. Why ischemia is not effective on a more widespread basis in the 50%–70% that are described as solitary only is unknown. The right-sided preference, as noted by Churg and Warnock,[422] if confirmed is interesting, and the only association suggested by this might be with aspiration-related events.

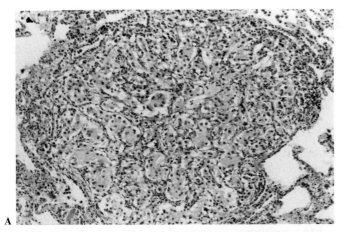

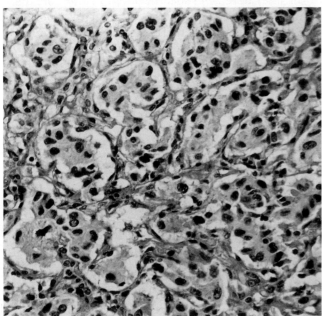

Fig. 33–85 A,B. Metastatic paraganglioma in lung. **A.** Small nodule of metastatic tumor shows distinct cell balls. H and E, ×100. **B.** Fibrous encapsulation of small nests of somewhat anaplastic cells. H and E, ×400.

However, aspiration has only been seen with certainty in only one case.

Other questions remain. Why do 84% of these cases occur in women? Those in men seem to occur in the same age spectrum and with the same multiplicity as those in women. They generally occur in the same spectrum of the disease, except that primary pulmonary hypertension and birth control pill-related thrombi are more common in women. In fact, more men have cardiovascular disease-related ischemia, and it would be anticipated they would be affected even more frequently. What is the connection of the pia-arachnoid-type cell characteristics as described by electron microscopy with those of other cells in the lung?

The location of chemodectoma-like bodies in the walls of small pulmonary veins and small venules is interesting. If they were a shunt cell, their location on the venous side seems inappropriate. Do they have some other role in possible local control, perhaps in a fashion similar to the glomus cell? Alterations in venous pressure are known to affect arterial supply and therefore easily result in shunting of arterial blood away from injured areas. For example, in severe chronic passive failure that lungs are described as being even more dry than usual. Histologically, there is a reactive pulmonary arterial hypertension, which appears to develop to an even greater degree than that caused by venous stasis. In some areas of bleb formation, the pulmonary arteries leading to this area are hypertrophic with concentric muscular hyperplasia, while vessels immediately adjacent in more normal lung parenchyma have normal caliber. It could be the cells forming these bodies serve as stretch receptors, as has been discussed by Kuhn and Askin.[423] Perhaps these bodies are not the receptors themselves, but some local hypertrophy or hyperplasia caused by such receptors. Their ultrastructural meningothelious appearance is enticing but leaves equal questions as to their source and the cell of origin's role, if any.

As Churg and Warnock[422] stated, "It is easy to rule out a number of possible origins for the so-called 'minute chemodectoma of the lung' but it is more difficult to assign a new one." This statement certainly could apply to several entities discussed in this chapter.

Tumors Reported as Primary Pulmonary Chemodectomas

Possible paraganglionic origin for presumed primary tumors in lung has been suggested in some case reports. Heppleston[427] in 1958 was the first to make such a suggestion, on the basis of a relatively slow-growing tumor observed for approximately 6 years. The patient was a coal miner and an achondroplastic dwarf. Although this tumor was shelled out, the patient was well in 3 years of follow-up. Fine capillaries permeated the tumor cells, and no mucin, glycogen, argentaffin, or chromatin reaction was present.

Fawcett and Husband[428] in 1967 described an apical lesion in a 66-year-old woman that suggested a similar possible origin. Their tumor was negative for chromatin, argentaffin, argyrophil, and autofluorescence tests. Goodman and Laforet[429] in 1972 reported two cases, one in a 69-year-old woman injured in an auto accident and another in a 43-year-old woman. The latter tumor contained focal silver-staining granules. All these authors were cautious in their diagnosis of a primary chemodectoma of lung.

Singh et al.[430] summarized these and other reported cases of possible primary pulmonary paragangliomas published to 1977. This review included three additional cases in English,[431–433] one of which was from Scandinavia[432]; two were in German,[434,435] and a report of two cases in French.[436] All these tumors occurred in asymptomatic people between the ages of 43 and 69 years and varied from 1 to 5 cm in diameter. Singh et al.[430] acknowledged the possible overlap of carcinoid tumors but thought their case could be distinguished by its intimate relationship to an artery. This tumor was 4.5 cm large, and described as "in the interlobular septum," but did have a branch of the pulmonary artery associated with it. The normal paraganglia elsewhere may (as with carotid body tumors) or may not (as with organ of Zuckerkandl tumors) be associated with larger vessels. As noted, normal paraganglia have only rarely been reported in human lungs.

Singh et al.[430] recognized that the high degree of vascularity, nesting tendency, and reticulin pattern with well-documented neurosecretory granules were suggestive of paraganglioma, but did not absolutely distinguish between carcinoid tumors and paragangliomas. They thought that carcinoid tumors should be more bronchial associated. Eliminating carcinoid tumors from the differential diagnosis remains a difficult problem. Theoretically one might suspect paragangliomas should not stain with epithelial markers, particularly cytokeratins, while carcinoid tumors should. I have seen a very nice and rather classical example of a large peripheral spindle cell carcinoid tumor that did not stain with either low or high molecular weight cytokeratin by standard immunoperoxidase techniques. If this tumor had the organoid appearance of polygonal cells it might suggest the appearance seen in chemodectomas, and this staining might be used to support this suggestion.

Although malignant behavior for paragangliomas outside the lung is reported in the range of 5%–10%,[437] higher in some studies,[438] this is only rarely reported in the lung. One case in a 38-year-old, noted to have a 5.3-cm subpleural nonargyrophilic, nonargentophilic tumor, had a 4.8-cm metastasis.[437] Because of these difficulties, in the differential diagnosis current investigators will certainly be suspicious of the various patterns of carcinoid tumors, acinic cell tumors, benign clear cell (sugar) tumors, glomus tumors, amelanotic melanomas, and possibly nerve sheath-derived tumors. Lack of neurosecretory features will eliminate most in this list. A cell ball arrangement ("Zellballen") pattern can be seen in many primary and secondary tumors, and has proven nonspecific, at least in the lung.

Glomus Tumor: Glomangioma of Lung

Depending on the cellularity and degree of vascularity, different authors use different terms somewhat synonymously for these low-grade lesions that are thought to be derived from the cell of a special arteriovenous shunt, the Sucquet–Hoyer canal. The glomus apparatus in this location is thought to affect blood flow and to be sensitive to temperature, at least in the extremities. These lesions are not well defined in the normal lung and are only occasionally seen in their hyperplastic form elsewhere. Outside the lung,[439] they are most often found in the extremities, particularly around the fingernails, including nail beds. They may occur in internal organs, including stomach and jejunum.

Glomus tumors are rare in the lung, and only a few have been described there[440–442] or in the trachea.[104,119,443–447] One had oncocytic change, a change that has been reported in glomus tumors in soft tissue.[448] An additional case may be of lung origin,[449] but was followed soon thereafter in a 19-year-old man by a deeply infiltrating gluteal tumor mass, with other metastases shortly thereafter. The latter case would represent a malignant glomus tumor or glomangiosarcoma,[450] whatever its origin. When referring to hemangiopericytoma, Stout and Murray[451] called them the nonorganoid form, and glomus tumors the organoid form, of perivascular growths.

Both descriptions of glomus tumors in lung indicate they are well circumscribed, multilobed, grey to tan to red-brown, with a slippery glistening surface and without necrosis; vascular spaces are sometimes seen grossly, however. Microscopically cells are between medium and small in size, rather monotonous, often having round-to-oval nuclei, with variable cytoplasmic borders, including some which are quite distinct, giving this pattern the name of "chicken wire" pattern. There is no nuclear molding, and mitoses are quite infrequent. The nucleoli are inconspicuous, and the cytoplasm is usually granular and eosinophilic but also may be clear. There may be some variations in cellularity, with well-preserved cells near the vascular spaces. The vascular spaces are ectatic and slightly irregular in shape, larger than those in hemangiopericytoma, without the acute angle divisions of "antler-like" spaces. The case illustrated in Fig. 33–86 has monotonous cells centered on a smaller vascular space, surrounded by a large amount of dense collagen. Tumor cells themselves do not appear to make up the lining of the lumen in many areas, but exceptions do occur. Microscopic necrosis or spin-

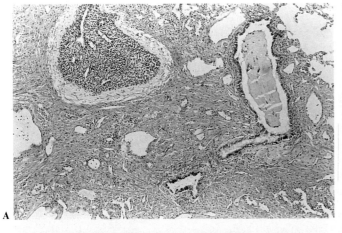

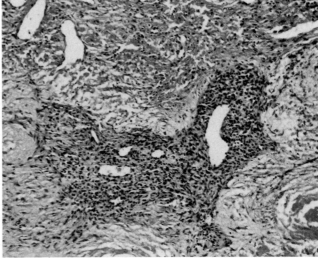

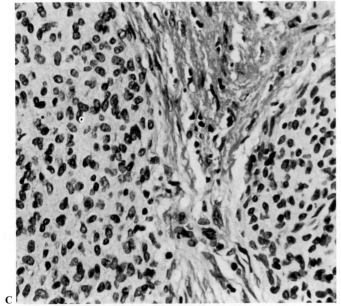

Fig. 33–86 A–C. Glomus tumor in lung. **A.** In focal area (*arrows*), small cells surround multiple vessels, and have elicited abundant spindle cell fibrous reaction entrapping bronchiole. H and E, ×50. **B.** Higher power view of some of these cells nested among dense collagen. H and E, ×75. **C.** Higher power view shows small cells, some with faint cytoplasmic borders. H and E, ×400.

dle cell change is not seen. Neurosecretory stains are negative and vimentin is positive.

Electron microscopic examination of these tumors in the lung[441] and brochus[443] show findings similar to those described elsewhere. The cells have smooth muscle features, including envelopment of individual cells by basal lamina, abundant pinocytotic vesicles, abundant intermediate filaments, and dense bodies and plaques. Nerve filaments are often in or near these tumor cells. They do not have neurosecretory granules.

The differential diagnosis includes hemangiopericytoma, which is usually slightly more pleomorphic in cellular characteristics, has the typical "antler-like" spaces (described previously), and does not have electron-dense bodies or plaques. Carcinoid tumors and true paragangliomas show identifiable neurosecretory features. Leiomyoblastomas or epithelioid leiomyosarcomas have more mitoses and more pleomorphism in

spindle cell areas, and they usually lack the typical ectatic vascular spaces found in glomus tumors.

Granular Cell Myoblastoma

Several reviews of this entity in the tracheobronchial system are available. Ostermiller et al.[452] added 3 cases to the literature, which contained 31 such cases by 1970. Oparah and Subramanian[453] added 2 cases to 42 in the literature by 1976. This series was expanded and additionally reviewed in 1983 by DeClercq et al.[454] The following facts are drawn from these series.

From 1.5% in one large institutional review[455] to about 10% in the literature[454] of the known granular cell myoblastomas in all sites involve the lower trachea and central bronchi down to the subsegmental bronchi. Three case reports of this lesion in the lung described nonbronchial-related coin lesion.[456-458] One had direct pulmonary extension from the bronchus.[459] Oparah and Subramanian[453] cautioned that these may raise the suspicion of metastatic granular cell myoblastomas to the lung from extrapulmonary sources; a case of metastasis to lung and pleura 5 and 6 years after primary excision from lip was reported by Klima and Peters[460] with another malignant case with pulmonary metastasis by Cadotte.[461] These lesions in the lung have so far always been benign, in contrast to 3%[455] to 6%[454,462,463] of lesions outside the lung, which are malignant.

These patients are generally in their thirties and forties, although one 8- and one 10-year-old patient have been described. The lesions in the tracheobronchial system usually present with symptoms of airway irritation and/or obstruction, including dyspnea, hemoptysis (blood-tinged sputum), and obstructive changes. Obstructive symptoms were present in 94% of one series.[452] One case was reported associated with hypercalcemia, which was cured following excision of the tumor.[464]

Granular cell myoblastomas occur in the right-main-stem bronchus in 59% of the cases, left-mainstem bronchus in 36% of cases, and in both bronchi in 5% of cases. These present as small crests or ridges, plaques, or polyps, and are generally in the range of 2 cm (Fig. 33–87). One tumor measured 6.5 cm.[452] Despite the large size of this one case, there was no evidence of untoward behavior of this large lesion. They are generally soft to friable to rubbery, yellow-tan to grey, and most often limited to the tracheobronchial wall. Overlying mucosa may be intact or may be focally ulcerated with associated bleeding. Ulceration occurs most often with pedunculated tumor polyps. Of all cases inside and outside the chest, about 20% have multiple lesions.[465] Of these, about 22% are multiple within the tracheobronchial system,[465-470] and there were even four multifocal bronchial cases reported from one institution.[469] The others occur with involvement of other organs, especially skin where the lesions may be multiple, but they also occur in tongue and esophagus. Of those that involve carina, about 40% occur with multiple pulmonary lesions, and in another 40% the carina is involved contiguous with a lesion in the main bronchus. Despite multicentricity, these act in a benign fashion. One peculiar case was reported with multiorgan involvement in a 29-week stillborn male. The infiltrate of abnormal cells was not as nodular expected, electron microscopy was done and showed abundant lysosomes. This case was S100 negative, and compared to congenital epulis lesions, only occurring systemically.[471]

Microscopically, these tumor masses are composed of monotonous large polygonal-to-elongated cells with granular cytoplasm that is also monotonous, without

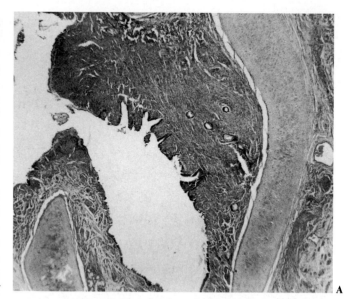

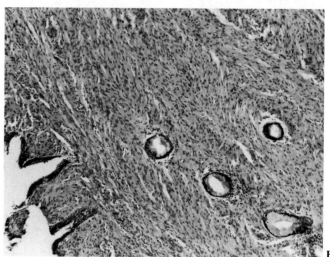

Fig. 33–87 A,B. Granular cell myoblastoma. **A.** Proliferation of cells distends submucosa in bronchus. H and E, ×50. **B.** These monotonous spindle cells, at low power, may be mistaken for fibroblasts, but delicately separate submucosal glands. H and E, ×250.

vacuoles or other variations, with eccentrically placed smaller nuclei, and no or only very rare mitotic figures (Fig. 33–88). The tumor cells infiltrate among submucosal glands and a third extend between fragments of bronchial cartilage; in only one case was there extension to involve adjacent lung.[472] Overlying squamous metaplasia occurs in some two thirds of the cases and sometimes it is atypical, but is not as often pseudoepitheliomatous in appearance as it is in mucosa or skin. As these are benign lesions, regional nodes and pleura are not involved. The granules are distinct, vary somewhat in

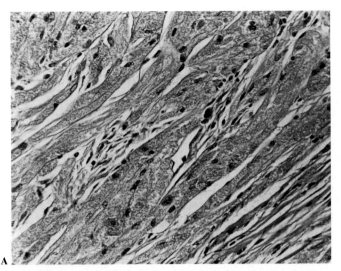
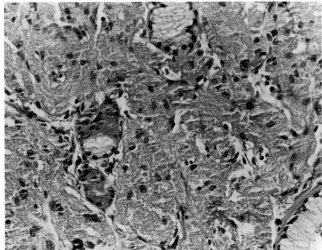

Fig. 33–88 A,B. Granular cell myoblastoma. **A.** Higher power shows granules cell in spindle cells. H and E, ×400. **B.** Granules are seen also in plump cells. H and E, ×400.

size and the larger ones stain with periodic acid–Schiff (PAS) and Alcian blue. By electron microscopy the granules vary in nature. The smaller granules contain packages of even smaller granules, and the larger granules appear to have mixed contents, including some with lysosomal characteristics.

In the lung there have been several case reports with these lesions associated with but usually separate from both primary pulmonary squamous carcinomas[473,474] and adenocarcinomas.[475] As with these tumors elsewhere, and even though it is less frequent, one must beware of the potential for exuberant reactive pseudoepitheliomatous hyperplasia, and distinguish this reaction from squamous carcinoma concurrent with myoblastoma.[476] As yet no malignancies have been observed to occur in the same region in the lung as the myoblastoma lesions.

The differential diagnosis of these lesions consists of other proliferations with large granular cells, including the inflammatory conditions of malakoplakia, Whipple's disease, and *Mycobacterium avium–intracellulare*, among others. As these are all basically histiocytic reactions, they have more fine vacuoles and more mixed plasma cells and lymphocytes, do not have the monotony of the cytoplasmic granular appearance as seen in granular cell myoblastoma, and are usually not too difficult to distinguish. Among the neoplastic proliferations that might be confused in the tracheobronchial tree are oncocytomas and oncocytic carcinoids. The granules in these lesions are finer and there is a larger nuclear-to-cytoplasmic ratio than in granular cell myoblastomas. Neurosecretory and S-100 stains and electron microscopic procedures will help in areas where there is difficulty. Most of these oncocytic tumors infiltrate in a more obliterative manner than the delicate approach of the granular cell myoblastomas.

These tumors in the lung and elsewhere are S-100 protein positive,[455] and this stain may be used to differentiate problem cases. Myoblastomas are now accepted as nerve sheath–Schwann cell derived, although cell cultures from a bronchial lesion appear unique from both Schwann cells and fibrohistiocytic cell lines, despite S-100 positivity in this cultured case.[477] Transbronchial biopsies may also be very suggestive of this entity, and cytology specimens, including sputa, washings, and brushings, may contain these cells and be at least suspicious for these lesions.[478]

Intraparenchmal Lymph Nodes

Lymphatic drainage of the lung is well monitored proximally by abundant nodes in the hilar region, and along ascending mediastinal routes (see Chapter 2, Anatomy). The lobar nodes are known to extend out to about the fourth-order bronchi, but nodes more distally are rare. Miller, in 1911,[479] 1924,[480] and again in 1947,[481] discussed increase in small aggregates of lymphoid tissue seen in older men, especially those with increased exposure to dust. He doubted, at least in his work, whether there were parenchymal nodes. Heller[482] in 1895 reported an early literature review of intraparenchymal nodes dating back to 1869. Kradin and associates[483] reviewed the 13 cases reported in the English literature from 1961 to 1974, and in 1975 added 10 well-studied cases of their own. The early cases were noted on lung specimens, and the first radiographic documentation of intraparenchymal lymph nodes was by Greenberg.[484]

Radiographically these appear as coin lesions, usually toward the periphery, and occasionally may have some finely stippled calcification.[481]

The incidence of intraparenchymal lymph nodes varies with the techniques used to detect them. Steele[485,486] noted four nodes in a review of 887 (about 1 in 222 cases, or 0.5%) solitary pulmonary nodules in man. Trapnell[487] did an extensive project, studying 92 lungs from 91 individuals at autopsy. These lungs were gas inflated, and specimen radiographs were done from several views. He could locate only one node (1% of cases) this way. He injected multiple pleural lymphatics with barium solution in 35 cases, and in 28 where deep lymphatic infiltration was achieved, specimen radiographs identified an additional five intraparenchymal lymph nodes (18% of successfully injected specimens), bringing his total to 6 of 92 cases (7%). The 18% positivity for the successfully injected specimen may be the most accurate incidence for whole lung specimens. Trapnell[487] noted that intraparenchymal lymph nodes highlighted by the injection technique were not identifiable even on review of the noninjected films. He proposed these were adjacent to non-air-bearing structures and therefore did not give distinct enough detail, even though they were actually large enough that he believed they probably should have been detected. My rough estimate is they have been seen in about 10% of surgical pathology-lobectomy specimens, if one is alert to their presence. Kradin and associates[483] have commented that, in the future, with newer radiographic techniques such as CT scan more small intraparenchymal nodules will be found and removed to exclude the possibility of cancer. They suggested that those nodes 0.6 cm and larger may be candidates for fine-needle aspiration cytology to (1) exclude cancer and (2) suggest this diagnosis.

When they are present, 35% of the reported cases of intraparenchymal lymph nodes prove to be multiple; in most of these just two nodes were detected, but an occasional case had four or five.[483] When multiple, they are in the same lobe 40% of the time and bilateral in most other cases. In the 16 cases reviewed of Kradin and associates,[483] six nodes were less than 0.5 cm, nine were 0.6–1.0 cm, and one was 1.5 cm in greatest dimension. Therefore, 60% of the nodes were 0.6 cm or greater, the size for possible aspiration. In their review of more recent cases reported in the literature, the largest reported node was 2.5 cm and two others were 2.0 cm. Therefore, most of the reported intraparenchymal lymph nodes are 1.6 cm or smaller. All were within 1 cm of the pleura, and were either adjacent to the pleura itself or in interlobular septa.

Intraparenchymal lymph nodes have been documented in the age group of "about 25"[487] or 30,[488] to 82

years of age,[487] but probably occur most often in older individuals because once the nodes develop they most likely persist. In all but one case (in which pigment in the lymph node was not described as present or absent), there was associated heavy pigmentation, and most occurred in men. In the series of Kradin and associates,[483] 80% occurred in men with a mean age of 56 years. All were tobacco smokers, and 6 of their 10 had exposure to either asbestos or nonfibrous silicates or both.

Grossly, these nodes are ovoid to round, occasionally flattened or discoid, or somewhat irregular in shape, and usually grossly benign-appearing nodes with abundant central carbon deposition. They have the usual 1- to 2-mm rim of tan material of lymphoid reaction with less pigmentation surrounding their pigmented cores. Their locations are predominantly subpleural, immediately adjacent to pleura or next to interlobular septa.

Microscopically, the nodes are usually subpleural and evenly contoured, and may be totally or only partially encapsulated (Fig. 33–89). Where there is a capsule there is often a subcapsular sinus. There is some organization with lymphoid material toward the periphery, and carbon and crystal deposition occurs more centrally as is seen in other nodes draining the lung. The lymphocytes cluster together and an occasional germinal center may be present. Lymphatic sinusoids are dilated within this lymphoid mass, and are often also dilated in adjacent lung, interlobular septa, and pleura. Polarization may reveal some small crystals suggestive of those associated with silica, and there may be silicotic-type scarring and nodule formation. In the Kradin et al. series,[483] small polarizable crystals were present along

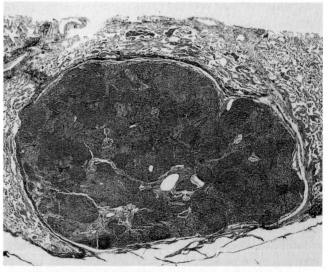

Fig. 33–89. Intraparenchymal lymph node. Subpleural encapsulated node, easily identified, with a few germinal centers and sinusoidal-type relationship. H and E, ×10.

with heavy carbon in 6 of 10 cases, and in 4 there were silicotic nodules present in these intraparenchymal nodes; however, only 1 had silicotic nodules in surrounding lung.

Dust exposure seems the most important stimulation for the appearance of these nodes. As these nodes function in the usual sense, they are subject to usual lymphangitic spread of disease. One such case also had involvement with metastatic poorly differentiated squamous carcinoma,[489] and in future cases we will probably find that sarcoid or other such pulmonary lymphangitic diseases may affect these intraparenchymal nodes.

The differential diagnosis radiographically consists of coin lesions in general. This list is long. The major concern is to eliminate the possibility of cancer. Histologically, once the benign well-structured nodal-like architecture is identified, there are not too many other lesions in the differential diagnosis. Other causes of lymphoid hyperplasia in the lung, such as reactive hyperplasias of the bronchus-associated lymphoid tissue (BALT), cause more reaction around bronchopulmonary rays. The infiltrates of pseudolymphoma and lymphoma are not well organized, and occur in lung parenchyma.

Intraparenchymal lymph nodes appear to be developmental, as they have not been described in children or very young adults. They seem to be stimulated by exposure to dusts. Their predominant occurrence in the lower half of the lungs is explained by the increased amount of lymphatic fluids produced in these lobes, especially when compared with the upper lobes,[490] despite the fact that the dust is in fact more damaging to the parenchyma of the upper lobes of the lung.

Rare Primary Tumors More Common Elsewhere or "Tumor Ectopias"

This section addresses a group of tumors described as primary in the lung because no other sources can be identified. This group, however, represents malignancies that are far more frequent in other sites, and their pulmonary metastases likewise are far more frequent than those described as primary in lung. As a group, these require thorough evaluation of these more frequent primary sites, and also helpful is an autopsy with no other tumor identified, or at least no other tumor in these more frequent extrapulmonary sites. This group includes melanoma, meningioma, ependymoma, thymoma, choriocarcinoma, and osteoclastic tumors. Some other items that might be included in this category, such

as endometrioma, are discussed elsewhere. Likewise, this section complements the section on tissue ectopias in the lung and thus might be called "tumor ectopias in lung," although some might reasonably object to that term.

Melanoma

Establishing a melanoma as a primary lesion in the lung is a very challenging and often impossible task. Regressing melanomas of the skin are a well-known source for regional lymph node and widespread metastases. In a large study by Das Gupta et al.[491] reported in 1963, 100 cases of 992 (10%) melanomas were found that at first review appeared to be without known primary. On thorough examination, only 37 (3.7%) remained in this category. Of these, 24 involved one node group only and 13 were widespread. None apparently was solitary in a visceral organ. (Also see discussion in Chapter 35, **Metastases to and from the Lung.**)

In a continuation of this large study, Das Gupta et al.[492] in 1964 noted the lungs are subject to metastatic melanoma more often than any other organ in an autopsy series of widespread metastases from melanoma. Metastatic melanoma to lung usually consists of multiple bilateral nodules varying between several millimeters and 2.5 cm and favoring the periphery of the lungs. These nodules are most common in areas of high blood flow, specifically in the lower lobes. In this series, 1 of 652 cases spread to the trachea and another to the bronchus. Forty-five (7% of total) spread to the lungs alone. None spread to the pleura alone. By 1969, Das Gupta et al.[493] had noted 2% of metastatic melanomas at autopsy spread to the bronchus. This is an important statistic, as the bronchus is the source of origin of those cases that are most likely primary in the lung.

Peripheral nodular melanomas should never be misinterpreted as primary melanoma. Different criteria have been offered by different authors[494–497] at different times in attempting to refine those most useful in making a diagnosis of primary melanoma of lung. This has more recently been reviewed.[498] To me the most reasonable of these criteria for suggesting this diagnosis during life appear to be the following: (1) absence of other past or present atypical-to-malignant pigmented lesions from any site; (2) a solitary lung lesion centered on a bronchus, with no evidence of other organ involvement; and (3) in situ atypical melanocytic change of bronchial mucosa adjacent to or overlying the major tumor mass (Fig. 33–90). See following further discussion. Long follow-up and long survival may also help support the suggestion of primary melanoma. Although some exceptions occur, many patients consid-

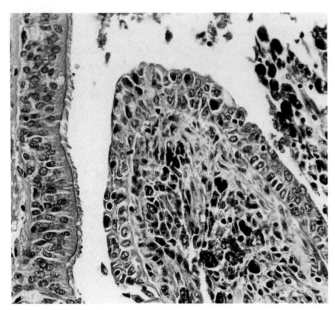

Fig. 33–90. Melanoma of bronchus. Atypical melanocytes replace mucosa in polypoid portion to right, with melanin in stromal macrophages. Contrast with ciliated columnar respiratory mucosa at left. H and E, ×400.

ered as having primary melanoma of the lung are dead within 1.5 years of diagnosis of their pulmonary tumors. In several cases, however, patients have survived 10[499,500] and 11[501] years post pneumonectomy without recurrent tumor elsewhere, yet in another case[499] a pulmonary lesion was diagnosed 31 years after a choroidal melanoma was excised. In yet another case,[500] 3 years after a melanoma from the left cheek was excised, a right-bronchial melanoma presented with hemoptysis. Recurrent hemoptyses required repeated cauterizations, and progressive involvement of the tracheobronchial system was identified during the next 10 years. At autopsy there were submucosal lesions in an area just below the larynx, in midtrachea, and both mainstem bronchi, each with overlying atypical melanocytic hyperplasia in the tracheobronchial mucosa. Perhaps this is a case of multiple primary melanomas, even though two of the three criteria just noted would not be supported.

Autopsy follow-up with thorough evaluation of all possible sites is also helpful. Several reported cases have tumor limited only to lung only or with only regional node spread. Obviously, very careful autopsies are required to exclude all sources.[502,503]

Some cases are as well documented as possible and probably are primary melanomas in the lung. Various authors have excluded different cases for different reasons, and these were reviewed by Taboada et al.[504] in

1972, Cagle et al.[505] in 1984, and Carstens et al.[506] in 1984. There has been only one case of possible primary pleural melanoma.[507] In the large series of metastatic melanomas by Das Gupta and Brasfeld,[492] the pleura alone was never involved by metastatic disease, and, as noted, it was involved only when widely disseminated melanoma was present in the adjacent lung.

One of the better histologic criteria used to suggest primary melanoma on mucous membranes, as in skin, is to identify atypical melanocytic hyperplasia in overlying or nearby bronchial mucosa[494] (see Fig. 33–90). Some have called this junctional or lentiginous change,[497,508] and some require this change to be associated with "dropping off" of nests of atypical melanocytes between the surface and the tumor mass.[509] This change is usually associated with squamous metaplasia, but also may be seen in thin glandular ciliated mucosa, with atypical cells present in the base of the mucosa.[510] This change in adjacent mucosa has been referred to by Salm[502] as the "melanoma flare." Other cases that appear to be primary have not always had this association, so its absence does not exclude a case as being considered a true primary melanoma.

Be careful not to be swayed by this finding in peripheral nodules of melanoma. I have seen a case of Pagetoid melanoma spreading in a peripheral bronchiole, adjacent to a 1.2-cm peripheral lung nodule in an older woman, who several months later was found to have rapidly growing bilateral inguinal node spread of melanoma from an undetermined source (Fig. 33–91). Primary bronchial melanomas are usually heavily pigmented, and there may be evidence of superficial ulceration and possible sources of hemorrhage. The tumors are polypoid in several cases, yet in others are flat and velvety. The major differential diagnosis is with metastatic melanomas, which may present with a large number of patterns (one of the "great imitators"); a more unusual one is illustrated in Fig. 33–92. Melanocytic carcinoid tumors must also be distinguished[511,512] (see Chapter 32). S100-positivity may be seen in granular cell myoblastomas in bronchi, and S100- and HMB-positivity are found in some benign clear cell "sugar" tumors of the lung. (See separate sections in this chapter.)

Melanin-containing cells have not been identified in normal bronchial mucosa, but most authors believe because the lungs are an outpouching of the endodermal tube and melanomas arise in the oropharynx, larynx, and esophagus, that melanocytes can occur, or at least there is the potential for their development, in the lungs as well as in the other unusual extracutaneous sites. Excluding the retina-choroid, most of the unusual sites are mucosal surfaces, as with the lung.

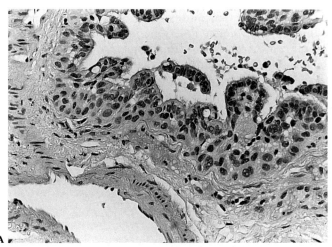
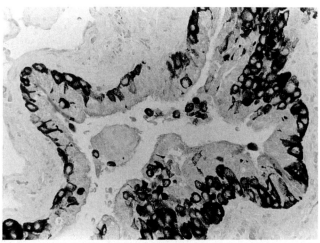

Fig. 33–91 A,B. Metastatic melanoma. Bronchiole is involved with "Pagetoid" spread of melanoma from adjacent, peripheral 1.2-cm solitary nodule of metastatic melanoma (see text). H and E, ×400. **B.** Human melanin black (HMB-45) by immunoperoxidase techniques highlights these cells, undermining negatively stained bronchiolar mucosa. ×400. (Original contributor, Dr. D. Bauermeister, Virginia Mason Clinic, Seattle, Washington.)

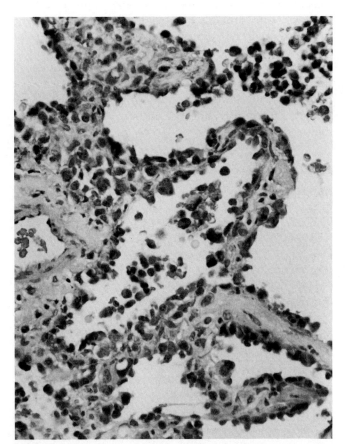

Fig. 33–92. Metastatic melanoma. Malignant larger cells are in interstitium and focally appear to be lining airways almost in a BAC pattern. H and E, ×400.

Meningiomas in Lung

About nine cases of presumed primary meningioma in lung have been reported.[513–519] Two reports concern two patients each[517,519]; another possible case was a 0.3-cm nodule in a patient with neurofibromatosis, including involvement of the bronchial systems, in whom a spinal cord meningioma was resected 1 year before death.[520] It is unclear whether this represents a metastasis or an independent primary. As with tumors that so often represent metastases, when a primary role is proposed, the more normal sources must be carefully examined, in this instance meninges of the brain and spinal cord. Also, an adequate follow-up should be included. The extent of any of this follow-up period is unclear and some propose it is never long enough. Complete autopsies documenting absence of tumor in these more usual sites is highly desirable if such cases are published. Most extracranial meningiomas are about the head and neck,[521] and the rare ones in the chest have been reported in the posterior mediastinum[522] and pleura[523] in addition to the lung.

Metastases from intracranial meningiomas do occur, usually following surgery or recurrences postoperatively, and in two series of 56[524] and 113[525] cases of metastasizing meningiomas the lung was involved in 60% and 61%, respectively.

The cases reported as primary in the lung have typical meningothelious appearance (Fig. 33–93) with whorls and often psammomatous calcifications, and no

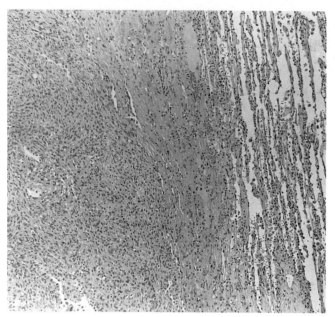

Fig. 33–93. Meningioma in lung. This field is border of metastatic meningioma. Those described as primary in lung often have psammatous calcification and meningothelious features, whereas this one is more fibrothelious. H and E, ×60.

mitoses or cellular pleomorphism. By electron microscopy, they have typical, highly interdigitated cell membranes and desmosomes, and by immunoperoxidase, are vimentin and epithelial membrane positive. They are solitary, usually round, vary from tan to light gray to dark gray, and are without necrosis.

Hoye et al.[526] has proposed a classification for extrapulmonary meningiomas to include (1) extracranial extension from intracranial primary meningiomas, (2) origin from arachnoid cells at the borders of the nervous system, such as the cranial foramens with exodus of cranial nerves, (3) totally detached extracranial ectopic meningiomas, and (4) metastases from benign appearing intracranial meningiomas. It might be wondered whether ectopic cells proposed in this second category might be related to small chemodectoma-like bodies discussed here, but in no case of proposed primary meningioma was there stimulation of these types of bodies nearby, as might represent a field effect.

Ependymoma of Lung

In 1992, Crotty et al.[527] reported a single case of a 2-cm, right-upper-lobe nodule typical of ependymoma, occurring only in the lung, with clinical evaluation of the central nervous system (CNS) being normal. Of interest, the patient had had a recent nodule in the right-upper lobe, somewhat more lateral, with hilar nodes

and superclavicular nodes being involved with tumor. The supraclavicular node was diagnosed as metastatic small cell carcinoma of lung some 30 months before, and radio- and chemotherapy yielded complete resolution of all tumor. The current tumor showed no evidence of recurrent nodal enlargement. The patient died 30 months later of a cerebral vascular accident in the distribution of the middle cerebral artery, and no autopsy was done. All the features of the tumor were typical of ependymoma. These authors noted that ependymomas are rare outside the CNS, and when they do occur they appear about the pelvis, externally around the soft tissues of the sacrococcygeal region, and within the pelvis, in and around the ovary, broad ligament, meso-ovarian, and uterosacral ligament. Two cases have been reported in the posterior mediastinum.[528,529] Ependymomas rarely metastasize outside the CNS, but when they do they most commonly involve the lung. Most cerebral ependymomas are intracranial in children and in the spinal cord and filum terminale in adults. Crotty et al.[527] noted that they cannot totally exclude origin in site(s) outside the lung as an autopsy was not obtained and another lesion might have been missed. Unfortunately, the original node biopsy of the patient's small cell carcinoma was compromised by poor preservation, but there was no evidence of glial fibrillary acidic protein, Leu-7, or S-100 proteins, all of which were present in the second nodule. Having two such nodules in the same location, temporally close to each other, is intriguing, and the authors discuss this possibility.

Intrapulmonary Thymoma

By 1989 about 14 cases of this entity had been published.[530–541] As with other "ectopic tumors," careful examination of the mediastinum must be included to exclude direct spread or metastases from a mediastinal thymoma (Fig. 33–94). Certainly ectopic thymomas have been reported in the neck and the thyroid.[538,542] They vary from small to 6 cm in diameter, and have been subdivided by Kalish[534] into peripheral and hilar, with most of the peripheral ones being on the right side and most of the central ones being on the left side, both for unexplained reasons,[535] with one exception each reported by Kung et al.[539] The histology usually is of lymphocyte predominant or mixed-type thymoma (Fig. 33–94B), and Fukayama et al.[541] showed two cases with TdT positivity, one of which stained with OKT6 and the other staining variably with this antigen, both markers of thymus-derived lymphocytes. In this last series, one case was multinodular in the pleura, but also was noted to apparently be in continuity with a deviated thymus; thus, the question of spread from mediastinal thymoma

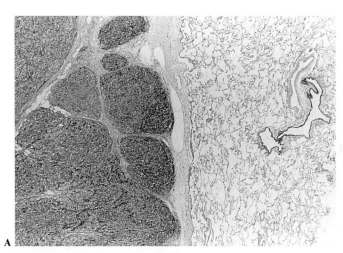

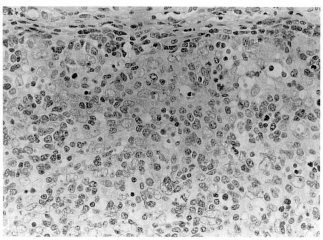

Fig. 33–94 A,B. Thymoma extending into lung. **A.** This represents a primary thymoma in mediastinum but is similar to those described as primary in lung. H and E, ×25. **B.** Patterns for tumor are similar to those in mediastinum, but its recognition in lung requires thinking of this possibility and appropriate evaluations. H and E, ×400.

cannot be excluded in this case. Patients are reported as having about an equal sex incidence, and their ages range from 14 to 74 years. Mechanisms such as ectopic fragments of thymus tissue developing thymoma or one-sided teratomatous development have been proposed. The differential diagnosis is with lymphoepithelial type of lung carcinomas[543,544] (also see Chapter 32). Of interest, at least in the first five cases of lymphoepithelial epithelioma-like carcinoma of lung, three had association with Epstein–Barr virus,[543] an occurrence so far undocumented with thymomas. T-Lymphocyte markers, as noted, may be helpful in difficult cases. Mixed-cell lymphomas should be separated by appropriate markers and/or electron microscopy.

Choriocarcinomas

A few cases have been described as presumed primary choriocarcinomas in the lung without identifiable genital sources[545–553] (Fig. 33–95). Pushchak and Farhi[550] noted 14 by 1987, with several more since.[551,552] These can occur in both men and women, and those in women can occur both in pregnant, recently pregnant or aborted, never pregnant, and postmenopausal states or in infancy. Possible theories of histogenesis include (1) origin from incompletely migrated germ cells, (2) metastases from genital primary tumors, and (3) origin from nongerm cells through neoplastic transformation.[550] A rare case has been described as primary large or giant cell carcinoma of the lung with human chorionic gonadotropin (HCG) production,[553–555] and at the same time metastases have been noted to undergo some peculiar large cell change and loss of trophoblastic differentiation.[556]

Osteoclastic Tumors

Giant cells in tumors in the lung can be true malignant cells, in which case they are large and generally pleomorphic, and are often seen in giant cell anaplastic carcinoma and focally in large cell or other carcinomas, and, at times, in sarcomas, both primary and secondary in lung. Syncytiotrophoblastic giant cells are seen in choriocarcinomas (see last section). Benign osteoclast-like (osteoclastic) giant cells, with multiple small round to slightly oval monotonous nuclei (Fig. 33–96), are identical to benign osteoclasts in bone and soft tissue by electron microscopy and staining with panhematopoetic or common leukocyte antigens and can occur within

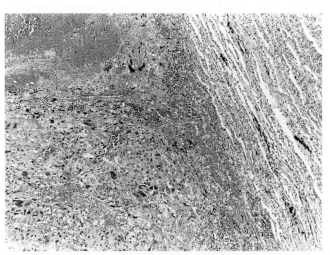

Fig. 33–95 Choriocarcinoma thought to be primary in lung. Necrosis is noted at top; syncytiotrophoblasts and cytotrophoblasts are seen in viable tumor. H and E, ×100.

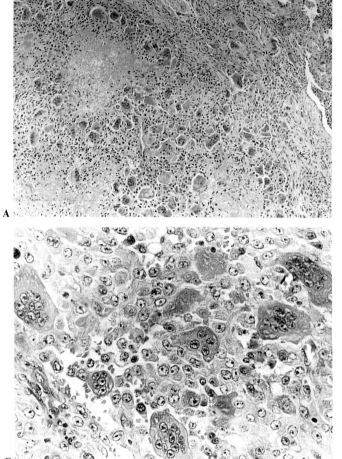

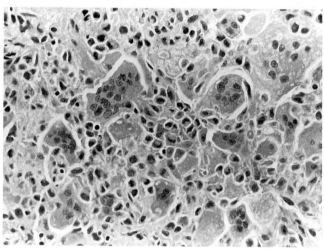

Fig. 33–96 A–C. Osteoclast giant cells in lung tumor. **A.** This is presumably a primary osteoclastoma in lung (see text) and shows typical benign osteoclastic giant cells in a bland background. H and E, ×100. **B.** Bland background and rather pycnotic-appearing cells are better shown at high power. All these cells stain with panhematopoetic antigen/common leukocyte antigen. H and E, ×400. **C.** Anaplastic carcinoma with benign osteoclast-like giant cells in its midst. Abundant mitoses outside this field, and this tumor pursued an aggressive course. Note larger mononuclear cell size, with higher nuclear-to-cytoplasmic ratio, than that seen in **B.** H and E, ×400.

malignant lung tumors.[556a] These have been seen in cancers of other sites, most often thyroid, pancreas, and breast, but also parotid gland, liver, ovary, uterine cervix, renal pelvis, soft tissue, heart, and skin.[557] These tumors usually are anaplastic, or the areas of osteoclasts are in anaplastic areas of more recognizable carcinomas. These are often adenocarcinomas, although rarely they are seen in nonkeratinizing squamous carcinomas, such as uterine cervix or lung, or in malignant mesenchymoma-MFH or epithelioid hemangioendotheliomas (see respective sections). Their presence in malignant tumors is more of interest than significance. They have now been proven to be benign histiocytic cells and appear to be a metaplastic host response to adjacent malignant cells. Because the tumors they are associated with are usually high-grade anaplastic and the patients have short survival, the benign histiocytic giant cell or osteoclastic reaction does not affect their behavior in any way.

Benign giant cell tumors of bone have pulmonary spread in 1%–2% of cases.[558] These contain similar benign osteoclasts, and the observer must be sure that the background small cells are typical of benign giant cell tumor of bone and do not represent smaller malignant anaplastic cells. In 1988, Bertoni et al.[559] added 6 cases, averaging 23 years in age (range, 19–30 years) to the cumulated world literature at that time of 39 cases with a mean age of 31.8 and range of 15–61 years. By that time there was a total of 26 men and 18 women, and most had undergone surgery previously for primary benign giant cell tumors of bone, some 4–54 months before the appearance of the lung lesions. Two had pulmonary nodules diagnosed at that time of surgery,[560,561] and only one had a lung nodule diagnosed before a sacral primary became known.[562] Through the courtesy of Dr. John Watts, I have seen an identical lesion in the lung without any bone tumor detected during follow-up of 3 years (see Fig. 33–96). About 85% of the patients with such spread from bone or soft tissue to the lung do well, and only a few in the literature have died of their pulmonary disease.[559]

No histologic characteristics in the primary soft tissue

or bony lesions help predict those that will become metastatic.[563] Benign giant cells in veins in the primary bone lesions have been identified in about a third of cases,[564–566] and spread appears to be mostly hematogenous, as the lungs most often are involved while lymph nodes have been involved in only one case.[567] Again, whether there is venous invasion identified does not affect the incidence of metastases-embolization. Caballes[568] nicely illustrated such vascular invasion in primary bone tumor sites.

As in the discussion of benign metastasizing leiomyomas, and perhaps endometriosis, in this chapter, and embolizing decidua in the following section and in the vascular chapter, Chapter 29, it is hard to know whether benign tissue that may continue to grow outside its source is simple evidence of embolization with persistence of implants at distal sites or truly represents metastases as noted earlier and in the other sections. These cells look identical to their sources and we are so far unable to sort them out as aggressive by mitoses or flow cytometry.

Tissue Ectopias

The category of ectopic tissue may either be lung in an ectopic location such as in diaphragm (Fig. 33–97), skin,[569] or other situations listed in Chapter 7, or it may be other benign tissues that are ectopically present in the lung. In the latter case, ectopic tissues in the lung can theoretically be derived from several sources, including embryologic remnants from nearby organ systems displaced during embryologic development, traumatic implantation from nearby sites, or embolization from other organ systems. Almost any tissue fragments can gain access to venous systemic blood and end up in the lungs, as is well illustrated in Chapter 29. However, most of these tissue fragments die, and apparently only a few appear to persist, under special conditions.

Microscopic fragments of endometrium with decidual tissue were first described by Park in 1954[570] in the lungs of a woman who died in the postpartum period. Other reports[571–573] have confirmed similar small residual fragments in and about pulmonary vessels. Cameron and Park[572] believed that some of the fragments seen in one of their cases were growing out from the vessel onto the alveolar septa and therefore were extravascular. Decidualization can be seen in some cases of metastasizing leiomyomas and in cycling endometriosis of the lung or pleura (Fig. 33–98). It was also a term used to describe one case[574] before the true epithelioid hemangioendothelioma nature of that case was known.

Endometriosis has been described in lung, bronchi, pleura, and diaphragm (Fig. 33–98) and has been reviewed by Spencer,[575] Hibbard et al.,[576] Karpel et al.,[577]

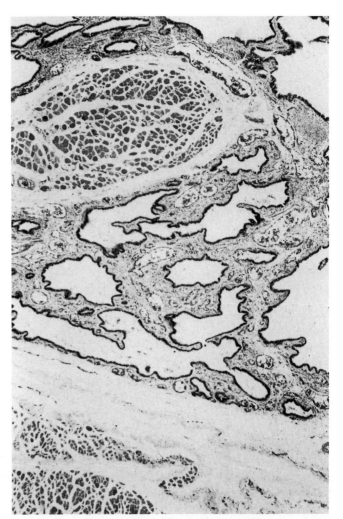

Fig. 33–97. Ectopic lung in diaphragm. Primitive lunglike spaces with cilia present admixed with muscle fibers of diaphragm. H and E, ×50.

Austin et al.,[577a] and Di Palo et al.[578] These cases are rare and according to Di Palo et al.[578] the first mention of these is attributed to Hart in 1912.[579] Schwartz in 1938[580] described recurrent hemoptysis with menses (catamenial hemoptysis) in a woman with inguinal node endometriosis. Pleural endometriosis was first described in 1939 by Buengeler.[581] By 1991 Foster et al.[582] summarized 65 cases of pulmonary endometriosis, 11 in lung parenchyma and 54 in pleura, and in 1985 a careful review of 87 thoracic cases was conducted by Karpel et al.[577] Four cases of parenchymal involvement have been reported from one center.[583]

These patients present with catamenial pneumothorax in 76% of the cases, hemothorax in 10%, hemoptysis in 8%, and asymptomatic mass(es) in 6%.[577] The number of recurrent pneumothoraces can be extraordinary, and as reviewed by Karpel et al.[577] these episodes are

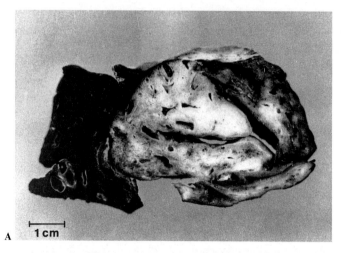

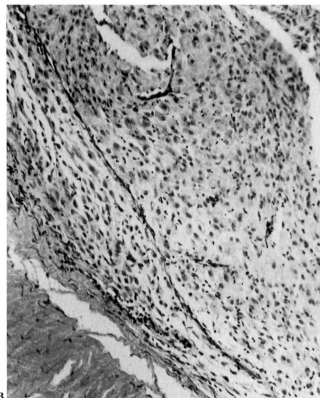

Fig. 33–98 A,B. Endometriosis. **A.** A 6-cm intraparenchymal right lower lobe endometrioma. (Courtesy of R. Fechner, University of Virginia Medical Center, Charlottesville, Virginia.[577a]) **B.** Decidual reaction in pleura. In ectopic sites of endometriosis, a decidual reaction may be all that is observed in plane of tissue sectioning, when seen at right time of cycle or during pregnancy. H and E, ×250.

probable in 2–42 times per patient, averaging 14, while clinically documented at 1–25 times per patient. Of these episodes, 95% are right-sided, and a few are bilateral, and only one is left-sided. Of interest, these are usually not associated with pleural effusion, pleural fluid, or documentation of pleural endometriosis. This is of interest in that catamenial hemothorax, although it occurs less often than pneumothorax, is always right-sided with extensive pelvic endometriosis, often with ascites.[577] Right-sided pleural involvement is most often thought to result from fluid spread through the diaphragmatic fenestra that are above the liver and its attachment to the diaphragm, thereby extending into the right pleural space.[584] Parenchymal involvement is probably hematogenous, and this, and bronchial involvement, are most often right-sided, with masses up to 6 cm.[585] One case had complete bronchial occlusion.[578] Foster et al.[582] noted that pleural involvement occurs in younger patients (mean age, 33.6) who have more pelvic endometriosis, than the parenchymal cases whose mean age is 39 years, with only 10% incidence of pelvic endometriosis, but with catamenial hemoptysis in 82% and catamenial pain and dyspnea in 18%.

Cytology has been helpful in making the diagnosis.[586,587] Benign columnar cells, and a few benign glands in a bloody and often hemosiderin-stained background, are very suggestive. Stromal cells look quite similar to alveolar macrophages or reactive mesothelial cells, and may not be of much help in diagnosis. Decidual change may occasionally be identified in cytologic and histologic specimens (Fig. 33–98).

Whether or not endometriosis is histologically proven, suppression of ovulation hormones has dramatically reduced the symptoms in many of these cases, and in some cases symptoms have returned after cessation of drugs. More recently, gonadotropin-releasing hormone agonists have shown some promise.[588]

Other Tissue Ectopias

Other tissue ectopias have occurred in the chest. Many authors suggest a congenital origin is detected early in life. There have been several cases with dissociated intrathoracic liver ectopias,[589–597] one of which was thought caused by trauma,[590] another in an infant with multiple congenital abnormalities,[597] and one of possible liver or adrenal gland origin is shown in Fig. 33–99. Pancreas has been described in a 2-month-old child[598]; gastrointestinal reduplication cysts and assorted fistulae are covered in Chapter 7. About 7 cases of splenosis pleura have been described[599] and are associated with trauma, as seen in the abdominal cavity. Perhaps at the time of rupture of the spleen there were also rents in the diaphragm that allowed fragments to pass through. Brain or neuroglial heterotopias had been described in about 16 cases[600–602] by 1992, 14 of which occurred with CNS disruption such as anencephaly or meningomyelocele, and one with mechanical CNS disruption.[602] It is

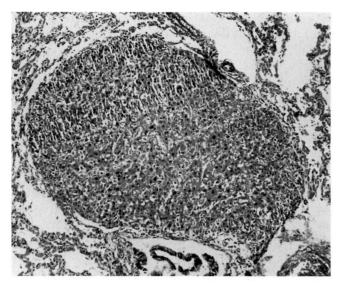

Fig. 33–99. Ectopic tissue in lung. Nodule of adrenal or liver tissue appears quite viable. (Courtesy of H. Spencer, Pulmonary Pathology Collection, London.) H and E, ×100.

though that free-floating fragments of brain cells implant in the lung.[602] The oldest reported case, in a 51-year-old man, was without brain problems or other congenital abnormalities.[603] Another presented with glial-lined pulmonary cysts, all right-sided, the largest 7 cm at 3 months of age; the patient has done well through follow-up at age 20.[601]

Teratoma

Teratomas are quite infrequent lesions in the lung, with only somewhat more than 20 cases of true intrapulmonary teratoma being noted by 1969[604] and 1978.[605] Cleotta,[606] in 1861, credited Mohr in 1839 with the first description of this lesion.

A moderate number of cases reported in the past appear to be mediastinal teratomas that extended into adjacent lung. These are much more frequent, and could present a problem in differential diagnosis. By 1944, Rusby[607] had collected 245 cases of anterior mediastinal teratomas, but by then only 7 or 8 truly intrapulmonary teratomas had been described,[608] for a ratio of lung-to-mediastinal teratomas of about 1:30. Also, teratocarcinomas metastasizing from germ cell neoplasms in other locations may occasionally present with mature elements only in the lung.[609] Therefore, one must exclude extension from both mediastinal teratomas and germ cell neoplasms elsewhere before diagnosing a primary pulmonary teratoma.[610]

Teratomas in the anterior mediastinum are often associated with thymic tissue, and are thought to be related to thymic derivation. Schlumberger,[611] in 1946, proposed that thymic rests may be incorporated with the outpouchings of the lung buds and account for such lesions in the lung. However, such thymic rests have not been identified in normal or nonteratomatous lesions, evidence needed to support this thesis.

It is interesting that most intrapulmonary teratomas occur in the left-upper lobe,[612] and some have occurred in the anterior segment, making one wonder about directly included fragments of thymus. It appears to me that a fair number of the seven reported cases of cystic pulmonary hamartomas with mixed mature tissue elements, six of which have occurred in the left-upper lobe, are actually teratomas.[613] A few teratomas have occurred on the right side.[614,615] Four have so far been described as endobronchial,[616–619] but only one has been seen endoscopically.[620] An occasional case connects with segmented bronchi. Bronchiectasis was seen in 2 cases,[617,621] one of which was extensive. Another occurred in the lung 10 years after excision of a mediastinal teratoma.[622]

Teratomas of lung occur in the age group 19–68 years,[605] except for one notable case reported by Pound and Willis[623] in which a large 9-cm lung tumor that presumably represented congenital origin was diagnosed in a 10-month-old infant. This had spread to regional nodes and represented one of the very rare cases of truly malignant pulmonary teratomas. As noted by Jamieson and McGowan,[619] this is the only definite case of such a malignant teratomatous lesion proven by metastases.

In an interesting case,[619] an infiltrate in the upper lobe, thought to be tuberculosis, was diagnosed at age 5 years and treated, and after slow resolution of the pulmonary infiltrate a perihilar mass persisted. At age 22 years, following 6 weeks of chest pain, cough, and hemoptysis, this perihilar mass was excised and found to be a teratoma that had changed little in size during 17 years. Rarely, the specific symptom of trichopytsis has been described with these lesions.[606,616]

Radiographically, including on CT scans, several clues may suggest this tumor but may be most helpful only in hindsight. These include calcifications[616] or lucencies within more solid densities. Some of the lucencies detected radiographically are caused by cavitation[617] and some by fat within the lesion.[605,608,624] These findings are not pathognomonic of teratoma of lung, as other lesions may also have lucent or cystic areas mixed with calcification, but confirming the densities of fat in these lesions, as in teratomas, is very suggestive of one of these types of masses or other fat-containing tumors. Their slow growth, where it has been documented,[619] may be contributory. Most often the diagnosis requires histologic examination.

Grossly, these tumors vary in texture and appearance, as does the spectrum of teratomas arising elsewhere, such as dermoid cysts of the ovary. Often cystic cavities are filled with either granular brown watery or flaky yellow debris. Most often identified grossly are sebum, fat, and possibly bone. Teeth have not so far been identified in these pulmonary lesions.

Microscopically, all three germ cell layers are present. The most common component is skin and its appendages (Fig. 33–100), and the cystic areas represent accumulated keratin and sebum. Fat is frequent, as are fragments of gastrointestinal or respiratory tract differentiation immediately adjacent to mucosa of other types in a mature but disorderly background. Thymus and pancreas are identified with some regularity.[619,620] Skeletal and smooth muscle, bone, cartilage and brain are also identified in some. About a third of these[610] have been called malignant, but this is based on the histologic appearance of immature cells, particularly stromal cells, and not on aggressive behavior. Only one case,[623] as noted, has been documented to actually have metastasized, and as already noted this case was exceptional in several ways.

Hamartomas (Benign Mesenchymomas)

The term "hamartoma" was coined by Albrecht in 1904[625] to indicate a tumor-like "malformation" composed of tissues normally found in a location, but with these normal-appearing tissues in excess or disarray. It was first used in reference to these lung lesions in 1934 by Goldsworthy.[626] The term has also been used to

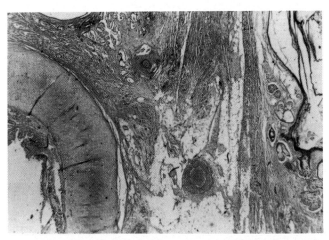

Fig. 33–100. Teratoma. At left is bronchus; at right is epidermis with skin appendage-bearing component of teratoma; at top is another glandular teratomatous area. Fat at middle lower is part of teratoma. H and E, ×50.

describe the entity of congenital cystic adenomatoid malformation, and as this entity, particularly as it is seen in children, is discussed in Chapter 7, it is not further addressed here. Another use of the term for the entity of mesenchymal cystic hamartoma, which is discussed separately. It is possible that the word hamartoma may be replaced for this latter entity in the future. Also note the reference to cystic pulmonary hamartomas in the previous **teratoma** section.

The remaining or "adult" hamartomas (also called "classic" or "local") are the most common benign tumor of lung, and, as noted in the introduction to this chapter, represented 100 of 130 (77%) of benign tumor masses in lung in one large series.[1] In another series of 721 thoracotomies done for treatment of lung tumors, 36 (5%) were benign, of which 21 (58% of the benign ones, 3% of the entire group) were hamartomas.[627] The incidence of pulmonary hamartomas in the general population was found to be 20 in 7,972 cases (about 1 in 400 or 0.25%) in a series of autopsies described by McDonald and associates[628] from Mayo Clinic in 1945. These lesions account for some 8% or so of solitary lung nodules,[629] and may be excised to exclude malignancy. Cartilage is present in 96%,[1,333] so it is understandable the name chondroma was originally used for these.[632] They are 1.7[630] to 4[631] times as common in men as in women in the parenchyma lesions, but are of more equal sex incidence in the central ones.[630] They occur mostly in the age group from late thirties to early seventies, with a peak in the late fifties and early sixties.[629,633] Several have been described in teenagers, and 1 was described as early as age 9.[634] These lesions have not been described at earlier ages; they are not seen in babies, and therefore are not congenital. A large 40-year series of 17 endobronchial and 147 intraparenchymal hamartomas from one institution was reviewed by Tomashefski[630] (see Table 33–7). Another large series of 136 cases of pulmonary hamartomas was presented in the French literature in 1985 by Malauzat et al.[635]

In the past, the glandular inclusions seen with these lesions caused considerable debate as to their tumorigenesis. Bateson, in several very nice sequential studies,[636–638] has shown that the glandular component is caused by metaplastic alveolar lining cells and entrapped bronchiolar cells. Several electron microscopic studies[639–641] are compatible with this theory. Intranuclear inclusions have also been seen in the lining cells, and probably represent surfactant as in alveolar and metaplastic lining cells.[640,641] Such entrapments occur in several low-grade primary pulmonary neoplasms and even in very low grade metastases. (See Table 33–7 and following discussion.)

Some authors make a distinction between peripheral

Table 33–7. Comparative features of endobronchial and parenchymal hamartomas

	Endobronchial (n = 17)	Parenchymal (n = 147)
Age		
Range	43–73 years	17–77 yrs
Mean	52.9 years	56.2 yrs.
Sex (M/F)	9/8	92/55
Involved lung (L/R)	13/4	43/45[a]
Size (maximum dimension)		
Range	0.3–3.4 cm	0.3–6 cm
Mean	1.4 cm	1.7 cm
Shape	Polypoid	Spherical
Epithelial clefts		
Internal	3 (18%)	127 (86%)
peripheral	2 (11.8%)	135 (93.1%)
Mesenchymal derivatives		
Cartilage	14 (82.4%)	141 (95.9%)
Percent Cartilage		
≥90%	3 (18%)	57 (39%)
75–90%	1 (6%)	44 (30%)
50–75%	3 (18%)	27 (18%)
10–50%	7 (40%)	9 (6%)
<10%	0	4 (3%)
None	3 (18%)	6 (4%)
Bone	2 (11.8%)	3 (2%)
Adipose tissue	14 (82.3%)	110 (74.8%)
Fibrous tissue	13 (76.4%)	108 (73.5%)
Fibroadenoma-like areas	1 (5.9%)	12 (8.8%)

[a] Data indicated for 88/147 patients. Modified with permission of Tomashefski JF, Jr. Benign endobronchial mesnchymal tumors: Their relationship to parenchymal pulmonary hamartomas. Am J Surg Pathol 1982;6:531–540.

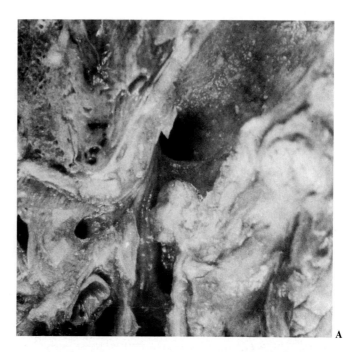

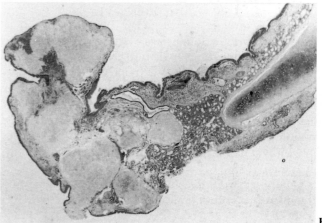

Fig. 33–101 A,B. Polypoid bronchial hamartoma. **A.** Grossly this nodular mass extends into major bronchus, from site of slight thickening of adjacent bronchial wall. **B.** Tissue section of same area as **A** shows multinodular areas of cartilage; this field shows unattached bronchial cartilage. H and E ×5.

intrapulmonary hamartomatous nodules and those in the more proximal bronchi and trachea, and use the glandular component to distinguish these (see following section on benign metastasizing leiomyomas for a similarly faulty argument), and also point to the frequent fusion of the cartilaginous proliferations in the tracheobronchial system with the native cartilaginous rings as distinguishing components. Both characteristics can be explained by the architecture in the areas where these arise. Both of these subsets of lesions occur in the same age group and can have the same mixture of components, or more monomorphic expression of these components. It therefore seems best to consider them the same type of lesion with some unique characteristics from their different location.[630,636] Different authors have estimated the number of central tracheobronchial hamartomas as 10%,[630,642,643] 15%,[644] and 19.5%[636] of the total number. The central or bronchial hamartomas are often polypoid (Fig. 33–101), and a few interfere with airflow and present with obstructive symptoms. Most of the central and peripheral lesions, however, are asymptomatic.

Radiographically, an occasional endobronchial ha-martoma may present as an air-displacing mass within the air shadow of the bronchi, but most often such lesions are detected because of symptoms leading to direct examination of these areas. The more peripheral ones are often subpleural and incidental on chest radiographs. Their radiographic characteristics have been well described by Bateson and Abbott[645] as sharply defined masses, often with lobulated borders, most often subpleural, and most often less than 3 cm in diameter (Figs. 33–102 and 33–103). Speckled calcification can be seen on radiographs, and in one series this was seen in 4 of 25 (16%) cases.[646] As smaller nodular

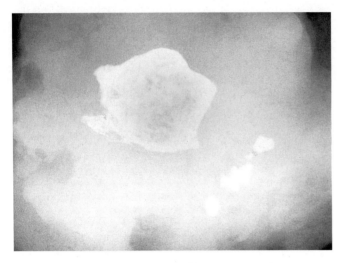

Fig. 33–102. Pulmonary hamartoma. Specimen radiograph shows major focus of calcification with several smaller ones. In largest one, there is increased density around the edge with some lucency in the center, so-called "popcorn" calcification. ×6. (Courtesy of Dr. Terrance Gleason, Providence Medical Center, Seattle, Washington.)

growths within the lesions are often found protruding in different directions, calcification in each of these protrusions may be seen as a "popcorn"-type calcification (see Fig. 33–102), but this occurs less frequently than originally believed.[647–649] Occasionally areas of lesser density, especially seen at the periphery of the nodules, may be seen radiographically and are compatible with fat tissue. (See also **Teratomas** elsewhere in this chapter.)

Computerized tomography (CT) has further refined the distinction of fat and cartilage, and has been effec-

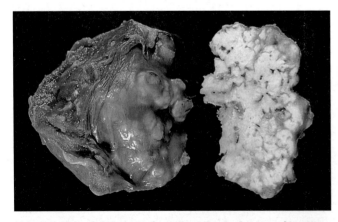

Fig. 33–103. Pulmonary hamartoma. A 3-cm pulmonary hamartoma is seen en face to left; its underside-cut appearance is shown to right. White serginous opacity is most cartilage. (Courtesy of Dr. T. Gleason, Providence Medical Center, Seattle, Washington.)

tively used by Siegelman et al.[650] in suggesting a hamartoma diagnosis. Their criteria include lesions 2.5 cm in diameter or less, with a smooth edge, with focal areas of fat alone, or fat admixed with areas of calcification. The presence of fat was most helpful, either alone (18 cases) or intermixed with calcification (10 cases). Seventeen cases did not have fat and could not be further classified by CT scans. Using these criteria, none of the 283 cases of primary carcinomas nor any of the 72 cases of metastatic carcinomas was confused with hamartomas.

Fine-needle aspiration with smear cytology and cell blocks suggested the diagnosis of hamartoma in 12 of 14 (86%)[647] and 59 of 61 (97%)[648] of cases. Some of these have been noted to enlarge while under radiographic surveillance. Jensen and Schiodt[651] and Weisel et al.[652] both estimated growth at about 0.5 cm in diameter per year. Sagel and Ablow[653] reported 1 case that grew from 1 to 2.6 cm over 1.5 years. Weinberger et al.[654] noted growth in an 11-year-old patient from 2 cm to 7 cm in maximum dimension over 3 years. This lesion was unusual in that it also encircled the hilar structures and required pneumonectomy for removal. (See possible malignancy, following.)

Grossly, these lesions vary from a few mm to 20 cm, but most are in the range of 1–3 cm (see Fig. 33–103). They usually "pop out" of the peripheral lung tissue, are rounded, and may have small smoothly contoured irregularities on their surface. The endobronchial hamartomas are often polypoid, either sessile or with a thin pedicle (see Fig. 33–101). Whether peripheral or central, they are usually well circumscribed from surrounding tissue and their texture is usually cartilaginous, although there may be areas that correlate with fat. The central lesions tend to develop predominantly cartilage, and the peripheral lesions are more an admixture of fibrous tissue, cartilage, and fat.

Microscopically, cartilage is present in most lesions (see Table 33–7), including 82% of endobronchial[630] (Figs. 33–101 and 33–104) and 96% of parenchymal ones[1,630] (Fig. 33–105), and appears more hyaline in the central lesions and more fibrohyaline in the peripheral ones. In those lesions that are predominantly cartilage, cartilaginous nests seem always to be surrounded by some cellular fibrous tissue, and often there are collections of mature fat cells (Fig. 33–105 and Table 33–7). Sometimes other tissue components are monotonous and compose the predominant mass without cartilage, such as occurs with lipomas, and possibly fibromas and myxomas (see following) of both lung and bronchi. Some consider the latter lesions discrete and others part of hamartomatous development. As both classifications are benign, which is chosen is up to the individual. I favor considering them within the spectrum of hamartomas. Rarely the fat cells have appeared atypical.[655]

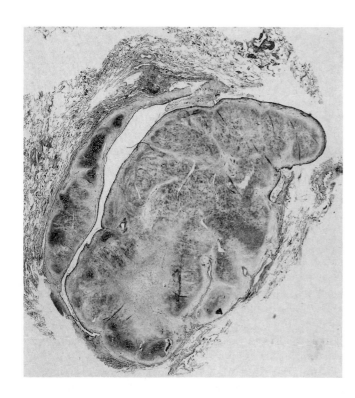

Fig. 33–104. Hamartoma of smaller airway. Predominantly cartilaginous mass, similar to that illustrated in Fig. 33–103 but in more peripheral airway. Focally there appears to be remnant bronchial cartilage. Previously this was a criterion for central airway "chondromas" as distinguished from pulmonary hamartomas (see text). H and E, ×15.

Fig. 33–105 A–D. Hamartomas. A. Cartilage, spindle fibrous cells, and focal fat. H and E, ×100. B. Cartilage with more abundant fat. H and E, ×50. C. Spindle cells entrapping metaplastic air spaces. H and E, ×100. D. Edge shows some chronic inflammation in fibrous tissue involvement of adjacent lung interstitium. H and E, ×100. (See following page for parts C and D.)

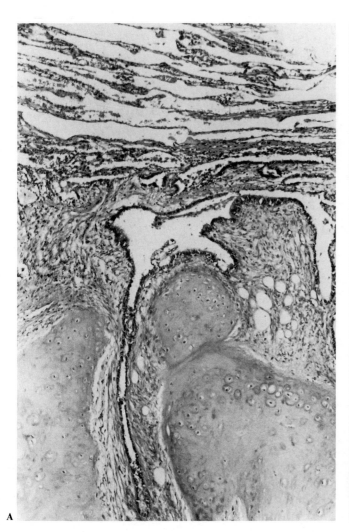

A

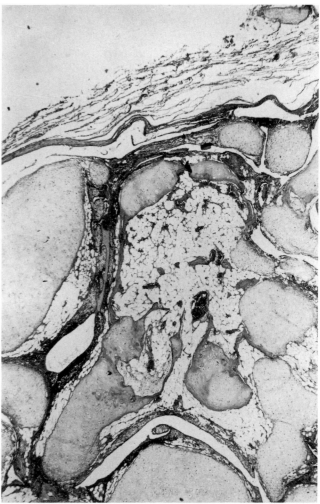

B

Rarely there may be bone, and occasionally entrapped vessels, bronchioles, or a small amount of smooth muscle.

Depending on the plane of section, one can find these lesions developing in the wall of bronchioles and occasionally of small bronchi (see Fig. 33–104). At times native cartilage is seen in the peripheral lesions, being enveloped by the new growth (Fig. 33–104). In the central lesions the cartilaginous proliferations of any size may or may not (Fig. 33–103) show fusion with the cartilaginous rings. The glandular component discussed can easily be traced from adjacent alveoli or adjacent bronchioles (Fig. 33–105), and the lining cells are cuboidal to low columnar and are sometimes distorted in their course within the lesions themselves, presumably as caused by irregularly proliferating mesenchyme. At times terminal bronchioles can be identified because of the cilia in their lining cells and some wisps of smooth muscle. Most of the time the lining cells appear more like metaplastic cells.

The theories of origin of these lesions have been discussed by Blair and McElvein.[646] Most now agree they are not congenital lesions, but the term hamartoma is still used to describe these and because of its familiarity is retained. It is recognized that the term carries with it the implication of congenital malformation. Whether these are reactive growths in response to some type of inflammation is unclear, but considering the number of episodes of pulmonary inflammation and the low incidence of hamartomas, and considering their solitary state compared to multifocal areas usually involved with inflammation, this is probably unlikely. Surrounding lung and bronchi are usually normal when these lesions are detected. More than likely they are benign neoplastic proliferations whose growth is determined by unknown factors. Tomashefski[630] refers to them as benign mesenchymomas of lung, which seems a fairly good term. Spencer has suggested that this may be the area of junction between peripheral lung growth and central lung growth, as discussed in the chapter section on blastomas. This is an interesting idea to explain their location, but the embryology does not seem to be supported by current thought.

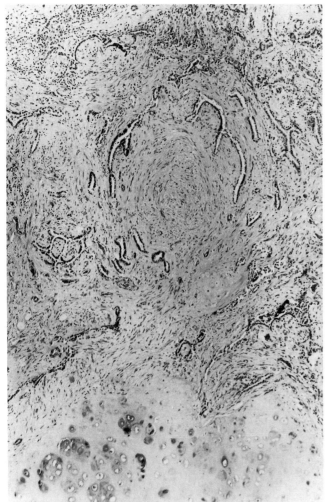

33-105C

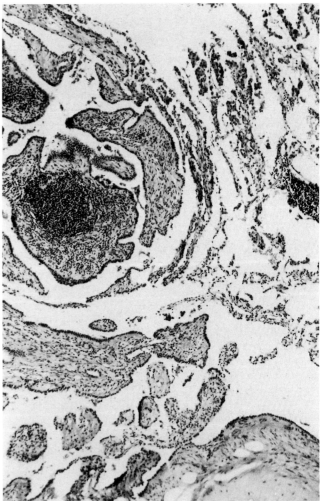

33-10

Only rarely are these lesions multiple,[657–659] and in some of these cases there is a lipoma along with a peripheral chondroma. There are occasional cases of multiple cartilaginous hamartomas, and these seem to be more frequent in association with Carney's syndrome.[660] This syndrome consists of epithelioid gastric smooth muscle tumors, either leiomyomas or leiomyosarcomas, functioning extraadrenal paragangliomas, and pulmonary chondromas. The association between these diverse proliferating tissues is unclear, but the syndrome appears now to be accepted as such, occurs predominantly in girls under the age of 20, and may have only two of the three lesions mentioned.[660]

Gabrail and Zara[661] found a high percentage of other abnormalities in 24 charts they reviewed. They particularly noted an increased incidence of other benign tumors, mostly outside the chest, and other developmental abnormality. In the latter group such items as inguinal hernias are included, and it is open to debate whether this is a developmental abnormality. I agree with these authors that more correlation is needed in a larger number of cases to determine the statistical significance of these assorted diseases. These authors note that many of the associated findings may overlap with Cowden's syndrome, but also that pulmonary hamartomas are not part of Cowden's multihamartoma syndrome.

There is a question whether any of these can become malignant.[662] There is an increased incidence of lung cancers in these patients, but whether this is related to increased incidence of chest x-rays and follow-up is unclear. One case was stable for 37 years and then underwent "explosive sarcomatous evolution,"[663] almost totally occupying a lower lobe. Another case documented a benign-appearing recurrence 5 years after tracheal chondroma was excised. Six years after that, chondrosarcoma developed at this site and the patient died of metastases 1 year later.[664] Given the challenge of diagnosing low-grade cartilaginous lesions in other sites, this may be a better example of such a problem. In only one study that I am aware of, clonality was evaluated in two cases of pulmonary hamartomas and of interest, both showed stromal cell chromosomal aberrations.[665]

Multiple fibroleiomyomatous hamartomas are a nonentity, and are discussed in the next section. A case of multiple small intrapulmonary fibrous nodules has been described in association with sclerosing mediatinitis.[666] In this case report, many small nodules composed of small collections of fibrocytes were found, and did not have the complexity of parts as seen in hamartoma. I have seen a case of multiple small amyloid nodules at first mistaken for multiple hamartomas. Considering the rarity of truly accepted cases of multiple hamarto-

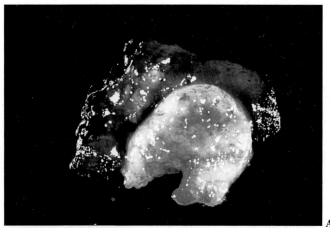

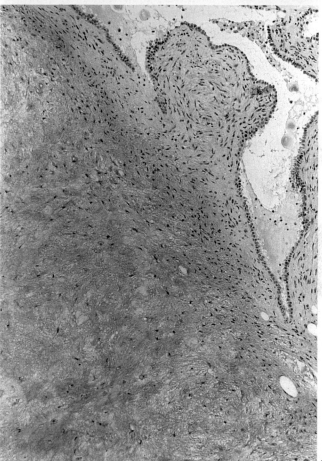

Fig. 33–106 A,B. Myxoma of lung. **A.** Grossly semitranslucent, gray-tan, well-circumscribed 1.2-cm nodule in lung. Nodule separated easily from the surrounding lung tissue (and the two pieces have been put back together for this picture). **B.** Same case as **A,** shows edge of tumor nodule, with entrapment of adjacent glands and fibrocellular reaction at top in periphery; dominant portion of the tumor is composed of loose mixoid tissue shown toward bottom left. H and E, ×100.

mas in lung, one must always be cautious in considering this diagnosis, especially when the lesions are not cartilaginous.

Myxomas

Rarely, discrete solitary benign lesions have been described as myxomas.[667] One has been described in the trachea as fibromyxoma.[668] Another case is illustrated in Fig. 33–106. As noted in the **Hamartoma** section, these may well be considered hamartomatous. Myxoid change in nerve sheath or lipid tumors is always a challenge, as maybe distinguishing embolizing cardiac myxomas. However, pulmonary myxomas are usually so bland and monotonous that their classification is not a problem.

Native Benign Smooth Muscle Lesions

In the classical sense, pulmonary hamartomas do not contain significant amounts of smooth muscle (see Table 33–7). A perhaps related, but distinct and perhaps reactive lesion is illustrated in Fig. 33–107. These consist of various sized proliferations of benign smooth muscle bundles in the interstitium of the lung, blending with or rising from native smooth muscle. These seem to center on centraicinar bronchioles. This may be a reactive stimulation of smooth muscle bronchiolar origin. Other areas of scarring can be associated with confluent smooth muscle proliferation (Fig. 33–108). Smooth muscle can be stimulated in pulmonary fibrosis, and some have referred to this as muscular cirrhosis of lung.[669,670] As reviewed by Spencer,[671] others have used that term to refer to the muscular proliferation in

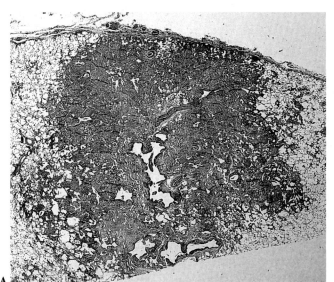

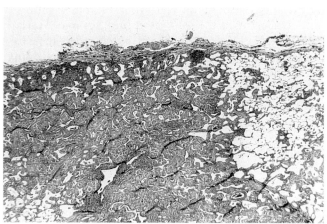

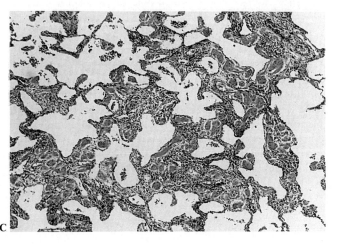

Fig. 33–107 A–C. Native benign modular smooth muscle proliferations. **A.** Large 1-cm nodule in periphery of lung apparently centers on bronchiole. H and E, ×16. **B.** High-power view of top-right corner of **A** at interface of this proliferation with pleura. H and E, ×50. **C.** Different case shows earlier lesion of smooth muscle proliferation located in the centriacinar and presumably peribronchilar region. H and E, ×100.

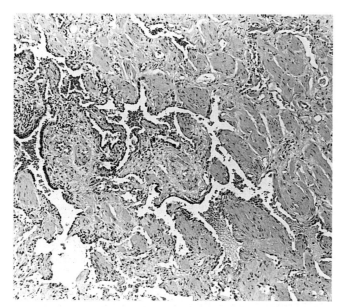

Fig. 33–108. Another case of benign smooth muscle proliferation occurred next to chronic cavity caused by aspirated broncholith. Note its benign appearance and entrapment of, or origin from, terminal bronchiolar region.

passive cardiac failure. (See also lymphangioleiomyomatosis, and leiomyomatosis-myofibromatosis at end of this chapter.)

Benign Metastasizing Leiomyomas

Until 1977, about 14 cases of multiple low-grade smooth muscle nodules in the lung had been described and previously called "fibroleiomyomatous hamartomas." They were summarized in 1977 by Horstmann et al.[672] These all occurred in women aged 30–74 years, with a mean age of 47 years, who were usually asymptomatic and had bilateral multiple nodules. Eight of these had histories of myomectomies or hysterectomies for leiomyomata. Four had no history available. One of these others had a benign tumor of her cervix removed years before, and the other had a benign cystic teratoma by abdominal radiograph.

Horstmann and associates[672] compared these lesions to a group of lung lesions called benign metastasizing leiomyomas, also all occurring in women, all of whom had a history of uterine leiomyomas. They could find no difference in the clinical, radiographic, or pathologic findings to substantiate separating these groups, and declared fibroleiomyomatous hamartomas a "non-entity." In the past, several other authors[673,674] have expressed concern about their inability to distinguish fibromyoleiomatous hamartomas and benign metastasizing leiomyomas.

Tench et al.[675] summarized 21 cases from the A.A. Liebow Pulmonary Pathology Collection in 1978. All were women aged 31–65, and all had undergone hysterectomy 3 to 20 years (mean, 10 years) previously. In 18 of 21 cases, benign leiomyomas were described in the uteri, but histologic slides of the uterine lesions were too infrequent for meaningful evaluation.

From background material in this study,[676] all but one had multiple bilateral nodules on chest radiographs; the other had a perihilar mass. Three of these patients had lung nodules detected 16, 19, and 20 years after their hysterectomies. These patients usually had lung nodules radiographically and pathologically that measured 0.3–4.0 cm in greatest dimension and were enucleated easily from the lung tissue. Some 94% of these cases histologically showed entrapment of metaplastic glandular lining cells.

Almost all the cases are asymptomatic, with rare exceptions. Two contrasting cases are mentioned. One, by Popock et al.,[677] a woman who at age 41 had her uterus removed for three large "leiomyomas" that had been present for some 15 years. She died 21 years later or 36 years after the detection of a large uterus of hemorrhagic pancreatitis. She had multiple, up to 2-cm lung nodules at the time of hysterectomy, which had grown to 5 cm at the time of autopsy and become predominantly cystic (Fig. 35–3). The patient had minimal pulmonary symptoms. A similar case was described by Uyama et al. in 1988,[678] with lesions noted for 20 years on the chest radiograph, gradually increasing in size; I estimated the largest to be about 11 cm from the photo of the chest x-ray. One protruded into the trachea causing some obstruction. The size would make one wonder if the classification sarcoma is more appropriate, but their slow growth would certainly indicate the low-grade behavior.

Some authors in the past used entrapped glandular spaces to try to separate the entity of fibroleiomyomatous hamartomas from more obvious benign metastasizing leiomyomas[678] (see below). Some leiomyomas and fibromas become so hyalinized as to make their cell of origin difficult to determine, yet still show air space entrapment. (See **Fibroma** section to follow.) As noted in Table 33–1, metaplastic alveolar lining and entrapped bronchiolar space lining cells are common in slowly growing lesions, and represent a background response and not an inherent component of the tumor. On careful serial section examinations, they were seen to be continuous with the lining of nearby air spaces.[680] Herrera et al.[681] studied these spaces by electron microscopy in a case of metastasizing smooth muscle tumor of lung that occurred 31 years after the patient had a hysterectomy for low-grade leiomyosarcoma. These authors found ultrastructural characteristics of entrapped alveoli and bronchiolar mucosa.

In 1979 Wolff and associates[682] further expanded the concept of metastasizing low-grade smooth muscle nodules in the lung in a report of six women and three men. They required the nodules of smooth muscle in the lung to have entrapped glandular spaces as described here, but this also is a good marker of low-grade growth. In five of six women, the uterus was identified as the source of leiomyomas, and for the other woman there is no history available. Of the three men, leiomyosarcomas were documented in saphenous vein, diaphragm, and probably the gluteal region. These authors carefully quantitated mitoses, both in the metastatic lesions and in the primary sites when tissue from primary lesions was available, using the mitotic counting methods of Kempson[683] and Norris.[684] Although mitoses are infrequent in the smooth muscle lesions of the lung, they could always identify them. Mitotic rate in the primary lesions varies, but many qualified as benign smooth muscle proliferations by the standard criteria.

Wolff et al.[682] reviewed all the cases in the literature that might qualify for this entity. The interested reader is referred to their paper[682] and that of Horstmann and associates[672] for specific references. The leiomyosarcomas arising in pulmonary arteries, and those in lung parenchyma proper, are considered separately under **Sarcomas.** See also leiomyomas in the following **Other Benign Mesenchymal Tumors.**

In the differential diagnosis of metastasizing low-grade smooth muscle tumors are plasma cell granulomas, especially when plump spindle cells are present, and hamartomas, when they are particularly fibroblastic, and primary leiomyomas. The first is differentiated by the increased number of plasma cells present and by documenting the basic cell as more a myofibroblast than pure smooth muscle cell. The spindle cells in each lesion appear different. Fibrous hamartomas are usually differentiated by their mixed tissue components and absence of smooth muscle. Primary leiomyomas should be considered as such only if solitary. The more diffuse smooth muscle proliferations of lymphangioleiomyomatosis and honeycombing with smooth muscle hyperplasia ("muscular cirrhosis") should cause no difficulty.

Are these lesions in the lung benign or malignant? Only since 1976 have pathologists begun to reliably use mitotic counting methods to determine low-grade or high-grade activity in uterine smooth muscle tumors. Even as done by both Wolff and associates[682] and Gal and associates,[685] many were benign or low grade by this method. One must then question whether sampling was adequate, whether the lesions became less mitotically active after an initial growth phase with metastases, or perhaps whether fragments of smooth muscle can embolize as such and not truly represent malignancy. One might use as an example the embolizing decidua

and fragments of endometriosis, as noted in the **Tissue Ectopias** section of this chapter. These lesions do continue to grow in most patients, but rarely threaten the patient's life. Because of the confusion with the term benign metastasizing leiomyomas, Horstmann and associates[672] support Steiner's[686] term of "metastasizing fibroleiomyoma." I believe as long as the reader is aware of the peculiarities of the term metastasizing leiomyomas, this is an acceptable term. As discussed, in light of their low mitotic rate, the possibility that benign tissues can embolize and grow in the lung needs to be considered as a potential route of spread. If so this might well be considered "embolizing leiomyomas." Gal and associates[685] in 1989 thoroughly reviewed the theories relating to benign metastasizing leiomyomas (BML) and favor a third theory, that of asynchronous smooth muscle proliferations in multiple sites. They use the conclusion of Zaloudek and Norris[687] that BMLs occur at an average age of 39, while uterine sarcomas occur at an average age of 52. Others support asynchronous evolution of these tumors, in part because their atypical locations, including nonhematogenous sites, avoid lung and liver.[688–690] Rarely benign metastasizing leiomyomas may present as a miliary pattern in lung.[691]

Horstmann and associates[672] noted hormonal sensitivity in their case of a 30-year-old woman who had multiple small pulmonary nodules bilaterally in early pregnancy, at which time she also had easily detected leiomyomas in her uterus. Both the lung and the uterine lesions became less apparent during pregnancy and during breast-feeding in the postpartum period, so much so that postpartum uterine exam could detect no leiomyoma, and her lung radiograph almost returned to normal. No follow-up beyond 6 months postpartum is given for this patient, and it would be interesting to know what happened to the pulmonary lesions. The uterus was removed at 6 months postpartum, and had multiple intramural and subserosal leiomyomas, varying from 1.3 to 2.5 cm in diameter. These were described as "extremely cellular." One was illustrated directly joining a vein lumen in the uterine wall. Mitotic rates were not quantitated.

Horstmann and associates[672] documented that these lesions in the lung in postmenopausal women tended to remain stable or progress slightly, again suggesting hormonal dependence. Regression has been seen following bilateral oophorectomy.[692] It now seems that hormonal manipulation, especially estrogen deprivation, may be effective therapy helping to control symptoms.[692] At times biopsy will show more hyalinized nodules, particularly in postmenopausal women. This hyalinization indicates their inactivity.

In 1982, Martin[693] proposed that benign metastasizing leiomyomas, intravascular leiomyomatosis, peritonealis disseminata, and lymphangioleiomyomatosis might all be better classified as leiomyomatosis, all occurring in reproductive-age women with tumorous growths enlarging with estrogen therapy, and treated with estrogen deprivation, usually in the background of a patient with leiomyomas of the uterus. Allen[694] in 1990 added to this list of entities other proliferations in women of reproductive age, which were all histologically bland and either contiguous or noncontiguous with local or distal spread and a tendency to differentiate in more than one Müllarian direction, including endometriosis, endosalpingiosis, endocervicocis, uterine stromal nodules, Müllerian adenofibroma, peritoneal gliomatosis, ectopic deciduosis, and low-grade endometrial stromal sarcomas. The implication is that these entities may all be benign metastasizing Müllerian tumors or uterine sarcomas. This is an interesting concept, and is further discussed in the following section on **Lymphangioleiomyomatosis.** I favor keeping the smooth muscle proliferations separate, but the reader is referred to both these authors.

Mesenchymal Cystic Hamartomas

This entity was described in five cases in 1986 by Mark.[695] Two of these cases have been previously published.[696,697] There were three women, aged 34, 42, and 54 years, and two males, a 28-year-old man and a 1.5-year-old boy. Four of the five tumors were multifocal, and all were slow growing, solid when small, and becoming cystic when they had reached 1 cm or so in diameter. The 34-year-old woman had a 8-cm umbilical cyst composed of similar tissue with atypical features and was the subject of a clinical pathological conference.[696] The 28-year-old man was the other separately reported case.[697] These patients presented with hemoptysis, pneumothorax, hemothorax, pleuritic pain, or mild moderate dyspnea. Initial chest radiograph showed one large cyst in three cases, multiple bilateral nodules in one, and a cyst and bilateral nodules in the other. Two who were initially thought to have unilateral disease became bilateral after many months, and the larger ones occasionally had fluid levels. CT scans helped highlight the cystic quality and also detected more lesions than were seen by plain films. All the patients are alive except for the oldest, who was 53 at the time of diagnosis, and who died 28 years later at age 81 of an auto accident, with no evidence of other tumor; no autopsy was done. Pathologically all five patients had cystic lung lesions ranging from 5 mm to 10 cm (see Fig. 33–109). In three cases the walls were thin and pliant, and in two they were thick and scarred. These were lined by either normal ciliated respiratory epithelium or bland epithelium with squamous metaplasia (see Fig. 33–109). These linings in the smaller lesions could be traced in continuity with the adjacent respiratory bronchioles. Tumor nodules less than 5 mm were mostly noncellular and nodular, but even then were associated with a plexiform airway configuration. Those 5 to 10 mm in diameter were nodular and cystic, and those larger than 10 mm were cystic. Only two patients had the entire spectrum of cysts, cystic nodules, and nodules.

The stroma lining these cysts was composed of smaller cells with a bland primitive mesenchymal appearance, and in between these cells and the cyst lining was a spared zone of collagen resembling a cambium layer (see Fig. 33–109). The outside of these walls was directly opposed to the lung tissue, and there was a variable degree of fibrous tissue, vessels, and hemosiderin. Focally, cellular 1- to 10-mm nodules grew off the larger cysts, and at times suggested papilla. The cysts contained blood in three cases, and the adjacent lung parenchyma had hemosiderin in all five. Thick-walled systemic arteries leading into these walls tended to infiltrate the outer portion of the tumor.

Follow-up has shown these to be of low aggressivity. Four of the five have had progressive cysts but only two had symptoms. The oldest person was followed 28 years; the other has been followed 2–4 years. One case was described in follow-up by Abrams et al.,[698] the one with the 8-cm umbilical nodule, and the initial history was given that she had benign uterine pathology and a hysterectomy.[696] On review of this pathology, however, it was noted that there was a low-grade endometrial stromal sarcoma extending into the round ligament, identical to both the umbilical and lung lesions. A similar companion case was presented by Abrams et al.[698] with a 1-cm cystic nodule in lung. Several other cases of metastatic low-grade microcystic endometrial stromal sarcomas in lung are presented in Chapter 35, but have a somewhat different appearance, and the whole group of uterine stromal sarcomas has recently been reviewed.[699] Both cases of Abrams et al.[698] were desmin positive. Of interest, the case by Holden et al.[697] has also been referred to as a possible benign fibrohistiocytic tumor (see following) and also as a cyst with hemangiomatous differentiation (see **Hemangioma** section).

Others that appear similar were described in the pediatric literature as malignant neoplasms arising in a cystic hamartoma,[700] as rhabdomyosarcoma,[701] or as blastomas of childhood.[241,702–704]

Follow-up of an additional case in Mark's original series[695] was noted by Manivel et al.[241] in a 1.5-year-old boy who died, presumably of tumor, but no other details were given. One case of Hedlund et al.[700] with

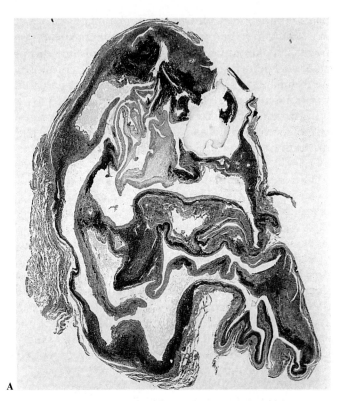

A

Fig. 33–109 A–C. Mesenchymal cystic hamartoma. **A.** Cystic nodule shows convoluted spaces with rim of hypocellular fibrous tissue surrounded by cambium layer of smaller darker cells. H and E, ×6. **B.** Higher power view of lower portion of **A.** H and E, ×18. **C.** Spaces are lined by cuboidal cells. Note varying density of cells, hypocellular zone near the cyst to right, smaller cell denser proliferation middle, and left separating a more spindle-like zone. H and E, ×100. (Courtesy of Dr. E. Mark, Massachusetts General Hospital, Boston, Massachusetts.)

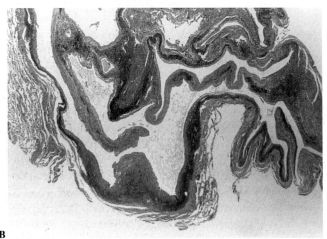

B

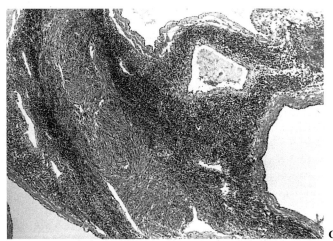

C

abundant mitoses was alive and free of tumor 12 years later. As noted, because of the small cells and cambium zone, some authors have called these rhabdomyosarcomas.[701]

Cystic Fibrohistiocytic Tumors

This is a recently described entity and as yet awaits definite confirmation or further broadening of its spectrum. Two cases were described by Joseph et al.,[705] who gave this lesion its name. The walls of the cyst were composed of storiform cells similar in appearance to those of dermatofibroma in skin. Both of their patients were adult men, one a 65-year-old with bilateral multiple "nodules" growing slightly during 2 years that focally were found to be cystic on open lung biopsy. The other case was a 30-year-old man with multiple and rather dramatic bilateral cysts, partially fluid filled, who underwent recurrent pneumothoraces and air emboli to the brain while flying on extended airplane flights. He was followed for 20 years with only slow enlargement. The authors referred to another possible case by Holden et al.[697] in a 21-year-old who had one cyst at the beginning of observation and within 2 years had multiple bilateral cysts. As noted in the preceding section, this case is also referred to in the mesenchymal cystic hamartoma and hemangioma section of this chapter.

The differential diagnosis of cystic lesions in adults are multiple. As reviewed by Joseph et al.,[705] these include necrotizing inflammatory reactions, postinfectious-type abscesses, cavitary pneumocystis or other cavity infections, bullous emphysema, cylindrical bronchiectasis, rarely pneumatoceles, which are much more common in younger patients, lung cysts, septic emboli, bland infarctions, eosinophilic granuloma, lymphangioleiomyomatosis, or other neoplastic lesions, including mesenchymal cystic "hamartoma," and some cases of papillomatosis or metastases such as cavitary sarcomas. They also may be cavitary vasculitis or autoimmune diseases such as rheumatoid nodules. The current entity is separated by the fibrohistiocytic-dermatofibromatous-type proliferation. The long follow-up in one and the age of the other of the two patients reported by Joseph et al.[705] would seem to dictate against postpneumocystis cavities in AIDS (see Chapter 6), and their growth and appearance of multiple lesions would seem to be unusual for other postinflammatory cysts.

"Alveolar Adenoma"

In 1986, Yousem and Hochholzer[706] published six cases that they chose to call "alveolar adenomas." The majority of their patients were asymptomatic older patients, with a mean age of 59 years. All lesions were solitary and appeared as noncalcified coin lesions on radiographs. Five were peripheral (three right-upper lobe, two left-lower lobe), and none had evidence of recurrence in a follow-up averaging 3.5 years. These were usually subpleural, well circumscribed but nonencapsulated, grey-white-tan, and finely cystic, sometimes with hemorrhage in some of the cysts (Fig. 33–110 and 33–111). They averaged 1.8 cm and easily "shelled out" from lung parenchyma.

These adenomas contain variously sized and contoured cystic spaces filled with granular or floccular material, occasionally with extravasated red cells. The interstitium shows some delicate to plump spindle cells, with some variation in cellularity between mild and moderate in degree (Fig. 33–110 and 33–111), in a loose background, containing a few mixed macrophages,

plasma cells, and lymphocytes. The lining of the cystic spaces is usually inapparent or squamoid, but may be more cuboidal and clear cell (Fig. 33–111). Centrally there may be some focal scars. No mucin is identified in the lining cells. There is no necrosis, and only a quite rare mitosis.

I believe the proliferating cell, like that of sclerosing hemangioma, is really a mesenchymal cell and the cystic spaces are incorporated alveolar spaces (see Table 33–1). I shall continue to use the proposed name tentatively doubting the epithelial nature of this entity, while awaiting more investigation. Some of these have been published in the past as "lymphangiomas."[707] The pulmonary lymphangioma term used in this way is distinguished from the dilated lymphatic spaces of a hygroma or mediastinal lymphangioma. (See lymphangiomatosis section toward the end of this chapter.) Their differential diagnoses are limited, and metastatic microcystic low-grade stromal sarcomas of uterus lead the list. Also, see chapter 35. The true nature of these nodular lesions is undetermined, but their characteristics are unique enough to establish a diagnosis.

Vacuolated Tumor

Occasionally, in a section on uncommon tumors, it is worthwhile to publish rare isolated cases and to mention others already in the literature such as the case of myoepithelioma mentioned above. A unique case is offered to see if any other cases similar to it are available for comparison. The case is that of a 32-year-old man who presented with an incidental finding of a 2-cm nodule in the right-lower lobe, which was well circumscribed, gray-pink and nodular, and 1 cm from the nearest pleural surface. Post excision he had been well for 17 months in follow-up of this case described by Clayton et al.[708] with accompanying electron microscopy. The vacuoles did not stain with fat or for mucosubstances, and the cells appeared more neoplastic than a reaction of lipoid pneumonia (Fig. 33–112). A well-defined basal lamina enclosed small groups of cells rather than individual tumor cells, and on that basis it was thought to be epithelial. At the time of publication no one immunohistochemistry was performed. The authors wondered whether it could be a alveolar type I cell tumor. During the discussion by an expert panel, others considered it mesothelial or possibly endothelial. I have had the opportunity to do a Factor VIII stain on this case and it was negative.

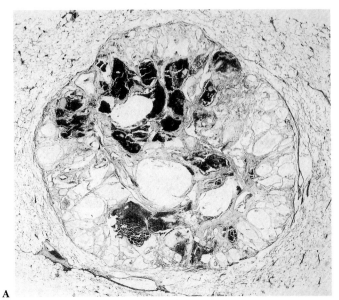

Fig. 33–110 A–C. "Alveolar adenoma." Spherical cystic lesion; some spaces are filled with clear fluid, other with blood (*darker areas*). H and E, ×15. **B.** Cysts are filled with flocculent material, and intervening stroma is delicate. H and E, ×100. **C.** Densest area of interstitial thickening in this example shows stellate interstitial cells mixed with some inflammatory cells. Focal cuboidal lining, perhaps metaplastic alveolar lining cells (see text) at upper left; squamoid lining to right. Note dilated capillaries in loose substance of tumor. H and E, ×400.

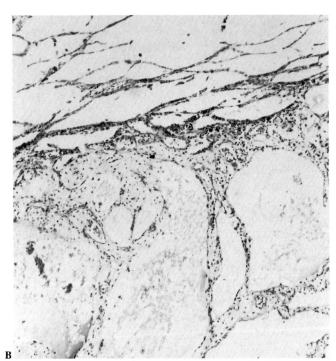

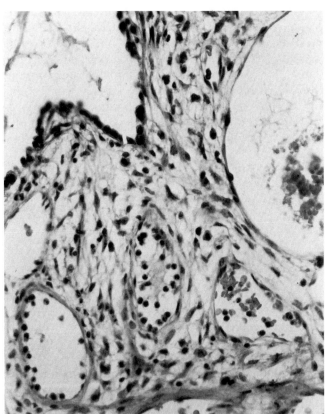

Other Benign Mesenchymal Tumors

Leiomyomas, fibromas, fibrous histiocytomas, lipomas, nerve sheath tumors, and hemangiomas are discussed here. These are the counterparts of those in soft tissue and elsewhere. They occur in the trachea, bronchi, and lung parenchyma, and it might well be argued in some that they represent one-sided overgrowth of supporting tissue other than cartilage, and therefore variances of hamartomas as noted. Those in the breathing tubes often lead to partial or complete obstruction with symptoms, and those of the lung parenchyma are often silent. These are thought to arise from the normal tissue of tracheobronchial and pulmonary parenchymal systems. An excellent review in 1969 by Miller[709] surveyed this general group of tumors. Sometimes the criteria to distinguish benign from malignant mesenchymal neoplasms are imperfect. These are very infrequent tumors, and appear to vary from slightly to definitely less frequent than their malignant counterparts.

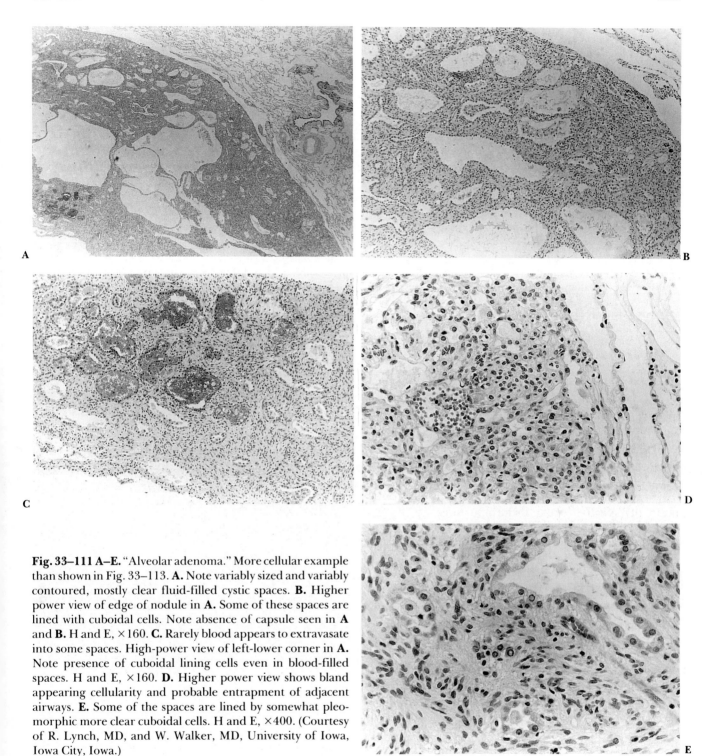

Fig. 33–111 A–E. "Alveolar adenoma." More cellular example than shown in Fig. 33–113. **A.** Note variably sized and variably contoured, mostly clear fluid-filled cystic spaces. **B.** Higher power view of edge of nodule in **A.** Some of these spaces are lined with cuboidal cells. Note absence of capsule seen in **A** and **B.** H and E, ×160. **C.** Rarely blood appears to extravasate into some spaces. High-power view of left-lower corner in **A.** Note presence of cuboidal lining cells even in blood-filled spaces. H and E, ×160. **D.** Higher power view shows bland appearing cellularity and probable entrapment of adjacent airways. **E.** Some of the spaces are lined by somewhat pleomorphic more clear cuboidal cells. H and E, ×400. (Courtesy of R. Lynch, MD, and W. Walker, MD, University of Iowa, Iowa City, Iowa.)

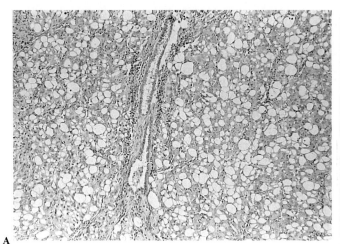

A

Fig. 33–112 A,B. Peculiar vacuolated tumor of undetermined histogenesis. **A.** Tumor cells contain variably sized intracellular spaces, giving appearance almost of "spider cells." Benign bronchiole in middle is innocently entrapped in center of this proliferation. H and E, ×30. **B.** Higher power view centering on same bronchiole as **A** shows some pleomorphism of cells and variation of cytoplasmic cystic spaces. Compare with Fig. 33–141. H and E, ×400.

Leiomyomas

Several excellent reviews of these particular tumors in the lower respiratory tract are available.[685,709–715] By 1969 Taylor and Miller[711] added 1 case to the 12 they found in the literature; by 1978 Orlowski et al.[712] collected 51 cases; and by 1983 Vera-Román et al.[713] added 1 case to 65 collected by this time. Other reviews were done by Yellen et al.[714] in 1984 and by White et al.[715] in 1985. Several series concentrated on leiomyomas of specific sites, including lung,[712,716] trachea,[717,718] or bronchi.[711,719] The reviews by Agnos and Starkey,[720] Yellin et al.,[714] and Gal et al.[685] contrast benign and malignant smooth muscle tumors of the lower respiratory tract.

By 1984, Yellin et al.[714] had documented 12 leiomyomas in trachea, 7 in central bronchi, 26 in small bronchi, and 29 that were considered parenchymal, as no bronchial association could be determined. In the trachea and major bronchi, 7 of the 10 in whom the gender was known were women. Most authors offer the caution that some of the parenchymal nodules in women may represent benign metastasizing leiomyomas, as just discussed in the preceding section. White et al.[715] suggested that women being considered for this diagnosis have their uteri carefully examined. Solitary metastases are difficult to distinguish. As noted later, some of these cases also occur in men who have leiomyosarcomas elsewhere. Solitary low-grade smooth muscle metastases are difficult to distinguish from primary leiomyomas in either sex (Fig. 33–113).

Tracheal leiomyomas range from 1 to 2.5 cm, while their malignant counterparts are from 2 to 5 cm.[714,719] Most leiomyomas of the trachea and bronchi present

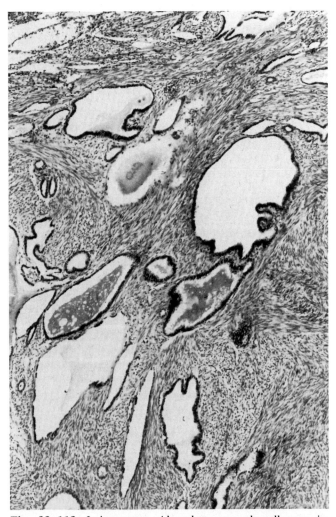

Fig. 33–113. Leiomyoma. Abundant smooth cells run in different directions, with entrapped or incorporated glandular spaces. H and E, ×100.

with irritative and obstructive symptoms of cough, hemoptysis, and shortness of breath. Asthma was present in some, as discussed in the **Tracheal Tumor** section (beginning of this chapter). One case presented with pneumothorax from air trapping.[720] Most of the peripheral intraparenchymal leiomyomas are asymptomatic, and in over 90%[715] are noted incidentally on chest radiographs done for other reasons.

One-third of all patients with bronchial or parenchymal leiomyomas are less than 20 years old, with the average age being in the mid-thirties. The tracheal leiomyomas have a mean age of 40.6 years, in contrast to leiomyosarcomas, which have a mean age of 50.[714]

Distinguishing leiomyomas from fibromas (Figs. 33–113 and 33–114), neurofibromas, or neurilemmomas by light microscopy alone is not always easy. Imperoxidase stains with discriminating antigens are proving most helpful in this concern. Electron microscopy also is of assistance in difficult cases.

Fibroma, Fibrous Tumor, and Fibrous Myxomas

Fibroma of the lung seems to have been a more frequent diagnosis in the past[721,722] than in more recent series. A lesion identified as a fairly large fibroma, pictured in Chapter 5 (Fig. 5–22), has caused bronchiectasis. This is an older case, and the microscopic slides were not available for review. Certainly some of these tumors today would be reclassified into other low-grade spindle cell proliferations, such as fibrous histiocytomas or neurofibromas. Those fibromas associated with the pleura are better called subpleural fibromas or fibrous tumors, and seem to be a special group; they are discussed in Chapter 34 and thus excluded from further discussion here. The term fibrous tumor, used in a rather generic manner, seems to be refocusing attention on these tumors whether in pleura,[723–725] peritoneum,[725,726] lung,[727] tracheobronchial tree,[728] mediastinum,[729] or upper respiratory tract.[730,731] This term incorporates the typical fibromas but allows for some greater variation. Also, calling something a fibroma sounds rather bland or "unfashionable" today.

Pulmonary fibromas have been described in the age group 24–84 years, and two-thirds of them occur in men.[709,722] Some of the endobronchial ones have been known to recur after endoscopic removal, and one case occurred with repeat obstructive symptoms in only 5 months from first removal.[721] Some of the deeper ones in trachea have been called invasive fibrous tumors.[728] Grossly, these tumors are dense and rubbery, and may have some trabeculae evident on cut section. They are generally spherical in whatever location they arise. Intermingling collagen and long spindle cells are seen, and occasionally these are slightly more cellular and may attain a "herringbone" pattern. The more cellular ones begin to raise the question of malignancy. The more hyalinized ones (Fig. 33–114) may overlap with similar changes in leiomyomas and other low grade spindle cell neoplasms and may also represent aging changes.

Paucicellular spindle cell tumors with abundant myxoid stroma have been called fibromyxomas or myxomas. One fibromyxoma of the trachea was described in 1985 by Pollak et al.[668] Perhaps closely related is the entity of a pulmonary myxoma, which was described by Littlefield and Drash[667] in 1959 (see earlier **Myxoma** section.) Some nerve sheath tumors may have myxoid change. Metastatic myxomas from heart are usually confined to or center on pulmonary arteries. I know of

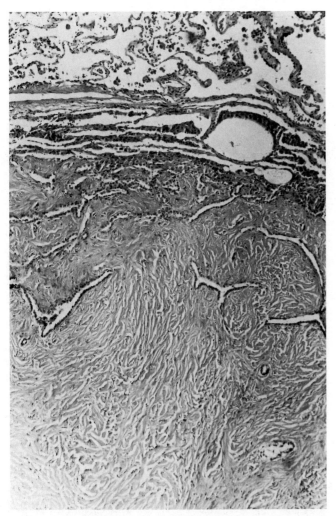

Fig. 33–114. Fibroma. Dense hyalinized tissue shows entrapment of adjacent airspaces, most noted at periphery of nodule. Compare with Figs. 33–105. H and E, ×100.

an interesting case of metastasizing/embolizing cardiac myxoma in a young Frenchman, who underwent more than 20 hospitalizations before a correct diagnosis of cardiac myxoma was made. By then, he had hypoxia from his multiple vascular emboli of this tumor.

Fibrous Histiocytoma

As in soft tissue, this and its malignant counterpart (malignant fibrous histiocytoma, MFH) are gaining favor as diagnosis in the lung[732] and tracheal-bronchial system.[733] The malignant lesion, MFH, is discussed separately in the following **Sarcoma** section, and there is no evidence that these lesions evolve from or through the benign histiocytomas. Fibrous histiocytomas in the lung or tracheal bronchial system overlap with those described as fibromas and fibrous tumors (see foregoing), and an occasional one overlaps with plasma cell granulomas, also already discussed. These lesions have the spectrum of storiform arrangement of some spindle cells in varying degrees of cellularity or fibrosis. Sometimes there is confusion between benign or malignant lesions in this category. A few are intermediate in grade with increased mitoses and overlap with the entity of invasive fibrous tumors such as described in the tracheal-bronchial system by Tan-Liu et al.[728] Some totally occlude bronchi in children.[734] Fibrous histiocytic lesions may occur in the trachea and seven of nine reported by 1990 were benign.[733] One in a 17-year-old woman was a low grade MFH.[735] Most were in young women and were polypoid in the upper third of the trachea for reasons that are unknown. Another in a postradiation-treated patient, was of higher grade.[736]

Fibrous histiocytomas have recently been included in the description of several series, including in 14 cases by Matsubara et al.[322] and 3 cases by Gal et al.[347] The Gal series[347] is in abstract form, but will be interesting when it is available, as it includes 15 cases of pulmonary inflammatory pseudotumor and 13 cases of MFH, suggesting a spectrum similar to that originally proposed by Sajjad et al.[737]

Lipomas

These lesions usually occur in the bronchi[738–744] (Fig. 33–115), less commonly in the trachea,[745,746] and an occasional one has been described in the lung parenchyma or subpleural zone.[738,747–748a] In the bronchi, they are submucosal and may be only submucosal (Fig. 33–115) or may be dumbbell shaped, extending between portions of bronchial cartilage. They may cause atelectasis. Twenty-five cases were reported by Plachta and Hershey[738] in 1962; 32 cases in the English literature were described by Crutcher et al.[742] in 1968, and another 2 were added by Billin et al.[743] by 1971. These

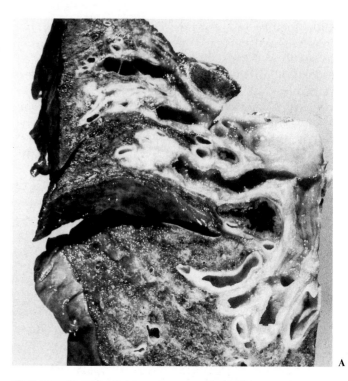

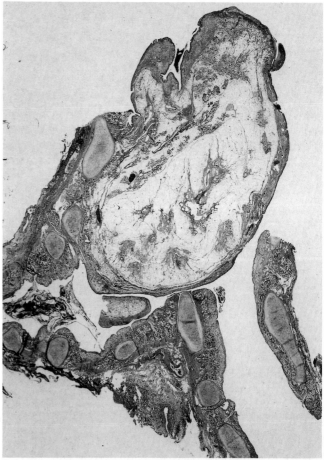

Fig. 33–115 A,B. Intrabronchial lipoma. **A.** Intrabronchial lipoma has caused atelectasis of upper lobe. **B.** Fat is predominant component of this lesion. H and E, ×10.

groups offer summary reviews. The reader is also referred to the series by MacArthur et al.[744] in 1977, and Schraufnagel[739] and Politis et al.,[741] both in 1979.

Most of these arise in the age group 40–60 years, with an age spectrum of 29–64 years. About 90% are in men, for unknown reasons. Sometimes these lesions have been noted to change in shape, becoming more flattened during deep inspiration and round again on expiration.[740,745,748] These lesions rarely appear different than water density, probably because they are surrounded by air.[747a] Computerized tomography (CT) and magnetic resonance imaging (MRI) can help to distinguish the fatty quality of these lesions, if they are large enough for detection.

One large, 6.5-cm lipomatous tumor was described as an atypical lipomatous hamartoma of the lung by Palvio et al.[748a] in 1985. This had minute islands of cartilage and bone and a small amount of epithelial clefts, and was considered atypical because of some atypical nuclei. Portions of cartilage have been described in other lipomas[743] and there is evidence some, if not all, may be in the family of hamartoma (see **Myxoma**).

Nerve Sheath Tumors

A neurofibroma in the bronchus in association with von Recklinghausen's disease was first described in 1914 by Askanazy.[749] In this setting they may be multiple, and as with diagnosing their malignant counterpart of neurosarcomas elsewhere, this is best done in the setting of neurofibromatosis.

Bartley and Arean[750] conducted a very nice review of intrapulmonary neurogenic tumors in 1965. They described 24 cases of neurofibromas and 8 cases of neurilemmomas that occurred either in lung parenchyma or bronchi. They also discussed the malignant counterparts. These tumors occur in the age range of 6–63 years. A more recent discussion is by Miura et al.[751]

Younger patients may be involved in the spectrum of neurofibromatosis, and pulmonary lesions in these cases were described by Unger et al.[520] These authors noted about 15% of these patients have respiratory system and thoracic involvement, but most of these have involvement of posterior mediastinum. These patients also have an increased amount of interstitial fibrosis over age 35, and slightly more than 20% of these patients suffer from this disease.[752,753] Unger et al.[520] noted by 1984 more than 30 cases of primary neurogenic tumors, either neurofibromas or neurilemmomas, had been reported in patients without von Recklinghausen's disease. They also noted a small meningioma in their case, and refer to the fact that the lung is the most common site of spread in cases of metastasizing meningiomas. (See separate earlier section on **Meningiomas**.)

Neurofibromas, neurilemmomas, and neuromas have a light microscopic appearance similar to that described elsewhere, and stain similarly with special stains and immunoperoxidase stains. Electron microscopy of one pulmonary case with typical findings was done by Silverman et al.[754] See **Sarcomas** for a malignant schwannoma.

Hemangiomas

Isolated hemangiomas usually arise in bronchial wall in newborns, children, and adults,[755–759] and are most convincingly neoplastic in newborns and children, where they represent a spectrum of capillary hemangiomas, often associated with similar lesions elsewhere. (See Chapters 7 and 8). In adults they may be reactive to irritation in the bronchial wall, either translumenal or transmural such as passage of a broncholith (Fig. 33–116). In adults these are usually cavernous and sometimes show thrombosis or reorganization (Fig. 33–116C). As with pyogenic granulomas evolving at times into capillary hemangiomas in skin, it is anticipated this reactive capillary variant of hemangioma might also be seen in bronchi in adults. I have seen an early lesion suggesting this in a biopsy site with a polypoid excrescence of granulation tissue.

At times, cystic lesions in lung may have linings that are rich in capillary vessels in both the newborn[760] and adults.[697] The latter case by Holden et al.[697] is also referred to in the sections on **Cystic Fibrohistiocytic Tumors** and **Mesenchymal Cystic Hamartoma**.

At times tangles of enlarged, thick-walled vessels represent portions of arterial-venous fistula, which are most commonly found in the mid- and lower lung fields. I have recently seen a case in a patient with submucosal tumor-like masses, which when biopsied led to rapid exsanguination.[761] Hemangiomas may also be associated with hereditary hemorrhagic telangiectasia, or Rendu–Oslu–Weber syndrome.

Sarcomas

In the past the term "pulmonary sarcomas" has included lymphomas and soft tissue type of sarcomas,[762,763] and even carcinosarcomas.[764] The lymphoproliferative disorders are covered in Chapter 31, the carcinosarcomas elsewhere in this chapter, and this section will concentrate on the counterpart of the soft tissue type of sarcomas.

As with carcinomas, the most common sarcoma in the lung is metastatic, and one must always be alert to this possibility. Primary sarcomas of the lung are usually solitary and can be large, and a fair number present asymptomatically. Metastatic sarcomas are more often

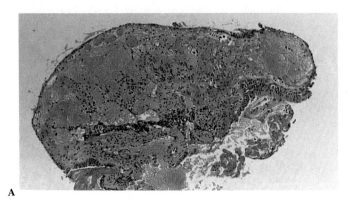

Fig. 33–116 A–C. Bronchial hemangiomas. **A.** Multiple thin-walled blood-filled spaces distend bronchiolar submucosa. H and E, ×40. **B.** High power view of spaces in **A** shows thin walls and red cell content. H and E, ×250. **C.** Different case showing various stages of thrombosis of dilated blood vessels in bronchus. H and E, ×20.

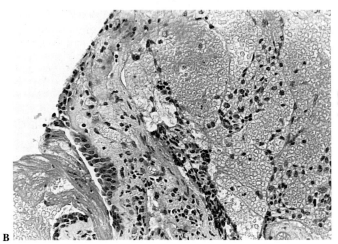

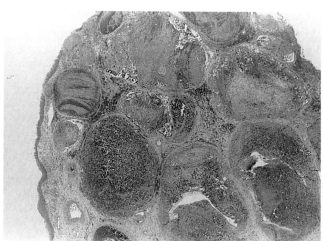

multiple. The source of metastatic sarcomas often can be detected, and it is extraordinary for it to remain silent. True primary pulmonary sarcomas are rare. Metastasizing sarcomas outnumber primary lung sarcomas, I would guess, by a factor of about 3000:1. Even Kaposi's sarcoma in AIDS usually only involves the lungs after skin and other visceral involvement, and might then be considered metastatic. (See separate section on Kaposi's sarcoma later in this chapter.) Because of AIDS, Kaposi's sarcoma has probably now become the number one sarcoma of any particular cell type in the lung in adults. Primary lung sarcomas occur in relationship to primary lung carcinomas in the same institute: 9 of 6,000 (0.15%) cases in Edinburgh,[765] 10 of 3,400 (0.29%) at Duke Medical Center,[766] and 22 of 5,712 (0.39%) at Memorial Hospital, New York City.[762] An incidence of about 1 in 500 (0.20%) has been quoted by Iverson,[767] and is an easy figure to remember. The average of the three series just mentioned is 1 in 371 (0.27%) cases. In relationship to total admissions in one small series, they represented 2 of 400,000 (0.005%), and in relationship to the number of operative specimens, 2 of 100,000 (0.002%).[463] In sequential autopsies

they occur in 1 in 8,000 (0.0125%)[768] and 1 in 7,272 (0.01375%) of cases.[769]

Several differences are apparent in comparing primary lung sarcomas and primary lung carcinomas. Sarcomas occur at a slightly younger age, do not usually metastasize outside the chest, and have a somewhat greater tendency to local recurrence and are much less often detected by exfoliated cell cytology specimens of lung or pleura than lung carcinomas.

Only a few institutions have a series large enough to offer meaningful comparison, and much of the material available in the literature consists of smaller case reports and review of literature findings. Lung sarcomas can be divided in several ways, including those that predominantly involve major vessels, those that are primarily endobronchial, and those that predominantly involve the lung parenchyma. In this chapter the sarcomas will be divided into the following three groups: (1) sarcomas arising from major vessels; (2) parenchymal and bronchial wall–endobronchial sarcomas; and (3) sarcomas derived from smaller vessels. The latter category is not commonly used, but is convenient for purposes of classification. The endobronchial lesions have some distinct characteristics but overlap those of parenchymal lesions, so these are discussed together.

Some additional generalizations about primary lung sarcomas are worth noting before discussing the individual groups and entities, although exceptions occur to each generalization. The smaller parenchymal sarcomas are usually asymptomatic, although some large ones may be also. Endobronchial tumors present fairly early because of respiratory compromise. These endobronchial tumors are usually lower grade tumors and have a good prognosis. Smaller sarcomas are usually grossly described as grey-white to yellow-grey, rubbery, and rather monotonous. Larger sarcomas are more often described grossly as having variegated color, with the periphery of the tumor more viable in appearance and the center more variegated from necrosis and hemorrhage. Grossly and radiographically detected calcification is infrequent, except in those specific tumors normally producing calcification such as chondrosarcoma and osteosarcoma. Most parenchymal sarcomas are described as round or lobulated and sharply contoured; they slightly compress the nearby lung parenchyma but do not have a capsule. These infrequently cavitate and only occasionally spread to regional nodes.

Spindle cell carcinomas have been variably classified depending on the techniques available, and many of the cases reported in the past may be reclassified into different subgroups today. Some of the subdivisions of sarcoma are based on only a few cases and therefore conclusions from this limited number of cases may be proven invalid in the future as larger series are accumulated.

Differentiation of some sarcomas from pleomorphic and spindle cell carcinomas and some carcinosarcomas will be a recurring challenge. Carcinosarcomas may be so predominantly sarcomatous that only after careful search and at times application of immunohistologic chemical techniques does the epithelial component become apparent. (See **Osteosarcoma** section.)

When symptomatic, most patients with sarcoma present with symptoms of chest pain, cough, and dyspnea, but hemoptysis and other related pulmonary problems are also sometimes seen. A peripheral sarcoma will usually exclude the central type described as major vessel or bronchial derived, but a central tumor does not exclude a parenchyma-derived sarcoma.

Primary Sarcomas of Larger Vessel Origin

These rare neoplasms most often arise in or adjacent to the pulmonary arterial trunk. Several good reviews are available.[770–774] They frequently extend more distally along the pulmonary arteries and may embolize to the lung parenchyma. Occasionally just one pulmonary artery is involved without involvement of the pulmonary trunk (Fig. 33–117). In some cases tumor extends into, or arises from, the right ventricle, and hence the broader term right outflow tract sarcomas is preferred by some. One case may have arisen in an arterial venous fistula near the right hilum,[775] and rare ones are thought secondary to past radiotherapy.[776,777]

These tumors present either as a pulmonary embolus or multiple smaller emboli, or with obvious right-heart failure, or they may present with ongoing progressive mysterious symptoms. Once a diagnosis is made, many of the symptoms are related to right-heart obstruction and compromised perfusion of one or both lungs, and/or embolization. CT and/or MRI scans and/or angiography are the best ways to detect these, but even with these, premortem diagnosis is only made in 50%–60% of the cases.[778,779] Even when these neoplasms are detected, surgery is only rarely curative.[774,778,780]

Mandelstamm[781] is credited with the first description of outflow tract–pulmonary artery sarcoma in 1932. Twenty-one cases were summarized by Wackers et al.[770] in 1969, 37 by Shmookler et al.[771] in 1977, 60 in 1980 by Bleisch and Kraus,[772] and 78 by 1985 by Baker and Goodwin,[773] who then summarized the 48 cases in English literature; the review of Bleisch and Kraus[772] covers those in the non-English literature. McGlennen et al.[774] in 1989 estimated about 100 cases had been reported, but it is still so rare that their experience with 4 cases over 15 years at a major medical center is considered a large series. The later reviews are the source of the facts given here.

Some 76% of the patients present with dyspnea, 60% with chest pain, 53% with cough, and others with assorted pulmonary obstructive and hypoxic symptoms suggested above. Many are not diagnosed until autopsy. Average survival after diagnosis in life is 12 months, and at the time of diagnosis 78% have metastases, including 67% with metastases to the lung itself with direct vascular spread and peripheral vascular emboli. Occasionally these tumors spread to regional nodes and outside the chest. Postsurgical recurrence is common, and no chemotherapy or radiotherapy has been proven to be effective. A rare patient may have symptoms for prolonged periods, and in one case this was 21 years.[772] The youngest patient was 15 years, and the oldest 81. Sixty percent occur in the 45- to 64-year-old group, most frequently in the 50- to 54-year-old group. Twice as many women as men are involved.

Grossly, the tumor masses most often involve the pulmonary trunk and may extend along the walls to involve either or both pulmonary arteries. They may extend in retrograde fashion and involve the pulmonic valve. Most are described as multinodular, firm, yellow-tan, and smoothly contoured, although possibly multilobulated. Some have grossly evident endovascular tu-

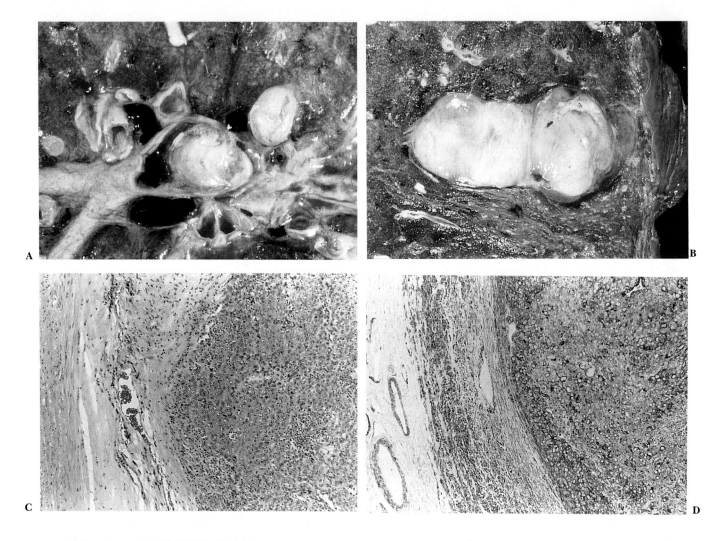

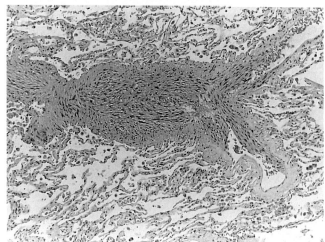

Fig. 33–117 A–E. Pulmonary artery sarcoma. **A.** Pulmonary artery sarcoma is limited right mainstem–peripheral pulmonary artery without more proximal involvement. Seen from hilar aspect in two vessels, there is still partial patency to left in larger. **B.** Tumor actually becomes larger in more peripheral artery, here approaching pleura. **C.** Muscle wall of pulmonary artery is seen to left, and tumor cells fill lumen. These cells are large and epithelioid, with some mixed inflammatory cell infiltrate. H and E, ×100. **D.** Desmin stain by immunoperoxidase highlights muscle coat of pulmonary artery and several smaller arteries toward left; tumor cells are regionally positive. ×100. **E.** Different case shows more spindle cell sarcoma arising in pulmonary outflow tract, here in its distal reaches seen extending into smaller branches of pulmonary artery. H and E, ×100. (**A–D,** courtesy of Dr. J. Bolen and **E.** Courtesy of Dr. K. Galagan, Virginia Mason Clinic, Seattle, Washington.)

mor polyps. Some of these have thrombus material attached to their ends. Occasionally there is evidence of recent embolization from such a site, both as an acute fracture line on the proximal tumor and a distally identified companion fragment. Some endovascular tumor resembles thrombus material throughout. Some are localized to a main pulmonary artery (see Fig. 33–117), while direct extension grossly is noted to the lungs in 56% of the cases, and sometimes this can be traced almost to the periphery. Although usually small, nodules of metastatic tumor as large as 3 cm may be present in the lung parenchyma, and these are often bilateral. The nodules may show associated bronchial and parenchymal invasion after spread through the vascular wall, but often they are contained within the vessels. There may be other densities that represent infarcts from either growing tumor or tumor emboli or thromboemboli plugging vessels.

Microscopically, these sarcomas can represent quite a spectrum of appearance, McGlennen et al.[774] nicely summarized the pathology of 100 cases. Some are quite cellular, others are hypocellular and more myxoid, while still others have a variegated pattern. Most commonly the sarcomatous elements are described as undifferentiated (34%), leiomyosarcomatous (20%), rhabdomyosarcomatous (6%), fibrosarcomatous (17%), chondrosarcomatous (4%), osteogenic sarcomatous (4%), MFH (2%), and 6% have mixed differentiation and are classified malignant mesenchymomas.[774] Less angiosarcoma differentiation is present than would be expected for origin in this organ, but this is also true for sarcomas arising in other large vessels, whether they be arteries or veins. Some of the primary chondrosarcomas in lung may belong to this vascular group.[781–783] A few of these sarcomas of major vessel origin have large to giant pleomorphic undifferentiated cells, sometimes being multinucleate. Three percent to 5% have definite mixed differentiated sarcoma components, and in one case in the pulmonary outflow, there was malignant chondroid and rhabdomyoblastic change[784]; the term "malignant mesenchymoma" may be preferred for some of these.

Microscopically, tumor may spread in a circumferential manner along the inner walls of the vessels (see Fig. 33–117). More distally there may be eccentric or concentric thickening by an admixture of tumor, fibrin, and collagen in varying proportions. In some places such thickenings appear to be collagen only, but on serial sections, nearby tumor is identified in the same vessels. A similar situation exists for carcinomatous emboli (see Chapter 35). Infarcted areas may show endovascular tumor toward their central apex of infarction, and sometimes these empty and result in cavities (Fig. 33–118). Tumor spread in these vessels often is

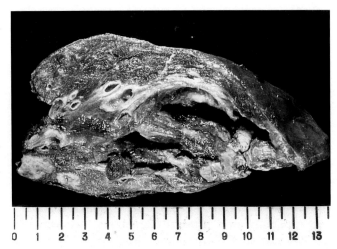

Fig. 33–118. Cavitary vascular sarcoma. Sarcoma remains as two nodules in left-lower portion of lung tissue and focally as nodules around cavitary wall. Patient was thought to have an abscess preoperatively.

contained in the vessels but can be seen extending through them, invading the bronchi and bronchioles, and occasionally showing lymphatic invasion.

Metastases from right outflow track sarcomas are logically most commonly identified in the lungs. The next most common sites are hilar and mediastinal nodes, and by direct extension the pleura, heart, diaphragm, and sometimes the liver. Extrathoracic sites of spread include brain, thyroid, kidney, adrenal gland, mesentery, jejunum, and omentum. Postoperative recurrence is most often in the field nearest the tumor, even in cases in which it appears the tumor was clearly excised at first operation.

Primary sarcomas of the main pulmonary vein are quite rare.[785,786] Five of the six reported cases by 1990 had left atrial obstruction.[786] It is also interesting to note that the seven cases of primary malignant fibrous histiocytoma (MFH) of heart all arose in the left atrium.[787] Sometimes sarcomas of pulmonary vein represent invasion of the vein by adjacent primary or secondary sarcomas or carcinomas, and occasionally emboli to distal sites have been described from these tumors, including massive emboli to peripheral-extremity vessels.[788] This is further discussed at the end of Chapter 35. Rarely, they are considered low grade.[789]

Parenchymal and Bronchial–Endobronchial Sarcomas

These sarcomas are discussed together because they often overlap in cell patterns. However, each seems to be otherwise rather distinct, with the endobronchial tumors presenting earlier with obstructive symptoms, with little extension into adjacent parenchymal areas, and a better prognosis.

Parenchymal sarcomas are those that are not grossly and predominately endovascular or endobronchial (Fig. 33–119). Patients with parenchymal sarcomas of less than 5 cm do well. Those with tumors near the hilum or in the immediate subpleural zone do less well. In the past many of these tumors were classified on the basis of light microscopy only, and had the predominant cell type of spindle cell sarcoma. The cases, classified as "leiomyosarcoma" and "fibrosarcoma" in the past, may not all conform to today's classification when electron microscopy and immunoperoxidase markers are applied. Newer tumor designations such as MFH are being applied more frequently.

The spindle cell group is discussed first, followed by the growing entity of malignant fibrous histiocytoma and other subdivisions of sarcoma. It must be remembered that there are no good histologic criteria for establishing primary versus secondary sarcoma of any type in the lung.

Spindle Cell Sarcomas

A large number of cases of primary spindle cell sarcomas have been studied at the Armed Forced Institute of Pathology (AFIP) by Guccion and Rosen.[790] In their review, published in 1972, they added 19 cases new cases classified as leiomyosarcoma to the 48 cases in the literature of primary leiomyosarcomas and added 13 new cases classified as fibrosarcomas to the 48 cases in the literature. Therefore 67 cases were so classified as leiomyosarcoma by 1972, and Wick et al.[791] in 1982 noted that about 84 cases were known by this date, for an addition of only about 17 more cases in 10 years. The AFIP series had autopsy followup in 21 of 26 cases (81%) compared to about 40% in the literature. Guccion and Rosen[790] divided each group into endobronchial and parenchymal tumors. They further subdivided the parenchymal tumors into those less than and greater than 10 cm in maximum dimension. Men were more often involved than women in each category in both the AFIP series and in the literature review. Primary bronchopulmonary fibrosarcomas in childhood and adolescence have a better prognosis than those in adults.[792] MFH group is discussed separately to follow.

Yellin et al.[714] in 1984 summarized the literature of lower respiratory tract smooth muscle tumors, including both leiomyomas (68 in number) and leiomyosarcomas (92) of lung, and leiomyomas (12) and leiomyosarcomas (7) of trachea. (Leiomyomas are discussed under **Other Benign Tumors** elsewhere in this chapter.) Their series of leiomyosarcomas had a male to female ratio of 2.45:1.

Endobronchial Types

Guccion and Rosen[790] in 1972 reported a total of 16 endobronchial fibrosarcomas and 8 endobronchial leiomyosarcomas. Again, these classifications were estab-

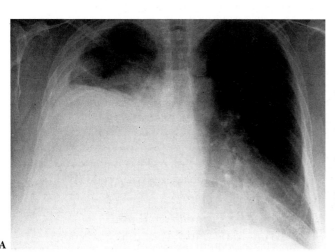

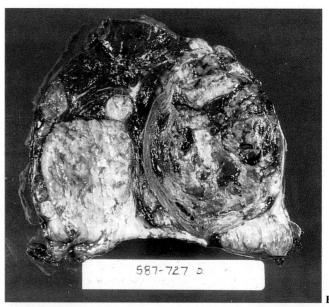

Fig. 33–119 A,B. Massive pulmonary hemangiopericytoma in right lung of 39-year-old woman.[817] **A.** Plain film of chest shows massive replacement of right mid- and inferior lung. Note pleural effusion around remaining upper lung field. **B.** Several extensions of tumor present multinodular effect. Multifocal necrosis is evident in larger two. (Courtesy of Dr. R. Schmidt, University of Washington, School of Medicine, Seattle, Washington.)

lished by use of light microscopy only, but of note, twice as many endobronchial sarcomas were in the category of fibrosarcoma as leiomyosarcoma. Seventy-five percent of the patients with endobronchial fibrosarcomas reported in their series were children or young adults, and for endobronchial leiomyosarcomas, 50% were in this age category. These tended to be lower grade histologically and to have a better prognosis. Most were contained within the bronchi, although a few showed focal infiltration. One was congenital and excised at 24 hours of age.[793] It seems best to eliminate the large parenchymal tumors with focal endobronchial protrusion from this category, and therefore by definition most of the tumor has to be endobronchial. See **Fibrous Histiocytoma** section also.

Parenchymal Types of Sarcomas

Many of these are spindle cell types. Men are more frequently involved, both in the AFIP and the literature review series,[790] with both the leiomyosarcomas and fibrosarcomas of lung parenchyma. These tend to occur in a slightly older age group than the endobronchial sarcomas, with 30 of 43 (70%) of the fibrosarcomas being over the age of 40, and 37 of 57 (65%) of the leiomyosarcomas in lung parenchyma being in patients over age 50. Exceptions do occur; 1 relatively large spindle cell sarcoma was noted in a newborn, and some were noted in patients in their twenties. The oldest patient was 93 years. In each of these groups a little fewer than half of the patients were asymptomatic, despite their sarcomas being at times very large. These authors considered under 10 cm as "relatively small" (see Fig. 33–119). Because of their large size, many of these tumors had the tendency to invade adjacent structures including chest wall, mediastinum, and diaphragm.

Guccion and Rosen[790] found mitotic rate was a helpful indicator in both types of spindle cell sarcomas to predict aggressive behavior. They noted 8 or fewer mitoses per 10 high-power fields acted as low grade, and 12 or more per 10 high-power fields acted aggressively, with the count between these two being an indeterminate zone. Their endobronchial tumors generally had less than 3 mitoses per 10 high-power fields.

Pathology of Spindle Cell Sarcomas

Grossly, the endobronchial sarcomas usually arise in larger bronchi, and are sometimes but not always contained in the wall (Fig. 33–120). Occasionally they are in lobar bronchi. They measure 1.0–2.5 cm, are soft, tan, and polypoid, and often occur with a stalk that allows

them to move around somewhat. They also often have superficial ulceration and hemorrhage.

The intraparenchymal sarcomas are usually large, and on cut surface have some nodularity or lobulation. The larger tumors often have necrosis and hemorrhage and are softer than the smaller ones. Some are friable and soft.

Microscopically, the spindle cell sarcomas follow the criteria as applied to soft tissue. As these criteria have changed somewhat because of advances in techniques, the reader is referred to the study of Guccion and Rosen[790] for their criteria given in 1972. In marginal cases today, a larger group might be left as just spindle cell sarcomas. In general, those classified as leiomyosarcomas by light microscopy have more cytoplasm, more pleomorphism of nuclei, and more streaming of cells (Figs. 33–121 and 33–122) or small fascicle formation, whereas the fibrosarcomas have less cytoplasm, less pleomorphism, and a greater amount of "herringbone" growth pattern. Electron microscopy or immunoperoxidase should be able to distinguish smooth muscle differentiation, as in soft tissues. Some subtle differences between pericytes, glomus cells, and smooth muscle cells are covered in their respective sections. As with spindle cell sarcomas elsewhere, when they reach a more pleomorphic form, caution should always be used in both their classification and their possible confusion with pleomorphic carcinomas.

Pleural-based spindle cell sarcomas are often confused with focal mesotheliomas (see Chapter 34). Many of the lesions described as solitary or localized fibrous mesotheliomas of pleura by Stout[794] and Foster and Ackerman[795] as localized mesotheliomas of pleura are (sub)pleural fibromas-fibrous tumors, both benign and malignant subtypes, or fibrosarcomas. See Chapter 34 for further discussion. Also see **Sclerosing Hemangiomas** section for reclassification of solitary epithelial mesotheliomas.

Differential diagnosis of both endobronchial and parenchymal sarcomas includes plasma cell granulomas, which usually have a greater admixture of inflammatory cells but may have abundant fibrosis and collagen deposition (see discussion elsewhere in this chapter, along with discussion in Chapter 8). Other entities include hemangiopericytomas with their distinctive vascular pattern (see elsewhere in this chapter), sarcomatous components of carcinosarcomas and sometimes blastomas, and occasionally cases of metastatic spindle cell melanomas or hypernephromas, pleomorphic or sarcomatoid carcinomas, either primary or secondary, and spindle cell carcinoid tumors. Distinction of malignant from their benign counterpart in lung is not as well defined as in uterus, but mitotic rate, pleomorphism, necrosis, and proven aggressiveness are helpful. Gal

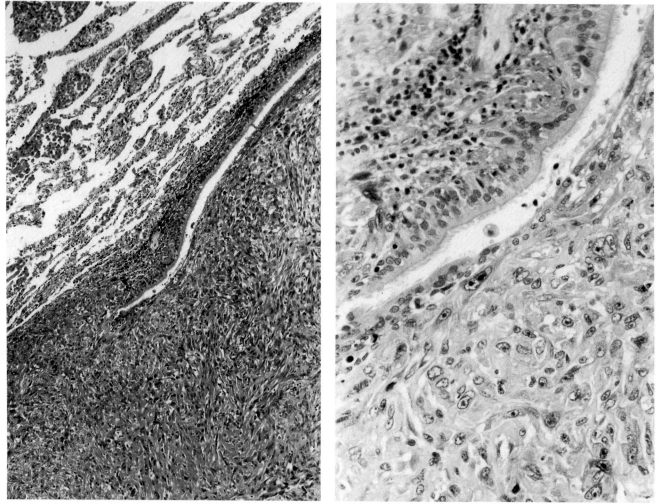

Fig. 33–120 A,B. Pleomorphic spindle cell sarcoma, probably leiomyosarcoma. **A.** Rather evenly contoured tumor abuts bronchus. H and E, ×50. **B.** High-power view of bronchial lining abutment from **A.** H and E, ×400.

et al.[685] suggested greater than 1 mitosis per 10 high power fields or any degree of hypercellularity and/or pleomorphism to be indications of potentially aggressive behavior, at least with smooth muscle tumors.

Malignant Fibrous Histiocytomas

Of interest, in all soft tissue locations, postradiation sarcomas are now most often classified as MFH.[813] An occasional case in the lung has multiple differentiated sarcomatous components, and some might classify this better as a malignant mesenchymoma. One such case was accompanied by benign osteoclasts. (See separate section addressing osteoclasts.) (Also see **Benign Fibrous Histiocytoma** for low-grade lesions.)

As in soft tissues,[796] malignant fibrous histiocytomas (MFH) in the lung has gained great favor as a diagnosis. As noted by Lee et al.,[797] many of the past series of

sarcomas in the lung did not list MFH as one of the cell types, but many of these series predate knowledge or classification of this tumors in soft tissue. In their review, Lee and associates[797] reclassified 5 of their 10 pulmonary sarcomas as primary malignant fibrous histiocytomas. They used the criteria of (1) demonstration of storiform, pleomorphic, or fascicular growth patterns; (2) predominantly spindle cell proliferation; (3) variable number of large cells resembling histiocytes, usually accompanied by pleomorphic multinucleate tumor giant cells; (4) absence of morphologic features of other sarcomatous differentiation; (5) absence of features to suggest anaplastic carcinoma; and (6) exclusion, as best as possible, of possible sources of metastasis from other locations.

So far, this sarcoma in the respiratory tract has been mentioned in the trachea,[735,736] pulmonary arteries,[776,798–800] and possibly radiation induced.[776] Others

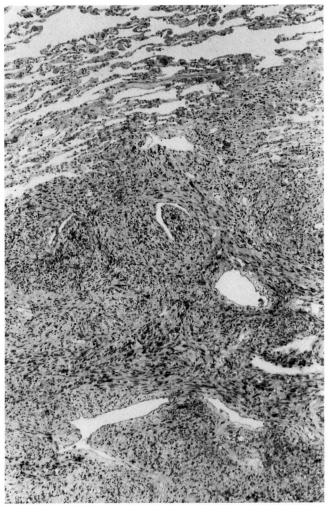

Fig. 33–121. Leiomyosarcoma. Pleomorphic spindle cells run in different directions. H and E, ×50.

occur in the lung.[737,797,801–810] One in lung directly invaded the aorta.[808] They are rare as a primary sarcoma in the lung; those in soft tissue far outnumber those in lung, and 75%–90% of those that are deep seated in soft tissue spread to lung.[796,811,812] In only 0.5% of those with lung spread are the primary tumors not yet undiscovered.

Yousem and Hochholzer in 1987[809] summarized 16 cases from the literature and added 22 cases of their own from the U.S. Armed Forces Institute of Pathology (AFIP). This is the largest series to date and is detailed here. In 1988 McDonnell et al.[810] summarized 12 cases in the lung. In Yousem and Hochholzer's large series,[800] there were 12 women and 10 men, aged 18–80 years, mean age, 52.3 years, and none with a past history of soft tissue sarcomas. More than 90% of the sarcomas were solitary, 4 had invaded the chest wall, and 50% had vascular invasion, the latter appearing to represent the route of metastases from the chest to brain, liver, and

kidney. Mitoses average 7 per 10 high-power fields, and osteoclast-like giant cells were seen in 3 (14%). Poor prognosis was associated with stage at diagnosis, with unresectability, and the subtypes of inflammatory or myxoid MFH. Of interest, size, location in lung, pleura or blood vessel invasion, infiltrative borders, necrosis, abnormal versus normal mitotic figures, or presence or absence of osteoclast-like giant cells did not predict behavior.

These tumors in the lung conform to their diagnostic patterns in soft tissue, and variant patterns are being described in a similar fashion as those in the soft tissues.[796,807,812] As always, one must exclude a source from outside the lungs, of which sarcomatoid renal cell carcinoma is one particularly similar one, with this pattern noted in 26 of 42 (62%) cases of primary sarcomatoid renal cell carcinoma in one series.[814] Some cases of spindle cell squamous carcinoma have been confused with these entities in the lung. In fact, of 14 patients with sarcomatoid carcinomas of the lung, Ro et al.[229] reported a malignant fibrous histiocytoma pattern in 9 (64%) of these tumors.

Grossly, the tumors are described as grey-yellow, and microscopically have varying degrees of spindled and storiform patterns, with pleomorphic cell areas, sometimes with multinucleate giant cells. Necrosis is frequent. Lymphocytes may be found scattered among tumor cells. As yet no inflammatory malignant fibrous histiocytoma pattern with polymorphonuclear leukocytes (PMNs) has been described in the lung. Some cases have myxoid areas, and in at least one this was dominant.[806] Mitoses are easily identified and are often atypical, perhaps relating to the highly aggressive nature of these tumors.

By electron microscopy, these tumors have histiocytic changes with cells with lysosomes and fat droplets in them and other cells with more fibroblastic and myofibroblastic differentiation. These should not have tonofilaments, well-formed desmosomes, intracellular lumens, secretory vacuoles, or basal lamina, as these would be indicators of poorly differentiated tumors of other types.[805]

Hemangiopericytoma

Hemangiopericytomas are thought to arise from pericytes that occur mostly around smaller vessels. The tumors probably arise in smaller caliber vessel as they do not encase larger vessels in the same way, but this is as yet unproven. Stout and Murray[451] first reported the entity of hemangiopericytoma in 1942.

Three excellent series have characterized this tumor in the lung. That by Meade et al.[815] in 1974 added 4 cases to the 24 reported in the literature. The series by

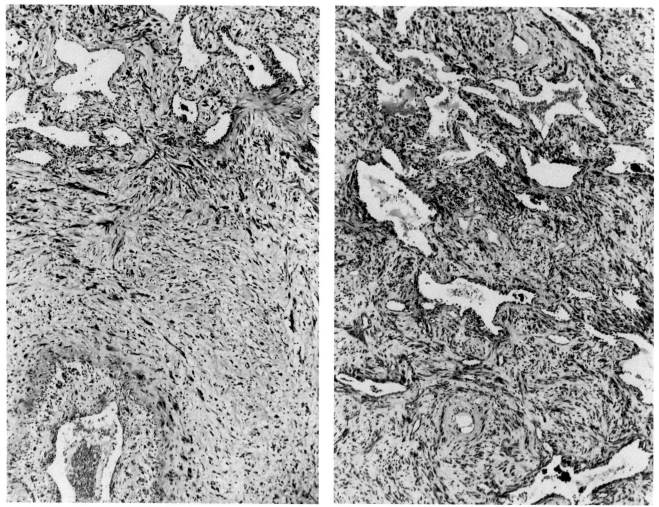

Fig. 33–122 A,B. Parenchymal leiomyosarcoma with vascular wall infiltration. **A.** Spindle cells involve intima and media of vessel, and extend into adjacent lung. H and E, ×250. **B.** Further interstitial spread of spindle cells. H and E, ×250.

Shin and Ho[816a] in 1979 added 2 cases to the review of 34 cases in the literature. A 1987 series by Yousem and Hochholzer[817a] principally discussed their large series of 18 cases seen in consultation, with little literature review. The literature now contains somewhat more than 60 cases of primary pulmonary hemangiopericytomas. The interested reader is referred to data and individual references in these three series, and these resources serve for many of the characteristics described here.

These tumors may be classified as low grade (called benign by some, and innocent by others) and high grade (called malignant by most). All should be considered potentially malignant, even though the criteria for malignancy are not well developed (but are covered toward the end of this section). These tumors occur in patients aged from 10 to 73 years at the time of diagnosis,[816a] and have about equal sex representation. Men have a

mean age of 42 at the time of diagnosis, and women a mean age of 50. Most cases occur in patients over age 30 and are in men, but a 17-year-old girl was noted to have a 24 cm, 650 gm tumor.[816] Another massive tumor, 17 cm in maximum dimension, occurred after radiation therapy and was reported by Rusch et al.[817] About 4 have been reported in the trachea where they may overlap with a glomus tumor.[818] It is estimated that about 1 in 10 hemangiopericytomas in all locations occurs in lung.[815]

Presenting complaints include hemoptysis, chest pain, dyspnea, cough, and only rarely pulmonary osteoarthropathy. The incidence of asymptomatic presentation in the literature is 44%, and in the series by Yousem and Hochholzer, 38%.[817a] Meade et al.[815] divided the patients by sex in their earlier series, and noted 52% of the women presented asymptomatically, compared with 33% of the men. Radiographically, these tumors are located centrally[816a] or periph-erally.[817a] They are rounded, usually with sharply de-fined contours, and are most often homogeneous with-out calcification. Sometimes they have been mistaken for thoracic aortic aneurysm.[816a] Fifty-eight percent of these tumors appear on the left side, particularly the left-lower lobe,[816a] but otherwise have been reported in all lobes and follow the general volume of tissue. They do not usually invade hilar structures, and gross endo-vascular invasion is rare. There is no radiographic evidence to help distinguish this neoplasm from others, and short of evidence of metastasis; there is no radio-graphic evidence to help differentiate between low- and high-grade tumors.

Grossly, these tumors are yellow-tan to grey-white with frequent necrosis and some hemorrhage (see Fig. 33–119). Despite their vascular origin, they are not bloody neoplasms when cut. This is related to the fact that the cell forming the tumor is not an endothelial cell. About 10% are multiple, usually with smaller nodules in the same lobe. Nodes are usually not involved. About 11% may be focally cystic, and an equal number show some endobronchial spread.

Microscopically, the most characteristic and required pattern for diagnosis is "antler-like" vascular spaces (see Fig. 33–123). These are usually acute angled bifurca-tions of sinusoidal spaces, which generally have a nar-row and elongated caliber, but sometime are more interdigitating while still retaining some of these quali-ties. There may be narrow collagen bands between the tumor cells and these spaces, or it may appear that tumor cells form these spaces. Necrosis is commonly seen in some 83% of cases.[817a]

The neoplastic cells are usually rather monotonous. These vary from the blander appearance of low-grade neoplasms in being round to oval, almost suggesting those of a glomus tumor, but often with indistinct cytoplasmic borders by light microscopy. The more aggressive ones have larger spindle cells that are some-times arranged perpendicular to vascular spaces and sometimes arranged more longitudinally (Fig. 33–123). When the cells are more spindled, the appearance of the H and E stained slide is strikingly blue, presumably from their high amount of nuclear DNA (Fig. 33–123A). The cytoplasm is generally less, whether in lower or higher grade lesions, than most sarcomas in the lung, and this also gives a very cellular appearance. More pleomorphic cells are usually seen only in high-grade lesions. Where there is some myxomatous change, as described below, there is a tendency to more cellular pleomorphism. Necrosis may highlight a pattern of vascular cuffing (Fig. 33–123C), but this is usually an artifact caused by preservation of cells near the vascular supply. Sometimes the stroma becomes hyalinized.

The borders of hemangiopericytoma with lung pa-renchyma are usually sharply defined. A fibrous cap-sule was present in 7 of 18 in one series (39%),[817a] and in other cases tumor stops at adjacent lung parenchyma with only minimal extension into adjacent alveolar septa. This is not a tumor that extends in serpentine fashion into adjacent lung parenchyma, as might be a pattern with small chemodectoma-like bodies or some other lesions.

Microscopically, the pleural elastica was involved in approximately 44% of the series by Yousem and Hochholzer.[817a] In the same series, vascular invasion was seen in 35% and smooth muscle and cartilage destruction of bronchi in 28%.

Reticulum stains were thought at one time to be characteristic of this lesion (Fig. 33–123D), but cross-over with appearances in other sarcomas made this unreliable as a unique characteristic. Electron micros-copy has shown these cells to have pinocytotic vesicles, intermediate filaments without dense bodies or plaques, and generally no other particularly distin-guishing characteristics. There has been confusion as to the cell of origin, and some believe they have character-istics of fibroblasts but are surrounded by basal lamina. Others believe these are modified smooth muscle cells, perhaps immature smooth muscle cells.[818a–820] Of in-terest, although smooth muscle differentiation is noted ultrastructurally, no alpha smooth muscle actin and only vimentin are present in this tumor whereas in glomus tumors both are present.[820] The pericyte in its tumorous form is difficult to define and separate from other tumors, and correlation with electron microcopy is often required. It has been suggested[818,821] that tumors being considered for this diagnosis by electron microscopy should at least show some areas or transi-tion to areas of more typical pericytes.

Prognosis is related to several factors. Somewhat helpful in this determination are the following: size greater than 5 cm (two-thirds of all), presence of necro-sis, mitotic rate more than 3 per 10 high power fields, and vascular invasion. Even more suggestive of malig-nant potential are size greater than 8–10 cm, pleural or bronchial wall invasion, unresectability, and symptoms including a history of hemoptysis. Recurrences are usually local and occur within 2 years of the primary excision. Metastases to distant sites, such as brain and bone, do occur but are not frequently seen. In the review of Shin and Ho,[816a] 7 of 34 (21%) metastasized. No insulin-like products with hypoglycemia have been described in this tumor of the lung, as have been described for it elsewhere.[822]

The differential diagnosis involves these entities in the lung that are cellular, and at least focally have "antler-like" vascular spaces. Solitary subpleural fibro-

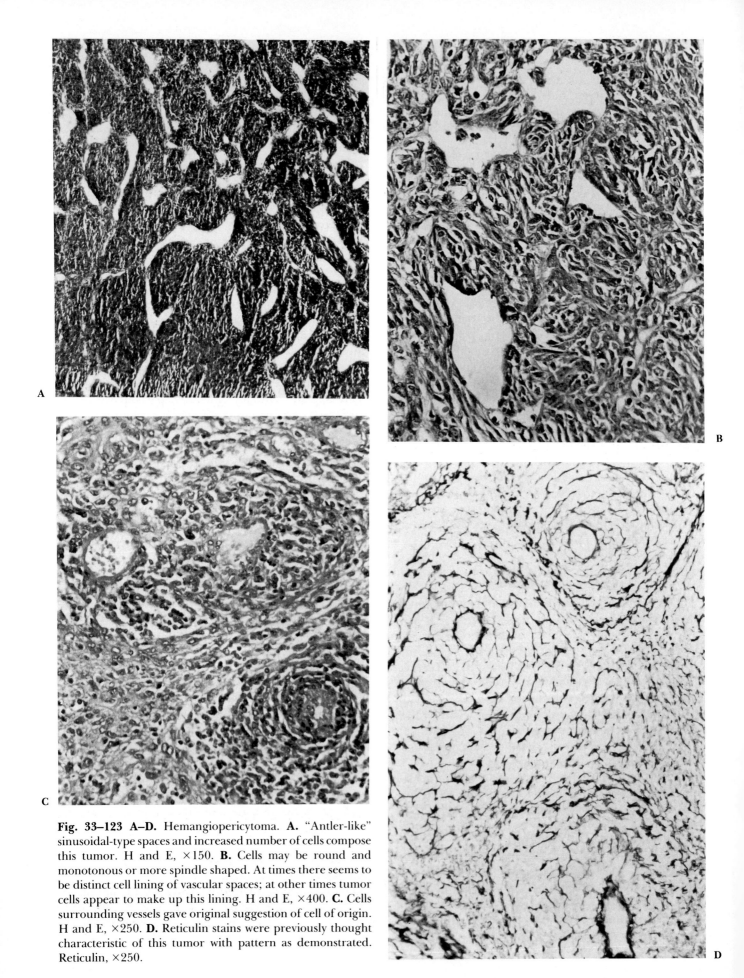

Fig. 33–123 A–D. Hemangiopericytoma. **A.** "Antler-like" sinusoidal-type spaces and increased number of cells compose this tumor. H and E, ×150. **B.** Cells may be round and monotonous or more spindle shaped. At times there seems to be distinct cell lining of vascular spaces; at other times tumor cells appear to make up this lining. H and E, ×400. **C.** Cells surrounding vessels gave original suggestion of cell of origin. H and E, ×250. **D.** Reticulin stains were previously thought characteristic of this tumor with pattern as demonstrated. Reticulin, ×250.

mas may have this pattern, which should be distinguished by the connection with the pleura and more collagen associated with individual cells. Peripheral carcinoid tumors, especially the spindle cell forms, should have neurosecretory features, and often have nearby basilar cell hyperplasia in bronchioles. I have seen metastatic melanoma have this pattern. Metastatic sarcomas such as synovial sarcomas should also be considered. Glomus tumors have cells in the size range of the low-grade hemangiopericytomas, but have more ectatic larger vascular channels, and by electron microscopy have characteristics of smooth muscle, including dense bodies and dense plaques.

Chondrosarcoma

These very rare primary sarcomas of lung were first described as enchondromas of lung, with the first description attributed to Wilks in 1862.[823] It is difficult to evaluate many of the early cases, as criteria were established only in the 1940s, to diagnose better differentiated chondrosarcomas. Some of the older cases may no longer qualify for this category. One must also be sure it is not a description of a large hamartoma or chondroma. In a 1972 review, Morgan and Salama,[824] using very restrictive criteria to eliminate chondrosarcomas of other sources possibly spreading to the lung, described eight cases in the lung, including two with pulmonary vascular invasion, one being predominantly in the pulmonary artery[781] and another involving the pulmonary vein[782]; this later case apparently spread to the pulmonary vein from a parenchymal tumor mass.

A few of these may be in the category of larger vessel chondrosarcomas, but some are most likely truly parenchymal. Others have been described in the tracheobronchial tree.[825,826] One must suspect metastases if the lesions are multiple. An early case described as chondrosarcomatosis of the lung was wisely eliminated from consideration by Morgan and Salama,[827] and is now known to be a case of epithelioid hemangioendothelioma of lung with dystrophic chondrification. (See following.)

Morgenroth et al.[826] in 1989 and Bailey and Head[828] in 1990 updated the known cases and reviewed four to six cases in the trachea, five or so in the major bronchi, and six to nine in the segmental or more peripheral bronchi. Bailey and Head[828] described a presumed primary pleural chondrosarcoma with lung or bony changes who was surviving 13 years later without tumor recurrence. On the other hand, Morgenroth et al.[826] noted a 6-cm chondrosarcoma of the left-lower-lobe bronchus, and this patient died 8 months later of massive mediastinal nodal spread. Another case recurred first at the bronchial line of excision several times before spreading to the mediastinum.[829] At times a period of slow growth is noted following a very rapid increase in tumor size.[824] In another series, most were dead within 6 months.[825] Pleural spread can occur from adjacent structures such as rib primaries.[830]

Five of the seven cases reviewed by Morgan and Salama[824] contained calcification or ossification in the chondrosarcomas. This finding is worthy of caution, as there is a radiographic dictate that calcified pulmonary coin lesions are benign.[831] In most cases this is true, but chondrosarcoma and osteosarcoma are notable exceptions.

Grossly, these tumors appear variegated and nodular, with some cartilaginous, translucent grey-white areas admixed with cystic areas, some with more densely calcified areas, and some with focal necrosis and hemorrhage. Microscopically, most are reported as rather well-differentiated chondrosarcomas. This is usually the only differentiation in the pulmonary tumors so classified. However, chondrosarcoma may be evident in other tumors, as is noted here.

Osteosarcoma

Osteoid differentiation may occur in pulmonary blastomas or carcinosarcomas, and may be a component of sarcomas with mixed differentiation, whether of larger vessel or parenchymal origin. Primary pulmonary osteosarcomas are quite rare. Reingold and Amromin[831a] in 1971 added 2 cases to the 3 they found in the literature. In a review of 18 pulmonary sarcomas from the Mayo Clinic in 1982 by Nascimento et al.,[832] 2 were so classified, and it was noted that each was a high-grade osteosarcoma.

A caution is noted here. Occasionally, on further sampling what were originally thought to be primary osteosarcomas showed epithelial areas, occurring in two of five cases reported by Colby et al.[233] and one of two reported by Loose et al.,[234] the latter being in a case where the epithelial nature was detected only in the mediastinal recurrence. (See also **Carcinosarcoma** section.) By 1990 there were a total of only about 10 cases without any malignant epithelial components,[241] and a few more of these might have been reclassified if the rare foci of cancer had been identified. This figure compares with a total of about 200 cases of extraskeletal osteosarcoma in all sites by 1987.[234] One was diagnosed by CT scan and pleural biopsy.[833]

These tumors vary in size from 4 cm to "massive." As one would expect, grossly these tumors are hard, pearly grey, and often have chalky-white opaque areas. Small cystic areas may occur. Microscopically, besides malignant osteoid and benign and malignant chondroid areas, areas of more monotonous spindle cells may intermix with some pleomorphic and more anaplastic areas. How many of these should be classified as true malignant mesenchymomas is not clear.

Malignant Mesenchymoma

Mixed mesenchymal differentiation may be present in several settings, as noted. Stout[834] defined malignant mesenchymoma as a mesenchymal neoplasm containing two or more distinct areas of mesenchymal differentiation besides fibrosarcoma pattern (Fig. 33–124). Only two cases have been published under this title in the lung, but perhaps some of those listed in the foregoing sections should be rightly considered for this designation. Certainly one case published as MFH of the trachea qualifies,[735] as do several in pulmonary arteries.[776,835–837] In the lung, the one case described by Kalus et al.[838] was perihilar, 4 cm in diameter, and entrapped the right-main bronchus, and contained osteosarcoma, chondrosarcoma, and rhabdomyosarcoma in addition to undifferentiated malignant areas. The adjacent nodes were not involved. This tumor was incompletely excised and the patient died 1 month later. At autopsy, tumor extended around the lower trachea and crossed the midline to involve the opposite mainsteam bronchus; there was no tumor elsewhere. This tumor spread is reminiscent of the case of Daniels et al.[825] presented in the **Chondrosarcoma** section. The other case in lung, a 6-cm subpleural mass in a 69-year-old man, is illustrated in Fig. 33–124 from a teaching exercise.[839]

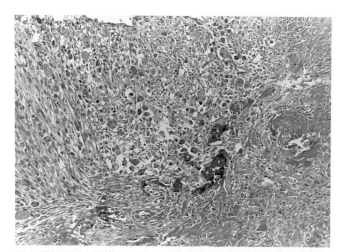

Fig. 33–124. Malignant mesenchymoma. Rhabdomyosarcoma is present in upper-center portion of field as plump rhabdoid cells; osteoid present in lower mid- and right field. Note also spindle cell proliferation toward left. H and E, ×200.

Rhabdomyosarcoma

Rhabdomyoblastic differentiation may be seen in the lung in several settings, including congenital cystic adenomatoid malformations, carcinosarcomas, and blastomas, and as a mixed component in some of the sarcomas just discussed, such as in the malignant mesenchymoma case. These are very rare primary lung sarcomas, and a total of 15 nonteratomatous cases in the lung and 3 in the lower trachea were reported in 1982 by Ericksson et al.[840] In a case reported by this group of authors, a patient died of asphyxia from a polypoid tumor. These authors noted only 3 other cases with endobronchial–tracheobronchial type tumors who died of suffocation could be found in the literatures; 1 was from a carcinosarcoma,[841] 1 an undifferentiated carcinoma,[842] and the other a lipoma.[843] The first described case of primary pulmonary rhabdomyosarcoma was in a 25-year-old man, and the tumor was described as being quite large.[844] Other more recent reviews are by Lee et al.[845] and Avignina et al.[846] A total of 6 cases have been reported in children up to 1987,[847,848] including only 3, or less than 3% from the Inter Group Rhabdomyosarcoma Study Group, even when considering those in the mediastinum.[847] Two cases in children presented with pneumothoraces.[847] For more information in sarcomas and pneumothoraces, see Chapters 8 and 35 and the section on **Cystic Mesenchymal Lesions** and **Mesenchymal Cystic Hamartoma.** It should also be noted that 6% of pulmonary artery sarcomas have rhabdomyosarcomatous differentiation.[772]

The gross description is similar to other noncalcified sarcomas. Microscopically, cross-striations are present in the cases described in the literature. The cells may be small, pleomorphic, straplike, or an admixture of these. Electron microscopy should contain definite striated muscle features. Desmin by immunoperoxidase techniques should help identify many of these tumors, as large fields can be surveyed for the rhabdomyoblastic differentiation.

Liposarcomas

These are extremely rare primary sarcomas of lung. Seven cases were reported by 1982 by Sawamura et al.[849] In this report, their case consisted of a 4-cm tumor that invaded both the adjacent bronchus and the pulmonary artery, and recurred 6 months later, causing the patient's death. At autopsy there was recurrent tumor only in the opposite pulmonary artery. The first case is ascribed to Latienda and Itoiz.[850] One has been described in pleura.[851] To date these tumors have occurred in four men and five women, with an age span of 9 to 59 years.

Histologically, some of the same problems are present with diagnosis of liposarcomas in the lung as in the soft tissue, and the interested reader is referred to the review of Sawamura et al.[849] and the individual articles for detail. Some of these cases may not stand up to modern criteria.

Neurosarcomas

In the large review of intrapulmonary neurogenous tumors by Bartley and Arean[750] mentioned in the other **Benign Tumor** section previously, 7 of 24 (29.1%) of the lesions classified as neurofibromas were malignant. In the category of nerve sheath tumors, only very rare malignancy was suggested (Fig. 33–125). As with some of the categories, some of the same problems with diagnosis in soft tissue, including diagnostic neurosarcomas, are prevalent in the lung. It has been suggested the safest way to make this diagnosis is only in the setting of classical neurofibromatosis.

Sarcomas of Smaller Vessel Origin

A certain group of pulmonary sarcomas seems best classified together as possibly derived from smaller vessel origin. These consist of angiosarcoma, Kaposi's sarcoma, and epithelioid hemangioendothelioma. Hemangiopericytoma perhaps should be included here but acts more like a parenchymal sarcoma, and thus is discussed in that section. More benign tumors, presumably of vessel wall, including perivascular chemodectoma-like bodies and glomus tumors, are described elsewhere in this section. Some of the benign and malignant smooth muscle proliferations in lung probably come from vessels. Several peculiar smooth muscle proliferations of vascular wall (LAM and intravascular leiomyomatosis-myofibromatosis) are discussed later in this chapter.

Angiosarcomas

As with other sarcomas already discussed, and perhaps even more so here, metastatic angiosarcoma is the most common form of this tumor seen in the lung. These may come from any sites where angiosarcomas arise including post mastectomy and other causes of vascular stasis, postirradiation fields, Thorotrast-exposed patients, and those arising independently in such areas as head, scalp, breast, and heart.[852,853] Spencer[854] wondered whether there is any truly primary angiosarcoma in lung. Even in a group of large pulmonary vessel sarcomas, only rarely are they classified as angiosarcoma. It is interesting the lung is not more subject to angiosarcoma, or, for that matter, other truly vascular neoplasms, considering how much of a vascular organ it is.

Three cases have been presented by Yousem[855] as "angiosarcoma presenting in the lung." These were all women between the ages of 22 and 30 at the time of diagnosis who presented with bilateral infiltrates without cardiac tumor identified. One patient later died, and no autopsy was done. The second had bilateral nodular parenchymal infiltrates and a right-atrial and right-ventricular tumor, including a possible tumor nodule in the liver, and was alive at 5 months. The third case had bilateral reticulonodular infiltrates, but on clinical evaluation had no malignancy elsewhere at the time of diagnosis. Three months later she had central nervous system and hepatic involvement, and died 1 month later. Again, no autopsy was performed. At least

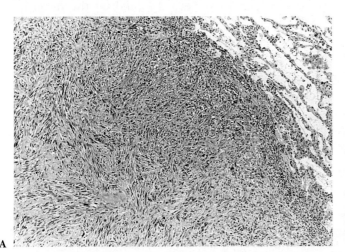
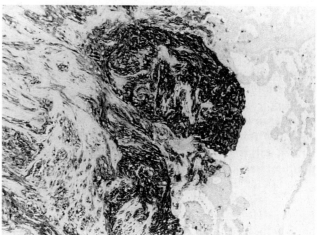

Fig. 33–125 A,B. Malignant schwannoma in lung. **A.** Pleomorphic large spindle cells form fairly even border. H and E, ×200. **B.** S100 stain by immunoperoxidase technique shows intense staining in many areas of tumor. ×400.

the second case must be considered definitely metastatic, and the other two are suspicious as being so. Because autopsies were not available in the other two cases, a full description of the extent of these lesions will remain unknown in these cases, and these authors acknowledged this with their choice of "presenting in" instead of "arising in" the lung in their title.

A more convincing but still unusual case was presented by Spragg et al.[852] in 1983. They reviewed the past literature and noted 10 possibly primary cases, but on close review many of these cases cannot be confirmed as primary pulmonary angiosarcomas. Only 2 cases are reported as most likely to represent primary angiosarcomas in their review.[856,857] Their added case was a 75-year-old man with bilateral diffuse pulmonary infiltrates, who at autopsy had diffusely hemorrhagic and heavy lungs, with the right lung weighing 2700 g and the left, 1700 g. This was a diffuse process with highly pleomorphic, malignant endothelial-appearing cells forming some thin-walled vascular-like spaces, but Factor VIII-related antigen by immunoperoxidase was negative in their case. An embolus of malignant cells, appearing to have come from vascular invasion in the lung, ended up in the femoral blood supply. The only other site of malignancy was a 0.3 × 0.1 cm presumed metastatic lesion in the submucosa of the colon. These authors argued reasonably that, due to the bulk of the disease in the lung, the lung was most likely the primary site. Their patient had a prior history of industrial exposure in South African copper mines.

One of the cases accepted by Sprague et al.[852] is from a case report in the Massachusetts General Hospital Weekly Clinicopathological Exercises. It was in a 48-year-old man who entered with hemoptysis and bloody pleural effusion and opacification of much of the right chest, with multiple bilateral nodules detected. When he died there were 1800 cc of blood and blood clot in the right side of the chest with only 200 cc in the left. After this was removed there was a large hemorrhagic necrotic mass present in the cardiophrenic angle. Microscopically, there was extensive tumor in the myocardium of the heart, along with 0.3- to 2.0-cm nodules throughout both lungs, in the pericardium, and focally in the posterior mediastinum. There was no malignancy outside the chest. It is possible that this case represents angiosarcoma of heart or serosa. The other case by Tralka and Katz,[857] published in 1963, may also not be definite.

As noted, the bulk of the evidence in the Sprague et al.[852] case would suggest lung primary. The negative Factor VIII stain is bothersome. If positive it would have helped confirm this as an angiosarcoma. Also no electron microscopy was reported in this case. These authors were kind enough to allow me to review the

malignant tumor in the lung. It is a high-grade diffuse pleomorphic round cell malignant tumor without other specific differentiation and is difficult to subtype this further, especially in view of the negative Factor VIII stain. I agree with Spencer that if there is a primary angiosarcoma of lung, it must be extraordinarily rare. A case of much more frequent metastatic angiosarcoma is shown in Fig. 33–126.

Kaposi's Sarcoma

This entity was described in 1872 by an Hungarian physician, Moricz Kaposi.[858] Classically it is a slowly growing skin and subcutaneous lesion on the extremities, usually lower extremities, of older individuals, usually men of Ashkenazi-Jewish or Mediterranean descent. These lesions tend to have low aggressive behavior, and an average lifespan of 8–14 years can be expected.[859] These patients usually die of another cause before significant disease develops.[860]

This topic is also discussed in Chapter 6, **Introduction to AIDS Pathology.** For historical purposes, in equatorial Africa, where in some areas Kaposi's sarcoma accounts for 10% of all pre-acquired immunodeficiency syndrome (AIDS) malignancies,[861] three forms of disease have been described.[862] There is the counterpart of the lower extremity localized disease, representing a nodular plaque form growing by slowly expansile growth. The second type is a localized but more aggressive infiltrative form, sometimes infiltrating bones and requiring amputation. The third form is more widespread and involves nodes, sometimes bilaterally, and rarely viscera, and has been called the generalized form. This last one is the condition most often affecting the lung in whatever circumstances it arises. As reviewed by Templeton,[862,863] there is a predominance of men in all of the subtypes listed here. In children the male-to-female ratio is 3:1, and in adults it is 10–20:1. Children usually have dissemination, including sometimes an extraordinary degree of involvement of nodes, and the disseminated form accounts for 4% of the total cases in males and 18% in females. Therefore, females tend to have a relatively greater degree of dissemination, but considering the heavy male predominance of this disease, men have more disseminated disease relative to absolute numbers in Africa. The sex ratio difference has not been explained in the past, but may relate to some of the factors discussed next in AIDS cases. About half the men in the African studies are in the age group of 15–45 years.

Kaposi's sarcoma (KS) next became known as an unusual tumor occurring in renal transplant patients. In this setting it coexists with an increased number of lymphomas, the most common secondary tumor. These

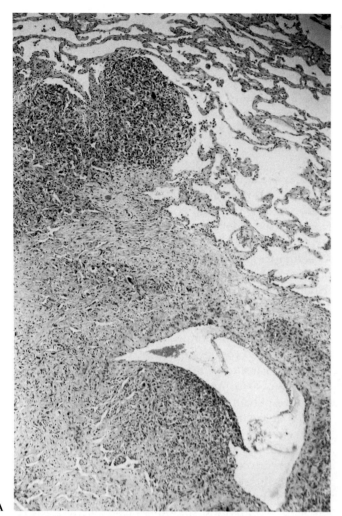

A

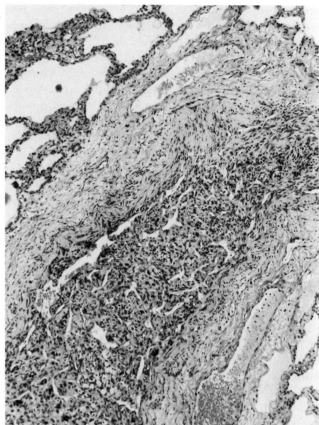

B

Fig. 33–126 A,B. Metastatic angiosarcoma to lung. **A.** Tumor cells in larger vessels at bottom extend as two nodules toward top. H and E, ×50. **B.** Intravascular malignant cells form irregular vascular spaces within confines of muscle coat of preexistent vessel. H and E, ×150.

patients have about a 400-fold increased risk of developing Kaposi's sarcoma compared with the general population in the United States, and this approaches an overall lifetime risk for transplant patients of 4%.[864,865] Of those who develop KS in this setting, 45% go on to have the disseminated disease.[866] Kaposi's sarcoma represented 3.2% of all malignancies that developed in renal transplant recipients in the Denver Transplant Tumor Registry, as reported by Penn.[866] In this group the male-to-female ratio was 2.3:1. Although somewhat rare, symptomatic lung involvement with the dissemination in both the more classical form of the disease, and renal transplant patients, has been described.[867–873]

In the early 1980s, AIDS has caused a rapid acceleration in reported cases of Kaposi's sarcoma involving the lung. These cases are most in keeping with the spectrum seen in the immunosuppressed group of renal transplant patients. About half exist as the sole lung disease, and half concur with one or more multiple

opportunistic infections, making it difficult to distinguish between pulmonary Kaposi's sarcoma and pulmonary infection clinically and radiographically.[874] Fever and cough are prevalent in pulmonary KS alone, even without infection. Pre- or concurrent infection is frequent, occurring in 79% of the cases in one series.[875]

To summarize some of the pertinent details from Chapter 6 including several nice reviews,[875–879] KS is the malignancy most frequently seen of any type in AIDS cases, occurring in 20%–25% of cases.[874] For contrast, the second most frequent malignancy in AIDS cases is lymphoma, occurring in 2%–5% of AIDS cases.[879] KS usually involves the lung after involvement of skin or gastrointestinal tract or other locations, and occurs in the lung in 20% of those cases in which it is involved elsewhere.[874] As it is usually not the first organ involved,[874–883] it may be considered a metastatic tumor in this setting. It is an unusual sarcoma in that it discretely follows lymphatic pathways in the lung, with nodal spread, and therefore may be a lymphangitic sarcomatosis counterpart of lymphangitic carcinomatosis.

In contrast to pre-AIDS KS, in AIDS there is a higher incidence of aggressive systemic spread in younger individuals, with increased incidence of lymphadenopathy and opportunistic infections, and a more lymphangitic, diffuse, and less nodular type of spread in the lung. Its incidence in AIDS cases, as with CMV, seems to be decreasing. Of the first 1000 reported AIDS cases, it was noted on initial presentation in one-third, whereas by 1987 this was so in only 10% of cases.[884] Within AIDS high-risk groups, KS has the highest incidence within the homosexual subset, significantly higher than among drug abusers, hemophiliacs, or heterosexual mates.[884] Perhaps because of this selectivity, KS does not appear to be a prevalent component of AIDS in children.[885]

Pulmonary Kaposi's sarcoma may be difficult to diagnose in life, but was so diagnosed in 2 of 70 (3%),[886] 1 of 19 (5%),[887] and 8 of 30 (6%)[888] of cases of AIDS, and with experience was done in 89% of a 1987 series[889] and in 5 of 7 (71%) by bronchoscopy.[890] At autopsy, pulmonary Kaposi's sarcoma in AIDS patients has been reported in 9 of 36 cases (25%),[891] 15 of 56 (27%),[892] 3 of 10 (30%),[893] 4 of 13 cases (31%),[894] 6 of 17 (35%),[895,896] and in 49 of 52 cases (94%).[897] The last series by Moskowitz et al.,[897] using the expanded criteria for diagnosing Kaposi's sarcomas, is discussed next. Pulmonary involvement with KS was unrelated to the length of time from diagnosis, severity, or progression of the mucocutaneous KS.[874]

Kornfeld and Axelrod[898] first reported KS presenting in the lung as the first manifestation of this disease in an AIDS case. Meduri et al.[896] and Rucker and Meador[899] reported other cases with particularly fulminant pulmonary involvement. Nash and Fligiel[895] noted a tendency for lesions to follow airways and vessels and to be in regional nodes. Ognibene and associates[874] and Meduri and associates[896] emphasized this pattern and also noted red to violaceous to blue visceral pleural plaques. Purdy et al.[880] clearly showed patterns of involvement in the lung were lymphangitic. Similar bright to dark red to violaceous lesions have been seen in the mucous membranes of the tracheobronchial tree, and are nicely illustrated with correlative histology and color photos of the in situ lesions by Pitchenick and associates.[900] Many patients with pulmonary KS develop hemoptysis, and a few have bloody pleural effusion.[880]

The lesions of Kaposi's sarcoma can be focal and can be quite difficult to diagnose, specifically in their early form. Even in the more obvious lesions in the bronchial mucosa, biopsies are often not diagnostic. Nash and Fligiel[901] noted, in two separately reported cases, that of

44 slides of lung tissue in their two cases of open lung biopsies, only 5 slides had focis of diagnostic tumor. Some believe that the diagnosis on small fragments of tissue is difficult at best and hazardous or impossible at worst.[874,896,901] Others think it is helpful if diagnostic areas are present,[880,890,897] and, as noted, accuracy of diagnosis seems to be significantly improving with experience.

Grossly, the surface of the lungs may show, in the visceral pleura, flat to slightly raised disk-shaped red to violaceous plaques (Fig. 33–127). These have not been described on the parietal pleura. A few changes have been noted in the lung parenchyma. Most striking is lymphangitic thickening by tumor, giving a red to red-blue discoloration about bronchopulmonary rays, sometimes appearing as fusion of bronchioles in accompanying pulmonary arteries, in interlobular septa, and focally thickening the pleura (Figs. 33–127 and 33–128). There are sometimes nodules of red to purple to grey tumor that vary in size up to 0.5 cm. These may coalesce to form larger tumor densities. The nodes may be involved by spongy red-to-grey material replacing the usual translucent tan architecture. Central carbon deposition, so common in these nodes, may also be disrupted. The tracheobronchial mucosa may have the plaques as described. In addition to Kaposi's sarcoma, there is also an admixture of other disease events, such as opportunistic infection (Fig. 33–127) and respiratory distress syndrome, and nonspecific changes that will add other densities to the gross findings.

Microscopically, lesions may be subtle, especially when focal. Attention should be paid to the areas of expected lymphatic routes. In the more solid regions, spindle cells are in loose fascicles with some tendency to form interdigitating fascicles (Figs. 33–128 and 33–129). There are slitlike spaces, often without identifiable endothelial cells and/or lining tumor, with abundant scattered red cells (Fig. 33–129) and some hemosiderin, both in these spaces and in the more solid part of the tumor. The smooth muscle of the bronchioles and pulmonary arteries may be infiltrated by tumor, giving it a thickened appearance, almost like granulation tissue. The larger bronchi show focal spindle cell and hemorrhagic proliferations in the involved submucosa (Fig. 33–130). Fairly extensive acute intraalveolar hemorrhage may be present, especially at the time of death. This background of acute hemorrhage can be confusing and may possibly obscure some of the lesions that would be more obvious without it. Movat's pentachrome stain is one stain that offers contrast between red cells and yellow connective tissue, with black elastic tissue, and may be of assistance in sorting these three components from the rather homogeneous eosinophilic counterstain of H and E. In the nodular

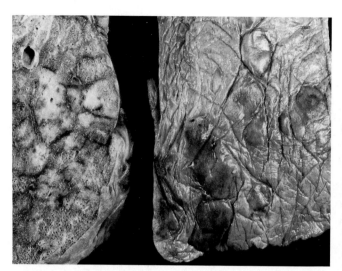

Fig. 33–127. Kaposi's sarcoma in AIDS case. On left is lung showing darkly colored accentuation of interlobular septa with lighter CMV pneumonia. On right are dome-shaped violaceous pleural nodules seen on visceral pleura. (Courtesy of R. Askins and W.B. Kingsley, Baylor University Medical Center, Dallas, Texas.)

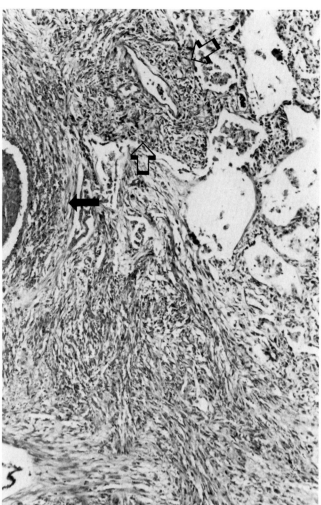

Fig. 33–129. Kaposi's sarcoma. Spindle cells separate cleftlike vascular spaces. Larger vessel shows involvement of vessel wall (*solid arrow*). Lymphangitic cuffing is present around smaller vessel (*open arrows*). (Courtesy of R. Askins and W.B. Kingsley, Baylor University Medical Center, Dallas, Texas.) H and E, ×250.

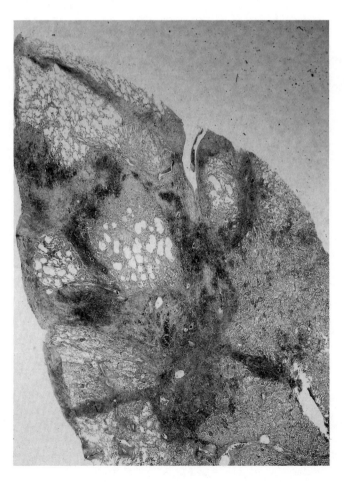

Fig. 33–128. Kaposi's sarcoma. Lymphangitic spread, appreciated at this low power, involves bronchopulmonary rays and interlobular septa along with focal pleural involvement. (Courtesy of R. Askins and W.B. Kingsley, Baylor University Medical Center, Dallas, Texas.) H and E, ×6.

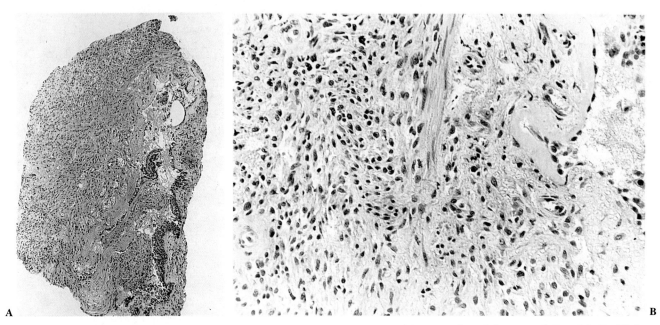

A   B

Fig. 33–130 A,B. Kaposi's sarcoma on transbronchial biopsy. **A.** Low power of bronchial wall with nodule spindle cells on one side and bronchial lumen on the other, with intact mucosa opposite the nodule, and sloughed mucosa but intact lamina propria on side toward nodule. H and E, ×25. **B.** Higher power view shows basal lamina of mucosa to the right in region of sloughed bronchial cells, with infiltration of Kaposi's sarcoma consisting of spindle cells nearby. H and E, ×200.

form recognition is easier, and approaches that described in the classical Kaposi's sarcoma, with more abundant spindle cells and vascular clefts. Mitoses are not prominent, but may be seen with careful examination. The tumor nuclei are elongated, moderately dark, and not greatly enlarged, but do show some anaplastic features. Intracytoplasmic hyalin bodies, thought possibly to represent a stage of erythrophagocytosis,[902] are present in a few cells on high-power examination. They tend to be in more epithelioid-appearing malignant cells. Necrosis in the tumor cells or distant lung is rarely caused by tumor, being more often the result of coexistent infection.

Another variant of the more typical Kaposi's lesions as described here has been called inflammatory, early, or polymorphous Kaposi's sarcoma. This has been described in skin in early lesions,[883,902,903] and represents a variant pattern, not necessarily a precursor to the more typical lesions.[880,897] This variant lesion consists of dilated vascular spaces with more pleomorphic cells lining them, and often are obscured by plasma cells, lymphocytes, macrophages, and some eosinophilic leukocytes. The same inflammatory reaction is seen in focal, and sometimes in more generalized, infiltrates in the interstitium of the lung. Focal collections of these inflammatory cells with blood should lead one to search these areas more carefully, and perhaps do serial sections if Kaposi's sarcoma is suspected. Of note, plasma cells in particular have been associated with these infiltrates. These lesions blend with areas of more typical KS, and were originally recognized in the skin because of this association.

Another variant, or part of the early lesion variant, is the cavernous-angiomatous pattern (Fig. 33–131), seen in pleural and interlobular septa, or around blood vessels.[904] Blood-filled thin-walled dilated channels are sometimes seen on only one side of a blood vessel, or focally in other lymphatic drainage areas, and should be a clue to this diagnosis. First of all, blood should not be in the lymphatic pathways. Second, in reactive states, the whole system should be involved equally. Dilated vessels filled with blood (Fig. 33–131C) may account for some of the pleural plaques seen from the surface (see Fig. 33–127). Similar changes may occur in nodes (Fig. 33–132) and elsewhere, both of the variant patterns and in more typical Kaposi's lesions. Early nodal spread is first seen in the subscapular sinus, again in keeping with this lymphangitic spread of this peculiar sarcoma. Thickening of a node capsule in an eccentric manner may suggest serial sections are warranted to detect Kaposi's sarcoma nearby. Nodes may be so involved as to have obliteration of germinal centers, subcapsular and interfollicular sinuses, and eventually of the medullary regions, leading to enlarged but lymphoid-depleted nodes.[894] Focally, KS may extend into adjacent fat near the nodes, or into fat adjacent to some of the

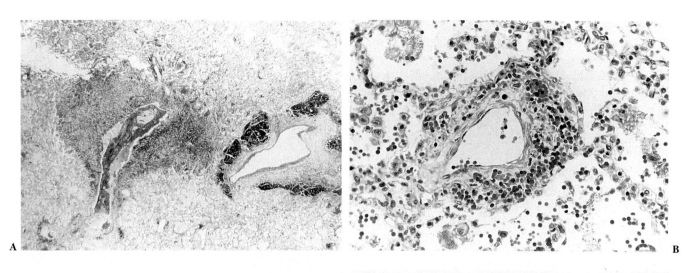

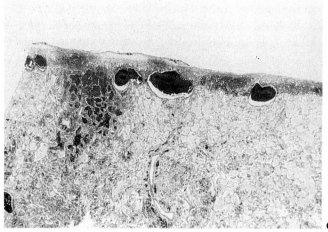

Fig. 33–131 A–C. Kaposi's sarcoma. **A.** Combination of smaller slitlike vessels of Kaposi's sarcoma presents as nodule to left and cavernous hemangiomatous pattern is seen to right. Note each is about vessel in lymphangitic pattern. H and E, ×25. **B.** Perivascular lymphangitic spaces filled with blood, even about this smaller vessel. Note spared zone to left-lower edge. H and E, ×400. **C.** Cavernous hemangioma pattern extends to pleura and accounts for some blood-filled bleb formation grossly seen in pleura in Figure 33–127. H and E, ×25.

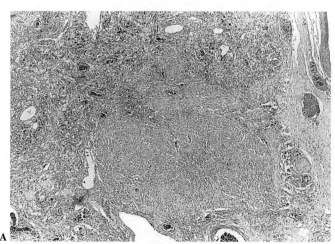

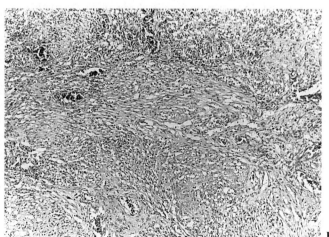

Fig. 33–132 A,B. Kaposi's sarcoma in bronchial lymph node. **A.** Spindle cell nodule is most compact in mid-lower portion of field but is also mostly replacing lymphocytes with only some carbon staining remaining in upper portion of field. H and E, ×32. **B.** Higher power field of interface between nodule and replacement of rest of node shows some cleftlike vascular spaces in nodule and capillary-type spaces above it. H and E, ×100.

more proximal main bronchi. Familiarity with these variations led to 94% of KS being recognized in autopsy lungs of AIDS cases in the series by Moskowitz et al.[897]

The atypical spindle cells that focally line cleft-shaped vascular spaces, and the increased red cells, in association with hemosiderin, plasma cells, and other mixed inflammatory cells, should help to distinguish Kaposi's sarcoma from fibrosarcoma, granulation tissue, and other fibroblastic proliferations. The hyaline droplets that are fairly characteristic for Kaposi's sarcoma are also helpful if identified. The lymphangitic distribution pattern is also useful, and is distinct from the intraalveolar organizing fibroblastic polyps, or Masson bodies, bronchiolitis obliterans, or other forms of fibrosis. Lymphangiomatosis, lymphangiectasia, lymphangioma, and other diluted lymphatics should be distinguished from dilated blood vessels by their nonred blood cells, clear to pink fluid contents, and by the absence of small slitlike spaces seen in KS. Hemangiomatosis causes dilatation of small round capillaries, and is further discussed in its own section. It is not usually accompanied by spindle cell, although some cellular proliferation can occur. Lymphangioleiomyomatosis (LAM) has rims of spindle cells, without vascular clefts, but also follows lymphatic pathways. LAM forms air cysts in the lung whereas KS does not. LAM only rarely shows acute bleeding or congestion. These two should only rarely be confused. A history of documented Kaposi's sarcoma elsewhere is very helpful.

Epithelioid Hemangioendothelioma

Epithelioid hemangioendothelioma is an unusual tumor that has now been well characterized in multiple sites. In the lung it usually presents as multiple bilateral nodules less than 2 cm in diameter (Figs. 33–133 and 33–134). Eighty percent of the cases are in women, 50% diagnosed before age 40. Cases have been documented to occur between ages 12 and 61.[309] Although one 93-year-old was believed to have this tumor, it is unclear from the case report whether this case is truly representative.[905] Considering all sites, the youngest affected patient was aged 4 years.[906] One 15-year-old girl had fairly extensive disease for her early age, with multiple lesions in the liver and lung and a bone lesion.[907]

The first mention of epithelioid hemangioendothelioma in the lung as an entity was a presentation of 20 cases by Dail and Liebow[908] in 1975. These cases were consultation cases seen by Dr. Liebow since 1962, and it was originally proposed that it was an unusual variant of bronchioloalveolar tumor with a high rate of intravascular spread, or intravascular BAT, abbreviated IV-BAT. This confusion was based on its multifocal bilateral nodular appearance and on a case with concurrent adenocarcinoma in the lung, with a typical bronchio-

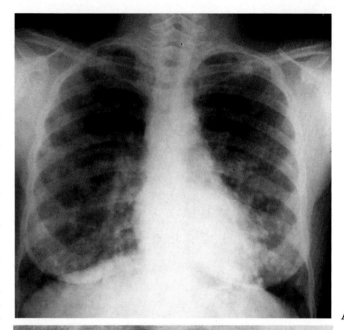

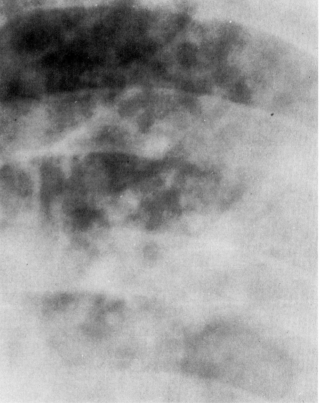

Fig. 33–133 A,B. Epithelial hemangioendothelioma. **A.** Chest radiograph of 13-year-old girl shows multiple bilateral nodules. (Reprinted with permission from *Cancer* 1983; 51:452–464.[309]) **B.** Close-up from 28-year-old man who was "relatively well."

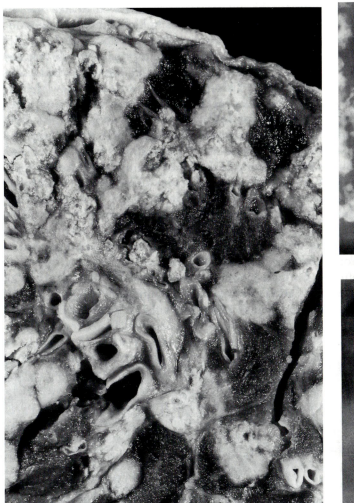

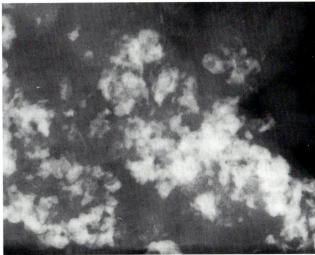

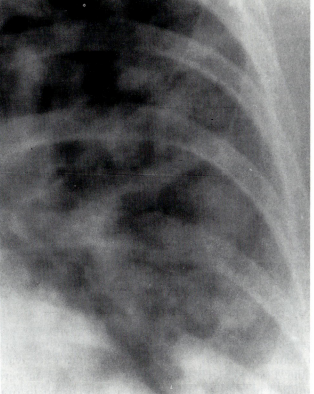

Fig. 33–134 A–C. Epithelioid hemangioendothelioma. Patient with 20-year survival. Nodules have focal calcification in roughened areas on gross **(A)** and specimen radiograph **(B)**. Chest radiograph **(C)** was taken 12 years before death! (Courtesy of R. P. Spark, MD, Tucson Medical Center, Tucson, Arizona).

loalveolar carcinoma pattern. On reflection, this latter occurrence was just a misleading independent primary (or metastatic) adenocarcinoma unrelated to the lesions under current discussion. There have been no other concurrent malignancies in the lung described with these cases.

As with many other rare or previously undescribed entities, comparisons with known disease processes occur first, followed by application of special techniques in trying to resolve the cell of origin. The tumor was first thought to have a chondroid appearance, and an early case was published by Smith et al.[827] in 1960 as chondrosarcomatosis of the lung. This same case was rejected by Morgan and Salama[824] as any type of typical chondrosarcoma, in their critical review article of primary chondrosarcomas of the lung in 1972. Its multifocal character was unlike any other chondrosarcoma. Another early case was published by Farinacci et al.[574] as "Deciduosis of the Lung," as it was discovered in a woman undergoing evaluation for an ectopic preg-

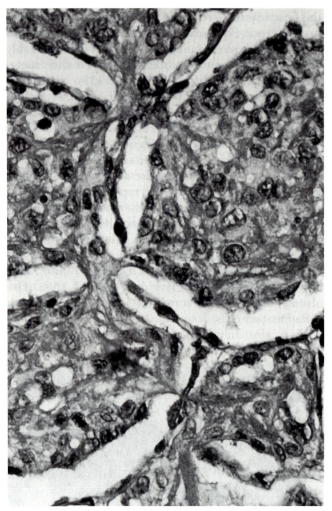

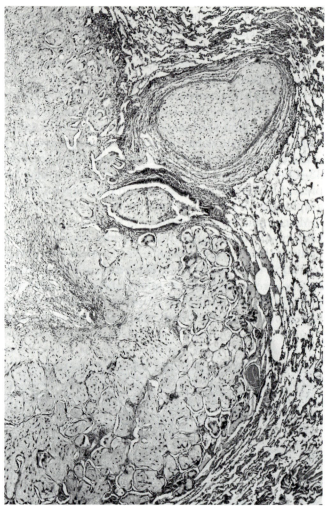

Fig. 33–137. Epithelioid hemangioendothelioma. Extension through pores of Kohn evident in multiple sites. Note focal vacuoles representing primitive vascular lumens. H and E, ×600.

Fig. 33–138. Epithelioid hemangioendothelioma. Tumor may extend in retrograde fashion into bronchioles and be in pulmonary arteries. Note rarely observed central focus of reabsorption of tumor in center of nodule. H and E, ×75.

There are low- and high-grade lesions. The low-grade lesions are easiest to diagnose because of their described conformation and their cytology (listed next). Special diagnostic techniques help confirm this tumor. The high-grade lesions are more difficult to diagnose with certainty, and must retain many of the described characteristics to be so classified, especially to avoid overlap with other sarcomas (see following discussion of differential diagnosis). In low-grade lesions there are exceptionally rare or no mitoses. Nuclei are oval to slightly irregular, slightly convoluted and bland appearing, and nucleoli are inconspicuous or small. Some nuclei have large eosinophilic cytoplasmic inclusions that are rather hyalinized, with only a rim of nucleus surrounding most of the inclusion.

Cytoplasm varies between being densely hyalinized (Fig. 33–138), finely granular, fibrillar (Fig. 33–137), or myxoid in nature. Cytoplasmic borders may also vary between being quite distinct, outlining polygonal cells or irregularly contoured cells, or being indistinct. The more myxoid is the background, the more distinct are the individual tumor cells and the more irregular are their cytoplasmic contours. Intracytoplasmic lumens, sometimes of fair size, are seen, and are an inherent and key part of the tumor when identified (Figs. 33–137 and 33–139 through 33–141). In some cases these are not obvious by light microscopy. Occasionally cytology specimens contain cells with similar features (Fig. 33–139). Factor VIII, Ulex, and CD34 stain positively both the cytoplasm of the tumor cells and these lumens. However, there is quite a degree of variability of staining in these lesions.[309]

In some tumors there is retrograde extension into terminal bronchioles by plugs of tumor (see Fig. 33–

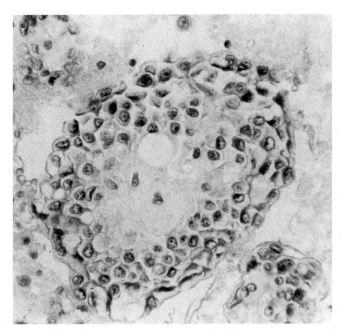

Fig. 33–139. Epithelioid hemangioendothelioma. Cytology specimens sometimes show clumps of cells with hyalinization and vacuoles. Papanicolaou stain, ×400.

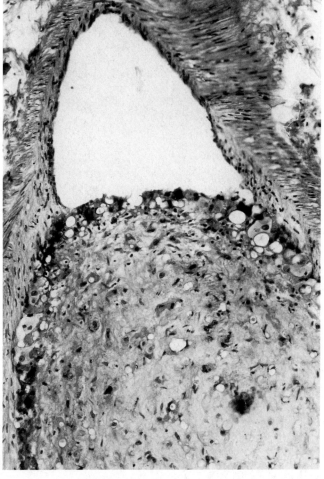

Fig. 33–140. Epithelioid hemangioendothelioma. Plugs of tumor may be in muscular arteries. Note vacuoles and background hyalinized effect. H and E, ×250.

138). Rarely these tumor plugs have been noted on bronchoscopy.[939] Sometimes pleural spread gives positive cytology with characteristic nodules (see Fig. 33–139). Vascular spread is also present in most lesions, often in the tumor nodules themselves, but at other times in vessels up to approximately 2 mm in diameter located away from identifiable nodules (Fig. 33–140). Elastic stains may help define involved vessels in the midst of the tumor nodules. Intraalveolar septal spread is rarely seen. Azumi and Churg[911] found this was most easily seen on 1-µm-thick plastic sections, but this is usually not apparent in paraffin sections. Rarely acute pulmonary hemorrhage has been described,[941] and, at least in the mediastinum, osteoclast-like giant cells have been reported.[942] (See separate section for more on osteoclasts.)

Lymphangitic spread has also been identified.[309,940] It may be in the form of elongated cells with eosinophilic cytoplasm, almost appearing as smooth muscle, or smaller groups of loosely cohesive cells that have an increased nuclear/cytoplasmic ratio and sometimes accentuate lymphatic spaces around the pulmonary artery, particularly thickening the wall. Sometimes this is seen as one-sided thickening of the vessel wall. The lymphatic spaces may be involved around the bronchopulmonary rays, interlobular septa, and pleura. The more lymphangitic spread there is, the worse the prognosis.

More aggressive tumors are usually more pleomorphic with greater variation in the nuclei, larger nuclei, hyperchromatic chromatin, and increased mitotic rate so that mitoses are found with only slight difficulty (see Fig. 33–141). These tumors are often associated with some degree of chronic inflammation. Multiorgan involvement is a bad prognostic sign, as is nonmalignant lymphadenopathy, at least as described by Dail et al.[309] in several cases.

Electron microscopy as described by Corrin et al.[916] and others* shows similar findings of cytoplasm, with

_____

*References: 309, 910, 911, 915, 931, 937.

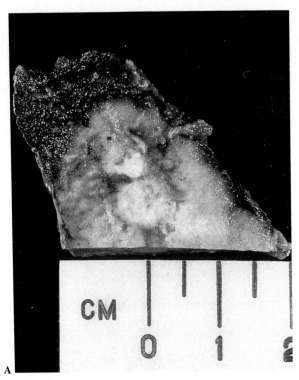

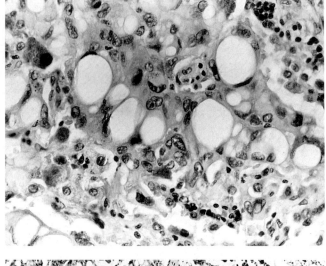

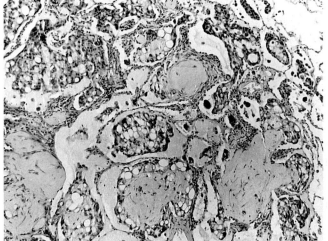

Fig. 33–141 A–C. Malignant epithelioid hemangioendothelioma. **A.** Solitary 5-cm tumor from upper lobe shows some central opaque necrosis. **B.** Edges of nodules show dense cores of hyalinization and are rimmed by tumor cells with abundant cytoplasmic vacuoles of varying size. H and E, ×100. **C.** Pleomorphic tumor cells are evident, with varying sized primitive lumens including very large ones. Mitoses are easily found. H and E, ×400. (Courtesy of Dr. J. Huehnergarth, Valley General Hospital, Renton, Washington.)

abundant intermediate filaments and corresponding reduction in other expected organelles (Fig. 33–142). The cytoplasmic membranes may have focal attachments with adjacent cells, described either as small desmosomes or as zonula adherens type. There are some pinocytotic vesicles along the cytoplasmic membranes. Although exceptions occur, usually there are no dense bodies or dense plaques as would be seen in smooth muscle. Cytoplasmic invaginations of intermediate filaments correspond with the nuclear inclusions seen grossly. The cytoplasmic lumens have delicate projections of tumor cell cytoplasm extending into them. Weibel–Palade bodies have been described in a fair number of these tumors, but also have been absent in otherwise acceptable lesions when studied by electron microscopy. The abundant filaments in the cell appear to give rise to the stroma. The basement membrane material is only partially around cells, usually away from the centers of the tumor nodules themselves, and against remnant interstitium. The filaments that compose the stroma also eventually have some collagen in them.

The differential diagnosis of this lesion in the lung consists of many lesions if one considers the diagnoses originally submitted in the series of 20 cases.[309] Practically speaking, the most common problems are with metastatic sarcomas of other types. Sarcomas, particularly leiomyosarcoma, chondrosarcoma, or osteosarcoma, can have micropolypoid filling of alveoli, but these tumor nodules usually rather rapidly eradicate the background lung architecture, become more spindle like, and somewhere in their mass give rise to their distinctive characteristics. In most of these cases mitoses are easily found. It is also unusual to have lung spread without being able to detect a primary source for most sarcomas. Very slowly growing metastases, such as in the entity of benign metastasizing leiomyoma, usually form more solid balls with entrapment of metaplastic spaces (see Table 33–1) but without preservation of the background architecture.

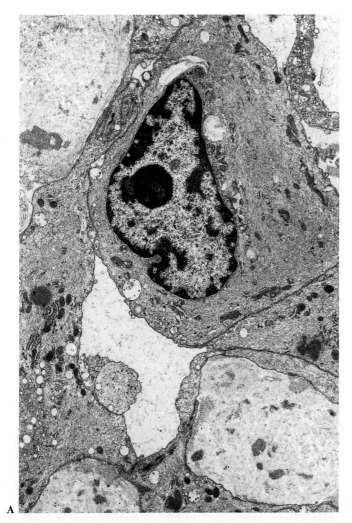

A

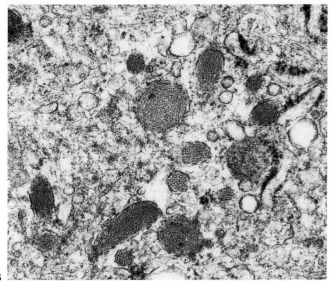

B

Fig. 33–142 A,B. Epithelioid hemangioendothelioma. **A.** Cells with abundant intermediate filaments; primitive vascular lumen. TEM, ×2,500. **B.** More organelles, seen focally, include typical Weibel–Palade bodies. TEM, ×10,000.

Another entity to be distinguished is sclerosing hemangioma. This is usually a solitary lesion, although in a few cases multiple lesions have been described. Sclerosing hemangiomas occur in women in 82% of the cases, a percentage very close to the 80% incidence in women of pulmonary epithelioid hemangioendotheliomas. The reader might also reflect on the 84% occurrence in women of small chemodectoma-like bodies (see that section, this chapter). Factor VIII and other vascular markers have been negative in the tumor cells of sclerosing hemangioma, and electron microscopy appears different in that there is no evidence of endothelial differentiation. Cytoplasmic extensions and interdigitations with other tumor cells there is also distinct (see **Sclerosing Hemangioma** segment). These tumors, by light microscopy, form larger papillae and denser areas of sclerosis, usually obliterating lung background. The proliferations carry with them a highly metaplastic (some believe neoplastic) alveolar type II cell covering, which causes confusion on electron micrographic and other studies. The micropolyps of epithelioid hemangioendothelioma lesions in the lung do not have a covering of reactive alveolar type II cells, and any lesions stimulating alveolar type II cell hyperplasia must be suspicious as not being this tumor.

As in other sites, the question of carcinomatous origin is valid because of the epithelioid appearance of this sarcoma, especially in those with distinct cytoplasmic borders and lymphangitic and nodal spread. Distinction must be made from the other epithelioid variants of vascular proliferation, including hemangiomas and angiosarcomas. An occasional case shows a more angiosarcomatous nature along with typical characteristics in the lung as described here.[943] The need for distinction from hemangioma in the lung is not as common as in other organs. When it occurs in liver, the tumor may be confused with sclerosing cholangiocarcinoma, and even venoocclusive disease. Part of the disparity in differential diagnosis in different organs results from host organ response.

No effective therapy is yet known for pulmonary epithelioid hemangioendothelioma. Various attempts have been made to treat symptomatic patients, but by this time they are usually preterminal. Radiotherapy effected temporary remission in one liver tumor associated with lung nodules, but the patient died soon thereafter. Mitotic rate of the usual lower grade lesions is so low that it may remain a difficult tumor to treat. The dense accumulation of stroma from the dying tumor cells may also mean that the mass effect of these lesions is not reversible to any degree, despite cell death, and only rarely has reabsorption of tumor been seen focally (see Fig. 33–138). Unlike most of these lesions in bone, soft tissue, or liver, lesions in the lungs cannot easily be resected because of the typical multiple and bilateral nodular infiltrates. Surgical excision was most effective in soft tissues of the extremities or for solitary internal tumors. Early experience with 10 transplantations for these tumors in liver is now seen to be unfavorable as recurrences are frequent.[921] In the lung, the surgeon often finds many more nodules than were radiographically appreciated.

These patients tend to be seen in one of two phases of their relationship to their tumors. One group dies within a year of diagnosis, these being the more symptomatic patients, with either more aggressive disease, or those toward the end of their natural course. However, a significant group may expect a longer life span. A boy 13 years old and a woman of 23 years at the time of diagnosis were alive and functioning well 20 years later despite very involved-looking chest radiographs.[309,924] Another patient (see Fig. 33–134) died 20 years after diagnosis of slow progression of her disease. At autopsy her right ventricle was 1.4 cm thick.[944] Death is usually from slow respiratory compromise, although one patient died with an acute pneumonia.[309]

The predominance of women, at least as this tumor involves the lung, suggests if these tumors may be stimulated by estrogen and should probably be estrogen or progesterone receptor positive, even though initial evaluations are conflicting. One case report by Nakatani and associates[931] in 1985 described some estrogen receptor positivity on tissue slides from a lung lesion in a 68-year-old man. These receptors were done on five formalin-fixed tissue in cases in one series by Ohori et al.[945] and were positive in only one, being negative in the other four. However, I suspect these may turn out to be positive on fresh or frozen receptor analysis.

In 1985, a series of five epithelioid hemangioendotheliomas in the liver were reported by Dean et al.,[946] all in women who were using birth control pills. This does not explain the many patients who were not on birth control pills in the series by Dail et al.,[309] nor does it explain the occurrence and growth in those patients (20%) who are men. Also summarized by Kelleher et al.[921] was that oral contraceptives were documented in only 15 of 40 (37.5%) of additional liver cases. Certainly estrogen and progesterone analysis should be done on these tumors, and if positive, antiestrogen therapy considered. The same therapies appear effective for lymphangioleiomyomatosis or benign metastasizing leiomyomas, but then these latter lesions occur almost predominantly in women (100% and 95% or so, respectively). Exposure to vinyl chloride was reported in one case in the liver[947] and one in the skin,[948] but does not appear to be a widespread association.

Vascular —omatosis of Lung

Although the following group of lesions does not technically form one or more tumor masses, this seems to be a good place to discuss them. They are an unusual group, and most are vascular related; some appear neoplastic, although in unusual ways. The lesions to be discussed include lymphangioleiomyomatosis, lymphangiomatosis, hemangiomatosis, and intravascular leiomyomatosis–myofibromatosis.

Lymphangioleiomyomatosis

This is a peculiar and rather spectacular disease. As noted in the introduction to this section, it is included in uncommon tumors, although it is not a tumor mass as such. Although it was originally described as lymphangioleiomyoma in the earlier literature, the reader of these earlier articles should not think that that represents a tumor mass. It is distinct from lymphangiomas such as cystic hygromas as occur in neck and mediastinum, and distinct from the entity of lymphangioma in lung and that variant which has more recently been given the name alveolar adenoma (see this discussed in the appropriate earlier section). The section following this discusses the entity of lymphangiomatosis, consisting of dilated lymphatic spaces without smooth muscle proliferation of their walls, and is distinct for classification purposes from the entity of lymphangiectasia, the latter being better described in newborns. The interested reader is referred to Chapter 7 for more on lymphangiectasia.

There is debate whether this is hamartomatous or truly neoplastic, and the areas involved are central in the body, being the mediastinal and periaortic lymph nodes, rarely clavicular and inguinal nodes, the main periaortic lymphatic duct-ductus lymphaticus-thoracic duct, and it also involves lungs but peculiarly not usually other organs. Only rarely are other organs in the thoracic cavity, such as pericardium, or abdomen, such as a ureter, involved.

This entity was first described within the syndrome of tuberous sclerosis by Lautenbacher in 1918.[949] It was described without the syndrome of tuberous sclerosis by two sets of authors in 1937, Burell and Ross[950] and von Stössel,[951] and was further discussed in 1942 by Rosendal.[952] Laipply and Sherrick[953] better described this disease and recognized its nonmalignant character, calling it "angiomyomatous hyperplasia" in 1958. In 1966, Cornog and Enterline[954] suggested this might be a multiple hamartomatous lesion. The earlier literature is well reviewed by these authors and by Harris et al.[955]

Two important larger series are available, one by Corrin et al.[956] published in 1975, noting 34 cases in the literature at that time and adding 23 previously unpublished cases. Taylor et al.[957] in 1990 reviewed 32 cases accumulated from the files at Mayo Clinic and Stanford; both these series are excellent and warrant careful review by the interested reader.

These patients were all women and generally of reproductive age (Table 33–8). Most were diagnosed at ages between 30 and 35 years, and pneumothorax, dyspnea, chylous pleural effusion, or hemoptysis were the usual presenting findings, easily explained by overproliferation of smooth muscle around lymphatic spaces in respiratory bronchioles, about venules and veins, and in lymphatic drainage, including in adjacent nodes (Fig. 33–143). The incidence of each of these findings is nicely contrasted with other interstitial diseases in the work by Carrington et al.[958] (Fig. 33–144). Pneumothorax (Fig. 33–145) was the major presenting finding in 53% and eventually occurred in 81% over the course of the disease in the series by Taylor et al.[957] and was present in 43% of the cases personally reviewed by them (see Table 33–8) and 35% of those in the literature before 1975 reviewed by Corrin et al.[956] Whether it has

become a more frequent presenting finding lately is unclear, but probably better detection techniques and access to health care allow for at least some of this increasing detection. Pneumothoraces are often multiple, and in this series by Carrington et al.[958] 22 episodes occurred in 4 patients.

Pleural effusion was not documented at presentation in any of the 32 cases of Taylor et al.,[957] but did occur eventually in 28% in this series. In the review by Corrin et al.,[956] effusion was initially present in 39% of the patients and in two-thirds throughout their course. Again, the reasons for these differences in the two series are unclear. Chylous pleural effusion may result when only regional nodes are involved without lung involvement, but pneumothorax by definition requires lung involvement. Nodes were involved with smooth muscle proliferation replacement of the lymphoid tissue in the mediastinum in 69% of the cases and in retroperitoneum in 50% of the cases with lung involvement in a series by Silverstein et al.,[959] and most of those with node involvement do have lung changes but not all. Chylous ascites occurred in 6% of the Taylor et al. series,[957] and rarely chyluria has been reported,[956,958,960] presumably because of involvement of the urinary tract, specifically ureter in its course near involved periaortic nodes. Rarely, chyloptysis has been also noted.[956,957] Hemoptysis can also occur and was noted in 38% of the Corrin series,[956] in 79% of the literature before 1975,[956] and in 44% of the series by Taylor et al.[957]

These presenting complaints can be explained by the involvement with overgrowth of smooth muscle from lymphatic walls. This is nicely seen in lymph nodes (Fig. 33–146), a location where lymphatic spaces and their walls are usually unrecognizable or difficult to detail, but with proliferating smooth muscle, the lymphoid tissues becomes quite atrophic and the nodes no longer function well as lymphatic drainage pathways, causing some obstruction and leading to the finding of chylous effusions. The thoracic duct is similarly involved. Within the lung, the smooth muscle proliferates around lymphatic walls and causes further obstruction to flow of chyle, especially those in respiratory bronchioles, and can lead to air-filled cyst formation. As the cysts form next to respiratory bronchioles, the respiratory bronchioles often loose their tethering effect of the adjacent lung tissue[960a] and airflow entrapment occurs with enlarging cysts. Cyst formation is accompanied by degeneration of parenchymal connective tissue, both collagen and elastic tissue,[961,962] in a fashion similar to cyst formation in emphysema[963] and histiocytosis.[964] Some of the cysts in the subpleural area may rupture and

Table 33–8. Clinical and radiographic findings in 32 women with lymphangioleiomyomatosis[a]

	At onset	During course
	Number of women (%)	
Symptoms		
Dyspnea		
Resting	0	13 (41)
Exertional	15 (47)	30 (94)
Cough	4 (12)	13 (41)
Chest pain	4 (12)	11 (34)
Chyloptysis	0	1 (3)
Hemoptysis	3 (9)	14 (44)
Findings		
Pneumothorax	17 (53)	26 (81)
Chylothorax	0	9 (28)
Wheezing	0	3 (10)
Chylous ascites	1 (3)	2 (6)
Chest radiography		
Normal	1 (3)	0
Reticulonodular change	15 (47)	30 (94)
Cysts or bullae	4 (12)	13 (41)
Effusion	0	9 (29)
Pneumothorax	17 (53)	26 (81)
Hyperinflation	0	8 (25)

[a]Reprinted with permission from Taylor JR, Ryu J, Colby TV, Raffin TA. Lymphangioleiomyomatosis: Clinical course in 32 patients. N Engl J Med 1990;323:1254–1260.

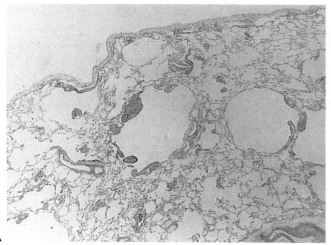

A

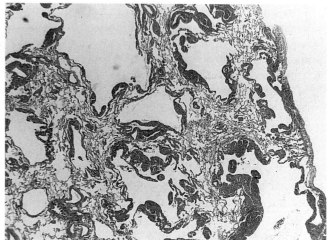

B

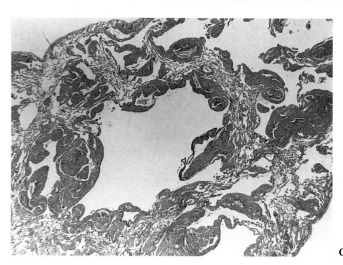

C

Fig. 33–143 A–C. Lymphangioleiomyomatosis. Three different cases have varying densities of muscle proliferation in cyst walls. Note relatively normal intervening lung parenchyma in each. **A.** Mild degree of smooth muscle proliferation, producing cysts around terminal bronchioles in center and subpleurally. H and E, ×50. **B.** Moderately–severe smooth muscle proliferation at first appears random until its relationship to lymphatic pathways is noted. H and E, ×50. **C.** Severe degree of muscle thickening. Note cysts are only moderately larger in comparison with A and B and that superimposition of focal thickenings of cyst walls could give a reticulonodular appearance on chest radiographs in **C.** H and E, ×50.

cause pneumothoraces. Lymphatic wall smooth muscle proliferation about venules and veins leads to their obstruction, causing bleeding and hemoptysis and hemosiderin deposits.

This is a disease rarely diagnosed before the age of 20, or after the age of 50 years, but a few exceptions occur at both extremes. In the series by Taylor et al.,[957] two patients were postmenopausal, aged 49 and 61, and of note both were receiving exogenous estrogens. In that series there was a 44-month delay in diagnosis after onset of symptoms. The symptoms at presentation during the course of the disease in this series are shown in Fig. 33–8.

Radiographic examinations of the chest most frequently show pneumothoraces, as this is the most common presenting finding. The lungs may be normal, this being described in only 1 of 32 cases (3%) in the Taylor series,[957] but, of note, these authors have described "clear lung fields" in most of those who are presenting with pneumothorax. This is in contrast to that illustrated in Fig. 33–145. Cysts may be outlined by slight

thickening around their edges. This was originally described on plain films as a reticular pattern, but with CT scan, was seen to be edge walls of cyst (see Figs. 33–143 and 33–145). Of interest, Kerley B lines on chest radiographs, indicating thickening of the interlobular septa, are not as frequently described as would be expected by the incidence of chylous pleural effusion. The cysts are dramatically shown by CT scan (Fig. 33–147), vary from small to large, involve all areas of lung fields, from superior to inferior and central to peripheral, and correlate with the gross findings nicely (Fig. 33–148). CT scans were more accurate in detecting cysts in several larger series[965–969] (Fig. 33–147). Air trapping has been documented by dynamic ultrafast high-resolution CT.[969] It has been questioned whether absence of cysts by CT scan exclude this disease, and certainly it is a sensitive procedure for suggesting it. Taylor et al.[957] suggested the jury is still out on this. I believe negative CT scans most likely do exclude this disease in all but the very earliest asymptomatic stages, when presumably those scans would not be ordered. The walls of the cyst

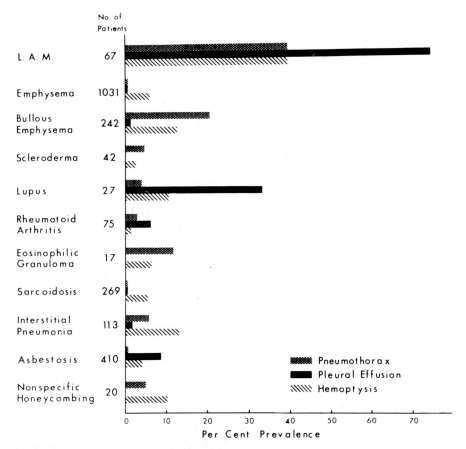

Fig. 33–144. Lymphangioleiomyomatosis (LAM). Incidence of pneumothorax, hemoptysis, and chyloud pleural effusion graphed in relationship to multiple other diseases. (Reprinted with permission from Am Rev Respir Dis 1977;116:977–995.[958])

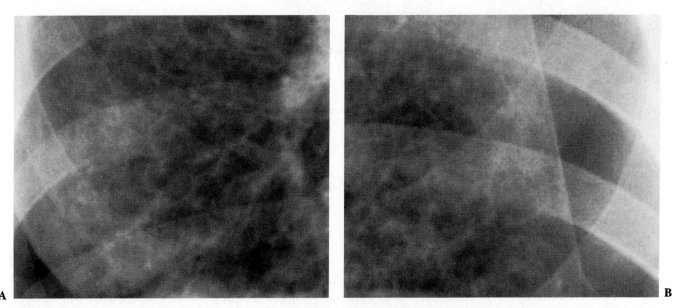

Fig. 33–145 A,B. Lymphangioleiomyomatosis; 25-year-old woman with biopsy-proven disease. Early cystic change is seen bilaterally. **A.** Expanded right lung. **B.** Pneumothorax is seen in left chest.

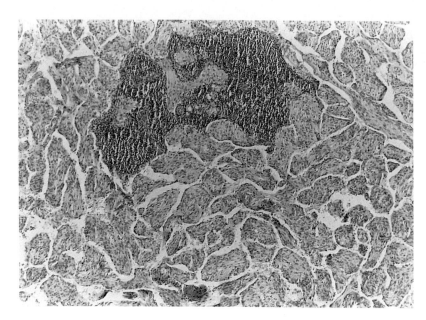

Fig. 33–146. Lymph node in lymphangio-leiomeiomytosis. Smooth muscle prolifera-tion of lymphatic wall in this pulmonary hilar lymph node has replaced all but small amount of lymphoid tissue. H and E, ×100. (Contributed by D. Runckel, MD, Salem Hospital, Salem, Oregon.)

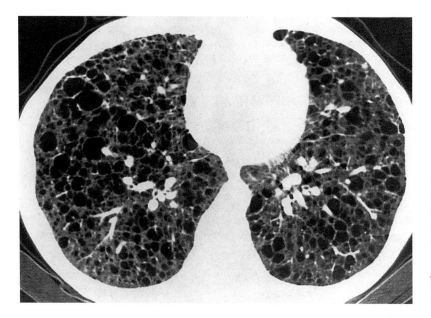

Fig. 33–147. Lymphangioleiomeiomytosis lung disease in tuberous sclerosis. High-resolution CT scan shows myriad thin-walled cysts throughout lungs. Intervening lung tissue is normal. Refer to Fig. 33–143 and correlate with Fig. 33–148. (Courtesy of Dr. J.D. Godwin, University of Washington School of Medicine, and reprinted with permission.[1069])

on CT scan vary from being imperceptible to 2 mm in thickness[968] and correlate with the findings by histology. Of interest, bronchography contrast material does not fill the cysts.[970,971] At times enlarged lymph nodes are seen with CT scans, having been described in 4 of 7 patients in one series,[965] while only 1 was suggested on plain film in this series. Also confirmed on CT scan are pneumothoraces, pleural fluid, and sometimes pericardial fluids.

Pulmonary function tests show obstructive changes earlier and a mixture of obstructive and restrictive changes later, with some diffusion defects that have been described as rather significant. Of interest, in the large series by Taylor et al.[957] the only ones presenting with restrictive defects were those having had tube thoracostomies or pleurodesis, but restriction developed later in others. The differential diagnosis by CT scan is with emphysema or cystic pulmonary histiocytosis X (eosinophilic granuloma)[972,973] (see differential diagnosis at end of this section).

The gross appearance of the lungs are quite characteristic. At surgery, there are multiple air-filled cysts forming protruding dome-shaped pleural changes, and the surgeon might describe a weeping of chylous fluid from the pleural surfaces. The nodes are rubbery, and the thoracic duct may be quite thickened, cigar shaped, and rubbery likewise. The lungs are essentially replaced by cysts of varying sizes, although in earlier involvement normal lung parenchyma between the cysts may be seen. These cysts vary usually from quite small to about 3 cm, although rarely isolated ones up to 6 cm have been described (see Fig. 33–148). In end-stage disease, the lungs are voluminous.

Microscopically there is a proliferation of plump spindle cell smooth muscle, sometimes with large and focally clearer leiomyoblastic-like cells. These outline spaces around terminal bronchioles, often with bronchiolar mucosa at one edge and a protrusion of the adjacent pulmonary artery into cysts. Figure 33–143 illustrates three different thicknesses of wall involvement; note however that cysts are present in all three. These smooth muscle proliferations can be focally identified around lymphatic spaces (Fig. 33–149 and 33–

150). Also, in some there is focally smooth muscle accentuation in the subpleural zone in the region of lymphatics, similar to the smooth muscle seen in lymph nodes (Fig. 33–151). Lymphatic spaces are dilated, and there can be variable degrees of hemosiderin and fresh blood, sometimes to rather extraordinary degrees. Occasionally there is iron encrustation of elastic tissue from this iron accumulation (see Chapter 22).

The smooth muscle proliferations stain vividly with smooth muscle actin. The clearer cells have glycogen in them on electron microscopy,[961,974,975] and stain focally human melanin black (HMB) 45 positive,[398] in a fashion similar to the smooth muscle focally showing this change in renal angiomyolipomas[397] (see earlier benign "sugar" cell tumor section). There may be lymphatic space dilatation in interlobular septa and around bronchopulmonary rays and in pleura. Occasionally there is intraalveolar edema, but this is less striking in the usual case than one would expect.

Open lung biopsies are often used to make the diagnosis. Because of the patchy nature of this disease, it

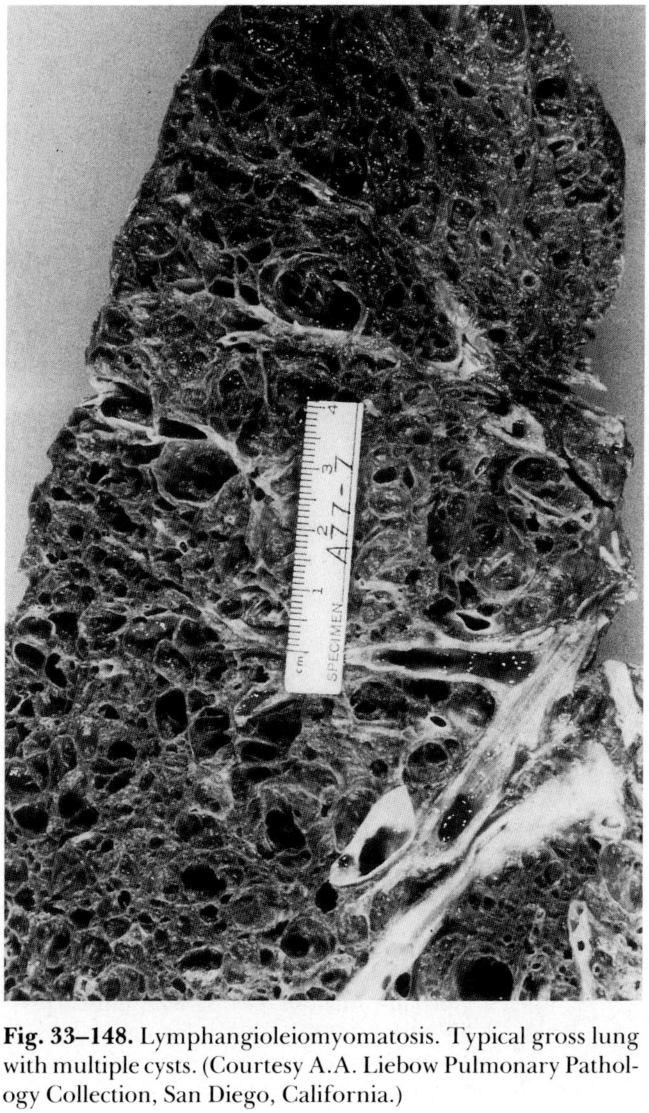

Fig. 33–148. Lymphangioleiomyomatosis. Typical gross lung with multiple cysts. (Courtesy A.A. Liebow Pulmonary Pathology Collection, San Diego, California.)

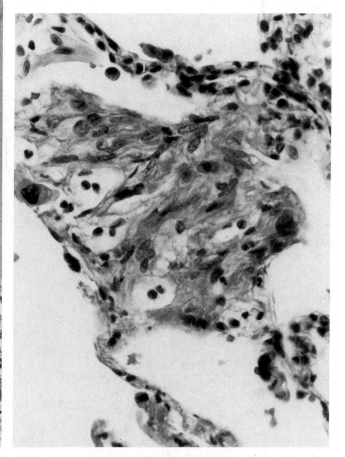

Fig. 33–149. Lymphangioleiomyomatosis. As linear portions of smooth muscle are cross sectioned, they appear as nodules on alveolar septa. Note atypia of cells. H and E, ×400.

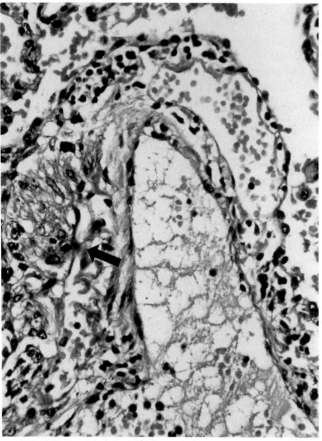

Fig. 33–150. Lymphangioleiomyomatosis. Note smooth muscle proliferation focally in lymphatic space around vessels (*arrow*). H and E, ×250.

would be expected that some transbronchial biopsies would not sample the characteristic lesions. However, if proliferating smooth muscle is present in a characteristic pattern, this diagnosis can be made.[950,976,977] In the series by Taylor et al.[957] of five transbronchial biopsies, all initially considered nondiagnostic, on a review by a skilled pulmonary pathologist, these were considered diagnostic in three and possibly another of the five.

Because these lesions occur predominantly in reproductive-age women, a role for estrogen stimulation has been hypothesized. Patients with this disease have been shown to have worsening effects with exogenous estrogen administration,[978–981] and several patients in the Taylor et al. series[957] who were postmenopausal were on estrogen replacement therapy. Also, this disease has been noted to worsen during pregnancy[982,983] and even during menses,[960a] and become somewhat better with menopause. As reviewed by Taylor et al.[957] receptor analysis has been done and the results are variable, some showing positivity for both receptors, some for one or the other and some have negative receptors. Of interest, it does not seem to matter for treatment purposes whether the patients are receptor positive or not.

Most consider this a hamartomatous change because of its peculiar central location. Allen in 1990[694] proposed that this, among other low-grade to benign predominantly female disorders outside the uterus, perhaps represented metastases. He did not define the source of proposed metastases in LAM, but most other lesions he discussed were from the uterus. Only one study of which I am aware cites six cases of smooth

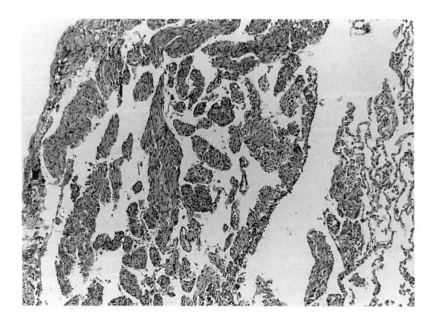

Fig. 33–151. Subpleural zone in lymphangioleiomyomatosis. Occasionally muscle proliferating in subpleural lymphatic spaces presents an accentuated subpleural zonal effect. Pleural space is to left. H and E, ×50.

Table 33–9. Lung disease in tuberous sclerosis and lymphangioleiomyomatosis

	Tuberous sclerosis	Lung disease with tuberous sclerosis	LAM
Age	<20	21–50	18–61
Sex	Male female	Female only	Female only
Family history	50%	20%–25%	—
Nodes involved	0	19%	67%
Chylothorax	0	6%	67%–74%
Pneumothorax	0	3%–50%	30%–43%
Mental retardation	46%–90%+	20%–45%	0
Seizures	70%–93%	20%–62%	0
Brain plaques	Many	55%	0
Skin lesions	60%–90%	84%–90%	0
Renal angio-myolipomas	40%–80%	73%–77%	15%
Complete triad	28%–Many	19%–52%	0

muscle proliferations in the uterus in eight cases of LAM.[984]

The lung changes in cases of tuberous sclerosis with lung disease are identical to lymphangioleiomyomatosis (LAM), and most now consider this a forme fruste of tuberous sclerosis.* Certainly there are multiple cases that show overlap (Table 33–9). Cases with tuberous sclerosis with lung disease are predominantly in women of reproductive age. Some have argued that this is a separate disease, and indeed those cases have less nodal involvement and less chylous pleural effusion than occur in typical LAM. I have wondered if the diseases are detected earlier because these patients generally are under closer medical observation, but in the Silverstein et al. review,[959] their average age of diagnosis was 33, identical to those in the large series by Taylor et al.[957] This remains unexplained but the pathology is identical and, with the exception of the degree of nodal involvement and pleural effusion, I think they should be considered synonymous. In those cases with tuberous sclerosis and lung involvement, it is interesting that the patients are older than the others who, when they have the full-blown spectrum of tuberous sclerosis, often die by the age of 20. Also, the general group of tuberous sclerosis has equal sex incidence and is diagnosed at an earlier age. The incidence of those with tuberous sclerosis having lung disease is generally quoted as 0.1%–1.0%,[990] and in a study of 355 patients at Mayo Clinic[991] followed with tuberous sclerosis, 49 have died, 40 from the effects of tuberous sclerosis, of whom 4 died of the effects of LAM from 10 (3%) of the total group who had this disease. More frequently death results from renal

disease from angiomyolipomas and/or cysts, and/or brain disease from involvement with tubers and/or seizures. In only one instance, of four generations involved with tuberous sclerosis, were a mother and a daughter both involved with lung disease–LAM.[990]

Also, in considering all cases of chylous pleural effusion,[992] this finding is much more frequent in secondary lymphomas or postoperative disruption of lymphatic drainage. It is estimated that 0.24%–0.5% of all postoperative thoracic surgical cases will have chylous pleural effusion.[992] The incidence of pneumothoraces in LAM is considered several orders in magnitude less than the incidence of spontaneous pneumothoraces.[957]

Rarely, LAM is associated with multiple other nontuberous sclerosis-associated-type abnormalities,[993] and in two cases there have been hyperplastic parathyroid tissue,[993,994] in another there were noncaseating granulomas,[995] and a rare one has hemopericardium.[996] These are all probably within the background spectrum of disease unrelated to this. Of course, overlap is more frequently seen with those entities which are a part of tuberous sclerosis (see Table 33–9).

Treatment has been directed originally at obliterating the causes for leaking of chyle, such as with pleural space obliteration, ligation, or resection of the main lymphatic drainage, or removal of hilar lymph nodes. These generally prove to be unsuccessful in slowing progressive deterioration. Radiation also is not helpful, and no known antitumor-type chemotherapy has been proved to be helpful.

Because of the sensitivity and stimulation by estrogen, more recent treatment attempts have been directed toward obliterating the estrogenic effect. Currently, it is recommended that methoxyprogesterone be given monthly for at least a year, followed by oophorectomy if this does not alter the course significantly.[957,997] Newer luteinizing hormone-releasing antagonists have also been suggested,[998] such as D-Try6-LHRH,[999] or goserelin.[1000] Tamoxifen and danazol have been tried but are not used very much, because they only reduce the estrogen to two- or fourfold the level of the post-oophorectomy state,[1001] and because some have suggested there may be increased incidence of pneumothoraces with this treatment.[1002] Lung transplantations have been done,[1003–1005] and it will be interesting to see whether there is any recurrence in transplanted lungs.

So far, therapies with methoxyprogesterone or oophorectomy are the standard of care,[957,997] but these have variable success, and those women who respond seem to produce an increased amount of chyle[957]; also, after a certain stabilization period, the patients tend to deteriorate. One interesting case of pelvic nodal involvement with lymphangiomyoma had a prolonged survival, 36 years after diagnosis, with the patient dying

*References: 955, 967, 970, 971, 985–989.

at age 89.[1006] It was presumed that the postmenopausal state allowed this stability in this case. It has previously been said that all patients die in 4 or 5 years,[959] and the most commonly quoted statistic by Corrin et al.[956] is that they are dead in 10 years. However, the recent series by Taylor et al.[957] shows some surprising survivability, in that all their patients who died did so within 5 years, and the others stabilized with the average survivorship being 8.7 years with no deaths after 5 years from time of diagnosis. This finding is at odds with the rest of the literature, but the number of cases is impressive and may reflect some effects of antiestrogen therapies.

There is little relationship between the initial chest radiograph appearance, presenting the symptoms, absence or presence of pleural fluid, and chance or rate of progression. However, documentation of an increasing lung volume is a bad indicator,[958] and most patients who respond have better exercise tolerance but often show no changes in their radiographic studies. This may relate to interstitial chyle accumulation.[957]

In the differential diagnosis, radiographically at least, are emphysema and pulmonary histiocytosis X (PHX) (eosinophilic granuloma or Langerhan's cell granulomatosis); both can form cysts, usually thin walled in emphysema, and usually representing cavities admixed with nodules in PHX, the latter characteristic helping to distinguish this disease from LAM. Both of these occur in smokers, have more of a mid- and upper-lung-field predominance, and PHX can occur in the same age group as LAM, but PHX is usually of equal sex incidence.

Also in the differential diagnosis of cysts is interstitial pulmonary fibrosis with honeycombing. In this instance, the fibrosis favors mid- and lower lung fields, and is worse in the subpleural zones (see Chapter 26); histologically, the cysts are filled with mucus, often representing dilated bronchioles with destruction of surrounding alveoli giving the appearance of "simplification of peripheral lung." There are more chronic inflammatory cells in the interstitium, PMNs are seen within the mucus of the dilated cystic spaces, and the interstitial tissue is composed of usually dense fibrous tissue, sometimes with younger, more myxomatous, components. There may be smooth muscle proliferation, but this is in discreet bundles in the interstitium itself; this has been termed "muscularization of lung" and appears to be a reaction of smooth muscle to contraction. Interstitial fibrosis can be patchy, but when seen often is more confluent, the cysts are not as delicate as those with LAM, and the stroma is spindle cell in LAM in contrast to fibrosis and inflammatory reactions in fibrosis. Also, toward end stage, these fibrotic lungs are often contracted whereas those of LAM are expanded; also, in LAM, the cysts are seen everywhere, are thin walled, and vary in caliber (see Fig. 33–148). The cysts in LAM are air filled and there is not the usual inflammatory reaction seen with fibrosis. The lung parenchyma is relatively normal between LAM cysts instead of densely fibrotic.

If veins are heavily involved, there may be some confusion with primary hemosiderosis or pulmonary venoocclusive disease, or other causes of chronic hemorrhage such as possibly Goodpasture's disease. Lymphatic space dilatation may suggest congestive heart failure or other forms of passive failure, or possibly lymphangiectasia in younger patients. The atypia in some of the proliferating myocytes has caused some to consider this to be sarcoma, but the distinctive cyst formation should allow this distinction. A few metastatic spindle cell sarcomas do cavitate but their walls are generally thicker and they are not limited to lymphatic walls. The entity of benign metastasizing leiomyomas was covered earlier in this chapter; some of these become very cystic, and distinction should also be made from the more newly recognized entity of cystic fibrohistiocytic tumor, which has a storiform lining.

Some of the cysts in pneumocystis have fibrotic linings, but more often occur in men and usually have association with pneumocystis (see discussions elsewhere in this chapter.) Also, in AIDS cases, Kaposi's sarcoma can involve younger people, and this can follow lymphangitic patterns but is associated with cleftlike vascular spaces with variable amounts of blood cells in them, and in some adjacent or nearby earlier hemangiomatous-type Kaposi's sarcoma lesions (see Kaposi's sarcoma earlier in this chapter). KS does not form the pulmonary cysts seen in LAM, and KS of the lung greatly favors men, although this may change in the future. The individual spindle cells in LAM are larger with more abundant cytoplasm, staining vividly with actin, in contrast to the endothelial markers such as CD34 that stain KS. Also, the proliferations in LAM are smooth muscle without small vascular spaces as are typical of KS.

This entity also needs to be distinguished from lymphangiomatosis, discussed in the section that directly follows.

Lymphangiomatosis

The term lymphangiomatosis has been applied to the spectrum of localized and systemic lesions involving dilated lymphatic channels. These entities include lymphangiectasias, whether congenital or developmental, hamartomatous proliferations, and reactive and perhaps neoplastic proliferations of varying degrees of aggressiveness.[1007]

Lymphangiectasia is most often a congenital pulmonary abnormality diagnosed in a stillborn or newborn and thought to be a persistence of dilated lymphatics in the fourteenth to twentieth week of intrauterine development.[1008] About a third are associated with cardiac anomalies, especially those retarding venous return, and this may be secondary to persistent increased lymphatic pressure.[1009] Others are associated with a wide variety of congenital defects, and in total, about 80% are associated with congenital defects. Spencer[1009] noted the absence of lymphatic valves in this disorder. (See Chapter 7 for more details in the congenital and early developmental state.) Lymphangiectasia may be more generalized or occur in adults, and in both circumstances may overlap with the disease of hemangiomatosis syndromes (see next section). Wagenaar et al.[1010] and Noonan et al.[1011] have suggested the classification of lymphangiectasias as essentially three variants: either limited to lung, with pulmonary and mediastinal involvement, or a generalized, and secondary to obstruction of pulmonary venous outflow.

Isolated lymphangiomas are congenital or developmental, and probably do not exist in the lung, but may affect lung function, and therefore are worth a brief review before discussing the entity of lymphangiomatosis. As reviewed by Enzinger and Weiss,[1008] those lymphangiomas that are congenital most often occur in the areas of primitive lymph sacs such as neck or axilla; 50%–65% are seen in newborns and infants. About 75% of cystic hygromas (see following definition) occur in the neck and 20% in the axilla.[1012] Only rarely has a case been described in the scalp with associated chylothorax.[1013] Those diagnosed in utero before 30 weeks gestation have a high rate of mortality and fetal death, and are usually detected during evaluation of polyhydramnios.[1014] These tumors have been subclassified depending on the size of spaces they produce. Those with grossly visible spaces of several millimeters to several centimeters have been called cystic lymphangiomas or cystic hygromas. Those with small but still dilated spaces are called cavernous lymphangiomas, and those composed of small-caliber vessels are called capillary lymphangiomas or lymphangioma complex or lymphangioma circumscripta; the latter are usually seen in the skin of adults and are not further discussed here. Bill and Sumner[1015] have proposed that larger spaces develop in areas of loose connective tissue, such as neck or axilla, while the cavernous congenital lymphangiomas develop in tighter areas; in infants, these most often occur in the oral cavity or skin. In a series of 61 cases of lymphangiomas by Enzinger and Weiss,[1008] only 5%–8% were in the mediastinum and 1% in the abdomen. Galifer et al.[1016] reviewed 139 cases in the abdomen in children. Another entity in the abdomen in adults that has been called cystic lymphangioma[1018] and occurs most commonly in the pelvic floor of young to

middle-aged women[1018–1020]; most of these now have been reclassified as cystic mesotheliomas.[1018,1019] Most recently it has been suggested that these represent reactive changes, and thus the term multilocular peritoneal occlusion cysts has been suggested.[1021]

Intrathoracic lymphangiomas have been described in the mediastinum and can either occur as extensions from cystic hygromas in neck, estimated to occur in about 10% of the cases,[1017] or as more isolated masses. Brown and associates[1021] have nicely reviewed 14 cases of mediastinal lymphangiomas from the Mayo Clinic and divided them by mediastinal compartment. The 5 cases in the superior mediastinum were in younger patients, average age 11 years (range, 3–27 years), and all but 1 extended from a large cervical or superclavicular location; the other focally extended into the neck by CT scans. Only 2 of the 5 could be completely removed because they extended in and around vital structures. All 5 deviated the trachea laterally. The 4 in the anterior mediastinum occurred in middle-aged individuals, average age 46 years (range, 27–63 years). Most were asymptomatic and overlapped in radiographic appearance with thymomas, lymphomas, and lymphadenopathies; these were easily excised. The 4 in the posterior mediastinum (average age, 54; range 31–76 years) divided into two equal groups, 2 with more simple masses, and the other 2 involving bone and extending below the diaphragm into the retroperitoneum. Their last case was so extensive in the mediastinum that it could not be subclassified; it invaded ribs, vertebra, and pleural space, and this 30-year-old man died of his disease. Some appear attached to the pericardium.[1022]

Brown et al.[1021] and Pilla et al.[1023] agree that 75% of mediastinal lymphangiomas that occur exclusively in the mediastinum occur in adults. Whether in infants, children, or adults, these are often associated with chyolous pleural effusions, bringing LAM into the differential diagnosis, and some are associated with bone lesions, often the ribs, but may be associated with extrathoracic bone such as the long bones of extremities. These overlap with hemangiomatosis of bone, which has been called disappearing bone disease or Gorham's syndrome, or osteolysis and angiomatosis.[1024] Multiple osteolytic lesions and chylothorax usually carry a poor prognosis.[1025] Other sites for lymphangiomas in the abdomen include spleen, liver, kidney, and pancreas.[1026]

The triad of soft tissue and bony hypertrophy of extremities, hemangiomas, and/or lymphangiomas and varicosities represents Klippel–Trenaunay syndrome. This may involve the thorax, and in a series of 42 cases, 12 such cases occurred in the thorax (29%), principally involving chest wall.[1027] Congenital absence of the cisterna chyli has been incriminated in some cases in the thorax.[1028] A large pleural-based lymphangioma has been described in a 33-year-old man, followed for 17 years with a recurrent chylothoraces, with tumor eventually surrounding both lungs and invading chest wall, vertebra, and diaphragm.[1029] I have seen a case of chest wall hemangiomatosis in a young man who had a cardiac output of 14 liters/min who eventually died with collapsed thoracic vertebra and cardiac failure.

CT scans show water density masses, sometimes highlighting cyst formation. The finding of chylous pleural effusion or ascites is very suggestive, although this may be associated with obstructing masses such as lymphomas (see discussion in LAM). Various attempts at therapy have included thrombosing or sclerosing agents, radiation, and surgery, all with variable results.

Wagenaar et al.[1010] reported three cases in young men, ages 13, 16, and 19 years, of intrapulmonary tumorous lymphangiectasia, limited to one or two lobes and the mediastinum. Each was asymptomatic. Their lymphatic cysts were thin walled and followed lymphatic channels; the cysts were up to 1.5 cm in diameter. The authors described sporadic smooth muscle in the walls of these lesions in men. There was no dilated or sclerotic veins, evidence of pulmonary hypertension, either primary or secondary, intraalveolar edema, or hemosiderosis that would indicate these lesions were secondary.

Swank and colleagues[1030] in 1989 reported a case of more diffuse pulmonary lymphangiomatosis mimicking lymphangioleiomyomatosis (LAM) in a 20-year-old woman. This was slowly progressive over 8 years. She was noted to have absence of involvement of lymph nodes or other organs; histology showed thick-fibrous-wall, dilated subpleural lymphatics, and it was specifically noted that there was no muscle in these walls. Of interest, despite this absence of muscle, she was treated in LAM with medroxyprogesterone and responded well.

Tazellar et al. in a 1992 abstract[1031] described six cases of diffuse pulmonary lymphangiomatosis, four in children aged 2–7 years, the others in adults aged 22 and 35. There were five males and one female; in none was there extrathoracic involvement. They described asymmetrically spaced bundles of smooth cells that stained for actin in four of six cases in desmin in three of six cases, reminiscent of those described by Wagenaar et al.[1010] these cases were all progressive, especially in children.

The pathology of lymphangiomatosis consists of usually generalized dilated lymphatics spaces occurring in the usual lymphatic pathways (Fig. 33–152). Long-standing cases may have very thickened walls (Fig. 33–152 A, B), may appear empty, or be filled with chyle

(Fig. 33–152 D), and occasionally have some spilled red blood cells in them.

There is confusion between the entities of lymphangiomatosis and some cases of cavernous hemangiomatosis in the lung.[1032–1037] Both are described as dilated, cavernous thick-walled spaces that follow lymphatic pathways around bronchopulmonary rays, and interlobular septa and pleura (see Fig. 33–152). Some are clearly empty or filled with chyle (Fig. 33–152D), and these should be identified as lymphangiomatosis. Others in the same route appear to have blood in them, and it is unclear whether this represents blood in transit or spillage into lymphatics.[1032] Koblenzer and Bukoruski[1033] proposed the name *angiomatosis* to avoid having to define which spaces are involved with contents of blood, as these are often identical in appearance.

I believe many cases of widespread cavernous hemangiomatosis in lung most likely represent lymphangiomatosis or pulmonary venoocclusive disease (see following). Also in the differential diagnosis is interstitial emphysema, in which the air bubbles do follow lymphatics at times, and at other times they seem to be in the interstitium eliciting metaplastic benign giant cell response. This disease is usually limited to newborn infants, often premature ones.

Hemangiomatosis

This section addresses the entity of capillary hemangiomatosis. (See the immediately preceding section on lymphangiomatosis and brief mention there of some cases of diffuse cavernous hemangiomatosis.[1032–1037]

Capillary hemangiomatosis of lung is an entity of some controversy, at least to my mind. Wagenvoort and cohorts[1038] first described such an entity in 1978 in a 71-year-old woman. By 1989, 14 cases had been reported[1039] including a small series of three patients by Faber et al.[1039] and four cases by Tron et al.[1040] These have involved patients in the age range 6–71 years mostly in the 20–40 year range.[1039] Some present with acute pulmonary symptoms, others hemoptysis and/or heart failure, and most die within 1–5 years. No therapy is known. Death usually occurs from pulmonary or cardiac failure. These reports described a multifocal, usually bilateral, widespread yet microscopically focal capillary engorgement, and a plexus of thin-walled dilated capillaries extending around and into vessels, both veins and arteries. The hallmark of the disease is capillaries that appear to fill veins and cause a secondary venous occlusion. All authors have carefully attempted to separate this from primary venoocclusive disease.

Most of the cases report similar findings of focal areas of capillary engorgement of the lung, sometimes associated with thick-walled, central or eccentric vessels, and

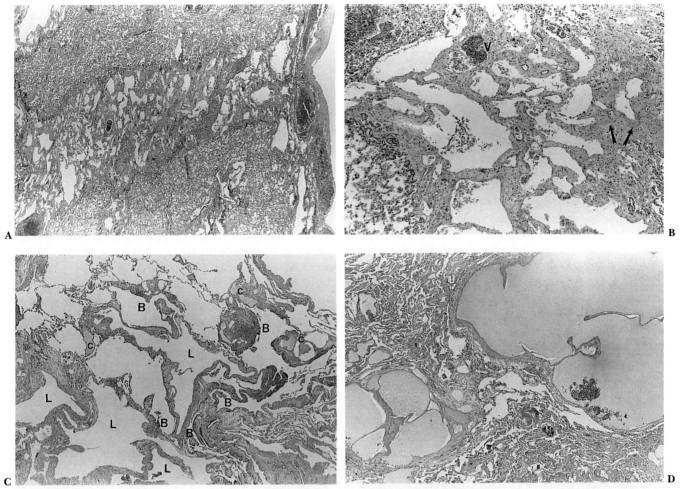

Fig. 33–152 A–D. Lymphangiomatosis. **A.** Low-power view of greatly dilated thick-walled lymphatic spaces in interlobular septum and adjacent pleura. H and E, ×50. **B.** Higher power view of widened channels and thickened walls; thickening is composed mainly of collagen, but *arrows* show remnant or proliferated fragment of smooth muscle. Note vein (V) at top. A small amount of blood has spilled into some of these spaces. H and E, ×100. **C.** At times fairly thick-walled cystically dilated lymphatic spaces (L) interdigitate in their native sites with terminal brochioles (B). Few dilated, more opaque lymphatics are seen (c). H and E, ×100. **D.** At times lymphatics are filled with fluid, and are not as thick walled or as proliferative as those seen in previous examples. H and E, ×100.

some identify an overgrowth of vessels that is thought characteristic.[1040] A secondary pulmonary hypertensive change is reported that involves thickening of the walls, both medial and with fibrointimal proliferation, but not the more severe degrees of pulmonary hypertension, specifically necrotizing, plexiform, or dilational lesions. Vascular tumors and/or proliferations were not described outside the lung in these patients. One report noted a rare familial occurrence.[1041]

By 1978, I had the opportunity to review 49 cases of primary pulmonary venoocclusive disease (PVO) of lungs, based on cases contained within the pulmonary consultation flies of A.A. Liebow, H. Spencer, and C.B. Carrington.[1042] At the time 31 had been published in the world's literature (see Table 33–10). The published cases were in younger individuals, average age 19, and we found them up to age 64 years, with a smaller percentage in youth. Perhaps this resulted from the type of case(s) referred for consultation, or because this disease is inherently challenging to diagnose, is much easier when the lesions are isolated in the pediatric population, and more complex as patients age and have heart failure and other complicating findings in the lung. Some present with acute episodes that are flu-like pneumonia (Fig. 33–153), and others have slowly progressive dyspnea. Most have widespread bilateral lesions (Fig. 33–153), and death is from pulmonary or cardiac failure. The dense areas are either small areas of venous infarcts with infarction of tissue around the periphery of the pulmonary lobule and with preserva-

Table 33–10. Pulmonary venoocclusive disease[a]

	This series (n = 49)	World literature (n = 31)
Age	6 months–64 years	2 months–48 years
	(average 27 years)	(average, 19 years)
	>48 years 12 (27%)	
	<17 years 7 (16%)	<17 years (55%)
Sex	25 M:22 F (53%)	17 M:14 F (55%)

[a] Reprinted with permission from Dail DH, Liebow AA, Gimelich JT. Carrington CD, Churg A. A Study of 43 cases of pulmonary veno-occlusion (PVO) disease (abstr.) of Lab Invest 1978;38:340.

tion of the central portion of the lobule (see Fig. 33–153), or areas of discrete congestion (see Fig. 33–154). There is usually back pressure-induced arterial hypertension, with muscular and fibrintimal thickening, but without necrotizing, plexiform, or dilatation lesions. The veins are best seen draining into interlobular septa, and within these septa themselves, they may show partial or complete occlusion (Fig. 33–154), at times appearing more cellular and spindle like, at other times more hyalinized appearing like old organized thrombi. The occlusion may be complete or partial with irregular nodules of thickening in the walls. Sometimes the vessels with incomplete and irregular thickening of their walls show a complete obstruction upstream in deeper sections. Arteries and veins can be difficult to distinguish on elastic stains as veins can become "arterialized" with a double elastic layer surrounding a smooth muscle proliferation in the media of veins. Sometime veins are quite thick walled and very muscular, yet located in intralobular septa (Fig. 33–154A). At times lymphatic dilatation is prominent (Fig. 33–154D) and can be confused with lymphangiomatosis.

The microscopic appearance varies depending on which of the multiple manifestations is most prevalent in a particular individual. The small areas of focal engorgement of capillary vessels is often exciting visually, especially compared to deflated vessels nearby (Fig. 33–155). These appear to be overly dilated, engorged, and very discrete. In pathology we are often left with deflated, fairly bloodless lung samples and thus do not truly know what normal capillary distension should be. A latex injection cast and histology section (see Fig. 2–25) in the normal anatomy chapter may be as close to in situ normal as possible. Many times there is a thickened, somewhat larger vessel in the vicinity of the discrete areas of congestion, sometimes misidentified as

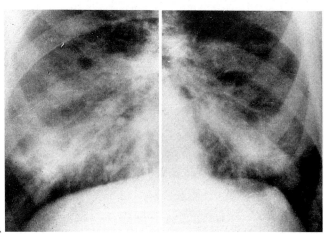
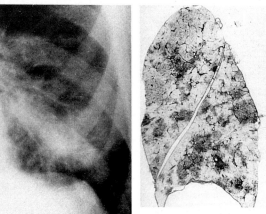
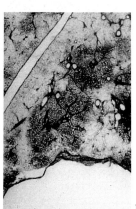
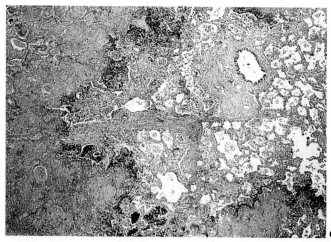

Fig. 33–153 A–C. Pulmonary venooclusive disease. **A.** Portions of bilateral lung on chest radiograph show focal infiltrates. **B.** Gough–Wentworth full mount sections show sections of both lungs have focal infiltrates–areas of congestion. **C.** Some infiltrates are accounted for by venous infarcts, with necrosis involving periphery of lobule. Note central portion of lobule is spared and pulmonary artery is mostly occluded by "backflow" arterial hypertension. (See text) H and E, ×25. (Courtesy of A.A. Liebow, Pulmonary Pathology Collection, La Jolla, California.)

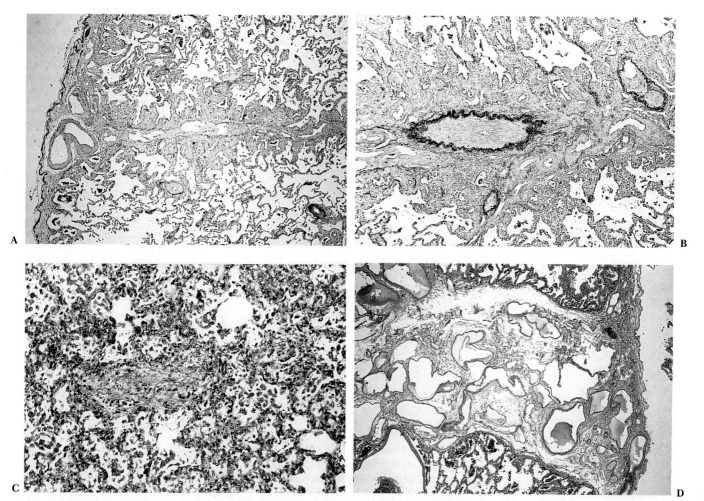

Fig. 33–154 A–D. Pulmonary venoocclusive disease–hemangiomatosis–lymphangiomatosis. **A.** Thickened pleural vessels and interlobular septum. Notice fibrotic reaction centers on interlobular septum and few small sclerotic veins nearby. VVG, ×25. **B.** Veins and interlobular septa are thickened, and central one is almost totally occluded. VVG, ×100.

C. Endo-thelial cell hyperplasia sometimes gives almost neoplastic appearance, also simulating interstitial cellular pneumonia. Note thickened vein in center of this reaction. H and E, ×100. **D.** Lymphatic spaces can become very dilated in venoocclusive disease, giving appearance of lymphangiomatosis. H and E, ×50.

an artery, but without accompanying bronchiole, and therefore most likely a vein (see Fig. 33–154). Sometimes step sections are needed to identify this. In this capillary hemangiomatous appearance, the vessels are usually thin walled, but at times approaches the thicker, small-caliber vessels of capillary hemangiomas as occur in young patients (Fig. 33–156D). Any time a discrete focus of capillary engorgement is present, one must search for an occluded venule or vein, because it is illogical to assume the rest of the lung's venous drainage is patent while one discrete focus stays distended without focal venous obstruction.

Varying degrees of fibrosis can occur in PVO and capillaries can proliferate in the areas of fibrosis, representing increased pressure attempts at collateralization. These vessels can extend around arteries and veins,

through their walls, and in their thickened intima (Fig. 33–156).

A pattern that is helpful in diagnosing PVO is interstitial thickening centered on an interlobular septum (Fig. 33–154 A, B). Sometimes this shows the capillary dilatation as illustrated, and at other times the vessels appear relatively empty and yet the interstitium appears to have too many stimulated cells in it. These can be traced to being endothelial cells in collapsed spaces, and their cellularity has been confused with cellular interstitial pneumonia or a neoplastic endothelial proliferation (Fig. 33–154C).

Backstream arterial hypertensive change in PVO has been confused with primary pulmonary hypertension. The lack of higher degrees of hypertensive injury and and funding venous hypertension changes should help

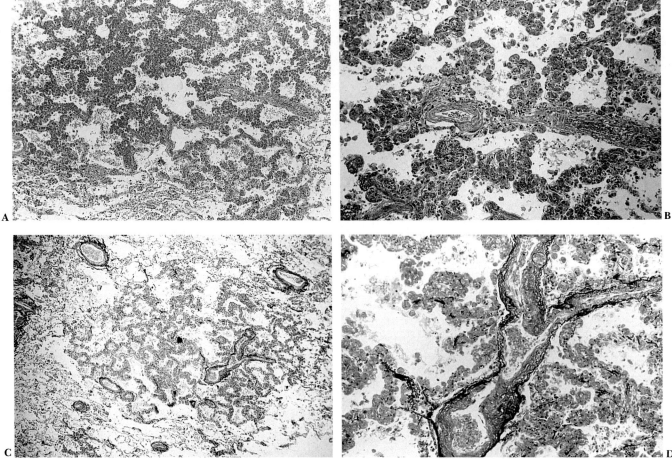

Fig. 33–155 A–D. Pulmonary venoocclusive (PVO)–disease hemangiomatosis. **A.** Discrete area of severe focal congestion. H and E, ×40. **B.** Vessel in center of **A** has thickened wall. Note degree of capillary engorgement. H and E, ×100. **C.** Same area as in **A,** with draining vessels better shown on elastic stain. VVG, ×40. **D.** "Y"-shaped vein from **C** shows regular thickening of its intima and wall with some duplication of elastic caused by increased pressure or obstruction. VVG, ×400.

separate this, and when present, venous infarcts are very helpful in indicating which part of the system is involved. As noted, these venous infarcts involve individual lobules, infarcting the peripheral portion of the lobules, and as noted preserving the central portion where the best oxygenated blood is still able to preserve tissue (see Fig. 33–153). These are distinctly separate from the wedge-shaped translobular arterial infarcts more commonly seen in lung with arterial emboli.

There can be excessive depositions of iron, leading to abundant iron-filled macrophages. Sometimes this deposits on elastic tissue, and is separately discussed in Chapter 22 under iron encrustation. An illustration shown there (Fig. 22–25) is from such a case of PVO. As iron encrusts, it can lead to foreign-body reaction with multinucleated giant cells, and some have confused this reaction with that from asbestos fibers, other dust, or injected or aspirated foreign material. At times it has been called "endogenous pneumoconiosis" (see Chapter 22).

Therefore, in PVO the admixture of these histologic appearances can lead to consideration of assorted entities in the differential diagnosis including angiomas-angiomatosis, interstitial cellular pneumonia, neoplastic endothelial cell proliferations, fibrosis of lung, hemosiderosis, Goodpasture's disease, chronic passive failure, pulmonary arterial hypertension, or lymphangiomatosis. In younger patients a proliferation of somewhat cellular areas within veins may overlap without intravascular leiomyomatosis-myofibromatosis. (See following). Usually the latter disease is more diffuse, has more obvious spindle cells, and is not so discretely centered on draining veins.

The venous drainage compartment of lung is probably one of the most overlooked portions of the lung anatomy in studying disease. I believe the entity of pulmonary venoocclusive disease is greatly underdiagnosed because of this difficulty, and because of the multiple masquerading presentations as described. In middle-aged and older individuals, the most common entity to be distinguished is chronic congestive heart failure. Pediatric pathologists are much more aware of

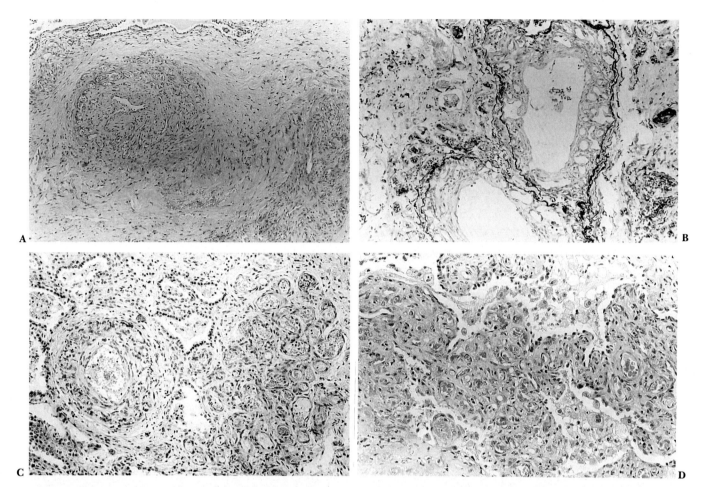

Fig. 33–156 A–D. Collateral vascular changes in pulmonary venooclusive disease. **A.** Two portions of thickened vein in widened interlobular septum with abundant fibrosis show some capillaries proliferating in vein walls, thickening their intimal coats. H and E, ×100. **B.** Capillary proliferation in intima is seen within this vein. Note some "arterialization" of vein wall with focal duplication of elastic. VVG, ×200. **C.** Small-caliber capillary proliferation inside thickened vessel to right is accompanied by larger caliber capillaries in lung to left. H and E, ×100. **D.** Capillary proliferation is adjacent to venous infarct, the latter seen just at bottom left. These capillaries can have thickened walls and focally contained thrombi, perhaps related to necrosis of infarct itself. H and E, ×200.

PVO, and as noted, their patients often have less distracting patterns in their lungs and the diagnosis is therefore easier and cleaner.

Pulmonary venooclusive disease radiographically can be suspected when there is a combination of a normal left atrium, normal left-sided heart valves, no reflex, normal injection fraction, normal-sized major pulmonary veins yet enlarged pulmonary arteries, perhaps Kerley B lines, and changes suggesting edema without vascular shunting to upper lobes. The wedge pressure can vary from classical left-sided heart failure. The wedge pressure in PVO is usually normal or low and not elevated as in congestive failure. When a small injection of saline is done with the measuring catheter in a wedged position, the pressure curve shows an immediate elevation but then tapers down to normal or low levels as the collateral flow drains off this increased pressure. This is one of the better diagnostic tests. As noted, left-sided cardiac and main pulmonary vein obstructions would lead to a persistent elevated pressure as all vessels are equally involved.

Is there a separate entity of pulmonary capillary hemangiomatosis, or is it solely one of the patterns of primary pulmonary venoocclusive disease? Certainly there is significant overlap in these two entities, as all authors agree and use the distinguishing characteristic of capillaries overgrowing and occluding veins stimulating a secondary venoocclusive pattern in capillary hemangiomatosis. It depends on whether the observer is a "lumper" or "splitter."

I favor this all being a part of primary pulmonary venoocclusive disease. There are too many overlapping patterns, and certainly capillary dilatation and capillary collaterization-overgrowth in and around vessels is one manifestation of PVO. The descriptions of pulmonary capillary hemangiomatosis note an increased amount of hemoptysis in the those patients compared with those of primary PVO, and I believe that is because this subset of

PVO has a greater number of capillary dilatational lesions that more frequently hemorrhage. An alternate choice, of course, is that I am not discriminating enough of this particular subset. Both cover the same age range, do not have established etiologies, have poor survivability, and are untreatable; also, many of the histologic findings overlap, so their similarities seem far greater than their uniqueness.

Intravascular Leiomyomatosis-Adult Myofibromatosis-Fibromyxoid

These sarcoma entities are considered together as there may be some overlap. Intravascular leiomyomatosis is a term most often used in the uterus, accompanying both vascular invasion-extension from a benign leiomeiomy-oma and primary smooth muscle proliferation originating in vascular walls within the myometrium. It is separate from the entity of intravascular fasciitis, a localized self-limited nonmalignant disorder that occurs mostly in children.[348,349] It may be part of the spectrum of myofibromatosis.[1043,1044]

The term intravascular leiomyomatosis is used here in a descriptive sense to highlight an unusual case. A 65-year-old woman had a normal chest radiograph 1 year before biopsy, with increasing soft nodular shadows during that time and decreasing pulmonary function tests.[1045] An open lung biopsy showed multiple nodules in pulmonary tissue, and it was noted that the pericardial sac also had similar nodules. She died suddenly 4 months later, and autopsy permission was only for transthoracic autopsy. She died of a pulmonary embolus, but both lungs were extensively infiltrated by 1- to 3-cm irregular nodules of firmness. These were

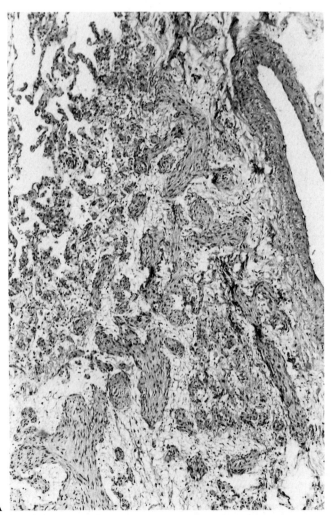

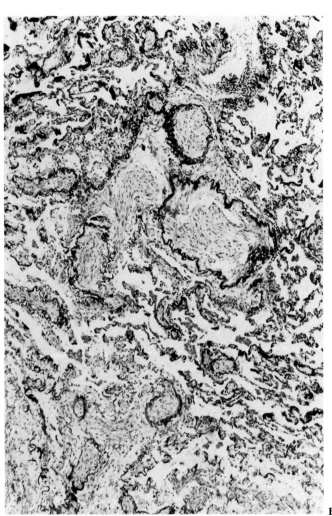

A

B

Fig. 33–157. Intravascular leiomyomatosis pattern. **A.** Bland-looking smooth muscle fills many small vessels around larger vessel. H and E, ×100. **B.** Intravascular location of some of this proliferation is identified with elastic stain. Elastic van Gieson, ×200.

also scattered over the pleura, and a transthoracic biopsy of the liver showed similar involvement. Such a case in an adult is unique in my experience.

The proliferating smooth muscle is seen in most of the structures radiating from the bronchopulmonary rays, around interlobular septa, in the interstitium and pleura (Fig. 33–157). The fascination in this case is that the smooth muscle proliferations appear so low grade, yet are so contained and yet extensive in the smaller vessel vascular system. If one considers proliferations with the ability to kill as malignant, then perhaps a better term for this is leiomyosarcomatosis, but these appear to be forming in their native sites of architecture like lymphangioleiomyomatosis, are neoplastic, but do not metastasize in the usual sense, as far as can be determined. More cases in adults will need to be described to further evaluate this disease.

The term myofibromatosis in adults may have some overlap with the entity recently described by Evans as low-grade fibromyxoid sarcomas.[1046,1047] These appear quite low grade histologically but do metastasize fairly rapidly and fairly extensively, often to lung. They seem to "break the rules" of usual sarcoma grading as related to predictive behavior as they are deceptively low grade in appearance.

An interesting case of fibromyxoid sarcoma is shared by Dr. J. Carlos Manivel.[1048] The patient, a 25-year-old man, had a right thigh mass with deep vein thrombosis. This was initially diagnosed as nodular fasciitis. The mass persisted for 7 months, and rebiopsy was done, which suggested the entity of musculoaponeurotic fibromatosis. Twelve months after initial leg biopsy, he had a right lung mass (Fig. 33–158). On review, the proliferation was similar in lung (Fig. 33–158) and leg

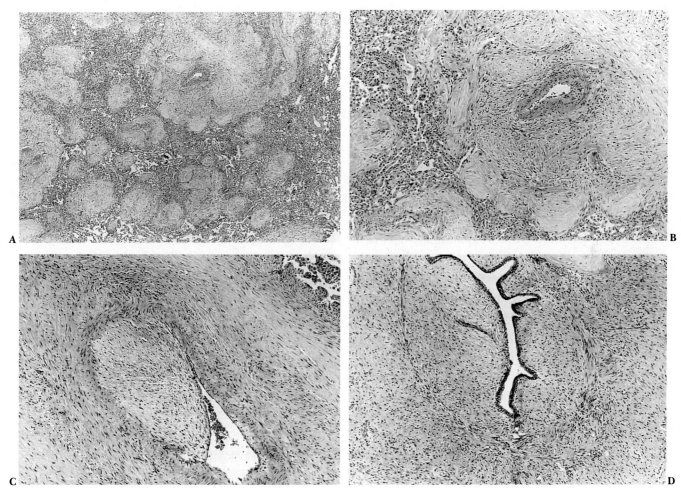

Fig. 33–158 A–D. Myofibromatosis–low-grade sarcoma. **A.** At first glance what appear to be random nodules in lung may well represent perivascular-lymphangitic spread. H and E, ×50. **B.** Higher power of the largest nodule in **A** shows this perivascular cuffing and mixed spindle cell and hyalinized response. H and E, ×100. **C.** Low-grade spindle cell proliferation surrounds vessel wall and infiltrates into lumen. In this field it appears to preserve muscle coat of native vessel wall. H and E, ×200. **D.** Similar involvement surrounds and infiltrates submucosa of bronchiole. Again, note preserved smooth muscle. H and E, ×100. (Courtesy of J. C. Manivel, University of Minnesota, Minneapolis, Minnesota.)

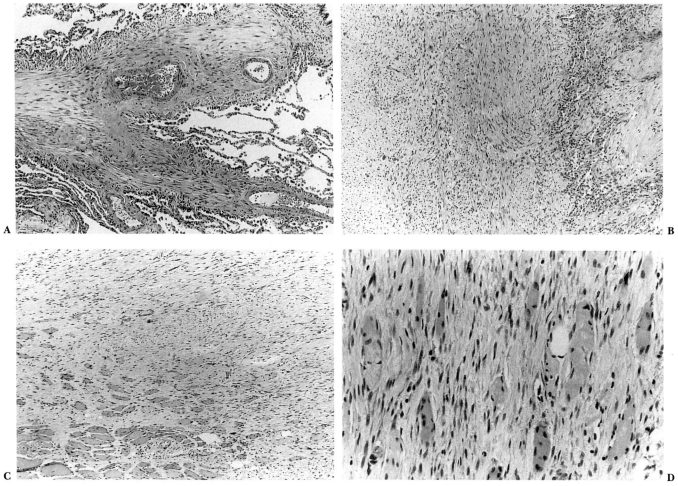

Fig. 33–159 A–D. Continuation of case seen in Fig. 33–154. **A.** Spindle cells extend around smaller vessels. H and E, ×200. **B.** Pleura is focally densely infiltrated by similar infiltrate to left. H and E, ×100. **C.** Preexistent thigh mass in this patient shows similar spindle cell neoplasm infiltrating skeletal muscle. H and E, ×100. **D.** These cells are seen better at higher power. H and E, ×400. (Courtesy of J. C. Manivel, University of Minnesota, Minneapolis, Minnesota.)

(Fig. 33–159). In the lung there is thickened pleura, with varying cellularity, sometimes densely hyalinized, sometimes moderately cellular. These areas extend around vessels, through their walls and into their lumens. They involve bronchi in a similar fashion. This proliferation is probably following lymphatic pathways in pleura, about vessels and bronchi. Its spread in a lymphangitic manner is unusual for sarcomas other than Kaposi's sarcoma.

References

1. Arrigoni MG, Woolner LB, Bernat PE, Miller WE, Fontana RS. Benign tumors of the lung. A ten-year surgical experience. J Thorac Cardiovasc Surg 1970;60:589–599.
2. Liebow AA. Tumors of the lowest respiratory tract. Washington DC: Armed Forces Institute of Pathology, 1952:11–148.
3. Liebow AA. Tumors of the lungs and trachea. In: Glenn WWL, Liebow AA, Lindskog GE, eds. Thoracic and cardiovascular surgery with related pathology. 3rd Ed. New York: Apppleton–Century-Crofts, 1975:325–404.
4. Carter D, Eggleston JC. Tumors of the respiratory tract. Washington DC: Armed Forces Institute of Pathology. 1980:51–58, 189–250, 284–297, 300–307, 321–327.
5. Mark EJ. Lung biopsy interpretation. Baltimore: Williams & Wilkins, 1984:117–229.
6. Spencer H. Pathology of the lung. 4th Ed. Oxford: Pergamon, 1985:837–1020, 1061–1083.
7. Dunnill MS. Pulmonary pathology. 2nd Ed. New York: Churchill-Livingstone 1987:403–441.
8. Churg A. Tumors of the lung. In: Thurlbeck WM, ed. Pathology of the lung. Stuttgart: Thieme, 1988:311–423.

9. Fraser RG, Paré JA, Paré PD, Fraser RS, Genereux GP. Diagnosis of diseases of the chest. Philadelphia: WB Saunders 1989;II:1327–1699.

10. Mackay B, Lukeman JM, Ordóñez NG. Tumors of the lung. Philadelphia: WB Saunders, 1991:285–322.

11. Colby TV, Lombard C. Yousem SA, Kitaichi M. Atlas of pulmonary surgical pathology. Philadelphia: WB Saunders 1991:59–132, 334.

12. Marchevsky AM, Koss MN. Tumors of bronchial gland origin. In: Marchevsky AM, ed. Surgical pathology of lung neoplasms. New York: Marcel Dekker 1990:289–323.

13. Gal AA, Koss MN, Marchevsky AM. Unusual tumors of the lung. In: Marchevsky AM, ed. Surgical pathology of lung neoplasms. New York: Marcel Dekker 1990:325–388.

14. Koss MN. Turmolike lesions of the lung. In: Marchevsky AM, ed. Surgical pathology of lung neoplasms. New York: Marcel Dekkeer 1990:389–432.

15. Corrin B. The lungs. 3rd Ed. London: Churchill Livingstone 1990:333–340, 373–418.

16. Norris CM. Tracheal obstruction. Laryngoscope 1949;59:595–620.

17. Acquarelli MJ, Ward NO, Hangos GW. Carcinoma of the trachea. Ann Otol 1967;76:843–850.

18. Daniel TM, Smith RH, Faunce H, Sylvest VM. Transbronchoscopic versus surgical resection of tracheobronchial granular cell myoblastomas: Suggested approach based on follow-up of all treated cases. J Thorac Cardiovasc Surg 1980;80:898–903.

19. Li W, Ellerbrock NA, Libshitz HI. Primary malignant tumors of the trachea. A radiologic and clinical study. Cancer (Philadelphia) 1990;66:894–896.

20. Grillo HC. The trachea—tumors, strictures and tracheal collapse. In: Glenn WW, Baue AE, Geha AS, et al., eds. Thoracic and cardiovascular surgery. New York: Appleton-Century-Crofts, 1983:308–325.

21. Houston HE, Payne WS, Harrison EG Jr, Olsen AM. Primary cancers of the trachea. Arch Surg 1969;99:132–140.

22. Shi ML, Fan KH, Zhou CW, Wu N, Shi ZH. X-Ray features of primary non-squamous cell carcinoma and other malignant neoplasms in the trachea and main bronchi: Analysis of 23 cases. Chung Hua Chung Liu Tsa Chih 1987;9:208–211.

23. Spizamy DL, Shepard JO, McLoud TC, Grillo HC, Dedrick CG. CT of adenoid cystic carcinoma of the trachea. AJR 1986;146:1129–1132.

24. Mayr B, Heywang SH, Ingrish H, Huber RM, Häussinger K, Lissner J. Comparison of CT with MR imaging of endobronchial tumors. J Comput Assist Tomogr 1987;11843–11848.

25. Hajdu SL, Huvos AG, Goodner JT, Foote FW Jr, Beattie EJ, Jr. Carcinoma of the trachea: Clinicopathologic study of 41 cases. Cancer (Philadelphia) 1970;25:1448–1456.

26. Gilbert JG, Mazzarella LA, Feit LF. Primary tracheal tumors in the infant and adult. AMA Arch Otolaryngol 1953;58:1–9.

27. Eschapasse H. Les tumeurs trachéales primitives. Traitement chirurgical. Rev Fr Mal Respir 1974;2:425–446.

28. Perel'man MI, Koroleva N. Surgery of the trachea. World J Surg 1980;4:583–591.

29. Weber AL, Grillo HC. Tracheal tumors: A radiological, clinical and pathological evaluation of 84 cases. Radiol Clin North Am 1978;16:227–246.

30. Grillo HC. Tracheal tumors: Surgical management. Ann Thorac Surg 1978;26:112–125.

31. Grillo HC. Tracheal surgery. Scand J Thorac Cardiovasc Surg 1983;17:67–77.

32. Xu L-T, Sun Z-F, Li Z-J, Wu LH, Wang ZZ. Tracheobronchial tumors: An eighteen-year series from Capital Hospital, Peking, China. Ann Thorac Surg 1983;35:590–596.

33. Xu L-T, Sun Z-F, Li Z-J, Wu LH, Zhang ZY, Yu XQ. Clinical and pathologic characteristics in patients with tracheobronchial tumors: Report of 50 patients. Ann Thorac Surg 1987;43:276–278.

34. Pearson FG, Todd TRJ, Cooper JD. Experience with primary neoplasms of the trachea and carina. J Thorac Cardiovasc Surg 1984;88:517–518.

35. Pollak ER, Nauheim KS, Little AG. Fibromyxoma of the trachea. Arch Pathol Lab Med 1985;109:926–929.

36. Hurt R. Benign tumors of the bronchus and trachea, 1951–1981. Ann R Coll Surg Engl 1984;66:22–26.

37. D'Aunoy R, Zoeller A. Primary tumors of the trachea: Report of a case and review of the literature. AMA Arch Pathol 1931;11:589–600.

38. Onizuka M, Doi M, Mitsui K, Ogata T, Hori M. Undifferentiated carcinoma with prominent lymphocytic infiltration (so-called lymphoepithelioma) in the trachea. Chest 1990;98:236–237.

39. Hilding AC. On cigarette smoking, bronchial carcinoma and ciliary action. III. Accumulation of cigarette tar upon artificially-produced deciliated islands in respiratory epithelium. Ann Otol 1956;65:116–130.

40. Hilding AC. Cigarette smoke and physiologic drainage of bronchial tree. Dis Chest 1961;39:357–362.

41. Schmitt FC, Zelandi-Filho C, Bacchi MM, Castilho ED, Bacchi CE. Adenoid cystic carcinoma of the trachea metastatic to the placenta. Hum Pathol 1989;20:193–195.

42. Briselli M, Mark GJ. Grillo HC. Tracheal carcinoids. Cancer (Philadelphia) 1978;42:2870–2879.

43. Wang N-S, Morin J. Recurrent endobronchial soft tissue tumors. Chest 1984;85:787–791.

44. Payne WS, Fontana RS, Woolner LB. Bronchial tumors originating from mucous glands: Current classification and unusual manifestations. Med Clin North Am 1968;48:945–960.

45. Conlan AA, Payne WS, Woolner LB, Sanderson DR. Adenoid cystic carcinoma (cylindroma) and mucoepidermoid carcinoma of the bronchus: Factors affecting survival. J Thorac Cardiovasc Surg 1978;76:369–377.

46. Spencer H. Bronchial mucous gland tumours. Virchows Arch [Path Anat] 1979;383:101–115.

47. Klacsmann PG, Olson JL, Eggleston JC. Mucoepider-

moid carcinoma of the bronchus: An electron microscopic study of the low grade and high grade variants. Cancer (Philadelphia) 1979;43:1720–1733.

48. Turnbull AD, Huvos AG, Goodner JT, Foote FW, Jr. Mucoepidermoid tumors of bronchial glands. Cancer (Philadelphia) 1971;28:539–544.

49. Enterline HT, Schoenberg HW. Carcinoma (cylindromatous type) of trachea and bronchi and bronchial adenoma; a comparative study. Cancer (Philadelphia) 1954;7:663–670.

50. Markel SF, Abell MR, Haight C, French AJ. Neoplasms of bronchus commonly designated as adenomas. Cancer (Philadelphia) 1964;17:590–608.

51. Olmedo G, Rosenberg M, Fonseca R: Primary tumors of the trachea. Clinicopathologic features and surgical results. Chest 1982;81:701–706.

52. Nomori H, Kaseda S, Kobayashi K, Ishihara T, Yanai N, Torikata C. Adenoid cystic carcinoma of the trachea and main-stem bronchus. J Thorac Cardiovasc Surg 1988;96:271–277.

53. Okura T, Shiode M, Tanaka R, Furukawa A, Kukita H. A case of peripheral adenoid cystic carcinoma (in Japanese). Nippon Kyobu Shikkan Gakkai Zasshi 1990;28:773–776.

54. Gallagher CG, Stark R, Teskey J, Kryger M. Atypical manifestations of pulmonary adenoid cystic carcinoma. Br J Dis Chest 1986;80:396–399.

55. Reid JD. Adenoid cystic carcinoma (cylindroma) of the bronchial tree. Cancer (Philadelphia) 1952;5:685–694.

56. Nascimento AG, Amaral ALP, Prado LAF, Kligerman J, Silveira TRP. Adenoid cystic carcinoma of salivary glands. Cancer (Philadelphia) 1986;57:312–319.

57. Matsuba HM, Spector GJ, Thawley SE, Simpson JR, Mauney M, Pikul FJ. Adenoid cystic salivary gland carcinoma. Cancer (Philadelphia) 1986;57:519–524.

58. Eby LS, Johnson DS, Barker HW. Adenoid cystic carcinoma of the head and neck. Cancer (Philadelphia) 1972;29:1160–1168.

59. Ishida T, Nishino T, Oka T, et al. Adenoid cystic carcinoma of the tracheobronchial tree: Clinicopathology and immunohistochemistry. J Surg Oncol 1989; 41:52–59.

60. Nguyen G-K. Cytology of bronchial gland carcinoma. Acta Cytol 1988;32:235–239.

61. Heilbrunn A, Crosby IK. Adenocystic carcinoma and mucoepidermoid carcinomas of the tracheobronchial tree. Chest 1972;61:145–149.

62. Wilkins EW, Darling RC, Soutter L, Sniffen RC. A continuing clinical survey of adenomas of the trachea and bronchus in a general hospital. J Thorac Cardiovasc Surg 1963;46:279–291.

63. Diaz-Jimenez JP, Canela-Cordona M, Meastre-Alacer J. Nd:YAG laser photoresection of low grade malignant tumors of the tracheobronchial tree. Chest 1990;97:920–922.

64. Lampe JL, Zatzkin H. Metastases of pseudoadenomatous basal cell carcinoma. Radiology 1948;53:379–385.

65. Grillet B, Demedts MD, Roelens J, Goddeeris P, Fos-

sion E. Spontaneous regression of lung metastases of adenoid cystic carcinoma. Chest 1984;85:289–291.

66. Larson RE, Woolner LB, Payne WS. Mucoepidermoid tumor of the trachea. Report of a case. J Thorac Cardiovasc Surg 1965;50:131–137.

67. Trentini GP, Palmieri B. Mucuoepidermoid tumor of the trachea. Chest 1972;62:336–338.

68. Leonardi HK, Jung-Legg Y, Legg MA, Neptune WB. Tracheobronchial mucoepidermoid carcinoma. J Thorac Cardiovasc Surg 1978;76:431–438.

69. Heitmiller RF, Mathisen DJ, Ferry JA, Mark EJ, Grillo HC. Mucoepidermoid lung tumors. Ann Thorac Surg 1989;47:394–399.

70. Yousem SA, Hochholzer L. Mucoepidermoid tumors of the lung. Cancer (Philadelphia) 1987;60:1346–1352.

71. Seo IS, Warren J, Mirkin D, Weisman SJ, Grosfeld JL. Mucoepideremoid carcinoma of the bronchus in a 4-year-old child: a high-grade variant with lymph node metastases. Cancer 1984;53:1600–1604.

72. Smetana HF, Iverson L, Swan LL. Bronchogenic carcinoma: an analysis of 100 autopsy cases. Milit Surg 1952;111:335–351.

73. Diaconitza G, Eskenasy A. Les tumeurs mucoépidermoïdes bronchopulmonaires. Etude anatomoclinique declinq cas opérés. Le Poumon et le Coeur 1974; 30:265–271.

74. Axelsson C, Burcharth F, Johansen A. Mucoepidermoid lung tumors. J Thorac Cardiovasc Surg 1973; 65:902–908.

75. Meckstroth CV, Davidson HB, Kress GO. Mucoepidermoid tumor of the bronchus. Dis Chest 1961; 40:652–656.

76. Reichle FA, Rosemond GP. Mucoepidermoid tumors of the bronchus. J Thorac Cardiovasc Surg 1966; 51:443–448.

77. Ozlu C, Christopherson WM, Allen JD, Jr. Mucoepidermoid tumors of the bronchus. J Thorac Cardiovasc Surg 1961;42:24–31.

78. Dowling EA, Miller RE, Johnson EM, Collier FCD. Mucoepidermoid tumors of the bronchi. Surgery 1962;52:600–609.

79. Healey WV, Perzin KH, Smith L. Mucoepidermoid carcinoma of salivary gland: Classification, clinical-pathologic correlation, and results of treatment. Cancer (Philadelphia) 1970;26:368–388.

80. Metcalf JS, Maize JC, Shaw EB. Bronchial mucoepidermoid carcinoma metastatic to skin: Report of a case and review of the literature. Cancer (Philadelphia) 1986;58:2556–2559.

81. Barsky SH, Martin SE, Matthews M, Gazdar A, Costa JC. "Low grade" mucoepidermoid carcinoma of the bronchus with "high grade" biological behavior. Cancer (Philadelphia) 1983;51:1505–1509.

82. Stafford JR, Pollock J, Wenzel BC. Oncocytic mucoepidermoid tumor of the bronchus. Cancer (Philadelphia) 1984;54:94–99.

83. Seo IS, Warfel KA, Tomich CE, Hull MT. Clear cell carcinoma of the larynx: A variant of mucoepidermoid carcinoma. Am J Otolaryngol 1980;89:168–172.

84. Stewart FW, Foote FW, Jr., Becker, WF. Mucoepidermoid tumors of the salivary glands. Ann Surg 1945;122:820–824.

85. Lack EE, Harris GBC, Erakles AJ, Vawter GF. Primary bronchial tumors in childhood. Cancer (Philadelphia) 1983;51:494–497.

86. Matsuo K, Irie J, Tsuchiyama H, Nakano M, Nakata T. A high-grade malignancy bronchial mucoepidermoid carcinoma with features of giant cell carcinoma. Acta Pathol Jpn 1986;36:293–300.

87. Green LK, Gallion TL, Gyorkey F. Peripheral mucoepidermoid tumour of the lung. Thorax 1991; 46:65–66.

88. Ferguson CJ, Cleeland JA. Mucous gland adenoma of the trachea: Case report and literature review. J Thorac Cardiovasc Surg 1988;95:347–350.

89. Weinberger MA, Katz S, Davis EW. Peripheral bronchial adenoma of mucus gland type. J Thorac Surg 1955;29:626–635.

90. Allen MS, Jr, Marsh WL, Jr., Greissinger WT. Mucus gland adenoma of the bronchus. J Thorac Cardiovasc Surg 1974;67:966–968.

91. Heard BE, Corrin B, Dewar A. Pathology of seven mucous cell adenomas of the bronchial glands with particular reference to ultrastructure. Histopathology 1985;9:687–701.

92. Ramsey JH, Reimann DL. Bronchial adenomas arising in mucous glands. Am J Pathol 1953;29:339–352.

93. Gilman RA, Klassen KP, Scarpelli DG. Mucous gland adenoma of bronchus. Am J Clin Pathol 1956;26: 151–154.

94. Kroe DJ, Pitcock JA. Benign mucous gland adenoma of the bronchus. Arch Pathol 1967;84:539–540.

95. Hegg CA, Flint A, Singh G. Papillary adenoma of the lung. Am J Clin Pathol 1992;97:393–397.

96. Rosenblum P, Klein RI. Adenomatous polyp of the right main bronchus producing atelectasis. J Pediatr 1935;7:791–796.

97. Emory WB, Mitchell WT, Jr, Hatch HG, Jr. Mucous gland adenoma of the bronchus. Am Rev Respir Dis 1973;108:1407–1410.

98. Matsuba K, Takazawa T, Thurlbeck WM. Oncocytes in human bronchial mucous glands. Thorax 1972; 27:181–184.

99. Sklar JL, Churg A, Bensch KG. Oncocytic carcinoid tumor of the lung. Am J Surg Pathol 1980;4:287–292.

100. Sajjad SM, Mackay B, Lukeman JM. Oncocytic carcinoid tumor of the lung. Ultrastruct Pathol 1980;1: 171–176.

101. Walter P, Waarter A, Morand G. Carcinöide oncocytaire bronchique. Virchows Arch [A] 1978;379:85–97.

102. Scharifker D, Marchevsky A. Oncocytic carcinoid of lung: An ultrastructural analysis. Cancer (Philadelphia) 1981;47:530–532.

103. Ghadially FN, Block HJ. Oncocytic carcinoid of the lung. J Submicrosc Cytol 1985;17:435–442.

104. Shin DH, Park SS, Lee JH, Park MH, Lee JD. Oncocytic glomous tumor of the trachea. Chest 1990;98: 1021–1023.

105. Stafford JR, Pollock J, Wenzel BC. Oncocytic mucoepidermoid tumor of the bronchus. Cancer (Philadelphia) 1984;54:94–99.

106. Fine G, Chang CH. Adenoma of type 2 pneumocytes with oncocytic features. Arch Pathol Lab Med 1991; 115:797–801.

107. Akhtar M, Young I, Reyes F. Bronchial adenoma with polymorphous features. Cancer (Philadelphia) 1974; 33:1572–1576.

108. Fechner RE, Bentinck BR. Ultrastructure of bronchial oncocytoma. Cancer (Philadelphia) 1973;31:1451–1456.

109. Black WC, III. Pulmonary oncocytoma. Cancer (Philadelphia) 1969;23:1347–1357.

110. Santos-Briz A, Terron J, Sastre R, Romero L, Valle A. Oncocytoma of the lung. Cancer (Philadelphia) 1977;40:1330–1336.

111. Böck P, Wuketich S, Gorgas K. Fine structure of a bronchial oncocytoma. Osterr Z Onkol 1977;4:14–18.

112. Warter A, Walter P, Sabountchi M, Jory A. Oncocytic bronchial adenoma. Virchows Arch [A] 1981;392: 231–239.

113. Cwierzyk TA, Glasberg SS, Virshup MA, Cranmer JC. Pulmonary oncocytoma. Acta Cytol 1985;29:620–623.

114. Nielsen AL. Malignant bronchial oncocytoma: Case report and review of literature. Hum Pathol 1985; 16:852–854.

115. de Jesus MG, Poon TP, Chung KY. Pulmonary onocytoma. NY State J Med 1989;89:477–480.

116. Fechner RE, Bentinck BR, Askew JB, Jr. Acinic cell tumor of the lung: A histologic and ultrastructural study. Cancer (Philadelphia) 1972;29:501–508.

117. Katz DR, Bubis JJ. Acinic cell tumor of the bronchus. Cancer (Philadelphia) 1976;38:830–832.

118. Gharpure KJ, Deshpande RK, Vishweshvara RN, Raghu CR, Bhargava MK. Acinic cell tumor of the bronchus (a case report). Indian J Cancer 1985;22:152–156.

119. Heard BE, Dewar A, Firman RK, Lennox SC. One very rare and one new tracheal tumor found by electron microscopy: Glomus tumour and acinic cell tumour resembling carcinoid tumours by light microscopy. Thorax 1982;37:97–103.

120. Yoshida K, Koyama J, Matsui T. Acinic cell tumor of the bronchial gland (in Japanese). Nippon Geka Gakkai Zasshi 1989;90:1810–1813.

121. Moran CA, Suster S, Koss MN. Acinic cell carcinoma of the lung ("Fechner Tumor"): A clinicopathologic, immunohistochemical and ultrastructural study of five cases. Am J Surg Pathol 1992;16:1039–1050.

122. Ellis GL, Corio RL. Acinic cell adenocarcinoma. A clinicopathologic analysis of 294 cases. Cancer (Philadelphia) 1983;52:542–549.

123. Grage TB, Lober PH, Arhleger SW. Acinic cell carcinoma of the parotid gland. A clinicopathologic review of eleven cases. Am J Surg 1961;102:765–768.

124. Eneroth CM, Hamberger CA, Jakobsson PA. Malignancy of acinic cell carcinoma. Ann Otol Rhinol Laryngol 1966;75:780–792.

125. Eneroth CM, Jakobsson PA, Blank C. Acinic cell carcinoma of the parotid gland. Cancer (Philadelphia) 1966;19:1761–1772.

126. Sidhu GS, Forrester EM. Acinic cell carcinoma: Long-term survival after pulmonary metastases. Light and electron microscopic study. Cancer (Philadelphia) 1977;40:756–765.

127. Miura K, Moringa S, Horiuchi M, Shimosata Y, Tsuchiya R. Bronchial carcinoid tumor mimicking acinic cell tumor. Acta Pathol Jpn 1988;38:523–530.

128. Payne WS, Schier J, Woolner LB. Mixed tumors of the bronchus (salivary gland type). J Thorac Cardiovasc Surg 1965;49:663–668.

129. Davis PW, Briggs JC, Seal RM, Starring FK. Benign and malignant mixed tumors of the lung. Thorax 1972;27:657–673.

130. Ushizima H, Fujiwara K, Yamaguchi T, Haitani K, Kakihara R, Suenaga Y. A case of lung cancer of malignant mixed tumor origin. Gan No Rinsho 1975;21:1330–1336.

131. Nakamura M, Shimosato Y, Kameya T, et al. Two cases of bronchial gland "mixed tumor" of the salivary gland type. Lung Cancer 1977;17:47–57.

132. Ebihara Y, Fukushima N, Asakuma Y. Double primary lung cancers: With special reference to their exfoliative cytology and to the rare, malignant "mixed" tumor of the salivary-gland type. Acta Cytol 1980;24:212–223.

133. Wright ES, Pike E, Couves CM. Unusual tumours of the lung. J Surg Oncol 1983;24:23–29.

134. Clarke PJ, Dunnill MS, Gunning AJ. Mixed tumours of the lung: A report of three cases. Br J Dis Chest 1986;80–87.

135. Sakamoto H, Uda H, Tanaka T, Oda T, Morino H, Kikui M. Pleomorphic adenoma in the periphery of the lung. Arch Pathol Lab Med 1991;115:393–396.

136. Mori M, Furuya K, Kimura T, Kitade M, Veda N. Mixed tumor of salivary gland type arising in the bronchus. Ann Thorac Surg 1991;52:1322–1324.

137. Kay S, Brooks JW. Benign mixed tumor of the trachea with seven-year follow-up. Cancer (Philadelphia) 1970;25:1178–1182.

138. Ma CK, Fine G, Lewis J, Lee MW. Benign mixed tumor of the trachea. Cancer (Philadelphia) 1979;44:2260–2266.

139. Sano T, Hirose T, Hizawa K, et al. A case of pleomorphic adenoma of the trachea. Jpn J Clin Oncol 1984;14:93–88.

140. Hemmi A, Hiraoka H, Mori Y, et al. Malignant pleomorphic adenoma (malignant mixed tumor) of the trachea. Report of a case. Acta Pathol Jpn 1988;38:1215–1226.

141. Wenig BM, Hitchcock CL, Gnepp DR. Metastasizing mixed tumor of salivary glands: A clinicopathologic and flow cytometric analysis. Am J Surg Pathol 1992;16:845–858.

142. Sim DW, Maran AG, Harris D. Metastatic salivary pleomorphic adenoma. J Laryngol Otol 1990;104:45–47.

143. Strickler JG, Hegstrom J, Thomas MJ, Yousem SA. Myoepithelioma of the lung. Arch Pathol Lab Med 1987;111:1082–1085.

144. Evans HL, Batsakis JG. Polymorphous low-grade adenocarcinoma of minor salivary glands: A study of 14 cases of a distinctive neoplasm. Cancer (Philadelphia) 1984;53:935–942.

145. Gnepp DR, Chen JC, Warren C. Polymorphous low-grade adenocarcinoma of minor salivary gland: An immunohistochemical and clinicopathologic study. Am J Surg Pathol 1988;12:461–468.

146. Tortoledo ME, Luna MA, Batsakis JG. Carcinoma ex pleomorphic adenoma and malignant mixed tumors: Histomorphologic indexes. Arch Otolaryngol 1984;110:172–176.

147. Schinella RA, Fazzini EP. Bronchial gland adenocarcinoma of the lung. Am Rev Respir Dis 1977;115 (Suppl.):160.

148. Hirata H, Noguchi M, Shimasoto Y, Uei Y, Goya T. Clinicopathologic and immunohistochemical characteristics of bronchial gland cell type adenocarcinoma of the lung. Am J Clin Pathol 1990;93:20–25.

149. Shimosato Y, Suemasu K, Suzuki A. Morphology of bronchial gland tumors, with special reference to adenocarcinomas (in Japanese). Gan No Rinsho 1973;19:170–179.

150. Kodama T, Shimosato Y, Kameya T. Histology and ultrastructure of bronchogenic and bronchial gland adenocarcinomas in relation to histogenesis. In: Shimosato Y, Melamed MR, Nettesheim P, eds. Morphogenesis of lung cancer. Vol. 1. Boca Raton: CRC Press, 1982:148–166.

151. Shimosato Y, Kodama T, Kameya T. Morphogenesis of peripheral type adenocarcinoma of the lung. In: Shimosato Y, Melamed MR, Nettesheim P, eds. Morphogenesis of lung cancer. Vol 1. Boca Raton: CRC Press, 1982:65–89.

152. Kimula Y. A histochemical and ultrastructural study of adenocarcinoma of lung cancer. Am J Surg Pathol 1978;2:253–264.

153. Mills SE, Garland TA, Allen MS, Jr. Low-grade papillary adenocarcinoma of palatal salivary gland origin. Am J Surg Pathol 1984;8:367–374.

154. Corio RL, Sciubba JJ, Brannon RB, Batsakis JG. Epithelial-myoepithelial carcinoma of intercalated duct origin. Oral Surg Oral Med Oral Pathol 1982;53:280–287.

155. Higashiyama M, Doi O, Kodama K, Tateishi R, Kurokawa E. Extramammary Paget's disease of the bronchial epithelium. Arch Pathol Lab Med 1991;115:185–188.

156. Zaino RJ. Paget's disease in a retroperitoneal teratoma. Hum Pathol 1984;15:622–624.

157. Batsakis JG. Tumors of the head and neck: Clinical and pathological considerations. 2d Ed. Baltimore: Williams & Wilkins, 1979:130–143.

158. Singer DB, Greenberg SD, Harrison GM. Papillomatosis of the lung. Am Rev Respir Dis 1966;94:777–783.

159. Lukens RM. Papilloma of the trachea: report of a case. Ann Otol 1936;45:872–874.

160. Kramer SS, Wehunt WD, Stocker JT, Kashima H. Pulmonary manifestations of juvenile laryngotracheal papillomatosis. AJR 1985;144:687–694.

161. Majoros M, Parkhill EM, Devine KD. Papilloma of the larynx in children: a clinicopathological study. Am J Surg 1964;108:470–475.

162. Al-Saleem J, Peale AR, Norris CM. Multiple papillomatosis of the lower respiratory tract: Clinical and pathologic study of eleven cases. Cancer (Philadelphia) 1968;22:1173–1184.

163. Font JH. Laryngotracheobronchial papillomatosis of children: report of a case. Arch Otolaryngol 1956; 64:270–274.

164. Rosenbaum HD, Alari SM, Bryant LR. Pulmonary parenchymal spread of juvenile laryngeal papillomatosis. Radiology 1968;90:654–660.

165. Runckel D, Kessler S. Bronchogenic squamous carcinoma in nonirradiated juvenile laryngotracheal papillomatosis. Am J Surg Pathol 1980;4:293–296.

166. Greene JG, Tassin L, Saberi A. Endobronchial epithelial papilloma associated with a foreign body. Chest 1990;97:229–230.

167. Kirchner JA. Papilloma of the larynx with extensive lung involvement. Laryngoscope 1951;61:1022–1029.

168. Ogilvie OE. Multiple papillomas of trachea with malignant degeneration: report of two cases. AMA Arch Otolaryngol 1953;58:10–18.

169. Sherwin RP, Laforet EG, Strieder JW. Exophytic endobronchial carcinoma. J Thorac Cardiovasc Surg 1962;43:716–730.

170. Moore RL, Lattes R. Papillomatosis of larynx and bronchi: case report with 34-year follow-up. Cancer 1959;12:117–126.

171. Spencer H, Dail DH, Arneaud J. Noninvasive bronchial epithelial papillary tumors. Cancer 1980;45: 1486–1497.

172. Laubscher FA. Solitary squamous cell papilloma of bronchial origin. Am J Clin Pathol 1969;599–603.

173. Helmuth RA, Strate RW. Squamous carcinoma of the lung in a nonirradiated, nonsmoking patient with juvenile laryngotracheal papillomatosis. Am J Surg Pathol 1987;11:643–650.

174. Bewtra C, Krishman R, Lee SS. Malignant changes in nonirradiated juvenile laryngotracheal papillomatosis. Arch Otolaryngol 1982;108:114–116.

175. Brach BB, Klein RC, Matthews AJ, Cook EW. Papillomatosis of the respiratory tract. Arch Otolaryngol 1975;104:413–416.

176. Cohen SR, Geller KA, Seltzer S, Thompson JW. Papillomatosis of the larynx and tracheobronchial tree in children. A retrospective study. Ann Otol 1989; 80:497–503.

177. Dallimore NS. Squamous bronchial carcinoma arising in a case of multiple juvenile papillomatosis. Thorax 1985;40:797–798.

178. Rhaman A, Ziment I. Tracheobronchial papillomatosis with malignant transformation. Arch Intern Med 1983;143:577–578.

179. Schouten TJ, van den Broek P, Cremers CWRJ, Jongerius CM, Meyer JW, Vooys GP. Interferons and bronchogenic carcinoma in juvenile laryngeal papillomatosis. Arch Otolaryngol 1983;109:289–291.

180. Solomon D, Smith RRL, Kashima HK, Leventhat B. Malignant transformation in non-irradiated recurrent respiratory papillomatosis. Laryngoscope 1985; 95:900–904.

181. Trillo A, Guha A. Solitary condylomatous papilloma of the bronchus. Arch Pathol Lab Med 1988;112:731–733.

182. Bejui-Thivolet F, Liagre N, Chignol MC, Chardonnet Y, Patricot LM. Detection of human papilloma virus DNA in squamous bronchial metaplasia and squamous cell carcinomas of the lung by in situ hybridization using biotinylated probes in paraffin-embedded specimens. Hum Pathol 1990;21:111–116.

183. Spencer H. Personal communication. London, 1977.

184. Assor D. A papillary transitional cell tumor of the bronchus. Am J Clin Pathol 1971;55:761–764.

185. Lemos L, Assor D. A group of papillary endobronchial tumors. Am J Clin Pathol 1976;65:265 (abstr).

186. Smith PS, McClure J. A papillary endobronchial tumor with a transitional cell pattern. Arch Pathol Lab Med 1982;106:503–506.

187. Daroca PJ, Jr., Robichau WH. Busaloid carcinoma of the bronchus. Surg Pathol 1985;2:339–344.

188. Brambilla E, Moro D, Veale D, et al. Basal cell (baseloid) carcinoma of the lung: A new morphotopic and phenotypic entity with separate prognostic significance. Hum Pathol 1992;23:993–1003.

189. Montes M, Allen H, Brennen JC. Bronchiolar apocrine tumor. Am Rev Respir Dis 1966;93:946–950.

190. Fantone JC, Geisinger KR, Appleman HD. Papillary adenoma of the lung with lamellar and electron dense granules: an ultrastructural study. Cancer 1982;50: 2839–2844.

191. Noguchi M, Kodama T, Shimosato Y, et al. Papillary adenoma of type 2 pneumocytes. Am J Surg Pathol 1986;10:134–139.

192. Kodama T, Biyajima S, Watanabe S, Shimasoto Y. Morphometric study of adenocarcinoma and hyperplastic epithelial lesions in the peripheral lung. Am J Clin Pathol 1986;85:146–151.

193. Mark EJ, Quay SC, Dickersin R. Papillary carcinoid tumor of the lung. Cancer 1981;48:316–324.

194. Kauffman SL, Alexander L, Sass L. Histologic and ultrastructural features of the Clara cell adenoma of the mouse lung. Lab Invest 1980;40:708–715.

195. Sato T, Kauffman SL. A scanning electron microscopic study of the type II and Clara cell adenoma of the mouse lung. Lab Invest 1980;40:28–36.

196. Travis W, Linnoila I, Horowitz M, Pass H, Ozols R, Gazdar A. Pulmonary nodules resembling bronchioalveolar carcinoma (BAC) in adolescent cancer patients [abstr.]. Mod Pathol 1988;1:94A.

197. Miller RR, Nelems B, Evans KG, Müller NL, Ostrow DN. Glandular neoplasia of the lung. Cancer (Philadelphia) 1988;61:1009–1014.

198. McElvaney G, Miller RR, Müller NL, Nelems B, Evans KG, Ostrow DN. Multicentricity of adenocarcinoma of the lung. Chest 1989;95:151–154.

199. Miller RR. Bronchioalveolar cell adenomas. Am J Surg Pathol 1990;14:904–912.

200. Nakanishi K. Alveolar epithelial hyperplasia and adenocarcinoma of the lung. Arch Pathol Lab Med 1990;114:363–368.

201. Rosen PP. Mucocele-like tumors of the breast. Am J Surg Pathol 1986;10:464–469.

202. Eck H, Haupt R, Rothe G. Die gut-und bosartigen Lungengeschwulste. In Henke F, Lubarsch O, eds. Handbuch der speziellen pathologischen Anatomic and Histologie; Berlin, Springer Verlag. 1969;11/4:59–61.

203. Sambrook-Gowar JFS. An unusual mucous cyst of the lung. Thorax 1978;33:796–799.

204. Dail DH. Uncommon tumors. In Dail DH, Hammar SP, eds. Pulmonary Pathology. New York: Springer-Verlag. 1988;865–866.

205. Dail DH, Hammar SP, Carter D. Tumors of the lung. Chicago: ASCP, (in press).

206. Morales CM, Traub B, Jenis E. Mucinous multilobular cyst carcinoma of the lung. ASCP Check Sample 1989;AP 89-11:1–4.

207. Urbanski JS, Larsen E, van Olm M. "Pseudomyxomatous" pulmonary adenocarcinoma: Morphologic variant with long clincal course. Lab Invest 1990;62:102A (Abstract).

208. Devaney K, Kragel P, Travis W. Mucinous cystadenocarcinoma of the lung: A tumor of low malignant potential. Am J Clin Pathol 1989;92:524 (Abstract).

209. Kragel PJ, Devaney KO, Meth BM, Linnoila I, Frierson HF, Travis WD. Mucinous cystadenoma of the lung. Arch Pathol Lab Med 1990;114:1053–1056.

210. Graeme-Cook F, Mark EJ. Pulmonary mucinous cystic tumors of borderline malignancy. Hum Pathol 1991;22:185–190.

211. Moran CA, Hochholzer L, Fishback N, Travis N, Koss MN. Mucinous (so-called colloid) carcinomas of lung. Mod Pathol 1992;5:634–638.

212. Donaldson JC, Kaminsky DB, Elliott RC. Bronchiolar carcinoma. Cancer 1978;41:250–258.

213. Liebow AA. Bronchioloalveolar carcinoma. Adv Intern Med 1960;10:329–358.

214. Hammar SP, MD, Seattle, WA. Personal communication, 1991.

215. Ishida T, Tateishi M, Kaneko S, et al. Carcinosarcoma and spindle cell carcinoma of the lung. Clinicopathologic and immunohistochemical studies. J Thorac Cardiovasc Surg 1990;100:844–852.

216. Ashworth TG. Pulmonary blastomas: A true congenital neoplasm. Histopathology 1983;7:585–594.

217. Kreyberg L, Liebow AA, Uehlinger EA. Histological typing of lung tumors. Geneva: World Health Organization, 1967.

218. Steele RH. Lung tumors: A personal review. Diagn Histopathol 1983;6:119–169.

219. Edwards CW. Pulmonary adenocarcinoma: Review of 106 cases and proposed new classifications. J Clin Pathol 1987;40:125–135.

220. Cagle PT, Alpert LC, Carmona PA. Peripheral biphasic adenocarcinoma of the lung: Light microscopic and immunohistochemical findings. Hum Pathol 1992;23:197–200.

221. Tsubota YT, Kawaguchi T, Hoso T, Nishino E, Travis WD. A combined small cell and spindle cell carcinoma of the lung. Report of a unique case with immunohistochemical and ultrastructural studies. Am J Surg Pathol 1992;16:1108–1115.

222. Cabarcos A, Gomez Dorronsoro M, Lobo Beristain JL. Pulmonary carcinosarcoma: A case study and review of the literature. Br J Dis Chest 1985;79:83–94.

223. Francis D, Jacobsen M. Pulmonary blastoma. Curr Top Pathol 1983;73:265–294.

224. Koss MN, Hochholzer L, O'Leary T. Pulmonary blastomas. Cancer (Philadelphia) 1991;67:2368–2381.

225. Herxheimer G, Reinke G. Carcinoma sarcomatodes (Pathologie des Krebses). Ergeb Allg Pathol 1912;16:280–282.

226. Bergmann M, Ackerman LV, Kemler RL. Carcinosarcoma of the lung. Review of the literature and report of two cases treated by pneumonectomy. Cancer (Philadelphia) 1951;4:919–929.

227. Moore TC. Carcinosarcoma of the lung. Surgery 1962;50:886–893.

228. Davis MP, Eagan RT, Weiland LH, Pairolero PC. Carcinosarcoma of the lung: Mayo Clinic experience and response to chemotherapy. Mayo Clin Proc 1984;59:598–603.

229. Ro JY, Chen JL, Lee JS, Sahin AA, Ordóñez NG, Ayala AG. Sarcomatoid carcinoma of the lung: Immunohistochemical and ultrastructural studies of 14 cases. Cancer (Philadelphia) 1992;69:376–386.

230. Diaconita G. Bronchopulmonary carcinosarcoma. Thorax 1975;30:682–686.

231. Coll R, Alberola C, Padilla J, Mayoyo E, Marco V. Un caso de carcinosarcoma de pulmon. Revision de la literature. Arch Bronconeumol 1981;17:63–66.

232. Addis BJ, Corrin B. Pulmonary blastoma, carinosarcoma and spindle-cell carcinoma: An immunohistochemical study of keratin intermediate filaments. J Pathol 1985;147:291–301.

233. Colby TV, Bilbao JE, Battifora H, Unni KK. Primary osteosarcoma of the lung: A reappraisal following immunohistologic study. Arch Pathol Lab Med 1989;113:1147–1150.

234. Loose JH. El-Naggar AK, Ro JY, Huang W-L, McMurtrey MJ, Ayala AG. Primary osteosarcoma of the lung: Report of two cases and review of the literature. J Thorac Cardiovasc Surg 1990;100:867–873.

235. Humphrey PA, Scroggs MW, Roggli VL, Shelburne JD. Pulmonary carcinomas with a sarcomatoid element: An immunocytochemical and ultrastructural analysis. Hum Pathol 1988;19:155–165.

236. Barnett NR, Barnard WG. Some unusual thoracic tumours. Br J Surg 1945;32:447–457.

237. Barnard WG. Embryoma of lung. Thorax 1952;7:229–301.

238. Spencer H. Pulmonary blastomas. J Pathol Bacteriol 1961;82:161–165.

239. Waddell WR. Organoid differentiation of the fetal lung. A histologic study of the differentiation of mammalian fetal lung in utero and in transplants. Arch Pathol 1949;47:227–247.

240. Fung CH, Lo JW, Yonan TN, Milloy FJ, Hakami MH, Changus GW. Pulmonary blastoma: an ultrastructural study with a brief review of literature and a discussion of pathogenesis. Cancer 1977;39:153–163.

241. Manivel JC, Priest JR, Watterson J, et al. Pleuropulmonary blastoma: The so-called pulmonary blastoma of childhood. Cancer (Philadelphia) 1988;62:1516–1526.

242. Askin FB. Pulmonary blastoma (editorial). Am J Clin Pathol 1990;93:167–175.

243. Askin FB, Rosai J, Sibley RK, Dehner LP, McAllister WH. Malignant small cell tumor of the thoracopulmonary region in childhood. A distinctive clinicopathologic entity of uncertain histogenesis. Cancer (Philadelphia) 1979;43:2438–2451.

244. Gibbons JRP, McKeown F, Field TW. Pulmonary blastoma with hilar lymph node metastases: Survival for 24 years. Cancer (Philadelphia) 1981;47:152–155.

245. Motlik K, Triska J. Bronchopulmonary carcinosarcomas. Acta Univ Carol [Med] (Praha) 1968;14:3–25.

246. Cornet E, Mussini-Montpellier J, Michaud JL, Lenne Y, de Lajartre AY. Le pneumoblastome. A propos de deux cas, revue de la litterature. Rev Fr Mal Respir 1975;3:143–156.

247. Davis PW, Briggs VC, Seal RME, Storring FK, Benign and malignant mixed tumours of the lung. Thorax 1972;27:657–673.

248. Souza RC, Peasley ED, Takaro T. Pulmonary blastomas. A distinctive group of carcinosarcomas of the lung. Ann Thorac Surg 1965;1:259–268.

249. Kern WH, Stiles QR. Pulmonary blastoma. J Thorac Cardiovasc Surg 1976;71:801–808.

250. Peacock MJ, Whitwell F. Pulmonary blastoma. Thorax 1976;31:197–204.

251. Roth JA, Elguezabal A. Pulmonary blastoma evolving into carcinosarcoma. A case study. Am J Surg Pathol 1978;2:407–413.

252. Bauermeister DE, Jennings ER, Beland AH, Judson HA. Pulmonary blastoma, a form of carcinosarcoma: a case of 24 years duration without treatment. Am J Clin Pathol 1966;46:322–329.

253. Siegel RJ, Bueso-Ramos C, Cohen C, Koss M. Pulmonary blastoma with germ cell (yolk sac) differentiation. Report of two cases. Mod Pathol 1991;4:566–570.

254. Cohen RE, Weaver MG, Montenegro HD, Abdul-Karim FW. Pulmonary blastoma with malignant melanoma component. Arch Pathol Lab Med 1990;114:1076–1078.

255. Michael H, Ulbright TM, Brodhecker CA. The pluripotential nature of the mesenchyme-like component of yolk sac tumor. Arch Pathol Lab Med 1989;113:1115–1119.

256. Kodama T, Shimosato Y, Watanabe S, Koide T, Naruke T, Shimose J. Six cases of well-differentiated adenocarcinoma simulating fetal lung tissues in pseudoglandular stage: comparison with pulmonary blastoma. Am J Surg Pathol 1984;8:735–744.

257. Manning JT, Jr., Ordóñez NG, Rosenberg HS, Walker WE. Pulmonary endodermal tumor resembling fetal lung. Arch Pathol Lab Med 1985;109:48–50.

258. Müller-Hermelink HK, Kaiserling E. Pulmonary adenocarcinoma of fetal type: alternating differentiation argues in favour of a common endodermal stem cell. Virchows Arch [A] 1986;409:195–210.

259. Korbi S, M'boyo A, Dusmet M, Spiliopoulos A. Pulmonary blastoma. Immunohistochemical and ultrastructural studies of a case. Histopathology 1987;11:753–760.

260. Heckman CJ, Truong LD, Cagle PT, Font RL. Pulmonary blastoma with rhabdomyosarcomatous differentiation: An electron microscopic and immunohistochemical study. Am J Surg Pathol 1988;12:35–40.

261. Berean K, Truong L, Dudley A Jr, Cagle P. Immunohistochemical characterization of pulmonary blastoma. Am J Clin Pathol 1988;89:773–777.

262. Yousem SA, Wick MR, Randhawa P, Manivel JC. Pulmonary blastoma: An immunohistochemical analysis and comparison with fetal lung in its pseudoglandular stage. Am J Clin Pathol 1990;93:167–175.

263. Nakatani Y, Dickerson R, Mark EJ. Pulmonary endodermal tumor resembling fetal lung: A clinicopathologic study of five cases with immunohistochemical and ultrastructural characterization. Hum Pathol 1990;21:1097–1107.

264. Huszar M, Herczeg E, Lieberman Y, Geiger B. Distinctive immunofluorescent labeling of epithelial and mesenchymal elements of carcosarcoma with antibodies specific for different intermediate filaments. Hum Pathol 1984;15:532–528.

265. Suster S, Huszar M, Herczeg E. Spindle cell squamous carcinoma of the lung: Immunocytochemical and ultrastructural study of a case. Histopathology 1987;11:871–878.

266. Matsui K, Kitagawa M. Spindle cell carcinoma of the lung: A clinicopathologic study of three cases. Cancer (Philadelphia) 1991;67:2361–2367.

267. Mark EJ. Lung biopsy interpretation. Baltimore: Williams & Wilkins, 1984:220–221.

268. Kradin RL, Young RH, Dickersin GIC, Kirkham SE, Mark EJ. Pulmonary blastoma with argyrophil cells lacking sarcomatous features (pulmonary endodermal tumor resembling fetal lung). Am J Surg Pathol 1982;6:165–172.

269. Tamai S, Kameya T, Shimosato T, Tsumuraya M, Wada T. Pulmonary blastoma: an ultrastructural study of a case and its transplanted tumor in nude mice. Cancer (Philadelphia) 1980;46:1389–1396.

270. Liebow AA, Hubbell DS. Sclerosing hemangioma (histiocytoma, xanthoma) of the lung. Cancer (Philadelphia) 1956;9:53–75.

271. Goorwitch J, Madoff I. Capillary hemangioma of the lung. Dis Chest 1955;28:98–103.

272. Katzenstein A-LA, Gmelich JT, Carrington CB. Scle-

rosing hemangioma of the lung: A clinicopathologic study of 51 cases. Am J Surg Pathol 1982;4:343–356.

273. Chan KW, Gibbs AR, Lio WS, Newman GR. Benign sclerosing pneumocytoma of the lung (sclerosing hemangioma). Thorax 1982;37:404–412.

274. Spencer H, Nambu S. Sclerosing hemangioma of the lung. Histopathology 1986;10:477–487.

275. Thomas A, Lee CN. Sclerosing haemangioma in Singapore. Ann Acad Med Singapore 1986;15:71–76.

276. Kimura H, Kusajima Y, Konishi I, et al. A case of sclerosing hemangioma of the lung and review of 196 cases in the Japanese literature. J Jpn Sco Clin Surg 1988;49:1403–1409.

277. Katzenstein A-LA, Weise DL, Fulling K, Battifora H. So-called sclerosing hemangioma of the lung: evidence for mesothelial origin. Am J Surg Pathol 1983;7:3–16.

278. Haimoto H, Tsutsumi Y, Nagura H, Kanashima N, Watanabe K. Immunohistochemical study of so-called sclerosing haemangioma of the lung. Virchow Arch [A] 1985;407:419–430.

279. Nagata N, Dairaku M, Ishida T, Sueishi K, Tanaka K. Sclerosing hemangioma of the lung: immunohistochemical characterization of its origin as related to surfactant apoprotein. Cancer (Philadelphia) 1985; 55:116–123.

280. Nagata N, Dairaku M, Sueishi K, Tanaka K. Sclerosing hemangioma of the lung: an epithelial tumor composed of immunohistochemically heterogenous cells. Am J Clin Pathol 1987;88:552–559.

281. Yousem SA, Wick MR, Singh G, et al. So-called sclerosing hemangiomas of lung: An immunohistochemical study supporting a respiratory epithelial origin. Am J Surg Pathol 1988;12:582–590.

282. Sugio K, Yokoyama H, Kanedo S, Ishida T, Sugimachi K. Sclerosing hemangioma of the lung: Radiographic and pathological study. Ann Thorac Surg 1992; 53:295–300.

283. Arean VM, Wheat MW, Jr. Sclerosing hemangiomas of the lung: a case report and review of the literature. Am Rev Respir Dis 1962;85:261–271.

284. Mori S. Sclerosing hemangioma of the lung. Dis Chest 1968;54:71–74.

285. Lee ST, Lee YC, Hsu CY, Lin CC. Bilateral multiple sclerosing hemangiomas of the lung. Chest 1992; 101:572–573.

286. Maezato K, Hitomi S, Kuwabara M. A case of multiple sclerosing hemangiomas of the lung and a review of the literature in Japan. (in Japanese) Nippon Kyobu Shikkan Gakkai Zasshi 1989;27:230–233.

287. Joshi K, Gopinath N, Shankar SK, Kumar R, Chopra P. Multiple sclerosing hemangiomas of the lung. Postgrad Med J 1980;56:50–53.

288. Noguchi M, Kodama T, Mornaga S, Shimosato Y, Saito T, Tsuboi E. Multiple sclerosing hemangiomas of the lung. Am J Surg Pathol 1986;10:429–435.

289. Tanaka I, Inoue M, Matsui Y, et al. A case of pneumocytoma (so-called sclerosing hemangioma) with lymph node metastasis. Jpn J Clin Oncol 1986;16:77–86.

290. Ogawa N, Maehara T, Satoh S, Nakatani Y, Misugi K.

Immunocytochemical analysis of progesterone and estrogen receptors of sclerosing hemangiomas of the lung (abstr.). Mod Pathol 1992;5:115A.

291. Aiba M, Hirayama A, Sakurada M, Suzuki T. So-called sclerosing hemangioma of the lung with nuclear inclusion bodies: Immunohistochemical study of a case. Acta Pathol Jpn 1988;38:873–881.

292. Kudo H, Morinaga S, Shimosato Y, et al. Solitary mast cell tumor of the lung. Cancer (Philadelphia) 1988;61:2089–2094.

293. Wang SE, Nieberg RK. Fine needle aspiration cytology of sclerosing hemangioma of the lung, a mimicker of bronchioloalveolar carcinoma. Acta Cytol 1986;30: 51–54.

294. Tengan I, Suemasu K, Eguchi K, et al. Benign tumors and tumor-like lesions (excluding adenomas) of the lung: Radiological and clinicopathological analysis of 48 cases. Jpn J Clin Oncol 1981;11:343–352.

295. Bahk YW, Shinn KS, Choi BS. The air meniscus sign in sclerosing hemangioma of the lung. Radiology 1978; 128:27–29.

296. Kennedy A. "Sclerosing hemangioma" of the lung: An alternate view of its development. J Clin Pathol 1973;26:792–799.

297. Haas JB, Unis EJ, Totten RS. Ultrastructure of sclerosing hemangioma of the lung. Cancer (Philadelphia) 1972;30:512–518.

298. Kay S, Still WJS, Borochovitz D. Sclerosing hemangioma of the lung: an endothelial or epithelial neoplasm? Hum Pathol 1977;8:468–474.

299. Hill GS, Eggleston JC. Electron microscopic studies of so-called pulmonary "slcerosing menangioma": report of a case suggesting epithelial origin. Cancer (Philadelphia) 1972;30:1092–1106.

300. Mikuz G, Szinicz G, Fischer H. Sclerosing hemangioma of the lung: case report and electron microscope investigation. Virchows Arch [A] 1977;385:93–101.

301. Heilman E, Feiner H. The role of electron microscopy in the diagnosis of unusual peripheral lung tumors. Hum Pathol 1978;9:589–593.

302. Koide T. Ultrastructural analysis of 7 cases of sclerosing hemangioma of the lung (Liebow) with a special reference to histogenesis. Haigan 1979;19:19–36.

303. Palacios JJN, Escribano PM, Toledo J, Garzon A, Larru E, Palomera J. Sclerosing hemangioma of the lung: an ultrastructural study. Cancer (Philadelphia) 1979; 44:949–955.

304. Alvarez-Fernandez E, Escalona-Zapata J. Sclerosing hemangioma of the lung: Histochemical, electron microscopic, tissue culture and time-lapse cinematographic study. Histopathology 1981;5:579–588.

305. Ng W-L, Ma L. Is sclerosing hemangioma of the lung an alveolar mixed tumor? Pathology 1983;15:205–211.

306. Fukayama M, Koike M. So-called sclerosing hemangioma of the lung: An immunohistochemical and ultrastructural study. Acta Pathol Jpn 1988;38:627–642.

307. Satoh Y, Tsuchiya E, Weng S-Y, et al. Pulmonary sclerosing hemangioma of the lung: A type II pneumocytoma by immunohistochemical and immunoelectron

microscopic study. Cancer (Philadelphia) 1989;64: 1310–1317.

308. Park YK, Yang MH. So-called sclerosing hemangioma of the lung—Two cases reported with ultrastructural study. J Korean Med Sci 1989;4:179–183.

309. Dail DH, Liebow AA, Gmelich JT, et al. Intravascular, bronchiolar, and alveolar tumor of the lung (IVBAT): An analysis of twenty cases of a peculiar sclerosing endothelial tumor. Cancer (Philadelphia) 1983;51: 452–464.

310. Eggleston EC. The intravascular bronchioalveolar tumor and the sclerosing hemangioma of the lung: Misnomers of pulmonary neoplasia. Semin Diagn Pathol 1985;2:270–280.

311. Singh G, Katyal SL, Ordóñez HG, et al. Type II pneumocytes in pulmonary tumors. Arch Pathol Lab Med 1984;108:44–48.

312. Alvarez-Fernandez E, Carretero-Albinana L, Manarguez-Palanca J. Sclerosing hemangioma of the lung: An immunohistochemical study of intermediate filaments and endothelial markers. Arch Pathol Lab Med 1989;113:121–124.

313. Huszar M, Suster S, Herczeg E, Geiger B. Sclerosing hemangioma of the lung: immunohistochemical demonstration of mesenchymal origin using antibodies to tissue-specific intermediate filaments. Cancer (Philadelphia) 1986;58:2422–2427.

313a. Ng W-L, Ma L. Is sclerosing hemangioma of lung an alveolar mixed tumor? Pathology 1983;15:205–211.

314. Lamovec J, Bracko M. Metastatic pattern of infiltrating lobular carcinoma of the breast: An autopsy study. J Surg Oncol 1991;48:28–33.

314a. Foster E, Ackerman L. Localized mesotheliomas of the pleura. The pathologic evaluation of 18 cases. Am J Clin Pathol 1960;34:349–364.

315. Chesney T McC. Placental transmagnification of the lung: A unique case with remarkable histopathological features. (ab Invest 1979;40:245–246.

315a. Fidler MY, Koomen M, Sebek B, Greco MA, Rizk CC, Askin FB. Placental transmogrification of the lung: A clinicopathologic study of three further cases (abstract). Mod Pathol 1993;6:130A.

316. Semeraro D, Gibbs AR. Pulmonary adenoma: A variant of sclerosing hemangioma of lung? J Clin Pathol 1989;42:1222–1223.

317. Bahadori H, Liebow AA. Plasma cell granulomas of the lung. Cancer (Philadelphia) 1973;31:191–208.

318. Spencer H. The pulmonary plasma cell/histiocytoma complex. Histopathology 1984;8:903–916.

319. Berardi RS, Lee SS, Chen HP, Stines GJ. Inflammatory pseudotumors of the lung. Surg Gynecol Obstet 1983;156:89–96.

320. Warter A, Satge D, Roeslin N. Angioinvasive plasma cell granuloma of the lung. Cancer (Philadelphia) 1987;59:435–443.

321. Pettinato G, Manivel JC, DeRosa N, Dehner LP. Inflammatory myofibroblastic tumor (plasma cell granuloma): Clinicopathologic study of 20 cases with immunohistochemical and ultrastructural observations. Am

J Clin Pathol 1990;56:533–546.

322. Matsubara O, Tan-Liu NS, Kenney RM, Mark EJ. Inflammatory pseudotumor of the lung: Progression from organizing pneumonia to fibrous histiocytoma or to plasma cell granuloma in 32 cases. Hum Pathol 1988;19:807–814.

323. Ishida T, Oka T, Nishino T, Tateishi M, Mitsudomi T, Sugimachi K. Inflammatory pseudotumor of the lung in adults: Radiographic and clinicopathological analysis. Ann Thorac Surg 1989;48:90–95.

324. Golbert SV, Pletnev SD. On pulmonary "pseudotumors." Neoplasma 1967;14:189–198.

325. Hartman GE, Shochat SJ. Primary pulmonary neoplasms in childhood: A review. Ann Thorac Surg 1983;36:108–119.

326. Shapiro MP, Gale ME, Carter BL. Variable CT appearance of plasma cell granuloma of the lung. J Comput Assist Tomogr 1987;11:49–51.

327. Monzon CM, Gilchrist GS, Burgert ED, et al. Plasma cell granuloma of the lung in children. Pediatrics 1982;70:268–273.

328. Usuda K, Saito Y, Imai T, et al. Inflammatory pseudotumor of the lung diagnosed as granulomatous lesion by preoperative brushing cytology: A case report. Acta Cytol 1990;36:685–689.

329. Sherwin R, Kern W, Jones J. Solitary mast cell granuloma (histiocytoma) of the lung. Cancer (Philadelphia) 1965;18:634–641.

330. Lund C, Sørenson IM, Axelsen F, Larsen K. Pulmonary histiocytomas. Eur J Respir Dis 1983;64:141–149.

331. Mohsenifar Z, Bein ME, Mott LJM, Tashkin DP. Cystic organizing pneumonia with elements of plasma cell granuloma. Arch Pathol Lab Med 1979;103:600–601.

332. Janigan DT, Marrie TJ. An inflammatory pseudotumor in the lung in Q fever pneumonia. N Engl J Med 1983;308:86–88.

333. Bishopric GA, d'Agay MF, Schlemmer B, Sarfati E, Brocheriou C. Pulmonary pseudotumor due to *corynebacterium equi* in a patient with the acquired immunodeficiency syndrome. Thorax 1988;83:486–487.

334. Kuzela DC. Ultrastructural study of a post inflammatory "tumor" of the lung. Cancer (Philadelphia) 1975;36:149–156.

335. Buell R, Wang N-S, Seemayer TA, Ahmed MN. Endobronchial plasma cell granuloma (xanthomatous pseudotumor): a light and electron microscopic study. Hum Pathol 1976;7:411–426.

336. Shirakusa T, Miyazaki N, Kitagawa T, Sugiyama K. Ultrastructural study of pulmonary plasma cell granulomas: Report of a case. Br J Dis Chest 1979;73:289–296.

337. Alvarez-Fernandez E, Escalona-Zapata J. Pulmonary plasma cell granuloma. An electron microscopic and tissue culture study. Histopathology 1983;7:279–286.

337a. Chen HP, Lee SS, Berardi RS. Inflammatory pseudotumor of the lung. Ultrastructural and light microscopic study of a myxomatous variant. Cancer (Philadelphia) 1984;54:861–865.

338. Muraoka S, Sato T, Takahashi T, Ando M, Shimoda H.

Plasma cell granuloma of the lung with extrapulmonary extension. Immunohistochemical and electron microscopic studies. Acta Pathol Jpn 1985;35:933–944.

339. Shirakusa T, Miyazaki N, Kitagawa T, Sugiyama K. Ultrastructural study of pulmonary plasma cell granulomas: Report of a case. Br J Dis Chest 1979;73:289–296.

340. Barbareschi M, Ferrero S, Aldovini D, et al. Inflammatory pseudotumor of the lung. Immunohistochemical analysis on four new cases. Histol-Histopathology 1990;5:205–211.

341. Wentworth P, Lynch MJ, Fallis JC, Turner JAP, Lowden JA, Conen PE. Xanthomatous pseudo-tumor of the lung: a case report with electron microscope and lipid studies. Cancer (Philadelphia) 1968;22:345–355.

342. Long FL, Nott DB, MacArthur EB. Xanthomatous tumors of the lung with identification of lipid content. Australas Ann Med 1970;19:362–365.

343. Toccanier MF, Exquis B, Groebli Y. Granulome plasmocytaire du poumon. Neuf observations avec étude immunohistochimique. Ann Pathol 1982;2:21–28.

344. Maier HC, Sommers SS. Recurrent and metastatic pulmonary fibrous histiocytoma/plasma cell granuloma in a child. Cancer (Philadelphia) 1987;60:1073–1076.

345. Fassina AS, Rugge M, Scapinello A, et al. Plasma cell granuloma of the lung (inflammatory pseudotumor). Tumori 1986;72:529–534.

346. Dorski JJ, Priebe CJ, Driessnack M, et al. Corticosteroids in the management of unresected plasma cell granuloma (inflammatory pseudotumor) of the lung. J Pediatr Surg 1991;26:1064–1066.

347. Gal AA, Koss MN, Hocholzer L, Hitchcock CL, Becker R, O'Leary T. Prognostic factors in pulmonary inflammatory pseudotumor and malignant fibrous histiocytoma. Mod Pathol 1992;5:113A (abstr.).

348. Patchefsky A, Enzinger FM. Intravascular fasciitis. Am J Surg Pathol 1981;5:29–36.

349. Nochomovitz LE, Orenstein JM. Inflammatory pseudotumor of the urinary bladder: Possible relationship to nodular faciitis. Two case reports, cytologic observations and ultrastructural observations. Am J Surg Pathol 1985;9:366–373.

350. Katzenstein A-LA, Maurer JJ. Benign histiocytic tumor of the lung: a light and electron microscopic study. Am J Surg Pathol 1979;3:61–68.

351. Bates T, Hull O. Histiocytoma of the bronchus. Am J Dis Child 1958;95:53–56.

352. Kauffman S, Stout A. Histiocytic tumors (fibrous xanthoma and histiocytoma) in children. Cancer (Philadelphia) 1961;14:469–482.

353. Engleman P, Liebow AA, Gmelich J, Friedman PJ. Pulmonary hyalinizing granuloma. Am Rev Respir Dis 1977;115:997–1008.

354. Drasin H, Blume MR, Rosenbaum EH, Klein HF. Pulmonary hyalinizing granulomas in a patient with malignant lymphoma, with development nine years later of multiple myeloma and systemic amyloidosis.

Cancer (Philadelphia) 1979;44:215–220.

355. Guccion JG, Rohatgi PK, Saini N. Pulmonary hyalinizing granuloma. Electron microscopic and immunologic studies. Chest 1984;85:571–573.

356. Schlosnagle DC, Check IJ, Sewell CW, Plummer A, York RM, Hunter RL. Immunologic abnormalities in two patients with pulmonary hyalinizing granuloma. Am J Clin Pathol 1982;78:231–235.

357. Chalaoui J, Gregoire P, Sylvester J, Lefebvre R, Amyot R. Pulmonary hyalinizing granuloma: a cause of pulmonary nodules. Radiology 1984;152:23–26.

358. Dent RG, Godden DJ, Stovin PGI, Stark JE. Pulmonary hyalinizing granuloma in association with retroperitoneal fibrosis. Thorax 1983;38:955–956.

359. Macedo EV, Adolph J. Pulmonary hyalinizing granulomas. J Can Assoc Radiol 1985;36:66–67.

360. Maijub AG, Giltman LI, Verner JL, Peace RJ. Pulmonary hyalinizing granuloma. Ann Allergy 1985;54:227–229.

361. Ikard RW. Pulmonary hyalinizing granuloma. Chest 1988;93:871–872.

362. Gans SJM, van der Elst AMC, Straks W. Pulmonary hyalinizing granuloma. Eur Respir J 1988;1:389–391.

363. Case records of the Massachusetts General Hospital (Case 6-1989). N Engl J Med 1989;320:380–389.

364. Patel Y, Ishikawa S, MacDonnell KF. Pulmonary hyalinizing granuloma presenting as multiple cavitary calcified nodules. Chest 1991;100:1720–1721.

365. Yousem SA, Hochholzer L. Pulmonary hyalinizing granuloma. Am J Clin Pathol 1987;87:1–6.

366. Personal communication, 1991, Rodney Schmidt M.D. University of Washington School of Medicine, Seattle, Washington.

367. Osborne BM, Butler JJ, Mackay B. Proteinaceous lymphadenopathy with hypergammaglobulinemia. Am J Surg Pathol 1979;3:137–145.

368. Eggleston JC. Sclerosing mediastinitis. In: Fenoglio CM, Wolff M, eds. Progress in surgical pathology. Vol. 2. New York: Masson, 1980:1–17.

369. Katzenstein A-LA, Mazur MT. Pulmonary infarct: An unusual manifestation of fibrosing mediastinitis. Chest 1980;77:521–524.

370. Goodwin RA, Nickell JA, Des Prez RM. Mediastinal fibrosis complicating healed primary histoplasmosis and tuberculosis. Medicine (Baltimore) 1972;51:227–246.

371. Schowengerdt CG, Suyemoto R, Main FB. Granulomatous and fibrous mediastinitis: A review and analysis of 180 cases. J Thorac Cardiovasc Surg 1969;57:365–379.

372. Ulbright TM, Katzenstein A-LA. Solitary necrotizing granulomas of the lung: Differentiating features and etiology. Am J Surg Pathol 1980;4:13–28.

373. Liebow AA, Castleman B. Benign "clear cell tumors" of the lung. Am J Pathol 1063;43:13a–14a (abstr.).

374. Liebow AA, Castleman B. Benign clear cell ("sugar") tumors of the lung. Yale J Biol Med 1971;43:213–222.

375. Andrion A, Mazzucco G, Gugliotta P, Monga G. Benign clear cell ("sugar") tumor of the lung. A light micro-

scopic, histochemical, and ultrastructural study with a review of the literature. Cancer (Philadelphia) 1985;56:2657–2663.

376. Gaffey MJ, Mills SE, Askin FB, et al. Clear cell tumor of the lung. A clinicopathologic, immunohistochemical, and ultrastructural study of eight cases. Am J Surg Pathol 1990;14:248–259.

377. Gaffey MJ, Mills SE, Zabo JR, Weiss LM, Gown AM. Clear cell tumor of the lung: Immunohistochemical and ultrastructural evidence of melanogenesis. Am J Surg Pathol 1991;15:644–653.

378. Gal AA, Koss MN, Hochholzer L, Chejfec G. An immunohistochemical study of benign clear cell ("sugar") tumor of the lung. Arch Pathol Lab Med 1991;115:1034–1038.

379. Sale GE, Kulander BG. 'Benign' clear-cell tumor (sugar tumor) of the lung with hepatic metastases ten years after resection of pulmonary primary tumor. Arch Pathol Lab Med 1988;112:1177–1178.

380. Nguyen GK. Aspiration biopsy cytology of benign clear cell ('sugar') tumor of the lung. Acta Cytol 1989; 33:511–515.

381. Kung M, Landa JF, Lubin J. Benign clear cell tumor ("sugar tumor") of the trachea. Cancer (Philadelphia) 1984;54:517–519.

382. Gerstl B, Tavaststjerna M, Smith JK, Hayman RB. The lipid and carbohydrate composition of pulmonary tumors. Am Rev Respir Dis 1966;84:23–27.

383. Becker NH, Soifer I. Benign clear cell tumor ("sugar tumor") of the lung. Cancer (Philadelphia) 1971;27:712–719.

384. Hoch WS, Patchefsky AS, Takeda M, Gordon G. Benign clear cell tumor of the lung: An ultrastructural study. Cancer (Philadelphia) 1974;33:1328–1336.

385. Sale GE, Kulander BG. Benign clear cell tumor of lung with necrosis. Cancer (Philadelphia) 1976;37:2355–2358.

386. Harbin WP, Mark GJ, Greene RE. Benign clear cell tumor ("sugar" tumor) of the lung: A case report and review of the literature. Radiology 1978;129:595–596.

387. Zolliker A, Jacques J, Goldstein AS. Benign clear cell tumor of the lung. Arch Pathol Lab Med 1979;103:526–530.

388. Fukuda T, Machinami R, Joshita T, Nagashima K. Benign clear cell tumor of the lung in an 8-year-old girl. Arch Pathol Lab Med 1986;110:664–666.

389. Ozdemir IA, Zaman N-U, Rullis I, Webb WR. Benign clear cell tumor of lung. J Thorac Cardiovasc Surg 1974;68:131–133.

390. Sidhu GS, Forrester EM. Glycogen-rich Clara cell type bronchioloalveolar carcinoma: Light and electron microscopic study. Cancer (Philadelphia) 1977;40:2209–2215.

391. Sale GE, Kulander BG. Benign clear cell ("sugar") tumor of lung. Arch Pathol Lab Med 1988;113:574.

392. Dail, DH. Benign clear cell ("sugar") tumor of lung (letter). Arch Pathol Lab Med 1988;113:573.

393. Nakanishi K, Kawai T, Suzuki M. Benign clear cell

tumor of the lung: A histopathologic study. Acta Pathol Jpn 1988;38:515–522.

394. Pea M, Bonetti F, Zamboni G, Martignoni G, Fiore-Donati L, Doglioni C. Clear cell tumor and angiomyolipoma. Am J Surg Pathol 1991;15:199–201.

395. Gaffey MJ, Mills SE. Clear cell tumor and angiomyolipoma. Author's reply (letter). Am J Surg Pathol 1991;15:201–202.

396. Termeer A, Arkenbout PM, Lacquet LK, Cox AI. Benign clear cell tumor of the lung: Intermediate filament typing as a tool in differential diagnosis. Eur Respir J 1988;1:288–290.

397. Pea M, Bonetti F, Zamboni G, et al. Melanocyte marker HMB-45 is regularly expressed in angiomyolipoma of the kidney. Pathology 1991;23:185–188.

398. Bonetti F, Pea M, Martignoni G, Zamboni G, Iuzzoliho P. Cellular heterogeneity in lymphangiomyomatosis of the lung. Hum Pathol 1991;22:727–728.

399. Unger PD, Hoffman K, Thung SN, Pertsemlides D, Wolfe D, Kaneko M. HMB-45 reactivity in adrenal pheochromocytomas. Arch Pathol Lab Med 1992; 116:151–153.

400. Zimmer C, Gottschalk J, Goebel S, Cervos-Navarro J. Melanoma-associated antigens in tumours of the nervous system: An immunohistochemical study with the monoclonal antibody HMB-45. Virchows Arch A Pathol Anat 1992;420:121–126.

401. Weeks DA, Chase DR, Malott RL, Mierau GW, Zuppan C, Chase RL. HMB-45 staining in renal angiomyolipoma and in other mesenchymal processes of vascular myogenous and fatty derivation (abstr.) Lab Invest 1991;64:9A.

402. Bonetti F, Pea M, Martignoni G, Mombello A, Colombari R, Zamboni G. False-positive immunostaining of normal epithelia and carcinomas with ascites fluid preparations of antimelanoma monoclonal and antibody HMB45. Am J Clin Pathol 1991;95:454–459.

403. Dupree WB, Langloss JM, Weiss SW. Pigmented dematofibrosarcoma protuberans (Bednar tumor): A pathologic, ultrastructural, and immunohistochemical study. Am J Surg Pathol 1985;9:630–639.

404. Gaffey MJ, Zarbo RJ, Weiss LM. PEC and sugar (Authors' reply). Am J Surg Pathol 1992;16:308.

405. Bonetti F, Pea M, Martignoni G, Zamboni G. PEC and sugar (letter). Am J Surg Pathol 1992;16:307–308.

406. Alvarez-Fernandez E, Folque-Gomez E. Atypical bronchial carcinoid with oncocytoid features. Its ultrastructure with special reference to its granular content. Arch Pathol Lab Med 1981;105:428–431.

407. Katzenstein A-L, Purvis R Jr, Gmelich J, Askin F. Pulmonary resection for metastatic renal adenocarcinoma: Pathologic findings and therapeutic value. Cancer (Philadelphia) 1978;41:712–723.

408. Middleton RG, Surgery for metastatic renal cell carcinoma. J Urol 1967;97:973–977.

409. Liebow AA. Tumors of the lower respiratory tract. Ser. 1. Washington DC: Armed Forces Institute of Pathology, 1952;17:79, 90.

410. Walter JB, Pryce DM. The histology of lung cancer. Thorax 1955;10:107–116.

411. Morgan A, Mackenzie D. Clear-cell carcinomas of the lung. J Pathol Bacteriol 1964;87:25–29.

412. Katzenstein A-LA, Prioleau PG, Askin FB. The histologic spectrum and significance of clear-cell change in lung carcinoma. Cancer (Philadelphia) 1980;45:943–947.

413. Edward C, Carlile A. Clear cell carcinoma of the lung. J Clin Pathol 1985;38:880–885.

414. Korn D, Bensch K, Liebow AA, Castleman B. Multiple minute pulmonary tumors resembling chemodectomas. Am J Pathol 1960;37:641–472.

415. Spencer H. Pathology of the lung. Oxford: Pergamon, 1962:690–692.

416. Zak FG, Chabes A. Pulmonary chemodectomatosis. JAMA 1963;183:887–889.

417. Barroso-Moguel R, Costero I. Some histochemical tests in Zak's chemoblastomatosis. Am J Pathol 1964;44:17a–18a.

418. Barroso-Moguel R, Costero I. Quimiorreceptores y otras estructuras intrapulmonares argentafines relacionadas con la regulacion de la circulacion pulmonar. Arch Inst Cardiol Mex 1968;38:337–344.

419. Costero I, Barroso-Moguel R, Martinez-Palomo A. Pleural origin of some of the supposed chemodectomoid structures of the lung. Beitr Pathol 1972;146:351–365.

420. Spain DM. Intrapulmonary chemodectomas in subjects with organizing pulmonary thromboemboli. Am Rev Respir Dis 1967;96:1158–1164.

421. Ichinose H, Hewitt RL, Drapanas T. Minute pulmonary chemodectomas. Cancer (Philadelphia) 1971;28:692–700.

422. Churg AM, Warnock ML. So-called "minute pulmonary chemodectoma": A tumor not related to paragangliomas. Cancer (Philadelphia) 1976;37:1759–1769.

423. Kuhn C, III, Askin FB. The fine structure of so-called minute pulmonary chemodectomas. Hum Pathol 1975;6:681–691.

424. Tu H, Bottomley RH. Malignant chemodectoma presenting as a miliary pulmonary infiltrate. Cancer (Philadelphia) 1974;33:244–249.

425. Pinkser KL, Messinger N, Hurwitz P, Becker NH. Cervical chemodectoma with extensive pulmonary metastases. Chest 1973;64:116–118.

426. Blessing MH, Hora BI. Glomera in der Lunge des Menschen. Z Zellforsch 1968;87:562–570.

427. Heppleston AG. A carotid body like tumour in the lung. J Pathol Bacteriol 1958;75:461–464.

428. Fawcett FJ, Husband EM. Chemodectoma of lung. J Clin Pathol 1967;20:260–262.

429. Goodman ML, Laforet EG. Solitary primary chemodectomas of the lung. Chest 1972;61:48–50.

430. Singh G, Lee RE, Brooks DH. Primary pulmonary paraganglioma: Report of a case and review of the literature. Cancer (Philadelphia) 1977;40:2286–2289.

431. Mostecky H, Lichtenberg J, Kalus M. A non-chromaffin paraganglioma of the lung. Thorax 1966;21:205–208.

432. Laustela E, Mattila S, Franssila K. Chemodectoma of the lung. Scand J Cardiovasc Surg 1969;3:59–62.

433. Lee YN, Hori JM. Chemodectoma of the lung. J Surg Oncol 1972;4:33–36.

434. Blessing MH, Borchard F, Lenz W. Glomustumor (sog chemodektom) der Lunge. Virchows Arch [A] 1973;359:315–329.

435. Stanulla H. Zur Kenntnis der Lungenchemodektome. Thorax Chir 1968;16:204–209.

436. Batime J, Roujeau J, Souguet R, et al. Chemodectomes solitaires intrapulmonaries (a propos de deux observations). J Fr Med Chirug Thorac 1972;26:279–289.

437. Lemonick DM, Pai PB, Hines GL. Malignant primary pulmonary paraganglioma with hilar metastases (letter). J Thorac Cardiovasc Surg 1990;99:563–564.

438. Enzinger FM, Weiss SW. Soft tissue tumors. (2d Ed.) St Louis: CV Mosby, 1988:836–860.

439. Enzinger FM, Weiss SW. Soft tissue tumors. 3d Ed. St. Louis: CV Mosby, 1988;581–595.

440. Hussarek M, Rieder W. Glomustumor der Luftrohre. Krebsarzt 1950;5:208–212.

441. Tang C-K, Toker C, Foris NP, Trump BF. Glomangioma of the lung. Am J Surg Pathol 1978;2:103–109.

442. Alt B, Huffer WE, Belchis DA. A vascular lesion with smooth muscle differentiation presenting as a coin lesion in the lung: Glomus tumor versus hemangiopericytoma. Am J Clin Pathol 1983;80:765–770.

443. Fabich DR, Hafez G-R. Glomangioma of the trachea. Cancer (Philadelphia) 1980;45:2337–2341.

444. Warter A, Vetter JM, Morand G, Philippe E. Tumeur glomique de la trachee. Arch Anat Cytol Pathol 1980;28:184–190.

445. Ito H, Motohiro K, Nomura S, Tahara E. Glomus tumor of the trachea: Immunohistochemical and electron microscopic studies. Pathol Res Pract 1988;183:778–784.

446. Kim YI, Kim JH, Suh J-S, Ham EK, Suh KP. Glomus tumor of the trachea: Report of a case with ultrastructural observation. Cancer (Philadelphia) 1989;64:881–886.

447. Rosai J. Ackerman's Surgical Pathology. 6th Ed. New York: CV Mosby, 1981:1441.

448. Slater DN, Cotton DWK, Azzopardi JG. Oncocytic glomus tumour: A new variant. Histopathology 1987;11:523–531.

449. MacKay B, Legha SS. Coin lesion of the lung in a 19-year-old male. Ultrastruct Pathol 1981;2:289–294.

450. Gould EW, Manivel JC, Albores-Saavedra J, Monforte H. Locally infiltrative glomus tumors and glomangiosarcomas: A clinical, ultrastructural, and immunohistochemical study. Cancer (Philadelphia) 1990;65:310–318.

451. Stout AP, Murray MR. Hemangiopericytoma: A vascular tumor featuring Zimmerman's pericytes. Ann Surg 1942;116:26–33.

452. Ostermiller WE, Comer TP, Barker WL. Endobronchial granular cell myoblastoma. Ann Thorac Surg 1970;9:143–148.

453. Oparah SS, Subramanian VA. Granular cell myoblas-

toma of the bronchus: report of two cases and review of the literature. Ann Thorac Surg 1976;22:199–202.

454. DeClerq D, Van der Straeten M, Roels H. Granular cell myoblastoma of the bronchus. Eur J Respir Dis 1983;64:72–76.

455. McSwain GR, Colpitts R, Kreutner A, O'Brien PH, Spicer S. Granular cell myoblastoma. Surg Gynecol Obstet 1980;150:703–710.

456. Poulet J, Cocheton J-J, Touretz L, Almosni M. Les localisations bronchotracheales des tumeurs a cellules granuleuses ou tumerurs d'Abrikossoff. Semin Hop Paris 1972;48:3325–3327.

457. Schulster PL, Khan FA, Azueta V. Asymptomatic pulmonary granular cell tumor presenting as a coin lesion. Chest 1975;68:256–258.

458. Teplick JG, Teplick SK, Haskin ME. Granular cell myoblastoma of the lung. Am J Roentgenol Radium Ther Nucl Med 1975;125:890–894.

459. Novi I. I tumori a cellule granulose (cosiddetti 'miomi mioblastici' di Abrikossoff): A proposito de un raro caso di tumore a cellule granulose del polmone ad evoluzione infiltrante. Arch Ital Chir 1958;83:333–336.

460. Klima M, Peters J. Malignant granular cell tumor. Arch Pathol Lab Med 1987;111:1070–1072.

461. Cadotte M. Malignant granular-cell myoblastoma. Cancer (Philadelphia) 1974;33:1417–1422.

462. Umansky C, Bullock WK. Granular cell myoblastoma of the breast. Am Surg 1968;168:810–817.

463. Robertson AJ, McIntosh W, Lamont P, Guthrie W. Malignant granular cell tumour (myoblastoma) of the vulva: Report of a case and review of the literature. Histopathology 1981;5:69–79.

464. Gabriel JR, Jr, Thomas L, Kondlapoodi P, Haque N, Chauhan PM. Granular cell tumor of the bronchus: A previously unreported cause of hypercalcemia. J Surg Oncol 1983;24:338–340.

465. Weitzner S, Oser JF. Granular cell myoblastoma of bronchus. Am Rev Respir Dis 1968;97:923–930.

466. Young CD, Gay RM. Multiple endobronchial granular cell myoblastomas discovered at bronchoscopy. Hum Pathol 1984;15:193–194.

467. Majumdar B, Thomas J, Gorelkin L, Symbas PN. Respiratory obstruction caused by a multicentric granular cell tumor of laryngotracheobronchial tree. Hum Pathol 1981;12:283–286.

468. Cooper JAD Jr, Arora NS. Multiple granular cell myoblastoma of the bronchial tree. South Med J 1982;75:491–492.

469. Redjaee B, Kumar Rohatgi P, Herman MA. Multicentric endobronchial granular cell myoblastoma. Chest 1990;98:945–948.

470. Ivantury R, Shah D, Ascer E, Srinivassan K, Heraud J, Rahman M. Granular cell tumor of larynx and bronchus. Ann Thorac Surg 1982;33:69–73.

471. Park SH, Kim TJ, Chi JG. Congenital granular cell tumor with systemic involvement: Immunohistochemical and ultrastructural study. Arch Pathol Lab Med 1991;115:934–938.

472. Sobel HJ, Marquet E. Granular cells and granular cell lesions. Pathol Annu 1974;9:43–79.

473. Hurwitx SS, Conlan AA, Gritzman MCD, Krut LH. Coexisting granular cell myoblastoma and squamous carcinoma of the bronchus. Thorax 1982;37:292–393.

474. Dabouis G, Nomballais MF, Naury B, Peltier P, Morineau JF, Corroller J. Tumeur d'Abrikossoff endolbronchique. Poumon Coeur 1979;35:211–216.

475. Gabriel JB Jr, Thomas L, Mendoza CB, Chauhan PM. Granular cell tumor of the bronchus coexisting with bronchogenic adenocarcinoma: A case report. Chest 1975;68:256–258.

476. Boath JB, Osborn DA. Granular cell myoblastoma of the larynx. Arch Otolaryngol 1970;70:279–293.

477. Alvarez-Fernandez E, Carretero-Albinana L. Bronchial granular cell tumor: Presentation of three cases with tissue culture and ultrastructural study. Arch Pathol Lab Med 1987;111:1065–1069.

478. Glant MD, Wall RW, Ransburg R. Endobronchial granular cell tumour. Acta Cytol (Baltimore) 1979;23:477–482.

479. Miller WS. The distribution of lymphoid tissue in the lung. Anat Rec 1911;5:99.

480. Miller WS. The pulmonary lymphoid tissue in old age. Am Rev Tuberc 1924;9:519.

481. Miller WS. The lung. 2d Ed. Springfield: Thomas, 1947;119–135.

482. Heller A. Über subpleurale Lymphdrusen: Zugleich ein Beitrag zur Lehr von den Staubinhalationskrankheiten. Dtsch Arch Klin Med 1895;55:141–145.

483. Kradin RL, Spirn PW, Mark EJ. Intrapulmonary lymph nodes: Clinical, radiologic and pathologic features. Chest 1985;87:662–667.

484. Greenberg HB. Benign subpleural lymph node appearing as pulmonary "coin" lesions. Radiology 1961;77:97–99.

485. Steele JD. The solitary pulmonary nodule: Report of a cooperative study of resected asymptomatic solitary pulmonary nodules in males. J Thorac Cardiovasc Surg 1963;46:21–39.

486. Steele JD. The solitary pulmonary nodules. Springfield: Thomas, 1964:180–181.

487. Trapnell DH. Recognition and incidence of intrapulmonary lymph nodes. Thorax 1964;19:44–50.

488. Shapiro R, Wilson G, Gabriele OP. Roentgen-ray diagnosis with intrapulmonary lymph nodes. Dis Chest 1967;51:621–624.

489. Greenfield H, Jelaso DV. Peripheral intrapulmonary lymph node metastasis. Br J Radiol 1965;38:955–956.

490. Goodwin RA, Des Prez M. Apical localization of pulmonary tuberculosis, chronic pulmonary histoplasmosis, and progressive massive fibrosis of the lung. Chest 1983;83:801–805.

491. Das Gupta T, Bowden L, Berg JW. Malignant melanoma of unknown primary origin. Surg Gynecol Obstet 1963;117:341–345.

492. Das Gupta T, Brasfield R. Metastatic melanoma. A clinicopathologic study. Cancer (Philadelphia) 1964;17:1323–1339.

493. Das Gupta TK, Brasfield RD, Paglia MA. Primary

melanomas in unusual sites. Surg Gynecol Obstet 1969;128:841–848.

494. Allen AC, Spitz S. Malignant melanoma: A clinicopathologic analysis of the criteria for diagnosis and prognosis. Cancer (Philadelphia) 1953;6:1–45.

495. Jensen OA, Egedorf J. Primary malignant melanoma of the lung. Scand J Respir Dis 1967;48:127–135.

496. Carter D, Eggleston JC. Tumors of the lower respiratory tract. Ser. 2. Washington DC: Armed Forces Institute of Pathology, 1980;17:220.

497. Allen MS, Jr, Drash EC. Primary melanoma of the lung. Cancer (Philadelphia) 1968;21:154–159.

498. Jennings TA, Axiotis CA, Kress Y, Carter D. Primary malignant melanoma of the lower respiratory tract: Report of a case and review of the literature. Am J Clin Pathol 1990;94:649–655.

499. Reed RJ, Kent EM. Solitary pulmonary melanomas: Two case reports. J Thorac Cardiovasc Surg 1964;48:226–231.

500. Rosenberg LM, Polanco GB, Blank S. Multiple tracheobronchial melanomas with ten-year survival. JAMA 1965;192:717–719.

501. Reid JD, Mehta VT. Melanoma of the lower respiratory tract. Cancer (Philadelphia) 1965;19:627–631.

502. Slam R. A primary malignant melanoma of the bronchus. J Pathol Bacteriol 1963;85:121–126.

503. Walter P, Fernandes C, Florange W. Melanome malin primitif pulmonaire. Ann Anat Pathol (Paris) 1972;17:91–99.

504. Taboada CF, McMurray JD, Jordan RA, Seybold WD. Primary melanoma of the lung. Chest 1972;62:629–631.

505. Cagle P, Mace ML, Judge DM, Teague RB, Wilson RK, Greenberg SD. Pulmonary melanoma; primary versus metastatic. Chest 1984;85:125–126.

506. Carstens PHB, Kuhns JG, Ghazi C. Primary malignant melanomas of the lung and adrenal. Hum Pathol 1984;15:910–914.

507. Smith S, Opipari MI. Primary pleural melanoma: A first reported case and literature review. J Thorac Cardiovasc Surg 1978;75:827–831.

508. Angel R, Prades M. Primary bronchial melanomas. J Louisiana State Med Soc 1984;136:13–15.

509. Gephardt BN. Malignant melanomas of the bronchus. Hum Pathol 1981;12:671–673.

510. Robertson AJ, Sinclair DJM, Sutton PP, Guthrie W. Primary melanocarcinoma of the lower respiratory tract. Thorax 1980;35:158–159.

511. Cebelin MS. Melanocytic bronchial carcinoid tumor. Cancer (Philadelphia) 1980;46:1843–1848.

512. Grazer R, Cohen SM, Jacobs JB, Lucas P. Melanin-containing peripheral carcinoid of the lung. Am J Surg Pathol 1982;6:73–78.

513. Kemnitz P, Spormann H, Heinrich P. Meningioma of lung: First report with light and electron microscopic findings. Ultrastruct Pathol 1982;3:359–365.

514. Chumas JC, Lorelle CA. Pulmonary meningioma. A light- and electron-microscopic study. Am J Surg Pathol 1982;6:795–801.

515. Zhang FL, Cheng XR, Zhang XS, Ding JA. Lung ectopic meningioma: A case report. Chin Med J 1983;96:309–311.

516. Strimlan CV, Golembiewski RS, Celko DA, Fino GJ. Primary pulmonary meningioma. Surg Neurol 1988;29:410–413.

517. Kodama K, Doi O, Higashiyama M, Horai T, Tateishi R, Nakagawa H. Primary and metastatic pulmonary meningioma. Cancer (Philadelphia) 1991;67:1412–1417.

518. Flynn DS, Yousem SA. Pulmonary meningioma: A report of two cases. Hum Pathol 1991;22:469–474.

519. Drlicek M, Grisold W, Lorber J, Hackl H, Wuketich S, Jellinger K. Pulmonary meningioma: Immunohistochemical and ultrastructural features. Am J Surg Pathol 1991;15:455–459.

520. Unger PD, Geller SA, Anderson PJ. Pulmonary lesions in a patient with neurofibromatosis. Arch Pathol Lab Med 1984;108:654–657.

521. Kepes JJ. Meningiomas in other unusual sites. In: Kepes JJ, ed. Meningiomas: Biology, pathology, and differential diagnosis. New York: Masson, 1982: 44–47.

522. Wilson AJ, Ratliff JL, Lagios MD, Aquilar MJ. Mediastinal meningioma. Am J Surg Pathol 1979;3:557–562.

523. Erlandson RA. Diagnostic transmission electron microscopy of human tumors. In: Erlandson RA, ed. Monographs in diagnostic pathology. Vol. 3. New York: Masson, 1982:125–128.

524. Karasick JL, Mullan SF. A survey of metastatic meningiomas. J Neurosurg 1974;39:206–212.

525. Stoller JK, Kavuru M, Mehta AC, Weinstein CE, Estes ML, Gephardt GN. Intracranial meningioma metastatic to the lung. Cleve Clin J Med 1987;54:521–527.

526. Hoye SJ, Hoar CS, Murray JE. Extracranial meningioma presenting as a tumor of the neck. Am J Surg 1960;100:486–489.

527. Crotty TB, Hooker RP, Swenson SJ, Scheithauer BW, Myers JL. Primary malignant ependymoma of the lung. Mayo Clin Proc 1992;67:373–378.

528. Doglioni C, Bontempini L, Iuzzolino P, Furlan G, Rosai J. Ependymoma of the mediastinum. Arch Pathol Lab Med 1988;112:194–196.

529. Nobles E, Lee R, Kircher T. Mediastinal ependymoma. Hum Pathol 1991;22:94–96.

530. McBurney RP, Clagett OT, McDonald JR. Primary intrapulmonary neoplasm (?thymoma) associated with myasthenia gravis. Report of a case. Proc Mayo Clin 1951;26:345–353.

531. Thorburn JD, Stephens B, Grimes OF. Benign thymoma in the hilus of the lung. J Thorac Surg 1952;24:540–543.

532. Crane AR, Carrigan PT. Primary subpleural intrapulmonary thymoma. J Thorac Surg 1953;25:600–605.

533. Horanyi VJ, Korenyi K. Intrapulmonary thymoma in children. Thoraxchir Vasc Chir 1955;3:245–249.

534. Kalish PE. Primary intrapulmonary thymoma. NY State J Med 1963;63:1705–1708.

535. Yeoh CB, Ford JH, Lattes R, Wylie RH. Intrapulmo-

nary thymoma. J Thorac Cardiovasc Surg 1966; 51:131–136.

536. Paplinski Z, Szyszko J. Intrapulmonary thymoma. Polski Przegl Chir 1967;39:343–346.

537. Gulya D, Khaidarly I. A case of benign thymoma of the lung. Grudn Khir 1968;10:1145.

538. Rosai J, Levine GD. Tumors of the thymus. Washington, D.C.: Armed Forces Institute of Pathology, 1976:1–43.

539. Kung I, Loke SL, So SY, Lam WK, Mok A, Khin MA. Intrapulmonary thymoma: Report of two cases. Thorax 1985;40:471–474.

540. Honma K, Shimada K. Metastasizing ectopic thymoma arising in the right thoracic cavity and mimicking diffuse pleural mesothelioma. An autopsy study of a case with review of literature. Wien Klin Wochenschr 1986;98:14–20.

541. Fukayama M, Maeda Y, Funata N, et al. Pulmonary and pleural thymoma: Diagnostic application of lymphocyte markers to the thymoma of unusual site. Am J Clin Pathol 1988;89:617–621.

542. Martin JME, Randhawa G, Temple WJ. Cervical thymoma. Arch Pathol Lab Med 1986;110:354–357.

543. Bégin LR, Eskandari J, Joncas J, Panasci L. Epstein–Barr virus-related lymphoepithelioma-like carcinoma of the lung. J Surg Oncol 1987;36:280–283.

544. Butler AE, Colby TV, Weiss L, Lombard C. Lymphoepithelioma-like carcinoma of the lung. Am J Surg Pathol 1989;13:632–639.

545. Kay S, Reed WG. Chorioepithelioma of the lung in a female infant. Am J Pathol 1953;21:555–561.

546. Hayakawa K, Takahashi M, Sasaki K, et al. Primary choriocarcinoma of the lung. Acta Pathol Jpn 1977;27:123–135.

547. Kalla AH, Voss EC, Reed RJ. Primary Choriocarcinoma of the lung (a case report). W Va Med J 1980;76:261–263.

548. Zapatero J, Bellon J, Baamonde C, et al. Primary choriocarcinoma of the lung. Presentation of a case and review of the literature. Scand J Thorac Cardiovasc Surg 1982;16:279–281.

549. Tanimura A, Natsuyama H, Kawano M, Tanimura Y, Tanaka T, Kitazono M. Primary choriocarcinoma of the lung. Hum Pathol 1985;16:1281–1284.

550. Pushchak MJ, Farhi DC. Primary choriocarcinoma of the lung. Arch Pathol Lab Med 1987;111:477–479.

551. Sullivan LG. Primary choriocarcinoma of the lung in a man. Arch Pathol Lab Med 1989;113:82–83.

552. Sridhar KS, Saldana MJ, Thurer RJ, Beattie EJ. Primary choriocarcinoma of the lung: Report of a case treated with multimodality therapy and review of the literature. J Surg Oncol. 1989;41:93–97.

553. Fusco FD, Rosen SW. Gonadotropin-producing anaplastic large-cell carcinoma of the lung. N Engl J Med 1966;275:505–515.

554. Hatch KD, Shingleton HM, Gore H, Younger B, Boots LR. Human chorionic gonadotropin-secreting large cell carcinoma of the lung detected during follow-up of a patient previously treated for gestational trophoblastic disease. Gynecol Oncol 1980;10:98–104.

555. Dailey JE, Marcuse PM. Gonadotropin-secreting giant cell carcinoma of the lung. Cancer (Philadelphia) 1969;24:388–396.

556. Mazur MT. Metastatic gestational choriocarcinoma. Unusual pathologic variant following therapy. Cancer (Philadelphia) 1989;63:1370–1377.

556a. Nakahashi H, Tsuneyoshi M, Ishida T, et al. Undifferentiated carcinoma of the lung with osteoclast-like giant cells. Jpn J Surg 1987;17:199–203.

557. Esmaili JH, Hafez GR, Warner TF. Anaplastic carcinoma of the thyroid with osteoclast-like giant cells. Cancer (Philadelphia) 1983;52:2122–2128.

558. Huvos AG. "Benign" metastasis in giant cell tumor of bone. Hum Pathol 1981;12:1151.

559. Bertoni F, Present D, Sudanese A, Baldini N, Bacchini P, Campanacci M. Giant-cell tumor of bone with pulmonary metastases: Six case reports and a review of the literature. Clin Orthop 1988;237:275–285.

560. Bertoni F, Present D, Enneking WF. Giant cell tumor of bone with pulmonary metastases. J Bone Joint Surg [Am] 1985;67A:890–900.

561. Jaffe HL. Giant cell tumor (osteoclastoma) of bone: Its pathologic delineation and the inherent clinical implication. Ann R Coll Surg Engl 1953;13:343–355.

562. Stargardter FL, Copperman LR. Giant cell tumour of sacrum with multiple pulmonary metastases and long-term survival. Br J Radiol 1971;44:976–979.

563. Dahlin DC. Bone tumors: General aspects and data on 6,221 cases. Springfield, Illinois: Charles C Thomas, 1978:99–115.

564. Sladden RA. Intravascular osteoclasts. J Bone Joint Surg [Am] 1957;39:346–357.

565. Hutter RVP, Worcester JN, Jr, Francis KC, Foote FW, Jr, Stewart FW. Benign and malignant giant cell tumors of bone. A clinicopathological analysis of the natural history of the disease. Cancer (Philadelphia) 1962; 15:653–690.

566. Pan P, Dahlin DC, Lipscomb PR, et al. "Benign" giant cell tumor of the radius with pulmonary metastasis. Mayo Clin Proc 1964;39:344–349.

567. Budzilovich GN, Truchly GI, Wilens SL. Tumor giant cells in regional lymph nodes of a case of recurrent giant-cell tumor of bone. Clin Orthop 1963;30:182–187.

568. Caballes RL. The mechanism of metastasis in the so-called "benign giant cell tumor of bone." Hum Pathol 1981;12:762–767.

569. Fraga S, Helwig EB, Rosen SH. Bronchogenic cysts in the skin and subcutaneous tissue. Am J Clin Pathol 1971;56:230–238.

570. Park WW. The occurrence of decidual tissue within the lung: report of a case. J Pathol Bacteriol 1954;47:563–570.

571. Hartz PH. Occurrence of decidua-like tissue in the lung. Am J Clin Pathol 1956;26:48–51.

572. Cameron HM, Park WW. Decidual tissue within the

lung. J Obstet Gynaecol Br Commonw 1965;72:748–752.

573. Lattes R, Shepard F, Tovell H, Wylie K. Clinical and pathologic study of endometriosis of the lung. Surg Gynecol Obstet 1956;103:552–558.

574. Farinacci CJ, Blauw AS, Jennings EM. Multifocal pulmonary lesions of possible decidual origin (so-called pulmonary deciduosis): Report of a case. Am J Clin Pathol 1973;59:508–574.

575. Spencer H. Pathology of the lung. 4th Ed. London: Pergamon, 1985:1011–1012.

576. Hibbard LT, Schumann WR, Goldstein GE. Thoracic endometriosis: A review and report of two cases. Am J Obstet Gynecol 1981;140:227–232.

577. Karpel JP, Appel D, Merav A. Pulmonary endometriosis. Lung 1985;163:151–159.

577a. Austin MB, Frierson HF Jr, Fechner RE, Callicott JH Jr. Endometrioma of the lung presenting as hemoptysis and a large pulmonary mass. Surg Pathol 1988;1:165–169.

578. Di Palo S, Mari G, Castoldi R, Standacher C, Taccagni G, Di Carlo V. Endometriosis of the lung. Respir Med 1989;83:255–258.

579. Hart C. Histologisch benigne Metastasen vom bau eines Adenymioms 22 jahre nach Extirpation eines tumors der Genitalien. Frankf Z Pathol. 1912;10:78.

580. Schwartz OH. In: Discussion of paper by Cousellor vs. Endometriosis, A clinical and surgical review. Am J Obstet Gynecol 1938;36:887.

581. Bungeler W, Fleury-Silveira D, Arg Cirug Clin Exp 1939;3:169–187.

582. Foster DC, Stern JL, Buscema J, Rock JA, Woodruff JD. Pleural and parenchymal pulmonary endometriosis. Obstet Gynecol 1981;58:552–556.

583. Svendstrup F, Husby H. Parenchymal pulmonary endometriosis. J Laryngol Otol 1991;105:235–236.

584. Slasky BS, Siewers RD, Lecky JW, Zajko A, Buckholder JA. Catamenial pneumothorax: The roles of diaphragmatic defects and endometriosis. AJR 1982;138:639–643.

585. Austin MB, Frierson HF, Fechner RE, Callicott JH, Jr. Endometrioma of the lung presenting as hemophysis and a large pulmonary mass. Surg Pathol 1988;2:165–169.

586. Granberg I, Willems JS. Endometriosis of lung and pleura diagnosed by aspiration biopsy. Acta Cytol (Baltimore) 1982;26:295–297.

587. Zaatara GS, Gupta PK, Bhagavan BS, Jarboe BR. Cytopathology of pleural endometriosis. Acta Cytol (Baltimore) 1982;26:227–232.

588. Espaulella J, Armengol J, Bella F, Lain JM, Calaf J. Pulmonary endometriosis: Conservative treatment with GnRH agonists. Obstet Gynecol 1991;78:535–537.

589. LeRoux BT: Heterotropic intrathoracic liver. Thorax 1961;16:68–71.

590. Gasser A, Wilson GL. Ectopic liver tissue mass in the thoracic cavity. Cancer (Philadelphia) 1975;36:1823–1826.

591. Hudson TR, Brown HN. Ectopic (supra-diaphragmatic) liver. J Thorac Cardiovasc Surg 1962;43:552–555.

592. Hansbrough ET, Lipin RJ. Intrathoracic accessory lobes of the liver. Ann Surg 1957;145:564–567.

593. Jimenez AR, Hayward RH. Ectopic liver: A cause of esophageal obstruction. Ann Thorac Surg 1971;12:300–304.

594. Kaufman SA, Medoff IM. Intrathoracic accessory lobe of the liver. Ann Intern Med 1960;47:353–356.

595. Sehdeva JS, Logan WB. Heterotopic (supra-diaphragmatic) liver. Ann Thorac Surg 1971;11:468–471.

596. Lasser A, WIlson GL. Ectopic liver tissue mass in the thoracic cavity. Cancer (Philadelphia) 1975;36:1823–1826.

597. Mendoza A, Voland J, Wolf P, Benirschle K. Supradiaphragmatic liver in the lung. Arch Pathol Lab Med 1986;44:1085–1086.

598. Kellett HS, Lipphard D, Willis RA. Two unusual examples of heteroplasia in the lung. J Pathol Bacteriol 1962;84:421–425.

599. Jariwalla AG, Al-Nasir NK. Splenosis pleurae. Thorax 1979;34:123–124.

600. Rakestraw MR, Masood S, Ballinger WE. Brain heterotopia and anencephaly. Arch Pathol Lab Med 1987;111:858–860.

601. Fuller C, Gibbs AR. Heterotopic brain tissue in the lung causing acute respiratory distress in an infant. Thorax 1989;44:1045–1046.

602. Kershisnik MM, Kaplan C, Craven CM, Carey JC, Townsend JJ, Knisley AS. Intrapulmonary neuroglial heterotypia. Arch Pathol Lab Med 1992;116:1043–1046.

603. King WI. Tumor (embryonal) of lung containing brain tissue. Med Bull Va 1938;15:181–183.

604. Gautam HP. Intrapulmonary malignant teratoma. Am Rev Respir Dis 1969;200:863–865.

605. Holt S, Deverall PB, Boddy JE. A teratoma of the lung containing thymic tissue. J Pathol 1978;126:85–89.

606. Cloetta. Über das Vorkommen einer Dermoidcyste in der Lunge. Virchow Arch Pathol Anat 1861;20:42–44. (As referred to by von Mohr. Medizinsche Zietung. Berlin, 1839:S130.)

607. Rusby NL. Dermoid cysts and teratomata of the mediastinum. J Thorac Surg 1944;13:169–222.

608. Ali MY, Wong PK. Intrapulmonary teratoma. Thorax 1964;19:228–235.

609. Synder RN. Completely mature pulmonary metastasis from testicular teratocarcinoma. Cancer (Philadelphia) 1969;24:810–819.

610. Gonzalez-Cruzzi F. Extragonadal teratomas. Washington DC: Armed Forces Institute of Pathology, 1982:184–186.

611. Schlumberger HG. Teratoma of the anterior mediastinum in the group of military age—a study of sixteen cases and a review of theories of genesis. Arch Pathol 1946;41:398–444.

612. Eckert VM, Garassimidis T. Intrapulmonales teratom.

Fallbericht und Literaturübersicht. Fortschr Med 1979;97:1051–1054.

613. Miura K, Hori T, Yoshizawa K, Hamaguchi N, Morita J. Cystic pulmonary hamartoma. Ann Thorac Surg 1990;49:828–829.

614. Trivedi SA, Mehta KN, Nanavaty JM. Teratoma of the lung: Report of a case. Br J Dis Chest 1966;60:156–159.

615. Gurkin KI, Sabar IR. Akcigerde (kalsifiye desmoid cyst) vaksasi munasebetile. Tip Fak Mec (Istanbul) 1955;18:17. (As referred to by Gautam HP.) Intrapulmonary malignant teratoma. Am Rev Respir Dis 1969;100:863–865.

616. Laffitte H. Embryome teratoide intra-pulmonaire. Exerese en un temps. Mem Acad de Chir (Paris) 1937;63:1076–1085.

617. Bateson EM, Hayes JA, Woo-Ming M. Endobronchial teratoma associated with bronchiectasis and bronchiolectasis. Thorax 1968;23:69–76.

618. Kravetz VM, Kamentsky MC, Efdaha PN, Ilivsky IP. Intrabronchial teratoma. Klin Khir 1976;8:54–55.

619. Jamieson MPG, McGowan AR. Endobronchial teratoma. Thorax 1982;37:157–159.

620. Day DW, Taylor SA. An intrapulmonary teratoma associated with thymic tissue. Thorax 1975;30:582–587.

621. Breatnach E, Weeks J. Unusual intrapulmonary tumor: A rare case of bronchiectasis. Chest 1990;97:197–198.

622. Prauer HW, Mack D, Babic R. Intrapulmonary teratoma 10 years after removal of a mediastinal teratoma in a young man. Thorax 1983;38:632–634.

623. Pound AW, Willis RA. A malignant teratoma of the lung in an infant. J Pathol 1969;98:111–114.

624. Collier FC, Dowling EA, Plott D, Schneider H. Teratoma of the lung. Arch Pathol 1969;68:138–142.

625. Albrecht E. Über Hamartome. Verh Dtsch Ges Pathol 1904;7:153–157.

626. Goldsworthy NE. Chondroma of the lung (hamartoma and chondromatosum polmonis). J Pathol Bacteriol 1934;39:291–298.

627. Mitsudomi T, Kaneko S, Tateishi M, Yana T, Ishida T, Sugimachi K. Benign tumors and tumor-like lesions of the lung. Int Surg 1990;75:155–158.

628. McDonald JR, Harrington SW, Clagett OT. Hamartoma (often called chondroma) of the lung. J Thorac Cardiovasc Surg 1945;14:128–143.

629. Jones RC, Cleve EA. Solitary circumscribed lesions of lung: Selection of cases for diagnostic thoracotomy. AMA Arch Intern Med 1954;93:842.

630. Tomashefski JF, Jr. Benign endobronchial mesenchymal tumors: Their relationship to parenchymal pulmonary hamartomas. Am J Surg Pathol 1982;6:531–540.

631. Koutras P, Urschel HC, Paulson DL. Hamartoma of the lung. J Thorac Cardiovasc Surg 1971;61:768–776.

632. Hart C. Über die rimaren chondrome der unge. Z Krebsforsch 1906;4:578.

633. Bateson EM. So-called hamartoma of the lung: A true neoplasm of fibrous connective tissue of the bronchi. Cancer (Philadelphia) 1973;31:1458–1467.

634. Carter D, Eggleston JC. Tumors of the lower respiratory tract. Series 2. Washington DC: Armed Forces Institute of Pathology, 1980:221–231.

635. Malauzat C, Malauzat F, Petit MA, Merlier M, Germouty J. Les hamartochondromes broncho-pulmonares (a propos de 136 cas, dont une seies homogene de 124 cas). Revue de la literature. Rev Pneumol Clin 1985;41:163–175.

636. Bateson EM. Relationship between intrapulmonary and endobronchial cartilage-containing tumours (so-called hamartoma). Thorax 1965;20:447–461.

637. Bateson EM. Cartilage-containing tumours of the lung: relationship between the purely cartilaginous type (chondroma) and the mixed type (so-called hamartoma). An unusual case of multiple tumours. Thorax 1967;22:256–259.

638. Bateson EM. Histogenesis of intrapulmonary and endobronchial hamartomas and chondromas (cartilage containing tumours). A hypothesis. J Pathol 1970;101:77–83.

639. Stone FJ, Churg AM. The ultrastructure of pulmonary hamartoma. Cancer (Philadelphia) 1977;39:1064–1070.

640. Incze JS, Lui PS. Morphology of the epithelial component of human lung hamartomas. Hum Pathol 1977;8:411–419.

641. Perez-Atayde AR, Seiler MW. Pulmonary hamartoma: an ultrastructural study. Cancer (Philadelphia) 1984;53:485–492.

642. Poirer TJ, Van Ordstrand HS. Pulmonary chondromatous hamartomas. Report of seventeen cases and review of the literature. Chest 1971;59:50–55.

643. Fudge TL, Oschner JL, Mills NL. Clinical spectrum of pulmonary hamartomas. Ann Thorac Surg 1980;30:36–39.

644. Hodges FV. Hamartoma of the lung. Dis Chest 1958;33:43–51.

645. Bateson EM, Abbott EK. Mixed tumors of the lung or hamartochondromas: A review of cases published in the literature and a report of fifteen new cases. Clin Radiol 1960;11:232–247.

646. Blair TC, McElvein RM. Hamartoma of the lung: a clinical study of 25 cases. Dis Chest 1963;44:296–302.

647. Hamper UM, Khouri NF, Stitik FP, Siegelman SS. Pulmonary hamartoma: diagnosis by transthoracic needle aspiration biopsy. Radiology 1985;155:15–18.

648. Sinner WN. Fine-needle biopsy of hamartomas of the lung. AJR 1982;138:65–69.

649. Crouch JD, Keagy BA, Starek PJK, Delany DJ, Wilcox BR. A clinical review of patients undergoing resection for pulmonary hamartoma. Ann Surg 1988;54:297–299.

650. Siegelman SS, Khouri NF, Scott WW, Jr, et al. Pulmonary hamartoma: CT findings. Radiology 1986;160:313–317.

651. Jensen KG, Schiodt T. Growth conditions of hamartoma of the lung: a study based on 22 cases operated on

after radiographic observation for from one to 18 years. Thorax 1958;13:233–237.

652. Weisel W, Glicklich M, Landis FB. Pulmonary hamartoma, an enlarging neoplasm. Arch Surg 1955;71:128–135.

653. Sagel SC, Ablow, RC. Hamartoma: On occasion a rapidly growing tumour of the lung. Radiology 1968;91:971–979.

654. Weinberger M, Kakos GS, Kilman JW. The adult form of pulmonary hamartoma. Ann Thorac Surg 1973;15:67–72.

655. Palvio D, Egeblad K, Paulsen SM. Atypical lipomatous hamartoma of the lung. Virchows Arch [A] 1985;405:253–261.

656. Spencer H. Pathology of the lung. 4th Ed. Oxford: Pergamon, 1985:1061–1083.

657. Jones EL, Lucey JJ, Taylor AB. Intrapulmonary lipoma associated with multiple pulmonary hamartomas. Br J Surg 1973;60:75–78.

658. King TE, Jr., Christopher KL, Schwarz MI. Multiple pulmonary chondromatous hamartomas. Hum Pathol 1981;13:496–497.

659. Bennett LL, Lesar MS, Tellis CJ. Multiple calcified chondrohamartomas of the lung: CT appearance. J Comput Assist Tomogr 1985;9:180–182.

660. Carney JA. The triad of gastric epithelioid leiomyosarcoma, functioning extra-adrenal paraganglioma, and pulmonary chondroma. Cancer (Philadelphia) 1979;43:374–382.

661. Gabrail NY, Zara BY. Pulmonary hamartoma syndrome. Chest 1990;97:962–965.

662. Hayward RH, Carabasi RJ. Malignant hamartoma of the lung: Fact or fiction? J Thorac Cardiovasc Surg 1967;53:457–466.

663. Basile A, Gregoris A, Antoci B, Romanelli M. Malignant change in a benign pulmonary hamartoma. Thorax 1989;44:232–233.

664. Salminen U-S, Halttunen P, Taskinen E, Mattila S. Recurrence and malignant transformation of endotracheal chondroma. Ann Thorac Surg 1990;49:830–832.

665. Fletcher JA, Pinkus GS, Weidner N, Morton CC. Lineage-restricted clonality in biphasic solid tumors. Am J Pathol 1991;138:1199–1207.

666. Magee JF, Wright JL, Dodek A, Tatassaura H. Mediastinal and retroperitoneal fibrosis with fibrotic pulmonary nodules: A case report. Histopathology 1985;9:995–999.

667. Littlefield JB, Drash EC. Myxoma of the lung. J Thorac Surg 1959;37:745–749.

668. Pollak ER, Naunheim KS, Little AG. Fibromyxoma of the trachea. Arch Pathol Lab Med 1985;109:926–929.

669. Liebon AA, Loring WE, Felton WL, II. The musculature of the lung in chronic pulmonary disease. Am J Pathol 1953;29:885–911.

670. Heppleston AG. The pathology of honeycomb lung. Thorax 1956;11:47–53.

671. Spencer H. Pathology of the lung. 4th Ed. Oxford: Pergamon, 1985;680.

672. Horstmann JP, Pietra GG, Harman JA, Cole NG, Jr., Grinspan S. Spontaneous regression of pulmonary leiomyomas during pregnancy. Cancer (Philadelphia) 1977;39:314–321.

673. Sargent EN, Barnes RA, Schwinn CP. Multiple pulmonary fibroleiomyomatous hamartomas. AJR 1970; 110:694–700.

674. Kaplan C, Katoh A, Shamato M, et al. Multiple leiomyomas of the lung: Benign or malignant. Am Rev Respir Dis 1973;108:656–659.

675. Tench WD, Dail D, Gmelich JT, Matanai N. Benign metastasizing leiomyomas: a review of 21 cases. Lab Invest 1978;38:367–368 (abstr.).

676. Matani N. San Diego, California. Personal communication, 1974.

677. Popock E, Craig JR, Bullock WK. Metastatic uterine leiomyomata: a case report. Cancer (Philadelphia) 1976;38:2096–2100.

678. Uyama T, Monden Y, Harada K, Sumitomo M, Kimura S. Pulmonary leiomyomatosis showing endobronchial extension and giant cyst formation. Chest 1988;94: 644–646.

679. Silverman JF, Kay S. Multiple pulmonary leiomyomatous hamartomas. Report of a case with ultrastructural examination. Cancer (Philadelphia) 1976;38:1199–1204.

680. Piccaluga A, Capelli A. Fibroleiomiomatosi metastatizzante dell'utero. Arch Ital Anat Istolog Patol 1967; 41:99–164.

681. Herrera GA, Miles PA, Greenberg H, Reinmann EF, Weisman IM. The origin of pseudoglandular spaces in metastatic smooth muscle neoplasm of uterine origin: Report of a case with ultrastructure and review of previous cases studied by electron microscopy. Chest 1983;83:270–274.

682. Wolff M, Silva F, Kaye G. Pulmonary metastases (with admixed epithelial elements) from smooth muscle neoplasms: Report of nine cases, including three males. Am J Surg Pathol 1979;3:325–342.

683. Kempson RL. Mitosis counting II (editorial). Hum Pathol 1976;7:482–483.

684. Norris HJ. Mitosis counting III (editorial). Hum Pathol 1976;7:483–484.

685. Gal AA, Brooks JSJ, Pietra GG. Leiomyomatous neoplasms of the lung: A clinical, histologic, and immunohistochemical study. Mod Pathol 1989;2:209–215.

686. Steiner PE. Metastasizing fibroleiomyoma of the uterus. Am J Pathol 1939;15:89–109.

687. Zaloudek C, Norris HJ. Mesenchymal tumors of the uterus. In: Kurman RJ, ed. Blaustein's pathology of the female genital tract. 3rd Ed. New York: Springer-Verlag, 1987:373–408.

688. Cho KR, Woodruff JD, Epstein JI. Leiomyoma of the uterus with multiple extrauterine smooth muscle tumors: A case report suggesting multifocal origin. Hum Pathol 1989;20:80–83.

689. Maltby JD, Misra JD, Knight FH. "Metastasizing leiomyoma" occurring as a mediastinal mass. Mo Med 1980;77:304–306.

690. Groeneveld ABJ, Bosma A, Ceelen TL, Kuouwenhoven TJ, Meuwissen SG. Progressive and fatal course of a patient with a multifocal leiomyomatous tumor. Am J Gastroenterol 1986;81:702–707.

691. Lipton JH, Fong TC, Burgess KR. Miliary pattern as presentation of leiomyomatosis of the lung. Chest 1987;91:781–782.

692. Clark DH, Weed JC. Metastasizing leiomyoma: A case report. Am J Obstet Gynecol 1977;127:672–673.

693. Martin E. Leiomyomatous lung lesions: A proposed classification. AJR 1983;141:269–272.

694. Allen PW. Benign metastasizing Mullerian tumors and uterine sarcomas. Surg Pathol 1990;3:3–17.

695. Mark EJ. Mesenchymal cystic hamartoma of the lung. N Engl J Med 1986;315:1255–1259.

696. Case Records of the Massachusetts General Hospital (Case 32-1985). N Engl J Med 1985;313:374–382.

697. Holden WE, Mulkey DD, Kessler S. Multiple peripheral lung cysts and hemoptysis in an otherwise asymptomatic adult. Am Rev Respir Dis 1982;126:930–932.

698. Abrams J, Talcott J, Corson JM. Pulmonary metastases in patients with low-grade endometrial stromal sarcoma: clinicopathologic findings with immunohistochemical characterisation. Am J Surg Pathol 1989;13:133–140.

699. Chan KL, Crabtree GS, Lim-Tan SK, Kempson RL, Hendrickson MR. Primary uterine endometrial stromal neoplasms. A clinicopathologic study of 117 cases. Am J Surg Pathol 1990;14:415–438.

700. Hedlund GL, Bisset GS, III, Bove KE. Malignant neoplasms arising in cystic hamartomas of the lung in childhood. Radiology 1989;173:77–79.

701. Ueda K, Gruppo R, Unger F, Martin L, Bove K. Rhabdomyosarcoma of lung arising in congenital cystic adenomatoid malformation. Cancer (Philadelphia) 1977;40:383–388.

702. Weinberg AG, Currarino G, Moore GC, Votteler TP. Mesenchymal neoplasia and congenital pulmonary cysts. Pediatr Radiol 1980;9:179–182.

703. Martinez JC, Pecero FC, Gutiérrez de la Pena C, et al. Pulmonary blastoma: Report of a case. J Pediatr Surg 1978;13:93–94.

704. Valderrama E, Saluja G, Shende A, Lanzkowsky P, Beckman J. Pulmonary blastoma: Report of two cases in children. Am J Surg Pathol 1978;2:415–422.

705. Joseph MG, Colby TV, Swensen SJ, Mikus JP, Gaensler EA. Multiple cystic fibrohistiocytic tumor of the lung: Report of two cases. Mayo Clin Proc 1990; 65:192–197.

706. Yousem SA, Hochholzer L. Alveolar adenoma. Hum Pathol 1986;17:1066–1071.

707. Wada A, Tateishi R, Terazawa T, Matsuda M, Hattori S. Lymphangioma of the lung. Arch Pathol Lab Med 1974;98:211–213.

708. Clayton F, Mackay B, Ayala AG, Diaz I. Vacuolated epithelial lesion in lung. Ultrastruct Pathol 1981; 2:303–307.

709. Miller DR. Benign tumors of lung and tracheobronchial tree. Ann Thorac Surg 1969;8:542–560.

710. Peleg H, Pauzner Y. Benign tumors of the lung. Dis Chest 1965;47:179–186.

711. Taylor TL, Miller DR. Leiomytoma of the bronchus. J Thorac Cardiovasc Surg 1969;57:284–288.

712. Orlowski TM, Stasiak K, Kolodziej J. Leiomyoma of the lung. J Thorac Cardiovasc Surg 1978;76:257–261.

713. Vera-Román JM, Sobonya RE, Gomez-Garcia JL, Sanz-Bondia JR, Paris-Romeu F. Leiomyoma of the lung: Literature review and case report. Cancer (Philadelphia) 1983;52:936–941.

714. Yellin A, Rosenman Y, Lieberman Y. Review of smooth muscle tumours of the lower respiratory tract. Br J Dis Chest 1984;78:337–351.

715. White SH, Ibrahim NBN, Forrester-Wood CP, Jeyasingham K. Leiomyomas of the lower respiratory tract. Thorax 1985;40:306–311.

716. Crastnopol P, Franklin WD. Fibroleiomyoma of the lung. Ann Surg 1957;145:128–132.

717. Sanders JS, Cornes VM. Leiomyoma of the trachea. Report of a case, with a note on the diagnosis of partial tracheal obstruction. N Engl J Med 1961;264:277–279.

718. Foroughi E. Leiomyoma of the trachea. Dis Chest 1962;42:230–232.

719. Agnos JW, Starkey GWB. Primary leiomyosarcoma and leiomyoma of the lung: Review of the literature and report of two cases of leiomyosarcoma. N Engl J Med 1958;158:12–17.

720. Shahian DM, McEnany MT. Complete endobronchial excision of leiomyoma of the bronchus. J Thorac Cardiovasc Surg 1979;77:87–91.

721. Sauk JJ, Pliego M, Anderson WR. Primary pulmonary fibroma. Minn Med 1972;55:220–223.

722. Corona FE, Okeson GC. Endobronchial fibroma. Am Rev Respir Dis 1974;110:350–353.

723. Briselli M, Mark EJ, Dickersin GR. Solitary fibrous tumor of the pleura: Eight new cases and review of 360 cases in the literature. Cancer (Philadelphia) 1981; 47:2678–2689.

724. England DM, Hochholzer L, McCarthy MJ. Localized benign and malignant fibrous tumors of the pleura: A clinicopathologic review of 223 cases. Am J Surg Pathol 1989;13:640–658.

725. El-Naggar AK, Ro JY, Ayala AG, Ward RM, Ordonez NG. Localized fibrous tumor of the serosal cavities: Immunohistochemical, electron-microscopic, and flow-cytometric DNA study. Am J Clin Pathol 1989;92:561–565.

726. Young RH, Clement PB, McCaughey WTE. Solitary fibrous tumors (fibrous mesotheliomas) of the peritoneum. Arch Pathol Lab Med 1990;114:493–495.

727. Yousem SA, Flynn SD. Intrapulmonary localized fibrous tumor: Intraparenchymal so-called fibrous mesothelioma. Am J Clin Pathol 1988;89:365–369.

728. Tan-Liu NS, Matsubara O, Grillo HC, Mark EJ. Invasive fibrous tumor of the tracheobronchial tree: Clinical and pathologic study of seven cases. Hum Pathol 1989;20:180–184.

729. Witkin GB, Rosai J. Solitary fibrous tumor of the mediastinum. Am J Surg Pathol 1989;13:547–557.

730. Zukerberg LR, Rosenberg AE, Randolph G, Pilch BZ, Goodman ML. Solitary fibrous tumor of the nasal cavity and paranasal sinuses. Am J Surg Pathol 1991;15:126–130.

731. Witkin GB, Rosai J. Solitary fibrous tumor of the upper respiratory tract: A report of six cases. Am J Surg Pathol 1991;15:842–848.

732. Viguera JL, Pujol JL, Reboiras SD, Larrauri J, DeMiquel LS. Fibrous histiocytoma of the lung. Thorax 1976;31:475–479.

733. Gonzalez-Campora R, Matilla A, Sanchez-Carrillo JJ, Navarro A, Galera H. 'Benign' fibrous histiocytoma of the trachea. J Laryngol Otol 1981;93:1287–1292.

734. Tagge E, Yunis E, Chopyk J, Wiener E. Obstructing endobronchial fibrous histiocytoma: Potential for lung salvage. J Pediatr Surg 1991;26:1067–1069.

735. Randleman CD, Unger ER, Mansour KA. Malignant fibrous histiocytoma of the trachea. Ann Thorac Surg 1990;50:458–459.

736. Louie S, Cross CE, Amott T, Cardiff R. Postirradiation malignant fibrous histiocytoma of the trachea. Am Rev Respir Dis 1987;135:761–762.

737. Sajjad SM, Begin LR, Dail DH, Lukeman JM. Fibrous histiocytoma of lung: A clinicopathologic study of two cases. Histopathology 1981;5:325–334.

738. Plachta A, Hershey H. Lipoma of the lung: Review of literature and report of a case. Am Rev Respir Dis 1962;86:912–916.

739. Schraufnagel DE, Morin JE, Wang NS. Endobronchial lipoma. Chest 1979;75:97–99.

740. Rosenberg RF, Rubinstein BM, Messinger NH. Intrathoracic lipoma. Chest 1971;60:507–509.

741. Politis J, Funahashi A, Gehisen J, DeCock D, Stengel BF, Choi H. Intrathoracic lipomas: Report of three cases and review of the literature with emphasis on endobronchial lipomas. J Thorac Cardiovasc Surg 1979;77:550–556.

742. Crutcher RR, Waltuck TL, Ghosh AK. Bronchial lipoma. J Thorac Cardiovasc Surg 1968;55:422–425.

743. Bellin HJ, Libshitz HI, Patchefsky AS. Bronchial lipoma: Report of two cases showing chondroitic metaplasia. Arch Pathol 1971;92:20–23.

744. MacArthur CG, Cheung DL, Spiro SG. Endobronchial lipoma: a review of four cases. Br J Dis Chest 1977;71:93–100.

745. Parrish RW, Banks J, Fennerty AG. Tracheal obstruction presenting as asthma. Postgrad Med J 1983; 59:775–776.

746. Bates CA, Rahamin J. Tracheal lipoma. Thorax 1989;44:980.

747. Shapiro R, Carter MG. Peripheral lipoma of the lung. Am Rev Tuberc Pulm Dis 1954;69:1042–1044.

747a. Madewell JE, Feigin DS. Benign tumors of the lung. Semin Roentgenol 1977;12:175–186.

748. Gramiak R, Koerner HJ. A roentgen diagnostic observation in subpleural lipoma. AJR 1966;98:465–467.

748a. Palvio D, Egeblad K, Paulsen SM. Atypical lipomatous hamartoma of the lung. Virchows Arch [Pathol Anat] 1985;405:253–261.

749. Askanazy M. Über schwer erkannbare Neurofibromatosen. Arb Geb Pathol Anat Bakt 1914;9:147.

750. Bartley TD, Arean VM. Intrapulmonary neurogenic tumors. J Thorac Cardiovasc Surg 1965;50:114–123.

751. Miura H, Kato H, Hayata Y, Ebihara Y, Gönüllü U. Solitary bronchial mucosal neuroma. Chest 1989;95: 245–247.

752. Israel-Asselain R, Chebat J, Sors C, et al. Diffuse interstitial pulmonary fibrosis in a mother and son with Von Recklinghausen's disease. Thorax 1965;20:153–157.

753. Bernabeu L, Gillon JC, Loison F, et al. Une cause rare de fibrose interstitielle diffuse: la maladie de Von Recklinghausen. Lille Med 1980;25:283–285.

754. Silverman JF, Leffers BR, Kay S. Primary pulmonary neurilemmoma: Report of a case with ultrastructural examination. Arch Pathol Lab Med 1976;100:644–648.

755. Paul KP, Borner C, Muller KM, Vogt-Moykopf I. Capillary hemangioma of the right main bronchus treated by sleeve resection in infancy. Am Rev Respir Dis 1991;143:876–879.

756. Shikhani AH, Jones MM, Marsh BR, Holliday MJ. Infantile subglottic hemangiomas: An update. Ann Otol Rhinol Laryngol 1986;95:336–347.

757. Harding JR, Williams J, Seal RM. Pedunculated capillary hemangioma of the bronchus. Br J Dis Chest 1978;72:336–342.

758. Masson RG, Altose MD, Maycock RL. Isolated bronchial telangiectasia. Chest 1974;65:450–452.

759. Burman D, Mansell PWA, Warin RP. Miliary haemangiomata in the newborn. Arch Dis Child 1967; 42:193–197.

760. Bowyer JJ, Sheppard M. Capillary haemangioma presenting as a lung pseudocyst. Arch Dis Child 1990;65:1162–1164.

761. Personal Communication, 1992, Dr. Corinne Fligner. King County Medical Examiner's Office, Seattle, WA.

762. Martini N, Hajdu SI, Beatie EJ Jr. Primary sarcoma of the lung. J Thorac Cardiovasc 1971;61:33–38.

763. Crane M, Sutton JP. Primary sarcoma of the lung. South Med J 1972;65:850–854.

764. Gebauer C. The postoperative prognosis of primary pulmonary sarcoma: A review with a comparison between the histological focus and other primary endothoracic sarcomas based on 474 cases. Scand J Thorac Cardiovasc Surg 1982;16:91–97.

765. Cameron EW. Primary sarcoma of the lung. Thorax 1975;30:516–520.

766. Lee JT, Shelburne JD, Linder J. Primary malignant fibrous histiocytoma of the lung: A clinicopathologic and ultrastructural study of five cases. Cancer (Philadelphia) 1984;53:1124–1130.

767. Iverson L. Bronchopulmonary sarcoma. J Thorac Surg 1954;27:130–148.

768. Mallory TB. Case records of the Massachusetts General Hospital No. 22441. New Engl J Med 1936; 215:837–839.

769. Ellis RC. Primary sarcoma of the lung with brain metastases. J Kansas Med Soc 1939;40:243–245, 253.

770. Wackers FJ, van der Schoot JB, Hampe JR. Sarcoma of the pulmonary trunk associated with hemorrhagic tendency: A case report and review of the literature. Cancer (Philadelphia) 1969;23:339–351.

771. Shmookler BM, Marsh HB, Roberts WC. Primary sarcoma of the pulmonary trunk and/or right or left main pulmonary artery: A rare cause of obstruction of right ventricular overflow. Am J Med 1977;63:263–272.

772. Bleisch VR, Kraus FT. Polypoid sarcoma of the pulmonary trunk: Analysis of the literature and report of a case with leptomeric organelles and ultrastructural features of a rhabdomyosarcoma. Cancer (Philadelphia) 1980;46:314–324.

773. Baker PB, Goodwin RA. Pulmonary artery sarcomas: A review and report of a case. Arch Pathol Lab Med 1985;109:35–39.

774. McGlennen RC, Manivel JC, Stanley SJ, Slater DC, Wick MR, Dehner LP. Pulmonary artery trunk sarcoma: A clinicopathologic, ultrastructural, and immunohistochemical study of four cases. Mod Pathol 1989;2:486–494.

775. Wang N-S, Seemayer TA, Ahmed MN, Morin J. Pulmonary leiomyosarcoma associated with an arteriovenous fistula. Arch Pathol 1974;98:100–105.

776. Shah IA, Kurtz SM, Simonsen RL. Radiation-induced malignant fibrous histiocytoma of the pulmonary artery. Arch Pathol Lab Med 1991;115:921–925.

777. Chowdbury L, Swerdlow MA, Jao W, Kathpalia S, Desser RK. Post-irradiation malignant fibrous histiocytoma of the lung. Am J Clin Pathol 1980;74:820–826.

778. Killebrew E, Gerbode F. Leiomyosarcoma of the pulmonary artery diagnosed preoperatively by angiocardiography. J Thorac Cardiovasc Surg 1976;71:469.

779. Lyerly HK, Reves JG, Sabiston DC, Jr. Management of primary sarcomas of the pulmonary artery and reperfusion intrabronchial hemorrhage. Surg Gynecol Obstet 1986;163:291–301.

780. Head HD, Flam MS, John MJ, Lipnik SS, Slater D, Stewart RD. Long-term palliation of pulmonary artery sarcoma by radical excision and adjuvent therapy. Ann Thorac Surg 1992;53:332–334.

781. Mandelstamm M. Über primäre Neubildungen des Herzens. Virchows Arch Pathol Anat 1923;245:43–54.

781a. Greenspan EB. Primary osteoid chondrosarcoma of the lung: report of a case. Am J Cancer 1933;18:603–609.

782. Lowell IM, Tuhy JE. Primary chondrosarcoma of the lung. J Thorac Surg 1949;18:476–483.

783. Moegen P. Über einen primären sarkomatosen Tumor der Pulmonalarterie mit ausgedehnten Metastasen in der rechten Lunge. Z Kreisl Forsch 1951;40:150–160.

784. Hagström L. Malignant mesenchymoma in pulmonary artery and right ventricle. Report of a case with unusual location and histologic picture. Acta Pathol Microbiol Scand 1961;51:87–94.

785. Wagenvoort CA, Heath D, Edwards JE. The pathology of the pulmonary vasculature. Springfield: Thomas, 1964:440–477.

786. Kaiser LR, Urmacher C. Primary sarcoma of the superior pulmonary vein. Cancer (Philadelphia) 1990; 66:789–795.

787. Laya MB, Mailliard JA, Bewtra C, Levin HS. Malignant fibrous histiocytoma of the heart. Cancer (Philadelphia) 1987;59:1026–1031.

788. Prioleau PG, Katzenstein A-LA. Major peripheral arterial occlusion due to malignant tumor embolism: Histologic recognition and surgical management. Cancer (Philadelphia) 1978;42:2009–2014.

789. Peters P, Trotter SE, Sheppard MN, Goldstraw P. Primary leiomyoma of pulmonary vein. Thorax 1992;47:393–394.

790. Guccion JC, Rosen SH. Bronchopulmonary leiomyosarcoma and fibrosarcoma: A study of 32 cases and review of the literature. Cancer (Philadelphia) 1972;30:836–847.

791. Wick MR, Scheithauer BW, Piehler JM, Pairolero PC. Primary pulmonary leiomyosarcomas: A light and electron microscopic study. Arch Pathol Lab Med 1982;106:510–514.

792. Pettinato G, Manivel JC, Saldana Mj, Peyser J, Dehner LP. Primary bronchopulmonary fibrosarcoma of childhood and adolescence: Reassessment of a low-grade malignancy clinicopathologic study of five cases and review of the literature. Hum Pathol 1989;20:463–471.

793. Jimenez JF, Uthman EO, Townsend JW, Gloster ES, Seibert JJ. Primary bronchopulmonary leiomyosarcoma in childhood. Arch Pathol Lab Med 1986;110:348–351.

794. Stout AP, Himadi GM. Solitary (localized) mesothelioma of the pleura. Ann Surg 1951;133:50–64.

795. Foster EA, Ackerman LV. Localized mesotheliomas of the pleura. The pathologic evaluation of 18 cases. Am J Clin Pathol 1960;34:349–364.

796. Weiss SW, Enzinger FM. Malignant fibrous histiocytomas: an analysis of 200 cases. Cancer (Philadelphia) 1978;41:2250–2266.

797. Lee JT, Shelburne JD, Linder J. Primary malignant fibrous histiocytoma of the lung: A clinicopathologic and ultrastructrual study of five cases. Cancer (Philadelphia) 1984;53:1124–1130.

798. Sleyster TJW, Heystraten FMJ. Malignant fibrous histiocytoma mimicking pulmonary embolism. Thorax 1988;43:580–581.

799. Pruszczynski M, Coronel CMD, Naudin ten Cate L, Roholl PJM, van der Kley AJ. Immunohistochemical and ultrastructural studies of a primary aortic intimal sarcoma. Pathology 1988;20:173–178.

800. Van Damme H, Vaneerdeweg W. Malignant fibrous histiocytoma of the pulmonary artery. Ann Surg 1987;205:203–207.

801. Viguera JL, Pujol JL, Reboiras SD, Larrauri JL, De-Miguel LS. Fibrous histiocytoma of the lung. Thorax 1976;31:475–479.

802. Bedrossian CWM, Verani R, Unger KM, Salman J.

Pulmonary malignant fibrosis: Light and electron microscopic studies of one case. Chest 1979;75:186–189.

803. Kern WH, Hughes RK, Meyer BW, Harley DP. Malignant fibrous histiocytoma of the lung. Cancer (Philadelphia) 1977;75:1793–1801.

804. Chowdhury LN, Swerdlow MA, Wellington J, Kathpalia S, Desser RK. Post-irradiation malignant fibrous histiocytoma of the lung: demonstration of alpha-1-antitypsin-like material in neoplastic cells. Am J Clin Pathol 1980;74:820–826.

805. Paulsen SM, Egeblad K, Christensen J. Malignant fibrous histiocytoma of the lung. Virchows Arch [A] 1981;394:167–176.

806. Silverman JF, Coalson JJ. Primary malignant myxoid fibrous histiocytoma of the lung: Light and ultrastructural examination with review of the literature. Arch Pathol Lab Med 1984;108:49–54.

807. Kearney MM, Soule EH, Ivins JC. Malignant fibrous histiocytoma: a retrospective study of 167 cases. Cancer (Philadelphia) 1980;45:167–178.

808. Laas J, Schmid C, Mugge A, Daniel W. Malignant fibrous histiocytoma of the lung infiltrating the descending aorta: A diagnostic chameleon necessitating an extended operation. (letter) J Thorac Cardiovasc Surg 1990;100:798–800.

809. Yousem SA, Hochholzer L. Malignant fibrous histiocytoma of the lung. Cancer (Philadelphia) 1987;60:2532–2541.

810. McDonnell T, Kyriakos M, Roper C, Mazoujian G. Malignant fibrous histiocytoma of the lung. Cancer (Philadelphia) 1988;61:137–145.

811. Pezzi CM, Rawlings MS, Esgro JJ, Pollock RE, Romsdahl MM. Prognostic factors in 227 patients with malignant fibrous histiocytoma. Cancer (Philadelphia) 1992;69:2098–2103.

812. Enjojii M, Hashimoto H, Tsuneyoshi M, Iwasaki H. Malignant fibrous histiocytoma: A clinicopathologic study of 130 cases. Arch Pathol Jpn 1980;30:727–741.

813. Laskin WB, Silverman TA, Enzinger FM. Postradiation soft-tissue sarcomas: An analysis of 53 cases. Cancer (Philadelphia) 1988;62:2330–2340.

814. Ro JY, Avala AG, Sella A, Samuels ML, Swanson DA. Sarcomatoid renal cell carcinoma: Clinicopathologic study of 42 cases. Cancer (Philadelphia) 1987;59:576–526.

815. Meade JB, Whitwell F, Bickford BJ, Waddington JKB. Primary haemangiopericytoma of lung. Thorax 1974;29:1–15.

816. Page AC, Wells IP, Clarke JT. Pleuropulmonary haemangiopericytoma masquerading as a post-infective encysted pleural effusion. Br J Dis Chest 1988;82:426–430.

816a. Shin MS, Ho K-J. Primary hemangiopericytoma of lung: radiography and pathology. AJR 1979;133:1077–1083.

817. Rusch VW, Schuman WP, Schmidt R, Laramore GE. Massive pulmonary hemangiopericytoma: An innovative approach to evaluation and treatment. Cancer (Philadelphia) 1989;64:1928–1936.

817a. Yousem SA, Hochholzer L. Primary pulmonary hemangiopericytoma. Cancer (Philadelphia) 1987;59:549–555.

818. Gavilán J, Rodriguez-Peralto JL, Tomás HD, Nistal M, Gavilán C, Burgos E. Hemangiopericytoma of the trachea. J Laryngol Otol 1987;101:738–742.

818a. Morales AR, Fine G, Pardo V, Horn RC, Jr. The ultrastructure of smooth muscle tumors with a consideration of the possible relationship of glomangiomas, hemangiopericytomas, and cardiac myxomas. Pathol Annu 1975;10:65–92.

819. Kuhn C, III, Rosai J. Tumors arising from pericytes. Ultrastructure and organ culture of a case. Arch Pathol 1969;88:653–663.

820. Schurch W, Skalli O, Lagace R, Seemayer TA, Gabbiani G. Intermediate filament proteins and actin isoforms as markers for soft-tissue tumor differentiation. III. Hemangiopericytomas and glomus tumors. Am J Pathol 1990;136:771–786.

821. Battifora H. Hemangiopericytoma: ultrastructural study of five cases. Cancer (Philadelphia) 1973;31:1418–1432.

822. Enzinger FM, Smith BH. Hemangiopericytoma: An analysis of 106 cases. Hum Pathol 1976;7:81–82.

823. Wilks S. Enchondroma of the lung. Trans Pathol Soc (London) 1862;13:27–28.

824. Morgan AD, Salama FD. Primary chondrosarcoma of the lung: Case report and a review of the literature. J Thorac Cardiovasc Surg 1972;64:460–466.

825. Daniels AC, George H, Strans FH. Primary chondrosarcoma of tracheobronchial tree. Arch Pathol 1967;84:615–624.

826. Morgenroth A, Pfeuffer HP, Viereck HJ, Heine WD. Primary chondrosarcoma of the left inferior lobar bronchus. Respiration 1989;56:241–244.

827. Smith EAC, Cohen RV, Peale AR. Primary chondrosarcoma of the lung. Ann Intern Med 1960;53:838–846.

828. Bailey SC, Head HD. Pleural chondrosarcoma. Ann Thorac Surg 1990;49:996–997.

829. Sun C-CJ, Kroll M, Miller JE. Primary chondrosarcoma of the lung. Cancer (Philadelphia) 1982;50:1864–1866.

830. Pandolfo I, Gaeta M, Blandino A, La Spada F, Casablanca G, Caminiti R. Costal chondrosarcoma with pleural seeding: CT findings. J Comput Assist Tomogr 1985;9:405–409.

831. Abeles H, Chaves AD. The significance of calcification in pulmonary coin lesions. Radiology 1952;58:199–202.

831a. Reingold IM, Amromin GD. Extraosseous osteosarcoma of the lung. Cancer (Philadelphia) 1971;41–498.

832. Nascimento AG, Unni KK, Bernatz PE. Sarcomas of the lung. Mayo Clin Proc 1982;57:355–359.

833. Connolloy JP, McGuyer CA, Sageman WS, Bailey H. Intrathoracic osteosarcoma diagnosed by CT scan and pleural biopsy. Chest 1991;100:265–267.

834. Stout AP. Mesenchymoma, the mixed tumor of mesenchymal derivatives. Ann Surg 1948;27:278–290.

835. Munk J, Griffel B, Kogan J. Primary mesenchymoma of the pulmonary artery: Radiologic features. Br J Radiol 1965;38:104–111.

836. Hagstrom L. Malignant mesenchymoma in pulmonary artery and right ventricle. Acta Pathol Microbiol Scand [A] 1961;51:87–94.

837. Hohbach CHG, Mall W. Chondrosarcoma of the pulmonary artery. Beitr Pathol 1977;60:298–307.

838. Kalus M, Rahman F, Jenkins DE, Beall AC, Jr. Malignant mesenchymoma of the lung. Arch Pathol 1973;95:199–202.

839. Listrom MB, Johnson FP, Black WC. Malignant mesenchymoma of the lung. Am Soc Clin Pathol AP Check Sample 1990;AP-I (4):1–4.

840. Eriksson A, Thunell M, Lundquist G. Pedunculated endobronchial rhabdomyosarcoma with fatal asphyxia. Thorax 1982;37:390–391.

841. Drurv RAB, Stirland RM. Carcino-sarcomatous tumours of the respiratory tract. J Pathol Bacteriol 1959;77:543–554.

842. Brunn H, Goldman A. Differentiation of benign from malignant polypoid bronchial tumors. Surg Gynecol Obstet 1940;71:703–722.

843. Penfold JB. Lipoma of the hypopharynx. Br Med J 1952;1:1286.

844. Helbing C, 1898, as quoted by Drennan JM, McCormack RJM. Primary rhabdomyosarcoma of the lung. J Pathol Bacteriol 1960;79:147–149.

845. Lee SH, Reganchary SS, Paramesh J. Primary pulmonary rhabdomyosarcoma: A case report and review of the literature. Hum Pathol 1981;12:92–96.

846. Avignina A, Elsner B, DeMarco L, Bracco AN, Nazar J, Pavlovsky H. Pulmonary rhabdomyosarcoma with isolated small bowel metastases: A report of a case with immunohistological and ultrastructural studies. Cancer (Philadelphia) 1984;53:1948–1951.

847. Allan BT, Day DL, Dehner LP. Primary pulmonary rhabdomyosarcoma of the lung in children: Report of two cases presenting with spontaneous pneumothorax. Cancer (Philadelphia) 1987;59:1005–1011.

848. Christ WM, Raney RB Jr, Newton W, Lawrence W Jr, Tefft M, Foulkes MA (for the intergroup Rhabdomyosarcoma Study Committee). Intrathoracic soft tissue sarcomas in children. Cancer (Philadelphia) 1982;50:598–604.

849. Sawamura K, Hashimoto T, Nanjo S, et al. Primary liposarcoma of the lung: Report of a case. J Surg Oncol 1982;19:243–246.

850. Latienda RI, Itoiz OA. Mixoliposarcoma del pulmón. Arch Soc Argent Anat Norm Pathol 1946;8:563–570.

851. Gupta RK, Paolini FA. Liposarcoma of the pleura: Report of a case with review of literature and views on histogenesis. Am Rev Respir Dis 1967;95:298–304.

852. Spragg RG, Wolf PL, Haghighi P, Abraham JL, Astarita RW. Angiosarcoma of the lung with fatal pulmonary hemorrhage. Am J Med 1983;74:1072–1076.

853. Maddox JC, Evans HL. Angiosarcoma of skin and soft tissues: A study of forty-four cases. Cancer (Philadelphia) 1981;48:1907–1921.

854. Spencer H. Pathology of the lung. 4th Ed. Oxford: Pergamon, 1985:1000.

855. Yousem S. Angiosarcoma presenting in the lung. Arch Pathol Lab Med 1986;110:112–115.

856. Case Record #40191, Massachusetts General Hospital. N Engl J Med 1954;250:837–843.

857. Tralka GA, Katz S. Hemangioendothelioma of the lung. Am Rev Respir Dis 1963;87:107–115.

858. Kaposi M. Idiopathisches multiples Pigmentsarkom der Haut. Arch Dermatol Syphiloe 1872;4:265–273.

859. Volberding D. Therapy of Kaposi's sarcoma in AIDS. Semin Oncol 1984;11:60–66.

860. Cox FH, Helwig EB. Kaposi's sarcoma. Cancer (Philadelphia) 1959;12:289–298.

861. Safai B, Good RA. Kaposi's sarcoma: A review in recent developments. Clin Bull 1980;10:62–69.

862. Templeton AC. Studies in Kaposi's sarcoma: postmortem findings and disease patterns in women. Cancer (Philadelphia) 1972;30:854–867.

863. Templeton AC. Kaposi's sarcoma. Pathol Annu 1981 (part 2):315–336.

864. Myers BD, Kessler E, Levi J, Pick A, Rosenfeld JB, Tikvah P. Kaposi's sarcoma in kidney transplant recipients. Arch Intern Med 1974;133:307–311.

865. Harwood AR, Osoba D, Hofstader SL, et al. Kaposi's sarcoma in recipients of renal transplants. Am J Med 1979;67:759–765.

866. Penn I. Kaposi's sarcoma in organ transplant recipient. Transplantation 1979;27:8–11.

867. Nesbitt S, Mark PF, Zimmerman HM. Disseminated visceral idiopathic hemorrhagic sarcoma (Kaposi's disease): Report of case with necropsy findings. Ann Intern Med 1945;22:601–605.

868. Stats D. The visceral manifestations of Kaposi's sarcoma. J Mt Sinai Hosp 1946;12:971–983.

869. Loring WE, Wolman SR. Idiopathic multiple hemorrhagic sarcoma of lung (Kaposi's sarcoma). NY State J Med 1965;65:668–676.

870. Guerrin JC, Ode L, Brunet H, Berard J. Maladie de Kaposi: a localisation pumonaire. Poumon Coeur 1967;23:341–347.

871. Martino A, Calvanese F, Esposito C, Fogliani V. Partecipazione delpolmone nella malattia di Kaposi. Arch Tisiol Mal Appl Respir 1968;23:721–740.

872. Dantzig PI, Richardson D, Rayhanzadeh S, Mauro J, Shoss R. Thoracic involvement of non-African Kaposi's sarcoma. Chest 1974;66:522–525.

873. Hanno R, Owen LG, Callen JP. Kaposi's sarcoma with extensive silent internal involvement. Int J Dermatol 1979;18:718–721.

874. Ognibene FP, Steis RG, Macher AM, et al. Kaposi's sarcoma causing pulmonary infiltrates and respiratory failure in the acquired immunodeficiency syndrome. Ann Intern Med 1985;102:471–475.

875. Garay SM, Belenko M, Fazzini E, Schinella R. Pulmonary manifestations of Kaposi's sarcoma. Chest 1987; 91:39–43.

876. White DA, Matthay RA. Noninfectious pulmonary complications of infection with the human immunode-

ficiency virus. Am Rev Respir Dis 1989;140:1763–1787.

877. McLoud TC, Naidich DP. Thoracic disease in the immunocompromised patient. Radiol Clin North Am 1992;30:525–554.

878. Ognibene FP, Shelhamer JH. Kaposi's sarcoma. Clin Chest Med 1988;9:459–465.

879. Heitzman ER. Pulmonary neoplastic lymphoproliferative disease in AIDS: A review. Radiology 1990;177:347–351.

880. Purdy LJ, Colby TV, Yousem SA, Battifora H. Pulmonary Kaposi's sarcoma: Premortem histologic diagnosis. Am J Surg Pathol 1968;10:301–311.

881. Hymes KB, Cheung T, Greene JB, et al. Kaposi's sarcoma in homosexual men: A report of eight cases. Lancet 1981;ii:598–600.

882. Kaposi's sarcoma and *Pneumocystis* pneumonia in homosexual men—New York City and California. MMWR 1981;30:305–308.

883. Gottlieb GJ, Ackerman AB. Kaposi's sarcoma: An extensively disseminated form in young homosexual men. Hum Pathol 1982;13:882–892.

884. Des Jarlais DC, Stoneburner R, Thomas P, Friedman SR. Declines in proportion of Kaposi's sarcoma among cases of AIDS in multiple risk groups in New York City. Lancet 1987;ii:1024–1025.

885. Joshi VV, Oleske JM, Minnefor AB. Pathologic pulmonary findings in children with acquired immunodeficiency syndrome: A study of ten cases. Hum Pathol 1985;16:241–246.

886. Marchevsky A, Rosen MJ, Chrystal G, Kleinerman J. Pulmonary complications of the acquired immunodeficiency syndrome: A clinicopathologic study of 70 cases. Hum Pathol 1985;16:659–670.

887. Friedman-Kien AE, Laubenstein LJ, Rubinstein P, et al. Disseminated Kaposi's sarcoma in homosexual men. Ann Intern Med 1982;96:693–700.

888. Stover DE, White DA, Romano PA, Gellene RA, Robeson WA. Spectrum of pulmonary diseases associated with the acquired immune deficiency syndrome. Am J Med 1985;78:429–437.

889. Fouret PJ, Touboul JL, Mayaud CM, Akoun GM, Roland J. Pulmonary Kaposi's sarcoma in patients with acquired immune deficiency syndrome. Thorax 1987;42:262–268.

890. Hamm PG, Judson MA, Aranda CP. Diagnosis of pulmonary Kaposi's sarcoma with fiberoptic bronchoscopy and endobronchial biopsy: A report of five cases. Cancer (Philadelphia) 1987;59:807–810.

891. Welch K, Finkbeiner W, Alpers CF, et al. Autopsy findings in the acquired immune deficiency syndrome. JAMA 1984;252:1152–1159.

892. Niedt GW, Schinella RA. Acquired immunodeficiency syndrome: Clinicopathologic study of 56 cases. Arch Pathol Lab Med 1985;109:727–734.

893. Reichert CM, O'Leary TJ, Levens DL, Simrel CR, Macher AM. Autopsy pathology in the acquired immune deficiency syndrome. Am J Pathol 1983;112:357–382.

894. Guarda LA, Luna MA, Smith JL, Mansell PWA, Gyorkey F, Roca AN. Acquired immune deficiency syndrome and postmortem findings. Am J Clin Pathol 1984;81:549–557.

895. Nash G, Fligiel S. Pathologic features of the lung in the acquired immune deficiency syndrome (AIDS): An autopsy study of seventeen homosexual males. Am J Clin Pathol 1984;81:5–12.

896. Meduri GU, Stover DE, Lee M, Myskowski PL, Caravelli JF, Zaman MB. Pulmonary Kaposi's sarcoma in the acquired immune deficiency syndrome: Clinical, radiographic and pathologic manifestations. Am J Med 1986;81:11–18.

897. Moskowitz LB, Hensley GT, Gould EW, Weiss SD. Frequency and anatomic distribution of lymphadenopathic Kaposi's sarcoma in the acquired immunodeficiency syndrome: an autopsy series. Hum Pathol 1985;447–456.

898. Kornfeld H, Axelrod JL. Pulmonary presentation of Kaposi's sarcoma in a homosexual patient. Am Rev Respir Dis 1983;127:248–249.

899. Rucker L, Meador J. Kaposi's sarcoma presenting as homogeneous pulmonary infiltrates in a patient with acquired immunodeficiency syndrome. West J Med 1985;142:831–833.

900. Pitchenick AE, Fischl MA, Saldana MJ. Kaposi's sarcoma of the tracheobronchial tree. Chest 1985;87:122–124.

901. Nash G, Fligiel S. Kaposi's sarcoma presenting as pulmonary disease in the acquired immunodeficiency syndrome: Diagnosis by lung biopsy. Hum Pathol 1984;15:999–1001.

902. Reynolds WA, Winkelman RK, Soule EH. Kaposi's sarcoma: A clinicopathologic study with particular reference to its relationship to the reticuloendothelial system. Medicine (Baltimore) 1965;44:419–443.

903. Tedeschi CG. Some considerations concerning the nature of so-called sarcoma of Kaposi. AMA Arch Pathol 1958;66:656–684.

904. Dail DH, Hammar SP, Carter D. Tumors of the lung. Chicago:ASCP Press, (in press).

905. Ekfors TO, Joensuu K, Toivio I, Laurinen P, Pelttari L. Fatal epithelial hemangioendothelioma presenting in the lung and liver. Virchows Arch [A] 1986;410:9–16.

906. Ellis GL, Kratochvil FJ III. Epithelioid hemangioendothelioma of the head and neck: A clinicopathologic and followup study of twelve cases. Oral Surg Oral Med Oral Pathol 1986;61:61–68.

907. Case Record #10-1990. A 15-year-old girl with multiple radiotolerant bony defects and multiple pulmonary nodules. N Engl J Med 1990;322:683–690.

908. Dail D, Liebow A. Intravascular bronchioloalveolar tumor (abstr.). Am J Pathol 1975;78:6a–7b.

909. Corrin B, Manners B, Millard M, Weaver L. Histogenesis of the so-called "intravascular bronchioloalveolar tumor." J Pathol 1979;128:163–167.

910. Weldon-Linne CM, Victor TA, Christ ML, Fry WA. Angiocentric nature of the "intravascular bronchioloal-

veolar tumor" of the lung. An electron microscopic study. Arch Pathol Lab Med 1981;105:174–179.

911. Azumi N, Churg A. Intravascular and sclerosing bronchioloalveolar tumor. A pulmonary sarcoma of probable vascular origin. Am J Surg Pathol 1981;5:587–596.

912. Ferrer-Roca O. Intravascular and sclerosing bronchioalveolar tumor. Am J Surg Pathol 1981;5:587–596.

913. Weldon-Linne CM, Victor TA, Christ ML. Immunohistochemical identification of factor VIII-related antigen in the intravascular bronchioloalveolar tumor of the lung. Arch Pathol Lab Med 1981;105:628–629.

914. Bhagavan BS, Murthy MSN, Borfman HD, Eggleston JC. Intravascular bronchioloalveolar tumor (IVBAT). A low-grade sclerosing epithelioid angiosarcoma of lung. Am J Surg Pathol 1982;6:41–52.

915. Pilotti S, Rilke F, Lombardi L, Pastorino V. Immunohistochemistry and electron microscopy of intravascular bronchioloalveolar tumor of the lung. Tumori 1983;69:283–292.

916. Corrin B, Harrison WJ, Wright DH. The so-called intravascular bronchioloalveolar tumour of lung (low grade sclerosing angiosarcoma): Presentation with extrapulmonary deposits. Diagn Histopathol 1983; 6:229–237.

917. Weiss SW, Enzinger FM. Epithelioid hemangioendothelioma: A vascular tumor often mistaken for a carcinoma. Cancer (Philadelphia) 1982;50:970–981.

918. Yousem SA, Hochholzer L. Unusual thoracic manifestations of epithelioid hemandioendothelioma. Arch Pathol Lab Med 1987;111:459–463.

919. Shirakusa T, Yoshida M, Tsutsui M, et al. Advanced intravascular bronchioloalveolar tumor and review of reports in Japan. Respir Med 1989;85:127–132.

920. Ishak KG, Sesterhenn IA, Goodman MZD, Rabin L, Stromeyer FW. Epithelioid hemangioendothelioma of the liver: A clinicopathologic and followup study of 32 cases. Hum Pathol 1984;15:839–852.

921. Kelleher MB, Iwatsuki S, Sheahan DG. Epithelioid hemangioendothelioma of liver: Clinicopathological correlation of 10 cases treated by orthotopic liver transplantation. Am J Surg Pathol 1989;13:999–1008.

922. Dietze O, Davies SE, Williams R, Portmann B. Malignant epithelioid haemangioendothelioma of the liver: A clinicopathological and histochemical study of 12 cases. Histopathology 1989;15:225–237.

923. Tsuneyoshi M, Dorfman HD, Bauer TW. Epithelioid hemangioendothelioma of bone: A clinicopathologic, ultrastructural and immunohistochemical study. Am J Surg Pathol 1986;10:754–764.

924. Weiss SW, Ishak KG, Dail DH, Sweet DE, Enzinger FM. Epithelioid hemangioendothelioma and related lesions. Semin Diagn Pathol 1986;3:259–287.

925. Meister P, Hoede N, Rumpelt H-J. Epithelioid hemangioendothelioma of the scalp. Pathol Res Pract 1985;180:220–226.

926. Rosai J, Gold J, Landy R. The histolcytoid hemangiomas: A unifying concept embracing several previously described entities of skin, soft tissue, large vessels, bone and heart. Hum Pathol 1979;10:707–730.

927. Kuo T-T, Hsueh S, Su I-J, Gonzalez-Crussi F, Chen J-S. Histiocytoid hemangioma of the heart with peripheral eosinophilia. Cancer (Philadelphia) 1985;55:2854–2861.

928. Silva EG, Phillips J, Langer B, Ordonez NG. Spindle and histiocytoid (epithelioid) hemangioendothelioma: Primary in lymph nodes. Am J Clin Pathol 1986; 85:731–735.

929. Taguchi T, Tsuji K, Matsuo K, Takebayashi S, Kawahara K, Hadama T. Intravascular bronchioloalveolar tumor: Report of an autopsy case and review of the literature. Acta Pathol Jpn 1985;35:631–642.

930. Gledhill A, Kay JM. Hepatic metastasis in a case of intravascular bronchioloalveolar tumor. J Clin Pathol 1984;37:279–282.

931. Nakatani Y, Aoki I, Misugi K. Immunohistochemical and ultrastructural study of early lesions of intravascular bronchioloalveolar tumor with liver involvement. Acta Pathol Jpn 1985;35:1453–1465.

932. Fukayama M, Nihei Z, Takizawa T, Kawaguchi K, Harada H, Koike M. Malignant epithelioid hemangioendothelioma of the liver, spreading through the hepatic veins. Virchows Arch [A] 1984;404:275–287.

933. Persaud V, Bateson EM, Bankay CD. Pleural mesothelioma associated with massive hepatic calcification and usual metastases. Cancer (Philadelphia) 1970;26:920–928.

934. Morgan AG, Walker WC, Mason MK, Herlinger H, Losowsky MS. A new syndrome associated with hepatocellular carcinoma. Gastroenterology 1972;63:340–345.

935. Ludwig J, Grier MW, Hoffman HN II, McGill DB. Calcified mixed malignant tumor of the liver. Arch Pathol Lab Med 1975;99:162–166.

936. Echevarria RA, Arean VM, Galindo L. Hepatic tumors of long duration with eventual metastases. Am J Clin Pathol 1978;69:624–631.

937. Verbecken E, Beyls J, Moerman P, Knockaert D, Goddeeris P, Lauweryns JM. Lung metastasis of malignant epithelioid hemangioendothelioma mimicking a primary intravascular bronchioloalveolar tumor. A histologic, ultrastructural and immunohistochemical study. Cancer (Philadelphia) 1985;55:1741–1746.

938. Huehnergarth J. Valley Medical Center, Renton, Washington. Personal correspondence, 1984.

938a. Pettinato G, Insabato L, DeChiara A, Forestieri P, Maruco A. Epithelioid hemangioendothelioma of soft tissue: Fine needle aspiration cytology, histology, electron microscopy and immunoshistochemistry of a case. Acta Cytol 1986;30:194–200.

939. Yook TS. St. Joseph Hospital, Mt. Clements, Michigan. Personal communication, 1981.

940. Wenisch HJC, Lulay M. Lymphogenous spread of an intravascular bronchioloalveolar tumor. Case report and review of literature. Virchows Arch [A] 1980; 387:117–123.

941. Carter EJ, Bradburne RM, Jhung JW, Ettensohn DB.

Alveolar hemorrhagic with epithelioid hemangioendothelioma. Am Rev Respir Dis 1990;142:700–701.

942. Lamovec J, Sobel HJ, Zidar A, Jerman J. Epithelioid hemangioendothelioma of the anterior mediastinum with osteoclast-like giant cells. Am J Clin Pathol 1990;93:813–817.

943. Clary C, Jacob C, Blaive B, Kermarec J. Tumeur bronchiolo-alveolaire intra-vasculaire I.V.B.A.T.: Etude d'une à tendance angiosarcomateuse. Ann Pathol 1985;5:107–114.

944. Spark RP. Tuscon Medical Center, Tuscon, Arizona. Personal communication, 1986.

945. Ohori MP, Yousem SA, Sonmez-Alpen B, Colby TV. Estrogen and progesterone receptors in lymphangioleiomyomatosis, epithelioid hemangioendothelioma, and sclerosing hemangioma of the lung. Am J Clin Pathol 1991;96:529–535.

946. Dean PJ, Haggitt RC, O'Hara CJ. Malignant epithelioid hemangioendothelioma of the liver in young women. Relationship to oral contraceptive use. Am J Surg Pathol 1985;9:695–704.

947. Gelin M, Van de Studt J, Rickaert F, et al. Epithelioid hemangioendothelioma of the liver following contact with vinyl chloride. Recurrence after orthotopic liver transplantation. J Hepatol 1989;8:99–106.

948. Davies MF, Curtis M, Howat JM. Cutaneous haemangioendothelioma: A possible link with chronic exposure to vinyl chloride. Br J Ind Med 1990;47:65–67.

949. Lautenbacher R. Dysembryomes métotypiques des reins, carcinose submiliere aiguë poumon avec emphysème généralisé et doulde pneumothorax. Ann Med Intern (Paris) 1918;5:435–450.

950. Burrell LS, Ross HM. A case of chylous effusion due to leiomyosarcoma. Br J Tuberc 1937;31:38–39.

951. von Stössel E. Über muskuläre Cirrhose der Lunge. Beitr Klin Tuberk 1937;90:432–442.

952. Rosendal T. A case of diffuse myomatosis and cyst formation in the lung. Acta Radiol 1942;23:138–146.

953. Laipply TC, Sherrick JC. Intrathoracic angiomyomatous hyperplasia associated with chronic chylothorax. Lab Invest 1958;7:387–400.

954. Cornog JL, Jr, Enterline HT. Lymphangiomyoma, a benign lesion of chylous lymphatics synonymous with lymphangiopericytoma. Cancer (Philadelphia) 1966;19:1909–1930.

955. Harris JO, Waltuck BL, Swenson EW. The pathophysiology of the lungs in tuberous sclerosis. A case report and literature review. Am Rev Respir Dis 1969;100:379–387.

956. Corrin B, Liebow A, Friedman PJ. Pulmonary lymphangiomyomatosis: A review. Am J Pathol 1975;79:347–382.

957. Taylor JR, Ryv J, Colby TV, Raffin TA. Lymphangioleiomyomatosis: Clinical course in 32 patients. N Engl J Med 1990;323:1254–1260.

958. Carrington CB, Cugell DW, Gaensler EA, et al. Lymphangioleiomyomatosis: Physiologic, pathologic, radiologic correlations. Am Rev Respir Dis 1977;116:977–995.

959. Silverstein EF, Ellis K, Wolff M, Jaretzki A, III. Pulmonary lymphangiomyomatosis. AJR 1974;120:832–850.

960. Gray SR, Carrington CB, Cornog JL, Jr. Lymphangiomyomatosis: Report of a case with ureteral involvement and chyluria. Cancer (Philadelphia) 1975;35:490–498.

960a. Sobonya RE, Quan SF, Fleishman JS. Pulmonary lymphangioleiomyomatosis: Quantitative analysis of lesions producing airflow limitation. Hum Pathol 1985;16:1122–1128.

961. Basset F, Soler P, Marsac J, Corrin B. Pulmonary lymphangioleiomyomatosis: Three new cases with electron microscopy. Cancer (Philadelphia) 1976;38:2357–2366.

962. Fukuda Y, Kawamoto M, Yamamoto A, Ishizaki M, Basset F, Magusi Y. Role of elastic fiber degeneration in emphysema-like lesions of pulmonary lymphoangiomyomatosis. Hum Pathol 1990;21:1252–1261.

963. Fukuda Y, Masuda Y, Ishizaki M, Masugi Y, Ferrans VJ. Morphogenesis of abnormal elastic fibers in lungs of patients with panacinar and centriacinar emphysema. Hum Pathol 1989;20:652–659.

964. Fukuda Y, Basset F, Soler P, Ferrans VJ, Masugi Y, Crystal RG. Intraluminal fibrosis and elastic fiber degradation lead to lung remodeling in pulmonary Langerhan's cell granulomatosis (histiocytosis X). Am J Pathol 1990;137:415–424.

965. Sherrier RH, Chiles C, Roggli V. Pulmonary lymphangioleiomyomatosis: CT findings. AJR 1989;153:937–940.

966. Rappaport DC, Weisbrod GL, Herman SJ, Chamberlain DW. Pulmonary lymphangioleiomyomatosis: High-resolution CT findings in four cases. AJR 1989;152:961–964.

967. Lenoir S, Bravner M et al. Pulmonary lymphangiomyomatosis and tuberous sclerosis: Comparison and radiographic and thin-section CT findings. Radiology 1990;175:329–334.

968. Müller NL, Chiles C, Kullnig P. Pulmonary lymphangioleiomyomatosis: Correlation of CT with radiographic and functional findings. Radiology 1990;175:335–339.

969. Stern EJ, Webb WR, Golden JA, Gamsu G. Cystic lung disease associated with eosinophilic granuloma and tuberous sclerosis: Air trapping at dynamic ultrafast high-resolution CT. Radiology 1992;182:325–329.

970. Green GJ. The radiology of tuberose sclerosis. Clin Radiol 1968;19:135–147.

971. Milledge RD, Gerald BE, Carter WJ. Pulmonary manifestations of tuberous sclerosis. Am J Roentgenol 1966;98:734–738.

972. Brauner MW, Grenier P, Mouelhi MM, Mompoint D, Lenoir S. Pulmonary histiocytosis X: Evaluation with high-resolution CT. Radiology 1989;172:255–258.

973. Moore ADA, Godwin JD, Müller NL, et al. Pulmonary histiocytosis X: Comparison of radiographic and CT findings. Radiology 1989;172:249–254.

974. Kane PB, Lane BP, Cordice JWV, Greenberg GM. Ultrastructure of the proliferative cells in pulmonary lymphangiomyomatosis. Arch Pathol Lab Med 1978;102:618–622.

975. Wolff M. Lymphangiomyoma—clinicopathologic study and ultrastructural confirmation of its histogenesis. Cancer (Philadelphia) 1973;31:988–1007.

976. Kuwabara H, Biyazima S, Osaka T, et al. A case of pulmonary lymphangiomyomatosis diagnosed by TBLB and treated with progesterone and oophorectomy. Nippon Kyobu Shikkan Gakkai Zasshi 1984;22:795–799.

977. Luna CM, Gené R, Jolly EG, et al. Pulmonary lymphangiomyomatosis associated with tuberous sclerosis. Treatment with tamoxifen and tetracycline-pleurodesis. Chest 1985;88:473–475.

978. Shen A, Iseman MD, Waldron JA, King TE. Exacerbation of pulmonary lymphangioleiomyomatosis by exogenous estrogens. Chest 1987;91:782–785.

979. McCarty KS, Mossler JA, McLelland R, Sieker HO. Pulmonary lymphangiomyomatosis responsive to progesterone. N Engl J Med 1980;303:1461–1465.

980. Kitzsteiner KA, Mallen RG. Pulmonary lymphangiomyomatosis. N Engl J Med 1981;304:978–979.

981. Sinclair W, Wright JL, Churg A. Lymphangiomyomatosis presenting in a post-menopausal woman. Thorax 1985;40:475–476.

982. Yockey CC, Riepe RE, Ryan K. Pulmonary lymphangioleiomyomatosis complicated by pregnancy. Kans Med 1986;87:277–278,293.

983. Banner AS, Carrington CB, Emory WB. Efficacy of oophorectomy in lymphangiomyomatosis and benign metastasizing leiomyoma. N Engl J Med 1981;305:204–209.

984. Urban T, Kuttenn F, Gompel A, Marsac J, Lacronique J. Pulmonary lymphangiomyomatosis. Follow-up and long-term outcome with antiestrogen therapy: A report of eight cases. Chest 1992;102:472–476.

985. Jao J, Gilbert S, Messer R. Lymphangiomyoma and tuberous sclerosis. Cancer (Philadelphia) 1972;29:1188–1192.

986. Monteforte WJ Jr, Kohnen PW. Angiomyolipomas in a case of lymphangiomatous syndrome: Relationship to tuberous sclerosis. Cancer (Philadelphia) 1974;34:317–321.

987. Stovin PGI, Lum LC, Flower CDR, Darke CS, Beeley M. The lungs in lymphangiomyomatosis and in tuberous sclerosis. Thorax 1975;30:497–509.

988. Valensi QJ. Pulmonary lymphangiomyoma, a probable forme fruste of tuberous sclerosis, report of a case and survey of the literature. Am Rev Respir Dis 1973;108:1411–1415.

989. Capron F, Ameille J, Leclerq P, et al. Pulmonary lymphangioleiomyomatosis and Bourneville's tuberous sclerosis with pulmonary involvement: the same disease? Cancer (Philadelphia) 1983;52:851–855.

990. Slingerland JM, Grossman RF, Chamberlain D, Tremblay CE. Pulmonary manifestations of tuberous sclerosis in first degree relatives. Thorax 1989;44:212–214.

991. Shepherd CW, Gomez MR, Lie JT, Crowson CS. Causes of death in patients with tuberous sclerosis. Mayo Clin Proc 1991;66:792–796.

992. Valentine VG, Raffin TA. The management of chylothorax. Chest 1992;102:586–591.

993. Cagnano M, Benharroch D, Geffen DB. Pulmonary lymphangioleiomyomatosis: Report of a case with associated multiple soft-tissue tumors. Arch Pathol Lab Med 1991;115:1257–1259.

994. Kreisman H, Robitaille Y, Dionne GP, PaRayew MJ. Lymphangiomyomatosis syndrome with hyperparathyroidism: A case report. Cancer 1978;42:364–372.

995. Huml JP, Borkgren MW, Henley LB, Fahey PJ. Pulmonary lymphangioleiomyomatosis associated with pulmonary parenchymal, hilar, and mediastinal noncaseating granulomas. Chest 1991;100:1726–1728.

996. Fahy J, Toner M, O'Sullivan J, FitzGerald MX. Haemopericardium and cardiac kamponade complicating pulmonary lymphangioleiomyomatosis. Thorax 1991;46:222.

997. Eliasson AH, Phillips YY, Tenholder MF. Treatment of lymphangioleiomyomatosis. A metaanalysis. Chest 1989;196:1352–1355.

998. Cutler GB, Hoffman AR, Swerdloff RS, Santen RJ, Meldrum DR, Comite F. Therapeutic applications of luteinizing-hormone-releasing hormone and its analogs. Ann Intern Med 1985;102:643–657.

999. Egsvogel MMM, Page PS. Lymphangiomyomatosis. Chest 1990;98:1045–1046 (letter).

1000. Rossi GA, Balbi B, Oddera S, Lantero S, Ravazzoni C. Response to treatment with analog of the luteinizing-releasing-hormone in a patient with pulmonary lymphangioleiomyomatosis. Am Rev Respir Dis 1991;143:174–176.

1001. Heldrum DR, Pardridge WM, Karow WG, Rivier J, Vale W, Judd HL. Hormonal effects of danazol and medical oophorectomy in endometrosis. Obstet Gynecol 1983;62:480–485.

1002. Hofford JM. Lymphangiomyomatosis. Chest 1990;98:1043–1044 (letter).

1003. Estenne M, de Francquen P, Wellens F, et al. Combined heart-and-lung transplantation for lymphangioleiomyomatosis. Lancet 1984;i:275.

1004. Wellens F, Estenne M, Goldstein J, Leclerc JL, De Francquen P, Primo G. Heart-lung transplantation for terminal pulmonary lymphangioleiomyomatosis. Transplant Proc 1985;17:225–226.

1005. Lizotte PE, Whitlock WL, Prudhomme JC, Brown CR, Hershon JL. Lymphangiomyomatosis (letter). Chest 1990;98:1044–1045.

1006. Bhattacharyya AK, Balogh K. Retroperitoneal lymphangioleiomyomatosis. A 36-year benign course in a postmenopausal woman. Cancer (Philadelphia) 1985; 56:1144–1146.

1007. Sathyavagiswaran L, Sherwin RP. Acute and chronic pericholangitis in association with multifocal hepatic lymphangiomatosis. Hum Pathol 1989;20:601–603.

1008. Enzinger FM, Weiss SW. Soft tissue tumors. 2d Ed. St. Louis: CV Mosby, 1988:614–637.

1009. Spencer H. Pathology of the lang. 4th Ed. Oxford: Pergamon, 1985;125–129.

1010. Wagenaar SJSC, Swierenga J, Wagenvoort CA. Late presentation of primary pulmonary lymphangiectasis. Thorax 1978;33:791–795.

1011. Noonan JA, Walters LR, Reeves JT. Congenital pulmonary lymphangiectasis. Am J Dis Child 1970; 120:314–319.

1012. Nanson EM. Lymphangioma (cystic hygroma) of the mediastinum. J Cardiovasc Surg (Torino) 1968;9:447–452.

1013. Thomas HM, Shaw NJ, Weindling AM. Generalized lymphangiomatosis with chylothorax. Arch Dis Child 1990;65:334.

1014. Langer JC, Fitzgerald PG, Desa D, et al. Cervical cystic hygroma in the fetus: Clinical spectrum and outcome. J Pediatr Surg 1990;25:58–61; discussion, 61–62.

1015. Bill AH, Jr, Sumner DS. A unified concept of lymphangioma and cystic hygroma. Surg Gynecol Obstet 1965;120:79–86.

1016. Galifer RB, Pous JG, Juskiewenski, Pasquie M, Gaubert J. Intra-abdominal cystic lymphangiomas in childhood. Prog Pediatr Surg 1978;11:173–238.

1017. Ricci C, Santoro E, Moretti M. II linfangioma cistico cervico-mediastinico e mediastinico: Rassegna della letteratura e presentazione di due casi personali. Arch Chir Torace 1964;21:57–90.

1018. Mennemeyer R, Smith M. Multicystic, peritoneal mesothelioma: A report with electron microscopy of a case mimicking ultra-abdominal cystic hygroma (lymph-angioma). Cancer (Philadelphia) 1979;44:692–698.

1019. Weiss SW, Tavassoli FA. Multicystic mesothelioma: An analysis of pathologic findings and biologic behavior in 37 cases. Am J Surg Pathol 1988;12:737–746.

1020. Ross MJ, Welch WR, Scully RE. Multilocular pertoneal inclusion cysts (so-called cystic mesotheliomas). Cancer (Philadelphia) 1989;64:1336–1346.

1021. Brown LR, Reiman HM, Rosenow EC, III, Gloviczki PM, Divertie MB. Intrathoracic lymphangiomas. Mayo Clin Proc 1986;61:882–892.

1022. Case 30-1980, Massachusetts General Hospital. N Engl J Med 1980;303:270–276.

1023. Pilla TJ, Wolverson MK, Sundaram M, Heiberg E, Shields JB. CT evaluation of cystic lymphangiomas of the mediastinum. Radiology 1982;144:841–842.

1024. Gorham LW, Wright AW, Shultz HH, Maxon FC. Disappearing bones: A rare form of massive osteolysis: Report of two cases with autopsy findings. Am J Med 1954;17:674–682.

1025. Rasaretnam R, Chanmugam D, Sabanathan K, Paul

1026. ATS. Cervico-mediastinal lymphangioma. Aust NZ J Surg 1976;46:378–381.

1026. Cutillo DP, Swayne LC, Cucco J, Dougan H. CT and MR imaging in cystic abdominal lymphangiomatosis. J Comput Assist Tomogr 1989;13:534–536.

1027. Telander RL, Kaufman BH, Gloviczki P, Stickler GB, Hollier LH. Prognosis and management of lesions of the trunk in children with Klippel–Trenaunay syndrome. J Pediatr Surg 1984;19:417–422.

1028. Servelle M, Noguès C. The chyliferous vessels. Paris: Expansion Scientifique Francaise, 1981;49–59.

1029. Carlson KC, Parnassus WN, Klatt EC. Thoracic lymphangiomatosis. Arch Pathol Lab Med 1987; 111:475–477.

1030. Swank DW, Hepper NGG, Folkert KE, Colby TV. Intrathoracic lymphangiomatosis mimicking lymphangioleiomyomatosis in a young woman. Mayo Clin Proc 1989;64:1264–1268.

1031. Tazelaar KH, Yousem S, Saldana M, Colby T. Diffuse pulmonary lymphangiomatosis (abstract). Mod Pathology 1992;5:114A.

1032. Rowen M, Thompson JR, Williamson RA, Wood BJ. Diffuse pulmonary hemangiomatosis. Radiology 1978;127:445–451.

1033. Koblenzer PJ, Bukowski MJ. Angiomatosis (hamartomatous hemolymphangiomatosis): Report of a case with diffuse involvement. Pediatrics 1961:28:61–76.

1034. Goodall JF, Stewart I. Cavernous haemangioma of the lung. Lancet 1958;i:242–243.

1035. Liebow AA. Tumors of the lower respiratory tract. Washington DC: Armed Forces Institute of Pathology 1952:112–118.

1036. Holden KR, Alexander F. Diffuse neonatal hemangiomatosis. Pediatrics 1970;46:411–421.

1037. Askin FB. Pulmonary disorders in the neonatal infant and child. In: Thurlbeck WM, ed. Pathology of the lung. Stuttgart: Thieme, 1988:117–119.

1038. Wagenvoort CA, Beetstra A. Spijker J. Capillary haemangiomatosis of the lung. Histopathology 1978;2:401–406.

1039. Faber CN, Yousem SA, Dauber JH, Griffith BP, Hardesty RL, Paradis IL. Pulmonary capillary hemangiomatosis: A report of three cases and a rcview of the literature. Am Rev Respir Dis 1989;140:808–813.

1040. Tron V, Magee F, Wright JL, Colby T, Churg A. Pulmonary capillary hemangiomatosis. Hum Pathol 1986;17:1144–1149.

1041. Langleben D, Heneghan JM, Batten AP, et al. Familial pulmonary capillary hemangiomatosis resulting in primary pulmonary hypertension. Ann Intern Med 1988;109:106–109.

1042. Dail DH, Liebow AA, Gmelich JT, Carrington CB, Churg A. A study of 43 cases of pulmonary veno-occlusive (PVO) disease (abstr.). Lab Invest 1978; 38:340.

1043. Enzinger FM, Weiss SW. Soft tissue tumors. St. Louis: CV Mosby, 1983:78–83.

1044. Roggli VL, Kim H-S, Hawkins E. Congenital generalized fibromatosis with visceral involvement: A case report. Cancer (Philadelphia) 1980;45:954–960.

1045. Cohen S. Kaiser Hospital, Panorama City, California. Personal communication, 1974.

1046. Evans HL. Low-grade fibromyxoid sarcoma: A report of two metastasizing neoplasms having a deceptively benign appearance. Am J Clin Pathol 1987;88:615–619.

1047. Evans HL. Low-grade fibromyxoid sarcoma: a report of 12 cases. Am J Surg Pathol 1993;17:595–600.

1048. Dr. J. Carlos Manivel, University, University of Minnesota. Personal communication, 1992.

CHAPTER 34

Pleural Diseases

SAMUEL P. HAMMAR

Embryology and Anatomy of the Pleura

Vertebrates have a complex system of body cavities of mesodermal origin called the pleural, pericardial, and peritoneal cavities. These cavities are lined by a flattened layer of cells referred to as mesothelium, and are referred to as serous cavities. Embryologically, the cavities develop from the coelomic cavity, which develops early in embryogenesis.[1] The lung buds initially grow into what is referred to as the pericardial-peritoneal cavity, which later develops into the pleural-pericardial cavity. The pleural-pericardial membrane separates the pleural cavity from the pericardial cavity, and the pleural-peritoneal membrane separates the pleural cavity from the peritoneal cavity (Fig. 34–1). An excellent description of the development of the coelomic cavity was published in 1890.[2] In the adult, the pleura is divided into the parietal pleura, which lines the inside of the thoracic cavity, and the visceral pleura, which covers the lung parenchyma (Fig. 34–2). The visceral and parietal pleura are connected at the hilum of the lung.

The pleural space measures approximately 10–20 μm in width,[3] and in most mammals the pleural space

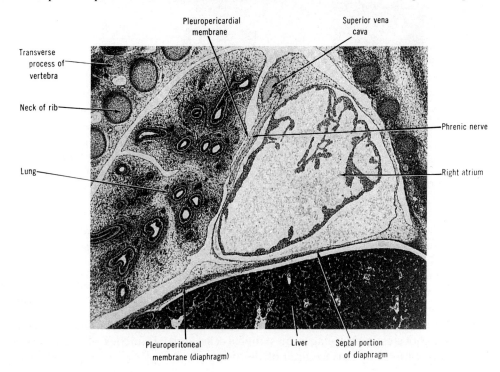

Fig. 34–1. Photograph of developing human embryo shows relationship of pleural, pericardial, and peritoneal cavities. (Reprinted with permission from Davies, J. Development of the respiratory system. In: Human Developmental Anatomy, New York, The Ronald Press Company, 1963.)

Transverse process of vertebra

Neck of rib

Lung

Pleuropericardial membrane

Superior vena cava

Phrenic nerve

Right atrium

Pleuroperitoneal membrane (diaphragm)

Liver

Septal portion of diaphragm

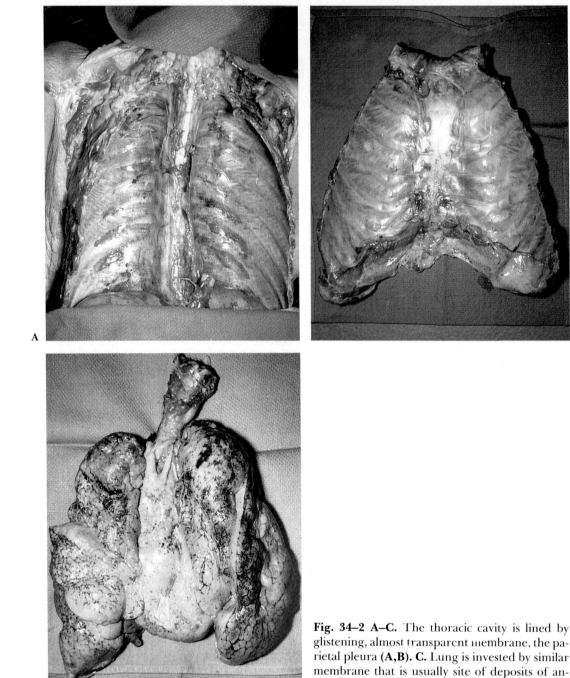

Fig. 34–2 A–C. The thoracic cavity is lined by glistening, almost transparent membrane, the parietal pleura (**A,B**). **C.** Lung is invested by similar membrane that is usually site of deposits of anthracotic pigment and other material.

contains a small amount of pleural fluid, which in normal conditions is approximately 0.1–0.2 ml/kg body weight.[3] The pleural fluid is a clear, colorless substance that contains a high concentration of glycosaminoglycans, primarily hyaluronic acid, and has a protein concentration of approximately 1.5 g/dl.[3] The pleural fluid normally contains a variety of cells, including monocytes, lymphocytes, macrophages, mesothelial cells, and rare neutrophils. The surface area of the two pleural cavities is approximately the same, and in a 70-kg man is about 2000 square cm.[3]

Blood Supply, Lymphatics, and Innervation of the Pleura

The costal pleura receives its blood supply from small branches of the intercostal arteries.[4] The mediastinal pleura is supplied by the pericardiophrenic artery, and the diaphragmatic parietal pleural is served by the superior phrenic and musculophrenic arteries.[4] The blood supply to the visceral pleura is controversial, but most likely is from branches of the bronchial artery.[4]

The visceral pleura has an extensive intercommunicating plexus of lymphatic channels that run over the surface of the lung toward the hilum, or communicate through the interlobular septa with peribronchial lymphatics which also flow to the hilum of the lung. The parietal lymphatic channels drain in various directions. The costal lymphatics drain centrally toward lymph nodes along the internal thoracic artery and toward the intercostal lymph nodes near the head of the ribs. Mediastinal parietal pleural lymphatics drain to the mediastinal nodes, and the lymphatics of the diaphragmatic pleura flow to the parasternal, middle phrenic, and posterior parietal pleura.[5]

Sensory nerve endings are found in the diaphragmatic and costal parietal pleura. Branches from the intercostal nerves supply the costal pleura and part of the diaphragmatic pleura. The central part of the diaphragm is innervated by branches of the phrenic nerve. The visceral pleura contains no nerve endings. Chest wall pain, which is a common symptom in mesothelioma, results from irritation and inflammation of the parietal pleura.[4]

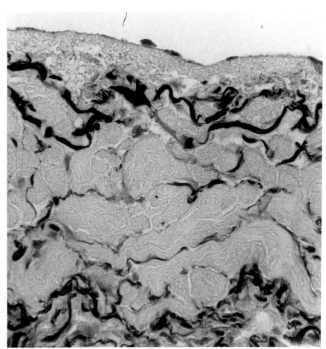

Fig. 34–3. Visceral pleura can be divided into five layers (see text), best seen with elastic tissue stain. ×550.

Histology of the Normal Pleura

The pleura can be divided into five layers: (1) innermost mesothelial cell layer, (2) submesothelial interstitial connective tissue layer, (3) inner thin elastic fiber layer, (4) outer interstitial connective tissue layer, and (5) thick elastic fiber layer[5] (Fig. 34–3). In the resting condition, the different layers of the pleura may be inconspicuous, and the mesothelial cells are only about 1 μm thick (Fig. 34–4). However, these cells are extremely reactive to any type of injury, and frequently undergo hypertrophy and hyperplasia to produce a much thicker mesothelial cell layer with a significantly increased number of mesothelial cells (Fig. 34–5). In the parietal pleura, the layers are not as distinct as in the visceral pleura, and the landmark that this author uses for parietal pleura is the fatty tissue that is present between the skeletal muscle of the chest wall and the connective-elastic tissue of the parietal pleura (Fig. 34–6).

Ultrastructure of the Pleura

The surface mesothelial layer is best appreciated by scanning electron microscopy, which shows the numerous microvilli that arise from these cells and project into the pleural space (Fig. 34–7).[6] In normal conditions, the microvilli measure about 0.1 μm in diameter and to

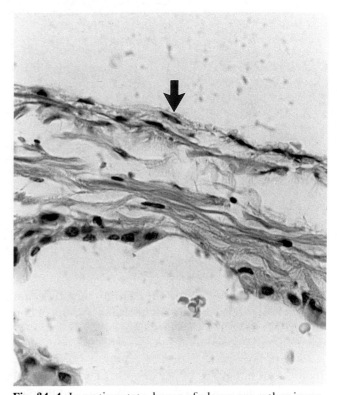

Fig. 34–4. In resting state, layers of pleura are rather inconspicuous. Note flattened appearance of mesothelial lining cells (*arrow*). ×300.

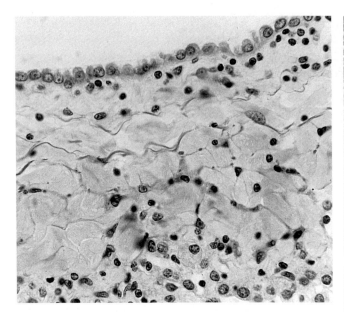

Fig. 34–5. Very slight irritation causes mesothelial cells to undergo hypertrophy and hyperplasia; pleura then becomes thicker. ×300.

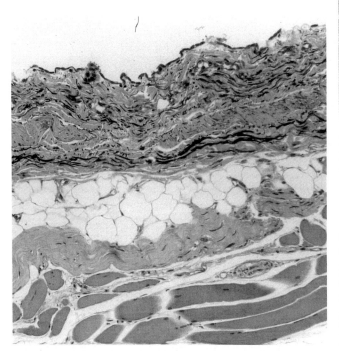

Fig. 34–6. Parietal pleura is also lined by mesothelial cells and contains elastic connective tissue stroma with layer of fat before chest wall skeletal muscle. ×125.

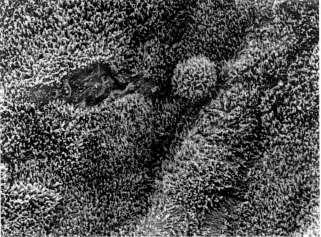

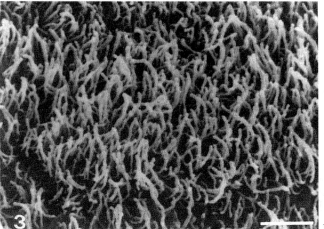

Fig. 34–7 A,B. Scanning electron micrographs of mesothelial lining of pleura show extensive microvillous surface. (Reprinted with permission from Gaudio et al., Chest 1988; 982:149–153.)

about 3 μm in length. When the pleura is injured and there is hypertrophy and hyperplasia of mesothelial cells, the number and length of the microvilli usually increase. The exact function of the microvilli is not entirely understood. At one time it was thought that they increased the absorptive surface of the visceral pleura, but later studies showed that the visceral pleura did not absorb pleural fluid to any significant degree.[3] Current thought is that microvilli serve as an increased surface area to release hyaluronic acid, which serves as a lubricant between the visceral and parietal layers of the pleura during movement of the lung in respiration.[3] The density of the microvilli is stated to be greater on the visceral mesothelial cells than on the parietal mesothelial cells. As described, the visceral and the parietal pleura have an extensive lymphatic network, although in the normal resting state, these lymphatic channels are inconspicuous. Although still considered somewhat controversial, openings between the mesothelial cells called "stomata" occur on the parietal surface and range between 2 and 12 μm in diameter[2,7,8] (Fig. 34–8). These

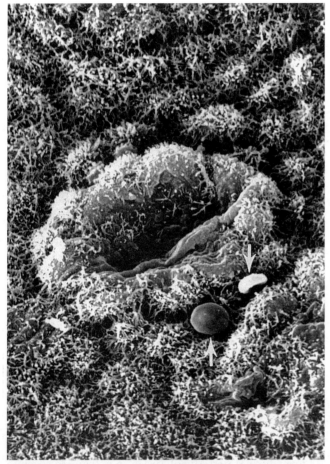

Fig. 34–8. Openings in mesothelium, called stomata. *Arrows* point to red blood cells. (Reprinted with permission from Whitaker et al. The pathobiology of the mesothelium. In: Henderson et al. *Malignant Mesothelioma.* New York, Hemisphere, 1992.)

stomata are stated to communicate directly with lymphatic lacuna. The stomata are thought to represent exit points for pleural fluid, protein, and cells that come from the pleural space.[7,9]

Pleural Fluid Formation

Pleural fluid formation has been discussed in detail by Sahn[3,10] and by Pistolesi et al.[11] The majority of pleural fluid is produced by the parietal pleura, and there is a dynamic interaction between production and resorption. As described by Sahn,[3] six mechanisms have been postulated for the accumulation of abnormal volumes of pleural fluid: (1) increase in hydrostatic pressure in the microvascular circulation; (2) decrease in oncotic pressure in the microvascular circulation; (3) decrease in pressure in the pleural space, (4) increased permeability of the microvascular circulation; (5) impaired

lymphatic drainage from the pleural space; and (6) movement of fluid from the peritoneal space.

The diagnostic techniques used in examining pleural fluid, and the significance of the findings, have been discussed in detail by Sahn[3] and by Light.[12]

Diagnostic Techniques to Evaluate Pleural Disease

Besides examining the characteristics of pleural fluid, closed and open pleural biopsies may be performed to diagnose pleural diseases. What type of biopsy, if any, depends on the clinical situation and the information needed. "Open" pleural biopsy is the standard against which closed pleural biopsy and thoracoscopic pleural biopsy are compared. As one might expect, open pleural biopsies have a higher diagnostic yield than closed pleural biopsies or thorascopic pleural biopsies. As is discussed later, this author believes that closed pleural biopsies and thorascopic pleural biopsies are often adequate for diagnosing mesothelioma. So long as an adequate tissue sample containing "diagnostic material" is obtained that can be studied by a variety of methods, a fairly accurate diagnosis is possible in a large percentage of cases.

The correct way of handling pleural tissue samples is determined to some degree by the clinical history of the patient being biopsied. It is important for the pathologist to communicate with the pulmonologist or surgeon who is performing the biopsy, to gain insight into the reason for doing the biopsy. For example, if the patient is thought to have an infectious pleuritis, a portion of the biopsy should be sent for culture. If the clinical diagnosis is cancer, then a portion of the specimen should be fixed in an electron microscopy fixative. In today's setting, most immunohistochemical tests can be performed on formalin-fixed, paraffin-embedded tissue, and no special fixation or processing is necessary. Ultrastructural evaluation also can be performed on formalin-fixed tissue, especially if the tissue is placed immediately into fixative.

Fine-needle aspiration biopsy specimens usually provide a small amount of tissue, which however can provide a great deal of information if appropriately handled. Most fine-needle aspiration biopsies are performed on masses thought to represent neoplasms. Small pieces of tissue obtained from such biopsies can be directly processed for electron microscopic examination or prepared as a cell block on which immunohistochemical analyses can be done. Rinses from the needle and the syringe can be directly put into fixative, centrifuged, and processed in a "Beem" capsule for electron microscopy.

Table 34–1. Causes of pleural effusion

Transudates
  Congestive heart failure
  Cirrhosis with ascites
  Nephrotic syndrome
  Hypoalbuminemia
  Peritoneal dialysis
  Atelectasis, acute
  Superior vena cava obstruction
  Subclavian catheter misplacement
  Early mediastinal malignancy
Exudates
  Parapneumonic effusion (bacterial pneumonia)
  Pulmonary infarction
  Malignancy (direct pleural involvement, late mediastinal
    involvement)
  Viral disease
  Connective tissue disease (lupus, rheumatoid, mixed)
  Tuberculosis
  Fungal disease
  Parasitic disease (*Entamoeba histolytica, Paragonimus westermani*)
  Gastrointestinal disease (pancreatitis, esophageal rupture,
    subphrenic abscess)
  Drug reaction (nitrofurantoin, methysergide)
  Asbestos
  Meigs' syndrome
  Postmyocardial infarction and postcardiac surgical operation
  Trapped lung
  Lymphatic abnormality
  Uremic pleurisy
  Atelectasis, chronic
  Chylothorax
  Sarcoidosis

Types and Causes of Pleural Effusions

Pleural effusions are frequently separated clinically into those that are transudates and exudates. Transudative pleural effusions are usually clear and straw colored, have a low protein concentration, and contain relatively few cells; in contrast, exudative pleural effusions have higher protein concentrations and usually numerous cells. Pleural fluid is sometimes described as serous (clear, straw-colored), sanguineous (bloody), or serosanguineous (slightly bloody but generally "thin"). Which tests should be performed on these samples, as for most clinical pathology specimens, depends on the clinical situation and the specific questions to be answered. The most common causes of pleural transudates and exudates are shown in Table 34–1. The causes and characteristics of pleural transudates are shown in Table 34–2; the most common cause is congestive heart failure. The causes and characteristics of pleural exudates are listed in Table 34–3. As shown, there are some overlapping features of both transudates and exudates, and it is sometimes the clinical history and knowledge of the patient that allow one to make a more specific diagnosis.

Nonspecific Pleural Changes

As previously stated, the pleura is an extremely reactive tissue, and it is perhaps not surprising that it undergoes a variety of nonspecific type changes. Pleural inflamma-

Table 34–2. Causes and characteristics of pleural transudates[a]

Disease	Clinical findings	Chest radiograph	Appearance	Cells/μl	Protein (g/dl)
Congestive heart failure	PND, orthopnea, rales, gallops, neck vein distension	Cardiomegaly, bilateral small–moderate PE of equal size	Serous	<1000 lymphocytes mesothelial	PF/S < 0.5 0.6–3.8
Cirrhosis	Stigmata of cirrhosis, clinical ascites	Normal heart size, small to massive right PE	Serous or hemorrhagic	<1000 lymphocytes mesothelial	PF/S < 0.5
Peritoneal dialysis	Renal failure, asymptomatic or acute dyspnea	Small bilateral PE, massive right PE	Resembles dialysate	<100 mononuclear	<1.0
Urinothorax	Urinary tract obstruction asymptomatic or acute dyspnea	Small–moderate PE, ipsilateral to obstructed kidney	Serous, odor of urine	<500 mononuclear	<1.0
Nephrotic syndrome	Edema	Bilateral PE of equal size frequently subpulmonic	Serous	<1000 mononuclear	<1.0
Atelectasis	Postoperative, lung cancer, mucous plug	Volume loss with small unilateral PE, lobar or complete lung collapse	Serous	<1500 mononuclear	PF/S < 0.5

[a] Abbreviations: PE, pleural effusion; PF/S, pleural fluid/serum; S, serum; PND, paroxysmal nocturnal dyspnea.

tion, increased vascularity, inflammation, and mild fibrosis are often associated with an underlying pneumonia or pulmonary infarct (Fig. 34–9). In a pulmonary infarct, there may be a relatively well-localized area of pleural reaction characterized by an increased vascularity, inflammation, and a layer of fibrin on the outer surface (Fig. 34–10). Mesothelial cell hypertrophy and hyperplasia (Fig. 34–11) are seen in almost all conditions that involve the lung parenchyma, such as idiopathic pulmonary fibrosis, asbestosis, and peripheral lung cancers, when that pulmonary condition is close to the pleural surface. Yokoi and Mark[13] reported on seven cases of primary carcinoma of the lung close to the pleural surface that were associated with atypical mesothelial cell hypertrophy and hyperplasia. In this author's experience this is a frequent finding, and not only hypertrophy and hyperplasia of the epithelial surface mesothelial cells, but sometimes proliferation of subserosal spindle cells, occur, by immunohistochemistry these subserosal cells express keratin, vimentin, and muscle-specific actin, and by electron microscopy have the ultrastructural features of myofibroblasts. Cases of idiopathic visceral pleural fibrosis have also been reported in which there is fibrous thickening of the visceral pleura, usually associated with varying degrees of inflammation.[14] Reactive eosinophilic pleuritis, a condition that may be confused with pulmonary eosinophilic granuloma, refers to an inflammatory process described in 1977 by Askin et al.[15] In their report, it was seen primarily in persons who had spontaneous pneumothoraces; specifically, in 22 of 57 cases. None of the patients had clinical or radiographic evidence of interstitial lung disease, and a follow-up of 20 patients from 6 months to 5 years showed no evidence of other conditions. Their paper was specifically written to distinguish that reaction from pulmonary eosinophilic granuloma, because the macrophages present associated with the eosinophils often had convoluted nuclei and the appearance of Langerhans' cells (see Chapter 17). This author has seen reactive eosinophilic pleuritis in all types of conditions, and believes that it is a relatively common and nonspecific reaction to injury. For reasons that are not clear, eosinophils are a common inflammatory cell in pleural disease and are seen in a variety of conditions.

Apical pleural fibrosis is seen in most cases of moderate to severe centrilobular emphysema, and is a relatively nonspecific fibrosis except that the fibrous tissue often has a more granular or less organized appearance than well-formed collagenous fibrosis (Fig. 34–12). Blebs that occur in the apical portion of the upper lobes as a result of emphysema also show nonspecific types of pleural reactions, with mesothelial hypertrophy and hyperplasia, submesothelial fibrosis, and varying degrees of inflammation (Fig. 34–13).

Infectious Pleuritis

Bacterial Infections

Bacterial-induced pneumonia often involves the peripheral portion of the lung and is characterized by a significant pleural neutrophil inflammatory infiltrate that initially may be associated with a sterile pleural effusion.[3] Approximately 60% of pneumococcal pneu-

Table 34–2. *Continued*

LDH (IU/liter)	Glucose (mg/dl)	pH	Other tests	Diagnosis	Comments
PF/S < 2/3 upper normal S 10–190	=S	7.45–7.55	—	Presumptive	Associated with pulmonary venous hypertension
PF/S < 2/3 upper normal S	=S	7.40–7.55	Radiolabeled tracer injected into ascitic fluid appears in chest	Presumptive, PF values similar to ascitic fluid	Incidence 6%, TCN pleurodesis effective if medical treatment fails
<100	300–400	>7.40	Radiolabeled tracer injected into ascitic fluid appears in chest	Protein <1.0 g/dl and glucose >300 mg/dl	Massive effusion usually occurs by 30 h after starting dialysis
<175	=S	7.0–8.0	CT scan	PF/S creatinine >1.0	Only cause of a low pH transudate, PF/S creatinine needs to be measured early
<100	=S	>7.40	—	Presumptive	30% have pulmonary embolism
PF/S < 2/3 upper normal S	=S	>7.40	—	Presumptive	Does not exclude curability in lung cancer

Table 34–3. Causes and characteristics of pleural exudates[a]
A.

Disease	Clinical findings	Chest radiograph	Appearance	Cells/μl	Protein (g/dl)
Parapneumonic effusion-uncomplicated	Pneumonia	Small–moderate ipsilateral, free-flowing PE	Turbid	10,000 PMNs	1.4–6.1
Parapneumonic effusion-complicated	Pneumonia	Moderate–large ipsilateral PE with tendency to loculation	Turbid or purulent	>20,000 (200–100,000) PMNs	>4.5
Tuberculosis	Acute or insidious cough, pleurisy, fever	Small–moderate unilateral PE pulmonary infiltrate (30%)	Serous	<5000 lymphocytes	>4.0
Actinomycosis	Chronic pneumonia, fever, cough	Consolidation unilateral PE and thickening, rib involvement	Serous or purulent	Moderate PMNs or lymphocytes	Exudate
Nocardiosis	Chronic pneumonia, fever, cough	Consolidation with cavitation, small–moderate PE	Serous or purulent	Moderate PMNs	Exudate
Aspergillosis	Remote pneumothorax therapy—cough, fever, weight loss, postop fever, purulent expectoration	Nodular pleural thickening, small–moderate PE, density lying free in pleural space postop-persistent air fluid level	Serous, serosanguinous, purulent, or black	Moderate lymphocytes mesothelials	Exudate
Blastomycosis	Chronic pneumonia, cough, fever, chest pain	Alveolar and interstitial infiltrates, pleural thickening, unilateral PE	Serous	180–3990 mononuclears or PMNs	4.2–6.6
Cryptococcosis	Chest pain, cough, fever; pneumonia vs. infarction	Peripheral alveolar infiltrate, small–massive unilateral PE	Serous or serosanguinous	Small–moderate lymphocytes	2.5–5.7

[a] Reprinted with permission from Sahn SA. The pleura. Am Rev Respir Dis 1988;138:184–234. Abbreviations: PE, pleural effusion; T/E, transudate or exudate; NHL, non-Hodgkin's lymphoma; PF/S, pleural fluid/serum; ILD, interstitial lung disease.

Table 34–3. *Continued*

B.

LDH (IU/liter)	Glucose (mg/dl)	pH	Other tests	Diagnosis	Comments
<700	=S	≥7.30	Blood culture	Presumptive	PE resolves without sequelae on appropriate antibiotics
>1000	<40	<7.10	Blood culture, CIE	Pus, + bacteriology ↓pH, ↓glucose and LDH	Requires chest tube drainage for resolution
<700	=S <60 (20%)	always <7.40 <7.30 (20%)	ADA, lysozyme promising	Presumptive-granuloma on pleural biopsy diagnostic-isolation of organism from PE or pleural tissue	Culture of pleural biopsy best diagnostic test with yield up to 80%
Exudate	—	—	—	Culture anaerobically from PE or sinus tracts	Sulfur granules can be identified in purulent fluid
Exudate	—	—	Sputum	Culture aerobically from PE, BAL or sputum	Steroids and alveolar proteinosis are predisposing factors
Exudate	—	—	Serum precipitins, antigens in PE	Culture from PE	Brown clumps of fungal hyphae suggest diagnosis, Ca oxalate crystals in PE suggest *A. niger* infection
>225	=S	≥7.30	Sputum	+PE smear, culture from PE, organism seen on pleural biopsy	Major pleural disease a poor prognostic sign
Exudate	=S	≥7.30	Antigen in PE	Culture from PE or pleural tissue, histology of pleural tissue	Normal host with localized pleuropulmonary disease can be observed

Table 34–3. Causes and characteristics of pleural exudates[a] (*continued*)
C.

Disease	Clinical findings	Chest radiograph	Appearance	Cells/μl	Protein (g/dl)
Coccidioidomycosis	Primary-fever pleurisy, cough; rupture of cavity—acute systemic toxicity or sub-acute chest pain, dyspnea	Unilateral moderate–large PE with infiltrate hydropneumothorax	Serous Turbid	1000–8000 lymphocytes PMNs	3.5–6.5
Histoplasmosis	Cough, fever, malaise, pleurisy	Subpleural infiltrate or nodule with small–moderate PE	Serous	Small–moderate lymphocytes eosinophilia	4.1–5.7
Paragonimiasis	Orientals—cough, fever, hemoptysis, isolated pleural disease; chronic asymptomatic PE	Diffuse infiltrates with unilateral small–massive PE	Turbid, white, yellow, or brown	<2000, eosinophilia	6.0–8.0
Amebiasis	Sympathetic effusion—insidious pleurisy, cough; rupture into pleural space—sudden chest pain, dyspnea, fever, cough	Small–moderate right PE elevated hemidiaphragm, plate-like atelectasis; large-massive right PE with contralateral mediastinal shift	Serous Brown pus	Moderate PMNs Moderate–large PMNs	
Echinococcosis	Acute chest pain, cough, fever, respiratory distress, shock	Moderate right PE, hydropneumothorax, elevated hemidiaphragm, RLL pneumonitis	Turbid	Moderate PMNs, eosinophils	Exudate
Viral	Acute chest pain following viral syndrome	Small unilateral PE with or without infiltrate, hilar adenopathy may be present	Serous	To 6,000 mononuclears	3.2–4.9
Mycoplasma	Cough, headache, myalgias	Small–moderate unilateral PE, lower lobe infiltrate	Serous	600–6,000 mononuclears	1.8–4.9
Legionellosis	Older, smoker, high fever, cough, CNS and GI symptoms	Unilobe alveolar infiltrate with progression, small–moderate unilateral PE	Turbid	Moderate PMNs	Exudate
Upper abdominal abscess	Fever, ↑WBC, upper abdominal pain, pleurisy in patient, postabdominal surgery	Elevated hemidiaphragm, small PE, gas within abscess cavity	Turbid	Moderate PMNs	Exudate
Hepatic abscess	Fever, chills, constitutional symptoms, RUQ pain in elderly with biliary tract disease or postop	Elevated hemidiaphragm, basilar infiltrates, abscess formation, small right PE	Turbid	Moderate PMNs	Exudate
Hepatitis	Hepatitis	Small right PE can be large and bilateral, no pulmonary infiltrates	Dark yellow	Few lymphocytes	3.0–5.0
Splenic abscess	Fever, abdominal pain, splenomegaly in patient with endocarditis	Small left PE, basilar infiltrates and atelectasis, contralateral mediastinal shift, elevated hemidiaphragm	Serous	Moderate PMNs	T/E
Esophageal perforation (spontaneous)	Severe retching or vomiting followed by chest pain and fever, subcutaneous air	Subcutaneous and mediastinal air, left pneumothorax early, left PE later	Early-serous Late-turbid, purulent	Moderate PMNs, Many PMNs	Exudate
Carcinoma	Dyspnea with exertion, cough, weight loss, appear chronically ill	Lung-unilateral moderate–large PE, primary lesion may be seen; extrathoracic primary-unilateral or bilateral moderate–large PE without other evidence of metastases	Serous-lymphatic obstruction; bloody-pleural invasion	2500–4000 lymphocytes, macrophages, mesothelials	4.0 (1.5–8.0)

Table 34–3. *Continued*

D.

LDH (IU/liter)	Glucose (mg/dl)	pH	Other tests	Diagnosis	Comments
Exudate	=S	≥7.30	CF titers	Culture from PE and pleural tissue, spherules in pleural tissue	Culture of pleural tissue has highest diagnostic yield; culture of PE usually positive
200–425	=S	≥7.30	CF titers	Culture from PE or pleural tissue, organism seen in pleural tissue	Treatment not necessary for acute histoplasma PE
>1000	<10	<7.10	CF titers, ova in sputum or stool	Ova in PE	With isolated pleural disease ova in PE only
Exudate	—	—	Serology, CT scan	Presumptive organism in PE, typical brownish pleural aspirate	Uncomplicated amebic empyema responds to early tube thoracotomy
Exudate	—	—	Casoni skin test, CF titers	Identification of scolices in PE or in pleural tissue	Requires emergency thoracotomy
Exudate	=S	≥7.30	Serology	Presumptive	May not have parenchymal infiltrates
Exudate	=S	≥7.30	Culture of sputum or pharyngeal secretions, serology	Presumptive	PE resolves in days-wk
Exudate	=S	≥7.30	Serology DFA and culture from sputum	Culture from PE	PE resolves with infiltrate on erythromycin
Exudate	>60	>7.20	CT scan, aspiration and culture of abscess	Presumptive	Drainage is definitive treatment, sterile PE resolves as abscess treated
Exudate	>60	>7.20	CT scan, aspiration and culture of abscess	Presumptive	Drainage is definitive treatment, sterile PE resolves with drainage of abscess
Exudate	=S	≥7.30	HBeAg, HBsAg, HBV	Presumptive	PE potentially infectious, resolves prior to resolution of hepatitis
T/E	=S	≥7.30	CT scan	Presumptive	Treatment is antibiotics and splenectomy
Exudate	=S	≥7.30 <7.30	Esophagram	pH 6.00, ↑amylase	With early diagnosis, prognosis good with primary closure
300, exudate by LDH only suggests malignancy	=S <60 (30%)	≥7.30 6.95–7.29 (30%)	CT scan, bronchoscopy, other biopsies	Cytology, pleural biopsy	Lung and breast most common, primaries, pleural fluid pH has prognostic and therapeutic implications

Table 34–3. Causes and characteristics of pleural exudates[a] (*continued*)
E.

Disease	Clinical findings	Chest radiograph	Appearance	Cells/μl	Protein (g/dl)
Lymphoma	Dyspnea with exertion, cough	Unilateral moderate–large PE without other findings	Serous	Few lymphocytes	Exudate
Mesothelioma	Males 6th–9th decade, asbestos exposure, chest pain, dyspnea with exertion	Large unilateral PE, absence of contralateral mediastinal shift, nodularity of pleura	Serous, bloody, viscous	<5000 (few 100–20,000) mononuclears	3.5–5.5
Rheumatoid pleurisy	Males 6th decade, moderate–severe arthritis, subcutaneous nodules, develop PE within 5 yr of onset of disease, chest pain or asymptomatic	Small–moderate unilateral PE, other evidence of rheumatoid lung (30%)	Turbid, yellow-green, debris	Few 100–15,000 acute-PMNs chronic-lymphocytes	Exudate to 7.3
Lupus pleuritis	Known lupus, pleuritic pain, pleural rub, fever, cough, dyspnea	Small–moderate bilateral PE, may have cardiomegaly, alveolar infiltrates or atelectasis	Serous, bloody	5000 (few 100–20,000) PMNs or mononuclears	Exudate
Postcardiac injury syndrome	Pleuritic pain, pericardial rub, fever, dyspnea, rales 3 weeks following pericardial injury	Left sided or bilateral small–moderate PE, left lower lobe pulmonary infiltrates	Serosanguinous, bloody	9500 (500–39,000) PMNs or mononuclears	3.7 (3.0–4.5)
Sarcoidosis	Stage 2 or 3 disease, chest pain or asymptomatic	Hilar adenopathy, interstitial disease, small–moderate unilateral PE	Serous, turbid, serosanguinous	100–7000 >90% lymphocytes	Exudate
Immunoblastic lymphadenopathy	Constitutional symptoms, diffuse lymph-adenopathy, hepatosplenomegaly	Bilateral interstitial infiltrates and mediastinal or hilar adenopathy, bilateral small–moderate PE	Serous	Few lymphocytes	Exudate
Pulmonary embolism	Pleuritic chest pain, tachypnea, rales, fever	Unilateral small–moderate PE, pulmonary infiltrate	Bloody or serous	100–50,000 PMNs or lymphocytes	Exudate, transudate (20%)
Pancreatitis	Acute abdominal pain, nausea, vomiting, fever	Unilateral, left-sided small PE (60%), right (30%), bilateral (10%), atelectasis	Turbid	1000–50,000 PMNs	Exudate
Pancreatic pseudocyst	Dyspnea, chest pain, cough, history of pancreatitis or alcoholism	Large–massive left PE without parenchymal infiltrates, may be right or bilateral	Serous, serosanguinous	Few to moderate mononuclears	Exudate
Asbestos pleural effusion	Asbestos exposure, asymptomatic (70%) chest pain	Small unilateral PE, pleural plaques (10%)	Serosanguinous	500–6000, PMNs mononuclears eosinophilia	4.7–7.5
Uremic pleural effusion	Uremia >1 year, fever, chest pain, cough, pleural rub	Unilateral moderate PE	Serosanguinous, bloody	80–3700 lymphocytes	2.1–6.7
Trapped lung	Remote history of pneumonia, hemo or pneumothorax asymptomatic	Unilateral small–moderate PE	Serous	Few mononuclears	T/E

Table 34–3. *Continued*

F.

LDH (IU/liter)	Glucose (mg/dl)	pH	Other tests	Diagnosis	Comments
Exudate	=S <60 (20%)	≥7.30 <7.30 (20%)	CT scan, lymph node biopsy	Cytology, pleural biopsy	Diagnosis more readily made by cytology or pleural biopsy in NHL than Hodgkin's; presence of PE poor prognostic sign
36->600	<60 (70%)	<7.30 (70%)	High levels of hyaluronic acid in PE supports Dx	Examination of tissue obtained at thoracoscopy or thoracotomy	Prognosis related to stage of disease at diagnosis and histologic variant
Frequently >1000	Initially <30 (67%) <50 (80%)	7.00 (80%)	Low complement; ↑ immune complexes in PE	Glucose, <30, pH 7.00, LDH >1000, RF ≥1:320	PE resolves over several months but may be recurrent and lead to trapped lung
Exudate	=S <60 (20%)	≥7.30 <7.30 (20%)	Low complement; ↑ immune complexes and ANA ≥1:160 in PE	LE cells in PE	Good response to steroids with resolution by 2 wk
202	>60	≥7.30	—	Presumptive	PE resolves in 1–3 wk spontaneously or with steroids
Exudate	=S	≥7.30	↑T lymphocytes with predominance of helper cells	Dx of exclusion; noncaseating granulomas on pleural biopsy, negative for fungi and AFB	PE resolves spontaneously or with steroids
Exudate	=S	≥7.30	Lymph node biopsy	Presumptive	Impaired lymphatic drainage or lymphocytic pleural infiltration most likely mechanisms
Exudate, transudate (20%)	=S	≥7.30	Lung scan, angiogram	Presumptive	PE apparent on admission, reaches maximum volume by 72 h
Exudate	=S	7.30–7.35	↑Serum amylase	PF/S amylase > 1.0	PE resolves as pancreatitis resolves
Exudate	=S	≥7.30	Ultrasound, CT may show pseudocyst and fistula	Amylase in PE, may be >100,000	Recurs rapidly following thoracentesis, surgery necessary for PE refractory to conservative Rx
Exudate	=S	≥7.30	—	Presumptive	PE resolves in 3–4 months, frequently is recurrent, diffuse pleural thickening may occur years after initial PE
102–770	=S	≥7.30	PF/S creatinine < 1.0	Presumptive	PE usually resolves over weeks with continued dialysis
T/E	=S	≥7.30	Pleural liquid pressure measurement	Presumptive	PE reaccumulates rapidly after thoracentesis, asymptomatic patient requires no RX

Table 34–3. Causes and characteristics of pleural exudates[a] (*continued*)
G.

Disease	Clinical findings	Chest radiograph	Appearance	Cells/μl	Protein (g/dl)
Meigs' syndrome	Postmenopausal, ascites and PE, chronic illness, dyspnea	Small–massive right PE	Serous	Few mononuclears	Exudate
Chylothorax	Dyspnea with exertion symptoms of underlying disease, most commonly lymphoma	Large unilateral PE without parenchymal disease	Milky, may be bloody, turbid or serous	2000–20,000 lymphocytes	Exudate
Lymphangio-myomatosis	Women of reproductive age, dyspnea, pneumothorax, chylothorax, hemoptysis	Interstitial lung disease with normal or increased lung volumes, chylothorax (75%), pneumothorax (40%)	Milky	2000–20,000 lymphocytes	Exudate
Yellow nail syndrome	40-year-old with yellow nails, lymphedema and respiratory tract involvement	Small–massive unilateral or bilateral PE	Serous	<1000 lymphocytes	>4.0
Radiation pleuritis	Pleuritic pain or asymptomatic PE from 2–6 months following >4000 rads, radiation pneumonitis	Small unilateral PE with loculations, radiation pneumonitis	Serosanguinous	Reactive mesothelials	Exudate
Endoscopic esophageal sclerotherapy	Chest pain following sclerotherapy, large sclerosant volume	Small unilateral (R or L) or bilateral PE within 48–72 h of procedure	Serosanguinous	100–38,000 PMNs, mononuclears	1.10–4.80
Dantrolene	Pleuritic pain and fever 2 months to 3 yr after beginning drug	Unilateral small PE without pulmonary infiltrates	Serosanguinous	Moderate eosinophils (36–66%)	Exudate
Methysergide	Recurrent chest pain, dyspnea, fever, pleural rub 1 month to 6 yr after drug started	Bilateral loculated PE	Serous, serosanguinous	<1000 mononuclears	Exudate
Amiodarone	Dyspnea, cough, constitutional symptoms, pleuritic pain, pleural rub after ingesting >100 g	Peripheral alveolar or interstitial infiltrates, pleural thickening, unilateral or bilateral small–massive PE	Serous, serosanguinous	<1000 macrophages, lymphocytes	2.8–3.7

Table 34–3. *Continued*
H.

LDH (IU/liter)	Glucose (mg/dl)	pH	Other tests	Diagnosis	Comments
Exudate	=S	≥7.30	CT scan, laparoscopy	Presumptive	Removal of ovarian neoplasm results in resolution of PE
Exudate	=S	>7.40	CT scan	Chylomicrons, triglycerides >110 mg/dl	Major complications malnutrition, immunologic compromise, radiation effective in lymphoma
Exudate	=S	>7.40	PFTs, lung biopsy	Chylothorax in women of childbearing age with ILD and normal lung volumes	Treatment symptomatic anecdotes with successful hormonal manipulation
>200	=S	7.40	—	Presumptive	Triad seldom appears simultaneously, chemical pleurodesis effective
Exudate	=S	7.40	—	Presumptive	PE persists for at least 4 months, may remain constant for years
77–1368	>100	≥7.30	—	Presumptive	Requires no specific therapy, resolves over days to weeks
Exudate	=S	≥7.30	Blood eosinophilia	Presumptive	Symptoms abate within days of stopping drug, CXR lags
Exudate	51 (one case)	—	—	Presumptive	Symptoms resolve quickly when drug stopped, CXR takes months to resolve and may not clear
128 (one case)	=S	7.43 (one case)	—	Presumptive	Pleural fluid macrophages containing foamy cytoplasm may be diagnostic

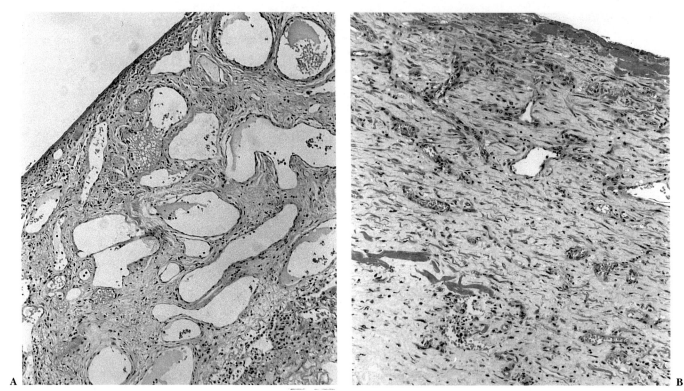

Fig. 34–9 A,B. Sections of visceral pleura show nonspecific increase in vascularity with mild inflammation and focal fibrin deposition. ×125.

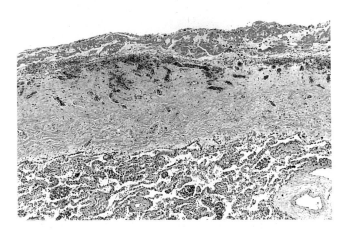

◁

Fig. 34–10. Pleura overlying wedge-shaped pulmonary infarct shows nonspecific increased vascularity, inflammation, fibrosis, and fibrin on outer surface, change referred to as fibrinous pleuritis. ×75.

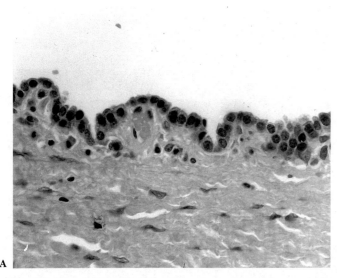

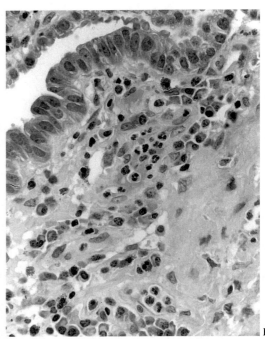

Fig. 34–11 A,B. Mesothelial cell hypertrophy and hyperplasia are nonspecific reactions seen in various conditions affecting underlying lung parenchyma. Sometimes cells show mild atypia. ×550.

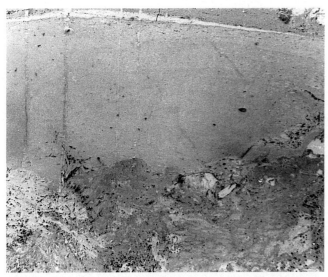

Fig. 34–12. This region of apical pleural fibrosis, sometimes referred to as apical pleural cap, is composed of more granular, less organized fibrous tissue. ×125.

monia cases and 40% of all bacterial-caused pneumonias are associated with an exudative pleural effusion.[16,17] If the condition is not treated, the bacteria can invade into and through the pleura, resulting in exudative pleural effusion and empyema (Fig. 34–14). The bacteria frequently activate the clotting system, causing a somewhat gelatinous type of pleural fluid that can serve as a lattice for organization and proliferation of fibroblasts. The most common causes of empyema in

North America are anaerobic bacteria, either alone or in concert with aerobic bacteria.[18,19] Gram-negative aerobes and *Staphylococcus aureus* are the next most frequent cause of empyema. The diagnosis of empyema should be made as rapidly as possible so that it can be adequately treated by drainage and antibiotic therapy as well as the instillation of streptokinase into the pleural fluid. Decortication of an organized empyema (Fig. 34–15) is sometimes necessary to control the pleural infection.

Tuberculous Pleuritis

Tuberculous pleuritis is a relatively infrequent condition in North America, with an incidence of about 1,100 cases per year.[20] Pleural effusion is commonly associated with this infection, and usually is serous or serosanguineous in nature, with a protein content greater than 4 g/dl. Tuberculous pleuritis occurs when a focus of tuberculosis below the visceral pleura ruptures into the pleural space.[21,22] These infections may be accompanied by a granulomatous inflammatory reaction, which occasionally can be identified by a closed pleural biopsy (Fig. 34–16).

Fungal Pleuritis

Primary fungal pleuritis is an uncommon condition, and in this author's experience is seen predominantly in people with a variety of malignant neoplasms (often lymphoma or leukemia) treated with chemotherapeutic

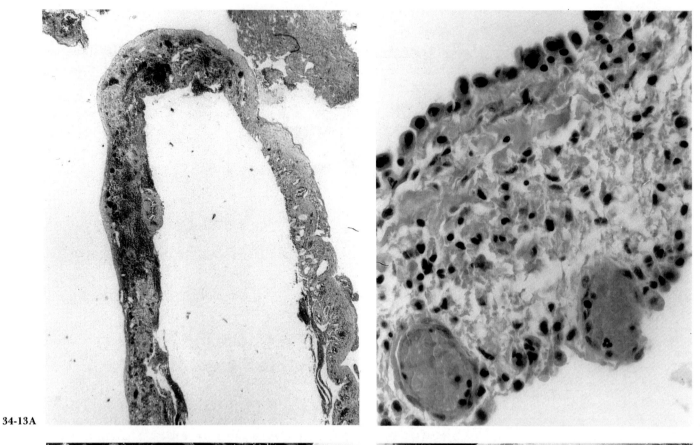

34-13A

34-13B

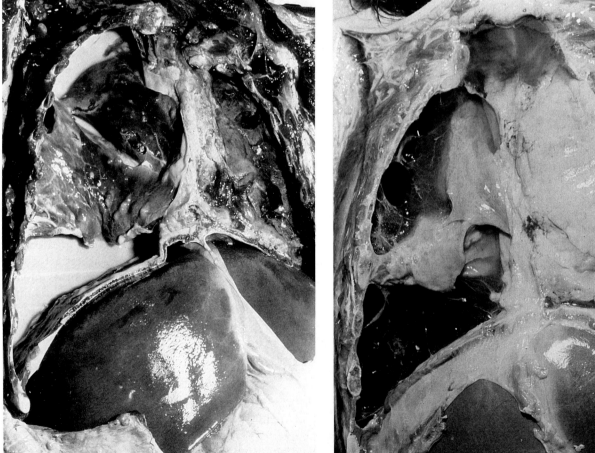

34-14A

34-14B

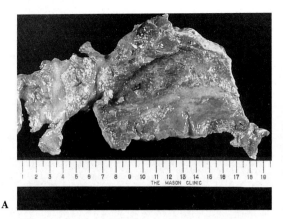

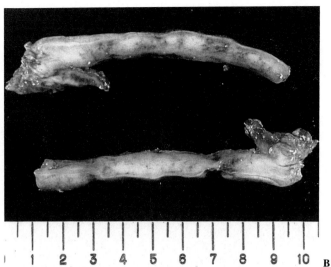

Fig. 34–15 A,B. Organized empyema produced 5- to 10-mm rind of moderately firm, greyish-white fibroinflammatory tissue. **A.** Flat surface of specimen. **B.** Cross section of decortication specimen.

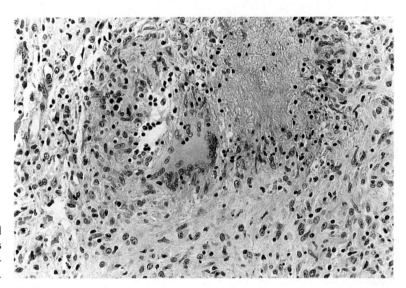

Fig. 34–16. Representative region from closed pleural biopsy shows necrotizing granulomatous inflammation. Acid-fast organisms were identified by Ziehl–Neelsen stain and by culture. ×330.

agents. It has also been described following lobectomy or pneumonectomy for tuberculosis or lung cancer, usually in association with a bronchopleural fistula.[3] Pathologically there are varying degrees of necrosis and inflammation, and the organisms are usually fairly easy to see, especially if they are large, like *Aspergillus* (Fig.

◁━━━━━━━━━━━━━━━━━━━━━━━━━━━━━━━━

Fig. 34–13 A,B. Apical pleural blebs resected from patient with centrilobular emphysema and pneumothorax are composed of fibroinflammatory-type tissue and often have layer of hypertrophied mesothelial cells on outer surface. **A,** ×25; **B,** ×550.

Fig. 34–14 A,B. Suppurative pleuritis with empyema is relatively rarely seen. **A.** Note pus in right pleural cavities. Cultures were positive for *Staphlococcus aureus*. **B.** coagulum covers left lung.

34–17). Most of the common fungi can be associated with pleuritis, and sometimes uncommon fungal organisms cause infection.[23]

Other Infectious Causes of Pleural Effusion and Pleuritis

A variety of other organisms occasionally infect the pleural fluid and cause pleuritis.[3] These include infections with *Entamoeba histolytica*, *Echinococcus granulosus*, *Mycoplasma pneumoniae*, *Coxiella burnetti*, *Legionella pneumophila*, *Actinomyces israelii*, *Nocardia asteroides*, *Pneumocystis*, and viruses such as adenovirus.[24] These infections are rare, and usually are not seen by pathologists in pleural biopsy specimens. As listed in Table 34–3, some of these infections produce changes in the pleural fluid that assist in their diagnosis.

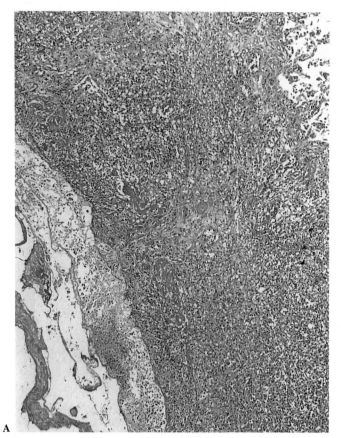

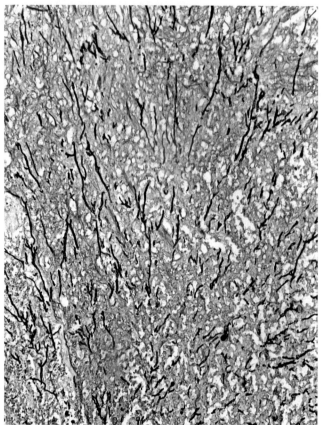

Fig. 34–17 A,B. Autopsy tissue section from patient with lymphoma who had been aggressively treated for lymphoma. In this case, *Aspergillus* infection was primarily in pleural distribution, sparing lung parenchyma. **A.** Note extensive acute pleural inflammation and necrosis. Organisms are difficult to see in H and E-stained sections but are readily seen in methenamine silver-stained sections **(B). A,** ×75; **B,** ×125.

Table 34–4. Drugs that may cause pleural disease

Nitrofurantoin
Dantrolene
Methysergide
Procarbazine
Methotrexate
Bromocriptine
Practolol
Amiodarone
Mitomycin
Bleomycin
Minoxidil

Drug-Induced Pleural Disease

Compared to the number of drugs that affect the lung parenchyma (see Chapter 23), relatively few cause changes in the pleura and/or a pleural effusion (Table 34–4).[3] In most instances biopsy specimens are not obtained from these patients, and only pleural fluid may be available for examination. In most cases these drugs also cause parenchymal lung disease, although some, such as methysergide, may cause severe visceral-parietal pleural fibrosis and chronic inflammation.

A variety of drugs, such as procainamide, Hydralazine, isoniazid, phenytoin, chlorpromazine, and quinidine, cause a lupus syndrome. Occasionally methyldopa, tetracycline, and penicillin produce a similar syndrome. These drugs often induce a pleural effusion and may be associated with a nonspecific, usually chronic type of pleuritis with pleural thickening. Methysergide (Sansert) is perhaps the drug most frequently recognized to cause a pleuropulmonary reaction. In the case seen by this author, the visceral-parietal pleura was markedly fibrotic and showed mild chronic inflammation (Fig. 34–18). Amiodarone has been reported to cause a pleural effusion that has some fairly characteristic features (see Chapter 23). The pleural toxicity caused by amiodarone appears to be dose related, and discontinuation of the drug and/or corticosteroid therapy usually results in resolution of the symptoms and/or pleural effusion.

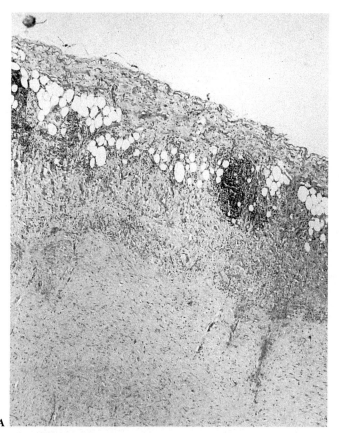

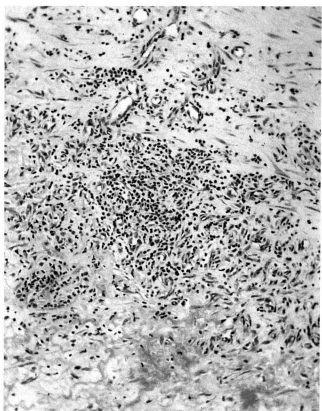

Fig. 34–18 A,B. Open pleural biopsy specimen from patient treated with Methysergide for several years. Visceral pleura was 2–3 mm thick and composed of relatively dense fibrous tissue, with sprinkling of chronic inflammation. **A,** ×75; **B,** ×330.

"Immunologic"-Associated Pleural Disease

Collagen Vascular-Induced Pleural Disease

Rheumatoid arthritis is associated with the highest incidence of pleural involvement of all the collagen vascular diseases.[25–27] Rheumatoid pleuritis is stated to occur in approximately 5% of patients with rheumatoid disease,[27,28] and may be associated with visceral-pleural fibrosis, rheumatoid nodules involving the visceral pleura (Fig. 34–19), or, occasionally, fibrosis and inflammation of the visceral and parietal layers of the pleura with adhesions. Autopsy studies suggest that pleural involvement in rheumatoid disease approaches 50%, although most patients are apparently asymptomatic. In contrast to the overall incidence of rheumatoid arthritis, symptomatic rheumatoid lung disease is more common in men than women, and that holds true for rheumatoid pleuritis as well. The typical patient who develops rheumatoid pleuritis is a male in the sixth decade with a pleural effusion within 5 years after the onset of rheumatoid disease. In most instances, patients with rheumatoid pleuritis have a high rheumatoid factor titer, and this antibody is usually present in the pleural fluid. The most striking consistent feature of rheumatoid pleural effusions are low pleural fluid glucose, low pH, and high LDH.

Involvement of the pleura in patients with systemic lupus erythematosus occurs to some degree in 50%–75% of patients diagnosed with lupus, and may be the presenting manifestation in as many as 5% of patients.[3] The changes in the pleura are nonspecific, and can consist of acute and chronic inflammation and fibrosis (Fig. 34–20). In most instances, the pleuritis is associated with an exacerbation of the basic disease. In contrast to the pleural fluid in rheumatoid pleuritis, in lupus pleuritis the pleural fluid glucose and pH are usually within normal limits. One can identify LE cells in the pleural fluid, although other serologic studies, such as DNA binding and extractable nuclear antigen (ENA) titers, will help clarify or prove the diagnosis of systemic lupus erythematosus.

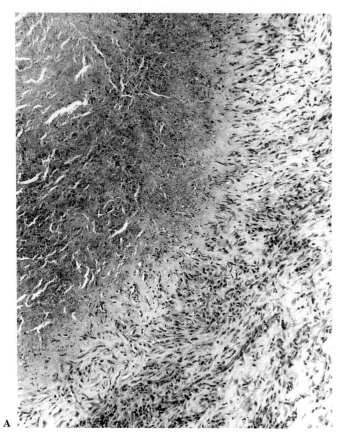

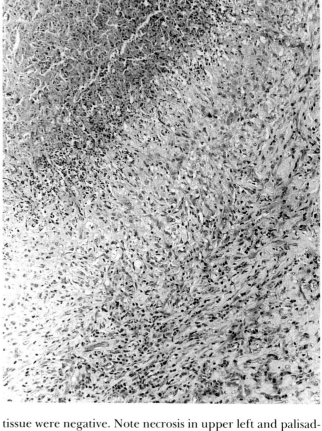

Fig. 34–19 A,B. Open lung-pleural biopsy shows necrotizing granulomatous process consistent with rheumatoid nodule. Patient had rheumatoid arthritis; cultures and special stains of tissue were negative. Note necrosis in upper left and palisading of inflammatory cells. **A** and **B,** ×125.

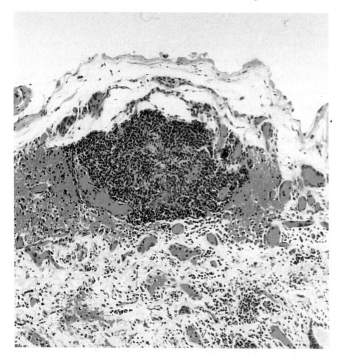

Fig. 34–20. Nonspecific chronic pleuritis in 35-year-old woman with systemic lupus erythematosus. ×125.

Sarcoidosis

Sarcoidosis is generally thought of as a nonnecrotizing granulomatous disease involving the lymph nodes and pulmonary parenchyma. Not infrequently, however, sarcoid can involve the pleura (Fig. 34–21), and in one retrospective study of more than 200 patients with biopsy-proven sarcoidosis, 10% had radiographic evidence of pleural thickening or effusion and 7% had evidence of pleural effusion.[29] Most patients with pleural involvement by sarcoid have at least radiographic stage II disease (See Chapter 19). The pleural fluid may be a transudate or an exudate, and often has an increased number of lymphocytes, specifically helper-inducer (CD4-positive) lymphocytes.

Wegener's Granulomatosis

As discussed in Chapter 29, Wegener's granulomatosis is characterized by a necrotizing granulomatous inflammatory process, typically involving the lungs, and also frequently involving the kidneys and other organ systems. As described by Mark et al.,[30] the basic pathogen-

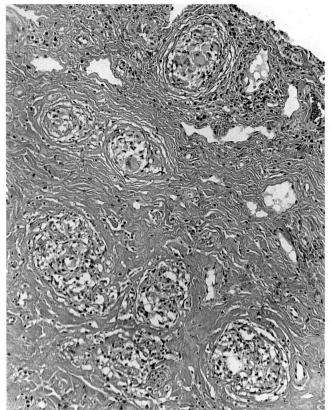

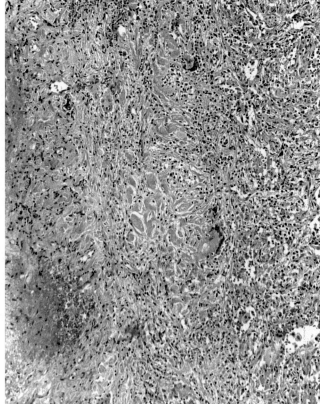

Fig. 34–22. This region of Wegener's granulomatosis shows a thickened visceral pleura due to fibrosis and a mixed inflammatory cell infiltrate. Note the multinucleated histiocytic giant cells. ×125.

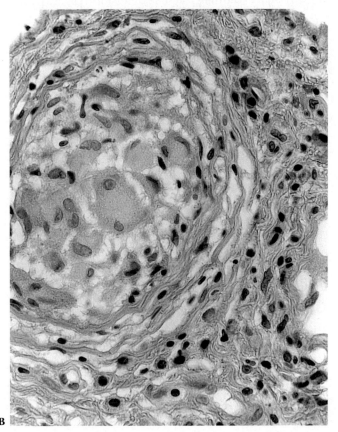

esis may be related to regions of necrobiosis of collagen that incite the inflammatory reaction. If these areas of necrosis and inflammation occur close to or in the pleural surface, one would expect an inflammatory reaction to be located in that region (Fig. 34–22). In some series,[31] pleural effusion has been observed in as many as 55% of cases, although in most instances the incidence is much less than that. The characteristic features of the pleural fluid in Wegener's granulomatosis have not been fully defined.

Post-Cardiac Injury Syndrome

Pleural pericarditis and parenchymal pulmonary infiltrates, occurring approximately 3 weeks following injury to the myocardium or pericardium, is referred to as

⟵————————————————————

Fig. 34–21 A,B. Open lung-pleural biopsy from patient with chest radiographic changes suggesting sarcoidosis. Note nonnecrotizing granulomata involving pleura. **A,** ×125; **B,** ×550.

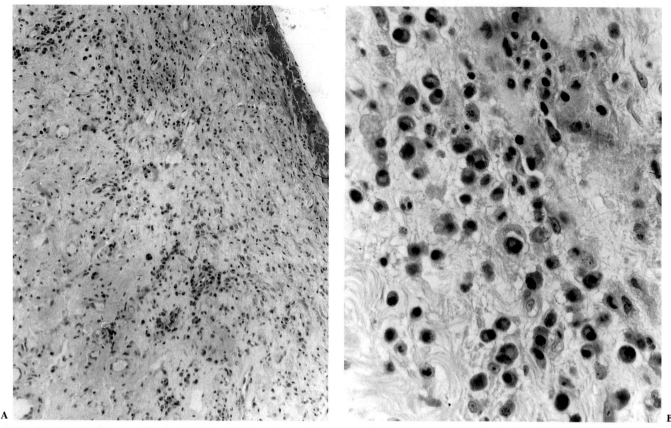

Fig. 34–23 A,B. Nonspecific chronic pleuritis in patient with post-cardiac injury syndrome. Most inflammatory cells are plasma cells. **A,** ×125; **B,** ×550.

the post-cardiac injury syndrome and is characterized by the onset of fever with the pleuropericarditis. The incidence of this syndrome varies approximately between less than 1% and 15%,[32,33] and is thought to be related to an immunologic reaction characterized by antibodies to myocardial tissue.[34,35] The pleuropulmonary manifestations are the most significant in this syndrome, and most patients present with pleuritic chest pain. Pleural fluid is characteristically a serosanguineous or bloody exudate, and may result in a chronic pleural thickening with varying degrees of inflammation (Fig. 34–23).

Hemothorax

Hemothorax refers to the presence of blood within the pleural cavity. It is occasionally seen as an almost invariably fatal complication of a ruptured thoracic aortic aneurysm or a traumatic rupture of the aorta. A moderate amount of blood causing a bloody pleural effusion can also be seen in other conditions, such as asbestos-induced pleural disease, tuberculosis, and a variety of neoplasms such as mesothelioma and primary lung

cancers invading the pleura. The pathologic features of these conditions will depend on the specific etiology.

Chylothorax

Chylothorax refers to an accumulation of milky fluid within the pleural cavity that has the features of lymph fluid, containing a high concentration of emulsified fats. Chylothorax occurs when the contents of the thoracic duct empty into the pleural cavity. Chylothorax can be bilateral, although is more commonly seen on the left side. It is most commonly associated with various malignancies arising within the thoracic cavity, most commonly lymphomas that cause obstruction of the major lymphatic ducts. Occasionally chylothorax can result from traumatic rupture of the thoracic; duct. It also is associated with lymphangioleiomyomatosis.

Pneumothorax

Pneumothorax refers to the presence of air or gas in the pleural cavities, and may be spontaneous, traumatic, or therapeutic. Spontaneous pneumothoraces are caused by abnormalities of the parenchyma that allow the escape of air into the pleural cavity. These may be caused by blebs associated with centrilobular emphysema, by an abscess cavity that communicates with the pleural space, or occasionally by asthma, which results in areas of overexpansion of the lung parenchyma that then ruptures.

Therapeutic pneumothorax was once commonly used to treat tuberculosis. Pneumothoraces occasionally occur during fine-needle aspiration biopsy attempts, and when inserting various catheters into the subclavian vein. Spontaneous idiopathic pneumothorax characteristically affects young persons, and usually occurs in the absence of any demonstrable pulmonary pathologic abnormality. Recurrent attacks are frequent and disabling, and often require surgical intervention to "roughen" the pleural surface with the hope of causing scarring and preventing further air leaks.

Pleural Neoplasms

In contrast to primary lung neoplasms, pleural neoplasms are uncommon. Pleural tumors are frequently associated with a pleural effusion; they may be difficult to diagnose and must be distinguished from primary or metastatic carcinomas involving the pleura and from benign reactive processes causing pleural thickening. A correct diagnosis is important so that appropriate therapy, although it may be only palliative, can be instituted. The most common and most important primary pleural neoplasm is mesothelioma, which has gained notoriety in recent years because of its etiologic relationship to asbestos exposure. Other neoplasms such as soft tissue sarcomas, leukemia-lymphoma, and metastatic carcinoma may also involve the pleura and must be differentiated from mesotheliomas. This part of Chapter 34 discusses pleural neoplasms, with the primary emphasis on mesotheliomas.

Mesothelioma

Definitions, History, and Incidence

Mesotheliomas are tumors derived from the serosal lining of the pleural, pericardial, and peritoneal cavities. They exhibit a wide variety of histologic patterns and may be confused with many other types of neoplasms. In years past, standard pathologic "doctrine" taught that the diagnosis of mesothelioma is a diagnosis of exclusion that can only be certain at postmortem examination. It is the author's opinion that immunohistochemical and ultrastructural analysis of pleural neo-

plasms can lead to an accurate diagnosis of mesothelioma and nonmesotheliomatous neoplasms in most cases.

Mesotheliomas are rare tumors, accounting for less than 1% of all cancer deaths in the world.[36] Two pleural tumors, possibly representing mesotheliomas, as noted by Chahinian[37] were described by Joseph Lieutaud in 1767 in a study of 3,000 autopsies. E. Wagner[38] recognized mesotheliomas as a pathologic entity in 1870. In 1924, Robertson[39] in an article entitled "Endothelioma" of the pleura, gave a thorough account of the early reports on the clinical and pathologic features of pleural neoplasms. He concluded that only sarcomas could be classified as primary malignant pleural tumors and that all epithelial-appearing neoplasms were metastases from an unrecognized or latent primary site. In 1931, Klemperer and Rabin[40] described five primary pleural neoplasms; four were localized and had mesenchymal features and one was diffuse, encasing the lung with a mixed epithelial and mesenchymal histologic appearance. Klemperer and Rabin divided primary tumors of the pleura into localized and diffuse forms, indicating that the localized tumors originated from the subpleural "aerolar" tissue, were low-grade malignancies, usually caused death by interference with the pulmonary circulation, and were potentially curable by surgical removal. They concluded that diffuse neoplasms of the pleura arose from the mesothelial cells lining the serosal surface and could exhibit an epithelial or mesenchymal histologic pattern.

Most cases of mesothelioma reported between 1940 and 1960 were localized.[41,42] in 1960 Wagner et al.[43] reported 33 cases of diffuse pleural mesothelioma in North Western Cape Province of South Africa. Of these 33 patients, 32 had a history of exposure to asbestos. Dr. Wagner recently recounted his experience with the discovery of mesotheliomas in South Africa.[44,45] A photograph of the initial case is shown in the preface of the book by Henderson et al. In 1965 Selikoff and colleagues[46] presented further evidence linking mesotheliomas to asbestos exposure by finding that 10 of 307 consecutive deaths in asbestos insulation workers were caused by diffuse mesothelioma. These two landmark reports were preceded by a report in 1943 by Wedler[47] of a diffuse mesothelioma in a person with asbestos exposure. Wedler[48] and Merewether[49] referred to tumors of the pleura in discussing cases of lung carcinoma in patients with asbestosis. It is possible that these neoplasms referred to as "tumors of the pleura" represented mesotheliomas. The first U.S. report of a diffuse mesothelioma with asbestos exposure was in 1947.[50] A pleural and a peritoneal mesothelioma associated with asbestosis were reported in the German literature in 1953 and 1954[51,52] and in 1960, Keal[53]

Table 34–5. Incidence of mesotheliomas[a]

Reference	Years surveyed	Location of population surveyed	Number of cases/million population/year
McDonald et al.[58]	1959–mid-1968	Canada	0.65 (males)
			0.35 (females)
Thériault and Grand-Bois[59]	1969–1972	Quebec	1.56 (males)
			0.74 (females)
Biava et al.[60]		Italy	21.4 (males)
Greenberg and Lloyd-Davies[61]	1967–1968	England, Wales Scotland	1.88 (males)
			0.42 (females)
McDonald and McDonald[62]	1960–1975	Canada	2.8 (males)
	1972	United States	0.7 (females)
Cutler and Young[63]	1969–1971	Metropolitan areas[b]	1.5 (males)
			0.7 (females)
Bruckman et al.[64]	1970–1972	Connecticut (United States)	1.7 (males)
			0.9 (females)
Churg[65]	1982	British Columbia	17 (males)
			1.9 (females)
McDonald and McDonald[67]	1950–1970	Eight cities	0.24% of 69,302 autopsies

[a] Incidence includes both pleural and peritoneal mesotheliomas, and in some instances mesotheliomas arising in ovary and male genital system.
[b] Atlanta, Birmingham, Dallas-Ft. Worth, Detroit, Pittsburgh, San Francisco-Oakland, Denver (United States).

reported the association of peritoneal mesotheliomas and asbestos exposure. Most mesotheliomas reported since 1970 have been diffuse; the localized form is rare.[54]

The history of the medical and legal aspects of asbestos-related lung disease was dicussed in detail by Motley[55] and Broudeur.[56,57] Information presented by these authors suggested that serious deleterious health effects of asbestos were known long before they were reported in the medical literature.

Because mesotheliomas are rare neoplasms, their exact incidence is unknown and varies among populations surveyed (Table 34–5). In 1970, McDonald et al.[58] reported a rate of 0.65 cases in men and 0.35 cases in women per million population per year in Canada. An incidence of 1.56 cases in men and 0.74 cases in women per million population per year were reported by Theriault and Grand-Bois[59] in Quebec, Canada, between 1969 and 1972. In Trieste, Italy, a shipbuilding city, Biava et al.[60] reported an incidence of 21.4 cases per million population per year in men. Greenberg and Lloyd-Davies[61] reported 1.88 cases in men and 0.42 cases in women per million population per year in England between 1967 and 1968. McDonald and McDonald[62] reported 2.8 cases in men and 0.7 cases in women per million population per year in North America between 1960 and 1972. An incidence of 1.5 cases in men and 0.76 cases in women per million population per year were reported between 1969 and 1971 by the Third National Cancer Survey[63] of seven metropolitan areas with a total population of 21 million. The Con-

necticut Tumor Registry[64] reported an annual mesothelioma incidence of 1.7 cases in men and 0.7 cases in women per million population per year between 1970 and 1972. Churg[65] reported a malignant mesothelioma rate of 17 cases in men and 1.9 cases in women per million population per year in British Columbia, Canada in 1982. The highest incidence in the world is currently in Australia, presumably a result of asbestos exposure at Wittenoon mine.[66]

The incidence of mesothelioma in autopsy series is considerably lower; McDonald and McDonald[67] summarized the incidence in six series from eight cities between 1950 and 1970. They tabulated 165 cases in 69,302 autopsies, an incidence of 0.24%.

Several studies[62,64,65] have documented an apparent increase incidence of malignant mesothelioma, especially in men, during the last several years. Hughes and Weill[68] estimated that 1,500 new cases of mesothelioma were diagnosed in the United States in 1986. The increased incidence of mesothelioma is probably related to the delayed effects of an increase in occupational exposure to asbestos. Selikoff et al.[46] reported that 10 of 307 deaths in asbestos insulation workers were caused by mesothelioma and that 8% of 17,800 workers in heat and frost insulation followed prospectively between January 1, 1967 and December 31, 1976 died of diffuse malignant mesothelioma.[69] As reviewed by Huncharek,[70] the incidence of mesothelioma is increasing at a rate of about 10% per year for U.S. males.

The author's experience has also suggested an increased incidence of mesothelioma that in part may

Table 34–6. Association of exposure to asbestos and incidence of mesothelioma

Reference	Number of cases	Sex distribution Male	Female	Cases associated with asbestos exposure Male	Female
Borrow et al.[74]	72	64	8	55/55 (100%)	5/5 (100%)
Cochrane and Webster[75]	70	70[a]		60/70[a] (99%)	
Tagnon et al.[76]	61	61	0	45/56 (80%)	
Whitwell and Rawcliffe[77]	52	40	12	35/40 (87.5%)	8/12 (67%)
Hammar et al.[78]	151	119	32	66/82 (80%)	10/22 (45%)
Taylor and Johnson[79]	30	23	7	17/23 (74%)	0/7 (0%)
Vogelzang et al.[80]	31	22	9	13/22 (60%)	2/9 (22%)
Newhouse and Thompson[81]	83	41	42	24/41 (59%)	17/42 (40%)
Peto et al.[82]	116	116	0	69/116 (59%)	
McDonald and McDonald[62]	557	395	162	188/344 (55%)	8/162 (5%)
Roggli et al.[83]	25	21	4	11/21 (52%)	0/4 (0%)
Oels et al.[84]	37	32	5	10/32 (31%)	0/5 (0%)
Brenner et al.[85]	123	84	39	16/84 (19%)	0/39 (0%)
Ratzer et al.[86]	31	21	10	4/31[a] (13%)	

[a] Gender not specified.

reflect an increased awareness by pathologists of this disease and of more accurate diagnostic methods such as electron microscopy and immunohistochemistry. Further, many or perhaps most cases of mesothelioma in the United States come to litigation, which has made the general public much more aware of this disease and in turn has caused heightened physician awareness.

Etiology

The association of asbestos exposure and the development of mesothelioma has been reviewed in detail.[71–73] Asbestos is the single most important causative agent of mesotheliomas. Numerous reports[74–86] have tabulated the percentage of mesothelioma cases associated with asbestos exposure (Table 34–6). The association between asbestos exposure and mesothelioma is greater in men than in women, and in many of the series very few women with mesothelioma have had a history of exposure to asbestos. The threshold amount of asbestos necessary to induce mesothelioma is unknown although in many reports[87,88] a dose–response relationship has been suggested; persons with a greater intensity and duration of exposure to asbestos have a higher incidence of mesothelioma. Small concentrations of asbestos may induce mesothelioma,[89,90] although positive proof of low-concentration-asbestos causation of mesothelioma is lacking because most adults in urban populations contain asbestos in their lungs.

Malignant mesothelioma can occur via household exposure to asbestos.[91] Vianna and Polan[92] reported a relative risk of 10 for such situations compared to matched controls unexposed to asbestos. Kane et al.[93] reported 10 cases of malignant mesothelioma in pa-

tients 40 years old or younger. In 7 of the 10 cases there was asbestos exposure, 2 occupational exposures and 5 household exposures. Cazzadori, et al.[94] reported a case of malignant pleural mesothelioma in a 37-year-old woman exposed to asbestos during childhood. From birth to age 10 she lived in a house next to an asbestos processing factory. Asbestos exposure was confirmed by finding 0.3 asbestos bodies/ml in her bronchoalveolar lavage fluid. Huncharek[70] pointed out that exposure to asbestos was no longer confined to asbestos industry workers and that there were nonoccupational hazards such as household and building occupant exposures. Dodoli et al.[95] reviewed death certificates of 39,650 persons between 1975 and 1988 in Leghorn and in 45,900 persons in La Spezia (Italy) between 1958 and 1988. A total of 262 cases of pleural mesothelioma were recorded, most of which occurred in persons occupationally exposed to asbestos in the shipbuilding industry. Thirteen cases of mesothelioma occurred in women who washed the asbestos-contaminated workclothes of their relatives, and 6 cases occurred in persons domestically exposed to asbestos, possibly from installing fireproof or nonconductive materials.

The exact mechanism whereby asbestos causes mesotheliomas is unknown. Stanton and Wrench,[96] Stanton et al.,[97] and Gross[98] have suggested that the physical characteristics of asbestos are more importat than its chemical characteristics in the causation of mesothelioma. Fibers that were long and thin, generally greater than 8 μm long and less than 0.25 μm wide with a length-to-width (aspect) ratio greater than 32 were found to be more tumorigenic than shorter and thicker fibers. However, in a study of asbestos fiber number and size from 10 patients with amphibole fiber-caused malignant pleural mesothelioma, Churg and Wiggs[99]

Table 34–7. Relationship of mesothelioma to type of asbestos

Reference	Type of asbestos exposed to	Setting of exposure	Total numbers of persons followed	Total number of deaths	Deaths due to mesothelioma	Percent of deaths due to mesothelioma
Weiss[100]	Chrysotile	Manufacturing plant	266	66	0	0
McDonald et al.[101]	Chrysotile ore	Mine	11,379	4,547	11	0.24
McDonald and Fry[102]	Factory A—Chrysotile	A—Asbestos textiles	A—3,747	A&B—2,341	A&B—1	A&B—0.04
	Factory B—Chrysotile	B—Textiles and friction products	B—4,959			
	Factory C—Crocidolite, amosite and Chrysotile	C—Asbestos textiles	C—5,175	C—1,429	C—18	C—1.26
Acheson et al.[103]	Leyland—Crocidolite	Gas masks	Leyland—757	Leyland—219	Leyland—5	Leyland—2.28
	Blackburn—Chrysotile	Manufacturing	Black.—570	Black.—177	Black.—1	Black.—0.56
Dement et al.[104]	Chrysotile	Asbestos textiles	1,261	308	1	0.32
Browne and Smither[105]	Factory A—Crocidolite, amosite and chrysotile	A—Asbestos textiles, insulation, friction products	A—10,000	A—Not given	A—120	
	Factory B—Crocidolite, amosite and chrysotile	B—Asbestos textiles and insulation	B—2,000	B—Not given	B—13	
	Factory C—Chrysotile and crocidolite	C—Asbestos insulation	C—6,000	C—Not given	C—4	
	Factory D—Amosite	D—Asbestos insulation	D—1,500	D—Not given	D—0	
	Factory E—Chrysotile	E—Asbestos textiles and friction products	E—15,000	E—Not given	E—0	
Berry and Newhouse[106]	Chrysotile Crocidolite—2 periods	Asbestos friction materials	13,460	1,638	8 (Occurred in those using crocidolite)	0.49

suggested that short wide amphibole fibers were also capable of inducing mesotheliomas.

Several studies[100–107] comparing the capacity of various types of asbestos to induce mesotheliomas have suggested that the commercial amphiboles, crocidolite and amosite, are more tumorgenic than chrysotile (Table 34–7).

In 1977, Weiss[100] reported on 264 men who worked in a chrysotile asbestos manufacturing plant producing asbestos papers and millboard, bound with starch or sometimes Portland cement. A total of 66 deaths were noted over a 30-year period, and none were caused by mesothelioma. McDonald et al.[101] obtained information on 11,379 persons who worked for at least a month in the mines and mills of Asbestos and Thetford Mines in Quebec and documented 11 deaths from mesotheliomas in a total of 4,547 deaths (0.24%). McDonald and

Fry[102] examined the incidence of mesothelioma in 13,881 persons who worked in three asbestos manufacturing plants in the United States, two of which used only chrysotile asbestos and one using crocidolite, amosite, and chrysotile. Of the 2,341 deaths that occurred in the two chrysotile plants, only 1 (0.04%) was caused by mesothelioma whereas 18 (1.26%) were reported in the plant that used crocidolite and amosite as well as some chrysotile. Acheson et al.[103] studied the number of deaths from mesotheliomas in two plants that manufactured gas masks during World War II. The plant that used chrysotile asbestos in the gas masks recorded only 1 death of 177 (0.56%) caused by mesothelioma whereas the plant employing crocidolite asbestos had 5 out of 219 (2.28%) deaths caused by mesothelioma. Dement et al.[104] reported 1 death in 308 (0.32%) recorded in 1,261 persons working in a

Table 34–8. Different mineral fibers and their various properties and their risks of causing mesothelioma, as found in epidemiologic studies[a]

Fiber	Risk of mesothelioma	Length–diameter ratio	Durability in biological tissue	Human exposure
Fibrous zeolite (erionite)	Very high	Very high	Very good	Only environmental
Amphiliboles				
Crocidolite	Very high	Very high	Very good	Occupational and environmental
Amosite	Fairly high	High, but lower than crocidolite	Good	Occupational
Tremolite	Probably high	As amosite	Good	Environmental
Anthophyllite	None	Fairly low	Good	Environmental (formerly occupational)
Serpentine				
Chrysotile	Low	Most fibers very short	Poorer than other asbestos	Occupational
Glass fibers	None	Low	Probably poor	Occupational

[a] Reprinted with permission from Hillerdal G, Br J Dis Chest 1983;77:321–343.

chrysotile textile manufacturing plant. Browne and Smither[105] in studying factors discriminating between pleural and peritoneal mesothelioma, found 120 cases of mesothelioma in 10,000 workers employed at an asbestos manufacturing plant extensively using crocidolite whereas no cases of mesothelioma were found in 15,000 workers employed in the plant that had only used chrysotile since its existence in 1902. Finally, Berry and Newhouse[106] reported 11 of 1638 (0.67%) deaths from mesothelioma in an asbestos plant manufacturing friction materials that had used primarily chrysotile except during two periods, 1929–1933 and 1939–1944, when crocidolite was specified in a contract for railroad blocks. Eight of the 11 workers who developed mesothelioma had been exposed to crocidolite. Two had been employed outside of the plant most of their lives and their mesothelioma could not be attributed to chrysotile. The other worker with mesothelioma had been intermittently exposed to crocidolite.

Churg et al.[108] examined the role of chrysotile in causing mesotheliomas by examining asbestos content of lung tissue from six long-term chrysotile miners and millers who had pleural mesotheliomas. The lung tissue from the mesothelioma patients contained both chrysotile and tremolite (also amosite in one patient), and the ratio of tremolite in lung tissue from patients with mesothelioma compared to lung tissue from control cases was 9.3 while the ratio of chrysotile in mesothelioma cases versus controls was only 2.8. Churg et al. concluded that chrysotile mine dust that contained both chrysotile and tremolite was capable of causing mesotheliomas in humans, but it was not clear whether chrysotile or the contaminating tremolite was responsible for inducing the mesotheliomas.

Despite this evidence that chrysotile seldom causes malignant mesotheliomas, cases of malignant-mesothelioma have been reported in which the only asbestos exposure was to chrysotile.[109,110] This author has seen 5 cases of malignant pleural mesothelioma in brake/clutch mechanics whose only known exposure was to chrysotile asbestos. More important was the report by Begin et al.,[111] who reviewed all cases of pleural mesothelioma seen and accepted by the Quebec Workmen's Compensation Board for related compensation of industrial disease. They identified 120 cases of pleural mesothelioma and divided the cases into three groups according to workplace asbestos exposure. Forty-nine cases originated in the mines and mills of the Quebec Eastern Township region, 50 cases from the manufacture and industrial application sector, and 21 cases from industries where asbestos was used as an incidental material. In the mining towns of Thetford and Asbestos, the incidence of mesothelioma was proportional to the workforce, suggesting that tremolite air contamination, which was 7.5 times higher in Thetford, was not a significant determinant in causing malignant mesothelioma. The incidence of mesothelioma in the chrysotile miners and millers was 62.5 cases per million population per year between 1980 and 1990, significantly above the rate found in the North American population, which was estimated to be between 2.5 to 15 cases per million in adult males. Begin et al.[111] concluded there was a significantly increased incidence of malignant mesothelioma in chrysotile miners and millers and that tremolite contamination was not a determining factor in causing mesothelioma in chrysotile workers. As discussed in Chapter 28, the issue of chrysotile toxicity is unsettled.

The proposed tumorigenicity of various types of asbestos and other fibers is summarized in Table 34–8, taken from the review article of Hillerdal.[112] In 1984 Peterson et al.[113] reviewed the nonasbestos causes of mesothelioma. This author has performed an extensive computer search of nonasbestos causes of mesothelioma and cannot find epidemiologic reports to support the nonasbestos etiologies of mesothelioma suggested by Peterson et al.[113] Potentially, malignant mesothelioma can develop at the site of pleural injury caused by almost any agent. Of particular interest has been a group of naturally occurring fibrous silicate minerals called zeolites. In 1975 and subsequent years, Baris and colleagues[114–118] reported that people living in Tuskoy and Karam, two small villages in central Turkey, had the highest incidence of mesothelioma in the world. In Karam, 21 of 50 deaths recorded in people over 20 years old during a 5-year period were caused by mesothelioma. People living in this region of Turkey were found to have very fine fibers of a zeolite called erionite in their sputum and lung tissue; these were not found in similar specimens of people living in other areas of Turkey. A search for asbestos in soil, rock, and water samples was negative, and it was hypothesized that airborne erionite fibers from building materials caused the mesotheliomas. Lillis[119] substantiated the findings of Baris et al.[114,115]; Sebastien and coworkers[120] demonstrated that 93% of ferruginous bodies from lung samples of two patients with malignant mesothelioma from Tuskoy were formed on erionite cores; and Wagner et al.[121] induced mesotheliomas in 38 of 40 rats innoculated with erionite. Rohl et al.,[122] however, were able to identify small amounts of tremolite and chrysotile in addition to erionite in environmental samples taken from Tuskoy and Karain. They also reported that erionite was found in environmental samples taken from villages with no reported cases of mesothelioma.

In 1985, Hillerdal and Berg[123] reported 2 patients who developed mesothelioma in regions of pleural scarring caused by tuberculosis that had been treated with intrapleural pneumothorax. They also reviewed the literature and found 20 additional cases of malignant tumors in pleural scars, 12 of which were squamous carcinomas. They indicated that squamous carcinoma was most common in scarring from chronic empyema and extrapleural pneumothorax.

Austin et al.[124] reported a malignant pleural mesothelioma in a 28-year-old woman who had a Wilm's tumor at age 4 that had been treated with nephrectomy followed by irradiation. The mesothelioma developed in the left pleural cavity, the same side as the Wilm's tumor. Austin et al. discussed the possibility of the tremor being related to irradiation and reviewed data from eight patients who developed mesothelioma and whom had received external irradiation. This case is of further interest because they performed asbestos analysis on the autopsy lung tissue and found the asbestos content to be within their "normal range" (0–20 asbestos bodies/gram of wet lung tissue). Anderson et al.[125] also reported a diffuse epithelial mesothelioma in a 16-year-old boy who at age 2 had received pulmonary irradiation for metastatic Wilm's tumor.

In 1985 Talerman et al.[126] reported a case of a diffuse malignant peritoneal mesothelioma in a 13-year-old girl and reviewed the literature identifying 41 previously reported cases of mesothelioma in children. Thirty-three of the 41 previously reported cases began in the pleura and 40 of the 41 children died 2 weeks to 21 months after diagnosis, a clinical course similar to that in adults. In many of the reported cases of mesothelioma in children a history of exposure to asbestos was not documented, although in their case and in 2 others reviewed there was no history of exposure to asbestos. Fraire et al.[127] independently reviewed slides available in 17 children previously diagnosed as having mesothelioma. Upon review, only 3 of these cases were confirmed as mesothelioma, and they concluded that mesothelioma in children may be rarer than suspected. Fraire et al.[128] conducted an extended evaluation of mesothelioma in childhood in 80 reported cases. Of the 80 cases, tissue slides were available for review in 22 cases, of which 10 were considered malignant mesothelioma, 9 nonmesothelial malignant tumors, and 3 malignant neoplasms of uncertain type. The authors found no relationship between childhood malignant mesothelioma and asbestos, radiation, or isoniazid. Lin-Chu et al.[129] reported a case of malignant mesothelioma in a 19-month-old female infant, the diagnosis confirmed by histochemistry and immunohistochemistry. In their review of the literature they found 3 other cases of malignant mesothelioma in infants. In their case, there was no information concerning exposure to asbestos.

Hereditary factors are considered potentially important in the development of mesothelioma. In 1985 Lynch et al.[130] described the occurrence of epithelial mesotheliomas in two brothers who had been exposed to asbestos, and reviewed the literature citing three other reports of familial mesothelioma. Ten of 11 family members in the four families reported had a definite history of exposure to asbestos. In 1984 Martensson et al.[131] reported two pairs of siblings, a brother and sister and two identical twin brothers, who developed malignant pleural mesotheliomas. Both pairs of siblings had an exposure to asbestos. We reported three brothers who had an asbestos insulation business; two developed mesotheliomas that arose in the pleura and the other brother had mesothelioma involving only the abdominal cavity.[132]

In our experience,[78] approximately 20% of men and 55% of women diagnosed as having pleural mesotheliomas give no history of exposure to asbestos or other potentially causative agents and no history of previous pleural injury.

Moalli et al.[133] have recently hypothesized that with respect to asbestos, repeated episodes of injury and regeneration of the pleura promote the development of

PROPOSED MECHANISM OF ASBESTOS CARCINOGENESIS

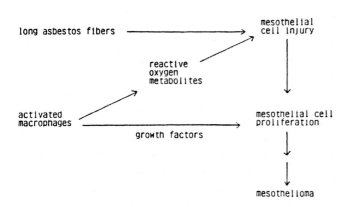

Fig. 34–24 Reprinted with permission from Maolli PA, Macdonald JL, Goodglick LA, Kane AB. Acute injury and regeneration of the mesothelium in response to asbestos fibers. Am J Pathol 1987;128:426–445.

mesotheliomas (Fig. 34–24). Adamson et al.[133a] studied the effect of intratracheal injection of crocidolite asbestos (long fibers, >20 μm) and chrysotile asbestos (short fibers, <1 μm) on DNA synthesis of pleural mesothelial cells in mice. They found up to 2% of pleural mesothelial cells showed DNA synthesis after long fiber (crocidolite) injection, and approximately 0.2% labeling of pleural mesothelial cells after short fiber (chrysotile) injection. Despite the increased proliferative activity of surface mesothelial cells and submesothelial spindle cells induced by long fiber asbestos, no asbestos fibers were identified morphologically in the pleural tissue. Adamson et al.[133a] suggested that asbestos-induced cytokines from activated interstitial macrophages diffuse across the interstitium and cause proliferation of mesothelial cells, which may be important in the generation of mesotheliomas and subpleural fibrosis. Although this mechanism of pleural injury is plausible, several reports demonstrating the presence of all type of commercial asbestos in human pleural tissue seemed to be ignored by these investigators. Also, the longest time from intratracheal injection of asbestos to sacrifice of the animals studied by the authors was only 16 weeks.

As reviewed by Muscat and Wynder,[134] there is no evidence that cigarette smoking is a factor in the development of malignant mesothelioma.

Mineralogy of Malignant Mesothelioma

Roggli et al.[135] determined asbestos body content of lung tissue from 25 cases of malignant mesothelioma

(19 pleural, 6 peritoneal) and compared the findings to the content of asbestos bodies in lung tissue from 50 consecutive adult autopsies and 4 cases of overt asbestosis. The 19 patients with pleural mesothelioma had between 29,700 and less than 1 asbestos body per gram of wet lung tissue. Nine patients with pleural mesothelioma had less than 20 asbestos bodies per gram of wet lung tissue, which was the upper limit seen in the general population with no occupational exposure to asbestos. The 6 patients with peritoneal mesothelioma had between 380 and less than 1 asbestos body per gram wet lung tissue, with 4 having 3.5, 1.2, and less than 1 (2 patients) asbestos bodies per gram wet lung tissue. As would be expected, the four patients with asbestosis had the highest concentration, ranging between 1,200 and 30,900 asbestos bodies per gram wet lung tissue. As determined by energy-dispersive x-ray analysis, 88 of 90 asbestos bodies analyzed had an amphibole core (amosite or crocidolite in 80/88 cases and anthophyllite or tremolite in 8/88 cases) with 2 asbestos bodies being formed on chrysotile cores. The malignant mesothelioma patients had an average lung asbestos body count intermediate between the patients with asbestosis, and the general population. The authors reviewed the literature concerning lung asbestos concentration in patients with malignant mesotheliomas and suggested hypotheses to explain the occurrence of malignant mesothelioma in the patients with no history of occupational exposure to asbestos and low (<20 asbestos bodies/g wet lung tissue) asbestos body counts: (1) There is no threshold level of asbestos exposure below which mesthelioma will not occur, and thus a certain small percentage of susceptible individuals will develop malignant mesothelioma in a society in which there is ubiquitous asbestos contamination of the environment. (2) Those individuals with low pulmonary asbestos body counts had undetected occupational or environmental exposure to submicroscopic asbestos fibrils or to chrysotile fibers, which do not readily form asbestos bodies. While there is evidence to suggest this is not the case, additional data are needed before this question can be answered with certainty. (3) Factors other than asbestos are responsible for causing malignant mesothelioma. As previously described, a handful of cases of malignant mesothelioma have been described in persons whose pleura was injured by agents other than asbestos. (4) Asbestos acts synergistically with other agents to produce mesothelioma, thus requiring a lower concentration of asbestos.

Tuomi et al.[136] evaluated lung asbestos fiber concentration from 23 patients (21 males and 2 females) with malignant mesothelioma diagnosed at the Helsinki University Central Hospital between January 1985 and December 1988. The patients with mesothelioma were interviewed personally concerning their work history, potential past occupational, domestic, and environmental exposure to asbestos, smoking history, injuries, and history of radiotherapy to the thorax. Occupational exposure to asbestos was classified into four categories: (1) definite exposure, group I: (2) probable exposure, group II; (3) possible exposure, group III; and (4) unlikely or unknown exposure, group IV. Of the 23 patients with malignant mesothelioma, 2 (9%) were placed in group I, 7 (30%) in group II, 6 (26%) in group III, and 8 (35%) in group IV. The concentrations of asbestos fibers in the patients with malignant mesothelioma ranged from 100,000 to 370 million fibers per gram of dry lung tissue. The highest concentrations were in the 2 group I patients (>100 million/g of dry lung tissue). Asbestos fibers consisting of amosite, crocidolite, athophyllite, and tremolite were found in 21 of 23 patients. In 1 patient no asbestos fibers were found, and in the other patient only silicate fibers were identified. Lung fiber burden of asbestos correlated relatively well with the work history of the patients. The authors had previously determined that a concentration of asbestos fibers more than 1 million per gram of dry lung tissue indicated occupational exposure. In group III patients (possible asbestos exposure), 3 of 6 (50%) had lung asbestos concentrations greater than 1 million fibers per gram of dry lung tissue, and in group IV patients (unlikely or unknown exposure to asbestos), 3 of 8 (38%) had greater than 1 million fibers per gram of dry lung tissue. The authors indicated that these three group IV cases emphasized caution when judging that a person has been occupationally exposed to asbestos. Based on the criteria that there was at least a possible history of occupational exposure to asbestos, or an asbestos fiber concentration of more than 1 million fibers per gram of dry lung tissue, 78% (18/23) of patients with mesothelioma had been exposed to asbestos at work. The authors stated their opinion that the causal significance of low concentrations of asbestos could not be evaluated for individual cases of mesothelioma although for medicolegal purposes such cases should be regarded as exposed to asbestos, because a positive history indicating exposure to asbestos could not be overruled by a "negative" lung fiber analysis.

Leigh et al.[137] performed long asbestos fiber analysis of lung tissue by analytical transmission electron microscopy and energy-dispersive x-ray analysis on 226 cases of malignant mesothelioma. The histologic type of these mesotheliomas was determined by a five-member expert panel of pathologists. The authors found a statistically significant trend between lung fiber content per gram of dry lung tissue from epithelial (low fiber content) through mixed to sarcomatous (high fiber content). Higher lung fiber content was found in peri-

toneal versus pleural mesotheliomas. The authors concluded that their findings were consistent with the hypothesis that there was progressive malignant change of mesothelial cells from an epithelial, through mixed, to sarcomatous neoplasm and that change was dose dependent. They further concluded that after an initial dose of asbestos had initiated the neoplastic change, continued exposure to asbestos further promoted de-differentiation of the tumor cells. The authors data also confirmed the findings of others, namely that epithelial mesotheliomas have a longer survival time than mixed or sarcomatous mesotheliomas. In their study, epithelial mesotheliomas had a median survival of 9 months, mixed mesotheliomas 7 months, and sarcomatous mesotheliomas 3.5 months.

Roggli et al.[137a] determined the types of asbestos fibers recovered from lung tissue in 94 patients diagnosed in the United States with malignant mesothelioma. Approximately one half of the patients were former asbestos insulators or shipyard workers. Amosite was identified in 81% of the cases, and represented 58% of all fibers 5 μm or greater in length. Tremolite, actinolite, and anthophyllite were found in 55% of cases and accounted for 10% of all fiber types. Chrysotile was found in 21% of the cases and comprised 3% of fibers exceeding 5 μm in length Crocidolite was found in only 16% of cases and accounted for 3% of fibers greater than 5 μm long. Roggli et al.[137a] concluded that to assert that crocidolite asbestos was the cause of most mesotheliomas in the United States was incorrect. Based on their data, they ranked asbestos fibers in terms of their relative importance in causing malignant mesothelioma in the United States as follows:

amosite > tremolite > chrysotile = crocidolite

Histologic Classification

The histologic classification of mesotheliomas is shown in Table 34–9. We do not recognize a benign epithelial

Table 34–9. Histologic classification of mesothelioma

Epithelial
  Tubulopapillary
  Epithelioid
  Glandular
  Large cell—giant cell
  Small cell
  Adenoid-cystic
  Signet ring
Sarcomatoid (fibrous, sarcomatous, mesenchymal)
Mixed epithelial-sarcomatoid (biphasic)
Transitional
Desmoplastic
Localized fibrous tumor of the pleura

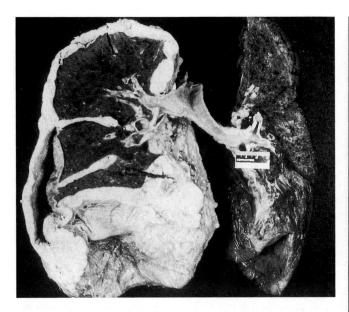

Fig. 34–25. Right lung is encased by thick rind of grayish-white tumor. Gross appearance characteristic of mesothelioma.

Fig. 34–26. Pleuropneumonectomy specimen. Lung was inflated via mainstem bronchus with formalin, fixed overnight, and then sectioned at 1-cm intervals from top to bottom. Note variable thickness of tumor and occasional space between visceral and parietal pleura.

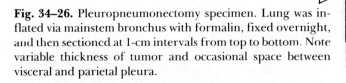

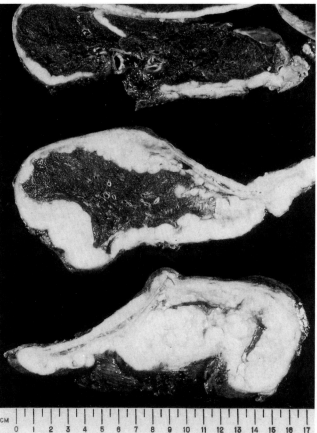

mesothelioma. As previously illustrated the pleura is a tissue capable of marked reactive proliferation, and in our opinion lesions classified as benign epithelial mesotheliomas represent hyperplasias rather than neoplasia. We do recognize a type of diffuse malignant mesothelioma that we believe is best classified as a "transitional" mesothelioma in that it has histologic features that are neither classically epithelial nor mesenchymal but between these two histologic patterns. Transitional mesotheliomas can be related to what we have termed the multipotential subserosal cell (see **Histogenesis**). The term "localized fibrous mesothelioma" has been replaced by "localized fibrous tumor of pleura."

Pathologic Features

Macroscopic Features

Diffuse malignant mesotheliomas of any histologic category grow by direct extension with encasement and infiltration of the lung (Fig. 34–25). It is difficult to determine if mesotheliomas begin in the visceral or parietal pleura, but frequently a space separates the involved pleural surfaces (Fig. 34–26). With time, most mesotheliomas invade the mediastinum, frequently encasing the trachea, esophagus, and great vessels (Fig. 34–27). They commonly invade the parietal and visceral pericardium and can encase the heart (Figs. 34–28 and 34–29). Mesotheliomas often directly invade into the pulmonary parenchyma, producing nodular masses (Figs. 34–30 and 34–31). This sometimes causes a nodular appearance on chest radiograph, occasionally even suggesting a primary tumor. Some epithelial mesotheliomas produce massive amounts of hyaluronic acid and form cystic spaces in the tumor and in the lung tissue where they invade (Fig. 34–32). These mesotheliomas can be described as "slimy."

Localized fibrous tumors of pleura are characteristically well demarcated and encapsulated masses that bulge into the pleural space (Fig. 34–33). They are composed of firm grayish-white fibrous tissue (Fig. 34–34).

Mesotheliomas do metastasize, most commonly to pulmonary parenchyma and bronchopulmonary-hilar and mediastinal lymph nodes, although sometimes it is impossible to determine whether involvement of these nodes resulted from metastasis or direct extension.

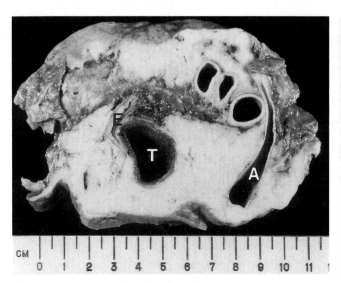

Fig. 34–27. Cross section through mediastinal structures shows encasement of trachea (T), esohagus (E), aorta (A), and vessels arising from arch of aorta near tumor.

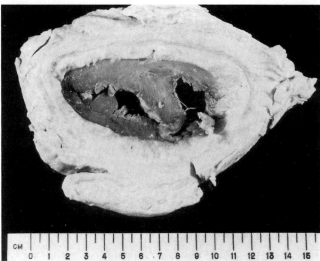

Fig. 34–28. Mesothelioma has directly invaded visceral and parietal pericardium, obliterating pericardial space and encasing heart.

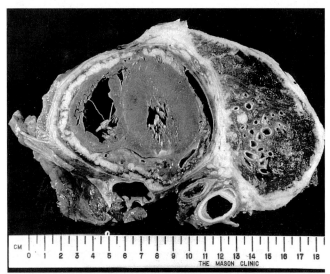

34-29

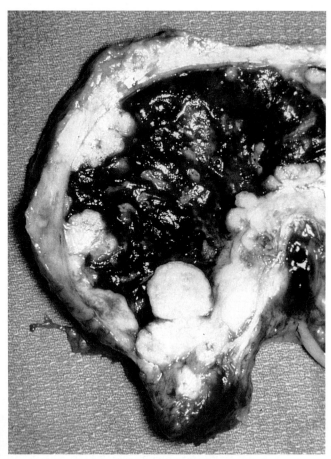

34-31

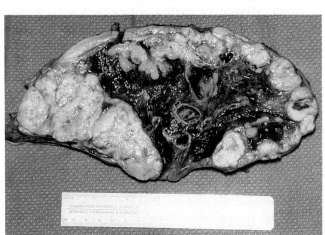

34-30

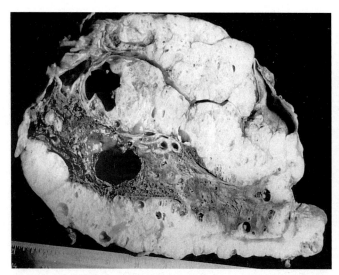

Fig. 34–32. Pleural mesothelioma was largest this author has ever seen, weighing approximately 5000 g and measuring 28 × 25 × 18 cm. Tumor was slimy and contained cystic spaces filled with gelatinous slimy material, representing hyaluronic acid; it compressed lung tissue and invaded into lung, with cystic lakes of hyaluronic acid in lung. (Photograph courtesy of J. Conrad Metcalf.)

Frequently, metastases to other more distant sites such as the adrenal gland occur (Fig. 34–35).

Most diffuse pleural mesotheliomas are associated with hyaline pleural plaques that involve the lateral and diaphragmatic parietal pleura (Fig. 34–36). Although these are often obscured on the side involved by tumor, in the "early" stages of some mesotheliomas they can be associated with nodular excrescences of tumor (Fig. 34–37).

Histologic Features

Mesotheliomas show a wide variety of histologic patterns and can resemble several other types of malignant neoplasms[138–142] (Table 34–9). In our opinion, immu-

◁—————————————————————

Fig. 34–29. Sagittal section through upper portion of left-upper lobe and heart. Mesothelioma is encasing lung and also encasing heart, obliterating pericardial cavity and growing into myocardiuum.

Fig. 34–30. Mesothelioma encasing lung and producing nodular pleural masses that are focally invading into lung parenchyma.

Fig. 34–31. Mesothelioma producing nodular masses that are invading pulmonary parenchyma. Sometimes these appear as nodular lung masses in chest radiographs, falsely suggesting diagnosis of primary lung cancer.

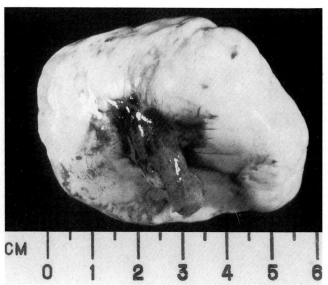

Fig. 34–33. Resected localized fibrous tumor of pleura. Tumor was attached to visceral pleura by fibrous pedicle.

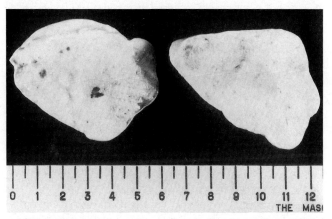

Fig. 34–34. Cut surface of tumor of Fig. 34–33 is composed of firm grayish-white fibrous tissue and appears encapsulated.

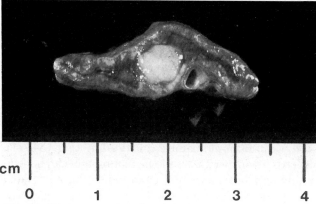

Fig. 34–35. Cross section through right adrenal gland shows 6-mm-diameter metastic tumor nodule.

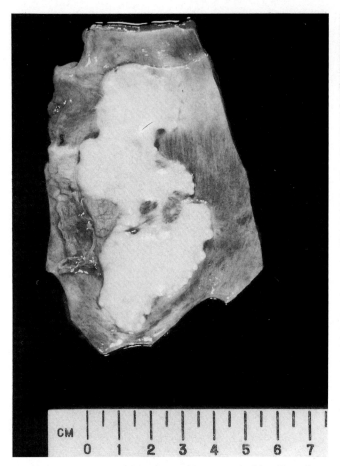

Fig. 34–36. Portion of diaphragm shows typical hyaline pleural plaque composed to pearly-white dense fibrous tissue that frequently shows calcification.

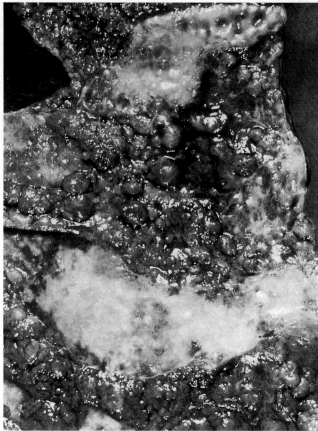

Fig. 34–37. Nodular xcresences of mesothelioma in association with two hyaline pleural plaques.

nohistochemical and ultrastructural analysis of percutaneous and open pleural biopsy-obtained tumor specimens or neoplastic cells in pleural fluid is sometimes necessary to make a specific diagnosis of mesothelioma.

Epithelial mesotheliomas are the most frequently diagnosed histologic type of mesothelioma, and the tubulopapillary pattern is the most common. Like all types of mesotheliomas, these usually obliterate the pleural space and encase the lung (Fig. 34–38). They are composed of relatively uniform cuboidal to polygonal cells with centrally located round nuclei, and form distinct papillary structures containing a fibrovascular core or small tubular structures when cut in cross section (Figs. 34–39 and 34–40). They may be associated with psammomatous calcification (Fig. 34–41), which is a nonspecific histologic feature and can be seen in any papillary neoplasm. Occasionally the individual tumor cells of a tubulopapillary mesothelioma are large and have large nuclei with prominent nucleoli (Fig. 34–42).

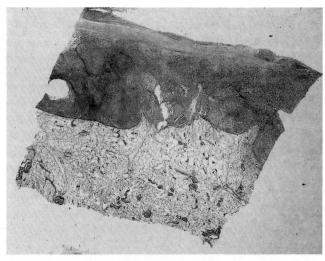

Fig. 34–38. Pleural tubulopapillary mesothelioma directly adherent to visceral pleural surface. ×4.

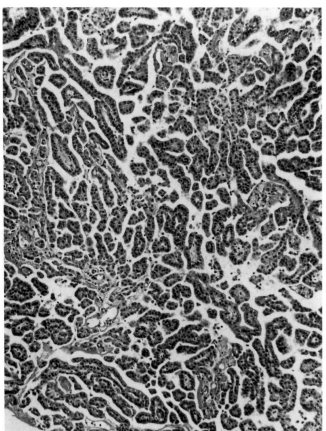

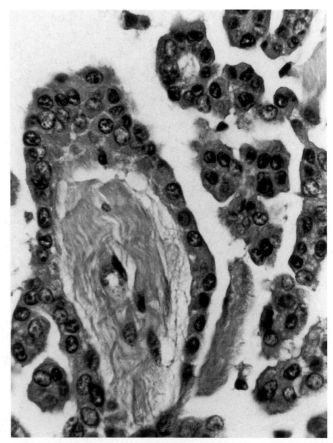

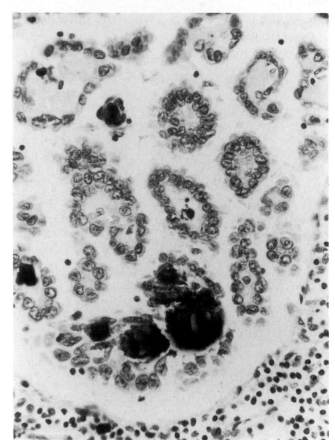

Fig. 34–39. Low-power microscopic appearance of tubulo-papillary mesothelioma. ×75.

Fig. 34–40. Enlarged region of tubulopapillary mesothelioma shows papillary structure with fibrovascular core. Note uniformity of tumor cells. ×550.

Fig. 34–41. Region of tubulopapillary mesothelioma metastatic in lymph node shows psammomatous calcification in tumor, a nonspecific finding that can be seen with any papillary neoplasm. ×300.

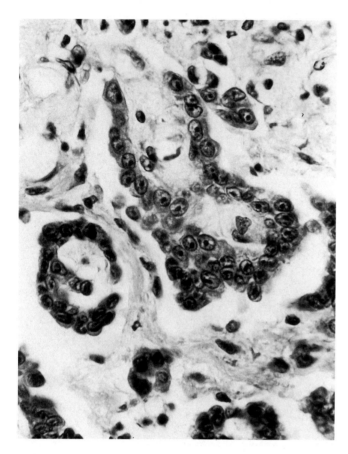

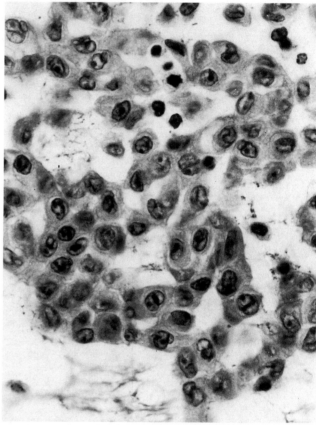

Fig. 34–42. Tumor cells forming some tubulopapillary mesotheliomas can be large and have large vesicular nuclei with prominent nucleoli. ×550.

Fig. 34–43. Epithelioid mesothelioma composed of relatively solid nests of large round cells with large vesicular nuclei and prominent nucleoli. ×550.

The next most frequent type of epithelial mesothelioma is often referred to as an epithelioid or histiocytoid mesothelioma. The tumor cells are usually round and occur in relatively solid sheets or nests (Fig. 34–43) and are sometimes associated with edematous myxoid stromal connective tissue (Fig. 34–44). These cells usually have round nuclei with large nucleoli and have abundant glassy eosinophilic cytoplasm in hematoxylin and eosin-stained sections. These cells usually stain with periodic acid–Schiff reagent because of cytoplasmic glycogen.

Epithelial mesotheliomas may form predominantly glandular structures that may vary in size and shape and be histologically identical to an adenocarcinoma (Fig. 34–45). This glandular pattern is not infrequently associated with a tubulopapillary or epithelioid pattern. Other forms of epithelial mesotheliomas exist. Rarely, an adenoid cystic pattern is seen (Fig. 34–46), and occasionally mesotheliomas are formed by uniform small cells with bland nuclei and a high nuclear cytoplasmic ratio (Fig. 34–47). In contrast to small cell mesotheliomas there are also mesotheliomas composed of large

pleomorphic cells that have a definite epithelial appearance (Fig. 34–48). Some epithelial mesotheliomas occur in relatively solid sheets and are composed of cells that show frequent cytoplasmic vacuoles analogous to signet ring cells (Fig. 34–49).

In our experience approximately 20% of epithelial mesotheliomas produce an acidic mucosubstance, hy-

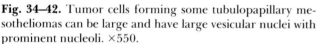

Fig. 34–44. Some epithelioid mesotheliomas are composed of nests of round cells embedded in myxomatous matrix. ×550.

Fig. 34–45. Some epithelial mesotheliomas are composed of uniform cells that form glands and may be confused with adenocarcinomas. ×300.

Fig. 34–46. An adenoid cystic pattern may be the dominant histologic appearance of some epithelial mesotheliomas. ×300.

Fig. 34–47. This mesothelioma is composed of uniform small round cells, an uncommon type of histologic pattern that may cause incorrect diagnosis. ×300.

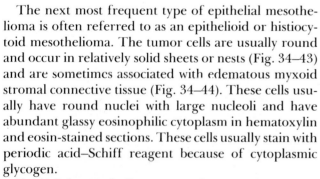

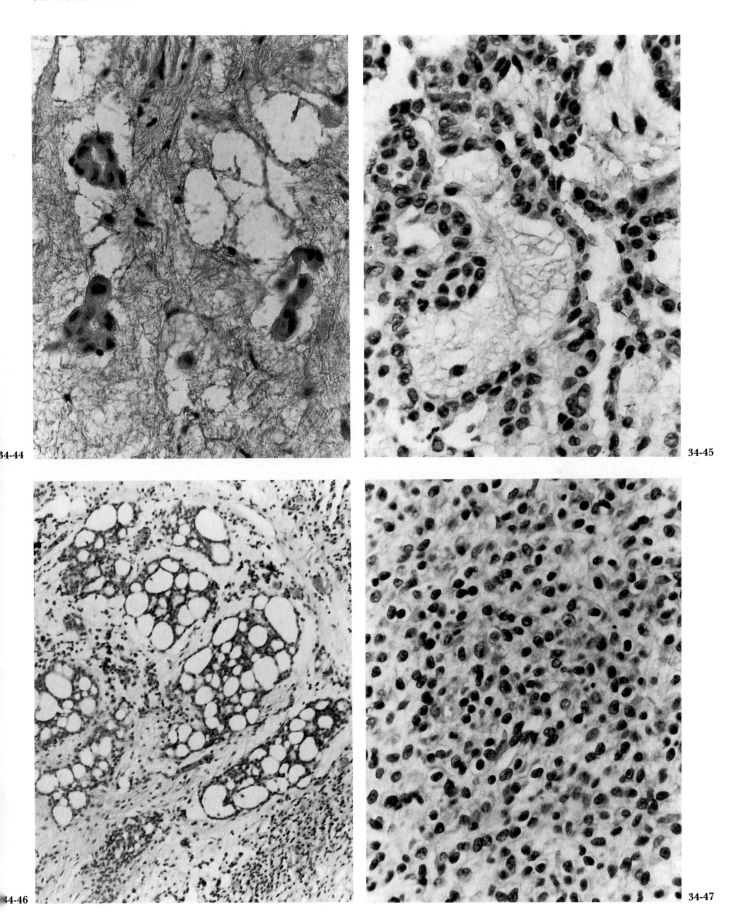

34-44

34-45

34-46

34-47

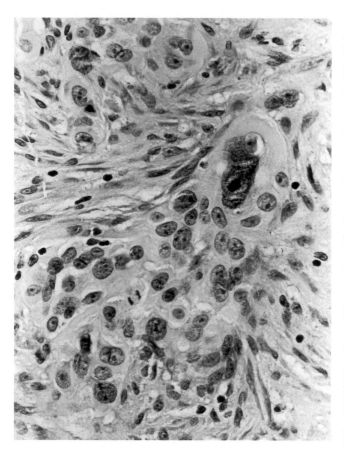

Fig. 34–48. In contrast to small cell epithelial mesotheliomas, some mesotheliomas are composed of large pleomorphic cells somewhat analogous to giant cell carcinoma of lung. ×550.

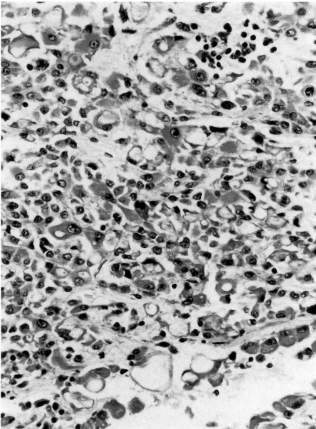

Fig. 34–49. Mesothelioma formed by cells that frequently show cytoplasmic vacuoles similar to those seen in signet ring adenocarcinoma. ×300.

aluronic acid, which can be demonstrated with an alcian blue or colloidal iron stain. Pretreatment of the tissue with hyaluronidase removes or decreases the staining reaction. The positive staining of mesotheliomas with acidic mucosubstance stains is characteristically seen between the cells, in intracellular lumens formed by the cells or in glands formed by the cells.

The hyaluronic acid frequently crystallizes (Fig. 34–50), which is best seen ultrastructurally (see following). In contrast, pulmonary adenocarcinomas contain intracellular mucosubstances that usually stain with a neutral mucosubstance stain such as periodic acid–Schiff diastase, or a slightly acidic mucosubstance stain such as Mayer's mucicarmine. Up to 5% of epithelial mesotheliomas show focal staining with Mayer's mucicarmine stain. Like the staining seen with alcian blue or colloidal iron, the mucicarmine staining is between cells, within intracellular lumens, or within glands, and is removed or decreased with pretreatment of tissue by hyaluronidase. The difference between mucosubstance production by epithelial mesotheliomas and pulmonary

adenocarcinomas is demonstrated best ultrastructurally (see following).

Like epithelial mesotheliomas, sarcomatoid mesotheliomas (fibrous or mesenchymal mesotheliomas) show a variation in histologic appearance (Fig. 34–51 A–F). Some resemble fibrosarcomas or leiomyosarcomas while others have an appearance suggesting a malignant fibrous histiocytoma or a pleomorphic sarcoma. Some sarcomatoid mesotheliomas show cartilaginous and/or osseus metaplasia.[143]

Desmoplastic mesotheliomas were first described in 1980[144]; they were first discussed in detail in 1982,[145] and are the most difficult histologic type of mesothelioma to diagnose. Macroscopically they resemble other mesotheliomas characteristically growing by local extension encasing the lung and occasionally invading the chest wall, lung, and other structures. The difficulty in diagnosing desmoplastic mesothelioma is because they resemble benign reactive pleural tissue characteristically seen in chronic pleuritis such as that caused by an organizing empyema or asbestos. If an adequate sample

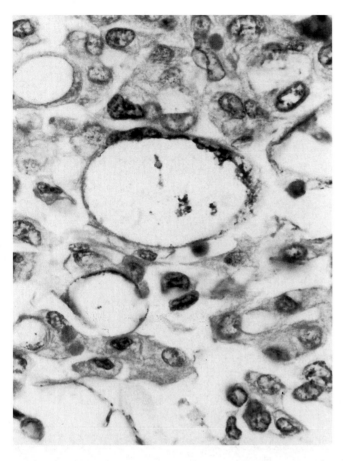

Fig. 34–50. Cytoplasmic vacuoles of these neoplastic mesothelial cells contain crystallized hyaluronic acid on inner aspect, better seen ultrastructurally (see Fig. 34–89). ×550.

of tissue is obtained for histologic analysis, stellate areas of necrosis (Fig. 34–52) and cellular atypia (Fig. 34–53) can be found in desmoplastic mesotheliomas and can help solidify the diagnosis. Clinical features such as chronic pain and radiographic evidence of invasion of the chest wall, lung, or bone by the tumor can help the pathologist make the correct diagnosis.

Transitional mesothelioma refers to a histologic type of mesothelioma that we believe has features transitional between epithelial mesotheliomas and sarcomatoid mesotheliomas. Some of the mesotheliomas described by Dardick et al.[146] as poorly differentiated would in our opinion fit in this category. They are composed of large polygonal to plump spindle-shaped cells occasionally arranged in nests or showing no distinct pattern (Figs. 34–54 and 34–55).

Biphasic or mixed mesotheliomas show histologic features of both epithelial and sarcomatoid mesotheliomas. These mesotheliomas may have an epithelial appearance in one region and a sarcomatoid pattern in another region, or can show both histologic patterns in

the same microscopic field and transitions between one form and the other (Fig. 34–56).

This histologic classification of mesotheliomas just described is an oversimplification of what exists, especially if one has larger tissue specimens, such as those obtained at autopsy or open biopsy, to examine. In general, the more sections taken the more histologic variation will be found (Fig. 34–57). It is not uncommon for a malignant mesothelioma to show a variety of epithelial and sarcomatoid patterns in the same tumor. Also, anaplastic mesotheliomas, composed of large undifferentiated-appearing cells, are relatively common (Figs. 34–58 and 34–59). In 1988, Henderson et al.[147] reported a type of mesothelioma they referred to as lymphohistiocytoid mesothelioma, which they described as a variant of a sarcomatoid mesothelioma characterized by an infiltrate of lymphocytes and histiocytes admixed with large, often slightly spindle-shaped cells (Fig. 34–60). As noted by these authors, this type of mesothelioma can be confused with a lymphoma unless one is familiar with the histologic pattern and appropriate ancillary studies, namely electron microscopy and immunohistochemistry, are performed on suspected cases.

This author has also seen other unusual variants of malignant mesothelioma that were not initially recognized as such or which raised a significant pathologic differential diagnosis, including mesothelioma. One case was a 74-year-old man with multiple parietal pleural nodules that histologically were composed of uniform, round-to-polygonal, medium-sized cells with clear cytoplasm (Fig. 34–61). These cells were PAS-, PASD-, and mucicarmine negative, but when studied ultrastructurally had the electron microscopic characteristics of an epithelial mesothelioma. No mitoses were noted, and the tumor showed no evidence of necrosis or hemorrhage.

Another case, a 69-year-old man, presented with a unilateral mass thought to be either a localized fibrous tumor of pleura or a primary pulmonary neoplasm. This mass was resected and was well demarcated and partially encapsulated. It was composed mostly of spindle-shaped cells but small tubular structures were scattered throughout (Figs. 34–62 and 34–63). The spindle-shaped cells expressed only vimentin, which would be the expected immunohistochemical staining result in localized fibrous tumors of the pleura. The epithelial cells forming the tubular structures immunostained for low- and high molecular weight keratin and were negative for CEA, Leu M1, B72.3, and Ber EP4 (see section on **Immunohistochemistry**). Ultrastructural examination showed these cells to exhibit epithelial mesothelial differentiation. In addition, when this patient's pleural cavity was closely inspected, one small white nodule was

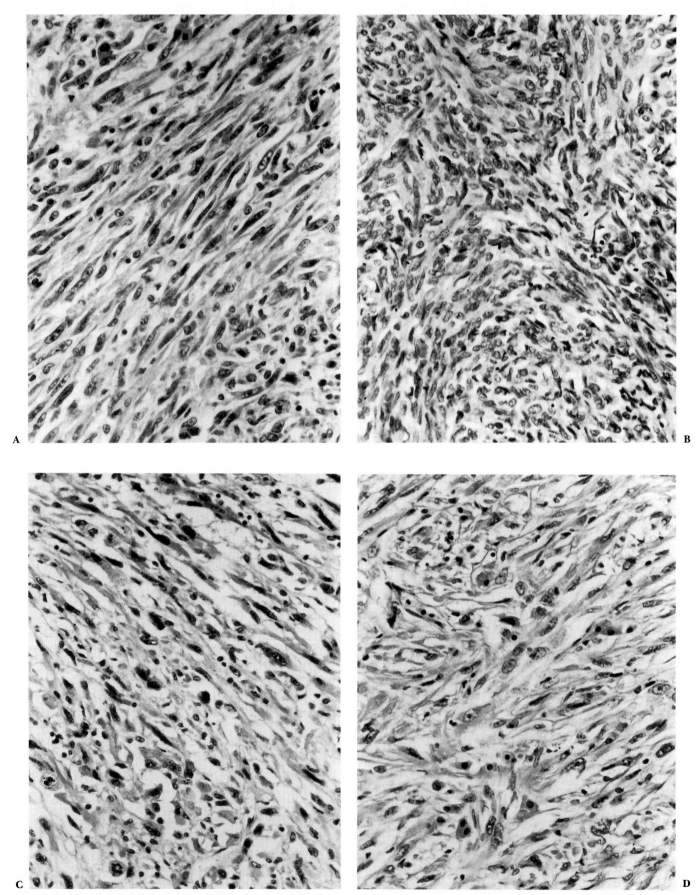

Fig. 34–51 A–F. Representative examples of sarcomatoid mesotheliomas show histologic growth patterns resembling fibrosarcomas, leiomyosarcomas, malignant fibrous histiocytomas, or pleomorphic sarcomas.

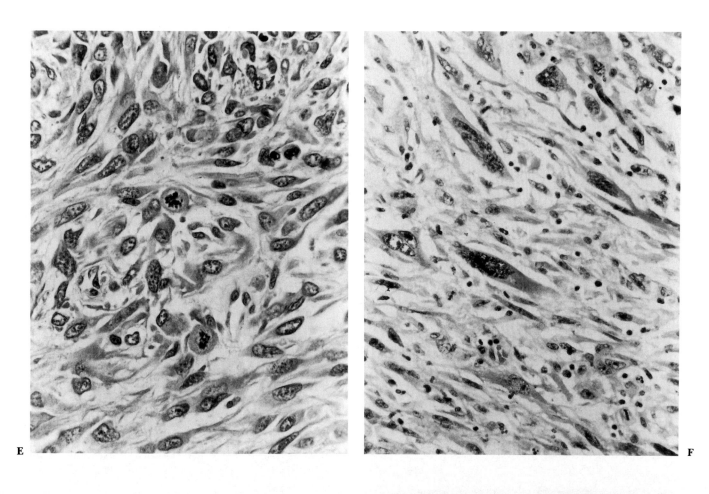

E

F

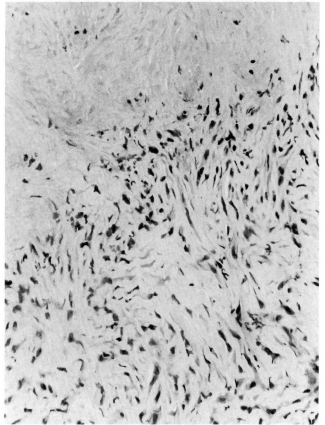

Fig. 34–52. Desmoplastic mesothelioma composed of mostly plump bland spindle cells shows region of geographic necrosis. ×300.

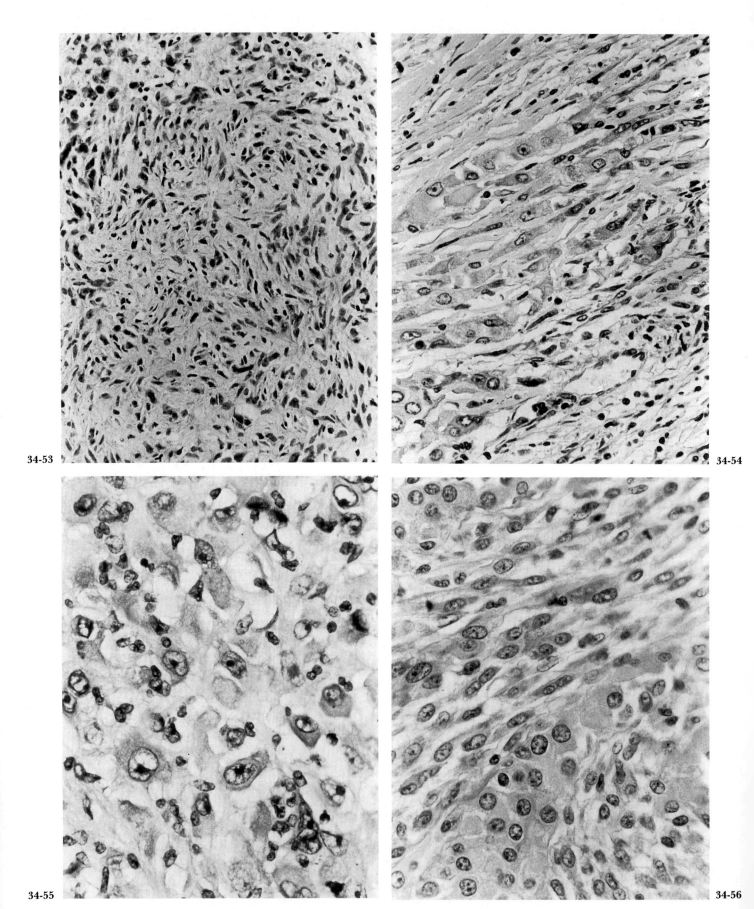

34-53

34-54

34-55

34-56

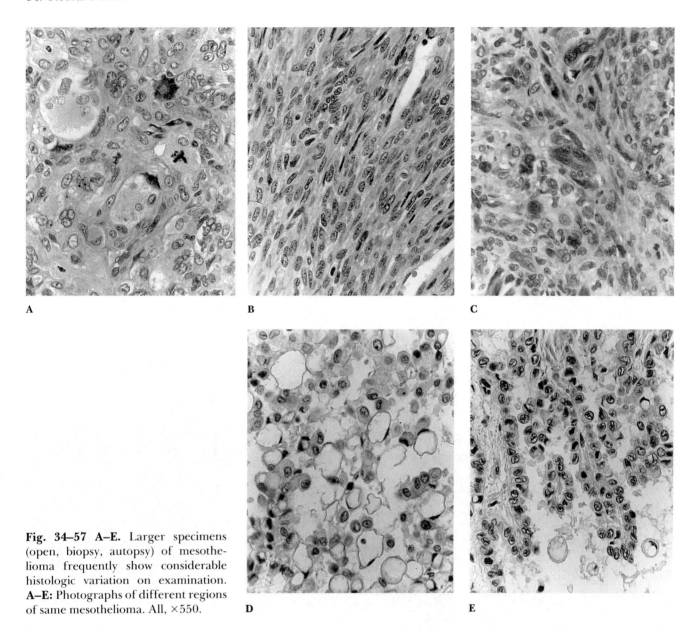

A

B

C

D

E

Fig. 34–57 A–E. Larger specimens (open, biopsy, autopsy) of mesothelioma frequently show considerable histologic variation on examination. **A–E:** Photographs of different regions of same mesothelioma. All, ×550.

Fig. 34–53. Desmoplastic mesothelioma shows regions of moderate cellularity with individual cell atypia and mitoses in some areas. ×300.

Fig. 34–54. Transitional mesothelioma formed by large polygonal to plump spindle-shaped cells. ×550.

Fig. 34–55. Cells of transitional mesothelioma are large and usually polygonal to somewhat elongate. ×775.

Fig. 34–56. Biphasic mesothelioma composed of round to polygonal epithelial cells in association with spindle-shaped tumor cells. ×550.

noted on the visceral pleura and another was found on the mediastinal parietal pleura. Both showed features of "early" and possibly in situ malignant epithelial mesothelioma.

This case raises two additional issues for pathologists. First, as described by Whitaker et al.,[2] surface mesothelial cells do have a "normal" turnover rate. Whitaker et al.[148] have described in situ malignant epithelial mesotheliomas, and this author has seen similar cases in which the surface epithelial mesothelial cells appear cytologically malignant and are usually associated with focal areas of infiltration (Figs. 34–64 and 34–65). Second, Meyer et al.[149] have described malignant tumors with histologic and immunohistochemical features of malignant mesotheliomas that have occurred as

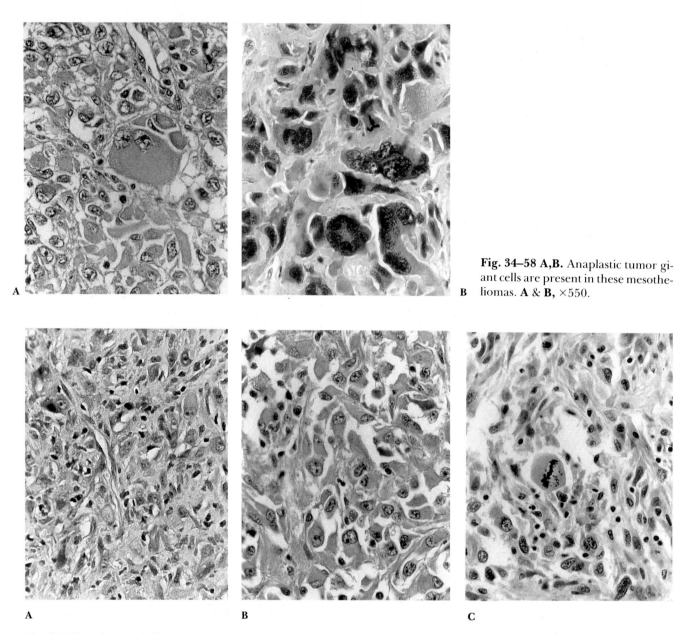

Fig. 34–58 A,B. Anaplastic tumor giant cells are present in these mesotheliomas. **A** & **B,** ×550.

Fig. 34–59 A–C. Mesotheliomas composed predominantly of large anaplastic tumor cells are relatively common. This histologic appearance does not exclude diagnosis of mesothelioma. ×550.

Fig. 34–60 A,B. This type of mesothelioma, referred to as lymphohistiocytoid mesothelioma, is variant of sarcomatoid mesothelioma; most of neoplastic cells are plump and spindle shaped. Neoplasm is heavily infiltrated by lymphocytes and histiocytes and can be confused with mixed lymphoma. **A,** ×55; **B,** ×550.

Fig. 34–61 A,B. Unusual mesothelioma composed of uniform cells with clear cytoplasm and round, medium-sized nucleoli neoplasm was confirmed to be epithelial mesothelioma by its ultrastructural features. **A,** ×125; **B,** ×300.

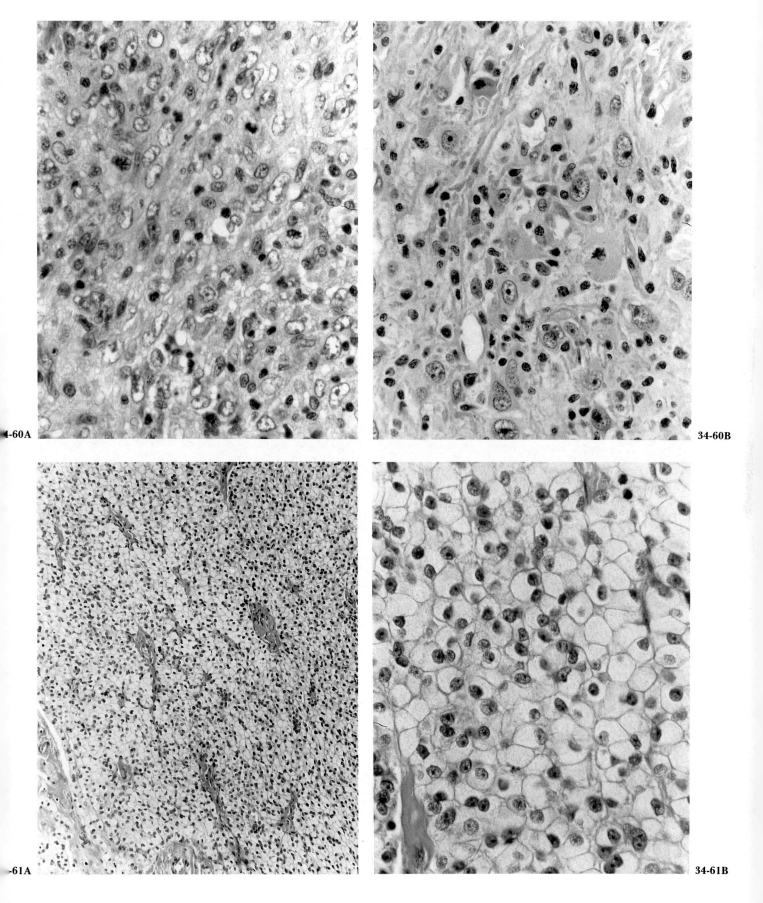

34-60A

34-60B

34-61A

34-61B

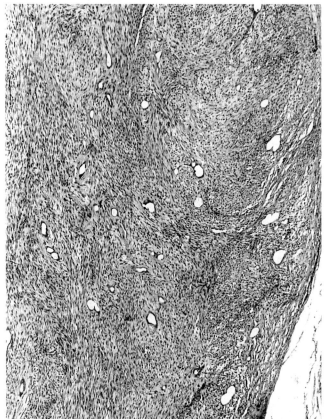

34-62A

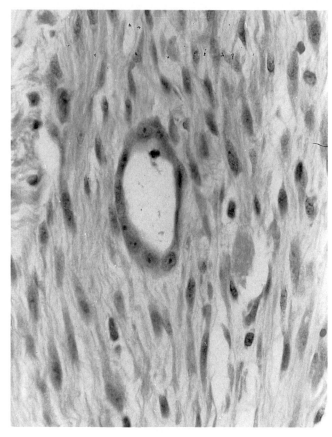

34-62

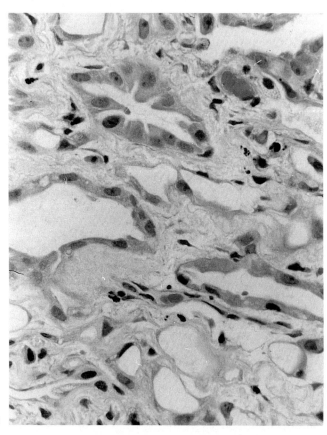

34-63

Fig. 34–62 A,B. Mesothelioma composed predominantly of relatively bland spindle-shaped cells with mesenchymal features. **(A).** Scattered among spindle-shaped cells were small tubular structures formed by epithelial cells that had immunohistochemical and ultrastructural features of epithelial mesothelioma. (This case was contributed by Susan D. Patterson, MD, and John W. Bolen, MD, Virginia Mason Medical Center, Seattle, Washington.) **A,** ×75; **B,** ×550.

Fig. 34–63. Patient whose unusual mesothelioma is shown in Fig. 34–62 had two small pleural nodules composed of tubular/glandular structures formed by mesothelial cells that were infiltrating pleura. ×550.

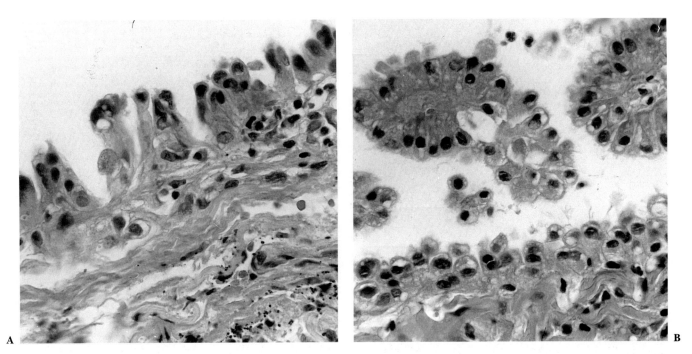

Fig. 34–64 A,B. Atypical mesothelial cells line visceral pleura and show focal papillary proliferation, a type of change reported as epithelial mesothelioma in situ. **A,** ×550; **B,** ×550.

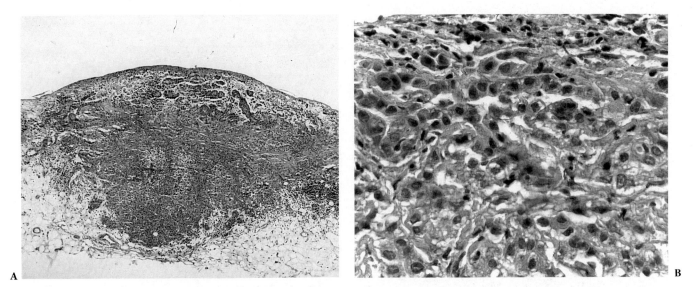

Fig. 34–65 A,B. In situ mesothelioma shown in Fig. 34–64 shows focal areas of infiltration. **A,** ×25; **B,** ×550.

isolated masses rather than extensively involving the pleura. This author has seen several such cases. This is important because it indicates that an isolated pleural tumor can represent a malignant mesothelioma.

Neoplasms that have been referred to in the past as localized fibrous mesotheliomas are typically well-encapsulated masses (Fig. 34–66) attached to the visceral pleura by a thin pedicle or located within the lung subpleurally. They can attain a large size and can be associated with hypoglycemia. The largest this author has seen weighed 1,500 g and measured 13 cm in greatest dimension. On cut section, these are usually tan or gray-tan and may have a nodular, whorled, or lobulated pattern. Brisselli et al.[150] reported 8 new cases and reviewed the features of 360 previously reported in the literature. They referred to these tumors as solitary fibrous tumors of the pleura. Doucet et al.[151] subsequently, described 12 such tumors in 10 patients, and

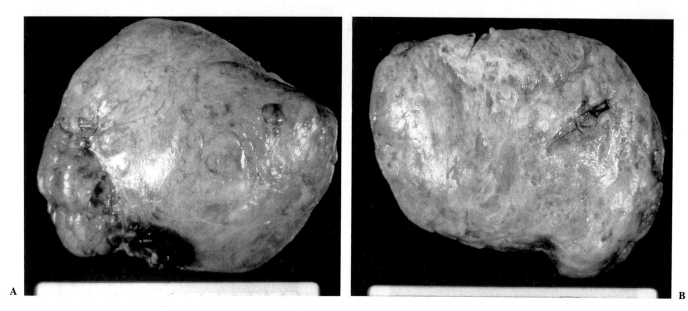

Fig 34–66 A,B. A. Localized fibrous tumor of pleural attached to visceral pleura by pedicle. **B.** Cut surface of tumor. (Photograph courtesy of Terrence H. Gleason, M.D.)

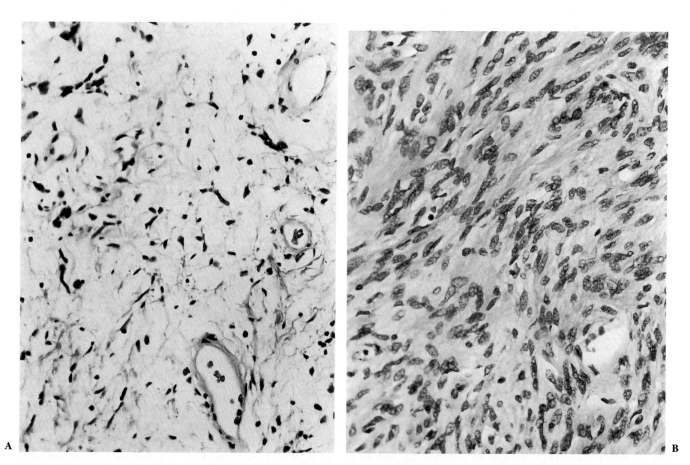

Fig. 34–67 A,B. A. Region of localized fibrous tumor of pleura composed of loosely separated benign-appearing spindle cells. **B.** Different region of same tumor seen in **A** shows increased cellularity but no mitotic activity. **A** and **B,** ×330.

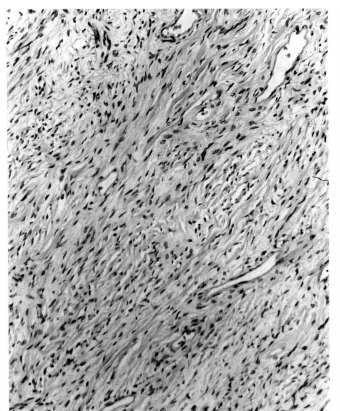

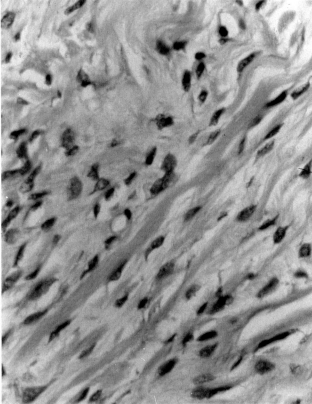

Fig. 34–68 A–C. Histologic appearance of resected neoplasm shown in Fig. 34–66. **A.** Tumor is composed of bland spindle-shaped cells with varying amounts of extracellular collagen. ×125. **B.** Higher magnification shows spindle-shaped cells and collagen. ×550. **C.** Immunohistochemically, spindle-shaped cells express vimentin (dark staining) in contrast to sarcomatoid mesotheliomas that characteristically express keratin and vimentin. ×550.

Carter and Otis[152] reported 17 fibrous tumors of the lung, of which 8 were localized fibrous tumors.

The largest, most complete study to date concerning localized fibrous tumors of the pleura was by England et al.,[153] who analyzed the clinical and pathologic features of 223 cases of localized benign and malignant fibrous tumors of the pleura. Histologically these are spindle cell neoplasms that show varying degrees of cellularity and collagen production (Figs. 34–67 and 34–68). The criteria used by England et al.[153] for malignancy included high cellularity, a mitotic rate of more than four mitoses per 10 high-power fields, pleomorphism, hemorrhage, and necrosis. Figure 34–69 shows an example of malignant fibrous tumor of the pleura occurring in a 27-year-old woman. Macroscopically, this tumor invaded into the chest wall and lung; histologically, it was cellular (Fig. 34–70) and had a

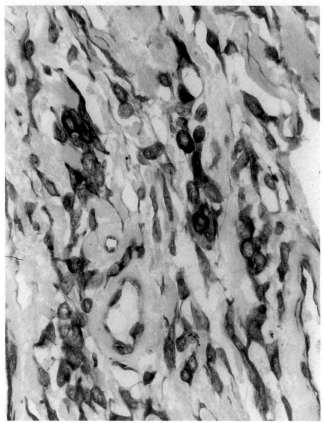

34-68A

34-68B

34-68C

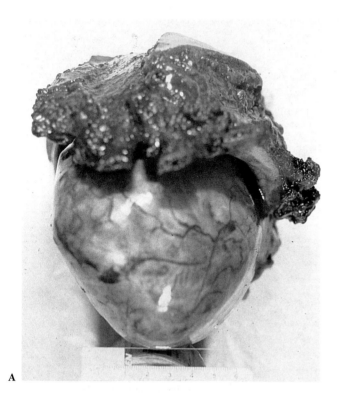

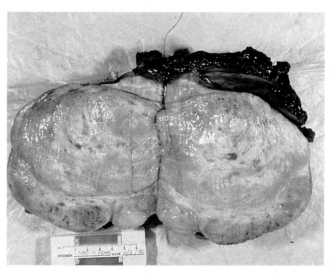

Fig. 34–69 A,B. A. Malignant localized fibrous tumor of the pleura is well encapsulated but is invading the attached portion of the chest wall. **B.** On cut section this malignant localized fibrous tumor of the pleuras was lobulated but overall similar to its benign counterpart. (Photographs courtesy of W.A. Franklin, MD, Department of Pathology, University of Colorado Health Sciences Center, Denver, Colorado.)

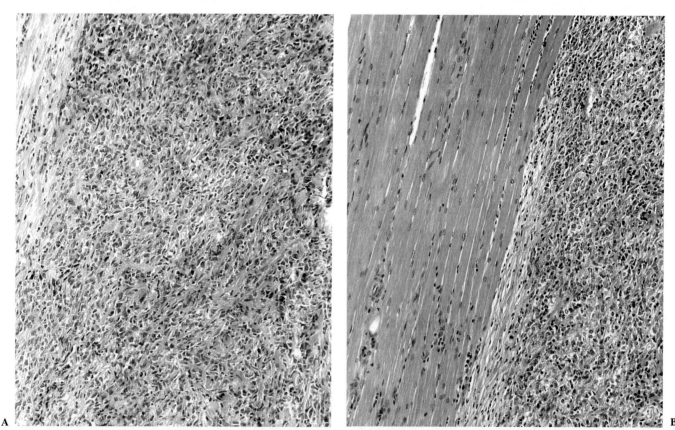

Fig. 34–70 A,B. A. This malignant localized fibrous tumor of pleura shows infiltration of chest wall muscle. ×125. **B.** Neoplasm was composed of plump spindle-shaped cells. ×125.

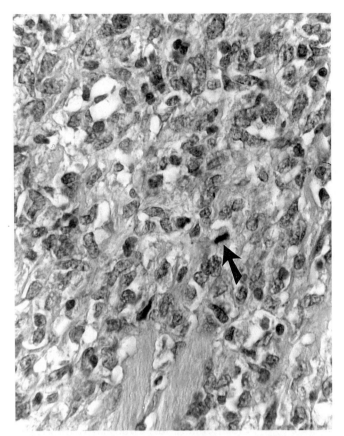

Fig. 34–71. Malignant localized fibrous tumor of pleura shows relatively frequent mitoses (*arrow*). ×550.

mitotic rate greater than four mitoses per 10 high-power fields (Fig. 34–71).

The reason for calling these tumors localized fibrous tumors of the pleura and not localized fibrous mesotheliomas is discussed in the sections on **Immunohistochemistry** and **Histogenesis,** which follow.

Histochemical Features of Mesotheliomas

Several standard histochemical tests for the demonstration of carbohydrate substances have been promoted as being useful in differentiating mesotheliomas from other malignant tumors, primarily pulmonary adenocarcinomas. The two main substances to be considered are mucin and glycogen. Mucin is a vague term and is frequently used synonymously with mucopolysaccharide, proteoglycan, glycosaminoglycan, mucosubstance, and glycoconjugate. Glycoconjugate is the term currently preferred by some;[154] we refer to them as mucosubstances. The protein portion of mucosubstances is synthesized in the rough endoplasmic reticulum, and the carbohydrate portion is added in the Golgi apparatus. Mucosubstances can be divided into highly acidic, weakly acidic, or neutral mucosubstance.

As already stated, approximately 20% of epithelial mesotheliomas produce highly acidic mucosubstances such as hyaluronic acid that can be identified with an alcian blue or Hale's colloidal iron stain. The presence of positive-staining material within cytoplasmic vacuoles, tubular lumina, or aggregates of epithelial cells that is removed with hyaluronidase is helpful in confirming the diagnosis of epithelial mesothelioma. A note of caution is that the stromal connective tissue surrounding nests of epithelial mesothelioma cells can be rich in hyaluronic acid and thus misinterpreted as a positive reaction.

Approximately 65%–70% of pulmonary adenocarcinomas show intracytoplasmic staining for neutral or weakly acidic mucosubstance that can be identified by periodic acid-Schiff reagent with diastase (PAS-D; pretreatment with diastase removes glycogen) or Mayer's mucicarmine (see Chapter 32). Another note of caution is that most pulmonary adenocarcinomas that show intracytoplasmic staining with periodic acid–Schiff diastase or Mayer's mucicarmine will also be alcian blue positive at pH 2.5; unlike most epithelial mesotheliomas showing this reaction, the positive-staining material is resistant to pretreatment with hyaluronidase.

Glycogen is present in the cytoplasm of epithelial mesothelioma cells in up to 50% of cases and readily stains with periodic acid–Schiff reagent. This is a nonspecific finding because primary pulmonary carcinomas such as pulmonary adenocarcinomas frequently contain glycogen, especially those showing degenerative changes (see Chapter 32). Many of the so-called clear cell carcinomas of the lung represent neoplasms whose cells contain significant amounts of glycogen, which is removed during processing and causes cytoplasmic clearing. In our experience, epithelial mesotheliomas containing significant quantities of glycogen usually do not exhibit a clear cell histologic pattern.

Ernst and Atkinson[155] reported 7 of 18 epithelial mesotheliomas to be mucicarmine positive. They attributed the positive staining reaction to hyaluronic acid. The review article on malignant mesothelioma by the U.S.-Canadian Mesothelioma Panel[156] illustrated a case of mucicarmine-positive mesothelioma and indicated this did not exclude the diagnosis of mesothelioma. MacDougall et al.[157] reported a case of malignant epithelial mesothelioma, the diagnosis documented by electron microscopy and immunohistochemistry that was mucicarmine- and PAS-D positive.

We[158] compared the histochemical and immunohistochemical staining reactions of ten epithelial mesotheliomas (diagnosis documented by ultrastructural examination) that were mucicarmine positive and compared them with 10 pulmonary adenocarcinomas. The adenocarcinomas were all primary "nodular" lung adenocarcinomas that were mucicarmine positive. We concluded that the mucicarmine and PAS-diastase staining reactions resulted from hyaluronic acid production by these neoplasms. When the tissue sections were pretreated with hyaluronidase, the intensity of staining reactions with mucicarmine and PAS-diastase usually decreased or disappeared. In some cases, the staining reaction was not completely eradicated. The electron microscopic correlates of mucicarmine positive mesotheliomas are discussed in the section on **Ultrastructural Features of Mesotheliomas.**

Benjamin and Ritchie[159] examined the staining results for glycogen and mucosubstance of 30 diffuse epithelial mesotheliomas. Tissue was fixed in formalin and processed using standard techniques. Tissue sections were stained with the World Health Organization Stain for mucin, periodic acid–Schiff reagent with and without diastase, Hale's colloidal iron stain with and without hyaluronidase, potassium hydroxide–periodic acid–Schiff technique, and alcian blue at pH 1.0 and 2.5. They found that 7 of the 30 mesotheliomas failed to stain by any method tested, and concluded that the staining reactions of epithelial mesotheliomas with mucopolysaccharide stains were too inconsistent to be of much value in diagnosing epithelial mesotheliomas.

Immunohistochemical Features of Mesotheliomas

Immunohistochemical techniques have contributed to our understanding of normal serosal tissue and mesotheliomas.

We employ a "battery" of commercially available antibodies to evaluate cases of suspected mesothelioma, including antibodies to different molecular weight cytokeratins, vimentin, human milk fat globule protein-2, carcinoembryonic antigen, Leu M1, B72.3, and Ber EP4, and use an avidin-biotin immunoperoxidase technique.[160]

Cytokeratins are a complex family of 20 different proteins ranging in molecular weight from approximately 40 to 68 kdaltons.[161,162] Any given epithelium usually contains from 2 to 10 different cytokeratin proteins, and the pattern of cytokeratin expression is dependent on cell type, cellular growth environment, stage of differentiation, and disease state. As a general rule, the lower molecular weight cytokeratin proteins are present in simple epithelia whereas the higher molecular weight cytokeratins are present in stratified squamous and complex epithelia. By employing a battery of monoclonal antibodies to different molecular weight cytokeratin proteins, one can characterize a given tissue type and/or tumor by its pattern of reactivity, that is, expressing only low molecular weight cyto-

keratin, high molecular weight cytokeratin, or a more complex combination pattern. Commercially available monoclonal antibodies generally recognize low molecular weight cytokeratins, high molecular weight cytokeratins, or represent a "cocktail" of several monoclonal antibodies designed to achieve a wide range of specificity. The intermediate filament vimention of 57 kdaltons is present in a wide range of mesenchymal cells, and several commercially available antibodies recognize it.

The immunohistochemical features of various types of mesotheliomas are shown in Table 34–10. Most types of epithelial mesotheliomas are decorated by antibodies against low and high molecular weight cytokeratin, epithelial membrane antigen, and human milk fat globule protein (Fig. 34–72 A–E).[163] In our experience they usually do not express carcinoembryonic antigen. The pattern of immunostaining for cytokeratin is often diffuse, although there may be some perinuclear accentuation using antibodies against high molecular cytokeratin, which correlates ultrastructurally with perinuclear tonofilaments (see following). As shown in Fig. 34–72, antibodies against epithelial membrane antigen and human milk fat globule protein-2 characteristically show localization in the cell membrane. In our experience, most small cell mesotheliomas and many large cell anaplastic varieties express vimentin (Fig. 34–73 A,B.). Sarcomatoid, transitional, and desmoplastic mesotheliomas characteristically express low molecular weight cytokeratin and vimentin (Fig. 34–74 A,B).[163–164] Some are also decorated by antibodies against high molecular weight cytokeratin (Fig. 34–75), epithelial membrane antigen (Fig. 34–76), and milk fat globule protein-2 (Fig. 34–77). As emphasized by Leong et al.,[165] epithelial mesotheliomas may show very "thick" cell membranes, when stained with epithelial membrane antigens. We have observed the same thick cell membrane immunostaining pattern with human milk fat globule protein-2 (Fig. 34–78).

This immunostaining pattern is helpful diagnostically in differentiating soft tissue sarcomas from these types of mesothelioma, because most soft tissue sarcomas, with the exception of synoviosarcoma and epithelioid sarcoma, express vimentin and/or desmin but do not contain low or high molecular weight cytokeratin.[166] The epithelial component of biphasic mesotheliomas shows the same immunostaining pattern as epithelial mesotheliomas, and the sarcomatoid region expresses vimentin and cytokeratin. As is explained in the section on histogenesis, because reactive serosal connective tissue cells also express cytokeratin and vimentin it is therefore not possible to use this immunostaining pattern to differentiate desmoplastic mesothelioma from reactive serosal tissue such as seen in cases of chronic fibrous pleuritis. In our experience, the cells

Table 34–10. Immunohistochemical features of malignant mesotheliomas

Lesion	LMWk	HMWk	Vimetin	EMA	HMFG-2	CEA	LeuM1	B72.3	BerEP4	HHF-35
Epithelial										
Tubulopapillary	+	+	±	±[a]	±[a]	−[b]	−[c]	−[d]	−[e]	−
Glandular	+	+	±	±[a]	±[a]	−[b]	−[c]	−[d]	−[e]	−
Epithelioid (histiocytoid)	+	+	±	±[a]	±[a]	−[b]	−[c]	−[d]	−[e]	−
Solid poorly differentiated	+	+	±[f]	±[g]	±[g]	−	−	−	−	−
Adenoid cystic	+	+	±	±[a]	±[a]	−[b]	−[c]	−[d]	−[e]	−
Signet ring	+	+	±	±[a]	±[a]	−[b]	−[c]	−[d]	−[e]	−
Sarcomatoid	+[h]	±[h]	+	−[i]	−[l]	−	−	−	−	±
Mixed-biphasic					·					
Epithelial	+	+	±	±[a]	±[a]	−[b]	−[c]	−[d]	−[e]	−
Sarcomatoid	+[h]	±[h]	+	−[i]	−[i]	−	−	−	−	±
Anaplastic (Pleomorphic)	+[j]	±	+	−[k]	−[k]	−	−	−	−	−
Transitional	+	±	+	−[k]	−[k]	−	−	+	+	−
Desmoplastic	+	±	+	−	−	−	+	+	+	±[l]

[a] In the positive cases, the pattern of immunostaining is in a cell membrane distribution.
[b] Up to 15% of cases of epithelial mesotheliomas show focal, usually low-intensity immunostaining.
[c,d] Rare cases of epithelial mesothelioma show immunostaining, usually focal.
[e] In one report, up to 20% of epithelial mesotheliomas show focal immunostaining.
[f] Vimentin may be expressed in any type of epithelial mesothelioma, but is more frequently expressed in the epithelial mesotheliomas that are more poorly differentiated.
[g] Infrequently positive.
[h] Despite what is published, some sarcomatoid mesotheliomas do not immunostain for keratin with commercially-available anti-keratin antibodies.
[i,j,k] Rare cases may be positive.
[l] Most cases are positive.
Abbreviations: LMWk, low molecular weight keratin; HMWk, high molecular weight keratin; EMA, epithelial membrane antigen; HMFG-2, human milk fat globule protein-2; CEA, carcinoembryonic antigen; LeuM1, CD15; B72.3, TAG-72; HHF-35, muscle-specific actin.

forming localized fibrous mesotheliomas express only vimentin (Fig. 34–79).

In 1983 Said et al.[167] studied patterns of localization of different molecular weight keratins in reactive mesothelial cells, mesotheliomas, and lung carcinomas. These investigators were unable to detect a 63-kdalton keratin in pulmonary adenocarcinomas and large cell undifferentiated carcinomas of the lung, whereas this protein was present in all reactive mesothelial cells, mesotheliomas, and in 8 of 17 squamous carcinomas of lung studied. Watts et al.[168] also observed difference in keratin species in exfoliated mesothelioma and adenocarcinoma cells. However, many commercially available antibodies developed against high molecular weight cytokeratins (34BE12; AE1/AE3) characteristically immunostain epithelial mesotheliomas and pulmonary adenocarcinomas. The intensity of the immunostaining for epithelial mesotheliomas in general is greater than for pulmonary adenocarcinomas, although in our experience this is variable.

Kahn and colleagues[169] reported a difference in the pattern of keratin intermediate filament distribution in benign and malignant mesothelial cells compared to adenocarcinomas. They reported that in mesothelial cells the keratin filaments were in a peripheral or perinuclear distribution whereas in adenocarcinomas they had an aborizing pattern. Their initial report in

1982 was followed by a more extensive report in 1986[170] in which they examined 10 adenocarcinomas, 10 carcinoids, and 4 mesotheliomas for the pattern of keratin distribution in the tumor cells using three monoclonal antibodies and three polyclonal antibodies to keratin. When they allowed the diaminobenzidine color reaction to proceed for less than 2 min, they identified a weblike pattern in adenocarcinomas, a punctate or crescentic pattern in the carcinoids, and a perinuclear pattern in mesotheliomas. Further experience is necessary to determine the diagnostic usefulness of their observations.

Blobel et al.[171] reported that epithelial mesotheliomas contained keratin 5, as demonstrated by immunohistochemistry, whereas pulmonary adenocarcinomas did not. The Moll et al.[172] study supported this observation by finding immunostaining for keratin 5 in 12 of 13 epithelial mesotheliomas using antibody AEH, whereas 21 pulmonary adenocarcinomas were negative or showed only focal staining in a few cases.

As listed in Table 34–10 and shown previously, vimentin intermediate filament is present in all sarcomatoid desmoplastic, and transitional mesotheliomas. Occasionally some epithelial mesotheliomas that are composed of small uniform cells or large cells express vimentin. Churg[173] reported vimentin in two alcohol-fixed mesotheliomas, one of which was a tubulopapil-

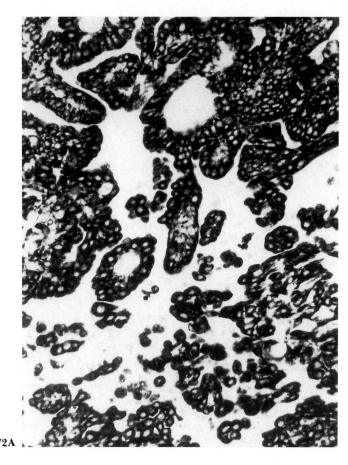

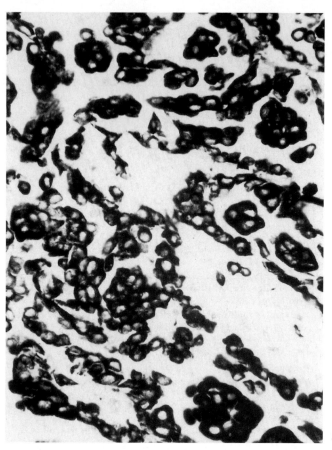

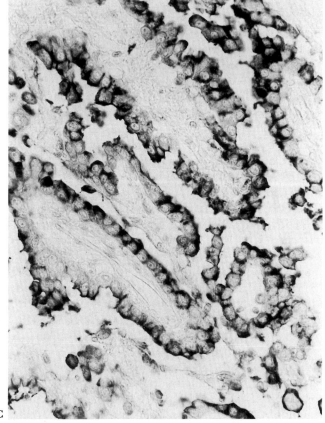

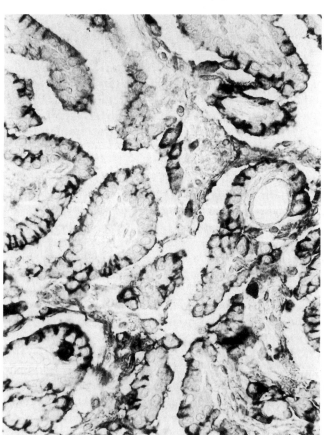

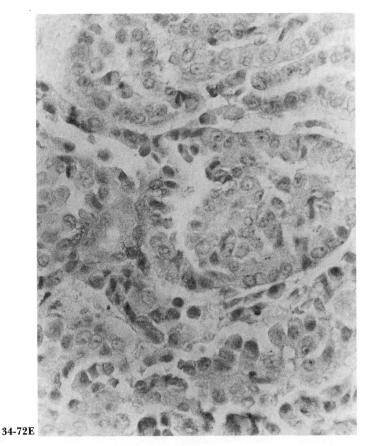

34-72E

Fig. 34–72 A–E. Immunohistochemical features of tubulo-papillary epithelial mesothelioma. **A.** Immunostaining for low molecular weight cytokeratin. **B.** Immunostaining pattern for high molecular weight cytokeratin. **C.** Immunostaining for epithelial membrane antigen; note localization in region of cell membrane. **D.** Immunostaining pattern for human milk fat globule protein is similar to staining pattern of epithelial membrane antigen. The immunostaining pattern for epithelial membrane antigen and human milk fat globule protein is most commonly in a cell membrane distribution. **E.** Negative immunostaining for carcinoembryonic antigen. Epithelioid and glandular mesotheliomas show identical results. ×300.

◁

Fig. 34–73 A,B. Immunostaining pattern of small cell epithelial mesothelioma in Fig. 34–27. **A.** Cells show intense diffuse immunostaining for low molecular weight cytokeratin. **B.** Tumor cells also show diffuse but less intense immunostaining for vimentin. ×300.

▽

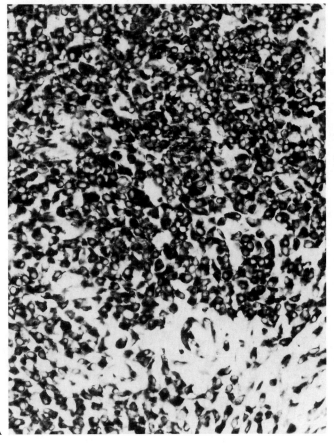

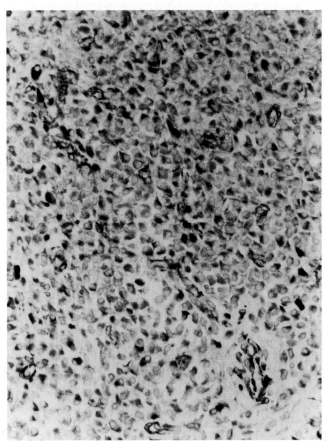

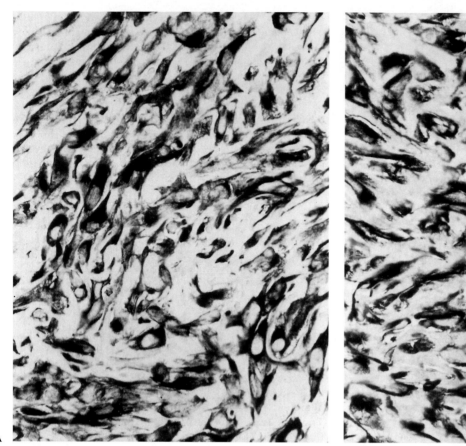

34-74A

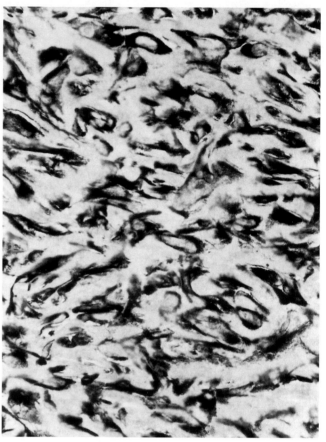

34-74B

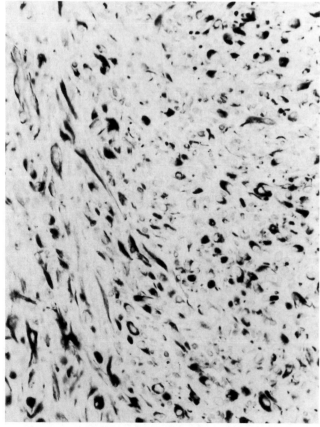

34-75

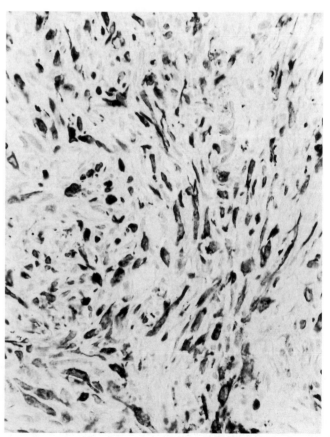

34-76

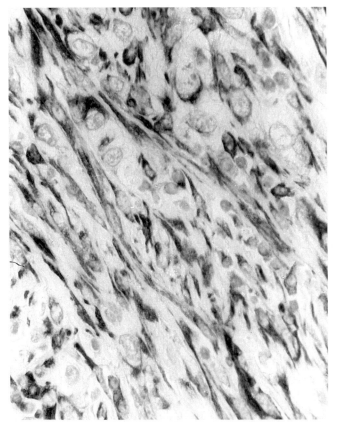

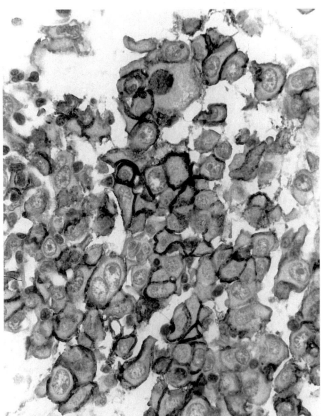

34-78A

Fig. 34–77. Sarcomatoid mesothelioma shows immunostaining of some tumor cells for human milk fat globule protein-2. ×330.

▷

Fig. 34–78 A,B. Poorly differentiated epithelial mesothelioma shows intense cell membrane immunostaining for human milk fat globule protein-2. This pattern makes cell membranes appear thick. **A,** ×300; **B,** ×550.

◁———————————————

Fig. 34–74 A,B. Immunostaining pattern of sarcomatoid mesothelioma in Fig. 34–51. **A.** Spindle-shaped cells show intense immunostaining for low molecular weight cytokeratin. **B.** Tumor cells also show intense immunostaining for vimentin. ×550.

Fig. 34–75. Region of transitional mesothelioma shows immunostaining for high molecular weight cytokeratin. ×550.

Fig. 34–76. Region of transitional mesothelioma shows immunostaining for epithelial membrane antigen. ×550.

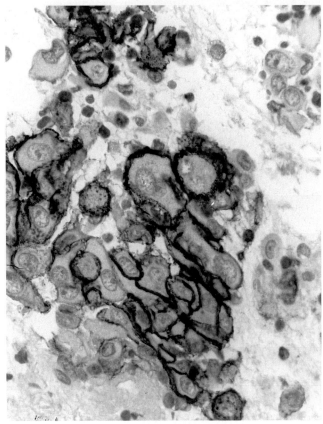

34-78B

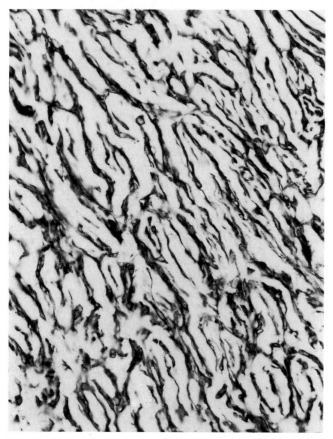

Fig. 34–79. Region of localized fibrous mesothelioma shown in Fig. 34–67 stains intensely for vimentin. ×300.

lary mesothelioma; Jasani et al.[174] also reported vimentin expression in 75% of 44 malignant mesotheliomas, including all histologic types. They also found vimentin in 46% of 24 pulmonary adenocarcinomas examined. Mullink et al.[175] also found that it was more common for epithelial mesotheliomas than for primary pulmonary adenocarcinomas to coexpress keratin and vimentin. We have observed several large cell indifferentiated carcinomas of the lung that have expressed vimentin and keratin, a finding similar to that reported by Upton et al.[176] (See Chapter 32). We have also found that about 30% of epithelial mesotheliomas express vimentin in formalin-fixed, paraffin-embedded tissue (unpublished observations).

Two other commercially available antibodies already mentioned, one against epithelial membrane antigen and the other against human milk fat globule protein-2, have been used in studying reactive mesothelial cells, mesotheliomas, and pulmonary adenocarcinomas. Epithelial membrane antigen and human milk fat globule protein are antigenically similar large glycoproteins. Marshall et al.[177] found that 12 of 16 mesotheliomas, 3 of 13 cases of reactive mesothelium, and 27 of 27 pulmonary adenocarcinomas expressed human milk fat globule protein. Loosli and Hurlimann[178] found 9 of 15 mesotheliomas and 5 of 5 pulmonary adenocarcinomas were decorated by antibodies against milk fat globule protein. In addition, we[179] found that 50 of 64 epithelial mesotheliomas showed immunostaining for epithelial membrane antigen and 45 of 65 were positive for human milk fat globule protein. We found only 2 of 13 cases of reactive mesothelial cells were positive for epithelial membrane antigen and human milk fat globule protein. In contrast, Battifora and Kopinski[180] initially reported that 12 mesotheliomas failed to express milk fat globule protein whereas 100% of breast, lung, and ovarian adenocarcinomas were intensely positive. They suggested that a negative milk fat globule protein was strong evidence for the diagnosis of an epithelial mesothelioma and was superior to a negative carcinoembryonic antigen in distinguishing pulmonary adenocarcinoma from mesothelioma. Their position has changed in that they initially considered the cell membrane staining by epithelial mesotheliomas to be a negative result but now consider the cell membrane immunostaining pattern to be characteristic of epithelial mesothelioma. In addition, they found that most pulmonary adenocarcinomas and other adenocarcinomas show cytoplasmic immunostaining with human milk fat globule protein. This author generally agrees with their observations with the exception that some (up to 20%) bronchioloalveolar cell carcinomas show a cell membrane immunostaining pattern for human milk fat globule protein-2 (Fig. 34–80).

Most investigators are in agreement that pulmonary adenocarcinomas and most other primary carcinomas of the lung show immunostaining for carcinoembryonic antigen. This oncofetal antigen has a molecular weight of approximately 200 kdaltons and has several different antigenic forms. The immunostaining results of carcinoembryonic antigen in mesotheliomas are variable[174,177,179–190] (Table 34–11). Mezger et al.[191] summarized carcinoembryonic antigen staining in epithelial mesotheliomas. Most of the mesotheliomas reported to express carcinoembryonic antigen showed a low intensity of immunostaining. This author has seen more than 15 epithelial mesotheliomas express carcinoembryonic antigen. In all instances, this immunostaining has been focal and of low to moderate intensity. Focal carcinoembryonic antigen immunostaining has been observed most commonly in those epithelial mesotheliomas that were mucicarmine positive, suggesting that the immunostaining reaction was possibly related to hygluronic acid.

Monoclonal antibody Leu M1 was first reported to react against lacto-*N*-fucose-pentosy III on cells of my-

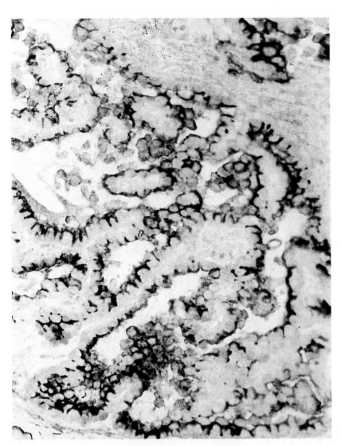

Fig. 34–80. Bronchioloalveolar cell carcinoma shows prominent cell membrane staining for human milk fat globule protein-2. ×300.

Table 34–11. Results of immunostaining of mesotheliomas for carcinoembryonic antigen

Reference	Cases examined	Cases positive	Cases negative
Wang et al.[81]	12	0	12
Whitaker and Shilkin[182]	40	0	40
Corson and Pinkus[183]	20	9	11
Kwee et al.[184]	7	0	37
Said et al.[185]	8	2	6
Ghosh et al.[186]	1	0	1
Holden and Churg[187]	22	8	14
Lee et al.[188]	43	15	28
Sheibani et al.[189]	28	2	26
Szpak et al.[190]	20	5	15
Jasani et al.[174]	44	0	44
Marshall et al.[177]	16	0	16
Hammar et al.[179]	65	1	64
Blattifora and Kopinski[180]	12	2	10
	368	44 (12%)	324 (88%)

elomonocytic origin. Leu M1 also immunostains Reed–Sternberg cells in some types of Hodgkins' disease. In 1985, Sheibani and Battifora[192] reported that Leu M1, also referred to as CD15, immunostained the tumor cells in a metastatic, poorly differentiated adenocarcinoma. In 1986, Sheibani et al.[195] performed an immunohistochemical analysis of 400 malignant neoplasms and found immunostaining in 105 of 179 adenocarcinomas for Leu M1, but no immunostaining in 18 epithelial mesotheliomas. Subsequently, they[194] studied the reactivity for Leu M1 in 50 primary pulmonary adenocarcinomas and 28 pleural epithelial mesotheliomas, finding a positive reaction in 47 (94%) of pulmonary adenocarcinomas and in none of the epithelial mesotheliomas. In another study,[195] they reported no immunostaining of tumor cells in 127 cases of malignant mesothelioma. However, Otis et al.[196] reported positive immunostaining of only 50% of the pulmonary adenocarcinomas they evaluated for Leu M1, a finding similar to what this author has observed. In addition we have observed several epithelial mesotheliomas that

have exhibited focal Leu M1 immunostaining (Figure 34–81).

Monoclonal antibody B72.3 is also used in distinguishing epithelial mesotheliomas from pulmonary adenocarcinomas. The antigen detected by B72.3 is called TAG-72 and has been isolated from a human cancer cell line. Szpak et al.[190] found B72.3 immunoreactivity in 19 of 22 (86%) pulmonary adenocarcinomas and in none of the 20 epithelial mesotheliomas they evaluated. In this author's experience, B72.3 has a low sensitivity with only approximately 20%–30% positive staining for pulmonary adenocarcinomas. We have also observed two epithelial mesotheliomas to show focal staining for B72.3 (unpublished observations).

A more recently developed, commercially available monoclonal antibody claimed to distinguish between epithelial mesotheliomas and pulmonary adenocarcinomas is designated Ber-EP4. Sheibani et al.[197] evaluated 83 adenocarcinomas and 120 epithelial mesotheliomas and found Ber-EP4 reactivity in 87% of adenocarcinomas and in only 1 epithelial mesothelioma. A subsequent report by Gaffey et al.[198] described focal and rarely diffuse immunostaining of mesothelioma tumor cells in 20% of epithelial mesotheliomas. Radosevich et al.[199] developed monoclonal antibody 44-3A6 from a human pulmonary adenocarcinoma cell line and in one study[188] reported strong immunostaining of neoplastic cells in 10 of 10 cases of pulmonary adenocarcinoma and focal work immunostaining of tumor cells in 10 of 43 epithelial mesotheliomas. Spagnolo et al.[200] evaluated immunohistochemical staining of cell block preparations of pleural fluid and fine-needle aspiration biopsy specimens from 24 cases of pulmonary adenocarcinoma and 36 cases of pleural

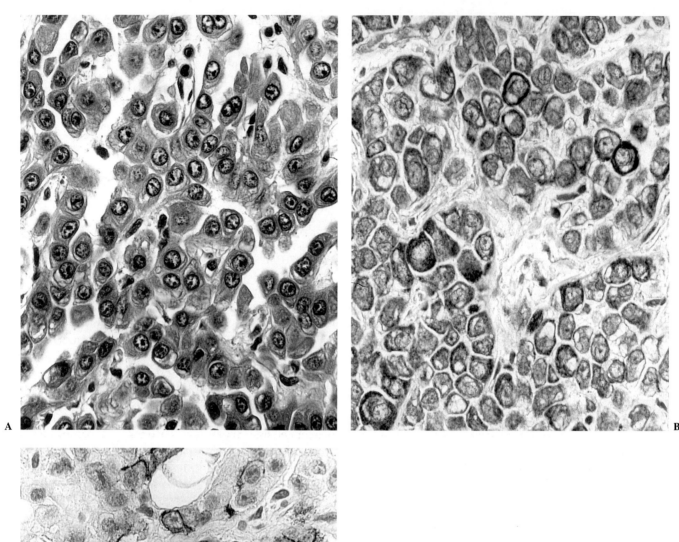

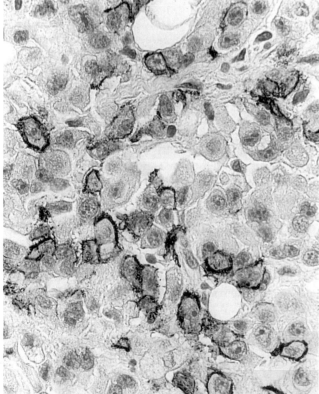

Fig. 34–81. "Solid" epithelial mesothelioma shows cell membrane and focal cytoplasmic immunostaining for Leu M1 of approximately 40% of neoplastic cells. **A,** ×550; **B,** ×550; **C,** ×550.

malignant mesothelioma with monoclonal antibody 44-3A6 and found positive immunostaining in 24 cases (100%) of pulmonary adenocarcinoma and 3 cases (8.3%) of epithelial mesothelioma.

Collins et al.[201] evaluated 31 cases of malignant mesothelioma and 48 pulmonary adenocarcinomas for the presence of thrombomodulin, a 575 amino acid of 75 kdaltons, using antithrombomodulin antibody. Thrombomodulin, which is normally found in a restricted number of cells including endothelial cells and mesothelial cells, was identified in all 31 cases of malignant mesothelioma and 4 (8%) cases of pulmonary adenocarcinomas, a sensitivity of 100% and specificity of 92% for mesotheliomas.

Jordan et al.[202] evaluated the usefulness of expression of blood group antigens Lewis[x] and Lewis[y] by immunohistochemistry using monoclonal antibodies against these two substances in differentiating epithelial mesotheliomas and pulmonary adenocarcinomas. All (18 of 18) adenocarcinomas showed diffuse, intense homogeneous and/or membranous immunostaining for Lewis[y] antigen and 78% showed variable immunostaining for Lewis[x] antigen. In contrast, 6 of 30 samples (20%) of mesothelioma showed focal granular cytoplasmic staining for Lewis[x] and 7 of 30 (23%) showed similar staining for Lewis[y] antigen. This author has no experience with these antibodies and cannot comment on their usefulness.

Noguchi et al.[203] evaluated the usefulness of antibodies against surfactant apoprotein, Lewis[a] antigen, and Tn antigen (precursor of Thomsen–Friedenreich antigen) to distinguish between 9 cases of malignant mesothelioma (epithelial and biphasic), 7 cases of adenomatoid tumor, and 21 cases of non-mucus-producing pulmonary adenocarcinoma. Lewis[a] antigen, Tn antigen, and surfactant apoprotein were detected in 76%, 62%, and 62%, respectively. Surfactant apoprotein and Tn antigen were not identified in any of the mesotheliomas; one mesothelioma expressed Lewis[a] antigen.

Kawai et al.[204] studied the expression of ABH blood group-related antigens and lectin Helix promatia agglutinin in 5 reactive mesothelial lesions, 29 mesotheliomas, (20 epithelial, 3 biphasic, 6 sarcomatoid), and 38 well-differentiated pulmonary adenocarcinomas. Reactive mesothelial proliferations and malignant mesotheliomas showed no immunostaining with antibody against ABH blood group antigens or binding with Helix promatia agglutinin. In contrast, 83% of pulmonary adenocarcinomas immunostained with the blood group antibody, and between 94% and 100% of those of blood group A or AB showed a positive reaction with Helix promotia agglutinin.

Wick et al.[205] evaluated the expression of non-Leu M1 myelomocytic antigens M1, LN1, LN2, and Mac 387 in 41 malignant epithelial mesotheliomas and 43 adenocarcinomas involving the pleural surfaces (pulmonary, "serous-surface papillary," and metastatic breast-adenocarcinomas). Three cases of peritoneal malignant epithelial mesothelioma and 1 pleural epithelial mesothelioma showed multifocal immunostaining for LN2 as did 39 of 43 adenocarcinomas. LN1 was expressed in 18 of 41 malignant mesotheliomas and 37 of 43 adenocarcinomas. None of the mesotheliomas or adenocarcinomas immunostained for Mac 387. In this author's opinion these other myelomonocytic markers are not specific enough to use in differentiating adenocarcinomas involving sersosal surfaces from peritoneal or pleural mesotheliomas.

Azumi et al.[206] used an immunoperoxidase technique to study 33 mesotheliomas and 37 adenocarcinomas for the presence of hyaluronate. Three of 37 adenocarcinomas and all mesotheliomas showed immunostaining for hyaluronate with 26 of 33 epithelial mesotheliomas showing a moderate to high-intensity reaction. The authors concluded that the demonstration of hyaluronate should be considered an important adjunct to be used with other immunohistochemical tests and electron microscopy, in diagnosing malignant epithelial mesotheliomas.

O'hara et al.[207] produced a monoclonal antibody designated ME1 that was reactive only in frozen sections and immunostained normal mesothelial cells and mesothelioma cells in 40 cases of malignant mesotheliomas. None of the 19 well to moderately differentiated adenocarcinomas showed immunostaining. The authors concluded that ME1 was the first monoclonal antibody to immunostain malignant mesothelial cells and was a useful reagent in differentiating pleural and peritoneal mesotheliomas from other types of neoplasms involving the serosal surfaces. Unfortunately, their antibody was reactive only in frozen-section material.

As reviewed by Sheibani et al.,[208] Dr. H. Battifora produced a monoclonal antibody designated HBME that appeared to immunostain the majority of epithelial mesotheliomas in formalin-fixed, paraffin-embedded tissue sections. In mesotheliomas, the pattern of immunostaining is in a cell membrane distribution (personal communication from Dr. Battifora, U.S./Canadian Mesothelioma Panel).

Rarely, unusual substances have been demonstrated immunohistochemically in malignant mesotheliomas. Okamoto et al.[209] described two unusual pleural neoplasms consistent with primary pleural mesotheliomas that contained anaplastic tumor giant cells that showed immunostaining for human chorionic gonadotropin. Both patients had high levels of serum human chorionic gonadotropin. McAuley et al.[210] evaluated a patient with malignant mesothelioma who had hypercalcemia and elevated plasma concentrations of parathyroid-like peptide. As a result of this observation, they evaluated nine epithelial mesotheliomas for the presence of parathyroid-like peptide and found abundant immunopositive cells in eight of nine cases. They also found strong cytoplasmic parathyroid-like peptide immunoreactivity in normal and reactive mesothelial cells. They concluded that parathyroid-like peptide immunoreactivity was common in normal, reactive and neoplastic mesothelial cells and that it might play a role in the production of hypercalcemia in those patients with mesothelioma who develop hypercalcemia. This author has seen two patients with malignant epithelial mesotheliomas, who developed inappropriate production of antidiuretic hormone and whose mesotheliomas showed immunostaining for vasopressin (unpublished observations).

Several other studies have shown the usefulness of immunohistochemistry in differentiating epithelial mesotheliomas from adenocarcinomas in tissue sections.[211–215] Similar studies have shown the effectiveness of performing such tests on cells in serous effusions.[216–220]

As shown in Table 34–10, sarcomatoid, transitional, desmoplastic, and anaplastic mesotheliomas coexpress keratin and vimentin. Rare cases may also express epithelial membrane antigen, and human milk fat globule protein. In this author's experience, about 30%–40% of desmoplastic mesotheliomas and 10% of sarcomatoid mesotheliomas express muscle-specific actin. The reason for this is explained in the section on **Histogenesis.**

As already mentioned, localized fibrous tumors of the pleura (sometimes referred to as localized fibrous mesotheliomas) show immunoreactivity only for vimentin.

A summary of the immunohistochemical findings is as follows: (1) Most epithelial mesotheliomas and pulmonary adenocarcinomas contain several different molecular species of keratin and also express epithelial membrane antigen and human milk fat globule protein: in epithelial mesothelioma, epithelial membrane antigen and human milk fat globule protein are expressed in cell membrane pattern whereas most pulmonary adenocarcinomas show a cytoplasmic staining location; (2) in general, all histologic types of mesotheliomas do not express carcinoembryonic antigen although the medical literature suggests that approximately 15% of epithelial mesotheliomas may express this antigen, usually showing a focal and weak immunostaining reaction; (3) most pulmonary adenocarcinomas and many other primary carcinomas of the lung express carcinoembryonic antigen; (4) sarcomatoid, desmoplastic, and transitional mesotheliomas characteristically coexpress keratin and vimentin. The literature reports that some

epithelial mesotheliomas also express vimentin as do some pulmonary adenocarcinomas and large cell undifferentiated carcinomas; (5) localized fibrous tumors of the pleura express vimentin but not keratin; (6) Leu M1 antigen is expressed in 50%–70% of pulmonary adenocarcinomas and in rare mesotheliomas (7) Ber EP4 is expressed in 50%–95% of pulmonary adenocarcinoma and focally in as many as 20% of epithelial mesotheliomas; (8) B72.3 is found in 20%–30% of pulmonary adenocarcinomas and rare epithelial mesotheliomas; and (9) Antibodies that may be relatively specific for epithelial mesotheliomas are being developed (e.g., HB-ME).

Ultrastructural Features of Mesotheliomas

Several reports in the medical literature have illustrated the ultrastructural features of mesotheliomas.[78,221–226] Similarly, the ultrastructural features of primary lung neoplasms have been described extensively (see Chapter 32). In my experience, epithelial mesotheliomas have ultrastructural features that can be used to differentiate them from pulmonary adenocarcinomas and other primary lung carcinomas; the converse is also true: Pulmonary adenocarcinomas and other primary lung carcinomas have electronmicroscopic characteristics that can be used to differentiate them from epithelial mesotheliomas. This does not mean that every epithelial mesothelioma or every primary pulmonary carcinoma looks identical by electron microscopy but that there are enough ultrastructural differences to allow their separation.

Ultrastructurally, tubulopapillary and other epithelial mesotheliomas are formed by cuboidal, polygonal, columnar, and round cells that are often connected to each other by well-formed desmosomes and junctional complexes (Fig. 34–82). Tumor cell nuclei are round, occasionally indented, and have medium-sized nucleoli. Their cytoplasm contains numerous mitochondria, short profiles of rough endoplasmic reticulum, and numerous intermediate filaments that are often aggregated into tonofilaments, which insert into large desmosomes connecting the cells together (Fig. 34–83). The most conspicuous ultrastructural feature of these cells are the numerous long, slender, sinuous microvilli that arise from the cell surface (Fig. 34–84). These are often referred to as bushy microvilli. The cells are characteristically separated from the fibrovascular tissue by a well-defined basal lamina that is often infolded and is associated with micropinocytotic vesicles in the cell membrane of the adjacent mesothelial cells (Fig. 34–85). Epithelioid epithelial mesotheliomas are composed of round cells that have ultrastructural features similar to those of tubulopapillary mesotheliomas. They

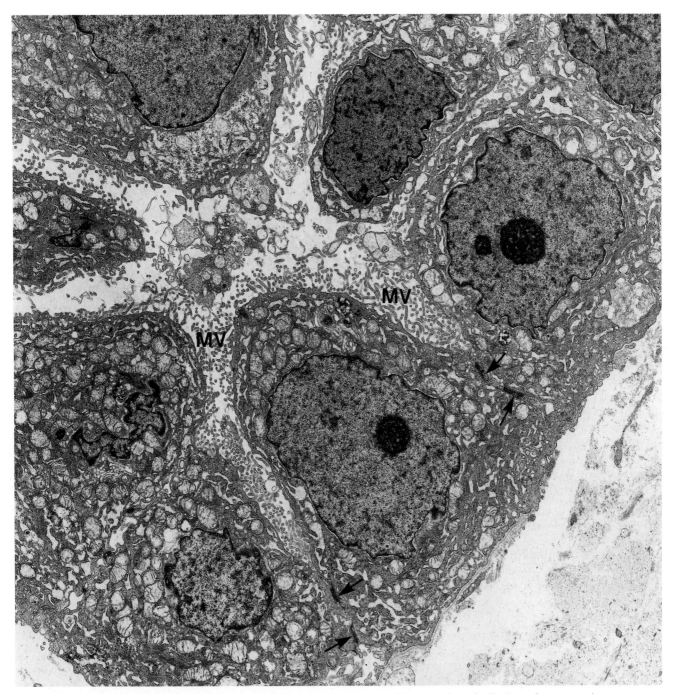

Fig. 34–82. Electron micrograph shows representative region of tubulopapillary mesothelioma. Tumor cells are similar in size and shape and are connected to each other by well-formed desmosomes (*arrows*). Round nuclei located near center of cell have medium-sized nucleoli. Cytoplasm contains numerous mitochondria and other organelles. Note microvilli (Mv) arising from cell surface. ×6,400.

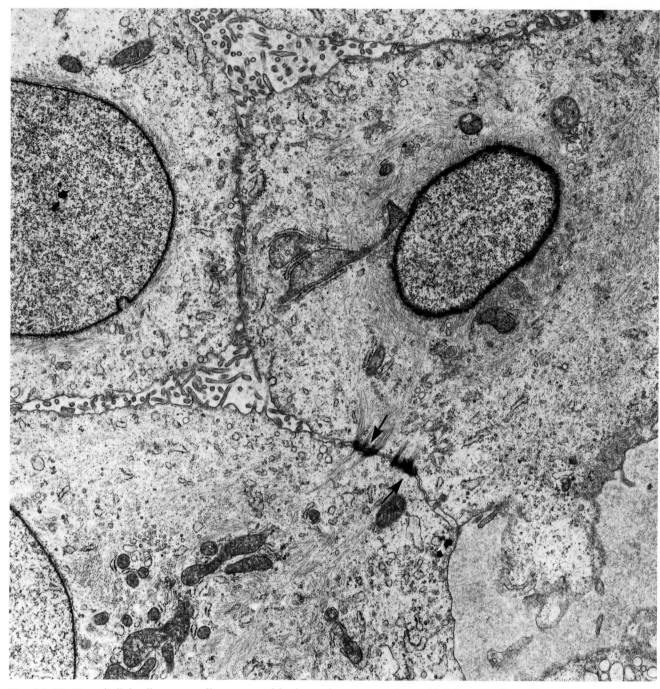

Fig. 34–83. Mesothelial cells are usually connected by large desmosomes into which intermediate filaments insert (*arrows*). ×10,600.

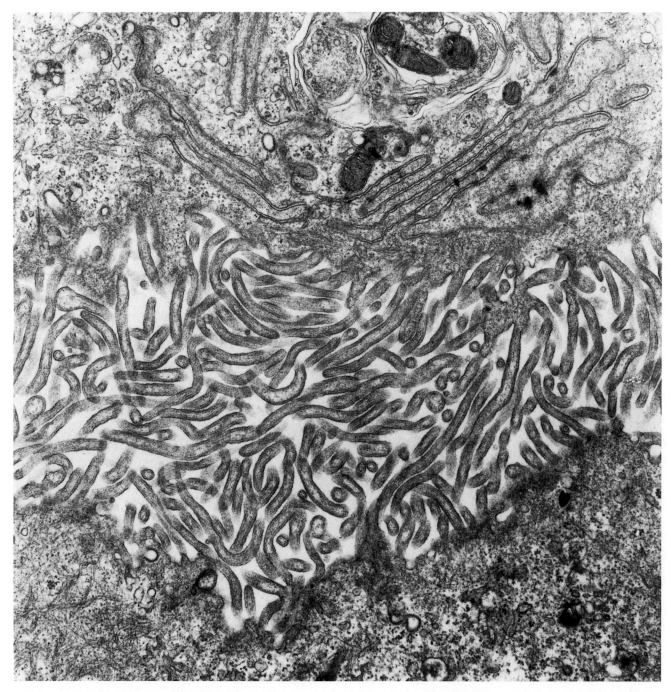

Fig. 34–84. Most characteristic feature of epithelial mesothelioma cells is long sinuous microvilli. These have length-to-width ratios averaging 10 to 15, significantly greater than length-to-width ratio of microvilli of pulmonary adenocarcinomas, and are not covered by a fuzzy glycocalyx. ×16,000.

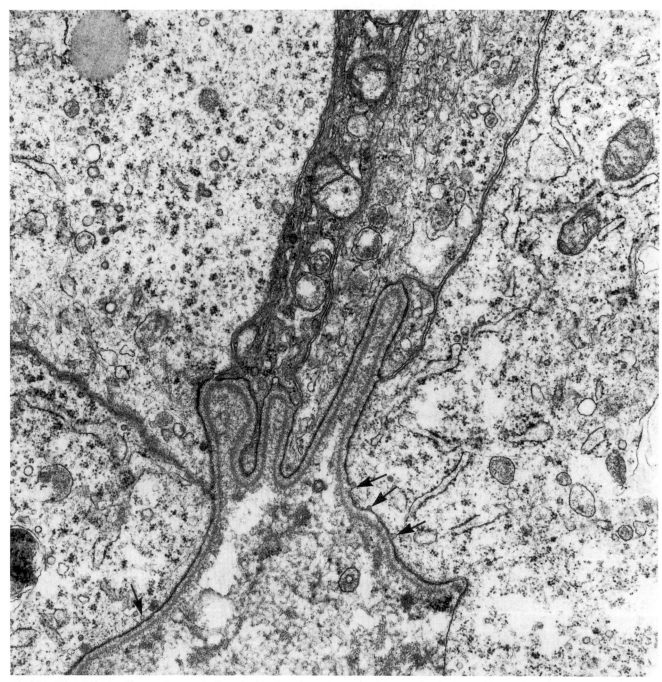

Fig. 34–85. Portions of several mesothelioma cells show invagination of their cytoplasm and investment by basal lamina (BL). Note micropinocytotic vesicles in cell membrane of tumor cells (*arrows*). ×25,500.

have long cell-surface microvilli, numerous cytoplasmic intermediate filaments including tonofilaments, and aggregates of cytoplasmic glycogen (Fig. 34–86). Small cell mesotheliomas have nonspecific ultrastructural features and lack cell-surface microvilli (Fig. 34–87).

As stated previously, about 20% of epithelial mesotheliomas produce a mucosubstance, hyaluronic acid,

that can be identified ultrastructurally as a medium electron-dense material associated with the cell microvilli (Fig. 34–88). This material is present in intracellular neolumens and often crystallizes (Fig. 34–89). It also may form scroll-like crystalline structures (Fig. 34–90). This "crystalloid" material probably represents hyaluronic acid.

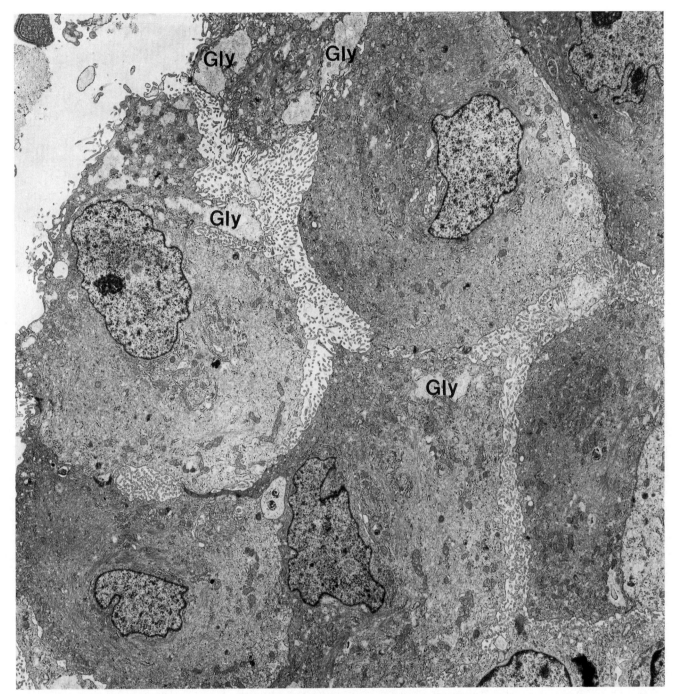

Fig. 34–86. Ultrastructural appearance of epithelioid mesothelioma. Cells are round with abundant intracellular intermediate filaments and aggregates of glycogen (Gly). Note long thin cell-surface microvilli (Mv). ×6,400.

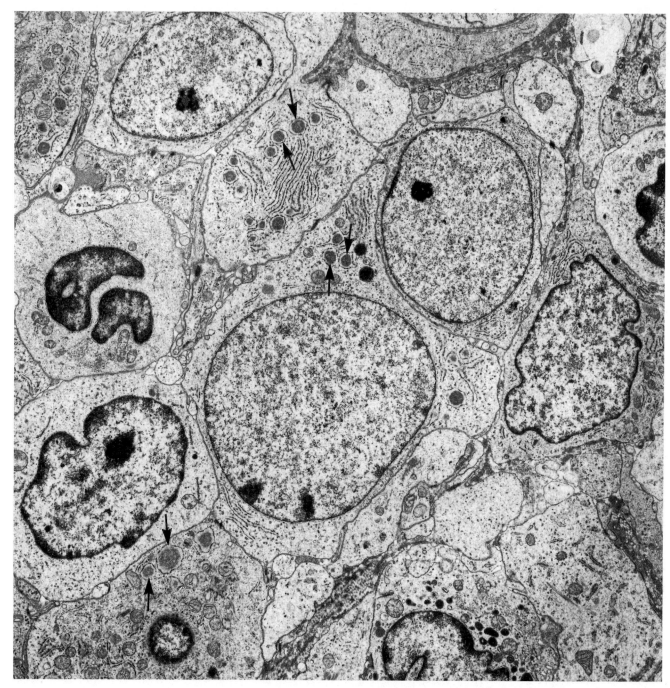

Fig. 34–87. Small cell epithelial mesotheliomas are composed of cells with nonspecific ultrastructural features. These cells are round to polygonal and contain some rough endoplasmic reticulum with some inspissated material in cisterna (*arrows*). ×6,400.

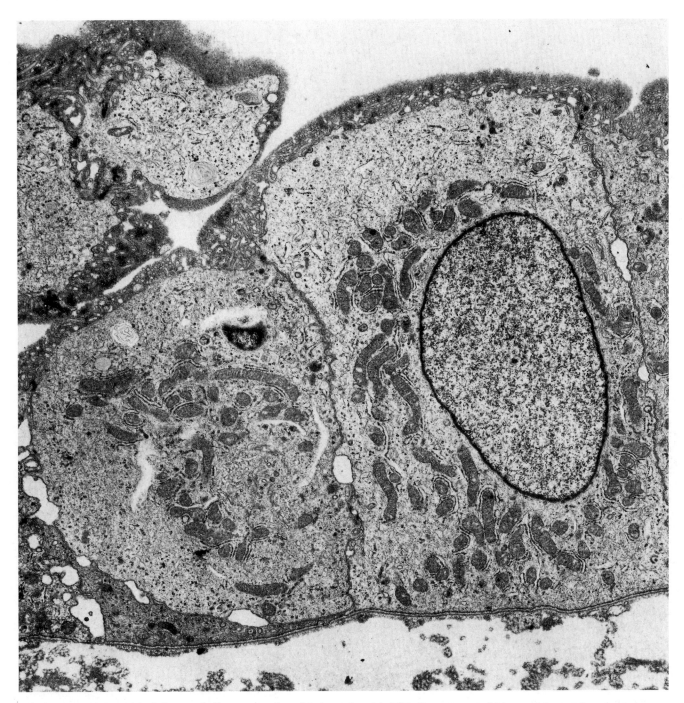

Fig. 34–88. Some epithelial mesotheliomas produce hyaluronic acid. This is not seen within cytoplasm of tumor cells but appears as medium electron-dense material on cell surface in which microvilli are "embedded." ×10,500.

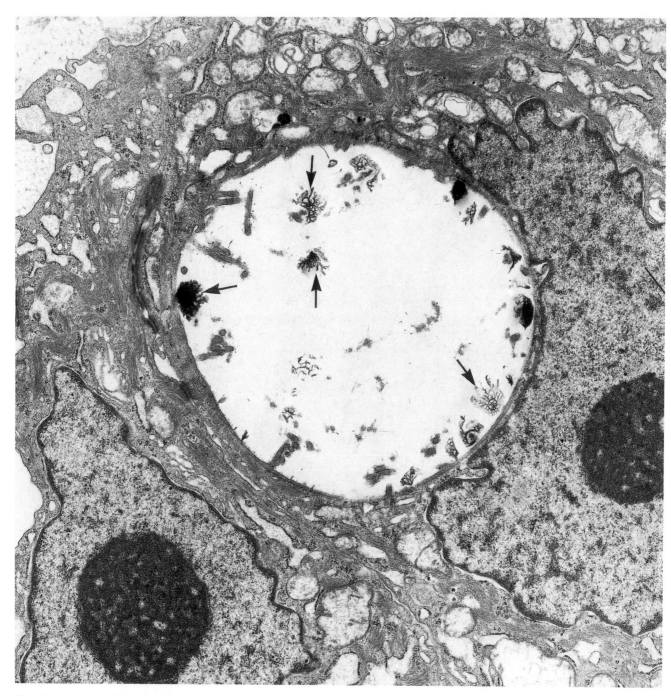

Fig. 34–89. Intracellular lumen in mesothelioma cell shows crystallized mucosubstance (*arrows*) that has fernlike appearance. ×16,000.

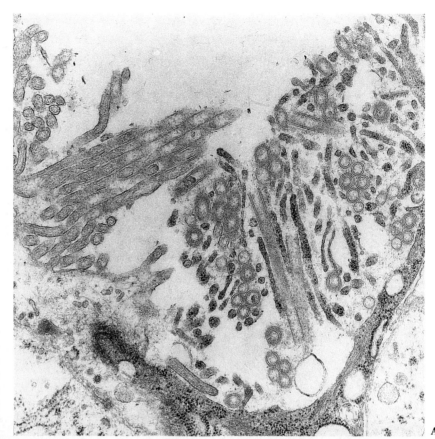

Fig. 34–90 A,B. A. In this hyaluronic acid-producing epithelial mesothelioma, hyaluronic acid crystallized to form hollow tubular structures with a scroll-like appearance on cross section. **B.** In cross-section, the hyaluronic acid crystals have a scroll-like morphology and resemble hollow chrysotile fibrils. **A,** ×42,000; **B,** ×69,000.

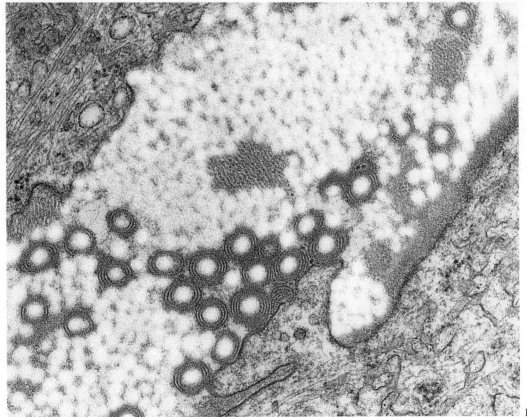

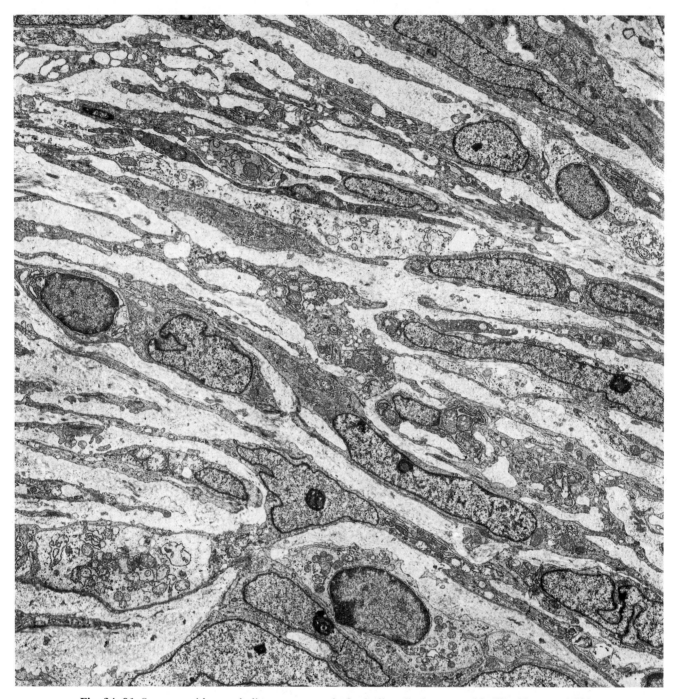

Fig. 34–91. Sarcomatoid mesothelioma composed of spindle cells that resemble fibroblasts. ×4,200.

Sarcomatoid mesotheliomas have variable ultrastructural features. The tumor cells may resemble fibroblasts (Fig. 34–91), containing short profiles of distended rough endoplasmic reticulum, a prominent golgi appartatus, and occasionally inspissated electron-dense material in the cisterna of the rough endoplasmic reticulum. Other sarcomatoid mesotheliomas show more variability in size and shape (Figs. 34–92 and 34–93) and not infrequently may show epithelial differentiation by the presence of well-formed intercellular junctions (Fig. 34–94) and basal lamina formation (Fig. 34–95) and tonofilaments (Fig. 34–96). They may even show a few microvilli arising from the cell surface (Fig. 34–97). Some desmoplastic and sarcomatous mesotheliomas have an ultrastructural appearance resembling myofibroblasts, containing peripherally located actin fila-

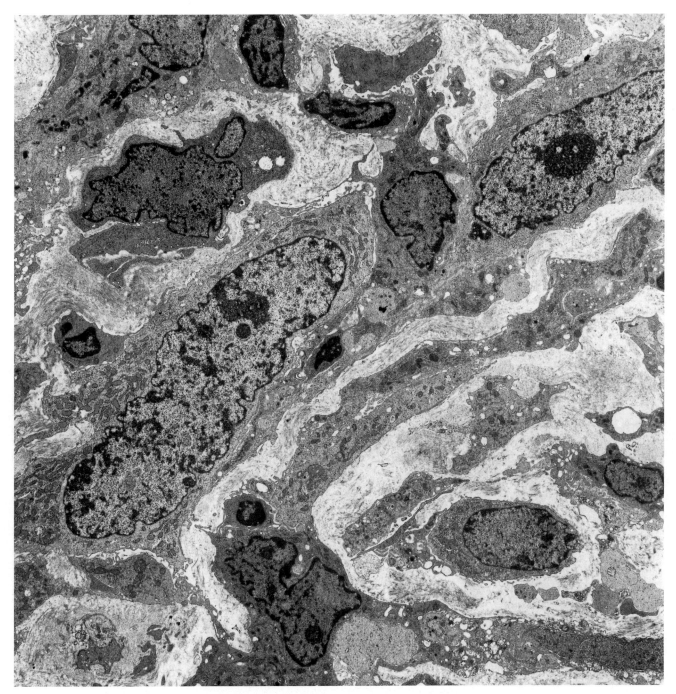

Fig. 34–92. Sarcomatoid mesothelioma shows more variability in size and shape of tumor cells. ×6,400.

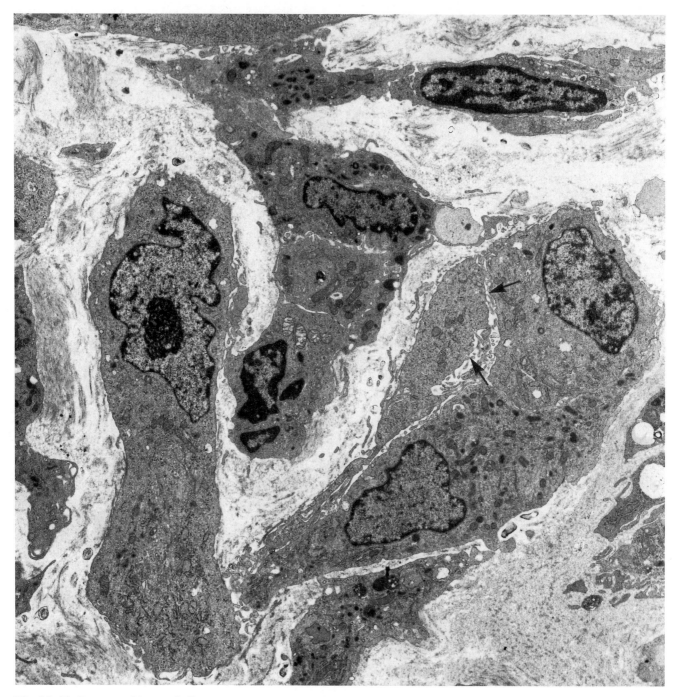

Fig. 34–93. Sarcomatoid mesothelioma composed mostly of spindle-shaped cells with large nuclei. An occasional cell shows a few cell-surface microvilli (*arrows*). ×6,400.

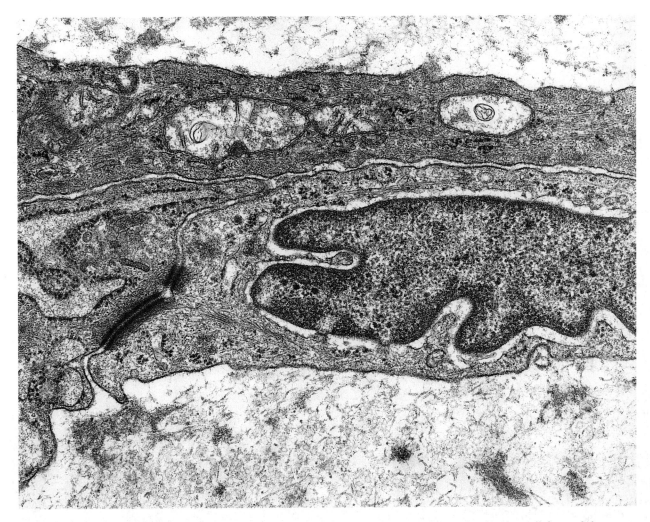

Fig. 34–94. Some neoplastic cells in this sarcomatoid mesothelioma are connected to each other by well-formed demosomes.

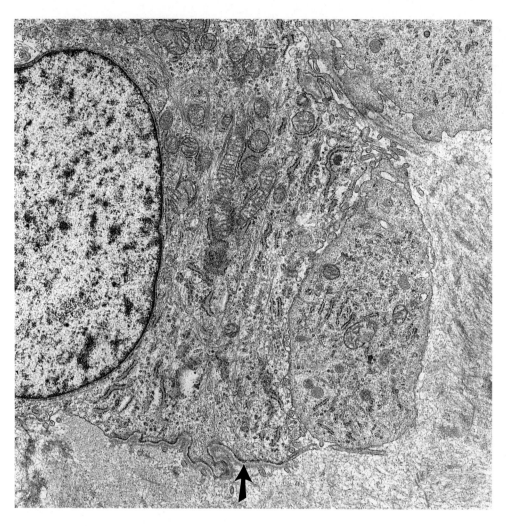

Fig. 34–95. Some neoplastic cells forming this sarcomatoid mesothelioma are surrounded by basal lamina (*arrow*). ×10,400.

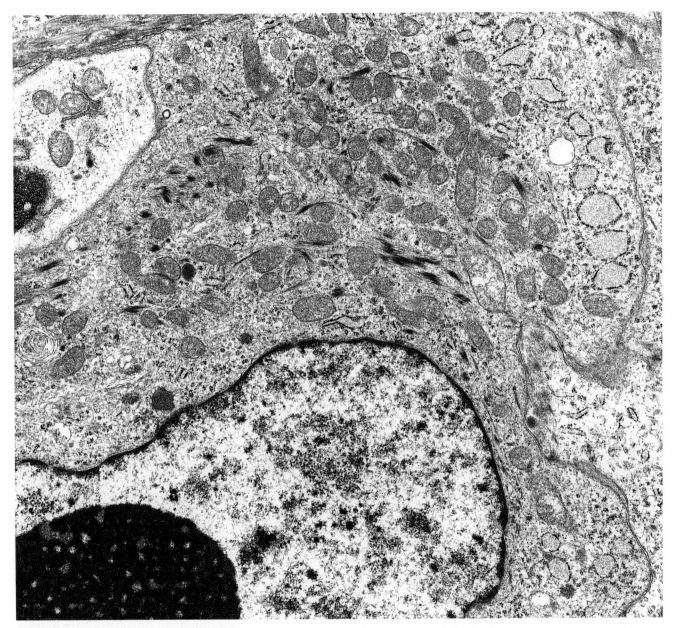

Fig. 34–96. In this sarcomatoid mesothelioma, many neoplastic cells contain aggregates of intermediate filaments in their cytoplasm, consistent with tonofilaments. ×16,000.

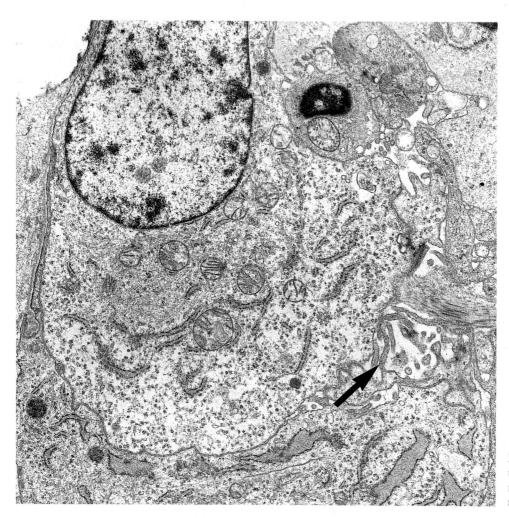

Fig. 34–97. In this sarcomatoid mesothelioma, a few tumor cells show microvilli (*arrow*). ×10,400.

ments and centrally located short profiles of rough endoplasmic reticulum[227] (Fig. 34–98). Desmoplastic mesotheliomas have variable ultrastructural features, being composed of cells that resemble fibroblasts or myofibroblasts.

Transitional mesotheliomas are composed of cells with electron microscopic features of both epithelial and mesenchymal cells. The tumor cells are frequently connected to each other by relatively well-formed intercellular junctions, have aggregated mitochondria, and have cytoplasmic intermediate filaments that may represent vimentin (Figs. 34–99 and 34–100). In some tumor cells, thin actin filaments are observed in association with the cell membrane. The tumor cells usually do not show the long, sinuous microvilli observed in epithelial mesotheliomas.

The epithelial component of biphasic mesotheliomas has the ultrastructural features of typical epithelial mesotheliomas with long bushy cell-surface microvilli and abundant intracellular tonofilaments and other organelles. The sarcomatoid portion is composed of cells with electron microscopic characteristics of sarcomatoid mesotheliomas. In transition zones, the tumor cells may have an ultrastructural appearance of transitional mesotheliomas with some cells expressing epithelial features and other cells sarcomatoid features.

Localized fibrous tumors of the pleura have a somewhat nondescript appearance, being composed of spindle-shaped cells with nondescript features. (Figs. 34–101 and 34–102). Many cells have processes that are closely associated with an adjacent cell process, and have relatively few cytoplasmic organelles, without the usual abundance of endoplasmic reticulum common to fibroblasts. With respect to localized fibrous tumors of the pleura Briselli et al.[150] found focal ultrastructural regions of "epithelial" differentiation in a study of 8 such neoplasms. Doucet et al.[151] also identified focal epithelial features by electron microscopy and reported that 1 of 10 localized fibrous mesotheliomas examined expressed cytokeratin immunohistochemically. Epstein and Budin,[228] however, reported that none of the 5 localized fibrous mesotheliomas they studied immuno-

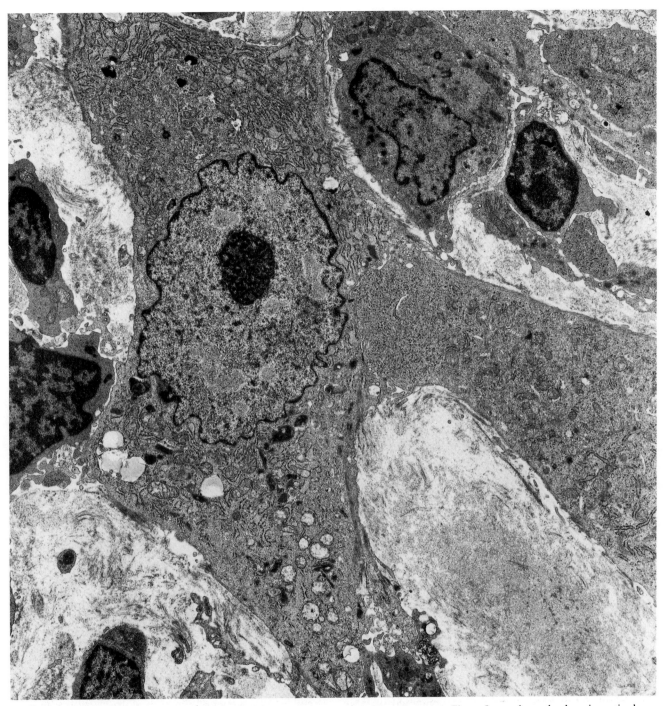

Fig. 34–98. Some cells of this sarcomatoid mesothelioma have ultrastructural features of myofibroblasts, with peripherally located thin filaments consistent with actin filaments and abundant short profiles of rough endoplasmic reticulum. ×6,400.

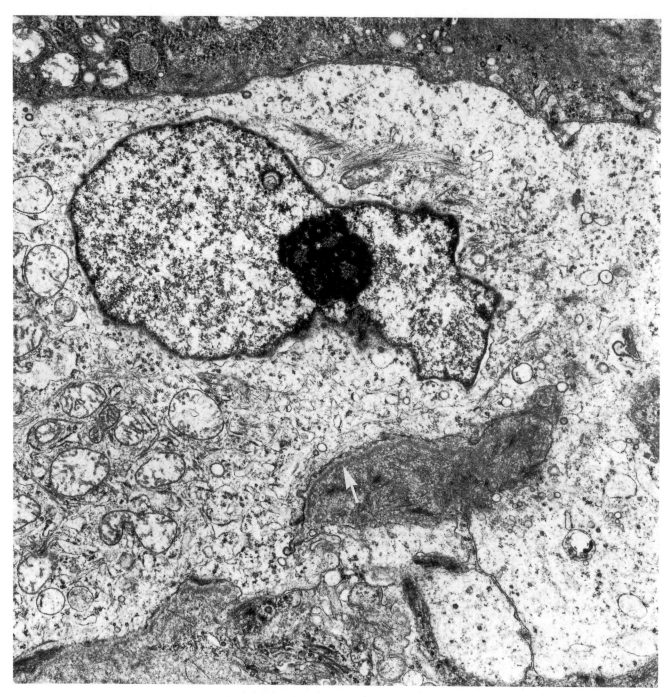

Fig. 34–99. Transitional mesothelioma composed of large polygonal cells with large nuclei and relatively nonspecialized cytoplasm. A few intermediate filaments in cell cytoplasm resemble tonofilaments. Note focal basal lamina (*arrow*). ×6,400.

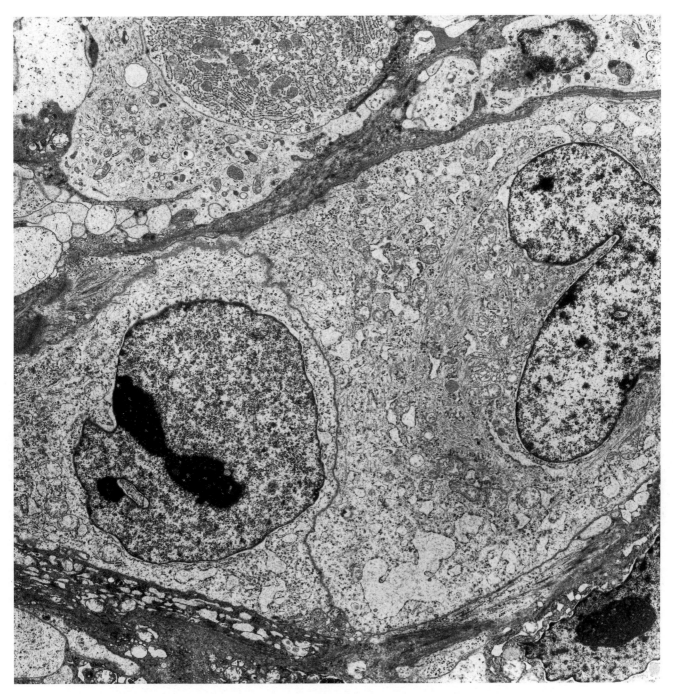

Fig. 34–100. Region of transitional mesothelioma with nondescript ultrastructural features. ×10,500.

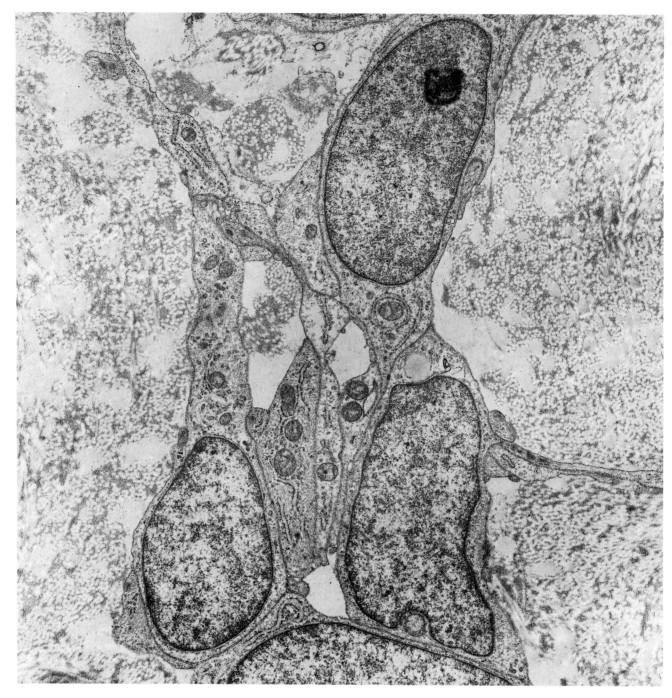

Fig. 34–101. Representative region of localized fibrous tumor of pleura; tumor cells are mostly spindle shaped but have long processes in association with processes from adjacent cells. ×6,400.

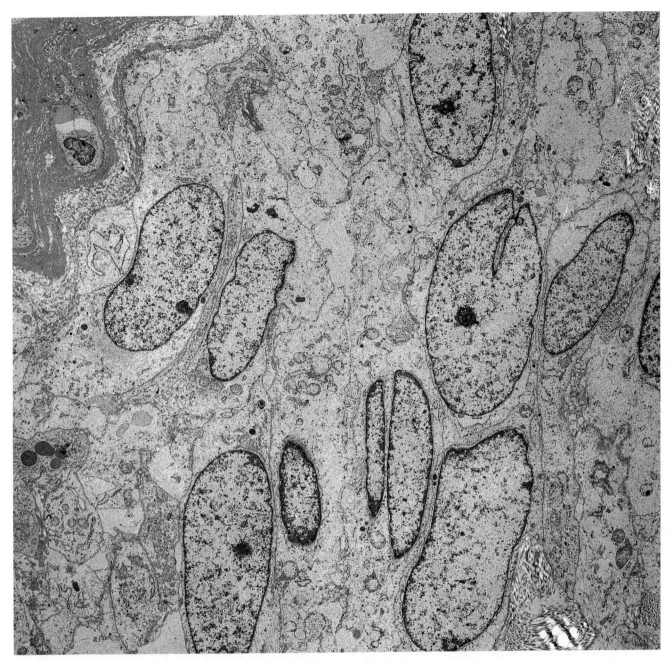

Fig. 34–102. This benign localized fibrous tumor of the pleura is slightly more cellular than the one shown in Fig. 34–101. The tumor cells contain few cytoplasmic organelles and are relatively unspecialized. ×4,100.

histochemically expressed cytokeratin or epithelial membrane antigen; Erlandson et al.[229] and el-Naggar et al.[230] reported finding only vimentin in the localized fibrous mesotheliomas they evaluated.

Most of the controversy concerning the ultrastructural features of mesotheliomas has centered around epithelial mesotheliomas, specifically with respect to whether they can be differentiated electron microscopically from pulmonary adenocarcinomas or other types of adenocarcinomas. Warhol et al.[231] and Warhol and

Corson[232] studied quantitatively the difference between the microvilli of epithelial mesotheliomas and pulmonary and breast adenocarcinomas. They found that the mean length-to-diameter ratio of epithelial mesothelioma microvilli was 15.7 whereas pulmonary adenocarcinoma microvilli had a length-to-diameter ratio of 8.7. Burns et al.[233] found similar results with a mean length-to-diameter ratio of 11.44 for seven epithelial mesotheliomas and 5.39 for three pulmonary adenocarcinomas. Warhol and colleagues also found

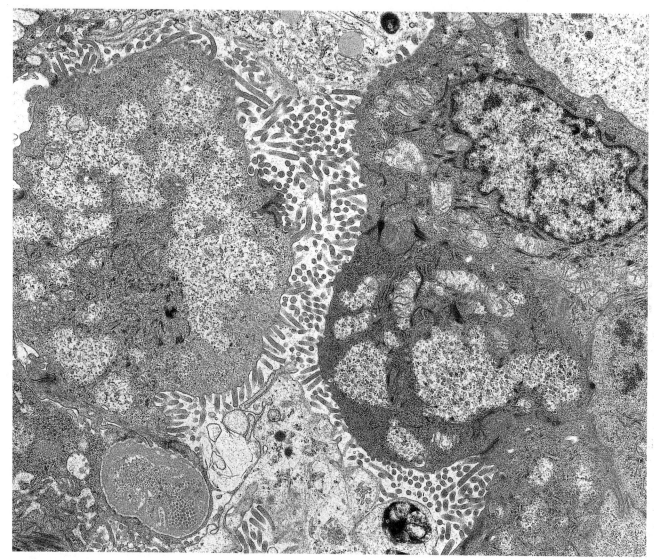

Fig. 34–103. Peripheral pulmonary adenocarcinoma had long slender microvilli resembling those seen in epithelial mesothelioma. ×10,400.

that epithelial mesotheliomas had more cytoplasmic tonofilaments than pulmonary adenocarcinomas. We[78,179] have emphasized the overall difference in the pattern of the microvilli of epithelial mesotheliomas and pulmonary adenocarcinomas. As shown, the microvilli of epithelial mesotheliomas are numerous, long, and sinuous, whereas the microvilli of pulmonary adenocarcinomas are often short, straight, and covered by a fuzzy glycocalyx (see Chapter 32). This author does not believe it is usually necessary to determine the length-to-width ratio of microvilli to tell the difference between epithelial mesothelioma and pulmonary adenocarcinoma. However, rare pulmonary adenocarcinomas exist that have relatively long microvilli and at first glance may resemble an epithelial mesothelioma (Fig. 34–103), but on closer inspection are covered by fuzzy microvilli

(Fig. 34–104), a finding incompatible with an epithelial mesothelioma.

There are also other ultrastructural differences between epithelial mesotheliomas and pulmonary adenocarcinomas. The cells forming both neoplasms are connected to each other by intercellular junctions. Where the tumor cells form glands, they are attached by junctional complexes and elsewhere are connected predominantly by desmosomes. As a general rule, the desmosomes connecting mesothelioma tumor cells are larger than those connecting pulmonary adenocarcinoma cells. This observation has been confirmed by a recently published semiquantitative study.[234]

As stated and shown previously, about 20% of epithelial mesotheliomas produce the mucosubstance hyalu-

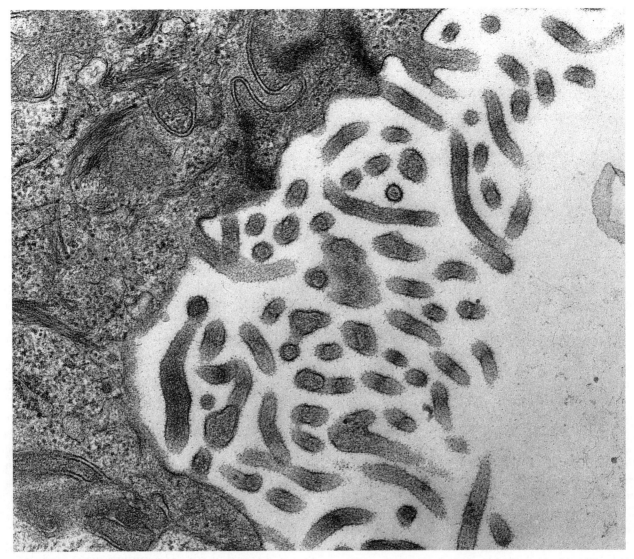

Fig. 34–104. At greater magnification, long microvilli of neoplastic cells shown in Fig. 34–104 were covered by fuzzy glycocalyx, a finding not seen in epithelial mesothelioma. ×50,600.

ronic acid, which can be identified ultrastructurally as a medium-electron-dense material in which the cell microvilli appear embedded. Hyaluronic acid-producing mesotheliomas do not contain mucosubstance granules in their cytoplasm, which is in contrast to the 60%–75% of pulmonary adenocarcinomas that are mucus producing and contain cytoplasmic mucus granules of variable size and density that are often associated with a prominent terminal web (see Chapter 32). Pulmonary adenocarcinomas of Clara cell or type II pneumocyte origin frequently contain cytoplasmic multivesicular bodies and lamellar bodies. These structures are not seen in epithelial mesotheliomas. A comparison of some of the ultrastructural features of epithelial mesotheliomas and pulmonary adenocarcinomas is shown in Table 34–12.

As described, the ultrastructural features of other types of mesotheliomas are more variable and less specific than epithelial mesotheliomas. Sarcomatoid mesotheliomas may be indistinguishable from soft tissue sarcomas, although they often show areas of epithelial differentiation.

Transitional mesotheliomas usually show cells with epithelial and mesenchymal features. The tumor cells usually do not have cell-surface microvilli but may contain cytoplasmic tonofilaments and be connected to each other by an occasional desmosome. As shown, some desmoplastic and sarcomatoid mesotheliomas may exhibit ultrastructural features of myofibroblasts containing short profiles of rough endoplasmic reticulum and peripherally located thin actin filaments.

Table 34–12. Comparison of the ultrastructural features of epithelial mesothelioma and pulmonary adenocarcinoma

Ultrastructural feature	Epithelial mesothelioma	Pulmonary adenocarcinoma
Microvilli	Long, sinuous, smooth	Short, usually straight; Covered by fuzzy glycocalyx
Intercellular junctions	Junctional complexes; Large desmosomes	Junctional complexes; Small desmosomes
Mucosubstance production	No mucosubstance granules in cytoplasm; Mucosubstance on cell surface; Crystallization	Mucus granules in cytoplasm; glycocalyceal bodies; mucus in gland lumen
Cytoplasmic intermediate filaments	Abundant; Often in a perinuclear distribution; Tonofilaments frequent	Common; often distributed throughout cytoplasm; tonofilaments variable
Cytoplasmic inclusions	Infrequent; some lysosomes	Frequent; multivesicular bodies and lamellar bodies frequent in bronchioalveolar cell carcinoma

Cytogenetic Abnormalities

Two recent reports discussed the cytogenetic abnormalities found in malignant mesotheliomas. Tiainen et al.[235] performed successful cytogenetic analyses on cells obtained from solid tumors and from pleural effusions in 34 of 38 patients with malignant mesothelioma. Clonal chromosomal abnormalities were detected in 25 patients, the majority being complex and heterogeneous with no chromosome abnormality specific to mesothelioma. Nine patients had normal karyotypes or nonclonal chromosomal abnormalities. Translocations and deletions involving a breakpoint at 1p11-p22 were the most common structural abnormality. The number of copies of chromosome 7 short arms was inversely correlated with survival, and a high concentration of asbestos fibers in the lung tissue was associated with partial or total losses of chromosomes 1 and 4, and a breakpoint at 1p11-p22.

Hagemeijer et al.[236] evaluated 40 confirmed cases of malignant mesothelioma in 90% of cases using malignant cells in pleural fluids. A normal karyotype was found in 9 cases, and complex karyotypic abnormalities were identified in 30 cases. The chromosomal changes were all complex and heterogeneous, with no consistent specific abnormality found. Two main patterns of nonrandom abnormalities were found: (1) loss of chromosomes 4 and 22, 9p and 30p in the most abnormal cases, corresponding to a hypodiploid and for hypotetraploid modal chromosome number; and (2) gain of chromosomes 7, 5, and 20 with deletion or rearrangement of 3p.

DNA Analysis and Proliferative Index in Malignant Mesothelioma

DNA concentrations or proliferative rates have been evaluated in reactive mesothelial cell proliferations and in malignant mesothelioma[231–238] (Table 34–13). Croonen et al.[237] evaluated malignant cells in 11 pleural fluids and two ascitic fluids from 6 patients with malignant mesothelioma, 5 proven by biopsy, and found DNA-euploid cells in 10 of 13 effusions. They concluded that mesotheliomas were usually DNA-euploid whereas most adenocarcinomas were aneuploid.

Cytophotometry was used by Hafiz et al.[238] to evaluate the DNA content of cells in Feulgen-stained sections of effusion specimens from 18 patients with malignant mesothelioma and 14 patients with reactive mesothelial proliferations, and found the mean DNA content of malignant mesothelial cells (30.5 ± 7.2) was significantly higher than the mean DNA content of reactive mesothelial cells (15.2 ± 2.9).

Friersson et al.[239] compared the DNA content in cell preparations made from 28 fresh effusion specimens that contained numerous proliferating mesothelial cells with ploidy profiles of cells obtained from 19 formalin-fixed, paraffin-embedded malignant mesotheliomas. Cytologically benign cells in the pleural fluid specimens were all DNA diploid. Malignant cells from 9 of 19 mesotheliomas were diploid, 7 contained an aneuploid population, and 3 had a flow cytometric pattern suggesting hyperdiploidy. The authors concluded that although only 53% of epithelial mesotheliomas were aneuploid, the finding of DNA aneuploid cells in an effusion specimen supported the diagnosis of malignant mesothelioma.

Burmer et al.[240] evaluated the DNA content of 46 cases of malignant pleural mesothelioma and found most to be DNA diploid with low to intermediate proliferative rates, whereas 85% of primary lung carcinomas were DNA aneuploid and had high proliferative rates.

Dazzi et al.[241] studied tumor tissue from 168 formalin-fixed, paraffin-embedded specimens from 70 patients with malignant pleural mesothelioma (31 epithelial, 21 sarcomatous, 18 mixed) by DNA analysis. They found that 38.6% of mesotheliomas were diploid and 61.4% were aneuploid; a higher percentage of the epithelial mesotheliomas were diploid. The authors found no significant difference in survival in the patients whose mesotheliomas were aneuploid versus diploid. Patients whose tumor showed an S-phase percent-

Table 34–13. DNA indices and proliferative rates of malignant mesotheliomas versus reactive mesothelial cells and other non-mesothelial malignant neoplasms

Study	Malignant mesothelioma					Reactive mesothelial cells					Non-mesothelioma malignant neoplasms				
	# of "cases"/ specimens	DNA index		S phase		# of "cases"/ specimens	DNA index		S phase		# of "cases"/ specimens	DNA index		S phase	
		Diploid	Aneuploid	≤6%	>6%		Diploid	Aneuploid	≤6%	>6%		Diploid	Aneuploid	≤6%	>6%
Croonen et al.[237]	13[a]	10	3[b]	ND	ND	45[a]	40	5[c]	ND	ND	29[a]	7[d]	22	ND	ND
Hafiz et al.[238]	18[e]	30.5±[f]	7.2[f]	ND	ND	14[e]	15.2[f]	±2.9[f]	ND	ND	—	—	—	—	—
Frierson et al.[239]	19[g]	9	10[i]	ND	ND	28[h]	28	0	ND	ND	—	—	—	—	—
Burmer et al.[240]	46[j]	30[k]	15[l]	23[m]	22[m]	—	—	—	—	—	31[n]	4[o]	27[o]	15[p]	15[p]
Dazzi et al.[241]	70[q]	3[r]	34[r]	19[s]	36[s]	—	—	—	—	—	—	—	—	—	—
Teirney et al.[242]	25[t]	u	u	ND	ND	11[t]	u	u	ND	ND	20[t]	—	20	ND	ND
El-Naggar et al.[243]	23[v]	18	6[w]	x	x	—	—	—	—	—	41[y]	5[z]	36[z]	aa	aa
Esteban & Sheibani[244]	45[bb]	30	5	cc	5[cc]	—	—	—	—	—	41[dd]	10	31	ee	ee

[a] Malignant cells in pleural/peritoneal fluids.

[b] Autopsy diagnosis was lung adenocarcinoma in two cases.

[c] In 2 of 54 cases there was an associated malignancy, but no evidence of malignancy on followup.

[d] In one case a primary tumor was not identified, and there was no evidence of recurrence or metastases.

[e] Cells in pleural or peritoneal fluid.

[f] Mean DNA content of 50 mesothelial cells in arbitrary absorbance units as determined by analysis of Feulgen-stained cells. TheDNA content of mesothelial cells was compared to the DNA content of lymphocytes.

[g] Deparaffinized malignant epithelial mesothelioma.

[h] Reactive cells in pleural or peritoneal effusions.

[i] None of the malignant epithelial mesotheliomas had multiple aneuploid peaks.

[j] Of the 46 mesotheliomas, 30 were epithelial, 5 were sarcomatous, and 11 were biphasic.

[k] Diploid or near-diploid.

[l] All but two of the aneuploid mesotheliomas exhibited a single aneuploid peak. No significant difference between percentage of aneuploid mesotheliomas according to histologic type.

[m] Only "fresh" tissue specimens were analyzed and one case could not be evaluated. Average S-phase for diploid mesotheliomas was 5.0% (17 cases) and 8.7% for aneuploid mesotheliomas (10 cases). No significant correlation between S phase and histologic subtype.

[n] 7 primary pulmonary adenocarcinomas, 6 primary poorly differentiated squamous carcinomas; 3 primary poorly differentiated carcinomas, not otherwise specified, 4 primary lung sarcomas, 3 metastatic sarcomas, 4 metastatic breast carcinomas, and 4 metastatic renal cell carcinomas.

[o] Non-mesothelioma malignant tumors that were diploid included 1 primary pulmonary adenocarcinoma, 1 metastatic renal cell carcinoma, 1 primary pulmonary sarcoma, and 1 metastatic sarcoma.

[p] One case could not be analyzed.

[q] 168 paraffinembedded tissue specimens from 70 patients with malignant pleural mesothelioma. 31 epithelial mesotheliomas, 21 sarcomatoid mesotheliomas and 18 biphasic mesotheliomas.

[r] 37 cases diploid or near-diploid, 34 cases aneuploid or multi-aneuploid.

[s] S phase % could be calculated in 55 cases. Range was 0.8–16.1%, median S phase was 6%.

[t] Feulgen stained nuclei of 100 tumor cells/reactive cells were measured using a DNA image analyzer. Lymphocyte nuclei were used as controls. Aneuploidy determined by measuring 5c exceeding rate (5cER), which was defined as the percentage of aneuploid cells having a DNA content >5 c where diploid = 2c. Previous studies suggested a 5cER or greater than 0.1 was malignant. In this study, a 5cER of 1 was used as a cut-off for malignancy.

[u] Information not given. Using the cut-off of 1 for 5cER (see (t)), 14 "mesothelial" cases were classified as benign, and 22 as malignant, which equated to a false-negative rate of 57% and a false-positive rate of 23%. All of the non-mesothelial tumors had a 5cER >1, which indicated they were aneuploid.

[v] All cases were of pleural origin and had epithelial histology. Tumor tissue from multiple blocks were analyzed.

[w] The mesotheliomas that were aneuploid exhibited a "solid" growth pattern.

[x] S + G_2M of 18 diploid mesotheliomas was 5.83 ± 2.62 SD. S + G_2M of 5 aneuploid mesotheliomas was 5.0 ± 1.23 SD.

[z] Of the 36 aneuploid pulmonary adenocarcinomas, 31 were well to moderately differentiated, and 5 were poorly differentiated. Of the 5 diploid pulmonary adenocarcinomas, 4 were well to moderately differentiated, and one was poorly differentiated.

[aa] SG_2M of 5 diploid pulmonary adenocarcinomas was 12 ± 7.48 SD. SG_2M for 36 aneuploid pulmonary adenocarcinomas was 16.42 ± 10.21 SD.

[bb] 31 epithelial mesotheliomas, 6 sarcomatoid mesotheliomas, 8 biphasic mesotheliomas. Five of the 45 mesotheliomas could not be analyzed because the histograms obtained were uninterpretable; 5 other cases of mesothelioma were excluded because the CVs were >9.

[cc] Not all cases could be analyzed; in most aneupoid mesotheliomas the S phase could not be determined. Five (17) of the diploid mesotheliomas had an S phase >10%.

[dd] All cases were pulmonary adenocarcinomas.

[ee] Nine of the diploid adenocarcinomas had an S phase >10%.

Abbreviation: ND, not done.

age greater than the median of 6% had a significantly shorter survival than those whose tumors had a lower S-phase percentage.

Tierney et al.[242] determined DNA cellular concentrations using DNA image analysis of Feulgen-stained tissue sections in a series of 56 pleural lesions, including reactive proliferations, malignant mesotheliomas, and metastatic tumors. Of the 36 cases of primary mesothe-lial lesions, data indicated that 11 were benign lesions and 25 were malignant mesotheliomas. As determined by pathologic diagnosis, there were 8 false-negative benign interpretations and 5 false-positive malignant interpretations. The authors concluded that mesothe-lial lesions appeared to have a wide range of ploidy values regardless of their biological behavior, and that ploidy could not be used as a reliable diagnostic index in diagnosing primary mesothelial tumors. With respect to metastatic neoplasms, DNA analysis was associated with no false positives or false negatives.

El-Nagar et al.[243] analyzed 23 ultrastructurally and immunohistochemically documented pleural epithelial mesotheliomas by flow cytometry and compared them with 41 pulmonary adenocarcinomas. Tumor tissue from multiple blocks was evaluated from each neoplasm to assess DNA heterogeneity. They found that 80% of pulmonary adenocarcinomas and 100% of pleural mesotheliomas showed a homogeneous DNA ploidy. The majority (78%) of epithelial mesotheliomas were diploid, whereas 88% of pulmonary adenocarcinomas were aneuploid. The proliferative fraction (S-phase percentage) of aneuploid adenocarcinomas was significantly greater than aneuploid epithelial mesotheliomas. These authors concluded that the DNA indices of epithelial mesotheliomas were significantly different than pulmonary adenocarcinomas.

Esteban and Sherbani[244] performed flow cytometric analysis on 45 malignant mesotheliomas and 41 pulmonary adenocarcinomas. Five cases of mesotheliomas were excluded because they had high coefficients of variation. Five cases (14%) of malignant mesothelioma were aneuploid with DNA indices between 1.2 to 1.9 (mean, 1.5), and 3 cases had increased S + G_2 M values. Of the aneuploid mesotheliomas, 4 were epithelial and 1 was sarcomatoid. In contrast to malignant mesotheliomas, 31 (75%) of pulmonary adenocarcinomas were aneuploid. The authors concluded that in view of the marked differences between DNA content in malignant mesotheliomas and pulmonary adenocarcinomas, ploidy analysis should be used in diagnostically difficult cases in which histochemistry, immunohistochemistry, and electron microscopy could not provide an unequivocal diagnosis.

This author agrees with the conclusion of Tierney et al.[242] that there is too much variability in DNA concentration in mesothelial lesions to be considered diagnostically useful.

Histogenesis of Mesotheliomas

Reactive nonneoplastic serosal tissue serves as a useful model for understanding the histologic, immunohistochemical, and ultrastructural features of mesotheliomas. Normal serosal tissue consists of a surface layer of mesothelium characterized by surface microvilli, laterally placed desmosomes, bundles of cytoplasmic tonofilaments, and basal lamina at the junction with the underlying connective tissue.[163] These surface cells express a wide range of different molecular weight cytokeratin proteins that are recognized by most commercially available monoclonal antibodies. The underlying connective tissue contains small vessels and scattered mesenchymal cells with the ultrastructural features of fibroblasts. Immunocytochemical studies reveal only the intermediate filament vimention.

An experimental model of rat serosal tissue[245] and our own studies[163] on human tissues have suggested that a subserosal connective tissue cell represents the proliferative cell in response to injury. We previously suggested the term multipotential subserosal cell, recognizing its unique ultrastructural and immunocytochemical phenotype. Serosal injury results in the loss of the surface mesothelial layer and the proliferation of the multipotential subserosal cell in the underlying connective tissue. Ultrastructural examination demonstrates the features of myofibroblasts with elongate processes, abundant rough endoplasmic reticulum, and peripherally arranged myofilaments. Despite the absence of ultrastructureal evidence of epithelial differentiation, immunocytochemical studies demonstrate actin and the co-expression of vimentin and low molecular weight cytokeratin. This contrasts to the typical immunocytochemical phenotype of myofibroblasts, which includes only actin and vimentin.[246,247] The multipotential subserosal cell is capable of surface mesothelial differentiation during which time surface microvilli, desmosomes, tonofilaments, and basal lamina are acquired concomitantly with the acquisition of high molecular weight cytokeratin and progressive loss of vimentin.

There are many phenotypic parallels between reactive nonneoplastic serosal tissue and mesotheliomas. Desmoplastic and sarcomatoid mesotheliomas resemble the multipotential subserosal cell. Both have the overall ultrastructural features of mesenchymal cells with variable quantities of rough endoplasmic reticulum, randomly dispersed 10-nm filaments consistent with vimentin, and small numbers of peripherally placed myofilaments. They likewise coexpress low molecular weight cytokeratin and vimentin. Diffuse epithelial mesotheliomas resemble surface mesothelium. They have long cell-surface microvilli, well-developed desmosomes, cytoplasmic tonofilaments, and basal lamina investments. Immunocytochemical characterization reveals a complex cytokeratin profile with a wide range of both low and high molecular weight cytokeratins. Mixed mesotheliomas resemble the multipotential subserosal cell in the spindled cell areas and surface mesothelium in the epithelial areas. The "transitional" mesotheliomas manifest morphologic and immunocytochemical features analogous to a stage of maturation between the two extremes. They may show subtle evidence of epithelial differentiation by light microscopy and feature ultrastructural observed tonofilaments, variably developed desmosomes, and rare surface microvilli while lacking the classic findings of an epithelial mesothelioma. Immunocytochemical studies also show a "transitional" pattern with the coexpression of vimentin and both low and high molecular weight cytokeratins.

In summary, the ability of normal serosal tissue to modulate its cell shape and intermediate filament expression lends considerable insight into the diversity of growth pattern exhibited by mesotheliomas.

Our hypothesis[163] concerning the histogenesis has recently been challenged by our Australian colleagues who believe that the variation in the histologic appearance of mesotheliomas probably results from surface mesothelial dedifferentiation. We cannot disprove their hypothesis but tend to favor our own, especially with respect to desmoplastic and sarcomatoid mesotheliomas that may show myofibroblastic differentiation. Our hypothesis is favored by Davila and Couch[248] who studied the role of mesothelial and submesothelial cells in matrix remodeling following pleural injury.

Other Pleural Neoplasms— Differential Pathologic Diagnosis

Metastatic neoplasms and peripheral pulmonary carcinomas frequently involve the pleura. Peripheral lung carcinomas, usually adenocarcinomas, may directly invade the pleura. Roberts[249] found 25 carcinomas of the lung for every mesothelioma, and O'Donnell and colleagues[250] reported a ratio of 5 lung carcinomas for every mesothelioma identified in asbestos workers. These statistics are probably correct, although this author sees far more pleural mesotheliomas than metastatic or invasive pleural cancers. In patients with metastatic carcinoma to the pleura, Chernow and Sahn[251] found that lung was the most common primary site (33%), followed by breast (20.9%) and stomach (7.3%). Almost 50% of these patients presented with unilateral pleural effusions, a clinical finding very common in mesotheliomas.

Babolini and Blasi[252] reported four cases of a neoplasm they referred to as the pleural form of primary lung cancer and cited other reported cases. Harwood et al.[253] reported six cases of a peripheral lung tumor that invaded the pleura and caused a desmoplastic reaction that simulated a mesothelioma. They referred to these neoplasms as pseudomesotheliomatous carcinomas and popularized this term. These neoplasms are discussed and illustrated in detail in Chapter 28 (Asbestos) because of their etiologic link to asbestos.

A histologic example of a pseudomesothelioma initially interpreted as a mesothelioma, is shown in Fig. 34–105. The tumor was composed of small tubules and

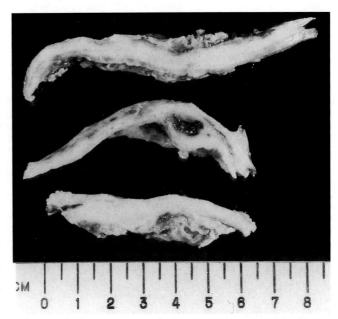

Fig. 34–105. Gross morphology of tumor that partially encased lung and had appearance consistent with mesothelioma.

glands and was surrounded by dense desmoplastic stromal tissue (Fig. 34–106). The tumor cells stained positive for Mayer's mucicarmine, showed intense immunostaining for carcinoembryonic antigen (Fig. 34–107), and had ultrastructural features of an adenocarcinoma. As discussed, a positive carcinoembryonic antigen in our experience strongly rules against the diagnosis of mesothelioma.

We also recently encountered a case of a 38-year-old cigarette-smoking man with a persistent pleural effusion. A pleural biopsy showed small nests of atypical cells associated with fibrous tissue. These cells showed weak immunostaining for carcinoembryonic antigen. An open lung biopsy showed a small peripheral lung adenocarcinoma, probably a bronchioalveolar cell carcinoma, that had directly invaded the parietal pleura (Fig. 34–108). In the open biopsy specimen the tumor showed intense immunostaining for carcinoembryonic antigen (Fig. 34–109).

Of concern to pathologists and clinicians is the accurate identification of malignant cells in pleural fluid and, in some instances, differentiation of reactive mesothelial cells from malignant mesothelial cells or other malignant cells. Our solution to this problem is to study abnormal cells in pleural fluid by electron microscopy and immunohistochemistry.

For electron microscopic examination, a sample of fluid is centrifuged and the cell pellet is fixed in modified Trump's fixative and processed as a tissue specimen. For immunohistochemical analysis, we prefer

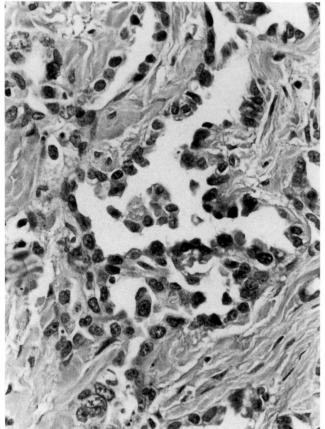

34-106

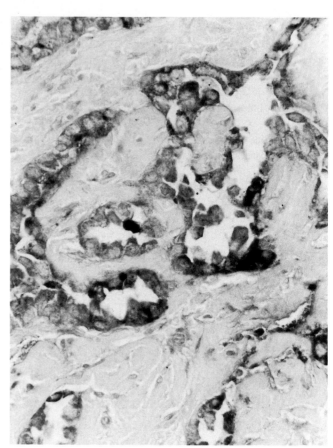

34-107

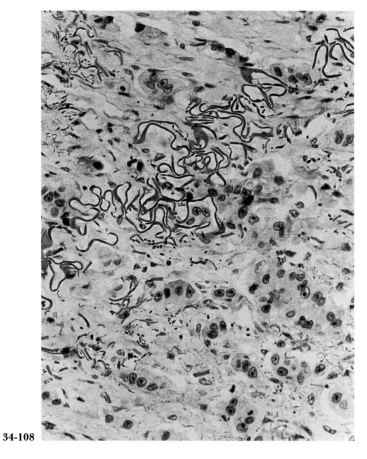

34-108

Fig. 34–106. Histologically, tumor shown in Fig. 34–105 is composed of small glands and tubules surrounded by desmoplastic stroma. ×300.

Fig. 34–107. Tumor cells show moderately intense immunostaining for carcinoembryonic antigen and are also positive for Mayer's mucicarmine. ×300.

Fig. 34–108. Small nests and cords of neoplastic epithelial cells invade through visceral pleural elastic tissue. ×300.

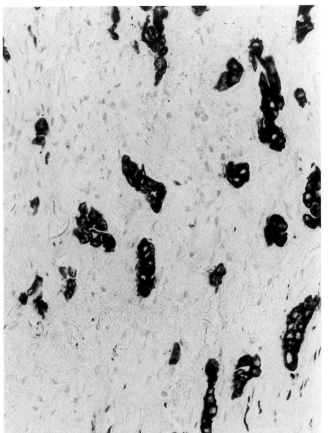

34-109

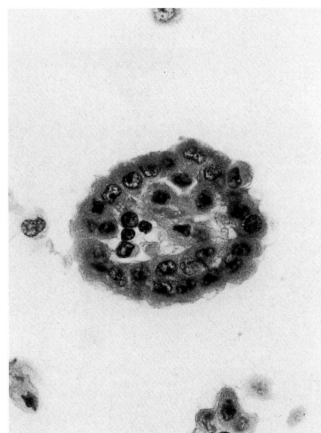

34-110

Fig. 34–109. Tumor cells show intense immunostaining for carcinoembryonic antigen and ultrastructurally have features of adenocarcinoma. ×300.

Fig. 34–110. Small papillary cluster of malignant cells identified in pleural fluid show similarity with those in Fig. 34–111. ×550.

Fig. 34–111. Small papillary cluster of malignant cells identified in pleural fluid shows similarity to those in Fig. 34–112. ×550.

───────────────────────────────▷

making a cell block and performing a battery of immunohistochemical tests, as described, on paraffin-embedded sections. Malignant mesothelial cells usually occur as papillary fragments or solid balls (Fig. 34–110), as do pulmonary adenocarcinomas and other adenocarcinomas (Fig. 34–111). When examined by electron microscopy, the malignant mesothelial cells have the same ultrastructural features as seen in tissue biopsy specimens (Fig. 34–112), whereas pulmonary adenocarcinomas and other carcinomas have ultrastructural features distinctly different from malignant and reactive mesothelial cells (Fig. 34–113). Immunohistochemically the adenocarcinoma cells in pleural fluid express carcinoembryonic antigen (Fig. 34–114) and other antigens

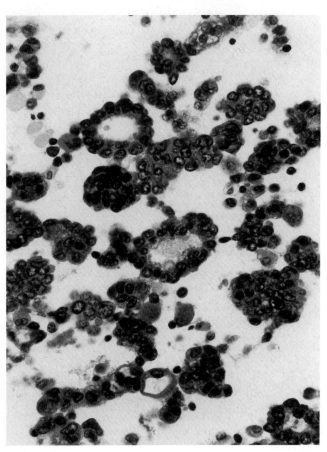

34-111

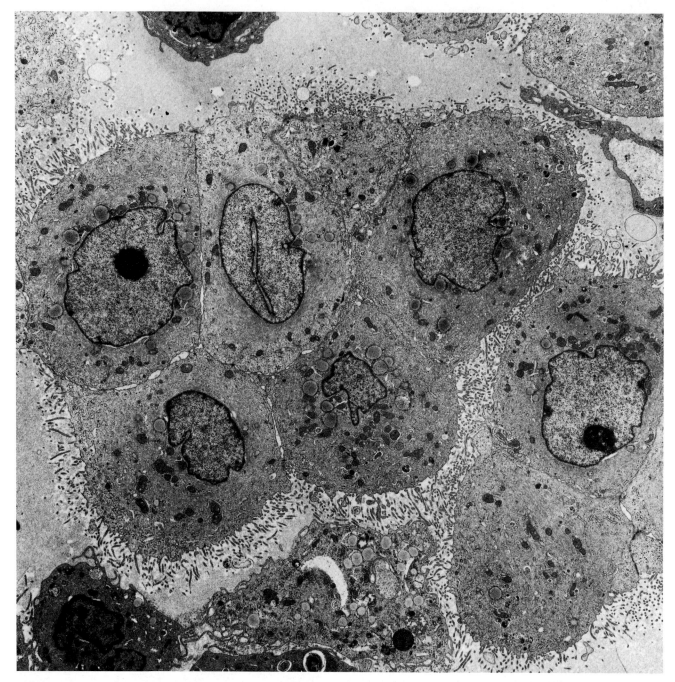

Fig. 34–112. Cells shown in Fig. 34–110 have ultrastructural appearance of malignant epithelial mesothelial cells. Note long cell-surface microvilli and numerous intermediate filaments in cytoplasm. ×4,100.

such as Leu M1, Ber EP4 and B 72.3, whereas the mesothelioma cells are usually negative for carcinoembryonic antigen and the other substances cited.

When studied by electron microscopy or immunohistochemistry, a reactive mesothelial cell is often difficult to impossible to distinguish from a malignant one in pleural fluid, although we believe that reactive me-

sothelial cells may have fewer cell-surface microvilli. As in tissue sections, reactive mesothelial cells usually do not express epithelial membrane antigen or human milk fat globule protein whereas malignant mesothelial cells do, characteristically in a cell membrane distribution. We routinely use carcinoembryonic antigen Leu M1, B 72.3, and Ber EP4 to differentiate reactive and

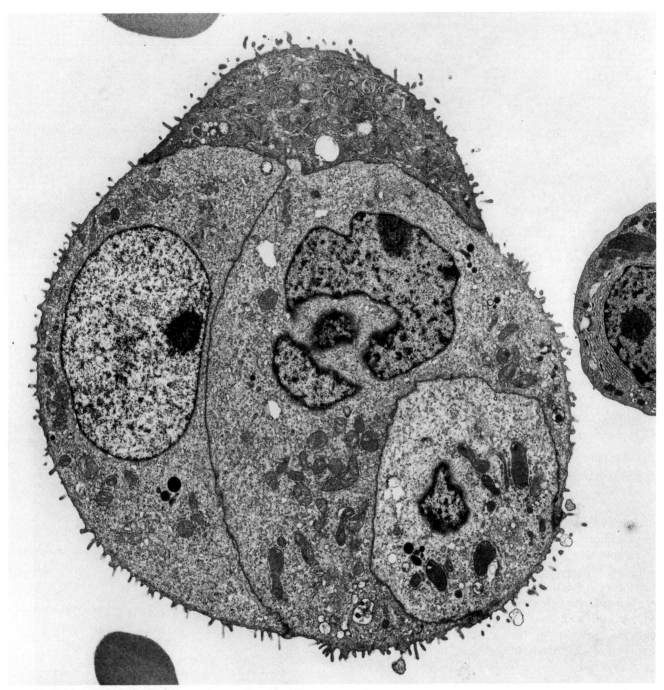

Fig. 34–113. Cells shown in Fig. 34–111 have ultrastructural appearance of pulmonary adenocarcinoma. Note short and relatively infrequent cell-surface microvilli. ×4,100.

malignant mesothelial cells in pleural fluid from adenocarcinoma tumor cells and other carcinoma cells. In our experience, reactive and neoplastic mesothelial cells are negative for these antigens whereas cells exfoliated from a pulmonary adenocarcinoma and many other types of carcinomas show immunostaining for one or more of them. Notable exceptions to this rule are metastatic renal cell carcinomas, thyroid carcinomas, ovarian carcinomas, and prostate carcinomas, which usually do not express carcinoembryonic antigen, Leu M1, M 72.3, and Ber EP4.

Soft-tissue sarcomas may rarely involve the chest wall in a diffuse manner and be confused with sarcomatoid mesotheliomas. Histologically it may be impossible to

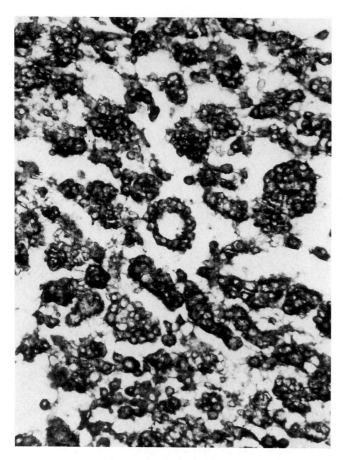

Fig. 34–114. Adenocarcinoma cells in pleural fluid show intense immunostaining for carcinoembryonic antigen. ×550.

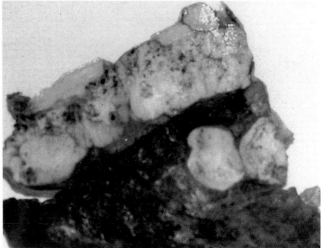

Fig. 34–115. Lung was focally surrounded by thick rind of tumor representing metastatic sarcomatoid renal cell carcinoma.

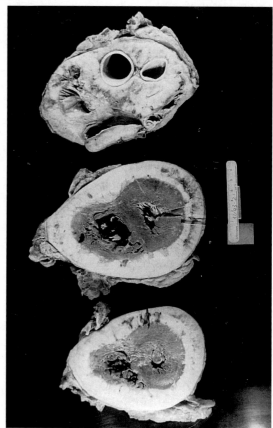

Fig. 34–116. Tumor encasing heart and great vessels has macroscopic appearance consistent with primary pericardial mesothelioma, although it represents metastatic melanoma.

differentiate spindle cell sarcomas from sarcomatoid mesotheliomas although, as shown, sarcomatoid mesotheliomas usually coexpress vimentin and cytokeratin whereas soft tissue sarcomas usually express only vimentin or combinations of vimentin, desmin, and muscle actin. Metastatic sarcomatoid renal cell carcinomas may mimic a sarcomatoid mesothelioma macroscopically (Fig. 34–115), histologically, and immunohistochemically. Immunohistochemically they coexpress cytokeratin and vimentin, just as do sarcomatoid mesotheliomas. Metastatic, amelanotic, spindle cell melanoma could be confused histologically with a sarcomatoid mesothelioma, and this author has seen one case that radiographically was stated to almost totally encase the lung. This author has also seen a metastatic melanoma simulate a pericardial mesothelioma (Fig. 34–116). Melanomas characteristically express S-100 protein and human melanoma black antigen-45 immunohistochemically, and ultra-structurally contain melanosomes in their cytoplasm.

Desmoplastic mesotheliomas are the most difficult mesothelioma to diagnose histologically. In many areas

they appear as reactive fibrous tissue but often have regions of geographic necrosis and marked cellular atypia, which are the two criteria used to differentiate them histologically from a reactive process. Clinically, patients with desmoplastic mesotheliomas usually present with chronic chest wall pain and may have radiographic evidence of invasion of chest wall, lung, or bone. It should be emphasized, however, that reactive benign pleural processes such as a chronic empyema can produce a markedly thickened pleura grossly and microscopically resembling a desmoplastic mesothelioma.

In 1984, three cases of angiosarcoma of serosal surfaces were described by McCaughey et al.[254] We have seen one case of a pleural angiosarcoma in a 34-year-old man. Histologically the tumor was quite pleomorphic but formed vascular-appearing spaces (Fig. 34–117). Ultrastructurally the tumor cells resembled endothelial cells and contained cytoplasmic Weibel–Palade bodies, characteristic markers for endothelial cells (Fig. 34–118). Immunohistochemically, the tumor cells showed immunostaining for vimentin and Factor VIII-related antigen and were negative for cytokeratin.

Lymphomas and leukemias can involve the pleura (see Chapter 31), and such involvement is occasionally used as a criterion of malignancy in pulmonary lymphoproliferative processes.

We recently encountered a malignant pleural neoplasm that was associated with dense fibrosis (Fig. 34–119) and histologically had the appearance of a squamous carcinoma (Fig. 34–120). A Mayer's mucicarmine stain showed focal positive staining material in some cells, thus suggesting a diagnosis of adenosquamous carcinoma. This tumor was thought to most likely represent a peripheral lung adenosquamous carcinoma invading the pleura and possibly represented a pseudomesotheliomatous carcinoma of the lung. However, Willen et al.[255] reported squamous cell carcinoma of the pleura following extrapleural pneumothorax for pulmonary tuberculosis. They described 10 patients who had been treated with extrapleural pneumolysis for pulmonary tuberculosis with the collapsed lung being maintained by repeated refills of air into the extrapleural space. Six patients developed squamous carcinoma in pleura, and 4 developed squamous metaplasia of the pleura between 8 months and 15 years after the cessation of refills of air; all had received more than 100 refills of air. Crome[256] described 4 cases of squamous metaplasia of the peritoneum, one of which was in a 39-year-old woman who had been treated for tuberculosis with pneumoperitoneum and multiple air refills. In 1981 Kwee et al.[257] reported a tumor in a 64-year-old man that they designated a primary adenosquamous mesothelioma of the pleura. Histologically, this tumor contained a distinct squamous component and also a glandular pattern in which the cells produced hyaluronic acid. Kwee et al.[257] mentioned that the neoplasm may have represented two separate neoplasms, an epi-

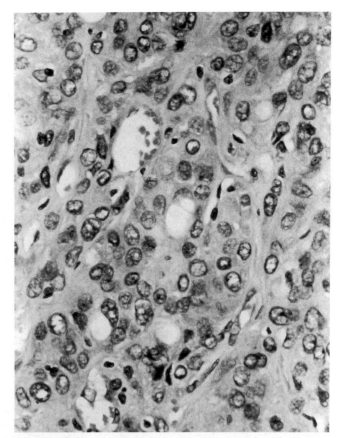

Fig. 34–117. This tumor, composed of large cells with large vesicular nuclei and prominent nucleoli that form spaces consistent with vascular spaces in some areas, is histologically consistent with angiosarcoma. ×550.

thelial mesothelioma and a squamous carcinoma, but thought this was unlikely because of the intimate relationship of the tumor and because both components were present in metastases.

Approach to the Diagnosis

Our approach to the diagnosis of pleural neoplasms is to accurately classify a neoplasm according to its histologic, immunohistochemical, and ultrastructural features. As shown in this chapter the histologic and cytologic features of epithelial mesotheliomas, pulmonary adenocarcinomas, and other carcinomas may be exceedingly similar. In this author's experience, a carcinoembryonic antigen is the single most useful immunohistochemical test to distinguish between an epithelial mesothelioma and pulmonary adenocarcinoma; mesotheliomas are consistently negative and pulmonary adenocarcinomas are almost always positive. The morphology of the microvilli is the most specific electron microscopic feature that distinguishes epithelial mesotheliomas from pulmonary adenocarcinomas; me-

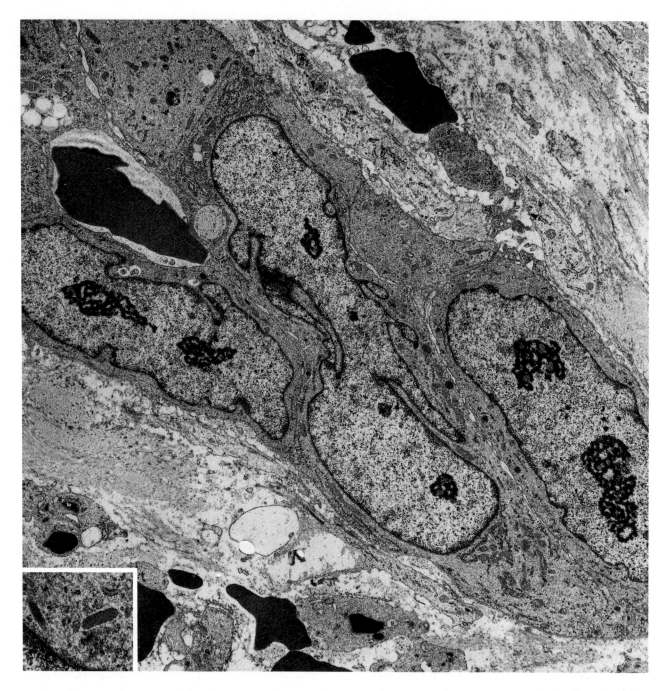

Fig. 34–118. Ultrastructurally, tumor cells contain numerous cytoplasmic intermediate filaments, presumably vimentin. ×6,400. Inset: Cytoplasmic Weibel–Palade bodies are pathog-nomonic markers of endothelial cells and were observed in these tumor cells. ×16,000.

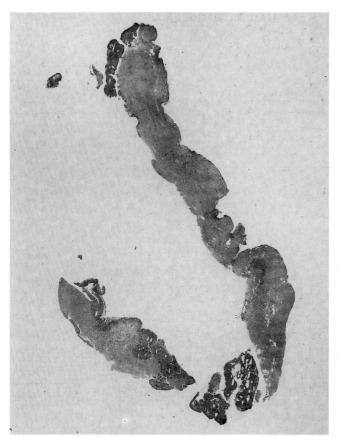

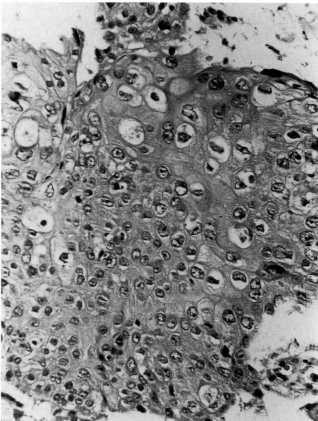

Fig. 34–119. Small nests of tumor associated with dense fibrous pleural plaque. ×4.

Fig. 34–120. Tumor cells associated with plaque exhibit mostly squamous features but also show focal intracellular mucin positivity, suggesting diagnosis of adenosquamous carcinoma, possibly primary in pleura. ×550.

sotheliomas have long slender bushy microvilli, and pulmonary adenocarcinomas usually have less frequent short stubby microvilli that are often covered by a fuzzy glycocalyx.

As we have shown, cells in pleural fluid may be examined by immunohistochemistry and electron microscopy as an aid to differentiating mesothelioma cells from other neoplastic cells. Karotype analysis has also been performed on cells cultured from pleural fluid.[258] As previously discussed, this technique can identify cells with chromosome abnormalities but cannot identify the origin of the abnormal cell and may be no more accurate than routine cytology in detecting malignant cells in pleural fluid.

Our approach to the diagnosis of mesothelioma is essentially identical to that described by Henderson et al.[259] with the exception that we usually do not perform histochemical tests (Fig. 34–121). These techniques can be applied to small "samples" of tumor including malignant cells in pleural fluid.

The concentration of hyaluronic acid in pleural fluid

and pleural neoplasms has been evaluated to determine if it is helpful in making a diagnosis of mesothelioma. The results have been controversial. Friman et al.[260] found an increased concentration of hyaluronic acid in pleural fluid in three cases of mesothelioma. Arai et al.[261] reported a hyaluronic acid concentration of 7 µg/ml in a case of diffuse mesothelioma. 14 ± 8.6 µg/ml in four cases of tuberculous pleurisy and 9.43 ± 5.13 µg/ml in seven cases of cancerous pleurisy. Other investigators[262–264] found similar variable results of hyaluronic acid concentration in pleural fluid.

In 1988, Pettersson et al.[265] reported their evaluation of hyaluronic acid concentration in pleural fluid from 85 patients with pleural effusions including 15 with malignant mesothelioma, 32 with other types of neoplasms, 31 with nonmalignant inflammatory disease, and 7 with congestive heart failure. Eleven of 15 (73%) patients with malignant mesothelioma and 7 of 31 (23%) with nonmalignant inflammatory conditions had pleural fluid hyaluronic acid concentrations greater than 100 mg/liter whereas all 32 patients with other

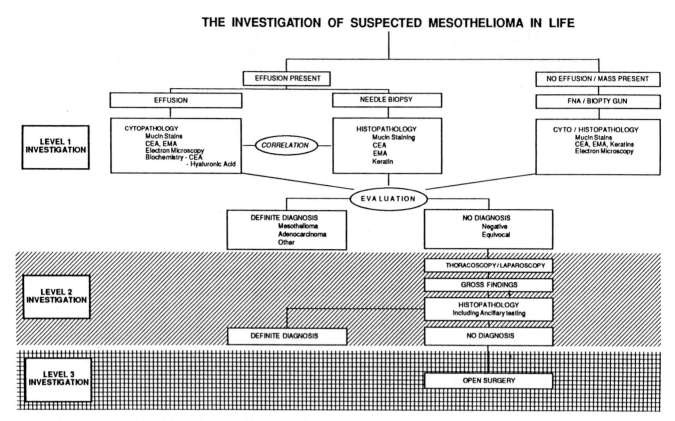

Fig. 34–121. Algorithm of scheme of investigation of various types of specimens in diagnosing mesothelioma in life. (Reproduced by permission from Henderson DW, Whitaker D, Shilkin KB. The differential diagnosis of malignant mesothelioma. In: Henderson DW, Shilkin KB, Langlois SLP, Whitaker D, eds., Malignant mesothelioma. New York: Hemisphere, 1992:184.)

types of cancers and the seven patients with congestive heart failure had hyaluronic acid concentrations less than 100 mg/L. The authors also evaluated the usefulness of pleural fluid carcinoembryonic antigen concentrations in differentiating malignant mesothelioma from other types of cancer. Four of 15 (27%) patients with malignant mesothelioma and 12 of 32 (38%) patients with other malignant neoplasms had carcinoembryonic antigen concentrations greater than 10 μg/liter. The authors concluded that, in pleural effusions associated with a malignant tumor, a high hyaluronic acid concentration and low carcinoembryonic antigen concentration in the pleural fluid suggested the diagnosis of malignant mesothelioma as opposed to other malignant neoplasms.

In a somewhat similar study, Hillerdal et al.[266] determined the hyaluronic acid concentration in serum and pleural fluid in 78 consecutive patients with pleural effusions. In 3 of 9 (33%) patients with malignant mesothelioma and 5 of 42 (12%) patients with metastatic malignant neoplasms, pleural fluid hyaluronic acid concentration was greater than 100 mg/liter. In addition, in 2 of 11 (1.8%) patients with cardiac disease,

3 of 4 (75%) patients with viral infection, 1 patient with a postinfectious effusion and 2 of 2 (100%) patients with benign asbestos-induced effusion had pleural fluid hyaluronic acid concentrations greater than 100 mg/liter. The serum hyaluronic acid concentrations were lower than those found in the pleural fluid, and there was no correlation between pleural fluid hyaluronic acid concentrations and serum hyaluronic acid levels. In contrast to the conclusion of Pettersson et al.,[265] the authors concluded that a high concentration of hyaluronic acid in pleural fluid was not specific for malignant mesothelioma and could be found in other malignant conditions and in benign diseases. They also concluded that a low pleural fluid hyaluronic acid concentration did not exclude the diagnosis of malignant mesothelioma.

In tissue specimens, Arai and colleagues[261] found at least 0.10 mg of hyaluronic acid per gram of dry tissue in four cases of mesothelioma, but only 0.02–0.03 mg of hyaluronic acid per gram of dry tissue in two cases of carcinomatous pleural tissue and in pleural tissue from two patients with asbestosis. Chiu et al.[267] isolated glycosaminoglycans from 21 mesotheliomas, 34 primary lung carcinomas, 12 carcinomas from other sites, and 4 soft tissue sarcomas. Hyaluronic acid was identified qualitatively in 20 of 21 mesotheliomas, approximately half of the lung carcinomas, and all of the soft tissue sarcomas. Quantitatively, hyaluronic acid constituted 45% of the total glycosaminoglycan in mesotheliomas and 28% of the total in carcinomas of the lung. The mean value of hyaluronic acid in mesotheliomas was significantly higher (0.74 mg/g) than lung adenocarcinomas (0.08 mg/g), but was not significantly higher than in soft tissue sarcomas (2.01 mg/g) or ovarian serous carcinomas (0.92 mg/g). They concluded that a hyaluronic concentration of greater than 0.4 mg/g dry tissue extract supported the diagnosis of mesothelioma when the alternative diagnosis was primary pulmonary adenocarcinoma.

Nakano et al.[268] also studied glycosaminoglycan concentration in five pleural mesotheliomas and contrasted it to that seen in one pulmonary adenocarcinoma. The average total amount of glycosaminoglycan was 7.9 times higher in the mesotheliomas than in the pulmonary adenocarcinoma, and hyaluronic acid and chondroitin sulfate were the main types of glycosaminoglycans found. They also found an increase in hyaluronic acid and chondroitin sulfate in pleural fluid from two patients with mesothelioma. Iozzo[269] reviewed the subject of proteoglycans and their role in neoplasia in 1985, having previously reported[270] that tissue extracts of mesotheliomas contain large amounts of chondroitin sulfate.

In this author's opinion, the most useful single "test" to differentiate epithelial mesothelioma from pulmonary adenocarcinoma is electron microscopy.[271] The ultrastructural features of moderately well-differentiated epithelial mesotheliomas are almost always distinct enough to separate them from a pulmonary adenocarcinoma often even when the tissue is removed from the paraffin block (Fig. 34–122).

Clinical Pathologic Correlations

Patients with pleural mesotheliomas and metastatic pleural neoplasms most commonly present with nonspecific symptoms and signs consisting of chest pain, dyspnea on exertion, cough, weight loss, and a pleural effusion. Physical examination is frequently nonspecific but may reveal dullness to percussion on the involved side if there is a pleural effusion, and distant breath sounds on the side of the pleural effusion by ascultation of the chest.

Antman[272] has adapted a clinical staging system from Butchart et al.[273] for patients with mesotheliomas according to the extent of disease, similar to that done for primary lung carcinoma (Table 34–14). In general there is a direct correlation with the stage of the disease

and survival. Antman reported that patients with stage I, II, and III disease survived a median of 16, 9, and 5 months, respectively, after diagnosis. In this author's experience, it is difficult to accurately stage mesotheliomas because they grow by direct extension and staging studies such as mediastinoscopy and computerized tomographic scans of the chest and other regions of the body are frequently not done or are difficult to interpret. Only at autopsy can disease extent be accurately evaluated.

Part of the problem of determining accurate anatomic stage of patients with malignant pleural mesothelioma is that systemic metastases are frequently not searched for because of the severity of symptoms caused by the pleural tumor, for example, chest pain and shortness of breath, and because of the poor prognosis and lack of adequate therapy for mesothelioma (see following). Mesothelioma is neoplasm that grows in a "spreading" manner and by direct invasion of adjacent tissues and organs. As a result, it is often thought to not metastasize. The exact opposite is true; mesotheliomas frequently metastasize. A summary of reports concerning the location and frequency of metastase is shown in Table 34–15.

In this author's experience, malignant pleural mesotheliomas most frequently metastasize to bronchopulmonary hilar, and mediastinal lymph nodes. The next most frequent site of metastases is to the opposite lung, usually the pleural surface and subpleural parenchyma. Sussman and Rosai[284] reported 6 cases in which lymphadenopathy was the initial manifestation of malignant mesothelioma. In 5 cases the mesothelioma was primary in the peritoneum and in the other case was a pleural primary. The involved lymph nodes were cervical in 4 cases, mediastinal in 1 and inguinal in 1. Another reported case[285] concerned a 42-year-old woman who presented with a skin rash and a left-sided neck mass proven by biopsy to be metastatic mesothelioma. Huncharek and Smith[286] reported finding lymph node involvement in 34 of 77 autopsy cases of malignant pleural mesothelioma with involvement of hilar and mediastinal nodes in 31 cases (41%). One patient had axillary lymph node involvement, one had supraclavicular lymph node involvement, and 6 patients had metastatic mesothelioma in abdominal lymph nodes. Kim et al.[287] also reported a case of a 52-year-old man with a malignant pleural mesothelioma diagnosed by axillary lymph node biopsy.

Uri et al.[288] reported a 62-year-old former shipyard worker with malignant pleural mesothelioma who developed diffuse contralateral nodular lung metastases that produced an unusual radiographic pattern. This author believes this represents lymphatic spread of tumor because it is common to see metastatic mesothelioma within lymphatic spaces (Fig. 34–123).

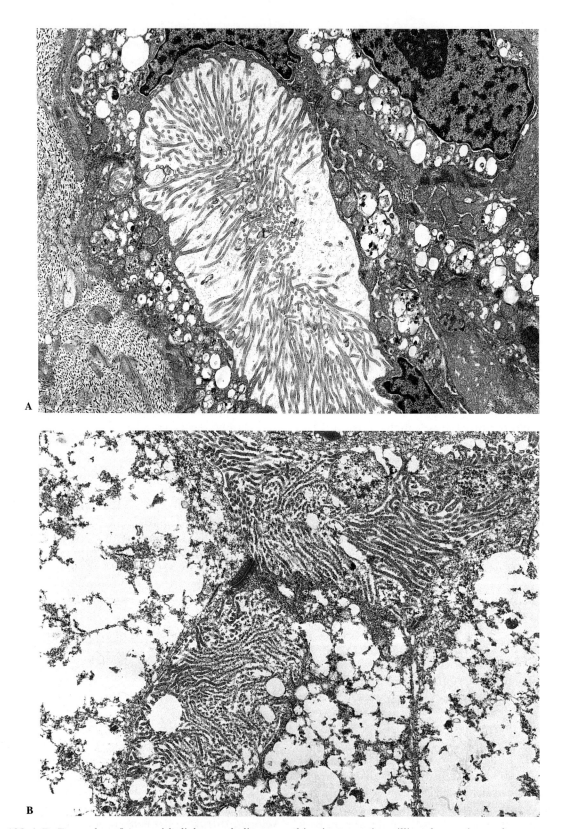

Fig. 34–122 A,B. Examples of two epithelial mesotheliomas diagnosed by examination of tumor tissue retrieved from paraffin block and studied by electron microscopy. Note long thin sinuous microvilli and prominent desmosomes in **B. A,** ×10,400; **B,** ×16,000.

Table 34–14. Pathologic staging of diffuse malignant mesothelioma of the pleura[a]

Stage I	Tumor confined within the "capsule" of the parietal pleura, i.e., involving only ipsilateral pleura, lung, pericardium and diaphragm.
Stage II	Tumor invading chest wall or involving mediastinal structures, e.g., esophagus, heart. Lymph node involvement inside the chest.
Stage III	Tumor penetrating diaphragm to involve peritoneum. Involvement of opposite pleura. Lymph node involvement outside the chest.
Stage IV	Distant blood-borne metastases.

[a] From Butchart et al.[278]

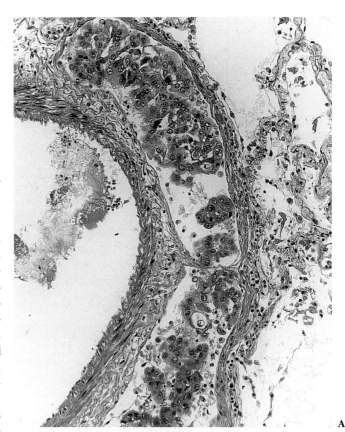

A

Brain metastases from malignant pleural mesothelioma have also been reported[288–292] but are uncommon and are usually diagnosed at autopsy. This author has seen three examples of brain metastases from pleural mesotheliomas. These mesotheliomas were relatively anaplastic. Chen[285] reported a peritoneal mesothelioma that presented as a Sister Joseph's nodule. This author has seen a case of a malignant pleural mesothelioma that presented as a periumbilical nodule, approximately 2 years before the patient's pleural mesothelioma was diagnosed (unpublished observations).

The treatment for diffuse malignant mesotheliomas and metastatic malignant neoplasms to pleura is generally unsuccessful. Chemotherapy, irradiation, and surgery have all been used as primary therapy. The median survival time in earlier reported series of mesotheliomas is 4–9 months after diagnosis and 8–14 months after the onset of symptoms.[274,294]

Several reports[295–302] have been published concerning prognostic factors and survival rates in patients with malignant mesothelioma since the first edition of this book. Most of these are summarized in Table 34–16.

Chailleux et al.[295] evaluated 167 cases of pleural mesothelioma diagnosed between 1955 and 1985 in the St. Nazaire region of France: 135 mesotheliomas were epithelial, 25 biphasic, and 7 sarcomatous; 131 (88%) were related to occupational exposure to asbestos. Eighty patients were treated, 14 by pleurectomy, 25 by partial pleurectomy, 4 by pleuropneumonectomy, and 42 with chemotherapy consisting of cisplatin alone, in cisplastin, adriamycin and bleomycin, cyclophosphamide alone, and other combinations. Survival from first symptoms was 54% at 1 year and 22% at 2 years with a median of 11 years. Survival from pathologic diagnosis was 39% at 1 year and 14% at 2 years with a median of

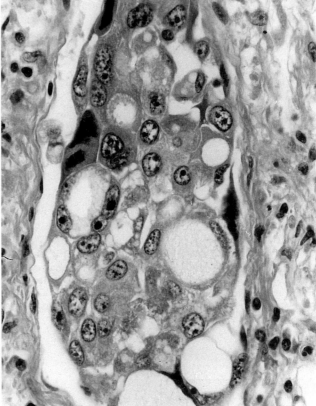

B

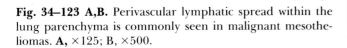

Fig. 34–123 A,B. Perivascular lymphatic spread within the lung parenchyma is commonly seen in malignant mesotheliomas. **A,** ×125; B, ×500.

Table 34–15. Location and frequency of metastases in malignant mesothelioma

	Roberts et al.,[274] 1976	Elmes et al,[275] 1976	Doward et al,[276] 1981	Roggli et al,[277] 1982	Chahinian et al,[278] 1982
Number of patients	32	377	32	24[g]	69[j]
Number autopsied	32[a]	148	21	23	14[k]
(Numer) and	(15)[b]	(48)[d]	(7)[e]	(21)	(11)
percent with metastases	47%	33%	33%	91%	79%
Number of evaluable patients with metastases	32	48	21	23	14
Location of metastases					
Thoracic lymph nodes	17	—	7	20	7
Extrathoracic lymph nodes	—	—	—	—	12
Contralateral lung and pleura	7	19	3	11[h]	19
Ipsilateral lung	—	—	—[f]	—	—
Liver	1	21	—	9	7
Peritoneum	5	—	5	2	8
Bone	1	—	5	4	3
Adrenal glands	3	—	—	7	3
Pericardium	2[c]	2[c]	2[c]	5	8
Myocardium	2[c]	2[c]	2[c]	—	3
Kidneys	5	—	4	4	1
GI tract	—	1	—	2	4
Spleen	—	—	—	—	6
Pancreas	—	2	—	2	2
Skin/subcutaneous tissue	—	—	—	1[i]	—
Brain	2	1	—	1	—
Pituitary	—	1	—	—	—
Urinary bladder	—	—	—	—	—
Gallbladder	—	—	—	1	—
Thyroid	—	—	1	1	—
Mesentery, omentum	—	—	—	2	—
Testes	—	—	—	—	—
Ovaries	—	—	—	—	—
Trachea	—	—	—	1	—
Uterus/adnexa	—	—	—	—	1
Brachial plexus and neck tissue	—	—	—	—	—
Bone marrow	—	—	—	—	1
Skeletal muscle	—	—	—	1	—

[a] The brain was not examined in some patients.

[b] Number indicates those cases with "distant" visceral metastases and excluded regional (thoracic) lymph node metastases.

[c] Metastases designated as "heart."

[d] Metastases referred to as hematogenous.

[e] Best estimate.

[f] Direct infiltration in 9 cases.

[g] Consisted of 19 patients with pleural mesothelioma and 5 patients with peritoneal mesothelioma. One patient (case 19) had a localized fibrous tumor of the pleura.

[i] Designated as chest wall metastases.

[j] Included 12 patients with peritoneal mesothelioma.

[k] Included 3 patients with peritoneal mesothelioma.

[l] Site of lymph node involvement not designated.

[m] Microscopic involvement of lymphatic vessels and veins.

[n] In 12 cases there was direct invasion of either mediastinal tissue, diaphragmatic muscle, or chest wall muscle.

[o] Thoracic lymph nodes included under mediastinal structures, that also included great vessels and myocardium. Not indicated if this was by direct invasion or metastasis.

[p] Other organs, not specified, were stated to be involved in 34 cases.

[q] Designated as "abdominal lymph nodes."

Table 34–15. *Continued*

Adams et al,[279] 1984	Solomons et al,[280] 1984	Krumhaar et al,[281] 1985	Huncharek et al,[282] 1989	Hulks et al,[283] 1989	Ruffie et al,[298] 1989	Totals
16	80	100	42	68	332	1172
16	10	100	42	40	92	538
(12)	(5)	82	(32)	(32)	(46)	(311)
75%	50%	82%[p]	76%	80%	50%	58%
16	52	100	42	40	92	480
5[l]	16[o]	51	19	14	37	193
—	—	18[q]	—	—	19	42
1[m]	15	26	16	12	15	144
16[m]	32	20	—	2	—	70
4	8	26	9	22	28	135
7	6	25	—	4	—	62
3	6	—	24	9	9	64
2	1	14	8	9	11	55
7	12	10[c]	—	10[c]	—	64
1	—	10[c]	—	10[c]	2	64
2	2	—	11	4	12	45
—	5	10	—	6	—	28
1	1	—	1	6	4	19
1	—	—	1	2	5	16
1	2	—	—	—	4	8
—	—	—	1	1	3	9
—	—	—	—	—	—	1
—	—	—	—	1	—	1
—	—	—	—	—	—	1
—	—	—	—	2	4	8
2	2	—	—	—	—	6
—	—	—	—	—	1	1
—	—	—	—	—	—	1
—	—	—	—	—	—	1
3	—	—	—	—	—	3
—	—	—	1	—	—	2
—[n]	—	—	—	—	1	2

10 months. No patient was alive 4 years after diagnosis. Patients treated by chemotherapy, surgery, or talc poudrage had a longer survival but there was no indication that one form of therapy was superior to another. One woman treated with cisplatin had a 15-month complete remission; no partial remissions were observed with chemotherapy. The histologic type of mesothelioma and a history of asbestos exposure had no predictive survival value. Patients less than 60 years old when the mesothelioma was diagnosed lived longer than those older than 60 years.

Antman et al.[296] evaluated 180 patients with malignant mesothelioma identified between 1965 and 1985, of which 136 were pleural, 37 peritoneal, 5 pericardial, and 2 testicular in origin. The median survival for those patients with pleural mesothelioma was 14–15 months. There was a significantly increased survival for those patients with a performance status between 0 and 1 (median, 31–32 months) versus those with a performance status >1 (median survival, 7 months), for those with epithelial histology (median survival, 17 months) versus sarcomatous histology (median survival, 7 months), for those with an absence of chest pain (median survival, 24 months) versus those with chest pain (median survival, 16 months), and those with an interval >6 months from the onset of symptoms (median survival, 16 months) versus those with an interval of <6 months from the onset of symptoms (median survival, 13 months) and possibly a better survival for those patients treated with chemotherapy or pleuropneumonectomy.

Alberts et al.[297] evaluated survival rates and prognostic factors in 262 patients diagnosed between 1965 and 1985 with malignant pleural mesothelioma who were

Table 34–16. Survival data and prognostic factors in malignant mesothelioma

Variable	Chailleux et al.[295]	Antman et al.[296]	Alberts et al.[297]	Ruffie et al.[298]
Number of patients	167	180	262	332
Age range	21–86	<20–<60	<40–>65	22–88
Mean age	62	NG	55	59
Men:Women	159:8	136:44	188:74	262:70
Location				
Pleural	166	136	262	332
Peritoneal	11[b]	37		
Pleural and peritoneal				
Other		5[c]		
Histologic type				
Epithelial	135	112	74	163
Sarcomatoid	7	24	36	53
Mixed	25	36	20	70
Not specified		5	131	46
Anatomic stage				
I	NG	111	201	56[d]
II	NG	32	34	96
III	NG	29	13	19
IV	NG	7	12	12
Survival range (mo) from first symptoms or diagnosis	<6–131	NG	1–60	1–174[f]
Median survival (mo)				
From first symptoms	13	NG	NG	NG
From diagnosis	10	15	9.6	1.4[j]–16.6[k]
Positive predictive factors for survival	Patients <60 years, treatment with chemotherapy; surgery, talc poudrage; delay in diagnosis >2 months from onset of symptoms	Epithelial histology, 0–1 performance status, absence of chest pain, interval of >6 mo from onset of symptoms and diagnosis; treatment with chemotherapy and pleurectomy	Good performance status; early stage of disease; female sex; duration of symptoms >6 mo at time of diagnosis; white race	Early stage of disease; lack of weight loss; epithelial or mixed histology

[a] Abbreviation: NG, not given.

[b] 11 cases stated to be present with extrathoracic involvement.

[c] Five testicular and two pericardial.

[d] Staging possible in 183 patients.

[e] Stage unknown in three patients.

[f] One patient with fibrosarcomatous mesothelioma stated to be alive at 14.5 years.

[g] One patient alive at 8 years, one patient dead after 7 years, and one patient surviving more than 5 years.

[h] Peritoneal mesotheliomas.

[i] Pleural mesotheliomas.

[j] Stage IV patients.

[k] Stage I patients.

[l] In the largest group of patients (76), median survival was 7.7 months.

[m] No therapy was found to be effective.

treated with chemotherapy only, radiotherapy only, radiotherapy and chemotherapy, or with decortication combined with chemotherapy and radiotherapy. The median survival for all patients from the time of diagnosis was 9.6 months, which was the same for all treatment groups. In a univariate analysis, favorable prognostic factors included good performance status, duration of symptoms >6 months at the time of diagnosis, early stage of disease, white race, and female gender. In a multivariate analysis, good performance status, white race, duration of symptoms, and stage of disease were significant favorable prognostic factors. The authors found that the stepwise addition of treatment modalities did not increase survival.

Ruffie et al.[298] performed a retrospective study of 332 patients diagnosed with malignant pleural mesothelioma between 1965 and 1984. The median survival was 9 months. Using univariate analysis, three

Table 34–16. *Continued*

Harvey et al.[299]	*Ribak & Selikoff*[300]	*Tammilehto*[301]	*Sridhar et al.*[302]
94	457	98	49
36–89	45–84	38–83	36–77
62	60	58	58
78:14	457:0	77:21	40:9
94	186	93	36
	271	5	10
			3
31	NG	36	25
16	NG	10	5
11	NG	52	7
34	NG	0	12
NG	NG	17	18[e]
NG	NG	61	19
NG	NG	14	6
NG	NG	1	3
<6–96[g]	1–>36	0–81	0–45
NG	7.4,[h] 11.4[i]	9	13
7.7[l]	NG	NG	10
Radical surgical therapy	None indicated[m]	Female sex; age ≤65; epithelial histology; early stage disease; low S phase; good performance status; lung asbestos burden <10⁶ fibers/g dry lung	Earlier stage disease; good performance status; longer duration of symptoms; absence of pain; combined surgery and chemotherapy

factors were found to have a significant effect on survival: (1) disease stage: stage 1, median survival 16.6 months, versus stage IV, 1.4 months; (2) weight loss: no weight loss, median survival, 10.5 months, versus weight loss, median survival, 4.8 months; and (3) histogical type: epithelial or mixed median survival of 9.9 and 9.2 months, respectively, versus sarcomatous median survival of 5.2 months. The authors found that there were no drastic differences in survival among groups of patients subjected to different therapeutic measures. Radical surgery and radiotherapy were found to be ineffective; there was a low response rate to chemotherapeutic agents.

Harvey et al.[299] also performed a retrospective analysis on 94 patients with malignant pleural mesothelioma treated at one institution between 1965 and 1988. Group I patients (*n* = 76) received supportive care only, including pleurodesis as needed. Group II patients (*n* = 9) were managed with debulking procedures including decortication and pleurectomy. Group III

patients (*n* = 7) were treated by extrapleural pneumonectomy. Median survival in group I patients was 231 days. Four patients in group I survived more than 2 years, and 1 patient who was treated with chemotherapy and tangential field external beam irradiation survived more than 5 years. Group II patients had a median survival of 360 days, and none were alive at the end of 2 years. Four of 7 group III patients expired within 6 months after treatment, although 1 patient died 7 years after therapy and one 36-year-old male was alive 8 years after diagnosis. The authors concluded that selected patients (7 young patients) benefit from radical surgery and that debulking may also extend survival.

Ribak and Selikoff[300] studied the clinical course of 457 consecutive fatal cases of pleural and peritoneal mesothelioma that occurred among 17,800 asbestos insulation workers observed prospectively from January 1967, to January 1987. In the pleural mesotheliomas, mean survival time was 11.4 months and median survival time 10 months. The mean survival time in

Table 34–17. Results of surgical resection for mesothelioma

Study	Year	Number of patients	Type of resection	Patients surviving (%)			Years of disease-free survival
				1 year	2 years	5 years	
Worn[303]	1974	186	Radical	75	34	9	Not specified
		62	"Palliative"	68	37	10	Not specified
Butchart et al.[273]	1976	29	Radical	30	30	3	3.5; 6
Wanebo et al.[304]	1976	33	Pleurectomy	NS*	30	15	2 to 5+[a]
DeLaria et al.[305]	1978	11	Radical	36	27	0	2; 4
Antman et al.[272]	1980	10	Pleurectomy	70	30	10	5

[a] In six patients. Reprinted by permission of *The New England Journal of Medicine* 1980; 303:200–202.

peritoneal mesothelioma was 7.4 months. The median survival time from diagnosis to death for patients with pleural mesotheliomas was 5 months and for peritoneal mesothelioma 2 months. The authors found no differences for survival time between various treatment modalities or between treated and untreated patients. The authors concluded that survival time in mesothelioma was short, most patients die within 1 year from the onset of symptoms and no effective therapy for malignant mesothelioma was available.

Tammilehto[301] prospectively studied 98 patients with histologically proven malignant mesothelioma, 93 pleural and 5 peritoneal, diagnosed between 1981 and 1990. Treatment consisted of surgery ($n = 15$), surgery and chemotherapy ($n = 11$), surgery and radiotherapy ($n = 14$), surgery chemotherapy and radiotherapy ($n = 28$), chemotherapy ($n = 3$), chemotherapy and radiotherapy ($n = 9$), radiotherapy ($n = 8$), and no treatment ($n = 10$). The median survival for all 98 patients calculated from the date of histologic diagnosis was 9 months with a range of 0–81 months. Eighteen patients were alive 2 years after diagnosis and 2 patients 5 years after diagnosis. By univariate analysis, good prognostic factors included age ≤ 65 years (11 months median survival versus 6 months median survival for those >65), female gender (13 months median survival versus 8 months for males), epithelial histology (median survival 14 months versus 2–5 months for sarcomatous histology), performance status WHO ≤ 1 (13 months median survival versus 3 months for WHO >1), stage I-IIA (11.5 months versus 5 months for stage IIB, III, and IV) and a diagnostic delay of more than 6 months from first symptom to histological diagnosis (14.5 months median survival versus 8 months for diagnostic delay of ≤ 6 months). Low S-phase fraction was associated with a better survival (16 months median survival) than a high S-phase fraction (median survival of 8 months), although DNA ploidy had no effect. Lung tissue fiber content of $<10^6$ fibers per gram of dry lung tissue was associated with a median survival of 26 months whereas a concentration $\geq 10^6$ fibers per gram of dry lung tissue showed a median survival of 13 months. Factors by multivariate analysis that were prog-

nostically favorable included good performance status (WHO ≤ 1), diagnostic delay of more than 6 months, epithelial histology, and clinical stage I or IIA. Although the patients who were treated with either surgery, chemotherapy, or irradiation appeared to survive longer this apparent increased survival was not significant when other factors were considered.

Sridhar et al.[302] evaluated survival rates and prognostic factors in 49 patients with malignant mesothelioma diagnosed between 1977 and 1991. The male-to-female ratio for patients with mesothelioma was 4:1, and the patients ranged in age between 36 and 77 years with a mean and median of 58 years. Asbestos exposure was identified in 75% of patients in whom a history was available. Most patients presented with Butchart stage 1–2 disease. Thirty-three patients were treated with a variety of combinations of chemotherapeutic agents, 14 were treated by various surgical modalities, and 10 patients received some type of radiation therapy. The median time from first symptom to diagnosis was 3 months. The median survival for pleural mesotheliomas was 13 months, and 15 months for peritoneal mesotheliomas from the onset of first symptom. Survival was longer in patients with earlier stage disease, a good performance status, a longer duration of symptoms, an absence of pain, and those who were treated with combined surgery and chemotherapy.

Antman[272] tabulated the results of surgical resection (Table 34–17) and has shown few patients survive more than 5 years and are disease free.

The experience at this author's previous institution to date with pleuropneumonectomy was variable. Two patients were alive with no evidence of disease 1.5 and 3 years after surgery, whereas two other patients were dead 5 and 7 months after surgery. The treatment for metastatic tumors to the pleura is also generally unsuccessful with survival times of usually less than 1 year.

Summary

In this chapter diseases of the pleura were discussed with an emphasis on pleural neoplasms, especially malignant mesothelioma. The histologic, immunohistochemical, and ultrastructural features of mesotheliomas were described in detail and are related to our concept of the histogenesis of mesotheliomas. The morphologic features of mesotheliomas were contrasted with other pleural tumors.

References

1. Davies J. Development of the respiratory system. In: Human developmental anatomy. New York: Ronald Press, 1963:135–143.
2. Minot C. The mesoderm and the coelom of vertebrates. Am Nat 1890;24:877–898.
3. Sahn SA. The pleura. Am Rev Respir Dis 1988;138:184–234.
4. Light RW. Anatomy of the pleura. In: Pleural diseases. 2d Ed. Philadelphia: Lea & Febiger, 1990:1–7.
5. Antony VB, Sahn SA, Mossman B, Gail DB, Kalica A. Pleural cell biology in health and disease. Am Rev Respir Dis 1992;145:1236–1239.
6. Gaudio E, Rendina E, Pannarale L, Ricci C, Marinozzi G. Surface morphology of the human pleura: A scanning electron microscopic study. Chest 1988;92:149–153.
7. Wang NS. The preformed stomas connecting the pleural cavity and lymphatics in the parietal pleura. Am Rev Respir Dis 1975;111:12–20.
8. Leak LV, Rahil L. Permeability of the diaphragmatic mesothelium: The ultrastructural basis for "stomata." Am J Anat 1978;151:557–594.
9. Courtice FC, Simmonds SJ. Physiological significance of lymph drainage of the serous cavities and lungs. Physiol Rev 1954;34:419–448.
10. Sahn SA. The differential diagnosis of pleural effusions. West J Med 1982;137:99–108.
11. Pistolesi M, Miniati M, Giontini C. Pleural liquid and solute exchange. Am Rev Respir Dis 1989;140:825–847.
12. Light RW. Clinical manifestations and useful tests. Pleural diseases. 2d Ed. Philaelphia: Lea & Febiger, 1990:39–73.
13. Yokoi T, Mark EJ. Atypical mesothelial hyperplasia associated with bronchogenic carcinoma. Hum Pathol 1991;22:695–699.
14. Buchanan DR, Johnston IP, Ken IH, Hetzel MR, Corrin B, Turner-Warwick M. Cryptogenic bilateral fibrosing pleuritis. Br J Dis Chest 1988;82:186–193.
15. Askin FB, McCann BC, Kuhn C. Reactive eosinophilic pleuritis: A lesion to be distinguished from pulmonary eosinophilic granuloma. Arch Pathol Lab Med 1977;101:187–191.
16. Light RW, Girard WM, Jenkinson SG, George RB. Parapneumonic effusions. Am J Med 1980;985–986.
17. Taryle DA, Potts DE, Sahn SA. The incidence and clinical correlates of parapneumonic effusions in pneumococcal pneumonia. Chest 1978;74:170–173.
18. Bartlett JG, Gorbach SL, Thadepalli H, Finegold SM. Bacteriology of empyema. Lancet 1974;i:338–340.
19. Varkey B, Rose HD, Kutty CPK, Politis J. Empyema thoracis during a ten-year period. Arch Intern Med 1981;141:1771–1776.
20. United States Department of Health Education and Welfare, Public Health Service. Center for Disease Control. Extrapulmonary tuberculosis in the United States. DHEW Publication (CDC) 78-8360. Washington, DC, 1978.
21. Stead WW, Eichenholz A, Stauss HK. Operative and pathologic findings in twenty-four patients with syndrome of idiopathic pleurisy with effusion, presumably tuberculosis. Am Rev Tuberc 1955;71:473–502.
22. Abrams WB, Small MJ. Current concepts of tuberculous pleurisy with effusion as derived from pleural biopsy studies. Scand J Respir Dis 1960;38:60–65.
23. Green WR, Bouchette D. Pleural mucormycosis (zyomycosis). Arch Pathol Lab Med 1986;110:441–442.
24. Mariuz P, Raviglione MC, Gould IA, Mollen MP. Pleural pneumocystis carinii infection. Chest 1991;99:774–776.
25. Rubin EH. Pulmonary lesions in "rheumatoid disease" with remarks on diffuse interstitial fibrosis. Am J Med 1955;19:569–582.
26. Sievers K, Aho K, Hurri L, Perttala Y. Studies of rheumatoid pulmonary disease: A comparison of roentgenographic findings among patients with high rheumatoid factor titers and with completely negative reactions. Acta Tuberc Scand 1964;45:21–34.
27. Walker WC, Wright V. Pulmonary lesions and rheumatoid arthritis. Medicine (Baltimore) 1968;47:501–519.
28. Horler AR, Thompson M. The pleural and pulmonary complications of rheumatoid arthritis. Ann Intern Med 1959;51:1179–1203.
29. Wilen SB, Rabinowitz JG, Ulrich S, Lyons HA. Pleural involvement in sarcoidosis. Am J Med 1974;57:200–209.
30. Mark EJ, Matsubara O, Jan-Liu NS, Fineberg R. The pulmonary biopsy in the early diagnosis of Wegener's (pathergic) granulomatosis: A study based on 35 open lung biopsies. Hum Pathol 1988;19:1065–1071.
31. Gonzalez L, VanOrdstrand HS. Wegener's granulomatosis. Radiology 1973;107:295–300.
32. Liem K, ten Veen JH, Lie KI, Feltkamp TEW, Durrer D. Incidence and significance of heart muscle antibodies in patients with acute myocardial infarction and unstable angina. Acta Med Scand 1979;206:473–475.
33. Toole JC, Silverman ME. Pericarditis of acute myocardial infarction. Chest 1975;67:647–653.
34. Engle MA, McCabe JC, Ebert PA, Zabriskie J. The post-cardiotomy syndrome and anti-heart antibodies. Circulation 1974;49:401–406.
35. Van Der Geld H. Anti-heart antibodies in the post-pericardiotomy and post-myocardial infarction syndromes. Lancet 1964;ii:617–621.
36. Aisner J, Wiernick PH. Malignant mesothelioma. Current status and future prospects. Chest 1978;74:438–443.
37. Chahinian AP. Malignant mesothelioma. In: Holland

JF, Frei E, III, eds. Cancer medicine. Philadelphia: Lea & Febiger, 1982:1744–1751.

38. Wagner E. Das tuberkelahnliche lymphadenom. Arch Heilk 1870;11:495–525.

39. Robertson HE. "Endothelioma" of the pleura. Am J Cancer 1924;8:317–375.

40. Klemperer P, Rabin CB. Primary neoplasms of pleura: report of 5 cases. Arch Pathol 1931;11:385–412.

41. Stout AP, Murray MR. Localized pleural mesothelioma: investigation of its characteristics and histogenesis by the method of tissue culture. Arch Pathol 1942;34:951–964.

42. Foster EA, Ackerman LV. Localized mesotheliomas of the pleura: The pathologic evaluation of 18 cases. Am J Clin Pathol 1960;34:349–364.

43. Wagner JC, Sleggs CA, Marchand P. Diffuse pleural mesothelioma and asbestos exposure in North Western Cape Province. Br J Ind Med 1960;17:260–271.

44. Wagner JC. The discovery of the association between blue asbestos and mesotheliomas and the aftermath. Br J Ind Med 1991;48:399–403.

45. Wagner JC. Asbestos and mesothelioma: A personal reminiscence. In: Henderson DW, Shilkin KB, Langlois SLP, Whitaker D, eds. Malignant mesothelioma. New York: Hemisphere, 1992:xvii–xxv.

46. Selikoff IJ, Churg J, Hammond EC. Relation between exposure to asbestos and mesothelioma. N Engl J Med 1965;272:560–565.

47. Wedler HW, Uber den Lungenkrebs bei Asbestose. Dtsch Arch Klin Med 1943;191:189–209.

48. Wedler HW. Uber den Lungonkrebs bei Asbestose. Deutsch Med Wochenschr 1943;69:575–576.

49. Merewether ERA. Annual Report of the Chief Inspector of Factories for the year 1947. His Majesty's Stationery Office, London. 1949:78–81.

50. Mallory TB, Castleman B, Parris EE. Case records of the Massachusetts General Hospital #33111. N Engl J Med 1947;236:407–412.

51. Weiss A. Pleurakrbs bei Lungenasbestose, in vivo morphologisch Geishert. Medizienische 1953;3:93–94.

52. Leicher F Primarer deckzellen Tumor des Bauchtells bei Asbestose. Arch Gewerbepathol Gewerbehyg 1954;13:382–392.

53. Keal EE. Asbestosis and abdominal neoplasms. Lancet 1960;ii:1211–1216.

54. Goodwin MC. Diffuse mesotheliomas with comment on their relationship to localized fibrous mesotheliomas. Cancer (Philadelphia) 1967;10:298–319.

55. Motley RL. The lid comes off. Trial 1980;15:21–24.

56. Brodeur P. Expendable Americans. New York: Viking, 1974.

57. Brodeur P. The asbestos industry on trial. I—A failure to warn. II—Discovery. III—Judgement. IV—Bankruptcy. New Yorker 1985;61:49–52+ (Je 10); 45–48+ (Je 17); 37–41+(Je 24); 36–38+ (Jl 1).

58. McDonald AD, Harper A, El Attar DA, McDonald JC. Epidemiology of primary malignant mesothelial tumors in Canada. Cancer (Philadelphia) 1970;26:914–919.

59. Theriault GP, Grand-Bois L. Mesothelioma and asbestos in the province of Quebec, 1969–1972. Arch Environ Health 1978;33:15–19.

60. Biava PM, Ferri R, Spacal B, et al. Cancro de lovora a Trieste: II mesothelioma della pleura. Sapere 1976;79:41–45.

61. Greenberg M, Lloyd-Davies TA. Mesothelioma register 1967–1968. Br J Ind Med 1974;31:91–104.

62. McDonald AD, McDonald JC. Malignant mesothelioma in North America. Cancer (Philadelphia) 1980;46:1650–1656.

63. Cutler SJ, Young JL. Third National Cancer Survey: Incidence data. Natl Cancer Inst Monogr 1975;41:442.

64. Bruckman L, Rubino RA, Christine B. Asbestos and mesothelioma incidence in Connecticut. J Air Pollut Control Assoc 1977;27:121–126.

65. Churg A. Malignant mesothelioma in British Columbia in 1982. Cancer (Philadelphia) 1985;55:672–674.

66. Ferguson D. Malignant mesothelioma—the rising epidemic. Med J Austral 1989;150:233–235.

67. McDonald JC, McDonald AD. Epidemiology of mesothelioma from estimated incidence. Prev Med 1977;6:426–446.

68. Hughes JM, Weill H. Asbestos exposure—quantitative assessment of risk. Am Rev Respir Dis 1986;133:5–13.

69. Selikoff IJ, Hammond EC, Seidman H. Mortality experience of insulation workers in the United States and Canada 1943–1976. Ann NY Acad Sci 1979;330:91–116.

70. Huncharek M. Changing risk groups for malignant mesothelioma. Cancer (Philadelphia) 1992;69:2704–2711.

71. Wagner JC. Mesothelioma and mineral fibers. Cancer (Philadelphia) 1986;57:1905–1911.

72. Rom WM, Lockey JE. Diffuse malignant mesothelioma: a review. West J Med 1982;137:548–554.

73. Legha SS, Muggia FM. Pleural mesothelioma: Clinical features and therapeutic implications. Ann Intern Med 1977;87:613–621.

74. Borow M, Conston A, Livornese L, Schalet N. Mesothelioma following exposure to asbestos: A review of 72 cases. Chest 1973;64:641–646.

75. Cochrane JC, Webster I. Mesothelioma in relation to asbestos fibre exposure. A review of 70 serial cases. S Afr Med J 1978;54:279–281.

76. Tagnon I, Blot WJ, Stroube RB, et al. Mesothelioma associated with the shipbuilding industry in coastal Virginia. Cancer Res 1980;40:3875–3879.

77. Whitwell F, Rawcliffe RM. Diffuse malignant pleural mesothelioma and asbestos exposure. Thorax 1971;26:6–22.

78. Hammas SP. Mesothelioma. In: Sheppard MN, ed. Practical pulmonary pathology. Kent: Edward Arnold (in press).

79. Taylor RA, Johnson LP. Mesothelioma: Current perspectives. West J Med 1981;134:379–383.

80. Vogelzang NJ, Schultz SM, Iannucci AM, Kennedy BJ. Malignant mesothelioma: The University of Minnesoto experience. Cancer (Philadelphia) 1984;53:377–383.

81. Newhouse ML, Thompson H. Mesothelioma of pleura and peritoneum following exposure to asbestos in the London area. Br J Ind Med 1965;22:261–269.

82. Peto J, Henderson BE, Pike MC. Trends in mesothelioma in the United States and the forecast epidemic due to asbestos exposure during World War II. In: Peto R, Schneiderman M, eds. Quantification of occupational cancer. Banbary Report 9. New York: Cold Spring Harbor Laboratory:51–69.

83. Roggli VL, McGavran MH, Subach J, Sybers HD, Greenberg SD. Pulmonary asbestos body counts and electron probe analysis of asbestos body cores in patients with mesothelioma: A study of 25 cases. Cancer (Philadelphia) 1982;50:2423–2432.

84. Oels HC, Harrison EG, Carr DT, Bernatz PE. Diffuse malignant mesothelioma of the pleura: A review of 37 cases. Chest 1971;60:564–470.

85. Brenner J, Sordillo PP, Magill GB, Golbey RB. Malignant mesothelioma of the pleura: review of 123 patients. Cancer (Philadelphia) 1982;49:2431–2435.

86. Ratzer ER, Pool JL, Melamed MR. Pleural mesotheliomas: Clinical experiences with thirty-seven patients. Am J Radiol 1967;99:863–880.

87. Newhouse ML, Berry G. Patterns of mortality in asbestos factory workers in London. Ann NY Acad Sci 1979;330:53–60.

88. Newhouse ML, Berry G. Predictions of mortality from mesothelial tumours in asbestos factory workers. Br J Ind Med 1976;33:147–151.

89. Epler GR, Gerlad MXF, Gaensler EA, Carrington CB. Asbestos-related disease from household exposure. Respiration 1980;39:229–240.

90. Chen W, Mottet NK. Malignant mesothelioma with minimal asbestos exposure. Hum Pathol 1978;9:253–258.

91. Anderson HA, Lils R, Daum SM, et al. Asbestosis among household contacts of asbestos factory workers. Am NY Acad Sci 1979;330:387–399.

92. Vianna NJ, Polan AK. Non-occupational exposure to asbestos and malignant mesothelioma in females. Lancet 1978;i:1061–1063.

93. Kane MJ, Chahinian P, Holland JF. Malignant mesothelioma in young adults. Cancer (Philadelphia) 1990;65:1449–1455.

94. Cazzadori A, Malesani F, Romeo L. Malignant pleural mesothelioma caused by non-occupational childhood exposure to asbestos. Br J Ind Med 1992;49:599.

95. Dodoli D, Del Nevo M, Fiumalbi C, et al. Environmental household exposure to asbestos and occurrence of pleural mesothelioma. Am J Ind Med 1992;21:681–687.

96. Staunton MF, Wrench C. Mechanisms of mesothelioma induction with asbestos and fibrous glass. J Natl Cancer Inst 1972;48:797–821.

97. Stanton MF, Layord M, Tegeris A, et al. Relation of particle dimension to carcinogenicity in amphibole asbestos and other fibrous minerals. J Natl Cancer Inst 1981;67:965–975.

98. Gross P. Is short fibered asbestos dust a biological hazard? Arch Environ Health 1974;29:115–117.

99. Churg A, Wiggs B. Fiber size and number in amphibole asbestos-induced mesothelioma. Am J Pathol 1984;115:437–442.

100. Weiss W. Mortality of a cohort exposed to chrysotile asbestos. J Occup Med 1977;19:737–740.

101. McDonald JC, Liddell FDK, Gibbs GW, Eyssen GE, McDonald AD. Dust exposure and mortality in chrysotile mining, 1910–75. Br J Ind Med 1980;37:11–24.

102. McDonald AD, Fry JS, Mesothelioma and fiber type in three American asbestos factories—preliminary report. Scand J Work Environ Health 1982;8(Suppl.):55–58.

103. Acheson ED, Gardner MJ, Pippard EC, Grime LP. Mortality of two groups of women who manufactured gas masks from chrysotile and crocidolite asbestos: A 40-year follow-up. Br J Ind Med 1982;39:344–348.

104. Dement JM, Harris RL, Symons MJ, Shy CM. Exposure and mortality among chrysotile asbestos workers. Part II. Mortality. Am J Ind Med 1983;4:421–433.

105. Browne K, Smither WJ. Asbestos related mesothelioma: Factors discriminating between pleural and peritoneal sites. Br J Ind Med 1983;40:145–152.

106. Berry G, Newhouse ML. Mortality of workers manufacturing friction materials using asbestos. Br J Ind Med 1983;40:1–7.

107. Acheson ED, Gardner MJ, Bennet C, Winter PD. Mesothelioma in a factory using amosite and chrysotile asbestos. Lancet 1981;ii:1403–1406.

108. Churg A, Wiggs B, Depaoli L, Kampe B, Stevens B. Lung asbestos content in chrysotile workers with mesothelioma. Am Rev Respir Dis 1984;130:1042–1045.

109. Rogers AJ, Leigh J, Berry G, Ferguson DA, Mulder HB, Ackad M. Relationship between lung asbestos fiber type and concentration and relative risk of mesothelioma: A case-control study. Cancer (Philadelphia) 1991;67:1912–1920.

110. Huncharek M. Brake mechanics, asbestos, and disease risk. Am J Forensic Med Pathol 1990;11:236–240.

111. Begin R, Gauthier J, Desmeules M, Ostiguy G. Work-related mesothelioma in Quebec, 1967–1990. Am J Ind Med 1992;22:531–542.

112. Hillerdal G. Malignant mesothelioma 1982: Review of 4710 published cases. Br J Dis Chest 1983;77:321–343.

113. Peterson JT, Jr., Greenberg SD, Buffler PA. Non-asbestos-related malignant mesothelioma: A review. Cancer (Philadelphia) 1984;54:951–960.

114. Baris YI. Pleural mesotheliomas and abestos pleurisies due to environmental asbestos exposure in Turkey: An analysis of 120 cases. Hacettepe Bull Med/Surg 1975;8:165–185.

115. Baris YI, Sahin AA, Ozesmi M, et al. An outbreak of pleural mesothelioma and chronic fibrosing pleurisy in the village of Karain/Urgup in Anatolia. Thorax 1978;33:181–192.

116. Artvinli M, Baris YI. Malignant mesotheliomas in a small village in the Anatolian region of Turkey: An epidemiologic study. J Natl Cancer Inst 1979;63:17–

22.

117. Baris YI, Saracci R, Simonato L, Skidmore JW, Artvinli M. Malignant mesothelioma and radiological chest abnormalities in two villages in central Turkey. Lancet 1981;i:984–987.

118. Artvinli M, Baris YI. Environmental fiber-induced pleuro-pulmonary diseases in an Anatolian village: An epidemiologic study. Arch Environ Health 1982;37:177–181.

119. Lillis R. Fibrous zeolites and endemic mesothelioma in Cappadocia, Turkey. J Occup Med 1981;23:548–550.

120. Sebastien P, Gaudichet A, Bignon J, Baris YI. Zeolite bodies in human lungs from Turkey. Lab Invest 1981;44:420–425.

121. Wagner JC, Skidmore JW, Hill RJ, Griffiths DM. Erionite exposure and mesotheliomas in rats. Br J Cancer 1985;51:727–750.

122. Rohl AN, Langer AM, Moncure G, Selikoff IJ, Fischbein A. Endemic pleural disease associated with exposure to mixed fibrous dust in Turkey. Science 1982;216:518–520.

123. Hillerdal G, Berg J. Malignant mesothelioma secondary to chronic inflammation and old scars: Two new cases and review of the literature. Cancer (Philadelphia) 1985;55:1968–1972.

124. Austin MB, Fechner RE, Roggli VL. Pleural malignant mesothelioma following Wilms' tumor. Am J Clin Pathol 1986;86:227–230.

125. Anderson KA, Hurley WC, Hurley BT, Ohrt DW. Malignant pleural mesothelioma following radiotherapy in a 16-year-old boy. Cancer (Philadelphia) 1985;56:273–276.

126. Talerman A, Montero JR, Chilcote RR, Okagaki T. Diffuse malignant peritoneal mesothelioma in a 13-year-old girl: Report of a case and review of the literature. Am J Surg Pathol 1985;9:73–80.

127. Fraire AE, Cooper S, Greenberg SD, Buffler PA, Langston C. Mesothelioma of childhood. Lab Invest 1987;56:25A.

128. Fraire AE, Cooper S, Greenberg SD, Buffler P, Langston C. Mesothelioma of childhood. Cancer (Philadelphia) 1988;62:838–847.

129. Lin-Chu M, Lee Y, Ho MY. Malignant mesothelioma in infancy. Arch Pathol Lab Med 1989;113:409–411.

130. Lynch HT, Katz D, Markvicka SE. Familial mesothelioma: review and family study. Cancer Genet Cytogenet 1985;15:25–35.

131. Martensson G, Larsson S, Zettergren L. Malignant mesothelioma in two pairs of siblings: Is there a hereditary predisposing factor? Eur J Respir Dis 1984;65:179–184.

132. Hammar S. Familial mesothelioma: A report of two families. Hum Pathol 1989;20:107–112.

133. Maolli PA, Macdonald JL, Goodglick LA, Kane AB. Acute injury and regeneration of the mesothelium in response to asbestos fibers. Am J Pathol 1987;128:426–445.

133a. Adamson IYR, Bakowska J, Bowden DH. Mesothelial cell proliferation after instillation of long or short asbestos fibers into mouse lung. Am J Pathol 1993;142:1209–1216.

134. Muscat JE, Wynder EL. Cigarette smoking, asbestos exposure, and malignant mesothelioma. Cancer Res 1991;51:2263–2267.

135. Roggli VL, McGavran MH, Subach J, Sybers HD, Greenberg SD. Pulmonary asbestos body counts and electron probe analysis of asbestos body cores in patients with mesothelioma: A study of 25 cases. Cancer (Philadelphia) 1982;50:2423–2432.

136. Tuomi T, Huuskonen MS, Tammilehto L, Vanhala E, Virtamo M. Occupational exposure to asbestos evaluated from work histories and analysis of lung tissues from patients with mesothelioma. Br J Ind Med 1991;48:48–52.

137. Leigh J, Rogers AJ, Ferguson DA, Mudler HB, Ackad M, Thompson R. Lung asbestos fiber content and mesothelioma cell type, site and survival. Cancer (Philadelphia) 1991;68:135–141.

137a. Roggli VL, Pratt PC, Brody AR. Asbestos fiber type in malignant mesothelioma: An analytical scanning electron microscopic study of 94 cases. Am J Ind Med 1993;23:605–614.

138. McCaughey WTE. Criteria for the diagnosis of diffuse mesothelial tumors. Ann NY Acad Sci 1965;132:603–613.

139. Kannerstein M, McCaughey WTE, Churg J, Selikoff IJ. A critique for the diagnosis of diffuse malignant mesothelioma. Mt Sinai J Med (NY) 1977;44:485–494.

140. Kannerstein M, Churg J, McCaughey WTE. Asbestos and mesothelioma: a review. Pathol Annu 1978:81–130.

141. Adams VI, Unni KK. Diffuse malignant mesothelioma of pleura: Diagnostic criteria based on an autopsy study. Am J Clin Pathol 1984;82:15–23.

142. McCaughey WTE, Kannerstein M, Churg J. Tumors and pseudotumors of the serous membranes. Washington, DC: Armed Forces Institute of Pathology, 1985.

143. Yousem SA, Hochholzer L. Malignant mesotheliomas with osseous and cartilaginous differentiation. Arch Pathol Lab Med 1987;111:62–66.

144. Kannerstein M, Churg J. Desmoplastic diffuse malignant mesothelioma. In: Fernoglio CM, Wolff M, eds. Progress in surgical pathology. New York: Masson, 1980:19–29.

145. Cantin R, Al-Jabi M, McCaughey WTE. Desmoplastic diffuse mesothelioma. Am J Surg Pathol 1982;6:215–222.

146. Dardick I, Al-Jabi M, McCaughey WTE, Srigley JR, van Nostrand AWP, Ritchie AC. Ultrastructure of poorly differentiated diffuse epithelial mesotheliomas. Ultrastruct Pathol 1984;7:151–160.

147. Henderson DW, Atwood HD, Constance TJ, Shilkin KB, Steele RH. Lymphohistiocytoid mesothelioma: A rare variant of predominantly sarcomatoid mesothelioma. Ultra Pathology 1988;12:367–384.

148. Whitaker D, Henderson DW, Shilkin KB. The concept of mesothelioma in situ: Implications for diagnosis and histogenesis. Semin Diagn Pathol 1992;98:151–161.

149. Myer J, Tazelaar H, Katzenstein L, et al. Localized malignant epithelioid and biphasic mesothelioma of the pleura: Clinicopathologic, immunohistochemical, and flow cytometric analysis of 3 cases. Mod Pathol 1992;5:679 (abstr).

150. Briselli M, Mark EJ, Dickersin GR. Solitary fibrous tumors of the pleura: Eight new cases and review of 360 cases in the literature. Cancer (Philadelphia) 1981;47:2678–2689.

151. Doucet J, Dardick I, Srigley JR, van Nostrand AWP, Bell MA, Kahn HJ. Localized fibrous tumour of serosal surfaces: Immunohistochemical and ultrastructural evidence for a type of mesothelioma. Virchows Arch [Pathol Anat] 1986;409:349–3653.

152. Carter D, Otis CN. Three types of spindle cell tumors of the pleura: fibroma, sarcoma and sarcomatoid mesothelioma. Am J Surg Pathol 1988;12:747–753.

153. England DM, Hochholzer L, McCarthy MJ. Localized benign and malignant fibrous tumors of the pleura: A clinicopathologic review of 223 cases. Am J Surg Pathol 1989;13:640–658.

154. Cook HC, Carbohydrates. In: Bancroft JD, Stevens A, eds. Theory and practice of histological techniques. New York: Churchill Livingstone, 1982:180–216.

155. Ernst CS, Atkinson BF. Mucicarmine positivity in malignant mesothelioma. Lab Invest 1980;42:113–114 (abstr).

156. McCaughey WTE, Colby TV, Battifora H, et al. Diagnosis of diffuse malignant mesothelioma: Experience of a US/Canadian mesothelioma panel. Mod Pathol 1991;4:342–353.

157. MacDougall D, Wang SE, Zidar BL. Mucin-positive epithelial mesothelioma. Arch Pathol Lab Med 1992;116:874–880.

158. Hammar SP, Bockus DE, Remington FL, Rohrbach KA. Mucicarmine positive mesothelioma: A histochemical, immunohistochemical, and ultrastructural comparison with micin-producing pulmonary adenocarcinoma (submitted to Ultra Pathol).

159. Benjamin CJ, Ritchie AC. Histological staining for the diagnosis of mesothelioma. Am J Med Technol 1982;48:905–908.

160. Hsu SM, Raine L, Fanger H. Use of avidin-biotin peroxidase complex (ABC) in immunoperoxidase techniques: A comparison between ABC and unlabeled antibody (PAP) procedures. J Histochem Cytochem 1981;29:577–580.

161. Sun TT, Eichner R, Nelson WG, et al. Keratin classes: Molecular markers for different types of epithelial differentiation. J Invest Dermatol 1983;81:109–115 (suppl).

162. Moll R, Franke WW, Schiller DL, et al. The catalogue of human cytokeratins: Patterns of expression in normal epithelia, tumors and cultured cells. Cell 1982;31:11–24.

163. Bolen JW, Hammar SP, McNutt MA. Reactive and neoplastic serosal tissue: A light-microscopic, ultrastructural and immunocytochemical study. Am J Surg Pathol 1986;10:34–47.

164. Montag AG, Pinkus GS, Coson JM. Immunoreactivity for keratin proteins in sarcomatoid diffuse malignant mesothelioma: A diagnostic discriminant among spindle cell tumors. Lab Invest 1985;52:44A.

165. Leong AS-Y, Parkinson R, Milios J. "Thick" cell membranes revealed by immunocytochemical staining: A clue to the diagnosis of mesothelioma. Diagn Cytopathol 1990;6:9–13.

166. Miettinen M. Keratin subsets in spindle cell sarcomas: Keratins are widespread but synovial sarcoma contains a distinctive keratin polypeptide pattern and desmoplakins. Am J Pathol 1991;138:505–513.

167. Said JW, Nash G, Banks-Schlegel S, Sassoon AF, Shintaku IF. Keratin in human lung tumors: Patterns of localization of different molecular-weight keratin proteins. Am J Pathol 1983;113:27–32.

168. Watts AE, Said JW, Shintaku IP, Sassoon AF, Banks-Schlegel S. Keratins of different molecular weight in exfoliated mesothelial and adenocarcinoma cells—an aid to cell identification. Am J Clin Pathol 1984;81:442–446.

169. Kahn HJ, Hanna W, Yeger H, Baumal R. Immunohistochemical localization of prekeratin filaments in benign and malignant cells in effusions: Comparison with intermediate filament distribution by electromicroscopy. Am J Pathol 1982;109:206–214.

170. Kahn HJ, Thorner PS, Yeger H, Bailey D, Baumal R. Distinct keratin patterns demonstrated by immunoperoxidase staining of adenocarcinomas, carcinoids and mesotheliomas using polyclonal and monoclonal anti-keratin antibodies. Am J Clin Pathol 1986;86:566–574.

171. Blobel GA, Moll R, Franke WW, Kayser KW, Gould VE. The intermediate filament cytoskeleton of malignant mesotheliomas and its diagnostic significance. Am J Pathol 1985;121:235–247.

172. Moll R, Dhovailly D, Sun T. Expression of keratin 5 as a distinctive feature of epithelial and biphasic mesotheliomas: An immunohistochemical study using monoclonal antibody AE14. Virchow Arch [B] Cell Pathol 1989;58:129–145.

173. Churg A. Immunohistochemical staining for vimentin and keratin in malignant mesothelioma. Am J Surg Pathol 1985;9:360–365.

174. Jasani B, Edwards RE, Thomas ND, Gibbs AR. The use of vimentin antibodies in the diagnosis of malignant mesothelioma. Virchows Arch [A] 1985;406:441–448.

175. Mullink H, Henzen-Logmans SC, Alons-van Kordelaar JJM, et al. Simultaneous immunoenzyme staining of vimentin and cytokeratins with monoclonal antibodies as an aid in the differential diagnosis of malignant mesothelioma from pulmonary adenocarcinoma. Virchows Arch [B] Pathol Anat 1986;42:55–65.

176. Upton MP, Hirohashi S, Tome Y, Miyazawa N, Suemasu K, Shimosato Y. Expression of vimentin in surgically resected adenocarcinomas and large cell carcinomas of lung. Am J Surg Pathol 1986;10:560–567.

177. Marshall RJ, Herbert A, Braye SG, Jones DB. Use of antibodies to carcinoembryonic antigen and human milk fat globule to distinguish carcinoma, mesothe-

lioma and reactive mesothelium. J Clin Pathol 1984;37: 1215–1221.

178. Loosli H, Hurlimann J. Immunohistological study of malignant diffuse mesotheliomas of the pleura. Histopathology 1984;8:793–803.

179. Hammar SP, Bolen JW, Bockus D, Remington F, Friedman S. Ultrastructural and immunohistochemical features of common lung tumors: An overview. Ultra Pathol 1985;9:283–318.

180. Battifora H, Kopinski MI. Distinction of mesothelioma from adenocarcinoma: An immunohistochemical approach. Cancer (Philadelphia) 1985;55:1679–1685.

181. Wang N-S, Huang S-N, Gold P. Absense of carcinoembryonic antigen-like material in mesothelioma: An immunohistochemical differentiation from lung cancer. Cancer (Philadelphia) 1979;44:947–954.

182. Whitaker D, Shilkin KB. Carcinoembryonic antigen in tissue diagnosis of malignant mesothelioma. Lancet 1981;i:1369.

183. Corson JM, Pinkus GS. Mesothelioma: Profile of keratin proteins and carcinoembryonic antigen: An immunoperoxidase study of 20 cases and comparison with pulmonary adenocarcinomas. Am J Pathol 1982;108: 80–87.

184. Kwee WS, Veldhuizen RW, Golding RP, et al. Histologic distinction between malignant mesothelioma, benign pleural lesion and carcinoma metastasis: Evaluation of the application of morphometry combined with histochemistry and immunostaining. Virchows Arch [A] 1982;397:287–299.

185. Said JW, Nash G, Tepper G, Banks-Schlegel S. Keratin proteins and carcinoembryonic antigen in lung carcinoma: An immunoperoxidase study of fifty-four cases with ultrastructural correlations. Hum Pathol 1983;14: 70–76.

186. Ghosh AK, Spriggs AL, Taylor-Papadimitriou J, Mason DY. Immunocytochemical staining of cells in pleural and peritoneal effusions with a panel of monoclonal antibodies. J Clin Pathol 1983;36:1154–1164.

187. Holden J, Churg A. Immunohistochemical staining for keratin and carcinoembryonic antigen in the diagnosis of malignant mesothelioma. Am J Surg Pathol 1984;8: 277–279.

188. Lee I, Radosevich JA, Chejfec G, et al. Malignant mesotheliomas: Improved differential diagnosis from lung adenocarcinomas using monoclonal antibodies 44–3A6 and 624A12. Am J Pathol 1986;123:497–507.

189. Sheibani K, Battifora H, Burke JS. Antigenic phenotype of malignant mesotheliomas and pulmonary adenocarcinomas: An immunohistologic analysis demonstrating the value of Leu M1 antigen. Am J Pathol 1986;123:212–219.

190. Szpak CA, Johnston WW, Roggli V, et al. The diagnostic distinction between malignant mesothelioma of the pleura and adenocarcinoma of the lung as defined by a monoclonal antibody (B72.3). Am J pathol 1986;122: 252–260.

191. Metzger J, Lamerz R, Permanether W. Diagnostic significance of carcinoembryonic antigen in the differen-

tial diagnosis of malignant mesothelioma. J Thorac Cardiovasc Surg 1990;100:860–866.

192. Sheibani K, Battifora H. Leu-M1 positivity not specific for Hodgkin's disease. Am J Clin Pathol 1985;84:682.

193. Sheibani K, Battifora H, Burke JS, et al. Leu-M1 in human neoplasms: An immunohistologic study of 400 cases. Am J Surg Pathol 1986;10:227–236.

194. Sheibani K, Battifora H, Burke J. Antigenic phenotype of malignant mesotheliomas and pulmonary adenocarcinomas: An immunohistologic analysis demonstrating the value of Leu M1 antigen. Am J Pathol 1986;123: 212–219.

195. Sheibani K, Azumi N, Battifora H. Further evidence demonstrating the value of Leu-M1 antigen in differential diagnosis of malignant mesothelioma and adenocarcinoma: an immunohistologic evaluation of 395 cases. Lab Invest 1988;58:84A.

196. Otis CN, Carter D, Cole S, Battifora H. Immunohistochemical evaluation of pleural mesothelioma and pulmonary adenocarcinoma. Am J Surg Pathol 1987; 11:445–456.

197. Sheibani K, Shin SS, Kezirian J, Weiss LM. Ber-EP4 antibody as a discriminant in the differential diagnosis of malignant mesothelioma. J Thorac Cardiovasc Surg 1990;100:860–866.

198. Goffey MJ, Mills SE, Swanson PE, Zarbo RJ, Shah AR, Wick MR. Immunoreactivity for BER-EP4 in adenocarcinomas, adenomatoid tumors, and malignant mesotheliomas. Am J Surg Pathol 1992;16:593–599.

199. Radosevich JA, Ma Y, Lee I, et al. Monoclonal antibody 44-3A6 in cell blocks in the diagnosis of lung carcinoma, carcinomas metastatic to lung and pleura, and pleural malignant mesotheliomas. Am J Clin Pathol 1991;95:322–329.

200. Spagnolo DV, Whitaker D, Carrello S, Radosevich JA, Rosen ST, Gould VE. The use of monoclonal antibody 44-3A6 in cell blocks in the diagnosis of lung carcinoma, carcinomas metastatic to lung and pleura, and pleural malignant mesothelioma. Am J Clin Pathol 1991;95:322–329.

201. Collins CL, Ordones NG, Schaefer R, et al. Thrombomodulin expression in malignant pleural mesothelioma and pulmonary adenocarcinoma. Am J Pathol 1992;141:827–833.

202. Jordan D, Jagurdar J, Kanedo M. Blood group antigens, Lewis[x] and Lewis[y] in the diagnostic discrimination of malignant mesothelioma versus adenocarcinoma. Am J Pathol 1989;134:931–937.

203. Noguchi M, Nakajima T, Hirohashi S, Akiba T, Shimosato Y. Immunohistochemical distinction of malignant mesothelioma from pulmonary adenocarcinoma with anti-surfactant apoprotein, anti-Lewis[a], and anti-Tn antibodies. Hum Pathol 1989;20:53–57.

204. Kawai T, Suzuki M, Torikata C, Suzuki Y. Expression of blood group-related antigens and helix promatia agglutinin in malignant pleural mesothelioma and pulmonary adenocarcinoma. Hum Pathol 1991;22:118–124.

205. Wick MR, Mills SE, Swanson PE. Expression of "my-

elomonocytic" antigens in mesotheliomas and adeno-carcinomas involving the serosal surfaces. Am J Clin Pathol 1990;94:18–26.

206. Azumi N, Underhill CB, Kagan E, Sheibani K. A novel biotinylated probe specific for hyaluronate: Its diagnostic value in diffuse malignant mesothelioma. Am J Surg Pathol 1992;16:116–121.

207. O'Hara CJ, Corson JM, Pinkus GS, Stahel RA. ME1: A monoclonal antibody that distinguishes epithelial-type malignant mesothelioma from pulmonary adenocarcinoma and extrapulmonary malignancies. Am J Pathol 1990;136:421–428.

208. Sheibani K, Esteban JM, Bailey A, Battifora H, Weiss LM. Immunopathologic and molecular studies as an aid to the diagnosis of malignant mesothelioma. Hum Pathol 1992;23:107–116.

209. Okamoto H, Matsuno Y, Noguchi M, et al. Malignant pleural mesothelioma producing chorionic gonadotropin: report of two cases. Am J Surg Pathol 1992;16:969–974.

210. McAuley P, Asa SL, Chiu B, Henderson J, Goltzman D, Drucker DJ. Parathyroid hormone-like peptide in normal and neoplastic mesothelial cells. Cancer (Philadelphia) 1990;66:1975–1979.

211. Warnock ML, Stoloff A, Thor A. Differentiation of adenocarcinoma of the lung from mesothelioma: periodic acid–Schiff, monoclonal antibodies B72.3 and Leu M1. Am J Pathol 1988;133:30–38.

212. Khoury N, Raju U, Crissman JD, Zarbo RJ, Greenawald KA. A comparative immunohistochemical study of peritoneal and ovarian serous tumors, and mesotheliomas. Hum Pathol 1990;21:811–819.

213. Wick MR, Loy T, Mills SE, Legier JF, Manivel JC. Malignant epithelioid pleural mesothelioma versus peripheral pulmonary adenocarcinoma: a histochemical, ultrastructural and immunohistologic study of 103 cases. Hum Pathol 1990;21:759–766.

214. Wirth PR, Legier J, Wright GL. Immunohistochemical evaluation of seven monoclonal antibodies for differentiation of pleural mesothelioma from lung adenocarcinoma. Cancer (Philadelphia) 1991;67:655–662.

215. Soosay GN, Griffiths M, Papadaki L, Happerfield L, Borrow L. The differential diagnosis of epithelial mesothelioma from adenocarcinoma and reactive mesothelial proliferation. J Pathol 1991;163:299–305.

216. Esteban JM, Yokota S, Husain S, Battifora H. Immunocytochemical profile of benign and carcinomatous effusions: A practical approach to difficult diagnosis. Am J Clin Pathol 1990;94:698–705.

217. Tickmon RJ, Cohen C, Varma VA, Fekete PS, De Rose PB. Distinction between carcinoma cells and mesothelial cells in serous effusions: Usefulness of immunohistochemistry. Acta Cytol 1990;34:491–496.

218. Nance KV, Silverman JF. Immunocytochemical panel for the identification of malignant cells in serous effusions. Am J Clin Pathol 1991;95:867–874.

219. Kuhlman L, Berghäuser K-H, Schäffer R. Distinction of mesothelioma from carcinoma in pleural effusions: An immunocytochemical study on routinely processed cytoblock preparations. Pathol Res Pract 1991;187:467–471.

220. Cibas ES, Corson JM, Pinkus GS. The distinction of adenocarcinoma from malignant mesothelioma in cell blocks of effusions: The role of routine mucin histochemistry and immunohistochemical assessment of carcinoembryonic antigen, keratin proteins, epithelial membrane antigen, and milk fat globule-derived antigen. Hum Pathol 1987;18:67–74.

221. Suzuki Y, Churg J, Kannerstein M. Ultrastructure of human malignant diffuse mesothelioma. Am J Pathol 1976;85:241–262.

222. Stoebner P, Bernaudin JF, Nebut M, Basset F. Contribution of electron microscopy to the diagnosis of pleural mesothelioma. Ann NY Acad Sci 1979;330:751–760.

223. Kay S, Silvergerg SG. Ultrastructural studies of a malignant fibrous mesothelioma of the pleura. Arch Pathol Lab Med 1971;92:449–455.

224. Wang N-S. Electron microscopy in the diagnosis of pleural mesotheliomas. Cancer (Philadelphia) 1973;31:1046–1054.

225. Bolen JW, Thorning D. Mesotheliomas. A light and electron-microscopical study concerning histogenetic relationships between the epithelial and mesenchymal variants. Am J Surg Pathol 1980;4:451–464.

226. Klima M, Bossart MI. Sarcomatous type of malignant mesothelioma. Ultrastruct Pathol 1983;4:349–358.

227. d'Andiran G, Gabbiani G. A metastasing sarcoma of the pleura composed of myofibroblasts. In: Fenoglio CM, Wolff M, eds. Progress in surgical pathology. New York: Mason, 1980:31–40.

228. Epstein JI, Budin RE. Keratin and epithelial membrane antigen immunoreactivity in nonneoplastic fibrous pleural lesions: Implications for the diagnosis of desmoplastic mesothelioma. Hum Pathol 1986;17:514–519.

229. Erlandson RA, Cordon-Cardo C, Melamed MR. Proposed classification of pleural neoplasms. Lab Invest 1986;54:19A.

230. el-Naggar A, Ward RM, Ro JY, Ayala AG, Ordonez NG. Fibrous tumor with hemangiopericytic pattern, so called "localized fibrous tumor of pleura." Lab Invest 1987;56:21A.

231. Warhol MJ, Hickey WF, Corson JM. Malignant mesothelioma: Ultrastructural distinction from adenocarcinoma. Am J Surg Pathol 1982;6:307–314.

232. Warhol MJ, Corson JM. An ultrastructural comparison of mesotheliomas with adenocarcinomas of the lung and breast. Hum Pathol 1985;16:50–55.

233. Burns TR, Greenberg SD, Mace ML, Johnson EH. Ultrastructural diagnosis of epithelial malignant mesothelioma. Cancer (Philadelphia) 1985;56:2036–2040.

234. Burns TRI, Johnson EH, Cartwright J, Jr., Greenberg SD. Desmosomes of epithelial malignant mesothelioma. Ultra Pathol 1988;12:385–388.

235. Tiainen M, Tammilethol L, Rautonen J, Tumoi T, Mattson K, Knoutila S. Chromosomal abnormalities

and their correlations with asbestos exposure and survival in patients with mesothelioma. Br J Cancer 1989; 60:618–626.

236. Hagemeijer A, Versnel MA, Van Drunen E, Moret M, Bouts MJ, van der Kwast TH, Hoogsteden HC. Cytogenetic analysis of malignant mesothelioma. Cancer Genet Cytogenet 1990;47:1–28.

237. Croonen AM, van der Valk P, Herman CJ, Lindeman J. Cytology, immunopathology and flow cytometry in the diagnosis of pleural and peritoneal effusions. Lab Invest 1988;58:725–732.

238. Hafiz MA, Becker RL Jr, Mikel UV, Bahr GF. Cytophotometric determination of DNA in mesotheliomas and reactive mesothelial cells. Anal Quant Cytol Histol 1988;58:120–126.

239. Frierson HF, Mills SE, Legier JF. Flow cytometric analysis of ploidy in immunohistochemically confirmed examples of malignant mesothelioma. Am J Clin Pathol 1988;90:240–243.

240. Burmer GC, Rabinovitch PS, Kulander BG, Rusch V, McNutt MA. Flow cytometric analysis of malignant pleural mesothelioma: relationship to histology and survival. Hum Pathol 1989;20:777–783.

241. Dazzi H, Thatcher N, Hasleton PS, Chattlerjee AK, Lawson AM. DNA analysis by flow cytometry in malignant pleural mesothelioma: Relationship to histology and survival. J Pathol 1990;162:51–55.

242. Tierney G, Wilkinson MJ, Jones JSP. The malignancy grading method is not a reliable assessment of malignancy in mesothelioma. J Pathol 1990;160:209–211.

243. El-Naggar AK, Ordone NG, Garnsey L, Batsakis JG. Epithelioid pleural mesotheliomas and pulmonary adenocarcinomas: A comparative DNA flow cytometric study. Hum Pathol 1991;22:972–978.

244. Esteban JM, Sheibani K. DNA ploidy analysis of pleural mesotheliomas: Its usefulness for their distinction from lung adenocarcinomas. Mod Pathol 1992;6:626–630.

245. Raftery AT. Regeneration of parietal and visceral peritoneum. An electron microscopical study. J Anat 1973; 115:375–392.

246. Schurch W, Seemayer TA, Legace R, Gabbiani G. Intermediate filament cytoskeleton of myofibroblasts: An immunofluorescence and ultrastructural study. Lab Invest 1984;50:52A.

247. Majno G. The story of the myofibroblast. Am J Surg Pathol 1979;3:535–542.

248. Davila RM, Couch EC. The role of mesothelial and submesothelial stromal cells in matrix remodeling following pleural injury. Am J Pathol 1993;142:547–555.

249. Roberts GH. Diffuse pleural mesothelioma. A clinical and pathological study. Br J Dis Chest 1970;64:201–211.

250. O'Donnell WM, Mann RH, Grosh JL. Asbestos, an extrinsic factor in the pathogenesis of bronchogenic carcinoma and mesothelioma. Cancer (Philadelphia) 1966;19:1143–1148.

251. Chernow B, Sahn SA. Carcinomatous involvement of the pleura: An analysis of 96 patients. Am J Med

1977;63:695–702.

252. Babolini G, Blasi A. The pleural form of primary cancer of the lung. Dis Chest 1956;29:314–323.

253. Harwood TR, Gracey DR, Yokoo H. Pseudomesotheliomatous carcinoma of the lung: A variant of peripheral lung cancer. Am J Clin Pathol 1976;65:159–167.

254. McCaughey WTE, Dardick I, Barr RJ. Angiosarcomas of serous membranes. Arch Pathol Lab Med 1983;107: 304–307.

255. Willen R, Bruce T, Dahlstrom G, Dubiel WT. Squamous epithelial cancer in metaplastic pleura following extrapleural pneumothorax for pulmonary tuberculosis. Virchows Arch [A] 1976;370:225–231.

256. Crome L. Squamous metaplasia of the peritoneum. J Pathol Bacteriol 1950;62:61–68.

257. Kwee WS, Veldhuizen RW, Golding RP, Donner R. Primary "adenosquamous" mesothelioma of the pleura. Virchows Arch [A] 1981;393:353–357.

258. Falor WH, Ward RM, Brezler MR. Diagnosis of pleural effusions by chromosome analysis. Chest 1982;81:193–197.

259. Henderson DW, Whitaker D, Shilkin KB. The differential diagnosis of malignant mesothelioma: A practical approach to diagnosis during life. In: Henderson DW, Shilkin KB, Langlois SLP, Whitaker D, eds. *Malignant Mesothelioma*, New York, Hemisphere, 1992;184.

260. Friman C, Hellström PE, Juvani M, Riska H. Acid glycosaminoglycans (mucopolysaccharides) in the differential diagnosis of pleural effusion. Clin Chim Acta 1977;76:357–361.

261. Arai H, Kang K, Sato H, et al. Significance of the quantification and demonstration of hyaluronic acid in tissue specimens for the diagnosis of pleural mesothelioma. Am Rev Respir Dis 1979;120:529–532.

262. Castor CW, Naylor B. Acid mucopolysaccharide composition of serous effusions. Cancer (Philadelphia) 1967;20:462–466.

263. Rasmussen KN, Faber V. Hyaluronic acid in 247 pleural fluids. Scand J Respir Dis 1967;48:366–371.

264. Thompson ME, Bromberg PA, Amenta JS. Acid mucopolysaccharide determination: A useful adjunct for the diagnosis of malignant mesothelioma with effusion. Am J Clin Pathol 1969;52:335–339.

265. Pettersson T, Fröseth B, Rista H, Klockars M. Concentration of hyaluronic acid in pleural fluid as a diagnostic aid for malignant mesothelioma. Chest 1988;94: 1037–1039.

266. Hillerdal G, Lindqvist U, Engström-Laurent A. Hyaluronan in pleural effusions and in serum. Cancer (Philadelphia) 1991;67:2410–2414.

267. Chiu B, Churg A, Tengblad A, Pearce R, McCaughey WTE. Analysis of hyaluronic acid in the diagnosis of malignant mesothelioma. Cancer (Philadelphia) 1984; 54:2195–2199.

268. Nakano T, Fujii J, Tamura S, et al. Glycosaminoglycan in malignant pleural mesothelioma. Cancer (Philadelphia) 1986;57:106–110.

269. Iozzo RV. Biology of disease. Proteoglycans: structure, function and role in neoplasia. Lab Invest 1985;53:

373–396.

270. Iozzo RV, Goldes JA, Chen W-J, Wight JN. Glycosaminoglycans of pleural mesothelioma: A possible biochemical variant containing chondroitin sulfate. Cancer (Philadelphia) 1981;48:89–97.

271. Hammar SP. *Mesothelioma*. In: Sheppard MN, ed. *Practical Pulmonary Pathology*, Mill Road, Hodder & Stoughton, in press.

272. Antman KH. Current concepts: Malignant mesothelioma. N Engl J Med 1980;303:200–202.

273. Butchart EG, Ashcroft T, Barnsley WC, Holden M. The role of surgery in diffuse malignant mesothelioma of the pleura. Semin Oncol 1981;8:321–328.

274. Roberts GH. Distant visceral metastases in pleural mesothelioma. Br J Dis Chest 1976;70:246–250.

275. Elmes PC, Simpson MJC. The clinical aspects of mesothelioma. Quart J Med 1976;45:427–429.

276. Doward AJ, Stack BHR. Diffuse malignant pleural mesothelioma in Glasgow. Br J Dis Chest 1981;75:397–402.

277. Roggli VL, McGavran MH, Subach J, Sybers HD, Greenberg SD. Pulmonary asbestos body counts and electron probe analysis of asbestos body cores in patients with mesothelioma. Cancer (Philadelphia) 1982;50:2423–2432.

278. Chahinian AP, Pajak TF, Holland JF, Norton L, Ambindar RM, Mandel EM. Diffuse malignant mesothelioma. Ann Intern Med 1982;96:746–755.

279. Adams VI, Unni KK. Diffuse malignant mesothelioma of pleura: Diagnostic criteria based on an autopsy study. Am J Clin Pathol 1984;82:15–23.

280. Solomons K. Malignant mesothelioma—Clinical and epidemiological features. S Afr Med J 1984;66:407–412.

281. Krumhaar D, Lange S, Hartman C, Anhuth D. Follow-up study of 100 malignant pleural mesotheliomas. Thorac Cardiovasc Surgeon 1985;33:272–275.

282. Huncharek M, Muscat J. Metastases in diffuse pleural mesothelioma: Influence of histological type. Thorax 1987;42:897–898.

283. Hulks G, Thomas JSJ, Waclawski E. Malignant pleural mesothelioma in western Glasgow, 1980–1986. Thorax 1989;44:496–500.

284. Sussman J, Rosai J. Lymph node metastasis as the initial manifestation of malignant mesothelioma: Report of six cases. Am J Surg Pathol 1990;14:819–828.

285. Case records of the Massachusetts General Hospital: Case 36-1990: N Engl J Med 1990;323:659–667.

286. Huncharek M, Smith K. Extrathoracic lymph node metastases in malignant pleural mesothelioma. Chest 1988;93:443–444.

287. Kim SB, Varkey B, Choi H. Diagnosis of malignant pleural mesothelioma by axillary lymph node biopsy. Chest 1986;91:279–281.

288. Uri AJ, Schulman ES, Steiner RM, Scott RD, Rose LJ. Diffuse contralateral pulmonary metastases in malignant mesothelioma: An unusual radiographic presentation. Chest 1988;93:433–434.

289. Kaye JA, Wang A, Joachim CL, Seltzer SE, Cibas E, Skarin A, Antman KH. Malignant mesothelioma with

brain metastases. Am J Med 1986;80:95–97.

290. Sridkar RS, Hussein A, Ganjei P, et al. Brain metastases in malignant pleural mesotheliomas. Case report and review of the literature. Am J Clin Oncol 1989;12:222–228.

291. Huncharek M, Muscat J. Cerebral metastases in pleural mesothelioma. Am J Clin Oncol 1990;13:180–181.

292. Falconieri G, Grandi G, DiBonito L, Bonifacio-Gori D, Giarelli L. Intracranial metastases from malignant pleural mesothelioma: report of three autopsy cases and review of the literature. Arch Pathol Lab Med 1991;115:591–595.

293. Chen KTK. Malignant mesothelioma presenting as Sister Joseph's nodule. Am J Dermatopathol 1991;13:300–303.

294. Antman KH, Blum RH, Greenberger JS, Flowerdew G, Skarin T, Canellos GP. Multimodality therapy for malignant mesothelioma based on a study of natural history. Am J Med 1980;68:356–362.

295. Chailleux E, Dabouis G, Pioche D, de Lajartre M, de Lajartre A-Y, Rembeaux A, Germaud P. Prognostic factors in diffuse malignant pleural mesothelioma: a study of 167 patients. Chest 1988;93:159–162.

296. Antman K, Shemin R, Ryan L, et al. Malignant mesothelioma: prognostic variables in a registry of 180 patients, the Dano-Farber Cancer Institute and Brigham and Women's Hospital experience over two decades, 1965–1985. J Clin Oncol 1988;6:147–153.

297. Alberts AS, Falkson G, Goedhals L, Vorobiof DA, Van Dor Merwe CA. Malignant pleural mesotheliom: a disease unaffected by current therapeutic maneuvers. J Clin Oncol 1988;6:527–535.

298. Ruffie P, Feld R, Minkin S, et al. Diffuse malignant mesothelioma of the pleura in Ontario and Quebec: A retrospective study of 322 patients. J Clin Oncol 1989;7:1157–1168.

299. Harvey JC, Fleischman EH, Kagan AR, Streeter OE. Malignant pleural mesothelioma: a survival pleural mesothelioma: a survival study. J Surg Oncol 1990;45:40–42.

300. Ribak J, Selikoff IJ. Survival of asbestos insulation workers with mesothelioma. Br J Ind Med 1992;49:732–735.

301. Tammilehto L. Malignant mesothelioma: Prognostic factors in a prospective study of 98 patients. Lung Cancer 1992;8:175–184.

302. Sridhar KS, Doria R, Raub WA, Jr., Thurer RJ, Saldana M. New strategies are needed in diffuse malignant mesothelioma. Cancer (Philadelphia) 1992;70:2969–2979.

303. Worn H. Moglichkeiten und Ergebnisse der chirugischen Behandlung des malignen Pleura mesothelioms. Thoraxchirurgie 1974;22:391–393.

304. Wanebo HJ, Martini N, Melamed MR, Hilaris B, Beattie EJ, Jr. Pleural mesothelioma. Cancer (Philadelphia) 1976;38:2481–2488.

305. DeLaria GA, Jensik R, Faber P, Kittle F. Surgical management of malignant mesothelioma. Ann Thorac Surg 1978;26:375–382.

CHAPTER 35

Metastases to and from the Lung

DAVID H. DAIL

Because metastastic neoplasms to the lung are the most common tumor found in the lung, this chapter concentrates on this problem. At the end of the chapter, a discussion of primary lung tumors and their own metastases is included, but for contrast and comparison they are mentioned throughout the discussion of secondary tumors arriving in the lung. In autopsy studies, the lungs are involved with metastases in 20%–54%[1-6] of cases of extrapulmonary malignancies, and in 15%–25%, the lung is the only site of such metastases.[1] Some selected excellent reviews of the basics of metastases,[7,8] their clinical, radiographic, and therapeutic details,[7,9] and their presence in the lung and pleura[7,9,10] are highly recommended for the interested reader.

The lungs are the organ system that acquires the most metastases of any system in the entire body. Perhaps this is related to several unique features of the lungs, for example, they receive the entire cardiac output every minute, they have the densest capillary bed in the body, they are the first capillary plexus met after most of the lymphatic drainage enters the venous system, and they consist of delicate membranes that may be beneficial for drawing on nearby oxygenated air for sustenance. There are perhaps other selective factors. In 1889, Stephen Paget[11] compared the apparent selectivity of hematogenously borne metastases to seeds needing to find the right soil, an idea that has become known as Paget's "seed and soil" theory. In 1928, James Ewing[12] proposed that metastases developed in the first organ to be exposed to drainage of fluids such as lymph or blood. As nicely reviewed by Zetter in 1990,[8] both theories are partially correct, and examples of direct flow, such as colon metastases to liver, and selective implantation, such as the liver as a destination of choroidal melanomas, are well known. Pulmonary neoplasms, whether primary or secondary, draw mostly on the bronchial artery supply, which is at high pressure, oxygenated, and part of the systemic supply. At the edge of growing tumor masses there is some sustenance from direct perfusion from adjacent alveoli or pulmonary venous or arterial blood, and the same sources may serve the establishment of early metastases.

Because of their overall frequency, carcinomas metastatic to the lung are the most common subgroup of malignancies, although lymphomas and sarcomas are also important and are also discussed. Virtually any malignancy may spread to the lungs, but most commonly such malignancies arise in breast, colon, stomach, pancreas, kidney, melanoma, prostate, liver, thyroid, adrenal glands, and male and female genital tracks, roughly in that order. By absolute numbers, adenocarcinomas far outnumber the other extrathoracic solid tumors that metastasize to lung.

The pathologist is often challenged with whether a tumor in the lung is primary or metastatic. If known, a history of malignancy outside the lung is certainly helpful. A comparison of the two tumors should be conducted. At times more than two tumors need to be compared. Electron microscopy, a battery of immunoperoxidase stains, and occasionally flow cytometry or the use of hormonal receptors, may help with this distinction. At other times, however, there is no way to distinguish them with absolute certainty. Specific immunoperoxidase markers are most helpful in distinguishing cancers of the prostate, thyroid, liver, germ cell, and melanocyte; more specific markers are certain to be developed. Estrogen and progesterone receptor analysis should be done when metastatic breast carcinoma is being considered. Some tumors, such as choriocarcinoma (Fig. 35–1) or osteosarcoma, are histologi-

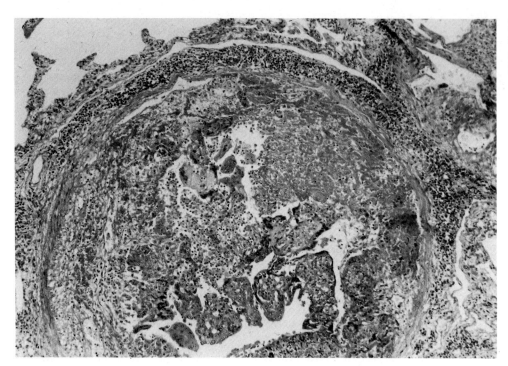

Fig. 35–1. Metastatic choriocarcinoma in pulmonary artery. Note syncytiotrophoblast formation.

cally unique and are found within blood vessels. This combination of unique histology and presence in vessels without a dominant lung tumor mass is very suggestive of metastatic tumor, and the tissue of origin can often be identified. There are rare cases of tumors, such as choriocarcinoma, that are generally metastatic and in which no primary can be found; when solitary, these are considered primary in the lung. Caution is always necessary in these cases; with choriocarcinomas, for example, sometimes only a small scar remains in the germinal system. Primary adenocarcinomas of the lung sometimes produce surfactant and have unique phospholipid profiles; when identified, they are helpful in identifying primary lung cancers. Other adenocarcinomas may have distinguishing characteristics; those from prostate have prostate-specific antigen and prostate acid phosphatase, and lower gastrointestinal trace cancers have unique mucin staining characteristics. Those with abundant desmoplasia might be suspected as coming from pancreas or biliary system, and knowing whether fat is present in a clear cell lung cancer may help distinguish primary clear cell carcinoma from metastatic renal cell carcinoma.

Tumors may spread to the lung by different routes. Hematogenous spread is most important, and includes direct tumor emboli. Tumor cells leaving their primary sites may gain access to venous blood by direct invasion, or secondarily by lymphatic spread with lymph drainage eventually entering venous blood. Occasionally tumors spread by direct extension, such as surface spread within the lung, or through chest wall, mediastinum, or

diaphragm, or via lymphatics permeating between these structures. Although direct extension to another organ is considered tumor spread, metastases usually imply discontinuous tumor deposits. Metastases in the lung may involve the lung parenchyma itself as nodules, either as solitary or multiple, either large or small, or may be a more diffuse interstitial infiltrate, the latter often suggesting vascular spread. Tumors may likewise involve bronchi in a nodular or diffuse fashion, and may embolize to large and small blood vessels, lymphatics, pleura, or hilar-mediastinal lymph nodes. Even peritoneal-venous shunting of malignant ascites can occur.[13] Each of these situations is discussed separately here.

The most common situation for metastatic lung tumors is presentation in patients with known extrapulmonary neoplasm. Bilateral pulmonary nodules, often of somewhat different sizes, favor the mid- to lower and peripheral lung fields, these areas being colonized presumably because of the volume of blood flow. The varying size nodules may relate to different times when metastatic deposits were established in the lung, or the varying quality of the "soil," the growth rate of individual cells that establishes different nodules, or other factors. Similarly sized nodules (Fig. 35–2) when seen throughout the lungs bilaterally may represent showers of tumor cells all of which originated about the same time.[9] The differential diagnosis of multinodular masses generally consists of various forms of vasculitis, synchronous or asynchronous primary tumors in the lung, or, if small, granulomatous disease or other in-

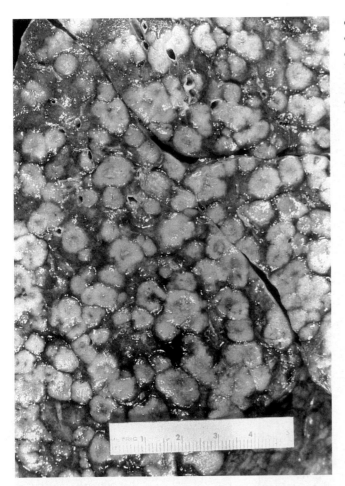

Fig. 35–2. Metastatic cholangiolar carcinoma. Multiple small nodules suggest "shower" of tumor cells perhaps occurring about the same time, in contrast to solitary or several larger or variably sized nodules of tumor, which suggest different ages of metastases (see text).

flammatory causes, or any combination of these. Further generalizations concerning metastases: they are usually smaller than lung primaries, measuring often less than 3 cm in diameter, grow more rapidly, are more peripherally located, and therefore may be less likely to be reached by the bronchoscope or biopsy forceps or have sloughed cells for cytology specimens. Exceptions to each of these generalizations occurs. In situ change may suggest a primary lung cancer, but is seen predominantly only in squamous carcinoma. Metastatic cancers can invade bronchial mucosa and should not be mistaken for an in situ change. It should be noted that some 3%–7% of patients with primary lung cancers have independent primary malignancies at some other bodily location[14]; the reverse is also detailed.

In one series,[15] up to 98% of the metastases were correctly identified as such. However, atypical presentations of metastatic disease to the lung can cause confusion with primary lung cancer. This confusion occurs most often when metastases are solitary, have cavitation, are centrally placed, including in an endobronchial location, or have hilar or mediastinal nodal involvement or an apical location invading the bronchial plexus, causing Horner's syndrome. Further ambiguity can occur when any of these occur with cell types that can also be seen in primary lung carcinomas, or when no extrathoracic tumor is documented. Once tumor is in the lung, whether it arose there or arrived there secondarily, it may spread to the lung vessels, including the lymphatics and venous routes but also the arterial routes, or extend by direct continuity such as with endobronchial spread or through the pleura, or by surface spread, such as in bronchioloalveolar carcinoma or metastases similating these carcinomas[16] (refer to Table 32–18). At times the tumor will follow a combination of routes. A miliary pattern of small nodules is seen most often with medullary carcinoma of the thyroid,[17] melanoma,[18] renal cell carcinoma, and at times ovarian carcinoma.[19] Diffuse interstitial pattern is typical of Kaposi's sarcoma (see Chapter 33) but certainly occurs with those metastases described next as having lymphangitic or vascular spread.

Solitary Metastases

Solitary metastases occur in 3%–9% of cases of all metastases to the lung.[13,20,21] This situation occurs most often with metastases from the colon, which account for 30%–40% of all cases,[20,21] breast, kidney, urinary bladder, nonseminomatous testicular sources, nasopharyngeal sources, and sarcomas.[20,22–27] Large cannonball metastases, generally considered to be larger than 5 cm, whether solitary of multiple, can occur especially with tumors arising in breast or kidney but can also be sarcomas or melanomas.[7] Solitary metastases in the absence of a known primary in one series was reported in only 0.4% of cases.[20] An independent lung primary must always be considered and excluded when considering a patient for metastatic disease. At times the primary lung tumors may be multiple and synchronous and may be of the same cell type or varying cell types. As summarized by Filderman et al.,[7] if a solitary lung nodule is detected in the face of extrathoracic malignancy, it is more likely to be a new primary than secondary deposits in cancers of the lung, breast, stomach, prostate, head, and neck,[27–29] is more often metastatic than primary in melanomas and sarcomas,[29,30] and of about equal incidence in carcinomas of kidney, colon, or testes.[29–31] Certain malignancies that arise in lung are typically multifocal and bilateral without a dominant tumor mass and include bronchioloalveolar

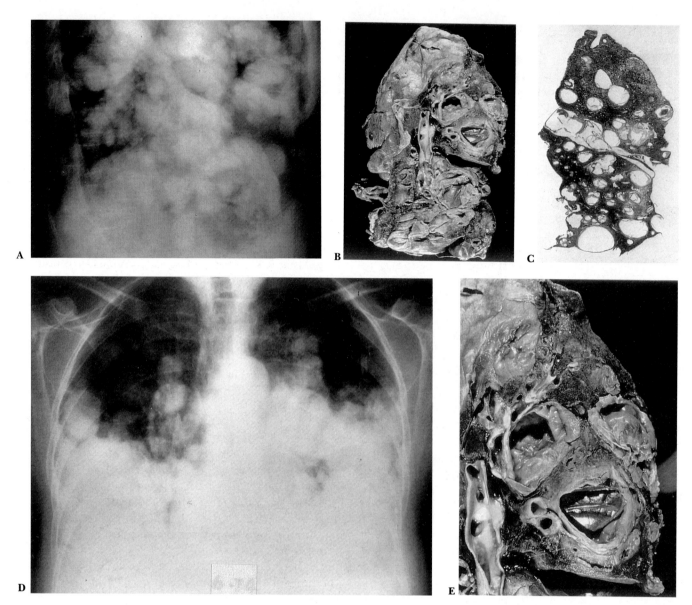

Fig. 35–3 A–E. Metastatic uterine leiomyomas, documented at death 21 years after multiple uterine leiomyomas up to 12 cm were removed. Note variable size and extent of cyst formation and thin walls. **A.** Lateral chest view. **B.** Autopsy specimen; similar orientation to **A. C.** Gough whole-mount section of lung from **B,** highlighting empty cystic metastases. **D.** Chest film shows increased tumors in mid- and lower lung fields. **E.** Closeup of gross cystic metastases. (From Pocock et al. Cancer (Philadelphia) 1976;38:2090–2100, with permission.)

carcinoma and epithelioid hemangioendothelioma. At times what appears to be a solitary tumor on plain chest radiograph is shown in different views, or by using different procedures such as CT scanning, to be multiple adjacent lesions. This may still be treated effectively as a solitary nodule in many cases, and in one study of sarcomas at least, patients having as many as five lesions did not have different survival than those with a solitary mass.[32] The term metastasectomy is used for resection of metastases.[32]

Cavitation

Cavitation can occur in 4% of metastatic disease and 9% of primary lung cancers.[33] It is most often seen in squamous cell carcinoma in either situation. The most frequent sources of squamous carcinoma metastases are head and neck in men, the genitourinary tract in women,[33] and the esophagus and rectum in either sex. Squamous carcinomas generally metastasize so rarely to the lung that finding such a lesion in the lung should be a good reason to suspect an independent primary cancer.[7] Other malignancies, such as sarcomas (Fig. 35–3) or adenocarcinomas, can cavitate, again either in primary or secondary forms.[33–36] At times cavitation of tumor masses peripherally has a role in establishing bronchopleural fistula, as is described next.

Endobronchial Metastases

Because they can be confused with centrally placed primary lung carcinomas, endobronchial metastases may be a particular challenge in distinguishing metastatic from primary disease (Fig. 35–4).[37] This is true especially when the metastatic lesions are adenocarcinomas, especially of a mucinous type. True primary bronchial adenocarcinomas are rare and often derive from bronchial glands.[38,39] Most primary lung adenocarcinomas are peripheral, and consequently their typical classification as one of the three types of bronchogenic carcinomas is usually erroneous. Indeed the term "bronchogenic" is somewhat confusing, and some would translate this as making a bronchus instead of being derived from one; thus the term might be better replaced by "bronchocentric" or perhaps best discarded entirely. Pathologists rarely use this term but all physicians learned it in medical school, and the term is carried forth for simplicity's sake especially among nonpulmonary physicians.

The incidence of endobronchial metastases varies; it was noted in 1.1% of bronchial tumor diagnoses by Bourke.[40] In the review by Braman and Whitcomb,[41] 2%–5% of patients dying of extrathoracic solid tumors have easily identifiable, significant tumor spread to central bronchi. In another series, it was 18%,[42] and when reviews are limited to only those specifying whether tumor was present or not in bronchi, or when microscopic spread is included, the percentage may be as high as 70%.[43] The most common sources for these tumors are breasts,[44,45] colon,[46] kidney,[47] rectum, melanoma, or sarcoma.[48] Other less frequent tumors include those from pancreas, prostate, choriocarcinoma, osteosarcoma, leiomyosarcoma, uterine cervix, ovary, skin, urinary bladder, penis, testes, stomach, larynx, or thyroid.[10,49–51] Sarcomas were found in one series[48] in 6 of 17 cases (35%). In another study by King and Castleman,[42] carcinomas and sarcomas had a relatively similar incidence of endobronchial spread once each tumor had established itself as metastatic in the lung. The trachea is a less common site of metastatic tumor involvement than bronchus,[52] but metastases to this site have been noted coming from breast, colon, and other locations.[52–54] Whether bronchial or tracheal in loca-

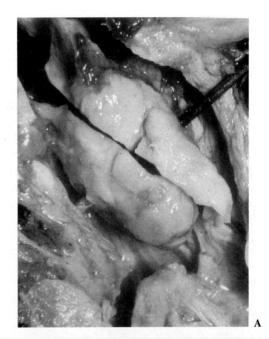

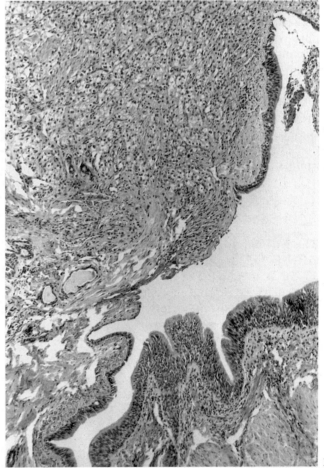

Fig. 35–4 A,B. Endobronchial metastatic hypernephroma. **A.** Probe elevates ovoid white tumor mass. **B.** Histology shows typical clear cell hypernephroma in bronchial submucosa that occurred 2 years after kidney cancer was excised.

tion, these tumors can often be biopsied through the bronchoscope.[40,55–57]

Possible mechanisms for endobronchial spread include hematogenous seeding, lymphatic spread, spread from immediately adjacent tumor in lung parenchyma, mediastinum, or nodes, or rarely by aerogenous routes.[41,42,45,48] It is possible a few metastases arise in the lung via spread from bronchial arteries, and perhaps a few rare ones in the central portions of nodes arise through nodal systemic arterial supply. Lymphangitic spread in bronchial walls can be detected with some regularity through the bronchoscope. As the tumor is "on the move" in this location, it may be a dilemma in the case of primary lung cancer whether to call a tumor in this site metastatic, with the possible misinterpretation as to whether the primary lesion, further out, is interpreted as metastatic. In such instances the pathologist should be careful in describing the fact that tumor spreading in bronchial wall may be related to primary lung cancer.

As with primary lung cancers, symptoms of endobronchial growth are cough, localized wheezing, dyspnea, or hemoptysis. Radiographically there may be separate lesions in lung parenchyma, postobstructive collapse, atelectasis, air-trapping, an obvious mass, or a CT scan or bronchoscopy documentation of a lesion in the endobronchus. Metastatic involvement to airways producing significant respiratory signs or symptoms or chest radiographic changes are reported to occur in less than 5% of those who die with solid extrapulmonary tumors.[41]

Vascular Metastases

This is an important route of spread, as most metastases arrive in the lung via the bloodstream (Figs. 35–1 and 35–5). As mentioned in the introduction, the lung is a particularly receptive organ because it receives the entire cardiac output, including most of the upstream lymph flow, and is a meshwork of delicate capillaries that easily entraps tumor cells and otherwise appears attractive to tumor growth. Tumors arising in whatever location, including the lung, may enter the circulation either directly through vascular penetration, or via the lymphatics, which then empty into the systemic venous circulation.

Most metastases in lung and other organs appear without endovascular tumor being identified (Fig. 35–6). This may be an artifact caused by not including the vessel of origin in the plane of sectioning or by obliteration of the vessel of origin by the neoplastic growth, or by origin from a small inapparent vessel, or perhaps spread by routes other than blood vessels. At other times a tumor may be seen extending around an artery that itself is filled with tumor (Fig. 35–6). This latter relationship, and those tumors that are purely endovascular, certainly appear to rise outside the site biopsied. One might expect to see individual tumor cells in the blood circulating in the lung, and certainly some such cells are seen in smaller caliber vessels. Some malignancies do present with abundant loosely cohesive cells, sometimes with such a tumor cell burden that cancer cells are identified even on peripheral blood smears; this has been called carcinoma cell leukemia, or carcinocythemia.[58–60] In the peripheral circulation, oat cell carcinomas from lung,[61–64] adenocarcinomas from breast,[58,65] and, less often, adenocarcinomas from intestine,[66] melanomas,[60] rhabdomyosarcomas,[67] or transitional cell carcinomas[60] have been thus identified.[58–60] Some lymphomas are also notorious for having leukemic phases, seen both in the peripheral blood and in the blood circulating through the lung. (See following discussion.)

The interested reader is referred to the basics of tumor metastasis, as well reviewed by Filderman et al.,[7] and the many steps a tumor cell must go through to both penetrate a blood vessel at its site of origin, live in the circulation, engraft, and grow to reestablish itself. Schmidt[68] in 1903 reviewed the nature of small emboli arriving in pulmonary vessels in humans and noted that blood and fibrin surround the tumor cells. Takahashi[69] and Iwasaki[70] in 1915, and Warren and Gates[71] in 1936, studied tumor emboli in experimental animals and noted that tumor cells that were entrapped by fibrin underwent degeneration and eventually became a focal fibrous scar in the intima.[72] Although carcinomas are most often involved, sarcomas can certainly undergo similar patterns of spread. Iwasaki in 1915,[70] Willis in 1934,[73] and others[74] later pointed out that tumor cells in distant blood vessels should not be interpreted as metastatic disease per se, as many tumor emboli die and never establish themselves.

Patients with vascular tumor embolization usually present with progressive shortness of breath, which may vary from acute to subacute. Winterbauer et al.[74] reviewed a series of 366 patients with carcinoma of the

Fig. 35–5 A–D. Metastatic pancreatic adenocarcinoma in many blood vessels of lung. **A.** Low power shows extent of blood vessel involvement without lymphatic spread. **B.** Intermediate power shows more solid, spindle-like appearance, almost appearing to be transitional cell. **C.** Higher power of more pleomorphic, large to giant cell variation in same case. **D.** Large, almost squamoid tumor cells in smaller artery focally extend into adjacent arterioles, appearing too large to pass through adjacent capillaries.

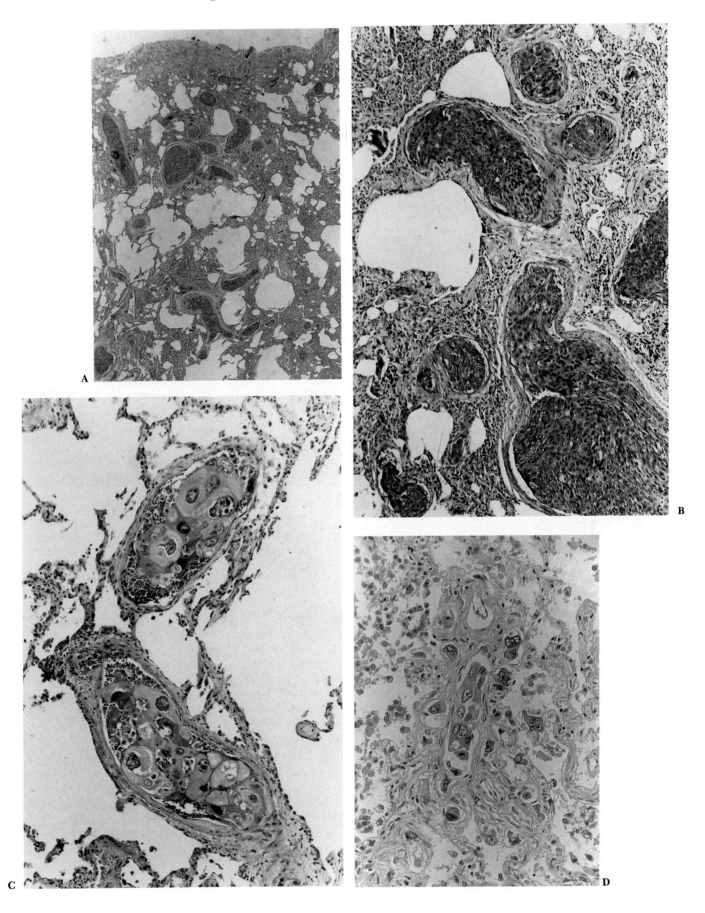

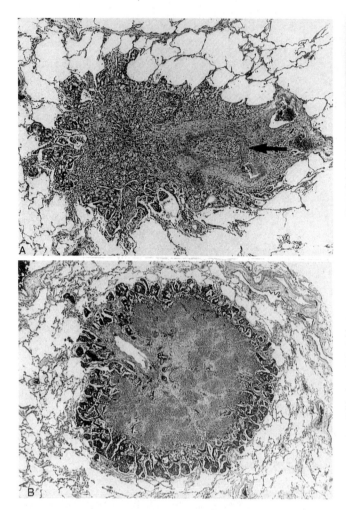

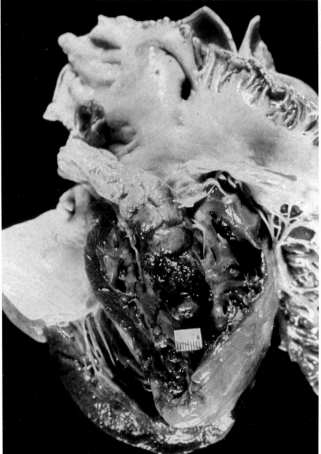

A

Fig. 35–6 A,B. Two variations of metastatic parenchymal tumor nodules. **A.** Muscular artery (*arrow*) is filled with tumor that extends into adjacent lung parenchyma. **B.** Apparently patent vessel, with extensive central necrosis of small tumor nodule, with viable tumor cells at edge, perhaps drawing nutrition from pulmonary vascular supply rather than bronchial supply (see text). (From Fraser et al. Diagnosis of diseases of the chest. Philadelphia: Saunders, 1989:1623–1699, with permission.)

breast, stomach, liver, kidney, or choriocarcinoma, and found 95 (26%) had some degree of tumorization of pulmonary vessels. In 30 (8%) this embolization was a significant factor contributing to the patient's death, and in 10 (3% of total, 10% of those with tumor emboli) these emboli were the direct cause of death. Although tumor emboli to lungs were first described in the early 1800s, these authors[74] found only 30 reported cases in the literature to 1967. Winterbauer and colleagues proposed a grading system based on the number and percentage of vessels involved on microscopic examination; in their 10 cases and 23 reviewed from the literature, 48% had associated pulmonary infarction and

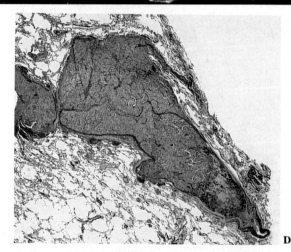

D

Fig. 35–7 A–F. Hypernephroma extending up inferior vena cava as tumor thrombus into right heart with lung metastases. **A.** In continuity, plug of tumor is seen extending into right ventricle with its tip above ruler. **B.** Tumor is still focally attached at junction of inferior vena cava and right atrium (*arrows*). **C.** Primary tumor has replaced right kidney, filling up inferior vena cava to right; liver is at top. **D–E.** Vascular embolus of hypernephroma to lung vessel and beyond. Elastic stain. **D.** Lower power. **E.** Higher power of point of transgression and spread around pulmonary artery elastic tissue.

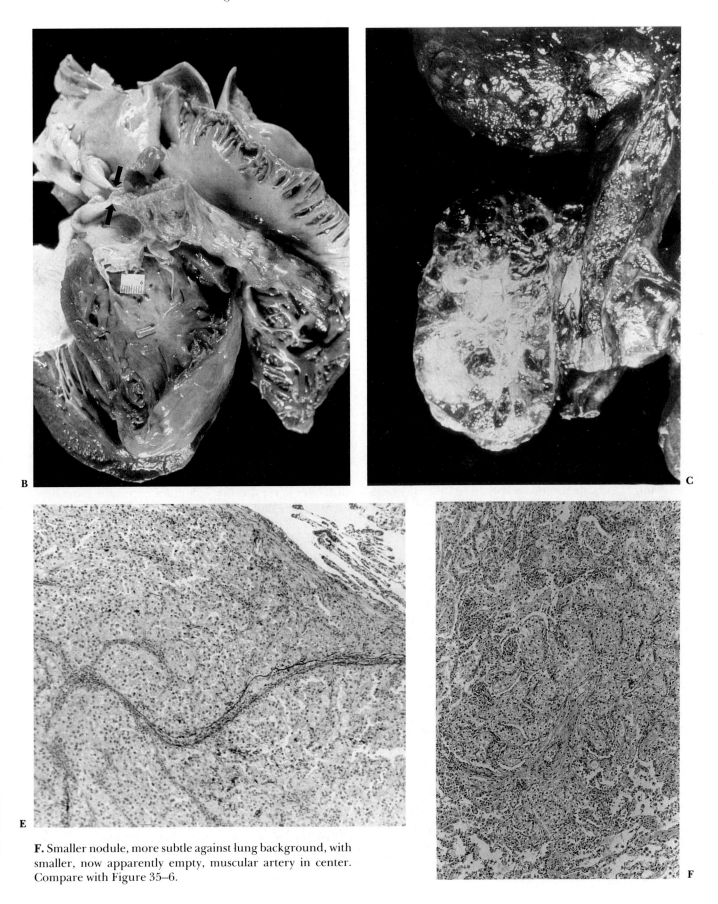

F. Smaller nodule, more subtle against lung background, with smaller, now apparently empty, muscular artery in center. Compare with Figure 35–6.

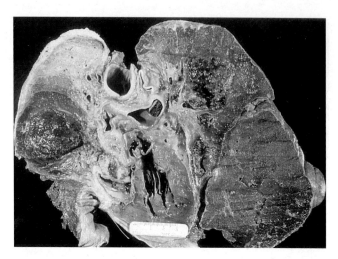

Fig. 35–8. Large fibrosarcoma in right lung–right hilum directly extends into right atrium; tumor extension into left lung is perhaps through embolization from right heart.

45% had evidence of pulmonary hypertension. Tumor emboli may lodge in either larger vessels or smaller vessels, and in their series at autopsy, about one-fourth had grossly identified tumor emboli, two-thirds of which were in the main or lobar pulmonary artery and one-third in the segmental arteries, and the remaining three-fourths had small artery or arteriole tumor obstruction. The liver was involved in 36% of the cases in their series[74] and in 50% in the series by Kane et al.[75] This might indicate secondary spread from the liver was feeding extensive pulmonary vascular spread. In the series by Kane et al.,[75] the spleen, which is rarely receptive to metastatic tumor, was involved in 37.5%. Tumor emboli present with dyspnea in some 50% of the cases,[75] cough in 8%–47%, pleuritic chest pain in 18%–28%, and/or hemoptysis in 5%–18%.[76–78]

Large vessel tumor embolization can lead to acute heart failure and other signs of a major acute embolus. Tumors giving rise to these are often connected with major systemic veins, with direct tumor extension into some part of this venous system; these most often include liver, kidney (Fig. 35–7), uterine smooth muscle tumors, and, rarely, primary inferior vena cava leiomyosarcoma, right-sided cardiac myxomas or right heart–pulmonary outflow tract sarcomas, and rare tumors directly infiltrating the right heart (Fig. 35–8) among other sources, such as pancreas. In smaller caliber vessels, which have potential for collaterals and shunting to less involved vessels, heart failure is generally more subacute than it is acute, but acute heart failure has certainly been described in this situation along with pulmonary hypertension.[7,74–93] Vessels with tumor emboli of any size may undergo thrombosis or fibrous obliteration, sometimes causing a pulmonary infarct

(Fig. 35–9). At times tumor emboli die leaving a thrombis, which may partially calcify (Fig. 35–10).

Tumors that spread to the smaller pulmonary vessels, generally those less than 2 mm in diameter, including arterioles and capillaries, are most often seen in cancers from breast, stomach, colon or rectum, liver, pancreas, uterus, cervix, choriocarcinoma, ovarian tumors, and prostate and urinary and gallbladder origins, as reviewed by Kane et al.[75] In this series by Kane et al.,[75] vascular emboli were noted in 2.4% of 1,085 consecutive autopsies for solid malignant neoplasms, and half of those involved had unexplained dyspnea; however, there was no significant difference in the mean percentage of small vessels involved within this group compared with those presenting without unexplained dyspnea. It is also interesting that there was no example of larger vessel tumor emboli in this large series. In the Soares et al.[89] series of 12 cases of tumor spread to pulmonary alveolar septal capillaries, including 9 tumors with origin outside the chest, 11 (92%) had other pulmonary vascular compartments involved, those being lymphatics in 9, arterioles in 7, and veins in 1; parenchymal tumor nodules were present in 5 of those 9 that were metastatic to lung and presumably in all the 3 arising in the lung. Only one of their cases had purely alveolar capillary spread, a case of squamous carcinoma of the cervix; this was compared to one other similar case reported by Abbondanzo et al.[84] in which the primary was in breast (Fig. 35–11). This figure also illustrates several other examples of tumor emboli to small vessels and capillaries, including melanoma and intravascular lymphoma and leukemia. Whether intravascular lymphoma, originally called malignant angioendotheliomatosis, is considered primary in any particular organ system is undetermined because it is considered primary in blood vessels themselves. It is in the differential diagnosis of intravascular malignancies, and may also be diagnosed by right-heart wedge catheterization (see Fig. 35–11F and following discussion).

Pulmonary veins may also be involved with leukemia (Fig. 35–11E) or tumors that are metastatic to lung as well as primary tumors arising there, and often represent one route for either tumor, once established in the lung, to move from that location. Venous spread is discussed more at the end of this chapter.

Lymphangitic Spread

It is generally accepted that about 6%–8% of metastases to the lung appear as lymphangitic disease[94–96] (Figs. 35–12 and 35–13). This has also been called lymphangitic, lymphangitis, or lymphangiosis carcinomatosis. Others have noted higher incidences, of 24%[97] to

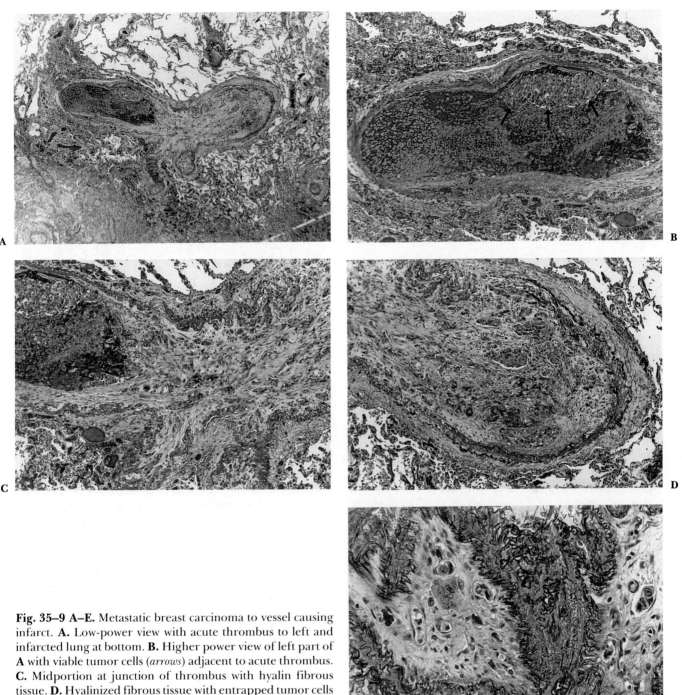

Fig. 35–9 A–E. Metastatic breast carcinoma to vessel causing infarct. **A.** Low-power view with acute thrombus to left and infarcted lung at bottom. **B.** Higher power view of left part of **A** with viable tumor cells (*arrows*) adjacent to acute thrombus. **C.** Midportion at junction of thrombus with hyalin fibrous tissue. **D.** Hyalinized fibrous tissue with entrapped tumor cells at right in **A**. **E.** High-power view of viable tumor cells in hyalinized connective tissue with some capillary ingrowth. Movat Pentachrome stain.

56%.[98] A summary of 275 cases by Yang and Lin[94] showed that 44% arose in the stomach, 23% in bronchus, 9% in breast, 5% in pancreas, and 4% each in uterus, colon-rectum, and prostate. In studying a single source, Goldsmith et al.[97] noted 24% of the patients with breast cancer had lymphangitic spread to the lungs, often with pleural effusion (see following). Breast cancer accounts for about half the cases of lymphangitic spread in North America (Fig. 35–12), while gastric carcinoma is expected to account for a high percentage in Japan.[99] Other metastatic tumors proven to cause this pattern are from ovary, cervix, thyroid,

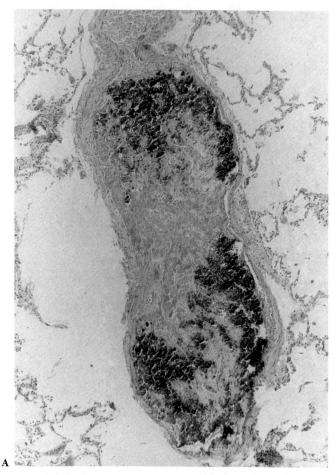

A

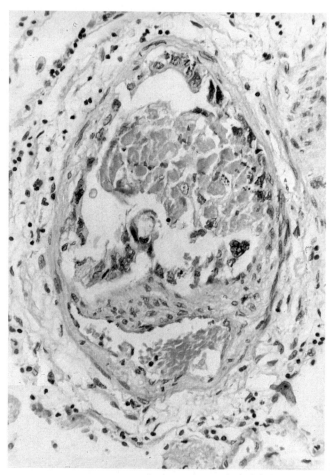

B

Fig. 35–10 A,B. Necrotic tumor thrombus from metastatic ovarian carcinoma is undergoing calcification; no viable tumor cells are seen in this vessel. **B.** Tumor nearby with ring of adenocarcinoma, encircling more acute thrombus. Note also older septum with smaller patent vessel at left.

liver, bladder, endometrium, nasopharanyx, esophagus,[94,95,100] and malignant carcinoid arising in the abdomen.[101] Certainly primary lung cancers can spread frequently via lymphatics as do lymphomas (Fig. 35–13E).

As many as 50% of the cases of histologically proven pulmonary lymphatic carcinomatosis present with normal radiographs[97,102] and CT scans increase this sensitivity, often showing a beaded appearance.[103–106] Perfusion scans may also highlight abnormalities in blood vessels.[88,107,108] Most cases are bilateral and diffuse but some are unilateral and focal, and these variations may depend on the source of the tumor and the route of spread in the lymphatics, as discussed later. About one-third have associated hilar or mediastinal node enlargement, and two-thirds have pleural disease.[94,100]

Lymphangitic tumor spread conveys a poor prognosis; about half the patients are dead within 3 months and 90% are dead within 6 months.[94] However, some rare cases have responded to treatment, including patients with breast,[109] prostate,[110] or ovarian carcinoma.[111]

The series by Yang and Lin,[94] who divided their 62 cases into four radiographic patterns, is of special note. The first pattern showed progressive linear infiltrates bilaterally without hilar enlargement or tumor masses, and all these cases proved to be cancers spreading from gastric adenocarcinoma. The presumed route of spread with this pattern was anteriorgrade through the diaphragm and pleural surfaces. The second group consisted of radiating linear lines from enlarged hilar masses, and this was found in association with gastric carcinoma in 25%, cervical carcinoma in 30%, breast carcinoma in 20%, and in fewer numbers, cancers from nasopharanyx, prostate, pancreas, and thyroid. This pattern was presumed to be due to retrograde lymphangitic spread from bilateral hilar node metastases. The third pattern represented a focal lymphangitic spread from one portion of the lung, and this was typical of a centrally placed primary lung carcinoma, often involving bronchus. Their fourth pattern consisted of radiating tumor from a parenchymal primary lung tumor that was not centrally placed. They note that

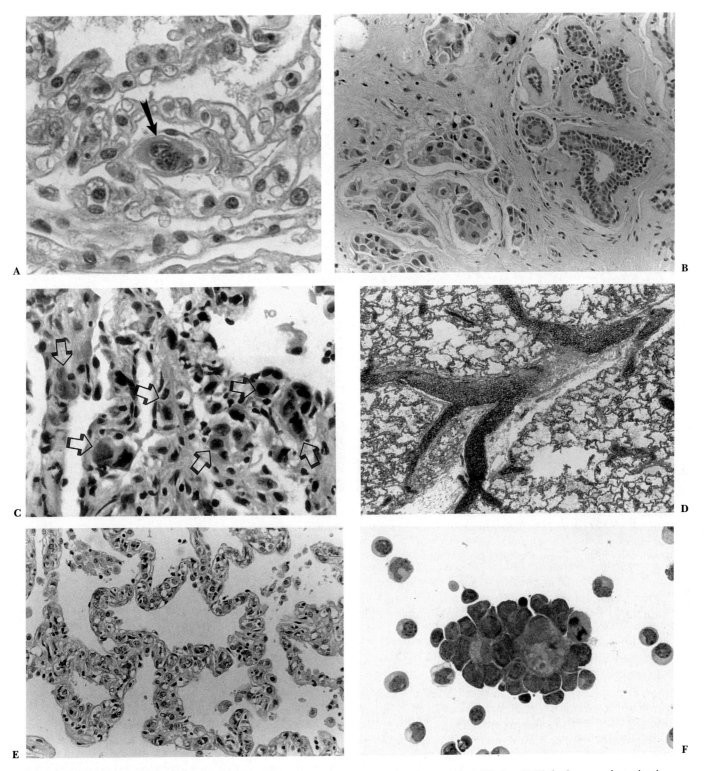

Fig. 35–11 A–F. Metastatic tumor in vessels. **A,B.** Adenocarcinoma of breast, in rare pulmonary capillaries (*arrow*) in **A. B.** Primary adenocarcinoma in breast in 38-year-old woman. **C.** Capillary spread of melanoma; loosely cohesive cells are most obvious in zones highlighted with *arrows* but account for some of cellularity elsewhere. **D.** Chronic myelogenous leukemia fills veins in interlobular septum. White count of patient was more than 500,000/ml. **E.** Intravascular lymphoma; large cells dilate alveolar septal capillaries. **F.** Right-heart catheterization in a case of intravascular lymphoma has obtained clump of malignant cells in fashion similar to which carcinoma is retrieved by similar procedure. (Original contributors: **A,B,** S. Patterson, M.D., Virginia Mason Clinic, Seattle, Washington; **E.** T. Colby, M.D., Mayo Clinic, Rochester, Minnesota; **F.** G. Kritzer, M.D., Virginia Mason Clinic, Seattle, Washington).

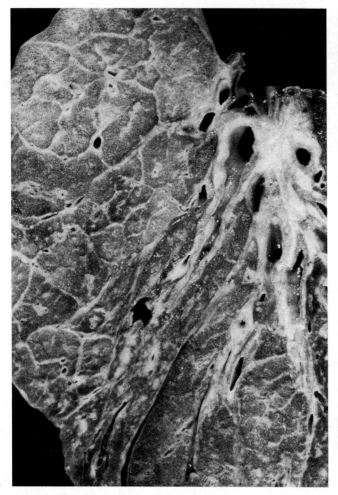

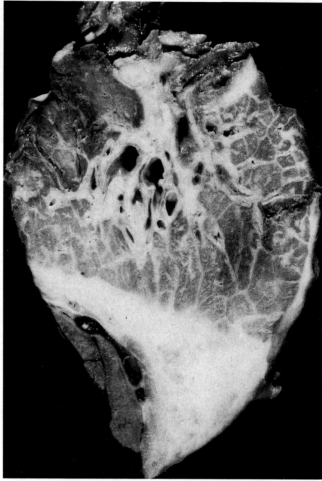

A   B

Fig. 35–12 A,B. Lymphangitic spread of breast cancer (from same case). **A.** Cancer cells highlight interlobular septa but also some bronchioles and bronchi, particularly in lower half. **B.** Extensive inferior pleural tumor plaque reflects dependent position, with extensive lymphangitic spread including bronchiolar encasement and lobar node involvement. Note lymphatics are not involved superiorly.

91% of all of the cases were adenocarcinomas. Lymphatic spread has also been found in primary lung carcinomas (see following). In a study of unilateral yet fairly widespread lymphangitic carcinoma by Youngberg,[112] associated adenopathy was seen in one-third of cases and pleura disease in two-thirds of cases. As already noted, nodes and pleura were also involved in similar frequencies in bilateral disease[94,100] and reflect lymphatic spread in both locations. (See following on pleural spread)

Three possible routes of lymphangitic spread have been described. The most likely one is via spread from adjacent blood vessels.[100,113] As noted in the first pattern of Yang and Lin,[94] direct lymphangitic invasion can also occur, particularly from gastric carcinoma and breast carcinoma (see Fig. 35–12), and yet retrograde lymphatic spread also occurs. As a further example of retrograde spread, I have personally seen one case of two right-sided synchronous lung cancers, an adenocarcinoma in the right-middle lobe with lymphangitic and hilar node spread, and a right-lower-lobe basilar compound tumor with a centrally placed well differentiated carcinoid tumor surrounded by a rim of keratinizing squamous carcinoma, with the surrounding lower lobe also showing lymphangitic spread of adenocarcinoma, presumably having occurred from retrograde spread. Adenocarcinomas in lymphatics may not form glands and may be more difficult to distinguish as adenocarcinoma, and may look more solid or squamoid in type (see Fig. 35–5). Some adenocarcinomas in lymphatics do, however, show a well-differentiated papillary or glandular pattern, sometimes with psammomatous calcifications or mucin production giving a fanciful appearance[9] (Fig. 35–14).

When tumor is confined to lymphatic spaces (see Figs. 35–13 and 35–14), there is little fibrin deposit or fibrosis or other evidence of organization. Nodular desmoplasia does occur with interstitial spread (Fig. 35–15); whether this is invasion first from lymphatic or blood vessels is difficult to tell, but I suspect it is most often from blood vessels. Blood vessels are often coexistently involved with metastatic cancer when lymphatics are so involved. In the series by Janower and Blennerhassett,[100] arterial involvement was noted in 20 of 23 cases (87%) with lymphatic spread, and in the series by von Herbay et al.,[86] lymphatics were involved in 18 of 21 (86%) cases when blood vessels were so involved. In the first series,[100] nodes were radiographically enlarged in only 5 of 23 (22%) and histologically positive in only 11 (48%), while all cases had extensive hematogenous spread of metastases to other organs, which supports hematogenous arrival. The true incidence of both vascular and lymphatic spread is underestimated because histologic sampling of lung, even at autopsy, is limited.

Although the favored and most probable thesis for lymphangitic spread is invasion from arteries, such spread is hard to document[86]; this probably occurs in small areas of interstitial invasion and desmoplasia (Fig. 35–15), where tumor cells gain access to the interstitium and then to lymphatics, respectively. The reader should remember that there are no lymphatics in the alveoli themselves, but tumor cells that gain entrance to the free alveolar spaces may perhaps reenter the interstitium around the terminal bronchioles in a fashion similar to dust reentry in this location in dust diseases. In contrast, multifocal primary bronchioloalveolar carcinoma of lung is thought to spread to multiple sites, including bilateral lungs, principally by an aerogenous surface route without lymphatic invasion. Multiple routes may be seen in the same case (Fig. 35–16).

Some, and perhaps many, cases that are clinically thought to represent lymphangitic carcinomatosis may represent vascular tumor emboli.[88,108] The technique of peripheral pulmonary vascular sampling by right-heart catheterization was described in 1985 by Masson and Ruggieri[114]; follow-up studies[115] confirmed that with some experience and care, tumor cells can be identified. Although these patients are considered histologically as having lymphangitic carcinoma solely or predominantly, a high yield on withdrawing a small amount of arterial-capillary or venous blood must indicate tumor cells are inside the blood vessels, or, less likely, accessible via direct or traumatic access to lymphatic routes from the blood system. Megakaryocytes are sought in this procedure to prove peripheral vascular sampling. This cell is chosen because it is a normal component of lung, and in fact the lung is the second richest source of megakaryocytes in the body after bone marrow.[116] In a study by Aabo and Hansen,[117] of 365 consecutive hospital autopsies were compared with 21 forensic autopsies, the latter in previously healthy individuals who died suddenly. Intravascular megakaryocytes were found in 95% of the hospital series and 67% of the forensic series in an average number of lung samples reviewed. The average number of megakaryocytes was 37 cm^2 in the hospital series and 4 cm^2 in the forensic series. Therefore, the stresses of events preceding death in a hospital appear to increase the number of megakaryocytes. These authors used 25 megakaryocytes cm^2 as the upper level of normal. This concentration is increased in myelofibrosis and may suggest extramedullary hematopoiesis in the lung, but it is also increased in intravascular coagulation, acute infections, bleeding, shock, cancer, and liver insufficiency, along with fever. An interesting companion study[118] of 55 cases of leukemia and 16 of multiple myeloma found an increased number of megakaryocytes in only one case in these diseases. (See also Chapter 31.) A recent study by Soares,[119] however, noted increased pulmonary megakaryocytes with tumor metastases to lung.

Intrathoracic Nodal Spread

It is logical that lymph nodes should be involved along with pleura when intraparenchymal pulmonary lymphatics are involved with tumor spread. As just discussed, nodal and pleural spread does not occur in as many cases as expected for the incidence of parenchymal lymphatic spread. When it does occur, such spread may be either from a primary or secondary tumor, then representing secondary and tertiary metastases, respectively.

Lymph node involvement in primary tumors is so valuable in cancer staging as to be one of the key findings here as elsewhere in the body. Certainly a unilateral lung mass and ipsilateral unilateral hilar nodal enlargement are considered cancer with spread until proven otherwise. Looking at metastases to the chest from a nodal viewpoint, in a series of 1,071 cases with various extrathoracic malignancies by McLoud et al.,[120] 25 patients (2.3%) showed nodal involvement on chest radiographs with 48% of these being from primary genitourinary malignancies, 32% from head and neck, 12% breast, and 8% melanomas. Tumor in nodes was accompanied by parenchymal involvement in 40% of this series, and the right paratracheal chain was involved most often (60%); unilateral hilar node involvement occurred in 32% and bilateral hilar node involvement in 28%. Subcarinal and posterior mediastinal lymph node involvement was uncommon, except in cases of testicular seminoma and, less often, other

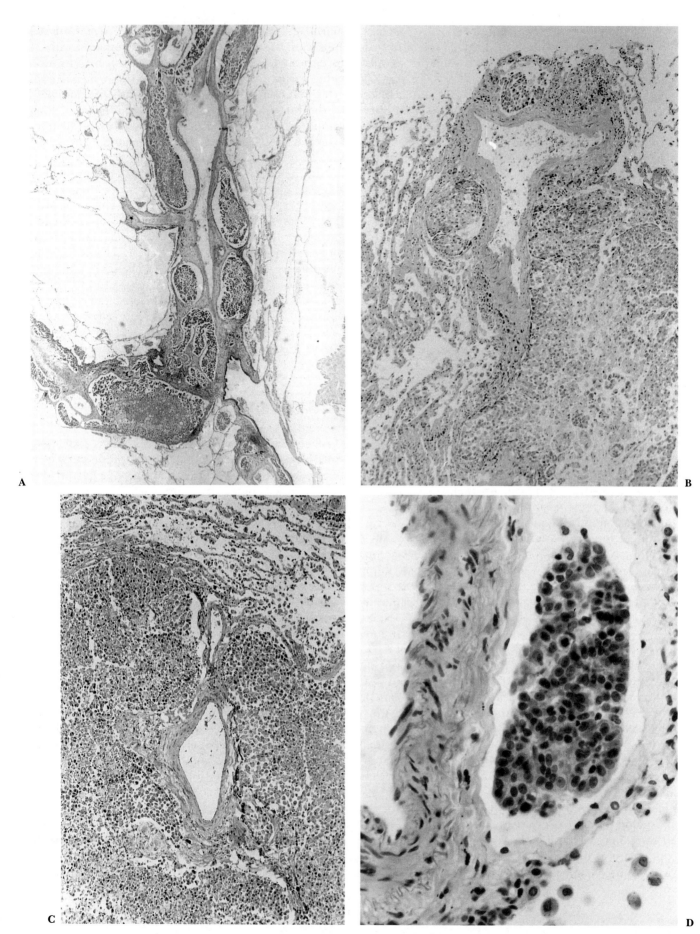

A

B

C

D

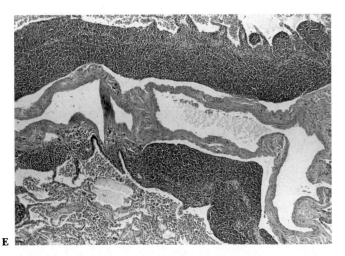

E

Fig. 35–13 A–E. Lymphangitic spread of malignancy. **A–C.** Same case of degenerating metastatic breast carcinoma in perivascular lymphatics. **A.** Low-power view. **B.** Higher power; note two smaller and one larger area of distension of perivascular lymphatics with tumor necrosis in larger areas. **C.** Extensive tumor encases vessel and appears as a nodule but represents lymphangitic spread. **D.** For contrast, mesothelioma is spreading in lymphatics with intact tumor cells. Note lack of reaction such as desmoplasia. **E.** Well-differentiated lymphocytic lymphoma spreads though pulmonary lymphatics.

◁ ——————————————————————————

testicular neoplasms. Such nodal spread is presumably in continuity along the periaortic nodes to account for this discrepancy.

Hilar or mediastinal nodal spread may represent tertiary spread from intraparenchymal lung metastases, but also may represent secondary spread by alternate routes. Lymphatic drainage from the retroperitoneum continues directly into the mediastinum via the ductus lymphaticus and other collateral spaces. Lympatic drainage into pleura may also occur via these routes with consequent movement of tumor cells via the pleural lymphatics to regional nodes.[121] The incidence of node involvement with metastatic melanoma to chest, similar to testis tumors, is unusually high (54%–55%).[122,123]

In the study by Winterbauer et al.[124] bilateral hilar adenopathy was found in 74 of 99 (74%) cases of sarcoid, 20 of 212 (9.4%) cases of lymphoma, 4 of 500 (0.8%) of primary lung cancer, and 2 of 1201 (0.2%) of extrathoracic malignancies. In this latter group, 354 had pulmonary metastases, indicating an incidence of these with pulmonary metastases of 2 of 354, or 0.6%. In the series by McLoud et al.[120] 40% of the cases had evidence of pulmonary vascular lymphatic involvement noting tumors spread to nodes occurred most often

from head and neck, testes, kidney, breast, melanoma, gastrointestinal tract, and prostate primaries.

Pneumothorax and Bronchopleural Fistula in Malignancies

Whether primary or secondary tumors are involved, if the tumor nodule is peripheral, there is a change of cavitation or erosion through to the pleura, producing a bronchopleural fistula. This may also occur via a postobstructive pneumonia, or air-trapping, and is more common in skeleton-derived tumors in children[125] than it is in the adult population,[118] with metastatic bone tumors accounting for 70% of such cases in one series.[125] It has been described with cavitary metastases such as squamous carcinoma, adenocarcinoma, or angiosarcoma.[126] As 80%–90% of bilateral multinodular metastases are peripheral and subpleural,[6,127] it is interesting this does not happen more often. In some cases metastatic tumor has been associated with bleb formation.[128]

Pleural Metastases

As has been noted, lymphatics run in pleura, and as with nodal spread it is not unusual to expect pleural spread with parenchymal lymphatic invasion (see Fig. 35–12). This may happen in an anteriograde or retrograde fashion, the latter secondary to obstruction or other causes of high pressure. This topic has been well reviewed by Filderman et al.,[7] and the following comments are drawn from this review.

Malignancy accounts for a significant percentage of pleural effusions, and this percentage increases with age. Chretien and Jaubert[129] collected 1,868 cases of pleural effusion from six series, including one of their own of 488 cases, in which there was an average malignancy of 42% (range, 24–80%). Sahn[130] collected nine series, for a total of 1,783 cases of malignant pleural effusion, and noted that 36% were from lung, 25% from breast, 10% from lymphoma, 5% from ovary, 2% from stomach, and 7% from unknown sources; similar findings were noted in another large review by Light.[131] Adenocarcinomas, whether from lung, breast, ovary, or stomach, lead the list of individual cell types, while other cell types are certainly included, including squamous carcinoma, small cell, or large cell undifferentiated from lung.

Interesting work on pleural spread in both secondary and primary lung cancers has been done by Cantó.[132–134] In primary lung cancers,[133] 14 of 22 squamous carcinomas (64%), 21 of 24 adenocarcinomas

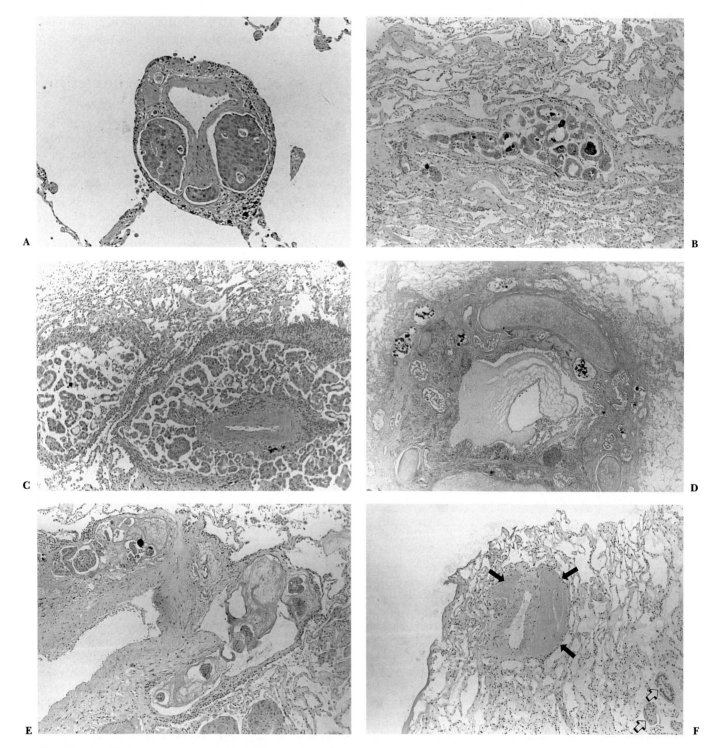

Fig. 35–14 A–F. Assorted patterns of carcinoma in lymphatics. **A.** More solid but still focally mucin-positive adenocarcinoma. Note apparent compression of blood vessels. **B.** Adenocarcinoma with preserved papillary and residual psammomatous calcifications. **C.** Larger perivascular collection of papillary adenocarcinomas. **D.** Psammomatous, cribiform, and mucinous qualities preserved in adenocarcinoma spreading through lymphatics in bronchial mucosa. **E.** A few tumor cell collections produce excess mucin in lymphatics. Note some tumor nodules in nearby lung at bottom. **F.** Same case of excess mucin-producing carcinoma as in **E** showing only pools of mucin-distended, perivascular lymphatic spaces (*solid arrows*); *open arrows* show few nests of tumor cells in nearby lung parenchyma.

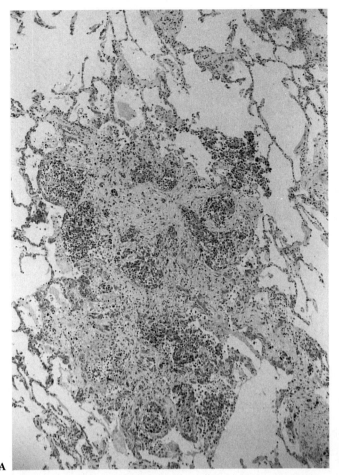

A

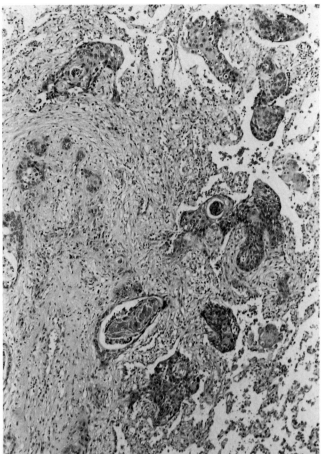

B

Fig. 35–15 A,B. Presumed route of endovascular to endolymphatic spread via fibrous nodules. **A.** Metastatic breast carcinoma in which 99% of tumor elsewhere in the lung is strictly endovascular; this field represents rare nodule of interstitial infiltration with desmoplasia, and nearby, outside this field, is only site of lymphatic spread that presumably extends from this nodule. **B.** Metastatic adenosquamous carcinoma with collapsed muscular artery lumen to left, tumor cells inside remnant lumen extending through wall and causing abundant fibrosis, and focally keratinizing squamous carcinoma extending into adjacent alveoli. Elsewhere, tubuloglandular pattern shows where lymphatic spread is more obvious; however, tumor is always associated with desmoplasia in this case in contrast to focal desmoplasia of case in **A.**

(87.5%), and 26 of 29 (89.6%) have pleural spread. A contrasting study of 126 metastatic breast carcinoma and malignant pleural effusion in 85 cases[134] showed the pleural space to be involved from the same side as the breast primary in 76.5% of cases and on the opposite side in 23.5%. When the contralateral side was involved, 80% represented spread from a left-sided chest wall primary to the right pleural space. These authors have shown that, whether primary lung cancer or metastic lesions, the dependent portion of the pleural space is most subject to tumor studding, with the largest nodules most inferior, suggesting earliest arrival or settling-implantation in the most dependent locations (see Fig. 35–12). Pleural fluid was positive for malignant cells in 43% of these histologically proven cases, of which 61% of the total were serous and 39% serohematic.

As also explained earlier, malignant cells may arrive in the pleural space from transdiaphragmatic chest wall or mediastinal lymphatics and from there be picked up by pleural lymphatics. Breast and gastric and hepatic tumors are good examples of such spread. In several series, women have malignant pleural effusions more often than men because their incidence of breast cancer is greater.[135] Although this is compensated by men's increased incidence of lung cancer, the ratio for malignant pleural effusions is still two women for each man.[135]

Malignant pleural effusions are usually moderate to large in volume, ranging from 500 to 2000 ml.[135,136] Not all pleural effusions in cancer patients are malignant, however, and the common pathway seems to be obstruction of the lymphatics; mediastinal lymph nodes

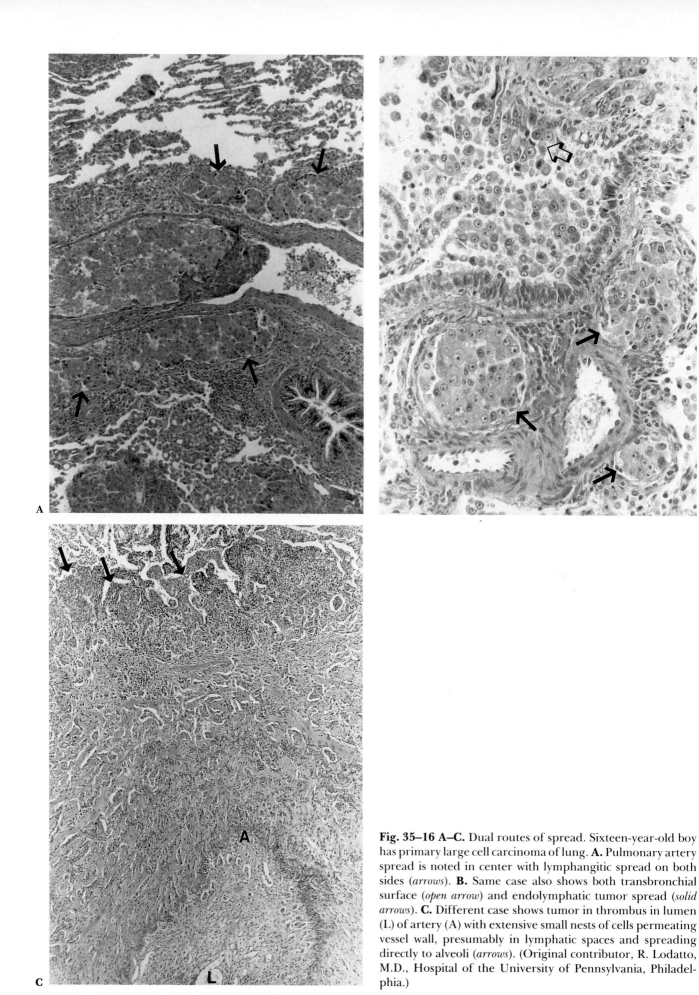

Fig. 35–16 A–C. Dual routes of spread. Sixteen-year-old boy has primary large cell carcinoma of lung. **A.** Pulmonary artery spread is noted in center with lymphangitic spread on both sides (*arrows*). **B.** Same case also shows both transbronchial surface (*open arrow*) and endolymphatic tumor spread (*solid arrows*). **C.** Different case shows tumor in thrombus in lumen (L) of artery (A) with extensive small nests of cells permeating vessel wall, presumably in lymphatic spaces and spreading directly to alveoli (*arrows*). (Original contributor, R. Lodatto, M.D., Hospital of the University of Pennsylvania, Philadelphia.)

involved with malignancy have a high percentage of pleural effusions.[135,137] Pulmonary infiltrates were seen in 40%, and evidence of pulmonary metastases, either in lung or mediastinal lymphadenopathy, was present in an additional 31% in the series reported by Chernow and Sahn.[135] That lymphatic metastases of cancer appear to be an important mechanism in effusion formation is shown by the fact that sarcomas, even when they are in the pleura, do not typically invade lymphatics[133] and do not have associated pleural effusion. Heart failure with chemotherapy and radiation treatment can affect lymph drainage in these cases. Of note, about 30% of Hodgkin's disease have pleural effusion,[133] but in some cases this results from obstructive lymphatic drainage in the mediastinum. Spread to pleura could be through distal arterial-capillary vascular supply, lymphatics in the lung, or directly through chest wall via pleural space, such as noted in the case of breast, liver, and stomach. A 78% incidence of malignant pleural effusions occurred in one series of hepatic metastases,[137] and this is thought to be a contributing source for tertiary spread to pleura.[74,137]

Special Situations in Metastases to Lung

As very nicely reviewed by both Filderman et al.[7] and Fraser et al.,[9] there are some characteristics of specific organ system metastases to lung that are worthwhile emphasizing. This should be considered a summary that is not all inclusive. We begin with two special situations, that of sarcoma and melanoma, and continue from the head region to the genital region.

Sarcomas

Sarcomas have a high incidence of spread to lung, especially after local recurrence. Clinically they have been detected in as many as 38% of cases[138,139] and at autopsy up to 95% of cases.[139–142] Sarcomas are usually nodular and multiple, can become quite large,[143,144] may cavitate or have endobronchial spread,[145] and may lead to spontaneous pneumothoraces[146–151] or present as thin-walled cysts.[152–154] Bone-derived sarcomas, especially in children,[125,155] when metastatic to lung[125,126,155,156] have an especially high frequency of bronchopleural fistulae and pneumothorax.

Melanoma

The majority of disseminated metastatic melanoma patients have spread to lung[157]; in one series,[123] 70% of 652 cases had pulmonary metastases, and in 7% the lungs were the only site of such metastases. They frequently have concurrent malignant pleural effusions and are usually multiple, being solitary in 20%–25%[122,157,158] of those cases with thoracic metastases. However, in a series of 200 melanomas with distant metastases, an asymptomatic pulmonary nodule was the first evidence of dissemination in 38% of cases.[159] A few are miliary, estimated to be 1.5% in one series[157] and 12% in another,[122] and lymphangitic spread occurs in some 8%.[122] A rare case as illustrated in Figure 33–92 appears to be interstitial-alveolar and almost simulates an adenocarcinoma. Most occur within 4–6 months of the diagnosis of the primary tumor. Some may be endobronchial[160] or, rarely, associated with diffuse pulmonary ossification.[161]

Not all solitary nodules in melanoma patients are metastatic melanoma. In one series, 16 of 49 patients (33%) with pulmonary resections for suspected melanoma had benign disease.[162] In a series by Patel et al.,[163] another primary neoplasm somewhere in the body was present in 7.4% of cases of metastatic melanoma. At autopsy, melanoma is usually present in multiple metastatic sites, involving only one site in less than 1% of cases in another series.[163] An unusually large and recent single institution series of 945 cases of pulmonary metastatic melanoma is by Harpole and associates.[158] See Chapter 33 for criteria for primary melanoma of lung.

Head and Neck

Squamous carcinomas, particularly those arising in the larynx, hypopharanyx, tonsillar fossa, and nasopharynx, account for many of the cases from head and neck sources that become pulmonary metastases. The incidence of this is from 12.3% to 40.7%,[164–167] and cervical nodes are usually involved with metastases in 65%–80% of cases[166,167] before lung lesions occur. The larynx and lung may have coexistent carcinomas, as was noted in one series[168] of 60 such cases and is further discussed in Chapter 33. These concur because of common tobacco and other environmental pollutant exposure. In one study[169] of lung lesions with head and neck cancers, 28% were benign, 19% metastatic, and 53% were primary lung tumors, so it is important to evaluate a lung nodule as a possible separate primary malignancy. Some salivary gland tumors can recapitulate those arising in bronchial glands (see Chapter 33 and Fig. 33–31). Metastatic adenoid cystic carcinomas in lung may be among those slow growing metastatic tumors.[170]

Thyroid

Follicular and anaplastic thyroid carcinomas can spread hematogenously in the course of the disease and enter the lung.[171–174] Depending on cell type, it is estimated that 15%–47% of thyroid carcinomas will eventually spread to lung[171,172,175–178]; the papillary variant most often involves lymph nodes first, is more indolent, and may grow slowly in the lung once it arrives there.[171,179] Metastases are often multiple but may be solitary or very small, and hilar and mediastinal nodes are involved in as many as 50% of the cases with lung metastases.[171] Thyroid carcinomas, especially the anaplastic, but also some papillary and follicular types, can directly invade the trachea.[180]

Breast

Breast origin has been mentioned in many of the metastatic patterns discussed here. This is attributed to the high incidence of cancer in the breast, its ability to frequently metastasize, its high frequency of being an adenocarcinoma, in addition to the proximity of the breast to the lung. Spread may be hematogenously or lymphatically, or by direct penetration of the chest wall and then lymphatically. About 50% of disseminated breast cancers have pleural effusions.[97,181] The sole manifestations of breast metastases were seen as lung metastases in 15% and as pleural metastases in 10%, in contrast to the high incidence of bone metastases as single-site metastases in 56%.[182] In another series, the lungs and pleura represented the initial sites of recurrence of breast cancer in 10% of cases.[183] Metastases are most often nodular, but they may also be lymphangitic, vascular, embolic, pleural with effusion, or endobronchial.[47,97,182–185] In one interesting series,[184] 3% of breast cancers had a solitary nodule in the lung at the time of diagnosis of the breast lesion, and of these 5% were benign, 43% represented metastatic breast cancer, and again 52% represented new primary lung cancers.

Liver

The lungs represent the most common site of liver metastases, which have been reported to occur in 37%–70% of cases in autopsy series[186–188] but are less often clinically detected.[189] These present as nodules, often multiple, but pleural effusions are common; there is a tendency for more nodules to be in the right-lower lobe, and a greater degree of effusion to occur in the lower lobes,[190] suggesting probable transdiaphragmatic spread. Occasionally these spread in a miliary pattern.[190] These tumors may also spread in continuity through the venous route directly, into the right heart as a large plug of tumor that may cause a major vessel embolus or as multiple smaller endovascular tumor emboli. The role of metastases in liver that then spread

in a tertiary manner to the pleural space and pleural lymphatics has already been emphasized.

Colon and Rectum

In general, 6%–47% of colorectal carcinomas have pulmonary metastases,[191] which may be nodular, either solitary or multiple, and involve hilar or mediastinal nodes or endobronchial or endotracheal sites.[192] Of note, some 30%–40% of all solitary metastases to lung are from colon and rectum.[20,23] Many cancers arising in these sites go through the portal circulation and spread to the liver before the lungs. Because collateral circulation from the left side avoids liver, and because the original disease is often at an advanced stage at time of discovery, the rectum and, less often, the left colon have a higher incidence of pulmonary spread than the rest of the colon.[191,193–198]

Pancreas

Pancreatic metastases usually first involve nodes, then liver, with spread to the lung thereafter. In an autopsy series of 104 patients, 62% had liver spread and 40% had lung spread.[199] Metastases may be nodular, both solitary and multiple, and incidence of lymphatic, pleural, and nodal spread is fairly high.[199] The nodular lesions can cavitate[199,200] or spread to endobronchus.[201] Tumors arising in the tail of pancreas more often have hilar and mediastinal node metastases than those that arise in the head and body.[199] The histology of these metastases, as with certain other glandular primaries, is not always clear-cut adenocarcinoma (see Fig. 35–5).

Renal Cell Carcinoma

Renal cell carcinoma spreads fairly frequently to the lung, perhaps because it frequently invades veins and then directly embolizes to lung as the next vascular network. It has been described in the lung in from 55%–75% of series,[202–206] and all types of pulmonary spread have been described including nodules, occasionally quite large, both large vessel and small vessel tumor emboli (see Fig. 35–5); endobronchial spread (see Fig. 35–4) is fairly common,[207–212] as is lymphatic hilar and mediastinal node spread, occasionally with bilateral hilar adenopathy.[202,213–215] Of interest, 30%–45% of patients with pulmonary spread have no symptoms referable to the primary kidney lesion.[203] Also, metastatic lesions in lung occasionally appear many years after the primary has been excised, sometimes up to 50 years later.[216] The main differential diagnoses in lung are with primary lung cancer with clear cell change or benign "sugar cell" tumors (see Chapter 33). Renal cell adenocarcinoma is often the most frequent recipient and lung the most frequent donor of tumor to tumor metastases.[217]

Ovarian Cancer

As many as 50% of ovarian cancers have intrathoracic spread, including lung parenchyma and pleura.[218–220] This is the highest rate of intrathoracic spread of any gynecological malignancy.[221,222] Pleural spread is most common, and is usually accompanied by malignant pleural effusion in to 39% of all cases, being positive in 77% of those with thoracic metastases.[219] Parenchymal spread occurs in 7%–39%,[219,223,224] often in continuity with pleural tumor nodules.[224] Solitary lesions may occur in 7%, lymphatic spread in 6%, and nodal spread in 11%,[208] with rare endobronchial spread.[225] Spread to the chest usually follows fairly extensive pelvic and peritoneal tumor,[219,220,226] and small vessel embolization to lung has sometimes been described with peritoneal–venous (LeVeen type) shunting for malignant ascites.[13,219] This has occasionally led to rapid death from respiratory failure with lung capillaries filled with tumor cells.[13,227–231]

Uterus

The cervix, endometrium, and myometrium are considered here. Invasive carcinoma of the cervix has been reported as spreading to lung in 5.8%[232] to 33%[233] of cases, averaging about 10%.[234] In a study by Sostman and Matthay,[235] cervical adenocarcinomas spread with an incidence of 20% and were stage independent while squamous carcinomas had an incidence of pulmonary spread of 4% and were stage dependent. The lung may be the sole site of metastatic cervical carcinoma in 12%[232,236] to 25%[237] of cases. Multiple nodules are usual,[104,235,237] but in as many as one-third of the cases may be solitary[236–239] and sometimes are quite large-"cannonball."[237] Cavitation[237,240] along with endobronchial spread* has been identified as well as lymphangitic spread.[94,243,244] At times hilar or mediastinal nodes are the only evidence of metastases,[245] and effusion may occur.[237]

Endometrial cancers spread very rarely to lung, having occurred in only 2.3% of 470 cases in one series with a 2- to 12-year follow-up.[246] Pulmonary spread usually occurs late, often after disease is evident elsewhere.

Uterine wall-derived smooth muscle tumors are frequent sources for spread to the lung. When a lower or

---

*References: 42, 48, 53, 241, 242.

higher grade smooth muscle nodule is found in the lung of a woman, the uterus frequently is the most likely source. The lower grade ones are referred to as "benign" metastasizing leiomyomas; the reader is referred to Chapter 33 and selected reviews.[247–249] Whether low or high grade, such nodules in lung are usually asymptomatic but rarely do lead to respiratory failure and death.[154,247,250] Metastases are usually nodular and bilateral, occasionally cystic,[150,247] but micronodular[251,252] and miliary[253] patterns and endobronchial spread[254] have been described. Some uterine-derived leiomyosarcomas or intravascular leiomyomas, as well as those primary in the inferior vena cava, extend up to and fill the inferior vena cava and make extend directly into the right heart, and even directly into pulmonary artery,[255] and they may break off as large tumor emboli.[256]

Endometrial stromal sarcomas when high grade often metastasize to lung. More recently, low-grade pulmonary metastases from these tumors have received attention[257,258] and occasionally show microcystic change or sex-cord-like differentiation,[259] even in their metastatic location (Fig. 35–17). Occasionally they are cystic, and confusion with cystic mesenchymal hamartoma is possible.[258] (See Chapter 33.)

Female Gestational Choriocarcinoma

These tumors frequently become nodules in the lung, either single or multiple[260,261] and sometimes reaching large size, or they can cause a diffuse miliary pattern[262–264] or vessel embolus, again often large in size.[263,265–267] Cavitation[268] and/or pneumothorax can occur.[269] In one series, pulmonary metastases occurred in 87% of cases.[263] Spontaneous regression can occur but more often is induced by chemotherapy, with only focal fibrosis or dystrophic calcification remaining.[263,270,271] Occasionally partially responding tumors can have unusual pathologic appearances[272] and thus rarely are mistaken for a primary large cell carcinoma of lung.[273]

Prostate

Prostate adenocarcinoma most often extends regionally to lymphatics first, or frequently directly to bone, before extending to the lung[274,275]; bone is almost invariably involved before lung,[276] but rare exceptions occur.[277,278] Clinically only 5%–15% of cases have lung metastases,[274,279,280] but autopsy series have noted 24%[279]–38%.[280] These may be solitary or multiple nodular metastases,[203,276] rarely with endobronchial spread,[51,281–284] lymphangitic spread,[285,286] or nodal

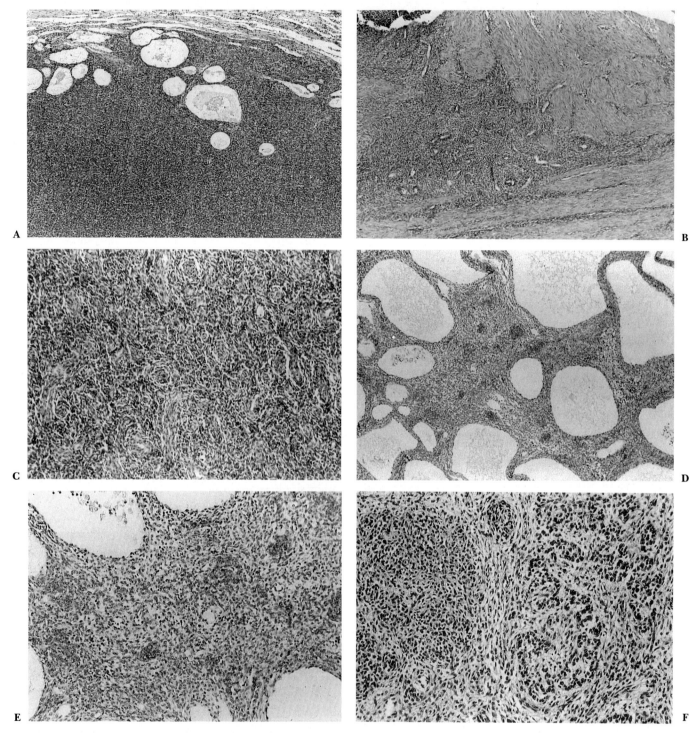

Fig. 35–17 A–F. Metastatic low-grade uterine stromal sarcoma: two different examples of solitary metastases many years after hysterectomy. **A–C.** Sixty-one-year-old woman with solitary 1.2-cm, right-lower-lobe nodule resected 13 years after hysterectomy. **A.** Lung lesion shows some incorporated cysts at edge that represent entrapped alveolar spaces. Note they disappear centrally; tumor is quite cellular. **B.** Uterine tumor shows edge with typical endolymphatic stromal myosis-type appearance. **C.** Higher power view of other portions of uterine tumor show more cellular but still low-mitotic-rate neoplasm, similar to that seen in lung in **A.** Note tendency toward whorls, also noted but not illustrated at higher power in lung nodule in **A. D–F.** Forty-seven-year-old woman with solitary 1.5-cm, right-lower-lobe nodule resected 11 years after hysterectomy. **D.** Lung with varying size cysts in tumor nodule and cellular stroma with focal tumor cell condensations. **E.** Higher power shows these condensations and rather bland appearance of stroma. **F.** Low-grade uterine stromal tumor focally has appearance of "ovarian sex cord-like" appearance.

spread.[287] Malignant pleural effusion has been noted in 14% of stage D prostate carcinomas.[287]

Testes

Seminomas usually evolve slowly, and spread through nodes sequentially before pulmonary spread.[288] Non-seminomatous tumors, however, are more rapidly growing and spread to the lung early by both hematogenous and lymphatic routes.[288–290] Choriocarcinoma spreads via venous routes solely. Single or multiple nodules are seen most commonly[291] and may occasionally be large, and endobronchial spread[292,293] has been identified. Although lymphatic spread in lung is unusual,[291] direct spread up the periaortic node chain appears to account for mediastinal node involvement without lung involvement,[120] this representing the most common manifestation of intrathoracic metastatic testes tumors.[294] Alpha-fetoprotein and human chorionic gonadotropin are often markers that help identify this tumor, either on serum analysis or by immunohistochemical tissue staining. Some of the nonseminomatous germ cell neoplasms mature into teratomas either spontaneously or after chemotherapy,[295,296] and other testicular neoplasms respond to therapy and may leave residual pulmonary cysts or lacunae.[297]

Metastases from the Lung

It is apparent, from the extent of the foregoing discussion, that metastases in lung may be difficult to distinguish from primary pulmonary tumors. Vice versa, primary tumors, must in certain situations, be distinguished from metastases and treated accordingly as independent primary cancer(s) in a patient with known malignancy elsewhere in the body. Some 3%–7% of patients with lung cancer have metachronous tumors in another location.[14] Some general principles have been covered; such central, solitary tumors with unilateral hilar node involvement are most often, but not always, primary carcinomas. Solitary metastases to lung do occur in some 3%–9% of cases,[3,20,21] and endobronchial metastases add potential for further confusion. Primary lung cancers can be peripheral in the zone(s) of the lung most often involved with metastases.

Synchronous or metachronous multiple unilateral or bilateral primary lung cancers can occur as discussed in a review[9] and in two large single institutional series,[298,299] and were metachronous in two-thirds of the series.[9,298]

Either primary or secondary tumors that grow in the lung can metastasize from the lung, following similar routes. Primary tumors often spread through lymphatics; this is an important step in staging cancers, and the regional nodes are the chain most often involved, followed by the upstream mediastinal nodes. Whether directly or via lymphatics, eventually hematogenous dissemination occurs, and in the case of lung cancer favors liver, adrenal glands, and bone, although almost any site in the body can be involved. Of interest, early unilateral spread to adrenal glands is usually to the ipsilateral adrenal, suggesting this is lymphangitic. Later, when generalized hematogenous spread has occurred, this is not true.[300] Because lung tumors are prevalent, they can spread to unusual sites,[301,302] such as the gastrointestinal tract, both male and female genital tracts including the placenta (Fig. 35–18), the choroid coat of the eye, or the bones of hands and feet.

Some primary lung tumors, once they have gone throughout the lymphatics and venous exit pathways from their primary site, similarly can reenter the lung directly as secondary tumor or as tertiary metastases from secondary involvement of other sites. In one series,[303] the opposite lung was involved with metastatic oat-cell carcinoma in 8% of cases. Certainly lung cancers can primarily enter their own lymphatic spaces anteriograde and drain to regional nodes, but such tumors can also spread back in to other portions of lung in a retrograde fashion because of obstructed nodes (see foregoing discussion of lymphatic spread). Although primary lung tumors typically spread to unilateral hilar lymph nodes, they spread to bilateral hilar nodes in 0.8% of cases, which compares to secondary tumors with pulmonary involvement that show this spread in 0.6% of the cases.[74] Primary lung cancers are also a significant cause of malignant pleural effusions, and in one series by Cantó,[133] 14 of 22 squamous carcinomas (64%), 21 of 24 adenocarcinomas (87.5%), and 26 of 29 small cell carcinomas (89.6%) and all 3 primary lung tumors (100%) not otherwise specified had malignant spread to pleura. Spread of primary lung cancer to pleural space is important in staging, and essentially means the lung cancer is incurable.[133]

In contrast, bronchioloalveolar carcinomas can spread aerogenously, and, despite their extensive spread, avoid the lymphatic pathways and regional nodes. As noted earlier, this tumor and epithelioid hemangiendotheliomas can present as multiple smaller nodules without a dominant tumor mass, and yet may still represent primary lung tumors. However, both may also represent patterns of secondary spread.

Primary lung tumors can invade both pulmonary arteries and veins. Gonzalez-Vitale and Garcia-Bunuel[85] discussed pulmonay artery embolization from primary lung cancers, finding this present in 3 of 133 cases (10%) of patients dying with non-oat-cell primary lung cancer. In the same series, venous spread occurred

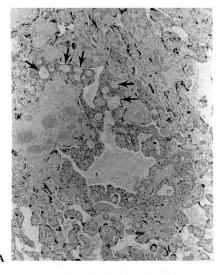

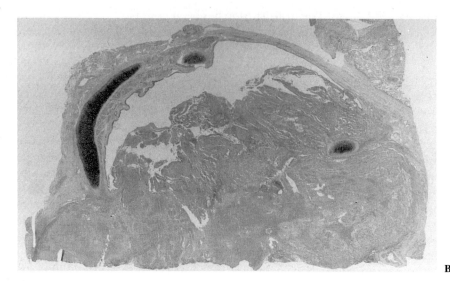

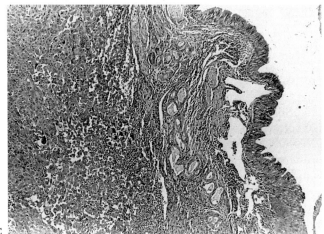

Fig. 35–18 A–C. Metastatic lung carcinoma to placenta. **A.** Placenta with small focus of metastatic carcinoma; focal mucin droplets highlighted with *arrows*. **B.** Primary lung tumor in this case is extending beneath bronchial mucosa. **C.** Higher power view of **B.** (Original Contributor, R. Lodatto, M.D., Hospital of the University of Pennsylvania, Philadelphia.)

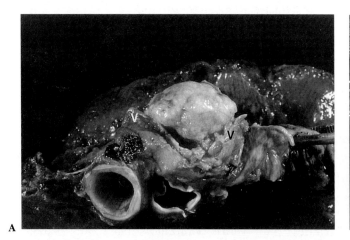

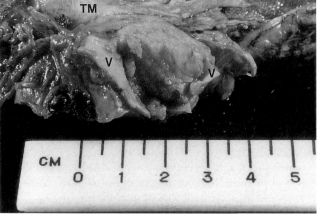

Fig. 35–19 A,B. Primary lung cancer extending into pulmonary vein. A 4.5-cm central primary pulmonary squamous carcinoma has invaded the central vein. **A.** Intact pneumonectomy specimen is viewed from hilum. Wall of vein (V) is noted around the tumor protruding into its lumen. Note main stem bronchus and main pulmonary artery below tumor. **B.** On the cut surface of the lung above is seen a portion of the primary tumor (TM).

in 79% and lymphangitic spread was noted in 84%. Adenocarcinoma showed this frequency in 16.5% of cases, compared to 5.8% for squamous carcinoma and 7.7% for large cell differentiated carcinomas. None of the bronchioloalveolar carcinomas did so. Coexistent lymphatic invasion occurred in 84% of the cases with vascular spread, focal in only 1% and diffuse in the others. When focal, it was seen in the areas coexistent with tumor emboli in vessels. Tumor embolization within the lung may occur in the absence of widespread metastases and was present in 9% of the cases in one series.[81] In my experience there seems to be an inordinate number of cases of primary adenocarcinoma of lung associated with scarring (so-called scar carcinomas), in which there is a thick-walled, compressed muscular artery in the middle of the scar appearing larger than it should for the territory it occupies and whose remnant luminal space contains tumor. The mechanism for this in unclear. Lung cancers are notorious for direct spread into adjacent structures, such as into the branchial plexus superiorly, producing Horner's syndrome, but also into the mediastinum, hilar structures, heart, pericardium, or other adjacent regions. Likewise, bony metastases from primary lung cancers are most often to ribs and vertebrae.

Massive malignant arterial emboli to systemic arteries are most often caused by lung cancer (Fig. 35–19), with only a rare case due to primary aortic cancer.[304,305] Of note, some of these tumor emboli from the lung come from metastatic lesions in the lung.[304] Occasionally a primary cardiac myxoma will cause a massive embolus, and paradoxical tumor emboli passing through patent foramen ovale, septal defects, or patent ductus arteriosum may also present a systemic arterial emboli. Rarely, nonpulmonary malignancies will directly penetrate the aortic wall and cause similar massive emboli to systemic vessels.[306]

References

1. Farrell JT, Jr. Pulmonary metastasis: A pathologic, clinical, roentgenologic study based on 78 cases seen at necropsy. Radiology 1935;24:444–451.
2. Abrams HJ, Spiro R, Goldstein N. Metastates in carcinoma, analysis of 1000 autopsied cases. Cancer (Philadelphia) 1950;3:74–85.
3. Rosenblatt MB, Lisa JR, Trinidad S. Pitfalls in the clinical and histological diagnosis of bronchogenic carcinoma. Dis Chest 1966;49:396–404.
4. Johnson RM, Lindskog GE. 100 cases of tumor metastatic to the lung and mediastinum. JAMA 1967;202:94–98.
5. Willis RA. The spread of tumours in the human body. London: Butterworths, 1973:167–174.
6. Crow J, Slavin G, Kreel L. Pulmonary metastasis: A pathologic and radiologic study. Cancer (Philadelphia) 1981;47:2595–2603.
7. Filderman AE, Coppage L, Shaw C, Matthay RA. Pulmonary and pleural manifestations of extrathoracic malignancies. Clin Chest Med 1989;10:747–807.
8. Zetter BR. The cellular basis of site specific tumor metastasis. N Engl J Med 1990;322:605–612.
9. Fraser RG, Paré JAP, Paré PD, Fraser RS, Genereux GP. Diagnosis of diseases of the chest. 3d Ed. Philadelphia: WB Saunders, 1989:1623–1699.
10. Marchevsky AM. Metastatic tumors of the lung. In: Marchevsky AM, ed. Surgical pathology of lung neoplasms. New York: Marcel Dekker, 1990:231–245.
11. Paget S. The distribution of secondary growths in cancer of the breast. Lancet 1989;i:571–573.
12. Ewing J. A treatise on tumors. 3d Ed. Philadelphia: WB Saunders, 1928.
13. Fildes J, Narvaez GP, Baig KA, Pai N, Gerst PH. Pulmonary tumor embolization after peritoneovenous shunting for malignant ascites. Cancer (Philadelphia) 1988;61:1973–1976.
14. Yesner R, Carter D. Pathology of carcinoma of the lung: Changing patterns. Clin Chest Med 1982;3:257–289.
15. Muller KM, Respondek M. Pulmonary metastases: Pathologic anatomy. Lung 1990;168(Suppl.):1137–1144.
16. Rosenblatt MB, Lisa JR, Collier F. Primary and metastatic broncho-alveolar carcinoma. Dis Chest 1967;52:147–152.
17. Hie J, Stenwig AE, Kullman G, Lindegaard M. Distant metastases in papillary thyroid cancer. Cancer (Philadelphia) 1988;61:1–6.
18. Dwyer AJ, Reichert CM, Woltering EA, Flye MW. Diffuse pulmonary metastasis in melanoma: Radiographic-pathologic correlation. AJR 1984;143:983–984.
19. Coppage L, Shaw C, Curtis AM. Metastatic disease to the chest in patients with extrathoracic malignancy. J Thorac Imag 1987;2:24–37.
20. Steele JD. The solitary pulmonary nodule. J Thorac Cardiovasc Surg 1963;46:21–39.
21. Toomes H, Delphendahl A, Manke H, Vogt-Moykopf I. The coin lesion of the lung: A review of 955 resected coin lesions. Cancer (Philadelphia) 1983;51:534–537.
22. Head JM. Surgery of pulmonary metastases. In: Choi WC, Grillo HC. eds. Thoracic oncology. New York: Raven Press, 1983:359–365.
23. Clagett OT, Woolner LB. Surgical treatment of solitary metastatic pulmonary lesion. Med Clin North Am 1964;48:939–943.
24. Paglicci A. Tumori metastatice del polmone; studio su 152 casi (Metastatic tumors of the lung: a study of 152 cases). Radiol Med (Tor) 1956;422:184–192.
25. Holmes EC, Ramming KP, Eiber FR. The surgical management of pulmonary metastases. Semin Oncol 1977;4:65–69.
26. Huth JF, Holmes EC, Vernon SE, Callery CD, Ramming KP, Morton DL. Pulmonary resection for metastatic carcinoma. Am J Surg 1980;140:9–16.

27. Cahan WG, Castro EB. Significance of a solitary lung shadow in patients with breast cancer. Ann Surg 1975;181:137–143.

28. Judson WF, Harbrecht PJ, Fry DE. Associated lung lesions in patients with primary head and neck carcinoma. Ann Surg 1973;178:703–705.

29. Saegesser F, Besson A, Kafai F. Pulmonary cold lesions and metastases. In: Saegesser F, Pettraral J, ed. Surgical oncology. Baltimore: Williams & Wilkins, 1970:539–610.

30. Cahan WG. Excision of melanoma metastases to lung: problems in diagnosis and management. Ann Surg 1973;178:703–709.

31. Cahan WG, Castro EB, Hajdu SI. The significance of a solitary lung shadow in patients with colon carcinoma. Cancer (Philadelphia) 1974;33:414–421.

32. Jablons D, Steinberg S, Roth J, Pittaluga S, Rosenberg SA, Pass HI. Metastasectomy for soft tissue sarcoma: Further evidence for efficacy and prognostic medicators. J Thorac Cardiovasc Surg 1989;97:695–704.

33. Dodd GD, Boyle JJ. Excavating pulmonary metastases. AJR 1961;85:277–293.

34. Aronchick JM, Palevsky HI, Miller WT. Cavitary pulmonary metastases in angiosarcoma. Diagnosis by transthoracic needle aspiration. Am Rev Respir Dis 1989;139:252–253.

35. Gilman JK, Sievers DB, Thornsvard CT. Malignant fibrous histiocytoma manifesting as a cavitary lung metastasis. South Med J 1986;79:376–378.

36. Wright FW. Spontaneous pneumothorax and pulmonary malignant disease—A syndrome sometimes associated with cavitating tumors. Clin Radiol 1976;27:211–222.

37. Trinidad S, Lisa JR, Rosenblatt MB. Bronchogenic carcinoma stimulated by metastatic tumour. Cancer (Philadelphia) 1965;16:1521–1529.

38. Schnilla RA, Fazzini EP. Bronchial gland adenocarcinoma of the lung. Am Rev Respir Dis 1977;115(suppl.):160 (abstr.).

39. Hirata H, Noguchi M, Shimosato Y, Uei Y, Goya T. Clinicopathologic and immunohistochemical characteristics of bronchial gland cell type adenocarcinoma of the lung. Am J Clin Pathol 1990;93:20–25.

40. Bourke SA, Henderson AF, Stevenson RD, Banham SW. Endobronchial metastases simulating primary carcinoma of the lung. Respir Med 1989;83:151–152.

41. Braman SS, Whitcomb ME. Endobronchial metastasis. Arch Intern Med 1975;135:543–547.

42. King DS, Castleman B. Bronchial involvement in metastatic pulmonary malignancy. J Thorac Surg 1943;12:305–315.

43. Seiler HH, Clagett T, McDonald JR. Pulmonary resection for metastatic malignant lesions. J Thorac Surg 1950;19:655–679.

44. Gerle R, Felson B. Metastatic endobronchial hypernephroma. Dis Chest 1963;44:225–233.

45. Schoenbaum S, Viamonte M. Subepithelial endobronchial metastases. Diagn Radiol 1971;101:63–69.

46. Furth J. Experiments on the spread of neoplastic cells through the respiratory passages. Am J Pathol 1946;22:1101–1107.

47. Albertini RE, Edberg NL. Endobronchial metastasis in breast cancer. Thorax 1980;35:435–440.

48. Fitzgerald RH. Endobronchial metastases. South Med J 1977;79:440–443.

49. Baumgartner WA, Mark JB. Metastatic malignancies from distant sites to the tracheobronchial tree. J Thorac Cardiovasc Surg 1980;79:499–503.

50. Shepherd MP. Endobronchial metastatic disease. Thorax 1982;37:362–365.

51. Lee DW, Ro JY, Sahin AA, Lee JS, Ayala AG. Mucinous adenocarcinoma of the prostate with endobronchial metastatis. Am J Clin Pathol 1990;94:641–645.

52. Garces M, Tsai E, Marsan RE. Endotracheal metastases. Chest 1974;65:350–351.

53. Coaker LA, Sobonya RE, David JR. Endobronchial metastases from uterine cervical squamous carcinoma. Arch Pathol Lab Med 1984;108:269–271.

54. Yeh TJ, Batayias G, Peters H, et al. Metastatic carcinoma to the trachea: Report of a case of palliation by resection and marlex graft. J Thorac Cardiov Surg 1965;49:886–892.

55. Mohsenifar Z, Chopra SK, Simmons DH. Diagnostic value of fiberoptic bronchoscopy in metastatic pulmonary tumours. Chest 1978;74:369–371.

56. Chuang MT, Padilla ML, Teirstein AS. Flexible fiberoptic bronchoscopy in metastatic cancer to the lungs. Cancer (Philadelphia) 1983;52:1949–1951.

57. Poe RH, Ortiz C, Israel RH, et al. Sensitivity, specificity and predictive values of bronchoscopy in neoplasm metastatic to the lung. Chest 1985;88:84–88.

58. Carey RW, Taft PD, Bennett JM, Kaufmann S. Carcinocythemia (carcinoma cell leukemia): An acute leukemia-like picture due to metastatic carcinoma cells. Am J Med 1976;60:273–278.

59. Lugassy G, Vorst EJ, Varon D, et al. Carcinocythemia: Report of two cases, one simulating a Burkitt lymphoma. Acta Cytol 1990;34:265–268.

60. Gallivan MVE, Lokich JJ. Carcinocythemia (carcinoma cell leukemia): Report of two cases with English literature review. Cancer (Philadelphia) 1984;53:1100–1102.

61. Dannaher CI, Yam LT, McKeown JM. Metastatic carcinoma with carcinocythemia mimicking leukemia. South Med J 1979;72:622–624.

62. Ejeckam GC, Sogbeing SK, McLeish WA. Carcinocythemia due to metastatic oat cell carcinoma of the lung. Can Med Assoc J 1979;120:336–338.

63. Solanki DI, McCurdy PR. Oat cell carcinoma mimicking leukemia. Postgrad Med 1980;68:213–216.

64. Finkel GC, Tishkoff GH. Malignant cells in a peripheral blood smear. N Engl J Med 1960;26:187–188.

65. Myerowitz RD, Edwards PA, Sartiano GP. Carcinocythemia (carcinoma cell leukemia) due to metastatic carcinoma of the breast: Report of a case. Cancer (Philadelphia) 1977;40:3107–3111.

66. Rappaport H. Tumors of the hematopoietic system. Washington, DC: Armed Forces Institute of Pathology, 1966:418.

67. Krause JR. Rhabdomyosarcoma presenting as carcinocythemia. South Med J 1979;72:1007–1008.

68. Schmidt MB. Die Verbreitungswege der Karzinome und die Beziehung generalisierter Sarkome zu den leukämischen Neubildungen. Jena: G Fisher, 1903, as quoted by Saphir.[72]

69. Takahashi M. An experimental study of metastatis. J Pathol Bacteriol 1915;20:1–13.

70. Iwasaki T. Histological and experimental observations on the destruction of tumor cells in the blood vessels. J Pathol Bacteriol 1915–16;20:85–105.

71. Warren S, Gates O. The fate of intravenously injected tumor cells. Am J Cancer 1936;27:485–492.

72. Saphir O. The fate of carcinoma emboli in the lung. Am J Pathol 1947;23:245–253.

73. Willis RA. The spread of tumours in the human body. London: Churchill, 1934.

74. Winterbauer RH, Elfenbein IB, Ball WC, Jr. Incidence and clinical significance of tumor embolization to the lungs. Am J Med 1968;45:271–290.

75. Kane RD, Hawkins HK, Miller JA, et al. Microscopic pulmonary tumor emboli associated with dyspnea. Cancer (Philadelphia) 1975;36:1473–1482.

76. Shriner RW, Ryu JH, Edwards WD. Microscopic pulmonary tumor embolism causing subacute cor pulmonale: a difficult antemortum diagnosis. Mayo Clin Proc 1991;66:143–148.

77. Goldhaber SZ, Dricker E, Buring JE, et al. Clinical suspicion of autopsy-proven thrombotic and tumor pulmonary embolism in cancer patients. Am Heart J 1987;114:1432–1435.

78. Chan CK, Hutcheon MA, Hyland RH, Walker Smith GJ, Patterson BJ, Matthay RA. Pulmonary tumor embolism: a critical review of clinical, imaging, and hemodynamic features. J Thorac Imaging 1987;2:4–14.

79. Fahrner RJ, McQueeney AJ, Mosley JM, Peterson RW. Trophoblastic pulmonary thrombosis with cor pulmonale. JAMA 1959;170:1898–1901.

80. Fanta CH, Compton CC. Microscopic tumour emboli to the lungs: A hidden cause of dyspnea and pulmonary hypertension. Thorax 1979;43:794–795.

81. Greenspan EB. Carcinomatous endarteritis of the pulmonary vessels resulting in failure of the right ventricle. Arch Intern Med 1934;54:625–644.

82. Marini JJ, Bilnoski W, Huseby JS. Acute cor pulmonale resulting from tumor microembolism. West J Med 1980;132:77–80.

83. Storstein O. Circulatory failure in metastatic carcinoma of the lung. A physiologic and pathologic study of its pathogenesis. Circulation 1951;4:913–919.

84. Abbondanzo SL, Klappenbach RS, Tsou E. Tumor cell embolism to pulmonary alveolar capillaries. Arch Pathol Lab Med 1986;110:1197–1198.

85. Gonzalez-Vitale JC, Garcia-Bunuel R. Pulmonary tumor emboli and cor pulmonale in primary carcinoma of the lung. Cancer (Philadelphia) 1976;38:2105–2110.

86. Yon Herbay A, Illes A, Waldherr R, Otto HF. Pulmonary tumor thrombotic microangiopathy with pulmonary hypertension. Cancer (Philadelphia) 1990;66:587–592.

87. Altemus LF, Lee RL. Carcinomatosis of the lung with pulmonary hypertension. Arch Intern Med 1967;119:32–38.

88. Crane R, Rudd TG, Dail D. Tumor microembolism: Pulmonary perfusion pattern. J Nucl Med 1984;25:877–880.

89. Soares FA, Landell GAM, de Oliveira JAM. Pulmonary tumor embolism to alveolar septal capillaries: A prospective study of 12 cases. Arch Pathol Lab Med 1991;115:127–130.

90. Soares FA, Landell GAM, de Oliveira JAM. Pulmonary tumor embolism from squamous cell carcinoma of the vulva. Gynecol Oncol 1990;38:141–143.

91. Soares FA, Landell GAM, de Oliveira JAM. Pulmonary tumor embolism to alveolar septal capillaries. Arch Pathol Lab Med 1992;116:187–188.

92. Durham JR, Ashley PF, Dorencamp D. Cor pulmonale due to tumor emboli. JAMA 1961;175:107–110.

93. Kupari M, Laitinen L, Hekali P, Luomanmaki K. Cor pulmonale due to tumor cell embolization. Acta Med Scand 1981;210:507–510.

94. Yang SP, Lin CC. Lymphangitic carcinomatosis of the lungs: The clinical significance of its roentgenologic classification. Chest 1972;62:179–187.

95. Harold JT. Lymphangitis carcinomatosa of the lungs. Q J Med 1952;21:353–360.

96. Minor GR. A clinical and radiologic study of metastatic pulmonary neoplasms. J Thorac Cardiovasc Surg 1950;20:34–42.

97. Goldsmith HS, Bailey HD, Callahan EL, Beattie EJ, Jr. Pulmonary lymphangitic metastases from breast cancer. Arch Surg 1967;94:483–488.

98. Fichera G, Hägerstrand I. The small lymph vessels of the lungs in lymphangiosis carcinomatosa. Acta Pathol Microbiol Scand 1965;65:505–513.

99. Thurlbeck WM. Neoplasia of the pulmonary vascular bed. In: Moser KM, ed. Pulmonary vascular disease. New York: Marcel Dekker, 1979;629–649.

100. Janower ML, Blennerhassett JB. Lymphangitic spread of metastatic cancer to the lung: a radiologic-pathologic classification. Radiology 1971;101:267–273.

101. Amundson DE, Weiss PJ. Hypoxemia in malignant carcinoid syndrome: A case attributed to occult lymphangitic metastatic involvement. Mayo Clin Proc 1991;66:1178–1180 (letter).

102. Trapnell DH. The radiological appearance of lymphangitic carcinomatosa of the lung. Thorax 1964;19:251–260.

103. Johkoh T, Ikezoe J, Tomiyama N, et al. CT findings in lymphangitic carcinomatosis of the lungs: Correlation with histologic findings and pulmonary function tests. AJR 1992;158:1217–1222.

104. Stein MG, Mayo J, Müller N, Aberle DR, Webb WR, Gamsu G. Pulmonary lymphangitic spread of carcinoma: appearance on CT scans. Radiology 1987;162:371–375.

105. Ren H, Hruban RH, Kuhlman JE, et al. Computed tomography of inflation-fixed lungs: The beaded sep-

tum sign of pulmonary meastases. J Comput Assist Tomogr 1989;13:411–416.

106. Munk PL, Muller NL, Miller RR, Ostrow DN. Pulmonary lymphangitic carcinomatosis: CT and pathologic findings. Radiology 1988;166(3):705–709.

107. Sostman HD, Brown M, Toole A, Bobrow S, Gottschalk A. Perfusion scan in pulmonary vascular/lymphangitic carcinomatosis: The segmental contour pattern. AJR 1981;137:1072–1074.

108. Green N, Swanson L, Kern W. Lymphangitic carcinomatosis: lung scan abnormalities. J Nucl Med 1976;17:258–260.

109. Schimmel DH, Julien PJ, Gamsu G. Resolution of pulmonary lymphangitic carcinoma of the breast. Chest 1976;69:106–108.

110. Heffner JE, Duffey DJ, Schwartz MI. Massive pleural effusions from prostatic lymphangitic carcinomatosis: resolution with endocrine therapy. Arch Intern Med 1982;142:375–376.

111. Fernandez K, O'Hanlan KA, Rodriquez-Rodriquez L, Marino WD. Respiratory failure due to interstitial lung metastases of ovarian carcioma reversed by chemotherapy. Chest 1991;99:1533–1534.

112. Youngberg AS. Unilateral diffuse lung opacity. Radiology 1977;123:277–281.

113. Morgan D. The pathology of subacute cor pulmonale in diffuse carcinomatosis of the lungs. J Pathol Bacteriol 1959;61:75–84.

114. Masson RG, Ruggieri J. Pulmonary microvascular cytology: A new diagnostic application of the pulmonary artery catheter. Chest 1985;88:908–914.

115. Masson RG, Krikorian J, Lukl P, Evans GL, McGrath J. Pulmonary microvascular cytology in the diagnosis of lymphangitic carcinomatosis. N Engl J Med 1989;321:71–76.

116. Scheinin TM, Koivuniemi AP. Megakaryocytes in the pulmonary circulation. Blood 1963;22:82–87.

117. Aabo K, Hansen KB. Megakaryocytes in pulmonary blood vessels. 1. Incidence at autopsy, clinicopathological relations especially to disseminated intravascular coagulation. Acta Path Microbiol Scand [A] 1978;86:285–291.

118. Hansen KB, Aabo K. Megakaryocytes in pulmonary blood vessels. 2. Relation to malignant hematological diseases especially leukemia. Acta Path Microbiol Scand [A] 1978;86:293–295.

119. Soares FA. Increased numbers of pulmonary megakaryocytes in patients with arterial pulmonary tumour embolism and with lung metastases seen at necropsy. J Clin Pathol 1992;45:140–142.

120. McLoud TC, Kalisher L, Stark P, Greene R. Intrathoracic lymph node metastases from extrathoracic neoplasms. AJR 1978;131:403–407.

121. Meyer KK. Direct lymphatic connections from the lower lobes of the lung to the abdomen. J Thorac Surg 1958;35:726–733.

122. Webb WR, Gamsu G. Thoracic metastasis in malignant melanoma. Chest 1977;71:176–181.

123. Das Gupta T, Brasfield R. Metastatic melanoma: A clinicopathological study. Cancer (Philadelphia) 1964;17:1323–1339.

124. Winterbauer RH, Belic N, Moores KD. A clinical interpretation of bilateral hilar adenopathy. Ann Intern Med 1973;78:65–71.

125. D'Angio GJ, Iannaccone G. Spontaneous pneumothorax as a complication of pulmonary metastases in malignant tumors of childhood. Amer J Roentgenol 1961;86:1092–1102.

126. Wright FW. Spontaneous pneumothorax and pulmonary malignant disease—A syndrome sometimes associated with cavitating tumors. Clin Radiol 1976;27:221–222.

127. Scholten ET, Kreel L. Distribution of lung metastases in the axial plane. Radiol Clin North Am 1977;46:248–265.

128. Samo RC, Carter BL. Bullous change by CT heralding metastatic sarcoma. Comput Radiol 1985;9:115–120.

129. Chretien J, Jaubert F. Pleural responses in malignant metastatic tumors. In: Chretien J, Bignon J, Hirsch A. eds. The pleura in health and disease. New York: Marcel Dekker, 1985;489–505.

130. Sahn SA. Malignant pleural effusion. In: Fishman AP, ed. Pulmonary diseases and disorders, 2d Ed. New York: McGraw-Hill, 1988:2159–2169.

131. Light RW. Tumors of the pleura. In: Murray JF, Nadel JA, eds. Textbook of respiratory medicine. Philadelphia: WB Saunders, 1988:1770–1780.

132. Cantó A, Rivas J, Saumench J, Morera R, Moya J. Points to consider when choosing a biopsy method in cases of pleurisy of unknown origin. Chest 1983;84:176–179.

133. Cantó A, Ferrer G, Romagosa V, Moya J, Bernat R. Lung cancer and pleural effusion. Clinical significance and study of pleural metastatic locations. Chest 1985;87:649–852.

134. Cantó-Armengod A. Macroscopic characteristics of pleural metastases arising from the breast and observed by diagnostic thoroscopy. Am Rev Respir Dis 1990;142:616–618.

135. Chernow B, Sahn SA. Carcinomatous involvement of the pleura: An analysis of 96 patients. Am J Med 1977;63:695–702.

136. Sahn SA. Malignant pleural effusions. Clin Chest Med 1985;6:113–125.

137. Meyer PC. Metastatic carcinoma of the pleura. Thorax 1966;21:437–443.

138. Cantin J, McNeer GP, Chu FC, et al. The problem of local recurrence after treatment of soft tissue sarcoma. Ann Surg 1968;168:47–53.

139. Jeffree GM, Price CHG, Sissons HA. The metastatic patterns of osteosarcoma. Br J Cancer 1975;32:87–107.

140. Marcove RC, Mike V, Hajek JV, et al. Osteogenic sarcoma under the age of twenty-one. J Bone Joint Surg [Am] 1970;52:411–423.

141. Scranton PE, DeCicco FA, Totten RS, et al. Prognostic factors in osteosarcoma. A review of 20 year's experience at the University of Pittsburgh Health Center Hospitals. Cancer (Philadelphia) 1975;36:2179–2191.

142. Vezeridis MP, Moore R, Karakousis CP. Metastatic pat-

terns in soft-tissue sarcomas. Arch Surg 1983;118:915–918.

143. Aronchick JM, Palevsky HI, Miller WT. Cavitary pulmonary metastases in angiosarcoma. Diagnosis by transthoracic needle aspiration. Am Rev Respir Dis 1989;139:252–253.

144. Gilman JK, Sievers DB, Thorsvard CT. Malignant fibrous histiocytoma manifesting as a cavitary lung metastasis. South Med J 1986;79:376–378.

145. Flynn KJ, Kim HS. Endobronchial metastasis of uterine leiomyosarcoma. JAMA 1978;240:2080.

146. Hinton AA, Sandler MP, Shaff MI, et al. Pulmonary nodules and spontaneous pneumothorax in an adolescent female. Invest Radiol 1984;19:479–483.

147. Lodmell EA, Capps SC. Spontaneous pneumothorax associated with metastatic sarcoma. Radiology 1949;52:88–93.

148. Thornton TF, Bigelow RR. Pneumothorax due to metastatic sarcoma. Arch Pathol 1944;37:334–336.

149. Shaw AB. Spontaneous pneumothorax from secondary sarcoma of lung. Br Med J 1951;1:278–280.

150. Sherman RS, Brant EE. An x-ray of spontaneous pneumothorax due to cancer metastases to the lungs. Chest 1954;26:328–337.

151. Dines DE, Cortese DA, Brennan MD, Hahn RG, Payne WS. Malignant pulmonary neoplasms predisposing to spontaneous pneumothorax. Mayo Clin Proc 1973;48:541–544.

152. Crow NE, Brogdon BG. Cystic lung lesions from metastatic sarcoma. Am J Roentgenol Radium Ther Nucl Med 1959;81:303–304.

153. Traweek ST, Rotter AJ, Swartz Azumi N. Cystic pulmonary metastatic sarcoma. Cancer (Philadelphia) 1990;65:1805–1811.

154. Pocock E, Craig JR, Bullock WK. Metastatic uterine leiomyoma. A case report. Cancer (Philadelphia) 1976;38:2090–2100.

155. Spittle MF, Heal J, Harmer C, White WF. The association of spontaneous pneumothorax with pulmonary metastases in bone tumours of children. Clin Radiol 1968;19:400–403.

156. Janetos GP, Ochsner SF. Bilateral pneumothorax in metastatic osteogenic sarcoma. Am Rev Respir dis 1963;88:73–76.

157. Chen JTT, Dahmash NS, Ravin CE, et al. Metastatic melanoma to the thorax: Report of 130 patients. AJR 1981;137:293–298.

158. Harpole DH, Jr., Johnson CM, Wolfe WG, George SL, Seigler HF. Analysis of 945 cases of pulmonary metastatic melanoma. J. Thorac Cardiovasc Surg 1992;103:743–750.

159. Balch CM, Soong SJ, Murad TM, Smith JW, Maddox WA, Durant JR. A multifactorial analysis of melanoma: prognostic factors in 200 melanoma patients with distant metastases. J Clin Oncol 1983;1:126–134.

160. Sutton FS, Jr., Vestal RE, Creagh CE. Varied presentations of metastatic pulmonary melanoma. Chest 1974;65:415–419.

161. Kayser K, Stute H, Tuengerthal S. Diffuse pulmonary ossification associated with metastatic melanoma of the lung. Respiration 1987;52:221–227.

162. Pogrebniak HW, Stovroff M, Roth JA, Pass HI. Resection of pulmonary metastases from malignant melanoma: Results of a 16-year experience. Ann Thorac Surg 1988;46:20–23.

163. Patel JK, Didolkar MS, Pickren JW, et al. Metastatic pattern of malignant melanoma: A study of 216 autopsy cases. Am J Surg 1978;135:807–810.

164. Demington ML, Carter DR, Meyers AD. Distant metastases in head and neck epidermoid carcinoma. Laryngoscope 1980;90:196–201.

165. O'Brien PH, Carlson R, Steubner EA, et al. Distant metastases in epidermoid cell carcinoma of the head and neck. Cancer (Philadelphia) 1971;27:204–307.

166. Papec R. Distant metastases from head and neck cancer. Cancer 1984;53:342–345.

167. Probert JC, Thompson RW, Bagshaw MA. Patterns of distant metastases in head and neck cancer. Cancer (Philadelphia) 1974;33:128–133.

168. Cahan WG, Montemayor PB. Cancer of the larynx and lung in the same patient. J Thorac Cardiovasc Surg 1962;44:309–320.

169. Malefetto JP, Kasimis BS, Moran EM, Wuerker RB, Stein JJ. The clinical significance of radiographically detected pulmonary neoplastic lesions in patients with head and neck cancer. J Clin Oncol 1984;2:625–630.

170. Lampe JL, Zatzkin H. Metastases of pseudoadenomatous basal cell carcinoma. Radiology 1948;53:379–385.

171. Massin J-P, Savoie J-C, Garnier H, Guiraundon G, Leger FA, Bacourt F. Pulmonary metastases in differentiated thyroid carcinoma. Study of 58 cases with implications for the primary tumor treatment. Cancer (Philadelphia) 1984;53:982–992.

172. Samaan NA, Schultz PN, Haynie TP, Ordonez NG. Pulmonary metastasis of differentiated thyroid carcinoma: Treatment results in 101 patients. J Clin Endocrinol Metab 1985;60:376–380.

173. Franssila KO. Prognosis in thyroid carcinoma. Cancer (Philadelphia) 1975;36:1138–1146.

174. McKenzie AD. The natural history of thyroid cancer. A report of 102 cases analyzed 10 to 15 years after diagnosis. Arch Surg 1971;102:274–277.

175. Rasmusson B. Carcinoma of the thyroid. Acta Radiol 1978;17:177–188.

176. Nemec J, Pohunková D, Zamrazil V, Röhling S, Zeman V. Pulmonary metastases of thyroid carcinoma. Czech Med 1979;2:78–83.

177. Høec J, Stenwig AE, Kullmann G, Lindegaard M. Distant metastases in papillary thyroid cancer. 1988;61:1–6.

178. Venkatesh YSS, Ordonez NG, Schultz PN, Hickey RC, Goepfert H, Samaan NA. Anaplastic carcinoma of the thyroid: A clinicopathologic study of 121 cases. Cancer (Philadelphia) 1990;66:321–330.

179. McGee AR, Warren R. Carcinoma metastatic from the thyroid to the lungs. Radiology 1966;87:516–517.

180. Tsumori T, Nakao K, Miyata M, et al. Clinicopathologic study of thyroid carcinoma infiltrating the trachea. Cancer (Philadelphia) 1985;56:2843–2848.

181. Fracchia AA, Knapper WH, Carey JT, et al. Intrapleural chemotherapy for effusion from metastatic breast carcinoma. Cancer (Philadelphia) 1970;26:626–629.

182. Cutler SJ, Asire AJ, Taylor SG. Classification of patients with disseminated cancer of the breast. Cancer (Philadelphia). 1969;24:861–869.

183. Winchester DP, Sener SF, Khandekar JD, et al. Symptomatology as an indicator of recurrent or metastatic breast cancer. Cancer (Philadelphia) 1979;43:956–960.

184. Casey JJ, Stempel BG, Scanlon EF, Fry WA. The solitary pulmonary nodule in the patient with breast cancer. Surgery 1984;96:801–805.

185. DeBeer RA, Garcia RL, Alexander SC. Endobronchial metastasis from cancer of the breast. Chest 1978;73:94–96.

186. Eppstein S. Primary carcinoma of the liver. Am J Med Sci 1964;247:43–50.

187. MacDonald RA. Primary carcinoma of the liver. A clinicopathologic study of one hundred eight cases. Arch Intern Med 1957;99:266–279.

188. Patton RB, Horn RC. Primary liver carcinoma. Autopsy study of 60 cases. Cancer (Philadelphia) 1964;17:757–768.

189. Levy JI, Geddes EW, Kew MC. The chest radiograph in primary liver cancer. An analysis of 449 cases. S Afr Med J 1976;50:1323–1326.

190. Tsai GL, Liu JD, Siauw CP, Chen PA. Thoracic roentgenologic manifestations in primary carcinoma of the liver. Chest 1984;86:430–434.

191. August DA, Ottow RT, Sugarbaker PH. Clinical perspective of human colorectal cancer metastasis. Cancer Metastasis Rev 1984;5:303–324.

192. Berg HK, Petrelli NJ, Herrera L, Lopez G, Mittelman A. Endobronchial metastasis from colorectal carcinoma. Dis Colon Rectum 1984;27:745–748.

193. Dionne L. The pattern of blood-borne metastasis from carcinoma of rectum. Cancer (Philadelphia) 1965;18:775–781.

194. Langer B. Cororectal cancer: Managing distant metastases. Can J Surg 1985;28:419–421.

195. Russell AH, Tong D, Dawson LE, Wisbeck W. Adenocarcinoma of the proximal colon. Sites of initial dissemination and patterns of recurrence following surgery alone. Cancer (Philadelphia) 1984;53:360–367.

196. Taylor FW. Cancer of the colon and rectum: A study of routes of metastases and death. Surgery 1962;52:305–308.

197. McCormack PM, Attiyeh FF. Resected pulmonary metastases from colorectal cancer. Dis Colon Rectum 1979;22:553–556.

198. Pihl E, Hughes ES, McDermott FT, Johnson WR, Katrivessis H. Lung recurrence after curative surgery for colorectal cancer. Dis Colon Rectum 1987;30:417–419.

199. Lisa JR, Trinidad S, Rosenblatt MB. Pulmonary manifestations of carcinoma of the pancreas. Cancer (Philadelphia) 1964;17:395–401.

200. Bunker SR, Klein DL. Multiple cavitated pulmonary metastases in pancreatic adenocarcinoma. Br J Radiol 1982;55:455–456.

201. Cassiere SG, McLain DA, Emory WB, Hatch HB, Jr. Metastatic carcinoma of the pancreas simulating primary bronchogenic carcinoma. Cancer (Philadelphia) 1980;46:2319–2321.

202. Greenberg BE, Young JM. Pulmonary metastasis from occult primary sites resembling bronchogenic carcinoma. Dis Chest 1958;33:496–505.

203. Latour A, Shulman HS. Thoracic manifestations of renal cell carcinoma. Radiology 1976;121:43–48.

204. Mountain CF. Pulmonary metastatic disease—Progress in a neglected area. Int J Radiat Oncol Biol Phys 1976;1:755–757.

205. Bennington JL, Beckwith JB. Tumors of the kidney, renal pelvis, and ureter. Atlas of tumor pathology. Second Series, Vol. 12. Washington, DC: Armed Forces Institute of Pathology, 1975:168.

206. Saitoh H. Distant metastasis of renal adenocarcinoma in patients with a tumor thrombus in the renal vein and/or vena cava. J Urol 1982;127:652–653.

207. Amer E, Guy J, Vaze B. Endobronchial metastasis from renal adenocarcinoma simulating a foreign body. Thorax 1981;36:183–184.

208. Gerle R, Felson B. Metastatic endobronchial hypernephroma. Dis Chest 1963;44:225–233.

209. Jariwalla AG, Seaton A, McCormack RJM, Gibbs A, Campbell IA, Davis BH. Intrabronchial metastases from renal carcinoma with recurrent tumor expectoration. Thorax 1981;36:179–182.

210. Merine D, Fishman EK. Mediastinal adenopathy and endobronchial involvement in metastatic renal cell carcinoma. J Comput Tomogr 1988;12:216–219.

211. Themelin D, Duchatelet P, Boudaka W, Lamy V. Endoscopic resection of an endobronchial hypernephroma metastases using a polypectomy snare. Eur Respir J 1990;3:732–736.

212. Noy S, Michowitz M, Lazebnik N, Baratz M. Endobronchial metastasis of renal cell carcinoma. J Surg Oncol 1986;31:268–270.

213. Reinke RT, Higgins CB, Niwayama G, et al. Bilateral pulmonary hilar lymphadenopathy. Radiology 1976;121:49–53.

214. King TE, Fisher J, Schwarz MI, Patzelt LH. Bilateral hilar adenopathy: An unusual presentation of renal cell carcinoma. Thorax 1982;37:317–318.

215. Kutty K, Varkey B. Metastatic renal cell carcinoma simulating sarcoidosis: analysis of 12 patients with bilateral hilar lymphadenopathy. Chest 1984;85:533–536.

216. Katzenstein A-LA, Purvis RW Jr, Gmelich JT, Askin FB. Pulmonary resection for metastatic renal adenocarcinoma. Cancer (Philadelphia) 1978;41:712–723.

217. Sella A, Ro JY. Renal cell cancer: Best recipient of tumor-to-tumor metastasis. Urology 1987;30:35–38.

218. Kerr V. Pulmonary metastases and ovarian cancer. Conn Med 1984;48:770–776.

219. Kerr VE, Cadman E. Pulmonary metastases in ovarian cancer. Cancer (Philadelphia) 1985;56:1209–1213.

220. Piatkowski Z. Distant metastases in cases of primary ovarian carcinoma. Pol Med J 1972;11:147–151.

221. Bernstein P. Tumors of the ovary. A study of 1,101 cases

of operations for ovarian tumor. Am J Obstet Gynec 1936;32:1023–1039.

222. Meigs JV. Cancer of the ovary. Surg Gynecol Obstet 1040;71:44–53.

223. Dauplat J, Hackner NF, Nieberg RK, Berek JS, Rose TP, Sagae S. Distant metastases in epithelial ovarian carcinoma. Cancer (Philadelphia) 1987;60:1561–1566.

224. Dvoretsky PM, Richards KA, Angel C, et al. Distribution of disease at autopsy in 100 women with ovarian cancer. Hum Pathol 1988;19:57–63.

225. Merrill CR, Hopkirk JAC. Late endobronchial metastasis from ovarian tumour. Br J Dis Chest 1982;76:253–254.

226. Smith JP, Day TG, Jr. Review of ovarian cancer at the University of Texas Systems Cancer Center M.D. Anderson Hospital and Tumor Institute. Am J Obstet Gynecol 1979;135:984–993.

227. Chew SY, Stemmerman GN. Fatal pulmonary tumor microembolism complicating peritoneovenous shunt. Hawaii Med J 1981;40:130–134.

228. Lokich J, Reinhold R, Silverman M, Tullis J. Complications of peritoneovenous shunting for malignant ascites. Cancer Treat Rep 1980;64:305–309.

229. Matt B, Oosterlee J, Spoos JA, White H, Lammer FB. Dissemination of tumor cells via LeVeen shunt. Lancet 1979;i:988.

230. Oosterlee J. Peritoneovenous shunting for ascites in cancer patients. Br J Surg 1980;67:663–666.

231. Smith RL, Sternberg SS, Paglia MA, Goldberg RB. Fatal pulmonary tumor embolization following peritoneovenous shunting for malignant ascites. J Surg Oncol 1981;16:27–35.

232. Carlson V, Delclos L, Fletcher GH. Distant metastases in squamous cell carcinoma of the uterine cervix. Radiology 1967;88:961–966.

233. Badib AO, Kurohara SS, Webster JH, et al. Metastasis to organs in carcinoma of the uterine cervix. Cancer (Philadelphia) 1968;21:434–439.

234. Tellis CJ, Beechler CR. Pulmonary metastasis of carcinoma of the cervix: A retrospective study. Cancer (Philadelphia) 1982;59:1705–1709.

235. Sostman HD, Matthay RA. Thoracic metastases from cervical carcinoma: Current status. Invest Radiol 1980;15:113–119.

236. Braude S, Thompson PJ. Solitary pulmonary metastases in carcinoma of the cervix. Thorax 1983;38:953–954.

237. D'Orsi CJ, Bruckman J, Mauch P, Smith EH. Lung metastases in cervical and endometrial carcinoma. AJR 1979;133:719–722.

238. Seaman WB, Arneson AN. Solitary pulmonary metastases in carcinoma of the cervix. Obstet Gynecol 1953;1:165–176.

239. Omenn GS. Pancoast syndrome due to metastatic carcinoma from the uterine cervix. Chest 1971;60:268–270.

240. Kirubakaran MG, Pulimood BM, Ray D. Excavating pulmonary metastases in carcinoma of the cervix. Postgrad Med J 1975;51:243–245.

241. Kennedy PS, Stockman G, Smith FE. Endobronchial metastasis from cervical cancer: A case report. Gynecol

Oncol 1976;4:340–344.

242. King TE Jr, Neff TA, Ziporin P. Endobronchial metastasis from the uterine cervix: Presentation as primary lung abscess. JAMA 1979;242:1651–1652.

243. Buchsbaum HJ. Lymphangitis carcinomatosis secondary to carcinoma of cervix. Obstet Gynecol 1970;36:850–860.

244. Kennedy KE, Christopherson WA, Buchsbaum HJ. Pulmonary lymphangitic carcinomatosis secondary to cervical carcinoma: A case report. Gynecol Oncol 1989;32:253–256.

245. Scott I, Bergin CJ, Müller NL. Mediastinal and hilar lymphadenopathy as the only manifestation of metastatic carcinoma of the cervix. J Can Assoc Radiol 1986;37:52–53.

246. Ballon SC, Donaldson RC, Growdon WA, et al. Pulmonary metastases in endometrial carcinoma. In: Weiss L, Gilbet HA, eds. Pulmonary metastasis. Boston: GK Hall, 1978;182.

247. Wolff M, Kaye G, Silva F. Pulmonary metastases (with admixed epithelial elements) from smooth muscle neoplasms. Am J Surg Pathol 1979;3:325–342.

248. Gal AA, Brooks JSJ, Pietra GG. Leiomyomatous neoplasms of the lung: A clinical, histologic and immunohistochemical study. Mod Pathol 1989;2:209–216.

249. Cho KR, Woodruff JD, Epstein JI. Leiomyoma of the uterus with multiple extrauterine smooth muscle tumors: A case report suggesting multifocal origin. Hum Pathol 1989;20:80–83.

250. Kaplan C, Katoh A, Shamoto M, et al. Multiple leiomyomas of the lung: Benign or malignant. Am Rev Respir Dis 1973;108:656–659.

251. Boyce CR, Buddhdev HN. Pregnancy complicated by metastasizing leiomyomas of the uterus. J Obstet Gynecol 1973;42:252–258.

252. Barnes HM, Richardson PJ. Benign metastasizing fibroleiomyoma. A case report. J Obstet Gynecol Br Commonw 1973;80:569–573.

253. Lipton JH, Fong TC, Burgess KR. Miliary pattern as presentation of leiomyomatosis of the lung. Chest 1987;91:781–782.

254. Flynn KJ, Kim H-S. Endobronchial metastasis of uterine leiomyosarcoma. JAMA 1978;240:2080.

255. Akatsuka N, Tokunaga K, Isshiki T, et al. Intravenous leiomyomatosis of uterus with continuous extension into the pulmonary artery. Jpn Heart J 1984;25:651–659.

256. Norris HJ, Parmley T. Mesenchymal tumors of the uterus. V: Intravenous leiomyomatosis. A clinical and pathologic study of 14 cases. Cancer (Philadelphia) 1975;36:2164–2178.

257. Dail DH. Pulmonary metastases of uterine stromal sarcoma: unique histologic appearance suggesting their source. Lab Invest 1980;42:110a (Abstr.).

258. Abrams J, Talcott J, Corson JM. Pulmonary metastases in patients with low-grade endometrial stromal sarcoma: clinicopathologic findings with immunohistochemical characterisation. Am J Surg Pathol 1989;13:133–140.

259. Clement PB, Scully RE. Uterine tumors resembling ovarian sex-cord tumors. Am J Clin Pathol 1976;

66:512–525.

260. Hendin AS. Gestational trophoblastic tumors metastatic to the lungs. Cancer (Philadelphia) 1984;53:58–61.

261. Kumar J, Ilancheran A, Ratnam SS. Pulmonary metastases in gestational trophoblastic disease: A review of 97 cases. Br J Obstet Gynecol 1988;95:70–74.

262. Tsao M-S, Schraufnagel D, Wang N-S. Pulmonary metastasis of choriocarcinoma with a miliary radiographic pattern. Arch Pathol Lab Med 1981;105:557–558.

263. Bagshawe KD, Noble MIM. Cardiorespiratory aspects of trophoblastic tumours. QJ Med 1966;35:39–54.

264. Burton RM. A case of chorion-epithelioma with pulmonary complications. Tubercle 1963;44:487–490.

265. Bagshawe KD, Garnett ES. Radiological changes in the lungs of patients with trophoblastic tumours. Br J Radiol 1963;36:673–679.

266. Carlson JA, Jr., Day TG, Jr., Kuhns JG, Howell RS, Jr., Masterson BJ. Endoarterial pulmonary metastasis of malignant trophoblast associated with a term intrauterine pregnancy. Gynecol Oncol 1984;17:241–248.

267. Bagshawe KD, Brooks WDW. Subacute pulmonary hypertension due to chorioepithelioma. Lancet 1959; 28:653–658.

268. Evans KT, Cockshott WP, de V Hendrickse JP. Pulmonary changes in malignant trophoblastic disease. Br J Radiol 1965;38:161–167.

269. Santhosh-Kumar CR, Vijayaraghauan R, Harakati MS, Ajarim DSS. Spontaneous pneumothorax in metastatic choriocarcinoma. Respir Med 1991;85:81–83.

270. Cockshott WP, de V Hendrickse JP. Pulmonary calcification at the site of trophoblastic metastases. Br J Radiol 1969;42:17–20.

271. Xu LT, Sun CF, Wang YE, Song HZ. Resection of pulmonary metastatic choriocarcinoma in 43 drug-resistant patients. Ann Thorac Surg 1985;39:257–259.

272. Mazur MT. Metastatic gestational choriocarcinoma: Unusual pathologic variant following therapy. Cancer (Philadelphia) 1989;63:1370–1377.

273. Hatch KD, Shingleton HM, Gore H, Younger B, Boots LR. Human chorionic gonadotropin-secreting large cell carcinoma of the lung detected during follow-up of a patient previously treated for gestational trophoblastic disease. Gynecol Oncol 1980;10:98–104.

274. Bumpus HC. Carcinoma of the prostate: A clinical study of one thousand cases. Surg Gynecol Obstet 1926;43:150–154.

275. Ware JL. Prostate tumor progression and metastasis. Biochim Biophys Acta 1987;907:279–298.

276. Varkarakis MJ, Winterberger AR, Gaeta J, et al. Lung metastases in prostatic carcinoma: clinical significance. Urol 1974;3:447–452.

277. Petras AD, Wollett FC. Metastatic prostatic pulmonary nodules with normal bone image. J Nucl Med 1983;24:1026–1027.

278. Saitoh H, Hida M, Shimbo T, Nakamura K, Yamaguta J. Metastatic patterns of prostatic cancer: correlation between sites and number of organs involved. Cancer 1984;54:3078–3084.

279. Mintz ER, Smith GG. Autopsy finding in 100 cases of prostatic cancer. N Engl J Med 1934;211:479–487.

280. Elkin M, Mueller HP. Metastases from cancer of the prostate: autopsy and roentgenological findings. Cancer 1954;7:1246–1248.

281. Scoggins WG, Witten JA, Texter JH, Hazra TA. Endobronchial metastasis from prostatic cancer in patient with renal cell carcinoma. Urology 1978;12:207–209.

282. Lali C, Gogia H, Raju L. Multiple endobronchial metastases from carcinoma of prostate. Urology 1983; 21:164–165.

283. Scherz H, Schmidt JD. Endobronchial metastasis from prostate carcinoma. Prostate 1986;8:319–324.

284. Kenny JN, Smith WL, Brawer MK. Endobronchial metastases from prostatic carcinoma. Ann Thorac Surg 1988;45:223–224.

285. Legge DA, Good CA, Ludwig J. Roentgenologic features of pulmonary carcinomatosis from carcinoma of the prostate. AJR 1971;11:360–364.

286. Mestitz H, Pierce RJ, Holmes PW. Intrathoracic manifestations of disseminated prostate adenocarcinoma. Respir Med 1989;83:161–166.

287. Apple JS, Paulson DF, Baber C, Putman CE. Advanced prostatic carcinoma: Pulmonary manifestations. Radiology 1985;54:601–604.

288. Skinner DG, Scardino PT, Daniels JR. Testicular cancer. Annu Rev Med 1981;32:543–557.

289. Bosl GJ, Geller NL, Cirrincione C, et al. Multivariate analysis of prognostic variables in patients with metastatic testicular cancer. Cancer Res 1983;43:3403–3407.

290. Prognostic factors in advanced non-seminomatous germ-cell testicular tumours: Results of a multicentre study. Report from the Medical Council Working Party on Testicular Tumours. Lancet 1985;i:8–11.

291. Bergman SM, Lippert M, Javapour N. The value of whole lung tomography in the early detection of metastatic disease in patients with renal cell carcinoma and testicular tumors. J Urol 1980;124:860–862.

292. Varkey B, Heckman MG. Diagnosis of a case of embryonal carcinoma by bronchial biopsy. Chest 1972;62:758–760.

293. Toner GC, Geller NL, Lin SY, Bosl GJ. Extragonadal and poor risk nonseminomatous germ cell tumors. Survival and prognostic features. Cancer (Philadelphia) 1991;67:2049–2057.

294. Williams MP, Husband JE, Heron CW. Intrathoracic manifestations of metastatic testicular seminioma: A comparison of chest radiographic and CT findings. AJR 1987;149:A73.

295. Mandelbaum I, Williams SD, Einhorn LH. Aggressive surgical management of testicular carcinoma metastatic to lungs and mediastinum. Ann Thorac Surg 1980; 30:224–229.

296. Vogelzang NJ, Stenlund R. Residual pulmonary nodules after combination chemotherapy of testicular cancer. Radiology 1983;146:195–197.

297. Charig MJ, Williams MP. Pulmonary lacunae: sequelae of metastases following chemotherapy. Clin Radiol 1990;42:93–96.

298. Deschamps C, Pairolero PC, Trastek VF, Payne WS.

Multiple primary lung cancers: Results of surgical treatment. J Thorac Cardiovasc Surg 1990;99:769–778.

299. Rosengart TK, Martini N, Ghosn P, Burt M. Multiple primary lung carcinoma: Prognosis and treatment. Ann Thorac Surg 1991;52:773–779.

300. Karolyi P. Do adrenal metastases from lung cancer develop by lymphogenous or hematogenous route? J Surg Oncol 1990;43:154–156.

301. Matthews MJ. Problems in morphology and behavior of bronchopulmonary malignant disease. In: Israel L, Chahanian P, eds. Lung cancer: Natural history, prognosis and therapy. New York: Academic Press, 1976;23–62.

302. Auerbach O, Garfinkel L, Parks UR. Histologic type of lung cancer in relation to smoking habits, year of diagnosis and sites of metastases. Chest 1975;67:382–387.

303. Hirsch FR. Histopathologic classification and metastatic pattern of small cell carcinoma of the lung. Copenhagen: Munksgaard, 1983.

304. Prioleau PG, Katzenstein A-L A. Major peripheral arterial occlusion due to malignant tumor embolism: histologic recognition and surgical management. Cancer (Philadelphia) 1978;42:2009–2014.

305. Heitmiller RF. Prognostic significance of massive bronchogenic tumor embolus. Ann Thorac Surg 1992;53:153–155.

306. Van Way CW, III, Lawler MR. Osteogenic sarcomatous emboli to the femoral arteries. Am J Surg 1969;117:745–747.

Index